Smith's
Textbook of
ENDOUROLOGY

Second Edition

Smith's
Textbook of
ENDOUROLOGY

Arthur D. Smith, MD

Gopal H. Badlani, MD
Demetrius H. Bagley, MD
Ralph V. Clayman, MD
Steven G. Docimo, MD
Gerald H. Jordan, MD
Louis R. Kavoussi, MD
Benjamin R. Lee, MD
James E. Lingeman, MD
Glenn M. Preminger, MD
Joseph W. Segura, MD

Second Edition

2007
BC Decker Inc
Hamilton • London

BC Decker Inc

P.O. Box 620, L.C.D. 1
Hamilton, Ontario L8N 3K7
Tel: 905-522-7017; 800-568-7281
Fax: 905-522-7839; 888-311-4987
E-mail: info@bcdecker.com
www.bcdecker.com

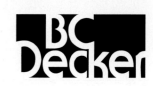

06 07 08 09/ LEGO/9 8 7 6 5 4 3 2 1

ISBN 1-55009-365-7
Printed in Italy by Legatoria Editoriale Giovanni Olivotto
Production Editor: Petrice Custance; Cover Designer: Lisa Mattinson

---

Sales and Distribution

United States
BC Decker Inc
P.O. Box 785
Lewiston, NY 14092-0785
Tel: 905-522-7017; 800-568-7281
Fax: 905-522-7839; 888-311-4987
E-mail: info@bcdecker.com
www.bcdecker.com

Canada
BC Decker Inc
50 King St. E.
P.O. Box 620, LCD 1
Hamilton, Ontario L8N 3K7
Tel: 905-522-7017; 800-568-7281
Fax: 905-522-7839; 888-311-4987
E-mail: info@bcdecker.com
www.bcdecker.com

Foreign Rights
John Scott & Company
International Publishers' Agency
P.O. Box 878
Kimberton, PA 19442
Tel: 610-827-1640; Fax: 610-827-1671
E-mail: jsco@voicenet.com

Japan
Igaku-Shoin Ltd.
Foreign Publications Department
3-24-17 Hongo
Bunkyo-ku, Tokyo, Japan 113-8719
Tel: 3 3817 5680; Fax: 3 3815 6776
E-mail: fd@igaku-shoin.co.jp

UK, Europe, Scandinavia, Middle East
Elsevier Science
UK, Europe, Scandinavia, Middle East, Africa
Elsevier Ltd.
Books Customer Services
Linacre House
Jordan Hill
Oxford
OX2 8DP, UK
Tel: 44 (0) 1865 474 010
Fax: 44 (0) 1865 474 011
E-mail: eurobkinfo@elsevier.com

Singapore, Malaysia, Thailand, Philippines, Indonesia, Vietnam, Pacific Rim, Korea
Elsevier Science Asia
583 Orchard Road
#09/01, Forum
Singapore 238884
Tel: 65-737-3593
Fax: 65-753-2145

Australia, New Zealand
Elsevier Science Australia
Customer Service Department
Locked Bag 16
St. Peters, New South Wales 2044
Australia
Tel: 61 02-9517-8999
Fax: 61 02-9517-2249
E-mail: customerserviceau@elsevier.com
www.elsevier.com.au

Mexico and Central America
ETM SA de CV
Calle de Tula 59
Colonia Condesa
06140 Mexico DF, Mexico
Tel: 52-5-5553-6657
Fax: 52-5-5211-8468
E-mail: editoresdetextosmex@prodigy.net.mx

Brazil
Tecmedd Importadora E Distribuidora
De Livros Ltda.
Avenida Maurílio Biagi, 2850
City Ribeirão, Ribeirão Preto – SP – Brasil
CEP: 14021-000
Tel: 0800 992236
Fax: (16) 3993-9000
E-mail: tecmedd@tecmedd.com.br

India, Bangladesh, Pakistan, Sri Lanka
Elsevier Health Sciences Division
Customer Service Department
17A/1, Main Ring Road
Lajpat Nagar IV
New Delhi – 110024, India
Tel: 91 11 2644 7160-64
Fax: 91 11 2644 7156
E-mail: esindia@vsnl.net

CONTRIBUTORS

Fernando Abarzua, MD
Department of Cell Biology and Urology
Okayama University Medical School
Okayama, Japan

Sidney C. Abreu, MD
Department of Laparoscopic and Robotic
    Surgery
Cleveland Clinic Foundation
Cleveland, Ohio

Jim M. Adshead, MA, MD, FRCS
Department of Urology
St. Mary's Hospital
London, England

Thomas E. Ahlering, MD
Department of Urology
University of California
Irvine, California

David M. Albala, MD
Department of Surgery
Duke University Medical Center
Durham, North Carolina

Michael A. Aleman, MD
Glickman Urological Institute
Cleveland Clinic
Cleveland, Ohio

Peter Alken, MD
Department of Urology
University Hospital
Mannheim, Germany

Samuel A. Amukele, MD
Department of Urology
New York Medical College
Valhalla, New York

Jason W. Anast, MD
Department of Urology
University of California
San Francisco, California

Kevin R. Anderson, MD
Department of Surgery
Yale University
New Haven, Connecticut

Rodney A. Appell, MD, FACS
Department of Urology
Baylor College of Medicine
Houston, Texas

Dean G. Assimos, MD
Department of Urology
Wake Forest University School of Medicine
Winston-Salem, North Carolina

Fatih Atug, MD
Department of Urology
Tulane University Health Sciences Center
New Orleans, Louisiana

Richard K. Babayan, MD
Department of Urology
Boston University School of Medicine
Boston, Massachusetts

Gopal H. Badlani, MD
Department of Urology
Long Island Jewish Medical Center
New Hyde Park, New York

Demetrius H. Bagley, MD
Department of Urology
Jefferson Medical College
Philadelphia, Pennsylvania

Linda Baker, MD, FAAP
Department of Urology
University of Texas Southwestern
Dallas, Texas

Laurence Baskin, MD
Department of Urology
University of California
San Francisco, California

Steven M. Baughman, MD
Department of Urology
Wilford Hall Medical Center
Lackland AFB, Texas

Darren T. Beiko, MD, FRCSC
Department of Urology
Queens University
Kingston, Ontario

Gary C. Bellman, MD
Department of Endourology
Kaiser Permanente Medical Center
Los Angeles, California

Ralph C. Benson Jr, MD
Department of Veterans Affairs Medical Center
West Palm Beach, Florida

Vincent G. Bird, MD
Department of Urologic Surgery
University of Miami
Miami, Florida

Jay T. Bishoff, MD, FACS
Department of Urology
Wilford Hall Medical Center
Lackland AFB, Texas

Jerry G. Blaivas, MD
Department of Urology
Cornell University Medical School
New York, New York

Michael L. Blute, MD
Department of Urology
Mayo Clinic
Rochester, Minnesota

Damien M. Bolton, MD
Department of Surgery
University of Melbourne
Melbourne, Australia

Nancy Brettschneider, BSN, CURN
Urology Nurse Clinician
Long Island Jewish Medical Center
New Hyde Park, New York

Jeffrey A. Cadeddu, MD
Department of Urology
University of Texas Southwestern
    Medical Center
Dallas, Texas

Douglas A. Canning, MD
Department of Urology
Children's Hospital of Philadelphia
Philadelphia, Pennsylvania

Patrick C. Cartwright, MD
Department of Urology
University of Utah
Salt Lake City, Utah

Wilfrido R. Castaneda, MD
Department of Radiology
Louisiana State University Medical Center
New Orleans, Louisiana

Erik P. Castle, MD
Department of Urology
Tulane University Health Sciences Center
New Orleans, Louisiana

R. Duane Cespedes, MD
Department of Urology
Wilford Hall Medical Center
Lackland AFB, Texas

David Chan, MD
Department of Urology
Johns Hopkins Medical Institutions
Baltimore, Maryland

Paramjit S. Chandhoke, MD, PhD
Department of Surgery and Medicine
University of Colorado Health
    Sciences Center
Denver, Colorado

Andy Y. Chang, MD
Department of Urology
Children's Hospital of Philadelphia
Philadelphia, Pennsylvania

Gary W. Chien, MD
Department of Surgery
University of Chicago
Chicago, Illinois

George K. Chow, MD
Department of Urology
Mayo Clinic
Rochester, Minnesota

Ralph V. Clayman, MD
Department of Urology
University of California
Irvine, California

Robin O. Cleveland, PhD
Department of Aerospace and Mechanical
    Engineering
Boston University
Boston, Massachusetts

Michael Conlin, MD
Department of Surgery
Oregon Health and Sciences University
Portland, Oregon

Douglas E. Coplen, MD
Department of Pediatric Urology
St. Louis Children's Hospital
St. Louis, Missouri

Hillary L. Copp, MD
Department of Urology
University of Virginia
Charlottesville, Virginia

Marlene Corujo, MD
Department of Surgery
Yale University School of Medicine
New Haven, Connecticut

Anthony J. Costello, MD
Department of Urology
The Royal Melbourne Hospital
Victoria, Australia

Sakti Das, MD
Department of Urology
University of California Davis Medical Center
Sacramento, California

Kim Davenport, MBChB, MRCS
Bristol Urological Institute
Southmead Hospital
Bristol, England

Rodney Davis, MD
Department of Urology
Tulane University Health Sciences Center
New Orleans, Louisiana

John D. Denstedt, MD, FRCSC
Department of Surgery
University of Western Ontario
London, Ontario, Canada

Mahesh Desai, MD
Department of Urology
Muljibhai Patel Urology Hospital
Gujarat, India

Steven G. Docimo, MD
Department of Urology
University of Pittsburgh School of Medicine
Pittsburgh, Pennsylvania

James F. Donovan Jr, MD
Department of Surgery
University of Cincinnati
Cincinnati, Ohio

Matthew D. Dunn, MD
Department of Urology
Norris Cancer Center
Los Angeles, California

Louis Eichel, MD
Department of Urology
University of Rochester School of Medicine
Rochester, New York

Alaa El-Ghoneimi, MD, PhD
Department of Pediatric Surgery
    and Urology
Hôpital Robert Debré
Paris, France

Assaad El-Hakim, MD, FRCS
Department of Urology
Cornell University Medical School
New York, New York

Michael Erhard, MD
Nemours Children's Clinic
Jacksonville, Florida

Gregory David Espenan, MS
Department of Diagnostic Radiology
Louisiana State University Medical Center
New Orleans, Louisiana

Andrew P. Evan, PhD
Department of Anatomy and Cell Biology
Indiana University School of Medicine
Indianapolis, Indiana

Michael D. Fabrizio, MD, FACS
Devine Tidewater Urology
Norfolk, Virginia

Rodolfo Favela-Camacho, MD
Department of Urology
University of Guadalajara
Guadalajara, Mexico

Agana Filipas, MD
Department of Urology
University of Hamburg
Hamburg, Germany

Antonio Finelli, MD, MSc, FRCSC
Glickman Urological Institute
Cleveland Clinic Foundation
Cleveland, Ohio

Margit Fisch, MD
Department of Urology
University of Hamburg
Hamburg, Germany

Brian Fong, MD
Department of Urology
Swedish Urology Group
Seattle, Washington

Israel Franco, MD, FACS, FAAP
Departments of Urology and Pediatrics
New York Medical College
Valhalla, New York

Daniel Franco-Carrillo
Department of Urology
University of Guadalajara
Guadalajara, Mexico

Russell M. Freid, MD
Lawrenceville Urology Clinical Research
Lawrenceville, New Jersey

Matthew T. Gettman, MD
Department of Urology
Mayo Clinic
Rochester, Minnesota

Inderbir S. Gill, MD
Department of Laparoscopic and Robotic
    Surgery
Cleveland Clinic Foundation
Cleveland, Ohio

Peter Gilling, FRACS
Department of Urology
Tauranga Hospital
Tauranga, New Zealand

Sarah K. Girardi, MD
Department of Infertility and Female Urology
North Shore University Hospital
Manhasset, New York

Ricardo R. Gonzalez, MD
Department of Urology
Weill Cornell Medical Center
New York, New York

Emanuel E. Gottenger, MD
Department of Veterans Affairs
Medical Center
West Palm Beach, Florida

Michael Grasso III, MD
Department of Urology
St. Vincent's Medical Center
New York, New York

Stavros Gravas, MD, FEBU
Department of Urology
University of Amsterdam
Amsterdam, The Netherlands

Mantu Gupta, MD
Department of Urology
Columbia University
New York, New York

Jorge Gutierrez-Aceves, MD
Department of Urology
University of Guadalajara
Guadalajara, Mexico

Nathan Lewis Hatfield
Department of Urology
Jefferson Medical College
Philadelphia, Pennsylvania

Sean P. Hedican, MD
Department of Surgery
University of Wisconsin Medical School
Madison, Wisconsin

Khai-Linh V. Ho, MD, FACS
Department of Urology
Mayo Clinic
Rochester, Minnesota

R. John D'A. Honey, MD, FRCSC
Department of Surgery
St. Michael's Hospital
Toronto, Ontario, Canada

Denis H. Hosking, MB, ChB, FRCSC
Department of Urology
University of Manitoba
Winnipeg, Manitoba

R. Guy Hudson, MD
Department of Pediatric Urology
Oregon University
Portland, Oregon

Stephen V. Jackman, MD
Department of Urology
National Naval Medical Center
Bethesda, Maryland

Daniel Janoff, MD
Department of Surgery
Oregon University
Portland, Oregon

Thomas W. Jarrett, MD
Department of Endourology and Laparoscopy
Johns Hopkins Medical Institutions
Baltimore, Maryland

Andrew B. Joel, MD
Department of Urology
University of California
San Francisco, California

Gerald H. Jordan, MD, FACS, FAAP
Department of Urology
Eastern Virginia Medical School
Norfolk, Virginia

Christopher J. Kane, MD
Department of Urology
University of California
San Francisco, California

Jihad H. Kaouk, MD
Glickman Urological Institute
Cleveland Clinic Foundation
Cleveland, Ohio

Aaron E. Katz, MD
Department of Urology
Columbia University
New York, New York

Sanjeev Kaul, MD, MCh
Department of Robotic Urology
Vattikuti Urology Institute
Detroit, Michigan

Louis R. Kavoussi, MD
Department of Urology
Johns Hopkins University School of Medicine
Baltimore, Maryland

Jonathan D. Kaye, MD
Department of Urology
Long Island Jewish Medical Center
New Hyde Park, New York

Keith W. Kaye, MD
Department of Urology
St. Lukes University Medical School
Belize, Central America

Francis X. Keeley Jr, MD, FRCS
Bristol Urological Institute
Southmead Hospital
Bristol, England

Hyung L. Kim, MD
Department of Urology
University of California
Los Angeles, California

Samuel C. Kim, MD
Methodist Urology
Indianapolis, Indiana

Jennifer Kirk, MSN, CPNP
Department of Urology
Children's Hospital of Philadelphia
Philadelphia, Pennsylvania

Bodo E. Knudsen, MD, FRCSC
Department of Surgery
Ohio State University Medical Center
Columbus, Ohio

Bradley P. Kropp, MD
Department of Urology
University of Oklahoma
Oklahoma City, Oklahoma

Hiromi Kumon, MD, PhD
Department of Urology
Okayama University Medical School
Okayama, Japan

Ramsay L. Kuo, MD
Department of Urology
Jefferson Medical College
Philadelphia, Pennsylvania

Pilar Laguna, MD, PhD
Department of Urology
University of Amsterdam
Amsterdam, The Netherlands

Jason S. Lai, MD
Department of Urology
Southwest Healthcare System
Murrieta, California

John S. Lam, MD
Department of Urology
University of California
Los Angeles, California

Ezekiel H. Landau, MD
Department of Pediatric Urology
Hadassah Hebrew University Medical Center
Jerusalem, Israel

Jaime Landman, MD
Department of Surgery
Washington University School of Medicine
St. Louis, Missouri

Benjamin R. Lee, MD
Department of Urology
Long Island Jewish Medical Center
New Hyde Park, New York

David I. Lee, MD
Department of Urology
Penn Presbyterian Medical Center
Philadelphia, Pennsylvania

Nina L. Lee, RN
Department of Surgery
Duke University Medical Center
Durham, North Carolina

Richard Lee, MD
Department of Urology
Weill Cornell Medical Center
New York, New York

Andrew J. LeRoy, MD
Department of Radiology
Mayo Clinic
Rochester, Minnesota

Raymond J. Leveillee, MD
Department of Urologic Surgery
University of Miami
Miami, Florida

Evangelos N. Liatsikos, MD, PhD
Department of Urology
University Hospital of Patras
Patras, Greece

John C. Lieske, MD
Department of Urology
Mayo Clinic
Rochester, Minnesota

James E. Lingeman, MD
International Kidney Stone Institute
Indianapolis, Indiana

Benjamin H. Lowentritt, MD
Department of Urology
Tulane University
New Orleans, Louisiana

Robert Marcovich, MD
Department of Urology
University of Texas Health Sciences Center
San Antonio, Texas

James A. McAteer, PhD
Department of Anatomy and Cell Biology
Indiana University School of Medicine
Indianapolis, Indiana

R. Clay McDonough III, MD
Department of Urology
Wilford Hall Medical Center
Lackland AFB, Texas

Elspeth M. McDougall, MD
Department of Urology
University of California
Irving, California

Freddy R. Mendez-Torres, MD
Department of Urology
Tulane University
New Orleans, Louisiana

Mani Menon, MD, FACS
Department of Urology
Vattikuti Urology Institute
Detroit, Michigan

Adam R. Metwalli, MD
Department of Urology
University of Oklahoma
Oklahoma City, Oklahoma

April Beeman Metwalli, JD
Department of Urology
University of Oklahoma
Oklahoma City, Oklahoma

Maurice Stephan Michel, MD, PhD
Department of Urology
University Hospital
Mannheim, Germany

Ronald A. Miller, MS, FRCS, FRGS
Department of Urology and Minimally
  Invasive Surgery
Whittington Hospital
London, England

Robert M. Moldwin, MD
Department of Urology
Long Island Jewish Medical Center
New Hyde Park, New York

Terri G. Monk, MD
Department of Anesthesiology
Washington University School of Medicine
St. Louis, Missouri

Debora K. Moore, MD
Minimally Invasive Urology of the Southwest
Las Palmas Medical Center
El Paso, Texas

Robert G. Moore, MD
Minimally Invasive Urology of the Southwest
Las Palmas Medical Center
El Paso, Texas

Michael E. Moran, MD
Capital Region Urologic Surgeons
Albany, New York

Timothy Mulholland, MD
Department of Urology
University of Oklahoma
Norman, Oklahoma

Ravi Munver, MD
Department of Urology
Hackensack University Medical Center
Hackensack, New Jersey

Rolf Muschter, MD, PhD
Department of Urology
University of Munich
Munich, Germany

Lance A. Mynderse, MD
Department of Urology
Mayo Clinic
Rochester, Minnesota

Stephen Y. Nakada, MD
Department of Surgery
University of Wisconsin Medical School
Madison, Wisconsin

Yasutomo Nasu, MD, PhD
Department of Urology
Okayama University Medical School
Okayama, Japan

Caleb P. Nelson, MD
Department of Urology
University of Michigan Medical School
Ann Arbor, Michigan

C.F. Ng, MD
Scottish Lithotriptor Centre
Western General Hospital NHS Trust
Edinburgh, United Kingdom

Thai T. Nguyen, MD
Department of Urology
University of Iowa College of Medicine
Iowa City, Iowa

Regina D. Norris, MD
Comprehensive Kidney Stone Center
Duke University Medical Center
Durham, North Carolina

Carol J. Olsen, RN, BSN
Long Island Jewish Medical Center
New Hyde Park, New York

Michael C. Ost, MD
Department of Urology
Long Island Jewish Medical Center
New Hyde Park, New York

Lane S. Palmer, MD, FACS, FAAP
Departments of Urology and Pediatrics
Albert Einstein College of Medicine
Bronx, New York

John M. Park, MD
Department of Urology
University of Michigan Medical School
Ann Arbor, Michigan

Donna W. Parsons, RN
Department of Surgery
Duke University Medical Center
Durham, North Carolina

Anup Patel, MS, FRCS
Department of Urology
St. Mary's Hospital
London, England

Rajen P. Patel, MD
Department of Urology
University of Pittsburgh School of Medicine
Pittsburgh, Pennsylvania

Ryan F. Paterson, MD
Department of Urology
University of British Columbia
Vancouver, British Columbia

David E. Patterson, MD
Department of Urology
Mayo Foundation
Rochester, Minnesota

Margaret S. Pearle, MD
Department of Urology
University of Texas Southwestern
    Medical Center
Dallas, Texas

Craig A. Peters, MD, FAAP, FACS
Department of Urology
University of Virginia
Charlottesville, Virginia

Ann M. Phillips, RN, BSN
Long Island Jewish Medical Center
New Hyde Park, New York

Peter A. Pinto, MD
Brady Urological Institute
Johns Hopkins Medical Institutions
Baltimore, Maryland

Jed Pollack, MD
Department of Radiation Oncology
Long Island Jewish Medical Center
New Hyde Park, New York

James Porter, MD
Department of Urology
Swedish Urology Group
Seattle, Washington

Glenn M. Preminger, MD
Department of Surgery
Duke University Medical Center
Durham, North Carolina

Sejal S. Quayle, MD
Department of Surgery
Washington University School of Medicine
St. Louis, Missouri

Danny M. Rabah, MD, FRCSC
Devine Tidewater Urology
Norfolk, Virginia

Raymond R. Rackley, MD
Glickman Urological Institute
Cleveland Clinic
Cleveland, Ohio

Ardeshir Rastinehad, DO
Department of Urology
Long Island Jewish Medical Center
New Hyde Park, New York

Rose Ravalli, MSN, CURN
Department of Urology
Long Island Jewish Medical Center
New Hyde Park, New York

Hassan Razvi, MD, FRCSC
Department of Urology
University of Western Ontario
London, Ontario, Canada

Omar M. Abdel Razzak, MBBCh, MSc, MD
Department of Urology
Cairo University
Cairo, Egypt

John C. Rewcastle, PhD
Department of Radiology
University of Calgary
Calgary, Alberta, Canada

Jean de la Rosette, MD, PhD
Department of Urology
University of Amsterdam
Amsterdam, The Netherlands

Matthew E. Rutter, MD
Department of Urology
Medical College of Ohio
Toledo, Ohio

Francisco J.B. Sampaio, MD
Department of Anatomy
State University of Rio de Janeiro
Rio de Janeiro, Brazil

Jaspreet Sandhu, MD
Department of Urology
Weill Cornell Medical Center
New York, New York

Charles D. Scales Jr, MD
Department of Surgery
Duke University Medical Center
Durham, North Carolina

Jonathan D. Schiff, MD
Department of Urology
Weill Cornell Medical Center
New York, New York

Peter Schulam, MD
Department of Urology
University of California
Los Angeles, California

Joseph W. Segura, MD
Department of Urology
Mayo Clinic
Rochester, Minnesota

Ojas Shah, MD
Department of Urology
New York University Medical Center
New York, New York

Arieh L. Shalhav, MD
Department of Surgery
University of Chicago
Chicago, Illinois

Andrew I. Shpall, MD
Department of Endourology
Kaiser Permanente Medical Center
Los Angeles, California

Douglas Skarecky
Department of Urology
University of California
Irvine, California

Steven J. Skoog, MD, FAAP, FACS
Department of Pediatric Urology
Oregon Health and Science University
Portland, Oregon

Arthur D. Smith, MD
Department of Urology
Long Island Jewish Medical Center
New Hyde Park, New York

Brent W. Snow, MD
Department of Urology
University of Utah
Salt Lake City, Utah

Howard M. Snyder III, MD
Department of Pediatric Urology
St. Louis Children's Hospital
St. Louis, Missouri

Andrea Sorcini, MD
Department of Urology
Lahey Clinic
Burlington, Massachusetts

W. Patrick Springhart, MD
Comprehensive Kidney Stone Center
Duke University Medical Center
Durham, North Carolina

Andrew P. Steinberg, MD
Department of Laparoscopic and Robotic
    Surgery
Cleveland Clinic Foundation
Cleveland, Ohio

Marshall L. Stoller, MD
Department of Urology
University of California
San Francisco, California

Stevan B. Streem, MD
Department of Urology
Cleveland Clinic Foundation
Cleveland, Ohio

Li-Ming Su, MD
Department of Urology
Johns Hopkins Medical Institutions
Baltimore, Maryland

Chandru P. Sundaram, MD, FRCS
Department of Urology
Indiana University School of Medicine
Indianapolis, Indiana

Roger L. Sur, MD
Department of Surgery
Duke University Medical Center
Durham, North Carolina

Ronald S. Sutherland, MD
Department of Surgery
Tripler Army Medical Center
Honolulu, Hawaii

Hubert S. Swana, MD
Department of Urology
University of California
San Francisco, California

Andrew H.H. Tan, MBChB, FRACS
Department of Urology
University of Western Ontario
London, Ontario

Yeh Hong Tan, MD, FRCS
Department of Urology
Duke University Medical Center
Durham, North Carolina

Alexis E. Te, MD
Department of Urology
Weill Cornell Medical Center
New York, New York

Joel Teichman, MD
Department of Urology
University of Texas
San Antonio, Texas

Atul A. Thakre, MD
Department of Surgery
Kesar SAL Medical College and
    Research Institute
Ahmedabad, Gujarat, India

Raju Thomas, MD
Department of Urology
Tulane University Health Sciences Center
New Orleans, Louisiana

T.J. Thompson, MD
Scottish Lithotriptor Centre
Western General Hospital NHS Trust
Edinburgh, United Kingdom

D.A. Tolley, MD
Scottish Lithotriptor Centre
Western General Hospital NHS Trust
Edinburgh, United Kingdom

Scott Troxel, MD
Department of Urology
University of Iowa
Iowa City, Iowa

Robert D. Tucker, PhD, MD
Department of Pathology
University of Iowa
Iowa city, Iowa

Ingolf A. Tuerk, MD, PhD
Department of Urology
Tufts University School of Medicine
Boston, Massachusetts

Osamu Ukimura, MD
Department of Laparoscopic and Robotic
    Surgery
Cleveland Clinic Foundation
Cleveland, Ohio

Brian A. VanderBrink, MD
Department of Urology
Long Island Jewish Medical Center
New Hyde Park, New York

John M. Varkarakis, MD
Department of Urology
Johns Hopkins Medical Institutions
Baltimore, Maryland

Ilya A. Volfson, MD
Department of Surgery
University of Medicine and Dentistry of New
    Jersey
Newark, New Jersey

Lennart Wagrell, MD
Department of Urology
University Hospital Uppsala
Uppsala, Sweden

David S. Wang, MD
Department of Urology
Boston University School of Medicine
Boston, Massachusetts

James C. Williams Jr, PhD
Department of Anatomy and Cell Biology
Indiana University
Indianapolis, Indiana

Lynn R. Willis, PhD
Department of Anatomy and Cell Biology
Indiana University School of Medicine
Indianapolis, Indiana

Howard N. Winfield, MD
Department of Urology
University of Iowa College of Medicine
Iowa City, Iowa

J. Stuart Wolf Jr, MD
Department of Urology
University of Michigan
Ann Arbor, Michigan

Michael Woods, MD
Department of Urology
Tulane University Health Sciences Center
New Orleans, Louisiana

E. James Wright, MD
Department of Urology
Johns Hopkins Medical Institutions
Baltimore, Maryland

Paulos Yohannes, MD
Department of Urology
Long Island Jewish Medical Center
New Hyde Park, New York

Filiberto Zattoni, MD
Department of Urology
University of Verona
Verona, Italy

Stephen A. Zderic, MD, FACS, FAAP
Department of Urology
University of Pennsylvania
Philadelphia, Pennsylvania

CONTENTS

PREFACE

As a surgical intern, I was taught that exposure was the single most important principle of the specialty. The incision, I was informed, must be large to permit an adequate view of the operative field. In one sense, nothing has changed: exposure of the surgical field is still paramount. Yet the way this exposure is achieved has changed dramatically. Various endoscopes and imaging techniques are now often used rather than scalpels. Paradoxically, these new approaches through small incisions give us better visibility because of the magnification provided by endoscopes. As a further benefit, the small incisions greatly reduce the morbidity of surgery.

This change has been part of the development of a new subspecialty known as endourology-closed controlled manipulation within the genitourinary tract. It might be said that endourology was launched in 1978. At that year's meeting of American Urological Association in Washington, DC, a poster illustrated several such techniques, primarily in high-risk patients in whom traditional surgery was not possible. Since then, the creative efforts of many urologists, radiologists, and engineers have vastly expanded the number of closed procedures, many of which have replaced traditional open operations even in low-risk patients. In the course of time all urologic procedures may prove amenable to endoscopy, and future surgical interns will no longer be cautioned about the need for large incisions.

These first two paragraphs were written as a preface to the first edition. In the past ten years, there has been a radical change in urology and now laparoscopic nephrectomy, nephroureterectomy and adrenalectomy have become mainstream urologic procedures while laparoscopic prostatectomy, cystectomy, and para-aortic node dissection are routinely performed.

The development of robotic surgery has shortened the learning curve for laparoscopic surgical training, because the flexibility of the robotic arms enables the urologist to suture more rapidly and with greater accuracy. This in turn encourages the urologist to tackle more demanding reconstructive and vascular procedures.

A goal of urology is to minimize the morbidity of our various therapies. It is obvious that the advent of smaller incisions with more effective access to the site of the pathology has revolutionized therapy. Technology has now introduced the capability for therapies that require yet smaller or no incisions, examples being percutaneous needle ablation of tumors using heat, cold or radioactivity. High frequency ultrasound applied without any incision is being used on prostatic and kidney tumors. Urologists are the physicians who are most familiar with urologic pathology and the natural progression of urologic conditions and ours must be the medical discipline that continues to treat these patients. Therefore it is essential that we embrace and perform these procedures.

This new edition differs from the first in many respects. New chapters have been introduced and the existing chapters have been updated. There are abundant colored illustrations and the book has been reformatted to comprise one large volume.

I would like to take this opportunity to thank Brian Decker for publishing this second edition expeditiously so that new information could be dispensed sooner. His team including Maria Reyes and Petrice Custance have been exceptionally helpful and accommodating.

The reader will greatly benefit from the wealth of experience evident throughout this textbook and I am grateful to all of the contributors for sharing their knowledge so generously.

Finally I would like to thank my wife Kay for all her support and help during the production of this new edition.

Arthur D. Smith, MD
August 2006

To those who have been responsible
for my professional training

D.J. (Sonny) du Plessis, Professor of Surgery
at the University of Witwatersrand,
who taught me the basic principles of surgery.

P.J. (Nol) van Blerk, Professor of Urology
at the University of Witwatersrand, who encouraged
and stimulated me to become a urologist.

Elwin Fraley, Professor of Urology
at the University of Minnesota, who nurtured
my interest in academic urology and
taught me to question established techniques.

Finally, I would like to acknowledge my colleagues
and patients who have challenged me to come up
with new solutions to many problems.

A.D.S

Part I

Basic Principles

Optics of Flexible and Rigid Endoscopes: Physical Principals

Richard K. Babayan, MD
David S. Wang, MD

Until the mid-1980s, urologists had relied almost exclusively on rigid optical endoscopes for visualization of the urinary tract. With the introduction of endourologic techniques, there arose a definite need for instruments capable of accessing the hidden reaches of the upper as well as the lower urinary tract. Adaptation of the flexible fiberoptic endoscopes used in the respiratory and gastrointestinal tracts filled the initial void. Later, as urologists became more familiar with the use of these flexible fiberscopes, purpose-built flexible cystoscopes and ureteropyeloscopes began to appear. This chapter will describe the physical principles involved in the manufacture and use of these different urologic endoscopes, discussing both their similarities and their differences and how these optical and mechanical variations affect the daily usefulness of flexible and rigid endoscopes.

RIGID ENDOSCOPES

HISTORY The history of rigid optical urologic endoscopes is well documented[1–3] and takes as its earliest predecessor the direct-vision urethral tube, through which candlelight was transmitted, as illustrated by Bozzini's Lichtleiter in 1806. By 1879 Nitze and Leiter had incorporated a simple lens system into the viewing tube, creating a rudimentary version of the modern cystoscope. Within the next decade, indirect illumination was replaced by heated platinum wires and later by incandescent light bulbs. Modern fiberoptic lighting was introduced in the 1960s and replaced the incandescent bulb, revolutionizing the manufacture of rigid endoscopes by providing not only more illumination, but also by making it safer, cooler, and less bulky. This use of cold fiberoptic illumination form of external light source has permitted the development of smaller-profile endoscopic shafts as well as more room within the shaft for instrumentation and irrigation channels. The other major developmental breakthrough in the twentieth century was the introduction of the Hopkins rod-lens system.[4] By replacing the thin relay lenses within the shaft of the telescope with long, contoured glass rods, Hopkins was able to increase light transmission ninefold over previous lens systems. This resulted in both an improvement in the refractive index and an increase in the viewing angle, while at the same time decreasing the profile of the telescope shaft (Figure 1-1).

PHYSICAL CHARACTERISTICS Much of the work by the endourologist involves structures that may be accessed by means of rigid endoscopes. These endoscopes differ from one another depending on the purpose for which they have been manufactured. Whether it is a nephroscope being passed through a dilated or sheathed percutaneous nephrostomy tract into the renal pelvis, or a ureteroscope that needs to be maneuvered through the urethra and bladder before entering the ureter, these rigid endoscopes are little more than sophisticated adaptations of the standard rigid cystoscopes that have been used by urologists for more than 100 years. The physical differences revolve around changes in diameter, length, and instrumentation channel. Very little difference exists insofar as rigid optics are concerned, regardless of whether one is referring to rigid nephroscopes, ureteroscopes, or cystoscopes. For nephroscopes and cystoscopes, which are of comparable working lengths, there is little impact on the optics during routine use. Rigid ureterorenoscopes, on the other hand, may have their optics severely impaired during routine passage. This tends to be related to both the caliber and the working length of the instrument as well as to the tortuosity of the anatomy through which the scope is being passed. For this reason, the newer, smaller-profile miniscopes incorporate a rigid shaft design by a flexible fiberoptic imaging lens, which will be described in detail elsewhere.

OPTICS Rigid endoscopes use a telescope that consists of a series of lenses along the shaft to relay a single optical image from the imaging lens at the distal tip of the endoscope back to the eye of the urologist as he peers into the ocular lens. In the early days of rigid optics, the image was transmitted back through the hollow tube of the telescope via thin relay and field lenses placed at precise distances within the air-filled assembly tube. In the late 1950s, Hopkins invented the rod-lens system, which reduced the air spaces between lenses with long rods of glass, ground, contoured, and polished at both ends with only short gaps of air in between. Once this endoscopic image is transported back through the telescope, it can be magnified at the ocular lens. The degree of magnification is to some extent dependent on the diameter of the viewing lens. Thus the size of the magnified image obtained through a small-caliber ureteroscope will always be smaller than that obtained from a larger bore cystoscope. The rod-

lens design allows for excellent clarity of vision and resolution as long as the shaft remains straight. If too much torque is placed on the shaft of the endoscope, as is often the case in the ureteroscope, the image may become distorted, commonly resulting in a half-moon appearance, or the lens may be damaged or come out of alignment if the shaft is bent too much. This problem has led manufacturers to merge flexible fiberoptics with a rigid shaft design in the creation of narrow-profile "miniscopes" for ureteroscopy.

In recent years, the addition of video cameras and monitor-based endoscopes has largely eliminated the discrepancy between images obtained from large versus smaller endoscopes. By projecting the image on a large TV monitor, the urologist not only benefits from the larger projected image, but also has the advantage of binocular as opposed to monocular viewing. Objective lenses with angles ranging from 0 to 120 degrees are available for use, depending on the task at hand. Traditionally, cystoscopes have been manufactured with interchangeable lenses, with the 30- and 70-degree lenses used most commonly within the bladder. The 0- and 5-degree lenses are favored for direct-vision internal urethrotomy of urethral strictures, whereas lenses varying from 12 to 30 degrees are preferred for transurethral prostate surgery. For rigid ureteroscopes and nephroscopes, the direct-vision lens is most often used, and rarely is it necessary to exchange lenses. Given the fact that most rigid nephroscopic and ureteroscopic procedures are performed within a confined space, virtually all of the smaller-profile rigid ureteroscopes and most working rigid nephroscopes are manufactured with permanent direct-vision lenses. Interchangeable lenses are available on larger ureteroscopes and some nephroscopes, but these are seldom used.

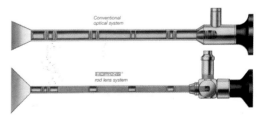

Figure 1-1 Traditional and Hopkins rod-lens design telescopes. Note how the profile has been reduced while the image size has been increased.

CONSTRUCTION Most cystoscopes use straight, direct-viewing telescopes. Access to the instrumentation channel is via angled ports inferior to the telescope (Figure 1-2). This system works well with flexible accessories, but precludes the use of removable rigid accessories such as stone graspers or forceps. To allow for easy entry and removal of rigid accessories, many rigid ureteroscopes and nephroscopes use a right-angle or offset-oblique ocular configuration so that the urologist can have direct access to the instrumentation port for the passage of rigid accessories without impairing the view of the scope (Figure 1-3). This is especially important for rigid nephroscopy in which the placement of large-caliber ultrasonic lithotripsy probes, stone graspers, and endopyelotomy knives requires a straight-line access to the instrumentation channel. With increasing use of video cameras, which have become smaller and less cumbersome, this is becoming less an issue. In the future, as the trend continues toward digital and electronic imaging, the need for a viewable ocular lens may be totally eliminated (Figure 1-4).

FLEXIBLE ENDOSCOPES

HISTORY The use of flexible fiberoptic endoscopes within the urinary tract is a relatively recent phenomenon. The first urologic cases involved the use of modified bronchoscopes in an attempt to retrieve residual stones from kidneys and ureters following open stone surgery via postoperative nephrostomy tube tracts. Later, as interventional techniques improved and percutaneous nephrostolithotomies were routinely being performed, purpose-built flexible nephroscopes appeared to help visualize areas of the upper urinary tract that were inaccessible to rigid scopes. Proper use of these new flexible instruments required the acquisition of a new skill, and endourologists found themselves practicing with the flexible nephroscope to view a familiar and easily approachable organ, the bladder. It soon became apparent that not only could one learn to use the flexible nephroscope by inserting into the bladder, but this technique also yielded a diagnostic view of the bladder itself that was equivalent to the standard rigid cystoscope and was a great deal more comfortable for the patient. Soon thereafter, purpose-built flexible cystoscopes began to be manufactured, and it is estimated that greater than 50% of all in-office diagnostic cystoscopy performed today is done with flexible instrumentation. The use of flexible ureteroscopes was somewhat slower to come

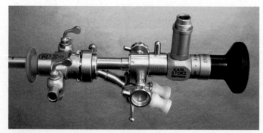

Figure 1-2 Typical rigid cystoscope design.

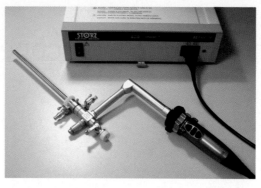

Figure 1-3 Rigid nephroscope with offset (right-angle) configuration of the eyepiece. A solid-state video camera is attached to the ocular lens. Note how the instrumentation port is unencumbered.

about, primarily because of the technical difficulties inherent in designing a small-caliber, flexible, deflectable ureteroscope capable of being easily passed up the ureter without the need for dilation of the ureteral orifice. The first available flexible ureteroscopes were significantly larger in diameter than their rigid counterparts. Their 12 French (F) tip profiles required significant ureteral dilatation, and passage of the scope into the renal pelvis and calices was often difficult. With improvements in engineering design, manufacturers were able to streamline the flexible ureteroscopes, allowing easier, less traumatic passage without causing significant deterioration of optics. Currently, flexible, deflectable ureteroscopes with diameters as small as 7F are available.

PHYSICAL CHARACTERISTICS Flexible instrument design differs significantly from rigid endoscope design in cost and complexity of construction. Flexible endoscopes are both costly and delicate. The basic design common to all flexible fiberoptic endoscopes is illustrated in Figure 1-5. Within the shaft are generally three fiberoptic bundles—two noncoherent bundles of fibers that transmit light and a single coherent bundle of glass fibers that constitutes the imaging bundle.[5] Unlike its rigid counterpart, the image obtained by the fiberoptic bundle is not a single image, but rather a composite matrix of each fiber within the bundle. The image obtained is analogous to a newspaper photograph—that is, it is composed of multiple dots merging into a single reconstructed image (Figure 1-6). This "honeycomb" effect, although not as high in resolution as the rigid rod-lens image, is certainly adequate for urinary endoscope, especially when one considers the lack of distortion of the image regardless of the number of turns or angles the flexible endoscope must make to reach its target. Each optical fiber in the bundle is approximately 8 micrometers in diameter and is composed of glass possessing a higher refractive index than the cladding that surrounds it (Figure 1-7). This composition allows for excellent light and image preservation over long distances and around significant flexion of the bundle. The coherent bundle consists of thousands of individual fibers with an identical arrangement of

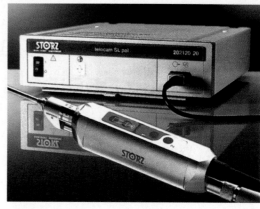

Figure 1-4 Videoendoscope. Note the lack of a direct-viewing ocular lens.

these fibers at each end of the bundle. Thus the exact image and orientation of each fiber is transmitted along the entire bundle to the ocular lens at the eyepiece. Even though the optical fibers are quite flexible, they are also quite delicate and may be damaged by excessive flexion, force, or pressure on the shaft of the scope. If an individual fiber is damaged on the optical bundle, it will be reflected within the composite image as a black dot, which will be incapable of transmitting light. Too many broken fibers will eventually lead to an indeterminate image.

Most flexible endoscopes possess the capability of active deflection in two directions, either up and down or side to side. This action is accomplished via a series of interlocking hinges within the distal shaft of the scope, which are connected to the deflecting lever in the handle via thin rods and pulleys that run the length of the shaft (Figure 1-8). The orientation of the irrigation/instrumentation port to the direction of maximum deflection varies with each manufacturer. Most flexible endoscopes are sufficiently torque stable so that the direction of the angle of flexion can be changed by rotating the shaft of the scope. All the new flexible endoscopes possess an area proximal to the active deflection where they will passively flex on contact with tissue. This ability to passively deflect allows retroflexion of the flexible cystoscope to

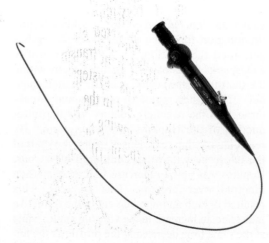

Figure 1-5 Typical flexible endoscope design.

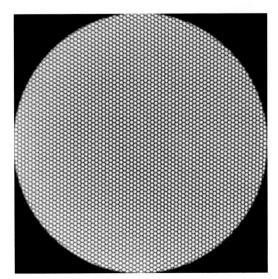

Figure 1-6 Magnified view of a composite image from a flexible fiberoptic imaging bundle.

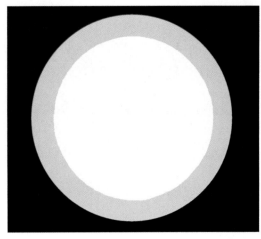

Figure 1-7 Magnified cross section of a single flexible glass fiber illustrating a central glass core with cladding of different optical refraction.

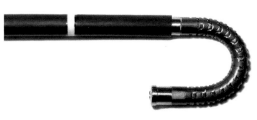

Figure 1-8 Tip of a flexible endoscope with the outer "skin" peeled away to reveal an active deflection mechanism.

view the bladder neck. It also allows flexible ureteroscopes to passively deflect off of the renal pelvis and enter lower and middle calices.

COMPOSITE SCOPES

As mentioned previously, a recent trend in rigid ureteroscopy has been to merge rigid shaft construction with flexible optics. The resulting "miniscopes" thus possess a small-profile rigid shaft with either one or two irrigation/instrumentation ports and a fiberoptic imaging bundle. The use of fiberoptics rather than the traditional rigid rod-lens design allows for the smaller shaft diameter and also eliminates the optical distortion when the shaft of the scope is torqued. These favorable characteristics more than compensate for any loss in resolution of the endoscopic image resulting from the fiberoptic imaging bundle.

DIGITAL ENDOSCOPES

Although significant advances in endoscopic optics have occurred within the last century, it is likely that traditional optical systems with direct-viewing lenses will be replaced by digital and electronic imaging. The endoscope of the future, whether rigid or flexible, will contain no viewing lens component. The traditional lenses will be replaced by charge coupled device (CCD) chips small enough to be mounted at the distal end of the shaft. Instead of a rod-lens design or fiberoptic viewing bundles, the CCD chip will relay digitized

viewing information via a single fiber back to a distant processor, which will reconstruct and enhance the image electronically on a television monitor. Not only will the quality of the image be superior to present-day optics, but also the reproduction of the images will not suffer any generational deterioration, as is the case with present-day analog imaging. The use of carbon fibers and materials such as nitinol and superelastic and superplastic steels are now used in construction of more durable scopes with better flexion capability. The space savings with the shaft of the scopes will allow for lighter weight and narrower contour designs as well as larger instrumentation channels.

At the present time, such technology has already been implemented, resulting in fully digital flexible cystoscopes. Such prototype digital cystoscopes contain no fiberoptic cables, which is distinctly different from conventional analog cystoscopes. Instead, the image viewed via the tip of the cystoscope is electronically and digitally transferred through a single cable and recreated on a television monitor. The picture generated

using such digital technology is superior to that of conventional cystoscopy. In addition, the digital technology eliminates the need for an additional light source and camera setup. The lack of bundled fiberoptic cables will allow for smaller-sized scopes, larger working elements, increased flexibility, and improved scope durability. Continued efforts are underway to adapt digital technology to flexible and rigid ureteroscopes. Such technology should allow for continued reduction in instrumentation size with improvement in instrument visualization and durability.

FUTURE TRENDS

Without question, technological improvements in endoscope design will continue to improve the urologist's ability to diagnose and treat pathologic conditions along the urinary tract. Future technology may also further improve visualization by incorporating three-dimensional imaging options, using two CCD chips to create stereoscopic images with true depth perception. At present, stereoscopic imaging modalities exist in laparoscopic and robotic surgery, and such technology could be applied to endoscopic equipment designed for the urinary tract. All these concepts involve technology that exists at present. The incorporation of these concepts into manufacturers' designs will emerge as the costs of technology decrease and the miniaturization of the CCD chips evolves. It is also conceivable that as digital technology progresses, endoscopes will be able to transmit images wirelessly, further simplifying the scopes and making them less cumbersome with better ergonomics.

In addition to improvements in image quality, it is probable that instruments of the urinary tract, particularly of the upper tract, will continue to decrease in size. Currently, for instance, ureteroscopy in pediatric patients can be more challenging than in adult patients because of the smaller anatomic size. However, continued refinements will likely lead to reduced-caliber instrument size without the loss of flexibility or scope durability.

REFERENCES

1. Nicholson P. Problems encountered by early endoscopists. Urology 1982;19:114–9.
2. Moore TT. The history of the development of urology as a specialty. J Urol 1993;10:99–120.
3. Buerger L. A historical survey of the development of modern urological instruments. Urol Cutaneous Rev 1931;35:1–25.
4. Hopkins HH. Optical principles of the endoscope. In: Berci G, editor. Endoscopy. New York: Appleton-Century-Crofts; 1976. p. 3–26.
5. Epstein M. Endoscopy: developments in optical instrumentation. Science 1980;210:280–5.

Care and Sterilization of Instruments

Donna W. Parsons, RN
Nina L. Lee, RN
Glenn M. Preminger, MD

The cleaning and maintenance of all surgical instruments and equipment are critical to provide safe and efficient patient care. But the care of endoscopic and other specialized endourologic instruments presents unique problems. Most rigid and flexible endoscopes are fragile, as well as costly, thereby necessitating appropriate cleaning and storage. The general operating room staff is often unfamiliar with specialized endourologic equipment such as intracorporeal lithotripsy devices, which warrant individualized care. New and unique endoscopes and other instruments are constantly being developed for use in the field of endourology before eventually being used in other minimally invasive surgical procedures. Therefore physicians and support staff should be familiar with appropriate care and maintenance of such specialized equipment.

This chapter discusses cleaning, disinfection, sterilization, maintenance, handling, and storage of the instruments used in urologic endoscopic surgery.

DECONTAMINATION

The two methods of decontamination currently being used in operating rooms and endoscopy suites are sterilization and disinfection. Sterilization involves total destruction of all microorganisms and bacterial spores using flowing or pressurized steam or chemical agents such as ethylene oxide. Alternatively, disinfection destroys or inhibits the growth of pathogenic microorganisms.

Medical devices that come in contact with patients in the operating room may be divided into the following categories: (1) critical items, which enter normally sterile tissue or the vascular system; (2) semi-critical items, which come in contact with mucous membranes or nonintact skin; and (3) noncritical items, which do not touch the patient but may come in contact with intact skin. Endoscopic equipment falls into the semicritical and noncritical categories, in which various sterilization methods may be used, as well as high-level disinfection (Table 2-1).

The method of sterilization depends on many factors, including the level of disinfection desired, time needed for adequate sterilization, and availability of backup instruments. Compliance with federal and institutional guidelines as well as manufacturers' recommendations must also be considered. The degree of decontamination achieved by the various methods of sterilization and disinfection is noted in Table 2-2.

Table 2-1 Classification of Endoscopic Equipment	
Semi-critical	**Noncritical**
Rigid endoscopes	Video cameras
Flexible endoscopes	Light cords
Ultrasound/electrohydraulic lithotripter probes	Electrical cords
Laser lithotripsy fibers	

STERILIZATION Steam Heat and moisture are used during steam sterilization to decontaminate endoscopic instruments. Temperatures of 1,208 to 1,458°C and adequate exposure times are necessary to ensure sterility of all bacterial spores. The steam must come in contact with all surfaces of the instruments and a "steam indicator" should be placed with the endoscope to ensure that sterility has been achieved.

Although steam sterilization is ideal for most metal surgical instruments, it cannot be used for heat-labile or moisture-sensitive instruments such as some delicate surgical instruments, large pieces of equipment, plastic and porous materials, and electrical instruments. Much of the endoscopic and intracorporeal lithotripsy equipment is of this type; therefore steam sterilization is not recommended for most endoscopic instruments.

Gas The preferred method of sterilization for most endoscopic equipment is gas sterilization using ethylene oxide. The ethylene oxide gas, in conjunction with humidity, facilitates bactericidal and sporicidal activity. Ethylene oxide gas is a severe local irritant; therefore lengthy aeration of gas-sterilized items follows the sterilization cycle. A "gas indicator" should be placed with these instruments to ensure that adequate sterilization has been achieved.

DISINFECTION Cold Soak High-level disinfection is achieved by soaking instruments in

Table 2-2 Decontamination Achieved and Time Required with Sterilization and Disinfection		
Type	Degree Achieved	Time
Steam	Sterilization	4–10 min
Gas	Sterilization	4 hr, aeration 8 hr
Cold soak	High-level disinfection	20–45 min
Automated soak	Sterilization/high-level disinfection*	20-min cycle
*		

solutions such as glutaraldehyde, which requires a minimum exposure time of 30 minutes, depending on manufacturers' as well as federal and institutional recommendations. Thorough rinsing of equipment with sterile water or saline solution is necessary before placing the items in the sterile field. The cold soak disinfection method for endoscopic equipment has been used for years because of its low cost and ease of use. Newer methods of soaking endoscopic instruments, however, have recently been developed.

Automated Soak Another method of high-level disinfection is automated soak using peracetic acid—a component of an equilibrium mixture of acetic acid, hydrogen peroxide, and water. This method uses a cold sterilant and is nontoxic. The sterilizer is a tabletop machine with external requirements of a water supply, sink drain, and 110 V of electricity (Figure 2-1). The machine is operated by push button, controlled by a computer, has self-diagnostic capabilities, and produces a printed document showing that the sterilization parameters of temperature and exposure time have been met during the sterilization cycle. Precleaned items are loaded into the sterilizer, and a container of peracetic acid is inserted into the machine. The unit is then cycled for automatic dilution, and the instruments are ready within 30 minutes.

COMPARISON OF METHODS The choice of decontamination method depends on the situation (Table 2-3). Gas sterilization is the preferred method for overnight decontamination because the equipment is processed and ready for early-start procedures, and sterility is guaranteed until the integrity of the wrapping or packaging is broken. Cold soak or automated soaking is recom-

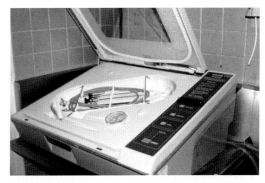

Figure 2-1 An automated soaking system (Steris, Mentor, Ohio) that uses peracetic acid to decontaminate rigid and flexible instruments.

Item	Steam	Gas	Cold soak	Automated (Steris)
Table 2-3 Choosing the Proper Method of Sterilization/Decontamination				
Rigid endoscopes (eg, sheaths, bridges, stopcocks)	Yes	Yes	Yes	Yes
Microlens	No	Yes	Yes	Yes
Flexible endoscopes	No	Yes	Yes*	Yes†
Light cords	No	Yes	Yes	Yes
Electrical cord (eg, electrohydraulic lithotripter, ultrasonic transducers)	No	Yes	Yes†	No
Laser fibers	No	Yes	Yes†	No
Cameras	No	Yes	Yes	Yes†

*Make sure gas/soak dial is properly set.
†Check manufacturer's recommendations.

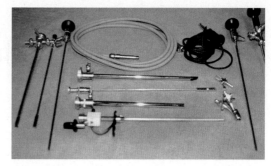

Figure 2-2 Sample of rigid endoscopes used for routine endourologic procedures. Also included are a light cord and an electrosurgical cord.

mended for rapid turnover of procedures, as all endoscopic equipment is considered either semicritical or noncritical. The chemical used for cold soak is highly toxic; therefore precautions must be taken to prevent splashing and contact with skin. Instruments must be thoroughly rinsed and all ports flushed with sterile water before use.

The chemicals used in the automated method are nontoxic; therefore, instruments can be taken directly from the sterilizer to the operating room. Sterile rinsing occurs as part of the processor's cycle. Minimum exposure times for the cold soak and automated methods can range from 20 to 45 minutes, which makes these methods advantageous for rapid turnover of procedures (see Table 2-2).

Steam sterilization should not be used because of the possibility of damage to the equipment. At our institution, gas sterilization is used in preparation for early-morning (first-case) procedures, and cold soak and/or automated soak are used for subsequent procedures. We have found that these methods work very well since the same equipment is not used every day; therefore, gas-sterilized equipment is ready for immediate use.

RIGID ENDOSCOPIC EQUIPMENT

Rigid endoscopes include cystoscopes, resectoscopes, nephroscopes, ureteroscopes, and laparoscopes (Figure 2-2). The cleaning process begins at the operating table where all residual matter (eg, blood, tissue, irrigation fluid) is rinsed off with sterile water or saline solution. All connection sites and interchangeable parts are disassembled and mechanically cleaned at a sink using sponges, soft brushes, mild detergent, and water. Thorough rinsing and drying of endoscopes is essential to prolong the life of the instruments and to prepare them for terminal gas sterilization.

RIGID LENS SYSTEM Rigid endoscopes require special handling because of the delicate nature of the glass ocular lens, the eyepiece, the fiberoptic light-cable connection, the shaft (which contains either a rod-lens or fiberoptic lens system), and the objective lens. Before the cleaning process is begun, the rigid endoscope must be inspected for damage. The scope is held by the heavy eyepiece, and the distal end is supported (Figure 2-3). Initially, the lens is cleansed with a mild detergent, water, and a soft cloth, after which it is cleaned

with 70% alcohol and reinspected for damage. The endoscope is then packaged for gas sterilization or decontamination using either cold soak or peracetic acid, depending on the manufacturer's recommendation. If gas sterilization is planned, the rigid lens system should be placed in a padded rigid box for protection during transport and sterilization (Figure 2-4).

ENDOSCOPIC SHEATHS The endoscopic sheath also requires special handling to avoid bending or denting of the shaft (Figure 2-5). The sheath is inspected for rough edges or metal burrs and the inner channels and working and irrigation ports are cleaned with soft brushes and rinsed thoroughly. Stopcocks are opened, cleaned with soft brushes and mild detergent, and rinsed well. The obturator should be inspected for smoothness and efficiency of the locking mechanism. Stopcocks and movable parts of the rigid endoscope are lubricated as needed with instrument milk to ensure smooth movement of these parts.

SINGLE-PIECE ENDOSCOPES Single-piece endoscopes such as nephroscopes, ureteroscopes, and laparoscopes should be cleaned in a similar fashion as rigid endoscopes (cystoscopes) and microlens systems. The lens should be carefully inspected for breakage or cloudiness. The sheath should be inspected for debris, denting, or rough surfaces. All channels and ports should be cleaned with water and a mild detergent using a soft brush, and the lens should be cleaned with 70% alcohol and dried with compressed air. All ports and channels should be opened before gas sterilization or soaking.

FIBEROPTIC LIGHT CORDS AND ELECTROSURGICAL CORDS

Fiberoptic cables may be cleaned with a mild detergent and water, and the distal and proximal ends are cleaned with 70% alcohol. The light cable should be inspected for damage by holding one end up to the light and observing the other end for black spots. The spots indicate broken fibers. The cords are then loosely peel-packed for gas sterilization, or they can be soaked in glutaraldehyde for the recommended institutional and federally regulated time. The cords can then be rinsed with sterile water and used on the sterile field. Many of the light cords currently on the

market can be flash sterilized for 10 minutes in an autoclave. The manufacturers' instructions for each particular light cord should be followed for appropriate sterilization methods.

FLEXIBLE ENDOSCOPIC EQUIPMENT

The flexible endoscopes used in endourology have a narrow outer diameter and working channels smaller than 2 mm. These scopes consist of an eyepiece connected to a flexible fiberscope that has one or two working/irrigation channels. The delicate fibers, small ports, and eyepiece make flexible endoscopes difficult to clean and maintain. Gentle handling and proper cleansing are required to maintain the integrity and life of flexible endoscopes (Figure 2-6).

Water should be suctioned through the working ports of the instrument immediately after use to remove debris. All channels and ports are opened and flushed with a mild detergent and water. The channel brush supplied by the manufacturer is inserted into the port and used to scrub the entire length of the endoscope. If any resistance is encountered during cleaning, the port can be flushed with water until the brush is easily inserted. The scope is rinsed with copious amounts of water until clear, and the outside jacket is cleaned with a mild detergent, water, and a soft cloth. The scope is air dried by blowing compressed air through the channel. It is now ready for gas sterilization or cold soaking as per the manufacturer's guidelines. After soaking in a glutaraldehyde bath, copious amounts of sterile saline solution must be used to flush out the glutaraldehyde to prevent irritation to the patient.

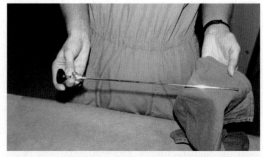

Figure 2-3 The rigid objective lens should be properly supported during the cleaning process. The lens is cleaned with a mild detergent and water and a soft cloth.

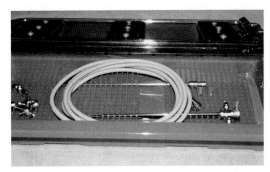

Figure 2-4 Both rigid and flexible endoscopes can be stored in specialized plastic containers during gas sterilization. Such sterilization/storage boxes can be equipped with specialized rubber supports to protect the delicate endoscopic equipment.

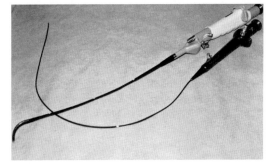

Figure 2-6 Flexible endoscopes require special handling because of the delicate nature of these specialized instruments.

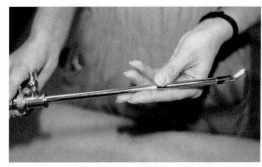

Figure 2-5 Endoscopic sheaths and obturators should also be handled with care to avoid bending or denting of the shaft. The obturator should cleanly slide through the endoscopic sheath.

LEAKAGE TESTING Flexible endoscopes should be periodically "leak tested" to determine the integrity of the scope. A leakage tester is usually supplied by the manufacturer (Figure 2-7). Testing should be performed according to the manufacturer's instructions and recommendations. Most manufacturers recommend that a leakage test be performed before immersion of the flexible endoscope to determine whether a significant defect in the working channel(s) or outside covering of the scope exists. After the absence of any major defects or leaks is confirmed, the flexible endoscope may be immersed in a shallow water bath to determine the loss of working port integrity in its watertight construction. If no leaks are noted, the endoscope can be safely soaked for disinfection.

VIDEO EQUIPMENT

The video camera operates as the eyes of the urologic surgeon, and special care must be taken to prevent damage and prolong the life of this essential piece of equipment. The video camera is cleaned with a mild detergent, rinsed with water, and dried with a soft cloth (Figure 2-8). Particular attention is given to the eyepiece; a soft, lint-free cloth and 70% alcohol are used for cleaning. Since video cameras may be considered noncritical items that normally do not come in contact with the patient, they can be wrapped with a plastic camera drape and placed on the sterile field (Figure 2-9). Another alternative is to sterilize the video camera using gas after placing it in a well-padded, sturdy container. The camera cord should be loosely wrapped in the box to avoid twisting or bending of the cable.

The optical coupler of the video camera should be cleaned and lubricated weekly. The quad ring within the coupler should be lubricated weekly with a few drops of mineral oil, taking care that the mineral oil does not come in contact with the lens surface. The camera can also be soaked in glutaraldehyde for a maximum of 2 hours. When using a cold soak, the connector plug should not be placed in the solution because the chemical may leak into the connector, damaging the delicate contents of the plug.

Other cables are cleaned with a mild detergent, rinsed with water, and dried with a soft cloth. They

are then loosely peel-packed for gas sterilization. Under no circumstances should a steam autoclave be used for the optical coupler or camera.

LITHOTRIPSY EQUIPMENT

ULTRASONIC LITHOTRIPTOR The ultrasonic lithotriptor consists of a sonotrode and a metal probe. The sonotrode and the metal probe should be separated using the special wrench supplied by the manufacturer (Figure 2-10). The sonotrode contains two channels: one for the suction tubing and the other containing the cord to the ultrasonic generator. After each use, the sonotrode should be cleaned with water and a nonabrasive detergent. The probe is removed and the suction channel cleaned with a cleaning stylet or cleaning pistol. The channel is dried with compressed air.

All nondisposable probes for ultrasonic lithotripsy should be carefully inspected for any damage to the interior surface of the probe material. The probe should be carefully inspected for dent-

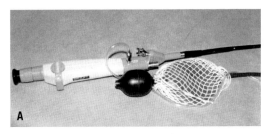

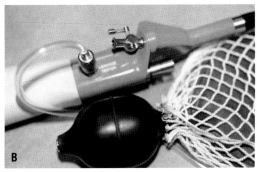

Figure 2-7 *A*, Leakage testing should be performed routinely on flexible endoscopes to prevent damage during disinfection and/or use. This type of testing ensures the integrity of the flexible endoscope channels. *B*, Close-up view of testing device.

ing, bending, or metallic burrs that may form on the distal tip of the probe. The probe is cleaned with a mild detergent and the channel brush is carefully inserted and maneuvered through the entire length of the probe. The probe is rinsed with water and dried with a soft cloth. The channel is then visually reinspected for scratches, denting, or grooves. The probes and transducer are then stored in an approved sterilizing container and gas sterilized.

The transducer may also be cold soaked; to avoid damaging the contents, however, the connector should not be immersed in the solution. Any grasping forceps used during ultrasonic lithotripsy should be cleaned with a mild detergent, rinsed with water, and dried with a soft cloth.

ELECTROHYDRAULIC LITHOTRIPSY With electrohydraulic lithotripsy, the electrical current travels through a nondisposable cable into a disposable, Teflon-coated probe. The probes are sized according to the location of the calculi. Larger probes (5 French and 9F) are usually used for bladder calculi, whereas smaller ones (1.9F and 3F) are used for ureteral stones. The connecting cable is cleaned with a soft cloth, moistened with water and a mild soap, and dried carefully with a soft cloth. The cable can then be gas sterilized. Most manufacturers do not recommend steam sterilization or cold soaking because this may damage the contents of the connecting cable. The electrohydraulic lithotripsy probes are disposable and should be discarded immediately after use.

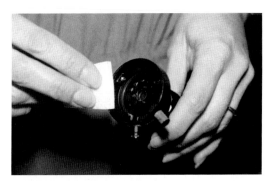

Figure 2-8 The video camera head should be cleaned with a mild detergent and dried with a soft cloth. The objective lens can be dried with an alcohol swab.

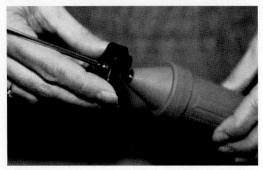

Figure 2-9 Video cameras may be placed in a camera drape since they are considered to be noncritical items.

LASER FIBERS Most laser fibers can be disinfected by immersion in a 2% solution of glutaraldehyde. The manufacturer's recommendations must always be followed for proper disinfection. Sterilization can be achieved using ethylene oxide following hospital sterilization procedures.

INSTRUMENT STORAGE

RIGID ENDOSCOPES Standard rigid urologic endoscopes should be stored in a carefully padded and approved rigid container to prevent damage during transport and gas sterilization (see Figure 2-4). Different types of sterilization/storage boxes are available and made primarily of either metal or plastic. Care must be taken to ensure that the rigid scopes fit securely in the foam rubber compartments.

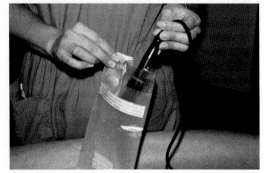

Figure 2-10 The ultrasonic lithotripsy probe should be disassembled from the sonotrode with the wrench supplied by the manufacturer prior to cleaning and decontamination.

FLEXIBLE ENDOSCOPES Flexible endoscopes should always be stored in the extended position without any bending or curling of the shaft. The fiberoptic fibers and internal cables that provide the flexibility of these scopes also make them susceptible to damage from bending or twisting. Moreover, caution should be exercised when storing flexible endoscopes in a box with a lid since it is possible to compress or break the optical fibers if the shaft is inadvertently compressed by the lid.

If the flexible scope is to be gas-sterilized, it should be placed in a carefully padded, rigid box for transport and sterilization. Special attention should be paid to specific manufacturers' guidelines on how to prepare these scopes for gas sterilization; some require a special "gas cap" placed on the specified port. The manufacturer's recommendations should always be followed for storage of each particular scope.

One method of storing flexible endoscopes is to place them vertically on a "wall hanger" (Figure 2-11). This system lessens the chance that the scope will be bent excessively or crushed and will prevent pooling of fluid, promote drying, and prevent early degeneration of the scope.

CONCLUSION

Endourologic instrumentation has changed rapidly as minimally invasive management of urologic diseases has expanded. Improved endoscopes, sophisticated fiberoptics, and advanced video systems facilitate the performance of endourologic procedures. However, the newer fiberoptic endoscopes, lithotripsy devices, and video equipment must be cleaned, sterilized, and properly stored to ensure their proper functioning. Diligent and careful handling of endourologic instruments will greatly prolong the life of this equipment and allow successful completion of minimally invasive urologic procedures.

At Duke University Medical Center, we use cold soak and the automated Steris system (Steris, Mentor, OH) because these methods allow for effective and rapid decontamination of instruments between patients. For instruments that are used infrequently or may be used for the first patient of the day, gas sterilization is an acceptable alternative.

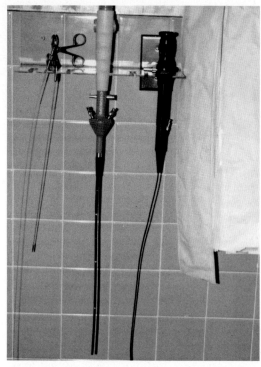

Figure 2-11 An optional means of storing flexible endoscopes is a plastic wall hanger. This method lessens the likelihood that the delicate flexible endoscopes will be damaged during storage.

REFERENCES

1. Association of Operating Room Nurses. Recommended practices for care of instruments, scopes and powered surgical instruments. In: AORN standard and recommended practices for perioperative nursing—1992. Denver, CO: AORN, 1992.
2. Association of Operating Room Nurses. Recommended practices for sterilization and disinfection. In: AORN standard and recommended practices for perioperative nursing—1992. Denver, CO: AORN, 1992.
3. Block SS. Disinfection, sterilization and preservation, 4th ed. Philadelphia: Lea & Febiger, 1991.
4. Froelich MR, Young EC. Care of endoscopic instrumentation. Today's OR Nurse 1993;15:21–26.
5. Kralovic RC. Influence of medical instruments design on sterilization assurance by users. In: Sterilization in the 1990's. Washington, D.C.: Health Manufacturers Association; 1989. pp 97–111.
6. Marousky RT. Troubleshooting the video endoscopy system. Today's OR Nurse 1993;15:31–34.
7. Perkins J. Principles and methods of sterilization and health sciences, 2nd ed. Springfield, Ill: Charles C Thomas, 1983.
8. Rutala WA. APIC guidelines for selection and use of disinfectants. Am J Infect Control 1990;18:99–117.

How to Protect Yourself and Others from Radiation

Wilfrido R. Castaneda, MD
Gregory David Espenan, MS

Imaging equipment in endourology typically uses radiation for image formation, guidance, and verification of catheter placement. Radiographic localization is also employed in lithotripsy for accurate patient positioning prior to stone fragmentation procedures. Radiation devices have been intimately involved in, and are central to, the development of numerous endourologic techniques. Thus, the endourologist is well acquainted with these devices. Despite this familiarity, however, he usually has little formal training in how the unit functions, the amount of radiation it produces, and methods used to minimize both operator and patient exposure.

By law, all parameters affecting image quality, reproducibility, and radiation output from each radiographic unit must be evaluated routinely to ensure optimal image quality while minimizing the patient's radiation dose. Radiation outputs for a set of machine parameters do not vary significantly among units; however, patient and operator doses do vary significantly as a result of the physician's imaging techniques. The endourologist can improve his imaging techniques, and by using simple, "common sense," as low as reasonably achievable (ALARA) techniques minimize both his and the patient's radiation exposure with no concurrent loss of image quality. The increased incidence of radiation-induced skin desquamation and depilation in patients who have undergone fluoroscopically guided procedures underscores the need to control the amount of radiation to which patients are exposed.[1] Skin erythemas have become more common as a result of the increasing length and complexity of fluoroscopic procedures.[2]

This chapter will give a brief overview of the basic principles of x-ray production, estimates of typical machine outputs and radiation fields, implementation of ALARA principles, and guidelines for maintaining patient exposure well below the erythema threshold and estimating typical exposures. In addition, imaging modalities and minor procedural and equipment modifications that offer significant reductions in exposure for both patients and physicians are discussed.

BASIC PRINCIPLES OF X-RAY PRODUCTION AND USE

A brief review of x-ray production will provide the foundation for understanding how to shield physicians, patients, and others from radiation during radiographic imaging. Figure 3-1 is a diagram of an evacuated glass tube and rotating anode x-ray system. The anode is made of a dense material capable of handling a high heat load without warping or vaporizing—the element tungsten is ideal for this purpose. The anode rotates at a high speed to assist in heat dissipation and to minimize focal spot vaporization (the focal spot is the point where impinging electrons are focused). In front of the rotating face of the anode is a cathode that liberates electrons when electric current is applied to its filament. When a filament current (in milliamperes [mA]) is applied to the cathode, electrons are liberated from the cathode in direct proportion to the current applied. In applying a large-voltage potential (kilovolt potential, or kVp) across the tube (usually a 50,000- to 100,000-volt potential difference, or 50 to 100 kVp), electrons liberated from the cathode are accelerated toward the anode.

Most of these electrons (.95%) merely produce heat in the anode. The remaining electrons produce both bremsstrahlung x-rays (or "braking" x-rays) and x-rays characteristic of tungsten. The majority of the radiation produced is of the bremsstrahlung type. Bremsstrahlung is a polyenergetic continuum of x-ray energies produced during the "slowing down" of the accelerated electrons as they interact with the electrons of the anode. A typical spectrum is shown in Figure 3-2. It can be noted from the figure that the average energy of the x-rays (photons) produced is one third of the maximum potential energy applied across the tube. The potential energy is increased

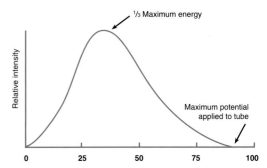

Figure 3-2 Energy distribution of a typical bremsstrahlung-produced x-ray spectrum.

or decreased to compensate for differences in patient thickness as the penetrability of the radiation is directly proportional to the average energy of the photons produced. That is, higher-energy x-rays will penetrate deeper into tissue and will also require more shielding. In increasing the potential energy, enough photons will traverse a thick patient to form an acceptable image. The potential energy is decreased for thinner patients so that the image is not "burnt out" by an overabundance of photons. By using the appropriate potential energy, an image that is useful for diagnostic or positioning purposes is made.

The tube has a lead-lined steel housing to prevent emanation of incoherent, stray, or "leakage" radiation. The housing incorporates shielding that reduces the dose to persons in the vicinity of the tube. A beryllium window in the tube allows only the focused x-rays to leave the tube. These x-rays exit the housing through a focal opening through the shield. As a result of the x-ray tube's thin window, the photons are only slightly attenuated (reduced in quantity) as they leave the tube.

As the distance from the focal spot increases, the size of the beam geometrically increases in diameter. To limit the beam size, the focused radiation is collimated (limited in size) by a lead-leaved collimator or fixed-lead "cut-outs." The collimator is used to reduce the area imaged to only that which is of clinical interest, reducing the size of the patient's irradiated area as well as lessening the radiation scattered from the patient into the room.

After reviewing the fundamentals of equipment function, it follows that the simple techniques listed below will reduce radiation exposure to both the operator and the patient:

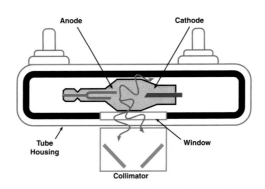

Figure 3-1 Diagram of a typical rotating anode x-ray tube with the main components indicated.

1. When attempting to obtain a diagnostic-quality image and the image is underpenetrated, given the choice between increasing the milliamperes (increasing the total number of x-rays) or increasing the potential energy (increasing the penetrability of the x-rays already present), the potential energy should always be increased first. Although increasing either potential energy or milliamperes will improve the image, increasing the milliamperes will significantly increase the radiation output, whereas increasing the potential energy will not.

2. The radiation output from the x-ray tube should have been evaluated within the past year by a qualified professional (generally a radiologic physicist). This person determines whether the unit's radiation output is within legal limits as well as optimal for each examination. In the case of radiographic imaging, outputs can be compared to national averages, or National Evaluation of X-ray Trends (NEXT) values. NEXT values are assessed by the Food and Drug Administration (FDA) Center for Devices and Radiological Health (CDRH). The CDRH updates these values every few years to allow a comparison of each facility with the national average. The average trend is downward since dose-reducing techniques are continually being implemented.

3. Collimating the image to the minimum size necessary for performing the work will reduce the amount of unnecessary radiation to which the patient and anyone else in the room is exposed.

TYPICAL OUTPUTS AND PRIMARY AND SCATTERED RADIATION FIELDS

Although many different manufacturers and vintages of x-ray equipment are used in endourology, the radiation necessary to produce radiographic and fluoroscopic images is quite consistent from unit to unit. The reason for this is that the speed of the film (the amount of radiation necessary to produce a latent image) and the light output of image intensifiers are consistent from one facility to another. For a typical patient, a good-quality anterior to posterior abdominal radiograph can be obtained by setting the unit to approximately 75 kVp and 20 mA (milliamperes multiplied by the time in seconds). For facilities where 200 speed film is used, this results in an average patient entrance skin exposure of 490 milliroentgens (mR); for 400 speed film, a "faster" film in widespread use, fewer milliamperes are needed, and an average exposure of 300 mR is encountered.[3] The average inhabitant of the United States receives approximately 300 mR per year from natural background radiation and man-made sources.[4]

Fluoroscopic outputs are promulgated by the FDA and evaluated and regulated by state agencies. Prior to 1995 there was a complicated two-tiered system dictating the maximum radiation outputs in the normal and boost modes. Fluoroscopic units were allowed unlimited radiation outputs in the boost mode and 5 R/min (5,000 mR/min) in the normal mode. All other units were limited to 10 R/min (10,000 mR/min). The current limits for all units are 10 R/min (10,000 mR/min) in the normal mode and 20 R/min (20,000 mR/min) in the boost mode. These upper limits are obtained at the maximum potential energy (usually 120 kVp) and milliampere settings (usually 2 mA) and are not typical for clinical images.

Typical fluoroscopic abdominal images are obtained at 70 to 80 kVp and 1 to 2 mA. This combination results in an average entrance skin exposure rate of 1 to 2 R/min. Poorly performing units or imaging of thick patients will cause outputs to approach 5 to 6 R/min to create optimal images. We will use 5 to 6 R/min as an example of a "worst case" scenario. Note that typical values will remain well below this value.

Radiation entering the patient is absorbed, scattered, or transmitted as a function of the density of the tissue it encounters. As a rough estimate, only 0.1% of the incident beam is scattered in the direction normal (90°) to the incident radiation. (For the sake of the previous example, this results in patient-scattered radiation of 5 to 6 mR/min at tableside, assuming there is no direct contribution from the primary beam imaging the patient or from x-rays leaking from the tube housing.) The contribution from tube leakage, scatter from machine components, and scatter from the patient comprises the secondary radiation field. The secondary radiation field is the one of most concern to persons in the room during fluoroscopic imaging. The secondary radiation field can be as high as 50 mR/hr at tableside for interventional techniques, but is routinely 10 to 15 mR/hr during abdominal imaging. The dose rate at tableside drops off rapidly as a function of distance, the specifics of which will be covered in the next section.

IMPLEMENTING THE PRINCIPLES OF THE ALARA APPROACH

The basis of the ALARA approach is that unnecessary exposure to radiation is to be avoided. This avoidance of exposure must be reasonable in that it does not hinder the performance of the task at hand, is not high in cost, does not increase the time necessary to perform the task, and offers a significant reduction in exposure. The basic principles of ALARA are time, distance, and shielding and they will be addressed in that order.

It is relatively simple to reduce the amount of time spent near a radiation field or to shorten the time that a fluoroscopy unit is on. It is possible to significantly reduce exposure by limiting the use of the fluoroscope to points during a procedure where it is actually needed for positioning or placement. Too often, there is a temptation to view even the smallest step in a procedure or to have the beam on continuously throughout the procedure. Considering the patient and operator exposures that were mentioned previously, it can easily be seen that total exposure adds up quickly. Reducing the amount of time spent in the vicinity of the patient also lessens the amount of radiation exposure for those performing and assisting in the procedure. Minimizing time does not hinder the procedure; the cost is low and a significant exposure reduction is achieved, thus meeting the criteria for ALARA.

Radiation "spreads out" in a three-dimensional space with a discrete or fixed number of photons spreading out into successively larger spaces. As a result, the area geometrically increases as a function of distance from the source (Figure 3-3). By doubling the distance from the source, the radiation is reduced to one fourth of its original intensity because the same number of photons are in a space that is four times larger. By tripling the distance, radiation is reduced to one ninth. This is the law of inverse square—that is, the resulting intensity is $1/radius^2$ times the initial intensity. Moving from an initial distance of 1 ft. to a distance of 2 ft. away from the table will result in a 75% reduction in dose. Concurrently, moving 3 ft. away will reduce the dose by 89%! As a rule of thumb, at a distance of 12 ft. the dose rate is near the level of natural background and is usually not measurable on radiation monitoring badges that are issued monthly or quarterly. Increasing the distance from the source is one of the least expensive and most dramatic ways to reduce the dose of radiation to which operating personnel are exposed.

In cases where time cannot be minimized or distance employed, shielding is used. Shielding, whether provided by lead aprons and thyroid shields or incorporated into room design, is a method of last resort. Effective shields are composed of dense materials (eg, lead) designed to effectively attenuate the radiation. As a result, personal shields tend to be bulky, stiff, and hinder work performance. New, lighter aprons have recently become available; these aprons only slightly compromise the effectiveness of the shield in favor of comfort. Lead aprons used to protect personnel during fluoroscopy contain an equivalent lead thickness of 0.5 mm of lead. For

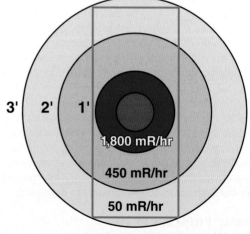

Figure 3-3 View from above the table showing typical dose rates as a function of distance from the source. Reduction in dose rates due to inverse square is dramatic.

the potential energy range most often encountered during fluoroscopy (ie, 70 to 100 kVp), the radiation is attenuated by between 99.5% and 96.5% of its initial value.[5] Lead aprons, gloves, and thyroid shields therefore provide excellent protection and should always be worn by those who work near the fluoroscopy table as a means of limiting the dose of radiation to which they are exposed. When fluoroscopy is performed, the radiation dosimetry badge is worn on the collar, outside the apron. The actual effective whole-body dose is up to 99% lower than the dose measured by the badge as a result of this technique. [6] Movable transparent lead shields and lead drapes can also provide additional protection to those who must work close to the source. This equipment has been shown to have only a minimal impact on the work being performed.

Equipment design and component positioning can significantly influence scattered radiation fields. The fluoroscopic image intensifier is lead-lined to minimize scattered radiation from the imaging chain, but with judicious placement can also reduce scattered radiation from the patient. When the tube is above the table, as in Figure 3-4, leakage from the tube and scatter from the patient are not attenuated, resulting in a higher than necessary dose rate at the tableside.

When the image intensifier is placed above the patient and the tube is shielded by the table, as in Figure 3-5, both leakage and scatter radiation are minimized. The inherent shielding in the image intensifier housing eliminates the scatter radiation and protects the user. From an ALARA standpoint, the equipment configuration in Figure 3-5 is preferred.

It seems logical at this point to expand on radiation dosimeters or, as they are more commonly referred to, "film badges." These devices record the amount of radiation exposure received by the wearer during the issue period. Without them there would be no measurement of improve-

ABOVE TABLE DESIGN

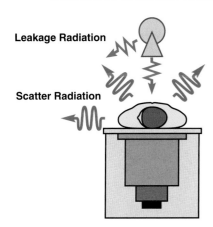

Figure 3-4 The position of the tube contributes significantly to operator exposure due to both leakage and scatter radiation. In this configuration the image intensifier does not assist in reducing operator exposure and tube leakage is not reduced by a second barrier.

ment in performance as ALARA principles are implemented. Neither would there be any individual specific records of exposure. Although not specifically required by law, radiation dosimeters are central to employee peace of mind and are considered to be inexpensive insurance against future damage claims for radiation-induced injuries. These badges can be had for as little as a dollar a badge per month.

The basic precepts of an effective ALARA program are to minimize time, maximize distance, and as a last resort to use effective shielding. By implementing these principles, a program can effect significant reductions in radiation exposure.

ERYTHEMA THRESHOLDS AND DOSE ESTIMATES

One of the very first effects of x-rays was discovered in the late 1890s. Pioneer radiologists, lacking other means and unaware of the danger, used reddening of their skin exposed to x-rays as a means of determining whether their x-ray units were functioning. As a result of this and other practices, more than 100 pioneer radiologists died of radiation-induced injuries within 20 years following the discovery of x-rays.

The radiation dose necessary to produce skin injury is variable and depends on several different factors but typical threshold doses are shown in Table 3-1.

Even typical dose rates can result in skin injury after less than 1 hour of fluoroscopy. The onset of this damage is delayed and cannot be sufficiently determined immediately after a procedure. Erythema is not usually noted unless the patient is asked specifically about these effects on follow-up.

As a result of this development, interventional departments have recently recognized the need to document the total fluoroscopic time in each patient's chart. When coupled with the unit's output for a typical procedure and multiplied by that value, it can be determined whether pointed follow-up of the patient is warranted or if the dose required for a procedure can be reduced. This documentation demonstrates that the physician is both conscientious and aware of possible adverse effects and the need to manage them. The FDA recommends the use of a qualified medical physicist to assist in the implementation of ALARA principles and documentation so that they do not adversely affect the clinical aspects of the procedure. The FDA also recommends establishing guidelines for standard procedures, determining each unit's radiation output, evaluating protocols and modifying them to limit cumulative absorbed doses, and assessing the potential for radiation injury for each protocol.

SPECIAL EQUIPMENT FOR MINIMIZING RADIATION EXPOSURE

A new generation of equipment has been designed with patient and operator dose reductions central

BELOW TABLE DESIGN

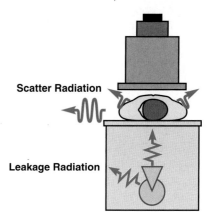

Figure 3-5 With the image intensifier above the table, the leakage radiation is reduced as the tube is shielded by an additional layer of material. As an added benefit, the image intensifier reduces the scattered dose to the user.

to its development. Two features have become available that reduce the dose of radiation delivered to the patient—pulsed fluoroscopy and digital imaging. Fluoroscopy units employ a video monitoring system to provide the user with live time images. In most video systems the screen is "refreshed" with a new signal 30 times per second. By coupling the output of the fluoroscope with the refresh rate, the beam can be pulsed off and on to coincide with the image formation with very little loss of resolution and up to an 80% reduction in dose.

Digital equipment eliminates the need for film; the information is electronically captured and manipulated in a computer. As a result, the image can be manipulated and enhanced, obviating the need for "retakes" and providing a sophisticated tool for dynamically evaluating patient organ function using videotape techniques. The images also become easily transferable by numerous electronic techniques, increasing the availability of results for those who need them.

Many manufacturers are incorporating passive radiation shielding into their equipment design to limit operator exposure. Improved movable leaded glass shields that are ceiling-mounted and well-balanced have become increasingly available. Unobtrusive personal dosimeters containing an alarm have also become available so that high-exposure techniques can be indicated, modified, and improved.

Table 3-1 Observed Effects of Typical Threshold Doses	
Threshold Dose	Observed Effect
300 R (300,000 mR)	Temporary depilation
600 R (600,000 mR)	Main erythema
1500-2000 R (1,500,000- 2,000,000 mR)	Moist desquamation, dermal necrosis, secondary ulceration
Adapted from Wagner LK, et al.[2]	

CONCLUSION

It is reasonable to assume that continuing efforts will be made to further protect users and reduce the amount of radiation exposure for both patients and the physicians involved in endourologic procedures. Individual techniques will always be the area with the most significant impact on dose reduction. Implementation of simple, common sense ALARA concepts—minimizing time, maximizing distance, and using shielding—can provide a significant reduction in both operator and patient radiation exposure. The establishment of standard, dose-minimized imaging protocols, documentation of total exposure time and estimated patient exposure, and purchase and cost-effective implementation of improved modalities are elements of an effective and focused radiation exposure control program.

REFERENCES

1. FDA Public Health Advisory. Avoidance of serious x-ray-induced skin injuries to patients during fluoroscopically guided procedures. Washington (DC): U.S. Government Printing Office; 1994.
2. Wagner LK, Eiffel PJ, Geise RA. Potential biological effects following high x-ray dose interventional procedures. J Vasc Intervent Radiol 1994;5:71–84.
3. FDA Center for Devices and Radiological Health. National evaluation of x-ray trends. Washington (DC): U.S. Government Printing Office; 1993.
4. National Council for Radiation Protection and Measurement. Ionizing radiation exposure of the population of the United States. Report No. 93. Bethesda (MD): NCRP; 1987.
5. National Council for Radiation Protection and Measurement. Structural shielding design and the evaluation for medical use of x-rays and gamma rays of energies up to 10 MeV. Report No. 49. Bethesda (MD): NCRP; 1976.
6. Niklason LT, Marx MV, Chan HP. The estimation of occupational effective dose in diagnostic radiology with two dosimeters. Health Phys 1994;67:611–5.

Video Imaging and Documentation

Glenn M. Preminger, MD

Roger L. Sur, MD

Charles D. Scales Jr, MD

April 4, 2015. Dr. Endo Maniac has just finished performing the virtual reality simulation of Mr. Jones's laparoscopic radical nephrectomy. Due to the large size of the renal tumor, Dr. Maniac imports images from the computed tomography and magnetic resonance imaging scans into the simulation package, allowing the computer to construct a patient-specific, three-dimensional (3D) surgical model. He simulates various laparoscopic approaches to remove the 15-cm upper pole renal mass. The data from the simulation will be accessed through the hospital's wireless network and used by the robotic assistant during the laparoscopic radical nephrectomy. After obtaining access, the kidney is successfully removed in 60 minutes with less than 50 cc blood loss. During the procedure, the surgeon wears a head-mounted display that provides a three-dimensional high definition image that has the capability of superimposing the real-time and radiologic images on the video displays. Moreover, images of adjacent structures are accessed from the image network and superimposed on the binocular video images to orient the operating surgeon as to potential injury to nearby organs.

Upon returning to his office, Dr. Maniac sits at his telepresence surgical console. He has been proctoring a urology resident at an outlying hospital and is now assisting in the performance of a laparoscopic ureteral reimplantation. After finishing the procedure, the data are stored on digital video disc (DVD) and later reviewed with the resident on the high definition television screen in the urology conference room. The surgeon then dictates the operative report using a voice recognition dictation system and selects video images to incorporate into the report. The patient's electronic medical record is updated, and a copy of the report is sent via fiber optic transmission to the referring physician.

Virtual reality surgical simulation; three-dimensional high-definition television; telepresence surgery; image processing; fiberoptic transmission—are these procedures and equipment just a dream, or technology that is right around the corner? Indeed, rapid advances in video technology and significant enhancements in video imaging make the aforementioned scenario plausible within the next few years. Much of the groundwork for these advanced imaging modalities has already been established. Anticipated improvements in technology and increasing con-

sumer applications should allow for a significant reduction in the cost of this advanced imaging equipment. These factors will allow the rapid introduction of this technology into the operating room and greatly facilitate our performance of minimally invasive endourologic procedures.

The following chapter will review the current state of the art of video imaging and documentation systems within endourology. Current advanced techniques will be discussed, along with new and innovative technologies that are just on the horizon. It is anticipated that this information will not only help readers to enhance their video imaging practices today, but also prepare them for tomorrow's tremendous innovations in advanced imaging modalities.

DIGITAL IMAGING

There have been a number of recent major improvements that have greatly enhanced video-endoscopic surgery.[1–3] These significant advances have been the development of the charge-coupled device (CCD) chip camera and the introduction of digital video imaging. Once an optical image is focused on the CCD chip, there is a conversion of the optical (light) image to an electronic signal.[4] This electronic information, which includes both color and light (luminance), can be scanned by a video monitor to produce an image on the screen.

Standard National Television Systems Committee (NTSC) video signals use a limited "bandwidth" that includes both the color and luminance information in a single, or "composite," signal. Problems with this format include "signal noise," which is caused by the camera having to first process color and luminance information separately and then combine the two pieces of information to create a video signal. This video noise, or "cross talk," may be the cause of decreased resolution, grainy images and loss of information around the edges of the video image. Moreover, this video noise will increase as additional copies of the videotape are produced.

With the advent of digital imaging, two newer video formats have been introduced.[5] The first format allows the color and luminance information to be carried as two separate signals. This "component" video signal is called Y/C, with Y standing for luminance (light brightness) and C referring to color. Also known as Super VHS (or S-VHS), this component signal contains less cross talk and,

therefore, appears cleaner and sharper than images generated by composite signals. The video signal in a Y/C format is carried by a single cable, as with the NTSC format, although the color and luminance information are still separated.

The final digital video format is known as RGB (Red-Green-Blue). This RGB format is also a component signal, yet it is distinct from the Y/C format in that the video information (color and luminance) is separated into four signals. These include a red, green, and blue signal as well as a timing signal. Each individual signal carries its own luminance information. Separation of the video signals is performed electronically in the camera head. The RGB format requires less electronic processing than do the NTSC or Y/C formats because the color and luminance information are separate from the start. Therefore, the RGB image quality is greatly enhanced compared to the other two formats. In contrast to the single-cable NTSC and Y/C formats, the RGB video signal is carried by four separate cables (red, green, blue, and sync). While most video monitors will accept standard NTSC video formats, a special (and more expensive) monitor is required to accept Y/C and RGB formats (Figure 4-1). The increased price, however, will result in a far superior image to standard NTSC formats.

In standard analog video processing (NTSC format), images or signals remain as voltages. Small errors in recording and reproducing these voltages are inevitable, and the errors accumulate with each generation of the video image (Figure 4-2A). Hence, multiple copies of an analog image will reveal a decrease in the quality of the video

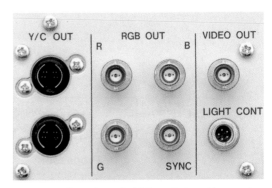

Figure 4-1 Rear view of a high-resolution video monitor that contains input access for composite National Television Systems Committee (NTSC), composite Y/C (digital), and component Red-Green-Blue (RGB) (digital) video signals.

pictures. In contrast, a digital converter changes all video signals into precise numbers (eg, 0 or 1) in the digital video formats (Y/C and RGB). Conversion to a digital signal gives the video image immunity to noise buildup or image quality degradation (Figure 4-2B). Moreover, image processing can be performed to enhance (and in some cases, alter) the digital video images. Once the video information has been digitized, it can be merged with other formats (eg, text, data, audio), transmitted or copied, with no loss of information.

STANDARD VIDEO SYSTEMS

The technical advantages created by video monitoring include binocular vision and magnification of the monitor images. Magnification may be as great as 20 times, depending on the initial optics system used. This enlarged image permits better inspection of detail and allows the operator, by virtue of the enlarged image size, to perform the procedure off the monitor rather than looking directly through the endoscope.[6] This approach significantly decreases operator strain because the surgeon no longer needs to conform his body to the angle of the viewing lens. Instead, the urologist can simply attach a video camera to the scope and manipulate the endoscope while standing comfortably and observing the video monitor.[3] Moreover, the upright position assumed by the urologist decreases the likelihood of coming in contact with potentially infected body fluids.

VIDEO CAMERAS All video systems are currently composed of a CCD solid–state-chip camera, a video processor (with or without a video recorder), and various video accessories. All of the chip cameras are fully immersible and shielded from electrical interference that may be created by cutting or coagulating currents during

endoscopic procedures.[7] The CCD chip high-resolution camera should have an automatic white balance feature, which allows one-touch color balance assuring true-to-life color reproduction. Additional features of the CCD camera may include a high gain option, which will boost the video signal to provide an exceptionally clear image, as well as a color bar option that allows the surgical team to adjust the monitors to represent accurate camera color prior to beginning the case.

Advances in CCD camera technology have significantly downsized current endoscopic video cameras, thereby allowing easier movement of the endoscope with the attached camera. With the recent significant improvements in CCD technology, tube cameras are no longer used due to their large size. When recording an actual endoscopic procedure, the camera may provide a VCR remote control switch for instant fingertip pausing of the recording device during documentation. Additionally, the camera head should be designed to prevent fogging between the coupling device and the camera head. All manufacturers can supply camera-head adapters for other endoscopic systems. Finally, the entire camera head cable and edge card could be designed to be cold-soaked in disinfectant solutions for easy sterilization between endoscopic cases.

As noted previously, CCD chip cameras have supplanted the tube cameras that were the first video systems on the market. A significant improvement in CCD camera technology has been the development of the three-chip camera, which contains three individual CCD chips for the primary colors—red, green, and blue (RGB). In addition to composite S-VHS and component signals, the three-chip cameras also provide an "uncoded" RGB signal (Figure 4-3). Color separation is achieved using a prism system overlying the chips.[8] This three-chip camera design pro-

vides improved color fidelity and enhanced image resolution. Moreover, three-chip cameras produce less cross talk due to the pure red-green-blue signals.[9,10] A digital converter captures each voltage signal as an image and translates the voltage values into numbers. The encoded numbers for each image element, or pixel, include information on color, light intensity, and contrast. These variables can then be modified using image-processing software within the camera.[11]

In theory, three-chip cameras produce better images than single-chip cameras. Despite the apparent advantages of three-chip cameras, some clinical comparisons have favored one-chip systems. Using normal video monitors, previous studies have implied that the resolution between the two cameras did not alter the visual perception of an image. Studies have found that digital contrast enhancement is a more important feature for endoscopic imaging than the number of camera chips. Three-chip cameras appeared to have no advantage over well-designed single-chip systems.[8,12,13] This apparent limitation may change, however, with the introduction of high-resolution digital monitors and high definition television (HDTV), as the amount of image information, and the degree of perception, are increased with these digital imaging modalities.[14]

Many of the CCD chip cameras (both single- and three-chip) contain electronic shuttering mechanisms that automatically adjust exposure time from 1/60 to 1/16,000 of a second (Figure 4-4). The advantage of such a sophisticated detection circuit is that the camera can react to varying light conditions almost instantaneously, thus reducing the flaring, "washout," and "blackout" that were noted with early video systems. Moreover, electronic shuttering mechanisms within the camera usually work more quickly than automatic light sources.

VIDEOENDOSCOPES A major advance in endoscopic systems has been the development of the digital videoendoscope. Miniaturization of chip technology now allows a CCD chip to be incorporated at the distal end of the endoscope (EndoEye) (Figure 4-5). Instead of relaying optical images from the objective lens at the distal end of the scope to a camera attached to the eyepiece, the image is immediately captured by the CCD chip, digitized and converted into electrical signals for transmission. This endoscope design has fewer interfaces, allowing the digital information to be directly transmitted to an image display unit with minimal image loss, interference, and distortion.[15,16] The creation of true videoendoscopes especially benefits the flexible laparoscope as well as the videoscope (Figure 4-6). As internal optics are not required in the long and flexible shafts of these instruments, durable deflection mechanisms can be used for the first time in laparoscopy, as well as to improve the durability of flexible endoscopes.[17,18] With no need to attach a camera head to the eyepiece of the scope, the videoscope cable can be secured to the light cord for attachment to the video system, providing a

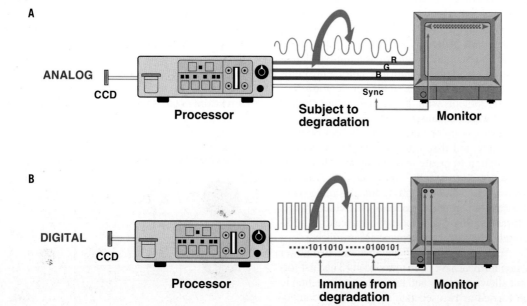

Figure 4-2 *A,* Representation of analog video imaging in which video signals remain as voltage waveforms. *B,* In contrast, digital video systems convert the analog video information to a digital format, which must then be converted back to analog information before it is viewed on the video monitor. Conversion to a digital signal gives the digital video image immunity to noise buildup or image quality degradation.

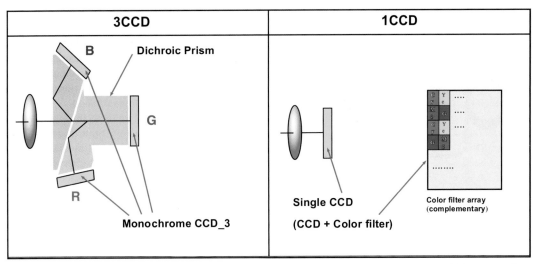

Figure 4-3 Schematic representation of three-CCD chip and one-CCD chip designs. Red, green, and blue sent to three separate CCDs by a prism. CCD = charge-coupled device. Photo courtesy of Olympus America, Melville, NY.

more lightweight and convenient setup. At present, this technology has only been incorporated into larger, rigid endoscopes (laparoscopes) and some flexible endoscopes (laparoscopes, bronchoscopes and cystoscopes),[19–21] but recent technologic advances have allowed miniaturization of CCD chips. One can expect to see such an integrated digital videoendoscope to replace smaller-caliber laparoscopes in the near future.

Another development in digital camera technology includes the use of a single monochrome CCD chip with alternating red, green, and blue illumination to form a color image rather than using three chips with three separate color filters. This design reduces the space requirements and takes advantage of established high-resolution monochrome CCD chip technology.[15] This design is currently used in a digital video cystoscope (CYF-V/VA, Olympus America, Mellville, NY). Such technology is currently being incorporated into digital laparoscopes as well.

VIDEO LIGHT SOURCES In addition to a CCD camera, a high-intensity light source, usually either halogen or xenon, should be used for appropriate illumination. Certain light sources have an automatic light sensing feature, which quickly adjusts the light output as required by the camera. This automatic light-adjustment feature is particularly helpful during endoscopic procedures, as the endoscope may be rapidly moved throughout the abdominal cavity or urinary tract, causing areas of too much or too little illumination. Light intensity will be automatically altered to maintain a preselected illumination level. As noted previously, some camera systems are equipped with an "automatic iris" system, which will electronically increase or decrease the aperture of the camera lens (see Figure 4-4). If the camera system is equipped with such a light-sensing feature, there is no need for an automatic light-adjusting light source. Newer CCD- or image–sensor-based endoscopic cameras feature electronic exposure. This system varies the effective exposure period (ie, light-gathering time) of the CCD as the live image is captured. Typical CCD exposure periods range from approximately 1/60 of a second to 1/10,000 of a second under very bright conditions. This electronic process can be used to maintain the brightness in the image. When the image brightness must be reduced to improve picture clarity, the image signal exposure period can be reduced electronically instead of adjusting the iris of the light source.

Shadows play an important role in depth perception and spatial orientation. Studies have demonstrated that endoscopic task performance improves significantly with video systems that provide proper illumination and appropriate shadows in the operative field.[22] Many of the current endoscopes employ a simple frontal illumination technique that produces an optically flat and shadowless image with resultant poor contrast. Newer illumination and imaging technologies provide shadow-inducing systems using a single-point or multipoint illumination system. One of these techniques employs the use of two independent illumination fiber bundles, with one fiber bundle ending at the front lens, as designed in conventional endoscopes, and the other fiber bundle ending behind the tip of endoscope. This configuration results in an improved image with better contrast due to shadow formation. Spatial orientation and perception between anatomic structures are considerably enhanced.[23]

VIDEO DOCUMENTATION SYSTEMS

The ability to make permanent copies of video-monitored cases is useful in documenting these procedures from both a medico-legal viewpoint and as a part of the patient's permanent medical record.[24] For example, video recording and/or hard copy acquisition of video images during laparoscopic varicocele ligation can document the preoperative image of the gonadal vessels and the postoperative appearance of the ligated gonadal veins. Hard copy pictures or video recording of some endoscopic procedures may also be an important adjunct during follow-up, if repeat endoscopic procedures are necessary. For example, stored video images of a patient with multiple superficial bladder tumors will allow the urologist the opportunity to review before and after images once treatment has been completed.

The ability to store sequential video images on an optical disc is another advantage of using video during endoscopy. One can provide the referring physician with prompt and detailed information regarding the surgical care of an individual patient. Video discs and hard copy technology now allow the presentation of patient data, graphic displays and video images on standard photographs, which can be placed in a patient's medical record. Enhanced digital printing technology is also available, which allows actual video images to be printed directly into an operative report.

One such system allows multiple video images to be stored during the endoscopic procedure. At the completion of the case, various video images can be selected and integrated directly into a dictated operative report (Figure 4-7). Such a report format proves invaluable for medico-legal purposes, as well as for dramatic documen-

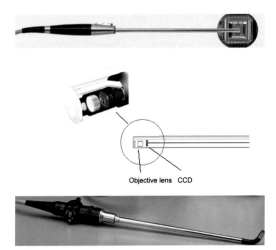

Figure 4-5 EndoEye technology. Flexible laparoscopy was enabled by this technology. Photo courtesy of Olympus America, Melville, NY.

Figure 4-4 Example of an electronic shuttering mechanism that will automatically adjust exposure times through the video camera. Note that the aperture can be manually set to *A*, an f-stop of 1,000 or, *B*, automatically adjusts to an f-stop of 30.

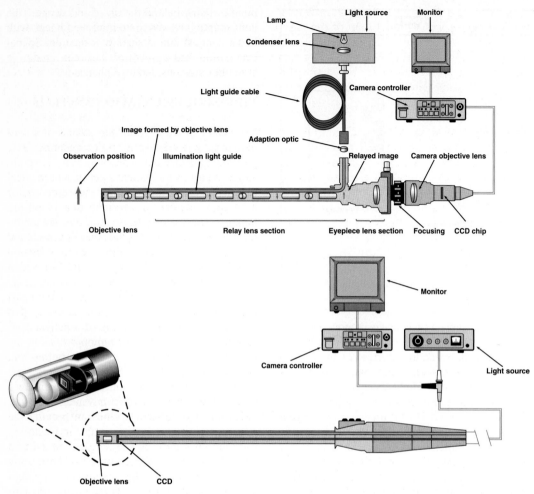

Figure 4-6 Traditional technology (*top*) compared with electronic transmission videoendoscopes (*bottom*). Photo courtesy of Olympus America, Melville, NY.

tation for the referring physician.

In addition, digitalization of video images permits specific endoscopic procedures to be brought "online" into a computer database system and further facilitates the use of a "paperless" medical record. Once the various video images are on the computer network, they can be recalled from any workstation linked to the network in the hospital. Moreover, one can use computer-manipulation (image processing) to further enhance the video images.[25]

HARD COPY PICTURES A printer generates an immediate, high-quality color photograph that can be used for documentation.[26] One, four, or nine separate pictures can be stored in the printer's memory and then reproduced on the same page, which allows one to document final results for the patient or referring physician or for use in the patient's permanent record. Some of these printers also contain character-generating capabilities, which allow one to add text to the video images.

DIGITAL IMAGE STORAGE Newer surgical video systems have integrated digital image-capture systems, allowing immediate capturing of still images from endoscopic procedures (Figure 4-8).[18] Alternatively, a less expensive digital

still-image capture adapter can be connected to endoscopic camera systems.[9] Digital still images can usually be recorded in Joint Photographic Experts Group (JPEG), tagged image file format (TIFF) or bitmap (BMP) formats. These digital images can be edited and optimized on the computer using various graphic software packages. Incorporating medical images into the patient's record, as well as creating an image library, can enhance urologic practice.[27,28] The quality of the digital image required depends on its purpose. Low-resolution images, in the range of 1 to 2 megapixels, can be used for e-mail attachments or *PowerPoint* presentations. A higher-quality image (from 3 to 4 megapixels) is more useful if a printed image is required. In cases where storage is not an issue, the image should be obtained at its highest resolution, thereby allowing for future image manipulation.

VIDEO RECORDING Recently, the majority of video recordings during endoscopic procedures were performed with conventional analog VHS or S-VHS formats, which could be digitally converted. The introduction of digital video recording devices now allows video footage to be recorded directly into a digital format (ie, Digital Video [DV], Moving Picture Experts Group [MPEG], and Audio Video Interleaved [AVI]). (Figure 4-9)

These video-capturing systems can be either part of an expensive commercial integrated video system, DV camera, DVD recorder, or a low-cost personal computer with digital video capture card.[29] Digital video editing may be performed on a personal computer using various editing programs (eg, *Adobe Premiere, Movie Maker*).

Smaller digital still images can be stored on different storage media (eg, SmartMedia, Compact Flash, Secure Digital, Multimedia card and Memory Stick) up to 1 gigabyte, depending on the media used. For larger files, especially video clips, Zip Disk (up to 750 megabytes [MB]), CD-ROM (up to 700 MB), and lately DVD (up to 17GB) can be used, but image storage can be an issue, especially with large numbers of digital files. Picture archiving and communication systems (PACS) are being developed to ultimately play an important role in "filmless" medical imaging in the near future.[30–32]

IMAGE TRANSMISSION

As we advance into the age of digital video imaging, images that have been "captured" can be immediately displayed, stored, printed or transmitted to various locations throughout the hospital or off-site. While video images can be transmitted over standard telephone lines, the narrow bandwidth of standard coaxial copper cable limits the quality of transmitted video images. Moreover, it is often difficult to transmit full motion video over standard telephone lines. Three newer modes of image transmission are being used in the communications industry and can, therefore, also be applied for the transmission of video images throughout the operating room, hospital or to distant sites.

FIBEROPTIC CABLE Fiberoptics has rapidly replaced coaxial cable and copper wire as the preferred mode of data transmission. It offers significant advantages over coaxial cable because it can

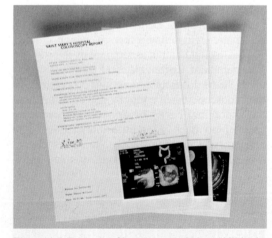

Figure 4-7 Example of image-processing capabilities by Med Images (Knoxville, TN) allowing various video images to be selectively incorporated into a dictated operative report. Digital printing technology allows incorporation of text, graphics, and video images to be printed on standard paper.

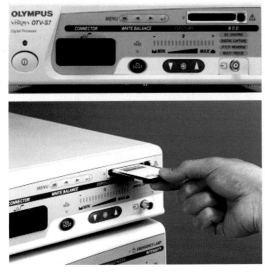

Figure 4-8 Still images and short video clips (depending on resolution) can be captured on a digital card. Direct digital video stream can be captured on a computer, digital camcorder, or digital recorder via an IEEE 1394 FireWire connector on the back panel. Photo courtesy of Olympus America, Melville, NY.

carry significantly more information in a small amount of space. For example, one fiber can carry upwards of 1.7 gigabits per second. This rate is thousands of times faster than data transmitted over standard coaxial cable. Moreover, optical fiber has a lower attenuation than coaxial cable and is not subject to electromagnetic interference.

The major advantage of optical fiber is that large amounts of digitized information (video, audio, data) can be rapidly transmitted.[24] This increased speed of transmission is especially important when dealing with the large amount of digital information contained in video images. While copper cable remains the primary mode of transmitting voice and data information today, the communications industry is rapidly replacing coaxial cable with fiberoptic conduits.

WIRELESS LOCAL AREA NETWORK Local area networks (LANs) using wireless fidelity (WiFi) have been introduced in the health care setting. These networks allow transmission of data and images to laptop and handheld computers throughout the patient care environment and often form the final link between a wired hospital network and the mobile user. The 802.11g standard, set by the Institute of Electrical and Electronics Engineers (IEEE), provides for data transmission at speeds up to 54 megabits per second (Mbps). At these transmission rates, digital still and video image transmission becomes practicable.[33]

The advantages of a wireless network are the ability to communicate with mobile users, ease of installation without the need for construction of a wired network, and flexibility for future technologic advancements. Disadvantages can include initial setup costs and the battery requirements of mobile workstations. Concerns have been expressed about interference of wireless devices with medical devices, but interference has only

occurred with a few devices and only when the medical device was within 10 cm of the LAN transmitter.[34] Wireless networks have been successfully used to transmit radiologic images for interpretation, as well as a live broadcast of a laparoscopic surgery to handheld computers for instructional purposes.[35–37]

SATELLITE COMMUNICATIONS The advent of satellite communications has also allowed the transmission of digitized video images to remote areas that are not linked by coaxial cable or fiberoptic conduit. Satellite communication currently allows the performance of teleconferencing and telemedicine, where voice and video images can be almost instantaneously transmitted to remote sites and allows interactive communication. It is believed that a combination of fiberoptic cable and satellite transmission systems could globally link distant operating rooms to major medical centers, thereby greatly facilitating performance of advanced endoscopic procedures. An experienced surgeon can assist or perform complex endoscopic procedures at the remote site (telepresence surgery).

VIDEO SYSTEM SETUP

VIDEO CART An essential part of any video system should be the video cart. This cart is an integral component for the entire system, which allows one to easily transport the video documentation system from one surgical suite to another (Figure 4-10). The video cart should have

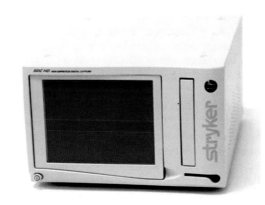

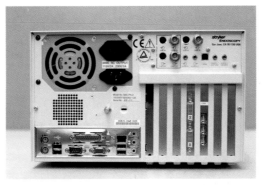

Figure 4-9 Direct DVD capture is possible, with storage in multiple formats (MPEG, AVI) offering flexibility for users. AVI = Audio Video Interleaved; DVD = digital video disc; MPEG = Moving Picture Experts Group. Photo courtesy of Stryker Endoscopy, San Jose, CA.()

room to hold the video camera electronics, the light source, and various recording devices such as a VCR, printer, or video disc recorder. Moreover, some video carts will also have room to hold the laparoscopic insufflator as well as electrocautery units. One should be able to adequately secure the cart during storage to prevent equipment loss. Finally, ensure that the video cart has the capability to hold CO_2 tanks, which will be needed during laparoscopic procedures.

VIDEO SETUP Traditionally, our standard operating room setup places the video cart, which contains a video camera and recorder, television monitor, and xenon light source, directly across from the operating surgeon. In addition, a second high-resolution video monitor will be placed on the other side of the table to be used by the assistants. If only one video monitor is available, it should be placed directly at the end of the operating table. All endoscopic procedures in our endoscopy suite and operating rooms are performed entirely off the video monitor(s).

With the advent of more current operating room designs, the fundamental differences between open and endoscopic or laparoscopic surgery have been recognized. Whereas, in the past, endoscopists and laparoscopists relied on mobile carts traveling from room to room, today, specialized rooms provide dedicated carbon dioxide lines, preventing the need to change tanks in mid-operation. Another issue relating to suboptimal operating room design is the effect of imperfect ergonomics on surgeon comfort from a musculoskeletal standpoint. Many recent studies have demonstrated significant stressors induced by laparoscopy on the surgeon. Many of these stressors are related to monitor placement, camera holding, trocar placement, and table position and height.[38–41] Operating room enhancements, such as ceiling-mounted monitors and designs focused on the endoscopic and laparoscopic sur-

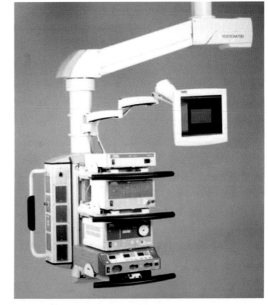

Figure 4-10 Video carts contain video camera electronics, light source, and various recording devices.

geons, allow for versatility in the ergonomics surrounding minimally invasive urologic procedures (Figure 4-11). Whether or not these specially designed operating rooms improve on musculoskeletal complications in surgeons has yet to be determined, but some studies indicate this is, in fact, the case and that overall operating room efficiency is improved as well.[42,43] A novel addition to the operating room of the future may incorporate high-resolution, binocular face-mounted devices, as have been explored at the bench level, thus providing less surgeon neck/back strain and improved visualization and satisfaction, compared to conventional standard video monitors.[44]

FUTURE DIRECTIONS OF ENDOSCOPIC VIDEO SYSTEMS

As previously noted, significant advances have been made in the development of video imaging technology for minimally invasive surgical procedures. A major limitation of current video systems, however, continues to be the two-dimensional images provided to the surgeon. Although the image quality itself is quite satisfactory, the lack of depth perception may impair delicate dissection or suturing during minimally invasive procedures, as one is relying on motion parallax and other indirect evidence of depth to judge the correct spatial relationship of the objects in the operating field. At times, one has to actually touch the tissues in order to gauge depth, thereby significantly reducing the speed and precision at which minimally invasive surgical procedures can be performed.

Moreover, as advanced reconstructive and minimally invasive surgical procedures are developed, some training opportunities become limited. This lack of "routine" cases makes it often times difficult for the medical student, house officer, and practicing physician to become familiar with more complex, minimally invasive surgical maneuvers. Therefore, a way to simulate such complex procedures would be beneficial to aid in the training of the endoscopic surgeon.

3D Video systems as well as high definition television have recently been introduced to significantly improve visualization during minimally

invasive surgical procedures. In addition, virtual reality techniques have been developed, which allow enhanced image processing of videoendoscopic procedures as well as the development of surgical simulations to aid in training of complex surgical maneuvers. The following sections will review these enhanced imaging technologies for endoscopic surgery.

3D VIDEO IMAGING   3D Video imaging enhances the ability to perform delicate endoscopic maneuvers, such as dissection or precise suturing.[45] Moreover, those who are observing have a better understanding of the surgical anatomy because of the 3D image.

Principles of 3D Stereoendoscopy   In normal human vision, depth perception is a factor taken for granted. Normally, the eyes will accommodate and converge in such a way that there is intersection of the visual axes of both eyes. This intersection is known as the point of fixation (Figure 4-12). When viewed by both eyes, lateral disparity causes the viewed object to be projected in slightly different orientations on the retina of the right and left eyes. The human brain interprets this disparity on a small region of the retinal fovea (called Panum's area) as depth information. The brain then fuses these images to give the perception of depth, and this effect is called stereopsis.[46]

Accommodation is the ability of the human eyes to clearly visualize objects which are both near and farther away. The eyes converge, and the lens increases its dioptic strength so that the object is brought into sharp focus on the retina. The nearest an object can be to the eye and still be in focus is called the near point, while the farthest it can still be in focus is called the far point. The region of depth is the area between the near and far points. This ability to accommodate is preserved when viewing objects with a 3D video system.

As noted, when viewing a particular object with binocular vision, one normally would perceive that object in three dimensions. If one eye is closed, one might note a "flattening" of the image. Owing to the capability of the "image center" within the brain to capture and recall images, the viewed object may appear with somewhat limited depth (ie, $2^1/2$D). This ability to visually process two-dimensional flat images off a standard video screen

and view them in a partial three-dimensional manner may be a significant factor in the ability of experienced endoscopic surgeons to adequately perform endoscopic surgical tasks. This innate ability to perceive standard flat video images in three dimensions is significantly reduced when the surgeon is confronted with a scene that has not been viewed before. Therefore, the introduction of 3D video systems should facilitate the performance of endoscopic surgical procedures, especially those that require intricate dissection or reconstructive techniques.

To mimic normal 3D vision, a three-dimensional video system must therefore convey separate offset images to each eye. The figure is captured in a slightly different orientation by the stereoendoscope and, after image processing by the brain, appears as a three-dimensional object (Figure 4-13). Any 3D video system must therefore incorporate the principles of stereopsis.[46,47] One potential limiting factor of 3D endoscopic systems is that the normal interpupillary distance for human vision is approximately 60 mm, while the maximum separation of two objective lenses in a standard 10-mm endoscope is approximately 8 mm. Various endoscopic designs, however, have accounted for this disparity, still allowing for adequate capture and display of three-dimensional images.

Stereoendoscopic Image Processing   Most of the three-dimensional stereoendoscopic video systems currently available have four basic principles of stereoendoscopic image processing in common: image capture, conversion of 60 Hertz (Hz) to 120 Hz images, presentation of left and right images on a single monitor, and separation of the left- and right-eye images.[48] While the components of the various 3D video systems may differ slightly, they each contain the same basic principles. The following sections will describe in more detail current stereoendoscopic equipment used for three-dimensional endoscopic surgery.

Stereo Laparoscope   Stereo laparoscopes are of two basic designs: a two-lens optical system or a single optical channel (Figure 4-14). The dual-lens systems individually capture slightly different images of the operating field, much like the right and left eye will capture slightly different views of a single image (Figure 4-15). The

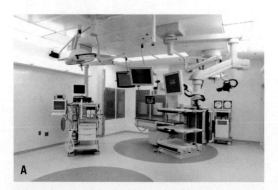 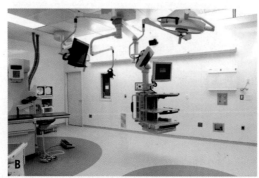 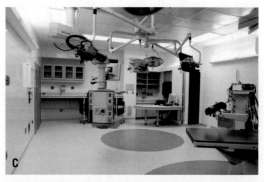

Figure 4-11 Endoscopic/laparoscopic operating room. *A*, Ceiling mounted flat panel monitors. Built-in endoscopy table with adequate room for laparoscopic applications. *B*, Touch panel control allowing for routing of different source images on different monitors. Wall plug in for C-arm integration with room monitors. Wall panel integrating operating room with audio-visual center allowing for video capture, integration with conference rooms, and teleconferencing. *C*, Ceiling mounted camera for external footage.

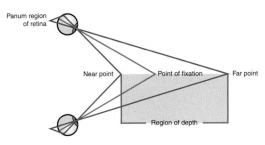

Figure 4-12 Basic aspects of stereoscopic vision in humans. The region of depth is defined as the distance between the near and far points of focus.

parallel optical channels then present the separate images to the left- and right-eye camera systems.

In contrast, the single optical channel design captures the image with a single objective lens at the distal end of the endoscope. At the proximal end of the endoscope, adjacent to the stereo camera, the image is split into separate left- and right-eye images. One advantage of this single optical channel design may be higher resolution and more light for the three-dimensional video image

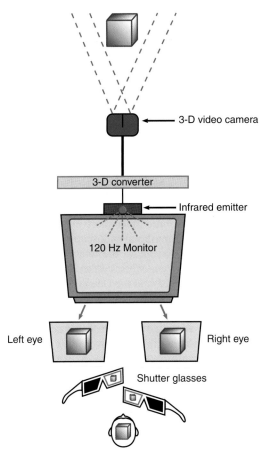

Figure 4-13 Principles of a 3D video system. Demonstration of stereo endoscopic image processing after image capture by a two-headed camera. The image is "seen" in slightly different orientations by the left- and right-eye cameras. The different views are displayed alternately on the 3D video monitor after passing through the 3D conversion processor. When viewed with "active" shutter glasses, the left eye receives information from the left camera and the right eye image is seen by the right eye. The image center of the brain processes this information as depth perception.

than presented by the smaller two optical systems contained in the dual optical channel endoscopes.

One final design option uses a "standard" single channel endoscope but provides a "universal optical converter" to produce a three-dimensional video image.[47] This design has the significant advantage of not requiring a stand-alone endoscope, which must be used to capture three-dimensional images, but can be used with any available endoscope, regardless of its diameter. Some individuals question the true three-dimensional nature of this 3D video image.

Image Splitter The single-channel three-dimensional video systems use a device to split the images captured by the left and right half of the single-lens endoscopes. In some systems, the image splitter is incorporated into the proximal end of the single-channel stereo endoscope. As noted previously, however, the universal adaptor system uses a stand-alone image splitter, which may be attached to the distal end of any available endoscope.

Stereo Camera Most 3D video systems contain a stereo camera head, which incorporates two separate CCD image sensors (usually half-inch CCD chips) that capture the images from the stereo laparoscope. These images from the stereo laparoscope are viewed by the left- and right-eye cameras, just as two separate images are presented to the left and right eyes during normal binocular vision.

Three-Dimensional Image Processing Most three-dimensional video systems contain a 3D conversion unit, which processes the images obtained from the left- and right-eye cameras. These conversion systems allow the left- and right-eye images to be alternately synchronized on a single stereoscopic monitor at 120 Hz

(60 Hz for each eye). If the images are presented slower than 120 Hz, one may notice substantial "flicker" on the video monitor. Moreover, slower speeds of video display may also cause vertigo.

The 3D video conversion systems will allow viewing of live three-dimensional procedures, recording of surgical cases in three dimensions with subsequent playback of these cases in three dimensions. While initial 3D video systems recorded left- and right-eye images on separate video recorders, current systems can capture both the left and right images on a single videotape. The left- and right-eye images are stored on a single "video frame," which greatly simplifies the recording, playback and editing of three-dimensional endoscopic images. The image processing unit and standard three-dimensional video monitor are both necessary to view the previously recorded endoscopic images.

Three-Dimensional Display The three-dimensional conversion system will sequentially display the left- and right-eye images on the 120 Hz 3D video monitor. However, in order to view the left- and right-eye images on a single monitor, the images must be separated. One method involves "active" liquid crystal display (LCD) shutter glasses. These glasses are synchronized by an infrared emitter located on top of the video monitor. As the left-eye image is projected on the video screen, the emitter will control the shutter glasses so that the right eye is closed and left eye open. Alternatively, when the right eye is open, the left side of the LCD glasses is blackened and the right eye image appears on the video screen. The advantage of this active system is that more light is projected to each eye and therefore the 3D image appears brighter. However, the active LCD shutter

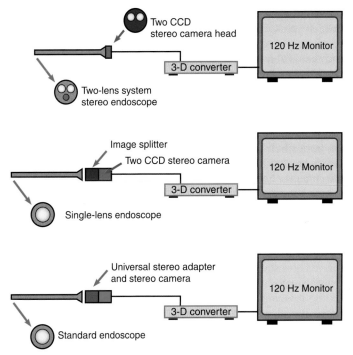

Figure 4-14 Three different designs for dual- and single-lens stereo endoscopic systems. The systems vary mainly with regard to the stereo endoscope: a two-lens scope, a single-channel scope with 3D conversion, or a "universal" stereo adapter that fits any standard endoscope.

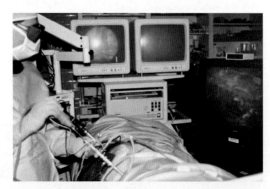

Figure 4-15 Close-up view of the distal end of an Olympus two-lens endoscope that contains separate viewing channels for the left- and right-eye images.

glasses require a battery, are somewhat heavy and quite expensive (approximately $1,000 [US]).

Alternatively, "passive" polarized glasses may be worn to view the left- and right-eye images from the single video monitor. This type of system requires a special polarizing filter on the video screen, which will "rotate" the left- and right-eye images in different orientations thereby allowing simultaneous viewing of the left and right images. The passive polarized glasses have the advantage of significantly cheaper cost than the active LCD shutter glasses and are more comfortable to wear, but the polarizing glasses present a slightly darker three-dimensional image than the active glasses.

An alternative to dual projection is the presentation of the two images independently to the left and right eye, much like looking through field binoculars. This technology is currently available as part of the robotic da Vinci Surgical System.[49]

Three-Dimensional Imaging with Electronic Processing The majority of 3D video systems use the "traditional" approach of dual-lens input to create 3D images. While the International Telepresence system noted above uses an optics interface between a single-lens endoscope and video camera, which splits the video image into two channels to create a stereoscopic effect, there is also a system that is able to create a 3D video image from standard monoscopic sources using electronic processing. This system is compatible with all single-camera endoscopic systems regardless of endoscope size or type.

The system uses time-multiplexing to create stereoscopic displays from single–video-channel outputs. In essence, time creates the third dimension.[50] Depth enhancement is obtained by spatially offsetting the left- and right-eye views as they are displayed on the video monitor. This form of "temporal" processing allows two different perspectives of a single video image to be produced at two different times. The sequential images are then displayed on a standard 3D monitor and separated with standard LCD (shutter) or polarized glasses. While it is unclear if such an electronically processed 3D video image presents true 3D vision, the primary benefit of such a system is that it can be used with standard video equipment currently available in the operating room. Therefore, such a system can be used with standard endoscopes and video cameras, obviating the need to purchase specialized 3D endo-

scopes or video systems (Figure 4-16). The existing camera signal is connected directly to a 3D processor, which converts the camera signal into a 3D stereoscopic image. This image is then viewed with the standard 3D video monitor.

Recording and Projection of 3D Video Images Early 3D video systems required two separate recorders to capture the left- and right-eye images. The majority of systems now use a three-dimensional conversion system, which will alternatively store the left- and right-eye images on a single videotape. This system design allows efficient capture of three-dimensional video footage for play-back at a later time.

There are three-dimensional video projectors available that will alternatively display left- and right-eye images on a large video screen (Figure 4-17). Such 3D video projectors are ideal for large group demonstrations and for educational purposes. As with separation of images during viewing on a three-dimensional video monitor, the 3D video projector can use active LCD shutter glasses or a passive polarized lens system.

Advantages Of 3D Videoendoscopy The increased depth of field afforded by three-dimensional endoscopic video systems facilitates intricate, minimally invasive surgical procedures.[51,52] Addition of a third dimension allows better recognition of tissue layers and may facilitate complex maneuvers, such as laparoscopic suturing or knot tying.[53] Indeed, skill tests assessing laparoscopic suturing and knot tying have demonstrated a 25% increase in speed and accuracy of these laparoscopic tasks when using a three-dimensional video system compared with a standard two-dimensional endoscopic video system.[54] Some investigations claim that three-dimensional video systems only facilitate surgical tasks in inexperienced laparoscopic surgeons. It appears that the reduction in time required to perform various minimally invasive surgical procedures may not be as dramatic in individuals who have a large amount of experience with standard 2D video systems during endoscopic surgery. Some studies suggest that a higher-resolution video system might be more advantageous than having 3D endoscopic imaging.[55–57] The major

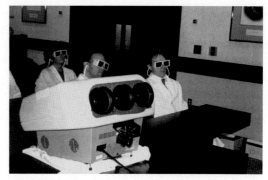

Figure 4-17 This 3D video projector by StereoGraphics may be used with either active or passive glasses. Such a 3D projector is ideal for educational purposes or large group demonstrations.

current use of 3D imaging systems is during laparoscopic, robotic surgical procedures, to allow for true stereoscopic imaging.[58–60]

Limitations of 3D Imaging Systems Late-model 3D videoendoscopic systems compared with the initial 3D components provide greatly improved three-dimensional viewing of minimally invasive surgical procedures. Yet they still provide reduced resolution and lower-light images as compared to standard single-chip or three-chip two-dimensional video cameras. The decrease in image brightness and resolution is due to the fact that most three-dimensional video systems use two optical channels that are significantly smaller than a single-lens system in a standard 10-mm laparoscope. Moreover, since most three-dimensional video systems incorporate two separate camera systems, the camera head is significantly larger than a single-camera system and, therefore, more cumbersome to work with during minimally invasive surgical procedures.

Cost continues to be a limitation of three-dimensional videoendoscopy. Most 3D video systems are two to three times more expensive than standard two-dimensional endoscopic video cameras. Moreover, except for the International Telepresence System which uses a three-dimensional endoscopic coupler, and the DeepVision 3D electronic processing system, most three-dimensional video systems are stand-alone units and therefore cannot be used with other endoscopic equipment.

While three-dimensional video imaging systems are more costly than conventional 2-dimensional video equipment, the enhanced depth perception produced by 3D endoscopes has been demonstrated to improve the performance of minimally invasive surgical procedures.[61] Three-dimensional imaging also facilitates the training of minimally invasive surgery and may lessen the learning curve of these technically demanding procedures. It is anticipated that three-dimensional video imaging will significantly improve the performance of current endoscopic procedures as well as facilitate the development of more advanced, minimally invasive surgical techniques.[45]

HIGH DEFINITION TELEVISION The development of high quality image display systems has

Figure 4-16 The major advantage of a 3D electronic processing system is that it may be used with standard endoscopes and video cameras, alleviating the need to purchase a specialized 3D endoscope or video system. Here the DeepVision system is being used during percutaneous stone removal.

become essential during endoscopic surgery. Previous studies have demonstrated that the inherent optical quality of most endoscopes and CCD camera exceeds the display resolution of standard television.[62] With the limited resolution of current analog NTSC, phase alternation line (PAL) and sequential color and memory (SECAM) monitors, there is a demand for higher-resolution image display systems. One such digital display system is high definition television (HDTV). The most common HDTV formats used in the United States are 720p and 1080i. The "p" represents progressive scanning, meaning that each scan includes every line for a complete picture, while the "i" signifies interlaced scanning with each scan including alternate lines for half a picture. These scan rates translate into a frame rate of up to 60 frames per second, twice that of conventional television monitors. HDTV offers greatly enhanced picture quality with improved image resolution. HDTV pixel numbers range from one to two million, compared to NTSC, PAL or SECAM's range of 300,000 to one million. The other significant feature of the HDTV format is its wider aspect ratio (the width-to-height ratio of the screen) of 16:9, compared with NTSC, PAL and SECAM screens, which have an aspect ratio of 4:3. Studies have suggested that the wider aspect ratio provides more information for the viewer, thereby enhancing both diagnostic and therapeutic interventions.[9,57] Current applications of high definition television in medicine include diagnostic and therapeutic maneuvers during endoscopic surgery. This increased resolution and clarity has been shown to greatly facilitate surgical performance.[9] In fact, some have likened the extremely high-resolution image afforded by HDTV to a three-dimensional video image. Although not a true 3D image, the increased video information provides the perception of depth.

The future application of high definition imaging (HDI) technology would improve endoscopic image resolution based on CCD chips. The European standard HDI chip resolution is

2,340,250 pixels, resulting in 1,250 horizontal lines. HDI has the advantage of resolution enhancement for image brilliance and the augmentation of secondary depth clues such as shadows. Other techniques under development for image resolution enhancement include the use of complementary metal oxide semiconductor (CMOS) technology to replace the CCD sensors.[23] Both CMOS and CCD imagers are manufactured in a silicon foundry; and the equipment used is similar. But alternative manufacturing processes and device architectures make the imagers quite different in both capability and performance. It is technically feasible, but not economical, to use a CCD processor to integrate other camera functions, like the clock driver and signal processing. These are normally implemented into secondary chips. Thus, most CCD cameras comprise several chips. On the other hand, one of the major benefits of CMOS cameras over the CCD design lies in the high level of product integration that can be achieved through virtually all of the electronic camera functions onto the same chips. Typically, a CMOS processor allows lower power usage and lower system cost.

The improved resolution and color separation of high definition imaging provides better diagnosis, and enhances the effect of secondary spatial cues, leading to easier orientation, particularly if the images are combined with improved illumination. Despite its current high cost, the price of HDTV cameras and monitors will continue to decline as newer HDTV products come onto the consumer market (Figure 4-18). With further optimization of size and weight of the camera system, HDTV can become a standard feature for endoscopic imaging and display during endoscopic and laparoscopic procedures.

VIRTUAL REALITY Endourologic procedures require specific training to achieve competency. Often, there are reduced training opportunities for residents due to a limited number of clinical cases. Moreover, ethical and cost issues may fur-

ther limit the use of animal or cadaver models for training purposes.[63–65] While hands-on training using bench models can successfully teach laparoscopic skills, it precludes the ability to vary clinical conditions.[66] Moreover, inanimate simulators lack the realistic feel of living tissue.

Advances in virtual reality (VR) simulation offer a practical tool for urologists to practice various endourologic procedures from the basic to the most complex in an inanimate but dynamic, life-like environment without risk to patients or ethical issues. Accurate reproduction of anatomic structures provides a realistic VR surgical simulation. Models should also provide appropriate tactile feedback and spatial cues.

As endoscopic procedures require little in the way of complex anatomic and tactile feedback, one of the earliest simulators in urology was a virtual reality ureteroscopy simulator (Immersion Medical, Gaithersburg, MD).[63,64,67] This simulator allowed urologists to explore the ureter and kidney for pathologic processes (specifically, stones and tumors). However, this early simulator was limited owing to lack of true anatomic representation and inadequacy in computer graphics. Advances in computing power, VR graphics and physical modeling techniques resulted in a new endoscopic simulator (URO Mentor system, Symbionix, Tel Aviv, Israel). This is a commercially available VR modular endoscopic simulator that provides virtual cystoscopy and ureteroscopy procedures using either rigid or flexible endoscopes. Real-time fluoroscopy with simulation of C-arm control and viewing of fluoroscopic images of injected contrast can also be simultaneously combined with endoscopic procedures. Various endourologic procedures, including cystoscopy, retrograde pyelography, insertion of guidewire, ureteral stenting, ureteroscopy, stone fragmentation, and fragment removal using various tools can be realistically simulated. Studies have demonstrated that use of this VR simulator resulted in more rapid acquisition of ureteroscopic skills in urologic trainees.[10,68–70] In fact, studies of both laparoscopic and ureteroscopic simulators demonstrated a significant reduction in the learning curve to perform both routine and complex endoscopic procedures. Endourologic skills can also be validated using VR simulation.[65,71]

Further advances in computer and software technology allowed VR simulation to become more realistic for the performance of laparoscopic procedures.[72–75] Similar to the aviation industry, VR simulation will likely be incorporated into the training, testing and credentialing of endourologists and laparoscopic surgeons over the next 5 to 10 years.

INTERNET AND TELEMEDICINE Telemedicine, defined as the use of electronic information and communication technologies to provide and support health care from a distance, has become an important aspect in patient care. Advances in digital imaging, high-speed computer connections, and the widespread availability of the Internet allowed a steady growth of telemedicine within

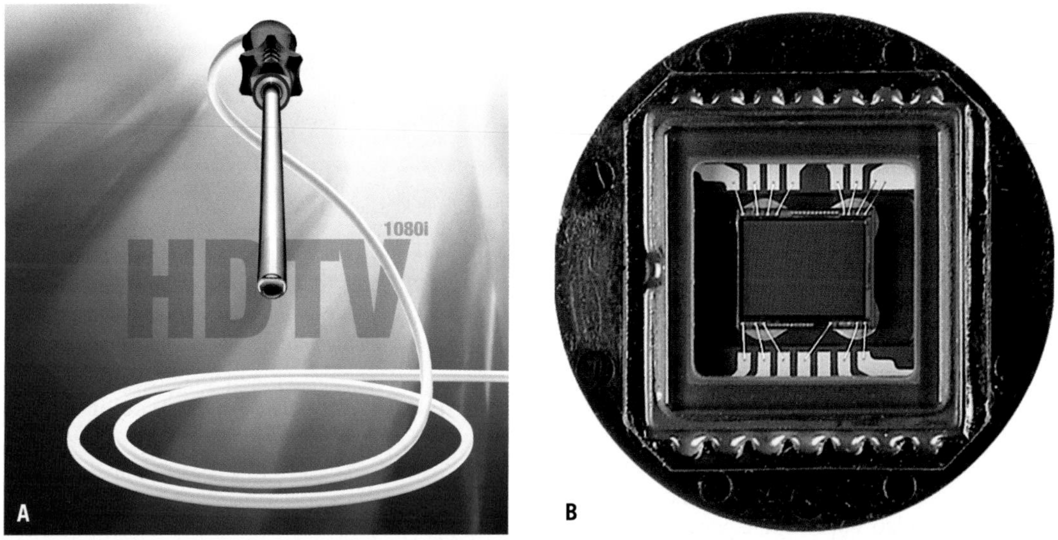

Figure 4-18 *A*, High definition (HD) endoscope offers improved resolution over traditional endoscopes. *B*, HD chip for endoscope. Photo courtesy of Olympus America, Melville, NY.

urology.[76] Digital images obtained from various sources, such as a digital still or video camera, scanner, computed tomography and magnetic resonance imaging can be exchanged over the Internet at high speeds using transmission modalities such as Integrated Services Digital Network (ISDN) at 128 kilobits per second, T1 lines at 1.54 Mbps, coaxial cable up to 6 Mbps, and Asymmetric Digital Subscriber Line (ADSL) at from 1 to 3 Mbps.[9,11,27] Two types of telemedicine systems emerged. The first is synchronous and real-time videoconferencing. In general, real-time motion requires that images are generated at a speed of 30 frames per second.[77] The advantage of "live" video teleconferencing is that it allows real-time interaction between physicians and patients with full-motion audio-visual images, developing a true physician-patient relationship. In addition, various medical centers can be linked with the teleconferencing facility to promote tele-education and tele-consultation. With proper equipment, digital images, including endoscopic pictures, pathologic slides, and radiologic images can also be transmitted in real time. The cost of real-time telemedicine systems and communication networks prevented the widespread use of this technology. For example, a teleconferencing system costing more than $80,000 (US)—not including the connection fee—could cost as much as $800 (US) per month.[77,78] Studies demonstrated that one could provide high-quality HDTV image-oriented telemedicine via ISDN lines or communication satellites, but at a minimum set up cost greater than $1,000,000 (US).[79]

Alternatively, telemedicine can also be accomplished using an asynchronous or "store-and-forward" system, whereby the information is transmitted via e-mail or the Internet. The recipients can review and respond to the information transmitted at their convenience, as the data have been stored in a locally accessible, computerized data storage and retrieval system. More surgical disciplines, including urology, are using this technology. Store and forward technology is also improving, with better software development and secure transmission of encrypted data over the Internet.[27] Despite lack of real-time interaction, these systems remain very effective and useful tools for medical care and endourologic training.[11]

Standardization of input devices for image data exchange is essential for telemedicine. The Digital Imaging and Communications in Medicine (DICOM) standard exists for radiological images, but there is no standard for other digital images, such as endoscopic still pictures or video clips. There is an urgent need for future standardization and integration of telemedicine hardware.[79]

The upcoming challenge for telemedicine lies within the decisions made about physician licensing requirements, regulation of telemedicine, reimbursement of consultations and protection of patient confidentiality.

Laparoscopic Applications Despite the shortcomings outlined above, telemedicine (and even telesurgery) have become reality. Kavoussi and colleagues in 1994 demonstrated their initial laboratory experience in telerobotic-assisted laparoscopic surgery.[41,80–84] Urological laparoscopic telesurgery has been performed in a clinical setting. In this study, five patients in Rome underwent laparoscopic procedures in a center where laparoscopy was only recently introduced.[85] In Baltimore, MD, a more experienced team oversaw the procedures in real time, offered advice, provided quality control, and even operated instruments remotely. The cases performed included a laparoscopic nephrectomy. Another laparoscopic radical nephrectomy was telementored from the United States to a surgical site in Singapore.[86] The first telerobotic percutaneous renal access was performed between Baltimore, MD, and Rome in 1998.[87] Non-urologic surgery, such as cholecystectomy, colonic resections, and Nissen fundoplication, have also been performed telesurgically.[88,89] This revolutionary approach to telemedicine has opened the door for more widespread applications of laparoscopic techniques, enhanced training, and improved patient care.

As one looks toward the 21st century, the future of telemedicine only looks brighter. Advances in digital imaging resolution and improvements in transmission bandwidth will make telesurgery and decision making through telemedicine more accurate. Technologic improvements will also lower the cost of imaging devices and the cost of using specialized telecommunications lines. These developments will make telemedicine systems even more affordable than they are today and greatly enhance the performance of laparoscopic procedures in urology.[80,84,86,90]

CONCLUSIONS

The application of video technology to endoscopic procedures provides several advantages in both the teaching and private practice settings not previously available to the urologist. Improved magnification and image quality facilitates performance of the procedure by the surgeon, as well as coordination of the assistants and ancillary personnel to provide a smoother, safer, and potentially shorter operation. Video monitoring facilitates teaching, both during and after the procedure, and provides preoperative patient education. The monitoring and recording of procedures allows case documentation and creates a permanent record for the patient's file. Video accessories provide immediate documentation for the patient's medical record, for use by the referring physician, or for the patient's own interest. Additionally, video and hard copy documentation provides an invaluable teaching aid for patients and medical personnel. Moreover, videoendoscopic procedures increase the safety of the procedure for the operating urologist.

The advent of endoscopic and laparoscopic urologic surgery demands that the urologist master video-based surgical procedures. Videoendoscopy will significantly enhance any endoscopic procedure with improved resolution and reduced operator strain. Video applications in urology have become an integral part of our daily practice during routine endoscopic and laparoscopic procedures.

It is also anticipated that three-dimensional video imaging, high definition television and virtual reality surgical simulation will rapidly be introduced into the entertainment and manufacturing industries. As increased applications are identified and more applications developed, it is anticipated that these types of advanced imaging technologies will be rapidly introduced into the medical and surgical fields.[91] Enhanced visualization afforded by three-dimensional imaging and high definition television will greatly facilitate the performance of endoscopic procedures. Moreover, telemedicine-assisted robotic surgery and virtual reality will also become a routine occurrence.[92–94] It appears that our scenario with Dr. Endo Maniac is right around the corner!

REFERENCES

1. Kennedy TJ, P. G. Impact of video on endourology. J Endourol 1987;1:75.
2. Litwiller DA, Preminger GM. Advances in electronic imagery for laparoscopy. J Endourol 1993;7:S195.
3. Preminger GM. Video-assisted transurethral resection of the prostate. J Endourol 1991;5:161.
4. Allhoff E, Bading R, Hoene E, et al. The chip camera: perfect imaging in endourology. AAJOURNAL262 1988;6:6.
5. Knyrim K, Seidlitz H, Vakil N, et al. Perspectives in "electronic endoscopy". Past, present and future of fibers and CCDs in medical endoscopes. Endoscopy 22 (Suppl) 1990;1:2.
6. Carr-Locke DL. Videoendoscopy in clinical application. Impact on teaching. Endoscopy 1990;22 (Suppl 1):19.
7. Flachenecker G, Fastenmeier K. High frequency interferences in video imaging systems during transurethral resection. AAJOURNAL262 1988;6:8.
8. Hanna G, Cuschieri A. Image display technology and image processing. World J Surg 2001;25:1419.
9. Kuo RL, Preminger GM. Current urologic applications of digital imaging. J Endourol 2001;15:53.
10. Weinberg DS. Digital imaging as a teaching tool for pathologists. Clin Lab Med 1997;17:229.
11. Kuo RL, Delvecchio FC, Babayan RK, et al. Telemedicine: recent developments and future applications. J Endourol 2001;15:63.
12. Aslan P, Kuo RL, Hazel K, et al. Advances in digital imaging during endoscopic surgery. J Endourol 1999;13:251.
13. Berci G, Wren SM, Stain SC, et al. Individual assessment of visual perception by surgeons observing the same laparoscopic organs with various imaging systems. Surg Endosc 1995;9:967.
14. Preminger GM, Delvecchio FC, Birnbach JM. Digital image recording: an integral aspect of video endoscopy. Stud Health Technol Inform 1999;62:268.
15. Boppart SA, Deutsch TF, Rattner DW. Optical imaging technology in minimally invasive surgery. Current status and future directions. Surg Endosc 1999;13:718.
16. Cuschieri A. Technology for minimal access surgery. Interview by Judy Jones. BMJ 1999;319:1304.
17. Afane JS, Olweny EO, Bercowsky E, et al. Flexible ureteroscopes: a single center evaluation of the durability and function of the new endoscopes smaller than 9Fr. J Urol 2000;164:1164.
18. Auge BK, Preminger GM. Digital cameras and documentation in urologic practice. AUA Update Series XXI, 2002.
19. Knyrim K, Seidlitz H, Vakil N. Current developments in electronic endoscopy. Endoscopy 1992;24 (Suppl 2):502.
20. Niwa H, Kawaguchi A, Miyahara T, et al. Clinical use of new video-endoscopes (EVIS 100 and 200). Endoscopy 1992;24:222.
21. Pelosi MA, Kadar N, Pelosi MA 3rd. The electronic video operative laparoscope. J Am Assoc Gynecol Laparosc 1993;1:54.
22. Emam TA, Hanna G, Cuschieri A. Ergonomic principles of task alignment, visual display, and direction of execution of laparoscopic bowel suturing. Surg Endosc 2002;16:267.
23. Schurr MO, Kunert W, Arezzo A, et al. The role and future of endoscopic imaging systems. Endoscopy 1999;31:557.
24. Huang HK. Image storage, transmission, and manipulation. Minim Invasive Ther Allied Technol 1992;1:85.
25. Fujino MA, Kawai T, Morozumi A, et al. Endoscopic image manipulation: state of the art. Endoscopy 1992;24 (Suppl 2):516.

26. Stroehlein JR, Barroso A, Glombicki A, et al. Documentation of fluoroscopic and endoscopic images using a color video printer. Gastrointest Endosc 1990;36:392.

27. Kuo RL, Aslan P, Dinlenc CZ, et al. Secure transmission of urologic images and records over the Internet. J Endourol 1999;13:141.

28. Kuo RL, Delvecchio FC, Preminger GM. Use of a digital camera in the urologic setting. Urology 1999;53:613.

29. Wurnig PN, Hollaus PH, Wurnig CH, et al. A new method for digital video documentation in surgical procedures and minimally invasive surgery. Surg Endosc 2003;17:232.

30. Arenson RL, Andriole KP, Avrin DE, et al. Computers in imaging and health care: now and in the future. J Digit Imaging 2000;13:145.

31. Fujino MA, Ikeda M, Yamamoto Y, et al. Development of an integrated filing system for endoscopic images. Endoscopy 1991;23:11.

32. Martinez R, Cole C, Rozenblit J, et al. Common object request broker architecture (CORBA)-based security services for the virtual radiology environment. J Digit Imaging 2000;13:59.

33. Yoshihiro A, Nakata N, Harada J, et al. Wireless local area networking for linking a PC reporting system and PACS: clinical feasibility in emergency reporting. Radiographics 2002;22:721.

34. Tan KS, Hinberg I. Effects of a wireless local area network (LAN) system, a telemetry system, and electrosurgical devices on medical devices in a hospital environment. Biomed Instrum Technol 2000;34:115.

35. Gandsas A, McIntire K, Park A. Live broadcast of laparoscopic surgery to handheld computers. Surg Endosc 2004;18:997.

36. Pagani L, Jyrkinen L, Niinimaki J, et al. A portable diagnostic workstation based on a Webpad: implementation and evaluation. J Telemed Telecare 2003;9:225.

37. Johnston WK 3rd, Patel BN, Low RK, et al. Wireless teleradiology for renal colic and renal trauma. J Endourol 2005;19:32.

38. Berguer R, Forkey DL, Smith WD. The effect of laparoscopic instrument working angle on surgeons' upper extremity workload. Surg Endosc 2001;15:1027.

39. Berguer R, Rab GT, Abu-Ghaida H, et al. A comparison of surgeons' posture during laparoscopic and open surgical procedures. Surg Endosc 1997;11:139.

40. Hemal AK, Srinivas M, Charles AR. Ergonomic problems associated with laparoscopy. J Endourol 2001;15:499.

41. Nguyen NT, Ho HS, Smith WD, et al. An ergonomic evaluation of surgeons' axial skeletal and upper extremity movements during laparoscopic and open surgery. Am J Surg 2001;182:720.

42. Herron DM, Gagner M, Kenyon TL, et al. The minimally invasive surgical suite enters the 21st century. A discussion of critical design elements. Surg Endosc 2001;15:415.

43. Kenyon TA, Urbach DR, Speer JB, et al. Dedicated minimally invasive surgery suites increase operating room efficiency. Surg Endosc 2001;15:1140.

44. Minnich DJ, Schell SR. Evaluation of face-mounted binocular video display for laparoscopy: outcomes of psychometric skills testing and surgeon satisfaction. J Laparoendosc Adv Surg Tech A 2003;13:333.

45. Durrani AF, Preminger GM. Three-dimensional video imaging for endoscopic surgery. Comput Biol Med 1995;25:237.

46. Zobel J. Basics of three-dimensional endoscopic vision. Endosc Surg Allied Technol 1993;1:36.

47. Mitchell TN, Robertson J, Nagy AG, et al. Three-dimensional endoscopic imaging for minimal access surgery. J R Coll Surg Edinb 1993;38:285.

48. Durrani AF, Preminger GM. Advanced endoscopic imaging: 3-D laparoscopic endoscopy. Surg Technol Int 1994;III:141.

49. Ballantyne GH. Robotic surgery, telerobotic surgery, telepresence, and telementoring. Review of early clinical results. Surg Endosc 2002;16:1389.

50. Garcia BJ, Greenstein RJ. True-stereoscopic video from monoscopic sources: the DeepVision system for minimally invasive surgery. Virtual Reality Systems Magazine 1994;1:52.

51. Birkett DH. 3-D imaging in gastrointestinal laparoscopy. Surg Endosc 1993;7:556.

52. Satava RM. 3-D vision technology applied to advanced minimally invasive surgery systems. Surg Endosc 1993;7:429.

53. Janetschek G, Reissigl A, Peschel R, et al. Chip on a stick technology: first clinical experience with this new videolaparoscope. J Endourol 1993;7:S195.

54. Babayan RK, Chiu AW, Este-McDonald J, et al. The comparison between 2-dimensional and 3-dimensional laparoscopic video systems in a pelvic trainer. J Endourol 1993;7:S195.

55. Herron DM, Lantis JC 2nd, Maykel J, et al. The 3-D monitor and head-mounted display. A quantitative evaluation of advanced laparoscopic viewing technologies. Surg Endosc 1999;13:751.

56. Hofmeister J, Frank TG, Cuschieri A, et al. Perceptual aspects of two-dimensional and stereoscopic display techniques in endoscopic surgery: review and current problems. Semin Laparosc Surg 2001;8:12.

57. van Bergen P, Kunert W, Buess GF. The effect of high-definition imaging on surgical task efficiency in minimally invasive surgery: an experimental comparison between three-dimensional imaging and direct vision through a stereoscopic TEM rectoscope. Surg Endosc 2000;14:71.

58. Chang L, Satava RM, Pellegrini CA, et al. Robotic surgery: identifying the learning curve through objective measurement of skill. Surg Endosc 2003;17:1744.

59. Dakin GF, Gagner M. Comparison of laparoscopic skills performance between standard instruments and two surgical robotic systems. Surg Endosc 2003;17:574.

60. Renda A, Vallancien G. Principles and advantages of robotics in urologic surgery. Curr Urol Rep 2003;4:114.

61. Chiu AW, Babayan RK. Retroperitoneal laparoscopic nephrectomy utilizing three-dimensional camera. Case report. J Endourol 1994;8:139.

62. von Orelli A, Lehareinger Y, Rol P, et al. High-definition true-colour television for use in minimally invasive medical procedures. Technol Health Care 1999;7:75.

63. Kuo RL, Delvecchio FC, Preminger GM. Virtual reality: current urologic applications and future developments. J Endourol 2001;15:117.

64. Preminger GM, Babayan RK, Merril GL, et al. Virtual reality surgical simulation in endoscopic urologic surgery. Stud Health Technol Inform 1996;29:157.

65. Shah J, Mackay S, Vale J, et al. Simulation in urology—a role for virtual reality? BJU Int 2001;88:661.

66. Matsumoto ED, Hamstra SJ, Radomski SB, et al. The effect of bench model fidelity on endourological skills: a randomized controlled study. J Urol 2002;167:1243.

67. Merril JR, Preminger GM, Babayan RK, et al. Surgical simulation using virtual reality technology: design, implementation, and implications. Surg Technol Int 1994;III:53.

68. Jacomides L, Ogan K, Cadeddu JA, et al. Use of a virtual reality simulator for ureteroscopy training. J Urol 2004;171:320.

69. Johnson DB, Kondraske GV, Wilhelm DM, et al. Assessment of basic human performance resources predicts the performance of virtual ureterorenoscopy. J Urol 2004;171:80.

70. Wilhelm DM, Ogan K, Roehrborn CG, et al. Assessment of basic endoscopic performance using a virtual reality simulator. J Am Coll Surg 2002;195:675.

71. Shah J, Darzi A. Virtual reality flexible cystoscopy: a validation study. BJU Int 2002;90:828.

72. Adrales GL, Park AE, Chu UB, et al. A valid method of laparoscopic simulation training and competence assessment. J Surg Res 2003;114:156.

73. Gettman MT, Kondraske GV, Traxer O, et al. Assessment of basic human performance resources predicts operative performance of laparoscopic surgery. J Am Coll Surg 2003;197:489.

74. Gornick ME, Eggers PW, Riley GF. Associations of race, education, and patterns of preventive service use with stage of cancer at time of diagnosis. Health Serv Res 2004; 39:1403.

75. Schijven MP, Jakimowicz J. The learning curve on the Xitact LS 500 laparoscopy simulator: profiles of performance. Surg Endosc 2004;18:121.

76. McFarlane N, Denstedt J. Imaging and the Internet. J Endourol 2001;15:59.

77. Goldberg MA. Teleradiology and telemedicine. Radiol Clin North Am 1996;34:647.

78. Crump WJ, Pfeil T. A telemedicine primer. An introduction to the technology and an overview of the literature. Arch Fam Med 1995;4:796.

79. Takeda H, Minato K, Takahasi T. High quality image oriented telemedicine with multimedia technology. Int J Med Inform 1999;55:23.

80. Byrne JP, Mughal MM. Telementoring as an adjunct to training and competence-based assessment in laparoscopic cholecystectomy. Surg Endosc 2000;14:1159.

81. Janetschek G, Bartsch G, Kavoussi LR. Transcontinental interactive laparoscopic telesurgery between the United States and Europe. J Urol 1998;160:1413.

82. Lee BR, Bishoff JT, Janetschek G, et al. A novel method of surgical instruction: international telementoring. World J Urol 1998;16:367.

83. Moore RG, Adams JB, Partin AW, et al. Telementoring of laparoscopic procedures: initial clinical experience. Surg Endosc 1996;10:107.

84. Rosser JC Jr, Herman B, Giammaria LE. Telementoring. Semin Laparosc Surg 2003;10:209.

85. Micali S, Vespasiani G, Finazzi-Agro E, et al. Feasibility of telesurgery between Baltimore, USA and Rome, Italy: the first five cases. J Endourol 1999;13:A145.

86. Lee BR, Png DJ, Liew L, et al. Laparoscopic telesurgery between the United States and Singapore. Ann Acad Med Singapore 2000;29:665.

87. Bauer J, Lee BR, Stoianovici D, et al. Remote percutaneous renal access using a new automated telesurgical robotic system. Telemed J E Health 2001;7:341.

88. Marescaux J, Leroy J, Rubino F, et al. Transcontinental robot-assisted remote telesurgery: feasibility and potential applications. Ann Surg 2002;235:487.

89. Rosser JC, Wood M, Payne JH, et al. Telementoring. A practical option in surgical training. Surg Endosc 1997;11:852.

90. Link RE, Schulam PG, Kavoussi LR. Telesurgery. Remote monitoring and assistance during laparoscopy. Urol Clin North Am 2001;28:177.

91. Satava RM. Robotics, telepresence and virtual reality: a critical analysis of the future of surgery. Minim Invasive Ther Allied Technol 1992;1:357.

92. Kavoussi LR, Moore RG, Partin AW, et al. Telerobotic assisted laparoscopic surgery: initial laboratory and clinical experience. Urology 1994;44:15.

93. Kuehnapfel UG, Neisius B. CAD-based graphical computer simulation in endoscopic surgery. Endosc Surg Allied Technol;1:181;1993.

94. Rininsland HH. Basics of robotics and manipulators in endoscopic surgery. Endosc Surg Allied Technol 1:154, 1993.

Intracorporeal Lithotriptors

Bodo E. Knudsen, MD, FRCSC
John D. Denstedt, MD, FRCSC

INTRACORPOREAL LITHOTRIPTORS

Extracorporeal shock wave lithotripsy (ESWL) has been the first-line therapy of choice at many centers for the treatment of ureteral stones and renal calculi less than 2 cm. However, with recent advances in both intracorporeal lithotripsy devices and the design of small-caliber flexible ureteroscopes, ureteroscopy is a reasonable alternative to ESWL and, in some cases, is the most appropriate first-line treatment. For stones located in the distal one-third of the ureter, cystine calculi, previous ESWL failures, and morbidly obese patients may be most effectively treated with ureteroscopy. New, advanced small-caliber ureteroscopes may be used without ureteral dilation, thus simplifying the procedure. Advances in technology have encouraged an increasingly prominent role for ureteroscopy lithotripsy in treatment of proximal ureteral and selected intrarenal calculi. Percutaneous nephrolithotomy (PCNL) is generally considered the most effective treatment option for renal calculi > 2 cm in diameter and for staghorn renal stones. Furthermore, PCNL with or without intracorporeal lithotripsy may also be considered a first-line option for patients with renal cystine calculi, previous ESWL failures, collecting system abnormalities likely to prevent successful stone evacuation (caliceal diverticulum, UPJ obstruction), or in patients having a body habitus precluding ESWL. Finally, intracorporeal lithotripsy, via either transurethral or percutaneous suprapubic approach, is the mainstay for treatment of bladder calculi. Open suprapubic removal of stones is rarely required. Indeed, open stone surgery is rapidly becoming a technique of historical interest as today's modern endoscopes and intracorporeal lithotripsy devices have allowed for even the most difficult stones to be treated with a minimally invasive approach. The various technologies, clinical outcomes, advantages and disadvantages of each device will be reviewed in this chapter (Table 5-1).

ELECTROHYDRAULIC LITHOTRIPSY

Electrohydraulic lithotripsy (EHL), developed in the late 1950s and first described by the physicist Yutkin, was the first modality of intracorporeal lithotripsy available for clinical use.[1,2] The principle behind EHL-induced stone fragmentation is based on the effect of an electrical discharge produced in a liquid medium. This electrical discharge vaporizes the surrounding fluid, creating a cavitation bubble that undergoes rapid expansion and collapse. The result of this phenomenon is a hydraulic shock wave that then collides with the stone to effect fragmentation.[3,4] The sequence from the time of electrical discharge to the creation of the hydraulic shock wave lasts 1/800 of a second.[5] The energy for any electrical discharge depends on the voltage and the capacity applied. Investigation has shown that the peak pressure and slope of the shock front depend solely on the voltage, whereas the pulse width is correlated with the capacity. Thus, by varying these parameters, the technique of EHL can be used to generate a wide range of patterns of shock waves with different peak pressures, rise times, and pulse widths.[6,7] It remains to be seen, however, whether a different type of shock wave transferring the same amount of energy has a different impact on various stones or on tissue. There are many electrohydraulic generators available, and in each case, the power output of the device can be carefully regulated (Figure 5-1). The electrohydraulic probe is connected via cable to the generator which, in turn, is activated by a foot pedal. Probe size has decreased significantly from the early 9 French and 5F probes to 3F and, more recently, to 1.9F in diameter (Figure 5-2).

The electrohydraulic lithotriptor has the narrowest margin of safety of all forms of intracorporeal lithotripsy. Bhatta and colleagues examined the effects of laser and EHL on the rabbit bladder and found EHL to be most likely to consistently produce bladder perforation.[8] Likewise Piergiovanni and colleagues, in comparing the tissue effects of a variety of lithotripsy devices in the pig model, found EHL to induce extensive tissue lesions secondary to heat.[9] As such, when intracorporeal EHL is performed, certain guidelines must be followed. The tip of the probe should be examined before it is inserted into the endoscope. The tip should be smooth, and the outer and inner layers of insulation should be intact. In all situations, the tip of the probe should extend 5 mm from the end of the endoscope to preclude any damage to the lens. The presence of a guidewire during EHL is safe as long as the probe is not fired directly on the guidewire. If there is any doubt, a 5F angiographic catheter can be used to cover the guidewire. During EHL, it is important that the flow of irrigant be rapid enough to permit a clear field of view and that ureteral distention be sufficient to avoid probe discharge on the urothelium. Traditionally, 1:6

Table 5-1 Comparison of Intracorporeal Lithotriptors					
Device	Mechanism of Action	Probe Size	Cost	Disposability	Tissue Safety
Electrohydraulic	Electrical discharge producing hydraulic shock waves	Flexible 1.9, 3, 5, and 9F probes	$10,000 to $15,000 (US)	Disposable probes $200 to $320 (US)	+
Ultrasound	Piezoelectrically generated ultrasonic waves	Rigid 2.5 – 5F solid or hollow probes	$15,000 – $20,000 (US)	Reusable probes $400 to $600 (US)	++
Pneumatic devices	Pneumatically driven, direct-contact "jackhammer"	Solid and semi-rigid, 0.8-, 2.5-, and 3-mm probes	$15,000 to $30,000 (US)	Reusable probes $400 to $620 (US)	+++
Combination ultrasound/ pneumatic device (Lithoclast Master/Ultra)	Piezoelectrically generated ultrasonic waves; pneumatically driven, direct-contact "jackhammer"	Rigid ultrasonic 3.3 and 3.8 mm; rigid pneumatic 0.8, 1.0, 1.6, and 2.0 mm	$39,500 (US) (Lithoclast Ultra)	Lithoclast Ultra: single use pneumatic $230 (US); three-time use ultrasonic $540 (US)	++
Holmium:YAG laser	Photothermal	200 to 1,000 μm (core size) semi-flexible probes	$45,000 to $150,000 (US) (requires maintenance contract)	Reusable and disposable fibers; $300 to $1,500 (US)	++

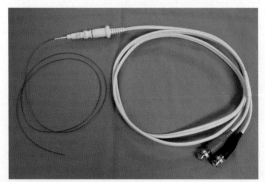

Figure 5-1 Electrohydraulic (EHL) generator.

normal saline solution has been recommended as the preferred irrigant; it has been reported, however, that the process works equally well in normal saline solution, thus simplifying preparation for nursing personnel and eliminating the hazards of using a hypotonic solution in the urinary tract.[10,11] Before the EHL generator is activated, the stone must be clearly visible, and the entire tip of the probe must be seen to rest on or < 1 mm from the center of the stone with no intervening urothelium. The goal of EHL is to break the stone into fragments that can be removed with grasping forceps or that are likely to pass spontaneously. Attempts to reduce the stone to fragments < 2 mm is generally not recommended since damage to the urothelium may occur. In addition, to enhance safety, it is our practice to initially set the generator on low voltage or power, which is gradually increased as necessary to effect adequate fragmentation. For intraureteral lithotripsy, the small 1.9F probes are preferred. Most manufacturers have discontinued production of the larger 5 and 9F probes. It is important that the probe not be overused, and after 10 discharges, the probe should be checked for wear. Overuse of the probe may result in its shedding insulation or the entire probe tip into the ureteral lumen, retrieval of which can be difficult.[12] As with other electrical therapeutic devices, certain precautions must be taken to avoid untoward events.[13] There have been several reports of medical personnel receiving electric shocks as a result of stray capacitance when the patient was touched during activation of the lithotriptor. For this reason, it is recommended that all operating room staff avoid touching the patient when the EHL unit is activated. It is also important to minimize patient contact with any grounded metal surfaces such as a Bovie pad during the procedure to avoid electrical burns. EHL should not be

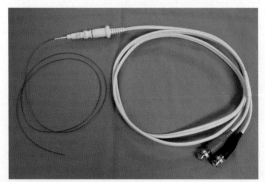

Figure 5-2 1.9 Fr electrohydraulic probe and cable.

used in patients with externally connected cardiac pacemakers. Finally, many older cystoscopes were manufactured with conductive eyepieces or lens-retaining rings, which have the potential to conduct the electrical current into the surgeon's eye. EHL should not be used under such circumstances, or alternatively, the eyepiece should be replaced with a nonconductive type.

The first EHL device, the URAT-1, was initially applied clinically to the treatment of bladder stones.[14] With experience, EHL was found to be a quick, effective, and relatively safe means of fragmenting vesical calculi. A number of authors have reported fragmentation rates of > 80% with a low incidence of complications.[2,15,16] Patients with a very large bladder stone burden or those with extremely hard stones may be resistant to EHL fragmentation and require use of another device, such as ultrasound or the Swiss Lithoclast.[17] Experience with EHL in the ureter preceded the development of ultrasound and laser lithotripsy.[18] These early investigators, however, did not have the benefit of endoscopic control. As such, initial experience with intraureteral EHL was complicated by extravasation, inconsistent stone fragmentation and, in animal studies, ureteral stricture.[19,20] In contradistinction, intraureteral EHL under endoscopic control has been found to be effective and safe. In their early work, Green and Lytton noted excellent fragmentation in 32 of 36 stones; 24 of their patients were evaluated radiographically 4 months to 4 years after intraureteral EHL, and no strictures were noted.[21] Additional early studies on the use of EHL reported that, by using a 5F electrohydraulic lithotripsy probe, there was a 6% incidence of ureteral perforation among 33 patients.[4] In contrast, Begun and colleagues noted no occurrence of ureteral perforation in 21 procedures, but in all their cases, a smaller 3F probe was used.[22] Subsequently, several groups have reported no immediate or long-term harmful side effects resulting from intraureteral EHL when performed under endoscopic control with 3F or smaller probes.[10,23] The development of a 1.9F probe facilitated the use of EHL with small-caliber, semi-rigid and flexible ureteroscopes. Elashry and colleagues reported their experience of treating 45 patients (32 ureteral and 57 renal) with small caliber endoscopes and a 1.9F EHL probe. They achieved an overall stone-free rate of 92% at a mean follow-up of 8.2 months. For previously difficult to treat lower-pole calculi, they achieved a stone-free rate of 87%.[24] During percutaneous nephrolithotripsy EHL is often less efficient than mechanical devices employing larger, rigid probes such as ultrasound or the Lithoclast. EHL in combination with flexible instruments, however, is often useful for fragmenting caliceal stones remote from the nephrostomy tract.[3]

EHL is the least expensive intracorporeal fragmentation method, with the generator costing approximately $10,000 to $15,000 (US). Disposable probes cost $200 to $320 (US), and the life span of an electrohydraulic probe is in the range of 20 to 60 seconds. The role of EHL for intracorpo-

real lithotripsy has declined significantly in recent years with the advent of the holmium:yttrium-aluminum-garnet (holmium:YAG) laser.

ULTRASONIC LITHOTRIPSY

In 1953, Mulvaney described the first attempt to destroy urinary calculi by ultrasonic waves.[25] More comprehensive were the experiments conducted 3 years later by Coates[26] and Lamport and Newman.[27] The latter tried unsuccessfully to disrupt urinary calculi in a water medium in vitro using ultrasound. The first effective uses of ultrasound for fragmentation of urinary calculi was reported from Germany[26,27,28–30] and subsequently from the United States.[31] Gasteyer described the use of a prototype device for fragmenting bladder calculi, but the probe design did not permit evacuation of fragments.[32] Concurrently, Hautmann and colleagues, in collaboration with Karl Storz Endoscopy of Tuttlingen, Germany, developed the "Aachen model" device, which incorporated the technical features that form the basis of all currently available units (Figure 5-3).[33]

Acoustic frequencies beyond the range of audibility of the human ear are called ultrasonic waves. These are mechanical waves covering a frequency range of 20,000 to 10^{10} cycles per second (Hz). Ultrasonic waves may be generated in different ways (eg, mechanically, thermally, electrostatically, magnetostrictively, and piezoelectrically). A high-frequency generator activated by a foot pedal applies a current to a piezoceramic crystal. This application of current causes the crystal to expand and contract, and results in vibratory energy at a frequency of approximately 23,000 to 27,000 Hz. The energy created is then transmitted along a solid or hollow probe and is converted to either horizontal or transverse vibration at the tip. This energy causes a drilling effect and results in fragmentation of the calculus. The fragmenting ability of the probe is strictly mechanical, and the effects of heat, cavitation, and shock waves are noncontributory factors.[34,35] Most ultrasonic lithotripsy devices rely on a system that suctions irrigation fluid through the center of the probe. (Figures 5-4 and 5-5) This serves to cool the instrument and also evacuates the small stone fragments that occur as a result of lithotripsy. Either the manufacturer's pump system or stan-

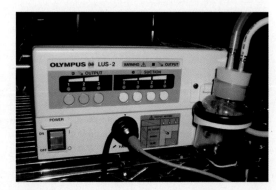

Figure 5-3 Ultrasonic generator and stone trap.

ultrasound generator

foot piece

piezoceramic elements

longitudinal vibration

ultrasound probe

suctional channel

acoustical end parts

Figure 5-4 Diagram of ultrasonic lithotriptor.

dard operating room suction is suitable. A variety of ultrasonic probe sizes are available, ranging from 2.5 to 6F in diameter. The smaller 2.5F probe, which is solid in design and relies on lateral vibration, can also be used with the smaller, rigid ureteroscopes. A potential drawback of the smaller probe is the fact that it contains no hollow center through which to aspirate fragments. Higashihara and Aso have reported on the use of a semiflexible 4.5F ultrasonic probe permitting use with flexible endoscopes.[36] Problems include the fact that endoscope deflection is limited to < 30°, and reported rates of fragmentation using ultrasound alone are 25%. Further refinements may result in a flexible ultrasonic probe that can be used effectively with both rigid flexible ureteroscopes.

The technique of ultrasonic lithotripsy is similar to that of other direct-contact rigid probes such as the Lithoclast. Although the relatively weak suction action of the probe may result in sufficient probe-stone apposition to cause fragmentation, direct probe contact on a calculus within the confines of the ureter or trapped against the urothelium of the kidney or bladder will allow more effective fragmentation. The rigid nature of the probe requires use of endoscopes with an end-on working channel and an offset lens system. Short bursts of ultrasonic probe activation are delivered in a direct-contact manner to the calculus, producing small particles that undergo simultaneous evacuation. In the case of larger calculi located in the bladder or kidney, working along cleavage lines can create larger fragments that may then be removed with grasping forceps. Longer periods of ultrasound activation in a clear field of view may also be used to achieve more rapid destruction of large stones, but there may be greater likelihood of significant probe heating under such circumstances. Probe overheating may be limited by not using pre-warmed irrigation fluids during the procedure. Hypothermia can be prevented by placing a forced-air warming blanket across the patient's upper torso.

In an extensive study, Terhorst and colleagues investigated the effect of a sonotrode generated at 20 to 25 kHz on the bladder wall of rabbits.[37] Even after exposure of up to 5 minutes, with the tip of the probe continuously in contact with the mucosa, the only alteration documented was edema of the mucosa with no lesions of the deeper layers of the bladder wall or perforations. Howards and colleagues also documented only minor urothelial alterations following direct probe activation in the canine model.[31] The only significant risk of injury that can be attributed to ultrasound is that related to the previously mentioned possibility of probe overheating and subsequent urothelial injury.[38] Clinically, thermal injury to surrounding urothelium can occur if irrigation is interrupted, allowing the probe tip to heat up. A single case of fatal venous air embolus during percutaneous nephrolithotripsy has also been reported, the result of a faulty connection between the aspiration and suction tubing.[39] Two cases of ultrasonic probe breakage requiring open surgery for removal of the burr tip have also been documented.[40] In general terms, clinical use of ultrasonic lithotripsy in both the lower and upper urinary tract has been found to be very safe.

Similar to EHL, the initial clinical experience with ultrasonic lithotripsy was in the treatment of vesical calculi. Hautmann and colleagues reported

on 10 years experience in treating 412 patients with bladder calculi with ultrasonic lithotripsy.[33] Many of the early operations were performed in the early 1970s with prototype devices, and a failure rate of 22% to 34% was reported. With technical advances, the failure rate improved to 1% during the final 100 operations. Two cases of bladder perforation occurred. Several additional groups have reported the successful use of ultrasonic lithotripsy, with a low incidence of complications, for vesical calculi.[17,41,42] As emphasized earlier, use of ultrasound requires a rigid cystoscope or nephroscope with an offset lens system and, in the case of bladder calculi, a working channel of sufficient size to accommodate a 4 to 6F hollow probe. With the advent of percutaneous and ureteroscopic techniques and their associated instrumentation, the use of ultrasonic lithotripsy was expanded to include calculi in the upper urinary tract. Ureteroscopic ultrasonic lithotripsy has been evaluated in a number of reports with success rates ranging from 69 to 100%.[43–46] With the larger hollow probes, a rigid ureteroscope of 9.5F or larger is required. The larger endoscopes often demonstrate greater utility in the distal, as opposed to the proximal, ureter, and this has been reflected in lower overall rates of success reported for proximal stones. The development of the 2.5F solid probe facilitated ultrasonic lithotripsy in the ureter because these devices lend themselves to use with smaller caliber ureteroscopes. Two large series have been published documenting treatment using the smaller, solid probe. In their series of 118 patients, Chaussy and colleagues reported a 96.6% complete fragmentation rate.[47] In a similar study carried out by Fuchs, success rates of 91, 94, and 98% for the upper, middle, and lower ureter, respectively, were reported.[48] Similar to electrohydraulic lithotripsy, the use of ultrasonic lithotripsy for ureteral calculi has declined significantly due to the advent of the holmium:YAG laser. The comparatively large size and rigid nature of ultrasound probes make it a cumbersome and relatively inefficient modality for intraureteral lithotripsy.

Since the first description of ultrasonic litholapaxy (lithotripsy) of staghorn calculi by Kurth and colleagues, the use of ultrasound in percuta-

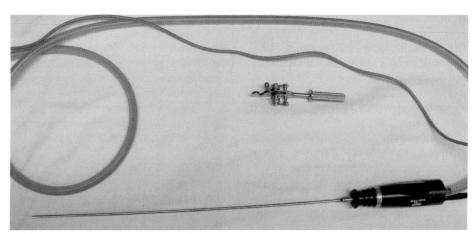

Figure 5-5 Ultrasonic handpiece and probe.

neous renal stone surgery has become widely practiced and highly regarded.[49] A number of investigators have found ultrasonic lithotripsy to be an effective method of destruction and percutaneous removal of large and staghorn renal calculi.[50–54] The advantages of ultrasound during percutaneous nephrolithotripsy include the ability to deal with a large stone burden rapidly and safely and the simultaneous evacuation of small stone fragments via the hollow probe.

Clayman effectively outlined, in the textbook *Techniques in Endourology*, his method of ultrasonic intracorporeal lithotripsy, which is summarized in the following paragraph.[55] The sonotrode, generator and suction should all be ensured to be functioning normally prior to placing the instrument through the nephroscope. Normal saline irrigation fluid should be used. The connections of the probe to the transducer should be tight, for efficient energy transfer. If the connection is loose, the instrument will either function suboptimally—or not at all. Some manufacturers include both a short and a long probe. A shorter probe is less likely to be clogged during the procedure with stone debris, but the length of the nephroscope may dictate the use of a longer probe. Continuous suction is used during the procedure to efficiently remove stone material as well as to aid the surgeon in maintaining good contact with the stone. Stronger suction will help prevent clogging of the probe, provided there is adequate irrigation. Direct contact with the stone is imperative for the ultrasound to function. The ultrasound probe should only be advanced under direct vision. It may be necessary to pin the stone to the back wall to ensure good contact, but care must be used when employing this technique so as to not perforate the collecting system with the rigid probe.

When the lithotripsy is first initiated, there is often very little working space, especially when the stone is occupying an entire calix. Care must be taken to keep to stone in direct vision to ensure no injury to surrounding tissue. Once the initial portion of the stone in fragmented, the working space increases, thus facilitating the procedure. The renal access sheath should be advanced over the nephroscope as more medial aspects of the stone are treated. This will help tamponade any bleeding vessels that may limit visibility. The suction should be periodically checked to ensure it is functioning well. Stone material may clog the sonotrode or the suction tubing. Not only will this impair the removal of the stone particles, but it may also result in overheating of the lithotripsy probe and decrease its efficiency.

The composition of the stone will often guide the technique used with ultrasonic lithotripsy. Stones that are very soft can often be very easily fragmented into small particles and completely "vacuumed" out. The goal is to not create a lot of small fragments that can migrate through the collecting system. The periphery of the stone is initially targeted, and a broad working front is created. The leading edges are systematically targeted until the stone has been completely removed. For stones that are of a harder composi-

tion, it is more efficient to reduce the stone to fragments that are just small enough to fit through the access sheath. The fragments are created by carving the stone with the ultrasound probe. Once a series of fragments are created, they are removed expeditiously with rigid, two-pronged non-toothed grasping forceps. Alternatively, a rigid, tipless nitinol stone basket (Perc NCircle, Cook Urological, Spencer, IN) may be employed. The rigid nitinol grasper is especially useful when multiple small stone fragments are present because multiple fragments can be captured and removed with each pass. After the stone burden is removed, a flexible nephroscope should be employed to systematically inspect the collecting system to ensure no stone material migrated to a calix that is inaccessible with the rigid nephroscope. A nitinol stone basket is used to remove any migrated fragments or stones remote from the nephrostomy access tract.

Liatsikos and colleagues compared the efficiency and efficacy of several intracorporeal ultrasonic lithotrites using plaster of Paris stone phantoms. The stone phantoms were immersed under water in a plastic container while continuous irrigation through a rigid nephroscope was performed.[56] The Storz ultrasound (Calcuson 27610020, Karl Storz) was determined in this study to have the lowest fragmentation time and highest efficiency of fragmentation when applied to three different stone phantoms. The other ultrasonic lithotrites tested and listed in order of best to worst performance were the Wolf (2270004), the Circon ACMI (USL 2000) and the Olympus LUS. An acknowledged flaw in the study design was a lack of standardization of the pressure applied to the phantom by the probes.

In an attempt to standardize the pressures applied to the stones, Kuo and colleagues designed an objective in vitro ultrasonic lithotriptor test system that eliminated any hand pressure on the probes. This was done by suspending the probes vertically and then placing a weight (62.7 g) on top of the probe in order to produce a constant force.[57] A total of 5 different ultrasonic devices were tested. The Olympus LUS-2 (Olympus, Inc., Melville, NY) and Circon-ACMI USL-2000 were the most efficient devices ($p < .05$). The remaining three devices tested in order of most to least efficient were the Karl Storz Calcuson, the Olympus LUS-1, and the Richard Wolf model 2271004.

Current cost of an ultrasound generator is approximately \$15,000 to \$20,000 (US). The transducers undergo wear and will require occasional replacement. The probes also undergo wear and require replacement periodically. A busy stone center would benefit with having two units available so that ,when the primary machine needs servicing, a backup machine is always on hand.

PNEUMATIC DEVICES

The first pneumatically driven intracorporeal lithotriptor, the Swiss Lithoclast, was developed through the collaborative efforts of the Departments of Urology and Medical Electronics at

Chur University Medical School and Electro Medical System le Sentier, respectively, both of Lausanne, Switzerland.[58] This device uses a direct-contact, solid, rigid probe to fragment stones under direct vision using mechanics similar to those of a pneumatic jackhammer. The Lithoclast consists of a generator (Figure 5-6), handpiece, and probe. Probes are available in a variety of sizes ranging from 0.8 to 3.0 mm and are connected to the handpiece, which contains a small metal projectile. The rigid nature of the probe limits the use of the Lithoclast to rigid or semirigid endoscopes; the variety of probe sizes, however, permits use of the device with any rigid endoscope having an end-on channel of suitable caliber. The handpiece is connected by flexible tubing to the generator which, in turn, is also connected to a dry, clean air supply. Either the hospital central air supply or a compressed air tank is a suitable source of compressed air. No special power supply is required to run the generator, which is portable and lightweight. The entire unit is activated by a foot pedal. On activation of the device, compressed air propels the metal projectile within the handpiece against the head of the probe at a pressure of 3 atmospheres and a frequency of 12 Hz. Repeated pounding of the probe tip against the stone results in breakage once the tensile forces of the stone are overcome. No heat is generated with activation of the device, and striking one's finger with the larger probes directly produces no discomfort. Preparing and assembling the Lithoclast for use is quick and simple, and both the probe and disassembled handpiece may be sterilized with gas or immersed for surgical sterilization/disinfection.

When using the Lithoclast, as with all methods of intracorporeal lithotripsy, accurate probe placement is necessary to prevent inadvertent tissue injury. Under endoscopic visual guidance, the Lithoclast probe is placed in direct contact with the stone. The foot pedal is then depressed, activating the unit. The Lithoclast has two operating modes: single-shot and continuous firing. We primarily employ the continuous firing mode. Firing the probe for 5 to 10 seconds at a time is then monitored under direct vision to ensure correct probe placement and to assess the effectiveness of fragmentation. The goal is to break stones into small fragments than can then be extracted with grasping instruments. Successful intracorporeal

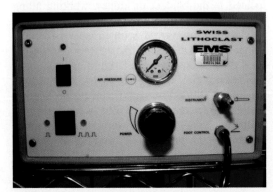

Figure 5-6 Swiss Lithoclast pneumatic generator.

lithotripsy with the Swiss Lithoclast is somewhat dependent on being able to pin the calculus against the urothelium and thus allow the jackhammer-like action of the probe to achieve the desired stone destruction. Such fixation is rarely difficult in the kidney or the bladder but may be problematic when working in the confines of the ureter, particularly when the ureter is capacious. Under such circumstances, the potential exists for retrograde displacement of the calculus. Possible solutions include trapping the calculus in a stone basket or proximal placement of a ureteral balloon occlusion catheter. The Stone Cone (Boston Scientific, Natick, MA) has also been shown to be effective in preventing the proximal migration of calculi during ureteroscopy employing a pneumatic lithotripsy device.[59,60]

Investigations of the tissue effects of the Lithoclast in animal models have demonstrated the safety of the device. In comparing the Lithoclast, EHL, holmium:YAG laser, and ultrasound, Piergiovanni and colleagues found that the Lithoclast produced the least macroscopic and histologic trauma to the urothelium.[61] We assessed the gross and microscopic histopathologic changes in a porcine model following direct probe activation on the wall of the ureter and bladder in both acute and chronic settings.[62] Immediately after probe firing, focal areas of hemorrhage were grossly visible in all bladders and ureters treated. Microscopic changes seen acutely in all animals included transmural edema, hemorrhage, and mucosal erosions at the sites of probe firing. No frank perforations of the bladder or ureteral walls were noted. Inspection of the sites of probe activation (in animals sacrificed 3 and 6 weeks after treatment) failed to reveal any grossly visible lesions. Similarly, histopathologic examination did not identify any evidence of surface urothelial loss, fibrosis, or other long-term damage related to use of the device. Animal data have thus confirmed the clinical experience with the Swiss Lithoclast in that the device appears to be associated with a relatively large margin of safety.

A number of reports in the literature have documented the versatility, efficacy, and safety of the Swiss Lithoclast in performing intracorporeal lithotripsy. The first clinical report by Languetin and colleagues in 1990 demonstrated the utility of the device in accomplishing endoscopic lithotripsy safely and in treating stones located at all levels of the urinary tract.[58] No ureteral perforations or mucosal injuries were noted, either endoscopically or on retrograde examinations. Hofbauer and colleagues, in an initial small series of 10 patients with cystine or calcium oxalate monohydrate ureteral calculi, reported 100% success in fragmenting stones to a size permitting successful extraction using a basket.[63] In a report from our own center, the Lithoclast successfully fragmented 94% of calculi with no evidence of intraoperative or long-term complications related to use of the device.[64] Failures in our series were related to the aforementioned difficulty in trapping ureteral stones in a capacious ureter to facilitate direct probe contact. More recently, Yinghao

and colleagues reported a successful fragmentation rate of only 69.7% utilizing the Swiss Lithoclast in 145 patients with ureteral stones, with five patients developing a ureteral perforation secondary to the procedure.[65]

Several authors have noted the utility of the device in managing patients with a large stone burden and thus have been particularly pleased with its usefulness in performing percutaneous nephrolithotripsy and endoscopic lithotripsy of bladder calculi.[17,66-69] In both situations, the advantage of the Lithoclast is related to its efficiency in fragmenting large and/or hard stones rapidly and safely.[66] The ability of the device to rapidly fragment large calculi is of importance in today's percutaneous nephrolithotripsy population. The Lithoclast is also particularly useful for clearing the initial calix of the stone rapidly and safely when securing access to a kidney harboring a large branched calculus. Several authors have reported on the utility of the Lithoclast as a method of intracorporeal lithotripsy for vesical calculi. A retrospective analysis of our experience with endoscopic lithotripsy of bladder calculi revealed that the Lithoclast was successful in fragmenting 85% of all stones treated, with no evidence of bladder wall injury or perforation.[17] Likewise, Shokeir described transurethral cystolitholapaxy using the Swiss Lithoclast in selected cases of vesical stones in children.[70]

One advance in intracorporeal lithotripsy was the development of a combination pneumatic and ultrasonic lithotrite, the Lithoclast Master (EMS, Bern, Switzerland) marketed by Boston Scientific, Natick, MA as the Lithoclast Ultra in the United States (Figure 5-7). The unit incorporates the efficient stone-fragmentation properties of the pneumatic lithotriptor with the rapid stone clearing ability of the ultrasonic lithotrite.

The pneumatic Lithoclast can be fitted with various probe sizes (0.8, 1.0, 1.6, and 2.0 mm) and has a repetition rate of up to 12 Hz. The 1.0 mm Lithoclast probe may be used in conjunction with the ultrasound probe (3.3 or 3.8 mm) (Figure 5-8). It runs through the hollow center of the ultrasound probe (3.3 or 3.8 mm), and the tip of the Lithoclast probe is positioned just within the ultrasound probe so as to ensure optimal contact of the ultrasonic probe with the calculus when the pneumatic probe is not activated. Positioning the pneumatic probe beyond the tip of ultrasonic probe will result in suboptimal performance of the ultrasound due to loss of direct contact with the stone. The unit is designed to allow for either separate activation of the Lithoclast and ultrasound or for combined activation. A foot pedal is used for activation. The control unit allows for adjustment of the pulse frequency (up to 12 Hz), number of pulses, and the pneumatic pressure level of the Lithoclast. Single- or continuous-pulse modes are available. The ultrasound power (up to 100%) and duty adjustment (10 to 100%) can also be set. Ultrasound frequency is 24 to 26 kHz. The hand piece containing the probes is relatively lightweight (340 g).[71] The pneumatic portion can be removed entirely, allowing Lithoclast to be used

just as an ultrasound device. Initial in vitro studies demonstrated the high efficiency of stone fragmentation using the combination pneumatic/ultrasonic lithotrite. Auge and colleagues reported a significantly faster mean time to fragment phantom stones with the combination pneumatic/ultrasound unit (7.41 minutes) versus the ultrasound (12.87 minutes) and the pneumatic lithotrites (23.76 minutes) used individually. Furthermore, the size of the fragments were significantly smaller for the combination device (1.67 mm) as compared to the ultrasonic (3.67 mm) or pneumatic lithotrites (9.07 mm).[72] Olbert and colleagues similarly reported that the simultaneous use of both the pneumatic and ultrasound components was significantly faster than using either individual modality alone in standardized in vitro conditions.[73]

Pietrow and colleagues randomized 20 patients undergoing percutaneous nephrolithotomy for symptomatic calculi to either a standard ultrasonic lithotrite (LUS-2) or to a combination pneumatic/ultrasound unit. The mean time for complete stone clearance was significantly faster for the combination unit (21.1 versus 43.7 minutes).[74]

It was reported by EMS that the tip amplitude (peak to peak) of the Lithoclast Master ultrasound probe when power is set to 100% was greater than previously available ultrasonic lithotripters (100 µm vs. 50 µm). It is speculated that the increased tip amplitude results in an increase in efficiency of the device, but at the expense of probe life. EMS now recommends routinely operating the Lithoclast Master/Ultra ultrasound at 50% power, which results in a tip amplitude of approximately 60 µm. Only when a particularly hard stone is encountered should the power be increased incrementally up to 100%. This should result in an increased lifespan of the probe.

The combination pneumatic/ultrasound lithotrite appears to be the most efficient device currently available for percutaneous nephrolithotomy and is our first-line lithotriptor. The starting settings used by the authors are 50% ultrasound power, 90% duty, 100% pneumatic power at 4 Hz. If the stone is not efficiently fragmented at these settings, the ultrasound power is incrementally increased by 10% until efficient lithotripsy occurs or 100% power is reached. The frequency of the pneumatic probe can also be increased to a maximum of 12 Hz. As the frequency is raised, however, the majority of the lithotripsy occurs via the pneumatic probe and not by the ultrasound.

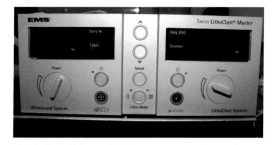

Figure 5-7 Swiss Lithoclast Master combination ultransonic/pneumatic generator.

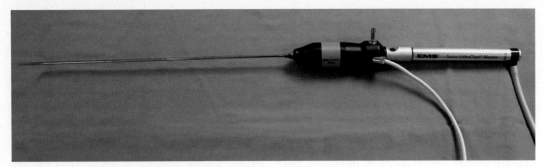

Figure 5-8 Swiss Lithoclast Master handpiece.

This can result in both an increase in the fragment size and number.

From an economic standpoint, the price of the pneumatic-based devices compares favorably with other intracorporeal lithotripsy devices. The cost of the generator is approximately $15,000 to $30,000 (US), and each reusable probe costs approximately $400 to $620 (US). No disposable items are used, which minimizes ongoing operating costs. The combination Swiss Lithoclast Ultra System has a list price in the United States of $39,500 (US). The single-use pneumatic probe cost is $230 (US) and the reusable (limited to 3 uses) ultrasonic probe is $540 (US). Outside of the United States, the pneumatic probes are sold as reusable devices.

LASER LITHOTRIPSY

A laser (light amplification by stimulated emission of radiation) is an optical source that emits photons in a coherent beam. An intense beam of light energy with a specific wavelength is created. Medical lasers first appeared in the early 1960s, and the first attempt at calculus destruction was carried out by Mulvaney and Beck in 1968 using a ruby laser.[75] Initial problems with excessive thermal energy limited the clinical applicability of their techniques. Continuous-wave lasers, such as CO_2 argon or neodymium:yttrium-aluminum-garnet (Nd:YAG), create constant energy, and as a result, the target area heats up, and thermal changes occur with use. Therefore, because of the large amounts of energy delivered in the vicinity (50 to 300 joules [J] with the ruby laser) and the inability to deliver CO_2 laser energy via an endoscope, it became obvious that further refinements were necessary. Advances in this area came from the work of Anderholm, Fair, and Yang, who demonstrated that it was possible to produce shock waves capable of fragmenting a stone without concomitant heat production.[76–78] In Anderholm's work, using a ruby laser system set at 7 J and 12 nanosecond (nsec) pulses, he was able to produce shock waves on the order of 34 kilobars, more than sufficient to fragment calculi. The next major advancement in technology involved the development of a Q-switched laser.[79] This system caused fragmentation via plasma production at the stone surface in contrast to the thermal action that occurred with previous lasers. A plasma is a rapidly expanding cavity of ions and electrons

that collapses rapidly after the laser pulse, thereby producing a mechanical shock wave. The Q-switched Nd:YAG laser emits at a wavelength of 1,064 nanometers, which is a wavelength at which calculi absorb poorly. By decreasing the pulse duration to the range of 8 to 10 nsec, a plasma can be formed, irrespective of absorption, as a result of the high-peak power densities created. The difficulty with such systems has been that the peak power density created by such ultrashort pulses is close to the damage threshold of quartz, thus resulting in fiber destruction. In addition, the energy that emerged from the tip of the laser fiber was non-focused and divergent; therefore, any separation of the stone from the fiber results in a falling off of the peak power density. Q-switched Nd:YAG lasers thus tend to be less efficient forms of intracorporeal lithotripsy systems and also do not have the same potential for miniaturization and flexibility as other laser systems. Hofmann and colleagues reported on clinical experience with a Q-switched laser with an 8 nsec pulse duration and a repetition rate of up to 50 Hz. Single-pulse energy of 35 to 50 millijoules (mJ) was delivered via a 600 nm quartz fiber.[80] The laser successfully fragmented 48 of 58 calculi (83%) as the sole modality of lithotripsy, with no reports of ureteral wall injury. Failures were associated with calcium oxalate monohydrate stone composition. Thomas and colleagues reported a less favorable experience in 31 patients, when laser lithotripsy with a Q-switched Nd:YAG system was successful in 17 of 31 patients (55%), without the need for other modalities.[81] Difficulties related to the delivery system, in particular, the large fiber diameter were emphasized. Interest in Q-switched Nd:YAG systems for lithotripsy waned with the advent of pulsed-dye systems for intracorporeal lithotripsy.

In 1987, using a flashlamp-pumped tunable dye laser, Watson and colleagues studied the variables of wavelength, pulse duration, and fiber diameter to determine the optimal combination.[82] The advantage of pulsed lasers over continuous-wave lasers is their ability to emit for a short duration. With brief pulse duration, laser power is high but cumulative heat production and resultant tissue injury is low. For a given delivered pulse energy, there is an inverse relationship between power density (watts/cm^2) delivered to the stone and pulse duration. As the pulse duration decreases, power density increases proportion-

ately. Similarly, as the cross-sectioned area of the optical fiber carrying the laser energy decreases and energy input remains constant, the power density will also increase. Any material, including an optical quartz fiber, has a characteristic laser power density threshold. Thus, it is apparent that there are limits to the energy levels than can be used with smaller diameter fibers. Larger diameter fibers permit higher levels of energy transmission but require larger working ports (therefore larger endoscopes) and are less flexible than their smaller counterparts. Watson and colleagues found the optimum pulse duration for fragmentation to be 1 μsec.[82] Several fiber diameters were tested, and it was found that the threshold energy at which fragmentation occurred was lowest with a 200 μm fiber. The tunable pulsed-dye laser is so named because its output wavelength can be adjusted by changing the dye in the reservoir. By selecting a specific green dye with a wavelength of 504 nm, it is possible to take advantage of the fact that this wavelength lies between the major absorption bands of hemoglobin. The result is that tissue does not absorb the wavelength as readily as the stone pigment, and thus, higher energies may be used without causing tissue injury. Two pulsed-dye laser systems have received clinical use. Fragmentation rates with pulsed-dye lasers have ranged from 64 to 100%.[83–85] The largest series was reported by Gautier and colleagues, who achieved a 73% complete fragmentation rate and a 25% partial fragmentation rate in 325 patients.[86] In another large study Dretler achieved successful fragmentation in 64% of 227 cases.[87] Treatment was completed either using EHL or by rapping fragments in a stone basket in an addition 28%. Segura and Patterson reported a 75% success rate in 36 patients. Most of their procedures required use of ancillary baskets, ultrasound, ESWL, or forceps extraction.[88] In contrast, Higashihara and colleagues achieved an 86% successful fragmentation rate in 28 patients with no additional therapy.[89] The primary advantage of pulsed-dye laser lithotripsy is that it has the lowest potential for causing ureteral or renal injury among all forms of intracorporeal lithotripsy. In addition, the laser fibers can be used for the entire duration of the procedure, in contrast to EHL probes, which have a limited life expectancy. A disadvantage of pulsed-dye laser lithotripsy compared with other modalities relates to the fact that the harder calculi, such as those composed of calcium oxalate monohydrate or cystine, may resist fragmentation. Among other disadvantages, the laser dye (which is toxic) requires regular changing, and safety goggles with green lenses, which can impair color perception, are required during its use. Furthermore, the laser units have an approximately 20-minute start-up cycle that occurs after being turned on and, being water-cooled, a fixed water supply is required, thus limiting portability.[90] Due to the development of the holmium:YAG laser, pulsed-dye laser is no longer used as an intracorporeal lithotripsy device for renal calculi.

In addition to the pulsed-dye laser, other wavelengths of laser have appeared and have been used with endoscopic lithotripsy systems. The alexandrite laser is a flashlamp-pumped, solid-state laser with an active medium that consists of an alexandrite monocrystal. The alexandrite laser operates at a wavelength at which stone and tissue absorption are poor. It may be optimum for dark calculi, such as biliary and calcium oxalate monohydrate stones. It is inefficient, however, for paler stones such as calcium phosphate. Despite these shortcomings, Weber and colleagues reported excellent success in fragmenting 26 of 27 calculi by means of an alexandrite system, with no apparent long-term complications on radiologic follow-up.[91] In a larger series, Pertusa and colleagues successfully fragmented 98 of 112 stones and reported no major ureteral wall injuries or fiber destruction.[92] These high success rates were not seen in all studies. Another report demonstrated only a 46% success rate using an alexandrite system in 30 patients. Multiple problems were encountered, including incomplete stone fragmentation, fiber burning, and technical problems related to laser calibration.[93] The alexandrite system is no longer widely utilized for the treatment of renal calculi.

The introduction of the holmium:YAG laser represented a major advance in the armamentarium of laser lithotripsy devices (Figure 5-9).[94] This laser operates at a wavelength of 2,100 nm in the near-infrared portion of the electromagnetic spectrum. Similar to other laser lithotriptors, it operates in a pulsed manner with pulses of 350 μsec in duration at a rate of 5 Hz, and up to 50 Hz in some lasers (VersaPulse PowerSuite, Lumenis, Santa Clara, CA). The laser delivers considerably higher energies per pulse than other commercial devices, ranging from 500 to 2,000 mJ. In preliminary ex vivo studies, Johnson and colleagues found that the holmium:YAG laser successfully fragmented urinary stones of varying sizes and composition.[95] Unlike the tunable dye lasers, the holmium wavelength is not selectively absorbed by common calculi. In fact, it is essentially color blind with respect to its target, fragmenting stones of varying color equally. The holmium:YAG laser has been shown to effectively fragment all types of urinary calculi regardless of composition.[96,97] The mechanism of stone fragmentation is due to chemical decomposition as a consequence of a dominant photothermal mechanism.[98] The stone fragments produced by the holmium:YAG laser have been demonstrated to be smaller compared to those produced by EHL, pneumatic lithotriptors, or pulsed-dye lasers.[99] The holmium:YAG is unique among laser lithotripsy devices, in that it is multipurpose and possesses cutting and coagulative properties for soft-tissue applications. Soft-tissue applications require significantly higher energy settings compared to those used to treat calculi. Regardless, the tissue effects demand a greater degree of caution (than is the case with other laser lithotriptors) to avoid ureteral wall injury. The effect of direct contact of the holmium laser fiber with the ureteral wall in a porcine model has been demonstrated. Using the lowest power setting of the laser (0.2 J, 5 Hz) it took only 1 to 2 pulses (less than one second) to create a full thickness perforation. As the distance from the tip of the laser fiber to the ureteral wall increased, however, the amount of energy required to perforate the ureter increased exponentially. At a distance of 2 mm the authors were unable to perforate the ureter despite maximal energy settings of 3.5 kJ at a power up to 26 watts.[100] The holmium:YAG is rapidly absorbed in water and has a depth of thermal injury of only 0.5 to 1.0 mm.[95,100,101]

The perforation rates in clinical studies utilizing the holmium:YAG laser for lithotripsy range up to 4%.[102–105] Perforations can occur when the laser is activated when it is not in direct vision. Treatment of impacted stones and drilling through a stone and encountering the back wall of the ureter can also result in perforation. The risk of perforation increases with high power settings, but because of the low (0.5 to 1.0 mm) depth of thermal injury, most perforations are small and can be managed with an indwelling stent. Matsuoka and colleagues reported a 3% incidence of ureteral perforation using the holmium:YAG laser in their series.[102] These were all managed in an indwelling ureteral stent for 1 to 2 weeks. Follow-up of 3 to 30 months revealed no long-term complications.

Guidewires and stone baskets can be damaged by the holmium:YAG laser.[106,107] The risk of damage to guidewires is minimized during ureteroscopy, where the laser fiber is typically operated in a parallel configuration to the guidewire. During percutaneous nephrolithotomy, the laser may be used in a manner where it is perpendicular to the guidewire, and therefore, the risk of damage to the wire is greater and appropriate care must be taken.[108] The holmium:YAG laser will easily cut through the twines of a stone basket. This may be used to a surgeon's advantage as reported by Teichman and colleagues, who described the release of an impacted stone basket by disassembling the basket and then reinserting the ureteroscope and freeing the basket by cutting an arm with the holmium:YAG laser.[109]

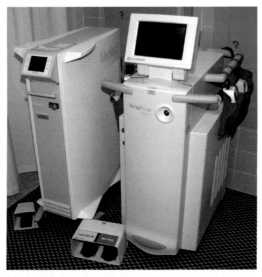

Figure 5-9 Holmium:YAG laser delivery systems.

A consequence of treating a uric acid calculus with the holmium:YAG laser is the production of cyanide.[110] Photothermal mechanisms coupling laser energy to the solid crystal lattice are responsible for the production of cyanide, and the amount of cyanide increases in proportion to the amount of holmium:YAG energy utilized.[111] A review of 18 patients with uric acid calculi who were treated with the holmium:YAG laser demonstrated no obvious significant toxicity.[112] Furthermore, there are no reports of cyanide toxicity resulting from holmium:YAG laser lithotripsy.[113] Although it appears that the production of cyanide is clinically insignificant, no upper safe limit has been established.

Many centers mandate the use of goggles or glasses that selectively block the holmium:YAG wavelength (2,100 nm) during intracorporeal lithotripsy with the laser. The rationale for this is twofold. Firstly, the goggles provide a physical barrier to the fiber should it inadvertently be broken and deflected towards the eye; secondly, the goggles filter out the holmium:YAG laser wavelength, and therefore, if the laser is fired directly at someone's eye, no harm should ensue. The depth of thermal penetration of the holmium:YAG laser, as previously noted, is only 0.5 mm to 1.0 mm. Therefore, any damage that may occur to the eye would likely only occur at the level of the sclera or cornea, and permanent blindness is unlikely.[114]

The clinical effectiveness of the holmium:YAG laser for treating urinary tract calculi has been reported in numerous series. Overall success rates for treating stones throughout the urinary tract range from 93 to 100%.[103,104,106,115,116] The largest series to date reported on holmium:YAG laser lithotripsy is 598 patients with urinary calculi. The overall stone-free rate was 97%. Stratified by location, the stone-free rate in the distal ureter was 98%, the mid-ureter was 100%, the proximal ureter was 97%, and the kidney was 84%. The complication rate was low at only 4%, and the need for secondary intervention was 6%.[115] These results demonstrate that the holmium:YAG laser is superior to pneumatic devices, EHL, and pulsed-dye laser for lithotripsy. The ability of the holmium:YAG laser to produce fragments less than 2 mm in size results in less of a need to resort to ancillary procedures, such as stone basketing, to remove the fragments, thereby shortening operative times. The holmium:YAG laser has clearly demonstrated its effectiveness as a powerful fragmentation device, resulting in a low incidence of complications with careful attention to technique (Tables 5-2 and 5-3).[95,115]

The holmium:YAG laser has been successfully and safely used as an intracorporeal lithotripsy device in children. Wollin and colleagues reported a series of 19 pediatric patients who underwent holmium:YAG laser lithotripsy for urinary calculi.[117] Fifteen were treated in a retrograde fashion, and 4 via percutaneous renal access. The overall success rate was 84% following one procedure, and 100% follow a two-stage procedure. No complications directly related to the laser were reported. Reddy and colleagues reported their experience in 8 pediatric patients.[118] Five patients were rendered stone-free after one procedure, and the remaining 3 patients required multiple procedures. Similarly, no complications were reported directly related to use of the holmium:YAG laser.

The holmium:YAG laser has been demonstrated in several studies to be a safe option for lithotripsy in patients who have a bleeding diathesis. One series reported the results of patients with bleeding diatheses who underwent holmium:YAG laser lithotripsy for upper urinary tract calculi. The bleeding diatheses were secondary to warfarin administration for various conditions in 17 patients, liver dysfunction in 3, thrombocytopenia in 4, and von Willebrand's disease in 1. The overall stone-free rate was 96%. No significant bleeding complications occurred when the holmium:YAG laser was the sole lithotripsy device. One patient, who was treated with a combination of the holmium:YAG laser and the electrohydraulic lithotriptor, developed a significant retroperitoneal hemorrhage and required a blood transfusion.[119] The use of the EHL was the probable cause of the bleeding, and it is therefore recommended that EHL not be used as an intracorporeal lithotripsy device in an anticoagulated patient.

Another advantage of the holmium:YAG laser is its apparent safety during pregnancy. Approximately 1 in 1,500 pregnancies are complicated by urolithiasis.[120,121] Furthermore, approximately 20 to 30% of the calculi will not pass spontaneously.[122] One report describes treating 8 pregnant women with a total of 10 symptomatic ureteral calculi, as well as two encrusted ureteral stents, with the holmium:YAG laser at a range of gestational ages.[123] Complete stone fragmentation and/or removal of the encrusted stent was reported in all the patients without encountering any obstetric or urologic complications. Holmium:YAG lasers offer the property of rapid absorption in water, thereby eliminating any energy transmission to the patient or the fetus. The ability to perform safe and effective intracorporeal lithotripsy in pregnant patients using the holmium:YAG laser reduces the need for undesirable ureteral stents and nephrostomy tubes during the pregnancy.

The initial starting settings for the fragmentation of ureteral calculi with the holmium:YAG laser is a pulse energy of 0.8 J at 8 Hz utilizing a 365 μm core-sized fiber. This minimizes the risk of stone migration. Should insufficient fragmentation occur, the pulse energy is raised to 1.0 J and the frequency to 10 Hz. Further increasing the pulse energy is rarely required for ureteral

Table 5-3 Keys to Successful Holmium:YAG Laser Lithotripsy

Check aiming beam prior to inserting fiber into scope to ensure that the fiber has been properly prepared.
Do not advance the fiber with the scope deflected. Doing so may damage the internal components of the ureteroscope.
Extend the fiber ≈ 3 mm beyond the tip of the endoscope to prevent damage.
Do not fire the laser unless the tip of the fiber is in direct view.
The end of the fiber must remain in contact with the stone for effective lithotripsy to occur.
Start with lower pulse energy and frequency settings. Increase these based on stone size, hardness, and location.
Create fragments less than 2 mm in maximal diameter.
Avoid firing the laser directly on guidewires or stone baskets.
Avoid firing the laser within 2 mm of the ureteral wall.
Attempt to avoid drilling through the stone to prevent back wall injury.
High pressure irrigation with 0.9% saline will facilitate visualization.

stones. The pulse frequency may be raised to 15 Hz for large calculi that can be safely targeting away from the ureteral wall. For intrarenal calculi, the initial setting used is pulse energy of 1.0 J at 10 Hz. The energy is delivered using a sub-300 μm core-sized fiber to allow for maximal irrigation and deflection of the flexible endoscope. For larger or resistant intrarenal calculi, pulse energy may be increased incrementally to 1.5 J and pulse frequency to 15 Hz as indicated.

There have been significant advances made in the development of flexible ureteroscopes that have revolutionized diagnostic and therapeutic procedures.[124,125] For example, the Storz Flex-X2 (Karl Storz, Tuttlingen, Germany) flexible ureteroscope is capable of 270° of primary deflection in either direction. The ACMI DUR-8 Elite (Southborough, MA), which is the first flexible ureteroscope to provide both primary and secondary active deflection, deflects to a maximum of ≈ 272° when both mechanisms are used. These highly deflectable ureteroscopes combined with small-caliber holmium:YAG laser fibers allow for lower-pole ureteroscopy and lithotripsy with success rates of 79 to 90%.[126,127] One significant limitation of the new small-caliber flexible ureteroscopes is their fragility and associated repair costs.[125,128,129] We have seen several holmium:YAG laser fibers fracture within the channel of a flexible ureteroscope while performing a procedure, and were concerned that laser fiber failures may be contributing to scope damage. A series of experiments were conducted evaluating the performance and safety of a number of commercially available holmium:YAG laser fibers (Sharplan 200, Lumenis Slimline 200 and 365, InnovaQuartz 273T and 400, Dornier Lightguide Super 200 and Dornier 400 micron) (Figure 5-10). Utilizing a Lumenis (Santa Clara, CA) 80W holmium:YAG laser, the fibers were bent to 180° with a diameter of 6 cm and ran the laser from 200 to 4000 mJ pulse energy to determine the minimum energy required to fracture the fiber. If the fiber did not fracture, the bending diameter was decreased by 1 cm and testing repeated until a bend diameter of 1 cm was reached. We determined that there was a significant difference in the amount of energy and the diameter of bend that it took to fracture different fibers (Table 5-4). All the testing was performed using brand new laser fibers. Future work will need to address whether other factors, such as

repeat use of the same fiber, sterilization, and cooling, affect failure rates.[130]

Although holmium:YAG laser lithotripsy has revolutionized intracorporeal lithotripsy, new laser delivery systems continue to be developed and tested for lithotripsy use. Erbium:YAG (Er:YAG) laser systems, which fragment calculi through a photothermal mechanism, have several theoretical advantages over existing holmium:YAG-based systems.[131] Er:YAG lasers operate at a wavelength of 2,940 nm, which is more efficiently absorbed by urinary calculi compared to the holmium:YAG wavelength of 2,100 nm. By more efficiently absorbing the laser energy, the calculi should fragment faster.[132] Teichman and colleagues compared the efficiency of these two laser systems by fragmenting human urinary calculi in an ex vivo laboratory setting. Er:YAG lithotripsy was found to be two to three times more efficient at ablating stones at the same energy settings than holmium:YAG lithotripsy.[133] At present, there is a lack of clinically useful fibers for lithotripsy available for Er:YAG lasers. Future advancement in the design of fibers should make the Er:YAG laser available for clinical urologic lithotripsy.

A short-pulsed Q-switched Frequency-Doubled Double-Pulse Nd:YAG laser (FREDDY) has been examined for lithotripsy of calculi. The FREDDY laser operates at dual wavelengths of

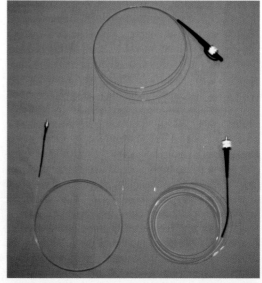

Figure 5-10 Small-core sized holmium:YAG laser optical fibers.

Table 5-2 Power Settings of the Holmium:YAG Laser for Lithotripsy

Stone Location	Energy (J)	Pulse Rate (Hz)
Ureteral	0.5 – 1.0	5 to 10
Intrarenal	1.0 – 1.5*	10 to 15
Bladder	1.0 – 2.0	10 to 20

*Lower energy settings are recommended during lower pole lithotripsy because of the risk of fiber and endoscope damage.

Table 5-4 Comparison of Holmium: YAG Laser Fibers

	Bend Diameter (cm)	Pulse Energy to Break Fiber (mJ)
Sharplan 200	1	600
Lumenis SL 200	1	4000
IQinc SureFlex 273T	1	200
Dornier LG Super 200	2	200
Lumenis SL 365	3	200
Dornier 400	3	200
IQinc 400	—	Did not break at max energy with 1 cm diameter bend

532 and 1,064 nm and emits very long pulses (1.0 to 1.4 μs) due to its resonator design, which results in very high pulse and shock wave intensity. In addition, the silica fiber used with this laser is highly flexible, with a core size of 280 μm, making it ideal for semi-rigid and flexible ureterorenoscopy. An in vitro study demonstrated that the FREDDY laser set at an energy of 90 mJ and pulse frequency of 10 Hz was able to efficiently fragment a range of human urinary calculi (whewellite, weddellite, uric acid, apatite, brushite and struvite). This study, however, did not make a direct comparison to existing holmium:YAG laser systems. The investigators also directly applied 2,000 pulses of 90 mJ laser energy directly to rabbit bladder mucosa to test the tissue safety of this laser. Histologic evaluation demonstrated light mucosal edema and hyperemia; light- to medium-grade bleeding was noted in the lamina propria mucosa, as well as punctiform coagulation necrosis of the epithelial layer. No perforations or lesions of the tunica muscularis were noted.[134]

The initial clinical experience with the FREDDY laser has shown it to be effective for middle and distal urinary calculi with a stone-free rate of 91% and 100%, respectively. For proximal ureteral calculi, however, the stone-free rate was only 62%.[135] Further prospective trials are needed to appropriately assess the efficacy and safety of this laser system.

The final evolution of laser lithotripsy may be the performance of a nonvisual procedure without endoscopy. Shah and colleagues reported preliminary experience with nonvisual laser lithotripsy by monitoring the feedback spectrum of plasma emission.[136] The concept of blind laser lithotripsy is attractive, since it obviates the problem of physical damage to the ureter produced by the ureteroscope. Furthermore, the high purchase and repair costs of the flexible ureteroscopes would be avoided. Difficulties to date include keeping the fiber on the stone and relocating fragments that occur as a result of lithotripsy.

The high initial purchase cost of the holmium:YAG laser has been an obstacle for some centers in acquiring the technology. The cost of a high powered (60 to 100 W) holmium:YAG laser ranges from approximately $110,000 to $150,000 (US). The holmium:YAG laser, how-

ever, has many treatment applications in urology other than just lithotripsy for stones. Tumor ablation, prostatic resection, and ureteral/urethral stricture incisions have all been successfully performed with this laser, thus helping to justify the cost.[96] But the advent of lower-powered holmium lasers (15 to 30 W), which are capable of performing all urologic procedures except prostatic resection, has significantly reduced the initial purchase price. Low-power holmium lasers range from approximately $45,000 to $150,000 (US) in price. The cost of the holmium:YAG laser fibers range between $300 to $1,500 (US). The majority of the fibers are reusable for approximately 20 cases,[127] although several manufacturers are marketing single-use, disposable fibers. The purchase price of the disposable fibers is approximately 50 to 60% less than reusable fibers, but because they are single-use only, the long-term cost is significantly greater.

CONCLUSION

Significant advances in intracorporeal lithotripsy have been made and have nearly obviated the need completely for open stone surgery. For percutaneous nephrolithotomy, the Lithoclast and the ultrasonic lithotriptor remain the mainstays for fragmentation. The advent of the Lithoclast Master/Ultra, which combines the two instruments into one, is an advance in terms of fragmentation efficiency. The holmium:YAG laser can be a useful adjunct during PCNL when a flexible nephroscope is employed to reach calculi that are inaccessible with a rigid nephroscope. EHL remains a useful fragmentation device in select cases, especially for caliceal calculi that cannot effectively be targeted with a laser optical fiber. The holmium:YAG laser has become the lithotrite of choice for ureteroscopic procedures. The ability of the holmium:YAG laser to efficiently fragment calculi of any composition, combined with a wide margin of safety, has resulted in its widespread adoption in urology. The advent of small-caliber, flexible ureteroscopes combined with small-core-sized holmium:YAG optical fibers has increased the urologists ability to treat intrarenal calculi. However, issues regarding the fracture of holmium:YAG laser fibers and associated high cost of ureteroscope repair remain a concern. Future advancements in laser and fiber design will hopefully address some of these concerns.

REFERENCES

1. Bulow H, Frohmuller HG. Electrohydraulic lithotripsy with aspiration of the fragments under vision—304 consecutive cases. J Urol 1981;126:454.
2. Rouvalis P. Electronic lithotripsy for vesical calculus with "Urat-1." An experience of 100 cases and an experimental application of the method to stones in the upper urinary tract. Br J Urol 1970;42:486.
3. Clayman RV. Techniques in percutaneous removal of renal calculi. Mechanical extraction and electrohydraulic lithotripsy. Urology 1984;23:11.
4. Green DF, Lytton B. Electrohydraulic lithotripsy in the ureter. Urol Clin North Am 1988;15:361.
5. Nasr ME. Studies on the fracture mechanism in urinary test concretions by lithotripter devices [dissertation]. Gainesville (FL): University of Florida; 1982.
6. Vorreuther R, Engelking R. Impact of voltage and capacity on

7. Vorreuther R. New tip design and shock wave pattern of electrohydraulic probes for endoureteral lithotripsy. J Endourol 1993;7:35.
8. Bhatta KM, Rosen DI, Flotte TJ, et al. Effects of shielded or unshielded laser and electrohydraulic lithotripsy on rabbit bladder. J Urol 1990;143:857.
9. Piergiovanni M, Desgrandchamps F, Cochand-Priollet B, et al. Ureteral and bladder lesions after ballistic, ultrasonic, electrohydraulic, or laser lithotripsy. J Endourol 1994;8:293.
10. Denstedt JD, Clayman RV. Electrohydraulic lithotripsy of renal and ureteral calculi. J Urol 1990;143:13.
11. Miller RA, Wickham JE. Percutaneous nephrolithotomy: advances in equipment and endoscopic techniques. Urology 1984;23:2.
12. Pelander WM, Kaufman JM. Complications of electrohydraulic lithotresis. Urology 1980;16:155.
13. Electrohydraulic lithotriptors (hazard). Health Devices 1982; 12:46.
14. Bergman B, Nygaard E, Osterman G, Tomic R. Vesical calculi. Experience of electrohydraulic lithotripsy with URAT I. Scand J Urol Nephrol 1982;16:217.
15. Angeloff A. Hydro electrolithotripsy. J Urol 1972;108:867.
16. Reuter HJ. Electronic lithotripsy: transurethral treatment of bladder stones in 50 cases. J Urol 1970;104:834.
17. Razvi HA, Song TY, Denstedt JD. Management of vesical calculi: comparison of lithotripsy devices. J Endourol 1996; 10:559.
18. Raney AM. Electrohydraulic ureterolithotripsy. Preliminary report. Urology 1978;12:284.
19. Raney AM, Handler J. Electrohydraulic nephrolithotripsy. Urology 1975;6:439.
20. Reuter HJ, Kern E. Electronic lithotripsy of ureteral calculi. J Urol 1973;110:181.
21. Green DF, Lytton B. Early experience with direct vision electrohydraulic lithotripsy of ureteral calculi. J Urol 1985; 133:767.
22. Begun FP, Jacobs SC, Lawson RK. Use of a prototype 3F electrohydraulic electrode with ureteroscopy for treatment of ureteral calculous disease. J Urol 1988;139: 1188.
23. Willscher MK, Conway JF Jr, Babayan RK, et al. Safety and efficacy of electrohydraulic lithotripsy by ureteroscopy. J Urol 1988;140:957.
24. Elashry OM, DiMeglio RB, Nakada SY, et al. Intracorporeal electrohydraulic lithotripsy of ureteral and renal calculi using small caliber (1.9F) electrohydraulic lithotripsy probes. J Urol 1996;156:1581.
25. Mulvaney WP. Attempted disintegration of calculi by ultrasonic vibrations. J Urol 1953;70:704.
26. Coats EC. The application of ultrasonic energy to urinary and biliary calculi. J Urol 1956;75:865.
27. Lamport H, Newman HF. Ultrasonic lithotresis in the ureter. J Urol 1956;76:520.
28. Terhorst B, Cichos M. [Ultrasonics for urinary calculi destruction (experimental studies)]. Biomed Tech (Berl) 1971;16:106.
29. Terhorst B, Lutzeyer W, Cichos M, Pohlman R. [Destruction of urinary calculi by ultrasound. II. Ultrasound lithotripsy of bladder calculi]. Urol Int 1972;27:458.
30. Terhorst B, Cichos M. [Ultrasonics in the disintegration of urinary calculi (clinical results)]. Biomed Tech (Berl) 1973;18:13.
31. Howards SS, Merrill E, Harris S, Cohn J. Ultrasonic lithotripsy: laboratory evaluation. Invest Urol 1974;11:273.
32. Gasteyer KH. [A new method of bladder calculi fragmentation: ultrasonic lithotripsy]. Urologe 1971;10:30.
33. Hautmann R. T. B. R. P. G. F. L. W. Ultrasonic litholapaxy of bladder stones - 10 years of experience with more than 400 cases. In: Ryall R, Brockis JG, Marshall V, editors. Urinary stones. New York: Churchill Livingstone; 1984. p. 120–4.
34. Lange PH. Diagnostic and therapeutic urologic instrumentation. In: Walsh PC, Gittes RF, Perlmutter AD, et al, editors. Campbell's urology, 5th ed. Philadelphia: WB Saunders; 1986. p. 510–40.
35. Wickham JEA, Miller RA, editors. Non-mechanical disruption of renal stones. In: Percutaneous renal surgery. Edinburgh: Churchill Livingstone; 1983. p. 75-107.
36. Higashihara E, Aso Y. Flexible ultrasonic lithotriptor and fiberoptic ureterorenoscope: a new approach to ureteral calculi. J Urol 1989;142:40.
37. Terhorst B, Cichos M, Versin F. Der Einfluss von electrodraulischer Schlagwelle und Ultraschall auf das Uroepithel. Urologe A 1975;14:41.
38. Clayman RV, McMurtry JM. Complications of ureteroscopic lithotripsy. Probl Urol 1987;1:593.
39. Hobin FP. Air embolism complicating percutaneous ultrasonic lithotripsy. J Forensic Sci 1985;30:1284.

40. Dalton JR, Brutscher SP. Two cases of ureteroscopy and attempted stone disintegration complicated by disruption of the burr tip of the ultrasonic probe. J Urol 1986;135:778.

41. Cetin S, Ozgur S, Yazicioglu A, et al. Ultrasonic lithotripsy of bladder stones. Int Urol Nephrol 1988;20:361.

42. el Fahiq S, Wallace DM. Ultrasonic lithotriptor for urethral and bladder stones. Br J Urol 1978;50:255.

43. Huffman JL, Bagley DH, Schoenberg HW, Lyon ES. Transurethral removal of large ureteral and renal pelvic calculi using ureteroscopic ultrasonic lithotripsy. J Urol 1983;130:31.

44. Ikemoto S, Sugimoto T, Yamamoto K, et al. Comparison of transurethral ureteroscopy and extracorporeal shock wave lithotripsy for treatment of ureteral calculi. Eur Urol 1988;14:178.

45. Kostakopoulos A, Sofras F, Karayiannis A, et al. Ureterolithotripsy: report of 1000 cases. Br J Urol 1989;63:243.

46. Marberger M. Disintegration of renal and ureteral calculi with ultrasound. Urol Clin North Am 1983;10:729.

47. Chaussy C, Fuchs G, Kahn R, et al. Transurethral ultrasonic ureterolithotripsy using a solid-wire probe. Urology 1987;29:531.

48. Fuchs GJ. Ultrasonic lithotripsy in the ureter. Urol Clin North Am 1988;15:347.

49. Kurth KH, Hohenfellner R, Altwein JE. Ultrasound litholapaxy of a staghorn calculus. J Urol 1977;117:242.

50. Alken P. Percutaneous ultrasonic destruction of renal calculi. Urol Clin North Am 1982;9:145.

51. Elder JS, Gibbons RP, Bush WH. Ultrasonic lithotripsy of a large staghorn calculus. J Urol 1984;131:1152.

52. Marberger M, Stackl W, Hruby W. Percutaneous litholapaxy of renal calculi with ultrasound. Eur Urol 1982;8:236.

53. Segura JW, Patterson DE, LeRoy AJ, et al. Percutaneous lithotripsy. J Urol 1983;130:1051.

54. Segura JW, Patterson DE, LeRoy AJ, et al. Percutaneous removal of kidney stones: review of 1,000 cases. J Urol 1985;134:1077.

55. Clayman RV. Ultrasonic lithotripsy. In: Techniques in endourology. Chicago: Year Book Medical Publishers; 1984. p. 239–54.

56. Liatsikos EN, Dinlenc CZ, Fogarty JD, et al. Efficiency and efficacy of different intracorporeal ultrasonic lithotripsy units on a synthetic stone model. J Endourol 2001;15:925.

57. Kuo RL, Paterson RF, Siqueira TM Jr, et al. In vitro assessment of ultrasonic lithotriptors. J Urol 2003;170:1101.

58. Languetin JM, Jichlinski P, Favre R, von Niederhausern W. The Swiss Lithoclast [Abstract]. J Urol 1990;143:179.

59. Desai MR, Patel SB, Desai MM, et al. The Dretler stone cone: a device to prevent ureteral stone migration-the initial clinical experience. J Urol 2002;167:1985.

60. Dretler SP. The stone cone: a new generation of basketry. J Urol 2001;165:1593.

61. Piergiovanni M, Desgrandchamps F, Cochand-Priollet B, et al. Ureteral and bladder lesions after ballistic, ultrasonic, electrohydraulic, or laser lithotripsy. J Endourol 1994;8:293.

62. Denstedt JD, Razvi HA, Rowe E, et al. Investigation of the tissue effects of a new device for intracorporeal lithotripsy—the Swiss Lithoclast. J Urol 1995;153:535.

63. Hofbauer J, Hobarth K, Marberger M. Lithoclast: new and inexpensive mode of intracorporeal lithotripsy. J Endourol 1992;6:429.

64. Denstedt JD, Eberwein PM, Singh RR. The Swiss Lithoclast: a new device for intracorporeal lithotripsy. J Urol 1992;148:1088.

65. Yinghao S, Linhui W, Songxi Q, et al. Treatment of urinary calculi with ureteroscopy and Swiss lithoclast pneumatic lithotripter: report of 150 cases. J Endourol 2000;14:281.

66. Denstedt JD. Use of Swiss Lithoclast for percutaneous nephrolithotripsy. J Endourol 1993;7:477.

67. Wollin, TA, Singal RK, Whelan T, et al. Percutaneous suprapubic cystolithotripsy for treatment of large bladder calculi. J Endourol 1999;13:739.

68. Teh CL, Zhong P, Preminger GM. Laboratory and clinical assessment of pneumatically driven intracorporeal lithotripsy. J Endourol 1998;12:163.

69. Wadhwa SN, Hemal AK, Sharma RK. Intracorporeal lithotripsy with the Swiss lithoclast. Br J Urol 1994;74:699.

70. Shokeir AA. Transurethral cystolitholapaxy in children. J Endourol 1994;8:157.

71. Hofmann R, Weber J, Heidenreich A, et al. Experimental studies and first clinical experience with a new Lithoclast and ultrasound combination for lithotripsy. Eur Urol 2002;42:376.

72. Auge BK, Lallas CD, Pietrow PK, et al. In vitro comparison of standard ultrasound and pneumatic lithotrites with a new combination intracorporeal lithotripsy device. Urology 2002;60:28.

73. Olbert P, Weber J, Hegele A, et al. Combining Lithoclast and ultrasound power in one device for percutaneous nephrolithotomy: in vitro results of a novel and highly effective technology. Urology 2003;61:55.

74. Pietrow PK, Auge BK, Zhong P, Preminger GM. Clinical efficacy of a combination pneumatic and ultrasonic lithotrite. J Urol 2003;169:1247.

75. Mulvaney WP, Beck CW. The laser beam in urology. J Urol 1968;99:112.

76. Anderholm NC. Laser generated stress waves. Appl Phys Letters 1970;16:113.

77. Fair HD Jr. In vitro destruction of urinary calculi by laser-induced stress waves. Med Instrum 1978;12:100.

78. Yang LC. Stress waves generated in thin metallic fibers by a Q-switched ruby laser. J Appl Phys 1974;45:2601.

79. Hofmann R, Hartung R. Use of pulsed Nd:YAG laser in the ureter. Urol Clin North Am 1988;15:369.

80. Hofmann R, Hartung R, Schmidt-Kloiber H, Reichel E. First clinical experience with a Q-switched neodymium:YAG laser for urinary calculi. J Urol 1989;141:275.

81. Thomas S, Pensel J, Engelhardt R, et al. The pulsed dye laser versus the Q-switched Nd:YAG laser in laser-induced shock-wave lithotripsy. Lasers Surg Med 1988;8:363.

82. Watson G, Murray S, Dretler SP, Parrish JA. An assessment of the pulsed dye laser for fragmenting calculi in the pig ureter. J Urol 1987;138:199.

83. Bagley DH, Grasso M, Shalaby M, Abass El-Akkad M. Ureteral laser lithotripsy using the pulsolith. J Endourol 1989;3:91.

84. Begun FP. Modes of intracorporeal lithotripsy: ultrasound versus electrohydraulic lithotripsy versus laser lithotripsy. Semin Urol 1994;12:39.

85. Dretler SP, Watson G, Parrish JA, Murray S. Pulsed dye laser fragmentation of ureteral calculi: initial clinical experience. J Urol 1987;137:386.

86. Gautier JR, Leandri P, Rossignol G, et al. Pulsed dye laser in the treatment of 325 calculi of the urinary tract. Eur Urol 1990;18:6.

87. Dretler SP. An evaluation of ureteral laser lithotripsy: 225 consecutive patients. J Urol 1990;143:267.

88. Segura JW, Patterson D. Use of the Candela laser in the ureter. Urol Clin North Am 1988;15:365.

89. Higashihara E, Horie S, Takeuchi T, et al. Laser ureterolithotripsy with combined rigid and flexible ureterorenoscopy. J Urol 1990;143:273.

90. Teichman JM, Johnson AJ, Yates JT, et al. Color vision deficits during laser lithotripsy using safety goggles for coumarin green or alexandrite but not with holmium:YAG laser safety goggles. J Urol 1998;159:683.

91. Weber HM, Miller K, Ruschoff J, et al. Alexandrite laser lithotriper in experimental and first clinical application. J Endourol 1991;5:51.

92. Pertusa C, Albisu A, Acha M, et al. In vitro lithotripsy with the Alexandrite laser. Eur Urol 1992;22:62.

93. Denstedt JD, Chun SS, Miller MD, Eberwein PM. Intracorporeal lithotripsy with the Alexandrite laser. Lasers Surg Med 1997;20:433.

94. Webb DR, Kocklburgh R, Johnson WF. The Versapulse holmium:YAG laser in clinical urology: a pilot study. Minim Invas Ther 1993;2:23.

95. Johnson DE, Cromeens DM, Price RE. Use of the holmium:YAG laser in urology. Lasers Surg Med 1992;12:353.

96. Wollin TA, Denstedt JD. The holmium laser in urology. J Clin Laser Med Surg 1998;16:13.

97. Grasso M. Experience with the holmium laser as an endoscopic lithotrite. Urology 1996;48:199.

98. Chan KF, Vassar GJ, Pfefer TJ, et al. Holmium:YAG laser lithotripsy: a dominant photothermal ablative mechanism with chemical decomposition of urinary calculi. Lasers Surg Med 1999;25:22.

99. Teichman JM, Vassar GJ, Bishoff JT, Bellman GC. Holmium:YAG lithotripsy yields smaller fragments than lithoclast, pulsed dye laser or electrohydraulic lithotripsy. J Urol 1998;159:17.

100. Santa-Cruz RW, Leveillee RJ, Krongrad A. Ex vivo comparison of four lithotripters commonly used in the ureter: what does it take to perforate? J Endourol 1998;12:417.

101. Nishioka NS, Domankevitz Y, Flotte TJ, Anderson RR. Ablation of rabbit liver, stomach, and colon with a pulsed holmium laser. Gastroenterology 1989;96:831.

102. Matsuoka K, Iida S, Inoue M, et al. Endoscopic lithotripsy with the holmium:YAG laser. Lasers Surg Med 1999;25:389.

103. Scarpa RM, De Lisa A, Porru D, Usai E. Holmium:YAG laser ureterolithotripsy. Eur Urol 1999;35:233.

104. Devarajan R, Ashraf M, Beck RO, et al. Holmium:YAG lasertripsy for ureteric calculi: an experience of 300 procedures. Br J Urol 1998;82:342.

105. Razvi HA, Denstedt JD, Chun SS, Sales JL. Intracorporeal lithotripsy with the holmium:YAG laser. J Urol 1996;156:912.

106. Grasso M. Experience with the holmium laser as an endoscopic lithotrite. Urology 1996;48:199.

107. Freiha GS, King DH, Teichman JM. Holmium:YAG laser damage to ureteral guidewire. J Endourol 1997;11:173.

108. Freiha GS, Glickman RD, Teichman JM. Holmium:YAG laser-induced damage to guidewires: experimental study. J Endourol 1997;11:331.

109. Teichman JM, Kamerer AD. Use of the holmium:YAG laser for the impacted stone basket. J Urol 2000;164:1602.

110. Teichman JM, Vassar GJ, Glickman RD, et al. Holmium:YAG lithotripsy: photothermal mechanism converts uric acid calculi to cyanide. J Urol 1998;160:320.

111. Zagone RL, Waldmann TM, Conlin MJ. Fragmentation of uric acid calculi with the holmium:YAG laser produces cyanide. Lasers Surg Med 2002;31:230.

112. Teichman JM, Champion PC, Wollin TA, Denstedt JD. Holmium:YAG lithotripsy of uric acid calculi. J Urol 1998;160:2130.

113. Corbin NS, Teichman JM, Nguyen T, et al. Laser lithotripsy and cyanide. J Endourol 2000;14:169.

114. Denstedt J, Haupt G, Leveillee R, et al. Intracorporeal lithotripsy. In: Segura J, Conort P, Khoury S, et al, editors. Stone disease. Paris: Health Publications; 2003. p. 213–47.

115. Sofer M, Watterson JD, Wollin TA, et al. Holmium:YAG laser lithotripsy for upper urinary tract calculi in 598 patients. J Urol 2002;167:31.

116. Gould DL. Holmium:YAG laser and its use in the treatment of urolithiasis: our first 160 cases. J Endourol 1998;12:23.

117. Wollin TA, Teichman JM, Rogenes VJ, et al. Holmium:YAG lithotripsy in children. J Urol 1999;162:1717.

118. Reddy PP, Barrieras DJ, Bagli DJ, et al. Initial experience with endoscopic holmium laser lithotripsy for pediatric urolithiasis. J Urol 1999;162:1714.

119. Watterson JD, Girvan AR, Cook AJ, et al. Safety and efficacy of holmium:YAG laser lithotripsy in patients with bleeding diatheses. J Urol 2002;168:442.

120. Meria P, Anidjar M, Hermieu JF, Boccon-Gibod L. [Urinary lithiasis and pregnancy]. Prog Urol 1993;3:937.

121. Rodriguez PN, Klein AS. Management of urolithiasis during pregnancy. Surg Gynecol Obstet 1988;166:103.

122. Evans HJ, Wollin TA. The management of urinary calculi in pregnancy. Curr Opin Urol 2001;11:379.

123. Watterson JD, Girvan AR, Beiko DT, et al. Ureteroscopy and holmium:YAG laser lithotripsy: an emerging definitive management strategy for symptomatic ureteral calculi in pregnancy. Urology 2002;60:383.

124. Grasso M, Bagley D. A 7.5/8.2 F actively deflectable, flexible ureteroscope: a new device for both diagnostic and therapeutic upper urinary tract endoscopy. Urology 1994;43:435.

125. Grasso M, Bagley D. Small diameter, actively deflectable, flexible ureteropyeloscopy. J Urol 1998;160:1648.

126. Grasso M. Ureteropyeloscopic treatment of ureteral and intrarenal calculi. Urol Clin North Am 2000;27:623.

127. Kourambas J, Delvecchio FC, Munver R, Preminger GM. Nitinol stone retrieval-assisted ureteroscopic management of lower pole renal calculi. Urology 2000;56:935.

128. Afane JS, Olweny EO, Bercowsky E, et al. Flexible ureteroscopes: a single center evaluation of the durability and function of the new endoscopes smaller than 9Fr. J Urol 2000;164:1164.

129. Landman J, Lee DI, Lee C, Monga M. Evaluation of overall costs of currently available small flexible ureteroscopes. Urology 2003;62:218.

130. Knudsen BE, Glickman RD, Stallman KJ, et al. Performance and safety of holmium:YAG laser optical fibers. J Endourol 2005;19:1092.

131. Chan KF, Lee H, Teichman JM, et al. Erbium:YAG laser lithotripsy mechanism. J Urol 2002;168:436.

132. Chan KF, Hammer DX, Choi B, et al. Influence of optical absorption on urinary calculus threshold fluence and ablation efficiency during infrared laser ablation. Proc SPIE 2000;3925:60.

133. Teichman JM, Chan KF, Cecconi PP, et al. Erbium:YAG versus holmium:YAG lithotripsy. J Urol 2001;165:876.

134. Zorcher T, Hochberger J, Schrott KM, et al. In vitro study concerning the efficiency of the frequency-doubled double-pulse Neodymium:YAG laser (FREDDY) for lithotripsy of calculi in the urinary tract. Lasers Surg Med 1999;25:38.

135. Ebert A, Stangl J, Kuhn R, Schafhauser W. [The frequency-doubled double-pulse Neodym:YAG laser lithotripter (FREDDY) in lithotripsy of urinary stones. First clinical experience]. Urologe A 2003;42:825.

136. Shah TK, Watson GM, Jiang ZX, King TA. Nonvisual laser lithotripsy aided by plasma spectral analysis: viability study and clinical application. J Urol 1993;149:1431.

Lasers

Joel Teichman, MD

Urologic applications of lasers have expanded tremendously since the first edition of this textbook. Lasers have expanded in their overall availability and applications, and in the sheer number of different types. An understanding of the basic science of lasers is integral to a urologist's ability to make best use of them. In this chapter, we will review the important aspects of laser basic science as it relates to urology, specifically with respect to laser wavelength, pulse duration, and delivery systems.

The word "laser" is an acronym for light amplification by stimulated emission of radiation. A laser consists of a box that contains an excitable medium, situated between two mirrors at opposite ends of the box (Figure 6A-1). The excitable medium is excited by an external energy source, which stimulates the medium to produce laser energy. On a molecular level, an electron can exist at two alternate energy levels. When the electron is excited from its baseline orbital to a higher orbital, the higher orbital is unstable, and the electron reverts to its baseline orbital; this return to baseline produces a quantum emission defined by the energy difference between electron orbits. Since the excitable medium is a homogenous material, the emitted wavelength is of a specific wavelength. Stimulated emission occurs when a photon collides with a high-energy electron and causes release of a second photon. These two photons then collide and produce additional photons of the same specific wavelength, and so on (Figure 6A-2). This process spirals as more and more electrons become excited, revert to baseline orbital, emit specific wavelength energy, and collide with other electrons and produce more energy. As mentioned above, the laser box has mirrors on both ends. Thus, emitted radiation reflects from both mirrors back into the box and excites the medium even further. The direction of the mirrors (opposite each other) amplifies the energy further and creates an axis or direction to the energy (in the direction of the mirrors) so that energy is traveling in the same direction. The emitted energy can escape the box only if one of the mirrors has a pinpoint opening (see Figure 6A-1). Thus, the laser energy travels in the same direction with minimal beam divergence, a physical phenomenon referred to as collimation. An additional feature of the dual mirror reflection is that the emitted energy is synchronized with respect to wavelength peaks and valleys, so that it is in phase. Thus, the energy that exits in the box through the pinpoint opening is of a specific wavelength, with all wavelengths in phase, and of

high collimation. This intense light is thus a relatively pure form of energy.

Lasers are named after the excitable medium that emits the specific wavelength. The excitable medium may be solid, liquid, or gaseous. Common examples are doped rods based on yttrium:aluminium:garnet (YAG), so that Nd:YAG is YAG doped by neodymium, while Ho:YAG is YAG doped by holmium. The external energy source to excite the medium may be electronic, chemical, or light. In most instances, the external source is electric (often a 220 V wall socket).

Lasers can produce an effect only where they are absorbed. Absorption depends largely on the wavelength, and the tissue's response to that wavelength. Absorption of a wavelength by a tissue depends on its optical absorption coefficient and optical scattering coefficient. The next absorption may be grossly conceptualized as the difference between these two coefficients. The depth of penetration and absorption characteristics are defined by fluence, which is defined by the distribution of optical energy per unit volume within water or tissue. For example, Nd:YAG is absorbed poorly and scatters widely through tissue. Thus, little energy per volume of tissue, or low fluence is achieved. Stated another way, the energy is distributed over a large volume of tissue, so heating is relatively low at any given location, producing the predominant effect of coagulation necrosis. Conversely, the CO_2 laser is highly absorbed by water. It has a narrow depth of penetration, and thus a high degree of fluence on tissue (which has high water content). Thus, a small volume of tissue absorbs the full impact on this

energy, and high heat is achieved, producing a thin volume of surface vaporization and minimal coagulation underneath the zone of vaporization.

LASER WAVELENGTHS

The absorption spectrum of tissue across the wavelengths relevant to laser applications is shown in Figure 6A-3. This curve results from the absorption spectrum of water combined with the absorption curves of pigments such as hemoglobin and melanin. The precise absorption curve of a specific tissue will vary with the presence of these pigments, but water will be a constant factor, particularly for endourology where irrigation is used.

Nd:YAG emits at 1,064 nm, in the near-infrared spectrum. The absorption of this wavelength is poor and scattering within tissue is intense. A low fluence is achieved. Bulk heating and thermal diffusion occur. The predominant effect is coagulation necrosis. Thermal diffusion is important, as it implies a low margin of safety. A urologist may use the Nd:YAG laser to irradiate a bladder tumor at the bladder dome, but in effect, thermal diffusion here could easily produce coagulation necrosis and perforation of adjacent small bowel. Several lasers are based on Nd:YAG. Q-switched Nd:YAG lasers add a swiveling mirrored apparatus to generate a short pulse duration and high peak power (see "Pulse Duration" below). The "FREDDY" laser is a frequency-doubled version of the Nd:YAG laser that produces half the wavelength, so that this Nd:YAG laser produces emitted light at 532 nm. Similarly, the KTP laser, based on potassium titranyl phosphate as the

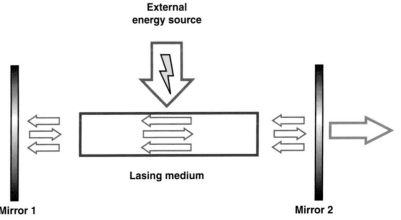

Figure 6A-1 A standard laser consists of a lasing medium, energized by an external energy source such as a flashlamp. Light oscillates between the mirrors, increasing in energy with each passage. Mirror 2 is partly transparent and the laser beam emerges as a high-quality beam of intense light energy.

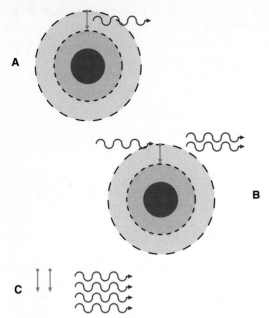

Figure 6A-2 Amplification process that occurs within the medium occurs because the photon released when an electron shifts from a higher to a lower energy level (then goes on to stimulate the emission of a hotter photon when it collides with a second energized electron (b). These photons cause the release of additional photons from other electrons at a higher energy level (c). The electrons become reenergized as a result of energy absorbed from the external energy source.

excitable medium, is placed in the cavity of a Nd:YAG laser, and again produces a frequency-doubled output at 532 nm. Lasers in this blue-green portion of the light spectrum are well absorbed by hemoglobin. Thus, the depth of penetration by tissue is low, as the energy is absorbed by blood. The KTP laser is especially useful for treating hemangiomas as the energy is relatively confined to the hemangiomas targeted. However, lasers in this blue-green spectrum, such as FREDDY or the pulsed dye (coumarin green) laser (504 nm) that are used primarily to fragment urinary stones have a high margin of safety.[1-3] These lasers are safe because any energy not absorbed by water or stone, and that inadvertently targets mucosa, produces little thermal effect because flowing blood acts as a "heat sink" so that the energy is removed with little local tissue injury.

Lasers in the mid-infared portion of the light spectrum include holmium:YAG (2,100 nm) and erbium:YAG (2,940 nm). These wavelengths are absorbed exceptionally well by water.[4,5] The CO_2 laser emits at 10,600 nm (far infrared) and is highly absorbed by water, too. Holmium, erbium, and C02 have high fluence, narrow depths of penetration, and predominant vaporization effects on tissue. Erbium and C02 produce little coagulation necrosis and are thus good lasers for surgical incision. Lasers such as holmium and erbium also produce an interesting problem for surgical use. Since they are highly absorbed by water, the energy is often absorbed by water before reaching the target tissue or stone. Thus, the separation distance between the optical fiber tip and target tissue is normally occupied by irrigation fluid (usually water or saline).

Thus, liquid becomes the initial target and vaporizes.[6] Water vapor transmits holmium:YAG wavelength more efficiently than water liquid, so that after an initial creation of a vapor bubble, laser energy is efficiently transmitted through the vapor "window" to the target stone or tissue.[7] The analogy is made to "parting the water," so that this phenomenon is called the "Moses effect."

A recent addition to laser technology has been semiconductor diode lasers. Previously, these compact lasers were employed by the entertainment industry (compact disc players, digital video disc players, laser discs). Diode technology is advantageous to conventional lasers in that diode lasers are smaller, and they require no flashlamp and mirrors. Thus, diode lasers should require low maintenance and be portable. These factors should eventually translate into lasers that are inexpensive to purchase and run, and may be transported easily between hospitals. Their limitation to date has been the inability to produce lasers at all desirable wavelengths of sufficient power to emulate their larger conventional laser counterparts. To date, some experience has been obtained with diode lasers in the 830 nm range wavelength for prostate applications.[8,9]

PULSE DURATION

A large impact of a laser's effect on tissue or stone is its pulse duration. A laser can be designed to emit a continuous beam in the same manner as a torch. This continuous wave emission can be interrupted in the same way that a torch can be flicked on or off. However, the rate of delivery of the laser energy (ie, power) remains constant as if it were emitting light continuously. The CO_2 laser is an example of a continuous wave laser.

In contrast to continuous wave lasers, a pulsed laser builds up the intensity of light by preventing any emission during the amplification of energy because light within the box travels mirror to mirror. The laser is then triggered to allow emission of energy at one instant. The duration of that instant and the total energy and power may be varied. In general, the shorter the pulse duration, the greater the potential to achieve high peak powers, because the total amount of energy is released within a minimal pulse duration. The pulsed-dye laser (coumarin green) is a laser with a pulse duration of 1.2 usec. It is an example of a flashlamp-pumped pulsed-dye laser. This short pulse duration means that energy is deposited quickly into water in front of the optical fiber with rapid accumulation of energy. This rapid accumulation produces "stress confinement," creating a high-energy vapor bubble or cavitation bubble.[10] The spherical cavitation bubble collapses symmetrically and synchronously, so the collapse releases a high-intensity acoustic pressure wave.[11,12] This pressure wave propagates circumferentially from the optical fiber tip. With sufficient peak pressure, a shock wave may be produced. Thus, the photoacoustic effect of this short pulse duration is due to the phenomenon whereby the laser energy is absorbed into the water, rather than the target tissue. The optical breakdown created by water absorption produces a secondary acoustic phenomenon. In this instance, the laser wavelength is relatively unimportant and the pulse duration is of paramount importance. In fact, the 504 nm wavelength was chosen because the difference in absorption coefficients of calculi and surrounding soft tissue was large; that is, this wavelength is absorbed more by tissue than stone. At a short pulse duration

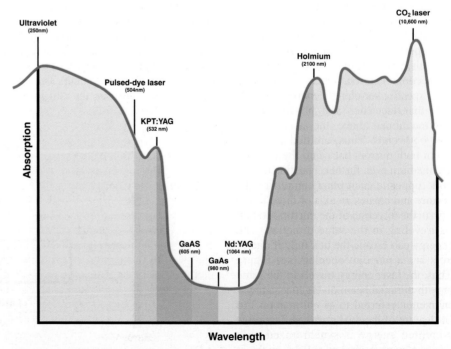

Figure 6A-3 Absorption spectrum for relatively unpigmented tissue showing the wavelengths of different lasers. Absorption is the inverse of penetration. Thus the Nd:YAG laser and GaAs semiconductor laser offer the greatest degree of tissue penetration. The holmium and CO_2 lasers offer the most absorption.

(1 usec approximately) and relatively slow repetition rate (5 Hz), little thermal effect was created. Similar photoacoustic effects can be produced by other lasers with short pulse durations using different wavelength emissions, such as Q-switched Nd:YAG or alexandrite. A Q-switch is a novel mirror apparatus within the laser box. The mirror at the end of the box opposite the pinpoint opening acts as a rotating shutter, as if one had constructed this mirror out of a venetian blind. The venetian blind is allowed to open and close continuously, so that only at the instant when the blind is closed, whereby the mirror is reflected directly at the opposite mirror, will amplification occur. Thus, emission through the pinpoint opening occurs only for that very brief pulse duration when the two mirrors face each other. Q-switched lasers can therefore produce high peak pressures with the capacity to create a plasma bubble on the stone surface.[11] High peak pressure is important in plasma generation, as the threshold energy required for plasma formation actually increases as pulse duration increases.[13] As pulse duration expands longer than 10 usec, the predominant effect is thermal, and photoacoustic properties become less important.[14] The holmium:YAG laser has a pulse duration of 250 usec and has a predominant photothermal effect both with stones and soft tissue.[6,15] In an experiment where holmium:YAG pulse duration was varied, at a pulse duration of 500 nsec, acoustic pressure waves were demonstrated, while at pulse durations longer than 1 usec, no significant pressure effects were observed.[14] Here again is a demonstration of how the pulse duration can be more important than the wavelength. As pulse duration expands longer than 200 usec, negligible photoacoustic properties are produced. As pulse duration expands longer than 20 msec, thermal effects are no longer confined to the target, but may be easily transmitted to adjacent tissue with unwanted coagulation and carbonization of surrounding tissue.[16] Thus, laser lithotripsy is best viewed as requiring a pulse duration either very short to create photoacoustic effects, or long enough to produce photothermal effects, but not so long as to risk adjacent tissue thermal injury.[17]

DELIVERY SYSTEMS

The delivery system can maximize the power density or diffuse the beam and reduce the power density. As well, delivery systems are not inert, and they sometimes may become unavoidable targets of the laser energy itself. Ideally, the delivery system should transmit the optical beam with no attenuation of energy and no loss of collimation. Invariably, loss of collimation and beam divergence occurs, as the emitted energy is coupled into an optical fiber. At this interface, the beam is reduced by an angle defined by the optical fiber characteristics (numerical aperture, or NA). According to Snell's law, the beam exiting the optical fiber at its output end is equal to sin (θ_0), where θ_0 is the half angle of beam divergence. This relation may be rewritten as θ_0 = arcsin (numerical aperture). For fibers with NA of 0.22 or 0.29 (common values of NA of commercially available optical fibers), the fibers have 0.167 and 0.221 acceptance angles, respectively, when normalized for water with a refractive index of 1.33.[7] Thus, beam divergence, despite initial laser collimation, reduces energy density and power density as separation distance between optical fiber tip and target tissue increase. This relationship is relevant for working on soft tissue. With holmium ablation of prostate, for example, vaporization is achieved with high power density when ablation is performed in contact mode. However, by withdrawing the optical fiber just off the prostate surface, power density is decreased and the laser is therefore "defocused," with more coagulation effect produced. Such defocusing allows the surgeon to use a laser with vaporization effect and transform it into a coagulation effect to control bleeding.

If the fiber tip is placed in direct contact with tissue or stone surface and ablation is performed over any length of time, invariably the fiber tip becomes damaged. Damage may result from ejected debris striking the optical fiber tip and producing microfractures, or as a result of surface carbonization, where the carbonized tip becomes the target of continued irradiation.[7,18] The optical output becomes markedly different when fiber tip damage occurs. In normal circumstances, where the optical output is from a clean, perfectly cleaved fiber, the output approaches a gaussian distribution. After fiber damage, the output is unpredictable, with loss of collimation, and inefficient ablation effects.[19] For holmium:YAG lithotripsy, fiber degradation becomes pronounced on calcium and struvite calculi at pulse energies > 1.0 J, with decreasing gains in lithotripsy efficiency as pulse energy is increased further.[20,21] A striking example of fiber degradation is from the alexandrite laser. This Q-switched laser has an ultrashort pulse duration and achieves high peak powers. The result is plasma production and laser-induced shock waves at the fiber tip. The fiber tip then becomes damaged by the high energy discharge of the shock wave. Shards of optical fiber can be left in the ureter as a result.

Optical fibers are not inert to the laser energy. In ideal circumstances, fibers are chosen for their perfect transmission of the wavelength involved, and are inexpensive. In reality, optical fibers are less than ideal.[22] The low-OH- silica fibers used for holmium:YAG transmission were chosen as they transmit over 99% of the input energy without internal absorption of the energy. However, when fibers are bent in a tight bending radius (such as lower pole ureteronephroscopy), there is a risk of energy accumulation at the site of maximal bend with fiber damage, fracture, and transmission of energy to the working channel of the ureteroscope.[23] At wavelengths above 2,500 nm, these same low-OH- silica fibers transmit less energy and become the targets of the laser energy itself. Erbium:YAG lithotripsy is currently constrained by lack of practical fibers

that can transmit the energy without fiber breakdown.[24] At the far infrared end of the spectrum, the CO_2 laser cannot be transmitted by current optical fibers, so that it generally is applied in a free beam mode.

Optical fibers can be configured to deliver the laser energy in an end-firing arrangement, where the beam exits in the same direction as the fiber (0° output). Most urologic laser applications have fibers with this type of output. Some delivery systems employ a mirror at the distal tip of the optical fiber to reorient the exit beam at various side-firing angles. Both Nd:YAG and Ho:YAG fibers exist with several angled fibers. These delivery systems are useful to produce different orientations. In circumstances where these angled fibers produce more direct perpendicular arrangement between beam and target, ablation is more efficient than with end-firing fibers.[25,26] A limitation of these angled fibers is that if the mirror becomes damaged (from ejected debris or surface carbonization), the mirror ceases to work properly and the output becomes inefficient.

APPLICATIONS

Lasers can be used to fragment calculi, coagulate tissue, incise tissue, weld tissue, and activate photoactive compounds for anticancer effects.

STONE FRAGMENTATION Currently, there are several lasers available for lithotripsy. These lasers include photoacoustic lasers such as the pulsed-dye, alexandrite, and FREDDY lasers, and photothermal lasers such as holmium:YAG and erbium:YAG lasers. In photoacoustic lasers, the laser energy is deposited rapidly in water or stone to create a high-energy vapor bubble or plasma.[11] In the case of vapor bubble collapse, fragmentation is similar to electrohydraulic lithotripsy. With plasma, fast plasma expansion produces internal pressure effects, similar to microwaving popcorn. Both types of photoacoustic phenomena produce irregular and unpredictable fragmentation. Stones are literally "ripped" apart as a result of pressure effects. Because the lasers have such short pulse durations, and the frequency is usually limited to 5 Hz or less, there is little risk of thermal energy accumulation and the margin of safety is high.

In contrast to short-pulsed duration lasers, holmium:YAG and erbium:YAG lasers have long pulse durations of 250 to 350 usec. Because of this long pulse duration, optical energy is deposited into water slowly relative to water absorption characteristics.[14] As a result, the holmium:YAG vapor bubble is pear-shaped, so it collapses asymmetrically with weak cavitation effects, minimal plasma formation, and negligible acoustic pressure waves.[6] The erbium:YAG laser similarly produces a vapor bubble that is torpedo-shaped, with similar weak cavitation effects, minimal plasma, and negligible acoustic pressure waves.[27] An interesting phenomenon associated with holmium and erbium lithotripsy is that their stone ablation craters are symmetric and consistent, whereas ablation effects of photoacoustic lasers are unpredictable.[7,27,28] Photoacoustic lasers and photothermal lasers differ in a number of respects. Photoacoustic laser fibers should be positioned just slightly off the stone surface to allow for maximal bubble expansion or plasma effect. In contrast, the holmium:YAG laser fiber should be positioned in contact or with as little separation distance between the fiber and stone surface as possible.[29] In addition, photoacoustic effects (from vapor bubble collapse) propagate circumferentially from the fiber tip. Thus, the fiber can be tangential or perpendicular to the stone surface with similar fragmentation outcome. In contrast, photothermal lithotripsy is directional, and enhanced lithotripsy occurs when the fiber beam is oriented perpendicular to the stone surface.[6,25–27,29] Another difference between photoacoustic and photothermal lasers is the size of fragments produced. Holmium and erbium lasers produce small fragments compared with pulsed-dye laser fragments.[30] Photoacoustic lasers produce more stone retropulsion than photothermal lasers. Because pressure waves are relatively weak with holmium or erbium, there is little stone retropulsion or recoil.[31,32] With holmium, retropulsion occurs as a result of ejected plume off the stone crater rather than the pressure wave effects of photoacoustic lasers. An interesting implication is that with holmium, retropulsion increases as a larger diameter optical fiber is used, despite having a lower power density than a smaller fiber.[32] Photoacoustic lasers have a high margin of safety. In contrast, photothermal lasers can easily vaporize, coagulate, and perforate a ureter if laser energy is applied to the ureter.[29,33] Photoacoustic laser may have difficulty fragmenting calcium oxalate monohydrate and cystine calculi, whereas photothermal lasers fragment all known stone compositions.[6,28,34–39]

PROSTATE COAGULATION

Lasers can be used to coagulate or vaporize prostate. For prostate, the holmium:YAG laser is well absorbed in water with a penetration depth less than 0.5 mm, so there is a predominant vaporization effect. Indeed, immediate tissue ablation or vaporization from holmium:YAG is the predominant effect on prostate.[40] Kabalin and colleagues showed that ablation craters in dog prostate from contact holmium:YAG ablation were predominantly vaporization with craters as wide as 2 cm. There was a small rim peripheral to the ablation crater where coagulation occurred. In contrast, continuous Nd:YAG irradiation (A = 1,064 nm) has greater tissue penetration, larger scatter, and decreased fluence, with resulting predominant thermal injury and coagulation.[41] The decreased fluence and greater tissue penetration occur as a result of the minimal absorption by water and body pigments. Thus, little vaporization occurs unless high-energy irradiation is performed for a prolonged period of time. In a study of dogs treated by Nd:YAG contact ablation, serial changes in the prostate histology were reported at 1 and 3 hours, and days 2, 4, and 7, and weeks 2,

3, 5, and 7 post-operatively.[42] At 1 and 3 hours, tissue disruption and hemorrhage separate a central coagulative necrosis from normal peripheral zone tissue. By day 1, this coagulation zone shows multiple areas of cavitation. In the ensuing weeks, these areas coalesce and form a large central cavity. By day 7, this central cavity is lined by a narrow zone of necrosis with macrophages and neutrophils. By 5 and 7 weeks, the central cavity is lined by transitional epithelium. These results demonstrate the thermal injury and delayed slough. Similar thermal injury, coagulation necrosis, and liquefaction changes are seen with interstitial delivery of Nd:YAG optical energy.[43,44] The KTP laser (532 nm) produces vaporization and coagulation effects intermediate between that observed by Nd:YAG and holmium:YAG lasers. The KTP wavelength is highly absorbed by hemoglobin, making it particularly advantageous for treating cutaneous and urethral hemangiomas.[45] Diode lasers such as the Indigo laser (A = 830 nm) use a diode pump and gallium-aluminumarsenide as the excitable medium. At this wavelength, diode lasers have similar tissue interactions as the Nd:YAG laser.[46,47]

REFERENCES

1. Nishioka NS, Kelsey PB, Kibbi A, et al. Laser lithotripsy: animal studies of safety and efficacy. Lasers Surg Med 1988; 8:357–62.
2. Watson G. The pulsed dye laser for urinary calculi in 600 patients. Proc SPIE 1990;1200:66–71.
3. Dretler SP. An evaluation of ureteral laser lithotripsy: 225 consecutive patients. J Urol 1990;143:267–72.
4. Jensen ED, van Leeuwen TG, Motamedi M, et al. Temperature dependency of the absorption coefficient of water for mid-infrared laser radiation. Lasers Surg Med 1994;14:258–94.
5. Frenz M, Pratisto H, Konz F, et al. Comparison of the effects of absorption coefficient and pulse duration of 2.12 urn and 2.79 urn radiation on ablation of tissue. IEEE J Quantum Electron 1996;32:2025–36.
6. Vassar GJ, Chan KF, Teichman JMH, et al. Holmium:YAG lithotripsy: photothermal mechanism. J Endourol 1999; 13:181–9.
7. Vassar GJ, Teichman JMH, Glickman RD. Holmium:YAG lithotripsy efficiency varies with energy density. J Urol 1998;160:471–6.
8. Greenberger M, Steiner MS. The University of Tennessee experience with the Indigo 830e laser device for the minimally invasive treatment of benign prostatic hyperplasia: interim analysis. World J Urol 1998;16:386–91.
9. Muschter R, de la Rosette JJ, Whitfield H, et al. Initial human clinical experience with diode laser interstitial treatment of benign prostatic hyperplasia. Urol 1996;48:223–8.
10. Jacques SL. Laser-tissue interactions: photochemical, photothermal, and photomechanical. Surg Clin North Am 1992;72:531–58.
11. Rink K, Delacretaz G, Salanthe RP. Fragmentation process of current laser lithotripters. Lasers Surg Med 1995;16:134–46.
12. Zhong P, Tong HL, Cocks FH, et al. Transient cavitation and acoustic emission produced by different laser lithotripters. J Endourol 1998;12:371–8.
13. Bhatta KM, Nishioka NS. Effect of pulse duration on microsecond-domain laser lithotripsy. Lasers Surg Med 1989;9:454–7.
14. Jansen ED, Asshauer T, Frenz M, et al. Effect of pulse duration on bubble formation and laser-induced pressure waves during holmium laser ablation. Lasers Surg Med 1996;18:278–93.
15. Schafer SA, Durville FM, Jassemnejad B, et al. Mechanisms of biliary stone fragmentation using the Ho:YAG laser. IEEE Trans Biomed Eng 1994;41:276–83.
16. Mulvaney WP, Beck CW. The laser beam in urology. J Urol 1968;99:112–5.
17. Watson G, Wickham JEA, Mills TN, et al. Laser fragmentation of renal calculi. Br J Urol 1983;55:613–6.
18. Grant SA, Soufiane A, Shirk G, Martin SW. Degradation-induced transmission losses in silica optical fibers. Lasers Surg Med 1997;21:65–71.
19. Lee H, Ryan RT, Teichman JMH, et al. Effect of lithotripsy on holmium:YAG optical beam profile. J Endourol 2003; 17:63–7 .
20. Kuo RL, Aslan P, Zhong P, Preminger GM. Impact of holmium laser settings and fiber diameter on stone fragmentation and endoscope deflection. J Endourol 1998;12:523–7.
21. Spore SS, Teichman JMH, Corbin NS, et al. Holmium:YAG lithotripsy: optimal power settings. J Endourol 1999;13:559–66.
22. Nazif OA, Teichman JMH, Glickman RD, Welch AJ. Review of laser fibers: a practical guide for urologists. J Endourol 2004;18:818–29.
23. Knudsen B, Stallman K, Denstedt JD, Teichman JMH. Comparison of 7 different laser fibers for holmium:YAG lithotripsy. [In preparation]
24. Lee H, Ryan RT, Teichman JMH, Welch AJ. Comparison of fibers for erbium:YAG lithotripsy. J Endourol 2006. [In press]
25. Teichman JMH, Rao RD, Glickman RD, Harris JM. Holmium:YAG percutaneous nephrolithotomy: the laser incident angle matters. J Urol 1998;159:690–4.
26. Teichman JMH, Rogenes VJ, McIver BD, Harris JM. Holmium:YAG cystolithotripsy of large bladder calculi. Urology 1997;50:44–8.
27. Chan KF, Lee H, Teichman JMH, et al. Erbium:YAG lithotripsy mechanism. J Urol 2002;168:436–41.
28. Teichman JMH, Vassar GJ, Glickman RD. Holmium:YAG lithotripsy efficiency varies with stone composition. Urology 1998;52:392–7.
29. Freiha GS, Glickman RD, Teichman JMH. Holmium:YAG laser-induced damage to guidewires: an experimental study. J Endourol 1997;11:331–6.
30. Teichman JMH, Vassar GJ, Bishoff JT, Bellman GC. Holmium:YAG lithotripsy yields smaller fragments than lithoclast, pulsed dye or electrohydraulic lithotripsy. J Urol 1998;159:17–23.
31. White MD, Moran ME, Calvano CJ, et al. Evaluation of retropulsion caused by holmium:YAG laser with various power settings and fibers. J Endourol 1998;12:183–6.
32. Lee H, Ryan RT, Teichman JMH, et al. Stone retropulsion during holmium:YAG lithotripsy. J Urol 2003;169:881–5.
33. Santa-Cruz RW, Leveillee RJ, Krongrad A. Ex vivo comparison of four lithotripters commonly used in the ureter: what does it take to perforate? J Endourol 1998;12:417–22.
34. Bhatta KM, Prien EL Jr, Dretler SP. Cystine calculi—rough and smooth: a new clinical distinction. J Urol 1989;142:937–40.
35. Dretler SP, Bhatta KM. Clinical experience with high power (140 mj.), large (320 micron) pulsed dye laser lithotripsy. J Urol 1991;146:1228–31.
36. Pearle MS, Sech SM, Cobb CG, et al. Safety and efficacy of the Alexandrite laser for the treatment of renal and ureteral calculi. Urology 1998;51:33–8.
37. Denstedt JD, Chun SS, Miller MD, Eberwein PM. Intracorporeal lithotripsy with the Alexandrite laser. Lasers Surg Med 1997;20:433–6.
38. Stark L, Carl P. First clinical experiences of laser lithotripsy using the partially frequency-doubled double-pulse neodym-YAG laser ("FREDDY") [abstract 1486]. J Urol 2001;165(supp):362A.
39. Sofer M, Watterson JD, Wollin TA, et al. Holmium:YAG laser lithotripsy for upper urinary tract calculi in 598 patients. J Urol 2002;167:31–4.
40. Kabalin JN. Holmium:YAG laser prostatectomy canine feasibility study. Lasers Surg Med 1996;18:221–4.
41. Kabalin JN, Terris MK, Mancianti ML, Fajardo LF. Dosimetry studies utilizing the Urolase right-angle firing neodymium:YAG laser fiber in the human prostate. Lasers Surg Med 1996;18:72–80.
42. Johnson DE, Price RE, Cromeens DM. Pathologic changes occurring in the prostate following transurethral laser prostatectomy. Lasers Surg Med 1992;12:254–63.
43. Johnson DE, Cromeens DM, Price RE. Interstitial laser prostatectomy. Lasers Surg Med 1994;14:299–305.
44. Cromeens DM, Price RE, Johnson DE. Pathologic changes following transurethral canine prostatectomy with a cylindrically diffusing fiber. Lasers Surg Med 1994;14:306–13.
45. Kennedy WA 2nd, Hensle TW, Giella J, et al. Potassium thiophosphate laser treatment of genitourinary hemangioma in the pediatric population. J Urol 1993;150:950–2.
46. Razvi HA, Muschter R, Anson K, et al. Alteration of laser-tissue interaction with the 805 nm diode laser indocyanine green in the canine prostate. Lasers Surg Med 1996;19:184–9.
47. Wyman A, Duffy S, Sweetland HM, et al. Preliminary evaluation of a new high power diode laser. Lasers Surg Med 1992;12:506–9.

Applications of Lasers in Endourology

Regina D. Norris, MD

W. Patrick Springhart, MD

Glenn M. Preminger, MD

Currently, there are several commercially available lasers that can be used to fragment calculi, seal tissue, coagulate tissue, cauterize tissue, ablate tissue, and activate photoactive compounds for anticancer effects.[1–5] The nature of laser-tissue interaction is determined by several physical properties, which include the tissue type, the laser wavelength, the laser power to be employed, and the mode of laser emission.

STONE FRAGMENTATION

The use of lasers in endourological approaches of intracorporeal lithotripsy for the treatment of calculi within the renal pelvis, ureter, and bladder has rendered open urolithiasis surgery virtually obsolete. The goal of laser lithotripsy is to provide stone fragmentation with minimal surrounding tissue injury. The various lasers employed differ in emission wavelength, pulse duration, pulse energy, fiber diameter, and therefore, in the mechanism of stone fragmentation and treatment efficiency.[6,7] Regardless of the type of laser employed, absorption of the laser energy by the stone initiates fragmentaion.[8]

The pulsed-dye laser with an emission wavelength of 504 nm was introduced in the 1980s for use in stone fragmentation. The pulse duration of 1 psec allowed for controlled stone fragmentation within the urinary tract. Because of the short pulse duration and the low frequency, usually 5 Hz or less, of the pulsed-dye laser, the energy was not well absorbed by water; therefore, there was significantly less thermal damage to the urothelium during lithotripsy.[9] The fragmentation efficiency of a pulsed-dye laser highly depends on the physical properties of the surface of the calculus, especially optical absorption. Therefore, this laser was not effective in treating calculi of harder composition, such as calcium oxalate monohydrate and cysteine stones.[10] The FREDDY (Frequency-Doubled Double-Pulse Nd:YAG [neodymium:yttrium-aluminum-garnet]) (World of Medicine, Berlin Germany) and alexandrite lasers have similar types of action, but their fragementation profiles are different from the pulsed-dye laser given their different emission wavelengths.

The FREDDY laser is a newly developed, short-pulsed, double-frequency solid-state laser, with 2 wavelengths at 532 and 1,064 nm.[11] This laser has been specifically designed to fragment urinary and biliary calculi. This laser is capable of producing very high pulse intensity owing to the partial frequency doubling of the infrared ray into the green range. Its mechanism of action is through the generation of a plasma bubble, which upon collapse generates a mechanical shock wave responsible for stone fragmentation. In comparison with the holmium laser, the FREDDY laser produces no thermal effects. In similarity to the pulsed-dye laser, the FREDDY is unable to break cystine stones, as cystine does not absorb the 532 or 1,064 nm wavelengths. Yet, current alterations of the FREDDY laser's output may allow fragmentation of cystine calculi in the future. The FREDDY has minimal absorption by water; therefore, it has a high safety profile for use within the urinary tract. When the FREDDY laser was activated with the fiber in direct contact with bladder mucosa of narcotized rabbits, the histologic changes were minimal even at maximum parameters of 90 mJ and 2,000 pulses.[12]

The holmium:YAG laser is currently the most widely utilized intracoporeal lithotripter, with its incorporation into urological practice in the mid-1990s. Although its energy is delivered in a pulsed mode, its mechanism of action seems to be mainly thermal. The emitted energy superheats water and creates a microscopic vaporization bubble at the tip of the delivery fiber. The implosion of the bubble creates a shock wave that is transmitted to the stone to induce fragmentation.[10,13,14] The pulse duration is considerably longer than that of the pulsed-dye laser, and the energy per pulse required to fragment stones is also much higher.

The holmium:YAG laser is capable of effectively fragmenting all stone types irrespective of composition, given its ability to be readily absorbed by water. Holmium laser lithotripsy along with small-caliber ureteroscopes allow for routine intrarenal ureteroscopic access to symptomatic renal stones and provide a reasonable alternative for the management of recurrent cystine calculi in patients who are not candidates for repeat percutaneous procedures.[15] The key to stone fragmentation with the holmium laser without collateral tissue injury is optimized with the laser fiber in contact with the surface of the stone, because the laser's energy is absorbed in the first 0.4 mm of substrate.[16] The fragmentation capability of the holmium laser also is impacted by various energy settings, frequency, and flexible fiber diameters. Small-diameter fibers (200 and 365 micron) in combination with semirigid or flexible ureteroscopes can be used effectively to treat upper urinary tract stones.[17] The 365-micron has been demonstrated to work best for the management of ureteral stones, as minimal endoscopic deflection is required to access these calculi. Because the 200-micron fiber is considerably more expensive, its use is reserved for fragmentation of intrarenal calculi, where maximum deflection is required during flexible ureterorenoscopy.[17]

If maximal deflection is still hampered by the laser fiber, as is the case in some lower-pole calculi, then a basket or grasper can be employed to displace the calculi into an upper-pole calyx or a less dependent position to facilitate easier fragmentation.[18–20] The ideal energy and frequency settings for the small fibers are < 1.0 J and 5 to 10 Hz.[17] Larger fibers (550 and 1,000 micron) can be used for managing bladder or renal calculi, as there is no need for significant fiber deflection.[17] The 550-micron fiber is preferred, as it is comparable in efficacy with the 1,000-micron fiber and is less expensive.[17] Energy and frequency can be maximized to 2.0 J and 15 Hz without damage to the fiber, but visibility can be affected by high frequencies.[17] Appropriate fiber selection and energy/frequency settings will allow access to most stones throughout the urinary tract, maximize fiber life, minimize fiber expense, and produce relatively small stone fragments allowing for easy passage.[17]

Improved laser technology and smaller caliber ureteroscopes have made it possible to successfully access and treat virtually any stone within the upper urinary tract in a relatively atraumatic fashion.[21] These advances in ureteroscopic instrumentation have reduced the morbidity associated with ureteroscopy and have expanded the role of ureteroscopy from simply a diagnostic tool to a therapeutic device with numerous indications.[22,23] However, since the development of the laser, electrohydraulic probes and additional lithotrites have been miniaturized to an extent that also allows them to be used via equivalent ureteroscopes. The laser has the advantage of being safer and more flexible than the electrohydraulic probe. The holmium laser is, however, considerably more expensive.

TISSUE COAGULATION

If the laser penetrates tissue with sufficient power delivered to heat the tissue to > 60°C, then the proteins become coagulated.[24] As the temperature rises, the tissue contracts with whitening and hemostasis. The temperature should not be allowed to rise so high that charring occurs if the intention is to maximize coagulative necrosis. Laser coagulation has been used to treat bladder tumors, renal tumors, secondary hepatic tumors, and the prostate.[25–28] This modality has the advantage of using fine fibers inserted into tissue to produce tumor necrosis.

BLADDER TUMORS The use of the photothermal effect of the laser for coagulation necrosis of exophytic superficial bladder tumors has been proposed as an alternative to the standard electrosurgical technique to minimize the morbidity associated with frequent resections. The Nd:YAG has been used to coagulate tumors of up to 2 cm in diameter. The dosimetry was established by Rothenberger and collegues, who used 40 watts for 4 seconds in overlapping regions of tumor.[29] The Nd:YAG laser allows for coagulation of the lesions as well as for treatment of the underlying tissue given its depth of penetration.[30] Small lesions can be coagulated completely in a single application of the Nd:YAG laser in free-beam mode, whereas larger lesions or exophytic lesions require initial coagulation of all visible tumor followed by physical dislodgement of the coagulated material to expose deeper layers of the tumor. The Nd:YAG has several limitations, which include the lack of tissue available for histologic evaluation and inability to determine the precise depth of tissue destruction, which may result in bladder perforation and bowel injury. The limited ability to coagulate bleeding tissue when used in a free-beam mode is because the laser beam is interrupted by the flow of blood.

The holmium:YAG laser can be used to vaporize the tumors and when used in contact, the laser fiber can be used to remove small bladder tumors. A series of 52 patients with recurrent papillary bladder tumors less than 3 cm were treated with the holmium:YAG laser under local anesthesia, and the procedure was found to be feasible for the vaporization of superficial bladder tumors and satisfactory for patients in terms of discomfort.[25]

The major advantages of laser coagulation include that it can be done safely in patients on anticoagulant therapy, requiring post-operative intravesical therapy, as well as those patients who may not tolerate formal anesthesia.[31,32] Overall, the laser is not appropriate for treatment of bladder tumors at first presentation, because the grade and stage must be established by means of standard electrical resection. The laser is not an alternative to radical surgery in cases of invasive bladder cancer; only in patients unfit for surgery can the laser offer a minimally invasive, palliative solution. The laser may also be used to treat recurrences under local anesthesia by injecting the anesthetic beneath the tumor base prior to resection or fulguration.

PROSTATIC APPLICATIONS

One of the most common applications for ablative lasers is the treatment of benign and malignant prostatic obstruction of the urethra. Laser prostatectomy has emerged as a viable surgical alternative for the management of symptomatic bladder outlet obstruction, and its clinical efficacy has been demonstrated in several studies.[33–35] The attractiveness of laser prostatectomy emerges from the idea that there is morbidity abatement, that is, less hyponatremia, hemorrhage, time to catheter removal, and physiological stress, as compared with the standard transurethral electrocautery resection. The Nd:YAG with contact tips or high-density power settings, the high-power potassium-titanyl-phosphate (KTP), and the holmium:YAG are the most frequently used lasers for prostatic ablative procedures.[36–38] The aim of the laser-prostatic tissue interaction is to produce a high-intensity thermal effect for the purpose of tissue ablation via vaporization.

The Nd:YAG lasers have been in use since 1990 for free-beam and contact-tip laser coagulation of the prostate.[24] The Nd:YAG laser has a wavelength of 1,064 nm and penetrates approximately 7 mm into tissue. Because of the large volume of affected tissue, heating occurs slowly and coagulation occurs beneath the base of the laser-induced crater. The predominant effect of the free-beam Nd:YAG laser is the production of coagulation necrosis with subsequent dissolution and sloughing of tissue over 6 to 12 weeks following the procedure.[24] Given this period of progressive tissue loss, there is no immediate effect on voiding symptoms, and the patient will experience gradual resolution and improvement of voiding symptoms. The progressive tissue loss is attributed to both direct thermal injury and ischemic injury to the prostatic transition zone.[39] Contact-tip technology of the Nd:YAG causes vaporization of tissue at the surface and coagulation at a deeper level, where less energy has been deposited—enough for coagulation, but not enough for vaporization.[24] Sapphire tips are fixed to the fiber end to absorb energy and become very hot, which in turn allows tissue cutting by vaporization.[24] The contact tip is positioned against the adenoma in order to create a furrow of vaporization, and the ridges between the furrows are then smoothed out to produce a TURP (transurethral resection of the protate)-like channel. A randomized controlled trial with 5-year follow-up of contact-tip Nd:YAG laser versus conventional TURP demonstrated that contact-laser patients had a lower median blood loss (39 mL vs 200 mL) and catheterization time (1 day vs 2 days).[40,41] Additionally, the rates of reoperation were roughly equal (18% vs 14.5%).[40,41] Contact-tip devices are less hemostatic, slower, and inefficient for glands > 40 grams when compared with free-beam Nd:YAG lasers.[24]

The KTP laser with a wavelength of 532 nm was introduced to combine the tissue-debulking characteristics of the conventional TURP with the favorable which the infrared beam has passed through the frequency-doubling KTP crystal which changes the wavelength to 532 nm, produces the characteristic green light of the KTP laser, and lends to its tissue cutting and vaporizing properties.[30] The KTP laser with tissue penetration of 0.3 mm to 1 mm can generate instant vaporization of cellular fluids with a simultaneous small rim of coagulation. A small series of 10 patients with 1-year follow-up who underwent KTP laser TURP demonstrated similar adenoma debulking, with prostate volume reduction of about 30% as compared with the conventional TURP.[43] One advantage of the KTP laser is that patients are treated on an ambulatory basis with less than 24 hours of urethral catheterization time.[43] The KTP laser has been used as an adjunct to the coagulation properties of the Nd:YAG in hybrid laser operating techniques with clinical outcomes similar to those of TURP in two randomized studies.[44,45] The major drawback to this technology is that no tissue can be retrieved for pathologic diagnosis.[24]

The holmium:YAG laser with a wavelength of 2,140 nm was first introduced as a tool for stone fragmentation. However, because of its ability to ablate, vaporize, and coagulate tissue, it has gained popularity for use in laser resection and enucleation of the prostate. The holmium:YAG laser wavelength is readily absorbed by water with a soft tissue penetration of only 0.4 mm. It can be used to cut tissue by vaporization and coagulate blood vessels simultaneously at a depth of 1 to 2 mm, generating much less histologic tissue damage as compared with other laser technologies.[46] Currently, holmium laser resection of the prostate uses the laser at exclusively high power settings of 80 to 100 W. A randomized controlled trial of the holmium:YAG versus conventional TURP demonstrated no significant difference between the two groups in AUA Symptom Score, peak flow rate, or quality-of-life score at 2 years.[47] Adverse events, including reoperations, incontinence, and loss of erectile potency were also similar.[47] The major advantages of holmium:YAG prostatectomy are direct-vision monitoring and simultaneous coagulation of encountered bleeding vessels, resulting in a relatively bloodless operation.[48] Tissue is coagulated by aiming at the blood vessel from a slight distance (defocusing) until the tissue blanches. With the holmium:YAG laser, obstructing prostatic tissue is removed immediately, thus making the resection of prostates up to 100 grams and enucleation of prostates up to 200 grams feasible.[49] The holmium:YAG laser prostatectomy can be learned by beginners because operative bleeding is rare and hyponatremia is unlikely to occur when physiologic saline is used for irrigation.

But a laser is not the only device that can produce coagulation. Microwaves, radiofrequency, cryotherapy, focused ultrasound, and even circulating hot water can induce coagulative necrosis. Furthermore, these methods can all be used without a general anesthetic. The interstitial application of lasers is mirrored by the interstitial insertion of an electrode for radiofrequency to induce coagulative necrosis. Therefore, if lasers are not to be replaced by other modalities that do not necessarily require a cystoscope, they must offer a more precise application.

TISSUE WELDING

Lasers can be used to weld tissue and have proven their efficacy in the laboratory setting when compared with more traditional methods of tissue approximation.[50–52] The technique relies on the fact that tissue when heated undergoes macromolecular structural alterations in electrostatic and covalent bonding between structural proteins, which form a weld on cooling.[53] The most common lasers used for urologic laser-assisted welds are the CO_2, Nd:YAG, argon, and holmium:YAG. The choice of laser depends on the characteristics of the recipient tissue, that is, degree of pigmentation, water content, depth, and thickness of the intended tissue closure. The laser has the advantage of being "nontouch" in comparison with other less costly methods of heating the tissue. The ideal laser is one that penetrates the tissue only superficially, while providing a sufficient seal of the tissue. Several other technologic advances, such as solder development, chromophore enhancement, and temperature control, have enhanced the application of laser tissue welding. Laser tissue welding has been applied on human subjects in open urologic surgery procedures such as vasovasotomy, urethral reconstruction (hypospadias repair, diverticulum, stricture or fistula), pyeloplasty, augmentation cystoplasty, and continent urinary diversion.

TISSUE CUTTING

Lasers can be used to incise tissue with extensive or minimal coagulation, depending on the parameters chosen. If a clean cut with minimal lateral coagulation is required, then the laser should be pulsed, and it should be used at as high a power density as possible and be absorbed readily by the tissue. A pulsed CO_2 laser is an ideal laser for producing a clean cut. However, a CO_2 laser cannot be transmitted via a fiber, and for endourologic applications, fiber delivery is essential. Alternatively, a charred fiber or contact tip could be used to produce wavelength conversion. Any laser when delivered through a narrow fiber to produce a high-power density can cause vaporization and charring with consequent cutting, provided that the fiber is in close contact with the tissue. Thus, one can use a pre-charred fiber with an Nd:YAG or a semiconductor diode laser, or one can use a contact tip coated with an infrared absorber. The laser can therefore be used to incise a urethral stricture, urethral valves, or an ureteropelvic junction (UPJ) obstruction. The advantage of using a laser in the urethra does not stem from any reduction in re-stenosis, which has not been established. It is, however, useful to have an instrument that cuts in an antegrade fashion rather than a cold knife, which cuts laterally.[54] The holmium:YAG laser has been demonstrated to be effective in the ablative treatment of traumatic bulbomembranous urethral strictures up to 2.5 cm in length.[55] The laser is particularly useful for very tight strictures, as the fiber can be easily maneuvered. In cases of UPJ obstruction both the holmium:YAG laser and the Nd:YAG laser have been used in a retrograde fashion through a ureteroscope. The laser has to be compared with cold-knife urethrotomy and electrical incision of the UPJ in a randomized controlled trial to determine its efficacy as compared with these methods.

ACTIVATION OF PHOTOSENSITIVE DRUGS

Photodynamic therapy (PDT) is based on the concept that laser irradiation can change an inert substance into an active one through a photooxidative process that damages proteins and nucleic acids in the cell.[56] In urology, hematoporphyrin derivative (HpD), which is activated by light at 630 nm, and Photofrin (Axcan Scandipharm Inc., Birmingham, AL) are used most commonly as photosensitizing agents predominantly for the treatment of transitional cell carcinoma of the bladder, either carcinoma in situ or recurrent superficial lesions unaffected by BCG.[57,58] Increased accumulation of photosensitizer in malignant cells may allow for more selective destruction of these cells as compared with normal cells. Complications of PDT include prolonged irritative urinary voiding symptoms and detrusor injury with resultant vesical fibrosis. Also, patients who undergo PDT should not be exposed to sunlight for 4 to 6 weeks after therapy, because the photosensitizing agents can be retained in the skin, with the risk of subsequent cutaneous damage.[16] More recently, the use of PDT for the treatment of prostate cancer is being evaluated; however, little is known about the effects of PDT on humans with prostate cancer, as an overwhelming majority of the current studies are conducted in animal models.[56] PDT is an experimental treatment, and even a preliminary evaluation will be possible only after the conclusion of clinical studies. Current studies are underway to investigate more efficacious photosensitizing agents, the optimal dose of photosenitizer, and the timing and amount of laser energy required for more selective destruction of malignant cells and to minimize the complication rate.

SELECTING A LASER

The lasers that are commercially available include combinations of lasers in one unit. The alternative strategy is to purchase a laser and then use different delivery devices to perform different functions. Table 6B-1 is a guide to the applications that correspond to the various lasers. Thus, for example, one can purchase a holmium laser and then have the capability to use lasers for all endourologic procedures. A low-power holmium laser (25W) supplies adequate fragmentation and incision power for virtually all endourologic cases.[59] The only current urologic application that cannot be performed with the low-power device is laser prostatic resection, which requires 80 to 100 W of power.[59] The reduced-power holmium laser should be considered as a low-cost alternative for the management of urinary tract stones, strictures, and urothelial tumors, especially in centers where laser prostatic resection is not performed.[59]

On the other hand, the only laser application that cannot be covered using a semiconductor or Nd:YAG laser with a full range of delivery devices is stone fragmentation. If one is seeking only to treat soft tissues and not stones, then one is faced with the choice of an Nd:YAG or a semiconductor diode laser. Diode lasers are small and are now in production with outputs of 60 W. They have no mirrors or flashlamps. However, the diodes can wear out. Decisions must be made on expenses over a 5-year period. Maintenance costs and warranties are obviously of key importance. The trend over the past few years is to place increasing importance on the delivery devices in laser applications. Some laser manufacturers have customized connectors on their fibers. The most useful connector is a standard mechanical adapter (SMA)-type connector, because it encompasses the widest range of fibers. Fortunately, many manufacturers can supply adapters so that SMA connectors can be used with their lasers. Thus, lasers rarely produce effects that cannot be produced by other modalities. Lasers have the advantage of being transmitted via very fine and flexible fibers that are well suited to endourology. No matter how many contortions a fiber is put through, the tip of the fiber straightens out from that curve. The penetration of laser light into tissue is more predictable than electrical energy, which is subject to the vagaries of conduction when the energy is unipolar. However, when all is said and done, the laser still must be justified in terms of cost. It is only when we have produced lasers in sufficient quantity that the cost of lasers will decrease. It is only when the cost of lasers decreases that we will see more

Table 6B-1 Guide to Lasers and Their Applications

Laser	Stone Fragmentation	Prostate Coagulation	Prostate Incision	Urethral Strictures and UPJ Stenosis
Pulsed-dye	++	N/A	N/A	N/A
Nd:YAG free beam	N/A	+++	N/A	+ (small fiber)
Nd:YAG with contact fibers and probes	N/A	+++	+++	+++
Semiconductor diode with contact fibers	N/A	+++	+++	+++
KTP Nd:YAG	N/A	+	+++	+++
Holmium:YAG	+++	+	+++	+++

N/A = not applicable; UPJ = ureteropelvic junction; + = fair; ++ = good; +++ = excellent.

widespread application of lasers in endourology. Cost issues are of increasing importance, and lasers rarely perform a task that cannot be performed by another cheaper modality.

REFERENCES

1. Lam JS, Greene TD, Gupta M. Treatment of proximal ureteral calculi: Holmium:YAG laser ureterolithotripsy versus extracorporeal shock wave lithotripsy. J Urol 2002;167:1972–6.
2. Sofer M, Denstedt J. Flexible ureteroscopy and lithotripsy with the holmium:YAG laser. Can J Urol 2000;7:952–6.
3. Razvi HA, Chun SS, Denstedt JD, Sales JL. Soft-tissue applications of the holmium:YAG laser in urology. J Endourol 1995;9:387–90.
4. Razvi HA, Denstedt JD, Chun SS, Sales JL. Intracorporeal lithotripsy with the holmium:YAG laser. J Urol 1996;156:912–4.
5. Bagley DH. Ureteroscopic laser treatment of upper urinary tract tumors. J Clin Laser Med Surg 1998;16:55–9.
6. Grocela J, Dretler SP. Intracorporeal lithotripsy: instrumentation and development. Urol Clin North Am 1997;24:13–23.
7. Watson GM. A survey of the action of lasers on stones. In : Steiner R, editor. Laser lithotripsy: clinical use and technical aspects. Berlin: Springer-Verlag; 1988. p. 15–24.
8. Welch AJ, Kang HW, Lee H, Teichman JM. Calculus fragmentation in laser lithotripsy. Minerva Urol Nefrol 2004;56:49–63.
9. Zhong P, Tong HL, Cocks FH, et al. Transient cavitation and acoustic emission produced by different laser lithotripters. J Endourol 1998;12:371–8.
10. Rink K, Delacretaz G, Salanthe RP. Fragmentation process of current laser lithotripters. Lasers Surg Med 1995;16:134–46.
11. Delvecchio FC, Auge BK, Brizuela RM, et al. In vitro analysis of stone fragmentation ability of the FREDDY laser. J Endourol 2003;17:177–9.
12. Zorcher T, Hochberger J, Schrott KM, et al. In vitro study concerning the efficiency of the frequency-doubled double-pulse Neodymium:YAG laser (FREDDY) for lithotripsy of calculi in the urinary tract. Lasers Surg Med 1999;25:38–42.
13. Rudhart M, Hrith A. Use of an absorbent in laser lithotripsy with dye lasers: in vitro study of fragmentation efficiency and jet formation. J Urol 1994;152:1005–8.
14. Bhatta KM, Rosen DI, Flotte TJ, et al. Effects of shielded or unshielded laser and electrohydraulic lithotripsy on rabbit bladder. J Urol 1990;143:857–60.
15. Kourambas J, Munver R, Preminger GM. Ureteroscopic management of recurrent renal cystine calculi. J Endourol 2000;14:489–92.
16. Floratos DL, de la Rosette JJ. Lasers in urology. BJU Int 1999;84:204–11.
17. Kuo RL, Asian P, Zhong P, Preminger GM. Impact of holmium laser settings and fiber diameter on stone fragmentation and endoscope deflection. J Endourol 1998;12:523–7.
18. Kourambas J, Delvecchio FC, Munver R, Preminger GM. Nitinol stone retrieval-assisted ureteroscopic management of lower pole renal calculi. Urology 2000;56:935–9.

19. Delvecchio FC, Preminger GM. Endoscopic management of urologic disease with the holmium laser. Curr Opin Urol 2000;10:233–7.
20. Auge BK, Dahm P, Wu NZ, Preminger GM. Ureteroscopic management of lower-pole renal calculi: technique of calculus displacement. J Endourol 2001;15:835–8.
21. Zheng W, Denstedt JD. Intracorporeal lithotripsy. Update on technology. Urol Clin North Am 2000;27:301–13.
22. Grasso M, Bagley D. Small diameter, actively deflectable, flexible ureteropyeloscopy. J Urol 1998;160:1648–54.
23. Bagley DH. Ureteroscopic surgery: changing times and perspectives. Urol Clin North Am 2004;31:1–4, vii.
24. Tan AH, Gilling PJ. Free-beam and contact laser soft-tissue ablation in urology. J Endourol 2003;17:587–93.
25. Jonler M, Lund L, Bisballe S. Holmium:YAG laser vaporization of recurrent papillary tumours of the bladder under local anesthesia. BJU Int 2004;94:322–5.
26. de Jode MG, Vale JA, Gedroyc WM. MR-guided laser thermoablation of inoperable renal tumors in an open-configuration interventional MR scanner: preliminary clinical experience in three cases. J Magn Reson Imaging 1999;10:545–9.
27. Amin Z, Donald JJ, Masters A, et al. Hepatic metastases: interstitial laser photocoagulation with real-time US monitoring and dynamic CT evaluation of treatment. Radiology 1993;187:339–47.
28. Staehler G, Hofstetter A. Transurethral laser irradiation of urinary bladder tumors. Eur Urol 1979;5:64–9.
29. Rothenberger K, Pensel J, Hofstetter A, et al. Transurethral laser coagulation for treatment of urinary bladder tumors. Lasers Surg Med 1983;2:255–60.
30. Absten GT. Physics of light and lasers. Obstet Gynecol Clin North Am 1991;18:407–27.
31. Kuo RL, Asian P, Fitzgerald KB, Preminger GM. Use of ureteroscopy and holmium:YAG laser in patients with bleeding diatheses. Urology 1998;52:609–13.
32. Watterson JD , Girvan AR, Cook AJ, et al. Safety and efficacy of holmium:YAG laser lithotripsy in patients with bleeding diatheses. J Urol 2002;168:442–5.
33. Cowles RS 3rd, Kabalin JN, Childs S, et al. A prospective randomized comparison of transurethral resection to visual laser ablation of the prostate for the treatment of benign prostatic hyperplasia. Urology 1995;46:155–60.
34. Meyhoff HH, Nordling J. Long term results of transurethral and transvesical prostatectomy. A randomized study. Scand J Urol Nephrol 1986;20:27–33.
35. Bruskewitz RC, Larsen EH, Madsen PO, Dorflinger T. 3-year followup of urinary symptoms after transurethral resection of the prostate. J Urol 1986;136:613–5.
36. Kabalin JN. Neodymium:YAG laser coagulation prostatectomy for patients in urinary retention. J Endourol 1997;11:207–9.
37. Barber NJ, Muir GH. High-power KTP laser prostatectomy: the new challenge to transurethral resection of the prostate. Curr Opin Urol 2004;14:21–5.
38. Gilling PJ, Cass CB, Cresswell MD, et al. The use of the holmium laser in the treatment of benign prostatic hyperplasia. J Endourol 1996;10:459–61.
39. Kabalin JN. Editorial: Laser Prostatectomy—what we have accomplished and future directions [editorial]. J Urol 1995;154:2093–5.
40. Keoghane SR, Lawrence KC, Gray AM, et al. A double-blind randomized controlled trial and economic evaluation of transurethral resection vs contact laser vaporization for benign prostatic enlargement: a 3-year follow-up. BJU Int

2000;85:74–8.
41. Keoghane S, Sullivan ME, Doll HA, et al. Five-year data from the Oxford Laser Prostatectomy Trial. BJU Int 2000;86:227–8.
42. Reich 0, Bachmann A, Schneede P, et al. Experimental comparison of high power (80 W) potassium titanyl phosphate laser vaporization and transurethral resection of the prostate. J Urol 2004;171(6 Pt 1):2502–4.
43. Hai MA, Malek RS. Photoselective vaporization of the prostate: initial experience with a new 80 W KTP laser for the treatment of benign prostatic hyperplasia. J Endourol 2003;17:93–6.
44. Carter A, Sells H, Speakman M, et al. A prospective randomized controlled trial of hybrid laser treatment or transurethral resection of the prostate, with a 1-year follow-up. BJU Int 1999;83:254–9.
45. Shingleton WB, Terrell F, Renfroe DL, et al. A randomized prospective study of laser ablation of the prostate versus transurethral resection of the prostate in men with benign prostatic hyperplasia. Urology 1999;54:1017–21.
46. Das A, Kennett KM, Sutton T, et al. Histologic effects of holmium:YAG laser resection versus transurethral resection of the prostate. J Endourol 2000;14:459–62.
47. Gilling PJ, Kennett KM, Fraundorfer MR. Holmium laser resection vs. transurethral resection of the prostate: results of a randomized trial with 2 years of follow-up. J Endourol 2000;14:757–60.
48. Le Duc A, Gilling PJ. Holmium laser resection of the prostate. Eur Urol 1999;35:155–60.
49. Gilling PJ, Cass CB, Malcolm A, et al. Holmium laser resection of the prostate versus neodymiuim:yttrium-aluminum-garnet visual laser ablation of the prostate: a randomized prospective comparison of two techniques of laser prostatectomy. Urolology 1998;51:573–7.
50. Bass L, Treat M, Dzaknoski C, Trokel SL. Sutureless microvascular anastomosis using the THC:YAG laser: a preliminary report. Microsurgery 1989;10:189–93.
51. Benson R. Tissue welding. In: Smith J Jr, editor. Lasers in urology surgery. 3rd ed. St. Louis: Mosby: 1993. p. 199–220.
52. White R, White G, Fujitani R, et al. Initial human evaluation of argon laser-assisted vascular anastomosis. J Vasc Surg 1959;9:542–7.
53. Poppas DP, Scherr DS. Laser tissue welding: a urological surgeon's perspective. Haemophilia 1998;4:456–62.
54. Matsuoka K, Inoue M, Iida S, et al. Endoscopic antegrade laser incision in the treatment of urethral stricture. Urology 2002;60:968–72.
55. Dogra PN, Ansari MS, Gupta NP, Tandon S. Holmium laser core-through urethrotomy for traumatic obliterative strictures of urethra: initial experience. Urology 2004;64:232–6.
56. Muschter R. Photodynamic therapy: a new approach to prostate cancer. Curr Urol Rep 2003;4:221–8.
57. Nseyo UO. Photodynamic therapy in the management of bladder cancer. J Clin Laser Med Surg 1996;14:271–80.
58. Nseyo UO, DeHaven J, Dougherty TJ, et al. Photodynamic therapy (PDT) in the treatment of patients with resistant superficial bladder cancer: a long-term experience. J Clin Laser Med Surg 1998;16:61–8.
59. Kourambas J, Delvecchio FC, Preminger GM. Low-power holmium laser for the management of urinary tract calculi, structures, and tumors. J Endourol 2001;15:529–32.

7

Monopolar and Bipolar Electrosurgery and Associated Problems

Robert D. Tucker, PhD, MD

Electrosurgery is the use of radiofrequency (RF) currents to both cut and coagulate tissue. Although electrosurgery is termed electrocautery by many physicians and operating room personnel, the two technologies differ greatly. In true electrocautery, a hot wire is used to coagulate bleeding vessels; electrocautery cannot cut tissue or work in a fluid medium. Electrosurgery employs alternating currents that pass from an active electrode through the patient and return to the generator. As the tissue resists the current flow, tissue heat is generated. It is this tissue heating that produces both the cutting and coagulating actions.

Two types of electrosurgery are employed in modern surgery: monopolar and bipolar. In monopolar electrosurgery the current flows from a small active electrode to the tissue at the surgical site, then flows through the patient to a large return electrode, typically on the patient's buttocks or thigh, where the current is collected and returned to the generator to complete the circuit. In bipolar electrosurgery, the large return electrode of the monopolar mode is replaced with a second small electrode; thus, current flows from one active electrode through the patient's tissue to the second active electrode, which is in very close proximity (ie, within several millimeters) and then returns to the generator to complete the circuit. Although monopolar and bipolar procedures require different instrumentation, the basic principles are similar.

Electrosurgery had its early beginning in 1891 when d'Arsonval found that RF alternating currents applied to tissue caused heating without muscle and nerve stimulation.[1] By 1900, Rivière had employed d'Arsonval currents for the coagulation of intractable ulcers.[2] The development of the vacuum tube in 1908 permitted the development of cutting waveforms as well as coagulating waveforms. This new electronic technology allowed the active pursuit of electrosurgical cutting and coagulating in various surgical procedures. In 1911, Clark (an American surgeon) routinely employed RF currents to excise benign and malignant tumors of the head, neck, breast, and cervix.[3]

Beer is credited with being the first to use electrosurgery endoscopically by placing an electrode through a cystoscope to remove tumors of the bladder neck.[4] Young improved the endoscopic application of electrosurgery by replacing the inner cutting tubular knife of a punch with a wire electrode to deliver current.[5] This design allowed water to be infused between the sheath and the electrode, thereby improving vision and cooling the instrument. Stevens and Bugbee are credited with performing the first electrosurgical endoscopic incision of the prostate in 1913.[6,7] The early resectoscope was developed in 1926 by Stern, who used a cutting loop consisting of a small ring of tungsten wire approximately 0.5 cm in diameter.[8] This loop was placed at right angles to the end of an insulted shaft and was connected such that the loop could be made to slide easily. The RF current was then delivered continuously under water to achieve dissection with decreased hemorrhaging.[8]

Although several groups developed generators capable of supplying both cutting and coagulating currents, it was William Bovie, a Harvard physicist, who pioneered the development of the first commercial electrosurgical generator.[9] With the aid of the Bovie generator, Cushing,[10,11] a neurosurgeon at Peter Brent Brigham Hospital, popularized the use of electrosurgery in the early 1930s.

Although many refinements have been made over the past 50 years since the commercialization of electrosurgery by Bovie, the basic physics and important variables have remained the same. The following section details the basic principles that produce the cutting and coagulating actions. While understanding the physics of electrosurgery aids in safely achieving the desired surgical effect, a rather substantial component of electrosurgery continues to be surgical art.

BIOPHYSICS OF ELECTROSURGERY

The surgical effect of RF currents is the result of tissue heating. In contrast with true electrocautery, tissue heating is not produced by conduction from a hot electrode; instead, heat is produced by passing alternating currents through the tissue, and as the tissue resists the flow of current, heat is produced. If heating is rapid and high temperatures are achieved, intracellular and extracellular fluids are vaporized, and a cutting action is produced. Should heat be produced more slowly, cells are desiccated, producing a coagulation action. The surgical characteristics of the heating are controlled, in part, by (1) the electrosurgical generator voltage and current output, (2) the waveform of the generator output, (3) the active electrode size, (4) the tissue resistance, and (5) the length of time the current is applied to the tissue.

Electrosurgical generators produce a voltage that alternates sinusoidally between positive and negative values at frequencies ranging from 500,000 to 3,000,000 cycles per second, or 500 kHz and 3 MHz. Voltage, measured in volts (V), is defined as the force necessary to push electrons or ions through a resistance. Several terms are associated with the generator output voltage: peak-to-peak voltage (V_{p-p}) and root mean square voltage (V_{rms}). Peak-to-peak voltage refers to the number of volts from the maximum to the minimum value, whereas V_{rms} refers to the average value of the voltage. Regardless of which measure of voltage is used to characterize an electrosurgical generator, the higher the voltage the greater the force that is available to push charged particles through a resistance, or in the case of electrosurgery, through the tissue. The flow of charged particles per second, either electrons or ions, is termed current (I) and is measured in amperes (A).

Each tissue type has a characteristic resistance (R) that is measured in ohms (Ω). The tissue resistance is inversely proportional to the number of charged particles in the tissue itself. For example, blood, which has a high electrolyte content, has a low resistance, typically 30 to 50 Ω/cm. Fat and bone have a high resistance of 1,000 Ω/cm or greater. Other tissues have intermediate values, for example, the liver with a high blood content has a resistance of approximately 150 Ω/cm and muscle has a resistance of between 200 and 500 Ω/cm . During electrosurgical action the resistance of the tissue at the operative site will vary dramatically; the initial tissue resistance may be a low value of 200 Ω/cm , but after several seconds of desiccation, the tissue resistance will rise to the 1,000 to 3,000 Ω/cm range.

The amount of tissue heating is proportional to the power (P) delivered to the tissue and is measured in watts (W). Power is equal to the current squared times the tissue resistance or $I^2 \times R$. This formula does not, however, take into account two critical electrosurgical variables, both of which are under the surgeon's control: the effect of area and the effect of time.

If an electrosurgical current is concentrated in a small area, such as a needle electrode, the heating effect is typically high, and a cutting action is produced; if this same current is passed through a large area, such as the ground pad or return electrode, there is little heating effect. Thus the current flow must be analyzed in terms of current flowing through a cross-sectional area (A) or current density (I/A). This modification yields a power formula of:

$$P = (I/A)^2 \times R.$$

Figure 7-1 demonstrates this effect. Current is concentrated at the application site and high temperatures are achieved. But as the current spreads through the tissue over a larger area, the temperature drops dramatically. Normal temperatures may be seen within a few millimeters of the surgical site as current spreads over a large volume of tissue. The diagram also demonstrates that thermal gradients are not uniform because tissue is anisotropic, and current follows paths of least resistance, such as blood vessels.

The concentration of current is an important variable directly under the surgeon's control. For a given electrode, the surgeon can vary the electrode-tissue contact and achieve different results. The electrode–tissue-contact pressure changes the resistance and, thus, the current flow. Traction on the tissue alters both the tissue resistance and the area of current flow. While based in science, these effects are part of the surgical art of utilizing electrosurgery.

To fully determine the extent of thermal tissue necrosis, the length of time that current flows through tissue must be considered. For example, 25 W of power applied to tissue by contact desiccation for 4 seconds will cause significantly greater tissue destruction than 25 W applied for only 1 second. The power times the activation time (t), or P × t, is termed energy (E) and is measured in joules (J); it is the total energy delivered to the tissue that correlates directly with the heat produced. Although the energy correlates directly with tissue necrosis,[12] the time course over which the power is delivered must be considered. If 100 J of energy is delivered to the tissue as 25 W for 4 seconds, the tissue necrosis will be readily apparent; if, however, the 100 J is delivered as 1 watt of power for 100 seconds, the tissue destruction may be imperceptible. Unfortunately, analysis of tissue destruction by energy considerations alone is simplistic and ignores the importance of current and power densities; even low levels of power delivered for short periods of time can cause tissue necrosis if delivered through a sufficiently small cross-sectional area.

Analysis of electrosurgical tissue destruction is further complicated by the rapid (microsecond-to-microsecond) changes that occur in the tissue. As the tissue heats, the resistance increases, thereby changing the paths of least resistance and the paths of current flow. This, in turn, modifies the thermal gradients; thus, the thermal analysis presented in Figure 7-1 should only be considered a single "snapshot." Changes in tissue resistance also change the typical generator output power; as tissue resistances increase, generator power output can drop dramatically. Figure 7-2 shows the monopolar power output of a generator set at 50 W; the power is not constant but varies with the tissue resistance. This effect is not true of all electrosurgical generators; several new generators maintain constant power output over a wide range of tissue resistance. Therefore, it becomes necessary for the surgeon to become familiar with the generators he or she employs in practice to achieve their desired effect without complications. Further complicating the analysis is the fact that generated heat is continuously removed from the surgical site by blood flow in vessels that have not been totally desiccated. It is obvious that a detailed microscopic picture of the effects of RF current on tissue is difficult at best.

The surgical effect of electrosurgery is also influenced by the generator waveform. Most generators provide separate monopolar waveforms for pure-cut, blended-cut, and coagulation actions, along with several bipolar waveforms. Unfortunately, terms such as cut waveform and coagulation waveform are misleading inasmuch as low-power settings in the cut mode produce excellent contact coagulation, and high-power settings in the coagulation mode will produce cutting action. Therefore selecting the appropriate waveform to achieve the desired surgical result requires some knowledge of the generator characteristics.

In general, cutting is produced by high tissue temperatures (> 100° C), whereas coagulation is produced by tissue heating between 70° and 100° C. Coagulation of blood can be achieved by either contact desiccation or fulguration. In contact desiccation, the active electrode is firmly in contact with the tissue. In fulguration, the electrode is not in contact with the tissue, but instead long sparks carry the RF current from the electrode to the tissue over distances of up to 10 mm.

Electrosurgical cutting requires the generation of small arcs from the electrode to the tissue; these arcs produce sufficiently high current density to provide rapid tissue heating and vaporization. Although the electrode may initially be in contact with the tissue, desiccation of the tissue will cause shrinkage, and then the initiation of arcs from electrode to tissue. These arcs are extremely small (submillimeter in length), tight, and compact compared to the arcs of coagulation waveforms.[13] To ionize air and produce arcs between electrode and tissue, the generator voltage must be greater than approximately 500 V$_{p-p}$. The typical cutting waveform is a pure sine wave (Figure 7-3A). Arcs from electrode to tissue will occur twice during each cycle at the minimum and maximum voltage of the sine wave. Generators typically use sine waves of 500 kHz to 3 MHz,

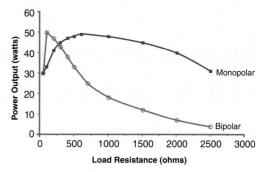

Figure 7-2 Monopolar and bipolar outputs of a typical multipurpose generator set at 50 W in both monopolar and bipolar modes. The power output of the generator is not constant but varies with the tissue resistance.

and therefore, arcs are produced at frequencies of 1 to 6 MHz. Currents used in cutting are approximately 0.1 A. Low-power, low-voltage (voltages < 500 V$_{p-p}$) cut waveforms provide excellent coagulation via contact desiccation. Even with low power, deep tissue desiccation can be produced with a longer application time. This effect emphasizes the misleading nature of the historical naming of cut and coagulation waveforms.

Most generators also provide for blended-cut waveforms; these waveforms use higher voltages than pure-cut waveforms to obtain increased lateral tissue coagulation. The waveforms are intermittent, that is, the generator supplies current for only part of each cycle. Blended waveforms typically supply current for only 50 to 80% of the activation period (Figure 7-3B).

Coagulation waveforms are modulated waveforms, that is, the generator supplies current for < 50% of the activation time (Figure 7-3C). Current is in the range of 0.5 A. These waveforms have large, peak-to-peak voltages, up to 10,000 V. When coagulation waveforms are employed with the active electrode in contact with the tissue, the high voltage causes deep tissue destruction. If sufficiently high voltages are used, sparking may also occur from electrode to tissue, which will produce tissue carbonization and coagulum adhesion to the electrode.

Modern generators also supply a fulguration or spray coagulation mode. This waveform is highly intermittent, with the generator supplying current only 5% of the activation time (Figure 7-3D). These waveforms are also high voltage (up to 10 kV) to produce long sparks between electrode and tissue. Operating in this mode, the active electrode does not touch the tissue, but instead, the high voltage causes air ionization and sparking. Fulguration uses relatively low current output (approximately 0.1 A) and thus leads to a thin layer of tissue necrosis with little depth of thermal damage.

Several new generators with microprocessor control have deviated from standard generators in that their voltage or power output is constant over a wide range of tissue resistances. This makes the surgical effect, or "feel," very consistent (eg, in cut mode, these generators will smoothly cut different tissues even at the interfaces between the

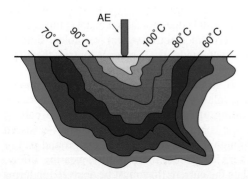

Figure 7-1 Diagram of thermal gradients in tissue under an active electrode (*AE*). As the current spreads over a larger area, causing a decrease in the current density, temperatures drop dramatically. Temperature gradients are also not uniform because the current follows paths of least resistance, such as blood vessels.

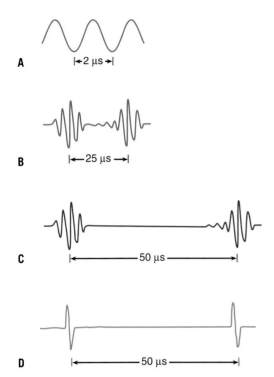

Figure 7-3 *A,* A typical cut waveform, which is a pure sine wave. *B,* A typical blended-cut waveform, which is intermittent with the generator supplying current for 50 to 80% of the activation period. Blended-cut waveforms use higher voltages than pure-cut waveforms to obtain increased lateral tissue coagulation. *C,* A typical coagulation waveform, which is modulated with the generator supplying current for < 50% of the activation period. Output voltages are higher than blended waveform voltages. *D,* A typical fulguration or spray coagulation waveform, in which the waveform is highly intermittent and the generator supplies current for only 5% of the activation period. Fulguration voltages are typically the highest of all waveform voltages.

tissues). These generators may also deposit more energy in the tissue than earlier models, which can affect tissue surrounding the surgical site. Changes in generator characteristics make it important for surgeons to understand each generator they use; this becomes problematic for surgeons practicing at several hospitals, which typically have different equipment. Surgeons taking the time to understand generator operating characteristics will be rewarded with enhanced surgical effect and fewer complications.

Most generators in use today include connections for bipolar electrosurgical output. Bipolar waveforms are usually pure sine waves, analogous to the monopolar cut waveform. Unlike monopolar cut waveforms, the bipolar voltages are substantially lower, usually not > 1,500 V_{p-p}. These low-voltage sine waves provide excellent contact desiccation. It should be noted that some generators provide bipolar waveforms similar to the pure-cut, blend-cut, and coagulation waveforms of the monopolar mode; this emphasizes the need for the surgeon to become familiar with the operating characteristics of the generator used.

The bipolar waveforms and voltage do not express the complete functionality. In the bipolar mode, the generator supplies less power into high resistances than monopolar outputs. Bipolar out-puts supply little current at tissue resistances of 0.1500 Ω, whereas monopolar outputs can supply significant power into the tissue resistances of several thousand ohms. Figure 7-2 shows the monopolar and bipolar power outputs of a typical generator versus the load or tissue resistance; although both outputs were set at 50 W, the generator power varied greatly with resistance. This functional difference was designed in part to prevent over-desiccation of tissue when using bipolar waveforms and to eliminate sparking.

New bipolar electrodes have been developed that are of special interest to endourologists. Bipolar TURP loops have been developed that effectively cut and coagulate tissue in a saline environment. These loops fit modified and specially designed resectoscopes. They eliminate the patient return electrode, localize the current flow to a volume about the loop and improve visibility over nonconductive irrigants. Another system applicable to the prostate can ablate (volumetrically remove) tissue in a saline environment. The bipolar electrode requires a specific generator that has feedback control of the output voltage to maintain the ablation effect. The active electrode is at the distal tip, and the return is a small cylinder on the shaft several millimeters away from the active electrode. When the electrode is energized in saline and not in contact with tissue, current flows from the tip through the saline to the return on the shaft. This flow vaporizes saline and forms a vapor pocket about the tip. When the tip is brought near tissue, the current arcs through the vapor to the tissue causing ablation; current returns to the cylindrical return electrode by tissue-saline paths.

COMPLICATIONS

During the past 50 years of widespread use of electrosurgery, generators have undergone many improvements to ensure safety and reduce the incidence of complications. The primary problem still encountered today is unintended burns. Two types of burns have been encountered: return-electrode and alternate-site burns. Various technologies have been developed that eliminate or greatly reduce the incidence of each of these types of burns.

Generators manufactured prior to 1970 were typically grounded—that is, the patient pad (return electrode or ground pad) was connected to the ground or earth. Therefore, if the patient came in contact with a grounded object, such as a metal ring stand or an ECG electrode that was also grounded, the current could flow from the active electrode through the patient to the unintended patient contact with the ground. This situation was responsible for many alternate-site burns.

In the early 1970s. isolated generators were developed that, in effect, placed resistance between the return electrode and the ground or earth. Therefore, the RF current no longer had a low-resistance path to the ground and the current would return preferentially to the generator. Such isolated generators significantly decreased the incidence of alternate-site burns under ECG electrodes or at sites where patients inadvertently came into contact with the ground. These generators, however, did not protect the patient from burns occurring under the return electrode. Return-electrode burns continued to occur if the electrode tissue contact area was decreased, and thus, the current density increased sufficiently to cause heating in the small contact area.

In the 1980s, most generators were produced with return-electrode monitoring (REM) systems, which decreased the incidence of even these burns. These monitoring systems indirectly measure the contact resistance between the return electrode and the patient's tissue. If the electrode contact area is decreased, the resistance increases and the generator is disabled. But even with REM systems, the occurrence of burns under the return electrode has not been eliminated during monopolar electrosurgery. Although rare, burns have continued to occur because non-REM return electrodes can be used with REM generators; in this event, the safety features of the REM circuitry are negated. To eliminate the occurrence of return-electrode burns with monopolar electrosurgery, it is necessary to make sure that a REM pad is used with a REM generator. These pads can be recognized by their two metal foil sections covered by conductive adhesive—in contrast to non-REM pads, which consist of a single metal foil covered by conductive adhesive. They are, of course, also marked on the package as REM-return electrodes.

Obviously bipolar electrosurgery, which does not employ a return electrode, also eliminates all return-electrode burns.

COMPLICATIONS ASSOCIATED WITH LAPAROSCOPY AND ENDOSCOPY The technologic advances previously discussed have ensured the relative safety of electrosurgery in open surgical procedures. But there are unique problems associated with the use of RF monopolar electrosurgery in closed spaces during laparoscopy and endoscopy.[14,15]

During laparoscopy, the electrosurgical active electrode is placed through a cannula (Figure 7-4). The surgeon's attention is focused on the 2 to 5 cm diameter zone 1. The surgeon does not typically view zone 2 or zone 3 during surgery. Therefore, the surgeon expects all of the electrosurgical current to flow from the tip of the active electrode in zone 1 to the patient's tissue. There are three situations in which the electrosurgical current can flow unintentionally to patient tissues in zone 2 or 3, or to the surgeon's hand in zone 4: insulation failure, capacitive coupling, and direct coupling. In any of these situations, the unintended current flow can lead to burns. Unfortunately, it is common for such burns to be out of the surgeon's field of view, and they remain undiscovered during laparoscopy and appear instead as post-procedural complications.

During endoscopy, the electrosurgical active electrode is placed through a flexible or rigid scope. Again, the surgeon's attention is focused on the small area analogous to zone 1 of laparoscopy. The remaining length of the scope is not

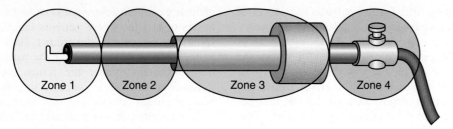

Figure 7-4 An active electrode placed through a cannula.

visible during surgery; therefore, insulation failure, capacitive coupling, and direct coupling could allow unintended current flow leading to burns. Although capacitive coupling has led to burns to the surgeon, and occasionally capacitive coupling burns from a resectoscope will occur in the patient, burns occurring during endoscopic procedures that can be attributed to these three mechanisms are uncommon.

INSULATION FAILURE Insulation failure of laparoscopic monopolar active electrodes can occur from the repeated use of reusable electrodes or from the physical trauma of placing electrodes through cannulas. Such insulation defects need not be large or even visible to pass 100% of the electrosurgical current to tissue.

Insulation failures in zone 2 will be outside the field of view of the laparoscope. Failures in this zone are potentially very dangerous to the patient; burns are not typically noticed during surgery but appear instead as postsurgical complications. Zone 3 insulation failures are also outside the field of view of the laparoscope but pose less risk to the patient. If the cannula is entirely nonconductive or plastic, the current from the zone 3 defect will not pass from the defect to the cannula. If, however, the cannula is all metal, the current will flow from the defect to the cannula and then to the patient's abdominal wall. This situation could lead to an abdominal wall burn or an external skin burn, which is, of course, a much less serious complication than an internal burn from a zone 2 defect. Long procedures during which a large amount of current is passed to the abdominal wall from a zone 3 defect will produce desiccation of any tissue that comes in contact with the metal cannula. It is theoretically possible that abdominal wall tissue resistance could become sufficiently high to allow current to flow from the distal tip of the metal cannula to moist internal tissue, which represents a path of less resistance.

Many surgeons believe that the use of disposable laparoscopic electrodes will prevent insulation failure. Although the electrodes may leave the factory with their insulation intact, damage can occur prior to, or during, a procedure. Even though standards have been set for the necessary electrical characteristics of the insulation, no such standards are required in terms of the insulation's capacity to withstand physical trauma such as scratching. Simple nonquantitative tests easily demonstrate that disposable insulation

from different manufacturers varies greatly in its ability to withstand trauma.

Electrode insulation failure in endoscopic procedures does not usually lead to serious patient complications. If the failure occurs outside the scope, sparking from the defect to the tissue is within the view of the surgeon, and the procedure can be stopped immediately and the electrode replaced. An electrode defect inside the scope is very unlikely to lead to patient injury. In flexible fiberoptic endoscopes or videoendoscopes, the metal frame of the scope is covered by an insulator. Therefore, any significant complications would require failure of both the active electrode insulation and the covering insulation of the flexible scope. Such failures must indeed be rare.

Insulation failure can also occur during transurethral resection of the prostate (TURP) and transurethral incision of the prostate (TUIP). The failure of these active electrodes can place electrosurgical current on the metal resectoscope. Because the conductive sheath is in contact with the entire length of the urethra, the large contact area leads to a low current density; thus, there is significantly less chance of a severe burn.

During an electrosurgical procedure, the surgeon should remember that any insulation failure that results in conduction of active electrode current through an unintended path decreases the amount of current available at the surgical site. This results in a perceptible decrease in the surgical cutting or coagulating capability, and if this decrease in function is noted, the electrode should be examined immediately for an insulation defect.

CAPACITIVE COUPLING Capacitive coupling is a basic law of physics that is poorly understood by physicians and engineers alike, and as a physical law, it cannot be eliminated from RF electrosurgery. Capacitive coupling is a phenomenon whereby any wire that carries RF current will induce stray current on any metal object in close proximity. This stray current is induced even though the current-carrying wire has intact insulation covering its surface.

Although this phenomenon does occur in open procedures, it is typically only a minor nuisance; but capacitive coupling is potentially extremely dangerous in laparoscopic monopolar procedures. Various situations lead to induced stray currents on metal objects near the active electrode, including an active electrode placed through a metal suction irrigator,[15] an active electrode placed through a metal cannula, or an active electrode placed

through an operative laparoscope. In these situations, each time the monopolar active electrode is energized, stray current will be induced on the suction irrigator, the cannula, or the laparoscope.

Higher generator voltages will lead to more stray current induced on nearby conductors; therefore, high-voltage coagulation or fulguration waveforms will produce higher capacitive coupled currents. Induced currents are also higher if the active electrode is energized while it is not in contact with the tissue (ie, open circuit activation); this is a result of the generator voltage being highest during open-circuit activation. Open-circuit activation can lead to five to ten times more stray power flowing through unintended paths. Significant currents exist, however, even with the active electrode in contact with the tissue as tissue resistance increases during desiccation, which in turn leads to increased generator voltage.

Higher stray current on a metal object will be produced the closer the metal object is to the active electrode. Thus, 5 mm metal cannulas will have higher induced stray currents than 11 mm cannulas inasmuch as their smaller diameter places the cannula in closer approximation to the active electrode. Although close proximity of the active electrode to the metal object helps to maximize the stray current, it is also necessary for the metal object to lie parallel to the active electrode. Therefore, a non-electrified grasper lying close and parallel to an active electrode will have stray current induced on it, while a grasper perpendicular to an active electrode will have little stray current.

Figure 7-5 shows the power on a 5-mm metal cannula versus a generator power setting with open-circuit activation. High-voltage coagulation waveforms produce the most induced power on a cannula; > 20 W of power is available on a 5-mm metal cannula for a generator setting of 50 W. Figure 7-6 shows the analogous situation with a

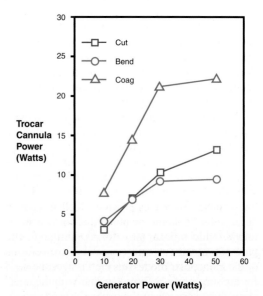

Figure 7-5 The power available by capacitive coupled current on a 5-mm metal cannula versus a generator power setting. The curves were obtained by open-circuit activation in pure-cut, blended-cut, and coagulation modes on a Valleylab Force 2 generator.

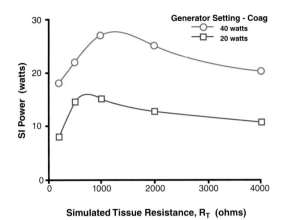

Figure 7-6 The maximum power available on a metal suction irrigator by open-circuit activation in coagulation mode with a generator set at 20 W and 40 W. The amount of power that can flow unintentionally to internal tissue varies with the tissue resistance. Most non-desiccated tissue resistances are < 1,500 ohms.

suction irrigator. At typical tissue resistances (2,000 Ω), a generator setting of 40 W in coagulation mode with open-circuit activation can produce nearly 30 W of power available from the suction irrigator. In both examples, the stray powers are high and could easily cause extensive unseen damage to internal viscera.

Laparoscopic capacitive coupled currents are not always dangerous; there is, however, one set of conditions that leads to an increased likelihood of unintended burns. This condition exists if an active electrode is placed through a hybrid cannula (that is, a metal cannula with a plastic abdominal wall anchor [Figure 7-7]). As the plastic abdominal anchor insulates the patient's abdominal wall from the metal cannula, any stray currents induced on the cannula will not flow to the abdominal wall. Should any internal organ touch the metal cannula, all stray current induced by capacitive coupling will unintentionally flow to the tissue. Analogous situations occur if an active electrode is placed inside a metal suction irrigator that has been introduced into the abdominal wall through a nonconductive (plastic) cannula or if an active electrode is used through an operative laparoscope that has been introduced into the abdomen through a nonconductive cannula. In either situation, the plastic cannula insulates the stray current from the patient's abdominal wall, potentially allowing the current to flow unintentionally to any internal tissue touching the suction irrigator or the operative laparoscope.

Flexible fiberoptic endoscopes and videoendoscopes also have capacitive-coupled stray currents induced on their metal frames when they are used with electrosurgery.[14,16] These induced currents, however, typically pose little problem to the patient but can cause burns to the endoscopist. Inasmuch as the metal framework of the endoscope is covered with insulating material, any burn would require a break in the insulation of the endoscope itself. Such a defect, regardless of how small, can allow capacitive coupled currents to flow to the patient, producing a burn if the power

density is sufficiently high. Usually these capacitive coupled currents flow from the metal frame of the endoscope to the operator, and occasionally, the operator may receive a small minor burn. This is especially true of older fiberoptic endoscopes where stray currents occasionally flow to the endoscopist via the eyepiece.

Resectoscopes present an increased burn risk to the patient compared to flexible endoscopes. As TURP and TUIP procedures employ high powers, the induced currents on the outer sheath of the resectoscope can be large. Routinely, these currents are spread over the entire urethra, and thus, current densities are very low and the likelihood of a burn is minimal. Occasionally small minor burns to the scrotum or the glands of the penis have occurred.

DIRECT COUPLING Direct coupling occurs whenever a monopolar active electrode touches another piece of metal, for example, a non-electrified grasper or the laparoscope. In this situation, the power density is usually sufficiently high to burn any tissue being held by the grasper. In the case of a laparoscope that has been introduced through a plastic cannula, the laparoscope will carry 100% of the electrosurgical current, and any tissue touching the scope has the potential to be burned. If the laparoscope has been introduced through an all-metal cannula, the currents would be transferred to the patient's abdominal wall rather than to internal viscera.

Direct coupling in endoscopic procedures rarely occurs. These procedures do not employ other metal instruments at the surgical site. Any direct coupling that could occur from the active electrode back to the endoscope is a result of insulation failure in the endoscope or electrode failure.

TECHNIQUE SOLUTIONS There are common-sense and technique solutions to minimize the potential for unintended laparoscopic burns. But even the most careful surgeon, using good techniques, will occasionally encounter unintended

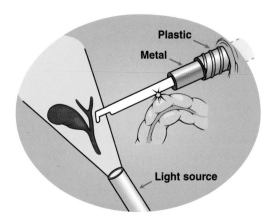

Figure 7-7 Diagram of a capacitive coupled bowel burn from a metal cannula. Capacitive coupled currents induced on the metal cannula are isolated from the patient's abdominal wall by a plastic abdominal wall anchor. As with most unintended, internal burns, this one occurs outside the field of view of the laparoscopist.

postsurgical complications during electrosurgery. The following suggestions are not intended to be the "best" techniques for all endourologic procedures—they are simply general guidelines. All surgeons must be familiar with their equipment and should be trained by qualified experts. There is no substitute for proper training and experience.

All active electrodes, either reusable or disposable, should be examined for insulation defects. Endoscopes, including resectoscopes, must be monitored for any defects in the covering and tip insulation. High-power settings, especially in the high-voltage coagulation or fulguration mode, should be used only when necessary. Contact coagulation employing the low-power cut mode should be used for contact coagulation. The electrode should be activated only when it is in contact with tissue (note that this contact activation is never possible during fulguration). Prolonged activation should be avoided.

All-metal or all-plastic cannulas should be used to introduce electrosurgical electrodes. Laparoscopes and resectoscopes should only be used with metal cannulas and metal sheaths, respectively. If a nonconductive plastic cannula is used to introduce a suction irrigator along with electrosurgery, the suction irrigator should be nonconductive.

Patients who have undergone electrosurgical procedures, either by laparoscopic or endoscopic access, should improve daily. In patients who respond poorly following surgery, the possibility of an electrosurgical complication must be considered.

TECHNOLOGY SOLUTIONS At present, there are two commercial technologies available that can further minimize unintended burns. The first one addresses the problems of insulation failure and capacitive coupling in monopolar laparoscopy. The system consists of 5- and 10-mm active electrodes with various tip designs that have integrated a shield into the electrode shaft. The shield is continuously monitored for both insulation defects and capacitive coupling; should a fault condition occur, the system deactivates the electrosurgical generator. Also available is a separate 7-mm shield, which can be introduced over existing 5-mm active electrodes. All potential complications from insulation failure or capacitive coupling in zones 2 and 3 are eliminated by the separate shield and the continuous monitoring system, whereas the integrated electrodes also monitor zone 4 or that portion of the electrode in the surgeon's hand. Although this system does not address endoscopic techniques, the use of this system will virtually eliminate all complications resulting from insulation failure and capacitive coupling in monopolar laparoscopic procedures.

The other technology that virtually eliminates all three problems (insulation failure, capacitive coupling, and direct coupling) is bipolar electrosurgery. Most bipolar electrodes are manufactured such that current is carried by two small insulated wires encased in a metal, insulated sheath; therefore, insulation defects in the sheath do not lead to complications because the sheath carries no RF currents. Capacitive coupling is also eliminated as the current flow in the bipolar connections occurs in two directions (ie, from the generator to the active electrode and from the active electrode to the generator). This flow is in opposite directions, and therefore, the induced currents are canceled. The likelihood of any direct coupling is also greatly reduced. If bipolar electrodes touch a metal object in the operative field—for example, a laparoscope—current simply flows from one electrode to the metal and returns to the generator via the second electrode. In this situation, current does not flow to the patient. Various bipolar electrodes are manufactured, such as hooks, needles, coagulators, biopsy forceps, snares, forceps, and scissors that mechanically cut and employ bipolar coagulation.

Bipolar electrodes have an added advantage over monopolar electrodes in that they typically cause less damage to surrounding tissue. Minimizing the amount of tissue necrosis may be particularly important when working in close proximity to delicate tissue, such as nerves, or during coagulation in hollow organs. These electrodes operate at significantly lower power settings than do monopolar electrodes, and therefore, the extent of lateral and deep tissue necrosis can be minimized.[12,17] If additional coagulation is needed, longer activation times may be employed to increase the amount of tissue necrosis. Bipolar electrodes also work well in conductive solutions, whereas monopolar electrodes require nonconductive solutions.

CONCLUSION

RF current has been used to cut and coagulate tissue for nearly a century, but technological innovations in generators and instruments have enabled the use of electrosurgery in new, minimally invasive procedures. These innovations, especially in generators, place added demands on surgeons to become familiar with their equipment. With minimally invasive procedures, poorly understood electrosurgical complications have arisen. Although analogous problems are seen in open procedures, the incidence of these complications is low and they are typically minor. In laparoscopy and endoscopy, however, electrosurgical complications can lead to serious morbidity, and even death. Various techniques can be employed to aid the surgeon in minimizing monopolar electrosurgical injuries, yet even good technique cannot prevent all electrosurgical complications. Two technologies are available to aid the surgeon in greatly decreasing the potential for post-procedural electrosurgical complications: an actively monitored shielding system for monopolar laparoscopic electrodes and the use of bipolar electrosurgery in laparoscopy and endoscopy. Although improved technology will aid surgeons in decreasing the potential for internal electrosurgical burns, there is no substitute for a well-trained, informed surgeon.

REFERENCES

1. d'Arsonval MA. Action physiologique des courants alternatifs. Soc Biol (Paris) 1891;43:283–6.
2. Rivière AJ. Action des courants de haute fréquence et des effleures du résonateur Oudin sur certaines tumeurs malignes. J Med Interne 1900;4:776–7.
3. Clark WL. Oscillatory desiccation in the treatment of accessible malignant growths and minor surgical conditions: A new electrical effect. J Adv Ther 1911;29:169–83.
4. Beer E. Removal of neoplasms of the urinary bladder. A new method employing high frequency (Oudin) currents through a catheterizing cystoscope. JAMA 1910;54:1768–74.
5. Young HH. A new procedure. Punch operation for small prostatic bars and contracture of prostatic orifice. JAMA 1913;60:253–7.
6. Stevens AR. On the value of cauterization of high frequency current in certain cases of prostatic obstruction. N Y Med J 1913;98:170–2.
7. Bugbee HG. The relief of vesical obstruction in selected cases. N Y State J Med 1913;13:410–7.
8. Stern M. Resection of obstructions at the vesical orifice. JAMA 1926;87:1726–9.
9. McLean AJ. The Bovie electrosurgical current generator: Some underlying principles and results. Arch Surg 1929;18:1863–73.
10. Cushing H. Meningiomas arising from the olfactory groove and their removal by the aid of electrosurgery. Lancet 1927;1:329–39.
11. Cushing H. Electrosurgery as an aid to the removal of intracranial tumors. With a preliminary note on a new surgical-current generator by W.T. Bovie. Surg Gynecol Obstet 1928 47:751–84.
12. Tucker RD, Kramolowsky EV, Bedell E, Platz CE. A comparison of urologic application of bipolar versus monopolar five French electrosurgical probes. J Urol 1989;141:662–5.
13. McLean AJ. Characteristics of adequate electrosurgical current. Am J Surg 1932;18:417–41.
14. Tucker RD, Voyles CR, Silvis SE. Capacitive coupled stray currents during laparoscopic and endoscopic electrosurgical procedures. Biomed Instrum Technol 1992;26:303–11.
15. Voyles CR, Tucker RD. Education and engineering solutions for potential problems with laparoscopic monopolar electrosurgery. Am J Surg 1992;164:57–62.
16. Barlow DE. Endoscopic applications of electrosurgery: A review of basic principles. Gastrointest Endosc 1982;28:73–6.
17. Tucker RD, Kramolowsky EV, Platz CE. In vivo effect of 5 French bipolar and monopolar electrosurgical probes on the porcine bladder. Urol Res 1990;18:291–4.

8

Sedoanalgesia: An Adjunct to Modern Endourology

Ronald A. Miller, MS, FRCS, FRGS

Sedoanalgesia was developed in response to the increasing demand for cost-efficient minimally invasive surgery, office surgery, and rapid complication-free recovery.[1] We have now used this technique involving topical injected local anesthetics in combination with systemic analgesics and sedatives in 8,000 procedures. In this chapter, the pharmacology of the drugs, techniques of administration, and management of patients undergoing endoscopic procedures using sedoanalgesia will be discussed.

Use of general, spinal, epidural, and local anesthetics in urologic procedures is well established. However, cardiopulmonary problems and the status of elderly and medically compromised patients, who constitute 33% of urologic patients, limit the use of standard anesthetic techniques, particularly for same-day surgery. Spinal and epidural anesthetics are contraindicated in patients with severe cardiac problems and restrict the early mobilization that is characteristic of same-day surgery. Although topical local anesthetics are commonly used, they are often unsatisfactory for procedures such as rigid therapeutic endoscopy. Not only do patients experience considerable discomfort, but they also are prone to severe anxiety symptoms,[2] which can exacerbate problems.

Sedoanalgesia (analgosedation monitored anesthetic care) was developed specifically for urologic procedures. This technique involves preoperative sedation using midazolam to ensure sedation, amnesia, relaxation, and anxiolysis. The therapeutic effects of midazolam can be complemented by systemic oral, rectal, or intramuscular analgesics. Low-trauma, low-profile instrumentation permits the administration of injectable local anesthetics; thus, the majority of lower urinary tract endoscopic procedures can be carried out in a calm and comfortable patient without the need for general or spinal anesthetics.

MIDAZOLAM

Midazolam, a short-acting benzodiazepine, is preferable to diazepam because of its shorter half-life (2 hours). Its effects are dose dependent and related to the number of benzodiazepine receptor sites occupied (Table 8-1).

The aim of sedoanalgesia is to produce a calm, anxiety-free patient and a degree of amnesia. The amnesiac effect is not dependable with the use of ideal doses; approximately 30% of patients will have either full or partial recall of the procedure. For this reason, effective local anesthesia is vital. The mean plasma half-life of midazolam is 2 to 3 hours in comparison with 24 to 48 hours for diazepam, for which the desmethyl derivative is an active metabolite. This makes midazolam ideal for ambulatory surgery. Because midazolam is water soluble, intravenous injection is not painful. Its onset of action, however, is slightly slower than that of diazepam. When it is injected intravenously, the peak effects are not achieved for approximately 5 minutes. Midazolam is considerably more potent than diazepam; approximately one-half to one-third of the dose is required to yield the same effect.

Midazolam may be administered orally, nasally, rectally, intravenously, or intramuscularly. The oral preparation is not licensed in the United Kingdom, however. I prefer intramuscular administration, which requires a lag period of 20 to 30 minutes to achieve the peak effect, but is far gentler and has a more gradual onset of sedation than intravenous administration, especially in patients who are elderly and infirm. The margin of safety and the beneficial effects of midazolam can be increased by intramuscular administration before the patient is brought to the operating room. Patients who are normally anxious and tense will therefore arrive calm, relaxed, and possibly asleep. In clinical practice, the dose ranges from 0.025 to 0.05 mg/kg body weight for intravenous administration and 0.05 to 0.12 mg/kg body weight for intramuscular administration. Typical doses are 2 to 5 mg intravenously and 5 to 8 mg intramuscularly.

For intravenous injection, a bolus injection of 2 to 3 mg of midazolam is usually given, supplemented by 0.05 mg progressively until the patient

Table 8-1 Dose-Related Effects of Midazolam	
Effect	Receptor Occupancy (%)
Low Dose	
Anxiolysis Anticonvulsan	20–30
Slight sedation Reduced attention Amnesia	25–50
High Dose	
Intense sedation Muscle relaxation Anesthesia	60–90

has reached the required level of sedation. Often the patient has already received the loading dose of intramuscular midazolam, which may not be sufficient. I therefore give incremental doses of 0.5 mg and wait at least 2 to 3 minutes to assess the effect.

The primary disadvantage of midazolam is that it causes respiratory depression, which is dose related and to some extent unpredictable. Thus, patients must be carefully monitored to ensure they do not become oxygen desaturated. Opioid drugs interact with midazolam and other benzodiazepines and potentiate their sedative and, therefore, their respiratory depressant effects. Although this synergism can be used to good effect, surgeons using sedoanalgesia without an anesthesiologist in attendance should avoid this combination. If opioids are used, midazolam in a dose of 15 to 20% of the normal range is appropriate. Oral analgesics such as acetaminophen or codeine and its nonsteroidal anti-inflammatory drug derivatives are more appropriate in this setting.

FLUMAZENIL

Flumazenil is a specific water-soluble benzodiazepine antagonist. It works by competitive antagonism at the benzodiazepine receptor sites. This remarkable drug will reverse the effects of midazolam, depending on the plasma concentration.[3,4] The minimal dose will reverse anxiolysis and mild sedation. The maximal dose will reverse muscle relaxation and deep sedation. The half-life of flumazenil is approximately 1 hour as opposed to 2 to 3 hours for midazolam. This suggests that resedation may follow reversal. However, the low dose of midazolam used during the procedure presents no clinical problem. Intramuscular administration is ideal since the patient is given midazolam approximately H hour prior to the operation, and the procedure is not likely to exceed the drug's action. Thus, by the time flumazenil is given for reversal, the half-life of midazolam has been decreased by H to 1 hour. Flumazenil at this stage has never been associated with resedation in my experience. My preference is to give flumazenil as a bolus injection of 0.5 mg in a 5 mL ampule. It takes between 45 and 160 seconds to reverse the effect of midazolam. Patients who are asleep become fully alert and oriented within approximately 1 minute. Flumazenil should be avoided in patients who are epileptic, and care should be taken in patients who are benzodiazepine abusers, since an acute withdrawal syndrome could be precipitated.

In emergency situations, flumazenil can be used for quick reversal when oxygen levels are falling to ensure a complication-free recovery in the critically ill patient.

ANALGESICS

Systemic analgesia is a critical component of sedoanalgesia. In recent years I have used nonsteroidal anti-inflammatory drugs for this purpose. They can be administered orally, intramuscularly, or intrarectally. For rectal administration, I routinely use diclofenac, but ketorolac is equally effective and can be added to the premedication regimen. The prolonged action of diclofenac ensures a smooth post-operative recovery. Although some have expressed theoretical concerns about prolonged bleeding times in endoscopic patients, I have not encountered this problem. Gastric intolerance must be taken into account in patients who have ulcers; in addition, its use should be avoided in asthmatic patients. Other oral opiate agents are all suitable, but they must be used with extreme caution because of their synergistic and respiratory depressive effects. The use of opiates should be confined to cases in which there is full anesthetic backup.

LOCAL ANESTHETICS

Both lidocaine and marcaine are incorporated into the sedoanalgesia regimen to produce local anesthesia.[5,6] Two percent lidocaine gel is used for surface urethral anesthesia. In our unit, we use Instillagel (Farco Pharma GmBH, Germany) or the accordion (Astra Pharmaceutical Products, Westborough, Mass.), both of which have excellent solubility that permits a thorough optical inspection of the lower urinary tract. If the endoscopic procedure is anticipated to be lengthy, 0.5% bupivacaine can be mixed with KY jelly or added to the urethral lidocaine instillation.[7,8] Approximately 15% of the total dose in the urinary tract is absorbed; however, this amount can reach 30% if the urinary tract is surgically breached. Plasma levels reach their maximum between 70 and 120 minutes. Much of the gel will be washed out by the irrigating fluids used during endoscopy. Therefore, I apply two 10 mL dosages of gel at approximately 10- to 15-minute intervals. The first dose will relax the sphincter area, and the second dose will lubricate the posterior urethra and enter the bladder itself. Bupivacaine and lidocaine are both cardiotoxic if injected in high doses. Toxic effects can be anticipated in the average adult when the plasma level exceeds 700 mg of lidocaine and 100 mg of bupivacaine. It is therefore safe to use 2 ampules containing 10 mL of 0.5% bupivacaine (50 mg each) and 2 to 3 ampules containing 10 mL of 1% plain lidocaine (100 mg each) for infiltration. If bupivacaine and lidocaine are combined, their effects can be potentiated; therefore, slightly smaller amounts should be used. Bupivacaine has a

longer action and longer onset of action. Conversely, lidocaine acts rapidly, but its effects last for only about 90 minutes. Therefore, a combination of the two has distinct advantages.

The maximal amounts of local anesthetic used for major endoscopic procedures such as transurethral prostatectomy in our unit are as follows:

- Two syringes of 10 mL lidocaine Instillagel preparation (urethra topical)
- 10 mL of 0.5% plain bupivacaine (subtrigonal)
- One ampule of 10 mL 1% plain lidocaine
- Two ampules of 1% lidocaine in a 1__:__400,000 adrenaline solution

In more than 1,000 procedures in which this regimen was used, no patients experienced complications. The operator/sedationist must, however, be prepared for anaphylactic and unexpected drug reactions, including cardiac effects, when these agents are used. The use of 1__:__400,000 adrenaline allows greater amounts of lidocaine to be used and also ensures hemostatic control, which is an important consideration during surgery. This can be achieved by using 5 mL of 1% lidocaine mixed with 5 mL of 1__:__200,000 of adrenaline and lidocaine to make 10 mL of a 1__:__400,000 adrenaline and lidocaine solution. All endoscopic injections must be made using a 10 mL syringe, since prostatic tissue resistance often precludes the use of a 20 mL syringe.

PRE-OPERATIVE PREPARATION

Ideally a pre-medication dose is given to ensure that the patient is calm and antibiotic coverage and systemic analgesia are adequate for the immediate post-operative period. The sedative component, midazolam, is given 20 to 30 minutes pre-operatively by intramuscular injection according to the dosage schedule listed in Table 8-2. In young patients, the typical dose is 5 to 8 mg, and in the elderly it averages 3 to 5 mg. A lower dose should always be used if there is any doubt, because it can always be supplemented if necessary. All patients receive oxygen at a rate of 4 L/min by nasal cannula, which dramatically reduces the chance of desaturation and enhances the safety of the procedure.

The use of rectal diclofenac for systemic analgesia prevents problems with gastric intoler-

Table 8-2 Recommended Doses of Midazolam*	
Midazolam Dose (mg/kg body weight)	Type of Patient
0.1–0.12	Young, fit, and anxious
0.1	Young and fit
0.075	Elderly and fit
0.025–0.5	Elderly and unfit

*Patients > 80 years of age should receive no more than 3 mg of intramuscular pre-medication. In patients with upper respiratory diseases, the dose should be reduced still further. When in doubt, a lower rather than a higher dose should be administered.

ance. Nonsteroidal anti-inflammatory drugs are contraindicated in patients with upper gastrointestinal ulceration and chronic indigestion and in patients with asthma. Alternatively, codeine derivatives and acetaminophen can be used.

Most of the endoscopic procedures performed in our unit are same-day or ambulatory surgery. This poses the risk of gram-negative septicemia in the early post-operative period. Patients are therefore given aminoglycoside antibiotics (80 mg gentamicin).

In male patients, 10 to 15 minutes before surgery 10 mL of lidocaine gel is applied to the urethra and a penile clamp is placed just above the corona of the glans to prevent the gel from leaking out. In patients suspected of having urethral strictures, the gel should be applied by the medical staff in the operating room. After being premedicated, the patient should be kept in a quiet, preferably darkened room to induce sleep or total relaxation before being taken to the operating room or endoscopy suite.

TECHNIQUE

The operating room lights should be dimmed to avoid startling the patient on arrival. After the patient's chart is reviewed, venous access is established. A pulse oximeter is attached to the patient's finger to monitor oxygen saturation and pulse rate. The surgeon in our unit now assumes full responsibility for the patient's welfare, and he should have a clear view of the readout throughout the procedure. The surgeon should be fully trained in cardiopulmonary resuscitation, and a trained assistant (doctor, nurse, technician, or anesthetic staff member) is designated to continuously check the patient's airway and level of consciousness. If an anesthetist is in attendance, he or she assumes this role.

The patient should be calm with his head resting on the pillow and the oxygen saturation level at 97 to 100%. Another tube of lidocaine gel is now applied to the urethra, which passes through the sphincter into the bladder. If the patient is still uncomfortable and anxious, more midazolam can be administered intravenously. We use 10 mg of midazolam in 5 mL vials (2.5 mL, or 5 mg, is drawn into a 10 mL syringe and diluted to 10 mL with normal saline solution). The 10 mL syringe now contains 5 mg of midazolam, or 2 mg/mL. Incremental doses of 1 to 2 mL are given until the patient is calm. Within 5 minutes, the action of midazolam should have taken full effect. Care should be taken not to oversedate the patient. The attendant can engage the patient in conversation to distract his attention from the procedure.

If the procedure is performed in the endoscopy suite, the environment should be warm, dark, quiet, and peaceful. Although some patients seem to like background music, we prefer that an attendant engage the patient in a nonprocedural-related conversation. Monitoring includes pulse oximetry and in major procedures blood pressure and ECG monitoring.

If an anesthetist is not present, the surgeon should be thoroughly familiar with the guidelines set forth by the Royal College of Surgeons concerning sedation[9]: "Sedation is a technique in which the use of a drug, or drugs, produces a state of depression of the central nervous system enabling treatment to be carried out, but during which communication is maintained such that the patient will respond to commands throughout the period of sedation. The drugs and techniques used for sedation should carry a margin of safety wide enough to render unintended loss of consciousness unlikely."

Anesthesia is defined as follows: "Any technique which exceeds this definition of sedation and where contact with the patient is lost may be regarded as general anaesthesia with all its attendant consequences and responsibilities."

Thus, any patient who does not respond to verbal commands is considered anesthetized and therefore legally should be under the care of an anesthesiologist. If the oxygen saturation rate falls as a consequence of oversedation, small doses of flumazenil can be used to "lighten" the patient. Medication is administered as 0.5 mg in a 5 mL syringe. We use 1 mL (ie, 1 mg) initially.

Elderly patients may have a paradoxical reaction to midazolam at higher doses and become agitated. This can be reversed with flumazenil administered as previously described.

All endoscopy suites must be fully equipped for cardiopulmonary resuscitation. Defibrillators, drugs, and suction apparatus must be checked regularly and maintained. Staff training for serious emergencies is essential.

THE MILLER INTEGRATED CYSTOSCOPE Both rigid and flexible endoscopy can be performed. In general, small, well-lubricated endoscopes are better tolerated than their larger equivalents. The Miller integrated cystoscope (GU Manufacturing, London, England) was specifically designed for this purpose.[10,11] This low-profile, smooth 17 French endoscope has a single 9F instrument irrigation channel (Figure 8-1). The channel and optical lens (10 degrees down, 110-degree field) are arranged so that the instruments leaving the instrument channel are under immediate optical control, unlike conventional rigid cystoscopes.

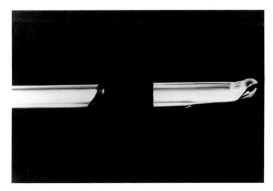

Figure 8-1 Left: Conventional 21F cystoscope. Right: Miller integrated cystoscope. Note the smooth contours of the 17F Miller integrated cystoscope and its terminal instrument port, which allows instrumentation to come under immediate optical control.

With the straight instrument channel, rigid, durable accessories can be used. Since the instrument is a single unit, it is easy to maintain and use. All accessories are passed down the instrument channel without the need for any assembly or dismantling. This precludes excessive endoscopic movements and ensures greater patient comfort.

Accessories include contoured stone, biopsy (Figure 8-2), and toothed forceps for stent removal; all of these forceps have scissor handles and action. A rigid insulated ball and knife diathermy probe permit coagulation cutting. Both forward-cutting and reverse-cutting (blades sharpened on reverse side) scissors can be used for cutting the ureteral orifice, tailoring stents, and opening urethral diverticula. The reverse-cutting scissors can be used to perform a 35F urethrotomy in female patients with minimal trauma. The scissors are opened in the bladder and drawn through the urethra in the open position and the urethra is cut with the back blade. The most important accessories are the Miller Endoneedles (Figure 8-3). The thin-bore Endoneedle allows trigonal and bladder infiltration of local anesthetic. It has a fine beveled point and a rigid stem. The thick-bore Endoneedle is more robust and can be used for prostatic injection of local anesthetic and for injection of Teflon and similar substances using pressurized syringes. The Birch-Miller Electrotest needle is an insulated needle with a sharp beveled tip that can be used for infiltration of local anesthetic. The block can be tested by diathermy current. This needle is especially useful for bladder tumor injections and bladder neck incisions.

In addition, the unique Miller Endoknife converts the instrument into an optical urethrotome at a fraction of the cost of conventional instruments. The knife has a disposable blade that can be rotated in both the 6- and 12-o'clock positions, unlike conventional instruments (Figures 8-4 and 8-5).

In an adequately relaxed patient, the external sphincter should be negotiated with ease. In a tense young patient, incremental doses of 0.5 mg midazolam may be necessary. Having the patient cough while hydrostatic pressure is being applied is also helpful. The endoscope can then be used in the traditional fashion. First the dome of the bladder is carefully inspected, since optical control will be lost as the bladder fills. This maneuver also precludes angulation of the telescope in the prostatic urethra, which is uncomfortable for the patient.

The instrument channel will accept double-J stents, ureteral catheters, and electrohydraulic and laser probes. It is ideal for the insertion of both metal and plastic endoprostatic stents and can also be used to retrieve stents with the aid of toothed grasping forceps.

If the bladder becomes full or at the conclusion of the procedure, it can be emptied with suction applied to the instrument channel or by gravity using abdominal pressure. The Miller integrated cystoscope cannot be used to wash the bladder out.

If areas of the urethra are not accessible, the Miller integrated cystoscope can be introduced suprapubically using a Bard Supracath set (Bard

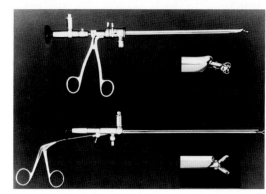

Figure 8-2 Top: Conventional cystoscope with biopsy forceps. Bottom: Miller integrated cystoscope with biopsy forceps. Insets: Close-up views show the infinitely preferable position of the biopsy forceps in the Miller integrated cystoscope. The biopsy forceps of the conventional cystoscope are at least 2 cm from the lens assembly itself.

Urological, Covington, Ga.). This is particularly useful in patients with stone-encrusted prostatic endostents. The stents can be freed from the bladder using electrohydraulic lithotriptors and withdrawn either through the bladder or via the urethra.

The entire lower urinary tract can be injected using the Miller integrated cystoscope and Endoneedle. In general, bleeding is undesirable when performing endoscopic procedures under sedoanalgesia, since the view will quickly become obscured because of the relatively small caliber of the Miller integrated cystoscope (Figure 8-6). For this reason, adrenaline solutions are preferred for the local anesthetic. I have noted that 20 mL of 1__:__400,000 adrenaline will not affect the ECG reading. In this regimen, 5 mL of 1% plain lidocaine is mixed in a 10 mL syringe with 5 mL of 1__:__200,000 adrenaline and lidocaine to yield a 1__:__400,000 solution. Two 10 mL syringes can be safely used.

A circumferential injection of 20 mL of 1__:__400,000 lidocaine and adrenaline around the base of the bladder tumor allows safe injection and resection using a 24 to 25F conventional resectoscope. In addition, it is possible to avoid the obturator response by deep injection of 1% plain lidocaine outside the bladder. Care must be taken to avoid injecting a vessel directly.

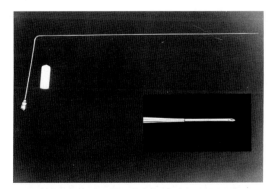

Figure 8-3 Miller Endoneedle. Inset: Note the hub on the needle itself. This is buried in the tissue and allows excellent subtrigonal injections beneath the mucosal surface of the bladder.

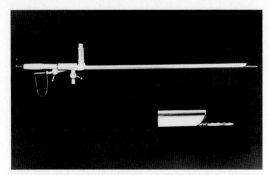

Figure 8-4 Miller Endoknife. Inset: Close-up view shows the blade of the knife, which can be rotated 360 degrees for cutting at both the 6- and 12-o'clock positions.

Although the Miller integrated cystoscope is ideal for most diagnostic and therapeutic endoscopic procedures performed under sedoanalgesia, it is contraindicated in patients with severe concurrent bleeding; these patients are unpredictable and conventional anesthesia is a wiser choice.

TRANSURETHRAL PROSTATECTOMY AND BLADDER NECK INCISION We have performed more than 600 transurethral prostatectomies using sedoanalgesia.[12,13] The general requirements are the same as described previously. Patients should be monitored by an anesthetist, since they are generally classified as ASA 3 or 4. An intravenous line should be placed and pulse, blood pressure, and heart rate monitored.

The Miller integrated cystoscope may be used for the procedure. The prostate is assessed and patients with prostate glands .40 g are excluded. Very large middle lobes with an extensive intravesicle component can be difficult to anesthetize adequately. In general, patients with complex glands should not undergo this procedure. Three syringes of local anesthetic are generally required. A fine-bore Endoneedle is used to inject 10 mL of 1% plain lidocaine or 10 mL of 0.5% bupivacaine into the trigone. The distribution is 3 mL lateral to the right ureteric orifice, 3 mL lateral to the left ureteric orifice, and 4 mL in the central trigonal area.

If the trigone remains sensitive, a supplemental injection of 10 mL bupivacaine or lidocaine can be given. Bupivacaine must not be injected intravenously since this can precipitate cardiac arrest.

The Miller integrated cystoscope is withdrawn into the prostatic cavity and 5 mL of 1__:__400,000 lidocaine and adrenaline is injected into the bladder neck at the 9- and 3-o'clock positions. The cystoscope is withdrawn further until the verumontanum is visualized and 5 mL is infiltrated into the floor of the bladder neck and prostate and 5 mL into the lateral lobes. The lidocaine and adrenaline solution is infiltrated again. Only 10 mL syringes can be used since the prostatic tissue is resistant to injection.

The external sphincter, which is still active in the conscious patient, is dilated to 28F using well-lubricated male sounds to overcome sphincter resistance to the resectoscope. This maneuver is also necessary in patients undergoing transurethral resection of bladder tumors. A 25 or 24F resectoscope is now used to perform a standard transurethral prostatectomy. Removal of slightly smaller chips requires less contact with the cutting loop. Prolonged exposure of the prostatic sidewall to the electrical discharge can lead to spreading of the current to the pelvic nerves, which can be painful. When sedoanalgesia is used, the patient may experience considerable discomfort if the operator breaches the capsule or is even working very close to the capsule as a result of current spread and nerve stimulation.

Passing a catheter at the close of the procedure requires meticulous technique, since sphincter activity is present in the conscious patient and the pelvic floor will tend to rise, which can cause the catheter to pass under the bladder through the thinned bladder neck region.

Ideal candidates for this procedure are elderly men in whom the resected weight is anticipated to be 10 to 30 g. If the procedure is prolonged, the patient can develop leg cramps, which can pose a serious problem. It is essential that the operating team be able to converse with the patient.

The local anesthetic injections can be quite uncomfortable. If the patient experiences excessive pain during the injections, it is wise to abandon the full procedure and limit the surgery to resecting the bladder neck, performing a bladder neck incision, or placing an endoprostatic stent. The alternative is conventional anesthesia, which should be a planned procedure.

The addition of small doses of rapidly acting opioids such as alfentanil can facilitate the procedure and prolong the analgesia. However, it is unsafe to use these agents without an anesthetist present.

During this procedure, blood and abdominal pressures may be elevated. There is a greater tendency for bleeding under such circumstances. Adrenaline counteracts this tendency and ensures excellent superficial hemostasis. At the conclusion of the procedure, blood and abdominal pressures stabilize as the patient recovers, in contrast to patients undergoing standard transurethral prostatectomy in whom coughing, straining, and restlessness cause pressures to rise. If hemostasis is maintained during the procedure, post-operative bleeding is extremely unlikely when the

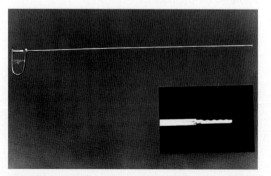

Figure 8-5 Disposable Endoknife with a spring handle. Inset: Close-up view shows how the blade can rotate within its inner tube.

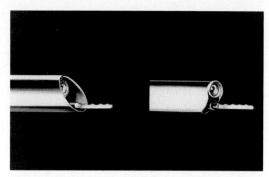

Figure 8-6 Left: Conventional urethrotome. Right: Miller integrated cystoscope. Note the difference in the caliber of the scopes.

operation is carried out under sedoanalgesia. In addition, high venous and abdominal pressures will counteract fluid absorption. The abdominal relaxation and relative hypotension as a consequence of low pelvic venous pressure associated with general and spinal anesthesia will encourage fluid absorption.

ALTERNATIVES TO TRANSURETHRAL PROSTATECTOMY Bladder neck incisions can be performed using the same anesthetic block described earlier. The insulated Endoknife and Miller integrated cystoscope are excellent tools for this purpose. Microwave hyperthermia, laser prostatectomy, balloon dilation, and radiofrequency heating are all facilitated by the prostatic nerve block.

URETHRAL STRICTURES: SPECIAL CONSIDERATIONS If a urethral stricture is present, the posterior urethra may not be fully exposed to the lidocaine gel. Pressurizing the lidocaine into the urethra may cause bruising and bleeding. In these cases, 10 mL of 1% lidocaine can be injected into the urethra along with an additional 10 mL of the gel and 1% lidocaine or 0.5% bupivacaine. Bupivacaine greatly aids in prolonging urethral anesthesia. Otherwise the stricture is released in the same fashion as under direct vision until the scar tissue is removed. Then dilators can be used to split the remaining tissue in the line of the previous incisions.

UPPER TRACT MANIPULATION It is standard practice in our unit to perform ureteral catheterization and obtain retrograde films under sedoanalgesia. The placement of double-J stents and difficult stone manipulations can, however, cause considerable patient discomfort. An opioid supplement is frequently necessary, and thus an anesthetist should be present. Semirigid and flexible ureteroscopy can also be performed under these circumstances. A mixture of 2% lidocaine gel and 0.5% bupivacaine is generally injected prior to manipulation. This mixture should be flushed out with 10 mL of 2% lidocaine after a few minutes to ensure a good endoscopic view.

URETHRAL MANIPULATIONS IN FEMALES Contrary to popular belief, endoscopic procedures in female patients can be challenging. Pre-medication with midazolam will relax the patient and facilitate endoscopy to some degree. The legs should be manipulated as little as possible and they should be supported rather than placed in the conventional lithotomy loops. In our unit, 2% lidocaine gel is applied to the inside of the urethra and the entire periurethral and vulval area. A topical 4% lidocaine spray is then used. Because this spray is alcohol based, it is essential to coat the vulval area with gel before use.

Before a urethrotomy is performed, 10 mL of bupivacaine is injected into the subtrigonal lesion followed by injection of 10 mL of lidocaine and adrenaline in the paraurethral area using a fine-bore needle. Otis urethrotomy and diathermy of the trigone and carbuncles can be performed with no patient discomfort. The reverse-cutting scissors are less traumatic than the conventional Otis instrument for performing urethrotomy. Patients usually experience little pain or voiding difficulties in the post-operative period. In a series of 300 patients operated on in our unit, only 4 were unable to void spontaneously after surgery.

POST-OPERATIVE CARE

Normally, patients recover spontaneously within H to 1 hour. This is especially desirable in patients who have undergone a major endoscopic procedure, since they will remain quiet and calm in the immediate post-operative period. Administration of flumazenil reverses the midazolam-induced sedation instantly. Although it may become necessary to use small perioperative doses of flumazenil to lighten sedation and reverse the agitation induced by midazolam in the elderly, the most important role of flumazenil is post-operative reversal of sedation. Its use is indicated in patients with low oxygen saturation rates and those with an ASA score of 3 or 4 in whom any degree of sedation may be detrimental. Reversal also has significant logistic and economic implications, enabling patients to leave the operating room without assistance or in a wheelchair without the need for bed rest. This is a radical departure from the usual post-operative scenario. Patients can be divided into four groups:

Push in (IM sedation)	Push out (no reversal)
Walk in (IV sedation)	Push out (no reversal)
Push in (IM sedation)	Walk out (IV reversal)
Walk in (IV sedation)	Walk out (IV reversal)

The push-in/push-out approach is conventional for elderly inpatients undergoing major endoscopic procedures such as transurethral prostatectomy in the operating room. It is also appropriate for elderly ambulatory patients whose health status is poor.[14] The walk-in/push-out approach is indicated in healthy young ambulatory patients who require a short post-operative stay in the recovery unit. The push-in/walk-out method is applicable for elderly, anxious, and unfit patients who have been sedated pre-operatively; it permits efficient post-ambulatory handling. In healthy young patients without catheters, a walk-in/walk-out approach can be used.

Endoscopic urologic procedures performed under sedoanalgesia dramatically change the customary post-operative dynamics and decrease staff requirements. No problems have been encountered in our experience with 3,000 patients who have remained in the recovery ward for H to 1 hour while oxygen is administered via nasal cannula. In the last 6,000 patients, the length of stay in the recovery unit was only 10 to 30 minutes.

The increasing number of ASA 3 and 4 patients being managed on an ambulatory basis makes written post-operative instructions and guidelines essential. Patients need to have someone available to accompany them home and offer support as needed. Patients should not drive for 24 hours or engage in strenuous activities for 48 hours. In a recent study of 2,100 ASA 3 and 4 patients over 80 years of age, we found that pain, hemorrhage, and infection posed no problem. Only 1 patient with a urethral prostatic stent was readmitted because of urinary retention.[15]

CONCLUSION

On average, 70% of urology patients are candidates for sedoanalgesia. The shortened anesthesia and recovery times are cost effective and permit a larger case load. As minimally invasive surgery expands, the use of sedoanalgesia will have greater applicability and will likely include all scrotal and genital surgery.

Staff training, careful patient monitoring, appropriate doses of midazolam, and the use of oxygen via nasal cannula are key to the success of this technique. Reversal with flumazenil makes for more efficient post-operative care and increases the margin of safety.

REFERENCES

1. Birch BRP, Anson KM, Miller RA. Sedoanalgesia in urology: a safe cost-effective alternative to general anaesthesia. A review of 1020 cases. Br J Urol 1990;66:342–50.
2. Birch BRP, Chakrabarty R, Miller RA. Anxiety in patients undergoing local anaesthetic cystoscopy. J Day Surg 1993;3:15–7.
3. Birch BRP, Anson KM, Gelister J, et al. The role of midazolam and flumazenil in urology. Acta Anaesthesiol Scand Suppl 1990;92:25–32.
4. Birch BRP, Anson KM, Clifford E, Miller RA. Day-case surgery: enhanced recovery with flumazenil. J R Soc Med 1990;83:436–8.
5. Lignocaine hydrochloride. In: Reynolds JEF, editor. The extra pharmacopoeia, 30th ed. London: Martindale; 1993. p. 1212–7.
6. Bupivacaine hydrochloride. In: Reynolds JEF, editor. The extra Pharmacopoeia, 30th ed. London: Martindale; 1993. p. 1209–11.
7. Dawkins G, Harrison NW, Ansell W. Urethral anaesthesia with topical bupivacaine. A role for longer-acting agents. Br J Urol 1995;76:484–7.
8. Birch BRP, Miller RA. Absorption characteristics of lignocaine following intravesical instillation. Scand J Urol Nephrol 1994;28:359–64.
9. Royal College of Surgeons of England. Guidelines for sedation by non-anaesthetists. June 1993, p 3.
10. Miller RA, Coptcoat M, Parry J, et al. The integrated cystoscope. An alternative to conventional and fibreoptic cystoscopy. Br J Urol 1987;60:128–31.
11. Miller RA. Development theory and design of urological endoscopes. In: Chisholm GA, editor. Scientific foundations of urology, 3rd ed. London: Heineman; 1988. p. 659–66.
12. Birch BRP, Gelister J, Parker C, Miller RA. Transurethral resection of prostate under local anaesthetic (sedoanalgesia). Experience in 100 cases. Urology 1991;38:113–8.
13. Birch BRP, Miller RA. Transurethral prostatectomy under local anaesthetic. In: Shah J, editor. Prostatic surgery. London: Blackwell Scientific; 1994. p. 131–41.
14. Briggs T, Anson KM, Jones A, et al. Urological day surgery in the elderly and medically unfit using sedoanalgesia: what are the limits? Br J Urol 1995;75:708–11.
15. Birch BRP, Miller RA. Walk-in, walk-out day case genitourinary surgery with sedation reversal: a survey of patient attitudes and morbidity. Br J Urol 1994;74:648–64.

9

Informed Consent and Related Legal Issues in Laparoscopic Surgery

April Beeman Metwalli, JD

Adam R. Metwalli, MD

James F. Donovan Jr, MD

The development of laparoscopy has resulted in new and exciting surgical procedures that offer a multitude of potential benefits to patients. Careful evaluation of laparoscopic surgical techniques in comparison with analogous open surgical procedures has revealed that patients who undergo laparoscopic surgery typically have decreased postoperative pain and morbidity, earlier hospital discharge, and a more rapid return to preoperative activity relative to their open surgery counterparts.[1–7] Beside the risks associated with any surgical procedure, laparoscopy entails specific disadvantages that must be considered. In addition to longer operating times, equipment costs and surgeons' fees may be higher, and injuries to major vascular structures, the gastrointestinal tract, or the urinary system may occur.[3,4,8] Familiarity with new instruments and surgical techniques requires specific training and additional practical experience. In addition to possible complications that are specific to laparoscopy, the experience of the laparoscopist has been strongly correlated with outcome, perhaps even more so than in open surgery.[9–11] Therefore, these issues must be discussed with potential candidates for laparoscopic surgery in order to obtain informed consent. The medicolegal doctrine of informed consent dictates that the relative advantages and disadvantages of laparoscopic surgery be discussed, as compared with alternative treatment, namely open surgical procedures.[12]

INFORMED CONSENT

The doctrine of informed consent is based on the premise that every human being has the right to determine what happens to his or her body. In the seminal 1914 case of Schloendorff versus Society of New York Hospital, Justice Benjamin Cardozo wrote, "Every human being of adult years and sound mind has a right to determine what shall be done with his own body; and a surgeon who performs an operation without his patient's consent commits an assault, for which he is liable in damages."[13] As the case law regarding informed consent has evolved, so too has the definition of what constitutes such consent. In 1994, the Supreme Court of Virginia summarized the need for specificity: "The law requires informed consent, not mere consent and the failure to obtain informed consent is tantamount to no consent."[14] Such disclosure compels the physician to provide, in layman's terms, three specific elements: the nature of the procedure; reasonable alternatives to the proposed treatment (including open and laparoscopic surgery, medical therapy, and no treatment); and the relative advantages and disadvantages of each alternative. Additionally, the physician is expected to assess the patient's level of understanding, and to discuss the acceptance of the intervention by the patient.[15]

DOCUMENTATION OF CONSENT The information provided that forms the basis of an informed consent must include the risks and benefits of the proposed procedure. It is crucial that the information be sufficient in scope to allow a reasonable person to render an informed decision based on a thorough explanation of the clinical situation and the treatment options available.[16] This entails a discussion of the disease and the consequences of nontreatment versus the benefits of the proposed treatment. Next, the physician must explain the proposed operation, its risks and benefits, and how it differs from other therapeutic approaches. Finally, a physician should inform the patient of alternative methods of treatment. Naturally, all information provided to the patient should be presented in terms easily understood by the layperson. Physicians should keep in mind that many states now apply the standard of a "reasonable patient" in cases involving the issue of informed consent. In practical terms, this means that the information given should be tailored to the understanding of a reasonable person, not to members of the medical community. While there is a national trend toward the use of the "reasonable patient" standard of informed consent, it is important to note that some jurisdictions still use the "reasonable physician" or "professional community" standard in determining what is material information for purposes of informed consent. This traditional standard requires only that a physician share with a patient the information a "reasonable and minimally competent physician" would disclose in a similar cirumstance.[17] Thus, it is in each physician's best interest to be familiar with the standards in effect locally.

Listing potential complications on the consent form serves to document that the patient was forewarned of possible complications. It is understood that such risks are inherent to the procedure and that their occurrence does not imply negligence. By documenting possible complications, however, the physician has not eliminated negligence or malpractice as a possible cause of the complications. Malpractice, negligence, and medical battery claims may still result and be pursued, separately or in conjunction with an action for inadequate informed consent.[18]

A routine preoperative discussion with a patient regarding the risks and benefits of a surgical procedure often provides the necessary information for a reasonable patient to make an informed decision. In a 2001 case involving a patient who underwent a laparoscopic hernia repair, the court found that the physician appropriately repaired the right-side hernia while the patient was already undergoing laparoscopic repair of his left-side hernia. The court held that since the repair to the right side did not differ significantly from the repair to the left side, the material risks, accordingly, were similar. To the surgeon's benefit was the evidence that prior to the procedure, while obtaining the patient's informed consent, the surgeon had made it clear that one of the benefits of laparoscopic hernia repair was the ability to see both sides and that he would look for other hernias. Thus, the court held that the patient had given his informed consent to the right, as well as the left side, hernia repair.[19]

There are specific circumstances that may constitute an exception to the general rule of full disclosure under the informed consent doctrine. One such exception is referred to as "therapeutic privilege." This privilege may be invoked when full disclosure would be detrimental to the patient because of his emotional or psychological state. The physician should carefully document the reasons for nondisclosure and discuss them with the patient's family members. In addition, if a patient specifically requests that he not be informed of possible complications or alternative therapies, he may waive his right to full disclosure.

The patient should be fully informed as to who will be performing the surgery and their qualifications and experience in laparoscopy.

Whether a surgeon has performed laparoscopic procedures in the past would obviously be "material" with respect to a patient's ability to give informed consent for surgery of this type. In the case of Johnson versus Kokemoor, the Supreme Court of Wisconsin ruled in favor of a patient who became a quardriplegic following surgery to clip an enlarging brain aneuryism. The patient, Ms. Johnson, argued that she had specifically asked her surgeon about his level of experience and that he had overstated the number of similar surgeries he had performed. (The surgeon told Ms. Johnson that he had performed dozens of the procedures, when, in fact, he had performed only nine in the preceding five years.) The court ultimately held that Ms. Johnson did not give informed consent because she did not have an accurate picture of the surgeon's experience and they ruled that the level of his experience was material.[20] As laparoscopic surgery is a relatively recent addition to the urologist's armamentarium, it is not unreasonable for a patient to inquire as to the individual surgeon's actual experience with a particular operation. Information regarding specific training, post-graduate courses, or practical experience in teaching laboratories should be offered voluntarily. Adherence to the highest ethical and fiduciary standards compels the surgeon to inform a patient if a proposed procedure has not been performed previously and/or if the scheduled operation is to be the surgeon's first attempt to use a newly acquired skill and/or technology.

Failure to provide informed consent implies that pertinent information allowing a rational decision regarding treatment was not provided. If one finds that a reasonable patient would have refused treatment if he or she had been more fully informed, then lack of informed consent has been established.

The conditions under which consent is obtained are an important consideration. Ideally, a detailed discussion can take place and questions can be answered in the surgeon's office during a preoperative visit. This avoids a hurried signature on an unfamiliar consent form in the preoperative holding room. The patient must not be under the influence of substances that might impair his judgment. In the case of a minor or an incompetent adult, the legal guardian must give informed consent. In emergency situations the physician must act within the constraints of time and the patient's clinical condition to provide information to the best of his or her ability.

COMPETENCE OF THE PATIENT   The competence of the patient is a very important element of valid informed consent. Consent is not deemed to be informed if the patient in question is not competent to weigh the information and make a decision.[21] Determining whether a patient possesses the capacity to make a reasonable, informed decision regarding their medical care is always a concern, but it may become even more paramount when elderly patients are weighing surgical options. Many older adults are completely competent to make their own medical decisions; however,

any physician whose practice encompasses elderly patients should be aware of the possibility of a dementing illness or other circumstance that make competent consent impossible. One in ten individuals over the age of 65 will develop Alzheimer's disease or a related dementia, and up to 50% of patients over 85 have some form of dementia.[22] This statistic only underscores the need for a thorough, unrushed explanation of proposed treatment to ensure that the physician meets his or her duty of care not only in providing the patient with the background necessary for an informed decision, but also in assesing the patient's competence.

ADDRESSING BENEFITS AND POSSIBLE COMPLICATIONS   With respect to laparoscopic procedures, the proposed operation should be explained and compared with alternative surgical options. Benefits of laparoscopic procedures may include improved cosmetic results, shorter hospitalization and quicker return to work, and decreased post-operative pain. On the other hand, patients need to know that general anesthesia is required, operative time may be longer, and there is a risk of bladder, bowel, or vascular injury.

Each procedure carries with it specific risks and the patient should be made aware of the relative frequency of these risks. It is of equal importance that the patient be apprised by the physician of the consequences should a complication occur. For example, lymphoceles can complicate pelvic lymph node dissection regardless of whether laparoscopic or open techniques are employed. Laparoscopic pelvic lymph node dissection may carry a higher risk of vascular injury that may necessitate conversion to an open procedure, thereby requiring a longer hospital stay and recovery period.

It is acceptable to estimate the frequency of such complications in general terms, such as common, uncommon, or rare. It is inadvisable to attempt to provide precise complication rates that might underestimate the true frequency of the complication. Patients also need to understand that complication rates are based on reports in the medical literature and not necessarily the personal experience of their particular operating surgeon or institution.

The condition of the individual patient must be considered when discussing specific complications. In a patient with multiple prior abdominal surgeries, the increased risk of intraperitoneal adhesions and possible bowel injury should be discussed and a description given of specific means by which this risk may be reduced (eg, performing open laparoscopy using the Hasson technique).

In addition to explaining complications to patients, the surgeon must be familiar with these complications and their appropriate management. Information regarding management of complications can be obtained from continuing medical education course materials, published books, and reports of successful management of such complications. Managing complications with innovative but unproven techniques may be tempting, but if they fail to resolve the complica-

tion or in fact worsen the complication, they may be interpreted as deviating from the standard of care, thereby constituting malpractice.

STANDARD OF CARE

Laparoscopic surgery is no different from other areas of medical care in that the physician will be judged with respect to the standard of care in the event of an adverse outcome. A specialist such as a urologist will certainly be held to national standards for that particular specialty, as regional variations in the standard are no longer commonly recognized. Generally, a "standard of care" presupposes that a physician will act as any reasonable and prudent individual might under a given set of circumstances.[23] In the case of laparoscopy, the "reasonably prudent" standard applies to physicians who are specially trained in the field of laparoscopy. To the point, increasingly this standard has been established by fellowship-trained laparoscopists, and this level of practice would have to be met by all physicians, irrespective of formal laparoscopic training. However, currently there are no nationally recognized standards by which physicians can be certified as competent in the use of laparoscopy. As laparoscopic procedures become more established in urologic practice, minimum training requirements for residency programs and perhaps for practicing urologists may be established by the American Board of Urology.

Generally, failing to provide the recognized standard of care can be legally viewed as negligence. There are three common errors that may lead to substandard care. Foremost is attempting to perform a procedure without adequate training. Typically, training for specific procedures occurs during residency with additional credentialing ongoing after completion of residency. For many physicians, new technologies such as laparoscopy must be learned through post-graduate courses. However, simply taking a course may not meet the standard of care to employ laparoscopic techniques in practice. Often, physicians will then undergo a mentoring period during which procedures are performed under the supervision of a more experienced practitioner. A second shortcoming that prevents proper treatment is failing to consult another physician when complications or problems arise. This error can occur intraoperatively or in the pre- or postoperative period. Finally, misrepresentation of experience or expertise with a particular procedure or technology would be considered negligent and not the appropriate standard of care.

CONCLUSION

In conclusion, the dialogue that leads to a patient's consent to laparoscopic surgery described herein is beneficial to both parties. The patient has participated in determining the course of treatment while becoming informed to the best of the physician's ability. The physician knows that the patient has gained an understanding of the relevant issues and has made a truly informed and responsible decision.

REFERENCES

1. Borten M, Friedman EA, editors. Laparoscopic complications: prevention and management. Toronto, Philadelphia: BC Decker: 1986. p. 449.
2. Ramos JR, Petrosemolo RH, Valory EA, et al. Abdominoperineal resection: laparoscopic versus conventional. Surg Laparosc Endosc 1997;**7:**148–52.
3. Berney T, Malaise J, Mourad M, et al. Laparoscopic and open live donor nephrectomy: a cost/benefit study. Transpl Int 2000;13:35–40.
4. Leventhal JR, Deeik RK, Joehl RJ, et al. Laparoscopic live donor nephrectomy—is it safe? Transplantation 2000;70:602–6.
5. Marubashi S, Yano H, Monden T, et al. The usefulness, indications, and complications of laparoscopy-assisted colectomy in comparison with those of open colectomy for colorectal carcinoma. Surg Today 2000;30:491–6.
6. Nguyen DB, Silen W, Hodin RA. Appendectomy in the pre- and postlaparoscopic eras. J Gastrointest Surg 1999; 3:67–73.
7. Rawlins MC, Hefty TL, Brown SL, Biehl TR. Learning laparoscopic donor nephrectomy safely: a report on 100 cases. Arch Surg 2002;137:531–4.
8. Mac Cordick C, Lecuru F, Rizk E, et al. Morbidity in laparoscopic gynecological surgery: results of a prospective single-center study. Surg Endosc 1999;13:57–61.
9. Perugini RA, Mason R, Czerniach DR, et al. Predictors of complication and suboptimal weight loss after laparoscopic Roux-en-Y gastric bypass: a series of 188 patients. Arch Surg 2003;138:541–6.
10. Higashihara E, Baba S, Nakagawa K, et al. Learning curve and conversion to open surgery in cases of laparoscopic adrenalectomy and nephrectomy. J Urol 1998;159:650–3.
11. Soutoul JH, Pierre F. [Medicolegal risks of celioscopy. Analysis of 32 cases of complications]. J Gynecol Obstet Biol Reprod (Paris) 1988;17:439–51.
12. Professional Liability Committee, American College of Surgeons. Professional liability/risk management: a manual for surgeons. Chicago: American College of Surgeons; 1991. p. 260.
13. Schloendorff v. Society of New York Hospital. In: NE, vol. 105. NY: 1914. p. 92.
14. Rizzo v. Schiller. In: VA: Supreme Court of Virginia, vol. 248. 1994. p. 155.
15. Mandell v. Maurer. In: OR App, vol. 150. 1997. p. 543.
16. Duttry v. Patterson. In: A. 2d, vol. 741. 1999. p. 199.
17. Rostolsky BM. Practice makes perfect: experience-related information should fall within the purview of Pennsylvania's doctrine of informed consent [comment]. In: Duq L. Rev., vol. 40, 2002. p. 543–60.
18. Even v. Bohle. In: LEXIS: Iowa App., vol. 1256. 2002.
19. Weiss v. Green. In: F. Supp. 2d, vol. 129, p. 742. 2001.
20. Johnson v. Kokemoor. In: NW 2d, vol. 545. 1996. p. 495.
21. Brown v. Murphy. In: NE 2d, vol. 664. 1996. p. 186.
22. Boustani M, Peterson B, Hanson L, et al. Screening for dementia in primary care: a summary of the evidence for the U.S. Preventive Services Task Force. Ann Intern Med 2003;138:927–37.
23. Sanfilippo JS, Smith S. Complications: what's the standard of care? Clin Obstet Gynecol 2003;46:31–6.

10

Patient Instructions and Nursing Care

Nancy Brettschneider, BSN, CURN
Rose Ravalli, MSN, CURN

Patients undergoing endourologic procedures require both medical and nursing expertise. Preoperative teaching begins at the time of diagnosis. A short lesson that makes use of diagrams or models will help patients understand the anatomy of the urinary tract and assist in educated mutual decision making.

At the time of the initial consultation, the appropriate endoscopic procedure is explained to the patient and any questions and concerns are addressed. Most often patients want to know how long the procedure will take, the length of hospitalization, the amount of pain they will have, and how long the recuperation period will be.

Prior to admission, a preoperative work-up is performed that includes a complete blood count, electrolyte measurements, urinalysis, and urine culture. If the culture is positive, the patient is treated preoperatively with antibiotics. Prothrombin time and partial thromboplastin time are determined if there is any history of bruising or bleeding. An electrocardiogram(ECG) and chest radiography are performed depending on the patient's age and medical history. On admission to the hospital, the patient's radiographs are reviewed again and informed consent is obtained.

PERCUTANEOUS PROCEDURES

NEPHROLITHOTOMY   Patients who had to undergo open lithotomies 20 to 25 years ago would have welcomed an endoscopic approach. Today this approach is commonplace, although it is difficult to minimize the patient's fears and anxieties. Most nephrolithotomy patients have no previous frame of reference and require the same pre-operative consideration.

The usual operative time for a percutaneous nephrolithotomy is approximately 2 hours. Patients with larger stones or staghorn calculi may require a longer intraoperative time or a second operative procedure. The patient is reassured that the procedure will be performed under general anesthesia. The basic details of cystoscopy, ureteral catheterization, and the percutaneous incision are explained. The patient is shown a sample nephrostomy tube so that he knows what to expect when he awakens in the recovery room and is told that the ureteral stent and urethral catheter will remain in place for at least 24 hours postoperatively. It is important that patients be advised that the percutaneous tube will be draining bloody urine and that length of hospitalization is about 4 days with approximately 1 week of recuperation at home.

Postoperatively, the patient will be returned to the nursing unit with an intravenous (IV) infusion catheter still in place. IV antibiotics will have been started intraoperatively based on preoperative urine cultures, and will be continued as long as the nephrostomy tube is in place.

The nurse is responsible for maintaining the urinary drainage systems (nephrostomy, ureteral, and urethral). Bags should be attached to the side of the bed or to an intravenous pole, always below the level of the bladder and coiled with a straight length of tubing entering the bag. This maintains gravity drainage and avoids the problems of wet dressings, flank pain, and obstructed catheters. Handwashing should precede any handling of the catheter and nonsterile gloves are donned to prevent nosocomial infection. A separate collection container is used for each patient to avoid cross-contamination. The emptying spouts should not touch the collection receptacle. The spouts of each bag should be swabbed with alcohol prior to being clamped shut. Unless contraindicated, a daily fluid intake of at least 64 ounces is encouraged to assist in keeping the drainage systems patent.

Color, patency, and output must be monitored. Oliguria, post-obstructive diuresis, and recurrent obstruction can all be assessed by observing output.[1] Care must be taken in managing the ureteral catheter and nephrostomy tube since they are not retention catheters kept in place by a balloon. The ureteral catheter will be attached to the Foley catheter with silk suture material. The nephrostomy tube, although sutured to the skin, can be easily dislodged if force is applied.

Patients should be observed for any signs of abdominal distention, diminished bowel sounds, and pain, since an iatrogenic tear of the renal pelvis may present as a paralytic ileus. Vital signs should be taken, lungs auscultated, and skin color observed to monitor for any signs of pneumothorax, hemorrhage, or shock. Flank pain is to be expected, but excessive pain that is unrelieved by analgesics is unusual and may be a sign of obstruction. The drug of choice is morphine sulfate, administered either intramuscularly or by a patient-controlled analgesia pump.

Dressings must be changed with care to avoid inadvertent tube dislodgment. Because the tract is larger than the tube, a small amount of leakage is to be expected. While the patient is hospitalized, the tube insertion site is swabbed with povidone-iodine prior to application of the dressing. For patients who go home with nephrostomy tubes, daily dressing changes are preferred. The site can

be cleansed with hydrogen peroxide rather than povidone-iodine to decrease the incidence of encrustation of sutures that can occur over time. We recommend patients shower with their dressings on to lessen the chances of tube dislodgment. Dressings should be changed after showering.

The use of split 4 × 4 inch gauze pads is discouraged because these dressings tend to adhere to the nephrostomy tube, making them difficult to remove, and they provide minimal support for the catheter. Rather, 4 × 4 inch gauze pads should be folded and placed around the tube in a picture-frame fashion. Then one 4 × 4 inch gauze pad is placed over this and secured with tape. In addition, the nephrostomy tube extension is secured with a piece of tape at the level of the thigh for extra security (Figure 10-1).

On post-operative day 1, ambulation is encouraged and a regular diet is resumed as tolerated. A nephrostogram is obtained 48 hours postoperatively. If there are no residual stones or fragments, the tube will be clamped. If the patient does not experience pain, leakage, or fever with the tube clamped, the nephrostomy tube is removed. Once it is removed, there will be some initial leakage from the open tract. Usually within 1 to 2 days the tract will close over by secondary intention. A urostomy appliance placed over the drainage site collects the urine and is easily emptied. Within 1 to 2 days, the site should be closed over. If the patient is afebrile, the intravenous infusion is discontinued and oral antibiotics are begun. If drainage persists for more than 3 days, cystoscopy and retrograde insertion of a ureteral catheter may be necessary. Oral antibiotics are continued for 5 days at home. The patient is seen 7 to 10 days later in the office. The percutaneous wound site is assessed. If the patient has recurrent stone disease, a metabolic work-up is indicated.

ENDOPYELOTOMY   Patients undergoing an antegrade endopyelotomy for a ureteropelvic junction obstruction have a similar pre- and postoperative course, except that they are discharged with a tube in place for 6 weeks. Discharge instructions must be precise and explicit, and whenever possible, a friend or relative of the patient should be present. The same basic guidelines apply to any patient discharged with a nephrostomy tube.

The dressing is changed at home, preferably on a daily basis. Gauze pads are folded in half and placed around the tube in a picture-frame fashion. If clamped, the tube is coiled around with a straight length coming out of the insertion site. A

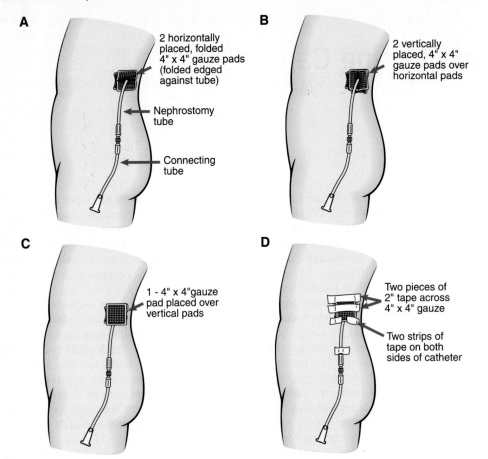

A — 2 horizontally placed, folded 4" x 4" gauze pads (folded edged against tube)

Nephrostomy tube

Connecting tube

B — 2 vertically placed, 4" x 4" gauze pads over horizontal pads

C — 1 - 4" x 4" gauze pad placed over vertical pads

D — Two pieces of 2" tape across 4" x 4" gauze

Two strips of tape on both sides of catheter

Figure 10-1 Dressing for nephrostomy tube insertion site after nephrolithotomy.

4 × 4 inch flat gauze pad is then placed over the coiled tube and secured with tape (Figure 10-2).

If a leaking tube must be connected to a drainage bag, the dressing remains the same, except that the catheter is enclosed on both sides with tape to prevent movement. The tape does not directly touch the tube. It is then secured lower down on the thigh, leaving a little slack (see Figure 10-1).

Gravity drainage must be maintained during the day as well as when the patient is reclining. Wet dressings are often the result of a kinked drainage tube or improper bag position. Connectors for attaching the nephrostomy tube to the leg bag are commercially available. In their absence, a connecting tube can be improvised by first cutting off the insertion end of a 22 or 24 French Foley catheter to the appropriate length. A Luer-Lok adapter is then fitted onto the proximal cut end of the catheter. This adapter will fit securely onto the nephrostomy tube and the other end will connect to either a leg bag or overnight drainage bag.[2]

Leg bags are used only when the patient is ambulatory. When the patient is lying down for more than 2 hours at a time, a night drainage bag is used. Bags should be cleansed daily with a solution of 1 part vinegar to 1 part cold water and then rinsed with cold water. Alternatively, soap and water can be used. Either a household funnel or a syringe can be used to pass the solution through. Bags can be draped over a hanger (with the spigots open) and left to dry.

Postoperative telephone triage is necessary for most patients who go home with an endopyelotomy tube. Generally the tube remains in place for 6 weeks. If significant leakage occurs around the tube, it should be connected to a drainage system. Patients are then instructed to clamp the tube again 2 days later. Reassurance is given that this will not affect surgical outcome. If there is still pain and leakage once the patient is hooked up to a drainage system, he is instructed to come into the office for irrigation, which is carried out by instilling 10 mL of normal saline solution into the tube. If this does not clear the tubing, another 10 mL of normal saline solution can be instilled and gently suctioned out. This should dislodge any mucous plug, sediment, or clot. If patency is not achieved, it may become necessary for the physician to reposition the tube under fluoroscopic guidance.

Patients should be told that minimal flank pain or drainage during micturition is normal, since the catheter extends from the kidney into the bladder. A detrusor contraction can cause retrograde expulsion of urine.

DISCHARGE INSTRUCTIONS Patients are discharged with an instruction sheet following any percutaneous surgery (Table 10-1). Intake of at least 64 ounces of fluid is encouraged if not otherwise contraindicated. Daily showering is permitted with the dressing in place, but direct shower pressure on the tube site must be avoided. Dressings must be changed immediately after the patient has showered. Strenuous activity and exercise are to be

avoided for 1 week. Stair climbing, walking, and sexual intercourse can be resumed. Oral antibiotics are given at home for 5 days. Hematuria is not unusual and patients should increase their fluid intake in an effort to clear this. Fever, gross hematuria that does not clear, and copious flank drainage are reasons to contact the physician.

After an endopyelotomy, patients are seen in the office 7 to 10 days later. At 6 weeks they return to the office for tube removal. Once the tube is removed, a urostomy appliance is placed over the site. Patients are told to remove the appliance when they have no leakage for at least 4 consecutive hours. They are given similar instructions when a percutaneous nephrostomy tube is removed. Two weeks later, intravenous urography is performed to assess the surgical outcome.

Patients are cautioned that after the removal of the tube, if they experience flank pain, fever, nausea, or vomiting, they must return to the hospital immediately for assessment and possible reinsertion of a nephrostomy tube.

URETEROSCOPY

The use of ureteroscopy with or without stone fragmentation has widely replaced ureterolithotomy. This procedure benefits the patient by reducing pain, edema, and bleeding and by shortening the period of convalescence.[3]

Postoperative nursing care includes careful observation of patients when they return to the nursing unit. Because ureteral manipulation causes edema, a ureteral stent will be left in place. If stone basket retrieval or lithotripsy has been performed, the patient will be left with an indwelling pigtail stent or a stent with a string coming out of the urethra for several weeks.

Based on the amount of edema postoperatively, the physician will decide when the ureteral catheter will be removed. The most common complication of ureteroscopy is ureteral perforation. If this occurs intraoperatively, the patient will still return to the unit with an indwelling pigtail stent to divert the urine. Vital signs and skin color should be monitored to detect any signs of infection or shock. Color and quality of urine as well as catheter patency should be recorded. Minimal bleeding is to be expected. Intravenous antibiotics are begun intraoperatively and continued for 12 to 24 hours.

After removal of the ureteral stent, ureteral spasms may occur, producing symptoms of colic. Analgesics and/or antispasmodic agents should be given at this time. The usual hospital stay is 1 to 2 days. Patients discharged home with an indwelling stent will return to the office in 10 to 14 days for cystoscopic removal.

DISCHARGE INSTRUCTIONS Discharge instructions include resuming a normal diet, increasing fluid intake, showering or bathing, and avoiding strenuous activity for 7 to 10 days (Table 10-2). Patients may resume walking, stair climbing, and sexual intercourse as soon as they feel able. Again,

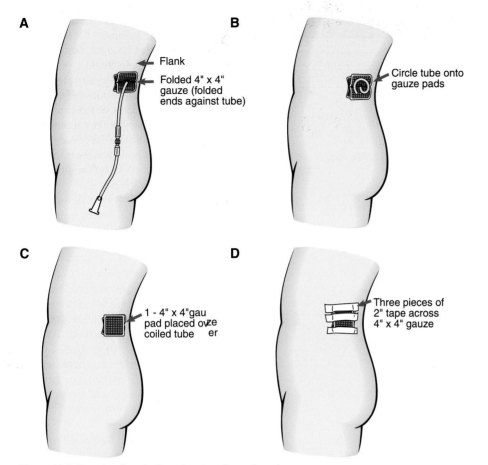

Figure 10-2 Dressing for tube insertion site after endopyelotomy.

they are sent home with a 5-day prescription of antibiotics. Hematuria is to be expected. This will clear with ingestion of fluids. A large amount of gross hematuria that does not clear or temperatures higher than 100.5°F must be reported.

LAPAROSCOPY

Laparoscopy is one standard of care for retroperitoneal surgery. This minimally invasive approach decreases post-operative pain, offers a smaller incision/scar, involves less blood loss, decreases hospital stay, and allows the patient to resume normal daily activities sooner. Known contraindications include coagulopathies, intestinal obstruction, abdominal wall infections, and suspected malignant ascites. Relative contraindications include morbid obesity, previous abdominal or pelvic surgery of an extensive nature, ascites, pregnancy, chronic obstructive pulmonary disease (COPD), and severe cardiac arrhythmias.

Pre-operatively, patients will have routine pre-admission testing. This will generally include a complete blood count (CBC), electrolyte panel, urinalysis, urine culture, chest radiograph, and ECG. Patients are to have nothing by mouth after midnight. Postoperatively, the patient will return to the nursing unit with a urethral catheter and an IV line in place. Depending on the procedure, they will have .5 to 1 cm incisions, most often covered with Steri-Strips. Vital signs are assessed and the lungs are auscultated. Monitoring hemodynamic status is critical since this may be the

first sign of internal hemorrhaging from blood vessel injury. Because bleeding can occur in the retroperitoneum, the abdomen must be assessed at least every 4 hours. In experienced hands, intra-

operative complications are less than 5%. Pain is to be expected, but should not be so severe that it cannot be relieved with medication. Even though the patient's incision may seem small, significant manipulation intraoperatively can cause postoperative pain. Monitoring for bowel or organ perforation as well as thermal injuries is imperative. Scrotal edema is common in pelvic laparoscopy as a result of insufflation of CO_2 intraoperatively.

A clear liquid diet is started on postoperative day 1 or the night of surgery and is advanced accordingly. The usual hospital stay for a laparoscopic adrenalectomy, laparoscopic nephrectomy, laparoscopic pyeloplasty cyst decortication, and radiofrequency ablation is about 1 to 2 days. On postoperative day 1, the urethral catheter is removed and intravenous antibiotics are discontinued. If the patient fails to void, a urethral catheter is temporarily reinserted. On discharge, patients may shower, climb stairs, and resume light activities.

With laparoscopic partial nephrectomy and a laparoscopic nephroureterectomy, the tumor is extracted within a specimen pouch/bag and a drain will be left in place in the flank. This needs to be monitored for amount and quality of drainage. Most likely this drain will be removed on day 2. Discharge home is usually on day 2 to 3.

The patient having a laparopscopic radical prostatectomy undergoes limited bowel prep. This prep consists of clear liquids, magnesium citrate the day before the surgery, and a Fleets saline enema the morning of the procedure to further clean the distal colon and rectum. At surgery, once the prostate gland is extracted within the pouch/bag, a drain is temporarily left in the abdomen. Following surgery, a urethral catheter

---

Table 10-1 Discharge Instructions Following Percutaneous Stone Extraction

Name_____

Nurse_____ Contact phone_____

Physician_____ Contact phone_____

Discharge Instructions Following Percutaneous Stone Extraction

Diet
Resume your usual eating habits.
Drink at least 6 to 8 glasses of fluid daily. If you experience urinary frequency, decrease your fluid intake after dinner.

Activity
You may shower with your dressing on with the force of the shower facing you.
Avoid strenuous activity and exercise until you receive permission from your physician, usually during your first office visit following surgery.
You may resume stair climbing and walking.
You may resume sexual relations.

Medication
If medication is prescribed, complete the full course.

Urination
Passing some blood in your urine is not unusual. Do not become alarmed. This should clear up as you increase your fluid intake.

Call Your Physician
If you have fever > 100.5°F.
If you see a large amount of blood in your urine that does not clear with increased fluid intake.
If you begin to drain urine from your flank (back) wound.
For an appointment to see your urologist 7 to 10 days following discharge from the hospital.

Table 10-2 Discharge Instructions Following Ureteroscopy

Name_____

Nurse_____ Contact phone_____

Physician_____ Contact phone_____

Discharge Instructions Following Ureteroscopy

Diet
Resume your usual eating habits.
Drink at least 6 to 8 (8 oz) glasses of fluid daily. If you experience urinary frequency, decrease your fluid intake after dinner.

Activity
You may shower or bathe daily.
Avoid strenuous activity and exercise until you receive permission from your physician, usually during your first office visit following surgery.
You may resume stair climbing and walking.
You may resume sexual relations.

Medication
If medication is prescribed, complete the full course.

Urination
You may have been discharged with an indwelling tube (stent) that runs from your kidney to your bladder. This tube was placed to facilitate the passage of stone fragments and urine. This stent will be removed by your urologist as an outpatient procedure. It may cause you to feel as though you have to urinate frequently or may cause a burning sensation in the bladder. These feelings will lessen with time. You may also continue to have blood in your urine.

Call Your Physician
If you have fever > 100.5°F.
If you see a large amount of blood in your urine that does not clear with increased fluid intake.
For an appointment to see your urologist 7 to 14 days following discharge from the hospital.

will remain in place for approximately 7 to 14 days. A cystogram is performed about 7 days post-op to confirm that the urethra and bladder neck have healed.

Laparoscopic surgery is much easier on the patient, but requires greater skill and technique on the part of the surgeon. As more surgeons receive specialized training and gain more experience in performing laparoscopic surgery, nursing care of these patients will become routine.

DISCHARGE INSTRUCTIONS Discharge instructions include resumption of a regular diet. Normal activities can be started within 3 to 5 days. Antibiotics are not usually continued postoperatively. Patients should monitor their trocar insertion sites for infection, swelling, and leakage. Subcutaneous emphysema can cause bloating and pain. This usually improves within a few days when the residual CO_2 is eliminated. Scrotal edema may persist for 1 to 2 weeks. This should be treated with elevation or a scrotal support when the patient is up and about.

If any pain persists that is unrelieved by mild analgesics, the patient should contact his physician. Fever, nausea, and vomiting are also indications that immediate care is necessary.

EXTRACORPOREAL SHOCK WAVE LITHOTRIPSY

Procedures that may precede or follow extracorporeal shock wave lithotripsy (ESWL) often involve endoscopy. Prior to ESWL, the patient undergoes the standard preadmission work-up. Laboratory requirements include a complete blood count, urinalysis, culture and sensitivity, and an ECG if the patient is over 40 years of age. It is important to explain renal anatomy so that the patient is familiar with the location of the stone in relation to the kidney.

Although there is no incision, patients must be informed that IV anesthesia is necessary for two reasons. Shock waves are painful and maintenance of proper patient positioning is essential. It is imperative that patients be made aware that stones are being fragmented but not removed. Passage of stone fragments through the urinary tract will occur postoperatively. Fluids will assist in their passage. Patients with a positive culture preoperatively will be treated with antibiotics.

For stones > 15 mm or those that have been pushed up from the ureter, a ureteral stent is inserted intraoperatively. This stent remains in place for 7 to 10 days or until the majority of fragments pass.

This is an ambulatory procedure; the patient recuperates for several hours in the postanesthesia care unit prior to being sent home. If the patient is sent home with an indwelling stent, antibiotics may be prescribed. Postoperatively, pain medication is prescribed. Complaints of bladder spasms, urgency, hematuria, and frequency are usually related to placement of the stent. If these symptoms are severe, an anticholinergic may be prescribed.

DISCHARGE INSTRUCTIONS ESWL is an ambulatory procedure that requires anesthesia, and patients are given specific instructions prior to discharge (Table 10-3). No driving, heavy lifting,

Table 10-3 Discharge Instructions Following Lithotripsy

Name_____

Nurse_____ Contact phone_____

Physician_____ Contact phone_____

Discharge Instructions Following Lithotripsy

You have completed treatment of your stone(s) with extracorporeal shock wave lithotripsy. Your stones have fragmented and will proceed to pass over the next several days to weeks. You have been given an anesthetic for the procedure, which may make you feel drowsy and weak. The anesthetic will require at least 24 hours to be eliminated from your system. Therefore for at least the next 24 hours we suggest:

1. No driving, no heavy lifting, no exercise, no sex, and no household work
2. No smoking or alcohol consumption
3. No important decision making

Your stone has fragmented and you should be aware that the fragments will pass during urination. The passage of fragments may cause discomfort such as flank pain, abdominal pain, nausea, and vomiting. There may also be blood in your urine. Any discomfort can usually be alleviated with the prescription for pain medication that you will be given at discharge. It is important for you to drink plenty of fluids (10 glasses per day) to help the stone(s) pass. The following symptoms should prompt you to call your physician:

1. Temperature higher than 100.5°F
2. Persistent or severe pain
3. Persistent vomiting
4. Bruising of the flank

If there is any problem contacting your physician, there will be a urologist on call 24 hours a day. The urologist can be reached at _____.

You may have been discharged with an indwelling tube that runs from your kidney to your bladder. This tube was placed to facilitate the passage of stone fragments and urine. This stent (tube) will be removed by your urologist as an outpatient procedure. It may cause you to feel as though you have to urinate frequently or may cause a burning sensation in the bladder. These feelings will lessen with time. You may also continue to have blood in your urine.

Please call the physician's office to make an appointment to be seen approximately 7 to 10 days from now. Arrive for your appointment 1 hour ahead of time, letting the secretary know that you will require an x-ray film prior to being seen.

exercise, sexual activity, or household work should be performed for 24 hours.

Passage of fragments may cause flank pain, abdominal pain, nausea, and vomiting. Mild hematuria is also to be expected. Pain should be relieved with analgesics. Fluid intake of at least 1,500 to 2,000 mL/day is indicated to ease the passage of stone fragments. Patients who awaken during the night to urinate are advised to continue

their fluid intake. In the event of temperatures higher than 100.5°F, persistent or severe pain, persistent vomiting, or flank bruising, it is important that the physician be notified.

All patients will undergo examination of the kidneys, ureter, and bladder on their follow-up office visit 7 to 10 days later. If a stent has been inserted, it will be removed by cystoscopy at that time.

REFERENCES

1. Bruton DS, Einhorn C, Readon LM, et al. Urinary calculi. In: Karlowicz KA, editor. Urologic nursing: principles and practice. Philadelphia: WB Saunders; 1995. p. 177–98.
2. Ravalli R, Smith AD. Nursing aspects of percutaneous stone extraction. In: Smith AD, Castañeda-Zúñiga WR, Bronson JG, editors. Endourology: principles and practice. New York: Thieme; 1986. p. 121–5.
3. Marshall B. Laser lithotripsy: a nursing perspective. Urol Nurs 1991;11:25–7.

11

Equipment, Instrumentation, and Operating Room Setup: Role of the Urology Nursing Team

Ann M. Phillips, RN, BSN

Carol J. Olsen, RN, BSN

Team collaboration and communication are essential to successful endourologic procedures. The entire staff must be thoroughly familiar with the equipment and instrumentation needed for specific procedures; they must ensure that instruments are functioning properly to avoid delays, and that the operating room setup meets the surgeon's specifications. In this chapter, we describe the responsibilities of the urology nursing team for setting up the equipment, instrumentation, and supplies, and for organizing the operating room for performing percutaneous nephrostomy, ureteroscopy, and laparoscopy.

PERCUTANEOUS NEPHROSTOMY

Several urologic procedures can be performed via percutaneous nephrostomy entry, such as percutaneous stone extraction (PSE), endopyelotomy, resection of renal tumors, and fulguration of caliceal diverticulum or renal cysts. This endoscopic approach allows the insertion of a rigid nephroscope to visualize the renal pelvis and the ureteropelvic junction of the upper urinary tract. The procedures require a similar room setup and standard preparation. Endourologic instrumentation and equipment will vary depending on the operative procedure.

OPERATING ROOM SETUP AND PATIENT PREPARATION The necessary equipment should be assembled in the operating room suite and its function assessed before the patient enters. The operating room setup should accommodate two table setups, the operating room table, the endoscopic video cart, the C-arm fluoroscope, and the anesthesia equipment (Figures 11-1 and 11-2). The nurses must have adequate room to set up equipment, to move about freely, to assist the anesthesiologist, and to perform nursing documentation. They must have access to the telephone.

The scrub nurse is responsible for assembling the two-part setup, which includes a cystoscopy setup and a standard percutaneous nephrostomy setup, each on a separate table (Figures 11-3 and 11-4). The components of the two setups are listed in Table 11-1. In the process of arranging the instrumentation, the scrub nurse must check the visual optics of the telescopes and nephroscope and the function of all other instruments on the sterile setups. Instrumentation and accessories on

these setups should be neatly arranged so that they are visible and easy to reach. It is not necessary for the scrub nurse to remain sterile during any of the percutaneous nephrostomy procedures.

The components of the standard percutaneous nephrostomy setup listed in Table 11-2 should be arranged in the order to be used, as shown in Figure 11-4. In the lower left corner of the table are the gown and gloves and the nephrostomy drape, 12-foot suction tubing, plastic fluoroscopic drape, Y irrigation tubing, light cable, camera, and Foley drainage bag. To the right of those components are the long 18-gauge needle with a stylet and the Amplatz renal dilator set. The renal dilators should be sequenced from 8 French to 30F, with French size clearly visible. The nephroscope is combined with a 26F working sheath, and a round rubber nipple is placed over the port to aid in the insertion of the operative forceps. The cup biopsy, peanut, and alligator forceps are laid out beside the nephroscope. The ultrasonic lithotriptor probe and wrench are also kept on the endourology tray and are included on the setup when a PSE is being performed. In the upper right-hand corner, a rolled towel contains plain 4 by 4 inch

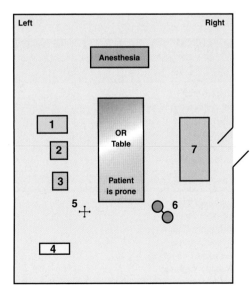

Figure 11-1 Operating room setup for right percutaneous nephrostomy. For left-sided procedures, the back table and fluoroscopy units are switched. 1 = fluoroscopy C-arm unit; 2 = fluoroscopy TV monitor; 3 = endoscopic video cart; 4 = cystoscopy setup; 5 = IV pole; 6 = double-suction apparatus; 7 = endourologic instrument setup.

gauze sponges for the dressing at the end of the procedure. The Kelly clamp, scissors, knife handle, Halsted clamp, toothed forceps, and needle holder are placed on the rolled towel. Lap pad sponges (with rings removed) are available on the setup. They are used to dry the patient's skin before the drape is adhered and to wash and dry the skin at the end of the procedure. A large basin is placed in the upper left corner of the table for sterile H_2O and, next to it, a small basin containing Hypaque solution. A 10-mL syringe and a 20-mL syringe for contrast injection should be placed in the small basin. The guidewires, .038 Teflon-coated and Saf-T-J (J-tipped, 100 cm), are placed in front of the two basins.

A contrast solution of 30% Hypaque (100 mL 50% Hypaque and 30 mL of H_2O) is mixed by the scrub nurse, drawn up in a 60-mL syringe, and passed off the field in an emesis basin. On completion of the two setups, the scrub nurse is available to assist the circulator nurse and other members of the urology team.

While the scrub nurse is preparing the sterile setup, the circulator nurse reviews the patient's chart. The circulator nurse acts as the patient's advocate, reviewing the operating room sequence with the patient, identifying the correct operative site and laterality, addressing any concerns the patient may have, and communicating with the patient's family. The availability of blood products for possible transfusion should be checked before the circulator nurse brings the patient into the operating room.

The patient is brought to the operating room and assisted onto the operating table, which is

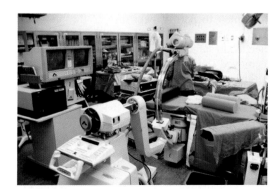

Figure 11-2 Operating room after setup for percutaneous nephrostomy.

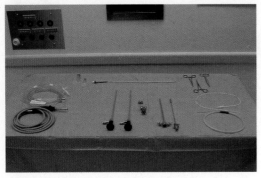

Figure 11-3 Back table cystoscopy setup.

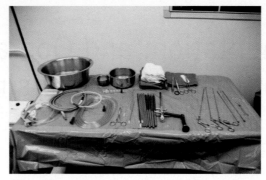

Figure 11-4 Percutaneous nephrostomy back table setup.

radiolucent for the region of the urinary tract. As a general practice, all patients undergoing any percutaneous nephrostomy procedure are given a general anesthetic.

PATIENT POSITIONING AND SKIN PREPARATION
After the endotracheal tube is secured, the patient is placed in a lithotomy position for cystoscopy. The patient's legs are raised slowly and simultaneously by two team members and positioned in gel-padded footrest stirrups, and the buttocks are extended over the table edge. Precautions must be taken to prevent pressure on the peroneal, saphenous, posterior tibial, popliteal, and sciatic nerves. Flexion, extension, and compression due to incorrect positioning of the legs can result in nerve damage, venous thrombosis, or sacroiliac joint dislocation. For a lengthy procedure, antiembolic stockings and compression sleeves are used to avoid pooling in the lower extremities and prevent thrombophlebitis in the post operative phase. Both arms should be secured on padded arm boards to prevent injury to the patient's fingers or hands when the table is raised or lowered. A cystoscopy is performed, and a 6F open-end ureteral catheter is inserted under C-arm fluoroscopy guidance to facilitate renal access. A 16F Foley catheter is inserted and attached to a drainage bag at the same time. Both catheters are tied with 2-0 silk to secure them in place. It is helpful to connect an empty syringe to the Luer-Lok adapter at the end of the ureteral catheter to prevent urine leakage. At the end of this procedure, both legs are slowly lowered simultaneously by two team members to prevent sudden hypotension.

The patient will be positioned on the abdomen to permit exposure of the posterior body. A minimum of four staff members are needed to safely position the patient. The patient is moved slowly and gently to allow the body to adjust to the position change. The positioning equipment (foam rubber pillow, foam rubber rolls, gel knee donuts, and arm boards) should be assembled and ready for use. The eyes, cheeks and ears, acromial process, breasts in women, genitals in men, patellas, and toes must be protected. The nurse assesses the integrity of the skin and makes sure that pressure points are properly padded (Figure 11-5). The anesthesiologist is responsible for the head and neck support and airway maintenance. A foam rubber pillow is placed under the head to prevent it from being angulated too much in relation to the trunk. The endotracheal tube is placed in the side slot of the foam pillow, making sure that the tube is unobstructed and free from kinks. This is monitored throughout the procedure by the anesthesiologist. The chest and abdomen are elevated on two foam rubber rolls that extend from the shoulder to the hip to reduce resistance to breathing. Gel knee donuts are covered with sheepskin placed inside the ring and are positioned between the knees and the operating room table to protect the bony prominences. A foam rubber roll is placed anterior to the ankles so that the feet and toes do not press on the table. The arms are flexed but must not be brought too far forward because of the risk of brachial palsy. They are secured on padded arm boards and the elbows are protected with sheepskin pads. A safety strap, or 3-inch adhesive tape, is secured across the knees and buttocks. At this time, the 2-0 silk tie securing the two catheters together is cut and discarded. The intravenous extension tubing is connected to the 60-mL syringe containing the Hypaque solution, and the tubing is primed. The nurse removes the empty syringe from the ureteral catheter and attaches the syringe and tubing to the Luer-Lok adapter of the ureteral catheter. The patient's buttocks and lower extremities are covered with a blanket to help maintain normal body temperature.

The purpose of the skin preparation is to remove microorganisms that can enter the surgical wound and cause infection. The solution for skin preparation depends on the hospital's preference. Starting at the incision site (below the twelfth rib) and working outward to include an extensive area surrounding the operative site, the area is thoroughly scrubbed for at least 5 minutes. A disinfectant topical solution is applied, and 70% alcohol is used to remove the disinfectant to enhance skin adherence for the nephrostomy drape.

X-RAY PRECAUTIONS All procedures are carried out under C-arm fluoroscopy, requiring that the staff wear x-ray gowns and thyroid collars. The x-ray gown should cover the front and back of the circulating personnel since they are in constant motion around the room. When the x-ray unit is turned on, team members are alerted so that they can adequately protect themselves. The C-arm exposure is absorbed by the patient, and if any rays escape, it is usually via the legs. Our hospital protocol requires that any personnel subjected to x-ray exposure wear an x-ray badge. On the first of each month, the badges are collected and sent to the radiology department, where they are forwarded to a company accredited by the National Institute of Standards and Technology. The following month, a written report is sent to the operating room with a radiation dosimetry report.

DRAPING, INSTRUMENTATION, AND OPERATIVE EQUIPMENT Nephroscopy requires an irrigant and some device to collect effluxing fluid. An adherent area on the nephrostomy drape is placed

Table 11-1 Back Table Setups for Percutaneous Nephrostomy	
Cystoscopy Setup (see Figure 11-3)	
Cystoscopy tray	Cystoscopy sterile drape pack
Single cystoscope tubing	Prep set
Surgilube	16F Foley catheter with 5-mL balloon
5-mL syringe	Foley drainage bag
6F open-end U catheter	.038 Teflon-coated guidewire
Gown and gloves	2-0 silk tie (to tie catheters together)
PSE Setup (see Figure 11-4)	
Endourology tray	20-mL syringe
Sterile table cover	10-mL syringe
Nephrostomy drape	Lap pads with no rings
Fluoroscope drape	Plain 4 by 4 inch pads
12 feet of suction tubing	No. 10 blade
Cystoscope Y tubing	2-0 silk FS needle
Universal camera drape (for ultrasonic lithotriptor)	No. 18 GA needle
Gown and gloves	Saf-T J 100-cm guidewire
Back basin (large) with water	.038 Teflon-coated guidewire
Small basin with 100 mL of 50% Hypaque and 30 mL water	Amplatz renal dilator
60-mL syringe with Hypaque solution	
PSE = percutaneous stone extraction.	

Table 11-2 Equipment and Supplies for Percutaneous Nephrostomy	
Sterile Instruments	
Endourology tray	Cystoscopy tray
0° wide-angle straightforward telescope	1 No. 30 and 70 telescope
26 F operating sheath	1 No. 22 cystoscope
Peanut grasping forceps	1 Albarran bridge
Alligator grasping forceps	1 light cable 1 scissors
Biopsy forceps	2 hemostats
Light cable	2 gray nipples
Water connector	**Urethrotome tray**
Round gray nipple	0° telescope
Kelly clamp	Working element
Straight Halsted clamp	21F sheath
No. 3 knife handle	Straight knife
Straight Mayo scissors	Sickle knife (J knife)
Medium needle holder	**Ureteroscopy tray**
Adult forceps with teeth	0° semirigid ureteroscope 6/7.5F
6/7-mm wrench	Flexible two-pronged grasping forceps
Ultrasonic lithotriptor probe	Flexible alligator forceps
	Flexible biopsy forceps
Equipment/Supplies	
Genitourinary imaging table	2 gel knee pads and 2 sheepskin pads
Stirrups and holders	1 gel bolster for under feet
X-ray gowns	Suction setup (double)
Adjustable IV pole with 4 hooks	Ultrasonic lithotriptor (generator box, foot pedal, transducer)
Sterile camera	1 3,000-mL bag of warm water (for cystoscopy)
Endoscopic cart	10 3,000-mL bags of warm saline solution
C-arm fluoroscope	2 50-mL bottles of 50% Hypaque
Face pillow	Multiple 3,000-mL bags of warm saline solution
2 foam chest bolsters	

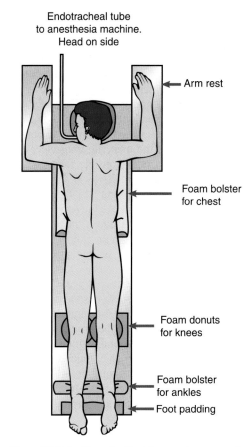

Figure 11-5 Position of patient for percutaneous nephrostomy approach.

directly over the puncture site to seal the skin; thus, any fluid that escapes goes onto the drape and runs down into a pocket connected to suction tubing that is attached to the double suction apparatus.

Normal saline irrigant in 3,000-mL bags is used throughout the procedure. Using an irrigant at room temperature can cause hypothermia and postoperative shivers. Heating the irrigant to body temperature promotes cardiovascular stability and allows the patient to remain warm during and after surgery. Warming cabinets are not the solution since the temperature of each bag cannot be controlled once it is removed from the cabinet. The ideal warmer is a system that keeps the irrigation solution at a controlled body temperature as it travels from the bag via the Y irrigation tubing and into the patient. The nursing team is responsible for monitoring the irrigation and changing the suction canisters. The irrigant is hung on a height-adjustable IV pole with four hooks. The pole (see Figure 11-1) is positioned next to the left end of the operating room table. The Y irrigation tubing is passed off by the surgeon, and the nurse connects it to the irrigation bags.

The endoscopic video cart (Figure 11-6) is positioned on the opposite side of the operative site, closer to the foot of the table. The surgeon will also pass off the light cable, and it is attached to the high-intensity light source. The light source is not turned on until the nephroscope is inserted into the patient. The C-arm fluoroscope is positioned over the patient, and the surgeon covers it with a sterile plastic fluoroscopic drape.

Before the nephroscope is inserted, the surgeon must enter the renal tract by a sequential dilation method. Using an 18-gauge trocar cannula needle under fluoroscopic guidance, the surgeon decides which pole of the kidney will be entered. Once the needle is in place, the stylet is removed and a guidewire is inserted. Following the renal dilation process, a dilator sheath will maintain patency for the insertion of the nephroscope. The light source is now turned on, and the camera is attached to the nephroscope, and a white balance check is performed to assure color quality. At this time, the specific operative treatment begins. Once renal access is secured, the surgeon will pass a guidewire through the ureteral catheter. At the surgeon's request, the ureteral catheter is removed via the urethra, and a clamp is placed at the end of the guidewire. At the end of the procedure, a nephrostomy tube is inserted. Before the tube is secured, a nephrostogram is obtained to check position and patency of the kidney and ureter. The tube is then secured with a 2-0 silk suture, and a drainage bag is attached to the end of the tube. A dry, sterile dressing is applied, the skin integrity is checked, and the patient is taken to the post-anesthesia care unit (PACU).

PERCUTANEOUS STONE EXTRACTION Percutaneous stone management was initially developed for high-risk patients who were poor candidates for surgery, but as the merits of this approach to stone disease became evident, it soon became the standard procedure for removing renal stones.

Smaller renal stones may be removed with a rigid alligator or peanut-type grasping forceps or a stone basket. Staghorn, hard, or large kidney

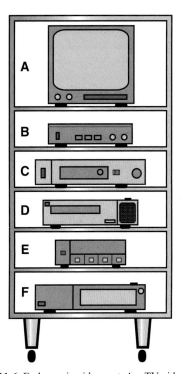

Figure 11-6 Endoscopic video cart. A = TV video monitor; B = camera unit; C = high intensity light source; D = super VHS or DVD recorder; E = ultrasonic lithotriptor generator; F = color video printer.

stones are first broken up with ultrasonic lithotripsy. The fragments are removed by grasping forceps or suction with the ultrasonic lithotriptor. The ultrasonic lithotriptor (Figure 11-7) consists of the generator power box, the transducer and rubber tubing that attaches to the foot pedal, a hollow ultrasonic probe, and a wrench. The probe and wrench found on the endourology tray are laid out on the sterile field, as well as a universal camera drape used to cover the unsterile transducer and tubing. The surgeon is responsible for attaching the probe to the transducer. To do so, the surgeon holds the camera drape (Figure 11-8) while the nurse inserts the transducer. As the surgeon tightens the probe onto the transducer, the nurse connects the suction tubing from the rubber tubing of the foot pedal to the double suction apparatus. A trap attached to the suction canister is used to collect the stone fragments. The foot pedal is placed by the surgeon's foot, the suction is turned on, and all connections are tested by the surgeon by stepping on the foot pedal with the probe tip held in water. A high-pitched sound signals that the equipment is ready. After the stones have been extracted, a 24F Malecot reentry or 14F Malecot nephrostomy tube is inserted. The stones are sent in a dry container for chemical analysis.

ENDOPYELOTOMY   Obstruction of the ureteropelvic junction may be treated by endopyelotomy. The advantages of endopyelotomy over open pyeloplasty are reduced operating time, less pain, shorter postoperative recovery time, and more rapid return to normal activities.

The endopyelotomy instrumentation consists of the basic percutaneous nephrostomy instruments with the addition of the urethrotome tray. The urethrotome is used with a cold knife (we use a sickle knife to open the ureteropelvic junction). At the end of the procedure a 14F Smith percutaneous endopyelotomy stent is inserted, and a drainage bag is attached.

RESECTION OF RENAL TUMORS AND FULGURATION OF CALICEAL DIVERTICULUM OR CYSTS
The instrumentation is the same as for endopyelotomy except that a resectoscope and loop electrode are used to resect or fulgurate. An electrosurgical unit with a foot pedal is needed, and the patient requires a grounding pad to be laced on a

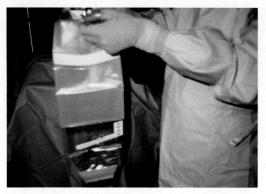

Figure 11-8 A camera drape is used to cover the ultrasonic lithotriptor transducer.

dry, non-hairy muscular area. The lateral thigh is the most common site for the pad application. The irrigant solution is changed to glycine when the surgeon is ready to resect or fulgurate. A 14F Smith percutaneous endopyelotomy stent is also needed at the end of these procedures.

URETEROSCOPY

A ureterolithotomy or open ureteral surgery was the standard procedure for removing stones and tumors until the late 1970s. These procedures required a hospital stay of 6 to 7 days, and recovery took approximately 6 to 8 weeks. Ureteroscopy has now become the standard method of visualizing the ureter and collecting system.

Ureteroscopy is performed for stone management, diagnosis of conditions such as hematuria and filling defects, treatment of upper ureteral obstruction and tumors at the ureteral orifices, biopsy or resection of ureteral tumors, and ureterotomy for ureteral strictures. Stone removal is the most frequent indication for ureteroscopy. Stones may be located in the ureter, or fragments may be left subsequent to extracorporeal shock wave lithotripsy.

OPERATING ROOM SETUP AND PATIENT PREPARATION   The scrub nurse is responsible for checking that the equipment and supplies are assembled and functional prior to the procedure (Table 11-3). She also oversees the operating room setup (Figure 11-9). Less equipment and

fewer supplies are needed for this procedure compared with the percutaneous nephrostomy setup. The primary equipment includes the radiolucent cystoscopy table, one-table setup, an endoscopic cart, the C-arm fluoroscope, and anesthesia equipment. Depending on the procedure, additional equipment may include the electrohydraulic lithotriptor unit, ultrasonic lithotriptor unit, laser, or electrosurgical unit.

The basic ureteroscopy setup on the back table consists of cystoscopy instruments, ureteroscopy tray, cystoscopy drape set, sterile plastic fluoroscope drape, Y irrigation tubing, open-end ureteral catheter, .038 Teflon-coated guidewire, 10- and 20-mL syringes for contrast injection, high-pressure inflation syringe, and a ureteral balloon dilator. As with any endourologic instruments, the visual ops of the telescopes should be checked before they are laid out and the function of each instrument assessed. The back table setup should be orderly and convenient for the urologist. The layout should be consistent with the order in which each component is to be used. In the lower left-hand corner are placed the gown and gloves, the cystoscopy drapes, Y irrigation tubing, light cable, camera and sterile plastic fluoroscopic drape. Next to these are the cystoscopy instruments (30° and 70° telescopes, small bridge with gray nipple, 21F and 23.5F cystoscopes, and Albarran bridge). To the right are the ureteroscopy instruments (0° semi-rigid ureteroscope and flexible forceps [two prong, alligator, and cup biopsy]). A 6F open-end ureteral catheter, .038 Teflon-coated guidewire and ureteral balloon dilator are placed at the upper right corner. The upper left-hand corner has a large basin of water, and next to it, a small basin filled with the 30% Hypaque solution. For the ureteroscopy procedures, the scrub nurse may set up the back table and then break scrub to be available to help other members of the urology team.

While the scrub nurse is preparing the back table setup, the circulator nurse checks the patient's chart and reviews the sequence of events with the patient. Concerns of the patient and family may be addressed at this time. The patient is transported into the operating room and assisted onto the radiolucent cystoscopy table. A regional or general anesthetic is usually administered,

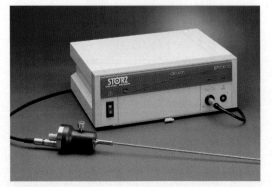

Figure 11-7 Ultrasonic lithotriptor generator with transducer, foot pedal, ultrasonic probe, and wrench.

Table 11-3 Equipment and Supplies for Ureteroscopy	
Sterile Instruments and Supplies	Equipment
Cystoscopy tray	Genitourinary imaging table
Ureteroscopy tray	X-ray gowns
Multiple 3,000-mL bags of warm saline solution	Adjustable IV pole with 4 hooks
Suction setup (double)	Endoscopic video cart
Two 50-mL bottles of 50% Hypaque	C-arm fluoroscope
Cystoscope Y tubing	Electrohydraulic lithotripsy machine
Sterile fluoroscope drape	Laser
Prep set	
Inflation syringe	
1 each 10-mL and 20-mL syringes	
100 mL of 50% Hypaque and 30 mL of water	
Cystoscopy pack	
Surgilube	

although some surgeons prefer general anesthesia and a muscle relaxant only.

PATIENT POSITIONING   For any ureteroscopy procedure, the patient is positioned in the lithotomy position using gel-padded footrest stirrups. Although most hospitals position both legs at equal heights, we keep the stirrup of the affected side lower than the other stirrup, and the leg in a straightened position (ie, if the right ureter is affected, then the right stirrup is lower and the right leg is straighter than the left). The contralateral leg is flexed and abducted to allow room for the operator. The ureteroscope must visualize the urethra, bladder, and kidney, and this position permits a straight path to the ureter and kidney. Both arms may be extended and secured on padded arm boards or tucked at the patient's sides with the drawsheet. Be sure the patient's hands and fingers are protected from injury when the table moves up or down.

INSTRUMENTATION AND OPERATIVE EQUIPMENT
There are a variety of ureteroscopes available for diagnosis and treatment of ureteral pathology. The rigid ureteroscope was the original instrument. It was followed by the flexible ureteroscope and more recently the semirigid short or long ureteroscope. All ureteroscopes have side ports that allow the introduction of ureteral catheters, flexible grasping and biopsy forceps, flexible scissors, stone baskets, laser probes, fulgurating electrodes, and lithotriptor probes.

Flexible ureteroscopes can access the entire collecting system without the need for dilation in many cases, and they permit the passage of 3F instrumentation (laser, extracorporeal shock wave lithotripsy probes, stone baskets, and cytology brushes) and simultaneous irrigation under sharp visualization. The flexible scopes are less traumatic and are used more frequently in the upper ureter or renal pelvis. Semirigid ureteroscopes have graduated diameters, such as 6 to 7.5F, which permit a sharper visual image and less traumatic access to an undilated ureter. The scope may be short or long and is available in sizes ranging from 6 to 9F. The 6F scope accommodates up to 3F instrumentation and the 9F up to 5F instrumentation. A second port allows the use of simultaneous irrigation.

Short scopes are used for strictures or stones in the lower ureter, and long scopes for middle and upper ureteral stones, strictures, or tumors.

To allow insertion of a semirigid ureteroscope, ureteral orifices are dilated using single or graduated metal bougies, coaxial plastic ureteral dilators, or a ureteral balloon dilator. The ureteral balloon dilator is inflated with a high pressure inflation syringe.

The ureteroresectoscope has a completely insulated beak. This is used for fulguration or resection of ureteral tumors or ureteral meatotomies. The cutting loop, knife, or hook electrode is connected to an electrocautery cord. For this instrument, the nurse must put a grounding pad on the patient and change the irrigant to water or

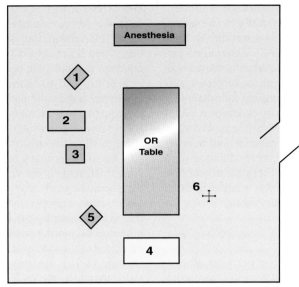

Figure 11-9 Operating room setup for ureteroscopy. 1 = endoscopic video cart; 2 = fluoroscopy C-arm unit; 3 = fluoroscopy TV monitor; 4 = instrument setup; 5 = laser or electrohydraulic lithotripsy unit; 6 = IV pole.

glycine. A cold knife may also be used with the ureteroresectoscope for ureterotomies. The function of the loop is to extend beyond the tumor before using the electrocautery. The tissue is then brought back inside the scope, and at that time, the coagulation is started and the tissue resected. If further coagulation is needed, a fulgurating electrode may also be used.

Electrohydraulic lithotriptors can disintegrate ureteral stones under direct vision via shock waves. Extracorporeal shock wave lithotripsy probes are available in 1F, 3F, and 5F sizes; these probes are flexible and can be inserted through a flexible scope. The probe is attached to a Y cable, which in turn, is attached to the electrohydraulic lithotriptor.

Because the fragments can obscure vision, the field must be kept clear with continuous irrigation. The irrigant also prevents overheating of the probe. More than one probe may be needed to reduce the size of the stone.

The pulsed-dye laser has been used to fragment stones since the early 1970s. The heat generated by the lasers at that time and later with the neodymium:yttrium-aluminum-garnet (Nd:YAG) laser caused extensive damage to soft tissues and to the fiber itself. As a result, the laser was abandoned for treatment of ureteral stones. Improvements in the pulsed-dye laser led to its reintroduction as a tool for treating stones. The laser lithotriptor uses a dye that is attracted to the stone (ureteral and fibrous) and is not absorbed by the tissue; therefore, no tissue damage occurs even when a stone is impacted. The laser is not fired continuously but is pulsated so that heat is not generated in the fiber. Current laser lithotripsy uses the holmium/Nd:YAG laser to fragment stones. A 200600 micron fiber is recommended for ureteral stones and a 200 400 micron fiber for kidney stones. A flexible ureteroscope allows for an optimal view and direct contact with the stone.

Stone baskets contain various numbers of flat or round wires and most are tipless, although some have filiform tips. Baskets of varying thicknesses, lengths, and other characteristics should be available as alternatives if one basket fails.

Disposable flexible rat-toothed, alligator, three-pronged, and cup biopsy forceps are available in different lengths (65 and 115 cm). Nondisposable types are rat-toothed, alligator, and cup biopsy forceps, which are found on the ureteroscopy tray.

Insertion of a ureteral stent and a Foley catheter is routine after ureteroscopy. Stenting diverts the urine so that the uroendothelial tissue can heal, and drains urine if obstruction results from edematous tissue, retained stone fragments, or a stricture. Choices include single or double pigtails and a pigtail with a nonabsorbable suture that comes outside the urethra for easy removal in the office. A flexible cystoscope can also be used to remove stents. Stents are composed of polyurethane and silicone. Some have Teflon coatings. A good selection of stents should be available to allow the endourologist to choose the one best suited to the patient.

PROCEDURE   Once the patient is positioned appropriately, skin preparation from the urethra to groin and perineum is performed. The patient is covered with cystoscopy drapes and the light cable, camera and Y irrigation tubing are passed off the field. The nurse connects the light cable to the light source, camera to camera box and turns the power on. The irrigation tubing is attached to irrigation bags (0.9% sodium chloride) after ensuring that irrigant temperature is equal to the normal body temperature. The C-arm fluoroscope is positioned over the patient and covered with the sterile plastic fluoroscope drape. Fluoroscopic precautions are maintained as described for percutaneous nephrostomy. The procedure begins with a cystoscopy and insertion of a ureteral catheter and guidewire. Contrast dye is injected, and the collecting system is observed by fluoroscopy. The ureteral anatomy is determined, and ureteroscopy is initiated. The ureter is dilated with a dilation device, depending on the surgeon's preference. The nurses are responsible for monitoring the irrigation and providing any additional equipment or supplies. At the end of the procedure, a ureteral stent or ureteral catheter and a Foley catheter are inserted for temporary drainage from the renal pelvis and to allow the ureter to heal. The patient is slowly repositioned to a supine position and transferred to the recovery room.

LAPAROSCOPY

Although the earliest laparoscopes were actually cytoscopes, urologic applications of laparoscopy have only recently been implemented. Pelvic lymph node dissection (PLND) is one of several urologic procedures now performed via laparoscope. The first laparoscopic nephrectomy was performed in June 1990 after the development of an impermeable surgical entrapment sack into which the entire kidney could be placed and an electrical tissue morcellator for fragmenting and evacuating the entrapped renal tissue. The procedures now being performed with a laparoscopic approach are nephrectomy (partial and radical), ablation of renal cyst, nephroureterectomy, pyeloplasty and radical prostatectomy.

The operating room preparation and setup, including equipment, supplies, and instrumentation, and perioperative procedures, are similar to that for PLND and nephrectomy but have their own distinctions and will be described separately (Table 11-4). Successful laparoscopy requires coordination, readiness, knowledge and experience, a team approach, adequate instrumentation, and equipment preparation. The members of the laparoscopy team include the surgeon, surgical assistant, camera operator, scrub nurse, circulator nurse, and anesthesiologist.

OPERATING ROOM SETUP The operating room suite should provide adequate space for equipment, instrumentation, and anesthesia components, and be equipped for conversion to open laparotomy should that become necessary. Safety is a priority in planning the arrangement of equipment during the perioperative phase. Once the equipment is arranged around the operating room table, there should be adequate walking space to allow the laparoscopy team to function.

One of the primary components of the operating room setup is the video monitor. The video cart should be positioned in line with the surgeon, laparoscope, and operative field to provide optimal visualization by the laparoscopic team. For procedures requiring one video monitor, it should be placed at the foot of the operating room table (Figure 11-10). For procedures requiring two video monitors, the mobile carts are positioned opposite each operator and diagonal to the head of the operating room table (Figure 11-11).

EQUIPMENT PREPARATION Equipment preparation is vital to the successful execution of a planned laparoscopic procedure. The video monitor, CO_2 insufflator with CO_2 tank, camera and control box, high-intensity light source, and DVD or VHS recorder are best stored on a mobile cart. This permits the laparoscopic team to monitor the insufflator and observe the procedure on the TV monitor, as well as anticipate the surgeon's needs. The mobile cart may also include a hard copy printer to produce documentation of the procedure for the patient's chart and for educational purposes. The cart allows for efficiency and coordination during the initiation of a laparoscopic procedure when the cords and tubing are being connected to their counterparts. The insufflator must be positioned on the second level of the cart,

or at eye level, so the digital readout is observable (Figure 11-12). The secondary mobile video cart will contain a TV monitor and the connecting cable for the carts.

The components of the mobile video cart are required to be tested either that morning or the day before the procedure (Table 11-5). The following checklist of equipment function and guidelines for preparation of equipment attached to the mobile cart may be helpful when checking each component:

1. Plug in video cabinet(s).
2. If two video cabinets are used, attach connecting cable.
3. Turn video monitor(s) power switch(es) on.
4. Turn insufflator power switch on.
5. Preset pressure to 15 mm Hg.
6. Open CO_2 tank and recheck volume.
7. Turn DVD or VHS recorder power switch on.
8. Attach camera to control unit, turn on, and check picture.

The availability of the remaining equipment must also be considered. Gas tanks should be checked for volume and adequate pressure. A backup CO_2 tank should be available. The nurses are responsible for ensuring that all equipment is properly functioning, clean, easily located, and available without delay during surgery.

INSTRUMENTATION AND OPERATIVE EQUIPMENT Laparoscopic instruments and operative equipment may be divided into two categories: disposable and non-disposable. The selection of disposable instrumentation has increased dramatically. The different types of instruments may be classified as grasping/dissecting, incisional, tissue

Table 11-4 Equipment for Laparoscopy
Mobile video cart
Video monitor
CO_2 insufflator
CO_2 tank
Camera, high-resolution, and control box
High-intensity light source
Super VHS or DVD recorder
Hard copy printer (optional)
Secondary video cart
Video monitor
Connecting cable
Electrosurgical unit with foot pedal
Double-canister suction apparatus
Pneumatic compression unit
Pressurized irrigation system
Multifunction operating room table
Mayo stand
Double-ring stand
Back table

Figure 11-10 Operating room setup for laparoscopic pelvic lymph node dissection. 1 = electrosurgical unit (located next to the primary surgeon); 2 = pneumatic compression unit; 3 = Mayo stand; 4 = double-ring stand; 5 = mobile video cart; 6 = CO_2 tank; 7 = double-suction apparatus; 8 = pressurized irrigator system; 9 = open laparotomy setup.

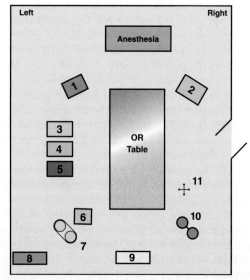

Figure 11-11 Operating room setup for right-sided laparoscopic nephrectomy. 1 = primary mobile video cart (located on the side where the kidney is to be removed); 2 = secondary mobile video cart; 3 = electrosurgical unit (located next to the primary surgeon); 4 = pneumatic compression unit; 5 = morcellator unit; 6 = Mayo stand; 7 = double-ring stand; 8 = open nephrectomy instruments; 9 = cystoscopy setup; 10 = double-suction apparatus; 11 = pressurized irrigator system.

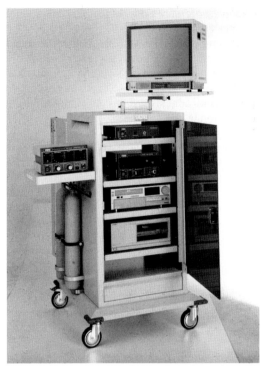

Figure 11-12 Mobile video cart containing laparoscopy equipment.

removal, clip appliers, and retractors. Prior to the laparoscopic procedure, the instruments should be checked to see that they are functioning properly.

As with traditional surgical instruments, rigid laparoscopic instruments have been designed to meet the needs of the surgeon. Endoscopic instruments meet the following specific surgical needs.

- They connect the operator's external actions to the action of the instrument within the peritoneal cavity.
- They are designed to remain closed unless overt action is applied by the operator (ie, they prevent inadvertent opening and/or damage to surrounding tissue).
- They are designed to be inserted and operated within the peritoneal cavity without leakage of air.

The standard sizes for laparoscopic instruments are 5 and 10 mm in diameter and 35 cm in length. The atraumatic grasping/dissecting instrument tips can be wide, narrow, blunt, or pointed (needle nose) with serrated edges. The traumatic tips that are toothed/clawed or spoon-shaped are best used for removing large amounts of tissue or fibrous tissue. The handles of these instruments also vary; they may be of an insulated, pistol mechanism, spring-loaded, or ratchet type. The instruments with insulated handles are connected to an electrosurgical unit to allow for coagulation of tissues. Other instruments, such as the Babcock, Allis, and right-angle graspers, copy the original clamps used for open surgical procedures and are useful for laparoscopic nephrectomy.

The most common incisional instrument used for these procedures is the endoscopic scissors. The tips may be serrated, curved, or hooked, and each type has specific functions. In contrast to other laparoscopic instruments, these scissors are available in reposable (partially reusable, partially disposable), disposable and reusable varieties. The reusable types naturally require sharpening after frequent use. The reposable scissors requires just the scissor tip to be replaced for each use. The disposable curved scissors has a rotating shaft and an electrosurgical connection. This pair of scissors allows for simultaneous coagulation and incising of tissue and is an important instrument for performing laparoscopic PLND and nephrectomy. Up-to-date technology has introduced an instrument that offers ultrasonic cutting and coagulation. The instrument tip is ultrasonically energized to allow for precise cutting and coagulation.

For PLND, tissue removal involves the nodal packets. The best instrument is the 10-mm spoon, or claw grasper with heavy teeth. For laparoscopic nephrectomy, the kidney is removed via an entrapment sack 5 by 8 mm in size. The sacks are impermeable to bacteria and tissue, and contain a drawstring about the neck. The drawstring is used to close the neck of the sack and also serves as a handle to pull the sack up through a 10-mm trocar site. Once the specimen is in the sack, it is further fragmented using an electrical tissue morcellator. The morcellator works in conjunction with a suction vacuum apparatus. The costly morcellator handpiece comes in a sterile package and should be opened only on the surgeon's request. The handpiece is designed with its own plastic drape to cover the unsterile component of the morcellator unit.

The occlusive clip applier and endoscopic retractors must be available whether or not they are used. Both are manufactured as disposable and non-disposable types. The occlusive clip applier is 10 mm in size and is used to ligate vessels or seal tubular structures such as the ureter. For retracting purposes, basic graspers may be used, but in certain procedures their width is inappropriate. A fanlike retractor may be essential during laparoscopic nephrectomy to keep some structures from obscuring the operative view.

The perioperative equipment necessary for laparoscopy includes the Veress needle or Hasson cannula, various trocar sheath units, trocar reducers, and a suction/irrigation system. The Veress needle used to create the pneumoperitoneum can be disposable or reusable. It varies in size, but the most common length for use in adults is 120 or 150 mm. A Hasson cannula may be used instead of the Veress needle in patients who have had previous abdominal surgery or those who are obese; this technique is called "open laparoscopy." The Hasson cannula has a blunt obturator and is secured to the fascia with two stay sutures of 0 silk or polypropylene. A G-inch strip of petrolatum gauze may be wrapped around the sheath to create an effective seal when necessary.

The trocar sheath units vary in size and length. The most common diameters are 5, 10/11, and 12-mm trocar units. The 5-mm trocars are used for instruments such as graspers or scissors and also for the 5-mm laparoscope. The 10- and 12-mm trocars are used for the 10-mm laparoscope, clip appliers, staplers, retractors (such as the fan retractor), and the tissue morcellator. The longer trocar sheaths (150 mm) may be used for patients with thick abdominal walls. The 5-mm instruments may be inserted through 10- and 12-mm trocar sheaths with the aid of a reducer. The reducer snaps onto the top of the trocar, allowing insertion of the instrument. Manufacturers have designed their own reducers, which are not interchangeable.

The suction/irrigation system functions to irrigate by controlled pressure, flushing away blood or tissue to enhance visualization of the abdominal cavity. Fluid and tissue are removed by the suction vacuum apparatus. The suction probe is available in different non-disposable and disposable styles. The probe may have a one-way stopcock or trumpet valve mechanism to control the irrigation and suction. One liter of saline solution with an anticoagulant and a broad-spectrum antibiotic of the surgeon's choice is recommended for irrigation.

PELVIC LYMPH NODE DISSECTION Following the operating room setup and equipment preparation (Table 11-6), the patient is assisted to the operating room table. The circulator nurse positions the patient supine and fastens a safety strap across the mid-thigh region. Thigh-high antiembolic stockings and pneumatic compression sleeves are applied. Tubing from the pneumatic compression unit is attached to the sleeves, and its power switch is turned on. Sheepskin pads are applied to both of the patient's heels to protect the skin.

The anesthesiologist inserts the endotracheal tube and initiates general anesthesia without using N_2O. After insertion of the nasogastric tube to decompress the stomach, a Foley catheter is inserted and connected to a drainage bag. The drainage bag is placed at the head of the table so that the anesthesiologist can assess urinary output.

The patient's arms are secured on each side with the drawsheet. A 3-inch adhesive tape is secured across the upper chest and upper thighs to prevent the patient from moving during differ-

---

Table 11-5 Preoperative Laparoscopy Equipment Function Checklist

Video cabinets plugged in
If two video cabinets, connecting cable attached
Video monitor(s) power switch on
Insufflator power switch on
CO_2 tank open
CO_2 tank contains adequate volume (gauge is in the green range)
Backup CO_2 tank in operating room
VHS recorder power switch is on
Camera attached to camera control box
Camera power switch on
Picture is clear and visible on monitor(s)
Light source power switch on
Light intensity is adequate
N_2O tank (for suction/irrigation) contains adequate volume
Electrosurgical unit digital panel functioning
Electrosurgical unit has foot pedal
Table functions in all positions

Table 11-6 Equipment for Laparoscopic Pelvic Lymph Node Dissection

Disposable Instruments/Supplies	Non-Disposable Instruments/Supplies
1 Veress needle	1 10-mm 0° objective lens
2 5-mm trocars	1 fiberoptic light cable
2 10/11-mm trocars	1 CO_2 insufflator tubing
1 10/11- to 5-mm trocar reducer	2 electrosurgical cords
1 suction/irrigation tubing and probe	2 5-mm atraumatic grasping forceps (blunt, wide type)
1 camera drape	1 5-mm atraumatic grasping forceps (needle-nose type)
1 10-mL syringe filled with normal saline solution	1 10-mm traumatic grasping forceps (claw type)
1 No. 15 blade	1 No. 3 knife handle
1 anti-fog solution	1 straight Mayo scissors
l electrosurgical scissors	1 needle driver
2 4-0 Vicryl PS-2 sutures 14 by 8 inch sponge pack	2 Adson forceps with teeth
1 marking pen	4 towel clips
1 small needle book	2 Kocher clamps
1 package /-inch adhesive strips	2 Kelly clamps
2 Band-Aids	2 Allis clamps
Have Available	2 curved Halsted clamps
1 Hasson cannula (blunt tip)	2 straight Halsted clamps
¹/4-inch petrolatum gauze	2 Army/Navy retractors
0 silk or 0 polypropylene suture	2 Senn retractors
1 occlusive clip applier	1 metal scope warmer (thermos)
1 5-mm 0° laparoscope	

ent table positioning, such as the lateral tilt and the 30° Trendelenburg's position. The table is hyperflexed to expose the pelvis during laparoscopy (Figure 11-13).

The electrosurgical grounding pad is placed on either thigh below the adhesive tape. Abdominal preparation includes shaving and cleansing the skin from the nipples to the pubic region with a povidone-iodine solution. The patient is draped with four towels, an adhesive plastic drape, and a wing laparotomy drape sheet. The abdomen must be dried before placement of the adhesive drape to ensure adherence.

After skin preparation and draping, the scrub nurse positions the Mayo stand at the foot of the sterile field and passes the light cable, CO_2 insufflator tubing, and suction/irrigation tubing off the end of the operating room table. The electrosurgical cautery cords are passed off the side of the sterile field where the surgeon is standing. Simultaneously, the circulator nurse brings the mobile video cart to the foot of the operating room table, and the double-ring stand is positioned next to the surgical assistant's right side. Initially, the CO_2 insufflator

tubing should be connected, and then the light cable, suction/irrigation tubing, and electrosurgical cords. The camera operator or surgical assistant may drape the camera at this point or during the insufflation period. The electrosurgical foot pedal is placed by the surgeon's foot, and the cut and coagulation controls are set. The recommended settings for both are in the 25- to 50-watt range.

After the Veress needle is inserted, the circulator nurse starts the CO_2 insufflation. The CO_2 insufflation tubing should be flushed with gas before it is attached to the Veress needle to remove air or residue. The flow dial is turned slowly at first and then may be increased with positive progression of insufflation. When the preset pressure of 15 mm Hg has been reached, the gas flow will spontaneously stop and the Veress needle is removed. The 10/11-mm trocar is passed to the surgeon for insertion and the 10-mm laparoscope is attached to the camera. At this time, the circulator nurse turns on the high-intensity light source to its maximum power. While the camera operator focuses on a white gauze sponge, the white balance button on the camera box is pressed. The automatic white a ance feature allows one-touch color balance, ensuring true-to-life color reproduction. The overhead lights may be dimmed to enhance the TV monitor. A metal graduated cylinder filled with very warm water and anti-fog solution should be on hand to clear the sterile field. The laparoscope may require defogging during the procedure.

Following the insertion of the primary trocar, two 5-mm trocars and another 10/11-mm trocar are inserted for the introduction of instruments into the abdominal cavity. The suction/irrigation setup should be prepared and ready for use. The spike end of the tubing is inserted into the irrigant solution, and the pressurized irrigator system is turned on. At the initial hookup, the tubing should be primed with irrigant and secured to the

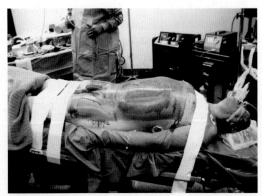

Figure 11-13 Position of patient for laparoscopic pelvic lymph node dissection.

drape. The pressure gauge of the N_2O tank should not measure .60 mm Hg.

After the nodal packets are removed and sent for frozen section analysis, the trocars are removed while hemostasis is maintained. The subcutaneous tissue is closed with an absorbable suture, and adhesive strips or Band-Aids are applied to the puncture sites.

LAPAROSCOPIC NEPHRECTOMY   The equipment and operating room setup differ from that used for PLND (Table 11-7). A secondary video monitor is placed on a mobile cart. The primary mobile video cart containing the camera is positioned on the same side as the kidney to be removed and diagonal to the head of the operating room table. The secondary mobile video cart is placed on the opposite side diagonal to the head of the operating room table. The scrub nurse prepares an additional cystoscopy setup for the initial part of the procedure. Instruments used for open nephrectomy as well as laparoscopy are essential components of the operating room setup (see Figure 11-11).

The patient is transferred to the operating room and positioned supine on a radiolucent cystoscopy table. Both arms are extended and secured on padded arm boards. A strap is fastened across the thighs to ensure patient safety. General anesthesia without N_2O is preferred for patients undergoing laparoscopic renal surgery. After the endotracheal tube is placed, a nasogastric tube is inserted to decompress the stomach.

The first part of the procedure involves cystoscopy and insertion of a ureteral occlusion balloon catheter. The patient's legs are positioned simultaneously in padded footrest stirrups. The C-arm fluoroscope is positioned, and the TV component is placed in view of the surgeon. A floppy-tip guidewire is inserted, and the ureteral occlusion balloon is introduced in the renal pelvis of the affected kidney under fluoroscopic visualization. The balloon catheter serves as a ureteral landmark for the affected kidney. At this time, a 16F Foley catheter with a 5-mL balloon is inserted and attached to a drainage bag. A ureteral drainage bag is attached to the balloon catheter. The two catheters are secured together with a 2-0 silk tie. The patient is repositioned in a supine position and prepared for transfer to a multifunction operating room table. A beanbag mattress covered with a sheet should be placed on the operating room table before moving the patient.

After the patient is transferred, thigh-high antiembolic stockings and pneumatic compression sleeves are applied. The flank area should be positioned over the kidney rest and the break in the table. The patient is placed in a lateral decubitus position, bringing the body to the edge of the operating room table. The ipsilateral arm (affected side) is positioned on a raised padded arm rest and the contralateral arm (unaffected side) is extended and positioned on a padded arm board. To protect the brachial plexus of the contralateral arm, an axillary roll is placed. Sheepskin pads are applied to both elbows to maintain the integrity of the skin. A pillow is placed between the legs, and the lower

Table 11-7 Equipment for Laparoscopic Nephrectomy

Disposable Instruments/Supplies	Non-Disposable Instruments/Supplies
1 Veress needle	1 10-mm 0° objective lens
3 5-mm trocars	1 fiberoptic light cable
1 10/11-mm trocar	1 CO2 insufflator tubing
1 12-mm trocar	2 electrosurgical cords
2 10/11- to 5-mm trocar reducers	2 5-mm atraumatic grasping forceps (blunt, wide type)
1 suction/irrigation tubing and probe	1 5-mm atraumatic grasping forceps (needle nose type)
1 camera drape	1 10-mm traumatic grasping forceps (claw type)
1 10-mL syringe filled with normal saline solution	2 endoscopic Babcock forceps
1 electrosurgical scissors	2 endoscopic right-angle forceps
1 anti-fog solution	1 No. 3 knife handle
3 occlusive clip appliers	1 straight Mayo scissors
1 retractor (fan type)	1 needle drive
1 No. 15 blade	2 Adson forceps with teeth
1 4 by 8 inch sponge	4 towel clips
1 marking pen	2 Kocher clamps
1 small needle book	2 Kelly clamps
1 package ½-inch adhesive strips	2 Senn retractors

Cystoscopy Setup

30° telescope	2 Army/Navy retractors
70° telescope	1 metal scope warmer (thermos)
20F cystoscope	**Have Available**
23F cystoscope	1 5 by 8 mm entrapment sack
Short bridge	1 sack introducer
Balloon catheter	1 10-mm tissue morcellator
Bentson guidewires	
16F Foley catheter with 5-mL balloon	
30% Hypaque	
Foley drainage bag	
2-0 silk tie	

leg is flexed 30° at the knee and hip with the upper leg remaining extended and slightly flexed (Figure 11-14). The knee, ankle, and foot should also be protected from undue pressure with sheepskin padding. The kidney region is exposed by raising the kidney rest, and the table is flexed. At this time, the beanbag mattress is connected to vacuum suction until it is firm and molded. Closing off the valve or leaving it connected to suction during the procedure keeps the beanbag firm. Finally, 3-inch adhesive tape is secured across the shoulders and hip area and fastened to the operating room table. The tubing from the pneumatic compression unit is attached to the sleeves, and the unit power switch is turned on. The two drainage bags are positioned at the head of the table so the anesthesiologist can monitor urinary output. The electrosurgical grounding pad is placed on the exposed thigh, and the body is examined to make sure that no part of the patient is touching metal.

The operative area is cleansed and disinfected with povidone-iodine solution. If necessary, the skin in the operative field is shaved. The full abdominal skin preparation includes the entire abdomen from the xiphoid process to the symphysis pubis and from just lateral to the contralateral rectus muscle to the posterior axillary line on the ipsilateral side. The patient is draped with four towels, an adhesive plastic drape, and a wing laparotomy drape sheet. The abdomen must be dry before the adhesive drape is applied to ensure adherence.

The scrub nurse positions the Mayo stand on the affected side and passes the light cable and

CO_2 insufflator tubing off the head of the table toward the primary video cart. The electrosurgical cautery cords are passed off the side of the sterile field where the surgeon is standing. At the same time, the circulator nurse positions the double-ring stand next to the scrub nurse and connects the CO_2 insufflator tubing and light cord. The scrub nurse passes the suction/irrigation tubing off the foot of the operating room table. The electrosurgical foot pedal is placed by the surgeon's foot and the unit is set as recommended for PLND.

After insertion of the Veress needle, the circulator nurse starts the CO_2 insufflator. The scrub

nurse flushes the tubing with gas before it is attached to the Veress needle to remove air or residue. The pressure is preset at 15 mm Hg, and the flow dial is turned slowly. With a positive progression of insufflation, the flow is increased until it reaches the preset pressure. Then the Veress needle is removed and the 10/11-mm trocar is prepared for insertion. Once inserted, the 10-mm laparoscope is attached to the camera. The circulator nurse then turns on the high-intensity light source to its maximum power. The camera must be white-balanced before the laparoscope is inserted into the abdominal cavity. The camera operator focuses on a white gauze sponge, and the circulator nurse presses the white balance button on the camera box. The overhead lights may be dimmed to enhance the TV monitors. Very warm water in a metal scope warmer with a rubber seal and anti-fog solution should be available to clean and defog the laparoscope lens throughout the procedure.

A total of five trocars are inserted for the introduction of instruments. The suction/irrigation setup should be assembled as described for PLND. For this procedure, it may be necessary to have more than one bag of irrigant available.

After the kidney is freed, the entrapment sack is prepared for insertion. The sack or bag is rolled around a metal introducer and inserted through the trocar. The kidney is placed in the sack and fragmented using a tissue morcellator. The circulator nurse and the scrub nurse prepare the tissue morcellator. After the morcellator unit is plugged in, the scrub nurse connects the suction tubing to the morcellator handpiece. The scrub nurse must make sure that the valve of the handle is turned off until the surgeon is ready to activate it. The foot pedal is placed by the surgeon's foot, and the valve is turned on by the surgeon once the kidney is in the entrapment sack.

Once the sack filled with renal tissue is removed, a check is made to ensure that all trocars have been removed and hemostasis is controlled. The anterior fascia at the 11-mm trocar sites is closed with No.1 absorbable braided suture. A subcuticular stitch is used to close the skin over

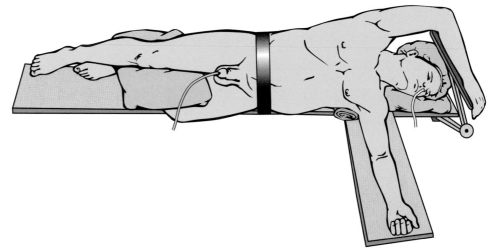

Figure 11-14 Position of patient for laparoscopic nephrectomy.

the 11-mm port sites, and tape strips are used to close the skin over the 5- and 11-mm port sites.[8]

REFERENCES

1. Gomella LG, Strup SE. The history of urologic laparoscopy: from cystoscope to laparoscope. In: Gomella LG, Kozminski M, Winfield HN, editors. Laparoscopic urologic surgery. New York: Raven Press; 1994. p. 9.

2. Clayman RV, McDougall EM. Laparoscopic renal surgery. In: Clayman RV, McDougall EM, editors. Laparoscopic urology. St. Louis: Quality Medical Publishing; 1993. p. 273.

3. Dorsey J. Operating room organization. Laser and advanced operative laparoscopy. Obstet Gynecol Clin North Am 1991;18:571.

4. Reichart M. Laparoscopic instruments. Patient care, cost issues. AORN J 1993;57:637.

5. Goldsteing DS, Chandhoke PS, Kavoussi LR. Laparoscopic equipment. In: Clayman RV, McDougall EM, editors. Laparoscopic urology. St. Louis: Quality Medical Publishing; 1993. p. 112.

6. Preminger G. Video systems for laparoscopic surgery. In: Gomella LG, Kozminski M, Winfield HN, editors. Laparoscopic urologic surgery. New York: Raven Press; 1994. p. 54.

7. Clayman RV, McDougall EM. Laparoscopic renal surgery. In: Clayman RV, McDougall EM, editors. Laparoscopic urology. St. Louis: Quality Medical Publishing; 1993. p. 279.

8. Kavoussi LR, Clayman RV. Laparoscopic renal surgery: nephrectomy, nephroureterectomy, and ureterolysis. In: Gomella LG, Kozminski M, Winfield HN, editors. Laparoscopic urologic surgery. New York: Raven Press; 1994. p. 157.

Part II

Percutaneous Surgery

12

Surgical Anatomy of the Kidney

Francisco J.B. Sampaio, MD

GENERAL ANATOMY

The kidneys are paired organs lying retroperitoneally on the posterior abdominal wall. Each kidney is of a characteristic shape, having a superior and an inferior pole, a convex border placed laterally, and a concave medial border. The medial border has a marked depression the hilum containing the renal vessels and the renal pelvis.

RENAL MORPHOMETRY   In adults, we found the left kidney larger than the right kidney, and this finding is in agreement with morphometric findings in fetal kidneys.[1] The right kidney presented a mean length of 10.97 cm, while the left kidney presented mean length of 11.21 cm. The right kidney presented 3.21 cm of mean thickness at the hilum, and the left kidney presented mean thickness of 3.37 cm.[2]

An interesting and worthwhile finding is that, in the same kidney, the superior pole has a greater width (mean = 6.48 cm) than the inferior pole (mean = 5.39 cm). We also found a statistically significant correlation between the kidney length and the stature of the individuals.[2]

POSITION OF THE KIDNEYS   Because the kidneys lie on the posterior abdominal wall, against the psoas major muscles, their longitudinal axis parallels the oblique course of the psoas (Figure 12-1). Moreover, since the psoas major muscle has a shape of a cone, the kidneys also are dorsal and inclined on the longitudinal axis. Therefore, the superior poles are more medial and more posterior than the inferior poles (see Figure 12-1). Because the hilar region is rotated anteriorly on the psoas muscle, the lateral borders of both kidneys are posteriorly positioned. It means that the kidneys are angled 30 to 50° behind the frontal (coronal) plane (Figure 12-2).[3]

PERIRENAL COVERINGS   The kidney surface is enclosed in a continuous covering of fibrous tissue called the renal capsule (or "true renal capsule"). Each kidney within its capsule is surrounded by a mass of adipose tissue lying between the peritoneum and the posterior abdominal wall and called the perirenal fat (see Figures 12-2 and 12-3). The perirenal fat is enclosed by the renal fascia (so-called fibrous renal fascia of Gerota or, in this textbook, Gerota's fascia). The renal fascia is enclosed anteriorly and posteriorly by another layer of adipose tissue, which varies in thickness, called the pararenal fat (see Figure 12-3).

The renal fascia comprises a posterior layer (a well-defined and strong structure) and an anterior layer, which is a more delicate structure that tends to adhere to the peritoneum (see Figures 12-2 and 12-3). The anterior and posterior layers of the renal fascia (Gerota's fascia) subdivide the retroperitoneal space in three potential compartments: (1) the posterior pararenal space, which contains only fat; (2) the intermediate perirenal space, which contains the suprarenal glands, kidneys and proximal ureters, together with the perirenal fat; (3) the anterior pararenal space, which unlike the posterior and intermediate spaces, extends across the midline from one side of the abdomen to the other. This space contains the ascending and descending colon, the duodenal loop and the pancreas (Figure 12-4).[3] Inferiorly, the layers of the renal fascia end weakly fused around the ureter (see Figures 12-3 and 12-5). Superiorly, the two layers of the renal fascia fuse above the suprarenal gland and end fused with the infradiaphragmatic fascia (see Figure 12-5). An additional fascial layer separates the suprarenal gland from the kidney (see Figure 12-5). Laterally, the two layers of the renal fascia fuse behind the ascending and descending colons. Medially, the posterior fascial layer is fused with the fascia of the spine muscles. The anterior fascial layer merges into the connective tissue of the great vessels (aorta and inferior vena cava) (see Figures 12-2 and 12-4).

These anatomic descriptions of the renal fascia show that right and left perirenal spaces are potentially separated, and therefore, it is exceptional that a complication of an endourologic procedure (eg, hematoma, urinoma, perirenal abscess) involves the contralateral perirenal space.[3]

KIDNEY RELATIONSHIPS WITH DIAPHRAGM, RIBS, AND PLEURA   The kidneys lie on the psoas and quadratus lumborum muscles. Usually, the left kidney is higher than the right kidney, being the posterior surface of the right kidney crossed by the 12th rib and the left kidney crossed by the 11th and 12th ribs (see Figure 12-1). The posterior surface of the diaphragm attaches to the extremities of the 11th and 12th ribs (Figure 12-6). Close to the spine, the diaphragm is attached over the posterior abdominal muscles and forms the medial and lateral arcuate ligaments on each side (see Figure 12-6). In this way, the posterior aspect of the diaphragm (posterior leaves) arches as a dome above the superior pole of the kidneys, on each side. Therefore, when performing an intrarenal access by puncture, the endourologist may consider that the diaphragm is traversed by all intercostal punctures, and possibly by some punctures below the 12th rib (Figure 12-7). Also, it can be expected that the pleura is transversed without symptoms in most intercostal approaches.[4]

Generally, the posterior reflection of the pleura extends inferiorly to the 12th rib; nevertheless, the lowermost lung edge lies above the 11th rib (at the 10th intercostal space) (see Figure 12-7). Regardless of the degree of respiration (mid- or full expiration), the risk of injury to the lung from a 10th intercostal percutaneous approach to the kidney is prohibitive.[4] Any intercostal puncture should be made in the lower half of the intercostal space, in order to avoid injury to the intercostal vessels above.

KIDNEY RELATIONSHIPS WITH LIVER AND SPLEEN   The liver on the right side and the spleen in the left, may be posterolaterally positioned at the level of the suprahilar region of the kidney, because at this point, these organs have their larger dimensions (Figure 12-8). Therefore, one may remember that a kidney puncture performed high in the

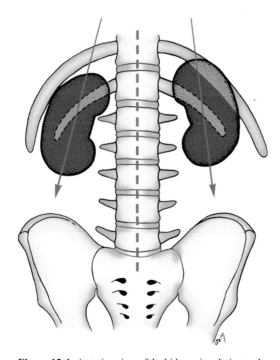

Figure 12-1 Anterior view of the kidneys in relation to the skeleton, shows that the longitudinal axes of the kidneys are oblique *(arrows)*, being the superior poles more medial than the inferior poles. The dashed line marks the longitudinal axis of the body. This figure also shows that the posterior surface of the right kidney usually is crossed by the 12th rib and the left kidney by the 11th and 12th ribs.

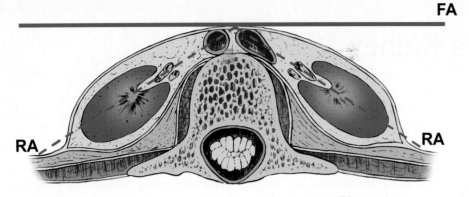

Figure 12-2 Superior view of a transverse section of the kidneys at the level of the 2nd lumbar vertebra shows that the kidneys are angled 30 to 50° behind the frontal (coronal) plane. *FA* = frontal plane of the body; *RA* = renal frontal (coronal) axis.

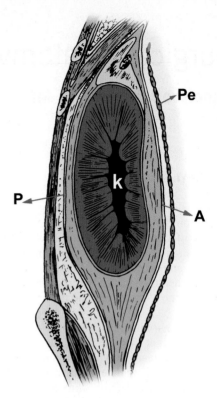

Figure 12-3 Lateral view of a longitudinal section through the retroperitoneum, reveals the posterior *(P)* and the anterior *(A)* layers of the renal fascia. *Pe* = peritoneum; *K* = kidney.

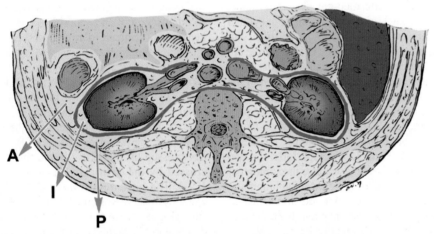

Figure 12-4 Superior view of a transverse section of the kidneys at the level of the 2nd lumbar vertebra shows the three compartments of the retroperitoneal space. *P* = posterior pararenal space, which contains only fat; *I* = intermediate perirenal space, which contains the suprarenal glands, kidneys and proximal ureters, together with the perirenal fat; *A* = anterior pararenal space, which unlike the posterior and intermediate spaces, extends across the midline from one side of the abdomen to the other, and contains the ascending and descending colons, the duodenal loop and the pancreas.

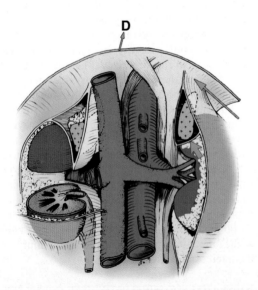

Figure 12-5 Anterior view of a schematic drawing of the renal fascia (Gerota's fascia) and the kidneys. This scheme depicts that the two layers of the renal fascia fuse above the suprarenal gland and end blended with the infradiaphragmatic fascia *(long arrow)*. Note a dependence of the fascia separating the suprarenal gland from the kidney *(short arrow)*. *D* = diaphragm muscle.

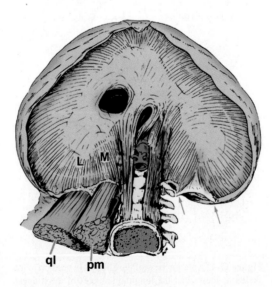

Figure 12-6 Schematic drawing of an inferior view of the diaphragmatic dome. The *arrows* point to the diaphragmatic attachments to the extremities of the 11th and 12th ribs. *M* = medial arcuate ligament, *L* = lateral arcuate ligament; *ql* = quadratus lumborum muscle; *pm* = psoas muscle.

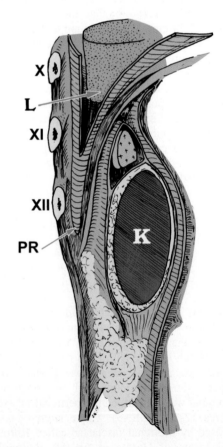

Figure 12-7 Schematic drawing from a lateral view of the kidney and its relationships with the diaphragm, ribs, pleura, and lung. *PR* = posterior reflection of the pleura, *L* = lower edge of the lung; *K* = kidney; *X* = 10th rib; *XI* = 11th rib; *XII* = 12th rib.

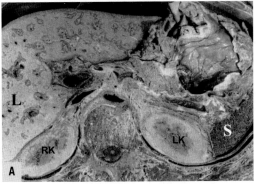 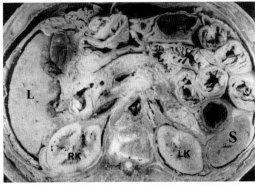

Figure 12-8 *A*, Inferior view of a transverse section through a cooled cadaver at the level of the suprahilar region of the kidney reveals that the liver *(L)* and the spleen *(S)* are posterolaterally positioned in relation to right *(RK)* and left *(LK)* kidneys. *B*, Similar section of that shown in *A*, performed at the level of the infrahilar region reveals that inferiorly, the liver *(L)* and the spleen *(S)* are more laterally positioned in relation to right *(RK)* and left *(LK)* kidneys.

abdomen has little space for the needle entrance.[4] If the intrarenal puncture is performed when the patient is in mid- or full inspiration, the risk to the liver and spleen is increased.[4] This knowledge is particularly important in patients with hepatomegaly or splenomegaly, on whom a computed tomography (CT) scan should be performed before puncturing the kidney.

KIDNEY RELATIONSHIPS WITH ASCENDING AND DESCENDING COLONS The ascending colon runs from the ileocolic valve to the right colic flexure (hepatic flexure), where it passes into the transverse colon. The hepatic colic flexure (hepatic angle), lies anteriorly to the inferior portion of the right kidney. The descending colon extends inferiorly from the left colic flexure (splenic flexure) to the level of the iliac crest. The left colic flexure lies anterolateral to the left kidney.

It is important to consider the position of the retroperitoneal ascending and descending colons. Occasionally, it was observed in the course of routine abdominal CT scan examinations, that the retroperitoneal colon is lying in a posterolateral or even a postrenal position.[5] Hence, in these cases, it is at great risk of being injured during the intrarenal percutaneous approach. This event (retrorenal colon) more commonly occurs with

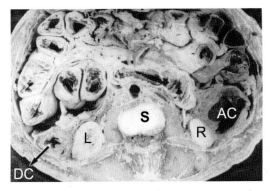

Figure 12-9 Superior view of a transverse section through a cooled cadaver at the level of the inferior poles of the kidney, reveals the ascending *(AC)* and descending *(DC)* colons lying in a posterolateral position in relation to right *(R)* and left *(L)* kidneys. *S* = spine.

regard to the inferior poles of the kidneys (Figure 12-9). In a controlled study, it was demonstrated by CT scan that, when the patient is in the supine position, the retrorenal colon was found in 1.9% of the cases. Nevertheless, when the patient assumes the prone position (the more frequent position used for percutaneous access to the kidney) the retrorenal colon was found in 10% of the cases.[5] Therefore, special attention should be given, under fluoroscopy and with the patient in the prone position, to detecting patients with retrorenal colon prior any invasive percutaneous renal procedure. This examination is especially important in the area of the inferior poles of the kidneys.[5]

INTRARENAL VESSELS **Intrarenal Arteries** To aid understanding of the next topics in this chapter, a brief summary on the classical anatomy and nomenclature of the renal artery and its branches is presented (Figure 12-10).

Generally, the main renal artery divides into an anterior and a posterior branch after giving off the inferior suprarenal artery. Whereas the posterior branch (retropelvic artery) proceeds as the posterior segmental artery to supply the homonymous segment without further significant branching, the anterior branch of the renal artery provides three or four segmental arteries. The segmental arteries divide before entering the renal parenchyma into interlobar arteries (infundibular arteries), which progress adjacent to the caliceal infundibula and the minor calices, entering the renal columns between the renal pyramids (see Figures 12-10 and 12-11).[6] As the interlobar arteries progress, near the base of the pyramids, they give origin (usually by dichotomous division) to the arcuate arteries (see Figures 12-10 and 12-11). The arcuate arteries give off the interlobular arteries, which run to the periphery giving off the afferent arterioles of the glomeruli (see Figure 12-11).[6]

Intrarenal Veins The intrarenal veins, unlike the arteries, do not have a segmental model. Moreover, in contrast to the arteries, there is free circulation throughout the venous system, providing ample anastomoses between the veins. These anastomoses, therefore, prevent parenchymal congestion and ischemia in case of venous injury.[7]

The small veins of the cortex, called stellate veins, drain into the interlobular veins that form a series of arches (Figure 12-12). Within the kidney substance, these arches are arranged in arcades, which lie mainly in the longitudinal axis. There are usually three systems of longitudinal anastomotic arcades and the anastomosis occur in different levels: between the stellate veins (more peripherally), between the arcuate veins (at the base of the pyramids) and between the interlobar (infundibular) veins (close to the renal sinus) (see Figure 12-12). We named these anastomoses as first order, second order, and third order, from periphery to center.[7] In previous works, we found three trunks (53.8%) and two trunks (28.8%) joining each other to form the main renal vein. Less frequently, we found four trunks (15.4%) and five trunks (1.9%).[7]

A detailed description of the kidney collecting system (pelviocaliceal system), as well as the anatomic relationships of the intrarenal arteries and veins with the kidney collecting system, which are of utmost importance for endourology, will be fully presented and discussed in the next topics of this chapter.

PELVIOCALICEAL SYSTEM: ENDOUROLOGIC IMPLICATIONS

ANATOMIC CLASSIFICATION Recent advances in endourology have revived interest in collecting system anatomy, since a full understanding of such anatomy is necessary to perform reliable endourologic procedures as well as uroradiologic analysis.[8–10] We have proposed a pelviocaliceal classification including all morphologic types of

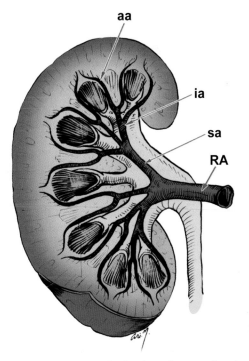

Figure 12-10 Schematic drawing of an anterior view from a right kidney, shows the branching of the renal arteries and their official nomenclature according to kidney regions. *RA* = renal artery; *sa* = segmental artery; *ia* = interlobar (infundibular) artery; *aa* = arcuate artery.

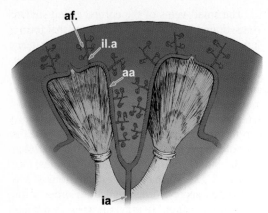

Figure 12-11 Schematic drawing of two adjacent pyramids and minor calices, depicts the renal vasculature from the level of the interlobar arteries to the glomerular level. *ia* = interlobar (infundibular artery); *aa* = arcuate artery; *il. a* = interlobular artery; *af.* = afferent arteriole of the glomerulus.

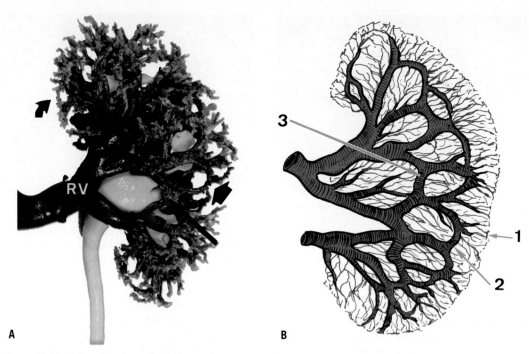

Figure 12-12 *A*, Anterior view of left kidney endocast of the pelviocaliceal system together with the venous vascular tree shows the three systems of longitudinal anastomotic arcades; from lateral (periphery) to medial (hilar): stellate veins *(curved arrow),* arcuate veins *(short arrow)* and interlobar veins *(long arrow)*. *RV* = renal vein. *B*, Schematic drawing shows the three orders of arcades: *1* = first order arcade; *2* = second order arcade; *3* = third order arcade.

collecting systems and we believe that such classification is interesting for endourologists, mainly for helping in unifying patients and procedures.[9]

Material of Investigation   We analyzed 140 three-dimensional polyester resin corrosion endocasts of the pelviocaliceal system, obtained from 70 fresh cadavers according to a technique described previously.[8] Figure 12-13 shows an endocast of the pelviocaliceal system together with a schematic drawing on which the basic elements of such a system are represented.

Basic Intrarenal Anatomy   The renal parenchyma consists basically of two kinds of tissue, the cortical tissue and the medullar tissue. On a longitudinal section (Figure 12-14), the cortex forms the external layer of renal parenchyma. The renal medulla is formed by several inverted cones, surrounded by a layer of cortical tissue on all sides (except at the apexes). As in longitudinal sections, a cone assumes the shape of a pyramid (see Figure 12-14), and the established expression for the medullar tissue is renal pyramid; the apex of a pyramid is the renal papilla. The layers of cortical tissue between adjacent pyramids are named renal columns (cortical columns of Bertin, see Figure 12-14).[8,10]

The cortical tissue comprises the glomeruli with proximal and distal convoluted tubules. The renal pyramids comprise the loops of Henle and collecting ducts; these ducts join to form the papillary ducts (about 20) which open at the papillary surface (area cribrosa papillae renalis, Figure 12-15) draining urine into the collecting system (into the fornix of a minor calix).

A minor calix is defined as the calix that is in immediate apposition to a papilla (see Figures 12-14 and 12-15). The renal minor calices drain the renal papillae and range in number from 5 to 14 (mean, 8); although the number of minor calices is widely varied, we found 70% of the kidneys presenting 7 to 9 minor calices.[8] A minor calix may be single (drains one papilla) or compound (drains two or three papillae) (see Figures 12-13 and 12-15). The polar calices often are compound, markedly in the superior pole (see

Figure 12-13). The minor calices may drain straight into an infundibulum or join to form major calices, which subsequently will drain into an infundibulum (see Figures 12-13 and 12-15). Finally, the infundibula, which are considered the primary divisions of the pelviocaliceal system, drain into the renal pelvis.

Classification of the Pelviocaliceal System
The analysis of 140 endocasts led us to a division

into two major groups (with two intermediate varieties into each major group). The division was based on superior pole, inferior pole and kidney midzone (hilar) caliceal drainage.

Group A   This group is composed of pelviocaliceal systems that present two major caliceal groups (superior and inferior) as a primary division of the renal pelvis and a midzone caliceal drainage dependent on these two major groups

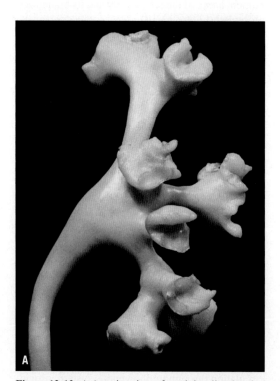

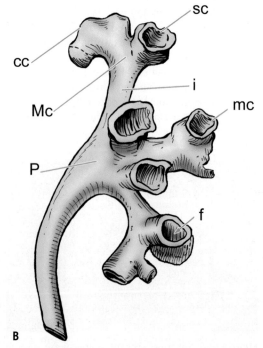

Figure 12-13 *A*, Anterior view of a pelviocaliceal endocast from a left kidney, obtained according to the injection-corrosion technique. *B*, Schematic drawing of the endocast shown in *A*, indicates the essential elements of kidney collecting system. *cc* = compound calix; *sc* = single calix; *mc* = minor calix; *Mc* = major calix; *f* = caliceal fornix; *i* = infundibulum; *P* = renal pelvis. Reproduced with permission from Sampaio FJB.[8]

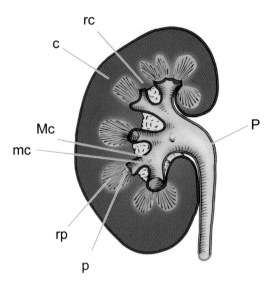

Figure 12-14 Schematic drawing of a longitudinal section of the kidney depicts the intrarenal structures. *c* = renal cortex; *rc* = renal column (cortical column of Bertin); *rp* = renal pyramid; *p* = renal papilla; *mc* = minor calix; *Mc* = major calix; *P* = renal pelvis. Reproduced with permission from Sampaio FJB.[8]

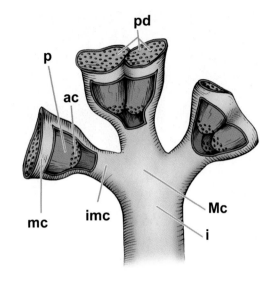

Figure 12-15 Schematic drawing representing the possibilities of minor calix arrangement. A single minor calix drains only one papilla and a compound minor calix drains two or three papillae. *p* = renal papilla; *pd* = papillary ducts; *ac* = area cribosa; *mc* = minor calix; *Mc* = major calix; *imc* = infundibulum of a minor calix (caliceal neck); *i* = infundibulum. Reproduced with permission from Sampaio FJB.[8]

system. In Figure 12-18B, we observe a cast presenting just the opposite aspect (both superior and inferior caliceal infundibula are short and thick); this kind of anatomic formation will certainly make easier the introduction and the manipulation of a nephroscope within the superior and inferior collecting systems.

COMPARATIVE ANALYSIS BETWEEN STANDARD PYELOGRAMS AND THE CORRESPONDING THREE-DIMENSIONAL COLLECTING SYSTEM ENDOCASTS Since the standard excretory urogram (intravenous pyelogram [IVP]) shows the collecting system in only one plane, it is extremely difficult for the practitioner to visualize and imagine this system in three dimensions, as it is in reality. A full understanding of pelviocaliceal anatomy is a prerequisite for successful endourologic interventions in the upper urinary tract as well as for interpreting IVPs and other imaging examinations.

Anatomic Background To assist endourologists in making a mental image of the collecting system in three dimensions and learning the exact spatial position of the calices, in 40 cases, before obtaining the pelviocaliceal system endocast, an iodinated contrast material was injected into the ureter to opacify the collecting system in order to obtain a pyelogram. After radiography, the contrast material was removed and the collecting system was filled with a polyester resin to obtain a three-dimensional endocast. These 40 kidneys enabled a comparative study between the radiographic images and their corresponding three-dimensional endocasts.

Findings and Clinical Implications The comparative study between pyelograms and

(62.2%) (Figure 12-16). Group A includes two different types (varieties) of pelviocaliceal systems.

Type A-I (45%)   The kidney midzone is drained by minor calices that are dependent on the superior or on the inferior caliceal groups, or even on both superior and inferior caliceal groups, simultaneously (see Figure 12-16A).

Type A-II (17.2%)   The kidney midzone is drained by crossed calices, one draining into the superior caliceal group and another draining into the inferior caliceal group, simultaneously (see Figure 12-16B). When we analyzed the endocasts that have crossed calices in the kidney midzone, we observed that the crossed calices (laterally) and the renal pelvis (medially) bound a region (space) that we designated the "interpelviocaliceal" (IPC) region (space) (see Figure 12-16B).

Group B   This group is composed of pelviocaliceal systems that present the kidney midzone (hilar) caliceal drainage independent of both the superior and the inferior caliceal groups (37.8%) (Figure 12-17). This group also includes two different types (varieties) of pelviocaliceal systems:

Type B-I (21.4%)   The kidney midzone is drained by a major caliceal group, independent of both the superior and the inferior groups (see Figure 12-17A).

Type B-II (16.4%)   The kidney midzone is drained by minor calices (one to four) entering directly into the renal pelvis (see Figure 12-17B). Such calices are independent of both the superior and the inferior caliceal groups.

The kidney collecting system is amply varied and is not symmetrical. We found pelviocaliceal systems with morphologic bilateral symmetry in the same individual in only 37.1% of the cases (26 pairs of kidneys).

Although our pelviocaliceal classification includes all morphologic types of calices and

renal pelves, in performing endourologic procedures, one must be aware that the collecting system anatomy is amply varied. In Figure 12-18A, for example, we observe a cast that reveals a very long and thin superior caliceal infundibulum; this anatomic formation will certainly cause difficulties in the introduction and manipulation of a nephroscope into the superior pole collecting

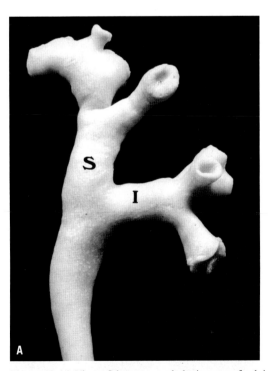

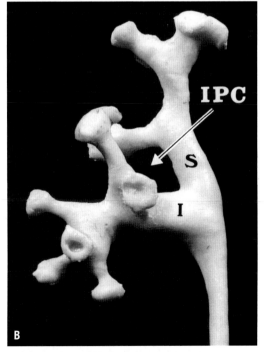

Figure 12-16 View of the two morphologic types of pelviocaliceal systems that constitute Group A. *A*, Type A-I: anterior view of a left pelviocaliceal cast shows the kidney midzone drained by calices dependent on the superior *(S)* and inferior *(I)* caliceal groups. *B*, Type A-II: anterior view of a right pelviocaliceal cast shows the kidney midzone drained by crossed calices, dependent on the superior *(S)* and inferior *(I)* caliceal group simultaneously. This cast shows the interpelviocaliceal space *(IPC)*. Reproduced with permission from Sampaio FJB.[8]

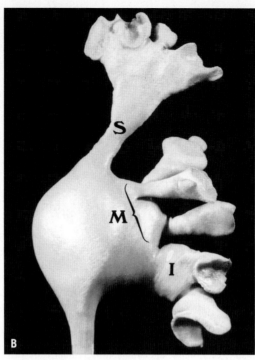

Figure 12-17 View of the two morphologic types of pelviocaliceal systems that constitute Group B. *A*, Type B-I: anterior view of a left pelviocaliceal cast shows the kidney midzone drained by a hilar major calix *(M)* independent of the superior *(S)* and inferior (I) major calices. *B*, Type B-II: anterior view of a left pelviocaliceal cast shows the kidney midzone drained by minor calices *(M)* entering straight into the renal pelvis, independent of both the superior *(S)* and inferior *(I)* caliceal groups. Reproduced with permission from Sampaio FJB.[8]

three-dimensional endocasts of the collecting system enabled a perception of some remarkable anatomic aspects of the kidney collecting system that are important for consideration by endourologists during endourologic procedures.

Presence of Perpendicular Minor Calices
In 11.4% of the cases (16/140 casts), we found a perpendicular minor calix draining directly into the renal pelvis or into a major calix (Figure 12-19). The minor calices perpendicular to the surface of the collecting system, which are seen in the casts, can be superimposed on other structures. Because of this fact, visualization of these calices radiographically can be difficult (Figure 12-20). Stones in such minor calices can be seen on standard anteroposterior radiographic images as if they were placed in the pelvis or in a major calix. Thus, one must consider this anatomic detail in cases of stones that do not alter renal function and that apparently are in the renal pelvis or in a major calix. In this situation, a complementary radiologic study with lateral and oblique films must be done to determine accurately the position and extent of the stones.[11,12]

When a stone is located in a perpendicular minor calix (see Figure 12-19) its removal presents additional difficulties for both extracorporeal shock wave lithotripsy (ESWL) and percutaneous nephrolithotripsy. Patients with stones in such calices are not good candidates for ESWL because these calices invariably present narrow infundibula (smaller than 4 mm in diameter); therefore, the discharge of the disintegrated stone fragments will be difficult.[13,14] Regarding the percutaneous removal, direct access into the calix containing the stone is an easy approach; nevertheless, it involves a puncture performed without

considering the arterial and venous anatomic relationships to the collecting system. This kind of puncture carries a great risk of injuring a vascular structure.[12] Therefore, in cases of stone in such calices, a variety of safe and refined accesses, techniques and instruments should be used.

Crossed Calices In 17.2% of the cases, the kidney midzone (hilar) was drained by crossed calices, one draining into the superior caliceal

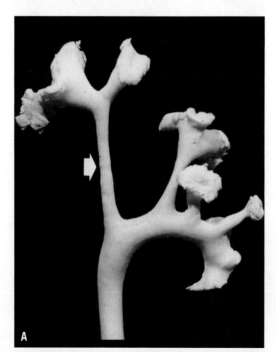
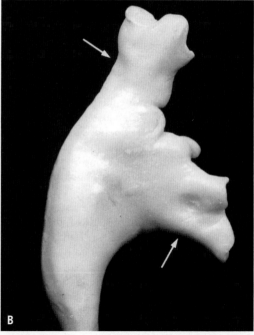

Figure 12-18 Anterior view of two left pelviocaliceal casts. *A*, This cast reveals long and thin superior caliceal infundibulum *(arrow)*. *B*, This cast reveals short and thick superior and inferior caliceal infundibula *(arrows)*. Reproduced with permission from Sampaio FJB.[8]

group and the other draining into the inferior caliceal group simultaneously. On the pyelograms, the crossed calices (laterally) and the renal pelvis (medially) outlined a radiolucent region that we termed the interpelviocaliceal region (see Figure 12-20A). In the three-dimensional endocasts, that same region is seen as if it were a space (see Figure 12-20B).[9,11,12]

The interpelviocaliceal space may have different shapes: like a lozenge (the most common), long and narrow, and even small and round, depending on the shape of the calices and the shape of the renal pelvis (Figure 12-21). Regardless of the form assumed by the interpelviocaliceal space, it is the result of crossed calices in the mid-kidney.

When the crossed calices were in the mid-kidney, the calix that drained into the inferior caliceal group was in ventral position in 87.5% of the cases,[9,11,12] (Figure 12-22). In some cases, even when radiographically the calix draining into the inferior group is apparently in dorsal position, we verified its ventral position on the endocast (see Figure 12-22). This constant spatial arrangement is noteworthy for endourologic maneuvers. If one intends to access the renal pelvis via crossed calix, or, contrariwise, intends to access a crossed calix via the renal pelvis, it is useful to remember that the calix draining into the inferior caliceal group is almost always in a ventral position. It is also worthy of note that detection of an interpelviocaliceal region on the pyelogram is an indirect sign of crossed calices in the kidney midzone.

Position of the Calices Relative to the Lateral Kidney Margin In 39 of 140 casts (27.8%), the anterior calices had a more lateral (peripheral) position than the posterior calices (Figure 12-23). In 27 casts (19.3%) the posterior calices were in a

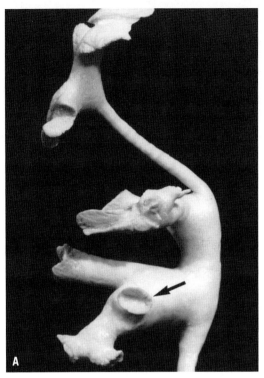 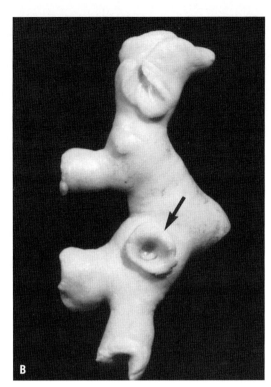 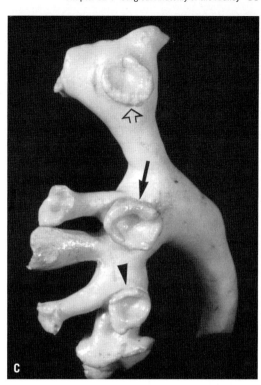

Figure 12-19 *A,* Anterior view of right pelviocaliceal endocast reveals perpendicular minor calix draining into the inferior caliceal group *(arrow). B,* Anterior view of right pelviocaliceal endocast reveals perpendicular minor calix draining into the inferior caliceal group *(arrow)* very close to the renal pelvis. *C,* Anterior view of right pelviocaliceal endocast reveals perpendicular minor calix draining into the renal pelvis *(arrow).* This cast also shows a perpendicular minor calix draining into the superior caliceal group *(open-arrow)* and a perpendicular minor calix draining into the inferior caliceal group *(arrowhead).* Reproduced with permission from Sampaio FJB.[12]

more lateral position than the anterior calices (Figure 12-24). In the majority of the cases (74 casts; 52.9%) the anterior and posterior calices had varied positions: superimposed or alternately distributed (in one region, the most lateral were the anterior calices, and in another region, the most lateral were the posterior calices) (Figure 12-25).

Since the place of choice to access the collecting system is through a posterior calix, much effort has been dispensed in an attempt to determine preoperatively which calices are anterior and which calices are posterior. Previous studies have presented contradictory results and have led to misunderstanding of this subject.[15] Since we described a kind of kidney collecting system,

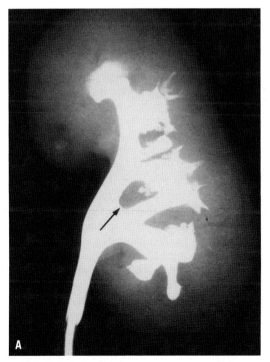 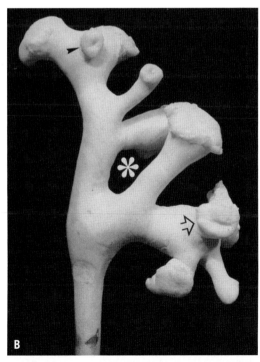 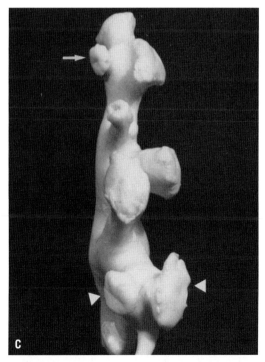

Figure 12-20 Comparative study between radiographic view of a left kidney and its corresponding three-dimensional cast. *A,* Anterior view of a retrograde pyelogram shows a radiographic image of the interpelviocaliceal region *(arrow). B,* Anterior view of the corresponding three-dimensional endocast. The *asterisk* demonstrates interpelviocaliceal space. The *arrowhead* shows a minor calix perpendicular and superimposed to the surface of a superior major calix, which cannot be seen on the pyelogram. *Open arrow* shows anterior minor calix superimposed on the posterior minor calix. On pyelogram, making a distinction between them can be difficult. *C,* Oblique view of the same case. The *arrow* shows a perpendicular minor calix into the superior caliceal group. *Arrowheads* demonstrate distinction between the anterior and posterior minor calices, which are superimposed on the pyelogram. Reproduced with permission from Sampaio FJB.[12]

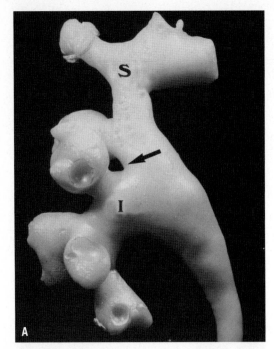
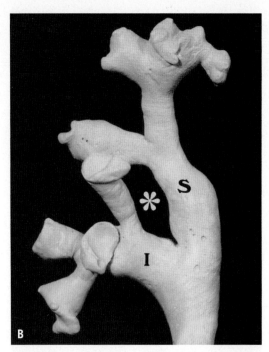
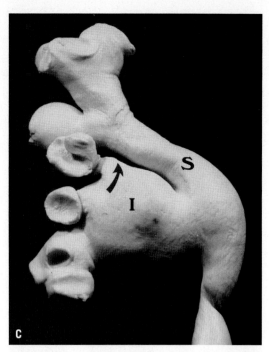

Figure 12-21 Anterior view of right pelviocaliceal endocasts demonstrating the different shapes that the interpelviocaliceal (IPC) space may assume. *A,* Small and round IPC space *(arrow). B,* Lozangic IPC space (most frequent shape), *asterisk. C,* Long and narrow IPC space *(arrow). S* = superior caliceal group; *I* = inferior caliceal group. Reproduced with permission from Sampaio FJB.[12]

found in the majority of the endocasts, on which the calices are disposed in varied positions (superimposed or alternately distributed), we may affirm that the position of the calices cannot be defined as more lateral or more medial. Considering the large variation of the calices (more than 50% in varied positions), we believe that precise determination of caliceal position becomes difficult with the

common radiologic methods, even using oblique and lateral views.[9,11] To solve this problem quickly and inexpensively, during endourologic procedures, with the patient in the prone position, injection of room air into the collecting system will rise to the more posterior portions of the collecting system, determining which calices are placed posteriorly (radiolucent contrast).[11,12,16]

Position of the Calices Relative to the Polar Regions and to the Kidney Midzone The superior pole was drained by a midline caliceal infundibulum in 98.6% of the cases (Figure 12-26). The midzone (hilar) was drained by paired calices that were arranged in two rows (anterior and posterior) in 95.7% of the cases (see Figure 12-26). The inferior pole was drained by paired calices arranged in two rows in 81 casts (57.9%) (see Figure 12-26A) and by a single midline caliceal infundibulum in 59 casts (42.1%) (see Figure 12-26B).

With regard to the caliceal drainage of the kidney polar regions, many investigators affirmed that there usually is only one caliceal infundibulum draining each pole.[3,10,14] In our study, the superior pole was drained by only one midline caliceal infundibulum in 98.6% of the cases. The inferior pole, however, was drained by paired calices arranged in two rows in 81 of 140 cases (57.9%) and by one midline caliceal infundibulum in 59 cases (42.1%) (see Figure 12-26). These results are important to endourology; it will be easier to access endoscopically a polar region drained by a single infundibulum, which usually has a suitable diameter, rather than a polar region drained by paired calices (see Figure 12-26). Because the inferior pole is drained by paired calices in 57.9% of the cases, one must keep in mind this anatomic detail in order to plan and perform the intrarenal access and the endoscopic procedures in the inferior pole. The caliceal drainage of superior and inferior poles is also of utmost importance in ESWL and was fully discussed in previous papers.[13,17] Concerning the kidney midzone (hilar) drainage, our results show that this region is drained by paired calices arranged in 2 rows (anterior and posterior) in 95.7% of the cases (see Figure 12-26). These

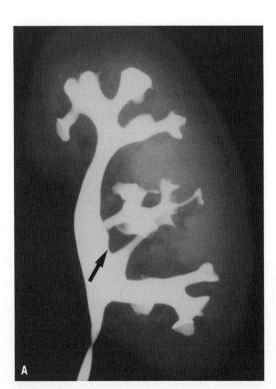
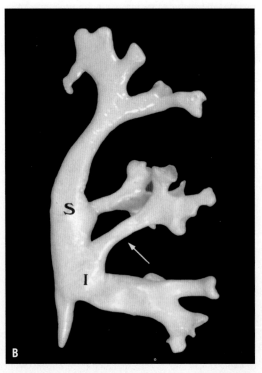

Figure 12-22 Comparative study between a retrograde pyelogram of a left kidney and its corresponding three-dimensional endocast of the pelviocaliceal system. *A,* Anterior view of a retrograde pyelogram shows radiographic image of interpelviocaliceal region *(arrow). B,* Anterior view of corresponding three-dimensional cast. *Arrow* shows that the calix draining into the inferior caliceal group is in ventral position (87.7% of the cases of IPC space). *S* = superior caliceal group; *I* = inferior caliceal group. Reproduced with permission from Sampaio FJB.[12]

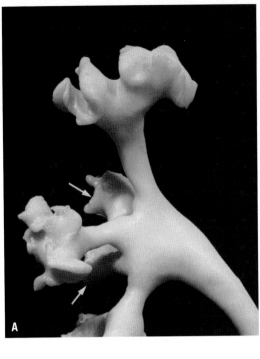

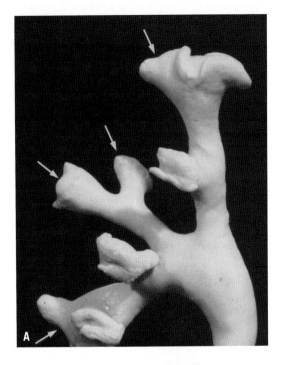

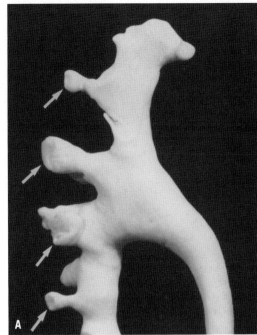

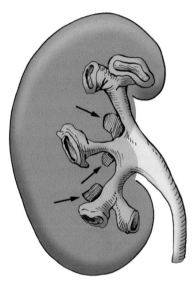

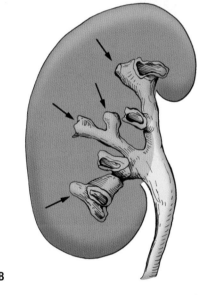

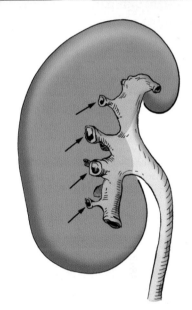

Figure 12-23 Position of the calices related to lateral margin of the kidney. *A,* Anterior view of right pelviocaliceal cast. This cast reveals that the anterior calices have a more lateral (peripheral) position than posterior calices *(arrows).* It means that the posterior calices are placed medially. *B,* Schematic drawing of the same case shown in *A,* demonstrates the peripheral calices in the anterior plane and the medial calices *(arrows)* in the posterior plane. Reproduced with permission from Sampaio FJB.[12]

Figure 12-24 Position of the calices related to lateral margin of the kidney. *A,* Anterior view of right pelviocaliceal cast. This cast reveals that the posterior calices *(arrows)* have a more lateral (peripheral) position than anterior calices. *B,* Schematic drawing of the same case shown in *A,* demonstrates the peripheral calices in the posterior plane *(arrows)* and the medial calices in the anterior plane. Reproduced with permission from Sampaio FJB.[12]

Figure 12-25 Position of the calices related to lateral margin of the kidney. *A,* Anterior view of right pelviocaliceal cast. This cast reveals that the calices in the anterior plane *(arrows)* are placed alternately relative to the lateral margin of the kidney. In one region, they are more lateral, and in another region, they are more medial. *B,* Schematic drawing of the same case shown in *A,* demonstrates the calices in the anterior plane *(arrows)* placed alternately relative to the lateral kidney margin. In one region, they are more lateral, and in another region, the calices in the posterior plane are more lateral. Reproduced with permission from Sampaio FJB.[12]

results should also be retained by endourologists to access and work in the mid-kidney.

ANATOMIC RELATIONSHIPS OF INTRARENAL VESSELS (ARTERIES AND VEINS) WITH THE KIDNEY COLLECTING SYSTEM: IMPORTANCE FOR THE INTRARENAL ACCESS BY PUNCTURE

Percutaneous nephrostomy is the procedure of choice for temporary drainage of urine and for gaining access to the kidney during numerous endourologic and interventional procedures. The development of new percutaneous techniques as well as the creation of a variety of working instruments, enabled the replacement of several open surgeries by percutaneous therapy (eg, renal abscess, caliceal diverticulum, infundibular stenosis, ureteropelvic junction obstruction, some cases of upper tract urothelial tumors, and even nephrectomy).[18–20] Percutaneous procedures are relatively invasive, and complications may occur. One of the most significant complications is vascular injury that occurs when the urologist is obtaining intrarenal access. This problem may have several cumbersome consequences, including intraoperative hemorrhage, hypotension, loss of functional renal parenchyma, arteriovenous fistula, and pseudoaneurysm.[21–25]

This section offers an anatomic depiction of refined details concerning intrarenal vessels and their relationships to the collecting system, showing how to perform safe percutaneous intrarenal access by keeping as many renal vessels as possible intact during puncture.

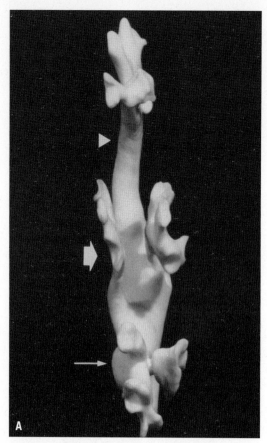

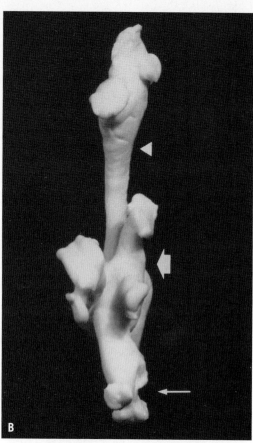

Figure 12-26 Position of calices related to the polar regions and kidney midzone. *A*, Lateral view of a left pelviocaliceal cast. The superior pole is drained by a single midline caliceal infundibulum *(arrowhead)*. The midzone (hilar) is drained by paired calices arranged in two rows *(short arrow)*; anterior and posterior. The inferior pole is drained by paired calices arranged in two rows *(long arrow)*. *B*, Lateral view of a right pelviocaliceal cast. The superior pole is drained by a single midline caliceal infundibulum *(arrowhead)*. The midzone is drained by paired calices arranged in two rows *(short arrow)*; anterior and posterior. The inferior pole is drained by only one midline caliceal infundibulum *(long arrow)*. Reproduced with permission from Sampaio FJB.[12]

MATERIAL STUDIED FOR THE ANATOMIC BACK-GROUND We analyzed 62 retrograde pyelograms and the corresponding three-dimensional polyester resin corrosion endocasts of the kidney collecting system, together with the intrarenal arteries and veins, from fresh cadavers.

The kidneys were punctured under fluoroscopic guidance and the endocasts obtained with the needles positioned in the place of puncture (Figure 12-27). For comparative analysis, we studied kidneys that had been punctured through a caliceal infundibulum and kidneys punctured through a caliceal fornix.

Intrarenal Access through an Infundibulum
Figure 12-13 highlighted the basic anatomy of the renal collecting system. Keeping those anatomic landmarks in mind, note that a puncture through an infundibulum (in any region of the kidney) presents clear hazards.[26]

Superior Pole Puncture is most dangerous through the upper-pole infundibulum because this region is surrounded almost completely by large vessels (Figure 12-28). Infundibular arteries and veins course parallel to the anterior and posterior aspects of the upper-pole infundibulum. In our series, injury to an interlobar (infundibular) vessel was a common consequence of puncturing the upper-pole infundibulum (67% of kidneys) (Figure 12-29); the injured vessel was an artery in 26% of those cases.

The most serious vascular accident in upper infundibulum puncture is a lesion of the posterior segmental artery (retropelvic artery). This event may occur because this artery crossed and is related to the posterior surface of the upper infundibulum

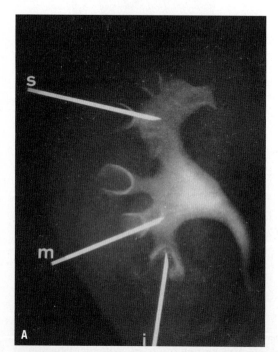

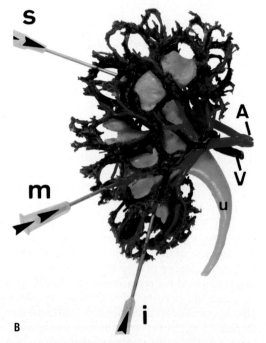

Figure 12-27 *A*, Anterior view of a retrograde pyelogram from a right kidney shows superior-pole *(s)*, mid-kidney *(m)*, and inferior-pole *(i)* punctures. These punctures were performed after polyester resin injections into the arterial and venous systems, while the resins were still in the gel state. Note that the injected resins are not opaque to x-rays. *B*, Anterior view of the corresponding corrosion endocast obtained after contrast removal and pelviocaliceal system injection with resin. The needles are maintained in their original places. s = superior-pole puncture; m = mid-kidney puncture; i = inferior-pole puncture. The arrowheads point out the tracts of the needles. A = renal artery; V = renal vein; u = ureter.

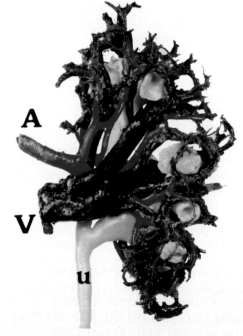

Figure 12-28 Oblique medial view of an endocast of arterial *(A)*, venous *(V)*, and pelviocaliceal systems from a left kidney reveals the upper infundibulum almost completely encircled by infundibular arteries and veins. This anatomic arrangement makes the upper-pole infundibular puncture especially dangerous. *u* = ureter.

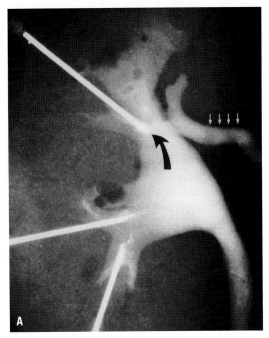

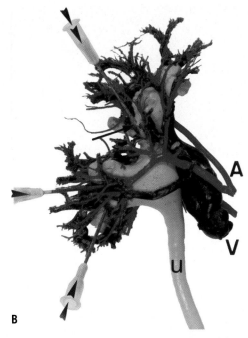

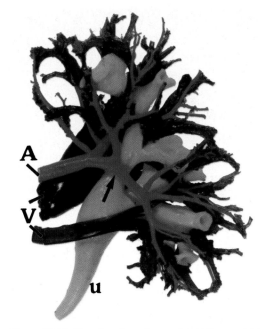

Figure 12-29 *A*, Posterior view of a retrograde pyelogram from a left kidney shows that a puncture performed through the upper-pole infundibulum injured an infundibular vein *(curved arrow).* Note the contrast material in the retropelvic vein *(short arrows).* *B*, Posterior view of the corresponding endocast reveals the site of lesion *(arrow). Arrowheads* point out the needle tracts. *A* = renal artery; *V* = renal vein; *u* = ureter. Reproduced with permission from Sampaio FJB, et al.[24]

Figure 12-30 Posterior view of an endocast from a right kidney reveals the posterior segmental artery (retropelvic artery) crossing the posterior surface of the upper infundibulum *(arrow). A* = renal artery; *V* = renal vein; *u* = ureter. Reproduced with permission from Sampaio FJB, et al.[24]

in 57% of the cases (Figure 12-30).[27] Figure 12-31 shows an upper infundibulum puncture in which the needle tract produced complete laceration of the posterior segmental artery. Because the posterior segmental artery (retropelvic artery) may supply up to 50% of the renal parenchyma, injury to it may result in significant loss of functioning renal tissue; in addition to causing hemorrhage.[28]

Middle Kidney Intrarenal access through the mid-kidney infundibulum produced arterial lesion in 23% of kidneys studied. The middle branch of the posterior segmental artery was injured more often than any other vessel.

Inferior Pole The posterior aspect of the lower-pole infundibulum is widely presumed by endourologists and interventional radiologists to be free of arteries. It is considered, therefore, to be a safe region through which to gain access to the collecting system and to place a nephrostomy tube. In about 38% of the kidneys examined, however, an infundibular artery is found in this region.[27] Thus, significant complications may develop as a consequence of a posterior approach through the supposedly vessel-free lower infundibulum.[22,25,26] In fact, we found an arterial injury in 13% of kidneys in which we had made a puncture through the lower-pole infundibulum.

Concerning the veins, in many kidneys that we studied, we found large venous anastomoses similar to collars around the caliceal infundibula (the so-called caliceal necks).[7] Puncture through the lower-pole infundibulum, therefore, also risks injury to a venous arcade (Figure 12-32). A venous lesion usually heals spontaneously, but consequent hemorrhage may be cumbersome during the procedure.

Our findings clearly demonstrate that percutaneous nephrostomy through an infundibulum

of a calix is not a safe route because this type of access poses an important risk of significant bleeding from interlobar (infundibular) vessels.

Infundibular puncture also creates the hazard of through-and-through (two-wall) puncture of the collecting system (Figure 12-33). Because major segmental branches of the renal artery, as

well as major tributaries of the renal vein, are positioned on the anterior surface of the renal pelvis, marked hemorrhage may occur as a result of an anterior through-and-through perforation. In addition, effective tamponade of anterior vessels that have been injured is difficult because they lie distantly in the nephrostomy tract.[24,26,29]

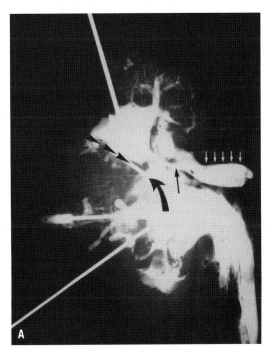

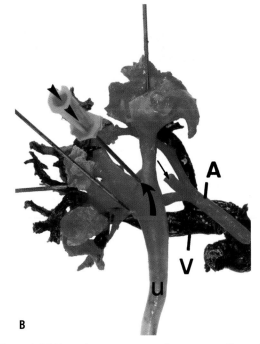

Figure 12-31 *A*, Posterior view of a retrograde pyelogram from a left kidney shows contrast medium extravasation and contrast material in the arterial system and in the main trunk of the renal artery *(short arrows).* The retropelvic artery was injured by the needle pointed by the *arrowheads.* The *curved arrow* shows the lesion site. *Straight arrow* points the retropelvic artery filled with contrast medium extravasated from the collecting system. *B*, Posterior view of the corresponding endocast reveals the retropelvic artery divided *(straight arrow)* and the needle responsible for the lesion *(arrowheads).* The *curved-arrow* reveals the lesion site. *A* = renal artery; *V* = renal vein; *u* = ureter. Reproduced with permission from Sampaio FJB, et al.[24]

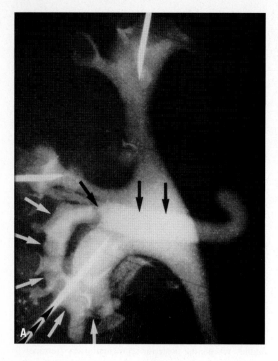

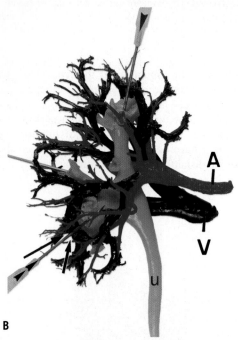

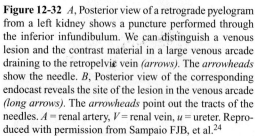

Figure 12-32 *A,* Posterior view of a retrograde pyelogram from a left kidney shows a puncture performed through the inferior infundibulum. We can distinguish a venous lesion and the contrast material in a large venous arcade draining to the retropelvic vein *(arrows).* The *arrowheads* show the needle. *B,* Posterior view of the corresponding endocast reveals the site of the lesion in the venous arcade *(long arrows).* The *arrowheads* point out the tracts of the needles. *A* = renal artery, *V* = renal vein, *u* = ureter. Reproduced with permission from Sampaio FJB, et al.[24]

Although the infundibular access is feasible in some circumstances, and must be considered in specific situations (some difficult anatomic cases for example), the surgeon must evaluate the risk of an arterial lesion, primarily in the superior pole and in the mid-kidney.[24]

Intrarenal Access Through the Renal Pelvis
Direct puncture of the renal pelvis for endourologic surgery should be excluded. Besides the fact

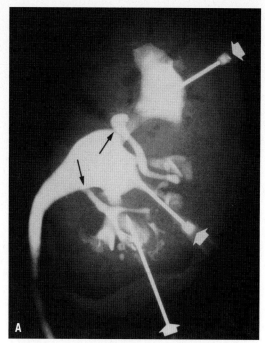

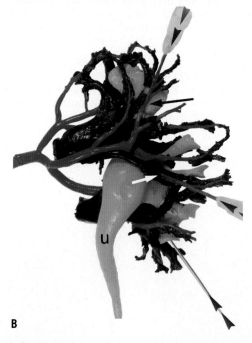

Figure 12-33 *A,* Posterior view of a retrograde pyelogram from a right kidney reveals superior, middle, and inferior punctures *(short arrows)* and the contrast material in the superior and inferior infundibular arteries *(black arrows).* *B,* Posterior view of the corresponding endocast reveals injury to an upper infundibular artery *(black arrow).* The mid-kidney puncture *(white arrow)* was a through-and-through (two walls) puncture and injured an anterior segmental artery. The injured vessel furnished the posteroinferior branch filled with contrast on the pyelogram. The *arrowheads* point out the tracts of the needles. *u* = ureter. Reproduced with permission from Sampaio FJB, et al.[24]

that the nephrostomy tube inserted at this site is easily dislodged and difficult to reintroduce during the operative maneuvers, renal pelvis puncture has a prohibitive and unnecessary risk of injuring a retropelvic vessel (artery and/or vein).[7,22,27]

Intrarenal Access through a Caliceal Fornix
When we made a puncture through a fornix of a

calix, venous injury occurred in fewer than 8% of the kidneys. These injuries occurred indiscriminately, in the upper-pole, mid-pole, and lower-pole calices. We did not detect any arterial lesions as a consequence of a fornical puncture.[24]

In conclusion, the high rate of vascular injury and the possibility of associated complications mean that a nephrostomy tube should not be placed through an infundibulum of a calix (Figure 12-34). On the other hand, and regardless of the region of the kidney, puncture and placement of a nephrostomy tube through a fornix of a calix is safe and must be the site chosen by the operator (Figure 12-35). Even in the superior pole, the intrarenal puncture through a caliceal fornix is harmless (Figure 12-36). In addition, when puncturing through a fornix of a calix, in case of lesion, the injury was always to a peripheral vessel, such as a small venous arcade (Figure 12-37).

VASCULAR ANATOMY AND INTRARENAL ENDOUROLOGIC SURGERY

The development of new endourologic procedures and instrumentation techniques as well as the conception of special operative instruments, allowed an important improvement in endourologic intrarenal surgery to treat numerous renal diseases and/or help the management of difficult cases in endourology.[19,20, 29, 30]

A serious and troublesome complication of endoscopic intrarenal operation is bleeding from an injured vessel.[29,30] To avoid such injury one must know the position of the intrarenal vascular structures in relation to the collecting system. With that knowledge, one must consider each specific kidney region with emphasis on the infundibular regions.[6,31]

MATERIAL STUDIED FOR THE ANATOMIC BACKGROUND We analyzed 82, three-dimensional polyester resin corrosion endocasts of the kidney collecting system together with the intrarenal arteries and 52 endocasts of the kidney collecting system, together with the intrarenal veins, obtained according to the injection-corrosion technique described previously.[7,11,27]

Regional Vascular Anatomy of the Kidney
Superior Pole The upper infundibulum is almost completely involved by segmental or interlobar (infundibular) arteries in 86.6% of the cases (Figure 12-38). In 84.6% of the cases, there was an anterior and a posterior venous plexus in close relationship to the upper infundibulum (Figure 12-39).

Middle Kidney The anterior aspect of the mid-kidney infundibulum of a major or a minor calix was in close relationship to a segmental or an infundibular artery in 65% of the cases (see Figure 12-38A). In the posterior aspect, in all cases, we found at least one mid-kidney infundibulum in close relationship to the mid-subdivision branch of the posterior segmental artery (retropelvic artery) (see Figure 12-38B).

Concerning the veins, the anterior aspect of a middle infundibulum was in contact with an ante-

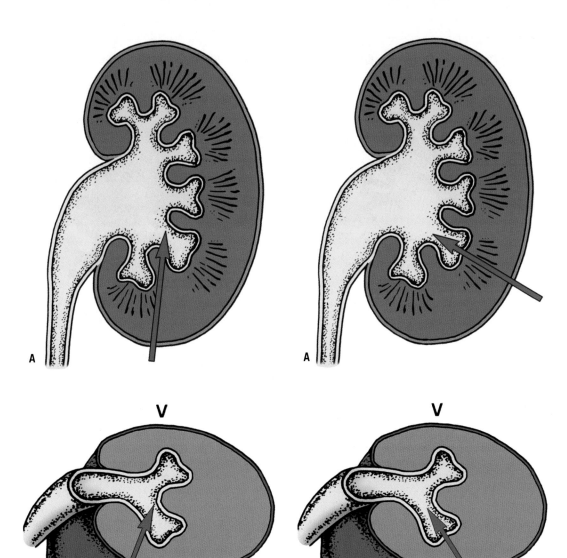

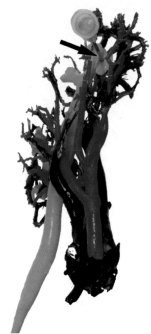

Figure 12-36 Superior view of an endocast from a left kidney shows that, even in the superior pole, a puncture through the fornix of a calix *(arrow)* is safe.

Figure 12-34 *A*, Posterior view of a longitudinal section of a right kidney demonstrates an intrarenal puncture performed through a caliceal infundibulum. This kind of puncture should not be performed because it presents a high risk of a vascular injury. *B*, Superior view of a transverse section of a kidney also demonstrates an intrarenal puncture through a caliceal infundibulum—not a recommended route. *V* = ventral region; *D* = dorsal region.

Figure 12-35 *A*, Posterior view of a longitudinal section of a right kidney demonstrates an intrarenal puncture performed through a caliceal fornix. This kind of puncture is safe and is associated with a very low incidence of vascular injury. *B*, Superior view of a transverse section of the kidney demonstrates an intrarenal puncture through a caliceal fornix—a route that is strongly recommended. *V* = ventral region; *D* = dorsal region.

Where to Incise the Kidney Collecting System Based on Vascular Anatomy If any intrarenal operation is necessary to free entrapped stones, to treat strictures and diverticula, to incise a narrowed infundibulum, to correct other anomalies that can cause stone formation, and even to facilitate the access for the rigid nephroscope to a specific calix,[29,30] the operator must visualize the

rior tributary of the renal vein in 71% of the cases. The posterior aspect of a middle infundibulum was in close relation to a posterior tributary of the renal vein in 21% of cases (see Figure 12-39).

The vascular relations to mid-kidney infundibula are amply varied because they follow the calices variations, which are large in this region.[8,27]

Inferior Pole In all cases, the lower infundibular anterior aspect of a major or a minor calix was in close relationship to a branch of the anteroinferior or the inferior segmental artery (see Figure 12-38A). Concerning the posterior aspect, in 38% of the cases, an extension of the posterior segmental artery itself was in close rela-

tion to the lower major caliceal infundibulum. In the other 62%, the posterior aspect of the lower major caliceal infundibulum was free from arteries; nevertheless, the posterior aspect of the lower-most minor calix infundibulum was related to an artery in all cases (see Figure 12-38B).

With respect to veins, the anterior aspect of at least one lower infundibulum was in contact with an intrarenal vein in all cases. The posterior aspect of a lower infundibulum was in close relationship to a large tributary of the renal vein in 21% of the cases (see Figure 12-39). In addition, in the inferior pole, a collar-like venous anastomosis around the minor calices infundibula (caliceal necks) is often found (see Figure 12-39).

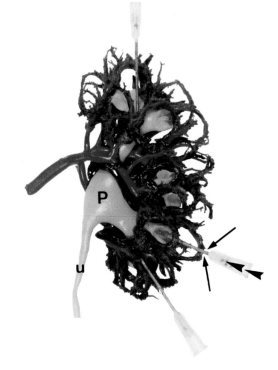

Figure 12-37 Posterior view of an endocast from a right kidney and an inferior puncture performed through a fornix of a calix. The *arrows* show a lesion to a small peripheral venous arcade. The *arrowheads* demonstrate the needle tract. *P* = renal pelvis; *u* = ureter.

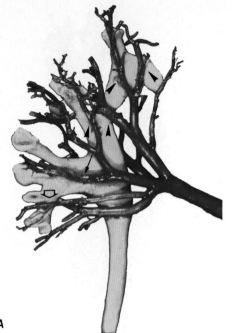

A

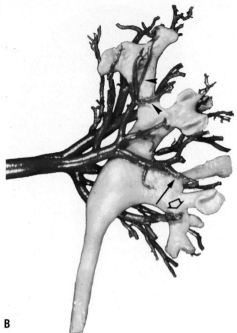

B

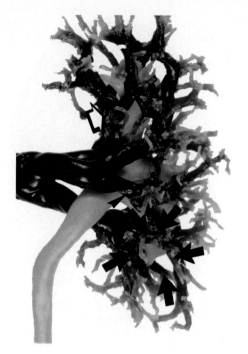

Figure 12-38 *A,* Anterior view of an endocast (pelviocaliceal system and arteries) from a right kidney shows the anterior surface of upper infundibulum in close relationship to segmental and interlobar (infundibular) arteries *(arrowheads).* The *arrow* points to an artery coursing in the anterior surface of mid-kidney infundibulum. The *open arrow* reveals the extension of the anteroinferior segmental artery close to the lower infundibulum anterior surface of a minor calix. *B,* Posterior view of the same cast shown in *A,* reveals infundibular arteries in close relationship to the posterior surface of the upper infundibulum *(arrowheads).* The *arrow* points to the mid-subdivision branch of the posterior segmental artery (retropelvic artery) crossing the posterior aspect of a mid-kidney infundibulum. The *open arrow* indicates an infundibular artery close to the posterior aspect of the infundibulum of the lowermost calix. Reproduced with permission from Sampaio FJB.[31]

Figure 12-39 Posterior view of an endocast (pelviocaliceal system and veins) from a right kidney reveals a large venous plexus in close relationship to the upper infundibulum *(short arrow).* The *arrowhead* points to the posterior aspect of the lower infundibulum in close relationship to a large vein. The *arrows* bound a collar-like venous anastomosis around the neck of the lower minor calix. Reproduced with permission from Sampaio FJB.[31]

arterial relations found more frequently in the area to be incised. It was established that one must examine the area under direct vision to be certain that there are no arterial pulsations,[29] and then a short incision to a depth of 1 to 2 mm may be made. If necessary (eg, the infundibulum remains thick), it is better to make a second incision in a different site than to deepen the first incision, due to the risk of injuring a large vessel.[29,31]

Even taking into account these technical recommendations, significant bleeding may occur during intrarenal endourologic surgery.[29,30] Also, arterial pulsations are not always readily identifiable endoscopically during surgery, mainly because patients may be hypotensive due to anesthesia.[6,31]

Although it is difficult to eliminate bleeding completely, maintenance of anatomic orientation during all steps of the procedure and a thorough knowledge of the relationship between the pelviocaliceal system and the vessels are imperative to reducing vascular complications, and improving on safe and efficient operations.

On the basis of the anatomic vascular background presented here, and considering that the circumference of an infundibulum is composed of four quadrants, we advise that the infundibular incision be done in the superior or in the inferior quadrant (Figure 12-40), because in general, these areas are not in relation to large vascular structures. Contrariwise, the posterior, and especially the anterior, aspects of infundibular surfaces are frequently related to intralobar (infundibular) vessels (see Figure 12-40). From

an anatomic standpoint, if more than one infundibular incision is necessary, we recommend the following sequence:

- The first incision in the superior quadrant.
- The second incision in the inferior quadrant.
- The third incision between the superior and the posterior quadrant.

- The fourth incision between the inferior and the posterior quadrant.
- The fifth incision in the posterior quadrant.
- Anterior incisions must be always avoided.

Because the free circulation throughout the venous system prevents parenchyma loss and ischemia, arteries are considered of utmost

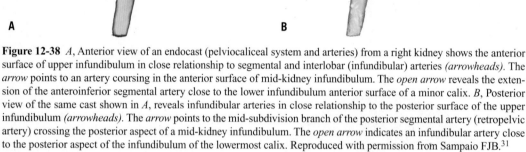
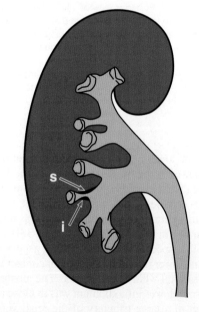
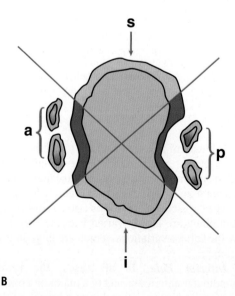

A

B

Figure 12-40 Schematic drawing of renal collecting system. *A,* anterior view of right kidney pelviocaliceal system points out the sites to be incised in infundibular stenosis; *s* = superior quadrant; *i* = inferior quadrant. *B,* Transverse section through an infundibulum shows the four quadrants that comprise the infundibular circumference and points out the preferred two areas to be incised (*s* = superior quadrant; *i* = inferior quadrant). This drawing also shows the anterior *(a)* and posterior *(p)* quadrants, which are usually closely related to vessels. Reproduced with permission from Sampaio FJB.[31]

importance in intrarenal endosurgery. Nevertheless, veins should be considered as well, because an injury to a large vein would result in important and troublesome back bleeding. Moreover, as the veins do not pulsate, they cannot be perceived through the nephroscope; therefore, knowledge of the anatomic relations between the veins and the collecting system is the only way to avoid venous lesion. If it is necessary to make an incision in the infundibulum (neck) of a minor calix, especially in the lower calices, the operator should remember that the regions close to the caliceal cups may be surrounded by venous collars (see Figure 12-39). In these cases, it is better to perform short radial incisions (up to 1 mm in depth) in the quadrants described previously, in order to avoid venous collar lesions.

VASCULAR ANATOMY OF THE URETEROPELVIC JUNCTION: IMPORTANCE FOR ENDOPYELOTOMY

Since its clinical introduction, the endoscopic treatment of ureteropelvic junction (UPJ) obstruction endopyelotomy has almost completely replaced open pyeloplasty for the treatment of UPJ obstruction.[32–37] It has a success rate comparable to the open surgery and is applicable to congenital and acquired conditions.[35–38] Nowadays, endopyelotomy is a common procedure for both primary and secondary UPJ obstruction.[39] In spite of the great success rate of laparoscopic pyeloplasty, endopyelotomy continues to be more commonly performed in academic centers.[40]

Because endopyelotomy is based on an intubated pyeloplasty (ureteropelvic incision followed by stenting for 1 to 6 weeks),[32,35–38,41] to achieve success, the endoscopist must incise the full thickness of the muscle at the stenotic wall of the UPJ until periureteral fat becomes visible. This deep incision must be carried out whether the approach is through a nephrostomy tract, by ureteroscopy, or with an Acucise catheter, and whether the instrument used to incise the stricture is a cold knife or an electrosurgical probe.[42]

Incising the UPJ until the perirenal space is entered obviously carries the risk of injuring a retroperitoneal vessel.[43–45] In fact, the most significant complication of this procedure is vascular injury that is followed by severe hemorrhage and/or formation of an arteriovenous fistula.[33,34,36,46–50] To protect the arteries from the lesion, it has been recommended to examine via intrarenal endoscopy the area to be incised for any arterial pulsation and to avoid incising this site. Nevertheless, arterial pulsations are not always readily identifiable endoscopically during surgery, mainly because patients may be hypotensive due to anesthesia.[31] In addition, because the veins do not pulsate, endoscopic examination of the area to be incised is not effective in avoiding a venous lesion.[7,31]

The risk of injuring a large vessel during endopyelotomy can be greatly reduced or even eliminated if the endourologist understands and keeps in mind the three-dimensional vascular relationships to the UPJ.[44,45,51] This section provides background on the vascular anatomy of the UPJ to be applied in performing endopyelotomy safely and efficiently.

VASCULAR BACKGROUND We analyzed 146 three-dimensional, polyester resin corrosion endocasts of the pelviocaliceal system, together with the intrarenal arteries and veins simultaneously in the same kidney.[45]

Anterior Vascular UPJ Relationships In 65% of the cases there was a prominent artery, or vein, or both vessels in close relationship with the ventral surface of the UPJ (Figures 12-41 and 12-42). Among these cases, in 45%, the relationship was with the inferior segmental artery (Figure 12-43).

Concerning patient selection for treatment of UPJ obstruction, it remains controversial whether it is important to diagnose anterior crossing vessels. Van Cangh and colleagues obtained preoperative digital angiography in patients prior to endopyelotomy and found an associated vessel in 39% of patients with UPJ obstruction.[52] These authors stated that the presence of an anterior crossing vessel with either mild or severe hydronephrosis resulted in a success rate of only 50% and 39%, respectively. More recently, Van Cangh and two other colleagues stated that significant risk factors for endopyelotomy failure are crossing vessels, degree of hydronephrosis, length of stricture and renal function.[53] Rehman and colleagues emphasized the importance of spiral CT angiography for delineating the renal vascular anatomy before open retroperitoneal UPJ obstruction repair.[54] They described two patients with repair failure of UPJ obstruction in whom anterior vessels were missed during open retroperitoneal surgery. Laparoscopic transperitoneal secondary dismembered pyeloplasty with posterior displacement of the crossing vessel was successfully performed in each case.

On the other hand, Smith[37] stated that this kind of study would be justified only if there were evidence that such vessels were etiologic

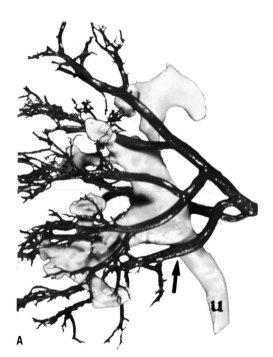

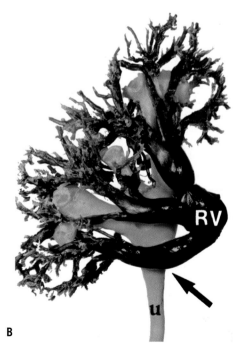

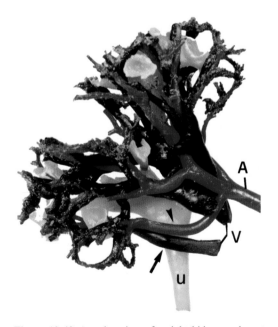

Figure 12-42 Anterior view of a right kidney endocast (pelviocaliceal system together with the intrarenal arteries and veins) reveals the anterior surface of the ureteropelvic junction in close relationship with the inferior segmental artery *(arrowhead)* and with a tributary of the renal vein *(arrow)*. *A* = renal artery; *V* = renal vein; *u* = ureter. Reproduced with permission from Sampaio FJB.[59]

Figure 12-41 *A*, Anterior view of a right kidney endocast (pelviocaliceal system together with the intrarenal arteries) shows a close relationship between the inferior segmental artery and the anterior surface of the ureteropelvic junction (UPJ) *(arrow)*. *B*, Anterior view of a right kidney endocast (pelviocaliceal system together with the intrarenal veins) shows a close relationship between a vein draining the lower pole and the UPJ *(arrow)*. *RV* = renal vein; *u* = ureter. Reproduced with permission from Sampaio FJB, and Favorito LA.[44]

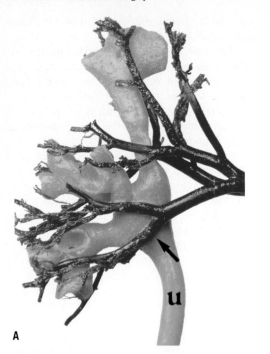

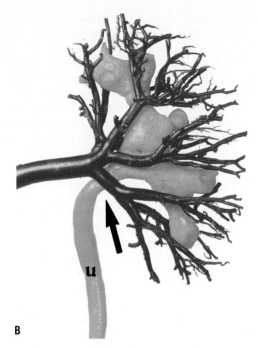

Figure 12-43 Anterior views of a right *(A)* and left *(B)* kidney endocasts (pelviocaliceal system together with the intrarenal arteries) reveal a close relationship between the inferior segmental artery and the anterior surface of the ureteropelvic junction *(arrows)*. u = ureter. Reproduced with permission from Sampaio FJB.[59]

in UPJ obstruction or if there were a risk of incising the vessel during endopyelotomy. More recently, Gupta and Smith stated that the current data suggest that the finding of crossing vessels preoperatively need not significantly influence the treatment rendered.[55] Corroborating that, Nakada and colleagues reported that helical computed tomography detected significant anterior or posterior crossing vessels in 38% of patients following successful endopyelotomy.[56] In their opinion, the adverse influence of the crossing vessel is not sufficient to justify the added expense of preoperative angiography, spiral CT or endoluminal ultrasound. Documenting the presence of a crossing vessel is inadequate to confirm that the vessel is causing obstruction. None of the current UPJ imaging techniques can distinguish crossing arteries that are the direct cause of obstruction from those that are not.[57,58] Therefore, in the absence of a prospective randomized trial comparing the results of open pyeloplasty and endopyelotomy, including the investigation of crossing vessels, the importance of imaging these crossing vessels before surgery is controversial.

It is worth pointing out that, in the 1994 Van Cangh and colleagues series, 39% of the patients presented a crossing vessel anteriorly to the UPJ, and these authors considered them anomalous arteries.[52] Considering these vessels anomalous is in disagreement with our extensive vascular anatomic studies.[43–45,59] Analyzing 280 endocasts of the pelviocaliceal system, together with the intrarenal arteries and veins, we found a close relationship between a normal artery (or vein, or both) and the anterior surface of the UPJ in 65.1% of the cases (see Figures 12-41 to 12-43).[45,59] In 45.2% of the cases, there was a close relationship between

the inferior segmental artery and the anterior surface of the UPJ when this vessel passed in front of this region to enter the inferior pole (see Figure 12-43).[45,59] This vessel is neither accessory nor aberrant, but, rather, a normal segmental artery that maintains a consistent anatomic relationship with the anterior surface of the UPJ without compressing the junction.[45,59,60] The mere presence of crossing vessels in the UPJ does not mean that they are necessarily obstructive.[37] We believe that an anomalous artery crossing the UPJ and causing

obstruction in 39% of patients, as described in 1994 by Van Cangh and colleagues[52] is a quite high incidence. It is possible that many of the vessels seen close to the UPJ during angiography and described as anomalous were normal segmental arteries. They may not cause the obstruction but rather increase the dilatation of a redundant renal pelvis previously obstructed by a primary muscular defect at the UPJ. In such a situation, the dilated renal pelvis balloons over the anterior crossing vessel, and the resulting angulation appears to worsen the obstruction.[45] Therefore, the exact role of crossing vessels in obstruction and the success of endopyelotomy are yet to be determined.[37,55]

With respect to the presence of multiple renal arteries, in 266 renal arterial pedicles analyzed, we found an inferior polar artery crossing anteriorly to the UPJ in only 6.8% of cases (Figure 12-44).[61] In only a few cases did this inferior polar artery pass close to the UPJ. Therefore, the presence of an anomalous vessel crossing the UPJ and causing obstruction is uncommon.

For patients with a crossing vessel and minimal to moderate hydronephrosis, laparoscopic clipping and incision of the crossing artery was reported.[52] Nevertheless, we emphasize that this approach should be precluded, because it results in loss of functioning renal parenchyma. It was well demonstrated and stressed that all renal arteries, even in case of multiple arteries, are terminal vessels; therefore, clipping the vessel will cause renal infarction.[28] As we have shown previously, the artery supplying the inferior pole of the kidney (inferior segment) represents from 7.4 to

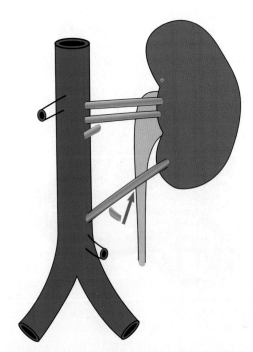

Figure 12-44 Schematic drawing of an anterior view of a left kidney showing an inferior polar artery *(arrow)* crossing anteriorly to the ureteropelvic junction (incidence of 6.8%).

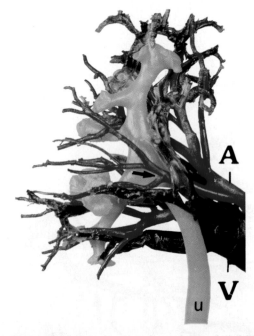

Figure 12-45 Posterior view of an endocast of a left kidney (pelviocaliceal system together with the intrarenal arteries and veins). A dorsal tributary of the renal vein *(arrowhead)* and the posterior segmental artery (retropelvic artery, *arrow*), are in close relationship to the posterior aspect of the ureteropelvic junction. *A* = renal artery; *V* = renal vein; *u* = ureter. Reproduced with permission from Sampaio FJB, and Favorito LA.[44]

38% of the total kidney area of functioning renal parenchyma (median area of the inferior segment = 22.6%).[28] For that reason, if one confirms that the UPJ obstruction is caused by a crossing artery, open surgery or a laparoscopic pyeloplasty with transposition of the crossing vessel should be proposed rather than clipping it.[59]

Posterior Vascular UPJ Relationships In 6.2% of cases, we found a direct relationship between a large vessel (artery or vein, or both) and the dorsal surface of the UPJ (Figure 12-45). In all cases in which an artery crosses the dorsal surface of the UPJ (3.5%), the vessel was the posterior segmental artery, also known as the retropelvic artery (Figures 12-45 and 12-46).

Most authors recommend that the UPJ be incised alongside its posterolateral aspect, but our findings evinced that this poses a serious risk of injuring a retropelvic vessel. In fact, even when the procedure is performed by experienced endourologists, the incidence of severe hemorrhage when the UPJ is incised posterolaterally is 12%.[36] A posterior or posterolateral incision at the UPJ stenosis also presents the possibility of injury to the posterior segmental artery (retropelvic artery) which, in addition to causing severe hemorrhage, can be associated with loss of a great portion of functioning renal tissue as a consequence of renal infarction. It is important to note that in some individuals, the posterior segmental artery supplies as much as 50% of the renal parenchyma.[28]

In addition to the 6.2% of vessels that had a direct dorsal relationship with the UPJ by crossing it just at the posterior surface, another 20.5% of cases were characterized by a vessel crossing less than 1.5 cm above the dorsal surface of the UPJ (Figure 12-47). This is of great importance to surgeons who perform endopyelotomy, because to

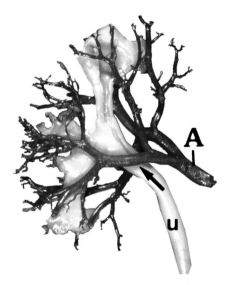

Figure 12-46 Posterior view of a left kidney endocast (pelviocaliceal system together with the intrarenal arteries) reveals the posterior segmental artery (retropelvic artery) in close relationship to the posterior aspect of the ureteropelvic junction *(arrow)*. A = renal artery; u = ureter. Reproduced with permission from Sampaio FJB, and Favorito LA.[44]

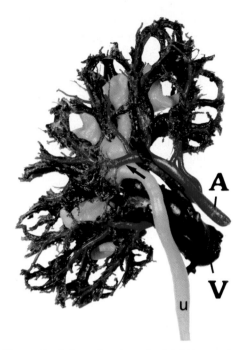

Figure 12-47 Posterior view of a left kidney endocast (pelviocaliceal system together with the intrarenal arteries and veins) reveals the posterior segmental artery (retropelvic artery) crossing less than 1.5 cm (0.5 cm) above the posterior aspect of the ureteropelvic junction *(arrow)*. A = renal artery; V = renal vein; u = ureter. Reproduced with permission from Sampaio FJB, and Favorito LA.[44]

achieve a patent UPJ it is generally necessary to extend the endoscopic incision into the healthy tissue for 1 to 2 cm on each side (above and below) of the UPJ stenotic zone. This means that the risk of injury to a dorsal vessel is especially great in posterior and posterolateral incisions.

Furthermore, the risk of injury to a vessel that crosses less than 1.5 cm above the UPJ is particularly high in cases of extensive fibrosis and scarring tissue at the UPJ, because under such circumstances, it is necessary to make a long incision, sometimes extending into the renal parenchyma.[45,60] Therefore, posterior and posterolateral incisions at the UPJ must be avoided.

Incision at the UPJ Stenosis Based on the Vascular Anatomy We recommend that the deep incision alongside the UPJ stenotic wall be done just laterally (Figure 12-48). An incision at this site, which we named the "nonvascular area" of the UPJ, avoids all important vessels that can be related anteriorly, posteriorly, or less than 1.5 cm above the posterior surface of the UPJ.[44,45,60]

Even in cases of extensive scar tissue at the UPJ and in cases of vessels that were transposed posteriorly in an earlier dismembered pyeloplasty, the lateral incision in the "nonvascular area" of the UPJ is safe and precludes preoperative angiographic examinations. Also, an unsuspected polar inferior artery crossing anteriorly or posteriorly at the UPJ[47,61] will be protected from injury.

Maintaining complete anatomic orientation under endoscopic vision is sometimes difficult. Consequently, it is our practice and our recommendation, to position the cutting instrument lat-

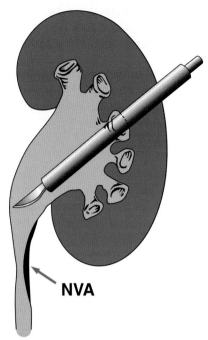

Figure 12-48 Anterior view of a schematic drawing from a left kidney shows the area to be incised in endopyelotomy *(arrow)* and the nonvascular area *(NVA)* of the ureteropelvic junction.

erally and under fluoroscopic guidance (Figure 12-49) before starting the incision at the UPJ. Such a maneuver assures the surgeon that the incision will be made precisely in the lateral aspect the nonvascular area of the UPJ.[49,60,62]

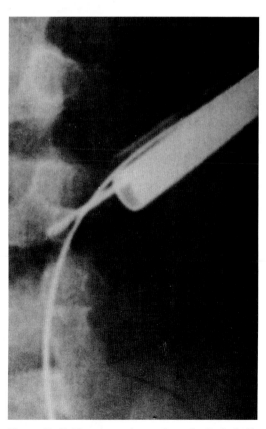

Figure 12-49 Note the cutting surface of a Sacks knife positioned laterally under fluoroscopic guidance during the procedure of endopyelotomy.

INTRARENAL ANATOMY FOR PERCUTANEOUS ACCESS TO THE URETEROPELVIC JUNCTION

For percutaneous endopyelotomy, usually a puncture through an upper pole or a midzone calix is recommended to establish a nephrostomy tract and directly visualize the UPJ to be incised.[36,63,64] Although a supracostal approach provides an excellent access to the UPJ, it involves the cost of an increased risk of pleural and adjacent organ perforation.[4] In our experience and based on the collecting system anatomy, in patients without previous renal surgery, we found that an upper-pole puncture is rarely necessary, and a midzone puncture is necessary in only one-third of cases. In most patients, an access through a lower-pole calix enables a frontal visualization of the UPJ.[65] The calix should be selected based on the angle that is formed between the caliceal infundibulum and the UPJ.

HOW TO DETERMINE THE ANGLE For evaluation of the angle, two lines must be drawn. The first line (y-axis) must link the central axis of the superior ureter with the central axis of the UPJ. The second line (x-axis) is the central axis of the calix being considered for puncture (Figures 12-50 to 12-52).

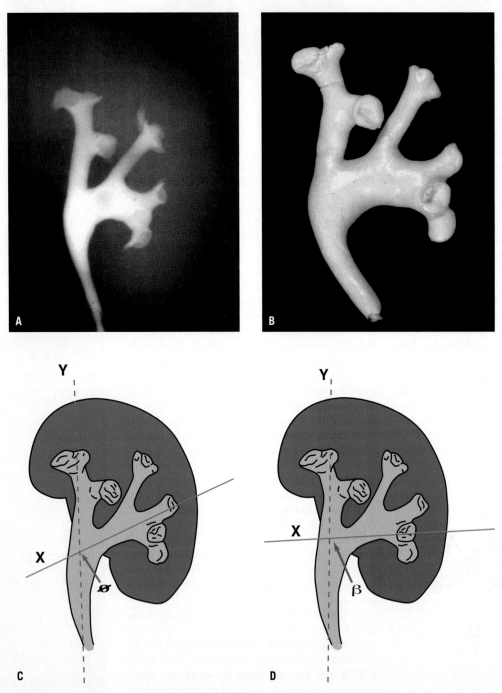

Figure 12-50 *A*, Anterior view of a retrograde pyelogram of a left kidney. *B*, Anterior view of three-dimensional polyester resin corrosion endocast of the same kidney. *C*, Schematic drawing of an anterior view of the same pelviocaliceal system, shows an access through an inferior-pole calix whose infundibulum forms an angle of greater than 90° (obtuse angle) with the ureteropelvic junction (UPJ). *Y* = first line linking the central axis of the superior ureter with the central axis of the UPJ. *X* = second line traced considering the central axis of the caliceal infundibulum chosen for intrarenal access. In this case, the angle formed *(θ)* measured 111°. This angle would allow easy frontal visualization of the UPJ. *D*, Another inferior-pole calix in the same kidney forms a less obtuse angle (β = 92°) but would still allow frontal visualization of the UPJ for percutaneous endopyelotomy.

After drawing these two lines, the angle formed by the intersection of the lines is measured with a protractor (see Figures 12-50 to 12-52). In clinical practice, however, we have found that the endourologist can simply deduce whether the angle is larger or smaller than 90° by examining the intersection of the lines.

HOW TO SELECT A CALIX FOR PUNCTURE An appropriate calix can be chosen based on the angle that is formed between the caliceal infundibulum

and the UPJ. If the chosen calix forms an angle equal to or greater than 90° with the UPJ, the intrarenal access through this calix will permit an easy and frontal visualization of the UPJ (Figure 12-53). Our anatomic studies showed that for about 70% of cases, it is possible to find at least one posterior lower calix where the infundibulum forms an angle of greater than 90° with the UPJ.

The angle formed between the UPJ and the caliceal infundibulum must be determined considering a specific chosen calix, because the

angle will vary in the same region of the kidney, depending on the calix chosen. That is, in one situation, the angle will be greater than 90° (98°, see Figure 12-51C), while in the same kidney, another calix may have an angle smaller than 90° (38°, see Figure 12-51D). Therefore, by selecting an appropriate calix based on the analysis of the angle, it is possible to access the UPJ through a lower calix in most cases.

In some cases (around 30%), it is necessary to puncture a midzone calix, because in these cases

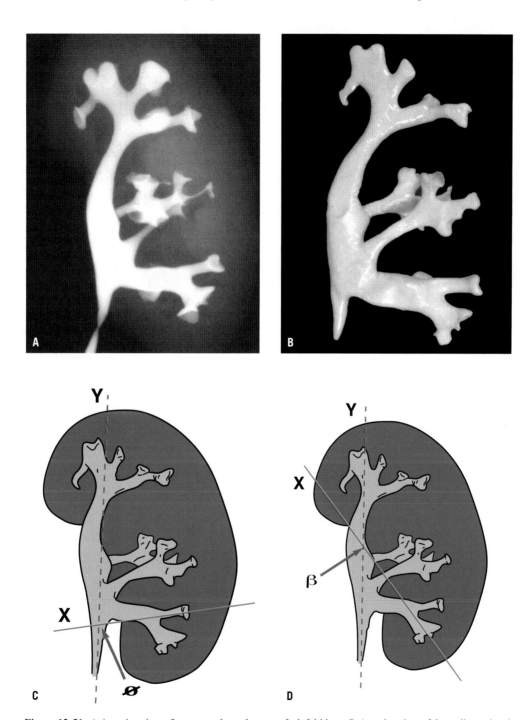

Figure 12-51 *A*, Anterior view of a retrograde pyelogram of a left kidney. *B*, Anterior view of three-dimensional polyester resin corrosion endocast of the same kidney. *C*, Schematic drawing of an anterior view of the same pelviocaliceal system, shows an access through an inferior-pole calix whose infundibulum forms an angle of greater than 90° (obtuse angle) with the ureteropelvic junction (UPJ). *Y* = first line linking the central axis of the superior ureter with the central axis of the UPJ. *X* = second line traced considering the central axis of the caliceal infundibulum chosen for intrarenal access. In this case, the angle formed *(θ)* measured 98°. This angle would allow easy frontal visualization of the UPJ. *D*, Another inferior-pole calix in the same kidney forms an acute angle (β = 38°) and would not allow frontal visualization of the UPJ for percutaneous endopyelotomy.

all lower caliceal infundibula form angles smaller than 90° with the UPJ (see Figure 12-52). Analyzing 208 pelviocaliceal systems, we have always found at least one midzone calix forming an angle equal to or greater than 90° with the UPJ.[65]

In cases with a history of previous open surgery, or even percutaneous surgery, an access through a midzone calix must be considered, because there is a high possibility of perinephric scarring. Depending on the pelviocaliceal anatomy, a middle calix puncture will offer easier access to the UPJ, avoiding the need for excessively inclining the scarred kidney, a maneuver that would result in intrarenal damage and bleeding.[66]

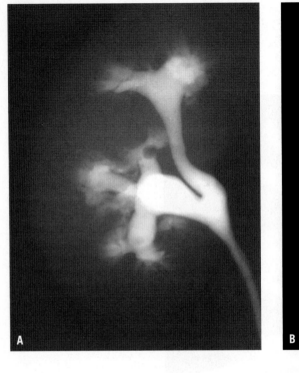

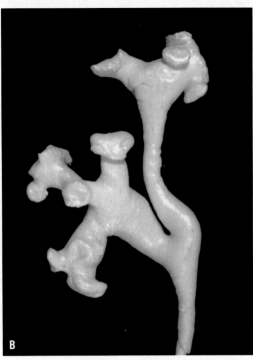

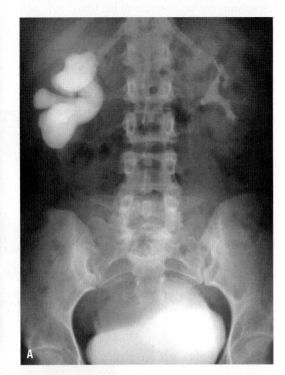

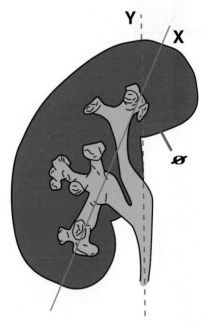

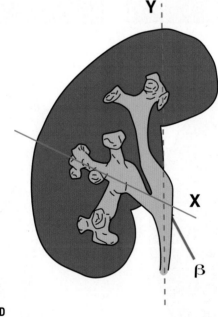

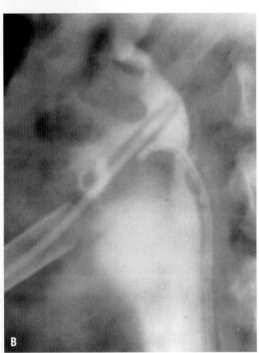

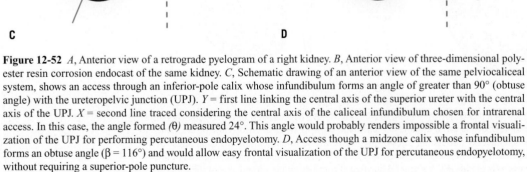

Figure 12-52 *A*, Anterior view of a retrograde pyelogram of a right kidney. *B*, Anterior view of three-dimensional polyester resin corrosion endocast of the same kidney. *C*, Schematic drawing of an anterior view of the same pelviocaliceal system, shows an access through an inferior-pole calix whose infundibulum forms an angle of greater than 90° (obtuse angle) with the ureteropelvic junction (UPJ). *Y* = first line linking the central axis of the superior ureter with the central axis of the UPJ. *X* = second line traced considering the central axis of the caliceal infundibulum chosen for intrarenal access. In this case, the angle formed *(θ)* measured 24°. This angle would probably renders impossible a frontal visualization of the UPJ for performing percutaneous endopyelotomy. *D*, Access though a midzone calix whose infundibulum forms an obtuse angle (β = 116°) and would allow easy frontal visualization of the UPJ for percutaneous endopyelotomy, without requiring a superior-pole puncture.

Figure 12-53 *A*, Intravenous pyelogram from a 30-year-old woman shows an ureteropelvic junction (UPJ) obstruction with a dilated pelviocaliceal system. *B*, Pyelogram performed through the nephrostomy tube immediately after endopyelotomy reveals contrast material extravasation through the incision in the UPJ. The Amplatz sheath is being withdrawn. The endopyelotomy was easily performed through an inferior-pole calix.

REFERENCES

1. Sampaio FJB. Analysis of kidney volume growth during the fetal period in humans. Urol Res 1992;20:271–4.

2. Sampaio FJB, Mandarim-de-Lacerda CA. Morphométrie du rein. Etude appliquée à l'urologie et à l'imagerie. J Urol (Paris) 1989;95:77–80.

3. Sampaio FJB. Renal anatomy: endourologic considerations. Urol Clin North Am 2000;27:585–607.

4. Hopper KD, Yakes WF. The posterior intercostal approach for percutaneous renal procedures: risk of puncturing the lung, spleen, and liver as determined by CT. AJR Am J Roentgenol 1990;154:115–7.

5. Hopper KD, Sherman JL, Luethke JM, Ghaed N. The retrorenal colon in the supine and prone patient. Radiology 1987;162:443–6.

6. Sampaio FJB. Relationships of intrarenal arteries and the kidney collecting system. Applied anatomic study. In: Sampaio FJB, Uflacker R, editors. Renal anatomy applied to urology, endourology, and interventional radiology. New York: Thieme Medical Publishers; 1993. p. 23–32.

7. Sampaio FJB, Aragão AHM. Anatomical relationship between the renal venous arrangement and the kidney collecting system. J Urol 1990;144:1089–93.

8. Sampaio FJB. Anatomic classification of the pelviocaliceal system. Urologic and radiologic implications. In: Sampaio FJB, Uflacker R, editors. Renal anatomy applied to urology, endourology, and interventional radiology. New York: Thieme Medical Publishers; 1993. p. 1–6.

9. Sampaio FJB, Mandarim-de-Lacerda CA. Anatomic classification of the kidney collecting system for endourologic procedures. J Endourol 1988;2:247–51.

10. Kaye KW, Goldberg ME. Applied anatomy of the kidney and ureter. Urol Clin North Am 1982;9:3–13.

11. Sampaio FJB, Mandarim-de-Lacerda CA. 3-Dimensional and radiological pelviocaliceal anatomy for endourology. J Urol 1988;140:1352–5.

12. Sampaio FJB. Basic anatomic features of the kidney collecting system. Three-dimensional and radiologic study. In: Sampaio FJB, Uflacker R, editors. Renal anatomy applied to urology, endourology, and interventional radiology. New York: Thieme Medical Publishers; 1993. p. 7–15.

13. Sampaio FJB, Aragão AHM. Inferior pole collecting system anatomy. Its probable role in extracorporeal shock wave lithotripsy. J Urol 1992;147:322–4.

14. Sampaio FJB. Renal collecting system anatomy: its possible role in the effectiveness of renal stone treatment. Curr Opin Urol 2001;11:359–66.

15. Kaye KW, Reinke DB. Detailed caliceal anatomy for endourology. J Urol 1984;132:1085–8.

16. Weyman PJ. Air as a contrast agent during percutaneous nephrostomy. J Endourol 1986;1:16–7.

17. Sampaio FJB, Aragão AHM. Limitation of extracorporeal shock wave lithotripsy in lower caliceal stones: anatomical insight. J Endourol 1994;8:241–7.

18. Elliott DS, Segura JW, Lightner D, et al. Is nephroureterectomy necessary in all cases of upper tract transitional cell carcinoma? Long-term results of conservative endourologic management of upper tract transitional cell carcinoma in individuals with a normal contralateral kidney. Urology 2001;58:174–8.

19. Murphy DP, Gill IS, Streem SB. Evolving management of upper-tract transitional-cell carcinoma at a tertiary-care center. J Endourol 2002;16:483–7.

20. Auge BK, Munver R, Kourambas J, et al. Neoinfundibulotomy for the management of symptomatic caliceal diverticula. J Urol 2002;167:1616–20.

21. Segura JW. The role of percutaneous surgery in renal and ureteral stone removal (Part 2). J Urol 1989;141:780–1.

22. Clayman RV, Surya V, Hunter D, et al. Renal vascular complications associated with the percutaneous removal of renal calculi. J Urol 1984;132:228–30.

23. Lee WJ, Smith AD, Cubelli V, et al. Complications of percutaneous nephro-lithotomy. AJR Am J Roentgenol 1987;148:177–80.

24. Sampaio FJB, Zanier JFC, Aragão AHM, Favorito LA. Intrarenal access: 3-dimensional anatomical study. J Urol 1992;148:1769–73.

25. Sampaio FJB. Intrarenal access by puncture. Three-dimensional study. In: Sampaio FJB, Uflacker R, editors. Renal anatomy applied to urology, endourology, and interventional radiology. New York: Thieme Medical Publishers; 1993. p. 68–76.

26. Sampaio FJB. How to place a nephrostomy, safely. Contemp Urol 1994;6:41–6.

27. Sampaio FJB, Aragão AHM. Anatomical relationship between the intrarenal arteries and the kidney collecting system. J Urol 1990;143:679–81.

28. Sampaio FJB, Schiavini JL, Favorito LA. Proportional analysis of the kidney arterial segments. Urol Res 1993;21:371–4.

29. Clayman RV, Hunter D, Surya V, et al. Percutaneous intrarenal electrosurgery. J Urol 1984;131:864–7.

30. Clayman RV, Castañeda-Zúñiga WF. Instrumentation for nephrolithotomy. In: Clayman RV, Castañeda-Zúñiga WR, editors. Techniques in endourology. A guide for the percutaneous removal of renal and ureteral calculi. Chicago: Year Book Medical Publishers; 1986. p. 185–237.

31. Sampaio FJB. Anatomic background for intrarenal endourologic surgery. J Endourol 1992;6:301–4.

32. Badlani G, Eshghi M, Smith AD. Percutaneous surgery for ureteropelvic junction obstruction (endopyelotomy): technique and early results. J Urol 1986;135:26–8.

33. Badlani G, Karlin G, Smith AD. Complications of endopyelotomy: analysis in series of 64 patients. J Urol 1988;140:473–5.

34. Clayman RV, Picus DD. Ureterorenoscopic endopyelotomy. Preliminary report. Urol Clin North Am 1988;15:433–8.

35. Clayman RV, Basler JW, Kavoussi L, Picus DD. Ureteronephroscopic endopyelotomy. J Urol 1990;144:246–52.

36. Meretyk I, Meretyk S, Clayman RV. Endopyelotomy: comparison of ureteroscopic retrograde and antegrade percutaneous techniques. J Urol 1992;148:775–83.

37. Smith AD. Editorial comment. J Urol 1991;146:1495.

38. Kletscher BA, Segura JW. Percutaneous antegrade endopyelotomy: review of 50 consecutive cases [Abstract]. J Urol 1994;151:371.

39. Streem SD. Contemporary intervention for UPJ obstruction: which one, when and how? Preface. Urol Clin North Am 1998;25:xiii–xv.

40. Marcovich R, Jacobson AI, Aldana JP, et al. Practice trends in contemporary management of adult ureteropelvic junction obstruction. Urology 2003;62:22–5.

41. Davis DM. Intubated ureterotomy: a new operation for ureteral and ureteropelvic strictures. Surg Gynec Obst 1943;76:513–4.

42. Kausik S, Segura JW. Surgical management of ureteropelvic junction obstruction in adults. Int Braz J Urol 2003;29:3–10.

43. Sampaio FJB. Relationship between segmental arteries and pelviureteric junction. Brit J Urol 1991;68:214–7.

44. Sampaio FJB, Favorito LA. Ureteropelvic junction stenosis: vascular anatomical background for endopyelotomy. J Urol 1993;150:1787–91.

45. Sampaio FJB. Vascular anatomy at the ureteropelvic junction. Urol Clin North Am 1998;25:251–8.

46. Cassis AN, Brannen GE, Bush WH, et al. Endopyelotomy: review of results and complications. J Urol 1991;146:1492–5.

47. Malden ES, Picus D, Clayman RV. Arteriovenous fistula complicating endopyelotomy. J Urol 1992;148:1520–3.

48. Segura JW. Editorial comment. J Urol 1992;148:782.

49. Streem SB, Geisinger MA. Prevention and management of hemorrhage associate with cautery wire balloon incision of ureteropelvic junction obstruction. J Urol 1995;153:1904–6.

50. Wagner JR, D'Agostino R, Babayan RK. Renal arteriroureteral hemorrhage: a complication of Acucise endopyelotomy. Urology 1996;48:139–41.

51. Sampaio FJB. Endopyelotomy, guided by meticulous anatomy. Contemp Urol 1994;6:23–6.

52. Van Cangh PJ, Wilmart JF, Opsomer RJ, et al. Long-term results and late recurrence after endopyelotomy: a critical analysis of prognostic factors. J Urol 1994;151:934–7.

53. Van Cangh PJ, Nesa S, De Groote P. Current indications for endopyelotomy. Braz J Urol 2000;26:54–63.

54. Rehman J, Landman J, Sundaram C, Clayman RV. Missed anterior crossing vessels during open retroperitoneal pyeloplasty: laparoscopic transperitoneal discovery and repair. J Urol 2001;166:593–6.

55. Gupta M, Smith AD. Crossing vessels. Endourologic implications. Urol Clin North Am 1998;25:289–93.

56. Nakada SY, Wolf JS Jr, Brink JA, et al. Retrospective analysis of the effect of crossing vessels on successful retrograde endopyelotomy outcomes using spiral computerized tomography angiography. J Urol 1998;159:62–5.

57. Frauscher F, Janetschek G, Helweg G, et al. Crossing vessels at the ureteropelvic junction: detection with contrast-enhanced color Doppler imaging. Radiology 1999;210:727–31.

58. Rouvière O, Lyonnet D, Berger P, et al. Ureteropelvic junction obstruction: use of helical CT for preoperative assessment—comparison with intraarterial angiography. Radiology 1999;213:668–73.

59. Sampaio FJB. The dilemma of the crossing vessel at the ureteropelvic junction: precise anatomic study. J Endourol 1996;10:411–5.

60. Sampaio FJB. Ureteropelvic junction anatomy. Atlas Urol Clin North Am. [In press]

61. Sampaio FJB, Passos MARF. Renal arteries: anatomic study for surgical and radiological practice. Surg Radiol Anat 1992;14:113–7.

62. Uflacker R. Percutaneous kidney procedures. Endopyelotomy. In: Sampaio FJB, Uflacker R, editors. Renal anatomy applied to urology, endourology, and interventional radiology. New York: Thieme Medical Publishers; 1993. p. 90–6.

63. Motola JA, Badlani GH, Smith AD. Results of 212 consecutive endopyelotomies: an 8-year follow-up. J Urol 1993;149:453–6.

64. Jarret TW, Smith AD. Endopyelotomy. In: Smith AD, editor. Controversies in endourology. Philadelphia: WB Saunders; 1995. p. 249–56.

65. Sampaio FJB. Percutaneous antegrade endopyelotomy: choosing a calyx to access the UPJ. Contemp Urol 1996;8:13–20.

66. Gumpinger R, Miller K, Fuchs G, Eisenberger F. Antegrade ureteroscopy for stone removal. Eur Urol 1985;11:199–202.

13

Pathophysiology and Evaluation of Obstructive Uropathy

John C. Lieske, MD

Urinary tract obstruction is important to diagnose since many cases are surgically correctable. It is also common, and accounts for up to 0.2% of all hospital admissions in the United States, and 2% of patients on chronic dialysis between the years of 1989 and 1993.[1] Hydronephrosis denotes dilatation of the urinary tract, whereas obstructive uropathy is the renal disease caused by impaired flow of urine or tubular fluid. In practice, it is often difficult to discern which hydronephrotic kidneys would benefit from surgical intervention, either because it is unclear if a dilated kidney is truly obstructed, or alternatively, whether a kidney is already so severely damaged that relief of obstruction would not allow any significant return of renal function.

This chapter will review the following topics:

1. Signs, symptoms and causes of renal obstruction.
2. The physiologic processes after the onset of renal obstruction that reduce glomerular filtration.
3. Causes of irreversible renal damage after prolonged renal obstruction.
4. Diagnosis of renal obstruction.
5. Treatment of renal obstruction.

SYMPTOMS, SIGNS, AND CAUSES OF RENAL OBSTRUCTION

Although kidney obstruction is sometimes discovered incidentally via imaging studies performed to evaluate unrelated problems, most cases come to medical attention because of specific clinical features. The main symptom that renal obstruction causes is pain. If the obstruction develops slowly, the resulting pain is often described as a dull loin ache. This pain is thought to result from stretching of the renal capsule, since the parenchyma itself is not innervated, and can be difficult to discriminate from mechanical low back pain. If the obstruction is more sudden and complete, or an acute diuresis is ongoing, this pain can become more severe and disabling. Ureteral colic, thought to be caused by smooth muscle spasm, is the most severe form of pain associated with renal obstruction, and is often quite intense and knife-like. Obstruction in the upper ureter often radiates to the loin, whereas obstruction in the lower third often radiates to the groin, labia, or testicle.

Signs of renal obstruction all relate to a decline in renal function and include hypertension or volume overload, as well as metabolic abnormalities such as acidosis or an elevated serum blood urea nitrogen, creatinine or potassium. Anuria can occur in complete bilateral renal obstruction, but it cannot be overemphasized that, in most cases, the obstruction is partial, and urinary volumes remain normal. Indeed, polyuria and polydipsia can be features of chronic obstructive uropathy due to an associated renal concentrating defect.

Obstruction can be classified anatomically in order to highlight potential causes, as listed in Table 13-1. Important levels of obstruction include the ureteropelvic junction, renal pelvis, the ureter, the bladder and ureterovesical junction, and urethra and bladder neck. At each level, causes can be intraluminal, intramural (intrinsic), or extramural (extrinsic).

RENAL PHYSIOLOGY AFTER OBSTRUCTION

In experimental animals, acute ureteral obstruction is followed by a transient increase in renal blood flow to the affected kidney.[2] Increased local production of prostacyclin and prostaglandin E appear to mediate this immediate vasodilation, which can be blocked by nonsteroidal anti-inflammatory agents such as indomethacin (Figure 13-1).[2–6] Increased production of nitric oxide (NO) also appears important.[7] Augmented renal blood flow, in turn, boosts intraglomerular pressures, partially offsetting the increased intratubular pressure and thereby helping to preserve glomerular filtration early after the onset of obstruction (Table 13-2). Three to five hours after the onset of obstruction, however, progressive vasoconstriction ensues, and within 24 hours, renal blood flow falls to values only 40 to 70% of those pre-obstruction (see Table 13-2). This secondary vasoconstriction appears to be mediated by increased production of angiotensin II (AII), thromboxane A_2 (TxA_2), antidiuretic hormone, endothelin and leukotriene, as well as decreased production of NO (see Figure 13-1).[2,8,9] In rats, this secondary vasoconstriction can be at least partially blunted using angiotensin

Table 13-1 Causes of Obstruction Classified According to Site			
Level	Intraluminal Causes	Intramural (Intrinsic) Causes	Extramural (Extrinsic) Causes
Renal pelvis and ureteropelvic junction	Renal stone/crystals; blood clots; sloughed tissue	Urothelial tumor; ureteropelvic obstruction; previous surgery/endourology; congenital duplications	Ovarian vein syndrome; bowel malignancy/inflammatory disease; pelvic malignancy; lymphocele; retroperitoneal fibrosis/lymphadenopathy/ hematoma
Ureter	Renal stone/crystals; blood clots; sloughed tissue	Primary megaureter; retrocaval ureter; retroiliac ureter; urothelial tumor; malacoplakia; ureteric stricture; previous surgery/endourology; congenital duplications	Retroperitoneal fibrosis/lymphadenopathy/hematoma; pelvic lipomatosis; pregnancy; endometriosis; ovarian vein syndrome; bowel malignancy/ inflammatory disease; pelvic malignancy; lymphocele
Ureterovesical junction	Renal stone; blood clots; sloughed tissue	Urothelial tumor; ureterocele; malacoplakia; vesicoureteral junction pathology (including valve, polyp, stricture); previous surgery/endourology	Pelvic lipomatosis; endometriosis; bowel malignancy/ inflammatory disease; pelvic malignancy; lymphocele; retroperitoneal fibrosis/lymphadenopathy/hematoma
Bladder	Renal stone; blood clots; sloughed tissue	Urothelial tumor; bladder cancer; malacoplakia; urinary diversions; previous surgery/endourology	Pelvic lipomatosis; endometriosis; bowel malignancy/ inflammatory disease; pelvic malignancy
Urethra and bladder neck	Renal stone; blood clots; sloughed tissue; bladder stone; prostatic stone	Bladder cancer; urethral stricture; previous surgery/endourology; neurogenic bladder	Phimosis; procidentia; prostate cancer; benign prostatic hyperplasia; pelvic malignancy; straddle injury; pelvic fracture

Adapted from Klahr S,[8] and O'Reilly PH.[37]

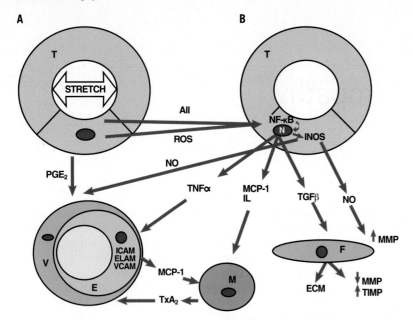

Figure 13-1 *A,* A simplified schema of the mechanisms that mediate interstitial fibrosis in obstructive uropathy. Increased stretch of tubular cells (T), perhaps driven by transmitted intratubular or interstitial pressure, is thought to trigger generation and release of PGE_2, AII, and ROS. PGE_2 appears to be an important mediator of the immediate vasodilatation that can increase renal blood flow early after obstruction. *B,* AII and ROS can both favor translocation of the transcription factor NF-κβ into the nucleus (N), which in turn, promotes synthesis and release of factors that mediate mononuclear cell recruitment and promote interstitial fibrosis. TNFα increases endothelial cell (E) expression of adhesion molecules that aid in monocyte accumulation (eg, VCAM), as well as the potent recruitment factor MCP-1. Once present in the interstitium, macrophages (M) are a rich source of fibrosis-promoting cytokines and TxA_2, thought to be an important mediator of constriction of vascular smooth muscle cells (V) that predominates 3 to 5 hours after the onset of obstruction. TGF-β1 is a key mediator of fibrosis, promoting fibroblast (F) proliferation, synthesis of extracellular matrix (ECM) components, decreasing production of matrix metalloproteinases (MMPs) and increasing production of tissue inhibitors of metalloproteinases (TIMPs). Increased production of NO by tubular cells via inducible nitric oxide synthase (iNOS) is thought to help counterbalance profibrotic factors, in part by allowing vasodilatation and increasing activity of MMPs. AII = angiotensin II; MCP-1 = monocyte-chemoattractant peptide-1; NF = nuclear factor; PGE_2 = prostaglandin E_2; ROS = reactive oxygen species; TGF = transforming growth factor; TNF = tumor necrosis factor; TxA_2 = thromboxane A_2; VCAM = vascular cell adhesion molecule.

converting enzyme (ACE) inhibitors, thromboxane synthase inhibitors, and V1-vasopressin receptor blockers.[9] Total body irradiation, which removes infiltrating macrophages, also reduces this secondary vasoconstriction and prevents the increase in local TxA_2 concentrations, suggesting these cells contribute importantly to the fall in renal perfusion.[10] Overall, within several hours after the onset of obstruction, transglomerular pressures (and glomerular filtration rate [GFR]) fall due to two factors: increased intratubular pressure as well as decreased intracapillary pressure, the latter mediated by vasoconstriction (see Table 13-2).

The initial signal that triggers changes in renal blood flow after obstruction appears to be mechanical stretch of tubular cells, produced by increased intratubular pressure and/or a rise in cortical interstitial pressure (see Figure 13-1).[10,11] How this stretch signal is transmitted and transformed into chemical events, such as the release of prostaglandins and angiotensin II, is unclear and might depend on the degree of obstruction and the volume status. Down-regulation of antioxidant proteins such as catalase, perhaps a direct result of mechanical stretch and resulting in increased local levels of reactive oxygen species (ROS), also appears to contribute to changes in tubular cell signaling pathway.[11]

CAUSES OF RENAL SCARRING
AFTER PROLONGED OBSTRUCTION

INTRODUCTION Renal interstitial fibrosis occurs as a consequence of longstanding obstructive uropathy.[10] Potential pathways are summarized in Figure 13-1. In experimental animals, infiltration by mononuclear cells, proliferation of interstitial cells, and increased interstitial extracellular matrix (ECM) have all been described. Under normal conditions, mononuclear cells are rare in the renal interstitium, especially the medulla, but macrophages and, to a lesser extent, T cells, appear there within four hours of obstruction and increase in number for the first 24 hours.[10,12] Although the factors that recruit mononuclear

cells to the interstitium are not entirely certain, an important one appears to be composed of lipid, and monocyte-chemoattractant peptide-1 (MCP-1) is a likely candidate for it.[10] Other factors, including transforming growth factor (TGF)-β1, osteopontin, intercellular adhesion molecule (ICAM)-1, vascular cell adhesion molecule (VCAM), and endothelial leukocyte adhesion molecule (ELAM)-1, are also overexpressed in the obstructed kidney and may participate in macrophage recruitment (see Figure 13-1).[10]

ANGIOTENSIN II AND TGF-β1 After the onset of renal obstruction, AII appears to be a key local mediator that not only promotes vasoconstriction but, over the longer term, renal interstitial scarring (Figure 13-2). Local release of kinins and NO may also be important.[13] Increased local concentrations of AII appear to promote TGF-β1 release by tubular cells, and this TGF-β1 accumulation can be blocked by ACE inhibition.[14] TGF-β1 is a key mediator of renal interstitial fibrosis because it is a chemoattractant for fibroblasts and promotes their proliferation.[15] This cytokine also stimulates fibroblast production of ECM proteins, including collagens type I, II, III, IV and V, fibronectin, thrombospondin, osteopontin, tenascin, elastin, hyaluronic acid, heparin sulfate, osteonectin, increases the activity of tissue inhibitors of metalloproteinases (TIMPs) thereby reducing matrix metalloproteinase activity, and stimulates production of ROS.[16] In the obstructed kidney, effects of AII may be mediated by translocation of nuclear factor (NF)-κβ into the nucleus.[17] Lending support for the central role of AII after obstruction is the list of events that can be at least partially blocked by ACE-inhibition, including increased ECM production, NF-κβ activation, fibroblast proliferation, and infiltration by mononuclear cells.[18]

MACROPHAGES AND ROS Early after obstruction the interstitium becomes infiltrated with macrophages.[18] Although T cells are also present, they do not appear necessary for fibrogenesis.[19] Macrophages, as well as tubular cells, are rich sources of mediators that can promote interstitial fibrosis. The net result appears to be an imbalance between ECM production and degradation. Another factor that may promote interstitial fibrosis is local oxidative stress. Tension stress, hypoxia, macrophage infiltration and cytokines can all alter the local redox state.[20] Recent studies have provided evidence suggesting oxidative stress indeed does occur within chronically obstructed kidneys,

Table 13-2 Hemodynamic Changes after Acute Obstruction					
Time	Vasoconstrictors	Vasodilators	Renal blood flow	Intratubular pressure	GFR
0–3 hours	AII	PGE, PGI, NO	Increased	Increased	No change or slight decrease
3–5 hours and later	AII, TxA_2, ADH, leukotriene B_4 endothelin	PGE, PGI, NO	Decreased	Increased	Marked decrease

AII = angiotensin II; GFR = glomerular filtration rate; PGE = prostaglandin E; TxA_2 = thromboxane A_2.

including higher levels of malondialdehyde, decreased reduced glutathione, increased oxidized glutathione, and increased expression of the counter-regulatory enzyme heme-oxygenase-1.[20] Local release of reactive oxygen species stimulates dissociation of NF-κβ, which can then translocate to the nucleus to induce transcription of genes that contribute to tissue inflammation, cellular proliferation and cellular differentiation.[10] The NF-κβ pathway can also be activated by a number of other factors unregulated after obstruction, including AII (see above) and tumor necrosis factor (TNF)-α.[17] NF-κβ stimulates production of MCP-1 (which promotes mononuclear cell recruitment), TNF-α, interleukins 1β, 2 and 6, inducible NO synthase (iNOS), and cycoloxygenase-2. Increased endothelial cell expression of adhesion molecules such as ICAM-1, in part stimulated by TNF-α, also promotes macrophage accumulation.[12,21]

Because of these observations, antioxidants have been investigated in experimental rat models of obstructive uropathy. Administration of probucol decreased renal levels of oxidized glutathione and reduced leukocyte infiltration of obstructed kidneys.[22] Similarly, *N*-acetyl cysteine reduced NF-κβ activation, expression of MCP-1 and VCAM-1, and infiltration of monocytes in rat models of obstructive uropathy,[23] and vitamin E reduced renal levels of malondialdehyde, TGF-β1 messenger ribonucleic acid (mRNA), and apoptotic cells.[24,25]

TNF-α   TNF-α appears to be a central mediator of the interstitial fibrosis and inflammation that can occur after obstruction.[10] Injury in general appears to up-regulate renal production of TNF-α, both by resident cells and infiltrating leukocytes.[8] In rats, TNF-α mRNA was more abundant in cortical tubules within 1 hour after ureteral obstruction.[8] This up-regulation was reduced 40% by the ACE inhibitor enalapril, suggesting that the increase was in part mediated by AII. Total body irradiation, which eliminates macrophage infiltration, did not alter the increased TNF-α production that occurs after obstruction. Therefore, macrophages were not the source, and tubular cell release of mediators (such as AII or ROS) directly triggered by physical stretch, may be more important (see Figure 13-1).

Local production of TNF-α has a myriad of effects. After binding to its cell surface receptor TNFR1, TNF-α stimulates production of chemotactic factors, including MCP-1 by mesangial cells and ROS by fibroblasts.[26] In cultured mesangial cells, TNF-α also up-regulates ICAM-1, ELAM-1 and VCAM-1.[10] Therefore, it appears that early up-regulation of TNF-α could set into motion a cascade of signals that promotes macrophage recruitment and interstitial inflammation within the obstructed kidney.

NO   Another key local mediator after obstruction appears to be NO. In obstructed rat kidneys, concurrent administration of L-NAME to block NO production ablates the rise in renal blood flow early after obstruction,[7] and L-NAME also abolishes the ability of ACE inhibitors to prevent pro-

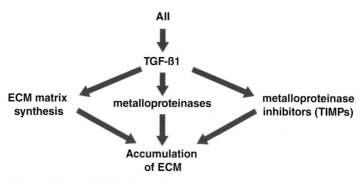

Figure 13-2 Potential roles by which angiotensin II (AII) promotes renal fibrosis after obstruction. By increasing local release of transforming growth factor (TGF)-β1, AII can favor accumulation of extracellular matrix via three complementary pathways.

gressive interstitial fibrosis longer term after obstruction.[10] These and other studies suggest the pathways by which ACE inhibition blocks interstitial inflammation may in part involve bradykinin-mediated NO generation. Conversely, administration of L-arginine to rats after renal obstruction, in order to boost local NO production, decreases interstitial fibrosis and ECM accumulation.[7]

Studies using knockout mouse models suggest that the role of NO may be more complex. Locally, NO is produced by tubular cells using iNOS, as well as the endogenous forms of the enzyme eNOS and nNOS. Although studies in one mouse knockout model suggested that iNOS-mediated NO production ameliorated renal fibrosis after obstruction,[27] another did not.[28] Further investigation using knockout mouse models suggested that NO produced by eNOS and or nNOS might be more important for limiting renal fibrosis after obstruction.[29] Taken as a whole, however, the current weight of evidence suggests that, after obstruction, up-regulated production of NO is beneficial and helps to limit renal fibrosis, although the specific pathways remain to be clarified.

APOPTOSIS   The eventual loss of renal mass and tubular atrophy that is observed after prolonged obstruction appears to be mediated, at least in part, by tubular cell apoptosis.[10,30,31] The number of apoptotic tubular cells in rat kidneys 35 days after obstruction was 30-fold higher than that observed in control kidneys.[30] Interestingly, this apoptotic surge was preceded by a rapid rise in renal mass and 60-fold increased tubular cell proliferation. Factors that may mediate both the proliferative and apoptotic changes include activation of the cell surface TNF-α receptor (TNFR1), and exposure to ROS.[31]

CONCLUSIONS   Studies elucidated previously unexpected mechanisms by which GFR falls after renal obstruction, and how chronically obstructed kidneys can become scarred and atrophic. Key mediators include prostaglandins, AII, ROS, NO and TNF-α, which in the end, produce fibroblast proliferation, ECM accumulation, and renal epithelial cell apoptosis. Physical stretch of tubular cells may trigger release of the key factors that initiate this cascade.

DIAGNOSIS OF RENAL OBSTRUCTION

Renal obstruction is diagnosed via imaging studies. The urinary sediment is typically normal, unless infection is superimposed.

ULTRASONOGRAPHY   Renal ultrasonography is often the initial screening study used to detect hydronephrosis.[32] Advantages include high sensitivity, as well as absent patient risk because ionizing radiation and contrast agents are not required.[33–35] Because functional obstruction can occur without hydronephrosis, a normal renal sonogram does not always rule out obstruction.[32] Examples where this scenario could operate include[36]:

1. Early obstruction when the collecting system is relatively noncompliant.
2. If the obstruction is incomplete, GFR may be impaired in the absence of marked hydronephrosis.
3. Clot or stone debris in the collecting system may distort the appearance of the dilated collecting system.
4. If the kidney is surrounded by fibrotic tissue (eg, from retroperitoneal fibrosis or postsurgical scarring), the renal collecting system may not dilate.
5. If renal function is markedly impaired secondary to severe parenchymal damage or poor renal perfusion (eg, with volume depletion), urine flow rates may be too reduced to result in significant hydronephrosis.

Conversely, kidneys can be hydronephrotic but retain normal function. A dilated renal collecting system without physiologic obstruction can arise as a result of pregnancy, vesicourethral reflux, relief after chronic obstruction, an extrarenal pelvis, and megacalyx.[37] The presence of normal renal function is one clinical indication that any hydronephrosis visualized on imaging studies may not be functionally significant. Overall, the sensitivity of renal ultrasonography for obstruction averages ≈90%, with a specificity of up to 98% (Table 13-3).

INTRAVENOUS UROGRAPHY   Intravenous urography was previously the preferred test to evaluate renal obstruction. Advantages include high sensitivity and specificity.[34,38] In addition, renal anatomy is much better visualized by intravenous urography, especially the ureters, and most often, the level of obstruction can be accurately determined. Cysts can also be easily discerned, whereas on ultrasonography, a dilated calyx can be hard to differentiate from a cyst. A rough estimate of renal function is also obtained, and distended but non-obstructed kidneys can be detected since they demonstrate good drainage of the contrast on later films. Additional information is also provided regarding calculi, necrotic papillae, and clots within the collecting system.

The major disadvantage of intravenous urography is the risk of contrast-induced nephrotoxicity. Risk factors for the development of contrast-induced acute renal failure include reduced renal function, diabetes, and amyloidosis.[34,40] If the detailed anatomic information that intravenous urography can supply is in fact required, it is important to institute measures that reduce the potential nephrotoxicity of intravenous contrast including, most importantly, volume expansion with 0.45% NS,[40] and possibly administration of N-acetyl cysteine.[41]

COMPUTED TOMOGRAPHY When compared to ultrasonography, computed tomography is of comparable sensitivity and specificity for detecting obstruction.[34] Disadvantages include cost and an exposure to radiation. A relative advantage is the possibility that important anatomic features, such as retroperitoneal fibrosis or lymphadenopathy, could be discerned if present.[34]

INTRARENAL DUPLEX DOPPLER ULTRASONOGRAPHY Although it is an excellent screening test, ultrasonography alone can lack sensitivity if the collecting system is obstructed but not dilated (eg, perirenal scarring), or specificity if collecting systems are dilated but not physiologically obstructed (eg, extrarenal pelvis).[36] Under these circumstances, intrarenal duplex Doppler ultrasonography is an excellent adjunctive test. As discussed above, within hours after the onset of obstruction, vasoconstriction of intrarenal arteries occurs. The resulting fall in renal blood flow can be detected via Doppler flow measurements and expressed quantitatively as a resistive index (RI).[42] Clinically, however, this technique is only useful if unilateral obstruction is suspected, since blood flow in the contralateral kidney serves as a control.

In a series of 23 patients with unilateral renal obstruction confirmed by excretory urogram, the mean RI in obstructive kidneys was 0.77 ± 0.07 as compared to 0.60 ± 0.04 in the non-obstructed side.[43] A difference in RI between kidneys of 0.1 was considered significant and, using this criterion, 20 of 23 obstructed patients were detected. The three false negative studies were attributed to pyelosinus extravasation (2 cases) and investigation too soon after the onset of obstruction (1 case). Since the fall in renal blood flow that occurs after obstruction takes hours to develop (see Table 13-2), it is recommended that Doppler ultrasonography be delayed at least six hours after the suspected onset. This technique requires experience on the part of the radiologist to perform and interpret accurately, and patient anatomy may preclude an interpretable signal. Doppler ultrasonography, however, is noninvasive, quick, and if available, can be quite useful in selected circumstances.

DIURETIC INTRAVENOUS UROGRAPHY Although intravenous urography provides good anatomic information, this technique often cannot evaluate function of a potentially obstructed kidney. In an attempt to provide this information, a loop diuretic can be administered intravenously at the beginning of the study.[44] If a kidney becomes visibly more hydronephrotic as result of the ensuing diuresis, it is likely that a functionally significant obstruction is present. If a patient experiences symptoms associated with visible hydronephrosis during the test, the kidney can also be implicated as a source of chronic pain. However, attempts to quantify the interpretation of diuretic intravenous urography and increase reliability by measuring the area of the renal pelvis, were disappointing. Although a negative study appeared diagnostic and correlated well with other tests, such as diuretic renography or pressure-flow studies, indeterminate or positive tests correlated poorly and were therefore of uncertain significance.[44] For this reason, as well as the inherent risks of a nephrotoxic contrast agent and ionizing radiation, diuretic urography is not often employed, especially given other test modalities.

DIURETIC RENOGRAPHY Diuretic renography was developed to circumvent many of the problems inherent in diuretic intravenous urography. In the standard approach, a bolus of radioactive tracer (typically ^{99m}Tc-MAG3 or ^{99m}Tc-DMSA) is injected intravenously and tracked as it is excreted by the kidney before and after a diuretic stimulus (eg, furosemide 0.5 mg/kg) that is given 20 minutes after the tracer ("F+20").[37] A gamma camera measures mean parenchymal transit time of the tracer. Time-activity curves are generated from different areas of the kidney: whole kidney, renal pelvis, bladder, and vacuolar pole. Subtraction of the renal pelvic curve from the whole kidney curve yields the renal parenchymal curve. The vascular curve is then subtracted from the whole kidney and parenchymal curves to remove activity related to recirculation. Normal mean parenchymal transit times are less than 4 minutes. Five excretion patterns have been described (Figure 13-3), including normal (Type I), dilated non-obstructed (Type III a), equivocal (Type III b), obstructed (Type II), and delayed decompression (Type IV).[37] The latter category (Type IV) was most recently described, and is believed consistent with, functional obstruction.

Timing of the diuretic dosage is potentially important. If the diuretic is administered 15 minutes before the tracer ("F-15"), the tracer will be excreted by the kidneys at the time of maximal diuretic effect.[45] This can potentially improve the diagnostic utility, by decreasing the equivocal response rate to 3% from 17%. Administering the diuretic simultaneously with the tracer has also been proposed ("F-0"), and appears to give comparable sensitivity and specificity to the traditional F+20 technique. A relative advantage for F-0, however, is decreased time for test completion ($\approx$20 min for F0 versus $\approx$40 min for F+20 or F-15). The F-15 technique appears to have maximal sensitivity when evaluating equivocal cases, for example a case with large dilated collecting systems. Importantly, the timing of diuretic administration has no influence on the ability to detect split renal function.

Three long-term studies confirm that even if a dilated collecting system is present, a normal diuretic renogram portends a good prognosis.[29,36,38] Between these three studies, approximately 200 patients with hydronephrosis but normal diuretic renography were prospectively followed for up to 5 years, and only one individual demonstrated a decline in glomerular filtration that required surgical intervention. Indeterminate studies are harder to interpret because some may indicate partial obstruction, but others may not. Additional studies are probably necessary in these cases.

Table 13-3 Modalities for Imaging Renal Obstruction

	Sensitivity	Specificity	Comments
Renal ultrasonography [32,34,35,61]	90%	93–98%	No patient risk; good screening test
Intrarenal duplex Doppler ultrasonography [32,43,62–65]	87–94%	88–99%	No patient risk; good adjunct to ultrasonography; can only evaluate unilateral obstruction
Intravenous urography [32,48]	70–97%	42–93%	Risk of contrast-induced nephropathy
Diuretic intravenous urography [38,44,48]	83%	86%	Risk of contrast-induced nephropathy; qualitative only; a positive test has poor predictive value.
Diuretic renography [29,37,45,49]	83–97%	85–93%	Current test of choice if results from ultrasonography are equivocal; a negative test portends an excellent long term prognosis
Perfusion pressure flow studies [38,47–50]	93–100%	79–97%	Invasive; most useful for dilated renal pelvis if diuretic urography is equivocal; does not correlate well with Diuretic renography
Computed tomography [34]	90%	93%	Sensitivity and specificity comparable to ultrasonography; increased anatomic detail

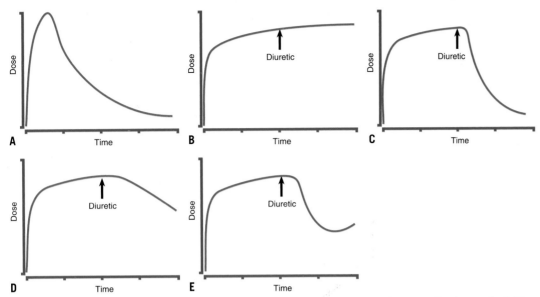

Figure 13-3 Diuresis renography responses. *A*, Type I, normal. *B*, Type III, obstructed. *C*, Type III a, hypotonic. *D*, Type III b, equivocal. *E*, Type IV, delayed decompression.

In the past, renal pelvis biopsy was sometimes performed at the time of pyeloplasty in order to obtain histologic information about the renal parenchyma.[29,46] In these samples, increased collagen deposition was taken as evidence of advanced fibrosis and scarring. Two studies indicate that results from diuretic renography correlate highly with the results of renal pelvis biopsy,[29,46] which is therefore rarely performed today (Table 13-4).

PERFUSION PRESSURE FLOW STUDIES Perfusion pressure flow study was popularized by Whitaker and often bears his name.[47] To perform this functional investigation, dilute contrast material is infused through a percutaneous nephrostomy tract proximal to the site of suspected obstruction, at a rate of 10 mL/min. Infusion is continued until the collecting system is full. Pressures > 22 mm H_2O are taken to indicate obstruction, whereas pressures < 15 mm H_2O are considered normal. Fluoroscopy allows visualization of dye passage and obstruction sites. Although perfusion pressure flow is considered the "gold standard," it is not clear that this invasive technique is truly superior to diuretic renography. In six trials where the two techniques were compared head-to-head, agreement was less than ideal.[29,38,47–50] Certain cases with a non-obstructed diuretic renogram nevertheless had an obstructed pressure perfusion flow study.[29,36,38,49] This lack of correlation makes the significance of an obstructed perfusion pressure flow study hard to determine, particularly in light of the above evidence that strongly suggests cases with a normal diuresis renogram have an excellent long-term prognosis. Other drawbacks of this technique include the invasive nature, exposure to ionizing radiation, and the fact that no information is provided regarding residual renal function.

CONCLUSIONS Renal ultrasonography is the screening test of choice, and if necessary,

Doppler ultrasonography evaluation of renal blood flow can improve sensitivity and specificity. The diagnostic test of choice if further evaluation of a hydronephrotic kidney is required is often diuretic renography.

If these noninvasive studies fail to provide a definitive answer, and the functional significance of an apparent obstruction remains equivocal, one pragmatic approach is to next pass a ureteral stent and monitor for improvement in renal function. Stents may be poorly tolerated, however, because they sometimes causes pain, hematuria, and dysuria, factors that obviously must be weighed when choosing whether to proceed or not. Percutaneous nephrostomies avoid some of these problems, but pose the risk of infection. It is important to remember that a thin renal parenchyma is always a relative contraindication to a percutaneous approach, owing to the risk of persistent leak after the tube is removed.

TREATMENT OF RENAL OBSTRUCTION

INDICATIONS FOR SURGICAL INTERVENTION All hydronephrotic kidneys require individual assessment and management. Asymptomatic patients without evidence of obstruction on imaging studies can be safely observed (see above discussion). On the other hand, even if renal function is preserved, surgical intervention should be considered for any symptomatic patients. In those patients who are observed, any evidence of renal functional deterioration would be an indication to reconsider the possibility of surgical intervention. The most vexing case might be that of the obstructed and poorly functional kidney. Especially if the renal cortex is thinned, the possibility that renal function may not improve—even if successfully relieved—must be factored against the surgical risk. The measurement of split renal function by renography, together with measurements of renal cortical thickness, is often used to gauge the potential for renal recovery. Studies confirmed that ^{99m}Tc-DMSA renal scintigra-

phy may be the best predictor of residual renal function after relief of obstruction, and suggested that surgical intervention might not be useful if the split function of the obstructed kidney is $< 10\%$ of the contralateral "good" kidney.[37,51] If surgical intervention is attempted as a therapeutic trial, it is important to remember that recovery can be delayed up to three months.

LONG TERM RESULTS AFTER SURGICAL RELIEF OF OBSTRUCTION Although there is significant variation from species to species, studies in dogs, rabbits, and rats suggest that no meaningful return of renal function can occur if a complete obstruction has been present more than 4 weeks.[52] In humans, the exact length of time that a complete obstruction can be present with at least some preservation of renal function is less clear because the timing and extent of blockage are often not known. Complete return of function is likely if the obstruction is present less than 3 weeks,[53] and partial return of function has been even observed when obstruction is present for much longer,[53–56] in one case perhaps as long as 1.5 years.[57]

Most functional recovery occurs in the first 7 to 10 days after relief of obstruction.[58,59] In general, it appears that tubular function recovers first, requiring days to weeks, whereas renal blood flow and GFR can continue to slowly improve over weeks, to as long as three months. Presumably, the length of time for recovery of renal function is required to reverse those pathways that produced the decline in the first place, including mononuclear infiltration. In most cases, however, if functional improvement is significantly delayed, partial recovery is the rule.

Under conditions of partial obstruction, and for a period after relief of obstruction, specific defects in tubular function are typically observed. These include a relative inability to conserve sodium, concentrate the urine, and excrete a potassium load.[58–60] In fact, this hyperkalemic renal tubular acidosis can be an early subtle sign of obstructive uropathy. Importantly, if the obstruction is unilateral, the normal kidney may mask these subtle defects. If an obstruction was complete enough to produce significant oliguria and/or anuria, a brisk post-obstructive diuresis often ensues after the obstruction is relieved. Contributing factors include a physiologic natriuresis of retained sodium and fluids, and an osmotic diuresis largely mediated by retained urea. In addition, the post-obstructed distal tubule is poorly responsive to antidiuretic hormone resulting in a transient form of nephrogenic diabetes

Table 13-4 Comparison of Diuresis Renography and Renal Pelvis Biopsy		
	Pelvic biopsy result	
Diuresis renogram result	Normal	Abnormal
Nonobstructed	6	0
Obstructed	0	18
Indeterminate	0	23
Technically unsatisfactory	0	6
Adapted from English PJ, et al,[29] and Lupton EW, et al.[46]		

insipidus.[60] During this period of post-obstructive diuresis the medullary osmotic gradient may be dissipated, thereby prolonging the period during which the urine cannot be maximally concentrated. A "medullary washout" is much more likely to occur if large amounts of intravenous fluids are administered during this recovery phase. In general, this post-obstructive diuresis is not likely to result in clinically significant volume depletion, and in most cases, the use of intravenous fluid should be modest rather that aggressive. Finally, it should be noted that, if the renal obstruction is unilateral, any post-obstructive diuresis is likely to be modest, if present at all.

CONCLUSIONS

Recent basic science advances have improved our understanding of the mechanisms that mediate the decline in renal function and the chronic scarring that can occur after renal obstruction. Newer radiologic techniques have likewise improved our ability to diagnose this condition, and discern those cases that might benefit from surgical intervention.

ACKNOWLEDGEMENTS

Special thanks go to Joanne Zimmerman and Dianne Kappas for secretarial assisitance. This work was supported by grants from the National Institutes of Health (R01 DK 53399 and R21 DK 607070) and the Ralph W. Wilson, Sr. Foundation.

REFERENCES

1. The scope and impact of kidney and urologic diseases. In: #90-583 NP, editor. National Kidney and Urologic Diseases Advisory Board. Long-Range Plan; 1990. Washington, DC. p. 7–35.
2. Klahr S, Pukerson ML. The pathophysiology of obstructive nephropathy: the role of vasoactive compounds in the hemodynamic and structural abnormalities of the obstructed kidney. Am J Kidney Dis 1994;23:219–23.
3. Yarger WE, Schocken DD, Harris RH. Obstructive nephropathy in the rat: possible roles for the renin- angiotensin system, prostaglandins, and thromboxanes in postobstructive renal function. J Clin Invest 1980;65:400–12.
4. Blackshear JL, Wathen RL. Effects of indomethacin on renal blood flow and renin secretory responses to ureteral occlusion in the dog. Miner Electrolyte Metab 1978;1:271–8.
5. Allen JT, Vaughan ED Jr, Gillenwater JY. The effect of indomethacin on renal blood flow and ureteral pressure in unilateral ureteral obstruction in awake dogs. Invest Urol 1978;15:324–7.
6. Gaudio KM, Siegel NJ, Hayslett JP, Kashgarian M. Renal perfusion and intratubular pressure during ureteral occlusion in the rat. Am J Physiol 1980;238:F205–9.
7. Morrissey JJ, Ishidoya S, McCracken R, Klahr S. Nitric oxide generation ameliorates the tubulointerstitial fibrosis of obstructive nephropathy. J Am Soc Nephrol 1996;7: 2202–12.
8. Klahr S. Obstructive nephropathy. Intern Med 2000;39: 355–61.
9. Purkerson ML, Klahr S. Prior inhibition of vasoconstrictors normalizes GFR in postobstructed kidneys. Kidney Int 1989;35:1305–14.
10. Klahr S. Obstructive nephropathy. Kidney Int 1998;54: 286–300.
11. Ricardo SD, Ding G, Eufemio M, Diamond JR. Antioxidant expression in experimental hydronephrosis: role of mechanical stretch and growth factors. Am J Physiol 1997;272:F789–98.
12. Klahr S. New insights into the consequences and mechanisms of renal impairment in obstructive nephropathy. Am J Kidney Dis 1991;18:689–99.
13. El-Dahr SS. The kininogen gene family in obstructive uropathy. Semin Nephrol 1998;18:633–40.
14. Kaneto H, Morrissey J, Klahr S. Increased expression of TGF-β1 mRNA in the obstructed kidney of rats with unilateral ureteral ligation. Kidney Int 1993;44:313–21.
15. Sharma K, Ziyadeh FN. The emerging role of transforming growth factor-beta in kidney diseases. Am J Physiol 1994; 266:F829–42.
16. Ohba M, Shibanuma M, Kuroki T, Nose K. Production of hydrogen peroxide by transforming growth factor-beta 1 and its involvement in induction of egr-1 in mouse osteoblastic cells. J Cell Biol 1994;126:1079–88.
17. Tham DM, Martin-McNulty B, Wang YX, et al. Angiotensin II is associated with activation of NF-κβ-mediated genes and downregulation of PPARs. Physiol Genomics 2002;11:21–30.
18. Diamond JR, Ricardo SD, Klahr S. Mechanisms of interstitial fibrosis in obstructive nephropathy. Semin Nephrol 1998;18:594–602.
19. Shappell SB, Gurpinar T, Lechago J, et al. Chronic obstructive uropathy in severe combined immunodeficient (SCID) mice: lymphocyte infiltration is not required for progressive tubulointerstitial injury. J Am Soc Nephrol 1998;9: 1008–17.
20. Kawada N, Moriyama T, Ando A, et al. Increased oxidative stress in mouse kidneys with unilateral ureteral obstruction. Kidney Int 1999;56:1004–13.
21. Ricardo SD, Levinson ME, DeJoseph MR, Diamond JR. Expression of adhesion molecules in rat renal cortex during experimental hydronephrosis. Kidney Int 1996;50: 2002–10.
22. Modi KS, Morrissey J, Shah SV, et al. Effects of probucol on renal function in rats with bilateral ureteral obstruction. Kidney Int 1990;38:843–50.
23. Klahr S. Urinary tract obstruction. Semin Nephrol 2001;21: 133–45.
24. Kuemmerle NB, Brandt RB, Chan W, et al. Inhibition of transforming growth factor β1 induction by dietary vitamin E in unilateral ureteral obstruction in rats. Biochem Molec Med 1997;61:82–6.
25. Chan W, Krieg RJ, Ward K, et al. Progression after release of obstructive nephropathy. Pediatr Nephrol 2001;16:238–44.
26. Meier B, Radeke HH, Selle S, et al. Human fibroblasts release reactive oxygen species in response to interleukin-1 and tumour necrosis factor-alpha. Biochem J 1989;263: 539–45.
27. Hochberg D, Johnson CW, Chen J, et al. Interstitial fibrosis of unilateral ureteral obstruction is exacerbated in kidneys of mice lacking the gene for inducible nitric oxide synthase. Lab Invest 2000;80:1721–8.
28. Huang A, Palmer LS, Hom D, et al. The role of nitric oxide in obstructive nephropathy. Pediatr Urol 2000;163:1276–81.
29. English PJ, Testa HJ, Gosling JA, Cohen SJ. Idiopathic hydronephrosis in childhood—a comparison between diuresis renography and upper urinary tract morphology. Br J Urol 1982;54:603–7.
30. Truong LD, Petrusevska G, Yang G, et al. Cell apoptosis and proliferation in experimental chronic obstructive uropathy. Kidney Int 1996;50:200–7.
31. Choi Y-J, Baranowska-Daca E, Nguyen V, et al. Mechanism of chronic obstructive uropathy: increased expression of apoptosis-promoting molecules. Kidney Int 2000;58: 1481–91.
32. Dodd GD III, Kaufman PN, Bracken RB. Renal arterial duplex Doppler ultrasound in dogs with urinary obstruction. J Urol 1991;145:644–6.
33. Ellenbogen PH, Scheible FW, Talner LB, Leopold GR. Sensitivity of gray scale ultrasound in detecting urinary tract obstruction. AJR Am J Roentgenol 1978;130:731–3.
34. Webb JA, Reznek RH, White FE, et al. Can ultrasound and computed tomography replace high-dose urography in patients with impaired renal function? Q J Med 1984; 53:411–25.
35. Malave SR, Neiman HL, Spies SM, et al. Diagnosis of hydronephrosis: comparison of radionuclide scanning and sonography. AJR Am J Roentgenol 1980;135:1179–85.
36. O'Reilly PH, Lupton EW, Testa HJ, et al. The dilated nonobstructed renal pelvis. Br J Urol 1981;53:205–9.
37. O'Reilly PH. Obstructive uropathy. Q J Nucl Med 2002; 46:295–303.
38. Kass EJ, Majd M, Belman AB. Comparison of the diuretic renogram and the pressure perfusion study in children. J Urol 1985;134:92–6.
39. Parfrey PS, Griffiths SM, Barrett BJ, et al. Contrast material-induced renal failure in patients with diabetes mellitus, renal insufficiency, or both. A prospective controlled study. N Engl J Med 1989;320:143–9.
40. Solomon R, Werner C, Mann D, et al. Effects of saline, mannitol, and furosemide to prevent acute decreases in renal function induced by radiocontrast agents. N Engl J Med 1994;331:1416–20.
41. Tepel M, van der Giet M, Schwarzfeld C, et al. Prevention of radiographic-contrast-agent-induced reductions in renal function by acetylcysteine. N Engl J Med 2000;343:180–4.
42. Shokeir AA, Provoost AP, Nijman RJ. Resistive index in obstructive uropathy. Br J Urol 1997;80:195–200.
43. Platt JF, Rubin JM, Ellis JH. Acute renal obstruction: evaluation with intrarenal duplex Doppler and conventional US. Radiology 1993;186:685–8.
44. Whitfield HN, Britton KE, Hendry WF, Wickham JE. Frusemide intravenous urography in the diagnosis of pelviureteric junction obstruction. Br J Urol 1979;51:445–8.
45. English PJ, Testa HJ, Lawson RS, et al. Modified method of diuresis renography for the assessment of equivocal pelviureteric junction obstruction. Br J Urol 1987;59:10–14.
46. Lupton EW, Testa HJ, O'Reilly PH, et al. Diuresis renography and morphology in upper urinary tract obstruction. Br J Urol 1979;51:10–14.
47. Whitaker RH, Buxton-Thomas MS. A comparison of pressure flow studies and renography in equivocal upper urinary tract obstruction. J Urol 1984;131:446–9.
48. Senac MO Jr, Miller JH, Stanley P. Evaluation of obstructive uropathy in children: radionuclide renography vs. the Whitaker test. AJR Am J Roentgenol 1984;143:11–5.
49. Hay AM, Norman WJ, Rice ML, Steventon RD. A comparison between diuresis renography and the Whitaker test in 64 kidneys. Br J Urol 1984;56:561–4.
50. Gonzalez R, Chiou R. The diagnosis of upper urinary tract obstruction in children: comparison of diuresis renography and pressure flow studies. J Urol 1985;133:646–9.
51. Thompson A, Gough DC. The use of renal scintigraphy in assessing the potential for recovery in the obstructed renal tract in children. BJU Int 2001;87:853–6.
52. Beer E. Experimental study of the effects of ureteral obstruction on kidney function and structure. Am J Urol 1912;8:171–6.
53. Earlam RJ. Recovery of renal function after prolonged ureteric obstruction. Br J Urol 1967;39:58–62.
54. Graham JB. Recovery of kidney after ureteral obstruction. JAMA 1962;181:993–4.
55. Brunschwig A, Barber HRK, Roberts S. Return of renal funciton after varying periods of ureteral occlusion: a clinical study. JAMA 1964;188:5–8.
56. Lewis HY, Pierce JM. Return of function after relief of complete ureteral obstruction. J Urol 1962;88:377–9.
57. Papaioannou AN, Brunschwig A. Return of renal function of a kidney not visualized on intravenous pyelogram for 1 1/2 years. Arch Surg 1965;90:367–70.
58. Better OS, Arieff AI, Massry SG, et al. Studies on renal function after relief of complete unilateral ureteral obstruction of three months' duration in man. Am J Med 1973;54:234–40.
59. Cohen EP, Sobrero M, Roxe DM, Levin ML. Reversibility of long-standing urinary tract obstruction requiring long-term dialysis. Arch Intern Med 1992;152:177–9.
60. Reyes AA, Robertson G, Klahr S. Role of vasopressin in rats with bilateral ureteral obstruction. Proc Soc Exp Biol Med 1991;197:49–55.
61. Fine LG, Ong AC, Norman JT. Mechanisms of tubulointerstitial injury in progressive renal diseases. Eur J Clin Invest 1993;23:259–65.
62. Talner LB, Scheible W, Ellenbogen PH, et al. How accurate is ultrasonography in detecting hydronephrosis in azotemic patients? Urol Radiol 1981;3:1–6.
63. Platt JF, Rubin JM, Ellis JH, DiPietro MA. Duplex Doppler US of the kidney: differentiation of obstructive from nonobstructive dilatation. Radiology 1989;171:515–7.
64. Platt JF, Rubin JM, Ellis JH. Distinction between obstructive and nonobstructive pyelocaliectasis with duplex Doppler sonography. AJR Am J Roentgenol 1989;153:997–1000.
65. Gottlieb RH, Luhmann Kt, Oates RP. Duplex ultrasound evaluation of normal native kidneys and native kidneys with urinary tract obstruction. J Ultrasound Med 1989;8:609–11.

14

Percutaneous Access, Tract Dilation, and Maintenance of the Nephrostomy Tract

Andrew J. LeRoy, MD

The development of techniques to establish safe and reliable percutaneous access into the renal collecting systems was a major factor in the wide clinical acceptance of endourologic procedures. A properly created nephrostomy tract has a wide range of subsequent applications from simple urinary drainage to intrarenal surgical procedures. As with all interventional procedures, a variety of technique descriptions have been published regarding percutaneous nephrostomy (PN) placement, tract dilation, and nephrostomy tract maintenance. Despite the subtle procedural differences emphasized in reports from various centers, central tenets are common to all reports and form the basis of this chapter.

Percutaneous nephrostomy evolved from the initial description of antegrade pyelography in the early 1950s. In 1955, Goodwin and colleagues described percutaneous nephrostomy for temporary relief of hydronephrosis.[1] The procedure languished until revived in the 1970s, primarily by European physicians.[2,3] Over the ensuing decade, percutaneous nephrostomy not only became a standard part of medical therapy, replacing surgical nephrostomy, but facilitated the introduction of endourologic procedures through the nephrostomy tract. The broad range of endourologic procedures introduced over the next two decades was dependent upon this maturation of percutaneous nephrostomy techniques, the development of acute tract dilation equipment and expertise, and the clinical utility of staged procedures through a well-maintained nephrostomy tract.

PROCEDURAL INDICATIONS

Percutaneous nephrostomy placement is the procedure of choice for decompression of obstructed kidneys in patients with supravesical obstruction of the urinary tracts. Nephrostomy drainage in that setting provides relief of azotemia, pain, or sepsis. The return of appropriate renal function after nephrostomy placement may take hours or days depending upon the acuity of the underlying obstruction, so life-threatening hyperkalemia from collecting system obstruction is better treated with hemodialysis, with nephrostomy placement to follow. In acutely ill patients with urinary tract obstruction requiring nephrostomy placement, complex intrarenal manipulations are often tolerated better and more successfully if simple nephrostomy insertion is effected, followed by several days of drainage prior to more complex intrarenal manipulations.

An established nephrostomy tract may be utilized for long-term nephrostomy drainage to divert urine away from ureteral leaks or fistulas. The nephrostomy tube also can be used to introduce appropriate medications, such as antifungal drugs to treat an upper tract yeast infection or chemotherapeutic agents for superficial transitional cell carcinoma.

A wide variety of manipulations can be performed within the urinary tracts through an established nephrostomy tract.[4] Procedures to manage urinary strictures include dilatation of ureteral strictures, ureteral stent insertion, incision of stenotic infundibula, and endopyelotomy. The most common interventional procedure performed through an established percutaneous nephrostomy tract in many practices is management of stone disease using percutaneous techniques. These more advanced techniques are discussed in subsequent chapters.

The primary contraindication to percutaneous nephrostomy creation is the presence of an uncorrectable bleeding diathesis. Most bleeding disorders can be corrected prior to tract creation with appropriate drug or blood product administration. Administration of clinically appropriate antibiotics may limit the development of sepsis following drainage of infected urinary tracts. The moral implications of percutaneous renal drainage to improve compromised renal function must be addressed in selected patients who suffer from untreatable malignancies or other terminal diseases.[5] In those situations, a thorough pre-procedural discussion with the patient and appropriate family members is an essential component of patient management.

PATIENT PREPARATION

The review of each patient by a urologic surgeon prior to intervention includes a frank discussion of procedural indications, goals, and concerns. An appropriate hemostasis evaluation, urine bacteriology assessment, and overall systemic appraisal are essential components of this consultation. The elective or emergency interventional nature of each individual patient's medical presentation determines the extent of this medical review.

The radiographic evaluation of patients prior to percutaneous renal access creation must be individualized also. Traditionally, a plain abdominal radiograph with tomograms of the kidneys was the initial examination to detect renal position and size, the number and location of renal calculi, and the overall abdominal status. In those patients undergoing elective percutaneous renal calculus removal, an intravenous urogram provides essential information about renal and stone anatomy as well as a baseline evaluation of renal function. Diagnostic ultrasound examination is performed in those patients with urographically detected abnormalities requiring further delineation or in those patients in whom primary urographic evaluation is likely to be suboptimal, including critically ill patients, those with poor renal function, or patients with a documented allergy to intravenous contrast material. In the past decade, computed tomography (CT) has become the primary abdominal diagnostic survey examination in patients with emergency or complex medical conditions. CT is also the best single radiographic test to detect urolithiasis and its complications and to display complex intra-abdominal anatomic variants.[6] The administration of intravenous contrast material in conjunction with serial CT scanning produces CT urography, which is an exquisite display of renal anatomy and function. Although a few authors have advocated pre-procedural CT scanning of the planned nephrostomy tract in all patients to avoid injury to adjacent intra-abdominal organs,[7] most practitioners use pre-procedural CT only in selected cases of body habitus deformity, splenomegaly, colonic malposition, or marked colonic distention (Figure 14-1). Magnetic resonance imaging (MRI) of the urinary tracts is less developed for clinical applications than CT. MRI does offer multiplanar evaluation of urinary abnormalities and their effects on renal function in patients in whom allergies to iodinated contrast agents preclude comprehensive CT exams. Radionuclide scanning techniques are helpful in the evaluation of altered renal function prior to planned endourologic procedures.

The establishment of an intravenous access line is an essential component of preoperative preparation. This facilitates the administration of intra-procedural analgesics and sedatives as well as rarely needed resuscitative medications. The administration of pre-procedural broad-spectrum antibiotics is practiced widely; those patients with known urinary tract infections are treated with infusions of bacteriologically specific antibiotics.

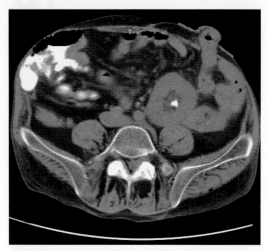

Figure 14-1 Computed tomography scan of the upper pelvis shows numerous bowel loops adjacent to the transplanted kidney in the left side of the pelvis. A safe tract into the kidney could not be created for removal of the infected renal stone.

The type of anesthesia administered during percutaneous renal access procedures must be customized to the individual patient and the local medical practice setting. Simple percutaneous nephrostomy for external urinary drainage is tolerated well by nearly all patients with adequate intravenous analgesia and sedation. The administration of a general anesthetic is often preferable for both simple and complex interventions in children or agitated adults. General anesthesia is also used commonly for the entire operation when percutaneous stone removal or other extensive endourologic manipulations are performed as an immediate continuation of the percutaneous access procedure. Because of the potential for the development of rare but life-threatening complications during percutaneous nephrostomy placement, this procedure should be performed in a facility that has full anesthesia, surgical, angiographic, and resuscitation services immediately available.

INSTRUMENTATION

IMAGING GUIDANCE The creation of a percutaneous access tract into the renal collecting system requires imaging equipment for guidance.[8] Initial percutaneous nephrostomy series all used fluoroscopic guidance for drainage tube placement. The development of high-quality C-arm configuration fluoroscopy equipment led to its use for percutaneous nephrostomy placement in angiographic suites or operating rooms. Fluoroscopic monitoring is essential for complex intrarenal catheter and guidewire manipulations, tract dilation, and residual stone evaluation during endoscopic stone removal. In most percutaneous stone therapy patients, primary fluoroscopic guidance for percutaneous nephrostomy placement is still preferred because of the high level of spatial accuracy afforded to the operator to achieve precise needle and guidewire positioning.[9]

The development of real-time diagnostic ultrasonography provided an alternative guidance system for urinary tract interventions. Percuta-

neous puncture of dilated renal collecting systems under ultrasonographic guidance has been widely adopted. The compromised visualization of intrarenal guidewire manipulations when monitored with ultrasonography is less critical in simple percutaneous nephrostomy drainage of dilated systems. Ultrasonographic guidance of percutaneous nephrostomy placement has obvious benefits in infants, pregnant women, and renal transplant recipients.[10]

The introduction of CT guidance of interventional procedures added another alternative for the management of complex cases. CT guidance for creation of a percutaneous renal access tract can be essential in patients with coexisting medical problems such as splenic enlargement, body habitus abnormalities like scoliosis, previous major intra-abdominal surgical interventions, or for grossly obese patients in whom ultrasonography and fluoroscopy are greatly compromised.[11] Percutaneous renal access creation under CT guidance is technically similar to other commonly performed CT-guided drainage procedures.[12] CT guidance is particularly useful in those patients with coexisting perinephric abnormalities, such as urinoma formation due to ureteral obstruction, in whom independent catheter drainage of the collecting systems and the urinoma can be effected simultaneously.[13]

Analogous to the introduction of CT-guided interventions several decades ago, several reports of magnetic–resonance-guided percutaneous nephrostomy placement have been published.[14] The clinical applications of this approach will evolve slowly because of the cumbersome nature of current magnetic resonance interventional activities, but the development of faster scanning techniques combined with better physical access to patients inside the scanning magnet are needed to support this evolution.

The electronics revolution of the past decade also has had an effect on PN guidance technology. Robotic systems have been developed for needle placement into the renal collecting systems, with the mechanical needle insertion depth and angulation based on fluoroscopic or CT-derived data sets.[15,16] Because of the prototype nature of these systems, active clinical implementation has been very limited. Other authors have described equipping standard C-arm fluoroscopy units with visible laser guidance systems as optical aids to enhance proper needle positioning.[17] Further developments of this type will certainly evolve, limited only by affordability, reliability, and clinical practice considerations.

Although the availability of all these imaging guidance technologies is necessary for the broad range of percutaneous nephrostomy insertion applications, the variable nature of patient presentations requires a customized approach for each patient. For uncomplicated renal drainage procedures, the ideal imaging guidance technique is the combination of initial percutaneous puncture guidance with real-time ultrasonography in a fluoroscopic suite, followed by fluoroscopic monitoring of needle catheter and

guidewire manipulations. The combined utilization of CT and fluoroscopy provides excellent nephrostomy-placement results in centers where these technologies have been integrated.[18] For endourologic stone therapy in patients with non-dilated collecting systems, fluoroscopic guidance of percutaneous access creation is preferred since ultrasonographic visualization and puncture of normal-sized calices is extremely difficult.

ACCESS EQUIPMENT A wide variety of equipment has been designed for creation of percutaneous access tracts into the urinary collecting systems. The commercially available access systems can be grouped into those that use a trocar with an insertable cannula or those that use needle-guidewire-catheter techniques.[19] In current practice, the trocar systems are almost never used. The wide popularity of the Seldinger–technique-based needle-guidewire equipment is based on its broad range of adaptability and physician familiarity with these systems from performing other interventional procedures.[20,21] There are two commonly used needle systems that differ primarily in access needle size. Definitive puncture of the renal collecting system with an 18-gauge needle permits the immediate introduction of a .035- or .038-inch guidewire into the collecting system. The rigidity of the 18-gauge needle is advantageous for accurately directing the needle tip as it is advanced through fascial planes. The 18-gauge needle tip is also readily identifiable with real-time ultrasonographic guidance. The alternative access needle system uses a 21-gauge primary access needle that accepts a stiff-bodied .018-inch guidewire. The use of a dedicated conversion catheter over this .018-inch guidewire permits subsequent introduction of a .035- or .038-inch guidewire into the collecting system for further manipulations.[22] The 21-gauge needle system has a number of advantages: (1) a theoretically decreased risk of renal parenchymal damage from this smaller needle during the repositioning passes required for precise access, (2) the better size match of this smaller needle with non-dilated calices, and (3) the straight nature of the access tracts that result from this needle's ability to resist torque. In contrast to the larger wires introduced through an 18-gauge needle, the soft tip of the .018-inch wire, which is an integral part of the 21-gauge needle system, rarely perforates the collecting system, even when manipulated through tight strictures or adjacent to tightly impacted stones.[23] The directionally torquable tip of this smaller wire also enhances the value of the 21-gauge needle system as a primary access set for all percutaneous nephrostomy placement applications.

A broad range of guidewires and catheters introduced for angiographic or endoscopic techniques are available commercially with only subtle distinctions in their individual capabilities. Soft J-tip wires are the least traumatic to the mucosa during manipulations within the urinary collecting systems. Stiffer shaft wires of .035- or .038-inch size are more valuable for initial tract dilation, endourologic instrument insertion, and tract maintenance applications. The standard wires used in urinary tract interventional procedures are Teflon-coated except for the hydrophilic-coated wires that are very valuable for passing through tight strictures or traversing tortuous pathways. Adapted from their original use in angiographic procedures, straight and angle-tipped catheters of 5 French to 7F sizes are used to stabilize guidewires along the percutaneous tract and within the collecting systems. Torquable angled catheters are invaluable for assisting the precise guidewire manipulations required to gain access around impacted stones or cross edematous, strictured areas in the central renal collecting systems or ureter. Small-caliber angiographic catheters are also used to maintain the established nephrostomy tract if tract dilation and endoscopic surgery are delayed after the access tract is created.

TECHNIQUE FOR CREATING ACCESS TRACTS

Prior to percutaneous needle insertion, the patient must be placed into the appropriate position. For most patients, this is either prone or prone oblique with the body side of the targeted kidney slightly elevated. These patient positions provide access to the posterolateral flank where the access tract originates. For practitioners using primarily fluoroscopic guidance, the operator's hands are out of the vertical x-ray beam with the patient prone. Ultrasonographic guidance of tract creation in a prone patient may be compromised by rib-generated artifacts, but real-time monitoring and transducer angulation techniques usually overcome that limitation. In those patients who cannot be turned prone, the supine oblique position can be used, with the body side of the targeted kidney elevated off the tabletop.[24] CT guidance of percutaneous nephrostomy placement is particularly advantageous in procedures in this position because the intra-abdominal structures and their relationships to the intended tract are defined precisely.

Thorough evaluation of the renal collecting system anatomy is essential prior to definitive percutaneous puncture for access tract creation.[25] The variations in caliceal and collecting system anatomy are well defined in another chapter (see Chapter 22, "Treatment of Caliceal Diverticula and Infundibular Stenosis"). If fluoroscopic guidance is used, the collecting system can be opacified either by direct percutaneous puncture with a 22-gauge needle followed by antegrade pyelography, injection of intravenous contrast material prior to puncture, or cystoscopic retrograde ureteral catheter placement with direct intrapelvic injection of contrast material.[26] Insertion of a retrograde ureteral balloon catheter makes subsequent access procedures less difficult because the collecting system also can be distended, facilitating percutaneous puncture. Retrograde ureteral catheter placement, however, does require an additional pre-nephrostomy pro-

cedure, usually accompanied by an additional patient repositioning from supine to prone. Fluoroscopic collecting system evaluation during antegrade or retrograde pyelography is essential for choosing the proper calix for definitive access puncture during nephrostomy tract creation. The subsequent injection of a small amount of carbon dioxide as a negative contrast agent into the opacified collecting system is helpful in delineating the posteriorly oriented calices prior to tract creation.[27] Carbon dioxide can also be used as the sole agent for pyelography in patients with life-threatening allergies to iodinated contrast materials (Figure 14-2). If ultrasonographic guidance is available for percutaneous nephrostomy placement in dilated systems, direct puncture of the appropriate calix obviates the need for initial collecting system opacification. If only the renal pelvis can be identified on ultrasonography, initial pelvic puncture with a 22-gauge needle permits antegrade pyelography prior to definitive caliceal puncture for percutaneous nephrostomy placement. With CT guidance of nephrostomy tract creation, the access needle can be placed directly into the collecting system without the need for prior opacification or intervention.

The ideal percutaneous access tract into the renal collecting system begins near the posterior axillary line. The skin puncture site may be more lateral in obese patients in whom the lateral segment of the colon is displaced ventrally. A more medial tract origination site often is uncomfortable for the patient, who invariably lies supine after the procedure, compressing the external portion of the nephrostomy tube into the back. A subcostal approach is desirable to prevent the complications associated with crossing the pleura, but the position of the kidney occasionally precludes this consideration and an intercostal approach must be used. Laterally initiated tracts that pass between the peripheral tips of the

eleventh and twelfth ribs technically are intercostal, but they are associated with far fewer complications than the vertical tracts that course directly ventrally between the medial aspects of those same ribs to enter the upper-pole calices.[28] The ideal tract courses through the posterolateral flank, through the renal parenchyma, into the tip of a posterolateral calix, and continues in a direct line into the middle of the renal pelvis. The transparenchymal portion of the tract stabilizes the nephrostomy tube and provides a seal around the tube, preventing urine extravasation into the perinephric tissues. Tract creation through a caliceal tip avoids the larger blood vessels that course around the renal pelvis and infundibula. Caliceal entry also offers the greatest possible working length of the tract within the central renal collecting system, which greatly aids subsequent endourologic manipulations.

The course of the nephrostomy tract reflects the purpose of its creation. Percutaneous nephrostomy placement for simple renal drainage is effective through nearly any tract, but patient comfort factors and the possibility of permanent nephrostomy drainage require tract creation along the idealized guidelines mentioned above. If a central renal pelvic stone is to be removed endoscopically, a direct tract to the mid-renal pelvis through any middle or lower-pole calix works well. Access tracts created specifically for endourologic procedures at the ureteropelvic junction (UPJ) or within the ureter preferentially enter the collecting systems through a middle-pole or upper-pole posterior calix since these give better endoscopic access to the surgical sites of interest.[29] The removal of targeted caliceal stones is

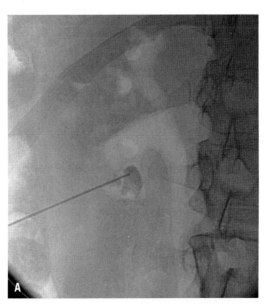
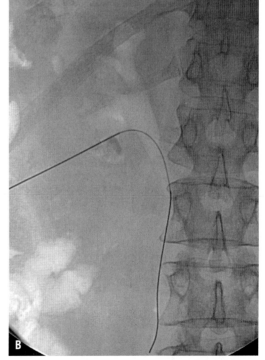

Figure 14-2 *A,* Antegrade pyelogram was done with carbon dioxide as a negative contrast material because of anaphylactic reaction to iodinated contrast media. *B,* The ESWL-resistant 1.5 cm stone was localized to the lower-pole calix, and then a guidewire was inserted across the ureteropelvic junction for tract stabilization prior to percutaneous stone removal. ESWL = extracorporeal shock wave lithotripsy.

greatly enhanced by direct access through the stone-bearing calix, and the tract must enter the calix peripheral to the stone to permit endoscopic success (Figure 14-3). Diverticular stones are best removed through a percutaneous tract that directly enters the diverticulum with a stabilizing guidewire advanced across the diverticular neck and then into the central renal collecting system.[30] Large staghorn calculi traditionally are approached through a stone-bearing middle-pole calix with subsequent advancement of the guidewire around the stone, across the UPJ, and into the ureter for tract stability (Figure 14-4). Creation of a second percutaneous tract into a stone-bearing lower- or upper-pole calix often facilitates removal of extensive stone volumes by development of multiple tracts during a single endoscopic stone removal procedure. In the past 5 years, many reports have favored creation of a single upper-pole access tract to effectively remove large branched renal stones.[31–33] This is often an intercostal tract, but the slight increase in complications from that route has been accepted to enhance stone removal efficiency.

Definitive access-tract creation is initiated by choosing the skin entry site on the posterolateral flank. In those patients in whom percutaneous nephrostomy is performed under intravenous sedation, local anesthetic medication is injected into the skin, subcutaneous tissues, the muscle, and facial layers of the body wall, and through the perinephric space to the renal capsule. The access needle is then advanced through the skin, the flank, and the renal parenchyma into the appropriate caliceal tip. The use of C-arm fluoroscopy assists in defining the three-dimensional tract. The same effect can be obtained by slight patient rotation and triangulation with fixed fluoroscopic units. If the definitive access puncture is made

under ultrasonographic guidance, real-time observation is essential to determine correct needle tip position. After the access needle tip enters the calix, the needle stylet is removed and a small amount of urine is aspirated to confirm the needle tip's intraluminal position. Small amounts of contrast material may be injected to confirm the intra-caliceal position of the needle tip if fluoroscopic guidance is used. A soft-tipped guidewire is then inserted into the needle and gently advanced beyond its tip. The wire is advanced carefully across the caliceal infundibulum and into the renal pelvis for stability. In collecting systems with dilated calices, the guidewire often curls within the punctured calix initially, requiring slight angulation on the external hub of the access needle combined with guidewire manipulations for the wire tip to leave the calix and enter into the renal pelvis. If the needle tip abuts the far wall of the punctured calix or lies within the wall of the calix, the guidewire often curls initially in the pericaliceal tissues. Tactile feedback during guidewire insertion combined with fluoroscopic guidewire tip observation is essential to avoid wire manipulations into the perinephric tissues.

Guidewire stabilization and intrarenal manipulation techniques greatly affect the subsequent success of nephrostomy tube placement and further endourologic procedures.[34] After the initial wire is advanced into the renal pelvis, much greater tract stability is achieved if the wire tip can be advanced across the UPJ and down the ureter. If that position cannot be achieved, a sufficient amount of wire can be coiled in the renal pelvis to prevent guidewire dislodgment with further catheter manipulations. After the access needle is removed from the guidewire, a variety of angiographic catheters can be inserted over the wire to achieve a more desirable final guidewire

position. The manipulations required to bypass impacted stones in the collecting system often require the use of small angled-tip catheters and hydrophilic-coated wires. Torquable guidewires with controllable tip deflection occasionally are also beneficial in performing complex intrarenal guidewire maneuvers.

Once the access tract has been created, tract dilation and endourologic procedures can follow immediately or at a later setting. Preservation of the tract with a nephrostomy tube during the inter-procedural interval provides both adequate urine drainage and tamponade of the acutely created tract. If the goal of percutaneous access creation is to provide external urinary drainage, serial fascial dilators are inserted over the working guidewire under fluoroscopic guidance, dilating the tract to a sufficient size to accept the nephrostomy tube. The insertion of a reserve guidewire into the tract is an essential component of endourologic procedures but is not needed for simple drainage tube placement. In most patients an 8 or 10F catheter is sufficient to provide temporary or long-term drainage. Locking loop catheters have attained near universal acceptance for initial external drainage applications because they are easily inserted over the working guidewire, and accidental dislodgment is rare after the retention loop is locked. For long-term nephrostomy drainage, the tract can be further dilated and standard Foley-type catheters can be inserted for drainage. Following final nephrostomy tube insertion and guidewire removal, the catheter is secured to the flank and a drainage bag attached.

SPECIAL SITUATIONS

Percutaneous access techniques must be altered for anatomic variations and subsequent endourologic procedural demands. Renal rotational

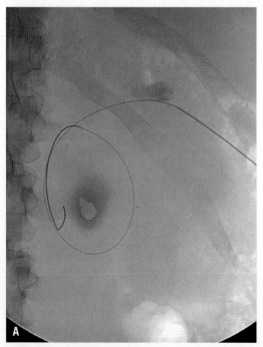
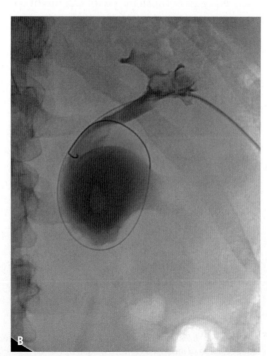
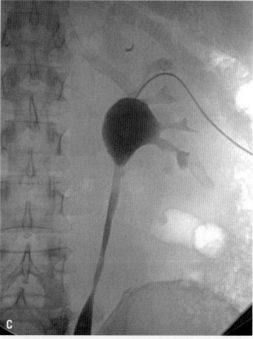

Figure 14-3 *A*, Percutaneous access tract was created by needle placement into the tip of the stone-containing upper-pole calyx. *B*, A guidewire was then inserted and coiled in the renal pelvis where a second stone was located. *C*, After the guidewire and catheter were manipulated down the ureter, the stable tract provided good endoscopic access for removal of both stones.

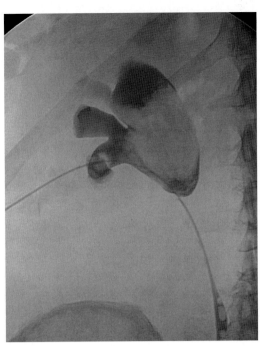

Figure 14-4 Large renal pelvic stone is completely accessible from a single nephrostomy tract, which enters through a stone-containing, lower posterior calix. To enhance tract stability for subsequent dilation and stone removal, the catheter was advanced down the ureter.

anomalies such as horseshoe kidneys position the renal parenchyma directly dorsally and the collecting system ventrally. The access tract to these kidneys is nearly perpendicular to the plane of the back, often in a paraspinous, relatively medial position. CT guidance of access tract creation in these patients may be necessary to avoid posteriorly positioned bowel loops (Figure 14-5). With the patient in the prone position, the operator must deal with the difficulties of precise needle visualization and guidewire manipulation at an unusual depth and orientation. The lack of mobility of these renal units as a result of their fixed vascular supply also requires a direct endoscopic approach for stone removal since comprehensive nephroscopy in these cases is markedly limited.

Percutaneous access to transplanted kidneys located in the usual iliac fossa position can be achieved through an extraperitoneal approach in nearly all cases. With the patient supine, the access tract is created from an external starting point medial to the anterior superior iliac crest. Ultrasonographic guidance is particularly valuable for percutaneous nephrostomy placement into these kidneys since an appropriate access calix usually can be localized ultrasonographically and directly punctured. CT guidance occasionally is needed to establish percutaneous access into a renal transplant when bowel loops lie between the anterior abdominal wall and the kidney. The full range of endourologic procedures can be performed on these transplanted renal units.[35–37]

Pelvic kidneys present a multitude of percutaneous access complexities. There are published reports of stone removal using combined transabdominal laparoscopic and transurethral retrograde access creation to pelvic kidneys.[38,39] The

risks of intraperitoneal blood and urine extravasation, vascular complications, and the technical complexity of such cases make it fortunate that these are rarely encountered situations.

Percutaneous nephrostomy placement in pediatric patients follows the same guidelines as in adults.[40–42] The primary added complexities in this setting are those of precise fluid management, temperature regulation, and the appropriate sizing of catheters and endourologic instruments. Long-term maintenance of nephrostomy access in an active child presents significant tube stabilization difficulties.

TRACT DILATION

After successful creation of a percutaneous access tract into the renal collecting systems, adequate tract dilation to accept endourologic instruments or a nephrostomy tube is the next major step for successful intervention. Techniques of access tract maintenance during surgical procedures, as well as in the postoperative period for follow-up examinations, are important determinants of overall endourologic procedure success rates.

All percutaneous access tracts can be slowly dilated with serial nephrostomy tube changes.[43] This tract dilation technique requires only that successively larger tubes be exchanged at regular intervals of weeks to months. This minimally invasive technique remains valuable in selected fragile or debilitated patients.

Prior to the development of percutaneous access techniques, nephrostomy tracts were created surgically. The initial insertion of large-caliber tubes was standard practice. With the development of Seldinger–technique-based percutaneous access tract creation, small drainage catheters were widely used. Rapid dilation of these acute tracts to accept endourologic equipment was necessary for the initial percutaneous stone removal techniques to be competitive with standard surgical pyelolithotomy. Acute dilation of nephrostomy tracts at the time of initial creation to sizes of 24 to 30F is now widely practiced and has proven to be safe and beneficial.

Acute dilation of nephrostomy tracts can be performed with a variety of instruments. The most widely used are serially introduced progressive fascial dilators, Amplatz renal dilator sets, metal coaxial dilators, and high-pressure balloon systems. These are all designed to be inserted over a working guidewire in the tract. Because of the risk of perinephric guidewire kinking with loss of the nephrostomy tract and laceration of the renal parenchyma, the utilization of all these dilator systems require fluoroscopic guidance.

Fascial dilator systems are used in a wide variety of angiographic and interventional procedures. The serially introduced catheters are commercially available in sizes from 3 to 30F, thus accommodating nearly all conceivable application requirements.[44] These sets are relatively inexpensive and easy to use. Because multiple catheter insertions are required, fluoroscopic guidance is important to prevent guidewire buckling during dilator inser-

tion (Figure 14-6). Since perinephric guidewire buckling is more common in grossly obese patients, this dilator set is not recommended for use in that group. Because these individual dilators are also somewhat flexible, this set is of limited value in dilating nephrostomy tracts that pass through dense postoperative scar tissue related to previous incisional flank surgery.[45] A theoretical disadvantage of these dilators is the generation of shearing forces by the angled dilator tips as the tract is wedged open with each larger dilator. These forces may be more likely to cause renal parenchymal tears with bleeding, but this effect has not been shown to be clinically important relative to other dilation techniques.

The Amplatz dilator set was developed to compensate for some of the deficiencies of the preexisting serial fascial dilators.[46] In the Amplatz system, an 8F angiographic catheter is initially inserted over the working guidewire. The progressively larger dilators then are inserted

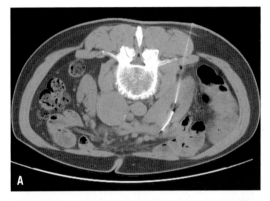

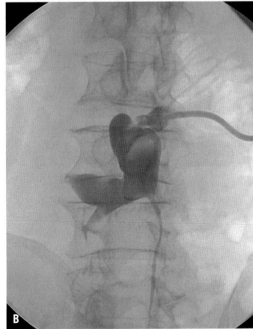

Figure 14-5 *A,* Computed tomography guidance was used to create a percutaneous nephrostomy tract into the upper-pole calix of a horseshoe kidney with a collecting system obstructed by a ureteropelvic junction stone causing pyelonephritis. *B,* Oblique fluoroscopic nephrostogram obtained 4 days later shows good drainage tube position. Percutaneous stone removal through this tract was successful.

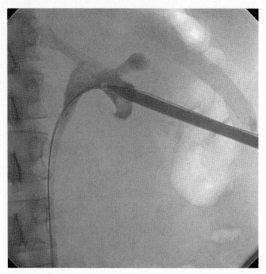

Figure 14-6 Acute tract dilation was performed by inserting a 26 French fascial dilator under fluoroscopic guidance into the lower-pole collecting system over the working guidewire. The reserve guidewire is in the same tract with the tips of both wires positioned in the bladder for tract maintenance.

serially over this guidewire and catheter combination. This additional obturator stiffness greatly reduces the risk of perinephric guidewire buckling. The individual Amplatz dilators are also relatively rigid, and in combination with the stiffer-working wire-catheter complex, they permit acute tract dilation through rigid perinephric scar tissue in nearly all patients. The commercially available equipment ranges up to size 30F. This is probably the most widely used tract dilation system because of its successful application in a broad range of patient presentations. Although there is the theoretical risk of increased renal parenchymal bleeding generated by the shearing forces of the angled catheter tips, this has not been shown to be a clinically important concern. An additional advantage of the Amplatz dilator set is the array of commercially available rigid working sheaths that can be immediately inserted over the appropriately sized dilator. These sheaths are used in many institutions to introduce various types of endourologic equipment through the acutely dilated tract.

Concentric metal dilator sets were developed by equipment manufacturers to facilitate introduction of their percutaneous nephroscopes. A central metal 8F rod is passed over the working guidewire until its leading tip is positioned within the renal pelvis. Tightly fitting metallic segments, each progressively increasing in size by about 4F, are advanced successively over the initial leader until their tips are stopped at the appropriate site within the collecting system by engineered external interlocking edges.[47] When the final dilator segment is inserted, the tract has been dilated to 24 or 26F, depending on the commercial unit used. This entire system is physically similar to extending and retracting a traditional automobile radio antenna. Because of the rigidity of this system, even the most dense perinephric scar tissue can be dilated successfully. This dilator system,

however, requires careful fluoroscopic observation since the entire rigid unit can be inserted too far, tearing the medial wall of the renal pelvis or the UPJ, or severely kinking the working guidewire. The other dilator sets have the potential for collecting-system injury, as well, but are less likely to do so because they are slightly more flexible than the metal set.

Balloon dilator technology was adapted from initial angiographic applications for use in access tract dilation (Figure 14-7). High-pressure balloons developing 15 to 30 atmospheres of pressure are available commercially, with balloon lengths up to 15 cm and diameters of 10 to 12 mm. With a single balloon inflation, the entire access tract is dilated.[48,49] Although these balloons are easy to use, generally they are more expensive than competing technologies. Balloons have been inconsistent in effectively dilating dense fascial tissue planes and retroperitoneal scar tissue, often requiring supplemental use of rigid dilators to complete the tract dilation. Balloon dilators possess the theoretical advantage of generating lateral compressive forces rather than angular shearing forces, which should reduce the risk of bleeding, although there is no clinical substantiation of this claim. Fluoroscopic monitoring of balloon inflation prevents initial balloon placement across the UPJ or other collecting system structures that would be affected adversely by balloon inflation to 30F.

Equipment used in urologic surgery for other applications has been modified by some practitioners for dilating percutaneous renal access tracts.[50–52] This equipment incises the perinephric tissues and renal parenchyma with urethrotome blades guided by passage of the urethrotome either visually along the tract of a previously placed percutaneous nephrostomy catheter or directly over a previously inserted per-

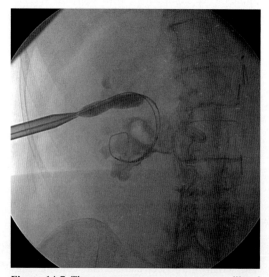

Figure 14-7 The percutaneous access tract was dilated with an inflated balloon with an Amplatz dilator/sheath back-loaded onto the balloon shaft for immediate sheath insertion. Because of postoperative distortion at the ureteropelvic junction limiting intrarenal wire manipulations, the working and reserve wires were coiled in the renal pelvis.

cutaneous access guidewire through a tip modification of the urethrotome. Deep fascial incision through the percutaneous tract with a scalpel also has been used to produce an opening adequate for subsequent large-caliber instrument placement. The disadvantage of these methods is their direct incisional nature, which is associated with an increased risk of serious renal hemorrhage from direct renal vascular laceration rather than the renal vascular compression produced by the other dilator systems.

Anesthesia requirements for nephrostomy tract dilation depend on the associated procedures performed. In many medical practices, nephrostomy tract creation, tract dilation, and endourologic surgery are performed as immediately sequential steps. General anesthesia is widely employed for this combination procedure. If tract dilation immediately follows access creation, but no subsequent intrarenal surgical manipulations are performed, intravenous sedation and analgesic administration generally are sufficient to ensure patient comfort. The dilation procedure itself usually requires less than 5 minutes, but this time may be extended in those patients with dense perinephric scar tissue that necessitates additional dilation maneuvers. The single inflation of a balloon dilation catheter is better tolerated than the serial insertion of multiple dilators if local anesthesia and intravenous sedation are used for tract dilation procedures. This advantage in patient comfort is negated by the use of general anesthesia.

Careful attention to the status of the working guidewire throughout all access tract dilation procedures is essential. A great mechanical advantage is gained if the tip of the working guidewire can be advanced across the UPJ and into the ureter. This stabilizes the kidney in the retroperitoneum and limits the amount of renal rotation produced by successive dilator insertion. The technique of routinely passing the tip of the guidewire completely down the ureter and into the urinary bladder also is helpful should small stone fragments pass into the ureter or if the need for ureteral stenting develops during subsequent endourologic maneuverings. Nearly any guidewire can be used for tract dilation, but stiff-bodied .035- or .038-inch wires are most commonly used. If a guidewire develops an acute angular kink during tract dilation maneuvers, or at any time during a subsequent endourologic procedure, immediate replacement with a fresh guidewire is recommended to prevent subsequent catheter manipulation problems.

The concept of introduction and maintenance of a second guidewire within the access tract was adopted by most early practitioners of endourologic procedures.[53] This reserve, or safety, guidewire continues to be an essential component of all tract dilation and intrarenal manipulative procedures. After the tip of the initial guidewire has been manipulated across the UPJ and into the ureter, a small vascular sheath (7 or 8F) is inserted over the guidewire into the collecting system under fluoroscopic guidance. When the obturator of this sheath is removed, a second guidewire is advanced through the sheath across the UPJ until the reserve wire tip enters the bladder. The vascular sheath is then removed and the tract dilation or endourologic procedure continues over the initial working guidewire. The reserve wire lies in the same tract as the working guidewire and subsequent instruments. Its presence is essential should the working guidewire become kinked or inadvertently dislodged. The reserve guidewire is then used with the small vascular sheath to reintroduce a fresh working guidewire, subsequently setting the reserve wire aside until it is needed again. The use of a reserve guidewire is inexpensive insurance to prevent the complete loss of an access tract during endourologic procedures.

Tract dilators advanced over the working guidewire must reach the calices to be effective, but further insertion may be harmful and should be monitored fluoroscopically. The tip of any dilator system should not be advanced across the UPJ to prevent collecting system tears.[54] The more rigid dilators can readily lacerate the medial wall of the renal pelvis if inserted haphazardly. Dilators are advanced only to the peripheral edge of large stones in the collecting systems. Caliceal or infundibular lacerations may result from utilizing large dilators adjacent to stones that are tightly adherent to the adjacent collecting system mucosa. Similarly, to avoid caliceal rupture, large dilators should not be passed beyond stones that fill calices. Serial dilators may be introduced rapidly; pausing between dilator exchanges has not resulted in any clinical differences in subsequent tract hemorrhage. If the patient's flank does not contain scar tissue, serial dilators can be introduced in 4 or 6F increments rather than in the 2F increments supplied in the commercial dilator sets. A recent report describes the insertion of a single large dilator to go from 8 to 28F without utilizing the intervening stepped dilators with good clinical success and without bleeding complications.[55]

The final size achieved during access tract dilation should correspond to the specific indication for tract creation as well as the final endourologic tool or nephrostomy tube to be inserted. For example, an access tract intended for simple renal drainage with a 10F nephrostomy tube does not need to be dilated to 30F. It is common practice to dilate tracts 2F sizes larger than the final tube to be inserted to eliminate all fascial resistance. Thus, introduction of a 24F nephrostomy tube or endoscope is readily accomplished through a tract dilated to 26F.

With the access tract successfully dilated, either endourologic equipment or a nephrostomy tube is introduced. For most endourologic procedures, a working sheath (such as an Amplatz sheath) or a rigid nephroscope is introduced into the kidney over the working guidewire. Fluoroscopic guidance is essential to confirm that the equipment is inserted through the parenchyma and into the collecting system to facilitate the best possible endoscopic visualization and optimize tract tamponade. Inadvertent over-insertion of any of these urologic instruments will likely cause laceration of a renal infundibulum or the pelvis. The choice of an appropriate nephrostomy tube to be inserted through an acute tract depends on the desired function of that tube. All nephrostomy tubes drain urine, but they also tamponade the acutely dilated structures along the course of the tract, thus reducing the risk of hemorrhage. Satisfactory percutaneous urinary drainage can be achieved through an 8 or 10F nephrostomy tube. Larger nephrostomy tubes are required following acute tract dilation to 24 to 30F. The most commonly used tubes are Foley-type urinary drainage catheters with a retention balloon near their tips. These soft tubes can be inserted over a guidewire by punching a small hole in the end of the catheter to accept the guidewire and then increasing the tube's longitudinal stiffness by inserting a central metal or plastic stiffening cannula down its center.[56] If a working sheath has been inserted, a large-caliber nephrostomy tube can be inserted through its central port prior to sheath removal. Thin-walled tear-away sheaths are commercially available in a large number of sizes to facilitate the introduction of soft, long-term nephrostomy catheters. Other widely used nephrostomy tubes include those with Malecot tips. A variation on the latter design is the reentry nephrostomy tube that adds an 8F angiographic catheter extension to the leading tip of the Malecot catheter. Designed to be inserted over the working guidewire with a central wing-collapsing stiffener, this catheter provides external urinary drainage with the Malecot tip in the renal pelvis while its catheter tip extends across the UPJ, maintaining access into the ureter.[57] In addition, many other nephrostomy tubes are available from commercial manufacturers with subtle design features developed by creative physicians to meet the needs of their individual practice situations.

After insertion through the flank, the nephrostomy tube is properly positioned under fluoroscopic guidance and secured to the flank. If further endourologic manipulations are planned within a couple of days, the reserve guidewire can also be secured in place. Alternatively, a small angiographic catheter can be inserted over the reserve wire with the catheter tip positioned in the mid- to low ureter and the reserve guidewire discarded. This facilitates reentry into the renal collecting system should the primary nephrostomy drainage tube be dislodged and also preserves access across the UPJ to the ureter should subsequent manipulations in those regions be needed. If long-term external drainage is desired without the need for ureteral access, the reserve wire can be removed after the nephrostomy tube is well positioned. The removal of the reserve wire and the abandonment of the inherent safety its presence provides is always the final decision made during nephrostomy tube insertion or at the end of an endourologic procedure.

TRACT MAINTENANCE

A properly positioned nephrostomy tube will provide adequate urine drainage unless it becomes displaced or obstructed. Prior to the introduction of self-locking loop nephrostomy tubes, spontaneous dislodgment of nephrostomy tubes inserted in an acute setting was reported in up to 15% of patients. The self-retaining design has reduced this complication to a rarity. Nevertheless, a tube of any design occasionally will be pulled out of its intended site accidentally and will cease functioning. Multiple complex external fixation devices have been designed to limit inadvertent nephrostomy tube displacement, but simple suture fixation to the skin is usually reliable. In chronic nephrostomy drainage settings, reinsertion of displaced tubes is usually a simple matter involving recannulation of the original tract and insertion of a fresh tube. This may require fluoroscopically guided manipulation of catheters and guidewires. Displacement of a small nephrostomy tube out of an access tract that is less than a week old often requires creation of a new acute tract since epithelialization of the original tract usually has not yet occurred. If recannulation is attempted within a short time period after actual tube dislodgment, the larger tracts used for endourologic access can usually be reestablished within 48 hours after their creation.

Obstruction of a properly positioned nephrostomy tube soon after initial tract creation most frequently is due to blood clot formation within the central renal collecting system. Because of the presence of urokinase, these clots readily lyse and pass through drainage catheters within 24 to 48 hours. Nephrostomy irrigation may help disrupt small blood clots but seldom is effective at completely clearing all clots from the collecting systems. This clot-induced tube obstruction is more common after initial tube insertion in patients with profound uremia or long-standing collecting system obstruction, and frequently extends the period prior to complete renal functional recovery.

Long-term nephrostomy drainage requires regular nephrostomy tube exchanges despite ongoing attempts to develop encrustation-resistant materials for nephrostomy tubes. Elective nephrostomy exchange prior to occlusion prevents bouts of clinical urosepsis related to the combination of tube obstruction and the presence of urinary bacterial colonization from the indwelling nephrostomy tube. In most patients, tube exchanges every 3 months are adequate, but some patients can tolerate 6-month intervals prior to tube occlusion. In metabolically active stone-forming patients and in pregnant women, the deposition of calculus material along the nephrostomy lumen may take only 4 to 6 weeks to cause tube occlusion between exchanges.

The technique of nephrostomy tube exchange is uncomplicated. For those nephrostomy tubes designed to be inserted over a guidewire, the old tube is exchanged for a fresh tube under fluoroscopic guidance over a guidewire. Large-caliber drainage tubes such as Foley catheters can be reinserted in well-epithelialized chronic tracts with minimal patient inconvenience or equipment requirements. Pre-procedural administration of antibiotics for a scheduled nephrostomy tube change limits the clinical impact of procedure-related bacteremia. Chronic administration of antibiotics in patients with nephrostomy tubes does not result in urine sterilization because of persistent bacterial colonization of the tube itself, but instead, frequently facilitates the growth of antibiotic-resistant bacteria and yeast infections that are clinically much more significant.

RESULTS

Percutaneous nephrostomy placement is successful in over 97% of patients in large series. Adequate urinary drainage can be achieved in nearly all patients, with occasional access failures in those patients requiring precise percutaneous access tracts for subsequent endourologic interventions. The primary causes of access attempt failures are: (1) the presence of nondistended renal collecting systems, (2) small obstructing infundibular stones with minimal caliceal dilation peripherally, (3) impacted large stones that prevent guidewire manipulations, and (4) obscuring of the precise location of the collecting systems by blood clot formation after initial needle insertion. In rare cases, percutaneous nephrostomy placement cannot be performed safely because of intra-abdominal anatomic variations such a postrenal positioning of the colon, marked splenomegaly with ventral displacement of the left kidney, or anomalous renal location.

COMPLICATIONS

Percutaneous access creation is a minor surgical procedure that is usually well tolerated. The major complications of percutaneous nephrostomy placement manifest as hemorrhage. All patients have initial hematuria following percutaneous nephrostomy placement, but this clears in 24 to 48 hours. Massive retroperitoneal hemorrhage is rare. Small subcapsular renal hematomas develop in less than 3% of patients, predominantly in those with long-standing collecting system obstruction. These collections usually have no clinical sequelae and resolve spontaneously.[58] Bleeding from iatrogenic arteriovenous-caliceal fistulas occurs in less than 1% of patients in large percutaneous nephrostomy series and is best managed by angiographic delineation and transcatheter embolization.

The other complications of percutaneous nephrostomy placement mirror those of percutaneous stone removal and are discussed in a later chapter (see Chapter 20, "Complications of Stone Removal"). Post-procedural complications are best imaged with CT and a nephrostogram. Small collecting system perforations heal quickly with adequate urinary drainage. Clinical sepsis results from percutaneous nephrostomy placement in patients with infected urine. Antibiotic administration before the procedure may lessen the severity of the clinical impact of bacteremia in this patient group, but it does not prevent sepsis completely. Prompt establishment of external urinary drainage with minimal intrarenal catheter manipulation reduces septic complications in this patient group.

It is difficult to separate the complications of acute tract dilation from those of nephrostomy tract creation or those of subsequent endourologic procedures through the nephrostomy tract.[59,60] Failure to adequately dilate a percutaneous renal access tract is nearly always the fault of the operator rather than the technique. In rare cases, marked perinephric scar tissue related to previous operation or infection may cause sufficient difficulty in the application of tract dilation equipment that the risk of renal parenchymal laceration or major collecting system disruption may preclude further dilation attempts. Even in those cases, a second attempt at tract dilation is nearly always successful following interval nephrostomy drainage. Other causes for rare failures nearly always are related to faulty technique, such as failure to insert a reserve guidewire, coupled with inadvertent dislodgment, or kinking of the working guidewire.

The other primary complications of tract dilation are loss of the acute percutaneous tract or major perforation of the renal collecting systems by the dilating equipment. Both of these are operator-related failures. Tract loss is caused by inadvertent dislodgment of the working guidewire combined with failure to insert a reserve wire. Collecting system lacerations result from vigorous dilator insertion without fluoroscopic monitoring, resulting in dilators disrupting the wall of the renal pelvis, the UPJ, or the upper ureter. Although these lacerations seldom require surgical repair, any planned intrarenal endourologic procedures must be delayed for 2 to 7 days to allow complete collecting system healing prior to further intervention.

CONCLUSION

Establishment of percutaneous renal access is a safe and reliable procedure. Accurate tract creation is an essential component of successful endourologic procedures. Precise access needle insertion followed by guidewire manipulations provides a stable tract for nephrostomy tube insertion, tract dilation, or complex nephroscopic interventions. Access-creation failures are rare and the complication rate is low.

Acute dilation of percutaneous renal access tracts is an important component of current endourologic techniques. These techniques are safe, simply accomplished in most patients, and provide properly sized tracts for acute or chronic percutaneous renal collecting system access. Careful attention to technique during dilator and guidewire manipulations produces good results with few complications. A properly created and well-maintained nephrostomy tract provides ready access to the renal collecting systems for a broad range of endourologic procedures.

REFERENCES

1. Goodwin W, Casey W, Woolf W. Percutaneous trocar (needle) nephrostomy in hydronephrosis. JAMA 1955;157:891–4.
2. Almgard LE, Fernstrom I. Percutaneous nephropyelostomy. Acta Radiol Diagn 1974;15:288–94.
3. Stables DP, Ginsberg NJ, Johnson ML. Percutaneous nephrostomy: a series and review of the literature. AJR Am J Roentgenol 1978;130:75–82.
4. Banner MP, Ramchandani P, Pollack HM. Interventional procedures in the upper urinary tract. Cardiovasc Intervent Radiol 1991;14:267–84.
5. Emmert C, Rassler J, Kohler U. Survival and quality of life after percutaneous nephrostomy for malignant ureteric obstruction in patients with terminal cervical cancer. Arch Gynecol Obstet 1997;259:147–51.
6. LeRoy AJ. Diagnosis and treatment of nephrolithiasis: current perspectives. [Comment]. AJR Am J Roentgenol 1994;163:1309–13.
7. Boon JM, Shinners B, Meiring JH. Variations of the position of the colon as applied to percutaneous nephrostomy. Surg Radiol Anat 2001;23:421–5.
8. Ramchandani P, Cardella JF, Grassi CJ, et al. Quality improvement guidelines for percutaneous nephrostomy. J Vasc Interv Radiol 2003;14:277–81.
9. Sandhu C, Anson KM, Patel U. Urinary tract stones—part II: current status of treatment. Clin Radiol 2003;58:422–33.
10. vanSonnenberg E, Casola G, Talner LB, et al. Symptomatic renal obstruction or urosepsis during pregnancy: treatment by sonographically guided percutaneous nephrostomy. Am J Roentgenol 1992;158:91–4.
11. Matlaga BR, Shah OD, Zagoria RJ, et al. Computerized tomography guided access for percutaneous nephrostolithotomy. J Urol 2003;170:45–7.
12. LeMaitre L, Mestdagh P, Marecaux-Delomez J, et al. Percutaneous nephrostomy: placement under laser guidance and real-time CT fluoroscopy. Eur Radiol 2000;10:892–5.
13. Titton RL, Gervais DA, Hahn PF, et al. Urine leaks and urinomas: diagnosis and imaging-guided intervention. Radiographics 2003;23:1113–47.
14. Hagspiel KD, Kandarpa K, Silverman SG. Interactive MR-guided percutaneous nephrostomy. J Magn Reson Imaging 1998;8:1319–22.
15. Cadeddu JA, Stoianovici D, Chen RN, et al. Stereotactic mechanical percutaneous renal access. J Endourol 1998;12:121–5.
16. Su LM, Stoianovici D, Jarrett TW, et al. Robotic percutaneous access to the kidney: comparison with standard manual access. J Endourol 2002;16:471–5.
17. Bilen CY, Asci R, Sarikaya S, et al. Laser-assisted fluoroscopic puncture: a new technique for accessing the kidney. J Endourol 2003;17:485–91.
18. Barbaric ZL, Hall T, Cochran ST, et al. Percutaneous nephrostomy: placement under CT and fluoroscopy guidance. Am J Roentgenol 1997;169:151–5.
19. Newhouse JH, Pfister RC. Percutaneous catheterization of the kidney and perinephric space: trocar technique. Urol Radiol 1981;2:157–64.
20. Soltes GD, Rainwater JR, Middlebrook MR, et al. Interventional uroradiology. World J Urol 1998;16:52–61.
21. Dyer RB, Regan JD, Kavanagh PV, et al. Percutaneous nephrostomy with extensions of the technique: step by step. Radiographics 2002;22:503–25.
22. Cope C. Conversion from small (0.018 inch) to large (0.038 inch) guide wires in percutaneous drainage procedures. Am J Roentgenol 1982;138:170–1.
23. LeRoy AJ, May GR, Bender CE, et al. Percutaneous nephrostomy for stone removal. Radiology 1984;151:607–12.
24. Shoma AM, Eraky I, El-Kenawy MR, El-Kappany HA. Percutaneous nephrolithotomy in the supine position: technical aspects and functional outcome compared with the prone technique. Urology 2002;60:388–92.
25. Sampaio F, Mandarim-de-Lacerda C. Three dimensional and radiological pelviocaliceal anatomy for endourology. J Urol 1988;140:1352–5.
26. Beckmann CF, Roth RA. Use of retrograde occlusion balloon catheters in percutaneous removal of renal calculi. Urology 1985;25:277–83.
27. Salomonowitz E, Castaneda-Zuniga WR, Lange PH, et al. Percutaneous renal stone removal. Use of carbon dioxide as contrast material. Radiology 1984;150:833–4.
28. Picus D, Weyman PJ, Clayman RV, McClennan BL. Intercostal-space nephrostomy for percutaneous stone removal. Am J of Roentgenol 1986;147:393–7.

29. Lee WJ, Badlani GH, Smith AD. Percutaneous nephrostomy for endopyelotomy. Am J Roentgenol 1987;148:189–92.

30. Auge BK, Munver R, Kourambas J, et al. Endoscopic management of symptomatic caliceal diverticula: a retrospective comparison of percutaneous nephrolithotripsy and ureteroscopy. J Endourol 2002;16:557–63.

31. Munver R, Delvecchio FC, Newman GE, Preminger GM. Critical analysis of supracostal access for percutaneous renal surgery. J Urol 2001;166:1242–6.

32. Radecka E, Brehmer M, Holmgren K, Magnusson A. Complications associated with percutaneous nephrolithotripsy: supra- versus subcostal access. A retrospective study. Acta Radiol 2003;44:447–51.

33. Kim SC, Kuo RL, Lingeman JE. Percutaneous nephrolithotomy: an update. Curr Opin Urol 2003;13:235–41.

34. Farrell TA, Hicks ME. A review of radiologically guided percutaneous nephrostomies in 303 patients. J Vasc Interv Radiol 1997;8:769–74.

35. Bosma RJ, van Driel MF, van Son WJ, et al. Endourological management of ureteral obstruction after renal transplantation. J Urol 1996;156:1099–100.

36. Fontaine AB, Nijjar A, Rangaraj R. Update on the use of percutaneous nephrostomy/balloon dilation for the treatment of renal transplant leak/obstruction. J Vasc Interv Radiol 1997;8:649–53.

37. Berger PM, Diamond JR. Ureteral obstruction as a complication of renal transplantation: a review. J Nephrol 1998;11:20–3.

38. Zafar FS, Lingeman JE. Value of laparoscopy in the management of calculi complicating renal malformations. J Endourol 1996;10:379–83.

39. Lee CK, Smith AD. Percutaneous transperitoneal approach to the pelvic kidney for endourologic removal of calculus: three cases with two successes. J Endourol 1992;6:133–5.

40. Jackman SV, Hedican SP, Peters CA, Docimo SG. Percutaneous nephrolithotomy in infants and preschool age children: experience with a new technique. Urology 1998;52:697–701.

41. Laurin S, Sandstrom S, Ivarsson H. Percutaneous nephrostomy in infants and children. Acad Radiol 2000;7:526–9.

42. Koral K, Saker MC, Morello FP, et al. Conventional versus modified technique for percutaneous nephrostomy in newborns and young infants. J Vasc Interv Radiol 2003;14:113–6.

43. Mazzeo VP Jr, Pollack HM, Banner MP. A technique for percutaneous dilatation of nephrostomy tracks. Radiology 1982;144:175–6.

44. LeRoy AJ, May GR, Segura JW, et al. Rapid dilatation of percutaneous nephrostomy tracks. Am J Roentgenol 1984;142:355–7.

45. Lynch W, Doust B, Golovsky D. Percutaneous dilatation of difficult nephrostomy tracts. Br J Urol 1992;70:455–6.

46. Rusnak B, Castaneda-Zuniga W, Kotula F, et al. An improved dilator system for percutaneous nephrostomies. Radiology 1982;144:174.

47. Alken P. The telescope dilators. World J Urol 1985;3:7–10.

48. Clayman RV, Castaneda-Zuniga WR, Hunter DW, et al. Rapid balloon dilatation of the nephrostomy track for nephrostolithotomy. Radiology 1983;147:884–5.

49. Won JH, Eshghi M. The use of one-step balloon and Amplatz sheath for dilation of the nephrostomy tract. J Endourol 1998;12(Suppl 1):115.

50. Davis BE, Noble MJ, Mebust WK. Use of the Collings knife electrode for percutaneous access in difficult endourology cases. J Urol 1991;145:257–62.

51. Morsy A, el Gammal M, Abdel-Razzak OM. Modified technique for dilatation of difficult nephrostomy tracts. Tech Urol 1998;4:148–51.

52. Goharderakhshan RZ, Schwartz BF, Rudnick DM, et al. Radially expanding single-step nephrostomy tract dilator. Urology 2001;58:693–6.

53. Dawson S, Papanicolaou N, Mueller PR, Ferrucci JT Jr. Preserving access during percutaneous catheterization using a double-guide-wire technique. Am J Roentgenol 1983;141:407.

54. Netto N, Lemos G, Fiuza J. Percutaneous nephrolithotomy in patients with previous renal surgery. Eur Urol 1988;14:353–5.

55. Frattini A, Barbieri A, Salsi P, et al. One shot: a novel method to dilate the nephrostomy access for percutaneous lithotripsy. J Endourol 2001;15:919–23.

56. Burkhalter JL, Morano JU. An alternative method for insertion of large nephrostomy catheters following percutaneous nephrolithotomy. J Urol 1986;135:14.

57. Khasidy LR, Smith AD. The re-entry nephrostomy catheter for endourological applications. J Urol 1985;133:165–6.

58. Lee WJ, Smith AD, Cubelli V, et al. Complications of percutaneous nephrolithotomy. Am Jo Roentgenol 1987;148:177–80.

59. Davidoff R, Bellman GC. Influence of technique of percutaneous tract creation on incidence of renal hemorrhage. [Comment]. J Urol 1997;157:1229–31.

60. Soble JJ, Streem SB. Prospective randomized comparison of percutaneous nephrostomy tract dilation techniques. J Endourol 1998;12(Suppl 1):115.

15

Retrograde Access

Denis H. Hosking, MB, ChB, FRCSC

Following the description in 1976 by Fernstrom and Johansson[1] of the removal of a renal calculus through a percutaneous nephrostomy tract, percutaneous nephrolithotomy virtually replaced open surgery in the management of renal calculi. One of the most technically demanding aspects of percutaneous nephrolithotomy is the establishment of a nephrostomy tract into an appropriate calix, often in an undilated collecting system.[2,3] Obese patients, patients who have undergone previous renal surgery, and patients with horseshoe kidneys may be particularly challenging. In addition, in patients with large or impacted calculi it may be difficult to pass a guidewire beyond the calculus down the ureter once the collecting system has been punctured. Under these circumstances, dilation of the nephrostomy tract is difficult and is associated with the risk of displacement of the guidewire. Before the introduction of extracorporeal shock wave lithotripsy (ESWL), almost all calculi were treated by percutaneous techniques, providing adequate opportunity for both urologists and radiologists to acquire and maintain the necessary skills for establishing a nephrostomy tract. With the advent of ESWL, fewer stones require percutaneous removal, and stones requiring percutaneous removal often represent a greater technical challenge in terms of nephrostomy placement than the typical stone formerly removed by percutaneous methods.

Retrograde techniques for establishing a percutaneous nephrostomy tract were first described in 1983.[4,5] These techniques of retrograde access are possibly a simpler method of establishing a percutaneous nephrostomy tract for those who do not have expertise in establishing a nephrostomy tract using conventional antegrade methods.

INDICATIONS

Retrograde access is indicated when a nephrostomy tract must be established in the absence of ureteric obstruction. It is therefore indicated in almost all patients undergoing percutaneous removal of renal calculi and is particularly useful in patients with undilated collecting systems and in those patients with large calculi occupying most of the collecting system.[6] Retrograde access can also be used in patients undergoing percutaneous endopyelotomy or other endourologic procedures such as percutaneous resection of superficial tumors of the renal pelvis and collecting system.

Retrograde access is not appropriate for the relief of renal obstruction as an emergency procedure, particularly in the presence of sepsis. Retrograde techniques are contraindicated in any patient with an abnormality of the lower urinary tract that prevents ureteric catheterization. The size of the catheters used for ureteric instrumentation makes retrograde access an unsuitable technique for use in children. Previous urinary diversion is a relative contraindication since it may be difficult to gain access to the ureter.

PATIENT PREPARATION

Several authors recommend that a preoperative intravenous pyelogram (IVP) should be obtained in all patients undergoing retrograde nephrostomy.[7–10] A pre-operative IVP may be helpful in determining that a calculus is in an unsuspected calyceal diverticulum, or identifying associated abnormalities such as ureteropelvic junction obstruction and horseshoe kidneys. Alternatively, in patients allergic to intravenous contrast agents, retrograde pyelography may be helpful in determining in advance the most appropriate calix or calices for nephrostomy placement and to rule out ureteric obstruction that might make retrograde access difficult or impossible. In obese patients, it may be difficult to visualize the calculus fluoroscopically at the time of surgery, making it helpful to determine the appropriate site for nephrostomy placement in advance of the procedure.

In patients with horseshoe kidneys and in patients with a dysmorphic body habitus, it is advisable to obtain a preoperative CT scan to determine the relationship of the kidney to other intra-abdominal organs. A preoperative ultrasound or CT scan may also be helpful for the same reason in patients in whom an upper caliceal nephrostomy tract is planned.[8] In my experience, a preoperative CT scan has not been necessary in patients with a normal body habitus and normal kidneys, irrespective of the calix used for nephrostomy placement.

Consent for retrograde nephrostomy is usually given in conjunction with consent for a procedure such as percutaneous nephrolithotomy. All patients should be advised of the risk of injury to other organs, in particular to the bowel.[11] Serious bleeding as a result of the creation of the nephrostomy tract is unlikely, but bleeding requiring transfusion is certainly possible following tract dilation and percutaneous nephrolithotomy.[12–14] Although failure to establish a nephrostomy tract is uncommon, obese patients, patients who have undergone previous open surgery involving the affected kidney, and patients with horseshoe kidneys should be advised that the creation of a suitable nephrostomy tract may not be possible.

PREOPERATIVE PREPARATION

Patients are prepared preoperatively primarily for the procedure performed in conjunction with retrograde nephrostomy. Bleeding disorders should be ruled out or corrected, and active urinary tract infections should be treated. Patients with infected renal calculi should receive preoperative antibiotics based on the sensitivities of the associated organisms. Prophylactic antibiotics are recommended in patients with sterile urine preoperatively.[8,9,15] Unless there is a history of allergy to penicillin or cephalosporins, cefazolin is a suitable choice.[15]

INSTRUMENTATION AND TECHNIQUES

Two basic techniques for performing retrograde nephrostomy were described initially, one by Lawson and colleagues[4] and the other by Hunter and colleagues.[5] Other authors have since reported modifications of the original techniques.[6,7,9,16,17] Over time, the Lawson technique has proven to be the more popular of the two, and most of the equipment required for this technique is available in kit form (Cook Urological, Spencer, IN). All procedures are performed under fluoroscopic control and usually under general anesthesia immediately prior to percutaneous nephrolithotomy. Some authors have reported that local anesthesia coupled with intravenous sedation is satisfactory.[5,7,8] The patient is in the lithotomy position with the ipsilateral hemipelvis and scapula elevated using appropriate supports (Figure 15-1). This elevates the area of the flank where the puncture wire will subsequently emerge, and also allows the bowel to fall away from the site of the proposed nephrostomy. An erasable mark on the skin just below the twelfth rib in the posterior axillary line allows rapid determination of the suitability of the site where the puncture wire will subsequently emerge. This mark makes it easy to determine whether the nephrostomy tract is excessively anterior or whether a supracostal course has been taken.

THE LAWSON TECHNIQUE The Lawson technique[4] and its modifications have been the subject of several reports.[9,10,16–18] The kit used for

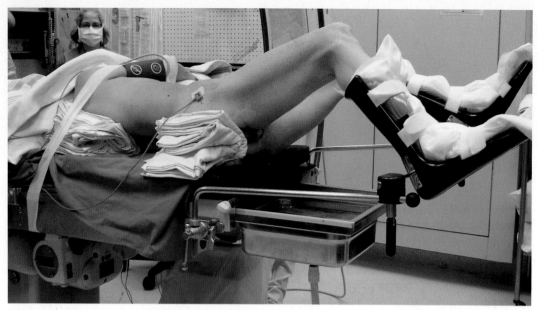

Figure 15-1 Patient positioning for right-sided retrograde nephrostomy.

this procedure (the Lawson-I Kit, 087000, Cook Urological) contains the following items:

- Floppy-tipped 145 cm 0.038-inch guidewire
- 85 cm 7 French polyethylene (Torcon) catheter
- 0.045-inch deflecting guidewire with three-ring handle
- 0.017-inch puncture wire and 3F Teflon puncture wire sheath
- Mitty-Pollack needle (22-gauge inner, 18-gauge outer needle)

In addition, the following items are needed:

- Cystoscopy equipment
- Radiographic contrast material
- Scalpel blade
- Two to three forceps
- 0.038-inch torque guidewire
- Fascia incising needle (optional)

After the patient is positioned, cystoscopy is carried out under sterile conditions. A floppy-tipped 0.038-inch guidewire (supplied) is passed up the ureter into the renal pelvis under fluoroscopic control (Figure 15-2). The 7F polyethylene catheter (supplied) is passed up the ureter over the guidewire and the guidewire is removed. Contrast material is then injected, opacifying the collecting system (Figure 15-3). If an impacted calculus or ureteric tortuosity prevents the passage of the guidewire or Teflon catheter, it may be possible to bypass the obstruction with a J-tipped wire or hydrophilic coated wire passed through the 7F catheter. A J-tipped wire or floppy-tipped hydrophilic coated wire is preferred since it is less likely to perforate the ureter or collecting system while attempts are made to negotiate it past the obstruction. In some cases, slight distention of the collecting system by contrast material may facilitate passage of the wire past an obstruction.

Once the collecting system has been opacified, the most appropriate calix for nephrostomy

placement is selected. The ideal calix allows the easiest access to the renal calculi, but in the case of retrograde nephrostomy, it also needs to allow the creation of the shortest, most horizontal nephrostomy tract possible. For this reason, in some patients lower-pole calices may not be suitable for retrograde nephrostomy placement. This is particularly important in obese patients in whom an excessively long nephrostomy tract may be created if the tract is not made as horizontal as possible. Therefore, in some patients, although the

lower calix might offer easier access to the stone, a middle or upper calix must be selected.

Although the nephrostomy tract tends to be shorter when a posterior calix is used, many authors agree that selection of a posterior calix is not essential.[8–10,18] A review of a study on caliceal anatomy by Kaye and Reinke reveals that the most lateral calices when viewed on an IVP will still usually be directed posterior to the midaxillary line because of the posterior rotation of the kidney.[19] Three reports on retrograde nephrostomy indicate that as long as the puncture wire exits posterior to the midaxillary line, tract dilation is no more difficult or dangerous to neighboring viscera.[9,10,18] Hunter and colleagues observed that whether originating from a posterior or anterior calix their retrograde nephrostomy technique appeared to provide a nephrostomy tract with a posterior pathway from the posterior fornix of a calix to the flank and allowed the nephrostomy tract to miss viscera.[8] My own observations based on over 1,500 retrograde nephrostomies over the past 18 years support those of Hunter and colleagues.

The 0.045-inch diameter deflecting wire is passed up the 7F polyethylene catheter and twist-locked to the base of the catheter. While an assistant steadies the cystoscope, the tip of the 7F catheter is deflected with the deflecting wire, and by advancing the catheter/wire combination it is usually possible to position the catheter in any pre-selected calix (Figure 15-4). In the case of staghorn or large branched renal calculi, it may not be possible to advance the catheter and deflecting wire into the desired calix. Passage of a J-tipped or

Figure 15-2 A guidewire is passed up the ureter into the renal pelvis under fluoroscopic control. From Hosking DH.[16]

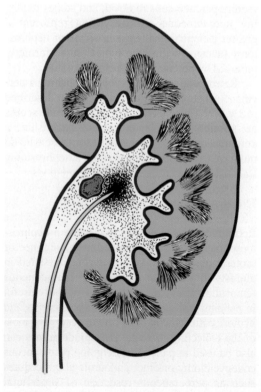

Figure 15-3 Contrast material is injected into the collecting system through the 7F polyethylene catheter. From Hosking DH.[16]

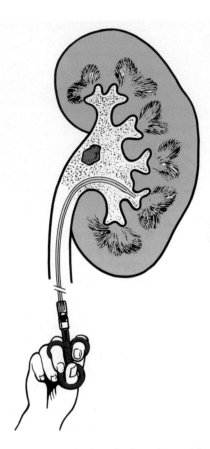

Figure 15-4 A deflecting wire is used to position the 7F catheter in a pre-selected calix. From Hosking DH.[16]

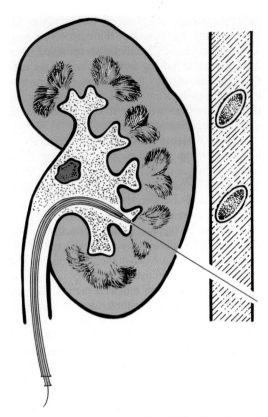

Figure 15-5 The puncture wire and sheath are inserted into the 7F catheter. The puncture wire is then advanced through the kidney, perinephric fat, and abdominal wall. From Hosking DH.[16]

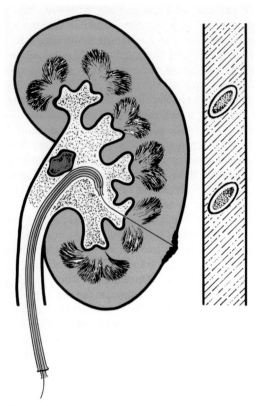

Figure 15-6 The Lawson puncture wire may not pass through perinephric scar tissue. Attempts to advance it under these circumstances will displace the 7F catheter from the calix. From Hosking DH.[16]

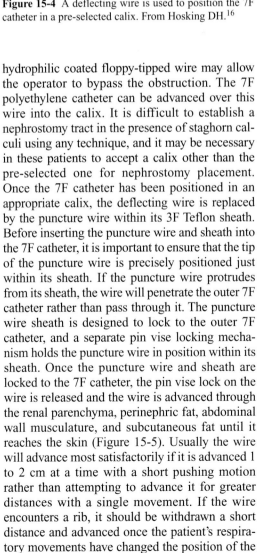

hydrophilic coated floppy-tipped wire may allow the operator to bypass the obstruction. The 7F polyethylene catheter can be advanced over this wire into the calix. It is difficult to establish a nephrostomy tract in the presence of staghorn calculi using any technique, and it may be necessary in these patients to accept a calix other than the pre-selected one for nephrostomy placement. Once the 7F catheter has been positioned in an appropriate calix, the deflecting wire is replaced by the puncture wire within its 3F Teflon sheath. Before inserting the puncture wire and sheath into the 7F catheter, it is important to ensure that the tip of the puncture wire is precisely positioned just within its sheath. If the puncture wire protrudes from its sheath, the wire will penetrate the outer 7F catheter rather than pass through it. The puncture wire sheath is designed to lock to the outer 7F catheter, and a separate pin vise locking mechanism holds the puncture wire in position within its sheath. Once the puncture wire and sheath are locked to the 7F catheter, the pin vise lock on the wire is released and the wire is advanced through the renal parenchyma, perinephric fat, abdominal wall musculature, and subcutaneous fat until it reaches the skin (Figure 15-5). Usually the wire will advance most satisfactorily if it is advanced 1 to 2 cm at a time with a short pushing motion rather than attempting to advance it for greater distances with a single movement. If the wire encounters a rib, it should be withdrawn a short distance and advanced once the patient's respiratory movements have changed the position of the

wire relative to the rib. I have found it helpful to request that the patient be kept in full expiration for a few seconds, which usually allows the wire to be passed just above the obstructing rib. Caution should be used in having the patient kept in full inspiration during passage of the puncture wire. Although this maneuver will almost certainly allow passage of the puncture wire below the rib, an excessively long nephrostomy tract may be created. In patients who have undergone previous surgery on the involved kidney, perinephric scar tissue may obstruct the progress of the puncture wire, causing the 7F catheter to be displaced from its calix (Figure 15-6). Occasionally it may be possible to overcome this problem by advancing the 7F catheter and embedding it in the renal parenchyma to provide additional support for the advancing puncture wire.

Once the puncture wire reaches the skin, it usually "tents" the skin rather than penetrates it (Figure 15-7). At this stage, if a mark has been placed on the skin previously, it can be used to determine whether the course of the wire is excessively anterior or cranial. If the wire emerges anterior to the midaxillary line, it should be withdrawn and a different calix selected for nephrostomy placement. After preparing the skin over the wire, a 3 to 4 mm incision is made to allow the wire to emerge. Different techniques have been described at this stage for the further development and dilation of the nephrostomy tract.

Spirnak and Resnick advance the puncture wire until 60 cm of wire exits from the flank.[18]

The puncture wire sheath is removed, and after cutting off the hub of the 7F polyethylene catheter, the cystoscope is removed. The 7F catheter is partially withdrawn down the ureter and the distal end is fixed to a Foley catheter. The patient is rotated into the prone position and the puncture wire is used as the guidewire for initial dilation of the nephrostomy tract.

Morrisseau and Trotter advance the puncture wire approximately 16 inches beyond the skin and commence tract dilation with the 18-gauge Mitty-Pollack needle supplied with the nephrostomy kit.[17] The Mitty-Pollack needle is then removed and a 6F dilator is passed over the puncture wire down the ureter until it hits the Lawson

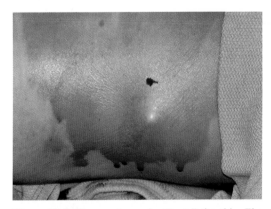

Figure 15-7 The puncture wire "tents" the skin. The black mark represents the posterior axillary line just below the twelfth rib.

7F catheter, which is partially withdrawn down the ureter. The puncture wire and 7F catheter are now removed and a 0.038-inch working safety wire is advanced through the 6F dilator down the ureter and curled in the bladder. A problem with the technique of Morrisseau and Trotter is that there is loss of control on one end of the nephrostomy wire, which might theoretically allow displacement of the wire during difficult dilation of the nephrostomy tract. This problem can be overcome by placing a forceps on the puncture wire to prevent it from accidentally being withdrawn, and under fluoroscopic control the 7F polyethylene catheter is advanced over the puncture wire and its sheath and through the renal parenchyma to the abdominal wall (Figure 15-8). It is important not to apply traction on the puncture wire during this maneuver or a severe laceration of the kidney could occur. Once the 7F catheter reaches the abdominal wall, traction on the puncture wire may pull the catheter through the abdominal wall. Frequently, however, traction on the puncture wire causes the 7F catheter to buckle at the level of the lumbar fascia. For this reason, I prefer to enlarge the defect in the lumbar fascia first with a fascial incising needle (No. 090070, Cook Urological). This simple instrument consists of an 18-gauge needle fixed to a small, blunt, diamond-shaped blade (Figure 15-9) that is passed over the puncture wire under fluoroscopic control through the abdominal wall until it reaches the tip of the 7F catheter. It is then withdrawn while gentle traction is placed on the puncture wire, thus advancing the catheter to the skin. The puncture wire and sheath are then withdrawn and a 0.038-

inch guidewire is advanced through the 7F catheter until it emerges at the cystoscope end. The cystoscope and 7F catheter are removed, leaving a guidewire passing from the flank to the urethral meatus, thereby establishing the nephrostomy tract. Clamps are placed on the guidewire at the urethral end to prevent it from being displaced during subsequent tract dilation.[16]

Obese Patients It is difficult to establish a nephrostomy tract in obese patients irrespective of the technique used. It is essential to create as horizontal a nephrostomy tract as possible, which usually dictates that a middle calix be used if at all possible. If a lower caliceal nephrostomy has to be created, a major concern is that the resulting nephrostomy tract will be excessively long. There are two maneuvers that may be helpful in these circumstances.

The first maneuver relies on the fact that the abdominal wall can alter the course of the puncture wire. The puncture wire is advanced to the abdominal wall while the patient is held in full expiration, keeping the kidney as high as possible. Once the abdominal wall musculature is penetrated by the puncture wire, respiration is resumed. As the kidney descends, there will be a tendency for the puncture wire traversing the abdominal wall musculature to adopt a more horizontal course, shortening the resulting nephrostomy tract. The second maneuver relies on an assistant indenting the fat just below the anticipated site of the emerging puncture wire. Once the puncture wire reaches the skin, the fat is released, carrying the puncture wire cranially, resulting in a shorter, more horizontal tract. In some excessively obese patients, the puncture wire can be advanced through the abdominal wall musculature, but the wire is not rigid enough to be advanced all the way to the skin. In these patients it may be possible to grasp the puncture wire in the subcutaneous fat under fluoroscopic control with a small forceps passed through a small skin incision.

Supracostal Nephrostomies It is not unusual for the puncture wire to emerge above the twelfth rib, and even above the eleventh rib, particularly when a middle or upper calix is used for the nephrostomy tract. Although supracostal nephrostomies have been associated with more postoperative pain than subcostal nephrostomies,[20,21] the risk of other significant complications is low.[22–25] Of the first 206 retrograde nephrostomies performed in our institution, 63 were supracostal. Pneumothorax was not identified in any of these patients.[26] Using antegrade techniques, Munver and colleagues reported no pneumothoraces in 72 patients undergoing supra-twelfth rib nephrostomy placement, but hemo- or pneumothorax was identified in 6 of 26 patients (23%) who underwent supra-eleventh rib nephrostomy insertion.[27] Also using antegrade techniques, Gupta and colleagues reported significant chest complications in 3 (5%) of 63 supracostal nephrostomies.[28] Use of a working sheath and postoperative placement of a large-bore (24 to 26F) nephrostomy tube have been

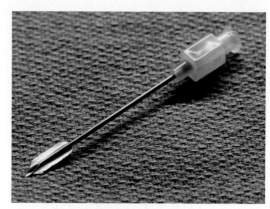

Figure 15-9 Fascial incising needle.

reported to be important in minimizing the risk of postoperative pneumo- or hydrothorax.[22,24,25,28] Although I always use a working sheath for percutaneous nephrolithotomy, I either use a 12F nephrostomy tube, or more commonly, place no tube postoperatively, and have rarely identified pneumothorax postoperatively. It is usually only possible to create a supracostal nephrostomy tract using retrograde techniques when the patient is in expiration, which may explain the low rate of pulmonary complications using this technique. Notwithstanding the low risk of complications, the anesthetist should be advised when a supracostal tract has been created so that air entry on the affected side can be monitored appropriately.

POSTOPERATIVE CARE

Most of the considerations regarding postoperative care relate to the endourologic procedure performed after retrograde access has been achieved. If a supracostal nephrostomy tract has been created, a postoperative chest radiograph is obtained to identify or rule out pneumothorax.

RESULTS

Irrespective of the technique used, most authors report a success rate for establishing a nephrostomy tract by retrograde techniques that ranges from 88 to 100%. In our first 206 attempted procedures, a nephrostomy tract was successfully established in 201, for a success rate of 98%.[26] A modification of the Lawson technique was used initially in all patients and was successful in 178 of 201 successful attempts, for a success rate of 89%. The Hawkins-Hunter system was used in the remaining 23 successful attempts. In 4 of our 5 failures, the reason for failure was inability to gain access to the renal pelvis, either because of excessive tortuosity of the upper ureter, or an impacted ureteric or renal pelvic calculus. Hawkins reported a 4% failure rate as a result of the inability to pass a catheter into the collecting system.[29] Leal reported 2 failures in 78 patients (2.6%).[7] In 1 patient the catheter was dislodged from the calix, and in 1 it was not possible to pass the guidewire through a tortuous ureteropelvic junction. Hunter and colleagues reported 3 failures (9.7%) in their first 31 attempted retrograde

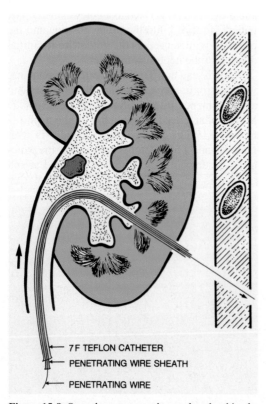

Figure 15-8 Once the puncture wire reaches the skin, the puncture wire sheath and the 7F catheter are advanced over the wire to the abdominal wall. From Hosking DH.[16]

— 7F TEFLON CATHETER
— PENETRATING WIRE SHEATH
— PENETRATING WIRE

nephrostomies.[8] In 2 patients, the needle could not be oriented in what was considered a safe direction, and antegrade nephrostomy was therefore performed. In 1 patient, bladder neck scarring prevented cystoscopy. Spirnak reported 2 access failures in 30 attempts (6.7%).[9] One of the 2 failures was considered to be caused by the nephrostomy tract being created above the twelfth rib. Morrisseau and Trotter reported no failure to establish a nephrostomy tract in 71 consecutive patients.[17] A modification of the Lawson system was used first in all their patients and was successful in 69 (97%). In a study on complex renal calculi, Bloom and Nieh reported 3 failures in 25 attempts (12%) because of access problems related to a tortuous ureter, an obstructing ureteropelvic calculus, and an obstructing infundibular calculus.[6] A kit for the Hawkins-Hunter system is unfortunately no longer available. This system was useful in patients who had perirenal scar tissue secondary to previous surgery. Establishing a nephrostomy tract in such patients is now more reliably achieved by antegrade techniques.

COMPLICATIONS

Most reports on complications include complications related not only to retrograde access, but also to the stone removal procedure usually performed at the same time. In our first 201 retrograde nephrostomies, 1 patient sustained a colon perforation, and in 2 patients, postoperative nephrostograms demonstrated intraperitoneal leakage of contrast material.[26] All 3 patients were successfully managed conservatively. In over 1,300 subsequent nephrostomies, there have been no further instances of bowel perforation. Four patients developed pneumothorax postoperatively, 1 requiring chest tube insertion. Hunter and colleagues reported 2 cases of pneumothorax and 2 episodes of hemorrhage requiring transfusion in their first 30 patients.[8] There were no episodes of hemorrhage in their last 15 patients, when 26F or larger nephrostomy tubes were used postoperatively. Stone removal was complete in 83% of their patients. Spirnak reported 1 colon perforation in 30 attempted nephrostomies.[9] Spirnak and Resnick reported that none of their patients required intraoperative or post-operative blood transfusions; they attribute this to the precise placement of the nephrostomy tract that the retrograde technique allows.[18] Leal reported that 8 of 85 consecutive patients required postoperative blood transfusion, but did not specify which patients had undergone retrograde nephrostomy.[7] Stone removal was complete in 87% of Leal's patients, 76 of whom underwent retrograde nephrostomy placement. Morrisseau and Trotter[17] reported that 1 of 71 patients required a postoperative transfusion. Stone removal was

successful in 86% of their patients. Hawkins reported that in his first 100 cases, 10 patients required blood transfusion.[29] Bleeding occurred late in the procedure during fragmentation of the stones. There were no cases of severe bleeding requiring embolization or nephrectomy. To date, there have been no studies comparing access success rates, stone removal rates, and complications in patients undergoing antegrade as opposed to retrograde access procedures.

CONCLUSION

The establishment of a nephrostomy tract using retrograde techniques does offer advantages over the more commonly used antegrade methods. In many institutions a retrograde pyelogram is performed as a preliminary step to antegrade nephrostomy. Establishing a nephrostomy tract using retrograde techniques is a relatively simple additional step if a retrograde pyelogram is necessary. Retrograde access is not a time-consuming procedure. In our first 201 successful nephrostomies, the mean procedure time for nephrostomy creation, including cystoscopy, was 27.9 minutes, with a range of 10 to 195 minutes and a median procedure time of 22 minutes.[26] Hawkins and colleagues report an average procedure time of about 30 minutes.[3]

Another advantage of retrograde nephrostomy is that the puncture needle is always directed from the inside to the outside, away from large blood vessels near the renal hilum, minimizing the risk of major hemorrhage secondary to major vessel injury at the time of tract dilation. In most of the techniques of retrograde nephrostomy, once a tract has been created, a guidewire, needle, or puncture wire traverses the entire urinary tract from the flank to the urethral meatus. This control over both ends of the wire eliminates the risk of accidental wire displacement, particularly at the time of tract dilation.

Finally, radiation exposure of the operator is minimized using retrograde access techniques. Because manipulation of the equipment occurs well away from the site of the nephrostomy, the operator is exposed to considerably less radiation than with antegrade techniques. Also, because the operator is not trying to puncture a small, moving, undilated calix, continuous fluoroscopy is not essential, reducing radiation requirements and potential exposure.

The description of techniques is quoted, in part, from Hosking DH.[30] Reprinted with permission of Thomson Healthcare Communications.

REFERENCES

1. Fernstrom I, Johansson B. Percutaneous pyelo-lithotomy. A new extraction technique. Scand J Urol Nephrol 1976; 10:257–9.
2. Banner MP, Stein EJ, Pollack HM. Technical refinements in percutaneous nephroureterolithotomy. AJR Am J Roentgenol 1985;145:101–7.
3. Hawkins IF, Hunter P, Leal G, et al. Retrograde nephrostomy for stone removal: combined cystoscopic/percutaneous technique. AJR Am J Roentgenol 1984;143:299–304.
4. Lawson RK, Murphy JB, Taylor AJ, Jacobs SC. Retrograde method for percutaneous access to kidney. Urology 1983;22:580–2.
5. Hunter PT, Hawkins IF, Finlayson B, et al. Hawkins-Hunter retrograde transcutaneous nephrostomy: a new technique. Urology 1983;22:583–7.
6. Bloom LS, Nieh PT. Retrograde nephrostolithotomy in management of complex renal calculi. J Urol 1991;145:706–9.
7. Leal JJ. Percutaneous removal of renal and ureteral stones with and without concomitant transurethral manipulation by a urologist using antegrade and retrograde techniques without a radiologist's assistance. J Urol 1988;139:1184–7.
8. Hunter PT, Finlayson B, Drylie DM, et al. Retrograde nephrostomy and percutaneous calculus removal in 30 patients. J Urol 1985;133:369–74.
9. Spirnak JP. Retrograde percutaneous nephrostolithotomy: an acceptable alternative to antegrade techniques. J Urol 1987;137:841–4.
10. Spirnak JP, Resnick MI. Retrograde percutaneous stone removal using modified Lawson technique. Urology 1987;30:551–3.
11. Morse RM, Spirnak JP, Resnick MI. Iatrogenic colon and rectal injuries associated with urological intervention: report of 14 patients. J Urol 1988;140:101–3.
12. Segura JW, Patterson DE, LeRoy AJ, et al. Percutaneous removal of kidney stones: review of 1000 cases. J Urol 1985;134:1077–81.
13. Lingeman JE, Coury TA, Newman DM, et al. Comparison of results and morbidity of percutaneous nephrostolithotomy and extracorporeal shock wave lithotripsy. J Urol 1987;138:485–90.
14. Roth RA, Beckmann CF. Complications of extracorporeal shock-wave lithotripsy and percutaneous nephrolithotomy. Urol Clin North Am 1988;15:155–66.
15. Spies JB, Rosen RJ, Lebowitz AS. Antibiotic prophylaxis in vascular and interventional radiology: a rational approach. Radiology 1988;166:381–7.
16. Hosking DH. Retrograde nephrostomy: experience with 2 techniques. J Urol 1986;135:1146–9.
17. Morrisseau PM, Trotter SJ. Retrograde percutaneous nephrolithotomy: urological treatment of a urological problem. J Urol 1988;139:1163–5.
18. Spirnak JP, Resnick MI. Retrograde percutaneous nephrostomy. Urol Clin North Am 1988;15:393–7.
19. Kaye KW, Reinke DB. Detailed caliceal anatomy for endourology. J Urol 1984;132:1085–8.
20. Carson CC. Complications of percutaneous stone extraction: prevention and treatment. Semin Urol 1986;4:161–9.
21. Coleman CC, Castaneda-Zuniga W, Miller R, et al. A logical approach to renal stone removal. AJR Am J Roentgenol 1984;143:609–15.
22. Forsyth MJ, Fuchs EF. The supracostal approach for percutaneous nephrostolithotomy. J Urol 1987;137:197–8.
23. Fuchs EF, Forsyth MJ. Supracostal approach for percutaneous ultrasonic lithotripsy. Urol Clin North Am 1990;17:99–102.
24. Narasimham DL, Jacobsson B, Vijayan P, et al. Percutaneous nephrolithotomy through an intercostal approach. Acta Radiol 1991;32:162–5.
25. Hulbert JC. Percutaneous extraction of difficult renal stones. Semin Urol 1986;4:139–47.
26. Hosking DH, Reid RI. The evaluation of retrograde nephrostomy in over 200 procedures. In: Walker VR, Sutton RAL, Cameron ECB, et al, editors. Urolithiasis: proceedings of the Sixth International Symposium on Urolithiasis. New York: Plenum Press; 1989.
27. Munver R, Delvecchio FC, Newman GE, Preminger GM. Critical analysis of supracostal access for percutaneous renal surgery. J Urol 2001;166:1242–6.
28. Gupta R, Kumar A, Kapoor R, et al. Prospective evaluation of safety and efficacy of the supracostal approach for percutaneous nephrolithotomy. BJU Int 2002;90:809–13.
29. Hawkins IF Jr. Retrograde percutaneous nephrostomy. Crit Rev Diagn Imaging 1987;27:153–65.
30. Hosking DH. Retrograde nephrostomy. Contemp Urol 1990; 1:4–9.

16

Nephroscopy

C. F. Ng
T. J. Thompson
D. A. Tolley

Nephroscopy is an important part of the urologic armamentarium. Percutaneous nephroscopy was first performed in 1941 when Rupel and Brown passed a rigid cystoscope through a drain track into the kidney of a patient and removed residual stone following open surgery.[1] Intraoperative nephroscopy, as practiced during open nephrolithotomy, used an L-shaped angled nephroscope specifically designed for the purpose of visualizing caliceal stone fragments.[2] However, the widespread use of endoscopic nephroscopy began with the introduction of percutaneous nephrolithotomy as a primary treatment of renal stones. This technique was pioneered in the early 1980s by Wickham and Kellet in the United Kingdom and Alken in Germany. A conventional rigid cystoscope was used initially. Purpose-designed nephroscopes with straight operating channels and either cranked or 45 degree offset optics were developed to allow the use of more effective rigid ancillary instruments for intrarenal surgery and the indications for the technique expanded rapidly. The intrinsic limitation of the rigid instrument was its inability to assess all parts of the collecting system through a single track, a problem unresolved by retro-viewing nephroscopes, which never gained popularity in daily clinical use. The problem was solved by the development of the flexible endoscope, thus giving the surgeon endoscopic access to the entire intrarenal collecting system, pelvis, and ureter, so allowing the urologist to perform a variety of endoscopic procedures in virtually every point of the urinary tract.

INDICATIONS FOR THE PROCEDURES

DIAGNOSTIC   The role of nephroscopy as an isolated diagnostic procedure has been largely superseded by advances in cross-sectional and ultrasound imaging and retrograde flexible pyelocalicoscopy. The future, however, may lie in the development of virtual nephroscopy as a noninvasive diagnostic tool for intrarenal pathology.[3]

THERAPEUTIC   The nephroscope is used to facilitate ablative and incisional procedures including:

Ablative
- Stone extraction, percutaneous nephrolithotomy (PCNL)
- Tumour ablation
- Removal of foreign body (eg, retained/encrusted stent)
- Ablation of renal cyst or caliceal diverticulum

- "Second-look" nephroscopy after previous PCNL

Incisional
- Endopyelotomy for ureteropelvic junction obstruction
- Incision of upper ureteric strictures
- Neo-calicopyelostomy for caliceal diverticulum

PATIENT PREPARATION

Careful preoperative planning will facilitate the intraoperative procedure. A detailed review of the intravenous urogram and a reconstructed view of computerized tomograms of the kidney will allow the urologist to familiarize himself or herself with the anatomy of the collecting system and will assist in the choice of caliceal access. The urine should be sterile wherever possible preoperatively, and antibiotic prophylaxis given in all cases. A preoperative course of appropriate antibiotics should be given in all cases where the urine is infected and urine cultures rechecked after antibiotic therapy to ensure urine is sterile.

Potential coagulopathy should be excluded. Particular attention should be paid to the patient's drug history, especially the use of aspirin or other antiplatelet drugs and coumarin. Aspirin should be discontinued at least 1 week before surgery. Patients on coumarin for significant clinical reasons should stop medication approximately 48 hours prior to surgery to allow the prothrombin time to normalize. The anticoagulant effect should then be maintained with subcutaneous shorter-acting heparins. Platelet count and prothrombin time must be checked before the operation. The heparin dose should be omitted immediately prior to the surgery, thus providing a window of normal blood clotting during which the therapeutic procedure can be performed. Additional tests (eg, bleeding time, specific factors, or inhibitors analysis) should be checked if clinically indicated and any abnormalities corrected preoperatively. Hematology advice should be sought in all patients with complex coagulopathy issues. Typing and screening of blood should be performed in all cases in case transfusion is required.

INFORMED CONSENT

The patient should be well informed about the details of his/her illness, the proposed treatment and outcome, the associated complications, and possible secondary procedures. For diagnostic nephroscopy, the nature of the suspected lesion and the reason for a percutaneous approach should be clearly stated. The implications of relevant pathologies and their subsequent management and prognosis should also be discussed. For therapeutic procedures, additional information about other surgical alternatives, including nontreatment, should also be outlined.

PREOPERATIVE PREPARATION

Access to the kidney is usually gained under general anesthesia via a nephrostomy track with patients in the prone or prone oblique position (Figure 16-1). Epidural anesthesia and occasionally local anesthesia can be used, particularly for secondary flexible nephroscopy. Both have the advantage of using the patient's cooperation to immobilize the kidney by breath-holding when nephroscopy is performed to remove retained stone fragments following previous PCNL.

The chest and pelvis must be well supported to avoid obstruction of venous return during operation in the prone position. Face, arms, breasts, genitalia, and other pressure points should be checked and protected from pressure. A splinting cushion is usually placed under the kidney to be operated on to reduce movement (Figure 16-2), thus facilitating the initial percutaneous puncture. Other positions, such as full-flank position[4] and supine position,[5] have been reported that may be beneficial in patients with severe cardiopulmonary disease and in those who are morbidly obese. In a recent prospective review of 130 patients receiving PCNL in either supine (53 patients) or prone (77 patients) position, there were no significant differences in overall success rate and complication rate between the two groups of patients.[6] In patients with severe skeletal deformities (eg, kyphoscoliosis) percutaneous nephroscopy, under local anesthesia, can be performed with the patient in the sitting position.

INSTRUMENTATION

Standard rigid nephroscopes are 19.5 to 27 French (F) in diameter and have rod lenses with offset eyepieces or fiberoptic bundles. Pediatric nephroscopes are also available. Flexible nephroscopes with an outer diameter around 15F are also manufactured, but in practical terms, the flexible cystoscope can serve this purpose just as well.

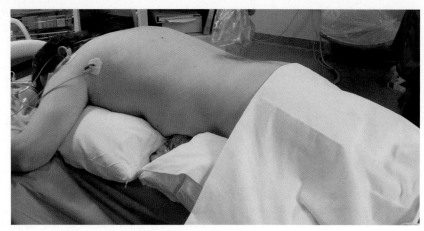

Figure 16-1 Patient put in prone position for percutaneous nephrolithotomy.

The use of rigid and flexible nephroscopes is complementary. Rigid nephroscopes usually afford a better view owing to the superior optics of the rod lens system and larger caliber irrigation channels. They also permit the passage of larger, stronger, and more powerful auxiliary instruments to facilitate procedures. Flexible nephroscopes enable access to otherwise inaccessible calices without the need for secondary caliceal puncture.

There has been increasing interest in the use of a smaller sized rigid nephroscope, introduced through a smaller track (the "mini-perc") from 13F to 20F.[7–9] The creation of a smaller percutaneous track is, in theory, less traumatic and may reduce morbidity. This benefit may not prove to be sufficiently advantageous in clinical practice for the procedure to become a standard of care, particularly in the light of developments in retrograde flexible pyelocalicoscopy.

STEP-BY-STEP DESCRIPTION OF OPERATIVE PROCEDURE

Percutaneous access should be planned so as to enter the most appropriate calix for successful completion of the surgical procedure with minimum complications. If difficulty is encountered because of such problems as bleeding, failure to place the working guidewire the collecting sys-

tem, or failure to advance the access sheath fully because of parenchymal scarring, then retrograde injection of methylene blue dye through the ureteral catheter can help the operator locate the collecting system.

Once the nephroscope and the sheath have entered the collecting system, the working guidewire can be removed if it hinders the manipulation of the nephroscope, but a safety guidewire should always be placed outside the access sheath using a dual lumen catheter during track dilatation and if possible placed in the ureter to reduce the risk of it being displaced accidentally. The collecting system can then be inspected systematically, except when it is completely filled with stone material.

Difficulty in locating or reaching the pathology may sometimes result in excessive bleeding. This is often due to applying excessive track torque on the kidney by rough use and levering of the rigid nephroscope. This may result in significant trauma to the renal parenchyma with resultant heavy bleeding. Therefore, it may be necessary to create another percutaneous track or, more usually, use a flexible nephroscope to avoid this problem. The decision will depend on the patient, the pathology, the anatomy of the collecting system, and the availability of instruments. The flexible nephroscope is placed through the sheath into the collecting system with or without the aid of a guidewire (Figure 16-3). The position of the air bubble and intraoperative fluoroscopy is helpful in confirming the exact position of the tip of the scope, as spatial orientation is more difficult in view of the endoscope's flexible nature. The intrarenal collecting system can then be inspected in a systematic fashion.

There is a risk of absorption and extravasation of irrigating fluid during the procedure and, therefore, only isotonic solutions should be used. Sterile normal saline is ideal for most situations, especially for stone surgery. If diathermy is required, 1.2% glycine or 3% mannitol should be used. All solutions should also be used at body temperature to avoid hypothermia. The effect of fluid absorption is not a major problem in many patients, but it may become clinically significant in patients with compromised cardiorespiratory

or renal function and also in children. In order to limit the amount of fluid absorbed, Miller and Whitfield advised that the height of the irrigation bag should be kept below 80 cm and an Amplatz open drainage system should be used. They also advised against prolonged intrarenal surgery when there is evidence of damage to the renal pelvis. In any event, the maximum endoscopy time should never be more than 2 hours.[10] In an in vitro kidney model, Low demonstrated that the use of larger caliber, shorter sheaths properly positioned in the collecting system can help to decrease the intrarenal pelvic pressure.[11] Meticulous attention to detail in this way is especially important during cases involving percutaneous removal of infected calculi and transitional-cell carcinoma to reduce risks of bacteremia and dissemination of cancer, respectively.

During secondary nephroscopy or other situations where a track of size greater than 15F is already well established, a flexible nephroscope can be passed into the kidney under direct vision along a guidewire after the nephrostomy tube has been removed. A working sheath is not necessary in this situation, but care must be taken to avoid creating a false passage and traumatizing the surrounding tissue. This procedure can be performed using local anesthetic instilled into the track and supplemented by analgesics.

Significant bleeding during the procedure may be due to tearing of the parenchyma during the dilatation of the track and can be controlled by tamponade using the access sheath. This generally results in complete cessation of bleeding within a few minutes. Troublesome bleeding from torn veins in the infundibulum can be cauterized, but occasionally, bleeding can be sufficient to impair the endoscopic view, rendering further surgery unsafe. The procedure should be abandoned at this point and a large-bore nephrostomy tube inserted. Occasionally, inflation of the balloon of a Foley catheter with no more than 5 mL of saline produces effective tamponade. The procedure can then be repeated in a few days time after the bleeding stops. Production of an arteriovenous fistula is a rare complication and its management is dealt with elsewhere.

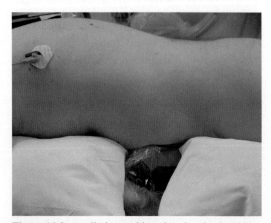

Figure 16-2 A splinting cushion placed under the kidney to be operated on.

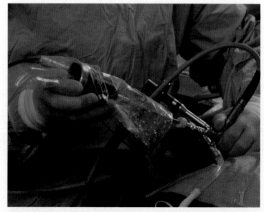

Figure 16-3 Working with a flexible nephroscope through the access sheath.

POSTOPERATIVE CARE

At the end of the procedure, an indwelling nephrostomy tube is left in place. Traditionally, a tube that is slightly smaller than the size of the percutaneous track is used to "stent" the tract. This serves the purpose of tamponade hemostasis as well as retaining access for a potential "second-look" procedure. Many factors influence the timing of removal of the tube, including the type of procedure, intraoperative complications (such as perforation of collecting system, and bleeding), as well as the need for a secondary procedure. For a simple, uncomplicated procedure, the tube can usually be removed in 1 to 2 days, after a clinical trial of clamping, with or without a prior check nephrostogram.

In some centers, including our own, smaller sizes of nephrostomy tubes (8–10F) are routinely used on the basis of better patient comfort.[12] For simple cases, "tubeless," that is, no placement of a nephrostomy tube, has been advocated.[13,14] In such situations, it is essential to be certain that meticulous hemostasis of the entry site into the kidney has been achieved. Some authors recommend withdrawal of the sheath under vision and electrocautery to any bleeding vessels. Also, one must be sure that no ureteral obstruction persists, because a nephrocutaneous fistula is likely to occur.

In the postoperative period, the patient should be monitored for bleeding. If significant parenchymal bleeding occurred intraoperatively, the hematocrit should be checked and blood transfusion may occasionally be necessary. In the event of early postoperative bleeding, control can be achieved by clamping the nephrostomy tube for a short period in the recovery room. This causes stasis and clotting of blood in the tube and intrarenal collecting system. As bleeding continues, the intrarenal pressure increases and provides tamponade to the bleeding site. Chest radiography should be performed if a pleural tear or perforation is suspected, especially when a supracostal approach has been used. Antibiotic therapy is continued postoperatively until all tubes are removed.

COMPLICATIONS

Simple diagnostic nephroscopy is generally an uncomplicated procedure, but may be associated with fever; infection, including septicemia; bleeding; fluid overload; perforation of intrarenal collecting system; and body injury related to poor positioning of the patient. Complications relating to percutaneous access and specific procedures carried out in conjunction with nephroscopy are discussed in the relevant chapters.

CONCLUSION

The role of percutaneous diagnostic nephroscopy is now less prominent because of advances in renal imaging and retrograde flexible pyelocalicoscopy. However, the need for competent and systematic nephroscopy during therapeutic percutaneous renal surgery confirms the importance of the technique and serves to emphasize that nephroscopy remains an essential, fundamental endourologic skill. Although therapeutic applications for retrograde flexible pyelocalicoscopy will undoubtedly increase, the limitations and availability of instrumentation and accessories in many parts of the world will ensure that percutaneous nephroscopic surgery remains an important part of endourologic practice for the foreseeable future.

REFERENCES

1. Rupel E, Brown R. Nephroscopy with removal of stone following nephrostomy for obstructive calculous anuria. J Urol 1941;46:177–82.
2. Vatz A, Berci G, Shore JM, et al. Operative nephroscopy. J Urol 2002;168:1914–6.
3. Takebayashi S, Hosaka M, Takase K, et al. Computerized tomography nephroscopic images of renal pelvic carcinoma. J Urol 1999;162:315–8.
4. Kerbl K, Clayman RV, Chandhoke PS, et al. Percutaneous stone removal with the patient in a flank position. J Urol 1994;151:686–8.
5. Valdivia Uria JG, Valle GJ, Lopez Lopez JA, et al. Technique and complications of percutaneous nephroscopy: experience with 557 patients in the supine position. J Urol 1998;160:1975–8.
6. Shoma AM, Eraky I, El-Kenawy MR, El-Kappany HA. Percutaneous nephrolithotomy in the supine position: technical aspects and functional outcome compared with the prone technique. Urol 2002;60:388–92.
7. Chan DY, Jarrett TW. Techniques in endourology: minipercutaneous nephrolithotomy. J Endourol 2000;14:269–72.
8. Monga M, Oglevie S. Minipercutaneous nephrolithotomy. J Endourol 2000;14:419–21.
9. Lahme S, Bichler KH, Strohmaier WL, Gotz T. Minimally invasive PCNL in patients with renal pelvic and calyceal stones. Eur Urol 2001;40:619–24.
10. Miller RA, Whitfield HN. Lithotripsy for renal stone disease. Br Med J 1985;291:967.
11. Low RK. Nephroscopy sheath characteristics and intrarenal pelvic pressure: human kidney model. J Endourol 1999;13:205–8.
12. Maheshwari PN, Andankar MG, Bansal M. Nephrostomy tube after percutaneous nephrolithotomy: large-bore or pigtail catheter? J Endourol 2000;14:735–7.
13. Goh M, Wolf JS Jr. Almost totally tubeless percutaneous nephrolithotomy: further evolution of the technique. J Endourol 1999;13:177–80.
14. Lojanapiwat B, Soonthornphan S, Wudhikarn S. Tubeless percutaneous nephrolithotomy in selected patients. J Endourol 2001;15:711–3.

17

Percutaneous Stone Extraction

Stevan B. Streem, MD

HISTORICAL CONSIDERATIONS

Rupel and Brown extracted an obstructing renal calculus via an operatively established nephrostomy tract in 1941.[1] In 1955, Goodwin and associates reported the use of percutaneous nephrostomy drainage for relief of obstruction and infection.[2] But removal of a renal calculus via percutaneous tract established specifically for that purpose was not performed until 20 years later when Fernstrom and Johansson used that technique successfully in three patients.[3] With the subsequent development of safe and effective means to fragment even large calculi, percutaneous stone extraction quickly gained acceptance as the procedure of choice for management of most patients requiring intervention for upper tract calculi in the late 1970s and early 1980s. During that time, any patient who would have otherwise required open lithotomy was considered a potential candidate for percutaneous extraction instead. Thus, the indications for this procedure were analogous to those for intervention for any stone, and included obstruction, pain, infection or hematuria associated with the stone, or active stone growth despite appropriate medical management.

INDICATIONS AND CONTRAINDICATIONS

While the introduction of both extracorporeal shock wave lithotripsy (ESWL) and ureteroscopic access to the calicealpyelocaliceal system have not significantly impacted the general indications for stone intervention, the indications for percutaneous extraction have narrowed and are now well defined. As summarized in Table 17-1, the contemporary indications for percutaneous stone extraction are essentially identical to the current contraindications to ESWL, and most of these indications are more relative than absolute. In general, the indications for percutaneous management of upper tract calculi currently include unusual body habitus precluding ESWL, obstruction distal to the stone, cystine stones, stones associated with upper tract foreign bodies, and large or otherwise complex stones. Relative indications include the presence of an implanted cardiac defibrillator, and a proximate calcified aortic or renal artery aneurysm. Finally, any patient who has failed ESWL can be considered for percutaneous management as a "salvage" procedure. In some of these settings, however, ureteroscopic management is also an option.

LeRoy and associates at the Mayo Clinic reported a contemporary experience with percutaneous stone management in the era of ESWL.[4] During one year at their tertiary care center, 143 patients with renal or upper ureteral calculi were treated percutaneously, during which time 854 patients were managed with ESWL. These authors, in reviewing their current indications and techniques for percutaneous management, noted that, despite the increased complexity of such cases, excellent results could still be achieved with acceptably low morbidity.

Currently, the only absolute contraindication to percutaneous stone extraction is an irreversible coagulopathy, though pregnancy poses additional considerations including, but not limited to, risk to the fetus of radiation exposure and anesthesia, and increased vascularity of the kidney as it pertains to a risk of bleeding. Percutaneous stone management should be applied to pregnant patients in extreme circumstances only.

PATIENT PREPARATION

The patient should be apprised of the potential risks and benefits of percutaneous nephrolithotomy versus the alternatives of ESWL, ureteroscopy, and open surgery. In these often complex cases, it is explained that percutaneous extraction may require more than one trip to the radiology or surgical suite, and even then the procedure may be unsuccessful, such that even open operative intervention may ultimately, albeit rarely, be required. In fact, the vast majority of patients will ultimately benefit from a successful percutaneous procedure with a relatively short hospital stay and greatly decreased period of convalescence compared to open operative intervention.[5–8]

Standard preoperative preparation includes assurance of the availability of blood for possible transfusion with a "Type and Screen," though preoperative cross-matching is rarely necessary. At times, the procedure may be performed under local anesthesia and appropriate intravenous sedation, though at our center, the vast majority of these procedures are done with general endotracheal anesthesia. Patients with urinary tract infection are treated with sensitivity-specific antibiotics on an outpatient basis for one to two weeks, then intravenously prior to the access and subsequent stone extraction. The need for prophylactic antibiotics in the face of a sterile urine is unproven, though our preference in this setting is a "short course" antibiotic protocol. Generally, a first generation cephalosporin is administered intravenously just prior to establishing percutaneous access, and this is continued for 48 hours following stone removal.

TECHNIQUE

STANDARD APPROACHES The technique of percutaneous stone extraction is specific to the size, location and chemical composition of the calculus. But the procedure is always performed with the same sequential steps, which include percutaneous access, dilation of the tract, stone fragmentation and extraction, and post-extraction drainage and tamponade of the tract.

The techniques of percutaneous access and tract dilation are described in the preceding chapter. As such, the techniques described herein begin with the assumption that access has been established and the tract dilated to a size large enough to accommodate a rigid nephroscope with or without a working sheath in place. Our preference, however, is to dilate the tract with a 30F balloon, backloaded with a 30F Amplatz working sheath. It is also assumed that a "safety wire" remains in place alongside the sheath with its distal tip coiled in the pelviocaliceal system or preferably, in the distal ureter. While "minipercs" have been described using smaller instrumentation, clinical studies thus far have shown no advantage to those techniques.[9]

The patient is in a prone-oblique position with the ipsilateral side elevated to approximately 20 degrees (Figure 17-1). For patients with horseshoe kidneys or analogous rotational anomalies, the contralateral side is elevated instead to allow a more medial rotation of the otherwise anteriorly projecting renal pelvis. This also allows a more lateral projection of the infundibula and calyces.

Actual stone extraction can be accomplished with a variety of techniques utilizing either direct vision through a nephroscope, fluoroscopic guidance, or both. At our center, the vast majority of percutaneous stone extractions are accomplished utilizing ultrasonic lithotripsy under direct vision through a rigid nephroscope. This approach was

Table 17-1 Indications for Percutaneous Management of Renal Calculi
Body habitus precluding ESWL
Cystine stones
Stones associated with distal obstruction
Stones associated with upper tract foreign bodies
Large or complex stones
Contraindication to ESWL
Failure of ESWL

first described by Alken and colleagues and Marberger and colleagues in Mainz, Germany, and Vienna, Austria[10,11] and popularized in the United States by Segura and associates at the Mayo Clinic[12] and Clayman and associates at the University of Minnesota.[13]

Light, suction, and irrigation attachments are made to the nephroscope. The nephroscope, with the obturator in place in most instances, is inserted through the working sheath (Figure 17-2). Once it is assured to be within the collecting system, the working wire can be removed while the safety wire is left indwelling alongside the Amplatz sheath. With rare exception, the irrigant of choice is normal saline. This prevents hyponatremia that may result from intravascular absorption when hyposmotic solutions are used.[14] Initially, vision may be obscured by blood clots that can be evacuated by adjusting the irrigation and suction from the sheath. Use of the ultrasound wand at this time can also help clear the calicealpyelocaliceal system of clots.

Stones less than 9 mm or 10 mm may be small enough to extract intact through an appropriately sized working sheath. These stones are simply grasped under direct vision utilizing rigid graspers, endoscopic forceps, or baskets passed via the working port (Figure 17-3). Most stones managed percutaneously today, however, are too large to be withdrawn intact, and the primary modality for management of these stones at most centers is ultrasonic lithotripsy.[15] The ultrasound wand (sonotrode) with its own suction attachment is introduced via the working channel of a rigid nephroscope (Figure 17-4). During this time, suction from the nephroscope sheath is turned down to prevent collapse of the renal pelvic wall. Under direct visual control, the tip of the sonotrode is impacted against the stone (Figure 17-5). Suction is then applied through the hollow sonotrode to hold the stone in place. This allows the fragments to be evacuated via the sonotrode as fragmentation proceeds. Fragments remaining that are too large to pass through the sonotrode channel can then be extracted utilizing any of the aforementioned grasping techniques under direct vision or by continuing the process of ultrasonic fragmentation.

While ultrasonic lithotripsy can efficiently fragment most calcium oxalate/phosphate, struvite, cystine, and uric acid stones, there are some stones that are physically too hard to fragment with this modality. For the most part, these will be large calcium oxalate monohydrate stones that often appear extremely dense and homogenous on plain x-rays, or some mixed calcium oxalate/uric acid stones. In such patients, intracorporeal electrohydraulic lithotripsy (EHL) with a small EHL probe has proven safe and extremely effective.[16] In these cases, the EHL probe is used to fragment the large stone into smaller pieces (Figure 17-6) which can be individually grasped and removed.

Alternative modes of intracorporeal lithotripsy that are also valuable in these cases include Holmium laser lithotripsy (Figure 17-7), or even more recently, combined ultrasonic and pneumatic lithotripsy.[17]

Figure 17-1 Prone-oblique position with the ipsilateral side elevated 10° to 20°. Reproduced with permission from Streem SB, Zelch MG, Risius B, Geisinger MA. Percutaneous extraction of renal calculi. Urol Clin North Am 1985;12:381.

Figure 17-2 Nephroscope with obturator in place is passed over a working wire fluoroscopic control. A safety wire is in place alongside the working wire.

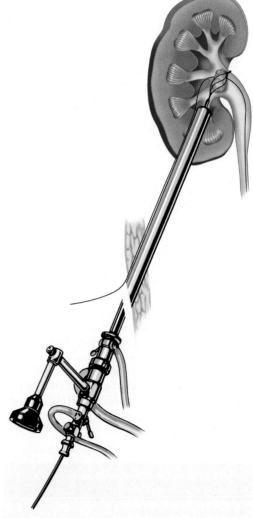

Figure 17-3 Relatively small stones can be extracted intact using baskets, forceps or graspers passed under direct vision via the working port of the nephroscope. Reproduced with permission from Streem SB, Zelch MG, Risius B, Geisinger MA. Percutaneous extraction of renal calculi. Urol Clin North Am 1985;12:381.

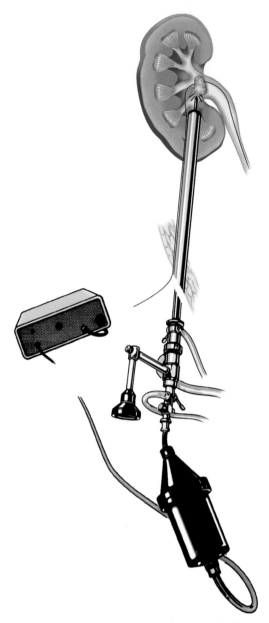

Figure 17-4 Larger stones require fragmentation for percutaneous extraction, and the primary modality utilized for this is ultrasound. The ultrasound wand (sonotrode) with its own suction attachment is introduced via the working channel of a rigid nephroscope. Reproduced with permission from Streem SB, Zelch MG, Risius B, Geisinger MA. Percutaneous extraction of renal calculi. Urol Clin North Am 1985;12:381.

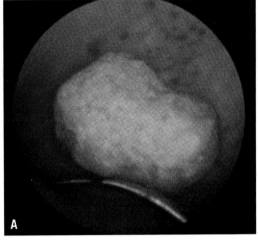 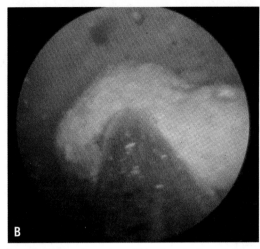

Figure 17-5 *A,* Nephroscopic view of a calculus in the renal pelvis. Note safety wire still in place in the pelvis and passing antegrade across the ureteropelvic junction. *B,* Nephroscopic view of calculus with sonotrode in place as fragmentation begins.

kets are ideal. The stone is then engaged and withdrawn intact (Figure 17-8). Alternatively, larger stones can be fragmented with a Holmium laser that allows intracorporeal lithotripsy via flexible instrumentation (Figure 17-9). EHL is a suitable alternative, though this modality is better applied to caliceal stones rather than ureteral stones.

When all accessible stone have been extracted as assured by visual and x-ray control, tamponade of the tract and nephrostomy drainage is instituted. If a working sheath has been used, a 22F or 24F nephrostomy tube is passed through it and positioned fluoroscopically with its tip in the renal pelvis. Our preference is to use the remaining safety wire to pass a 5F pyeloureteral catheter adjacent to the nephrostomy tube with its distal tip in the distal one-third ureter, and the proximal end coiled at skin level (Figure 17-10). This is secured in place as a safety precaution that allows rapid access back to the calicealpyelocaliceal system should that be required prior to elective removal of the nephrostomy tube. If a working sheath has not been used, a second wire is passed via the nephroscope under direct vision, or by using a 9F introducing set passed over the remaining safety

wire. The placement of a second "working" wire now allows passage of the nephrostomy tube. To summarize this precaution, a safety wire or pyeloureteral catheter is left in place undisturbed from the time the nephroscope is first inserted until the time the nephrostomy tract is mature, or until the nephrostomy tube is ready for removal.

Recently, the concept of "tubeless" percutaneous surgery has been introduced. This procedure requires the placement of a ureteral stent and Foley catheter in all patients, but may have the advantage of decreasing overall hospital stay. The author has no personal experience with this approach, which has been recommended primarily for otherwise uncomplicated procedures.[19]

TECHNIQUES FOR SPECIFIC INDICATIONS
Unusual Body Habitus Precluding ESWL
One of the most challenging indications for percutaneous stone extraction is encountered in patients in whom an unusual body habitus precludes successful ESWL. This occurs most frequently in those patients with morbid obesity. While some such patients can be successfully treated with ESWL,[20] in general, patients weigh-

Visualization, fragmentation, engagement and extraction of infundibular or caliceal calculi lying at acute angles to the percutaneous tract will generally require flexible nephroscopy.[18] Although flexible nephroscopy may be successful during the initial percutaneous procedure, at times, even a small amount of bleeding can obscure vision. As such, flexible nephroscopy may be more successful when performed via mature tract 2 to 3 days following the primary procedure.

The flexible nephroscope is passed through the Amplatz working sheath under direct vision with fluoroscopic control. When the stone is visualized, a flexible grasping forceps, prongs or basket is passed through the working sheath of the nephroscope. In this situation, tipless nitinol bas-

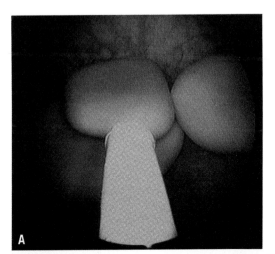 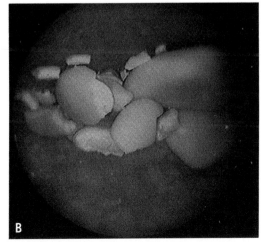

Figure 17-6 *A,* Nephroscopic view of multiple large calculi with EHL probe in place. *B,* Fragmentation of stones is evident after only a few EHL pulses.

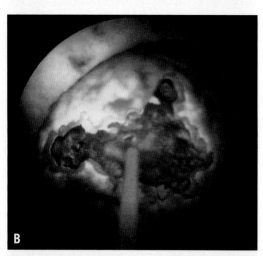

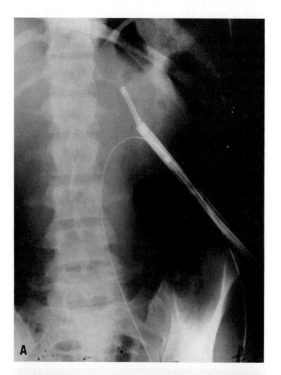

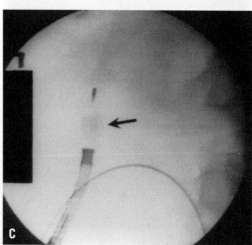

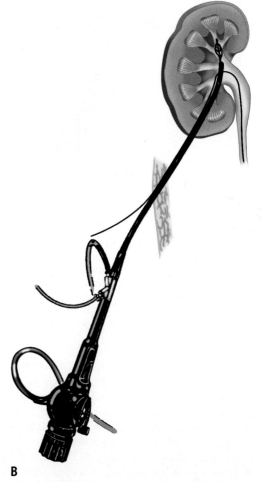

mentation and extraction of the stone may be severely hampered by limitations in the length of available instrumentation (Figure 17-11). In our experience, this can be overcome by allowing the tract to mature for several days following the initial dilation and placement of a large caliber nephrostomy tube. In most cases, maturation of the tract allows the kidney to fall back posteriorly closer to the skin level such that access with standard nephroscopic instrumentation can then be accomplished. Additionally, a mature tract can be used to pass readily available alternative instruments, such as standard rigid cystoscopes that are longer than most available nephroscopes, or flexible instruments that also have a longer working length. Fortunately, some manufacturers now offer "obese set" instrumentation, including working sheaths and rigid nephroscopes of significantly longer length.

One alternative that has been proposed for percutaneous management of such patients is the use of a flank position. One advantage of this position is that it may result in less restriction of respiratory-dependent chest wall movement. This also facilitates ventilation and anesthesia access. Additionally, a flank position allows the abdominal pannus to fall anteriorly. This may decrease the amount of tissue to traverse to allow easier access to the kidney.[21]

Despite the difficulties inherent in percutaneous stone management in morbidly obese patients, in experienced hands there is little difference in overall success rates and ultimate morbidity when comparing obese and non-obese patients.[22]

An analogous contraindication to ESWL regarding body habitus considerations occurs in those patients with severe scoliosis or body contractures preventing adequate positioning of the stone for ESWL. In such patients, access is again a major consideration because of the altered anatomy. Because the kidney in such patients may be located relatively anteriorly, another consideration in providing safe access is prevention of injury to adjacent solid or hollow viscera. We

Figure 17-7 *A*, Holmium laser lithotripsy has replaced EHL at most centers, including ours. *B*, Nephroscopic view of a renal pelvic stone with a 500 micron Holmium laser in place.

ing more than 300 pounds cannot be positioned adequately to get their stone either to the focal point or within the "powerpath" of an extracorporeally generated shockwave. In these patients, essentially all phases of percutaneous stone management are more difficult due to the patient's size. Both percutaneous access and tract dilation are more difficult, at least in part because the fluoroscopic image will be compromised. Once an adequate tract has been established, actual frag-

Figure 17-8 *A*, Radiographic view of flexible nephroscope in place through a working sheath. *B*,* Diagramatic representation of stone basket extraction via a flexible nephroscope. *C*, Fluoroscopic control of stone basket extraction via flexible nephroscope. *Reproduced with permission from Streem SB, Zelch MG, Risius B, Geisinger MA. Percutaneous extraction of renal calculi. Urol Clin North Am 1985;12:381.

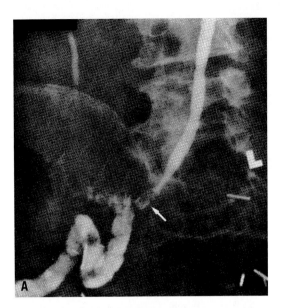

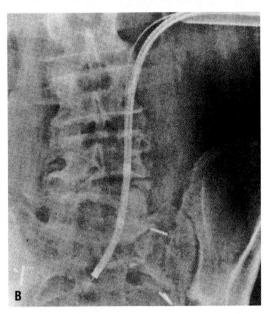

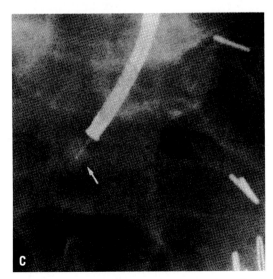

Figure 17-9 *A,* Antegrade nephrostogram reveals an obstructing stone at the left ureteroileal anastomosis in this patient with a urinary diversion. *B,* Flexible ureteroscope has been passed in an antegrade fashion to the level of the stone for subsequent laser lithotripsy. *C,* Note laser fiber in place abutted against the stone.

recently reported the use of computed tomography (CT) guided access in patients with complicated anomalies.[23] This technique can be invaluable for many patients with anomalies such as severe scoliosis, postrenal colon, or pelvic kidneys as illustrated in Figure 17-12.

Cystine Stones While small cystine stones may be managed successfully with ESWL,[24] in our experience, most cystinuric patients requiring intervention have large stones that fragment poorly with that modality. Fortunately, cystine stones are very amenable to ultrasonic lithotripsy (Figure 17-13). Currently, percutaneous ultrasonic nephrolithotomy remains the preferred approach for the majority of cystinuric patients requiring intervention.[25] But ureteroscopic management is now also being applied with increasing frequency to this group of patients.

Upper Tract Foreign Bodies The increasingly frequent use of self-retaining internal stents, nephrostomy tubes and dilating balloons in urologic practice has led to a corresponding increase in the number of patients with upper tract foreign bodies. The endoscopic management of bladder and urethral foreign bodies has long been a mainstay of urologic practice, and these principles are now being applied to management of patients with upper tract foreign bodies.[26] In many patients, these foreign bodies can be managed ureteroscopically in a retrograde fashion. However, a ureteroscopic approach may be precluded by a prior urinary diversion, formation of large calculi on the foreign body, or simple failure of ureteroscopic access. When ureteroscopic management is contraindicated or has failed for any of these reasons, a percutaneous approach is indicated. Site of access to the foreign body is chosen as for any stone, and this depends on its size and location. Standard nephroscopic instrumentation, including rigid forceps, graspers, and baskets may be utilized in conjunction with fragmentation of associated stones by intracorporeal lithotripsy with ultrasound or the Holmium laser (Figure 17-14).

Distal Obstruction Successful ESWL requires spontaneous passage of stone fragments. Therefore, obstruction distal to a stone remains a contraindication to ESWL as primary therapy. In most affected patients, the obstruction will relate to the ureter or ureteropelvic junction (UPJ), though the same principle applies to stones in caliceal diverticula, or stones associated with significant infundibular narrowing or true stenosis. Percutaneous management of these patients provides an ideal opportunity to both remove the stone and provide permanent relief of obstruction.

UPJ Obstruction The role of endopyelotomy for patients with UPJ obstruction is discussed in detail elsewhere (see Chapter 89, "Management of UPJ Obstruction: Laparoscopic Pyeloplasty in Children"). However, stone disease is encountered with relative frequency in association with UPJ obstruction. In these patients, percutaneous stone extraction with simultaneous endopyelotomy is an excellent alternative to open lithotomy and pyelo-

plasty.[27] Percutaneous stone extraction is performed in a standard manner and should precede the actual internal incision of the UPJ to prevent extravasation of irrigant or even loss of stone fragments during intracorporeal lithotripsy. Another caveat for this procedure is that the percutaneous access itself is best accomplished via superolateral calyx or infundibulum that allows direct endoscopic visualization of the UPJ with rigid instrumentation (Figure 17-15). At the completion of the stone extraction and endopyelotomy, an endopyelotomy stent is left indwelling for 4 to 6 weeks. Our preference is to use a tapered 10/7F stent for this.

Infundibular Stenosis or Narrowing Stones in calyces drained by long, narrow infundibula or truly stenotic infundibula respond well with percutaneous management. The best approach to such stones is a direct one to the involved calyx. Often times, subsequent access through the involved infundibulum cannot be obtained until the stone is extracted. Therefore, both the working and safety wires may be coiled in the involved calyx. Once the nephroscope is introduced, the infundibulum may be visualized under direct vision. Once such access is obtained, the infundibulum can be dilated using either sequential fascial dilators or a dilating balloon under direct vision, fluoroscopic control, or both. Following complete stone extraction and dilation of the infundibulum, a large-caliber nephrostomy

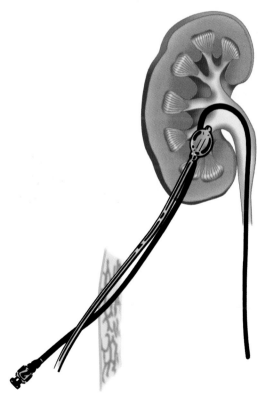

Figure 17-10 Tamponade and drainage of the tract is accomplished utilizing a 22F or 24F Foley nephrostomy tube. A 6F pyeloureteral catheter is left alongside as a safety precaution. This allows rapid access back to the collecting system should that be required for any reason. Reproduced with permission from Streem SB, Zelch MG, Risius B, Geisinger MA. Percutaneous extraction of renal calculi. Urol Clin North Am 1985;12:381.

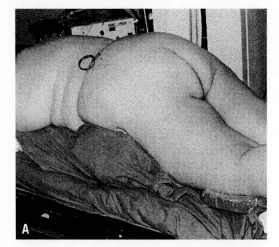

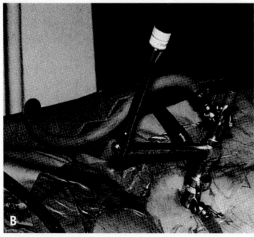

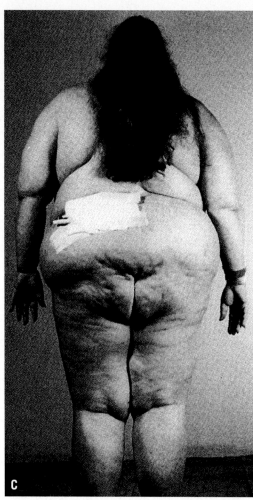

Figure 17-11 *A*, Positioning of a patient for percutaneous stone extraction in the setting of a body habitus that precludes ESWL. *B*, Nephroscope is in place in this patient all the way to its hub. At such times, standard instrumentation may not provide immediate access to the renal calculi. *C*, Despite the problems inherent in percutaneous stone extraction in such patients, the "end" result can still be rewarding.

tube is left indwelling across the infundibulum into the renal pelvis (Figure 17-16).

Caliceal Diverticula Stones in caliceal diverticula are often amenable to a percutaneous approach with techniques analogous to those described for patients with stenotic infundibula.[28,29] The best candidates are those in whom the diverticulum is posterior in the collecting system as determined by a CT scan (Figure 17-17). Again, ideal access involves direct puncture of the caliceal diverticulum in which the working and safety wires are coiled. Following nephroscopic removal of the stone, the diverticular neck may be better visualized for direct passage of a wire and subsequent dilatation (Figure 17-18). An excellent adjunct to help identify the diverticular neck in these patients is cystoscopic placement of an open-end ureteral catheter to the renal pelvis at the outset of the procedure. During nephroscopic examination of the diverticulum, methylene blue can be injected in a retrograde fashion to allow ready identification of the diverticular neck.

Cardiac Pacemakers and Defibrillators: Proximate Calcified Arterial Aneurysms The presence of a cardiac pacemaker or implanted defibrillator is no longer an absolute contraindication to ESWL.[30,31] The presence of an implanted defibrillator, however, often precludes that treatment because the stone can be obscured from vision in at least one plane. As such, percutaneous management becomes a primary modality for many of these patients. Likewise, the presence of a proximate calcified aortic or renal artery aneurysm has been considered a contraindication to ESWL, and therefore, an indication for percutaneous extraction. Several studies however, suggest that even these patients, when properly selected, may be treated safely with ESWL.[32–34] When ESWL is considered inappropriate in any of these cases, percutaneous management can be accomplished in a straightforward fashion using standard techniques described earlier.

Large or Complex Calculi For patients with large, extensively branched, or otherwise complex stones, a percutaneous approach alone may be used definitively.[35–37] The best candidates for percutaneous management of large stones are those in whom the stone burden is primarily central (Figure 17-19).

For patients with more extensively branched or complex stones, two or more percutaneous tracts can be used for definitive treatment (Figure 17-20).

Even very large and complex stones can be managed with percutaneous monotherapy (Fig-

ure 17-21). Multi-tract treatment is being used for these stones with increasing frequency at most centers, including ours.

Percutaneous management can also be used as a primary approach for debulking prior to adjunctive ESWL as part of a planned combination

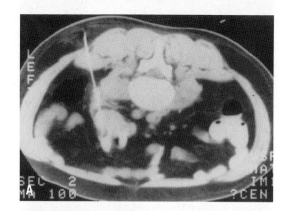

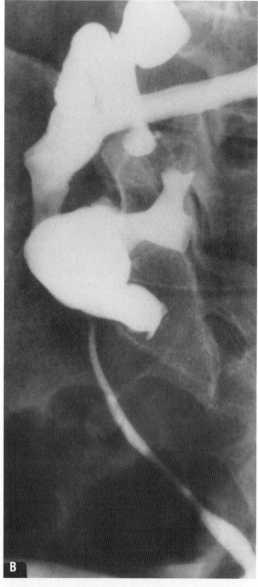

Figure 17-12 *A*, Computed tomography guided percutaneous access to a left pelvic kidney. Note the anterior location of the kidney and multiple loops of bowel interposed posteriorly. *B*, Nephrostogram shows access to the upper infundibulocalyx in this pelvic kidney. Again note the anterior location of the kidney.

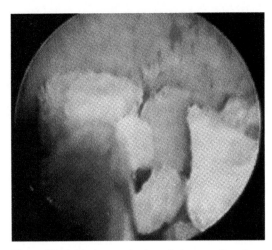

Figure 17-13 Nephroscopic view of a large cystine stone, which has been easily fragmented with ultrasound.

rate that ensures a sustained diuresis. For those patients with documented urinary infection associated with the stone disease, specific antibiotic therapy is continued intravenously for at least 48 to 72 hours in the hospital, and then orally at least until the first follow-up visit. In those patients with sterile urine initially, prophylactic antibiotic coverage can be discontinued within 48 hours of uncomplicated stone extraction.

A nephrostogram is generally obtained 48 hours following stone removal. Any residual fragments seen on this study that appear accessible to the percutaneous tract can be managed by repeat rigid or flexible nephroscopy that can often be performed with light intravenous sedation. If there are no residual stones, and no obstruction or extravasation are noted on the nephrostogram, the pyeloureteral catheter is

removed. The nephrostomy tube is then clamped for 12 to 24 hours and removed if there has been no flank pain, fever or significant drainage around the tube. The patient can then be discharged with a light dressing and allowed to return to full pre-hospitalization activity and employment 10 days following the procedure.

In those cases where extravasation or obstruction is noted on the initial nephrostogram, the nephrostomy tube is left to drainage and serial studies obtained until the problem resolves. Ureteral obstruction noted at this time is usually the result of blood clots that will lyse, or edema that should subside spontaneously. Occasionally, obstruction can result from small stone fragments in the ureter that will often pass spontaneously, or may be managed with antegrade or retrograde manipulation.

approach (Figure 17-22).[38–41] In such cases, the initial percutaneous procedure reduces the stone burden for subsequent ESWL. Furthermore, these patients often have infection-related struvite stones, so that placement of a large caliber nephrostomy tube at the termination of the percutaneous procedure prevents obstruction with the potential for bacteremia and sepsis during passage of fragments subsequent to the ESWL. A secondary percutaneous procedure is generally done through the mature tract within 48 hours of the ESWL to hasten clearance of stone fragments and allow early nephrostomy tube removal.

FAILED ESWL

Almost any patient who has failed ESWL can be managed successfully with a percutaneous approach as a "salvage" procedure. Failure of ESWL in these patients may have resulted because the stone was physically too hard for adequate extracorporeal fragmentation. Alternatively, ESWL may have been used for a patient in whom the stone burden was excessive at the outset. In these cases, the initial procedure should generally be percutaneous nephrostomy drainage to allow recovery of function and treatment of any associated infection. Once the patient has been stabilized, tract dilation and stone manipulation proceed in a standard fashion. Often times, patients who have failed ESWL have many associated ureteral fragments. Following management of the pyelocaliceal stones, the ureteral fragments can be extracted in an antegrade or retrograde fashion, or with a combined approach (Figure 17-23).

POSTOPERATIVE CARE

An accurate estimate of irrigation and output is imperative during and following the procedure. Generally, 20 mg furosemide is given intravenously at the termination of the percutaneous procedure. Vital signs are monitored closely and serial blood counts are obtained as determined by the course of the procedure. For approximately 24 hours postoperatively, intravenous fluids are administered at a

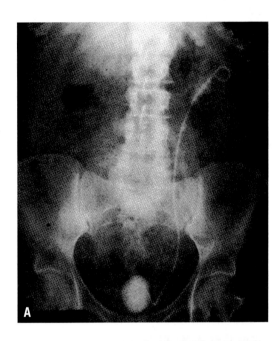

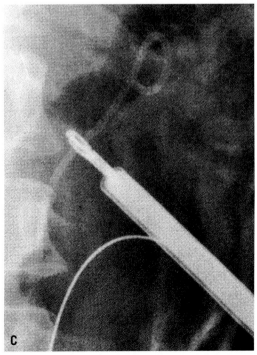

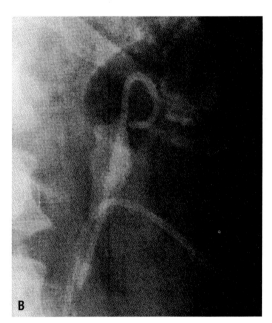

Figure 17-14 *A*, Plain x-ray reveals a left-sided internal stent with a large renal pelvic and bladder calcification. *B*, The bladder stone and distal part of the stent had been removed leaving only the proximal end of the stent and the large renal pelvic calcification. Percutaneous access is accomplished as for any renal pelvic stone. *C*, Following ultrasonic fragmentation and evacuation of the calcification associated with the stent, the stent is removed under direct vision with rigid forceps via the nephroscope. Reproduced with permission from Troy RB, Streem SB, Zelch MG. Percutaneous management of upper tract foreign bodies. J Endourol 1994;8:43.

RESULTS

Percutaneous nephrolithotomy is a well-established procedure with proven safety and efficacy. In a community setting, nearly 90% of targeted stones can be successfully removed[42] while at tertiary care centers, this figure approaches 100%.[43–45] Early morbidity remains acceptably low, even for complex stones or in complex patients.[4,22] Furthermore, patients can expect early return to pre-hospitalization employment and recreational activities, especially in comparison to open operative intervention.[5–8] Most importantly, morphologic and functional studies have repeatedly shown that percutaneous nephrolithotomy has little, if any, clinically significant deleterious effect on renal function,[46–51] even in patients with preexisting renal insufficiency or anatomically solitary kidneys.[52,53]

CONCLUSIONS

The contemporary indications for percutaneous management of upper-tract calculi have narrowed since the introduction of ESWL and flexible ureteroscopic access to the pyelocaliceal system. In fact, patients with upper-tract stones are often treated percutaneously only when ESWL is contraindicated or has failed. Despite the increasing complexity of the patients and stones managed percutaneously, rates of residual stones, complications, and morbidity remain acceptably low, especially in comparison to the alternative of open operative intervention.

Percutaneous management of renal calculi is a safe, well-established part of the urologic armamentarium that is almost universally applicable whenever ESWL is contraindicated or has failed.

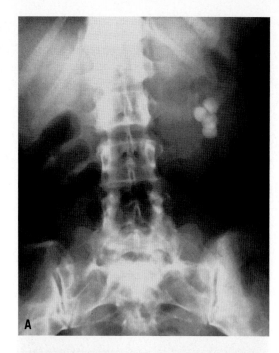
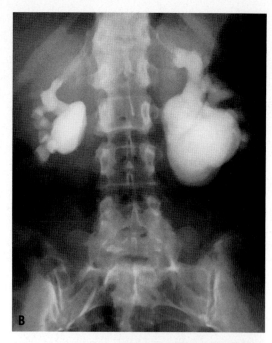
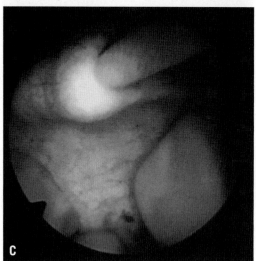
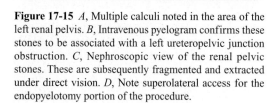
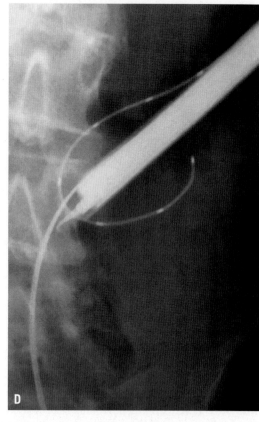

Figure 17-15 *A*, Multiple calculi noted in the area of the left renal pelvis. *B*, Intravenous pyelogram confirms these stones to be associated with a left ureteropelvic junction obstruction. *C*, Nephroscopic view of the renal pelvic stones. These are subsequently fragmented and extracted under direct vision. *D*, Note superolateral access for the endopyelotomy portion of the procedure.

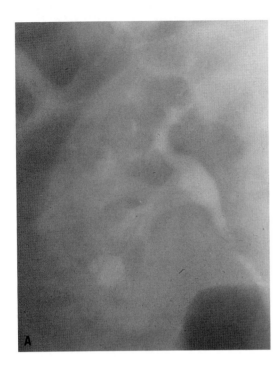

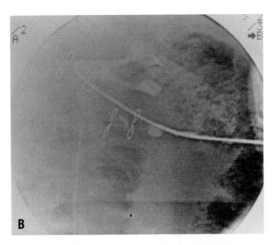

Figure 17-16 *A*, Large lower lateral caliceal stone was associated with a long, narrow infundibulum precluding successful treatment with ESWL. *B*, Optimal access is directly to the involved calyx (fluoroscopic view). *C*, Percutaneous ultrasonic fragmentation of the caliceal calculus. A safety wire remains in place across the involved infundibulum. *D*, Following stone extraction, the narrow infundibulum is dilated under fluoroscopic control with fascial dilators or a balloon catheter.

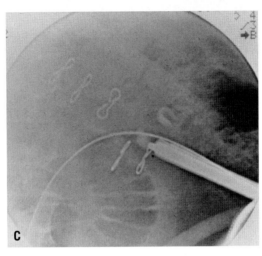

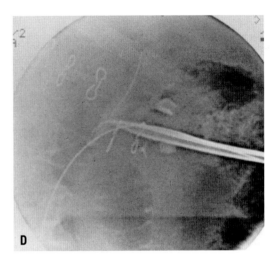

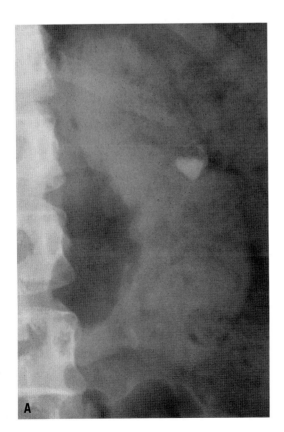

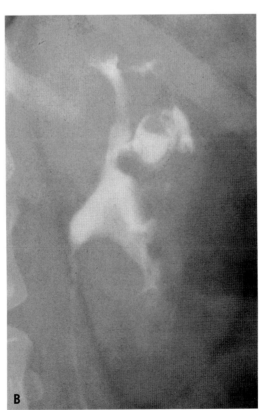

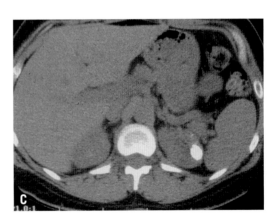

Figure 17-17 *A*, Plain film reveals "milk of calcium" suggestive of stone-filled caliceal diverticulum. *B*, Pyelogram confirms this as caliceal diverticular stone. *C*, Computed tomography confirms posterior location, making this ideally suited to a percutaneous approach.

Figure 17-18 *A*, Multiple stones suggestive of a caliceal diverticulum of the right kidney. *B*, Pyelogram confirms stones in a caliceal diverticulum. *C*, Optimal percutaneous access is directly into the diverticulum. *D*, Stones removed percutaneously from this caliceal diverticulum. *E*, Following extraction of the stones, the diverticular neck is dilated. Nephrostomy drainage is in place across the dilated diverticular neck with the tip of the nephrostomy tube now in the renal pelvis. *F*, Follow-up pyelogram confirms resolution of the stones and diverticulum.

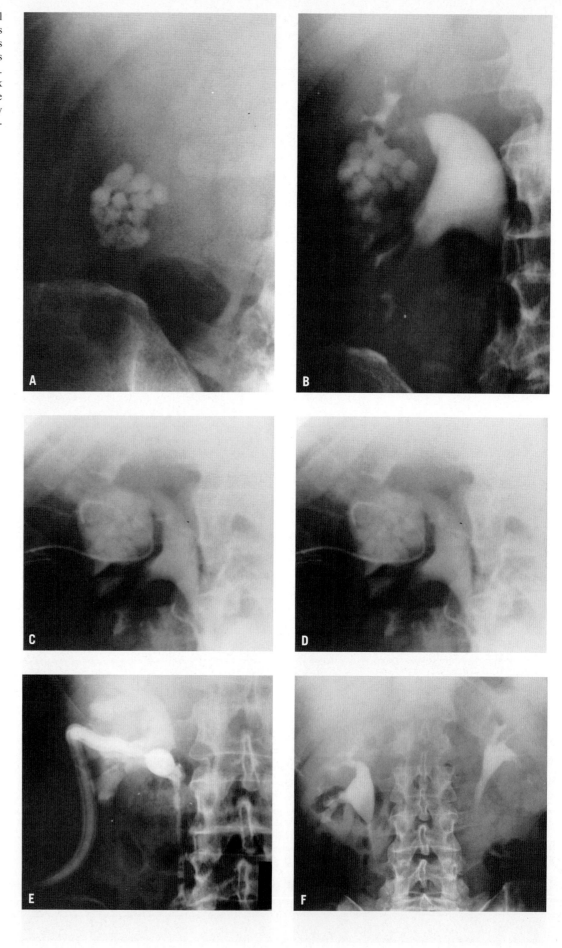

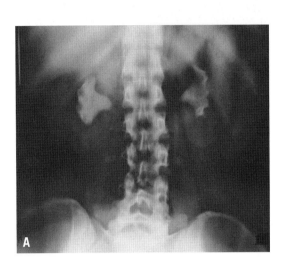

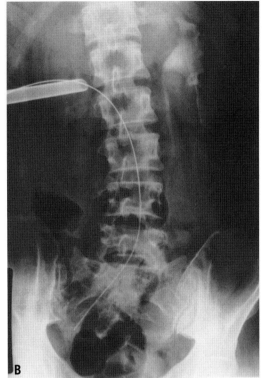

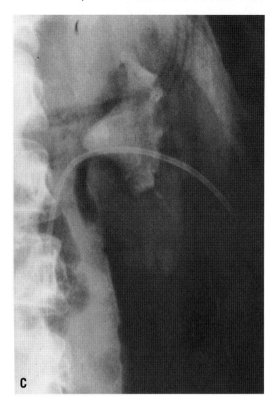

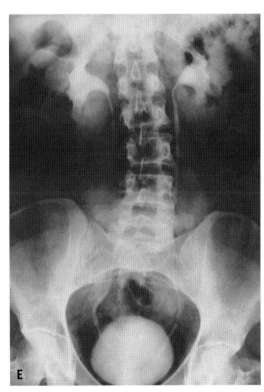

Figure 17-19 *A*, Plain x-ray reveals bilateral staghorn calculi with a "central" stone burden. *B*, Percutaneous management of right staghorn calculus via single tract. *C*, Simultaneous bilateral treatment can be performed safely in select cases. Access to the left sided stone, again via single tract, is seen here. *D*, Plain x-ray one month following percutaneous management of bilateral staghorn calculi reveals a stone-free result. *E*, Intravenous urogram confirms an excellent anatomic and functional result.

Figure 17-20 *A*, For this branched stone with a duplex configuration, adequate access is better achieved via two tracts. *B*, Nephroscope is in place for management of the lower aspect of the stone. Note access via the upper pole that will be used for management of that portion of the stone.

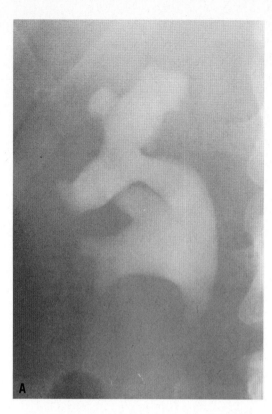

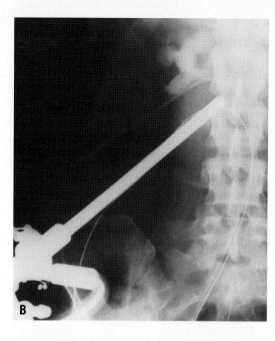

Figure 17-21 *A*, Plain film reveals large, fully mature branched calculus. *B*, Seven tracts were required for complete stone clearance. *C*, Plain film following this complicated muti-tract approach confirms a stone-free result.

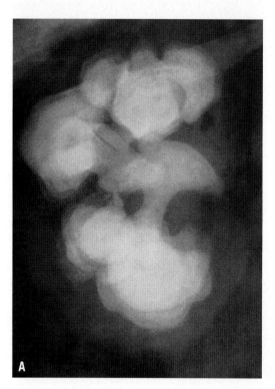

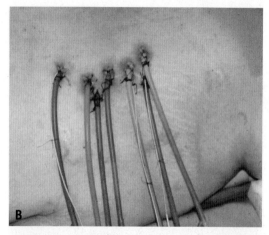

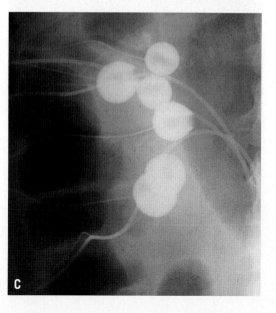

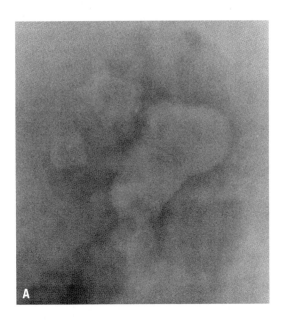

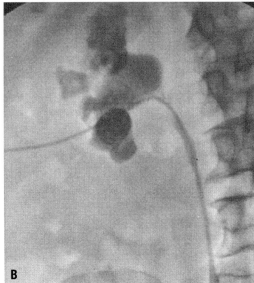

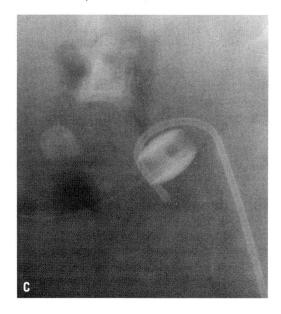

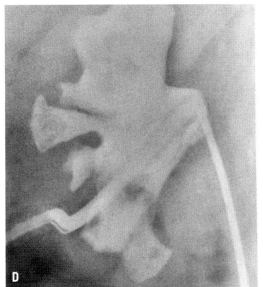

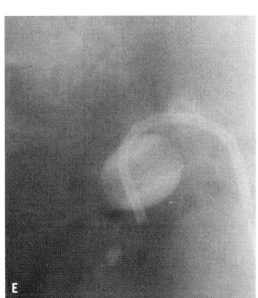

Figure 17-22 *A,* Large, complex, staghorn calculus filling the pelvis and essentially all infundibula and calyces. *B,* Single access for debulking of the stone prior to planned shock wave lithotripsy. *C,* Plain x-ray following debulking reveals a few remaining inaccessible caliceal calculi. *D,* Nephrostogram at this time confirms the inaccessible location of the remaining calculi to this tract. Complete percutaneous management, however, would require at least two more tracts. *E,* As an alternative to further percutaneous management, the remaining inaccessible calculi have been managed with ESWL. Note excellent fragmentation. *F,* Twenty-four hours later, the previously inaccessible gravel has now become accessible and is removed via the mature tract under local anesthesia. *G,* Follow up nephrostogram confirms an excellent anatomic result.

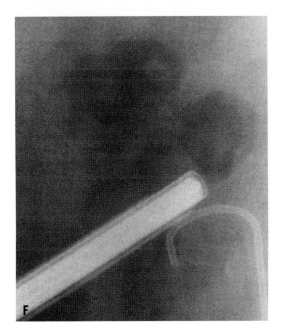

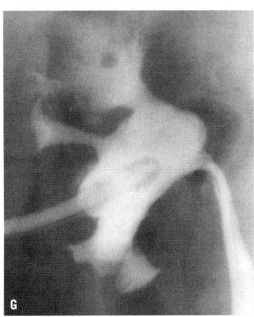

Figure 17-23 *A*, Large renal calculus. This stone burden precludes successful management with ESWL. *B*, Following ESWL, the patient was referred with stone fragments completely filling the upper collecting system. A stent that had been placed pre-ESWL had migrated distally. *C*, Management of this complication requires initial percutaneous drainage. This allows recovery of function and subsequent access for management of the pyelocaliceal and upper ureteral stone fragments. *D*, Remaining ureteral stones can be managed ureteroscopically. During this time, fragments may migrate back to the renal pelvis, and these are then removed via the mature percutaneous tract.

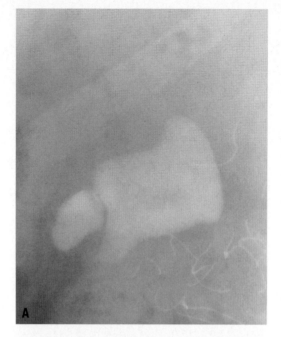
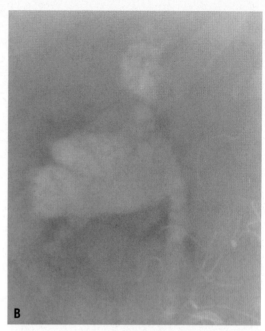
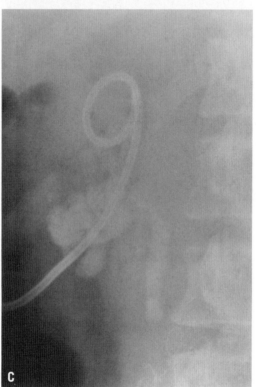
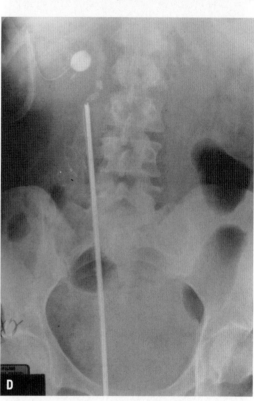

REFERENCES

1. Rupel E, Brown R. Nephroscopy with removal of stone following nephrostomy for obstructive calculous anuria. J Urol 1941;46:177.

2. Goodwin WE, Casey WC, Woolf W. Percutaneous trocar (needle) nephrostomy in hydronephrosis. J Am Med Assoc 1955;157:891–4.

3. Fernstrom I, Johansson B. Percutaneous pyelolithotomy: A new extraction technique. Scand J Urol Nephrol 1976;10:257–9.

4. LeRoy AJ, Segura JW, Williams HJ Jr, Patterson DE. Percutaneous renal calculus removal in an extracorporeal shock wave lithotripsy practice. J Urol 1987;138:703–6.

5. Preminger GM, Clayman RV, Hardeman SW. Percutaneous nephrostolithotomy vs open surgery for renal calculi. A comparative study. JAMA 1985;254:1054–8.

6. Brannen GE, Bush WH, Correa RJ, et al. Kidney stone removal: Percutaneous versus surgical lithotomy. J Urol 1985;133:6–12.

7. Burns JR, Hamrick LC, Keller FS. Percutaneous nephrolithotomy in 86 patients: analysis of results and costs. South Med J 1986;79:975–8.

8. Brown MW, Carson CC III, Dunnick NR, Weinerth JL. Comparison of the costs and morbidity of percutaneous and open flank procedures. J Urol 1986;135:1150–2.

9. Feng MI, Tamaddon K, Mikhail A, et al. Prospective randomized study of various techniques of percutaneous nephrolithotomy. Urology 2001;58:345–50.

10. Alken P, Hutschenreiter G, Gunther R, Marberger M. Percutaneous stone manipulation. J Urol 1981;125:463–6.

11. Marberger M, Stackl W, Hruby W. Percutaneous litholapaxy of renal calculi with ultrasound. Eur Urol 1982;8:236–42.

12. Segura JW, Patterson DE, LeRoy AJ, et al. Percutaneous stone removal of kidney stones: preliminary report. Mayo Clin Proc 1982;57:615–9.

13. Clayman RV, Surya V, Miller RP, et al. Percutaneous nephrolithotomy: extraction of renal and ureteral calculi from 100 patients. J Urol 1984;131:868–71.

14. Schultz RE, Hanno PM, Wein AJ, et al. Percutaneous ultrasonic lithotripsy: Choice of irrigant. J Urol 1983;130:858–60.

15. Kuo RL, Paterson RF, Siqueira TM Jr, et al. In vitro assessment of ultrasonic lithotriptors. J Urol 2003;170:1101–4.

16. Clayman RV. Techniques in percutaneous removal of renal calculi. Mechanical extraction and electrohydraulic lithotripsy. Urology 1984;23:11–9.

17. Auge BK, Lallas CD, Pietrow PK, et al. In vitro comparison of standard ultrasound and pneumatic lithotrites with a new combination intracorporeal lithotripsy device. Urology 2002;60:28–32.

18. Lange PH, Reddy PK, Hulbert JC, et al. Percutaneous removal of caliceal and other "inaccessible" stones: Instruments and techniques. J Urol 1984;132:439–42.

19. Limb J, Bellman GC. Tubeless percutaneous renal surgery: Review of first 112 patients. Urology 2002;59:527–31.

20. Thomas R, Cass AS. Extracorporeal shock wave lithotripsy in morbidly obese patients. J Urol 1993;150:30–2.

21. Kerbl K, Clayman RV, Chandhoke PS, et al. Percutaneous stone removal with the patient in a flank position. J Urol 1994;151:686–8.

22. Carson CC III, Danneberger JE, Weinerth JL. Percutaneous lithotripsy in morbid obesity. J Urol 1988;139:243–2456.

23. Matlaga BR, Shah OD, Zagoria RJ, et al. Computerized tomography guided access for percutaneous nephrostolithotomy. J Urol 2003;170:45–7.

24. Bhatta KM, Prien EL Jr, Dretler SP. Cystine calculi-rough and smooth: A new clinical distinction. J Urol 1989;142:937–40.

25. Streem SB. Medical and surgical management of cystine stones. Problems in Urology 1993;7:523.

26. Troy RB, Streem SB, Zelch MG. Percutaneous management of upper tract foreign bodies. J Endourol 1994;8:43–7.

27. Motola JA, Badlani GH, Smith AD. Results of 212 consecutive endopyelotomies: an 8-year followup. J Urol 1993;149:453–6.

28. Hulbert JC, Reddy PK, Hunter DW, et al. Percutaneous techniques for the management of caliceal diverticula containing calculi. J Urol 1986;135:225–7.

29. Bennett JD, Broan TC, Kozak RI, et al. Transdiverticular percutaneous nephrostomy for caliceal diverticular stones: J Endourol 1992;6:55.

30. Cooper D, Wilkoff B, Masterson M, et al. Effects of extracorporeal shock wave lithotripsy on cardiac pacemakers and its safety in patients with implanted cardiac pacemakers. Pacing Clin Electrophysiol 1988;11:1607–16.

31. Chung MK, Streem SB, Ching E, et al. Effects of extracorporeal shock wave lithotripsy on tiered therapy implantable cardioverter defibrillators. Pacing Clin Electrophysiol 1999;22:738–42.

32. Carey SW, Streem SB. Extracorporeal shock wave lithotripsy for patients with calcified ipsilateral renal arterial or abdominal aortic aneurysms. J Urol 1992;148:18–20.

33. Vasavada SP, Streem SB, Kottke-Marchant K, Novick AC. Pathological effects of extracorporeally generated shock waves on calcified aortic aneurysm tissue. J Urol 1994;152:45–8.

34. Deliveliotis C, Kostakopoulos A, Stavropoulos N, et al. Extracorporeal shock wave lithotripsy in 5 patients with aortic aneurysm. J Urol 1995;154:1671–2.

35. Clayman RV, Surya V, Miller RP, et al. Percutaneous nephrolithotomy: an approach to branched and staghorn renal calculi. JAMA 1983;250:73–5.

36. Snyder JA, Smith AD. Staghorn calculi: Percutaneous extraction versus anatrophic nephrolithotomy. J Urol 1986;136:351–4.

37. Winfield HN, Clayman RV, Chaussy CG, et al. Monotherapy of staghorn renal calculi: a comparative study between percutaneous nephrolithotomy and extracorporeal shock wave lithotripsy. J Urol 1988;139:895–9.

38. Schulze H, Hertle L. Graff J. et al. Combined treatment of branched calculi by percutaneous nephrolithotomy and extracorporeal shock wave lithotripsy. J Urol 1986;135:1138–41.

39. Kahnoski RJ, Lingeman JE, Coury TA, et al. Combined percutaneous and extracorporeal shock wave lithotripsy for staghorn calculi: an alternative to anatrophic nephrolithotomy. J Urol 1986;135:679–81.

40. Streem SB, Geisinger MA, Risius B, et al. Endourologic "sandwich" therapy for extensive staghorn calculi. J Endourol 1987;1:253.

41. Segura JW, Preminger GM, Assimos DG, et al. Nephrolithiasis Clinical Guidelines Panel summary report on the management of staghorn calculi. The American Association Nephrolithiasis Clinical Guidelines Panel. J Urol 1994;151:1648–51.

42. Bass RB Jr, Beard JH, Looner WH, et al. Percutaneous ultrasonic lithotripsy in the community hospital. J Urol 1985;133:586.

43. Reddy PK, Hulbert JC, Lange PH, et al. Percutaneous removal of renal and ureteral calculi: experience with 400 cases. J Urol 1985;134:662–5.

44. Segura JW, Patterson DE, LeRoy AJ, et al. Percutaneous removal of kidney stones: review of 1,000 cases. J Urol 1985;134:1077–81.

45. Lee WJ, Smith AD, Cubelli V, Vernace FM. Percutaneous nephrolithotomy: analysis of 500 consecutive cases. Urol Radiol 1986;8:61–6.

46. Mayo ME, Krieger JN, Rudd TG. Effect of percutaneous nephrostolithotomy on renal function. J Urol 1985;133:167–9.

47. Marberger M, Stackl W, Hruby W, Kroiss A. Late sequelae of ultrasonic lithotripsy of renal calculi. J Urol 1985;133:170–3.

48. Webb DR, Fitzpatrick JM. Percutaneous nephrostolithotripsy: a functional and morphological study. J Urol 1985;134:587–91.

49. Chatham JR, Dykes TE, Kennon WG, Schwartz BF. Effect of percutaneous nephrolithotomy on differential renal function as measured by mercaptoacetyl triglycine nuclear renography [Discussion 525–526]. Urology 2002;59:522–5.

50. Schiff RG, Lee WJ, Esghi M, et al. Morphologic and functional changes in the kidney after percutaneous nephrostolithotomy. AJR Am J Roentgnol 1986;147:283–6.

51. Geterud K, Henriksson CH, Pettersson S, Zachrisson BF. Computed tomography after percutaneous stone extraction. Acta Radiol 1987;28:55–8.

52. Chandhoke PS, Albala DM, Clayman RV. Long-term comparison of renal function in patients with solitary kidneys and/or moderate renal insufficiency undergoing shock wave lithotripsy or percutaneous nephrolithotomy. J Urol 1992;147:1226–30.

53. Liou LS, Streem SB. Long-term renal functional effects of shock wave lithotripsy, percutaneous nephrolithotomy and combination therapy: a comparative study of patients with solitary kidney [Discussion 36–37]. J Urol 2001;166:36.

18

Percutaneous Treatment of Ureteral Stones

Christopher J. Kane, MD

Jason W. Anast, MD

Marshall L. Stoller, MD

INDICATIONS

Percutaneous nephrolithotomy (PCNL) was introduced in the 1970s by Fernstrom and Johansson.[1] Throughout the 1980s, the technique was refined by the pioneers of endourology[2,3] and was a major advance over open surgery for the treatment of renal and ureteral stones. Over the past two decades, enhancements to percutaneous instrumentation have paralleled technical advances through the development of smaller fiberoptic endoscopes, flexible endoscopes, and new intracorporeal lithotrites, improving the efficacy and safety of percutaneous management. The treatment of upper ureteral stones changed dramatically, however, with the advent of extracorporeal shock wave lithotripsy (ESWL)[4] and ureteroscopy.[5]

The American Urological Association ureteral stones guidelines describe the recommendations for the management of ureteral calculi.[6] The majority of small ureteral stones (< 5 mm) will pass spontaneously.[7] Distal ureteral stones under 1 cm in diameter can be treated successfully with either extracorporeal shock wave lithotripsy or ureteroscopy. Over 1 cm distal ureteral stones are usually approached ureteroscopically, but ESWL may be appropriate in some cases. For proximal ureteral stones under 1 cm, either ESWL or ureteroscopy is appropriate, with endoscopy employed for ESWL failures. Stones > 1 cm can be treated with ESWL, although success rates fall and re-treatment rates increase in this size range. Ureteroscopy in the proximal ureter now achieves high stone-free rates with minimal morbidity.[8] For select patients with larger stones in the proximal ureter, antegrade percutaneous management may be the most efficient and appropriate treatment. We'll review the clinical situations in which percutaneous management is most commonly employed.

Large proximal ureteral stones, particularly those over 1.5 cm and impacted, are candidates for percutaneous treatment. (Figure 18-1). Percutaneous treatment can often be performed with intact stone removal, avoiding the likelihood of residual fragments and repeat procedures. The attractiveness of the definitive nature of the procedure must be weighed against the increased pain and morbidity of percutaneous treatment when compared to ureteroscopy. One of the advantages of percutaneous treatment is that the urologist is working through the dilated portion of the urinary tract and can therefore use larger endoscopes and remove larger stones and fragments.

Occasionally patients have distal ureteral abnormalities that make retrograde access difficult or impossible. Examples are those with previous crossed trigonal ureteral implantations for vesicoureteral reflux or preexisting ureteral strictures. In these cases, antegrade passage of stone fragments after ESWL and retrograde access with a ureteroscope is difficult, making percutaneous management attractive.

Failed ESWL cases are often first managed by ureteroscopy, but failed ureteroscopy cases may be amenable to an antegrade approach. Very hard stones such as cysteine or calcium oxalate monohydrate are more likely to fail ESWL (Figure 18-2). Depending on the intracorporeal lithotrite available, most hard stones can be effectively treated with ureteroscopy. In situations where ureteroscopy fails, however, an antegrade percutaneous approach is appropriate. At times, multiple retrograde access attempts may lead to ureteral injury or perforations distal to the stone. Percutaneous access may allow retrieval of stone fragments through the uninjured and dilated upper ureter.

Patients who have had a percutaneous nephrostomy tube placed to manage severe obstruction or infection proximal to an obstructing stone may also be ideal candidates for antegrade treatment.[9,10] Since a major part of the morbidity of percutaneous treatment of ureteral stones is related to obtaining access, patients with preexisting nephrostomy tracts are then exposed only to the morbidity of tract dilation and a 1 cm incision. The benefit may be more definitive treatment, with less need for re-treatment when compared to ureteroscopy.

One of the most common current indications for percutaneous management of ureteral stones is preexisting renal stone burden (Table 18-1). For patients with both renal and ureteral stones, options include ESWL or ureteroscopy of the ureteral stone first followed by appropriate treatment of the renal stone burden based on stone size, location, and patient anatomy. For patients with renal stone burdens who are good candidates for PCNL (ie, those with stones > 2.5 cm, lower-pole stones > 1.5 cm, or cysteine stones), percutaneous management of both renal and ureteral stones is ideal.

Although treatment of ureteral stones in children now parallels that in adults, small or young children with large proximal ureteral stone burdens may be well approached percutaneously.[11]

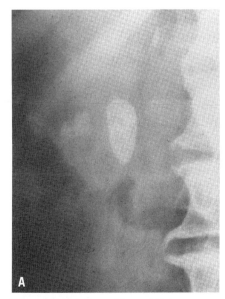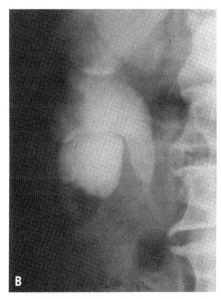

Figure 18-1 *A*, Scout film and *B*, intravenous pyelogram showing a large calculus, which is best treated by a percutaneous approach.

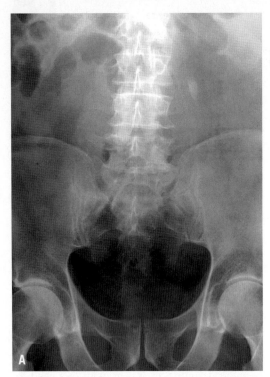 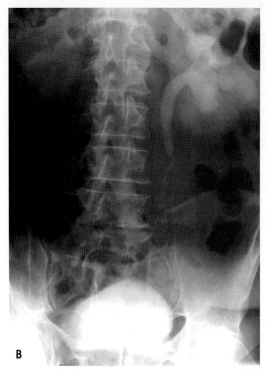

Figure 18-2 *A*, Scout film and *B*, intravenous pyelogram showing an upper ureteral stone that failed extracorporeal shock wave lithotripsy and was successfully treated percutaneously.

Multiple retrograde access attempts through very small caliber ureters can be technically difficult and treatment of large stone burdens with this technique may be inefficient. The morbidity of percutaneous treatment must be balanced with the morbidity of repeated retrograde access and perhaps repeat procedures or auxiliary procedures such as ESWL.

PATIENT PREPARATION

Assessment of current stone burden can be accomplished by different radiographic techniques. Intravenous pyelography (IVP) has been the traditional imaging study of choice because it reveals stone size and location and allows gross assessment of renal function and degree of obstruction. Non-contrast computed tomography (NCCT) replaced IVP as the imaging study of choice for patients with acute renal colic.[12,13] NCCT allows precise assessment of stone burden and gives indirect information concerning renal function (parenchymal thickness) as well as degree of obstruction (secondary signs of obstruction). It is limited in its assessment of intrarenal caliceal anatomy. In spite of that limitation, we often omit additional imaging other than NCCT prior to percutaneous management. When obtaining percutaneous access, a retrograde ureteral catheter is placed to facilitate percutaneous puncture, and intrarenal caliceal anatomy and puncture location is assessed at that juncture. If preoperative caliceal anatomy detail is desired prior to percutaneous puncture, IVP or retrograde pyelography should be obtained. For patients with impaired renal function or parenchymal loss on imaging, nuclear renal scintigraphy should be considered. Renal scan with MAG3 or DTPA can

assess differential renal function and degree of obstruction.[14] For nonfunctioning kidneys, laparoscopic nephrectomy may be more appropriate than complex stone treatment.

The patient's general health status should be assessed prior to any surgical intervention. Important preoperative information includes medical and surgical history with particular attention to cardiovascular risk factors. Where appropriate, anesthesia and medical assessment prior to general anesthesia is beneficial. Patients with extreme obesity or severe pulmonary disease may not tolerate the prone position typically employed for PCNL. Very obese patients may be better served with ureteroscopy than with percutaneous management, depending on the specific circumstances.[15] Patients with prior abdominal surgery, particularly procedures involving the retroperitoneum, colonic mobilization or renal or ureteral procedures, should have abdominal computed tomography (CT) prior to PCNL. CT allows visualization of the planned percutaneous approach to ensure colon or other intra-abdominal organs are not within the percutaneous tract.

Appropriate laboratory assessment includes a urinalysis and urine culture to exclude urinary infection or colonization. Serum electrolytes with serum creatinine for global renal function assessment. A complete blood count may be indicated in patients at risk for anemia and those with renal insufficiency. Clotting parameters should be assessed in patients with a history of bleeding diathesis, hepatic insufficiency, and prior medications affecting clotting factors or platelet dysfunction.

Preexisting urinary tract infection should be treated prior to percutaneous management. We usually use culture-directed oral antibiotics on an

outpatient basis prior to and throughout the period of stone manipulation and postoperatively until catheters are removed. In a patient with a negative preoperative urine culture, a single preoperative intravenous cephalosporin is given with further antibiotics directed by the clinical situation. If the patient has an intraoperative or postoperative fever, the antibiotics are continued until resolution or until all catheters are removed.[16]

INFORMED CONSENT

Informed consent should include a discussion of risks, benefits, expectations, and alternatives to the planned procedure. The alternatives are ESWL, ureteroscopy, open or laparoscopic surgery, and observation. Typically, when an antegrade percutaneous approach is considered, the patient or their stone may not be a good candidate for one or more of the alternatives. Open surgery is now very rare and is only contemplated after failed endoscopic management, simultaneous open surgery for a concomitant illness, or in select staghorn stones with intrarenal caliceal dilation.[17]

The expectations also depend on the clinical situation. For patients with a large proximal ureteral stone only, the patient can expect a 60- to 90-minute surgery, a 90% or higher stone-free rate, a Double-J ureteral stent postoperatively, and a brief period with a nephrostomy tube (up to 24 hours). Most patients go home on the first postoperative day without a nephrostomy tube. We typically remove the stent with a flexible cystoscope in the office in one to two weeks. Alternatively, if an antegrade ureteral stent is not placed, we remove the open-ended ureteral catheter on postoperative day one and clamp the nephrostomy tube that afternoon. If the patient tolerates the clamped tube, we either remove it on postoperative day two or send the patient home with a nephrostomy tube to be removed in the office. The chance of the patient requiring a blood transfusion is under 5%. It is important for patients to expect the possibility of gross hematuria occurring, which may wax and wane in intensity, for several weeks. If a patient has a more complex situation, such as a staghorn stone with a proximal ureteral stone, we alter our discussion of expectations to include a longer hospitalization, increased imaging post-procedure, and possible secondary procedures.

The benefits of the antegrade percutaneous approach are a definitive procedure with high

Table 18-1 Indications for Percutaneous Treatment of Ureteral Stones
Failed ESWL or ureteroscopy
Preexisting nephrostomy tube
Renal and ureteral stone burden
Distal ureteral stricture or access problem
Large proximal ureteral stones
Large proximal ureteral stones in children
ESWL = extracorporeal shock wave lithotripsy.

stone-free rates, low need for repeat or auxiliary procedures, and relatively low morbidity.

The potential risks or complications are numerous, although the most serious complications are fortunately rare. Potential complications include bleeding requiring transfusion, pulmonary injury, or hydro- or hemothorax, and injury to adjacent structures such as the colon, spleen, liver, duodenum, and pancreas. Fortunately, most adjacent organ injuries can be managed nonoperatively.[18] Injury to subcostal blood vessels is more likely with supracostal upper-pole punctures, although it is still rare.[19] Hydrothorax and pneumothorax are also more common in supracostal punctures, although they can usually be managed with simple aspiration or tube thoracostomy.[20,21] Ureteral perforations can occur and may contribute to future ureteral stricture formation, although the greatest risk factor for ureteral stricture appears to be stone impaction.[22] Extruded stone fragments can occur and may affect the appearance of future radiographs.[23] Sepsis can occur and is more common if struvite stones are treated; the incidence depends on the clinical situation and definition. Fever occurs in about 20% of patients undergoing PCNL. True sepsis, with tachycardia and hypotension is more rare, at less than 1% incidence, but may have serious sequelae.[24] The risk of cardiovascular complications such as perioperative myocardial infarction (MI), stroke, deep venous thrombosis (DVT), and pulmonary embolism (PE) depend on a patient's specific risk factors. Postoperative pneumonia, likewise, is rare, but the specific risk is unique depending on preexisting pulmonary and functional status.

PREOPERATIVE PREPARATION

The patient is without food after midnight the evening prior to the procedure. A formal bowel preparation is not necessary. If the preoperative urine culture is sterile, the patient receives a single preoperative dose of an intravenous first generation cephalosporin. Since transfusion is rare, perioperative autologous blood donation is not cost-effective and is not recommended.[25]

We perform urologist-obtained percutaneous access in the operating room. The sequence of events is different in cases where an interventional radiologist obtains access. The radiologist obtains access and nephrostomy tube placement either with ultrasonography or after percutaneous opacification of the collecting system. They typically do not use a ureteral catheter. The patient then arrives in the operating room with a nephrostomy tube in place and can be positioned prone after induction of general anesthesia.

For urologist-obtained access, the patient is placed in the lithotomy position and cystoscopy is performed with placement of an open-ended ureteral catheter or ureteral occlusion catheter. In cases of normal distal ureteral anatomy, fluoroscopy is not required for this portion of the procedure. If there is unusual ureteral anatomy, fluoroscopy may be helpful.

After the ureteral catheter is placed, it is taped to an indwelling Foley catheter. Intravenous extension tubing is connected to the open-ended catheter, and a 60 cc syringe with radiographic contrast material is connected for opacification of the collecting system.

The patient is then positioned prone on preplaced chest rolls on the fluoroscopically equipped operating room (OR) table. The patient is carefully padded and secured to the table. Other techniques of patient placement have been described, including performing the entire procedure, including ureteral catheter placement, with the patient in prone split-leg position.[26] Supine percutaneous nephrolithotomy has also been described, although it is not commonly performed in most centers.[27]

INSTRUMENTATION

Percutaneous access is achieved with a 20 gauge Chiba needle that allows a 0.035-inch removable core J-tipped guidewire to be passed into the collecting system. We use a 6 French and 8F fascial dilator followed by a 10F safety wire introducer catheter. A second guidewire is placed into the collecting system. Numerous wires are available as "working" wires with floppy tips and stiff (though slippery) middle portions. Examples include the Zebra or Lunderquist (Microvasive) wires.

Tract dilation is usually performed at our center with 30F radial balloons (Microvasive Nephromax or Cook) over which a 34F Amplatz sheath is passed into the collecting system. Although the cost of balloon dilation may be higher, it is faster and may be less traumatic than sequential dilation. Alternatives for dilation include the Amplatz sequential dilators, Alken metal dilators, or the laparoscopic radial dilator system.[28]

The 27F rigid nephroscope is available from many endourologic manufacturers and can be used without its outer sheath, which decreases its effective diameter but also reduces the volume of irrigation flow. Semirigid ureteroscopes from 7F through 11F can be used to bypass narrow infundibula or the ureteropelvic junction (UPJ). If lower-pole access is obtained, flexible nephroscopy is usually required. Our preference is a 15 or 16F flexible nephroscope, available from numerous manufacturers.

Rigid lithotrites include ultrasonic, pneumatic, and combination ultrasonic/pneumatic lithotrites (Swiss Lithoclast, LUS-2, and Lithoclast Ultra; EMS, Nyon, Switzerland). Auge and colleagues compared their performance in vitro and found smaller fragment size and more rapid stone clearance for the combination device.[29] The advantage of rigid lithotrites is that they have suction capabilities and large lumens; the disadvantage is that they can't be used in flexible instruments and require larger diameter access.

The most commonly used flexible lithotrites include electrohydraulic lithotripsy (EHL) and holmium:YAG laser. The holmium:YAG laser is our preferred flexible lithotrite since it is available in small sizes, allows good scope deflection, is effective against all stone types, and causes little ureteral trauma if employed carefully.

While a wide array of rigid graspers is available, we commonly use three-prong graspers. Many flexible baskets are also available, but we use tipless nitinol baskets most frequently. They have the advantage of being soft, allowing good scope deflection, are precise and relatively atraumatic, and allow easy stone engagement and disengagement.

If we leave a nephrostomy tube in place after the procedure, we typically use an 18 to 22F Foley catheter with a 5 cc balloon and the tip cut off to the level of the drainage holes. We find that councill-tipped catheters are often too long, resulting in the tip pressing on the medial portion of the renal pelvis. Others prefer 8F or 10F Cope tubes, re-entry Malecott catheters, or nephroureteral stents. If we leave the patient tubeless, we place an antegrade 6 or 7F Double-J ureteral stent. Internal stenting after PCNL has the disadvantage of requiring a second office procedure for removal, but may have the advantage of shorter hospitalization and less pain.

STEP-BY STEP DESCRIPTION OF PROCEDURE

After induction of general anesthesia, the patient is placed in the lithotomy position and sterilely prepped and draped for cystoscopy. Cystoscopy is initiated, and an open-ended 6F ureteral catheter or ureteral balloon catheter is inserted to the level of the stone. A Foley catheter is placed, and the stent is secured to it with tape and fastened to IV extension tubing and a syringe filled with contrast. The patient is placed in the prone position and carefully padded and secured.

After sterilely prepping and draping the patient, fluoroscopy is carried out with retrograde filling of the collecting system. The ideal calix is chosen and is usually a middle posterior calix. We place a mark on the patient's back corresponding to the position of the stone and draw a line on the patient's back that represents the optimal angle of penetration. A puncture incision is made on the line 6 to 10 cm from the stone mark, and the access needle is passed in the direction of the target calix under fluoroscopic guidance. When the needle is near the renal parenchyma, an oblique fluoroscopic image is obtained noting whether the original needle pass is superficial or deep. The fluoroscopy head is returned to the upright position, the depth of the needle is adjusted, and the process is repeated until the puncture path is correct in both the upright (posterior-anterior) and the oblique position. Entry into the calix is performed, the core of the needle is removed and urine/contrast drainage is confirmed. A wire is then passed into the collecting system under fluoroscopic guidance. While it is ideal for the wire to pass easily down the ureter, this is not imperative, and ureteral manipulation at this point is not stressed.

The incision is enlarged to 11 to 12 mm, followed by sequential fascial dilation to 8F, and then placement of a 10F safety wire introducer

Table 18-2 Percutaneous Nephrolithotomy Series with Ureteral Stone Cases

Article	Stone Location	Patients	Stone-Free after One Procedure (after Repeat Procedure) [after Treatment with Other Modality]	% Stone-Free	Median Postoperative Stay (days)	Major Complications	% Complications	Comments
Clayman, 1984[2]	U, M, L	44	4 (31)	9.8 (70)	11.8*	Bleeding requiring transfusion (4), extravasation (13), perirenal hematoma (1)	41	* Total hospital days
Bush, 1985[39]	U	37	30 (35)	81 (94)	5.3	Ureteral perforation (12) six requiring stent, pseudoaneurysm at nephrostomy site (1), reflux pyelitis (1)	38	
Gumpinger, 1985[40]	U, M	22	22	100	4	Ureteral perforation (1) with stent	4.5	
Kellett, 1985[41]	M	6	6	100	2.3	None	0.0	
Reddy, 1985[33]	U, M, L	68	65 [67]	98 [99]	–	–	–	
Segura, 1985[3]	U, M	195	172 (175) [195]	88 (90) [100]	–	–	–	
Beckmann, 1986[42]	U, M	44	42 [44]	95 [100]	–	Ureteral perforation (1)	2.2	Overnight ureteral dilation successful in 12 of 13
Harewood, 1986[43]	U, M	20	19 [20]	95 [100]	4.5	Ureteral stricture (1), arteriovenous fistula (1)		
Kahn, 1986[44]	U, M, L	60	57 [59]	95 [98]	2.6	Bleeding requiring transfusion (1), urosepsis (1), pyelonephritis (1), ureteral avulsion (1), ureteral perforation (2)	10	25 cases had two-step procedure (tract maturation)
Lingeman, 1986[45]	?	5	5	100	–	–	–	All stones pushed up to kidney fluoroscopically
Baba, 1987[46]	U, M	50	33 (47) [50]	66 (94) [100]	–	Ureteral perforation (4)	8.0	
Coptcoat, 1987[47]	U	4	4	100	–	–	–	
Streem, 1988[32]	U, M	29	25	83	5.1	Ureteral stenosis (1)	0.5	Better outcome when proximal ureter dilated (p = .01)
Henricksson, 1989[48]	?	108	108	100	–	–	–	
Liong, 1989[49]	U	19	19	100	5	Ureteral perforation (7) all stented, one with pleural effusion, pneumonia (1)	43	
Tan, 1989[50]	U, M	34	31[34]	91[100]	6.5	Pelvis/ureter perforation (2), extravasation (1), ureteral stenosis (3)	18	9 patients with 2-stage procedure; Pts. from 1986 to '87
Anselmo, 1990[9]	U	17	16 (17)	94 (100)	–	Ureteral perforation (1), stented	5.9	8 patients had previous nephrostomy tube
Berkhoff, 1990[51]	U	7	6 (7)	83 (100)	4	None	0.0	
Srivasrava, 1992[52]	U	29	23 [27]	79 [93]	6.2	Ureteral perforation (4), all stented, one case leading to stricture	13.8	5 patients had two-step procedure
Kahn, 1993[53]	U, M	9	9	100	–	Bleeding requiring transfusion leading to chronic renal insufficiency (1)	11.1	
Tan, 1995[54]	?	36	36	100	–	–	–	Pts. from 1988 to '92
Kumar, 1996[55]	U	86	66 (74) [83]	77 (86) [97]	8.8	Ureteral perforation (7), bleeding requiring transfusion (3), ureteral stricture (1)	12.8	
Mor, 1997[11]	U	2	2	100	–	–	–	Pediatric cases
Toth, 2001[56]	U, M	51	50 [51]	98 [100]	3	Retroperitoneal hematoma (1)	1.9	Method: direct perc. of ureter
Total		982	850 (909) [956]	86.6 (92.6) [97.4]	6.0		14.1	
Total before 1990		745	624 (691) [724]	86.2 (92.8) [97.2]	6.5		17.0	
Total since 1990		237	208 (218) [232]	87.8 (92.0) [97.9]	5.6		9.0	

L = lower; M = middle; Pts. = patients; U = upper; ? = unknown.

catheter and a second wire. The safety wire is secured with a clear sterile dressing. Balloon dilation to 30F is performed, and a 34F outer diameter Amplatz sheath is passed over the balloon into the collecting system. The balloon is then deflated and removed.

Rigid nephroscopy is performed initially to remove any blood clots and visualize the collecting system. An antegrade ureteral wire is now placed. If the ureteral stone has been chronically impacted, this may be difficult and may require lubricious wires. Irrigation through the ureteral catheter may dislodge the stone into the UPJ where it can be grasped or treated. If the stone is not visible with the rigid nephroscope, then flexible nephroscopy is performed with holmium:YAG laser lithotripsy, and fragment removal with a tipless nitinol basket. When the patient is stone-free, careful flexible nephroscopy is performed throughout the entire collecting system to ensure that no residual stones are present. The region of ureter previously involved with stone is inspected. If there are perforations or significant trauma, or if the patient is a candidate for a tubeless procedure, then an antegrade 6F ureteral stent is placed under fluoroscopic guidance. This maneuver usually requires removing the retrograde ureteral catheter that was placed at the beginning of the procedure.

If desired, a nephrostomy tube is placed through the Amplatz sheath, the catheter is sutured into position, an antegrade nephrostogram is performed, and the final wire is removed. A sterile dressing is placed, and the nephrostomy tube and Foley catheter are placed to gravity drainage. We often give a 12.5-gm dose of intravenous mannitol at the completion of the procedure, which seems to minimize venous bleeding and encourage diuresis. The patient is repositioned into the supine position and awakened from anesthesia.

POSTOPERATIVE CARE

The patient's diet is advanced as tolerated, and most patients take a regular diet by the morning of the first postoperative day. Intravenous ketorolac is used for two or three postoperative doses, and the patient is then placed on oral narcotics. Intravenous narcotics are available but usually not necessary. If the patient has both a nephrostomy tube and a retrograde ureteral access catheter in place, the ureteral catheter is removed the morning of the first postoperative day, and the nephrostomy tube is clamped. If the patient tolerates that procedure, then the nephrostomy tube can be removed in the afternoon. If no nephrostomy tube was left, then the patient can go home on postoperative day one.

If a patient had significant intracorporeal lithotripsy or had concomitant renal stone treatment, then an NCCT is performed to identify residual fragments and the need for additional procedures. Residual fragments are present in up to 32% of patients after PCNL for renal stones.[31]

Patients go home with oral narcotics, stool softeners and, if indicated, a short course of oral antibiotics. They follow up in the office in 7 to 14 days for flexible cystoscopy and stent removal. Imaging with a renal ultrasound, IVP or NCCT is performed three months postoperatively or sooner if the patient is symptomatic. Since most patients requiring percutaneous management of ureteral stones have some factor that makes them high risk for ureteral stricture (stone size, duration, failed treatments, impaction), postoperative imaging is important.

RESULTS

Stone-free rates after percutaneous antegrade treatment of ureteral stones since 1990 are 88% after the first procedure and near 100% when including subsequent or auxiliary procedures (Table 18-2). Streem and colleagues suggested that upper ureteral stones with proximal ureteral dilation had better outcomes (94%; 16 of 17 patients) compared to cases without ureteral dilation (43%, 3 of 7 patients).[32] Reddy and colleagues examined the outcome of 68 patients with stones in the upper, mid- and lower ureter and found that all of their failures were in the lower-ureter group.[33] Today, most of the mid- and distal ureteral stones in their series would have been treated with ESWL or ureteroscopy.

It is encouraging that, in the post-ESWL and ureteroscopy era, the performance of percutaneous antegrade treatment has remained high. Currently, only the most challenging stones are treated with this modality. The reason for the high performance in these challenging situations is due to multiple factors. Improvements in flexible endoscopes, videoendoscopy, improved basket technology, and perhaps most significantly, the versatility of the holmium:YAG laser[34] have all had a role. Typically, patients now have brief hospitalizations and go home without percutaneous nephrostomy tubes. Transfusion rates are low. Inpatient narcotic requirements are diminished with the enhanced use of intravenous ketorolac.

COMPLICATIONS

Complications due to percutaneous antegrade treatment of proximal ureteral stones parallel those from PCNL for renal stones. The rate of major complications since 1990 is nearly half the rate reported before 1990, likely reflecting improvements and standardization of techniques and instrumentation as earlier outlined. The possible complications are numerous, as outlined in the consent section of this chapter. Fortunately, most complications are rare.[35] The most common complication after PCNL is fever. In a retrospective review of 69 PCNL procedures, Cadeddu and colleagues found the incidence of fever over 38°C to be 28%.[24] All their patients had negative preoperative urine cultures and received perioperative antibiotics. None suffered sepsis, and

fever was not correlated to hospitalization. Surprisingly, fever was also not related to stone composition. These findings were in contrast to Troxel and Low who found that postoperative fever was correlated to stone composition in a group of 31 patients.[36] Intrarenal pressures did not correlate with fever in their series.

Another common complication is renal pelvis or ureteral perforation, occurring in up to 13% of cases in post-1990 series (see Table 18-2). Usually, this is noticed visually or with extravasation during contrast injection, and resolves without sequelae with drainage in most patients. Perforation at the site of stone impaction, however, has been associated with stricture formation in impacted ureteral calculi.[22] Roberts and colleagues found a 24% risk of ureteral stricture formation in patients whose stones had been impacted for over 2 months.[22]

Blood transfusions are now necessary in fewer than 5% of patients after PCNL. Therefore, autologous pre-donation is not recommended.[25]

Injury to intercostal blood vessels (< 2%) and pulmonary complications (5 to 10% of supracostal access) are both more common in patients with supracostal access.[37] Supracostal access is still favored by some because of the more direct route to the ureter and the higher likelihood of treating upper ureteral stones with a rigid nephroscope.[20]

Finally, injury to adjacent organs such as the colon occurs in less than 1% of cases and may be more common in patients with prior retroperitoneal surgery. Fortunately, most cases can be managed nonoperatively.[38] Ureteral avulsion and requirement for urgent open surgery or nephrectomy are described as rare complications that occur in less than 1% of patients.

CONCLUSION

Percutaneous treatment of ureteral stones is usually a secondary treatment. Common indications include failed endoscopy, existing nephrostomy, renal and ureteral stone burden and very large upper ureteral stones. Mid- or upper-posterior caliceal approach offers the most direct access to the upper ureter.

A variety of rigid and flexible scopes and lithotrites can be used to treat and remove the stone. Select patients can be treated with internal stenting and without postoperative nephrostomy tubes. Careful follow-up is important to ensure the early identification of a ureteral stricture.

REFERENCES

1. Fernstrom I, Johansson B. Percutaneous pyelolithotomy. A new extraction technique. Scand J Urol Nephrol 1976;10:257–9.
2. Clayman RV, Surya V, Miller RP, et al. Percutaneous nephrolithotomy: extraction of renal and ureteral calculi from 100 patients. J Urol 1984;131:868–71.
3. Segura JW, Patterson DE, LeRoy AJ, et al. Percutaneous removal of kidney stones: review of 1,000 cases. J Urol 1985;134:1077–81.
4. Drach GW, Dretler S, Fair W, et al. Report of the United States cooperative study of extracorporeal shock wave lithotripsy. J Urol 1986;135:1127–33.

5. Blute ML, Segura JW, Patterson DE. Ureteroscopy. J Urol 1988;139:510–2.
6. Segura JW, Preminger GM, Assimos DG, et al. Ureteral Stones Clinical Guidelines Panel summary report on the management of ureteral calculi. The American Urological Association. J Urol 1997;158:1915–21.
7. Miller OF, Kane CJ. Time to stone passage for observed ureteral calculi: a guide for patient education. J Urol 1999;162:688–91.
8. Lam JS, Greene TD, Gupta M. Treatment of proximal ureteral calculi: holmium:YAG laser ureterolithotripsy versus extracorporeal shock wave lithotripsy. J Urol 2002;167:1972–6.
9. Anselmo G, Bassi E, Fandella A, et al. Antegrade ureterolitholapaxy in the treatment of obstructing or incarcerated proximal ureteric stones. Br J Urol 1990;65:137–40.
10. Pearle MS, Pierce HL, Miller GL, et al. Optimal method of urgent decompression of the collecting system for obstruction and infection due to ureteral calculi. J Urol 1998;160:1260–4.
11. Mor Y, Elmasry YE, Kellett MJ, Duffy PG. The role of percutaneous nephrolithotomy in the management of pediatric renal calculi. J Urol 1997;158:1319–21.
12. Miller OF, Rineer SK, Reichard SR, et al. Prospective comparison of unenhanced spiral computed tomography and intravenous urogram in the evaluation of acute flank pain. Urology 1998;52:982–7.
13. Miller OF, Kane CJ. Unenhanced helical computed tomography in the evaluation of acute flank pain. Curr Opin Urol 2000;10:123–9.
14. Sfakianakis GN, Cohen DJ, Braunstein RH, et al. MAG3-F0 scintigraphy in decision making for emergency intervention in renal colic after helical CT positive for a urolith. J Nucl Med 2000;41:1813–22.
15. Andreoni C, Afane J, Olweny E, Clayman RV. Flexible ureteroscopic lithotripsy: first-line therapy for proximal ureteral and renal calculi in the morbidly obese and superobese patient. J Endourol 2001;15:493–8.
16. Dogan HS, Sahin A, Cetinkaya Y, et al. Antibiotic prophylaxis in percutaneous nephrolithotomy: prospective study in 81 patients. J EndoUrol 2002;16:649–53.
17. Kane CJ, Bolton DM, Stoller ML. Current indications for open stone surgery in an endourology center. Urology 1995;45:218–21.
18. Goswami AK, Shrivastava P, Mukherjee A, Sharma SK. Management of colonic perforation during percutaneous nephrolithotomy in horseshoe kidney. J EndoUrol 2001;15:989–91.
19. Thilagarajah R, Allen CM, Meganathan V, Whitfield HN. Subcostal artery laceration during percutaneous nephrolithotomy: an unusual complication. J Urol 2000;163:1513–4.
20. Gupta R, Kumar A, Kapoor R, et al. Prospective evaluation of safety and efficacy of the supracostal approach for percutaneous nephrolithotomy. BJU Int 2002;90:809–13.
21. Munver R, Delvecchio FC, Newman GE, Preminger GM. Critical analysis of supracostal access for percutaneous renal surgery. J Urol 2001;166:1242–6.
22. Roberts WW, Cadeddu JA, Micali S, et al. Ureteral stricture formation after removal of impacted calculi. J Urol 1998;159:723–6.
23. Dretler SP, Keating MA, Riley J. An algorithm for the management of ureteral calculi. J Urol 1986;136:1190–3.
24. Cadeddu JA, Chen R, Bishoff J, et al. Clinical significance of fever after percutaneous nephrolithotomy. Urology 1998;52:48–50.
25. Stoller ML, Lee KL, Schwartz BF, Viele MK. Autologous blood use in percutaneous nephrolithotomy. Urology 1999;54:444–9.
26. Grasso M, Nord R, Bagley DH. Prone split leg and flank roll positioning: simultaneous antegrade and retrograde access to the upper urinary tract. J Endourol 1993;7:307–10.
27. Shoma AM, Eraky I, El-Kenawy MR, El-Kappany HA. Percutaneous nephrolithotomy in the supine position: technical aspects and functional outcome compared with the prone technique. Urology 2002;60:388–92.
28. Goharderakhshan RZ, Schwartz BF, Rudnick DM, et al. Radially expanding single-step nephrostomy tract dilator. Urology 2001;58:693–6.
29. Auge BK, Lallas CD, Pietrow PK, et al. In vitro comparison of standard ultrasound and pneumatic lithotrites with a new combination intracorporeal lithotripsy device. Urology 2002;60:28–32.
30. Feng MI, Tamaddon K, Mikhail A, et al. Prospective randomized study of various techniques of percutaneous nephrolithotomy. Urology 2001;58:345–50.
31. Pearle MS, Watamull LM, Mullican MA. Sensitivity of noncontrast helical computerized tomography and plain film radiography compared to flexible nephroscopy for detecting residual fragments after percutaneous nephrostolithotomy. J Urol 1999;162:23–6.
32. Streem SB, Hall P, Zelch MG, et al. Endourologic management of upper and mid ureteral calculi: percutaneous antegrade extraction vs transurethral ureteroscopy. Urology 1988;31:34–7.
33. Reddy PK, Hulbert JC, Lange PH, et al. Percutaneous removal of renal and ureteral calculi: experience with 400 cases. J Urol 1985;134:662–5.
34. Teichman JM, Rao RD, Glickman RD, Harris JM. Holmium:YAG percutaneous lithotripsy: the laser incident angle matters. J Urol 1998;159:690–4.
35. Rudnick DM, Stoller ML. Complications of percutaneous nephrostolithotomy. Can J Urol 1999;6:872–5.
36. Troxel SA, Low RK. Renal intrapelvic pressure during percutaneous nephrolithotomy and its correlation with the development of postoperative fever. J Urol 2002;168:1348–51.
37. Kekre NS, Gopalakrishnan GG, Gupta GG, et al. Supracostal approach in percutaneous nephrolithotomy: experience with 102 cases. J Endourol 2001;15:789–91.
38. Gerspach JM, Bellman GC, Stoller ML, Fugelso P. Conservative management of colon injury following percutaneous renal surgery. Urology 1997;49:831–6.
39. Bush WH, Brannen GE, Lewis GP, Burnett LL. Upper ureteral calculi: extraction via percutaneous nephrostomy. AJR Am J Roentgenol 1985;144:795–9.
40. Gumpinger R, Miller K, Fuchs G, Eisenberger F. Antegrade ureteroscopy for stone removal. Eur Urol 1985;11:199–202.
41. Kellett MJ, Wickham JE, Payne SR. Combined retrograde and antegrade manipulations for percutaneous nephrolithotomy of ureteric calculi: "push-pull" technique. Urology 1985;25:391–2.
42. Beckmann CF, Roth RA, Luedke MD. Upper and midureteral calculi: percutaneous extraction with an occlusion balloon catheter. Radiology 1986;159:643–5.
43. Harewood LM, Cleeve LK. The visual endourological removal of ureteric calculi. Med J Aust 1986;145:574–9.
44. Kahn RI. Endourological treatment of ureteral calculi. J Urol 1986;135:239–43.
45. Lingeman JE, Sonda LP, Kahnoski RJ, et al. Ureteral stone management: emerging concepts. J Urol 1986;135:1172–4.
46. Baba S, Marumo K, Honda TA, et al. Balloon dilation of edematous ureteral segment in percutaneous urethrolithotripsy for long-term impacted calculi. J Endourol 1987;1:227.
47. Coptcoat MJ, Webb DR, Kellett MJ, et al. The treatment of 100 consecutive patients with ureteral calculi in a British stone center. J Urol 1987;137:1122–3.
48. Henriksson C, Geterud K, Grenabo L, et al. Percutaneous renal and ureteric stone extraction. Report on the first 500 operations. Scand J Urol Nephrol 1989;23:291–7.
49. Liong ML, Clayman RV, Gittes RF, et al. Treatment options for proximal ureteral urolithiasis: review and recommendations. J Urol 1989;141:504–9.
50. Tan EC, Tung KH, Foo KT, et al. Antegrade ureteroscopy and ultrasonic lithotripsy in the treatment of difficult upper and middle ureteric stones. Ann Acad Med Singapore 1989;18:55–8.
51. Berkhoff WB, Meijer F. Percutaneous antegrade fiberoptic ureterorenoscopic treatment of ureteral calculi. J Urol 1990;144:628–30.
52. Srivastava A, Ahlawat R, Kumar A, et al. Management of impacted upper ureteric calculi: results of lithotripsy and percutaneous litholapaxy. Br J Urol 1992;70:252–7.
53. Kahn RI. Percutaneous approach for uretreral stones. Probl Urol 1993;7:547–55.
54. Tan HM, Liew RP, Chan CC, et al. Multimodal approach in the management of 1163 ureteric stone cases. Med J Malaysia 1995;50:87–92.
55. Kumar V, Ahlawat R, Banjeree GK, et al. Percutaneous ureterolitholapaxy: the best bet to clear large bulk impacted upper ureteral calculi. Arch Esp Urol 1996;49:86–91.
56. Toth CS, Varga A, Flasko T, et al. Percutaneous ureterolithotomy: direct method for removal of impacted ureteral stones. J Endourol 2001;15:285–90.

19

Chemolysis of Urinary Calculi

Russell M. Freid, MD
Arthur D. Smith, MD

The treatment of urolithiasis has changed dramatically over the past several decades. The advent of percutaneous nephrolithotripsy (PCNL), extracorporeal shock wave lithotripsy (ESWL), and other endourologic techniques is largely responsible for the new management protocols. Currently, open renal surgery for nephrolithiasis is rarely necessary. Likewise, the use of chemolysis for stone dissolution has declined dramatically. Although its indications have diminished, chemolysis should not be discounted as a useless technique from the past.

Since the first report of chemolysis by Crowell in 1924,[1] countless others have successfully used this method of eliminating all forms of urinary lithiasis. Any urologist who treats stone disease should be familiar with the fundamentals of chemolysis therapy and its potential role in the management of urinary calculi. Dissolution therapy can be quite valuable in appropriately selected clinical scenarios. Patients with residual fragments may be rendered stone-free, thus reducing the potential for recurrences. Likewise, patients unfit for other therapy may undergo primary dissolution with minimal risk.

Chemolysis can be accomplished through either systemic or local administration of the active agent. Systemic treatment includes both oral and intravenous routes, whereas local treatment refers to the actual instillation of the solution into the urinary tract. This local or direct irrigation chemolysis is the most effective dissolution therapy to eradicate urinary lithiasis. The principles of safe and effective therapy are rather simple for the practicing urologist, but even minor errors in technique can result in catastrophic complications. Therefore, it is essential that all nursing staff fully comprehend the details of the technique as well as its potential dangers. Furthermore, an informed patient will serve as the best early warning system that a potential problem is developing.

STONE ANALYSIS

The decision to use direct chemolysis in a particular instance is dependent on the stone composition. Obtaining stone fragments for analysis before irrigation guarantees proper choice of irrigant. These can be obtained percutaneously when establishing a tract for a nephrostomy tube, retrograde via endoscopic instrumentation, or noninvasively if fragments are passed. When stones are not available for analysis, the ultimate success of chemolysis is jeopardized. However, it is possible to determine their composition with a reasonable degree of certainty.

Analysis of a prior stone from a given patient is a good indicator of the type of stone on recurrence. Otnes[2] reviewed stone analyses in 70 patients with two or more episodes of renal calculi and found a predominant pattern. Overall, two-thirds or more of patients with recurrent stones continue to form the same type of calculi (Table 19-1). Calcium stone formers will continue to form calcium-based (calcium oxalate/phosphate) stones more than 90% of the time. Cystine stone formers likewise will continue to produce this type of stone in nearly all recurrences. Other clues to the type of stone present can be found on routine laboratory studies. For instance, urine cultures positive for *Proteus* would suggest the possibility of struvite calculi. Low urine pH is supportive of uric acid stones. Serum chemistries should be checked as well for any abnormalities.

Radiologic investigations correctly identify and distinguish the various stone types with a high degree of accuracy.[3] Plain films and intravenous urograms provide a general estimate of a stone's opacity. Computed tomography (CT) scans, however, have been far more useful in distinguishing stone types. Hounsfield unit measurements vary widely for different stones, thus enhancing the scan's discriminatory ability (Table 19-2). Several investigators have demonstrated the high accuracy of stone identification with CT scan.[4,5] Therefore, if prior stone analysis, laboratory data, and radiologic evaluation are carefully considered, chemolysis may proceed in the absence of current stone analysis.

TECHNIQUES OF IRRIGATION

Once direct chemolysis is planned, the appropriate irrigation system is chosen. Multiple configurations are available for direct chemolysis (Table 19-3). Although certain irrigation systems are advantageous, any one can be used as long as the safety guidelines described by Nemoy and Stamey are observed.[6]

The most simple and least invasive system is a single ureteral catheter that is advanced to the renal pelvis or past a ureteral stone. The danger of this method is the limitation on outflow around this stent through the ureter. Further compromise of this outflow will result in rapid elevation of intrapelvic pressures and the incipient potential complications. An innovative technique using this system while avoiding high pressures has been described by Kuwahara and colleagues.[7] These investigators use a computer-controlled, pressure-monitoring intermittent pump (Figure 19-1A). This infuses fluid for 1 minute, holds for 30 seconds, and then drains for 9 seconds. If the pressure increases beyond the preset limit (15 cm H_2O), the infusion stops. If the pressure increase is sustained for 5 seconds, the drainage valve opens. In limited clinical trials this system was safe and effective, but it is not widely available because of the expense of the specialized computer pump and its limited potential for use. Without such a pump, a single ureteral catheter for irrigating is not recommended.

The addition of a single nephrostomy tube to the prior system provides a path for sufficient outflow (Figure 19-1B). However, the patient is practically immobile as a result of the irrigation inflow through a ureteral catheter traversing the urethra and bladder. Reversing the flow gives the patient more mobility (especially if the ureteral catheter is a double pigtail) at the expense of decreased outflow, thus limiting its utility. Therefore this system is reserved for patients with small stones expected to dissolve in a short period of time (eg, uric acid).

More effective systems are those that include dual nephrostomy tubes (Figure 19-1C). Standard 16 French or 18F Malecot catheters provide excellent inflow and outflow with minimal elevations in intrapelvic pressure. Such a configuration is versatile and can be used in most patients.

Table 19-1 Recurrent Stone Composition		
Initial Episode		Recurrences in Same Class
Uric acide and cystine	78%	
Struvite	65%	
Calcium oxalate	50%	91% recurrence rate with any calcium-based stone
Calciaum phosphate	70%	91% recurrence rate with any calcium-based stone
Calcium oxalate phosphate	65%	91% recurrence rate with any calcium-based stone
Adapted from Otnes B.[2]		

Table 19-2 CT Diagnosis of Urinary Calculi

	Hounsfield Units
Uric acid	540 ± 107
Struvite	651 ± 108
Cystine	703 ± 69
Calcium oxalate/phospate	$> 1,023$

Adapted from Mitcheson HD, et al.[5]

In those with large staghorn calculi, however, consideration should be given to ensuring unobstructed passage of fragments through the ureter. This is especially true for struvite stones, which tend to form large, irregular pieces on fragmentation.[8] An endopyelotomy stent (14 to 8.2F) works nicely in this setting because it provides excellent two-way outflow, keeps the ureter patent, and decreases the volume of fragments that enter the ureter (Figure 19-1D). An alternative arrangement is two nephrostomy tubes and a double-pigtail ureteral catheter.

Two coaxial techniques of irrigation have been described. A renal pelvic lavage set that allows inflow and outflow through one nephrostomy site is available (Figure 19-1E).[9] Once in place, an inner 6.3 or 8.3F pigtail catheter is directed at the stone for inflow. Outflow, which is limited, occurs through the surrounding sheath and down the ureter. This system allows for easier repositioning to irrigate different areas of the pelvis. The second coaxial technique of irrigation works well for upper ureteral stones[10,11] (Figure 19-1F). It is set up by inserting either a 5F ureteral or angiogram catheter over a wire through the lumen of an 18F Foley catheter, which serves as a nephrostomy tube. The small inner catheter, which provides inflow, can be advanced so its tip is adjacent to the stone, whereas the Foley catheter provides outflow. This is an effective method for dissolving upper ureteral stones. A three-way Foley catheter has also been used successfully for renal pelvic irrigations.[12]

Each of the systems described must have a means to measure intrapelvic pressure. The most common method is a central venous pressure (CVP) manometer connected to the inflow limb of the irrigation line. Although nursing staff find this easy to set up and use, there are several disadvantages. The system remains open and is therefore subject to contamination or overflow spills. Since there is no alarm or automatic shutoff for high pressures, frequent monitoring is required. A far better alternative is a closed continuous infusion pump available from IVAC (San Diego, CA). This pump provides a continuous display of the intrapelvic pressure and will sound an alarm and shut off if the preset limit is exceeded. This device is a valuable investment for those centers where chemolysis is used on more than a rare occasion.

Once the tubes are placed, there should be a 24-hour interval to allow the tract to seal prior to irrigating. For difficult nephrostomy punctures, multiple nephrostomy tubes, or struvite stones, a pre-irrigation nephrostogram is indicated to rule out extravasation. If urine cultures are negative, saline irrigations may commence at 30 mL/hr. If the patient stays afebrile and free of flank pain with acceptable irrigation pressures, the rate is doubled each 2 to 4 hours until the target rate of 120 mL/hr is reached. The saline irrigation is continued for 12 to 24 hours as a trial run prior to beginning the proper irrigant. Irrigation with the active solution is again begun at a low rate and titrated up to 120 mL/hr while observing closely. Some claim that warming the solution increases its effectiveness.[13–15] Although this has not been proven, a warmed solution is beneficial for patient comfort and avoidance of hypothermia.

During chemolysis, a schedule of laboratory and radiologic tests should be followed. A complete blood count and serum chemistry can be done every 2 to 4 days. Urine cultures should be done every 2 days in most cases. For struvite stone, when irrigating with Renacidin or Suby's solutions, daily urine cultures and serum magnesium levels should be checked. The progress of dissolution is followed with abdominal x-ray films or tomograms twice weekly or with nephrostograms for uric acid stones. Irrigation is continued for 24 to 48 hours after no fragments are visible. The urine is strained throughout the irrigation process to collect all fragments. Foley catheter drainage is not necessary during irrigations, although it may provide relief of urinary frequency, nocturia, or bladder irritation when these are troublesome.

Throughout the process of dissolution, appropriate antibiotic coverage should be provided. In general, a first-generation cephalosporin or sulfa preparation is acceptable. Of course, culture-specific coverage should be instituted for positive urine cultures, and broader coverage used for struvite stones.

Deep vein thrombosis prophylaxis is required as well. Although these occur infrequently,[16,17] one study reported a 3% incidence with several patients progressing to pulmonary emboli.[18] Ambulation several times daily is mandatory. Low-dose subcutaneous heparin (5,000 U twice daily) is begun immediately on initiation of therapy. Elastic stockings and sequential calf compression boots are added for bedridden patients and those with limited mobility.

TYPES OF CALCULI

STRUVITE Struvite renal stones account for 10 to 15% of all urinary calculi in the United States. These stones afflict about 8% of all spinal cord injury patients and 4.7 to 30% of patients with ileal conduits.[19–21] They are composed of magnesium ammonium phosphate and varying amounts of carbonate appatite, which crystallizes in the presence of urease-producing bacteria. This enzyme is produced by more than 45 different microorganisms but protei are identified in 72% of isolates from stone formers.[22]

The hydrolysis of urea to ammonium, hydroxide, and bicarbonate is catalyzed by urease through the following reaction:

Table 19-3 Guidelines for Direct Irrigation Chemolysis

Contraindications to Starting or Continuing Irrigation
Positive urine culture
Patient is febrile
Persistent flank pain
Intrapelvic pressure > 25 cm H_2O
Extravasation of irrigation fluid

Adapted from Nemoy NJ, Stamey TA.[6]

Urease
$$H_2N—C—NH_2 —> CO_2 + 2NH_3 \, H_2O$$
$$\underset{2}{N H_3} + H_2O —>?NH_4^+ + OH$$

These products alkalinize the urine (pH > 7.2) which, in the presence of trivalent phosphate, results in struvite crystal formation.

The significant morbidity associated with infection stones was highlighted by Griffith and colleagues with the term "stone cancer," referring to the downhill course of patients with untreated struvite calculi.[23] Priestley and Dunn noted a 41% 15-year survival in patients with unilateral stones managed nonoperatively.[24] Patients with bilateral branched stone disease had only a 50% 5-year survival. The improved survival with treatment is illustrated by the review of 125 patients by Blandy and Singh.[25] These patients were treated by extended pyelolithotomy and had a 10-year mortality rate of only 7.2%.

Efforts to eradicate such stones often have suboptimal success rates. Early forms of therapy, which provide one basis for comparison, include anatrophic nephrolithotomy and pyelolithotomy. The incidence of retained fragments following these procedures for staghorn calculi ranges from 12 to 36%.[6,19,26–29] A long-term stone recurrence rate of 22% is among the best reported for these therapies.[30] Persistence of infection was esti-

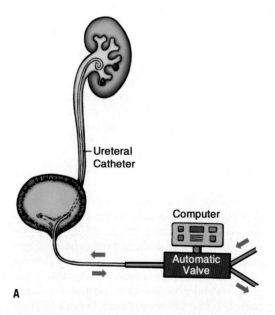

Figure 19-1 Irrigation configurations for direct chemolysis. *A*, Retrograde ureteral catheter with computer-driven inflow/outflow.

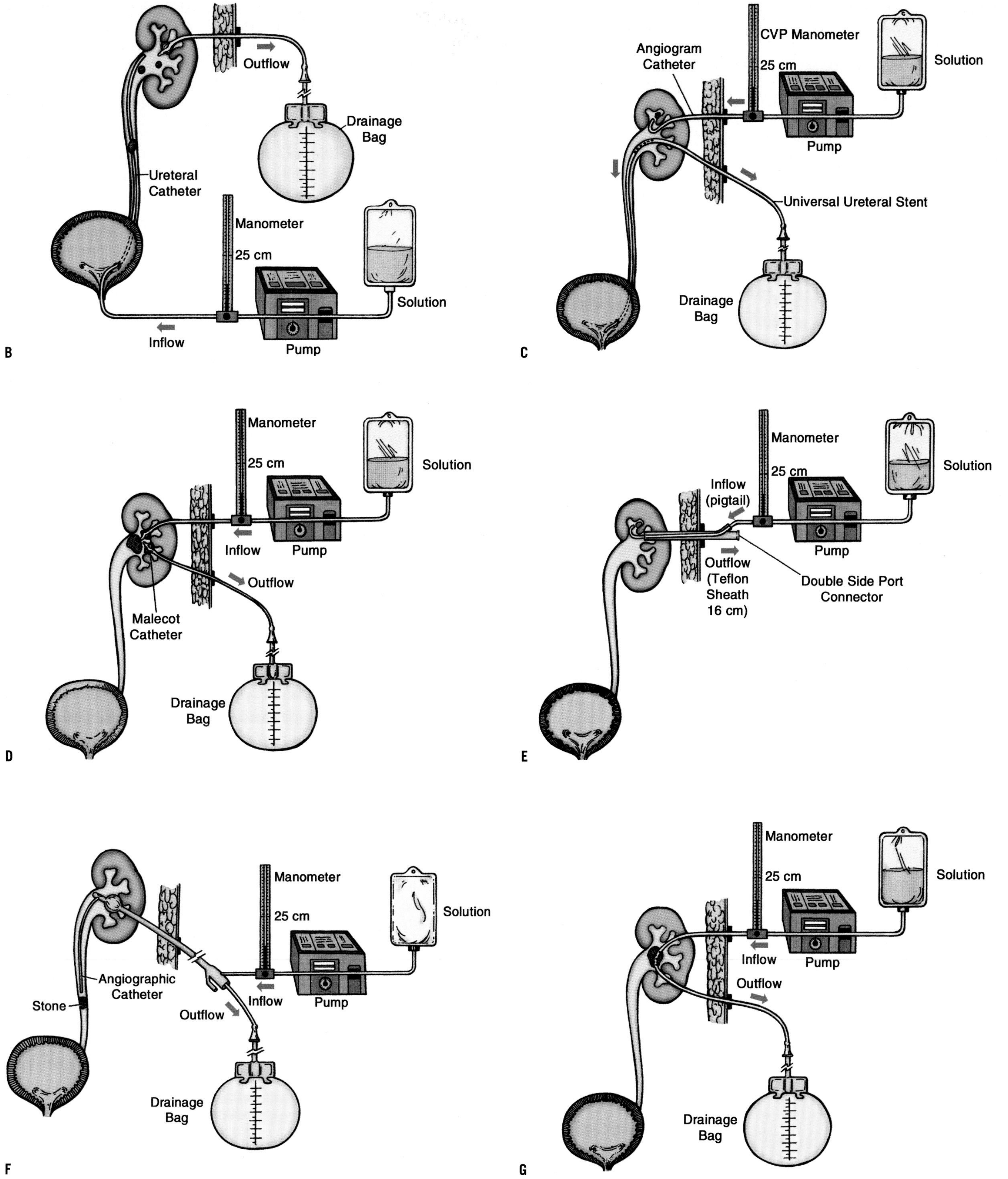

Figure 19-1 *Continued, B,* Retrograde ureteral catheter inflow and nephrostomy outflow. *C,* Dual nephrostomy irrigation. *D,* Nephrostomy inflow and universal/endopyelotomy stent drainage. *F,* Coaxial technique of ureteral catheter through Foley catheter. *G,* Circle tube for chemolysis.

mated to occur in approximately 40% and is believed to be responsible for many of the stone recurrences.[31] The presence of small stone particles with embedded bacteria serves as a nidus for rapid recurrences.

PCNL and ESWL, either combined or as monotherapies, have largely replaced open surgery for the treatment of struvite calculi. ESWL monotherapy, although least invasive, often requires multiple treatment sessions to reach a stone-free rate of 40 to 74%.[32–35] Numerous reports have demonstrated percutaneous lithotripsy to be more effective as a monotherapy,[35–43] but multiple sessions were likewise required to achieve the 68 to 90% stone-free rate. Combining the two modalities has yielded comparable stone-free rates (59 to 100%) at the expense of multiple procedures and increased hospital stays.[44–50] Furthermore, most of the follow-up figures given are for a period of 3 months, an interval too short to fully appreciate subclinical fragments. Therefore, even in the best of hands, a significant percentage of patients will have residual fragments, and thus, the potential for early recurrence. Long-term follow-up of 66 patients with residual struvite calculi was presented by Williams.[51] Nearly one-third of retained fragments passed over a mean follow-up of 18.5 years, whereas 47% required further surgery, and the remainder persisted asymptomatically.

Chemolysis is therefore a potentially valuable technique in combating struvite stone disease. Oral chemolysis is available primarily in the form of urease inhibitors. The most commonly used agent, acetohydroxamic acid (AHA), was identified as an irreversible inhibitor in 1964.[52] Furthermore, it acts synergistically with several antibiotics, sterilizing the urine more rapidly. Its clinical usefulness has been demonstrated in double-blind placebo-controlled studies,[53–55] but serious side effects (dose-related, reversible) precluded its use in approximately 20% of patients.[56] Most commonly reported are hemolytic anemia, neurosensory deficits, and thrombophlebitis. Headache, gastrointestinal upset, weakness, and flushing sensation after alcohol ingestion have also been reported.[57] At a dose of 250 mg orally three times daily, AHA can be expected only to halt further stone growth, although anecdotal reports of dissolution have been published.[56,58] The dose should be reduced to 250 mg orally twice daily for mild renal impairment, and it is contraindicated in patients with severe renal insufficiency (creatinine clearance < 20 mL/min, serum creatinine > 2.5) and in pregnancy. The efficacy and safety of many other urease inhibitors have been evaluated in an attempt to find a more ideal agent, but none has proven more advantageous than AHA.[59–65]

Other methods of oral chemolysis of struvite stones have been reported. Lewis and colleagues described a case of complete resolution of infected stones with 10 weeks of oral dicloxacillin sodium therapy only.[66] This once again reiterates the crucial role of infection in the pathogenesis of these stones. Dietary restrictions described by Shorr and Carter attempt to limit the amount of substrate for stone formation.[67] This low-phosphorous (500 mg), low-calcium diet supplemented with aluminum hydroxide gel as an intestinal phosphate binder resulted in partial or complete dissolution in 23% of stones in their series. Its use has not been popularized, however, because significant calcium abnormalities may occur with prolonged use of aluminum hydroxide preparations.[68] Therefore, systemic oral chemolytic agents are seldom effective in reducing stone burden on their own. Rather they can be thought of as adjunctive agents that can be used in select patients to maximize the effects of other therapies and minimize the recurrence rate.

Direct chemolysis of struvite calculi is a far more effective method of dissolution. The first application of direct chemolysis to struvite calculi was described by Suby and Albright[69] and Suby and colleagues.[70] The initial solution was found to be too irritating to the epithelium for clinical use. However, the addition of magnesium led to Suby's solution G, which has similar efficacy but decreased mucosal irritability. In 1959, Mulvany modified this solution and created hemiacidrin (Renacidin) (Table 19-4).[71] This multi-electrolyte solution contains citric, malonic, and gluconic acids in the form of esters, salts, anhydrides, and lactates. These acids provide hydrogen ions and citrate to form soluble complexes with phosphate (phosphoric acid) and calcium (calcium citrate) from the stone. In addition to reducing irritation, the magnesium undergoes ion exchange with stone calcium, thereby enhancing dissolution. The acidic pH of Suby's solutions G (4.0) and M (4.4) and Renacidin (4.0) is equally responsible for their clinical effectiveness. The solubility of struvite is markedly increased at a pH < 5.5.

Adherence to proper technique in chemolysis of struvite calculi is of the utmost importance. Severe complications and several deaths were reported in the early experience with chemolysis.[16,72–75] The perpetual source of bacteria from within the stone makes systemic sepsis the most frequent severe problem. In fact, the clinical courses and postmortem findings in many of the published complicated cases are consistent with sepsis rather than direct toxicity from the agents.[6] Further analysis of these case reports reveals numerous breaches in proper technique. Irrigations were continued despite fevers in multiple patients. Absence of pressure vents resulting in intrapelvic pressures as high as 80 cm H2O was also identified as a possible factor. Poor renal outflow in those patients irrigated through a single ureteral stent is another violation of proper technique that took place in some of these cases marred by severe complications. In response to these early cases, the United States Food and Drug Administration withdrew approval for use of these agents above the bladder. Despite their continued widespread use and the individual places to reapprove upper tract use,[76] there has been no reversal of this ruling, although permission to restudy this application has been granted.[77]

Safe and effective dissolution treatments nevertheless continue. The guidelines outlined earlier should be followed, with emphasis on adequate outflow drainage. The ideal system would include dual nephrostomy tubes (inflow and outflow) and an indwelling ureteral catheter securing unobstructed passage of fragments. This can be accomplished through a variety of configurations using combinations of simple nephrostomy tubes, circle tubes, universal stents, and other ureteral stents (see Figures 19-1C, 19-1D, and 19-1G). Inflow through a ureteral stent with no other means for outflow is to be condemned.

Treatment of bladder calculi is also effective with these agents. This is carried out by instilling 30 to 50 mL of Renacidin through a Foley catheter and then clamping it for 30 minutes. This is repeated four to six times daily for stones or three times daily for encrustations. Continuous bladder irrigation with a three-way Foley catheter is an alternative. A cystogram to rule out reflux, although recommended, is not essential in these patients.

Maintenance of a sterile urinary tract, while nearly impossible, is a worthy goal in all patients. Antibiotics appropriate for the preirrigation urine cultures should be begun. Chemolysis is initiated only in the presence of negative repeat cultures. Frequent (every 24 to 48 hours) surveillance cultures should be obtained throughout therapy. If febrile episodes occur despite negative urine and blood cultures, actual stone fragments should be cultured. These results are an integral part of the treatment regimen since the stones may harbor different organisms in their interstices than those found in the urine in up to 87% of cases.[6,78]

Table 19-4 Composition of Suby's Solutions and Renacidin

Compound	Suby's Solution		Renacidin
	G	M	
Citric acid (gm)	32.3	32.3	28.2
Magnesium oxide (gm)	3.8	3.8	0
Sodium carbonate (gm)	8.84	8.84	0
Calcium carbonate (gm)	0	0	1.0
D-Gluconic acid (gm)	0	0	5.0
Magnesium hydrocarbonate (gm)	0	0	14.8
Magnesium acid-citrate	0	0	2.5
Water (mL)	1,000	1,000	1,000
pH	4.5	4.0	4.0

Numerous investigators have attempted direct dissolution of struvite calculi (Table 19-5). Several have used dissolution as the primary means of stone eradication, whereas others have applied dissolution techniques in an adjuvant fashion to be used on residual fragments after a debulking procedure. Prophylactic irrigation in the absence of apparent residual calculi has also been advocated by some.[6,76,79] A review of the chemolysis literature shows that the variability in methodology between reports impairs making a direct comparison. The adjunctive procedures range from anatrophic nephrolithotomy to ESWL. The stone burdens among patients are diverse, as are the specific techniques of stone irrigation.

Certain generalizations can be made from the data. Both primary and adjuvant direct chemolysis of struvite calculi can be accomplished with moderate success. Adjuvant chemolysis, mainly as a result of the smaller stone burden, was on average slightly more successful (77 vs. 68%) and took a shorter length of time (9 vs. 14 days) than primary chemolysis in evaluable patients cited in Table 19-5. Renal stones were the targets in the majority of the studies, but bladder stones have been effectively treated.[13] Patients with urinary tract diversions, while afflicted with a disproportionate number of struvite stones, had equal success with dissolution as those with intact urinary tracts.[6,77,80] Furthermore, the complication rate in this population appears to be no worse than in those with normal anatomy.

Although long-term follow-up is limited, it is clear that chemolysis greatly reduces the recurrence rates of both urinary tract infections and calculi over surgery alone. Griffith calculated the postsurgical calculus recurrence rate for struvite stones to be 30% within 6 years.[31] In Silverman and Stamey's review the rate ranged from 20 to 52% at a similar average follow-up.[22] The recurrent infection rate presumably parallels that of calculi formation since they are integrally related. Table 19-6 shows significantly lower recurrence figures for patients receiving chemolytic therapy. The review of the Stanford experience by Silverman and Stamey is especially noteworthy.[22] Their mean follow-up in 40 patients was 8 years and they recorded a 2.5% and 17% recurrent calculi and infection rate, respectively. The basis of their success is their "total therapeutic program," which includes surgical debulking, aggressive culture-specific antimicrobial treatment, and definitive postsurgical chemolysis guided by precise radiographic monitoring (nephrotomograms at 5 mm intervals). The extra effort of such an approach is certainly justifiable considering the results obtained.

The clinical results of chemolysis do not come without a price. In addition to systemic sepsis, Renacidin and Suby's solutions have been implicated as the cause of numerous other complications. The release of large amounts of viable bacteria from the stones is presumably responsible for a number of infectious processes. Several cases of epididymitis, perirenal abscesses, and pyelonephritis have been reported.[73,74,81] These once again highlight the importance of appropriate antimicrobial coverage and proper technique. Some advocate adding neomycin directly to the irrigation solution.[14]

Fungal urinary tract infections have been reported in several patients, none of whom developed fungal sepsis.[76,77,82] It appears that the environment created with easy portals of entry (eg, nephrostomy tube, Foley catheter, ureteral catheter), struvite stones, irrigation fluid in the renal pelvis, and broad-spectrum antimicrobial therapy allow for initiation and establishment of fungal infection. Replacing the irrigation fluid with amphotericin B (50 mg/500 mL H_2O) at a rate of 125 mL/hr generally clears the funguria in less than 72 hours. Chemolysis irrigation resumes when urine cultures are negative for 24 hours. Fortunately, the common systemic side effects of amphotericin B are not observed in this route of administration.

Despite modifications of the solutions using extra magnesium, considerable mucosal irritability is still observed in many patients. In mild cases, the mucosa grossly has a roughened friable appearance. Microscopically, mucosal edema is present. When further advanced, mucosal ulceration and necrosis are evident with a corresponding microscopic appearance of epithelial sloughing and transmural infiltration with polymorphonuclear leukocytes.[16,74] These changes have been noted radiologically as linear or nodular edema and spiculation on nephrostograms in up to one-third of patients.[83,84,85] If such findings are noted, cessation of therapy for 2 to 3 days is indicated. This will often allow mucosal healing and reversal of the radiologic findings if implemented early enough. Further testament to the irritating effects of these acidic solutions are the frequent reports of painful chemical cystitis.[82,86] This condition usually resolves if a Foley catheter is inserted for drainage. In cases refractory to this measure, the irrigation is changed to normal saline solution for 24 to 48 hours and resumed if the cystitis resolves.

Early concern over direct toxic effects from struvite dissolution agents has not been realized. Direct intravenous infusion of Renacidin has been carried out in dogs.[87,88] Although lethal in one animal, the predominant effects were that of systemic acidosis and hypermagnesemia proportional to the amount infused. Even severe violations in technique in humans would result in absorption of relatively small quantities of solution as compared to the dogs.[72,73,80,89] However, numerous instances of hypermagnesemia have been reported. Although occurring primarily in patients with severe renal impairment, magnesium toxicity has been reported in patients with normal renal function.[90] Epithelial erosions, urinary infection, and increased irrigation pressures are factors that certainly contribute to elevated serum levels.

Table 19-5 Results of Direct Chemolysis of Struvite Calculi				
Irrigating Solution	Primary (1°) or Adjuvant (2°) Therapy	Dissolved/ Attempted	Duration of Irrigation (days)	Comment
Suby's Solution G				
Suby and Albright[69]	1°	3/7	10–90	
	2°	1/1		
Smith et al[10]	1°	2/2	5–9	Patients had ileal conduits
	2°	1/1	NA	
Renacidin				
Mulvaney[13]	1°	17/31*	N/A	Kidney/bladder/ureteral stones
Russell[154]	1°	2/2	10–13	
Kohler[74]	1°	4/5	14–115	
	2°	4/6	12–120	
Nemoy and Stamey[6]	1°	3/3	12–30	Prophylactic irrigation used
	2°	4/4	1–14	
Dretler et al[80]	1°	6/8	7–20	
Brock et al[80]	1°	3/4	2–9	Patients had ileal conduits
Rudman et al[57]	1°	2/2	14–17	9% recurrence at 66-mo follow-up
	2°	18/21	2–26	
Dretler and Pfister[83]	1°	16/23	6–45	
Palmer et al[153]	1°	7/9	6–68	Outpatient Rx performed
	2°	7/9	3–30	
Blaivas et al[84]	2°	8/11	2–21	
Jacobs and Gittes[86]	2°	7/11	2/22	
Nemoy and Stamey[156]	2°	2/2	8–15	
Kleine et al[82]	2°	8/9	4–34	
Silverman and Stamey[22]	2°	5/11	4.5(avg)	
Spirnak et al[157]	2°	9/11	2–8	ESWL 1.2 times per kidney
Angermeier et al[79]	2°	3/3	1–8	ESWL & PCNL irrigation with pressure control pump
Totals	1°	65/96	14(avg)	
	2°	77/100	9(avg)	

*Includes partial dissolutions. ESWL = extracorporeal shock wave lithotripsy; N/A = not applicable; PCNL = percutaneous nephrolithotripsy; Rx =

Table 19-6 Patterns of Recurrence Following Successful Hemiacidrin Irrigation of Struvite Calculi

		% Incidence of Recurrence		
Series	No. of patients	Stones	Infection	Mean follow-up (mo)
Nemoy and Stamey[6]	14	0	0	34
Jacobs and Gittes[86]	12	0	8	17
Royle and Smith[28]	28	25	27	42
Low[158]	14	14	28	22
Silverman and Stamey[22]	40	3	17	84
Sant et al.[76]	22	9	14	66

Hypermagnesemia (normal 1.7 to 2.7 mg/dL) is usually mild, and patients are asymptomatic, but signs of toxicity should be monitored. At levels of 5 to 6 mg/dL there may be mental confusion, nausea, and a decrease in deep tendon reflexes. At 7 to 9 mg/dL, respirations slow, hypotension occurs, and the PR, QT, and QRS intervals on the electrocardiogram are prolonged. At higher levels, respiratory paralysis, asystole, and coma may result.[91,92] These effects are much more likely to occur in patients with renal insufficiency because the kidneys are the primary route of magnesium excretion. Therefore, Suby's solutions and Renacidin are contraindicated in patients with a creatinine clearance < 10 mL/min.

Hypermagnesemia should be detected early with daily serum magnesium levels and frequent monitoring of deep tendon reflexes. Rapid initiation of treatment will greatly reduce the complications. Intravenous infusion of saline solution followed by furosemide (Lasix) will cause a dilutional drop in serum magnesium and initiate diuresis, causing a further reduction. One ampule of calcium gluconate is added to each liter of saline solution for mild cases (< 5 mg/dL). For more severe cases, one ampule is administered immediately over 5 to 10 minutes. Furthermore, oxygen, cardiac monitoring, and intensive nursing care should be provided. Hyperphosphatemia has been reported in one instance as well.[73]

URIC ACID Uric acid calculi constitute 5 to 13% of all urinary lithiasis.[93] The majority of these stones are formed in patients with idiopathic uric acid lithiasis,[94] but 10 to 25% of patients with primary gout and 30 to 40% of those with secondary gout due to myeloproliferative disorders have uric acid stones.[95] These stones are generally radiolucent because of their low density (0.226 gm/mL). They are also relatively soft in response to therapeutic fragmentation efforts and as measured by Dretler's "stone fragility index."[96] These characteristics make uric acid calculi amenable to dissolution therapy. They have been successfully dissolved by oral, intravenous, and direct chemolytic techniques, all using urinary alkalinization as the mechanism of action.

The stones have a pKa of 5.35 in urine at 378°C and are thus 50% dissociated at this pH.[91] At higher pH levels, the more soluble dissociated form predominates. For instance, at a pH of 5.0, the solubility of uric acid is 6 to 8 mg/100 mL, whereas at a pH of 7.0, the solubility is 158 mg/100 mL. For dissolution of these stones to occur, the pH of the urine should be 6.5 for systemic agents, or higher for direct irrigating agents. The choice of route for chemolysis depends on the size of the stone and its clinical significance. For asymptomatic uric acid calculi 1 cm or smaller, oral chemolytic therapy is the treatment of choice. Success rates of 80% or greater have been reported with this method alone.[97,98] However, several months may be required for complete dissolution in even the most compliant patient. Renal function in the affected kidney must be good for oral therapy to be effective. For larger or symptomatic stones and in patients who cannot tolerate the alkalinizing therapy, alternative forms of treatment are indicated.

Systemic alkalinization is generally achieved with oral therapy. The most popular agent is sodium bicarbonate, and the dose is 650 to 1,000 mg three to four times daily. An alternative preparation, if the sodium load is too great, is potassium citrate administered as 15 to 30 mEq three to four times daily. This reportedly decreases the formation of calcium stones in patients undergoing alkalinization.[99] The carbonic anhydrase inhibitor acetazolamide is an additional alkalinizing agent often useful in these patients. A dose of 250 or 500 mg is taken at bedtime to maintain urine alkalinity during sleep. Regardless of the method chosen, urine pH should be monitored with nitrazine paper or more accurate pH strips to optimize therapy.

Serum and urine uric acid levels are also important to follow, especially in those with recurrent calculi. The upper limit of serum levels is 7.0 mg/dL for men and 5.5 mg/dL for women. Upper limits for uric acid excretion are 750 to 800 mg/d in males and 650 to 700 mg/d in females. Treatment in addition to urinary alkalinizers is indicated in both hyperuricosemia and hyperuricosuria. Allopurinol is the mainstay of such therapy. This drug inhibits the enzymes xanthine oxidase and hypoxanthine oxidase and the resultant production of uric acid. The dosage is 100 to 300 mg daily, which should be halved in the event of renal insufficiency. As a single agent, allopurinol has been reported to result in stone dissolution with long-term therapy.[100] Side effects of allopurinol occur in approximately 20% of patients and include gastrointestinal distress, rash, fever, bone marrow suppression, hepatitis, toxic epidermal necrolysis, and vasculitis.[57] For mild reactions, a dose reduction of 50% will usually be sufficient, but 5% of patients will require termination of the drug.[57,101] Reduction of dietary intake of purines, although controversial, is usually effective in reducing uric acid excretion as well.[102]

Intravenous alkalinization is more effective than the oral route. Urinary pH is elevated quicker, higher, and more reliably. This technique, however, is typically reserved for hospitalized patients with acute episodes of colic and obstruction. One-sixth molar lactate solution has been demonstrated to dissolve uric acid stones even when they are causing ureteral obstruction.[103] This solution contains the racemic salts of sodium lactate, which are metabolized to bicarbonate and glycogen in 1 to 2 hours, providing a large acid neutralizing capability.[104] If this solution is unavailable, lactated Ringer's solution with one to two ampules of sodium bicarbonate added per liter is an acceptable alternative. The infusion rate (usually 50 to 100 mL/hr) is titrated to a urinary pH of 7.0 to 7.5, which occurs within 4 hours.[105] Extreme care must be exercised in hypertensive or cardiac patients because of the large sodium load in these solutions. Although effective, this technique should not be used in place of definitive therapy for totally obstructing stones.

Large-volume stone disease from uric acid is much less responsive to systemic alkalinization. A primary debulking procedure, using either ESWL or PCNL, is the initial procedure of choice. If a large amount of residual fragments are present or the patient is not a candidate for these procedures, direct chemolysis is a viable option. The most common alkalinizing irrigants are sodium bicarbonate solution (pH 7.0 to 9.0), tromethamine (THAM, pH 8.6), and THAM-E (pH 10.5). All three agents are effective, and each has advantages and disadvantages. Sodium bicarbonate solution is inexpensive and prepared easily by adding two to four ampules (44 mEq each) to each liter of irrigant solution (normal saline solution or water). With this solution, there is no value in increasing the final urinary pH > 7.5. In fact, higher elevations may be detrimental to stone dissolution because phosphatic and sodium urate encrustations may form a coating on stones.[91,105]

The THAM solutions do not appear to cause such mineral deposits. Therefore, when using these agents, the urinary pH can be raised even further. This has been shown in animal models to result in more rapid stone dissolution than sodium bicarbonate.[106] In fact, in vitro studies show that the dissolution rate was almost four times greater with THAM.[107] This effect appears to be primarily the result of increased solubility of the matrix component of the stones rather than directly on uric acid.[108] THAM-E is slightly more effective than THAM because of its higher pH.[108] Animal studies of urothelial toxicity, however, indicate that this pH is also responsible for more irritation and potential damage to the epithelium.[109] Therefore, for uric acid chemolysis, THAM appears to be the agent of choice.[98] The addition of 1.5% acetylcysteine solution to THAM has been reported for uric acid chemolysis, but does not appear to increase the effectiveness reliably.[107]

The high success rate of systemic alkalinization is duplicated by direct chemolysis of uric acid stones. This technique eradicates uric acid calculi rapidly (usually in less than 10 days) in over 90% of the cases (Table 19-7). All solutions are effective, but THAM appears to dissolve stones more rapidly. Chemolysis of uric acid calculi should not exclude other therapy. Allopurinol and oral alkalizers used in conjunction with direct chemolysis enhance stone destruction. Furthermore, vigorous hydration to force a diuresis of 2 L of urine daily is an important component of multimodal therapy. Overall, oral, systemic, and direct chemolysis coupled with ESWL and PCNL have essentially eliminated open surgical management of uric acid nephrolithiasis.

CYSTINE   Cystine urolithiasis continues to be one of the most challenging therapeutic dilemmas in urology. Such stones are formed almost exclusively in individuals with autosomal recessive cystinuria. Between 3% and 59% of those who are homozygous for the trait will produce stones.[110–112] The frequency of cystine calculi in heterozygotes, although reported, is less certain.[113] Most stone formers excrete more than 400 mg of urinary cystine per day.[114] The first calculus occurs at an average patient age of 22.6 years.[112] These individuals have abnormal transport mechanisms of ornithine, lysine, and arginine, which are inconsequential. The only clinically significant defect is that of cystinuria. Overall, these stones represent only 1 to 3% of all urinary calculi.[93]

The early management of cystine stones was predominantly by the open surgical approach. The recurrent nature of large stones is evidenced by the fact that male and female patients underwent an average of 3.4 and 2.8 open surgeries, respectively, prior to the introduction of dissolution therapy.[114] The uniform crystalline structure, which lacks radial or circumferential laminations, makes these stones extremely resistant to fragmentation procedures.[96] They have the lowest value of all urinary calculi in Dretler's "stone fragility index" despite having a very low density surpassed only by uric acid.[96] Stone-free rates of only 31%, 41%, and 55% have been obtained with ESWL, PCNL, and combined therapy, respectively.[115] The high retreatment rate for PCNL with cystine stones is approximately 50%, compared to 12.5% for other calculi.[35,43]

Cystine, like uric acid, is much more soluble in alkaline than acidic urine. It is composed of two cysteine molecules joined by a disulfide bond (Figure 19-2). The pK_a of cystine's amino group is 8.3. At a urinary pH of 6.0, cystine's solubility is 300 mg/L, whereas at a pH of 8.0, it is 800 to 1,200 mg/L.[91] A pH of approximately 7.5 or greater is required to prevent the formation of new stones.[112] The dissolution of cystine stones requires a pH elevation and splitting of the disulfide bond. These can be accomplished through either oral therapy or direct chemolytic therapy.

D-Penicillamine, the first oral agent used for cystine stones, was introduced in this role in

Table 19-7 Results of Direct Chemolysis of Uric Acid Calculi

Irrigating Solution	Dissolved/ Attempted	Duration of Irrigation (days)
Chemolysis Alone		
Sodium bicarbonate	11/11	3–21[11,73,159–162]
THAM	3/3	7–10[163]
Sodium lactate	3/3	7–14[164]
ESWL and Chemolysis		
Sodium bicarbonate	5/8*	2–7[165]

* Three patients had only small clinically insignificant fragments. ESWL = extracorporeal shock wave lithotripsy.

1963.[116] This drug is a disulfide exchange resin that facilitates separation at the disulfide bond through the thiol exchange reaction forming mixed disulfides (penicillamine disulfide-cysteine).[117] This complex is 50 times more soluble than cystine.[57] Furthermore, D-penicillamine decreases urinary excretion of cystine. The dose of D-penicillamine is 1 to 2 gm daily, administered in four divided doses, which is begun once a smaller dose is tolerated. The effectiveness of this agent is determined by assessing urine cystine content with either the sodium cyanide-nitroprusside test or amino acid analysis.[118] The drug's frequent severe side effects require cessation of therapy in up to 50% of patients.[119,120] These reactions include (1) hematologic changes (leukopenia and thrombocytopenia), (2) gastrointestinal disturbances, (3) skin rashes with fever and pruritus, (4) proteinuria and nephrotic syndrome, (5) neuropathies, and (6) abnormalities of taste and smell. The addition of pyridoxine (vitamin B_6, 25 mg twice daily) is recommended by some to reduce the incidence of neurologic complications.[117,121] D-Penicillamine has been reported to dissolve even large stones when combined with alkalinization. For instance,

in a Mayo Clinic study, 10 of 21 patients had complete dissolution in 24 to 41 months with combined hydration, alkalinization, and D-penicillamine.[112] Nevertheless, the length of treatment required and its potential for side effects severely limit its usefulness.[122]

α-Mercaptopropionylglycine (MPG) is a second disulfide exchange resin that was introduced in 1968.[123] This medication has fewer side effects than D-penicillamine and appears to be more effective.[120,124,125] As with penicillamine, fever, skin rashes, malaise, and gastrointestinal disturbances are the most common adverse reactions.[125] A reversible dose-dependent proteinuria is occasionally noted as well.[125] The usual dose of MPG is 600 to 1,800 mg daily in four divided doses. With prolonged use, the dose requirements may rise.[126] The goal of therapy is a reduction of urinary excretion of cystine to 200 to 300 mg or less daily.[112,125] Simultaneous treatment with oral sodium bicarbonate increases the effectiveness of this preparation because the disulfide exchange reaction is more active at higher pH levels. As a single agent, without sodium bicarbonate, MPG has been shown to increase urinary pH.[127] Although often better than D-penicillamine, MPG has limited efficacy in primary oral chemolytic therapy of cystine stones. Partial and complete dissolution rates range from 14 to 31% and 19 to 47%, respectively.[125,128] The duration of therapy is quite lengthy, ranging from 22 to 51 months.[125]

Acetylcysteine has been used orally as well.[129] The usual dose in adults is 0.7 gm four times daily (20 to 500 mg/kg/d). Side effects in humans are rare. In limited trials, complete dissolution was noted in one of six cases, whereas partial dissolution was found in two of six cases. Like the other agents, limited efficacy is seen after long-term oral therapy with acetylcysteine. There is some evidence that it may even increase urinary excretion of cystine.[98]

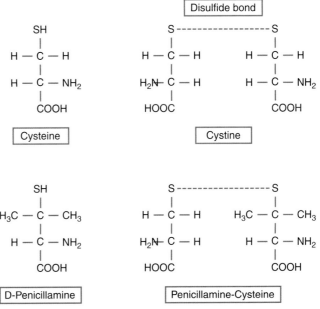

Figure 19-2 Chemical structure of cystine and related compounds.

Overall, oral acetylcysteine, MPG, and D-penicillamine are much more effective in preventing the formation of cystine calculi than dissolving them. When used for direct chemolysis, however, they are more potent dissolution agents. Their mechanisms of action are identical, regardless of how they are administered. During direct irrigation, however, the solution bathing the stone will have a much higher concentration of the active agent. The pH of the solution is likewise more easily controlled, thereby facilitating the thiol exchange reaction. Table 19-8 illustrates the multiple combinations of irrigating agents and adjunctive procedures that have been used to eliminate cystine stones.

In 1979, N-acetylcysteine (NAc) and sodium bicarbonate were first used by Smith and colleagues[130] with complete calculous dissolution in one patient in 26 days. In this report, 60 mL of 20% NAc and 300 mg of sodium bicarbonate were added to each liter of normal saline solution to form a 1% NAc solution initially, which was then doubled later in the therapy. In that same year, Crissey and Gittes[131] used THAM-E and successfully dissolved a ureteral calculus in 5 days but failed to dissolve a staghorn calculus. Stark and Savir[132] successfully dissolved residual cystine stones after pyelolithotomy with D-penicillamine irrigation. However, the duration of treatment was 6 months. Hayase and colleagues[133] used MPG irrigation for an average of 49 days and successfully dissolved one bladder stone and residual fragments after four pyelolithotomies. Others have used these agents with moderate degrees of success.[134,135–139]

Comparison of these reports to determine which agent is most efficacious is a futile task. There is far too much variability in technique, stone burden, and adjuvant therapy to draw any conclusions. Several investigators have attempted to solve this problem with in vitro testing of cystine chemolysis.[140,141,142,143] Evaluation of NAc alone indicates that a 2% (0.3 M) solution is the most effective.[140,141,143] The solutions tested were buffered from the original pH of NAc (2.0) to 7.5 to 10.6. The dissolution rates in the higher pH range were tenfold greater than those at the lower pH levels. THAM-E (pH 10.2 to 10.6) alone was slightly less effective than 2% NAc buffered to a similar pH with sodium bicarbonate.[142,143] Using THAM-E as the buffering agent did not improve dissolution rates over the sodium bicarbonate/NAc solutions at a comparable pH.[141,143] However, calcium phosphate salts are more likely to occur with sodium bicarbonate, thus impeding further dissolution.[106] Therefore, although not entirely clear, some suggest that, despite its higher cost, the best solution is 0.3 M NAc in THAM-E.[98]

The overall role that chemolysis has in the management of cystine stones has been examined.[91,114,144] Chemolysis alone would require lengthy durations of irrigation for all but the smallest stones. It has been estimated that approximately 9 days are required to dissolve a 1 cm cystine calculus. The addition of ESWL and PCNL

Table 19-8 Results of Direct Chemolysis of Cystine Calculi

Irrigating Solution	Dissolved/Attempted	Duration of Irrigation	Adjunctive Treatment, etc.
THAM-E	0/3[133]	25–37 days	3 partial dissolution, 1 nephrolithotomy
	1/2[131]	5 days	1 ureteral, 1 renal stone
THAM-E with/without n-acetylcysteine	3/9[144]	–	3 partial dissolution, ESWL with/without PCNL
	7/11[134]	6–42 days	1 partial dissolution
	2/2[166]	3–9 days	Surgery with/without ESWL
N-Acetylcysteine + sodium bicarbonate	1/1[130]	26 days	
	1/1[140]	30 days	
Mercaptopropionylglycine	5/5[151]	24–88 days	1 pyelolithotomy, 1 bladder stone, urokinase added to irrigant
Penicillamine	1/1[132]	6 mo	1 pyelolithotomy

greatly diminishes irrigation times since they reduce the stone burden and increase the surface area of the remaining fragments. Stones < 1.5 cm may be treated initially with ESWL (Figure 19-3). If successful fragmentation occurs, repeat ESWL or medical management may be sufficient follow-up therapy. Otherwise chemolysis alone or combined with PCNL is appropriate. For stones > 1.5 cm, PCNL is the initial procedure of choice. Residual calculi, which are likely to remain, can be effectively treated with chemolysis and additional PCNL or ESWL sessions. Simultaneous oral therapy should be implemented in all cases.

If the stones appear extremely resistant to therapeutic measures, the possibility of a mixed stone should not be overlooked. Hydroxyapatite, struvite, calcium oxalate, and calcium phosphate contaminants have been present in 14 to 46% of cystine calculi analyzed in some studies.[112,145,146] Prompt recognition of these additional components should guide therapy accordingly. For instance, Koide and colleagues[147] successfully used ESWL when cystine calculi in three patients were noted to contain predominantly hydroxyapatite. Coexistent urinary tract infections have been documented in 29 to 34% of patients with cystine stones as well.[112,148] Thus antibiotic coverage is an integral part of the therapeutic regimen. In summary, although cystine urinary calculi continue to present a formidable challenge to urologists, successful eradication without open surgery may be accomplished with chemolytic techniques in conjunction with minimally invasive fragmentation procedures.

CALCIUM OXALATE Calcium oxalate stones, while constituting the vast majority of all renal calculi, are the least amenable to chemolysis. The strong acids required to dissolve this compound cannot be safely used in humans. Therefore, attempts at dissolving these stones have been limited to the use of chelation agents. Ethylenediaminetetraacetic acid (EDTA) is the most commonly used solvent. Calcium from within the stone binds this substance and is therefore leached from the stone. The overall effectiveness of EDTA and other chelation agents has been tested at a variety of concentrations and pH levels.[148–150] EDTA is among the strongest calcium chelators tested. For maximal activity, a pH of 8.0 to 8.5 and

a concentration of 0.03 M are required,[148–150] but significant mucosal injury has been reported when irrigating with this type of solution.[151]

Nevertheless, EDTA-based solutions have been used with moderate success in humans. The greatest amount of work in this area has been done by Timmermann and Kallistratos.[18,148,152] In their initial 125 patients, a complete dissolution rate of 66% was reported, whereas the remainder had partial dissolution. Their next 135 patients had a complete dissolution rate of 46% which, when combined with the first 125, gives a rate of complete stone dissolution of over 50%. Patients with recurrent stones had 100% complete dissolution if they were treated within 6 months of formation. These investigators also used 0.25% lyophilized papain to dissolve the matrix component of the stones. Others have had similar success with EDTA-based solutions but with far fewer patients.[15]

EDTA solutions are not widely used primarily because they are irritative and noxious to the urothelium. Kallistratos[148] described the following techniques to reduce this toxicity:

1. Maintain the purity of the compounds in the solution.
2. Begin irrigating with dilute EDTA solutions and gradually increase the concentration.
3. Warm the solution to body temperature.
4. Add potassium ions to the solution.
5. Control intrarenal pressures carefully.

Direct endoscopic examination with biopsy in several cases failed to reveal significant changes in the urothelium when these measures were followed. The potential anticoagulating effect of EDTA is believed to be responsible for hematuria in some cases.[15] Overall, in its current state, chemolysis for calcium oxalate stones is limited at best. Some claim that there is no role for EDTA solutions in this capacity because of the potential for urinary tract damage.[98]

CONCLUSION

Chemolysis is a useful modality for treating urolithiasis when applied appropriately. With adherence to proper technique, the safety of this method remains high. Struvite, uric acid, and cystine stones respond reasonably well to the currently available agents. Chemolysis is much

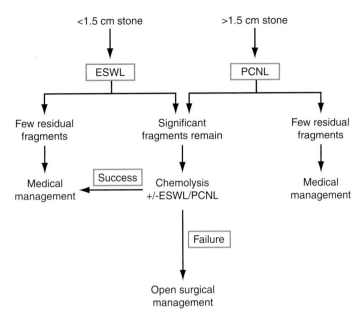

Figure 19-3 Management algorithm for cystine calculi.

less useful for calcium oxalate stones. The lengthy duration of treatment is the biggest drawback of direct irrigation chemolysis in this era of cost containment. However, successful outpatient treatments have been reported with few complications.[12,153] Therefore, as long as urinary stones continue to afflict man, chemolysis is likely to retain its limited but important role in their management.

REFERENCES

1. Crowell AJ. Cystine nephrolithiasis: report of case with roentgenographic demonstration of disintegration of stone by alkalinization. Surg Gynecol Obstet 1924;38:87.
2. Otnes B. Crystalline composition of urinary stones in recurrent stone formers: quantitative observations on the crystalline composition of urinary stones. Scand J Urol Nephrol 1983;17:179.
3. Van Ardsdalen KN, Banner MP, Pollack HM. Radiographic imaging and urologic decision making in the management of renal and ureteral calculi. Urol Clin North Am 1990; 17:171.
4. Federle MP, McAninch JW, Kaiser JA, et al. Computed tomography of urinary calculi. Am J Radiol 1981;136:255.
5. Mitcheson HD, Zamenhof RG, Bankoff MS, et al. Determination of the chemical composition of urinary calculi by computerized tomography. J Urol 1983;130:814.
6. Nemoy NJ, Stamey TA. Surgical, bacteriological, and biochemical management of "infection stones." JAMA 1971;215:1470.
7. Kuwahara M, Kambe K, Takahashi K, et al. Intermittent irrigation system for dissolution of renal calculi monitored by computer. J Urol 1982;128:1379.
8. Kahn SR, Hackett RL, Finlayson B. Morphology of urinary stone particles resulting from ESWL treatment. J Urol 1986;136:1367.
9. Hare WSC, McOmish D. Nephrostomy lavage set for dissolving renal stones. Radiology 1982;144:932.
10. Smith AD, Reinke DB, Miller RP, et al. Percutaneous nephrostomy in the management of ureteral and renal calculi. Radiology 1979;133:49.
11. Hedgcock MW, Eisenberg RL, Williams RD. Antegrade catheter technique to dissolve uric acid ureteral calculi. Urology 1982;19:407.
12. Kubota N, Koide T, Takemoto M, et al. Successful renal stone dissolution by long-term irrigation. Eur Urol 1981;7:312.
13. Mulvaney WP. The clinical use of Renacidin in urinary calcifications. J Urol 1960;84:206.
14. Mulvaney WP, Henning DC. Solvent treatment of urinary calculi: refinements in technique. J Urol 1962;88:_145.
15. Heap GJ, Perrin DD, Cliff WJ. Dissolving urinary stones with a chelating agent. Med J Aust 1976;1:714.

16. Auerbach S, Mainwaring R, Schwartz F. Renal and ureteral damage following clinical use of Renacidin. JAMA 1963;183:61.
17. Goldstein HH. The dissolution of staghorn calculi. Med Soc NJ 1961;58:409.
18. Timmermann A, Kallistratos G. Modern aspects of chemical dissolution of human renal calculi by irrigation. J Urol 1966;95:469.
19. Comarr AE, Kawaichi GK, Bors E. Renal calculosis of patients with traumatic cord lesions. J Urol 1962;87:647.
20. Kracht H, Buscher HK. Formation of staghorn calculi and their surgical implications in paraplegics and tetraplegics. Paraplegia 1974;12:98.
21. Koff SA, Lappides J. Altered bladder function in staghorn calculus disease. J Urol 1977;117:577.
22. Silverman DE, Stamey TA. Management of infection stones: the Stanford experience. Medicine 1983;62:44.
23. Griffith DP, McCue P, Lee H, et al. Stone cancer-palliative treatment with acetohydroxamic acid. World J Urol 1983; 1:170.
24. Priestley JT, Dunn JH. Branched renal calculi. J Urol 1949; 61:194.
25. Blandy JP, Singh M. The case for a more aggressive approach to staghorn stones. J Urol 1976;115:505.
26. Smith MJV, Boyce WH. Anatrophic nephrotomy and plastic calyraphy. J Urol 1968;99:521.
27. Marshall VR, Lavengood RW, Kelly D. Complete longitudinal nephrolithotomy and the Shorr regimen in the management of staghorn calculi. Ann Surg 1965;162:366.
28. Royle G, Smith JC. Recurrence of infected calculi following postoperative renal irrigation with stone solvent. Br J Urol 1976;48:531.
29. Pappathanassidus S, Swinney J. Results of partial nephrectomy compared with pyelolithotomy and nephrolithotomy. Br J Urol 1966;38:403.
30. Russell JM, Harrison LH, Boyce WH. Recurrent urolithiasis following anatrophic nephrolithotomy. J Urol 1981;125:471.
31. Griffith DP. Struvite stones. Kidney Int 1978;13:372.
32. Pode D, Caine M, Pfau A, et al. Shock-wave treatment for stones in the kidney and ureter: the Jerusalem experience. Israel J Med Sci 1987;23:243.
33. Cochran ST, Barbaric ZL, Mindell HJ, et al. Extracorporeal shock wave lithotripsy: impact on the radiology department of a stone treatment center. Radiology 1987;163:655.
34. Riehle RA, Fair WR, Vaughan ED Jr. Extracorporeal shockwave lithotripsy for upper urinary tract calculi—one year's experience at a single center. JAMA 1986;255:2043.
35. Winfield HN, Clayman RV, Chaussy CG, et al. Monotherapy of staghorn renal calculi: a comparative study between percutaneous nephrolithotomy and extracorporeal shock wave lithotripsy. J Urol 1988;139:895.
36. Lee WJ, Snyder JA, Smith AD. Staghorn calculi: endourologic management in 120 patients. Radiology 1987;165:85.
37. Young AT, Hulbert JC, Cardella JF, et al. Percutaneous nephrostolithotomy: application to staghorn calculi. Am J Roentgenol 1985;145:1265.

38. Kerlan RK, Kahn RK, Laberge JM, et al. Percutaneous removal of renal staghorn calculi. Am J Roentgenol 1985; 145:803.
39. Adams GW, Oke EJ, Dunnick NR, et al. Percutaneous lithotripsy of staghorn calculi. Am J Roentgenol 1985; 145:797.
40. Krieger JN, Rudd TG, Mayo ME. Current treatment of infection stones in high risk patients. J Urol 1984;132:874.
41. Culkin CJ, Wheeler JS, Nemchausky BA, et al. Percutaneous nephrolithotomy in the spinal cord injury population. J Urol 1986;136:1181.
42. Snyder JA, Smith AD. Staghorn calculi: percutaneous extraction versus anatrophic nephrolithotomy. J Urol 1986;136:351.
43. Segura JW, Patterson DE, LeRoy AJ, et al. Percutaneous removal of kidney stones: review of 1,000 cases. J Urol 1985;134:1077.
44. Gilhuis R, Carpentier PJ. Treatment of staghorn calculus by percutaneous lithotripsy followed by ESWL [Abstract]. J Urol 1987;137(Part 2):279.
45. Streem SB, Zelch MG, Risius B, et al. Planned endourologic "sandwich" therapy for extensive staghorn calculi [Abstract]. J Urol 1987;137(Part 2):280.
46. Schulze H, Hertle L, Graff J, et al. Combined treatment of branched calculi by percutaneous nephrolithotomy and extracorporeal shock wave lithotripsy. J Urol 1986;135: 1138.
47. Dickinson IK, Fletcher MS, Bailey MJ, et al. Combination of percutaneous surgery and extracorporeal shockwave lithotripsy for the treatment of large renal calculi. Br J Urol 1986;58:581.
48. Eisenberger F, Rassweiler J, Bub P, et al. Differentiated approach to staghorn calculi using extra-corporeal shock wave lithotripsy and percutaneous nephrolithotomy: an analysis of 151 consecutive cases. World J Urol 1987;5:248.
49. Kahnoski RJ, Lingeman JE, Coury TA, et al. Combined percutaneous and extracorporeal shock wave lithotripsy for staghorn calculi: an alternative to anatrophic nephrolithotomy. J Urol 1986;135:679.
50. Scharfe T, Alken P, Muller ST. Combined treatment of staghorn calculi by PNL and ESWL [Abstract]. J Urol 1986;135(Part 2):298.
51. Williams RE. Long term survey of 538 patients with upper urinary tract stones. Br J Urol 1963;35:416.
52. Fishbein WN, Carbone PP. Acetohydroxamate inhibition of bacterial urease in vitro and in vivo. Clin Res 1964;12:453.
53. Griffith DP, Khonsari F, Skurnick JH, et al. A randomized trial of acetohydroxamic acid for the treatment and prevention of infection-induced urinary stones in spinal cord injury patients. J Urol 1988;140:318.
54. Williams JJ, Rodman JS, Peterson CM. A randomized double-blind study of acetohydroxamic acid in struvite nephrolithiasis. N Engl J Med 1984;311:760.
55. Griffith DP, Lee H, Longuet R, et al. Double-blind clinical trial of Lithostat (acetohydroxamic acid) in the palliative treatment of infection-induced urinary stones (unpublished data).
56. Griffith DP, Moskowitz PA, Carlton CE Jr. Adjunctive chemotherapy of infection induced by staghorn calculi. J Urol 1979;121:711.
57. Rudman D, Afforah H, Tuttle EP, et al. Medical management of the patient with renal calculi. AUA Update Series 1983;2: No. 9.
58. Rodman JS, Williams JJ, Peterson CM. Partial dissolution of struvite calculus with oral acetohydroxamic acid. Urology 1983;22:410.
59. Martelli A, Buli P, Spatafora S. Clinical experience with low dosage of propionohydroxamic acid (PHA) in infected renal stones. Urology 1986;28:373.
60. Andersen JA. Benurestat, a urease inhibitor for the therapy of infected ureolysis. Invest Urol 1975;12:381.
61. Javor A, Frang D, Nagy Z. Applicability of biosuppressin as an urease inhibitor. Int Urol Nephrol 1984;16:191.
62. Millner OE Jr, Andersen JA, Appler ME, et al. Flurofamide: a potent inhibitor of bacterial urease with potential clinical utility in the treatment of infection induced urinary stones. J Urol 1982;127:346.
63. Kobashi K, Takebe S, Numata A. Specific inhibition of urease by N-acylphosphoric triamides. J Biochem 1985;98:1681.
64. Takeuchi H, Kobashi K, Yoshida O. Prevention of infected urinary stones in rats by urease inhibition. A new hydroxamic acid derivative. Invest Urol 1980;18:102.
65. Takeuchi H, Okada Y, Kobashi K, et al. Treatment of infected urinary stones in rats by a new hydroxamic acid, "N-(pivaroyl)glycinohydroxamic acid." Urol Res 1982;10:217.
66. Lewis GA, Schaster GA, Cooper RA. Dissolution of renal calculi with dicloxacillin. Urology 1983;22:401.

67. Shorr E, Carter AC. Aluminum gels in the management of renal phosphatic calculi. JAMA 1950;144:1549.

68. Lotz M, Zisman E, Bartter FC. Evidence for a phosphorus-depletion syndrome in man. N Engl J Med 1968;278:409.

69. Suby HI, Albright F. Dissolution of phosphatic urinary calculi by the retrograde introduction of a citrate solution containing magnesium. N Engl J Med 1943;228:81.

70. Suby HI, Suby RM, Albright F. Properties of organic acid solutions which determine their irritability to the bladder mucous membrane and the effect of magnesium ions in overcoming this irritability. J Urol 1942;48:549.

71. Mulvaney WP. A new solvent for certain urinary calculi. J Urol 1959;82:546.

72. Cato AR, Tulloch AGS. Hypermagnesemia in a uremic patient during renal pelvis irrigation with Renacidin. J Urol 1974;111:313.

73. Fostvedt GA, Barnes RW. Complications during lavage therapy for renal calculi. J Urol 1963;89:329.

74. Kohler FP. Renacidin and tissue reaction. J Urol 1962;87:102.

75. Ries SW, Malament M. Renacidin: a urinary calculi solvent. J Urol 1962;87:657.

76. Sant GR, Blaivas JG, Meares EM Jr. Hemiacidrin irrigation in the management of struvite calculi: long-term results. J Urol 1983;130:1048.

77. Fam V, Rossier AB, Yalla S, et al. The role of hemiacidrin in the management of renal stones in spinal cord injury patients. J Urol 1976;116:696.

78. Lerner SP, Gleeson MJ, Griffith DP. Infection stones. J Urol 1989;141:753.

79. Angermeier K, Streem SB, Yost A. Simplified infusion method for 10% hemiacidrin irrigation of renal pelvis. Urology 1993;41:3.

80. Brock WA, Nachtsheim DA, Parsons CL. Hemiacidrin irrigation of renal pelvic calculi in patients with ileal conduit diversion. J Urol 1980;123:345.

81. Mischol JR, Windbolz E. Instrumental chemolysis of renal calculi: indications and dangers. J Urol 1971;105:607.

82. Kleine RS, Cattolica EV, Rankin KN. Hemiacidrin renal irrigation: complications and successful management. J Urol 1982;128:241.

83. Dretler SP, Pfister RC. Percutaneous dissolution of renal calculi. Ann Rev Med 1983;34:359.

84. Blaivas JG, Pais UM, Spellman RM. Chemolysis of residual stone fragments after extensive surgery for staghorn calculi. Urology 1975;6:680.

85. Cunningham JJ, Friedland GW, Stamey TA. Radiologic changes in the urothelium during Renacidin irrigation. J Urol 1973;109:556.

86. Jacobs SC, Gittes RF. Dissolution of residual renal calculi with hemiacidrin. J Urol 1976;115:2.

87. Mulvaney WP. The hydrodynamics of renal irrigations: with reference to calculus solvents. J Urol 1963;89:765.

88. Rosen DI, Nemoy NJ, Wolf PL, et al. Intravenous infusion of Renacidin in dogs. Invest Urol 1971;9:31.

89. Jenny DB, Goris GB, Urwiller RD, et al. Hypermagnesemia following irrigation of renal pelvis: cause of respiratory depression. JAMA 1978;240:1378.

90. Fassler CA, Rodriguez RM, Badesch DB, et al. Magnesium toxicity as a cause of hypotension and hypoventilation. Occurrence in patients with normal renal function. Arch Intern Med 1985;145:1604.

91. Dretler SP. Chemolysis of urinary calculi. AUA Update Series 1986;5: No. 21.

92. Randall RE, Cohen DN, Spray CC, et al. Hypermagnesemia in renal failure: etiology and toxic manifestations. Ann Intern Med 1964;61:73.

93. Prien EL. Crystallographic analysis of urinary calculi: a 23-year study. J Urol 1963;89:917.

94. Kursh ED, Resnick MI. Dissolution of uric acid calculi with systemic alkalinization. J Urol 1984;132:286.

95. Strauss MB, Welt LG. Diseases of the Kidney, 2nd ed. Boston: Little, Brown; 1971. p. 987.

96. Dretler SP. Stone fragility—a new therapeutic distinction. J Urol 1988;139:1124.

97. Uhlir K. The peroral dissolution of renal calculi. J Urol 1970; 104:239.

98. Rodman JS, Vaughan ED Jr. Chemolysis of urinary calculi. AUA Update Series 1992;11: No. 1.

99. Sakhaee K, Nicar M, Hill K, et al. Contrasting effects of potassium citrate and sodium citrate therapies on urinary chemistries and crystallization of stone forming salts. Kidney Int 1983;24:348.

100. Wasko R, Frankenfield BA. Allopurinol dissolution of renal uric acid calculi. JAMA 1968;205:177.

101. Meno M, Krishman CS. Evaluation and medical management of the patient with calcium stone disease. Urol Clin North Am 1983;10:4.

102. Cifuentes L, Rapado A, Hodgkinson A, eds. Urinary calculi. International symposium on renal stone research. Basel, Switzerland: S Karger; 1973. p. 89.

103. Lewis RW, Roth JK, Polanca EJ, et al. Molar lactate in the management of uric acid renal obstruction. J Urol 1981; 125:87.

104. Libert MH, Wart F. Management of uric acid renal obstruction by intravenous lactate. Eur Urol 1985;11:22.

105. Petritsch PH. Management of uric acid lithiasis. Emirates Med J 1979;1(Suppl):73.

106. Sadi MV, Saltzman N, Feria G, et al. Experimental observations on dissolution of uric acid calculi. J Urol 1985;134: 575.

107. Burns JR, Gauthier JF, Birdwell F. Dissolution kinetics of uric acid calculi. J Urol 1984;131:708.

108. Ismail SI, Tawashi R. Effect of the organic matrix on the dissolution of uric acid stones. Eur Urol 1980;6:237.

109. Chernesky CE, Rodman JS, Reckler J, et al. Urothelial injury to the rabbit bladder from alkaline irrigants useful in the treatment of uric acid stone. J Urol 1987;138:893.

110. Dent CE, Senior B. Studies on the treatment of cystinuria. Br J Urol 1955;27:317.

111. Linari F, Marangella M, Fruttero B, et al. The natural history of cystinuria: a 15-year follow-up in 106 patients. In: Smith LH, Robertson WG, Finlayson B, editors. Urolithiasis: clinical and basic research. New York: Plenum Press; 1981. p. 145–154.

112. Dahlberg PF, VanDenBerg CJ, Kurtz SB, et al. Clinical features and management of cystinuria. Mayo Clin Proc 1977;52:533.

113. Wilken B, Smith A, Gaha TJ, et al. Screening for metabolic diseases in New South Wales. Med J Aust 1973;1:1129.

114. Singer A, Sakti D. Cystinuria: a review of the pathophysiology and management. J Urol 1989;142:669.

115. Martin X, Salas M, Labeeuw M, et al. Cystine stones: the impact of new treatment. Br J Urol 1991;68:234.

116. Crawhall JC, Scowen EF, Watts RWE. Effect of penicillamine on cystinuria. Br Med J 1963;1:588.

117. Bartter FC, Lotz M, Thier S, et al. Cystinuria. Ann Intern Med 1965;62:796.

118. Hambraeus L. Comparative studies of the value of two cyanide-nitroprusside methods in the diagnosis of cystinuria. Scand J Clin Lab Invest 1963;15:657.

119. Halperin EC, Thier SO, Rosenberg LE. The use of D-penicillamine in cystinuria: efficacy and untoward reactions. Yale J Biol Med 1981;54:439.

120. Pak CYC, Fuller C, Sakhaee K, et al. Management of cystine nephrolithiasis with alpha-mercaptopropionylglycine. J Urol 1986;136:1003.

121. Jaffe IA, Altman K, Merryman P. The antipyridoxine effect of penicillamine in man. J Clin Invest 1964;13:1869.

122. VanDuzteren GR, Wuggelinkhuizen J. Dissolution of bilateral staghorn cystine renal calculi. Arch Dis Child 1979;54:795.

123. King JS Jr. Treatment of cystinuria with alpha-mercaptopropionylglycine: a preliminary report with some notes on column chromatography of mercaptans. Proc Soc Exp Biol Med 1968;129:927.

124. MacDonald WB, Fellers FX. Penicillamine in the treatment of patients with cystinuria. JAMA 1966;197:396.

125. Koide T, Konoshita K, Takemoto M, et al. Conservative treatment of cystine calculi: effect of oral alpha-mercaptopropionylglycine on cystine stones, dissolution and/or prevention of stone recurrences. J Urol 1982;128:513.

126. Hautmann RE. Cystine stone therapy with alpha-mercaptopropionylglycine: ten years of experience with forty-two patients. In: Smith LH, Robertson WG, Finlayson B, editors. Urolithiasis: clinical and basic research. New York: Plenum Press; 1981. p. 139–143.

127. King JS, Wainer A. Treatment of cystinuria with alpha-mercaptopropionylglycine: a preliminary report with some notes on column chromatography of mercaptans. Proc Soc Exp Biol Med 1968;129:927.

128. Lotz M, Potts JT, Holland JM, et al. D-Penicillamine therapy in cystinuria. J Urol 1966;95:257.

129. Mulvaney WP, Quilter T, Mortera A. Experiences with acetylcysteine in cystinuric patients. J Urol 1975;114:107.

130. Smith AD, Lange PH, Miller RP, et al. Dissolution of cystine calculi by irrigation with acetylcysteine through percutaneous nephrostomy. Urology 1979;13:422.

131. Crissey MM, Gittes RF. Dissolution of cystine ureteral calculus by irrigation with tromethamine. J Urol 1979;121:811.

132. Stark H, Savir A. Dissolution of cystine calculi by pelviocalyceal irrigation with D-penicillamine. J Urol 1980;124: 895.

133. Hayase Y, Fukatsu H, Segawa A. The dissolution of cystine stones by irrigation with tiopronin solution. J Urol 1980; 124:775.

134. Dretler SP, Pfister RC, Newhouse JH, et al. Percutaneous catheter dissolution of cystine calculi. J Urol 1984;131:216.

135. Tseng CH, Talmalker YB, Tank ES, et al. Dissolution of cystine calculi by pelviocaliceal irrigation with tromethamine-E. J Urol 1982;128:1281.

136. Boyce WH. Organic matrix of human concretions. Am J Med 1968;45:673.

137. Elomaa I, Karanen SL, Kairento AL, et al. Seasonal variation of urinary calcium and oxalate excretion, serum 25-(OH)-D₃ and albumin level in relation to renal stone formation. Scand J Urol Nephrol 1982;16:155.

138. Otnes B. Observations on urinary stone weight correlated with composition. Scand J Urol Nephrol 1983;17:191.

139. Berkhoff WBC, Van Haga JJW, Roodvoets AP. Outpatient percutaneous chemolitholysis of cystine stones. Br J Urol 1987;60:180.

140. Schmeller NT, Holger K, Schuller J, et al. Combination of chemolysis and shock wave lithotripsy in the treatment of cystine renal calculi. J Urol 1984;131:434.

141. Saltzman N, Gittes RF. Chemolysis of cystine calculi. J Urol 1986;136:846.

142. Singh A, Marshall FF, Chang R. Cystine calculi: clinical management and in vitro observations. Urology 1988;31:207.

143. Burns JR, Hamrick LC. In vitro dissolution of cystine urinary calculi. J Urol 1986;136:850.

144. Kachel TA, Vijan SR, Dretler SP. Endourological experience with cystine calculi and a treatment algorithm. J Urol 1991;145:25.

145. Shaw DG, Sutor DJ. Cystine stone dissolution. Br J Radiol 1972;45:664.

146. Evans WP, Resnick MI, Boyce WH. Homozygous cystinuria—Evaluation of 35 patients. J Urol 1982;127:707.

147. Koide T, Toshiaki Y, Tamaguchi S, et al. A strategy of cystine stone management. J Urol 1992;147:112.

148. Kallistratos G. Litholytic agents with bacteriostatic properties in conservative treatment of urolithiasis. Eur Urol 1975;1:261.

149. Verplaetse H, Verbeeck RMH, Minnaert H, et al. Screening of chelating agents for chemolysis. Eur Urol 1986;12:190.

150. Ziolkowski F, Perrin D. Dissolution of urinary stones by calcium-chelating agents: a study using a model system. Invest Urol 1977;15:208.

151. Kane MH, Rodman JS, Horten B, et al. Urothelial injury from ethylenediaminetetraacetic acid used as an irrigant in the urinary tract. J Urol 1989;142:1359.

152. Timmermann A, Kallistratos G. Chemotherapy in nephrolithiasis. Israel J Med Sci 1971;7:689.

153. Palmer JM, Bishai MB, Mallon DS. Outpatient irrigation of the renal collecting system with 10 percent hemiacidrin: cumulative experience of 365 days in 13 patients. J Urol 1987;138:262.

154. Russell M. Dissolution of bilateral renal staghorn calculi with Renacidin. J Urol 1962;88:141.

155. Dretler SP, Pfister RC, Newhouse JH. Renal-stone dissolution via percutaneous nephrostomy. N Engl J Med 1979; 300:341.

156. Nemoy NJ, Stamey TA. Use of hemiacidrin in management of infection stones. J Urol 1976;116:693.

157. Spirnak JP, DeBaz BP, Green HY, et al. Complex struvite calculi treated by primary extracorporeal shock wave lithotripsy and chemolysis with hemiacidrin irrigation. J Urol 1988;140:1356.

158. Low AI. The use of hemiacidrin in the management of staghorn calculi. In: Brockis JG, Finlayson B, editors. Urinary calculus. Littleton (MA): PSG Publishers; 1981. p. 427.

159. Hardy B, Klein LA. In situ dissolution of ureteral calculus. Urology 1976;8:444.

160. Spaters RF, Linke CA, Barbaric ZL. The use of percutaneous nephrostomy and urinary alkalinization in the dissolution of obstructed uric acid stones. Radiology 1978;129:629.

161. Eason AA, Sharlip ID, Spaulding JO. Dissolution of bilateral uric acid calculi causing anuria. JAMA 1978;240:670.

162. Nummi P. Dissolution of uric acid stones by local lavage. Scand J Urol Nephrol 1973;7:172.

163. Gordon MR, Carrion JM, Politano VA. Dissolution of uric acid calculi with THAM irrigation. Urology 1978;12:393.

164. Ansari ER, Kazim E, Husain I. Management of the choked ureter in obstructive renal failure due to uric acid lithiasis. J Urol 1982;128:257.

165. Lee YH, Chang LS, Chen MT, et al. Experience with percutaneous nephrostomy, extracorporeal shock wave lithotripsy and chemolysis in the treatment of obstructive uric acid stones. Eur Urol 1991;19:208.

166. Aabech J, Andersen JT. Treatment of cystine stones: combined approach using open pyelolithotomy, percutaneous pyelolithotripsy, extracorporeal shock wave lithotripsy and chemolysis. Scand J Urol Nephrol 1993;27:415.

20

Complications of Percutaneous Renal Surgery

Ojas Shah, MD

Dean G. Assimos, MD

Percutaneous renal surgery (PRS) is an established urologic procedure that is used to treat patients with a variety of conditions, including nephrolithiasis, ureteropelvic junction (UPJ) obstruction, infundibular and ureteral strictures, and transitional cell carcinoma (TCC). Refinements in technology and increasing surgical experience with PRS have generally resulted in its safe and effective execution. Nevertheless, PRS in essence is controlled renal trauma, and therefore, complications may occur. Prompt recognition of such complications and institution of appropriate treatment will generally limit morbidity. The various complications associated with PRS, their treatment, and methods of prevention are herein reviewed.

HEMORRHAGE

INTRAOPERATIVE Transfusion-dependent hemorrhage has been reported to occur in 1 to 34% of individuals subjected to PRS.[1-4] It may manifest during the procedure or in the postoperative period. Patients are certainly concerned about receiving a blood transfusion. The risks for this have been linked to surgical technique, surgical experience, preoperative anemia, and older patient age.[4] Certain measures can be taken to limit this complication. The collecting system should be accessed through a posterior calyx along the direction of the infundibulum to avoid blood vessels coursing adjacent to the infundibulum.[5] The posterior calyx providing the most direct access to the targeted stone is chosen. This route is typically along the avascular intersegmental plane. The tract should only be dilated up to the peripheral aspect of the collecting system. One group reported that balloon dilation has a significantly lower risk of provoking bleeding compared with coaxial dilation, while others have not found this to be true.[6,7] The renal pelvis may be perforated and hilar vessels lacerated if dilation is directed too far medially. Stoller and colleagues reported that renal pelvic perforation is a risk factor for excessive blood loss during percutaneous nephrostolithotomy (PCNL).[4] If a working sheath is used, it must be kept in the collecting system to limit parenchymal bleeding. Excessive angulation/torquing of the working sheath and instruments may damage blood vessels and renal parenchyma and thus should be avoided. Flexible nephroscopy or creation of an additional nephrostomy tract should be performed instead. Lam and associates found that use of multiple access tracts and improved flexible endoscopic skills decreased transfusion requirements in their patients with staghorn calculi subjected to PCNL.[8] When visibility is significantly diminished because of bleeding, one should assess for malpositioning of the working sheath. If the sheath is malpositioned and bleeding persists after redirecting the sheath into the targeted portion of the collecting system, or if the tube is properly positioned and hemorrhage continues, the procedure should be terminated.

Most intraoperative bleeding is thought to be from venous sources. Heavy venous bleeding should be suspected when a high volume of dark-colored blood drains from the tract after fluid irrigation is stopped. Injection of contrast into the collecting system in this setting will sometimes demonstrate opacification of the renal venous system. There are various approaches for managing this problem. Inflation of a 30 French dilating balloon in the tract for 10 to 20 minutes with subsequent placement of a large nephrostomy tube is usually successful. An alternative is initial placement of a large nephrostomy tube that is subsequently clamped for 1 to 2 hours. This allows the blood to clot and tamponade the injured vein. Some feel that simultaneous administration of diuretic therapy hastens the tamponade process.[9] If these measures are not successful, the use of a specialized nephrostomy tamponade catheter should be considered (Kaye, Cook Urological, Spencer, IN). The peripherally located balloon is inflated in the tract while urine drains through the inner core of this device. It is typically left inflated for 2 to 4 days.[10,11] Significant injuries of the main renal vein can also be controlled using a tamponade approach. Gupta and colleagues reported successful management of this complication in 4 patients by inflating a Council balloon catheter adjacent to the point of venous injury.[12]

High-volume arterial bleeding should be suspected if the effluent is bright red or has a pulsatile flow. The aforementioned approach can be utilized, but angiography and selective or superselective embolization may be necessary if these measures are not successful.

In patients with high volume intraoperative bleeding, subsequent percutaneous procedures should generally not be undertaken until at least 1 to 2 weeks later. There should be no evidence of ongoing hemorrhage. Angiography and embolization may be required if such hemorrhage recurs.

POSTOPERATIVE Bleeding can occur in the immediate postoperative period, at the time of percutaneous nephrostomy tube removal, or several days to weeks later.[1,2,13-15] Serious perioperative bleeding, requiring intervention other than tamponade, occurs in approximately 1% of patients.[7,15] If high-volume bleeding from the tract is present, initial management should include finger tamponade of the tract site and subsequent placement of a tamponade catheter or the largest nephrostomy catheter that the tract will permit. The latter catheter should then be occluded. These maneuvers are optimally done under fluoroscopic guidance. The patients are placed on bedrest and administered blood transfusions as necessary. Renal arteriography should be performed when bleeding persists, especially with the continued need for blood transfusion or hemodynamic instability due to hemorrhage.

The most common causes of delayed bleeding are laceration of segmental renal vessels, and development of an arteriovenous fistula or pseudoaneurysm.[1-3,14] Kessaris and colleagues reported that 17 of 2,200 patients (0.8%) who underwent PRS over a 10-year period required angiography and embolization for uncontrolled significant bleeding.[15] Twenty-four percent of these patients presented in the immediate postoperative period (< 24 hours), 41% in the early postoperative period (2 to 7 days), and 35% in the late postoperative period (> 7 days). Superselective or selective angiographic embolization of such lesions, using Gianturco coils, absorbable gelatin sponges, or platinum microcoils, is generally quite successful (Figure 20-1). The bleeding site may sometimes be obscured by the nephrostomy catheter, which can be removed to allow angiographic localization. Kessaris and colleagues reported success in 15 of 17 such cases, and Patterson and associates in 7 of 7 cases with selective or superselective embolization.[14,15] Open surgical exploration with partial or total nephrectomy may be necessary if the aforementioned measures are unsuccessful.[1,2]

Perinephric hemorrhage can also occur intraoperatively and postoperatively (Figure 20-2).

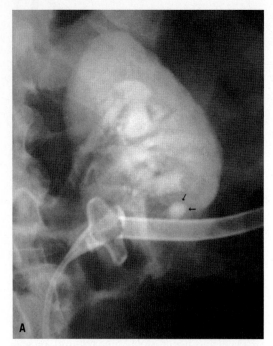 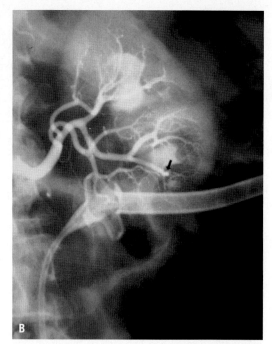

Figure 20-1 *A*, Delayed film of a renal arteriogram demonstrating a pseudoaneurysm (*arrows*). *B*, Renal arteriogram performed after embolization of injured vessel with Gianturco coils.

Difficulty accessing the kidney and malpositioning of the working sheath outside of the renal parenchyma or capsule may lead to this problem. This should be suspected if the patient has a decreasing postoperative hemoglobin level while urine from the bladder and nephrostomy tube appears relatively clear. Sandwich therapy with extracorporeal shock wave lithotripsy (ESWL) and subsequent second-look PCNL is a potential risk factor since subcapsular or perinephric hemorrhage from ESWL may increase with further tract and collecting system manipulation. A computed tomography (CT) scan should be performed if this diagnosis is suspected.

COLLECTING SYSTEM

EXTRAVASATION   Extravasation occurs with perforation of the collecting system or ureter when the access sheath is outside the collecting system. Lee and associates reported radiographic demonstration of extravasation in 7% of 582 cases.[16] Perforation should be suspected if retroperitoneal fat and other perirenal structures are visualized, or if the patient's abdomen or flank becomes distended. If the treatment is almost completed, it may be possible to finish the procedure with low flow irrigation, providing the patient is stable. Extrarenal stone fragment migration is a potential problem, however. This could also have oncologic implications in patients undergoing PRS for treatment of transitional cell carcinomas of the renal collecting system. Most perforations will heal with antegrade ureteral stent placement and nephrostomy tube drainage. Some larger rents may not heal, and open surgery may be necessary. Lee and colleagues reported this occurred in < 1% of patients.[16] If extravasation is due to malposition of the working sheath, this usually corrects with sheath repositioning.

Secondary signs of fluid extravasation are diminished backflow of irrigant via the access sheath, or discrepancy in the inflow-outflow fluid ratio. Management depends on the amount of extravasation. Small amounts of extravasation will resolve spontaneously with nephrostomy tube drainage. Large fluid collections (or urinomas) may develop, which usually resolve spontaneously. CT or ultrasound-guided drainage, however, may be necessary if persistent ileus, fever, respiratory compromise, or excessive abdominal distention develop.[17] Open surgical drainage is reserved for the extremely rare cases in which the aforementioned measures are unsuccessful.

STRICTURE   The development of ureteral stricture after PRS is quite rare; the reported incidence is less than 1%. The proximal ureter and UPJ are the areas most susceptible.[1,2] Strictures may result from inflammation due to stone impaction or from procedural trauma, including intracorporeal lithotripsy. Patients with a cutaneous urinary diversion and proximal ureteral calculi may be at increased risk for developing strictures secondary to an intense inflammatory response (obliterative pyeloureteritis) resulting from infection and other local factors.[18] Patients who develop strictures may be asymptomatic, and this underscores the importance of obtaining routine postoperative imaging in patients at risk for this complication.[19]

The majority of patients developing ureteral strictures can be managed successfully with an endourologic approach. Open surgical reconstruction may be required, however, for those failing the former or having extensive strictures.

INFUNDIBULAR STENOSIS   Infundibular stenosis can also rarely occur after PRS.[2,20,21] Parsons and associates reported a 2% incidence of infundibu-

lar stenosis following PRS. They found that prolonged operative time, a large stone burden requiring multiple procedures, and extended postoperative nephrostomy tube drainage were independent risk factors for this occurrence.[22] This problem usually manifests within one year after PRS (Figure 20-3). An endourologic approach for management of such patients should initially be considered. Observation is a consideration for asymptomatic patients without evidence of renal functional impairment of the involved kidney.

RETAINED FOREIGN BODIES   The tip on an ultrasound probe, electrohydraulic lithotripsy (EHL) electrode, stent, angiographic catheter, stone basket, guidewire, laser fiber, or other instrument may become dislodged in the collecting system and should be removed because infection, a granulomatous reaction, or new stone formation may otherwise occur. Fluoroscopy can be used to help identify the foreign body, which can then be extracted with a rigid or flexible nephroscope. Replacing instruments before instrument fatigue develops helps limit this occurrence. If the retained object is recognized after nephrostomy tube removal, retrograde ureteroscopic extraction should be initially considered. Percutaneous extraction may be required if the former is unsuccessful.

The tips of nephrostomy tubes, such as Malecot catheters, may become entrapped in the renal collecting system due to ingrowth of fibrous and inflammatory tissue. Koolpe and Lord described successful management of this problem with endoscopic removal of this restrictive tissue performed through another nephrostomy tract.[23]

EXTRARENAL STONE FRAGMENT MIGRATION   The consequences of extrarenal stone fragments are generally not of clinical significance provided the urine and stone are not infected, and the stone material does not become embedded in the submucosa.[24,25] Retrieval should usually not be attempted because this may enlarge the perforation.

SEEDING OF THE TRACT   Patients undergoing percutaneous treatment of TCC usually undergo a staged procedure to ensure completeness of

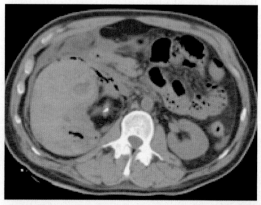

Figure 20-2 Right perinephric hematoma (the opacity is a stent within the proximal ureter).

tumor eradication. A second endoscopic evaluation is performed through the established tract after approximately 1 to 2 weeks with removal of any residual tumor burden. Risk of seeding of the tract can be minimized by correct placement of the sheath, performing low-pressure resection, and having low-pressure postoperative drainage (appropriately sized nephrostomy tube and urethral catheter). The three reports of tract seeding by Sengupta and Harewood, Sharma and associates, and Huang and colleagues were not in the context of a percutaneous resection of a tumor, but occurred after long-term nephrostomy tube drainage of obstructive, poorly differentiated cancer with parenchymal and perirenal fat invasion.[26–28] The only case of tract seeding following percutaneous resection of an upper tract tumor was reported by Fuglsig and Krarup and occurred in a patient with poorly differentiated, high-stage, locally advanced disease with renal fossa involvement at diagnosis.[29] Percutaneous resection should usually not be considered in this type of patient; although it might be considered for palliation. Percutaneous treatment of low-grade, low-stage, upper tract TCC has been established with long-term follow-up without seeding of the tract, either with or without adjunctive measures to prevent such an occurrence.[30–32]

URETERAL AVULSION Ureteral avulsion is an extremely rare complication, occurring in less than 0.2% of cases, which usually results from attempts at antegrade basketing of large, impacted ureteral stones.[16,33] This complication mandates prompt open surgical exploration. Percutaneous nephrostomy drainage may be used as a temporizing measure to allow patient stabilization.

NEPHROCUTANEOUS FISTULA Fistula formation between the renal collecting system and the skin is rare.[34] Prolonged postoperative drainage from the nephrostomy tract is usually caused by distal obstruction secondary to ureteral edema, an obstructing stone, blood clot, or stricture. Fistula drainage will usually cease after stone removal, placement of an indwelling Double-J stent in cases of ureteral edema, or treatment of the stricture. Very rarely will it be necessary to induce healing of the fistula tract by electrocautery in addition to the aforementioned measures.

DAMAGE SECONDARY TO ENERGY SOURCES Advances in the design of lithotripsy and ablative energy sources have allowed more efficient PRS. The potential for energy-related complications, however, should not be underestimated; intracorporeal damage from these sources can range from minor to extensive. A thorough knowledge of each individual energy source is necessary prior to its use. Additionally, it is extremely important that each source be used only when complete visualization of the operative field is attained.

Ultrasonic lithotripsy is a commonly used energy source for percutaneous nephrolithotomy.[33] The collecting system and ureter may be perforated with this device, especially if excessive pressure is applied to these tissues. If the probe is clogged with debris, instrument overheating occurs, which could result in thermal injury.

EHL is still used for PCNL but less commonly owing to the availability of newer devices with better safety profiles.[35] The most common complications associated with EHL are perforation of the collecting system and bleeding, which are managed as previously discussed.

The holmium laser is used as a lithotrite, for incision of strictures, and for ablation of upper tract tumors with a high rate of success. Holmium laser energy use has been reported to have a high safety profile.[36] Hemorrhage, perforation of the collecting system and ureter, and thermal injury may occur, the latter two potentially causing stricture formation. Such an occurrence can be minimized with careful technique and use of appropriate energy settings. Explosions within the collecting system have also been reported due to thermal interaction with hydrogen gas.[37]

Pneumatic lithotriptors and hybrid devices (pneumatic/ultrasound) are used during PCNL.[38–40] There is a small risk of perforation and hemorrhage with their use, but that can be limited with the aforementioned measures.

Electrocautery and electroresection can be used during PRS. It is important to ensure that the patient is properly grounded to prevent cutaneous thermal burns. Only nonconductive materials should be in contact with the collecting system and ureter. If not, current dispersal could result in significant thermal injury of these structures. Hemorrhage is another possible complication that can be minimized by maintaining proper orientation with respect to adjacent vascular structures. There is also the potential for a fluid absorption syndrome, which can be limited by using the lowest irrigation pressure allowing adequate visualization, limiting resection time, and using sterile glycine as an irrigant.

INJURY TO ADJACENT STRUCTURES

LUNG AND PLEURA The lung and pleura are the perirenal structures at greatest risk for injury during PRS, although lung parenchymal injury is rare.[1,2] Most of these injuries occur when a supracostal approach is used because of the proximity of the ribs with these structures.[41,42] These anatomic relationships were noted by Hopper and Yakes, who studied 43 randomly selected patients during maximal inspiration and expiration using CT and predicted that the pleura and lung would be traversed during full expiration with an 11th or 12th rib approach, 86% and 29% on the right side, and 79% and 14% on the left.[43] Fortunately, clinically significant injuries occur less frequently than their predictions. Pneumothorax has been reported in 0 to 4% and hydrothorax in 0 to 8% of individuals subjected to supracostal access.[44,45] Munver and associates performed an analysis of supracostal access for PRS. They compared complications associated with supracostal access to those occurring with an infracostal approach.[41] Approximately 33% of their

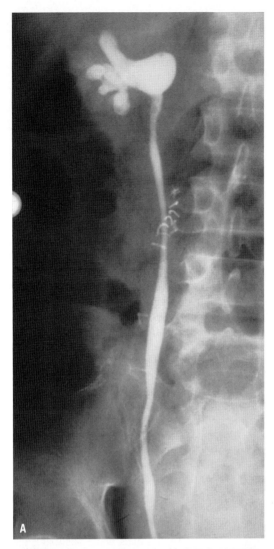

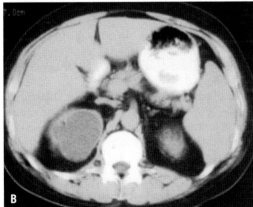

Figure 20-3 *A,* Postoperative computed tomography scan demonstrates dilated right upper pole calyx. *B,* Subsequent retrograde pyelogram reveals no communication to the upper pole collecting system caused by infundibular stenosis.

upper pole access cases required a supracostal approach. Of the supracostal approaches, 73.5% of the tracts were above the 12th rib, and 26.5% were above the 11th rib. The overall complication rate for supracostal access was 16.3% (supra-11th, 34.6%; supra-12th, 9.7%). Eighty-seven percent of the intrathoracic complications occurred with supracostal access that included hemothorax/hydrothorax in 4% of supracostal access tracts, nephropleural fistula in 2%, and pneumothorax in 1%.[41] A working sheath is recommended with a supracostal approach since the sheath provides a barrier to the influx of fluid and air into the pleural cavity if the parietal pleura is violated. Routine intraoperative chest fluoroscopy is recommended at the termination of PRS to evaluate for obvious hydrothorax or pneumothorax. Routine postoperative chest radiography is not necessary when fluoroscopy is normal and the patient has no signs of pulmonary compromise.[46]

Patients with a small-volume pneumothorax or hydrothorax can be observed when there are no signs of pulmonary compromise. Aspiration or tube thoracostomy may be required for large pneumo- or hydrothoraces or patient instability (Figure 20-4). Thoracoscopy or formal thoracotomy may be required if the aforementioned measures are unsuccessful, especially if a complex loculated pleural effusion or empyema develop. The intercostal vessels may be lacerated during supracostal access, resulting in hemothorax. Tube thoracostomy and open surgical thoracotomy may be necessary if this occurs. Nephropleural fistula should be suspected if thoracic fluid persists after tube thoracostomy (Figure 20-5). It will usually resolve after placement of an internalized ureteral stent.[47]

COLON Colonic perforation is an extremely rare complication of PRS; reported in less than 1% of cases.[16,33,48–51] This low incidence is attributed to the colon rarely being retrorenal (Figure 20-6). Hadar and Gadoth, and Sherman and associates found that the colon was postrenal in approximately 0.6% of individuals when analyzing the position of the colon with respect to the kidneys using CT.[52,53] Patients at higher risk for colonic injury are those with congenital anomalies such as horseshoe kidney and other forms of renal fusion and ectopia, and those with colonic distention due to jejunoileal bypass, partial ileal bypass, neurologic impairment, and "institutional" bowel. CT should be considered in high-risk groups to detect the presence of postrenal colon, and CT-guidance can be used in these patients to direct percutaneous access.[54]

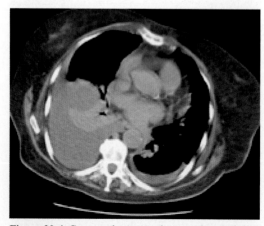

Figure 20-4 Computed tomography scan demonstrating right hydrothorax. The patient was subsequently treated with tube thoracostomy.

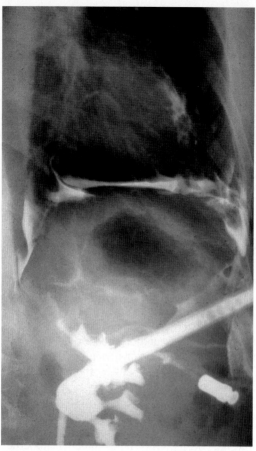

Figure 20-5 Nephrostogram demonstrating nephropleural fistula.

Colonic perforation can cause serious infectious complications when the perforation occurs intraperitoneally, or if diagnosis and management are delayed. Colonic penetration should be suspected if the patient has intraoperative diarrhea or hematochezia, signs of peritonitis, or passage of gas or feculent material through the nephrostomy tract. This complication may remain undetected, however, until a postoperative nephrostogram demonstrates contrast entering the colon.

The majority of colonic injuries can be managed conservatively if the penetration is retroperitoneal and the patient does not have signs of peritonitis or sepsis.[55] An indwelling Double-J ureteral stent is inserted, and the nephrostomy tube is pulled back into the colon. The patient is given broad-spectrum antibiotic therapy and placed on a low-residue diet. A contrast study is performed through the colostomy tube after 7 to 10 days and the tube is removed if there is no evidence of a nephrocolic fistula.[49,51] Open surgical management is required in patients with transperitoneal perforation, peritonitis, or sepsis and in those who fail conservative management.

DUODENUM The second and third portions of the duodenum are retroperitoneal and are somewhat anterior to the lower pole and pelvis of the right kidney. This structure may be injured during access if a needle, guidewire, or dilator perforates the renal pelvis or lower pole collecting system and penetrates the duodenum. Very few cases of

this complication have been reported, and its occurrence is rarer than colonic perforation.[56] It is usually diagnosed when communication with the duodenum is demonstrated on an intraoperative or postoperative nephrostogram. Open surgical management may be required if the perforation is large or if the patient has sepsis or peritonitis. Success with nonoperative management has been reported in less compromised settings. Patients are treated with antibiotics, placed on nasogastric suction, and administered parenteral hyperalimentation. The nephrostomy tube is positioned correctly to ensure adequate drainage. A nephrostogram and upper gastrointestinal radiographic study are performed 10 to 14 days later to determine whether the fistula has closed.

LIVER AND SPLEEN INJURY Because of the cephalad position of the spleen, there have been very few reports of splenic injury during PRS.[57,58] Hopper and Yakes also analyzed the relationship between the kidney, spleen, and lower ribs.[43] They noted that the spleen should not be traversed if an 11th to 12th rib supracostal approach to the upper pole collecting system is undertaken during expiration; there is a 13% risk if performed during inspiration. The risk increases to 33% if a 10th to 11th rib approach is used. The risk is also increased in patients with splenomegaly, and CT should be performed in these cases to determine whether safe access is possible and to assist with nephrostomy tube placement. Splenic injury can cause significant internal bleeding and hypovolemic shock. The diagnosis is established with ultrasonography or CT. Although some patients with splenic laceration can be managed non-operatively, the majority will require splenectomy secondary to significant hemorrhage.[1,2,58]

The liver is far less susceptible to injury than the spleen. Hopper and Yakes reported the risks of injury during an 11th to 12th rib intercostal approach was minimal and would occur in only 14% of patients if a 10th to 11th rib route was taken during inspiration.[43] Hepatomegaly places the patient at increased risk for this complication. Therefore, such patients should be evaluated with a preoperative CT scan. CT-guided access may help prevent this injury in select

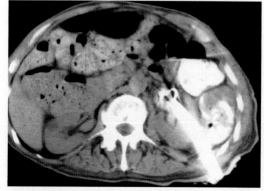

Figure 20-6 Computed tomography scan demonstrating a nephrostomy tube traversing the posterior aspect of the descending colon.

patients with hepatomegaly. If this is diagnosed postoperatively, the nephrostomy tube should be left in place 7 to 10 days to allow for tract maturation. The tube can be carefully removed at this interval but immediately reinserted if there is high-volume bleeding from the tract. Retrograde placement of an internalized ureteral stent at the time of nephrostomy tube removal has been recommended by some in an effort to avoid a reno-biliary fistula.

CHYLURIA   Perforation of the collecting system during PRS may result in disruption of adjacent renal lymphatics, which could lead to chyluria.[59] Management consists of optimizing urinary drainage and administration of total parenteral hyperalimentation until chyluria resolves. Somatostatin administration has some effectiveness in the management of such patients.[60] Refractory cases require renal pedicle lymphatic disconnection that can be performed with an open surgical or laparoscopic approach.[61,62]

MEDICAL COMPLICATIONS OF PERCUTANEOUS RENAL SURGERY

INFECTION AND SEPSIS   It is mandatory that patients with urinary tract infections (UTI) be treated with appropriate antibiotic therapy before PRS. The risk of sepsis from intravasation of bacteria via pyelovenous or pyelolymphatic backflow during PRS in the setting of inadequate antibiotic therapy is significant. Antibiotic therapy for patients with UTI is generally started at least one week before PRS. Results of urine cultures from patients with struvite stones are not predictive of stone bacteriology.[63,64] The antibiotic agent employed should have activity against the cultured urinary organism and have a broad spectrum to increase the likelihood of effectiveness against the usually unknown urease-producing stone organism. Stone culture is recommended in these cases since it will aid in the choice of postoperative antibiotic therapy. Prophylactic antibiotic therapy has been recommended by some investigators to further limit the risk of sepsis. Inglis and Tolley performed a prospective, randomized study and found that prophylactic antibiotic therapy reduced the risk of infectious complications in patients with sterile urine and noninfectious calculi.[65] Rao and colleagues demonstrated that patients without bacteriuria undergoing percutaneous stone removal may still develop bacteremia, endotoxemia, and increased release of tumor necrosis factor.[66]

Purulent urine may sometimes be unexpectedly encountered at the time of accessing the collecting system. If this occurs, treatment should be postponed, the renal collecting system drained, urine from the targeted kidney cultured, and appropriate antibiotic therapy administered.

Sepsis has been reported to occur in 0.6% to 1.5% of patients undergoing percutaneous stone removal.[1,2,33,67] Antibiotic therapy, fluid resuscitation, and the administration of steroids and pres-

sors may all be required in treatment of the septic patient. Evaluation of the patient with a CT scan should be considered if the aforementioned measures are unsuccessful to assess for complications that may be contributing to the septic event.

FLUID OVERLOAD   Irrigating fluid is used in PRS, and patients may absorb high volumes of fluid if extravasation or venous injury occurs. Careful intraoperative patient monitoring helps detect this problem. A discrepancy in input and output of irrigation fluid, unexpected hypertension, and hypoxemia are signs and manifestations of this problem. Sterile normal saline solution should be used as an irrigant, except when electrocautery and electroresection are undertaken, to limit the development of hyponatremia. Using the lowest irrigating pressure that will permit adequate visualization, discontinuing the procedure when perforation of the collecting system is encountered, and limiting the duration of PRS can limit this occurrence. The administration of diuretics and other agents may be required for managing the hypervolemic patient.

HYPOTHERMIA   Core body temperature decreases during PRS. Hypothermia may occur as a result of intraoperative heat loss from vasodilation related to anesthesia, length of the procedure, exposed body surface, low ambient room temperature, and use of room temperature irrigant. The potential consequences are impaired platelet function, altered enzymatic drug clearance, and postoperative shivering causing up to a 400% increase in oxygen consumption.[68] The latter problem places patients with compromised cardiac reserve at risk for myocardial ischemia and cardiac arrhythmia. The use of warmed irrigating fluid and proper coverage of patients (blankets, heat-preserving surgical drapes, bear huggers) helps limit hypothermia.

POSITIONING RELATED COMPLICATIONS   Brachial plexus damage, shoulder dislocation, other forms of peripheral nerve injury, and cutaneous trauma can occur with PRS. It is essential that appropriate positioning and padding be employed to prevent these complications. Prompt neurologic evaluation should be obtained if neuropraxia is suspected. These injuries usually resolve over time, and physical therapy plays a major role in the management of such patients.

AIR EMBOLISM   Air embolism is an extremely rare complication that may occur after injection of air or carbon dioxide in the collecting system to identify a posterior calyx or if there is reversal of airflow in an ultrasonic lithotriptor.[69] Patients may manifest with hypoxemia, cardiac instability, or circulatory arrest. A machinery type of cardiac murmur may also be present. Management consists of placing the patient in a left lateral decubitus position with the head and thorax tilted downward. A central venous access line is placed through which the air can be aspirated.

DEEP VENOUS THROMBOSIS (DVT) AND PULMONARY EMBOLISM   The incidence of DVT after PRS is 1 to 3%.[33,70] Prevention is directed toward identifying patients at risk, taking appropriate preventive measures with thromboembolic disease prevention stockings and sequential compression devices, and encouraging early postoperative ambulation. If postoperative DVT does occur, management is aimed at preventing extension of the thrombus and embolic events.[71] Anticoagulation in the immediate postoperative period following PRS is somewhat risky, and therefore, an inferior vena cava filter may need to be placed to prevent pulmonary embolism. This may not be necessary, however, in patients with a mature nephrostomy tract where anticoagulation is reasonably well tolerated.

MORTALITY   Postoperative death is extremely rare and has been reported in 0.1 to 0.3% of patients subjected to PRS.[16,33] The majority of these deaths have resulted from myocardial infarction and pulmonary embolism occurring in high-risk patients. Careful preoperative screening, invasive monitoring, and avoidance of hypotension, excessive hemorrhage and hypothermia may aid in preventing mortality in such patients.

RENAL PARENCHYMAL DAMAGE/DETERIORATION OF RENAL FUNCTION   Several studies have demonstrated that uncomplicated PRS produces negligible renal damage. Lechevallier and colleagues evaluated patients before and after PCNL with single–photon-emission CT, and demonstrated that small scars, usually involving < 4% of renal cortical mass, developed in the treated area.[72] Ekelund and colleagues evaluated patients with pre- and postoperative intravenous pyelography, nuclear renography, and CT, which demonstrated maintenance of renal function and the development of small, discrete parenchymal scars.[73] Urivetsky and colleagues evaluated patients with urinary enzyme studies before and after PCNL and reported no change in enzyme activity.[74] Patients with staghorn calculi may be at increased long-term risk of renal functional deterioration. Teichman and associates reported that 25% of such patients subjected to PCNL had renal functional deterioration. Factors associated with this outcome included solitary kidney, recurrent calculi, hypertension, complete staghorn stone, urinary diversion, and neurogenic bladder.[75]

Loss of a kidney is exceedingly rare with PRS. Acute renal loss is usually the result of uncontrollable hemorrhage. This has been reported to occur in only 0.1 to 0.3% of cases.[33,67] Meta-analysis of the literature on percutaneous removal of staghorn calculi indicated that the long-term risk of renal loss is 1.6%.[76]

CONCLUSIONS

Complications of PRS are usually avoidable with proper patient selection, preparation, and operative technique. Knowledge of potential complications, prompt recognition, and institution of the appropriate therapy will minimize the impact of these complications.

REFERENCES

1. Roth RA, Beckmann CF. Complications of extracorporeal shock-wave lithotripsy and percutaneous nephrolithotomy. Urol Clin North Am 1988;15:155.
2. Lang EK. Percutaneous nephrostolithotomy and lithotripsy: a multi-institutional survey of complications. Radiology 1987;162:25.
3. Clayman RV, Surya V, Hunter D, et al. Renal vascular complications associated with the percutaneous removal of renal calculi. J Urol 1984;132:228.
4. Stoller ML, Wolf JS Jr, St Lezin MA. Estimated blood loss and transfusion rates associated with percutaneous nephrolithotomy. J Urol 1994;152:1977.
5. Mahaffey KG, Bolton DM, Stoller ML. Urologist directed percutaneous nephrostomy tube placement. J Urol 1994;152:1973.
6. Soble JJ, Streem SB. Prospective randomized comparison of percutaneous nephrostomy tract dilation techniques. J Endourol 1998;12:S115A.
7. Davidoff R, Bellman GC. Influence of technique of percutaneous tract creation on incidence of renal hemorrhage. J Urol 1997;157:1229.
8. Lam HS, Lingeman JE, Mosbaugh PG, Steele RE, Knapp PM, Scott JW, Newman DM. Evolution of the technique of combination therapy for staghorn calculi: a decreasing role for extracorporeal shock wave lithotripsy. J Urol 1992;148:1058.
9. Fuchs GJ, Moody JA, Gutierrez-Aceves J, Barbaric ZL. Complications of percutaneous renal surgery: prevention, recognition and management. In: Taneja SS, Smith RB, Ehrlich RM, editors. Complications of urologic surgery, 3rd ed. Philadelphia: WB Saunders; 2001. p. 277.
10. Kaye KW, Clayman RV. Tamponade nephrostomy catheter for percutaneous nephrostolithotomy. Urology 1986;27:441.
11. Kerbl K, Picus DD, Clayman RV. Clinical experience with the Kaye nephrostomy tamponade catheter. Eur Urol 1994;25:94.
12. Gupta M, Bellman GC, Smith AD. Massive hemorrhage from renal vein injury during percutaneous renal surgery: Endourological management. J Urol 1997;157:795.
13. Sacha K, Szewczyk W, Bar K. Massive haemorrhage presenting as a complication after percutaneous nephrolithotomy (PCNL). Int Urol Nephrol 1996;28:315.
14. Patterson DE, Segura JW, LeRoy AJ, et al. The etiology and treatment of delayed bleeding following percutaneous lithotripsy. J Urol 1985;133:447.
15. Kessaris DN, Bellman GC, Pardalidis NP, Smith AG. Management of hemorrhage after percutaneous renal surgery. J Urol 1995;153:604.
16. Lee WJ, Smith AD, Cubelli V, et al. Complications of percutaneous nephrolithotomy. AJR Am J Roentgenol 1987;148:177.
17. Carson CC, Nesbitt JA. Peritoneal extravasation during percutaneous lithotripsy. J Urol 1985;134:725.
18. Zagoria RJ, Assimos DG, Yap MA, Dyer RB. Obliterative pyeloureteritis: a complication of stone disease in patients with urinary conduit diversion. J Urol 1993;150:961.
19. Meretyk S, Albala DM, Clayman RV, et al. Endoureterotomy for treatment of ureteral strictures. J Urol 1992;147:1502.
20. Weir MJ, Honey JD. Complete infundibular obliteration following percutaneous nephrolithotomy. J Urol 1999;161:1274.
21. Buchholz NP. Double infundibular obliteration with abscess formation after percutaneous nephrolithotomy. Urol Int 2001;66:46.
22. Parsons JK, Jarrett TW, Lancini V, Kavoussi LR. Infundibular stenosis after percutaneous nephrolithotomy. J Urol 2002;167:35.
23. Koolpe HA, Lord B. Eccentric nephroscopy for the incarcerated nephrostomy. Urol Radiol 1990;12:96.
24. Verstandig AG, Banner MP, Van Arsdalen KN, Pollack HM. Upper urinary tract calculi: extrusion into perinephric and periureteric tissues during percutaneous management. Radiology 1986;158:215.
25. Evans CP, Stoller ML. The fate of the iatrogenic retroperitoneal stone. J Urol 1993;150:827.
26. Huang A, Low RK, deVere White R. Nephrostomy tract tumor seeding following percutaneous manipulation of a ureteral carcinoma. J Urol 1995;153:1041.
27. Sengupta S, Harewood L. Transitional cell carcinoma growing along an indwelling nephrostomy tube track. Br J Urol 1998;82:591.
28. Sharma NK, Nicol A, Powell CS. Track infiltration following percutaneous resection of renal pelvic transitional cell carcinoma. Br J Urol 1994;73:597.
29. Fuglsig S, Krarup T. Percutaneous nephroscopic resection of renal pelvic tumors. Scand J Urol Nephrol 1995;172 (Suppl):15.
30. Smith AD, Orihuela E, Crowley AR. Percutaneous management of renal pelvic tumors: a treatment option in selected cases. J Urol 1987;137:852.
31. Streem SB, Pontes EJ. Percutaneous management of upper tract transitional cell carcinoma. J Urol 1986;135:773.
32. Patel A, Soonawalla P, Shepherd SF, et al. Long-term outcome after percutaneous treatment of transitional cell carcinoma of the renal pelvis. J Urol 1996;155:868.
33. Segura JW, Patterson DE, LeRoy AJ, et al. Percutaneous removal of kidney stones: review of 1,000 cases. J Urol 1985;134:1077.
34. White EC, Smith AD. Percutaneous stone extraction from 200 patients. J Urol 1984;132:437.
35. Denstedt JD, Clayman RV. Electrohydraulic lithotripsy of renal and ureteral calculi. J Urol 1990;143:13.
36. Grasso M. Experience with the holmium laser as an endoscopic lithotrite. Urology 1996;48:199.
37. Andrews PE, Segura JW. Renal pelvic explosion during conservative management of upper tract urothelial cancer. J Urol 1991;146:407.
38. Kostakopoulos A, Stavropoulos NJ, Picramenos D, et al. The Swiss lithoclast: an ideal intracorporeal lithotripter. Urol Int 1995;55:19.
39. Granata M, Costanzo V, Condorelli S, et al. Percutaneous lithotripsy: How to make it safer. Personal experience. Minerva Urol Nefrol 2002;54:173.
40. Denstedt JD, Eberwein PM, Singh RR. The Swiss lithoclast: a new device for intracorporeal lithotripsy. J Urol 1992;148:1088.
41. Munver R, Delvecchio FC, Newman GE, Preminger GM. Critical analysis of supracostal access for percutaneous renal surgery. J Urol 2001;166:1242.
42. Gupta R, Kumar A, Kapoor R, et al. Prospective evaluation of safety and efficacy of the supracostal approach for percutaneous nephrolithotomy. BJU Int 2002;90:809.
43. Hopper KD, Yakes WF. The posterior intercostal approach for percutaneous renal procedures: risk of puncturing the lung, spleen, and liver as determined by CT. AJR Am J Roentgenol 1990;154:115.
44. Forsyth MJ, Fuchs EF. The supracostal approach for percutaneous nephrostomy. J Urol 1987;137:197.
45. Picus D, Weyman PJ, Clayman RV, McClennan BL. Intercostal-space nephrostomy for percutaneous stone removal. AJR Am J Roentgenol 1986;147:393.
46. Pearle MS, Corwin TS, Mullican MA. Comparison of intraoperative chest fluoroscopy, chest radiography and chest CT for detecting hydropneumothorax after percutaneous nephrostolithotomy (PCNL). J Endourol 2000;14:A86.
47. Redorta JP, Gassol JMB, Vilaseca AP, et al. Renopleural fistula after percutaneous nephrostolithotomy. Urol Int 1988;43:104.
48. Vallancien G, Capdeville R, Veillon B, et al. Colonic perforation during percutaneous nephrolithotomy. J Urol 1985;134:1185.
49. Neustein P, Barbaric ZL, Kaufman JJ. Nephrocolic fistula: a complication of percutaneous nephrostolithotomy. J Urol 1986;135:571.
50. Morse RM, Spirnak JP, Resnick MI. Iatrogenic colon and rectal injuries associated with urological intervention: report of 14 patients. J Urol 1988;140:101.
51. Appel R, Musmanno MC, Knight JG. Nephrocolic fistula complicating percutaneous nephrostolithotomy. J Urol 1988;140:1007.
52. Sherman JL, Hopper KD, Greene AJ, Johns TT. The retrorenal colon on computed tomography: a normal variant. J Comput Assist Tomogr 1985;9:339.
53. Hadar H, Gadoth N. Positional relations of colon and kidney determined by perirenal fat. AJR Am J Roentgenol 1984;143:773.
54. Matlaga BR, Shah OD, Zagoria RJ, et al. Computerized tomography guided access for percutaneous nephrostolithotomy. J Urol 2003;170:45.
55. Gerspach JM, Bellman GC, Stoller ML, Fugelso P. Conservative management of colon injury following percutaneous renal surgery. Urology 1997;49:831.
56. Culkin DJ, Wheeler JS Jr, Canning JR. Nephro-duodenal fistula: a complication of percutaneous nephrolithotomy. J Urol 1985;134:528.
57. Goldberg SD, Gray RR, St Louis EL, Mahoney J, Jewett MA, Keresteci AG. Nonoperative management of complications of percutaneous renal nephrostomy. Can J Surg 1989;32:192.
58. Kondas J, Szentgyorgyi E, Vaczi L, Kiss A. Splenic injury: a rare complication of percutaneous nephrolithotomy. Int Urol Nephrol 1994;26:399.
59. Thrasher JB, Snyder JA. Post-nephrolithotomy chyluria. J Urol 1990;143:578.
60. Campieri C, Raimondi C, Dalmastri V, et al. Posttraumatic chyluria due to lymphorenal fistula regressed after somatostatin therapy. Nephron 1996;72:705.
61. Hemal AK, Gupta NP. Retroperitoneoscopic lymphatic management of intractable chyluria. J Urol 2002;167:2473.
62. Zhang X, Ye ZQ, Chen Z, et al. Comparison of open surgery versus retroperitoneoscopic approach to chyluria. J Urol 2003;169:991.
63. Ohkawa M, Tokunaga S, Nakashima T, et al. Composition of urinary calculi related to urinary tract infection. J Urol 1992;148:995.
64. Fowler JE Jr. Bacteriology of branched renal calculi and accompanying urinary tract infection. J Urol 1984;131:213.
65. Inglis JA, Tolley DA. Antibiotic prophylaxis at the time of percutaneous stone surgery. J Endourol 1988;2:59.
66. Rao PN, Dube DA, Weightman NC, et al. Prediction of septicemia following endourological manipulation for stones in the upper urinary tract. J Urol 1991;146:955.
67. Moskowitz GW, Lee WJ, Pochaczevsky R. Diagnosis and management of complications of percutaneous nephrolithotomy. Crit Rev Diagn Imaging 1989;29:1.
68. Roberts S, Bolton DM, Stoller ML. Hypothermia associated with percutaneous nephrolithotomy. Urology 1994;44:832.
69. Cadeddu JA, Arrindell D, Moore RG. Near fatal air embolism during percutaneous nephrostomy placement. J Urol 1997;158:1519.
70. Lee WJ, Smith AD, Cubelli V, Vernace FM. Percutaneous nephrolithotomy: analysis of 500 consecutive cases. Urol Radiol 1986;8:61.
71. Patel A, Fuchs GJ. Air travel and thromboembolic complications after percutaneous nephrolithotomy for staghorn stone. J Endourol 1998;12:51.
72. Lechevallier E, Siles S, Ortega JC, Coulange C. Comparison by SPECT of renal scars after extracorporeal shock wave lithotripsy and percutaneous nephrolithotomy. J Endourol 1993;7:465.
73. Ekelund L, Lindstedt E, Lundquist SB, et al. Studies on renal damage from percutaneous nephrolitholapaxy. J Urol 1986;135:682.
74. Urivetsky M, Motola J, King L, Smith AD. Impact of percutaneous renal stone removal on renal function: assessment by urinary lysozyme activity. Urology 1993;33:305.
75. Teichman JM, Long RD, Hulbert JC. Long-term renal fate and prognosis after staghorn calculus management. J Urol 1995;153:1403.
76. Segura JW, Preminger GM, Assimos DG, et al. Nephrolithiasis Clinical Guidelines Panel summary report on the management of staghorn calculi. The American Urological Association Nephrolithiasis Clinical Guidelines Panel. J Urol 1994;151:1648.

21

Percutaneous Treatment of Ureteropelvic Junction Obstruction

Khai-Linh V. Ho, MD, FACS
George K. Chow, MD
Joseph W. Segura, MD

Ureteropelvic junction (UPJ) obstruction may result from functional or anatomic abnormalities leading to decreased urinary flow from the renal pelvis to the ureter that could cause symptoms or renal damage. Congenital abnormalities of ureteral musculature or lumen, structural anomalies with high insertion, kinks, or extrinsic narrowing of the lumen, can all lead to UPJ obstruction. Acquired processes such as postoperative or inflammatory stricture, stone disease, or neoplasm may give a similar obstructive picture at the UPJ.[1,2] While most cases are congenital, UPJ obstruction may clinically manifest at any age.[3]

With reported success rates exceeding 90%, open pyeloplasty for UPJ obstruction is the standard to which other treatments are compared.[4,5] Less invasive alternatives, despite their slightly lower success rates, are now considered fist-line therapy for most patients due to the advantages of significantly reduced length of hospital stays and postoperative recovery time.[4,6,7]

Endourologic treatment of UPJ obstruction is based on the principle of full-thickness incision, stenting and drainage, and healing by secondary intent to an adequate caliber of a narrowed ureteral segment. This concept was first reported in 1903 by Albarran (ureterotome externe) and popularized by Davis in 1943.[8–10] Due to the excellent results achieved with open pyeloplasty, the potential of the intubated ureterotomy was not fully realized until refinement of endoscopic instrumentation and percutaneous technique. In 1983, Wickham and Kellet introduced percutaneous management of UPJ obstruction (pyelolysis) in the United Kingdom.[11] Subsequently, Smith renamed the procedure (endopyelotomy) and reported the first series in the United States.[12] Since then, further improvement in technology has allowed the retrograde treatment of UPJ obstruction with direct incision or with a fluoroscopically aided hot wire balloon with similar efficacy as antegrade endopyelotomy.[13–17] While the results of these techniques are roughly equivalent, antegrade endopyelotomy allows the opportunity to treat associated stones and to control the length, depth, and position of the incision at the UPJ.

PRESENTATION AND DIAGNOSIS

Patients with UPJ obstruction present with a wide variety of symptoms. Those who are sympto-matic often complain of a long history of intermittent abdominal or flank pain, nausea, and vomiting. Symptoms can be exacerbated by self-induced or iatrogenic diuresis (Dietl's crisis). Patients may also present with hematuria, either spontaneous or in association with minor trauma, urinary tract infections, renal stones, and occasionally with hypertension and azotemia.[3] Atypical presentations with testicular pain, pyeloduodenal fistula, and early satiety and weight loss have been reported.[18]

The evaluation of patients suspected to have UPJ obstruction should elucidate the anatomic site and functional significance of the blockage. The classic findings on excretory urography are delayed excretion of contrast, dilation of calices and renal pelvis, and narrowing of the UPJ. Parenchymal thinning may be present in chronic cases. On delayed films, there may be retention of the contrast, and if seen, the ureter should be of normal caliber. If possible, patients should be evaluated while they are symptomatic, or a diuretic urogram can be performed to increase diagnostic accuracy.

Ultrasonography or computed tomography (CT) may be useful when allergy or renal dysfunction precludes intravenous contrast, nonvisualization of the affected collecting system on EXU occurs, and in differentiation of acquired causes of obstruction such as radiolucent calculi or urothelial tumors.

If studies are equivocal, a diuretic renal scan may quantify the obstruction and give differential renal function. In patients with poor renal function, the diuretic response may be inadequate, rendering the test invalid. In kidneys with marginal function, a trial of drainage with repeat assessment may help clarify treatment options.

Retrograde pyelography (RPG), usually performed at the time of surgery in order to avoid the risk of introducing infection in an obstructed system, can demonstrate the length of narrowing. Indwelling ureteral stent placement for marginal kidney function, persistent infection, or rarely, for assessing the impact of an unobstructed collecting system on the patient's symptoms, may be preceded by RPG.

Alternatively, placement of a percutaneous nephrostomy may allow decompression of the system and the performance of pressure-flow studies (Whitaker test).[2]

PATIENT SELECTION

While open pyeloplasty can be applied to various etiologies of UPJ obstruction, endopyelotomy only addresses intrinsic abnormalities and therefore may be influenced by several factors. This might be the reason that open pyeloplasty enjoys a 10 to 20% higher success rate.[5–7] Characterization of prognostic factors is important to achieve better patient selection and lower failure and complications rates. The following factors have been reported to influence endopyelotomy success.

PRIMARY VERSUS SECONDARY UPJ OBSTRUCTION Initially, percutaneous endopyelotomy was used in order to avoid the potentially difficult open treatment of failed pyeloplasty. Experience with endopyelotomy in primary UPJ obstruction has proven almost as equally successful as in secondary cases. Gupta and colleagues reported an 82% and 89% success rate for their patients treated with antegrade endopyelotomy for primary and secondary UPJ obstruction, respectively.[19] The differences between the two groups were statistically significant. Hoening and colleagues analyzed the impact of the initial procedure on outcome of secondary intervention with antegrade endopyelotomy and the hot wire balloon device.[20] They found that a second endopyelotomy for failed initial endopyelotomy was associated with a 71% subjective and 55% objective success rate. Those patients who initially failed open surgery had an 88% subjective and 71% objective success rate. While the success rates tended to be higher in their patients who failed an open pyeloplasty, a statistically significant difference was not seen between the two groups. Shalhav and associates also obtained similar results with primary and secondary UPJ obstruction, with and without stones, treated by antegrade and retrograde endopyelotomy.[21] Success rates of endopyelotomy for primary and secondary obstruction of 62 to 94% and 67 to 100% for have been reported.[19,22–26]

HIGH URETERAL INSERTION High-insertion UPJ obstruction is uncommon, with a reported average incidence of 7.8% (5.9 to 14.3%).[27] Traditionally, this variant has been considered a potential factor for endopyelotomy failure.[28–30] Shalhav and colleagues, in a multi-series review, found a 78% success rate for high-insertion UPJ obstruction; this included an objective and subjective success rate of 70% and 80%, respectively, in their patient cohort.[27] Chow and associates reported no statistically significant difference in success rates between 60 patients treated with endopyelotomy for high insertion (78.9%), equivocal insertion (87.5%), or dependent ureteral insertion (76%).[31] Endopyelotomy may be an effective treatment for this variant by forming a more dependent insertion through incision of the common ureteropelvic wall.[32]

AGE   Open pyeloplasty remains the procedure of choice for the treatment of primary UPJ obstruction in young children. In older preadolescent children with good kidney function, mild to moderate hydronephrosis, and no crossing vessels, endopyelotomy would be a reasonable alternative to open surgery. Endopyelotomy as initial treatment is recommended for adolescent children with the same clinical picture. Patients with secondary obstruction following open pyeloplasty benefit from endourologic intervention regardless of age, although the procedure can be technically challenging in young children.[33] Endopyelotomy conveys success rates to the elderly similar to the adult group.[34,35]

LENGTH OF STRICTURE   Although there have be reports of successful management of strictures longer than 2 cm or obliteration of the UPJ,[36,37] these entities are considered contraindications to endourologic procedures and should be treated by open pyeloplasty. Success rates with endopyelotomy in these cases have been consistently poor.[6,15,30,38,39]

DEGREE OF HYDRONEPHROSIS AND RENAL FUNCTION   The degree of hydronephrosis and renal function are important prognostic factors for endopyelotomy. Gupta and colleagues found a statistically significant correlation between the degree of hydronephrosis and likelihood of endopyelotomy failure.[19] Patients with massive hydronephrosis had a 50% rate of failure, compared with only 4% for those with moderate hydronephrosis. Furthermore, patients with poor renal function had lower success rates (54%) than those with moderate function (80%) or good function (92%).[19] Danuser and coworkers also reported that mean preoperative pyelocaliceal volume was significantly higher in patients with failed endopyelotomy than in those with a successful one.[40] Patients with pyelocaliceal volume less than 50 mL had an 87% success rate, and those with greater than 100 mL had a 69% rate. Preoperative absolute renal function, as well as percentage of total renal function in the affected renal unit, was significantly lower in their patients who failed treatment.[40] Lam and associates compared treatment outcome between antegrade versus retrograde endopyelotomy.[41] With the antegrade approach, success rates of 100%, 92.6%, 80.2%, and 66.7% were found in patients with mild, moderate, severe, and massive

hydronephrosis, respectively. They also noted that antegrade endopyelotomy was statistically more successful than retrograde endopyelotomy in patients with high-grade hydronephrosis (66.7 vs. 20.0%; $p = .046$) and believe that UPJ will be more easily identified, incised, and drained antegrade when the UPJ is massively hydronephrotic. Several authors, however, believe that renal pelvis redundancy frequently will be self-correcting if adequate drainage is provided, and consider endopyelotomy an option in UPJ obstruction with high-grade hydronephrosis.[38,42,43] Hatsuse and colleagues reported an 83.3% success rate with endopyelotomy in the setting of massive hydronephrosis.[37] Likewise, treatment of poorly functioning kidneys may improve symptoms and function. Shalhav and colleagues showed a 78% subjective and objective success rate for 6 primary and 3 secondary cases with renal function between 14% and 25% treated with antegrade and retrograde endopyelotomy.[21] Interestingly, 3 patients had severe and another 3 had massive hydronephrosis. On follow-up renal scan, 4 patients had improvement and 1 had stabilization of function.[21] Another group reported subjective and objective success rates of antegrade endopyelotomy performed on kidneys with a glomerular filtration rate (GFR) less than 15 mL/min were 62% and 31%, and those with GFR between 15 and 25 mL/min were 90% and 76%, respectively. Statistically significant improvements in GFR and clearance of tracer was seen in 38% and 31%, respectively, of the former group, and 57% and 76%, respectively, of the latter.[44]

CROSSING VESSELS   The effect of lower pole crossing vessels on endourologic therapy is controversial.[6,19,24,43,45] Crossing vessels have been shown to have a statistically significant negative influence on the outcome of endopyelotomy.[45] Van Cangh and colleagues performed preoperative angiography on patients with symptomatic UPJ obstruction and treated them with antegrade endopyelotomy regardless of the result.[45] They found 39% of the patients had vessels in close proximity to the UPJ. Analysis of their results showed that the presence of crossing vessels reduced the final success rate to 42% from 86%. When crossing vessels occurred in combination with high-grade hydronephrosis, the success rate was 39% contrasted to a 95% rate with no crossing vessels and only moderate hydronephrosis present. The importance of these prognostic factors was confirmed in an updated series. The success rate decreased to 33% and 82% with and without crossing vessels, respectively. Crossing vessels were present in 67% of failures, but in only 18% of successful cases. Vessels of significant size were found in 83% of patients undergoing open surgery for endopyelotomy failure.[24] Knudsen and associates explored 18 of their 24 patients who failed antegrade endopyelotomy and also found that 83% had significant crossing vessels.[46]

Significantly sized (> 2 mm diameter) lower-pole crossing vessels are found in about 50% (33

to 79%) of adult patients with UPJ obstruction, yet success rates of greater than 80% have been reported for endopyelotomy.[47] Thus, not all crossing vessels are significant causes of obstruction. Gupta and coworkers reviewed 401 antegrade endopyelotomies performed over a 12-year period.[19] Fifty-four of 60 failures were explored, and crossing vessels were found in 13 (24%) of the cases. Severe extrinsic fibrosis was the most common finding as a cause of failure, while crossing vessels were potential factors of failure in only 4% of their total cases. Failure was strongly correlated with marked hydronephrosis and poor initial renal function.[19] Nakada and colleagues examined 16 patients with spiral CT scan 2 years after successful retrograde endopyelotomy; 38% of these patients were found to have a crossing vessel.[48]

Long-term success with antegrade endopyelotomy can be achieved in the presence of crossing vessels, but significant involvement of the UPJ with crossing vessels may reduce the success rate of endopyelotomy. When an entanglement is suspected on standard tests, it can be reliably proven using spiral CT or endoluminal ultrasonography.[49–51] To date, there are no preoperative diagnostic procedures that predict which crossing vessels will impact on the success of the endopyelotomy, but in cases of secondary UPJ obstruction and ectopic or malrotated kidneys, imaging may be helpful in suggesting the safest place to make the endopyelotomy incision.[33]

INDICATIONS AND PREPARATION

Surgical intervention should be reserved for patients with symptomatic UPJ obstruction, renal function deterioration, upper tract stones or infection, and rarely, causal hypertension. Close follow-up with repeat testing is warranted for asymptomatic patients with an obstruction of uncertain significance. For patients with caliceal or free-floating renal pelvic stones and UPJ obstruction, percutaneous stone treatment and endopyelotomy may be managed simultaneously. When obstruction is associated with an impacted UPJ stone, a period of nephrostomy drainage after stone removal may resolve the obstruction.[52]

Obstructed kidneys that have extensive stone burden, radiographically proven non-function, or failed repeated interventions, may best be treated with nephrectomy provided that the contralateral kidney is normal.

Absolute contraindications to percutaneous endopyelotomy are active infection and untreated coagulopathy. Sterile urine should be documented at the time of definitive intervention. If urinary tract infection cannot be cleared with antibiotics, the obstructed system should be drained with internal stenting or nephrostomy.

Patients should have a complete history and physical examination. Preoperative evaluation and appropriate laboratory tests should be used to optimize the patient for surgical intervention. A frank and thorough discussion with the patient should take place regarding the risks and benefits of selected treatment options tailored to the patient's anatomic and functional findings. Patients should be informed that any endourologic intervention for UPJ obstruction would probably yield results inferior to open pyeloplasty, and that a secondary procedure may be required. Patients should also understand that there is a small risk of bleeding that may require transfusion; as such, patients are "typed and screened".

INSTRUMENTATION

At the authors' institution, percutaneous endopyelotomy is performed with standard endoscopic and nephroscopic equipment. Only the Sachse cold knife is particular to the procedure.

TECHNIQUE

ACCESS Percutaneous access for endopyelotomy is similar to that used for stone removal, but to facilitate the use of rigid instruments at the UPJ, access should be through a lateral mid- or upper-pole calix. Lower-pole access for endopyelotomy has been reported.[53] Access across the UPJ is accomplished via cystoscopy, guidewire, and open-ended ureteral catheter placement into the renal pelvis with the patient in a prone position on a split-leg table. This may be done in lithotomy position and the patient repositioned prone for access. The ureteral catheter is secured to a urethral catheter and used to opacify the collecting system and guide percutaneous access. Alternatively, a wire may be passed into the bladder in an antegrade fashion fluoroscopically when the tract is initially established or by nephroscopy after tract dilation and sheath placement. Identification of the UPJ in this instance may be difficult if it is pinpoint or located in an unexpected position. Once access is gained, a wire is passed through the ureteral catheter and brought out of the sheath, achieving through-and-through access. Another, more rigid, working wire is placed into the bladder alongside the safety wire. Stones should be removed before the endopyelotomy incision is made so that stone fragments do not migrate into the peripyeloureteral tissue causing localized obstruction from fibrosis or granuloma formation.[54,55]

ENDOPYELOTOMY The classic description of antegrade endopyelotomy used a posterolaterally directed, full-thickness, intraluminal incision of the UPJ with a cold-knife urethrotome under direct vision.[11] At the authors' institution, antegrade endopyelotomy is performed with a wire-guided Sachse cold cutting knife that is honed in the hospital machine shop prior to each use to assure a precise incision. Prior to the incision, the UPJ is balloon-dilated with a 12F ureteral balloon if it is deemed too narrow to accommodate smooth passage of the knife (Figure 21-1). Small mucosa tears are sometimes seen after dilation, and an attempt to incorporate the tear into the endopyelotomy incision is made.

A better understanding of anatomic relationships between the collecting system and surrounding vasculature has led to the incision now being made in a purely lateral fashion.[56] The lateral position is determined by orienting the cutting knife with the lateral position of the patient's flank and referencing the radiographic studies. This may be a complicated task in malrotated kidneys. Visually guided adjustments are made according to the encountered anatomy as studies using endoluminal ultrasonography have demonstrated vessels lateral to the UPJ.[57–59]

The endopyelotomy knife is deployed over the guidewire, under direct vision. The incision should extend 1 to 2 cm into the renal pelvis to approximately 1 cm distal to the area of obstruction (Figure 21-2). Direct vision allows for control of location and depth of incision and the antegrade endopyelotomy incision can be lengthened with precision. Crossing vessels, distinguished as pulsations, can also be avoided. Visualization of fat and retroperitoneal tissue ensures that a full thickness incision of the renal pelvis and ureteral wall has been made. Scarring may make determination of proper depth of the incision difficult in cases of secondary UPJ obstruction.

Numerous other modifications of the original technique and cutting instruments have been described. The transpelvic approach first incises the renal pelvis laterally or posterolaterally so the ureteropelvic junction can next be incised from the outside inward.[37,53,60] The invagination modification uses a retrograde ureteral balloon inflated just beneath the UPJ.[25] The balloon is advanced cephalad such that the UPJ is brought into the renal pelvis, and a double layer of tissue (the renal pelvis and ureteral wall) is incised over the balloon. This method should avoid incision of a crossing vessel.

In the "stent first/hot knife" modification, the stent is passed before performing the endopyelo-

tomy incision using an acorn tip Bugbee electrode or Collins knife with a pure cutting current.[61] The advantages of this technique are that it eliminates the concern about avulsing the UPJ during placement of a stent following the incision, and that placement of the stent better defines the UPJ obstruction allowing a more precise incision.

Electrocautery may be used to point coagulate small bleeding periureteral vessels as well as incise the UPJ, but tips should be 250 to 400 μ as use of larger tips was associated with increased local acute inflammation and peri-incisional injury.[62] When using electrocautery, care must be taken to insulate wires or use nonconductive wires.

PERCUTANEOUS ENDOPYELOPLASTY Percutaneous endopyeloplasty accomplishes a Fengerplasty type of repair of the UPJ by approximation of a full-thickness longitudinal endopyelotomy incision, á la Heineke–Mikulicz pyloroplasty, performed through a percutaneous tract. Initially described by Oshinsky and colleagues, modified 3-0 PDS ski needles and laparoscopic needle drivers were used through the working channel of the nephroscope to close the longitudinal incision transversely.[63] This was technically demanding, and enthusiasm for the procedure waned. The modification by Gill and associates uses a 5F Bugbee electrode to incise the UPJ.[64] They recommended the incision be no longer than 3 cm in order to optimize endoscopic closure and to prevent postoperative UPJ diverticulum formation. Laparoscopic shears are used to undermine the distal aspect of the incision, creating adequate tissue mobilization and aiding percutaneous suturing. Suturing is facilitated with the use of a modified 5-mm SewRight 5SR (LSI Solutions, Rochester, NY) laparoscopic suturing device with 2-0 polyglactin 910 acid sutures. This device is placed through the working channel of the

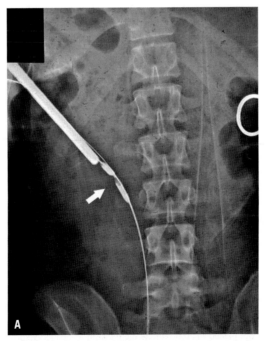
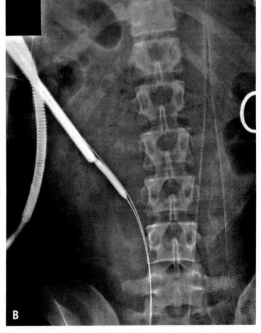

Figure 21-1 Balloon dilation of a UPJ obstruction to accommodate the endopyelotome. *A*, Arrow depicts the "waisting" of the obstruction. *B*, The obstruction is dilated to 12F.

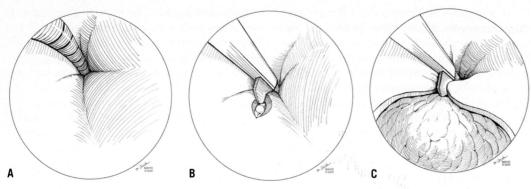

Figure 21-2 *A*, A guidewire is passed through the UPJ into the bladder. *B*, The cold knife is passed over the guidewire to incise the UPJ. *C*, Retroperitoneal tissue, peripelvic fat, and normal caliber ureter should be seen after the incision. Reproduced with permission from Gettman MT, Segura JW. Percutaneous management of ureteropelvic junction obstruction. Atlas Urol Clin 2003;11:165.

nephroscope, and the first suture is placed aligning the horizontal closure; additional interrupted sutures are placed to achieve a watertight closure. The suture is tied extracorporeally, and the knots are placed intraluminally with a knot pusher under direct vision (Figure 21-3). Potential advantages over conventional endopyelotomy include wider caliber reconstruction of the UPJ, full-thickness healing with primary intent, minimal urinary extravasation, and shorter stenting duration.[64]

STENT PLACEMENT At the authors' institution, a 26-cm 8F or 8.5F standard stent is placed with fluoroscopic and visual guidance after antegrade endopyelotomy for a duration of 6 weeks. A 22F nephrostomy is also placed. A 5F Double-J stent is used to stent the endopyeloplasty and a 20F nephrostomy tube drains the kidney.[64]

Size and duration of stenting has for many years been based on the work of Davis and colleagues and Oppenheimer and Hinman.[10,65] Their work showed that 6 weeks after intubated ureterotomy with 12F to 16F stents, reconstitution of the muscular layer was 90% complete through a combination of wound contracture and smooth muscle regeneration. Animal and clinical studies, however, have shown that smaller stents and a shorter duration of stenting may provide equivalent, or even superior results.

Increasingly, smaller easier-to-place ureteral stents are being used after endopyelotomy. Moon and colleagues failed to demonstrate any difference in ureteral healing in a porcine model after endoureterotomy and stenting with 7F or 14/7F stents.[66] Hwang and associates found no significant difference in results between the use of 14/7F and 6F after endopyelotomy or endoureterotomy in 41 patients.[67] Kletscher and colleagues achieved success in 95% of 21 patients stented with an 8F or 8.5F stent after endopyelotomy, compared to 85% of 26 patients stented with a 14/7F endopyelotomy stent;[35] the difference was not statistically significant. Interestingly, Danuser and coworkers reported using a 27F nephrostomy over a 14/8.2F external stent after antegrade endopyelotomy, with removal of the 27F portion after 2 to 3 weeks, leaving the external stent for an additional 3 to 4 weeks.[23] At 24 months of follow-up, success with this method of stenting was 93%, compared to 71% with 6 weeks of stenting with a 14/8.2F external stent alone.

While complete restoration of the ureteral musculature takes at least 6 weeks, it is unknown whether the stent needs to be present for the entire duration. Kerbl and associates randomized 14 minipigs treated with endoureterotomy to 7F stent placement for 1, 3, and 6 weeks.[68] Twelve weeks after stent removal, it was found that stent-

ing for 1 week provided results as good as stenting for 3 or 6 weeks. In the 1-week group, success rates for longer strictures were significantly better than the other groups. Abdel-Hakim used a 7F stent in 5 patients for 4 days, and in two patients for 5 weeks.[69] At a follow-up of 3 to 10 months, all patients were considered cured. Kuenkel and Korth reported that stenting for 3 weeks produced superior results to stenting for 6 weeks in 143 endopyelotomies.[70] Kumar and colleagues showed that stenting for 2 weeks was as effective as for 4 weeks in successful endopyelotomy.[71] Thus, the size and optimal time for post-endopyelotomy stenting remains unclear.

There appears to be no difference in efficacy between internal and external stents. Though the internal stent is better tolerated than the external stent, stent exchange or percutaneous nephrostomy drainage may be necessary if the stent becomes occluded. A rare complication of the internal stenting for endopyelotomy is migration of the proximal coil out of the incision into the retroperitoneum. A percutaneous tube was not placed at the end of endopyelotomy in 26 patients, with a reported 88.5% success rate.[72]

POSTOPERATIVE CARE

The nephrostomy tube is usually removed after 24 to 48 hours, with or without a brief trial of clamping or a nephrostogram. Patients are discharged after 48 to 72 hours, but some are released earlier. External endopyelotomy stents, if used, are capped after 48 hours. A daily suppressive dose of antibiotics is given while the stent is indwelling. Most patients are able to return to normal levels of activity one week after surgery. Patients return in 4 to 6 weeks for stent removal. An excretory urogram with or without a diuretic renogram should be obtained 6 to 8 weeks later. Patients are followed at periodic intervals to assess signs and symptoms of obstruction. Antegrade endopyelotomy is considered successful if the patient is asymptomatic and if postoperative studies show improved drainage.

The ureteral stent was removed 2 to 4 weeks following percutaneous endopyeloplasty in the nine patients with primary UPJ obstruction. All patients had an excretory urogram 2 weeks after stent removal and a diuretic renal scan at 3 months postoperatively. A success rate of 100% was reported at a mean follow-up of 4 months.[64]

RESULTS

Excellent success rates have been achieved by many, but some long-term reports suggest that the procedure may not be as durable as once thought (Table 21-1). Generally, most treatment failures occur early in the postoperative period. Kletscher and coworkers reported that all failures occurred in the first 2 months after endopyelotomy; a third of the failures were only found on radiographic screening.[35] Gupta and colleagues reported that 92% of failures occurred in the first year after surgery.[19] Others have reported higher incidences of late failures or

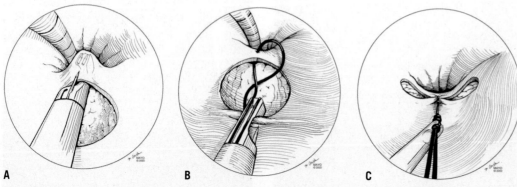

Figure 21-3 *A*, After the endopyelotomy incision is made, endoshears are used to elevate the ureteral margin in order to place the medial suture. *B*, The suture is passed through the lateral ureteral margin and tied extracorporeally. *C*, The knot is placed intraluminally with a knot pusher. Additional sutures are placed to approximate the incision as needed. Reproduced with permission from Gettman MT, Segura JW. Percutaneous management of ureteropelvic junction obstruction. Atlas Urol Clin 2003;11:165.

TABLE 21-1 Results of Antegrade Endopyelotomy

Study	No.	Method of Incision	Stent Size (Fr)	Stent Duration (wk)	Success Rate (%)			Mean Follow-up (range)
					Overall	1°	2°	
Ono et al[60]	22	Cold-knife	10–16	3–4	95	94	100	13 (4–26)
Meretyk et al[62]	23	Electrocautery/Cold-knife	14/7	6.5	78	75	82	22 (2–39)
Kletscher et al[35]	50	Cold-knife	8 or 8.5 or 14/7	6	88	90	82	12 (4–74)
Brooks et al[5]	13	Cold-knife	7 or 14/7	4–6	77	N/S	N/S	20 (4–53)
Van Cangh et al[24]	123	Cold-knife	10–12	6	71	68	83	62 (6–153)
Korth et al[80]	286	Cold-knife	Prime stent	3–6	73	80	67	20 (6–120)
Gallucci and Alpi[53]	46	Cold-knife	5 or 6	3	80	80	N/A	N/S
Combe et al[25]	49	Hot-knife	12/7	6	78	75	85	16 (3–36)
Gupta et al[19]	401	Cold-knife	12 or 14/8.2	6	85	82	89	51 (6–144)
Khan et al[81]	220	Cold-knife	8–12	6	86.7	N/S	N/S	N/S
Shalhav et al[21]	83	Electrocautery	7 or 14/7	4–6	83	89	77	32
Danuser et al[23]	77	Cold-knife or scissors	14/8.2	6; 27F removed after 2–3 wks	70	N/S	N/S	67 (2–118)
	55		27/14/8.2		94	N/S	N/S	23 (2–52)
Hatsuse et al[37]	107	Cold-knife	16/6	3	90	93.5	83	58
Lam et al[41]	64	Cold-knife, scissors, or Acucise	6	6	81.3	84.6	66.7	37 (5–76)
Knudsen et al[46]	80	Cold-knife or holmium	12/6	4–6	67	65	74	55 (16–138)
TOTAL	1699				81	81	81	

N/A-not applicable; N/S-not specified

recurrences. Van Cangh and associates found 7 of the 18 failures (39%) occurred after 1 year;[24] one occurred 6 years postoperatively. Knudsen and colleagues reported that their mean time to failure was 15 months (range, 1 to 79 months), and that 9 of their 26 failures (35%) presented more than one year after endopyelotomy.[46] Albani and colleagues reported an overall success rate of 74% for antegrade and retrograde endopyelotomy;[73] the results were not stratified according to treatment modality. They found that 9 of their 33 failures (27.3%) became evident only after one year postoperatively. Furthermore, the Kaplan-Meier estimate of long-term success was only 63% at 36 months. These findings may be explained by a strict surveillance protocol of objective testing at regular intervals. The late failure rate of antegrade endopyelotomy and its predisposing risk factors are not known. Thus, long-term follow-up is recommended to diagnose late failures.

The advantages of percutaneous endopyelotomy, compared to open pyeloplasty, are shorter operative times and length of hospitalization, less postoperative pain, and decreased length of convalescence.[4,5] While these advantages are important, the treatment outcomes of antegrade endopyelotomy are consistently lower than open pyeloplasty. Careful patient selection may allow results attained with endopyelotomy to be equivalent to open surgery. Using duplex ultrasonography, endoluminal ultrasonography, or spiral CT scans, antegrade endopyelotomy performed on select patients with favorable anatomy yielded success rates comparable to open surgery.[59,74]

Treatment options for failed endopyelotomy include repeat endopyelotomy, either antegrade or retrograde, and laparoscopic or open dismembered pyeloplasty. Hoenig and associates found a trend toward better success rates for endopyelotomy after failed prior open pyeloplasty than for failed prior endopyelotomy.[20] Similarly, Ng and

colleagues reported a 71.4% success rate for endourologic management of failed primary open intervention compared to only 37.5% after failed primary endopyelotomy.[75] Thus, open or laparoscopic pyeloplasty is generally offered to patients who have failed endopyelotomy. Though some have reported that plastic repair after endopyelotomy is slightly more difficult compared to primary cases, the results are not compromised and should exceed 95%.[19,75–77]

COMPLICATIONS

Aside from complications related to anesthesia and percutaneous access to the kidney, those inherent to antegrade endopyelotomy are infrequent. Significant hemorrhage from vascular injury is the most worrisome complication of endopyelotomy. Fortunately, this is uncommon, and transfusion rates range from 1% to 9% for antegrade endopyelotomy.[6,19,24,35,70] Differentiating bleeding attributed to dilation of the percutaneous access and that of the endopyelotomy incision is difficult. Intraoperative and postoperative management is akin to that of bleeding complication from percutaneous nephrolithotomy. If conservative measures fail, selective angiographic embolization is invariably successful. All attempts should be made to avoid pulsations during visualization of the UPJ and to redirect the incision if vessels are seen. Arteriovenous fistulae following antegrade endopyelotomy have been reported.[62,78] This may have occurred with access rather than endopyelotomy.

Urosepsis can occur in 2% to 4% of patients undergoing endopyelotomy.[79] Precautions such as ensuring preoperative sterile urine, perioperative, and prophylactic antibiotics while the patient is stented may lower complications related to infection.

Stent-related complications include stent irritation, migration, calcification and obstruction.

These may require stent manipulation or replacement. Other major complications include ureteral avulsion and ureteral necrosis (related to peelaway sheath use or overzealous incision), urinoma, and inadvertent incision on infundibular narrowing or renal pelvis.[79]

SUMMARY

Antegrade endopyelotomy is the treatment of choice for UPJ obstruction with stones and is a good alternative for those who have failed open surgery. Antegrade endopyelotomy in carefully selected patients may provide success rates approaching open pyeloplasty. Presently, with long-term results inferior to open intervention, the limited disability, minimal morbidity, and relative ease in application associated with antegrade endopyelotomy keep it a viable treatment option. Percutaneous endopyeloplasty is a promising technique that may overcome problems with healing of the UPJ by secondary intent, but further clinical experience and longer follow-up are needed.

REFERENCES

1. Anderson KR, Weiss, RM. Physiology and evaluation of ureteropelvic junction obstruction. J Endourol 1996;10:87–91.
2. Wolf JS Jr, Siegel CL, Brink JA, et al. Imaging for ureteropelvic junction obstruction in adults. J Endourol 1996;10:93–104.
3. Lowe FC, Marshall FF. Ureteropelvic junction obstruction in adults. Urology 1984;23:331–5.
4. Karlin GC, Badlani GH, Smith AD. Endopyelotomy versus open pyeloplasty: comparison in 88 patients. J Urol 1988;140:476–8.
5. Brooks JD, Kavoussi LR, Preminger GM, et al. Comparison of open and endourologic approaches to the obstructed ureteropelvic junction. Urology 1995;46:791–5.
6. Motola JA, Badlani GH, Smith AD. Results of 212 consecutive endopyelotomies: an 8-year follow-up. J Urol 1993;149:453–6.
7. Streem SB. Percutaneous endopyelotomy. Urol Clin North Am 2000;27:685–93.
8. Albarran J. Operations plastiques et anastomoses dans le traitment des retentions de viem. Theses DeParis 1903.
9. Davis DM. Intubated ureterotomy: a new operation for

ureteral and ureteropelvic stricture. Surg Gynecol Obstet 1943;76:513–23.

10. Davis DM, Strong GH, Drake WM. Intubated ureterotomy: experimental work and clinical results. J Urol 1948; 59:851–62.

11. Wickham JEA, Kellet MJ. Percutaneous pyelolysis. Eur Urol 1983;9:122–4.

12. Badlani G, Eshghi M, Smith AD. Percutaneous surgery for ureteropelvic junction obstruction (endopyelotomy): technique and early results. J Urol 1986;135: 26–8.

13. Inglis JA, Tolley DA. Ureteroscopic pyelolysis for pelvi-ureteric junction obstruction. Br J Urol 1986;58:250–2.

14. Gerber GS, Kim JC. Ureteroscopy endopyelotomy in the treatment of patients with ureteropelvic junction obstruction. Urology 2000;55:198–203.

15. Preminger GM, Clayman RV, Nakada SY, et al. A multicenter clinical trial investigating the use of a fluoroscopically controlled cutting balloon catheter for the management of ureteral and ureteropelvic junction obstruction. J Urol 1997;157:1625–9.

16. Nadler RB, Rao GS, Pearle MS, et al. Acucise endopyelotomy: assessment of long-term durability. J Urol 1996; 156:1094–7.

17. Faerber GJ, Richardson TD, Farah N, et al. Retrograde treatment of ureteropelvic junction obstruction using the ureteral cutting balloon catheter. J Urol 1997;157:454–8.

18. Tebyani N, Candela J, Hetal P, et al. Ureteropelvic junction obstruction presenting as early satiety and weight loss. J Endourol 1999;13:445–6.

19. Gupta M, Tuncay OL, Smith AD. Open surgical exploration after failed endopyelotomy: a 12-year perspective. J Urol 1997;157:1613–9.

20. Hoening DM, Shalhav AL, Elbahnasy AM, et al. Impact of etiology of secondary ureteropelvic junction obstruction on outcome of endopyelotomy. J Endourol 1998;12:131–3.

21. Shalhav AL, Giusti G, Elbahnasy AM, et al. Adult endopyelotomy: impact of etiology and antegrade versus retrograde approach on outcome. J Urol 1998;160:685–9.

22. Gill HS, Liao JC. Pelviureteric junction obstruction treated with Acucise retrograde endopyelotomy. Br J Urol 1998; 82:8–11.

23. Danuser H, Hochreiter WW, Ackerman DK, et al. Influence of stent size on the success of antegrade endopyelotomy for primary ureteropelvic junction obstruction: results of 2 consecutive series. J Urol 2001;166:902–9.

24. Van Cangh PJ, Nesa S, Galeon M, et al. Vessels around the ureteropelvic junction: significance and imaging by conventional radiology. J Endourol 1996;10:111–9.

25. Combe M, Gelet A, Abdelrahim AF, et al. Ureteropelvic invagination procedure for endopyelotomy (Gelet technique): results of 51 consecutive cases. J Endourol 1996;10:153–7.

26. Conlin MJ, Bagley DH. Ureteroscopic endopyelotomy at a single setting. J Urol 1998;159:727–31.

27. Shalhav AL, Ciusti G, Elbahnasy AM, et al. Endopyelotomy for high insertion ureteropelvic junction obstruction. J Endourol 1998;12:127–30.

28. Segura JW. Endourology. J Urol 1984;132:1079–84.

29. Ramsay JWA, Miller RA, Kellett MJ, et al. Percutaneous pyelolysis: indications, complications and results. Br J Urol 1984;56:586–9.

30. Perez LM, Friedman RM, Carson CC. Endoureteropyelotomy in adults. Urology 1992;39:71–6.

31. Chow GK, Geisinger MA, Streem SB. Endopyelotomy outcome as a function of high versus dependent ureteral insertion. Urology 1999;54: 999–1002.

32. Karlin G, Badlani G, Smith AD. Percutaneous pyeloplasty for congenital ureteropelvic junction obstruction. Urology 1992;39:533–7.

33. Figenshua RS, Clayman RV. Endourologic options for management of ureteropelvic junction obstruction in the pediatric patient. Urol Clin North Am 1998;25:199–209.

34. Horgan JD, Maidenberg MJ, Smith AD. Endopyelotomy in the elderly. J Urol 1993;150:1107–9.

35. Kletscher BA, Segura JW, LeRoy AJ, et al. Percutaneous antegrade endopyelotomy: review of 50 consecutive cases. J Urol 1995;153:701–3.

36. Lopatkin NA, Martov AG, Gushchin BL. An endourologic approach to complete ureteropelvic junction and ureteral strictures. J Endourol 2000;14:721–6.

37. Hatsuse K, Ono Y, Kinukawa T, et al. Long-term results of endopyeloureterotomy using the transpelvic extraureteral approach. Urology 2002;60:233–7.

38. Brannen GE, Bush WH, Lewis GP. Endopyelotomy for primary repair of reteropelvic junction obstruction. J Urol 1988;139:29–32.

39. Van Cangh PJ, Jonon JL, Wese FX, et al. Endoureteropyelotomy: percutaneous treatment of ureteropelvic junction obstruction. J Urol 1989;148:775–83.

40. Danuser H, Ackermann DK, Bohlen D, et al. Endopyelotomy for primary ureteropelvic junction obstruction: risk factors determine the success rate. J Urol 1998;159:56–61.

41. Lam JS, Cooper KL, Greene TD, et al. Impact of hydronephrosis and renal function on treatment outcome: antegrade versus retrograde endopyelotomy. Urology 2003;61: 1107–12.

42. Smart WR. An evaluation of intubated ureterotomy with a description of surgical technique. J Urol 1961;85:512–24.

43. Cassis A, Brannen GE, Bush WH, et al. Endopyelotomy: review of results and complications. J Urol 1991;146:1492–5.

44. Kapoor R, Zaman W, Kumar A, et al. Endopyelotomy in poorly functioning kidney: is it worthwhile? J Endourol 2001;15:725–8.

45. Van Cangh PJ, Wilmart JF, Opsomer RJ, et al. Long term results and later recurrence after endoureteropyelotomy: a critical analysis of prognostic factors. J Urol 1994;151:934–7.

46. Knudsen BE, Cook AJ, Watterson JD, et al. Percutaneous antegrade endopyelotomy: long-term results from one institution, Urology 2004;63:230–4.

47. Gupta M, Smith AD. Crossing vessels at the ureteropelvic junction: do they influence endopyelotomy outcome? J Endourol 1996;10:183–7.

48. Nakada SY, Wolf JS Jr, Brink JA, et al. Retrospective analysis of the effect of crossing vessels on successful retrograde endopyelotomy outcomes using spiral computerized tomography angiography. J Urol 1998;159:62–5.

49. Kumon H, Tsugawa M, Hashimoto H, et al. Impact of 3-dimensional helical computerized tomography on selection of operative methods for ureteropelvic junction obstruction. J Urol 1997;158:1696–700.

50. Kumar PV, Joshi HB, Timoney AG, et al. Endoluminal ultrasonography with reusable probe: preliminary results. J Endourol 2002;16:667–71.

51. Parkin J, Evans S, Kumar PV, et al. Endoluminal ultrasonography before retrograde endopyelotomy: can the results match laparoscopic pyeloplasty? BJU Int 2003;91: 389–91.

52. Rutchik SD, Resnick MI. Ureteropelvic junction obstruction and renal calculi: pathophysiology and implications for management. Uro Clin North Am 1998;25:317–21.

53. Gallucci M, Alpi G. Antegrade transpelvic endopyelotomy in primary obstruction of the ureteropelvic junction. J Endourol 1996;10:127–32.

54. Streem SB. Percutaneous endopyelotomy. Urol Clin North Am 2000;27:685–93.

55. Giddens JL, Grotas AB, Grasso M. Stone granuloma causes ureteropelvic junction obstruction after percutaneous nephrolithotomy and antegrade endopyelotomy. J Urol 2000;164: 118–9.

56. Sampaio FJB, Favorito LA. Ureteropelvic junction stenosis: vascular anatomical background for endopyelotomy. J Urol 1993;150:1787–91.

57. Bagley DH, Liu J, Goldberg BB, et al. Endopyelotomy: importance of crossing vessels demonstrated by endoluminal ultrasonography. J Endourol 1995;9:465–7.

58. Bagley DH, Liu J, Goldberg B. Endoluminal sonographic imaging of the ureteropelvic junction. J Endourol 1996; 10:105–10.

59. Conlin MJ. Results of selective management of ureteropelvic junction obstruction. J Endourol 2002;16:233–6.

60. Ono Y, Ohshima S, Kinukawa T, et al. Endopyeloureterotomy via a transpelvic extraureteral approach. J Urol 1992;147: 352–5.

61. Savage SJ, Streem SB. Simplified approach to percutaneous endopyelotomy. Urology 2000;56:848–50.

62. Meretyk I, Meretyk S, Clayman RV. Endopyelotomy: comparison of ureteroscopic retrograde and antegrade percutaneous techniques. J Urol 1992;148:775–83.

63. Oshinsky GS, Jarrett TW, Smith AD. New technique in managing ureteropelvic junction obstruction: percutaneous endoscopic pyeloplasty. J Endourol 1996;10:147–51.

64. Gill IS, Desai MM, Kaouk JH, et al. Percutaneous endopyeloplasty: description of a new technique. J Urol 2002;168: 2097–102.

65. Oppenheimer R, Hinman F Jr. Ureteral regeneration: contracture vs. hyperplasia of smoth muscle. J Urol 1955;74: 476–84.

66. Moon YT, Kerbl K, Pearle MS, et al. Evaluation of optimal stent size after endourologic incision of ureteral strictures. J Endourol 1995;9:15–22.

67. Hwang T, Yoon J, Ahn J, et al. Percutaneous endoscopic management of upper ureteral stricture: size of stent. J Urol 1996;155:882–4.

68. Kerbl K, Chandhoke PS, Figenshau, et al. Effect of stent duration on ureteral healing following endoureterotomy in an animal model. J Urol 1993;150:1302–5.

69. Abdel-Hakim AM. Endopyelotomy for ureteropelvic junction obstruction: is long-term stenting mandatory? J Endourol 1987;1:265–8.

70. Kuenkel M, Korth K: Endopyelotomy: long term follow-up of 143 patients. J Endourol 1990;4:109–15.

71. Kumar R, Kapoor R, Mandhani A, et al. Optimum duration of splinting after endopyelotomy. J Endourol 1999;13:89–91.

72. Limb J, Bellman GC. Tubeless percutaneous renal surgery: review of the first 112 patients. Urology 2002;59:527–31.

73. Albani JM, Yost AJ, Streen SB. Ureteropelvic junction obstruction: determining durability of endourological intervention. J Urol 2004;171:579–82.

74. Pardalidis NP, Papatsoris AG, Kosmaoglou EV. Endoscopic and laparoscopic treatment of ureteropelvic junction obstruction. J Urol 2002;168:1937–40.

75. Ng CS, Yost AJ, Streem SB. Management of failed primary intervention for ureteropelvic junction obstruction: 12-year, single-center experience. Urology 2003;61:291–6.

76. Jabbour ME, Goldfischer ER, Klima WJ, et al. Endopyelotomy after failed pyeloplasty: the long-term results. J Urol 1998;160:690–3.

77. Motola JA, Fried R, Badlani GH, et al. Failed endopyelotomy: implications for future surgery on the ureteropelvic junction. J Urol;1993:821–3.

78. Malden ES, Picus D, Clayman RV. Arteriovenous fistula complicating endopyelotomy. J Urol 1992;148:1520–3.

79. Bellman, GC. Complications of endopyelotomy. J Endourol 1996;10:177–81.

80. Korth K, Kuenkel M, Karsch J. Percutaneous endopyelotomy and results: Korth technique. J Endourol 1996;10:121–6.

81. Khan AM, Holman E, Pasztor I, et al. Endopyelotomy: experience with 320 cases. J Endourol 1997;11:243–6.

22

Treatment of Caliceal Diverticula and Infundibular Stenosis

Raymond J. Leveillee, MD

Vincent G. Bird, MD

Many things have changed since the first edition of this textbook. Advances in fiberoptics, introduction of the holmium:yttrium-aluminum-garnet (holmium:YAG) laser for treatment of soft tissue and stones, improvements in fiberoptic scope design and durability, as well as increased utilization of laparoscopy for renal surgeries have rendered many areas of the genitourinary tract previously treated by open surgery or percutaneous approaches less common. In this chapter, we will discuss the etiology, significance, and treatment options for two relatively uncommon pathological conditions: caliceal diverticula and intrarenal obstructions such as focal hydrocalicosis (also known as hydrocalix) due to infundibular stenosis. As these two entities can appear identical radiographically, it is important to understand their etiology in order to best diagnose and treat them optimally.

Focal renal dilatations are rare occurrences and are often confused with localized cystic lesions discovered incidentally during radiologic examination. We present in this chapter on caliceal diverticula and infundibular stenosis a description of radiographically similar lesions to be considered in the differential diagnosis, the anatomic basis for these two entities, the proposed etiologies, and the clinical significance of each of them. In addition, complications resulting from untreated and treated caliceal diverticula and infundibular stenosis will be discussed. Particular emphasis will be placed on the percutaneous endourologic approach to these relatively rare conditions. Additional comments on the Laparoscopic approach can be found in Chapter 57, "Renal Surgery: Benign Disease, Cyst Ablation, and Calicealectomy".

CALICEAL DIVERTICULA

Caliceal diverticula (or pyelocaliceal diverticula) are nonsecretory, urothelial lined cavities that passively fill with urine from adjacent portions of the collecting system. They were first described by Rayer in 1841 as "eventrations of the upper collecting system, lying within the renal parenchyma and communicating with the main collecting system via a narrow channel."[1,2] They form during the fifth to eighth weeks of embryologic life due to an incomplete reabsorption of third- to fourth-order ureteral buds. The majority branch off the calices, but some may branch off

the renal pelvis or infundibulum, thus leading to the terms "caliceal" and "pyelocaliceal" diverticula. They are uncommon findings on intravenous urograms (IVU), the incidence being between 2.1 to 6.0 per 1,000 IVUs in adults and 3.3 per 1,000 IVUs in the pediatric age group.[3,4] This similarity in incidence suggests a congenital origin.[5] Calculi are present in 9.5 to 50% of cases, although not all calculi within diverticula require treatment.[3,6,7] They occur with equal frequency in males and females and show no predilection for unilaterality. A composite of several series demonstrates that they can occur in any region of the kidney but are more common in the upper polar region, occurring about twice as often at that site (Table 22-1).[3-6,8,9] The significance of this propensity for an upper-pole location is evident when one considers the etiology as well as percutaneous or retrograde access and treatment.

Unlike simple renal cysts, which are lined by cuboidal epithelium, caliceal diverticula are lined by transitional epithelium and communicate directly with the main collecting system by narrow communications.[10,11] They do not communicate, however, with any collecting tubules nor papillae, thus any urine contained within them enters only in a retrograde fashion. They have been classified by Wulfsohn as type I if they communicate with a minor calix or infundibulum and type II if they connect with a major calix or directly with the renal pelvis.[2] An alternative classification was offered by Dretler,[12] in which the categorization is based on the patency of the ostium and the length of the diverticular neck.

1. Open mouth, short neck
2. Closed mouth, short neck
3. Closed mouth, long neck
4. Obliterated neck

A third classification system was proposed by Hulbert and colleagues, which is based on radiographic criteria and technical characteristics (Figure 22-1).[9] Because the epithelial lining is nonsecretory, caliceal diverticula do not produce urine; they do, however, contain urine, which flows passively in a retrograde direction into them via narrow ostia. For this reason, they are sometimes seen only on delayed films of an IVU or by relatively higher-pressure retrograde pyelography. The diameters of the ostia vary; thus, some fill and drain relatively easily, whereas others may not fill at all unless considerable filling pressure is exerted. The sizes of the diverticula are on the order of 0.5 to 2.0 cm, although they have been known to become quite large, occasionally achieving sizes up to 7.5 cm (Figure 22-2).[13]

DIFFERENTIAL DIAGNOSIS OF FOCAL RENAL DILATATIONS Caliceal diverticula must be differentiated from other "cystic diseases" of the kidney such as cortical, serous, hemorrhagic, parapelvic, or tuberculous cysts, or other focal

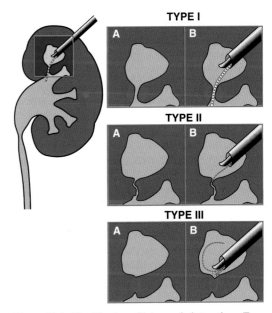

Figure 22-1 Classification of intrarenal obstructions. Type I: Narrowing through which a guidewire can be passed. Type II: Narrowing that is patent radiographically but through which a guidewire cannot be passed. Type III: Totally obliterated lumen/ostium. Adapted from Hulbert JH, Hunter DW, Castaneda-Zuniga WR, et al. Classification of and techniques for the reconstruction of stricture in the region of the ureteropelvic junction. J Urol 1988;140:468.

Table 22-1 Incidence and Location of Caliceal Diverticula within the Kidney		
Location	Right	Left
Upper	51	46
Middle	27	27
Lower	20	10
Totals	98	83

Adapted from Middleton AW Jr, et al,[3] Michel W et al,[4] Timmons JW, et al,[5] Williams G, et al,[6] Kottasz S and Hamvas A,[8] and Hulbert et al.[97]

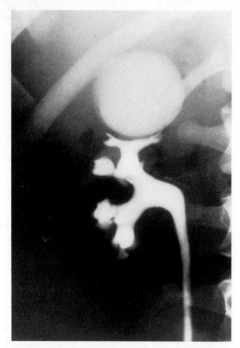

Figure 22-2 Retrograde pyelogram demonstrating a very large (7.5 cm) diverticulum containing calculous material. Large diverticula (> 2 cm) such as these should be fulgurated at the time of percutaneous stone extraction to ensure coaptation of sidewalls and optimal collapse.

support of his argument, he notes that, in 32 out of 250 patients with urinary tract infection and documented VUR, 23 also had radiographic evidence of caliceal diverticula. He does not, however, list radiographic criteria for these lesions, and classifies them as "caliceal diverticulum, pyelogenic cyst, or hydrocalix."[24]

A more widely accepted view is that caliceal diverticula are congenital structures[2,3,6,7,25,26] rather than acquired ones.[14–16]They occur during the fifth to eighth weeks of embryologic life due to non-degeneration of the third- and fourth-order divisions of the ureteral buds. This pattern of dichotomous branching of the ureteral bud with multiple subdivisions is best described by Wulfsohn,[2] who theorizes that some branches are normally absorbed. The caliceal diverticulum is the result of an incomplete reabsorption of one of these branches, and by the nature of this malabsorption, these structures lack communication with functioning glomeruli.

DIAGNOSIS, COMPLICATIONS, AND CLINICAL SIGNIFICANCE

The diagnosis of caliceal diverticula is often made by IVU and can be confirmed by retrograde pyelography, although this is not often necessary (Figure 22-5). Because there is no com-

munication with functional parenchyma, they can only fill in a retrograde manner. Depending on the diameter and length of the ostium, this retrograde filling may not occur immediately, and delayed filling seen on IVU is a hallmark of this entity. In addition, the lack of overlying parenchyma can be noted on intravenous tomography and/or computerized tomography (CT). If discovered incidentally, it must be differentiated from a tuberculous cavity or acquired hydrocalicosis, such as from secondary infundibular stenosis (scar, inflammation, edema, amyloidosis, or tumor). This distinction may be extremely difficult if only ultrasonography or CT is used.[27,28]

Although the vast majority of caliceal diverticula are asymptomatic, those associated with symptoms have provided the impetus for endourologic treatment approaches. Pain in combination with caliceal diverticula is by far the most commonly reported complaint and occurs in approximately 50% of patients. Associated symptoms such as hematuria occur in approximately 20% of cases,[14] whereas pyuria has been reported in up to 25% to 66% in some series.[8,29]

Calculi within diverticula occur with an incidence of from 9.5 to 50%.[3,6,7] The narrow neck of the diverticulum rarely allows these stones to pass.

caliceal obstructions.[11,14–17] Hydrocalicosis, a generic term that does not imply causation, is a cystic dilatation, or hydronephrosis, of a major calix due to infundibular obstruction (Figures 22-3 and 22-4).[18] Infundibular stenosis can be acquired or congenital and will be discussed in greater detail later in this chapter (see "Infundibular Stenosis"). The acquired forms may have an intrinsic cause such as inflammation, scar tissue, stone, clot, or tumor. Extrinsic obstruction can be secondary to the tumor or, as described by Fraley in 1966, from an intrarenal crossing vessel with resultant focal hydronephrosis, nephralgia, and microhematuria.[19]

ETIOLOGY AND EMBRYOLOGY

Most sources believe that caliceal diverticula are congenital structures rather than acquired ones. Several authors describe anecdotal case reports in which the ostium becomes completely occluded on follow-up studies of previously documented caliceal diverticula. They speculate that caliceal diverticula are the precursors of renal cysts.[20–22] Conversely, Reiss speculates that they are the result of simple cyst or abscess rupture into the collecting system.[23] Histologic examination reveals that the inner linings of diverticula (transitional cell) are not at all like simple renal cysts (simple cuboidal), thus making a common link highly unlikely.[10] It is more likely that, in the cases noted above, sealing off of the ostium may have occurred spontaneously, secondary to inflammatory changes, or the opening may be too fine to identify.[2] Amar speculated on the role of intrapelvic pressure secondary to vesicoureteral reflux (VUR) and infection causing local renal damage as leading to the formation of caliceal diverticula in children.[24] In

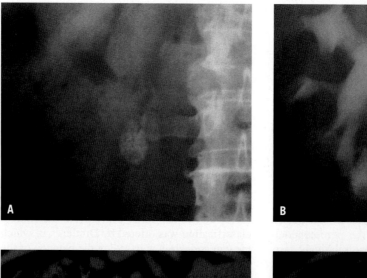

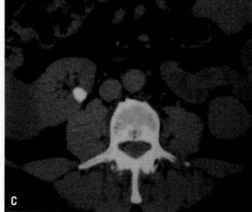

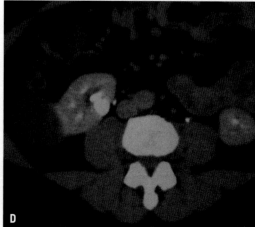

Figure 22-3 *A*, Plain abdominal film in a 61 year old asymptomatic male. *B*, IV Urogram film at 10 minutes demonstrates rapid filling via very narrow ostium (Arrow). *C*, Non-contrast and *D*, excretory phases of computerized tomography. Note the lack of overlying parenchyma (ie, dimpling) seen around the stone. This finding may give a clue as to the etiology and help to distinguish a caliceal diverticulum containing stone from a hydrocalix.

Recurrent urinary tract infection,[30] ureteral obstruction,[26] spontaneous rupture,[31] [32] abscess formation,[33–35] xanthogranulomatous pyelonephritis,[36] [37] and rupture of the kidney[38] have been reported and demonstrate that caliceal diverticulum, although often a benign radiographic finding, is not a negligible condition. Severe complications arising from them, however, are relatively uncommon. Auringer and Sumner also have reported focal renal uptake of radiotracer within a caliceal diverticulum on a bone scan.[39] One must be aware of this occurrence so that it is not confused with a blastic or metastatic lesion.

TREATMENT OPTIONS   The majority of caliceal diverticula are asymptomatic. Of those that are symptomatic, less than 50% will require operative intervention.[5,6,11,40] Most can be left alone or observed. Indications for operative intervention, whether calculi are present or not, include chronic pain secondary to the diverticulum, recurrent urinary tract infection, gross hematuria, or evidence of progressive renal damage.[5] When it comes to surgical intervention for symptomatic caliceal diverticula there are several treatment options available to patients, which we will discuss below. The choice of procedure usually is dictated by the actual location of the diverticulum within the kidney. Because the majority of these are located in the upper third of the kidney, many of these may be amenable to a retrograde ureterorenoscopic approach.[3–6,8,9] The standard treatment is endoscopic surgery with fulguration and/or marsupialization with dilation of the neck of the diverticulum. In the following section we will discuss patient selection, preoperative and intraoperative steps, post-operative course, results, as well as risks involved with each of the procedures available including: open, percutaneous, uretero-renoscopic, and laparoscopic surgery.

Open Surgery   Traditional open surgery involved three basic approaches with the overall goals of eradication of the diseased portion and conservation of as much normal renal tissue as possible. The first of these approaches involved unroofing of the diverticulum and excision of the entire lining, with obliteration of the communication to the collecting system using fine absorbable sutures. The cavity left behind was often packed with perirenal fat or omentum, and stents were not used.[7,41] Drawbacks to this approach included significant bleeding and loss of viable parenchyma when multiple hemostatic sutures were used.[6] The second approach was a simple or partial nephrectomy, but no parenchymal sparing is achieved with this method.[6,17,42] Prather and Newman and colleagues reported good results with the third method, which consisted of excision of the dome and upper portions of the diverticulum followed by dilating and stenting the communicating channel.[10,43] Each of these methods is effective in removing calculi and ablating the diverticulum; the invasiveness of each approach, however, and the prolonged convalescence afterward are obvious disadvantages.

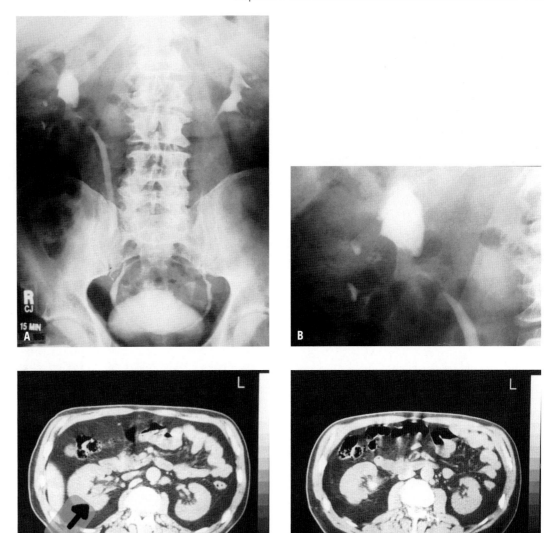

Figure 22-4   *A*, IVU demonstrating right upper-pole hydrocalix with filling defect in upper infundibulum and renal pelvis in a 65-year-old man with microhematuria and dull flank pain. This focal hydrocalix needs to be distinguished from caliceal diverticula. *B*, Close-up view of upper pole hydrocalix. *C*, CT scan without contrast of same patient demonstrating dilated calix. *D*, Lower cut reveals a uric acid calculus that was unresponsive to urinary alkalinization therapy. Subsequently, this stone was treated with percutaneous nephrostolithotomy.

Percutaneous Renal Surgery   Percutaneous renal surgery was developed by invasive radiologists and urologists working in close collaboration.[44–46] It required the development of C-arm fluoroscopy to allow accurate puncture of the renal collecting system through the avascular line of the kidney. The basic principles of closed controlled manipulation of the urinary tract (ie, manipulation over a guidewire) and the use of dilating catheters and balloons to widen and enhance safe access to the collecting system were developed in response to the need to remove kidney stones. As facility and skill with the management of stones by the percutaneous route improved, more complex clinical situations were addressed. One example of this is the percutaneous treatment of caliceal diverticula. Percutaneous techniques have enabled us to manage caliceal diverticula less invasively, not only for the removal of stones that may be within them, but also for the obliteration of the diverticulum itself. In an acute setting, percutaneous techniques are also useful for drainage of abscesses or for balloon dilation of the neck of a non–stone-containing diverticulum.[34,35,47] The location of the diverticulum within the kidney and its relationship to the calices are important considerations when using a percutaneous endourologic approach. If the diverticulum lies posteriorly, puncture will be more straightforward since the diverticulum or the adjacent posterior calix can be punctured directly. If the diverticulum is located anteriorly, then creating continuity from the diverticulum to the calix is more challenging. Our experience and that of others has indicated that success in managing and obliterating the diverticulum is more likely to occur if the diverticulum can be punctured directly.[9,29,48,49]

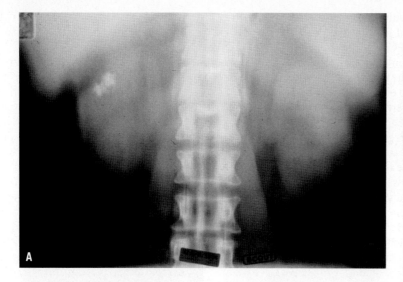

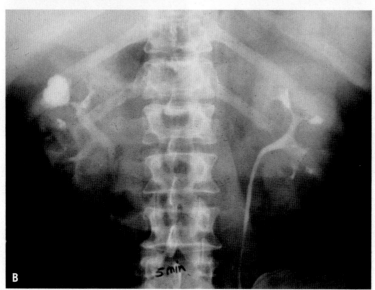

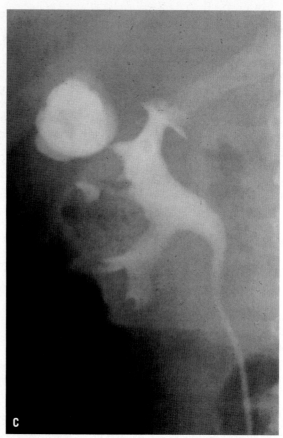

Figure 22-5 *A,* Scout tomogram of IVU in a patient with microscopic hematuria and chronic flank discomfort revealing a cluster of calcified material consistent with renal calculus. *B,* After the administration of intravenous contrast, retrograde filling of the upper pole diverticulum demonstrates that it contains stones. *C,* Close-up view showing the very narrow ostium connecting the diverticulum to the minor calix.

Ureterorenoscopic Surgery Other alternative minimally invasive techniques for the management of stones in caliceal diverticula and of caliceal diverticula themselves, including ureterorenoscopic surgery combined with extracorporeal shock wave lithotripsy (ESWL) or laser lithotripsy and laparoscopic surgery, have been reported (Figure 22-6).[50–52] The retrograde approach was actually first described over 50 years ago by Beneventi, who used metal dilators to stretch narrowed infundibula and necks of caliceal diverticula with fairly good results.[53]

Also known as retrograde intrarenal surgery (RIRS) the significant improvements in flexible ureteroscopes, as well as ureteral access sheaths and balloon dilators, over the past decade has afforded the ureteroscopist an opportunity to extend his or her reach into the domain of the renal pelvis and extremes of the collecting system. While most would agree that the best results with treatment of caliceal diverticula involves ablation of the sidewalls and opening the neck via an antegrade direct approach, philosophically, the retrograde approach falls in line with the "indirect" renal approach as outlined below.

Laparoscopic Renal Surgery At the publication of the first edition of this textbook, the concept of laparoscopic treatment of symptomatic caliceal diverticula was just being introduced.[54,55] Surprisingly, there have been few additional reports substantiating this approach, for which the authors are strong proponents. We will describe all three endoscopic approaches in the following section in greater detail.

PATIENT PREPARATION The patient is prepared as for any other surgical procedure. After the induction of anesthesia, the patient is placed prone on the fluoroscopy or operating table with the appropriate flank prepared and draped, as is typical for any percutaneous procedure. The placement of a retrograde catheter prior to the procedure is of great assistance in facilitating puncture since it allows both opacification and distention of the collecting system. As the diverticulum frequently communicates with the collecting system by only a very fine ostium, significant infusion of contrast through the retrograde catheter may be required in order to bring about opacification of the diverticulum itself.

TECHNIQUE Direct Approach The relationship of the diverticulum to the calices can be seen on a preoperative CT scan (indicating either an

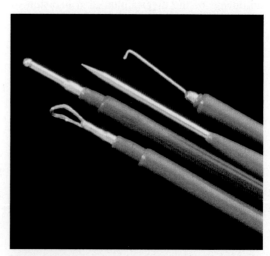

Figure 22-6 Enlarged view of several tip configurations available for performing various intrarenal electrosurgical procedures (available in 3 French and 5F sizes from Cook Urological, Spencer, Ltd.).

anterior or posterior location of the diverticulum), on oblique films and tomograms during intravenous pyelography, or by use of a rotational C-arm fluoroscope at the time of puncture to observe the movement of the diverticulum in relation to the other calices (parallax effect). If the diverticulum is located posteriorly, then puncture and management tend to be more straightforward. The diverticulum may be punctured and a floppy-tipped guidewire (0.035 cm) passed into the diverticulum. The wire may then be passed, with or without the assistance of an angled angiographic catheter, through the ostium and into the main part of the collecting system, with subsequent manipulation down the ureter. Once the wire has been positioned distally, a second working wire is placed for added safety. Tract dilation and access to the diverticulum can then

be achieved with relative ease similar to the techniques utilized for typical percutaneous nephrostolithotomy (PCNL). Any calculi in the diverticulum can then be removed under endoscopic control, and the narrow ostium into the collecting system can be either dilated or incised (or both).

Small diverticula do not usually require fulguration, since the trauma of dilation alone is enough to bring about obliteration. If the diverticulum is 2.5 cm in diameter, then fulguration of the wall of the diverticulum using either electrocautery or a laser enhances contracture and resolution of the diverticulum (see Figures 22-2 and 22-7). Percutaneous drainage for a period of up to 2 weeks may be required to allow collapse of the diverticulum to the size where obliteration will be inevitable as granulation occurs around the tube and traumatized lining.[48,56] Stenting for much

shorter periods (48 to 96 hours) has been shown to be effective if fulguration is performed simultaneously along with stone removal.[29,49,57]

On initial puncture of the diverticulum, if a guidewire cannot be manipulated through the ostium and into the collecting system (as is often the case), then a more difficult dilation of the tract can be achieved by carefully coiling several loops of the guidewire within the diverticulum (Figure 22-8) and dilating the tract with this rather tenuous access to the kidney (see Figure 22-7). Care must be taken not to attempt to coil too much wire within, as this may cause the diverticulum to rupture. Subsequent removal of the contents of the diverticulum may then enable passage of the wire into the collecting system under endoscopic guidance. Retrograde passage of carbon dioxide, air, or methylene blue mixed

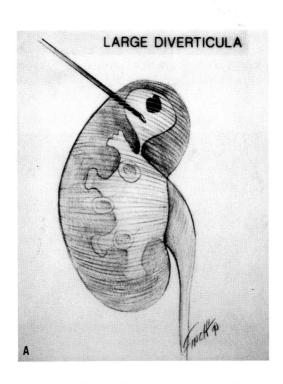

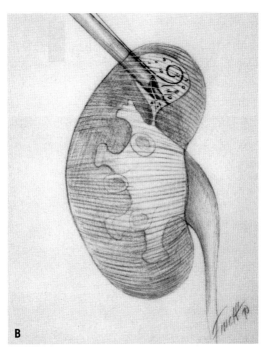

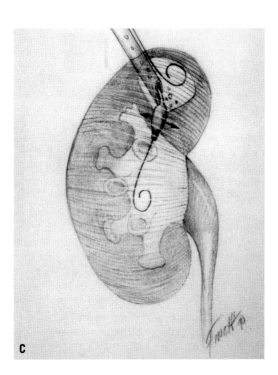

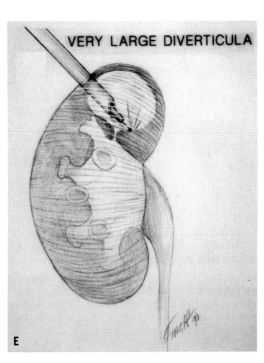

Figure 22-7 Direct approach to large diverticula demonstrating *A*, puncture, *B*, stone extraction, *C*, balloon dilation of ostium, and *D*, stenting with 22-F nephrostomy tube. *E*, Very large diverticula (> 2 cm) are probably best treated using electrocautery or a neodymium:yttrium-aluminum-garnet (Nd:YAG) laser to fulgurate the inner lining prior to tube placement.

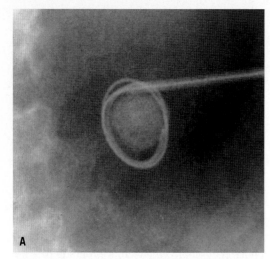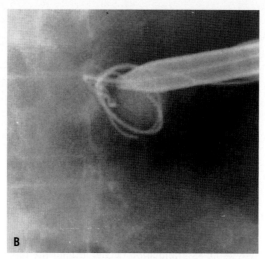

Figure 22-8 Direct puncture into a caliceal diverticulum containing a calculus. Note that the working wire is *A*, coiled for several loops, *B*, prior to tract dilation. Extreme care must be exercised to preserve access to the freshly created nephrostomy tract.

with iodinated contrast often helps the operator delineate the site of the ostium (Figure 22-9). On occasion, the use of a percutaneous needle passed directly through the diverticulum and into the calix may facilitate establishment of communication so that standard dilation as previously described can be performed.[58–60] Long-term patency of 60% at 2-year follow-up has been reported for these "neoinfundibula" that are stented for 8 weeks.[58]

An alternative approach was proposed by Monga and colleagues, whereby no attempt is made at all to traverse the ostium.[61] They instead directly punctured the diverticulum and, after visual inspection and/or stone removal, fulgurated the lining of the cavity with a "rollerball" electrode. They used a balloon nephrostomy for 48 hours and demonstrated complete cavity obliteration at mean follow-up of 38 months. Anteriorly located caliceal diverticula pose a more difficult problem. Here, direct puncture into the diverticulum requires a deep puncture, and once the wire is in the diverticulum, in effect, it must be negotiated backward into the collecting system. A number of options may bring about successful management. Initially, one must puncture the diverticulum directly, coil a wire into it as described above, and place the nephrostomy tract after dilation. Once entered, it may then be evacuated of its contents and the ostium located with the use of a flexible instrument. Considerable deflection of the flexible nephroscope may be required to accomplish this task. Use of the C-arm fluoroscope and simultaneous endoscopy may facilitate this maneuver, and the infusion of retrograde contrast, methylene blue (see Figure 22-9), or even the passage of a wire up through the retrograde catheter may be required to aid identification of the ostium and guidance of a wire through it. If the ostium has become obliterated, then very careful incision in the area of the ostium under endoscopic and fluoroscopic control may permit opening the calix so that a wire can be passed and safer access to the collecting system established (see Figures 22-9

and 22-10). Anteriorly located caliceal diverticula remain a special problem and require particular skill by both endourologists and invasive radiologists, often working in collaboration. It is in these situations that it is often advisable to seek an alternate approach.

Indirect Approach The direct approach as described above has been outlined and has the advantage of not only permitting removal of the contents of the diverticulum, but also destruction of the diverticulum itself. The alternative is to approach the diverticulum indirectly, that is, through a calix separate from that where the diverticulum arises (Figures. 22-11 and 22-12). Once access has been established to the collecting system, a flexible nephroscope can be used to identify the narrow opening of the ostium to the caliceal diverticulum so that a wire can then be passed through it and the opening either incised or dilated to reveal the contents. The disadvantage of this technique, however, is that it may be more difficult to obliterate the diverticulum, although use of a laser fiber or a small coagulating electrode through the flexible nephroscope is feasible. Indirect puncture may be desirable in patients in whom diverticula arise from the upper pole of the kidney where a direct supracostal puncture may be required. In our experience,

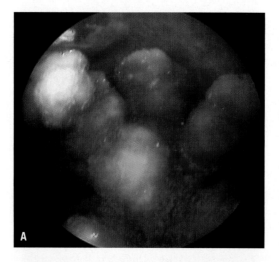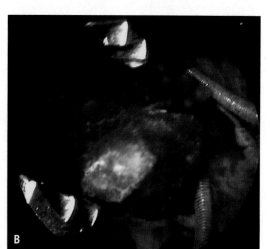

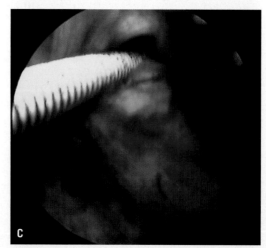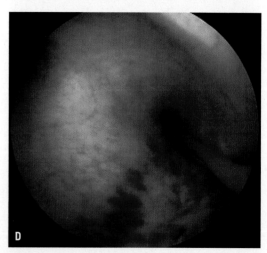

Figure 22-9 *A*, Endoscopic view on entering caliceal diverticula via direct puncture. *B*, Grasping forceps entering from the left extracting stone fragments after initial ultrasonic lithotripsy has caused fragmentation. (Note at right the guidewire coiled within lumen of diverticulum.) *C*, After all of the stony debris has been removed, methylene blue is injected into the renal pelvis via pre-placed retrograde catheter. Ostium of diverticula is thus identified and a guidewire is placed antegrade into the collecting system. *D*, View through the dilated diverticular neck demonstrating the ureteropelvic junction from above.

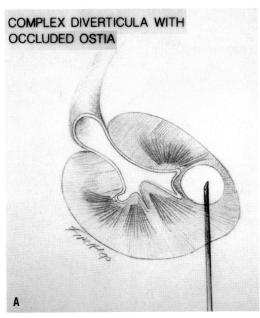

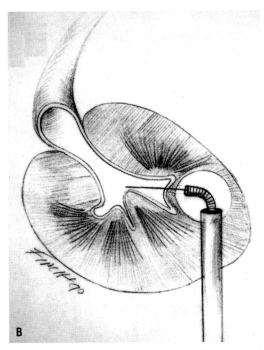

Figure 22-10 *A*, Direct approach to complex diverticula with occluded ostia demonstrating puncture. *B*, Perforation of the wall into main collecting system using the back (stiff) end of the guidewire. This is accomplished under direct visual and fluoroscopic control and is technically quite demanding. This approach should be performed only by those with considerable experience.

such punctures can be performed quite safely, although postoperative pain may be greater.[62] These techniques permit caliceal diverticula and their complications to be managed successfully with less invasive techniques than in the past. If the puncture, however, is above the eleventh rib, we would suggest alternative approaches as described below.

RESULTS OF PERCUTANEOUS REMOVAL AND DIVERTICULAR OBLITERATION
Very few series have looked critically at the long-term results of various approaches. Stone-free rates with the percutaneous approach, whether direct, direct with neoinfundibulum, or indirect, are on the order of 84 to 95%.[63–65] Obliteration of the "cavity" occurs less frequently, with approximate success of 70% (range 68 to 76%).[63,64]

RESULTS OF PERCUTANEOUS REMOVAL VS. ESWL
Despite the subsequent success of ESWL, percutaneous techniques appear to be more successful in removing stones completely from within diverticula since the narrow ostium is unlikely to allow easy passage of stone fragments after shock wave treatment (Table 22-2). Considerable controversy surrounds the preferred management of these rare occurrences. The diverticulum and the resultant urinary stasis are believed to be the underlying pathophysiology, not the calculi contained within per se.[29,48,49] Simply removing the calculi without widening the communication to the main collecting system, or better still, obliterating the diverticulum by destroying its lining, would appear to be suboptimal.

Results with ESWL show very low stone-free rates after treatment using several different lithotriptors (see Table 22-2). Stone-free rates of

0% to 25% with variable symptom-free rates of 36% to 86%, have been reported.[29,66–71] The follow-up in series reporting the highest symptom-free rates are relatively short:(Psihramis and Dretler, 5 5.9 months[66]; Ritchie and colleagues, 5 117 days[68]). Jones and colleagues[29] noted that, on extended follow-up (35 months), patients initially rendered symptom-free subsequently became symptomatic and required re-treatment. Only Streem and colleagues[72] achieved stone-free rates in excess of 25% when treating caliceal diverticular stones with primary ESWL. This group was able to attain such good results because of careful patient selection for ESWL vs. percutaneous removal. Only those patients with small calculi (1.5 cm) in diverticula with radiographically demonstrable patent ostia were offered ESWL (ie, Dretler type I).[12] They achieved a stone-free rate of 58% and a symptom-free rate of 86% initially, although recurrent stone growth was demonstrated in one patient during the follow-up, and six of nine patients (67%) with infection presumed to be secondary to the diverticulum developed recurrent infections.

Overall, although percutaneous nephrostolithotomy is an invasive procedure, it provides much higher stone-free and symptom-free rates when compared to ESWL (see Table 22-2).* More important, a percutaneous approach eliminates the primary pathologic condition (ie, the diverticulum) more than 80% of the time, something that ESWL cannot address. When the diverticulum persists, the possibility of recurrence of symptoms and new calculous formation is not insignificant. Although some authors advocate trying ESWL first and then using percutaneous procedures when this fails, this may not be optimal utilization of resources.[70,71,73]

URETERORENOSCOPIC SURGERY

The retrograde approach to treatment of symptomatic caliceal diverticula that contain stones has become more popular and more feasible owing to technical advances over the past decade. The continued improvements made in miniaturized flexible ureterorenoscopes, the advent of the holmium:YAG laser energy source, and the introduction of atraumatic tipless nitinol stone baskets have expanded the role of retrograde intrarenal surgery.[74,75]

The retrograde approach to the kidney is best handled with a thorough appreciation for the serpentine course of the ureter and a healthy respect for the limitations of the rigid or semirigid ureteroscope. The ureter is not a straight muscular tube, but instead undergoes a tortuous course from deep pelvis to pelvic inlet, over the iliac vessels on up to the renal pelvis. In virtually all cases, when intrarenal surgery is attempted via the retrograde direction, a flexible ureterorenoscope should be utilized.

At one time, the treatment was thought to be limited to upper and, occasionally, middle poles of the kidney. This approach, initially reported in 1989 by David and Fuchs, can provide effective symptom free relief.[76] Significant advances in flexible, miniaturized ureteroscopes with features of increased bidirectional flexibility, reinforced shafts, and both passive and active secondary deflection ability, have given surgeons the ability to reach virtually every calix and cavity in the urinary tract (Figure 22-13).[77]

PATIENT SELECTION Individuals who have symptomatic caliceal diverticula that are felt to be within the reach of a flexible ureteroscope are considered for RIRS at the current time. Although percutaneous management of the caliceal diverticular calculi is attractive because it allows simultaneous stone removal and fulguration of the cavity, it can be difficult when diverticula are located anteriorly. According to Dretler, "There is no conclusive evidence that fulgurating the nonsecretory mucosa of a diverticulum will obliterate its cavity…"[78] It is for this reason that the retrograde approach was designed. The best candidates for retrograde approach, therefore, are those with upper-pole diverticula with an angle of view approaching 90°, so that any attempts at incision to widen the neck of the diverticulum perpendicular to the infundibulum can be made. Those without stones are probably best treated, and then those with smaller stone as well as small caliceal volumes. The goal should be to widen the neck such that low-pressure reflux occurs between the diverticulum and the main part of the kidney to which it communicates.

INFORMED CONSENT Risks would include all those that pertain to ureterorenoscopy as it would for any other indication, such as ureteral perforation, submucosal wire passage, stricture formation, and bleeding. Bleeding as it pertains to caliceal diverticular incision is probably the greatest

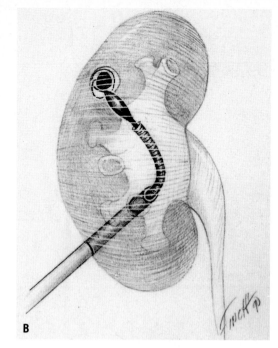

INDIRECT APPROACH TO
CALYCEAL DIVERTICULA

A

B

Figure 22-11 Indirect approach to diverticulum containing calculi demonstrating *A*, retrograde placement of a wire into the cavity, *B*, balloon dilation of the ostium, and *C*, basketing, grasping, or lithotripsy of calculus (1 to 3). No tube is left traversing the diverticular neck after stone extraction. Diverticula treated in this way often persist after stone removal (see Table 22-2).

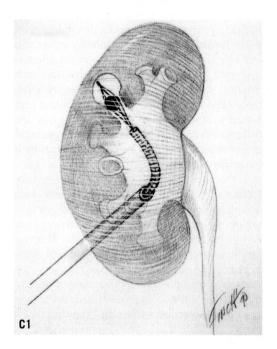

C1

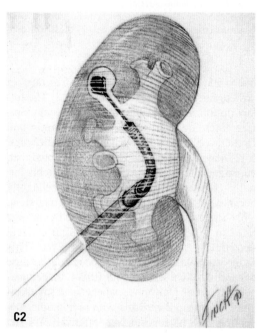

C2

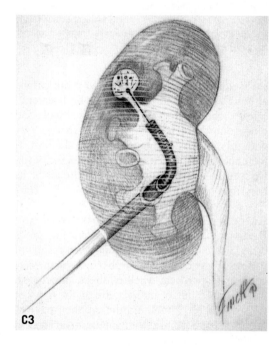

C3

risk because these entities can occur anywhere within the intrarenal collecting system and, thus, they may be in close proximity of the interlobar and interlobular arteries and veins. Because caliceal diverticula can sometimes harbor stagnant, infected urine, bacteremia and sepsis are possible risks. The literature on technique and risks is quite sparse due to the rareness of this entity.

TECHNIQUE AND RESULTS Interestingly there are very few reports of actual technique in the literature. After the initial report by Fuchs in 1989, Grasso and colleagues described their indications and techniques for combined retrograde and simultaneous antegrade (percutaneous) puncture of the diverticulum in 3 of 4 patients (4 out of 5 kidneys).[74] All patients underwent balloon dilation of the infundibular neck. Only one patient

had incision of the neck, with significant hemorrhage and transfusion resulting. No mention was made of the type of device used to incise the ostium. They used a 7.5 French ureteroscope and cannulated the "pinpoint" orifice initially, then used an angiographic balloon prior to entering the diverticulum. If the stone volume was small, then the stones were treated entirely retrograde. If the stone volume was large then a "snare" was placed into the cavity and a percutaneous puncture was made into that area. No long-term results are reported. Only a few scattered case reports have followed in the literature until Batter and Dretler reported their series of 26 patients in 1997.[78] They treated 14 upper, 5 middle and 7 lower symptomatic caliceal diverticula, the majority presenting with flank pain (81%), and urinary tract infection (54%). Only three had no stones. Their technique

included balloon dilation in all, and 6 cases where a Greenwald electrode was used to incise the neck. They reported no bleeding complications and no attempt was made to fulgurate the cavity. They were able to successfully enter and treat 84% of upper or middle diverticula, but only 29% (2 of 7) lower ones. It is possible that, with advancements in laser technology and continued endoscope improvements, these numbers will increase. They reported long-term follow-up of 45 months with 100% in whom they could enter retrograde as being symptom-free.

In two series in which this modality was employed as the sole treatment modality, it was successful in less than 2/3 of patients (2 of 5 [40%]; 18 of 26 [66%]).[74,78] This led Shalhav and colleagues to state that the ureteroscopic treatment of symptomatic stones containing caliceal diver-

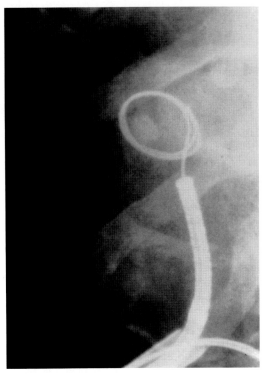

Figure 22-12 Fluoroscopic view of the indirect approach to a caliceal diverticulum containing a calculus via lower-pole calix. Alternatively, a retrograde ureterorenoscopic approach has also been described.

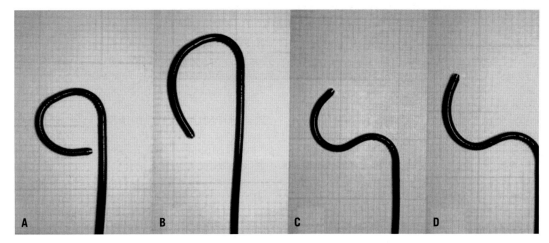

Figure 22-13 Advances in flexible ureteroscope designs include active dual deflection of both primary and secondary points. This allows for several different configurations and allows access to most intrarenal locations(DUR-8 Elite, ACMI Corporation, Stanford, CT).

ticula with respect to symptom- and stone-free rates are "inferior to the percutaneous approach."[64] This approach is probably best reserved for middle-pole, upper-pole and renal pelvis diverticula with small stone burdens (< 1 cm).

The only other significant series was published by Auge and colleagues, who retrospectively compared 17 patients with symptomatic caliceal diverticula treated in a retrograde fashion (URS), with 22 patients treated in a more traditional way (percutaneous nephrolithotomy [PNL]).[60] They like the other groups utilized balloon dilation from below, electrohydraulic lithotripsy (EHL) prior to 1997, and then started to incise the neck utilizing the holmium:YAG laser for simultaneous lithotripsy. The patients for whom an ostium could not be found were treated at the same setting with a percutaneous procedure often performing a neoinfundibulum with direct needle puncture through the diverticular wall. Utilizing stone-free and pain-free rates they found suboptimal treatment with URS. Thirty-five percent were symptom-free at 6 weeks in the URS group versus 86% for PNL, and only 19% were stone-free (URS) versus 78% for PNL. Their conclusion was that "PNL should be considered the primary modality for managing these difficult processes."

LAPAROSCOPIC RENAL SURGERY

The laparoscopic approach to treatment of symptomatic caliceal diverticula was first introduced in 1993 and is reserved for special circumstances.[54 55] These include those inaccessible via percutaneous or retrograde approach, such as in anteriorly located diverticula, those adjacent to the renal hilum, making percutaneous puncture somewhat risky, or those located in ectopic kidneys. Laparoscopically assisted PCNL was initially proposed to treat stones in malrotated or ectopic kidneys[79–81] and has been proposed by some to treat middle and lower caliceal diverticula, especially when they are anterior.[82,83] Another indication would be when other treatments, such as ureteroscopy, have failed, or when the stone burden is large in an anterior location.[84] Still others advocate this approach regardless of location.[85]

PATIENT PREPARATION   A thorough review of the radiographs is paramount to proper patient selection. A CT scan is essential to properly diagnose and plan the surgical approach. Because the diverticula contain stagnant urine and may harbor bacteria, a sterile preoperative urine culture is a must. The area to be incised typically is fibrotic and away from normal parenchyma, therefore, bleeding is expected to be minimal. A crossmatch of blood is usually not necessary. A bowel preparation is optional and is not routinely performed at our institution. A clear liquid diet the day prior to surgery is suggested, as well as broad spectrum preoperative antibiotics.

TECHNIQUE   We perform all of our laparoscopic caliceal diverticulectomies via transperitoneal approach under general anesthesia using carbon dioxide insufflation. Prior to positioning for laparoscopy, we perform rigid cystoscopy with the patient in a "frog-leg" position for retrograde placement of a 5F ureteral catheter. This catheter is used after the diverticulum has been incised in order to help identify the neck (ostium). An orogastric tube as well as a bladder catheter are placed,

Series	ESWL	No. of Patients	Device	Stone Free (%)	Symptom Free (5)	PNL	No. of Patients	Stone Free (5)	Symptom free (5)
Wilbert et al[98]	Yes	16	N/A	20	N/A	No	–	–	–
Psirhamis and Dretler[66]	Yes	10	HM-3*	20	70	No	–	–	–
Ritchie et al[68]	Yes	20	Wolf†	25	75	No	–	–	–
Garcia et al[69]	Yes	13	N/A	0	36	No	–	–	–
Kriegmair et al[70]	Yes	10	N/A	10	N/A	Yes	13	77	N/A
Jones et al[29]	Yes	26	HM-3*	4	36	Yes	24	87.5	100
Hendrikx et al[71]	Yes	15	Lithostar‡	13	60	Yes	16	80	80
Streem and Yost[72]	Yes	19	HM-3*	58	86	Yes	6	N/A	N/A
Hulbert et al[48]	No	–	–	–	–	Yes	10	100	100
Hulbert et al[97]	No	–	–	–	–	Yes	18	100	100
Thurhoff and Alken[99]	No	–	–	–	–	Yes	16	–	93
Hedelin et al[56]	No	–	–	–	–	Yes	13	77	69
Ellis et al[57]	No	–	–	–	–	Yes	10	100	87.5
Bellman et al[50]	No	–	–	–	–	Yes	20	95	100

Table 22-2 Comparison of ESWL and percutaneous nephrostolithotomy for symptomatic caliceal diverticula containing calculi

* HM-3 (Dornier, Kennesaw, Ga.).

†Wolf Piezolith (Kinittlingen, Germany).

‡Lithostar (Siemans Medical Systems, Erlangen, Germany)

N/A = information not available

and the patient is placed in a 45° posterior oblique position supported with a conformable beanbag device and securely fastened to the operating table. The ipsilateral arm is supported over the torso with a Krause arm hanger, or alternatively, can be supported with rolled sheets or pillows. After the establishment of pneumoperitoneum, the large bowel is mobilized medially by releasing the lateral attachments with scissors or Harmonic scalpel (Ethicon Endo-Surgery, Cincinnati, OH).

Whereas the goal of endoscopic management is widening of the diverticular neck to allow free reflux between the cavity and the main collecting system with or without fulguration of the cavity, the objective of the laparoscopic approach is to isolate the cavity from the rest of the kidney. This is best accomplished via incision of the lining of the neck and then oversewing the neck along with electro-fulguration of the cavity. Omental fat can be placed into the cavity if the defect is large.

After exposure of the kidney, Gerota's fascia is incised, perirenal fat is dissected off of the capsule of the kidney, and the renal surface is inspected. It is not necessary to perform a hilar dissection. The diverticulum can often be readily identified by noting a dimpling on the surface of the kidney where there is lack of cortical tissue (Figure 22-14). Intraoperative use of endocavitary ultrasonography or fluoroscopy is helpful to localize the diverticulum.[84,86] A circumscribing or cruciate incision is then made over the diverticulum, and stones can be extracted with graspers or suction. If they are numerous, they can be placed into an entrapment sac for subsequent removal (Figure 22-15). Redundant portions of the diverticulum can be sharply excised, and the cavity itself fulgurated using electrocautery or the Argon Beam Coagulator. Thus, the diverticulum has been marsupialized. Not all authors suture the ostium nor feel it is necessary. Injection of sterile dilute methylene–blue-stained saline is next injected retrograde via the previously placed ureteral catheter to help identify the ostium, which can be oversewn with absorbable suture. At this time, a pedicled omental flap or perirenal fat with Gerota's fascia can be affixed to the cavity to aid in scar-

ring and prevent a fistula. Alternatively, some have reported successful use of synthetic tissue glue to seal the ostium[85] (Figure 22-16). A closed suction drain is left and placed via dependent trocar site. Final wound closure and management are then similar to any laparoscopic procedure.

POSTOPERATIVE COURSE

Not all authors leave drains or stents. Most patients remain in the hospital for brief periods (< 48 hours), as one would expect for comparable laparoscopic surgery, but a wide range has been reported (3 to 6.6 days).[55,85,87] We remove the Foley catheter on postoperative day 1, and the closed suction drain approximately 3 days later if the output remains low.

RESULTS

Less than 15 cases have been reported worldwide with the largest series being 5 from the Cleveland Clinic.[54,55,84–88] A retroperitoneoscopic method has been described and is the most widely published approach, but since the most favorable location for a laparoscopic technique is in those diverticula located on the anterior surface of the kidney, a transperitoneal approach is favored by us.[84–88] Proponents of a retroperitoneal approach say that potential urine leak favors their method. In the few series, however, urine leak has not been reported and is likely due to adequate drainage being provided. Resolution of pain, infection, and stone-free rates have been reported to be equal to open surgery, with only one report of recurrence of the diverticulum.

MAIN COMPLICATIONS AND HOW TO AVOID THEM

Complications that can be expected with this approach are failure to identify the diverticulum, intraoperative bleeding, injury to the bowel, and urinary fistula. Bowel dissection is carried out utilizing ultrasonic shears (Laparosonic Coagulating Shears, Ethicon, Cincinnati, OH; Autosonix, U.S.

Surgical Corporation, Norwalk, CT) to minimize risk of injury. A retrograde ureteral catheter is placed for injection of methylene blue dye for ostial identification and aids placement of an internal ureteral stent at the end of the procedure if one is used, although this is optional. This stent, as well as a Jackson–Pratt-type wound drain, should help minimize postoperative urinoma and fistula formation. The small number of cases reported utilizing these techniques is a testament to the very highly successful and safe alternative endoscopic techniques, rather than any shortcomings of the laparoscopic approach. Percutaneous approaches have been highly successful with stone-free rates of 95% and resolution of the diverticulum (obliteration or improved drainage) of 80 %.[9,49,64] The operative times and length of hospital stays are comparable. Because equipment charges should be less, the cost of the percutaneous approach should be less; therefore, some feel it should be the procedure of choice for most situations.[89] Residual diverticula have been reported in 20 to 33% of cases.[87] Residual diverticula are a potential source of future stones, infection, and symptom recurrence; therefore, an argument can be made for a laparoscopic approach, with its higher likelihood of complete obliteration. One must keep in mind that the percutaneous approach attempts to increase the diameter of the ostium and would not be expected to have the same "obliteration" potential. We reserve the laparoscopic approach for those diverticula with large volume, anterior location, or those that fail endoscopic treatment.

INFUNDIBULAR STENOSIS

Infundibular stenosis as a distinct entity is uncommon. It exists in both an acquired and congenital form, with the latter being even more rare.[90,91] Cases of infundibular stenosis often present radiologically as a dilated calix (ie, a hydrocalix) They are often diagnosed by intravenous urography and confirmed on retrograde ureteropyelography. Related pathologies, such as renal transitional cell carcinoma, should be ruled

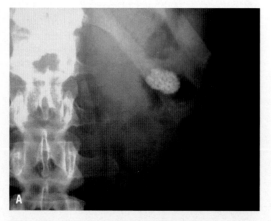
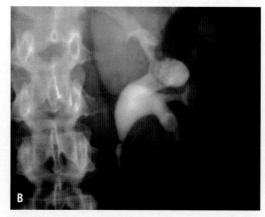
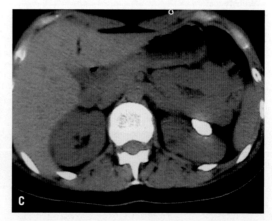

Figure 22-14 *A*, Scout film from IVP. *B*, Ten-minute film demonstrating mid-polar location. *C*, CT scan demonstrating anterior location. Note very little overlying parenchyma making "indirect approach" somewhat risky for perforation. This situation is handled well with laparoscopic approach.

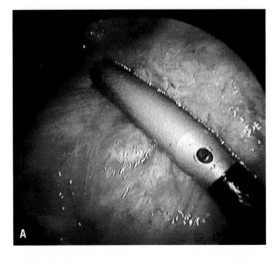

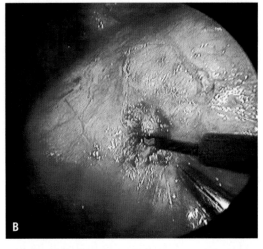

Figure 22-15 *A*, Use of intraoperative laparoscopic ultrasonography is helpful in locating the diverticulum containing stones. *B-D*, Once the diverticulum is marked it is opened with a hook electrode and the stones are removed piecemeal with graspers. *E*, In this instance, there are several dozen which are being placed into an entrapment sac for subsequent en masse removal.

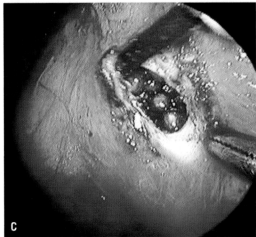

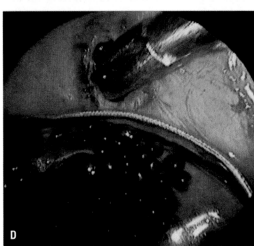

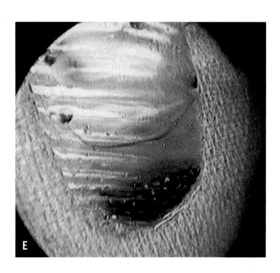

out, and are identified through imaging/visualization and biopsy of the region in question. If the diagnosis is still in question, it can be clarified with use of computerized tomography, which also demonstrates the specific relationship of this entity to the surrounding renal anatomy. In addition to anatomic imaging, functional testing, in the form of diuretic scintirenography, is useful in demonstrating the obstructive nature of this entity. A stenosed infundibulum due to edema as a result of stones may often be seen, but after

removal or treatment of the stones, the stenosis most often resolves as the edema subsides. These types of stenosis should not require any additional treatment other than the successful management of the stone. Nonetheless, in a minority of situations, stones and related manipulations may give rise to the acquired form of this entity. Parsons and colleagues noted that significant infundibular stenosis may occur as a complication (2%) after percutaneous nephrolithotomy.[92] In their series, the presence of this condition was

associated with prolonged operative time, a large stone burden requiring multiple removal procedures, and extended postoperative nephrostomy tube drainage. The authors also noted that stenosis generally occurred in areas corresponding to previous sites of percutaneous access.

Acquired forms of infundibular stenosis, both extrinsic and intrinsic, affecting the pyelocaliceal infundibulum, are both rare and variable. Extrinsic compression may occur from a variety of causes (Figures 22-17 and 22-18). A crossing

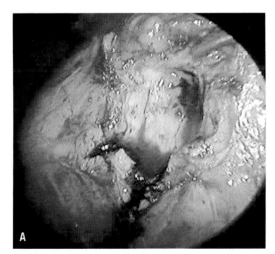

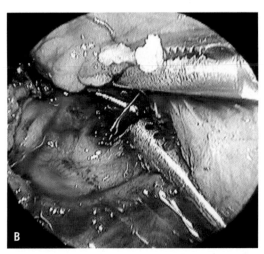

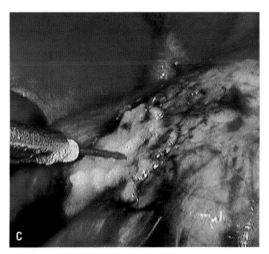

Figure 22-16 *A*, Retrograde injection of dilute methylene blue stained saline helps to identify the ostium which is then, *B*, oversewn with absorbable suture. *C*, Use of tissue sealant is optional.

upper-pole vessel may give rise to the well-known condition of infundibular stenosis and pain characterized as Fraley syndrome, and dilation of the infundibulum as a way of resolving the symptoms has been reported.[19] In this situation, however, the more traditional approach of infundibuloplasty and transposition of the infundibulum seems more likely to provide long-term relief of both obstruction and symptoms.[19] The other secondary causes of infundibular stenosis include extrinsic malignancy from metastases to the kidney or intrinsic conditions affecting the wall of the infundibulum itself, such as neoplasms, chronic inflammatory diseases such as tuberculosis, or chronic scarring as a result of long-standing trauma due to some agent, resulting in stenosis in a fashion similar to that of long-standing impacted urinary calculi.

The congenital form of this disease process is quite rare indeed, and is believed to be associated with hypertrophy of the muscular layer of the infundibulum, or to abnormal collagen deposition within the infundibular muscular layer. On pathological examination, widespread areas of cystic dysplasia have been noted proximal to the stenosis, which lends evidence to the existence of this entity as being clearly separate from the acquired form.[91]

Indications for treatment of infundibular stenosis are similar to those for caliceal diverticula, and include signs and symptoms of infection, obstruction, chronic pain, decreased renal function, and hematuria. Specific secondary causes, such as tuberculosis and lymphoma also certainly require disease-specific treatment. In addition, for cases without an obvious secondary cause, discerning between the congenital and acquired form of infundibular stenosis may be of importance, in that there is evidence, although only from relatively small numbers of patients, that surgical treatment of the congenital form is rarely of benefit, whereas failure to treat those with the acquired form will result in progressive hydronephrosis/hydrocalix and loss of renal function.[90,91,93] The congenital form of this disease process is believed to be associated with hypertrophy of the muscular layer

of the infundibulum, or to abnormal collagen deposition within the infundibular muscular layer. As stated previously, widespread areas of cystic dysplasia have been noted proximal to the stenosis. Husmann and colleagues noted that progressive hydronephrosis only occurred occasionally (24% of patients) in this patient group.[91] In contrast, the acquired form of this disease entity, often due to a chronic inflammatory process initiated by a variety of aforementioned entities, frequently results in progressive hydronephrosis and renal deterioration if left untreated.[94]

Management is very similar to that for a caliceal diverticulum regarding how access is obtained, in terms of either an antegrade (direct) or retrograde (indirect) direction (Figures 22-19 and 22-20).[44,45] In contrast to treatment for caliceal diverticula, these entities should not be fulgurated, because they are covered by a transitional cell lining that is in communication with urine-producing tubules. Unlike treatment of caliceal diverticula, for which obliteration of the cavity is an end point, the goal here is to provide adequate drainage into the main collecting system.[58]

TREATMENT OF INFUNDIBULAR STENOSIS

Patient Preparation *Informed Consent* After evaluation and proper diagnosis have been made, the treating urologist should have a thorough discussion with the patient. This discussion should include the various treatment options available to the patient, and what their relative success rates are, given the specific situation. The patient should be informed about the risks of the procedure, which are primarily related to anesthesia, bleeding, and infection. The patient should also be informed that it may be necessary to have some type of nephro-uretero catheter for a prolonged period of time. The potential morbidities of this catheter placement should also be discussed.

Preoperative Preparation Standard preoperative testing should be performed. This should include a urine culture to rule out active urinary tract infection. Any active urinary tract infection should be treated preoperatively. Prothrombin time, partial thromboplastin time, and platelet count are

routinely obtained for percutaneous procedures and procedures involving an intrarenal incision, as both of these surgical maneuvers somewhat rely on the patient's own coagulation system for maintenance of hemostasis. A type and crossmatch for blood products is also usually obtained.

Technique The choice of technique to be used for treatment of infundibular stenosis often depends on a combination of factors: severity of stenosis noted on radiologic imaging, operator experience with antegrade and retrograde approach, facilities and equipment available, and variations of anatomy that may preclude or mitigate against one of the approaches. It is critical that the urologist has a full understanding of where the incision will be made, and how this incision relates to the renal arterial anatomy (Figure 22-21). It is important to realize that, if an incision is used to treat this entity, it is made parallel to the longitudinal axis of the infundibulum, and may be in close proximity to significant intrarenal arterial blood supply. Treatment approaches here are differentiated according to the relative difficulty associated with crossing the stenosed segment (see Figure 22-1), but other aforementioned factors certainly may also influence the treatment approach.

Narrowing through which a Guidewire Can Be Passed In this patient group, an antegrade or retrograde approach may be chosen. Amongst other factors, the decision may depend on the specific intrarenal anatomy relating to the case in question. The retrograde approach, which is certainly the less invasive approach, has more often become an option in select patients (intrarenal location of ostium appears accessible and suitably oriented for ureteroscope and its particular characteristics relating to deflectability/passage of working elements [ie, laser fiber]). The increasing practicality of this approach is due to the evolution of ureteropyeloscopes, which have improved maneuverability, optics, and working channels.

In the retrograde approach, when the ostium in question is properly identified, a guidewire should be passed through the narrowed infundibulum. One should place a second wire for additional safety. Balloon dilatation may be performed first to create more working space (Figure 22-22). Cutting can be achieved with electrosurgical instruments such as the Greenwald, or Hulbert (Cook Urological, Spencer, IN) electrodes. If an electrosurgical instrument is utilized, appropriate settings for the electrosurgical generator are in the vicinity of 50 to 75 watts on a "pure cutting" mode. It is advisable to insulate the safety wire by using a ureteral catheter over it to preclude exposed bare wire. If the coagulating probe comes into contact with a bare wire, electrical current will be conducted along the entire course of the wire guide, leading to significant risk of ureteral, urethral, or external genital thermal injury!! If minor venous oozing should occur, one should avoid the temptation to use the cautery within the kidney. Overuse of the coagulating current may lead to worsening of bleeding as larger diameter vessels may be cut into, and will likely lead to tis-

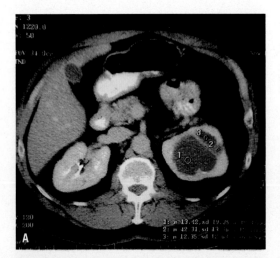
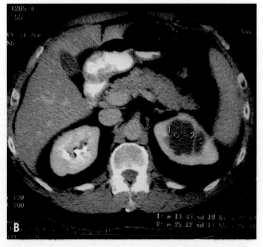

Figure 22-17 *A–B*, Computerized tomography demonstrates that an intrarenal parapelvic cyst is compressing this infundibulum. Note the presence of septations.

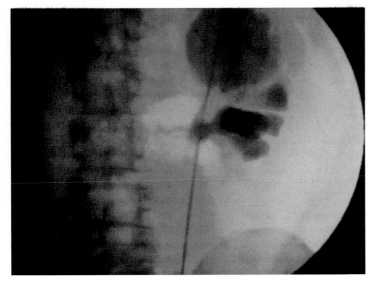

Figure 22-18 At time of retrograde injection, this patient appears to have narrowing of the infundibulum serving the upper pole of the kidney.

sue injury and fibrosis/restenosis. Acute arterial injury should be recognized and consideration for angio-embolization should be given without delay. More recently, the holmium:YAG laser, which possesses both cutting and coagulating properties, has been successfully employed for the incision in these cases.[95] A 200 μ fiber can be used. Its small diameter usually does not greatly impede the deflectability of the ureteroscope. After a cut has been made, one can then dilate over a wire to enhance the depth of the incision in one plane throughout the whole length of the stenosed segment. The incised infundibulum can then be balloon-dilated and stented. A large-bore stent (8 to 8.5F) or endopyelotomy stent (eg, 14/7F or 10/7F) may be used. There is no preponderance of evidence in the literature that supports the use of a tube of any particular diameter.

In the antegrade approach, after puncture of the calix, a guidewire can be passed through the narrowed infundibulum and down the ureter, gen-

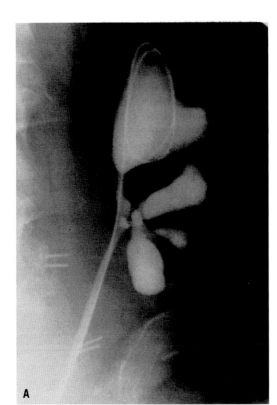

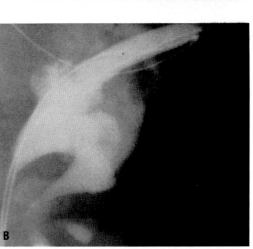

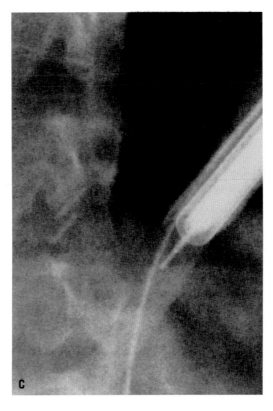

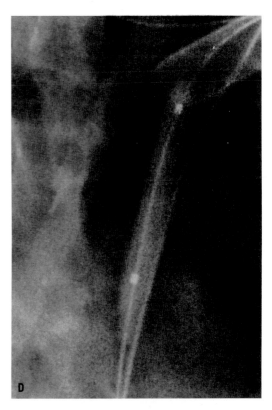

Figure 22-19 *A*, Retrograde ureteropyelogram of upper pole infundibular stenosis (type I) with placement of a guidewire into the dilated pyocalix. *B*, Antegrade puncture into dilated calix, *C*, with incision and then, *D*, subsequent balloon dilation prior to placement of 14/7 French universal stent for several weeks.

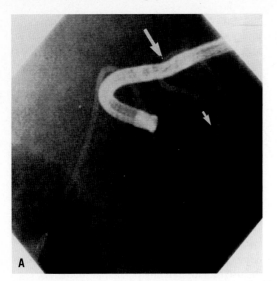
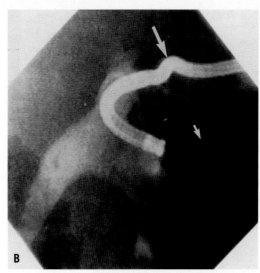
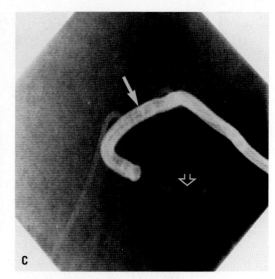

Figure 22-20 Fluoroscopic view of symptomatic renal caliceal calculus contained within an anterior middle calix with a stenotic infundibulum. This particular stone was unresponsive to ESWL and was approached percutaneously. *A*, Flexible nephroscopy (large arrow) entering through upper pole posterior calix. Calculus is identified by small arrow. *B*, Nephrostogram demonstrates a very tightly stenotic infundibulum located between the tip of the nephroscope (large arrow) and calculus (small arrow). *C*, Balloon dilation of the infundibulum prior to stone basket extraction. Balloon is seen with "waist" identified by open arrow.

erally without difficulty (Figure 22-23). Subsequent dilation of a tract into the kidney enables the operator to inspect the calix endoscopically, and to incise carefully through the infundibulum away from any obviously pulsatile areas. In a similar fashion, the stenosis can often be successfully cut with the use of the holmium:YAG laser. Subsequent stenting with a nephrostomy tube with side holes on either side of the obstruction for a period of 4 weeks is considered appropriate to maximize the chance of resolution. The authors generally use a large-bore nephrostomy catheter (24F Malecot re-entry catheter; Microvasive, Boston Scientific, Natick, MA) in this situation, though, once again there is no definitive evidence that supports use of any particular caliber of catheter. In order to assist with drainage of the obstructed calix we usually cut additional drainage holes proximal to the Malecot wings of the catheter, lest the tube may actually occlude the drainage of the calix. It is for this reason that we do not routinely employ Foley-catheters as nephrostomy tubes. Although inexpensive, they provide inferior drainage of the kidney and cannot be modified as such.

Narrowing that is Patent Radiographically but through which a Guidewire Cannot Be Passed A more difficult situation is encountered if a guidewire cannot be passed through the stenosed segment. As such, these cases must often be handled through an antegrade approach, possibly with the placement of a retrograde ureteral catheter as well. Thorough preoperative planning for this and more difficult cases is imperative. In these instances, it may still be possible for contrast to pass through the stenosed segment, and this can be observed on fluoroscopy. Infusion of contrast or, better still, methylene blue from below through a retrograde catheter may enable the operator to observe the site of the opening. A very delicate incision in this area may allow subsequent passage of the wire once some of the stenosed segment has been opened.[79] Once

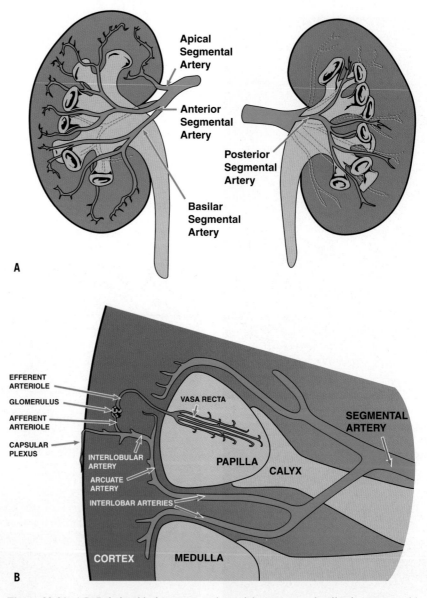

Figure 22-21 *A-B*, Relationship between renal arterial anatomy and collecting system. (*A*, From Kabalin JN: Surgical anatomy of the retroperitoneum, kidneys, and ureters. In: Campbell's urology, 7th ed. . *B*, From Spirnak JP, Resnik MI. Kidney and ureteral stone surgery. In: Gillenwater JY, et al. Adult and pediatric urology. 2nd ed. 1991. p. 619.)

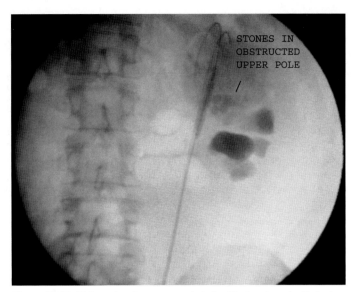

Figure 22-22 This patient has upper pole infundibular stenosis. He had an episode of acute obstruction by one of many calculi within the upper pole segment. In a retrograde approach guidewires are advanced into this obstructed upper pole segment.

access across the stenosis has been secured, treatment is carried out with incision, dilation, and stenting as previously described.

Totally Obliterated Lumen/Ostium This situation is the most challenging. When neither a guidewire nor contrast will pass through the stenosed segment, this difficult situation can still be managed successfully, but will often require the combined simultaneous use of both endoscopy and C-arm fluoroscopy. A guidewire passed up through a retrograde catheter to the point of stenosis from below will also be helpful. Manipulation of this wire from below, while the operator observes the other side of the stenosed segment with the nephroscope, may make it feasible to cut down through the stenosed segment onto the wire. Once again, after access has been secured, treatment with incision, dilation, and stenting is carried out as previously described. The use of the additional maneuvers described here requires considerable skill, delicate instruments, and a precise three-dimensional knowledge of the location within the kidney. This principle of "stereotactic surgery" requires the use of combined endoscopy and C-arm fluoroscopy for successful management. Another variation in this scenario is the use of simultaneous endoscopy using light/dark contrast techniques to identify and cross the region in question, which requires two skilled endoscopists. Although these situations are rarely encountered, resolution can be successfully achieved by skilled endourologists. Despite successful management, the factors that will influence long-term success are the length of the stenosed segment, the degree of fibrosis or scarring around the stenosed segment, and indeed, the etiology of the stenosis.

RESULTS OF TREATMENT OF INFUNDIBULAR STENOSIS The rarity of this problem has resulted in little documentation and long-term follow-up of treatment involving this patient group. Short strictures with minimal scarring tend to be associated with good results. Long strictures with dense scarring or with other peri-infundibular encasements are less likely to be treated successfully.[9] Such patients may require more invasive management if percutaneous techniques are not successful and may involve open surgery to perform an infundibuloplasty, uretero-calicostomy, or conceivably, a partial nephrectomy.[96] Cases involving a narrowing through which a guidewire cannot be readily passed are more likely to recur after treatment. Long-term internal stenting may also be an acceptable solution in selected cases. An open operation is often technically demanding and may be quite complicated, possibly resulting in nephrectomy.

CONCLUSION

The caliceal diverticulum and infundibular stenosis are diagnosed by IVU or retrograde pyelography and, unless symptomatic or detrimental to the kidney, do not require treatment. Indications for treatment include signs and symptoms of infection, chronic pain, decreased renal function, and hematuria. The role of ESWL in the treatment of intrarenal nooks containing stones is limited. The management of these two complex intrarenal problems has dramatically changed with the advent of more advanced retrograde endoscopic and antegrade percutaneous endoscopic techniques. Both entities can be successfully negotiated and addressed by these minimally invasive techniques. In properly selected patients, both techniques are safe and effective. The savings economically and the benefits to the patients in terms of shorter hospital stays, reduced analgesia requirements, and shorter convalescence with an earlier return to the work force, are considerable. As the laparoscopic approach has become more refined, it has also proven to be effective in certain situations, such as the treatment of the anteriorly located mid-pole and lower-pole caliceal diverticulum. Laparoscopic approaches offer very little over percutaneous and retrograde ureterorenoscopic approaches for the majority of these intrarenal cavities.

REFERENCES

1. Rayer P. Traits des maladies des reins. Bailliere: Paris 1841; 3:507.
2. Wulfsohn MA. Pyelocaliceal diverticula. J Urol 1980;123:1–8.
3. Middleton AW Jr, Pfister RC. Stone-containing pyelocaliceal diverticulum: embryogenic, anatomic, radiologic and clinical characteristics. J Urol 1974;111:2–6.
4. Michel W, Funke PJ, Tunn UW, Senge T. Pyelocalyceal diverticula. Int Urol Nephrol 1985;17:225–30.
5. Timmons JW Jr, Malek RS, Hattery RR, Deweerd JH. Caliceal diverticulum. J Urol 1975;114:6–9.
6. Williams G, Blandy JP, Tresidder GC. Communicating cysts and diverticula of the renal pelvis. Br J Urol 1969;41:163–70.
7. Yow RM, Bunts RC. Calyceal diverticulum. J Urol 1955; 73:663–70.
8. Kottasz S, Hamvas A. Review of the literature on calyceal diverticula, a hypothesis concerning its etiology and report of 17 cases. Int Urol Nephrol 1976;8:203–12.
9. Hulbert JC, Hunter D, Castaneda-Zuniga W. Classification of and techniques for the reconstitution of acquired strictures in the region of the ureteropelvic junction. J Urol 1988;140:468–72.
10. Prather G. Calyceal diverticulum. J Urol 1941;45:55.
11. Abeshouse BS. Serous cysts of the kidney and their differentiation from other cystic diseases of the kidneys. Urol Cutaneous Rev 1950;54:582–602.
12. Dretler SP. A new useful classification of calyceal diverticula. J Endourol 1992;6 (Suppl):81.
13. Hulbert JC, Lapointe S, Reddy PK, et al. Percutaneous endoscopic fulguration of a large volume caliceal diverticulum. J Urol 1987;138:116–7.
14. Abeshouse BS, Abeshouse GA. Calyceal diverticulum: A report of sixteen cases and review of the literature. Urol Int 1963;15:329–57.
15. Braasch W. Renal cysts simple and otherwise. J Urol 1944;51:1.
16. Banker RJ, Card WH. Calyceal diverticula. J Urol 1954;72: 773–6.
17. Wyrens RG. Calyceal diverticula or pyelogenic cysts. J Urol 1953;70:358–63.
18. Spigos DG, Zaitoon MM, Darwish ME, Sassoon H. Hydrocalycosis. A report of two cases. Radiologe 1980;20:596–9.

Figure 22-23 Stentstones. This patient was treated with an antegrade approach. Note the stenosed infundibulum (with wire and catheter across it), with stones in the obstructed segment.

19. Fraley EE. Vascular obstruction of superior infundibulum causing nephralgia. A new syndrome. N Engl J Med 1966;275:1403–9.

20. Amesur NRH. Para-pelvic cysts of the kidney. Indian J Surg 1963;25:45.

21. Mosli H, MacDonald P, Schillinger J. Caliceal diverticula developing into simple renal cyst. J Urol 1986;136:658–61.

22. Nicholas JL. An unusual complication of calyceal diverticulum. Br J Urol 1975;47:370.

23. Reiss MD. Traumatic rupture of renal cortical cyst into the calyceal system. Am J Roentgenol Radium Ther Nucl Med 1967;101:696–9.

24. Amar AD. The clinical significance of renal caliceal diverticulum in children: relation to vesicoureteral reflux. J Urol 1975;113:255–7.

25. Mackie GG. Abnormalities of the ureteral bud. Urol Clin North Am 1978;5:161–74.

26. Sandler CM, Toombs BD. "Ballooned" calyceal diverticulum with ureteral obstruction. J Can Assoc Radiol 1980;31:123–5.

27. Gardner KD Jr, Castellino RA, Kempson R, et al. Primary amyloidosis of the renal pelvis. N Engl J Med 1971;284:1196–8.

28. Goldman SM, Fishman EK, Hartman DS, et al. Computed tomography of renal tuberculosis and its pathological correlates. J Comput Assist Tomogr 1985;9:771–6.

29. Jones JA, Lingeman JE, Steidle CP. The roles of extracorporeal shock wave lithotripsy and percutaneous nephrostolithotomy in the management of pyelocaliceal diverticula. J Urol 1991;146:724–7.

30. Latiff A. Case profile: calyceal diverticulum causing recurrent urinary tract infection. Urology 1981;17:621.

31. Ulreich S, Lund DA, Jacobson JJ. Spontaneous rupture of a calyceal diverticulum during urography. AJR Am J Roentgenol 1978;131:337–8.

32. Taari K, Lindell O, Mankinen P, Markkola A. Shoulder pain due to rupture of a calyceal diverticulum as an acute sign of prostatic hyperplasia. Br J Urol 1994;73:458–9.

33. Deshmukh AS, Mancini AA, Sood SK. Calyceal diverticulum rapidly progressing to renal abscess. Urology 1975;05:380–2.

34. Ramchandani P, Soulen RL, Kendall AR, Davis JA. Percutaneous management of a pyelocaliceal diverticular abscess. J Urol 1985;133:81–3.

35. Savion M, Sibi J, Segal S, Zohav M. Percutaneous drainage of a giant pyelocaliceal diverticular abscess in pregnancy. Eur J Obstet Gynecol Reprod Biol 1987;26:349–52.

36. Siegel MJ, McAlister WH. Calyceal diverticula in children: unusual features and complications. Radiology 1979;131:79–82.

37. DeMarco RT, Cain MP, Davis MM. Xanthogranulomatous pyelonephritis associated with a congenital caliceal diverticulum. Urology 2001;57:168.

38. Costas S, Van Blerk PJ. Pyelocaliceal diverticula and rupture of the kidney. Br J Urol 1990;65:111–3.

39. Auringer ST, Sumner TE. Calyceal diverticulum. Focal renal uptake on bone scan. Clin Nucl Med 1992;17:142.

40. Devine CJ Jr, Guzman JA, Devine PC, Poutasse EF. Caliceal diverticulum. J Urol 1969;101:8–11.

41. Noe HN, Raghavaiah NV. Excision of pyelocaliceal diverticulum under renal hypothermia. J Urol 1982;127:294–6.

42. Engel W. The late results of partial nephrectomy for calyectasis with stone. J Urol 1947;57:619.

43. Newman HR, Lowman RM, Waters LL. The problem of calyceal diverticulum. Surg Gynecol Obstet 1952;94:77–82.

44. Clayman RV, et al. Percutaneous nephrolithotomy: extraction of renal and ureteral calculi from 100 patients. J Urol 1984;131:868–71.

45. Lange PH, et al. Percutaneous removal of caliceal and other "inaccessible" stones: instruments and techniques. J Urol 1984;132:439–42.

46. Reddy PK, et al. Percutaneous removal of caliceal and other "inaccessible" stones: results. J Urol 1984;132:443–7.

47. Kremers PW, Beckmann CF, Bihrle W 3rd. Percutaneous balloon dilatation in treatment of infected pyelocaliceal diverticulum. Urology 1988;32:29–32.

48. Hulbert JC, et al. Percutaneous techniques for the management of caliceal diverticula containing calculi. J Urol 1986;135:225–7.

49. Bellman GC, Silverstein JI, Blickensderfer S, Smith AD. Technique and follow-up of percutaneous management of caliceal diverticula. Urology 1993;42:21–5.

50. Fuchs GJ, David RD. Flexible ureterorenoscopy, dilatation of narrow caliceal neck, and ESWL: a new, minimally invasive approach to stones in calyceal diverticula. J Endourol 1989;3:255.

51. Fuchs GJ, David RD. Retrograde intra-renal surgery-Indications and results. J Endourol 1992;6:S80.

52. Mikkelson D, Kavoussi LR Clayman RV, et al. Advances in flexible deflectable ureteronephroscopy (FDU): intrarenal surgery [Abstract]. J Urol 1989;141:192.

53. Beneventi F. Its relief by retrograde dilatation. Am J Surg 1943;61:244.

54. Gluckman GR, Stoller M, Irby P. Laparoscopic pyelocaliceal diverticula ablation. J Endourol 1993;7:315–7.

55. Ruckle HC, Segura JW. Laparoscopic treatment of a stone-filled, caliceal diverticulum: a definitive, minimally invasive therapeutic option. J Urol 1994;151 122–4.

56. Hedelin H, et al. Percutaneous surgery for stones in pyelocaliceal diverticula. Br J Urol 1988;62:206–8.

57. Ellis JH, et al. Stones and infection in renal caliceal diverticula: treatment with percutaneous procedures. AJR Am J Roentgenol 1991;156:995–1000.

58. Lang EK. Percutaneous infundibuloplasty: management of calyceal diverticula and infundibular stenosis. Radiology 1991;181:871–7.

59. Al-Basam S, Bennett JD, Layton ZA, et al. Treatment of caliceal diverticular stones: transdiverticular percutaneous nephrolithotomy with creation of a neoinfundibulum. J Vasc Interv Radiol 2000;11:885–9.

60. Auge BK, Munver R, Kourambas J, et al. Endoscopic management of symptomatic caliceal diverticula: a retrospective comparison of percutaneous nephrolithotripsy and ureteroscopy. J Endourol 2002;16:557–63.

61. Monga M, Smith R, Ferral H, Thomas R. Percutaneous ablation of caliceal diverticulum: long-term followup. J Urol 2000;163:28–32.

62. Young AT, et al. Percutaneous extraction of urinary calculi: use of the intercostal approach. Radiology 1985;154:633–8.

63. Landry JL, et al. Long term results of percutaneous treatment of caliceal diverticula. Eur Urol 2002;41:474–7.

64. Shalhav AL, et al. Long-term outcome of caliceal diverticula following percutaneous endosurgical management. J Urol 1998;160:1635–9.

65. Donnellan SM, Harewood LM, Webb DR. Percutaneous management of caliceal diverticular calculi: technique and outcome. J Endourol 1999;13:83–8.

66. Psihramis KE, Dretler SP. Extracorporeal shock wave lithotripsy of caliceal diverticula calculi. J Urol 1987;138:707–11.

67. Wilbert D. Calyceal diverticular stones: is ESWL worthwhile [Abstract]? J Urol 1986;135:183.

68. Ritchie AW, Parr NJ, Moussa SA, Tolley DA. Lithotripsy for calculi in caliceal diverticula? Br J Urol 1990;66:6–8.

69. Garcia Reboll L, et al. [Extracorporeal shockwave lithotripsy: an alternative treatment for lithiasis of caliceal diverticula]. Actas Urol Esp 1992;16:467–70.

70. Kriegmair M, et al. [Diverticular calculi of the kidney calices—extracorporeal shockwave lithotripsy, percutaneous extraction or open surgery]. Urologe A 1990;29:204–8.

71. Hendrikx AJ, Bierkens AF, Bos R, et al. Treatment of stones in caliceal diverticula: extracorporeal shock wave lithotripsy versus percutaneous nephrolitholapaxy. Br J Urol 1992;70:478–82.

72. Streem SB, Yost A. Treatment of caliceal diverticular calculi with extracorporeal shock wave lithotripsy: patient selection and extended followup. J Urol 1992;148:1043–6.

73. Wulfsohn MA. Extracorporeal shockwave lithotripsy of calyceal diverticula calculi. J Urol 1988;140:835.

74. Grasso M, Lang G, Loisides P, et al. Endoscopic management of the symptomatic caliceal diverticular calculus. J Urol 1995;153:1878–81.

75. Chong TW, Bui MH, Fuchs, GJ. Calyceal diverticula. Ureteroscopic management. Urol Clin North Am 2000;27:647–54.

76. David R. Flexible ureteroenoscopy, dilation of narrow caliceal neck, and SWL: a new minimally invasive approach to stones in caliceal diverticula. J Endourol 1989;3:3.

77. Lobik L, Lopez-Pujals A, Leveille RJ. Variables affecting deflection of a new third-generation flexible ureteropyeloscope (DUR-8 elite). J Endourol 2003;17:733–6.

78. Batter SJ, Dretler SP. Ureterorenoscopic approach to the symptomatic caliceal diverticulum. J Urol 1997;158:709–13.

79. Eshghi AM, Roth JS, Smith AD. Percutaneous transperitoneal approach to a pelvic kidney for endourological removal of staghorn calculus. J Urol 1985;134:525–7.

80. Figge M. Percutaneous transperitoneal nephrolithotomy. Eur Urol 1988;14:414–6.

81. Toth C, Holman E, Pasztor I, Khan AM. Laparoscopically controlled and assisted percutaneous transperitoneal nephrolithotomy in a pelvic dystopic kidney. J Endourol 1993;7:303–5.

82. Danjou P. Nephrolithotomie percutanee par voie anterieure transabdominale guidee par laparoscopie pour le traitment d'un calcul intradiverticulaire. Prog Urol 1997;7:7a.

83. Brunet P, Meria P, Mahe P, Danjou P. Laparoscopically-assisted percutaneous nephrolithotomy for the treatment of anterior calyceal diverticula. BJU Int 2000;86:1088–9.

84. Miller SD, Ng CS, Streem SB, Gill IS. Laparoscopic management of caliceal diverticular calculi. J Urol 2002;167:1248–52.

85. Hoznek A, et al. Symptomatic caliceal diverticula treated with extraperitoneal laparoscopic marsupialization fulguration and gelatin resorcinol formaldehyde glue obliteration. J Urol 1998;160:352–5.

86. Van Cangh PJ, Abi Aad AS, Lorge F, et al. Laparoscopic nephrolithotomy: the value of intracorporeal sonography and color Doppler. Urology 1995;45:516–9.

87. Harewood LM, et al. Extraperitoneal laparoscopic caliceal diverticulectomy. J Endourol 1996;10:425–30.

88. Curran MJ, Little AF, Bouyounes B, et al. Retroperitoneoscopic technique for treating symptomatic caliceal diverticula. J Endourol 1999;13:723–5.

89. Ramakumar S, Segura JW. Laparoscopic surgery for renal urolithiasis: pyelolithotomy, caliceal diverticulectomy, and treatment of stones in a pelvic kidney. J Endourol 2000;14:829–32.

90. Kelalis PP, Malek, RS. Infundibulopelvic stenosis. J Urol 1981;125:568–71.

91. Husmann DA, Kramer SA, Malek RS, Allen TD. Infundibulopelvic stenosis: a long-term followup. J Urol 1994;152:837–40.

92. Parsons JK, Jarrett TW, Lancini V, Kavoussi LR. Infundibular stenosis after percutaneous nephrolithotomy. J Urol 2002;167:35–8.

93. MacMahon HE. Hypertrophic infundibular stenosis of the calyces of the kidney. Hum Pathol 1974;5:363–4.

94. Bodner DR, Caldamone AA, Resnick MI. Acquired infundibular stenosis. Urology 1987;29:19–21.

95. Kim HL, Gerber GS. Use of ureteroscopy and holmium: yttrium-aluminum-garnet laser in the treatment of an infundibular stenosis. Urology 2000;55:129–31.

96. Gupta CL, et al. Ureterocalycostomy for postpyelolithotomy stenosis after failure of intubated infundibuloplasty. Urology 1980;16:190–3.

97. Hulbert. 1988;

98. Wilbert. 1986;

99. Thurhoff , Alken. 1988;

23

Treatment of Renal Cysts

Matthew T. Gettman, MD
Joseph W. Segura, MD

Cystic diseases of the kidney are common uro- logic findings that can be broadly classified as having a congenital or acquired etiology. In many instances, cystic diseases of the kidney are inci- dentally discovered, yet a variety of clinical pre- sentations can also contribute to the diagnosis. For example, most patients with simple renal cysts are completely asymptomatic and therefore require no additional intervention. On the other hand, many patients with congenital cystic disor- ders not only require intervention targeted directly to the renal cysts but also careful treat- ment of associated medical problems. As such, treatment of renal cysts rests on an accurate diag- nosis of the cystic disorder and assessment of the patient's presenting complaints. This chapter dis- cusses radiographic imaging, clinical indications, and therapeutic options for cystic diseases of the kidney (Table 23-1).

IMAGING STUDIES

Increased utilization and technologic advances in abdominal imaging have improved detection of incidental renal masses and renal cystic disor- ders. Among cystic renal disorders, the most common incidental finding is a simple renal cyst. When performing abdominal computerized tomography (CT) for non-urologic indications, simple renal cysts are incidentally discovered in 20 to 24% of patients.[1,2] In addition, the inci- dence of renal cystic disorders characteristically increases with age.[3] Retrospective studies have shown that –up to 6% of patients < 40 years old, 18 to 19% of patients 40 to 60 years old, and 31% of patients > 60 years will have incidentally dis- covered simple renal cysts on CT scan.[1,2] In fact, the prevalence of simple renal cysts is reported to increase more than sevenfold from the fourth to eighth decade of life.[3] Laucks and McLachlan[1] initially reported that the incidence of simple renal cysts is similar among men and women, but subsequent contemporary studies reported an increased incidence in men.[3,4] The incidence of other renal cystic disorders may also show a predilection for men. For example, Ishikawa and colleagues reported that men with end-stage renal disease (ESRD) are predisposed to an ear- lier and more progressive course with acquired renal cystic disease.[5]

The incidence of simple renal cysts, however, appears to be the same in both the left and right kidney. Furthermore, among patients with renal cysts, 52% will have multiple cysts, and 35% will

have bilateral cysts. In addition, two-thirds of all simple cysts have a diameter of < 2 cm.[2] In a prior autopsy study, Kissane[6] noted that 50% of patients older than 50 years have benign renal cysts. This apparent discrepancy between CT scans and autopsy studies is explained by the fact that 48% of these autopsy cysts were < 1 cm in diameter and thus too small for detection by CT. Indeed, sensi- tivity of imaging does appear to impact the reported incidence of renal cysts. In a comparison of renal cyst detection rates between ultrasonogra- phy (US) and magnetic resonance imaging (MRI), MRI detected an increased number of simple renal cysts predominantly because of its increased sen- sitivity for detecting cysts < 1 cm in diameter.[4] Of 528 screened patients, 330 patients (63%) had at least one renal cyst on MRI and 315 patients (60%) had cysts of < 1 cm in diameter.

Data regarding the interval growth of renal cysts remains incompletely understood. Based on results of a longitudinal health screening pro- gram with abdominal US, Terada and colleagues calculated the mean increase in size and rate of enlargement for renal cysts as 2.8 mm and 6.3% yearly, respectively.[3] In fact, they reported that simple cysts grew significantly more rapidly in patients < 50 years old (rate of enlargement = 3.94 mm/year) in comparison to patients > 50 years old (rate of enlargement = 1.84 mm/

year). The researchers also reported a yearly growth rate of 2.18 mm for simple cysts in com- parison to a yearly growth rate of 6.93 mm for multiloculated cysts.[3] Laucks and McLachlan also reported that renal cysts increase in size, number, and incidence with age.[1] Likewise, Nascimento and colleagues found that cyst diam- eter significantly increased with age.[4] Other lon- gitudinal studies have reported contradictory data, yet these conclusions may be related to the sensitivity of available imaging technology or to specific definitions of cyst growth. For instance, in 1989 Holmberg and Hietala published longitu- dinal data on 14 renal cysts that were followed for a minimum of 3 years.[7] Using contemporary imaging at that time, 7% of the cysts were found to have decreased in size, 64% were unchanged, and 29% had increased in size. Among 34 patients with solitary renal cysts followed for 3 to 86 months (mean = 29 months) with serial US, Dalton and colleagues reported 65% of patients had no increase in cyst size or complexity, whereas 35% exhibited an increase in size or complexity.[8] In following cyst size, however, the authors stated an interval change in diameter of 3 mm was insignificant and within the bounds of observational error. Based on these criteria, no patient was reported to have a significant increase in cyst size. The authors concluded that significant changes in the appearance of renal cysts tend to occur in the degree of complexity rather than in cyst diameter.

In addition to simple renal cysts, other cystic renal disorders can also be diagnosed on the basis of radiographic imaging. In comparison to simple renal cysts, the natural history of other cystic renal disorders is often better understood and, in fact, the incidental discovery of these diseases is less common given the frequency of associated med- ical problems and related symptomatology. While modern imaging has made evaluation of the kid- neys more detailed and often times more com- plex, technologic advances have also improved the ability to categorize cystic renal lesions for presence of worrisome malignant features.

In 1986, Bosniak described a classification system using predominantly CT or US findings that distinguishes renal masses as benign or sus- picious for malignancy (Table 23-2).[9] Category I lesions represent simple renal cysts and approxi- mately 80% of cystic renal lesions belonging to this class.[10] On ultrasonography, benign cysts are anechoic with smooth, sharply marginated walls and evidence of good through transmission. On

Table 23-1 Cystic Diseases of the Kidney

Acquired
Simple cysts
Complicated cysts
Parapelvic cysts
Renal Sinus cysts
Multilocular cystic nephroma
Multicystic dysplastic kidney
Acquired renal cystic disease (ARCD)
Caliceal diverticulum
Medullary sponge kidney
Cystic renal cell carcinoma
Cystic Wilms tumor

Congenital
Autosomal dominant polycystic kidney disease (ADPKD)
Autosomal recessive polycystic kidney disease (ARPKD)
Familial juvenile nephronophthisis (medullary cystic disease)
Tuberous sclerosis
von Hippel-Lindau disease
Jeune's syndrome (asphyxiating thoracic dystrophy)
Zellweger syndrome
Meckel's syndrome

Table 23-2 Bosniak Classification of Renal Cysts				
Feature	I	II	III	IV
Wall	Thin	Thin	More than thin	Nodular or thick
Calcifications	None	Few or thin	Irregular	Coarse
Septations	None	Few or thin	More than a few	Numerous or thick
Density	0–20 Hounsfield units	0–20 Hounsfield units	0–20 Hounsfield units	More than 20 Hounsfield units
Enhancement	None	None	None	Present

CT scan, benign cysts exhibit sharp margination and demarcation from surrounding renal parenchyma, a smooth and thin wall, homogeneous water density contents (0 to 20 Hounsfield units), and no enhancement following the administration of intravenous contrast.[11]

Category II lesions include lesions with thin, smooth septa and minimal mural or septal calcification. High-density cysts (cysts that contain proteinaceous fluid or blood breakdown products and an x-ray density greater than water) are also included in this category as long as they are smooth, round, homogeneous, sharply demarcated, < 3 cm in diameter, and do not enhance with intravenous contrast. To adequately evaluate the cyst's outer wall, at least one-fourth of the cyst's circumference must be extrarenal.[12] If the high-density cyst is < 3 cm in diameter, then ultrasonography must be used to confirm the above properties. Although these lesions are characteristically considered benign, equivocal cases are denoted with the category II F classification. Category II F (F for follow-up) are evaluated with repeat scanning 3 to 6 months after the initial diagnosis and then on an annual basis.[11] Category II F lesions with demonstrated interval changes are treated as malignant lesions and require surgical exploration.

Category III lesions represent cystic lesions in which the possibility of malignancy cannot be ruled out radiographically. These lesions may have septa that are numerous, thick, irregular, enhancing, or attached to thickened regions of the cyst wall. Category III cysts may also contain extensive, thick, or irregular calcifications. These indeterminate lesions are classically associated with a 50% risk of malignancy. Approximately 5 to 8% of all cystic renal lesions are categorized as Bosniak III lesions.[11] Examples of category III lesions include large hemorrhagic cysts, multilocular cystic nephromas, multiloculated cysts, and densely calcified cysts.

Category IV lesions are complex cystic masses that contain obvious non-cystic components. They may have irregular margins or contain solid, enhancing tissue. This category includes cysts with adjacent solid tumors and solid tumors within the cysts. These lesions must be considered malignant until proved otherwise. While the diagnosis of cystic renal cell carcinoma is relatively uncommon, these cancers are usually identified at earlier stages, have slower growth, and are associated with a better prognosis than conventional renal cell carcinoma.[13–15]

With the Bosniak classification system, the diagnosis of category I and category IV lesions is most straightforward. Distinguishing features of category II and especially category III lesions can be more problematic. In fact, Aronson and colleagues[16] retrospectively compared the preoperative radiographic evaluations and the surgical pathology reports of 16 category II to IV renal cysts. They found that all category II lesions were benign, all category IV lesions were malignant, and that the seven category III lesions were split between three benign cysts and four malignant lesions. Curry and colleagues also evaluated the usefulness of the Bosniak classification system among 82 pathologically confirmed cystic renal lesions.[17] Between two experienced uroradiologists, all category I, II, and IV lesions were correctly categorized, and 29 of 49 category III lesions (59%) were found to be malignant. Nonetheless, the usefulness of the Bosniak system has been questioned in other series. For example, investigators have noted the presence of renal cell carcinoma in lesions determined to be Bosniak category II cysts.[18–20] Furthermore, in the reports by Wilson and colleagues and Koga and colleagues, all observed category III lesions (classically associated with a 50% risk of malignancy) were found to be malignant at renal exploration.[18,20]

Technical factors related specifically to the imaging test, the issue of interobserver variability, and specific characteristics of the radiographic image can influence classification of cystic renal lesions.[11,17] Siegel and colleagues had three radiologists independently review 70 pathologically proven cystic renal masses.[21] The radiologists agreed on the Bosniak classification in only 59% of cases. Of concern, 11 of 70 lesions (16%) were classified as Bosniak I or II by one radiologist and as Bosniak III or IV by at least one other radiologist. The most interobserver variability was noted for Bosniak II and III lesions. The authors concluded the Bosniak classification is useful, but distinguishing Bosniak II and III lesions is problematic, and interobserver variation is a concern. Siegel and another group evaluated the role of interobserver variability in the determination of enhancement of renal lesions.[22] Among simple and complicated cysts, observer concordance rates were 100% and 90%, respectively. Agreement about smaller lesions (diameter of 1.0 to 1.5 cm) was most problematic. A technical factor that can influence accurate classification of especially small simple renal cysts is pseudoenhancement.[23] Pseudoenhancement is an artifactual increase in the measured attenuation of a simple renal cyst after administration of contrast. For instance, Heneghan and colleagues found in an experimental model that pseudoenhancement can be a more significant problem when using a multidetector helical CT as opposed to a single detector helical CT.[23] On the other hand, Bae and colleagues found that pseudoenhancement was not a big issue for cysts larger than 1.0 cm in diameter.[24] In fact, the authors reported that none of the cysts greater than 1.0 cm in diameter were demonstrated to have greater than a 10–Hounsfield-unit increase in attenuation. Differentiating high-density cysts from renal neoplasms can also be problematic for CT scanning. In this regard, Macari and Bosniak recommended use of delayed CT (time delays of 15 to 240 minutes) as a way to differentiate cystic lesions (associated with no change in attenuation) versus tumor (associated with de-enhancement on delayed CT).[25] Israel and Bosniak also evaluated the prognostic importance of calcification within cystic renal lesions and found that even extensive calcification of a cystic renal mass is not as important in the diagnosis as the presence of soft-tissue enhancement.[26]

Other radiologic tests can be used to categorize cystic renal lesions.[27,28] For instance, Chicoskie and colleagues found MRI helpful in determining the presence of infected renal cysts in autosomal dominant polycystic kidney disease (ADPKD) patients.[28] MRI and US can also be useful in characterizing complex renal cysts. Among 55 complex renal lesions in 37 patients, Balci and colleagues noted mural irregularity, mural masses or nodules, increased mural wall thickness, and mural wall enhancement on MRI as independent factors significantly associated with malignancy.[29] In another report, contrast-enhanced Doppler US was shown to increase diagnostic accuracy in comparison to non-contrast Doppler US or contrast CT.[30]

The ability of imaging to provide prognostic information regarding cystic renal lesions, although not perfect, is an especially important clinical development. Prior to the advent of modern imaging and modern classification systems, space-occupying lesions of the kidney were frequently evaluated with invasive diagnostic testing if not treated immediately with nephrectomy. Since excretory urography could not reliably differentiate solid renal tumors from cystic lesions, urologists had little choice except to presume that these masses posed a significant risk of malignancy and remove them using open surgery. Unfortunately, the majority of these masses were benign, thereby subjecting the patient to unnecessary morbidity and possible mortality. With the later development of fluoroscopic and ultrasound-guided cyst aspiration and cystography, the ability to differentiate suspicious and solid renal lesions from benign cysts became possible. Ultimately, the ability to provide prognostic information was proven entirely using diagnostic imaging. For instance, Holmberg and colleagues compared ultrasonography, CT, arteriography, urography, and cyst cytology or fine-needle biopsy in evaluating 101 renal masses in 99 patients with the diagnosis confirmed by cytologic or histologic evaluation.[31] Renal ultrasonography showed a 96% sensitivity, whereas CT scans were 100% sensitive for renal cell carcinoma. Arteriography, cyst fluid cytology, and fine-needle aspirates provided no additional diagnostic value. These types of early comparative studies helped provide a foundation of classifying renal lesions solely on the basis of radiographic criteria. Nonetheless, CT-guided biopsy of indeterminate cystic renal lesion continues to be performed. Lang and colleagues performed cyst aspiration and biopsy of 199 patients with Bosniak IIF and III cystic renal lesions.[32] The diagnostic sensitivities for malignancy, benign cysts requiring intervention, and benign complex cysts were .71, .87, and .91, respectively. The fact that only 20 of 28 malignancies were accurately diagnosed on the basis of cytology and biopsy, however, is concerning. Furthermore, prior studies showed that, even when renal biopsies are performed on solid renal lesions, the results are unreliable.[33] As such, we would recommend that complex cystic lesions in most patients should not be evaluated with cyst aspiration and biopsy. Cyst aspiration and biopsy may be considered for patients who are poor surgical candidates, but all other patients with complex worrisome cystic lesions should undergo surgical evaluation.

INDICATIONS

Therapeutic interventions for renal cystic diseases depend on the specific disease entity and the appearance on radiographic imaging. For example, treatment recommendations for a patient with symptomatic ADPKD versus a patient with simple renal cysts can be vastly different. Furthermore, treatment recommendation for patients with ADPKD can also be radically different depending on the patient's location in the spectrum of disease (ie, normal renal function vs. ESRD). Indeed, the indications for any intervention depend on both the pathologic condition that produced the cyst and the symptoms caused by the cyst. Generally, symptoms that represent valid indications for intervention include (1) pain, (2) infection, (3) hypertension secondary to cyst encroachment on renal vessels or cyst compression of renal parenchyma itself, (4) segmental or global hydronephrosis secondary to cyst encroachment on the renal collecting system, (5) relief of respiratory embarrassment, especially in pediatric patients, and (6) presence of malignant features. In reality, the overwhelming majority of procedures performed on simple cysts are undertaken for pain relief. The treatment of these symptomatic cysts is directed not only towards cyst drainage but also towards the prevention of cyst fluid reaccumulation. In addition to solitary simple renal cysts, other cystic renal diseases can also require intervention for one or more of the previously discussed indications.

Ongoing evidence suggests that destruction of renal cysts has no adverse or beneficial effect on renal function. After the first reported unroofing of renal cysts by Rovsing in 1911,[34] cyst unroofing was considered a procedure that would help prolong renal function in ADPKD patients.[35] In the late 1950s and 1960s, however, three studies were published that appeared to show that unroofing of renal cysts resulted in a decreased glomerular filtration rate.[36–38] These studies, however, were severely limited by small cohort size (11 patients in all three studies) and by the lack of an accurate preoperative renal function assessment.[39] In addition, the studies were designed only to show that unroofing of renal cysts does not improve renal function, not that decortication is harmful to renal function. Elzinga and colleagues[39] subsequently reported a prospective study involving 30 patients with ADPKD in which the rate of declining renal function was determined prior to open cyst-reduction surgery. In this study, no significant change in renal function was observed with cyst decortication.

The physiologic effects of percutaneous cyst aspiration for benign renal cysts have also been investigated. In their study, Holmberg and colleagues percutaneously aspirated renal cysts in 19 kidneys and measured the single kidney glomerular filtration rate (SKGFR) of the treated kidneys and the contralateral non-punctured kidneys prior to puncture and again at 5 days and 6 months after aspiration.[40] Two of the 19 cysts (10%) were associated with some degree of collecting system obstruction, and in these kidneys, there was a 3% and 12% increase in SKGFR after cyst aspiration. In the remaining 17 kidneys, there was neither a significant increase nor decrease in SKGFR as a result of the cyst aspiration. It should be noted that the SKGFR was not significantly different for the two groups of kidneys before or after puncture. In addition, on 6-month ultrasonography evaluation, all cysts had regained from 40% to 114% of their original volume (mean recovery of 75%). No relationship was found between the change in cyst size and the change in SKGFR. Thus, studies by Elzinga and colleagues and Holmberg and colleagues suggest that renal cysts that do not obstruct the intrarenal collecting system have no effect on overall renal function.[39,40]

PAIN Pain is the most common presentation of symptomatic renal cysts, especially in patients with ADPKD. For example, approximately 60% of ADPKD patients have chronic pain that can be disabling or lead to narcotic dependence.[41]

Cyst-related pain is believed to be either secondary to stretching of the renal capsule as cysts enlarge, bleeding into the cyst, or the weight of the enlarged kidney pulling on the renal pedicle.[42] Prior to treating a patient with painful benign renal cysts, other sources of pain must be ruled out, such as obstruction of the collecting system by stone, clot, or neoplasm. The majority of acute pain episodes are self-limited and may be managed with narcotics or non-narcotic medications. If the pain persists despite adequate medical therapy, therapeutic intervention should be considered.

In general, good pain control has been obtained with any technique that will prevent the cyst from reforming. Elzinga and colleagues[39] reported a prospective study in which 30 patients with ADPKD underwent open cyst reduction surgery. After 2 years, 62% of these patients were pain-free. In 1993, Elzinga and colleagues[42] reported another prospective study in which, using ultrasound guidance, 11 patients with disabling pain from ADPKD underwent percutaneous aspiration of three to five dominant cysts in each symptomatic kidney. Dramatic pain relief was obtained in all 11 patients; it recurred, however, in 10 patients within 6 months. Follow-up ultrasonography suggested that this recurrence of pain was secondary to reaccumulation of fluid within the cysts. Six of the 10 patients with recurrent pain underwent open cyst reduction, and 70% were pain-free at 18 months.

INFECTION Infection is an uncommon indication for patients with benign renal cystic disease[43,44] but significantly more common in patients with ADPKD.[28] Both the diagnosis and treatment of these infections are complicated by the characteristics of the cysts themselves. Despite symptoms of pyelonephritis such as flank pain, anorexia, fever, and elevated leukocyte count, the diagnosis may be delayed because the cysts may not communicate with the renal collecting system,[45] and therefore, urinalysis, urine gram stain, and urine culture may remain negative. In fact, the delayed diagnosis of an infected renal cyst can increase the risk of severe secondary infections such as bacterial meningitis, retroperitoneal/lower extremity abscess, peripelvic abscess, septicemia, and death.[45–47]

Once cyst infection is suspected, treatment with antibiotics can be even more difficult. Most antibiotics penetrate renal cysts poorly, especially cysts of the distal nephron.[48] Thus, infected renal cysts frequently fail to respond to antibiotic therapy. The fluoroquinolones (ie, levofloxacin, ciprofloxacin) and trimethoprim-sulfamethoxazole (TMP-SMX) have been shown to obtain adequate bactericidal levels in cysts[45] and are therefore the antibiotics of choice for infected cysts. However, if infection persists for longer than 2 or 3 weeks despite appropriate antibiotic therapy, aspiration or percutaneous drainage is necessary.

Percutaneous aspiration or drainage of infected renal cysts is complicated by the difficulty of identifying the infected cyst or cysts. Patients with ADPKD have numerous cysts in each kidney, frequently with varying densities resulting from prior hemorrhage into the cysts. In addition, more than one cyst may be infected at a time. Diagnostic tests, such as indium-tagged leukocyte scans, can provide general information regarding the size and location of the infected cyst, but frequently the information provided by the scan is inadequate to definitively identify the affected cyst. Abdominal CT may show thickening or irregularity of the cyst wall, increased cyst attenuation, or thickening of the renal fascia in the presence of cyst infection. Unfortunately, the same signs can also be seen with a hemorrhagic cyst. If serial CT scans show these changes developing while the patient is symptomatic, then there is a significant chance the cyst is infected. Recently, MRI has provided useful information that can differentiate infected versus non-infected renal cysts.[28]

Chapman and colleagues[49] reported a case in which percutaneous cyst puncture was used to drain an infected renal cyst in a 31-year-old man with ADPKD. Fortunately, this patient had recently had a CT scan of the abdomen performed for a similar infection. One cyst was noted to have enlarged 300% from the previous study. This cyst was aspirated three times while the patient was treated with parenteral antibiotics. Cyst aspirate cultures were positive for *Staphylococcus aureus* (as opposed to the usual gram-negative organisms that are found in these patients), which was probably related to his known intravenous drug abuse. The third aspiration finally brought defervescence, and the patient was cured after a 4-week course of parenteral antibiotics. Although percutaneous aspiration is certainly a useful technique in treating pyocysts, it should be noted that the procedure may be futile if multiple cysts are infected or the infected cyst is multiloculated.

Some ADPKD patients with infected cysts ultimately will require more invasive management techniques such as laparoscopic decortication. Hemal and colleagues successfully used retroperitoneoscopic techniques for treatment of two ADPKD patients with infected cysts.[50] Both patients had immediate improvement in symptoms after treatment and a quick recovery with limited morbidity. The investigators especially favored a retroperitoneal laparoscopic approach when treating infected cysts so as to prevent bacterial contamination of the abdomen. For similar reasons, Nadu and colleagues also recommended a retroperitoneal approach when performing nephrectomy for presumed infection in ADPKD kidneys.[51] In a case of a 39-year-old man with an Aspergillus-infected kidney, the authors performed retroperitoneal nephrectomy in 80 minutes and safely removed the kidney using morcellation techniques after the kidney had been placed into a laparoscopic retrieval bag.

Hydatid disease can also present as a cystic renal mass. Echinococcosis can affect any visceral site, but the incidence of renal involvement is only about 2 to 4%. Ameur and colleagues reported on 34 patients with renal hydatid cysts treated between 1980 and 2001.[52] The most common presenting complaint was pain (63%) followed by hematuria (31%), mass (26%), fever (23%), and hydatiduria (11%). In the majority of cases, treatment consisted of open resection of the prominent cyst dome. In 9% of cases, treatment was complicated by urinary fistula (2 patients) or recurrent infection (1 patient). While conservative open surgery is the procedure of choice for renal echinococcosis, extensive damage to the renal parenchyma warrants nephrectomy in 14 to 25% of cases.[52–54]

RENIN-MEDIATED HYPERTENSION Hypertension is rarely caused by a simple benign renal cyst, but it is a common finding in patients with ADPKD.[55,56] Schwarz and colleagues suggest that there are two probable etiologies for this hypertension.[56] The first possibility is a parapelvic cyst (simple cyst arising from renal parenchyma near the hilum) or peripelvic cysts (multiple small cysts probably arising from ectasia of renal hilar lymphatics) impinging on the renal hilum and compressing one or more branches of the renal artery, resulting in renin release and hypertension. The second possibility is that a large renal cyst surrounds and compresses some portion of the renal parenchyma, again causing ischemia, renin release, and hypertension. Pedersen and colleagues also hypothesized that renin-mediated hypertension could occur by simple cyst expansion that would ultimately cause renal ischemia and renin release.[55] In a case-control study of 115 patients with incidental renal cysts compared to age and sex-matched controls, the authors found that systolic and diastolic blood pressures were significantly higher in patients with renal cysts.

In their review of the literature, Schwarz and colleagues found 42 reported cases of symptomatic parapelvic and peripelvic cysts.[56] In those cases in which blood pressure was reported, 59% of patients were hypertensive, and this hypertension resolved or improved in 60% following cyst aspiration, cyst resection, or nephrectomy. Schwarz and colleagues also reported a case in which new-onset hypertension was reversed by percutaneous drainage of a large parapelvic renal cyst and subsequent open marsupialization into the peritoneal cavity. Serum renin levels were elevated preoperatively but normalized following surgery. Two years later, the patient was normotensive and had no cysts on ultrasonography. Ekici and colleagues described another hypertensive patient with bilateral pararenal cysts who ultimately had improvement in hypertension following bilateral pararenal cyst marsupialization.[57] In addition, Bongu and colleagues noted the development of hyperreninemia and hypertension in an ESRD patient with ACRD.[58] The patient acutely developed hypertension refractory to pharmacotherapy after bleeding into one of the renal cysts, which ultimately impinged on the renal hilum and created a Page kidney. Following nephrectomy, the patient had normalization of the blood pressure. Lezrek and colleagues noted correction of both hypertension and erythrocytosis after laparoscopic drainage of a 15-cm renal cyst arising from the left kidney.[59] Thus, surgical cyst decompression appears to be justified when suspicious renal cysts are associated with renin-mediated hypertension, and arterial disease is not suspected.

Surgical intervention for hypertension in ADPKD has not been shown to be nearly as effective as it has been for simple renal cysts. In the prospective study by Elzinga and colleagues in which 30 patients with ADPKD underwent open cyst reduction surgery, 18 patients were hypertensive.[39] Postoperatively, a statistically significant decline in blood pressure was noted, but only 1 of 18 patients who were hypertensive preoperatively remained normotensive at 1-year follow-up. Uemasu and colleagues reported comparable findings in their small series of three ADPKD patients whose cysts were treated with percutaneous sclerotherapy using minocycline hydrochloride.[60] Because of the poor durability of cyst decompression in treating hypertension in patients with ADPKD, hypertension alone does not justify surgical intervention for ADPKD.

COLLECTING SYSTEM OBSTRUCTION Compression and obstruction of the renal calices, renal pelvis, or ureter are rare complications of simple renal cysts. Some renal cystic diseases, such as multilocular cystic nephroma, have a predilection to extend into the collecting system and have even been associated with spontaneous rupture into the renal pelvis.[61,62] Cysts that lie near or within the renal hilum can obstruct one of these structures if they possess adequate turgor.[63] In addition to urinary obstruction, renal cysts have also been reported to cause gastrointestinal obstruction.[64] In 1978, Hinman reported three patients with collecting system obstruction secondary to renal cysts.[63] One of these three also had ADPKD. The obstruction was relieved in all three by open unroofing of these cysts. Subsequently, Amar and Das reported six cases in which benign renal cysts compressed the renal collecting system, resulting in obstruction and declining renal function.[65] In all six cases, the cysts were unroofed during an open surgical procedure. In five of the six patients, significant improvements in renal function and radiographic appearance were achieved. In the remaining patient, only mild radiographic improvement was noted. Thus, decompression is warranted to relieve collecting system obstruction by renal cysts. The location of the cystic renal abnormality, however, appears important to the development of symptoms. For instance, Brown and colleagues reported on a 78-year-old man with a 25-cm left renal cyst that only caused symptoms of abdominal fullness as opposed to associated problems of hypertension or renal obstruction.[66]

RELIEF OF RESPIRATORY DISTRESS DUE TO MASS EFFECT Multicystic dysplastic kidney is one of the most common abdominal masses found in neonates.[67] Occasionally, the multicystic kidney is so large that it compresses adjacent organs and impinges on the thoracic cavity, preventing full expansion of the lungs.[68] Two cases have been reported in which infants with multicystic kidney disease were born in respiratory distress, intubated, and then treated with urgent percutaneous cyst aspiration. In the first case, cyst aspiration resulted in only transient improvement, and the child underwent open nephrectomy.[68] In the second case, the cyst aspiration resulted in a durable improvement in respiratory status, and the infant was dismissed from the hospital without open surgery. When the child was 2 months old, however, a nephrectomy was performed for persistently protuberant abdomen and bowel displacement. From these cases, it appears that percutaneous cyst aspiration is a reasonable first step in the treatment of respiratory distress due to multicystic dysplastic kidney.

MALIGNANT FEATURES The presence of malignant features is the most important indication for intervention. For patients with renal cystic lesions, initial classification of the cystic abnormality should be performed noninvasively using the system proposed by Bosniak. If the cyst falls into category III or IV, there is a significant chance of malignancy, and these lesions should be approached using accepted oncologic approaches. The vast majority of renal cysts fall into Bosniak classes I (80%) or II, and most of these are asymptomatic.[12] These lesions are considered benign and do not warrant any further therapy unless they become symptomatic. Patients with equivocal Bosniak IIF lesions (ie, hyperdense cysts, increased calcification) do require careful radiographic follow-up. If these cysts are noted to have interval growth or change in configuration, they should be considered malignant and should be explored.

TREATMENT OPTIONS

The traditional therapy for symptomatic benign renal cysts has consisted of open cyst drainage and decortication or even nephrectomy. These traditional approaches, however, can obviously be associated with unnecessary morbidity (ie, nephrectomy for benign cyst). In 1967, Kropp and colleagues[70]reported a postoperative complication rate of 30% among a series of 126 patients who underwent open surgical exploration for what proved to be benign renal cysts. The majority of these complications were minor, but 3% of patients suffered one or more major complications, including death (1.5%), myocardial infarction (1.5%), wound disruption (1%), wound infection (6%), sepsis (2%), and hemorrhage requiring transfusion (1.5%). In addition, hospitalization and recovery from the traditional open surgery are prolonged. Among ADPKD patients undergoing bilateral open cyst decortication, Flemming and Barry reported a mean hospitalization of 9 days,[71] and Elzinga and colleagues reported a mean hospitalization of 6 days.[39]

Advances in CT and ultrasonography have allowed renal cysts to be classified as benign without open exploration. Concomitant advances in endoscopy, laparoscopy, and nephroscopy have allowed the development of percutaneous (minimally invasive) techniques for treatment of symptomatic renal cysts. These new techniques can offer several advantages over open surgery with the possibility of decreased length of hospital stay, improved convalescence, and reduced risk of complications.

The currently available techniques, in addition to open surgery for cystic renal lesions, include simple cyst aspiration, cyst aspiration in combination with cyst sclerosis, endoscopic marsupialization techniques (antegrade and retrograde access techniques) percutaneous resection, and laparoscopic treatment. Recommended choice of therapy is based on the specific type of presenting cystic renal lesion as well as specific patient-related factors.

TECHNIQUE AND RESULTS

SIMPLE CYST ASPIRATION/SCLEROTHERAPY In many instances, first-line therapy for symptomatic simple renal cysts remains cyst aspiration in combination with sclerotherapy. Early on, many patients were treated with cyst aspiration alone. In the absence of cyst sclerotherapy, however, cyst reaccumulation with symptom recurrence is common. In one series of 52 patients with symptomatic cysts, 50% of cysts were completely reconstituted at a mean follow-up of 2.8 years.[72] In the series of 20 cyst aspirations reported by Ohkawa and colleagues only 5% of cysts were less than 50% of their original size, and 70% of cysts were unchanged or had increased in size at 3-month follow-up.[73]

The instillation of a sclerosing agent into a renal cyst following percutaneous aspiration significantly reduces the rate of recurrence. Many agents have reportedly been used for this purpose, including glucose, phenol, ethanol, iophendylate, morrhuate sodium, lipidol, povidone-iodine, tetracycline, n-butyl cyanoacrylate, laureth 9 (also called polidocanol), and bismuth phosphate.[7,74–78] An early basis for sclerotherapy was provided in a study by Holmberg and Hietala.[7] They randomized 159 patients with 181 cysts into three groups: observation, aspiration, or sclerotherapy with bismuth phosphate. The observation group showed virtually no change in their cysts over 36 months of observation. Initially, the aspiration group had a reduction in cyst size, but after 24 months, there were no significant differences in cyst size for the observation group and the aspiration group. At 3-year follow-up, 44% of bismuth phosphate-treated cysts were undetectable, and an additional 53% were diminished in size. An experimental phase of the study in the porcine model also showed no adverse effects of sclerosing agent on the renal parenchyma.

The technique of renal cyst puncture is usually performed under ultrasound guidance and followed by fluoroscopic evaluation and cystography. Subsequently, the sclerosing agent is instilled into the cyst and left in situ or aspirated after a specified period of time. Some protocols require multiple treatments, and others leave a nephrostomy tube or stent in place.[79,80] Response rates of 77% to 97% have been reported. Reports suggest that multiple sclerotherapy treatments may increase success of treatment.[81–86] With the exception of peripelvic cysts, the complication rate of 4% to 14% is similar to that of puncture and aspiration alone.

While ethanol is the increasingly favored agent for sclerotherapy, the specific choice of sclerosing agent does not appear critical to the success of treatment.[75,80–86] In an early report, Bean treated 26 patients (34 cysts) using 95%

ethanol left indwelling for 10 to 20 minutes and reported a 97% success rate for single-session therapy.[87] The single patient failing treatment had a very large cyst. Among 24 patients treated with a combination of ethanol and tetracycline, Liatsikos and colleagues reported a 96% success rate at 20 months follow-up after single-session therapy.[75] Paananen and colleagues reported significant decreases in cyst diameter and a 75% rate of symptom resolution after single-session sclerotherapy performed with 99% ethanol.[86] In an attempt to improve success rates, multiple sessions of ethanol sclerotherapy have been recommended.[84,85] For instance, Bozkurt and colleagues favored successive ethanol treatments, especially for patients with large symptomatic renal cysts.[82] Likewise, Delakas and colleagues managed 68 patients with two repeated ethanol sclerotherapy sessions and noted complete and partial regression rates of 84% and 12%, respectively, at a mean follow-up of 30 months.[81] Furthermore, Chung and colleagues noted success rates of 95% for patients undergoing repeated sessions of ethanol sclerotherapy versus a 57% success rate for patients undergoing single-session treatment.[83]

Successful treatment has also been reported with other sclerosing agents. Ongoing experience with povidone-iodine suggests safety for this as a sclerosing agent.[74,76,79] Gelet and colleagues described percutaneous stenting of symptomatic renal cyst and consecutive sclerosing treatments with povidone-iodine.[79] Nephrostomy tubes were removed approximately 4 to 5 days after sclerotherapy. At 1-year follow-up, a 70% rate of complete cyst resolution was reported. Of note, 2 of 10 patients became septic postoperatively—the first occurred during hospitalization, and the second, 3 months after sclerosis. Criticism of this technique has centered on the 4- to 5-day course of nephrostomy tube drainage and the associated risks of infection. Ohkawa and colleagues reported a series of 141 patients who had symptomatic benign renal cysts, which were aspirated under ultrasound guidance, imaged, injected with 100 or 200 mg minocycline hydrochloride, and followed up at 1, 3, 6, and 12 months.[73] They found that the maximum reduction in cyst size occurred at 3 months and then leveled off. At 3-month follow-up, 44.8% of cysts had resolved, 31.8% were reduced by 50% or greater, 18.2% were reduced by less than 50%, and only 5.2% were unchanged or increased in size. Minor complications such as pain or fever occurred in 12.8% of patients. These same symptoms occurred in 10% of patients treated with aspiration alone. Small amounts of the compound were found in the urine and the serum; thus use of minocycline hydrochloride is contraindicated in patients with a hypersensitivity to tetracyclines.

Reports of complications involving peripelvic cysts support avoidance of sclerotherapy in the treatment of these cysts. Camancho and colleagues[88] described a case in which a peripelvic cyst in an otherwise normal kidney was aspirated and then injected with iophendylate (Pantopaque). Subsequently, the patient developed severe flank pain and was found to have a new ureteropelvic junction obstruction. Dismembered pyeloplasty was necessary to correct the obstruction. At the time of surgery, the cyst was found to be tightly contracted and densely adherent to the renal pelvis. It is possible that the cyst was densely adherent prior to sclerotherapy or that the sclerosing agent caused these dense adhesions. Lang also found an increased complication rate with this particular sclerosing agent.[89] In addition, two nephrectomies have been reported following peripelvic cyst aspiration and sclerotherapy with the agent lipidol.[90] Thus, based on these reports, peripelvic cysts should not be subjected to sclerotherapy.

Most authors state that, with the exception of peripelvic cysts, sclerotherapy should be attempted in the treatment of benign renal cysts before more invasive procedures are performed.[91] In addition, most investigators require a cyst aspirate cytologic specimen to be obtained prior to any form of percutaneous cyst resection, and sclerotherapy can be attempted at this time. Some authors, however, disagree with these conventions and believe that laparoscopic resection should be the first treatment option for easily resected anterior lesions.[92]

ENDOSCOPIC MARSUPIALIZATION TECHNIQUES
Both antegrade and retrograde endoscopic marsupialization techniques have been described, yet there has been limited enthusiasm for these techniques. The theoretical basis of antegrade endoscopic marsupialization was based on endoscopic management of a recurrent urinoma in a 33-year-old female after partial nephrectomy.[93] After failed attempts of treatment with fluid aspiration, sclerotherapy, and even open surgery, the authors created a communication between the urinoma and collecting system via an antegrade access. This tract was then dilated and stented. The nephrostomy tube was later exchanged for a Double-J stent placed in antegrade fashion that originated in the urinoma and ended in the bladder. By 3-month follow-up, the urinoma had resolved and the stent was removed. While this procedure was performed for a urinoma, the authors suggested the technique could treat select patients with symptomatic renal cysts. To date, an additional experience with the antegrade marsupialization technique has not been reported.

Limited experience also exists for a similar retrograde endoscopic marsupialization procedure initially reported by Kavoussi and colleagues in 1991 for an obstructing peripelvic cyst.[94] Successful marsupialization was performed ureteroscopically by cutting a 3-cm longitudinal incision between the posterior wall of the renal pelvis and the cyst with electrocautery. The interior of the cyst was then inspected and fulgurated. A Double-J stent was left indwelling for 1 week. At 3-month follow-up, excretory urogram revealed no cyst recurrence and no residual obstruction. Liaconis and colleagues described

another successful case of ureteroscopic decompression of a cystic renal lesion using the holmium:YAG laser.[95] In other patients treated with endoscopic marsupialization, cyst recurrence has not occurred at a follow-up of 2 years.[96]

Although the concept of draining a renal cyst into the renal pelvis using percutaneous endoscopic or ureteroscopic techniques is appealing, limitations to the technique have been raised. First, the technical demands of the procedure are much greater than that of simple cyst aspiration and sclerosis. The technique also requires entry into the renal collecting system, and therefore, predisposes the patient to urine leak. Furthermore, the renal cyst must be directly abutting the renal pelvis where the cut is to be made for these procedures to be successful. In addition, the risk of vascular injury is always present.[94] Finally, the need for either prolonged Double-J stenting or a nephrostomy tube is a limitation.

PERCUTANEOUS RESECTION Percutaneous resection of benign renal cysts is more similar to the open surgical unroofing procedures than the endoscopic marsupialization techniques (Figure 23-1). Nonetheless, interest in percutaneous treatment of renal cysts has also been limited. In contrast to endoscopic marsupialization, the cyst does not need to be immediately adjacent to the renal pelvis. Percutaneous resection also avoids the multiple trocar sites, extensive dissection, and technical difficulty associated with laparoscopy.[97] Resection is performed with the nephroscope and scissors or a resectoscope and loop electrocautery. The nephroscope can be placed in one of three positions to facilitate cyst resection: (1) traditional transparenchymal position with the tip of the nephroscope inside the cyst, (2) nephroscope placed directly into the exophytic portion of the cyst, or (3) nephroscope placed adjacent to the cyst in an extraparenchymal location. Before percutaneous resection is attempted, the cyst should be percutaneously punctured and aspirated for cytologic examination. Some authors also place a ureteral stent prior to resection. Cystography is performed, or methylene blue is injected into the cyst, at this time to demonstrate that the cyst does not communicate with the renal pelvis. If the fluid obtained is consistent with a benign cyst and there is no communication with the renal collecting system, cyst wall resection and cauterization is performed.

Gelet and colleagues described six cases of symptomatic benign renal cysts in which a standard transurethral resectoscope was used to resect the cyst wall under epidural anesthesia.[79] The parenchymal portion of the cyst was subsequently cauterized. Drains were left in place, and the patients were generally dismissed from the hospital in 4 to 5 days. At follow-up, 66% of these six patients had no recurrence on imaging studies and all were asymptomatic. There were no complications.

Plas and Hübner reported a series of 10 patients who underwent long-term follow-up

after percutaneous resection.[98] The indications for treatment included flank pain in 6, caliceal compression in 3, and ureteral compression in 1. Percutaneous resection with a resectoscope was performed under local anesthesia and sedation. All resections began with ultrasound-guided cyst puncture, aspiration, and cytologic evaluation of the aspirate. If the cyst fluid was cloudy, then the procedure was abandoned. Bulb drainage was used postoperatively for 2 or 3 days. There were no complications. At an average follow-up of 46 months (range, 26 to 66 months) 50% were cyst-free, 20% showed residual cysts, and 30% had developed a distinct new cyst. All 10 patients were asymptomatic. The longest resection required 45 minutes. All patients were hospitalized until the drains were removed, but the authors believe this procedure could be performed on an outpatient basis.

Percutaneous resection is superior to all of the previous nonsurgical techniques because the cyst wall is resected, and thus, cyst fluid is less likely to reaccumulate. In addition, instruments are used that are familiar to the urologist. Disadvantages are that, as the cyst is resected, the cavity collapses, impairing visualization of the remaining cyst wall, and the irrigant may extravasate and could theoretically cause hyponatremia.[55] Plas and Hübner note, however, that electrolyte imbalances and postoperative bleeding have not been reported.[98] In addition, a drain is frequently left in place for 2 to 5 days postoperatively.[98]

LAPAROSCOPIC APPROACH The laparoscopic approach to renal cystic disorders will be discussed in detail in Part V (see Part V, "Basic and Procedural Laparoscopy"). Laparoscopic procedures used in the management of cystic renal disorders include cyst decortication, peripelvic cyst excision, partial nephrectomy, and nephrectomy. Briefly, laparoscopic cyst decortication can be performed via transperitoneal or retroperitoneal approach. The objective of laparoscopic cyst decortication is treatment of all visible cysts. Ideally, to prevent symptom recurrence the cyst walls are resected and the base of the lesion examined and then fulgurated. The results of laparoscopic renal cyst resection are similar to those obtained by percutaneous cyst resection. Laparoscopy has also been used for patients with Bosniak category II to IV cystic renal lesions and for patients with symptomatic ADPKD or ACRD on dialysis or after transplantation. At the present time, there does not appear to be enough evidence to recommend laparoscopy as the therapy of choice for management of complex renal cysts.[11]

OPEN SURGERY Open surgery is still warranted for definitive management of select patients with cystic renal lesions. While open surgery is less commonly employed nowadays for treatment of simple renal cysts and patients with symptomatic polycystic kidneys, open cyst decortication procedures remains straightforward and efficacious.[71] Open nephrectomy also remains a treatment for

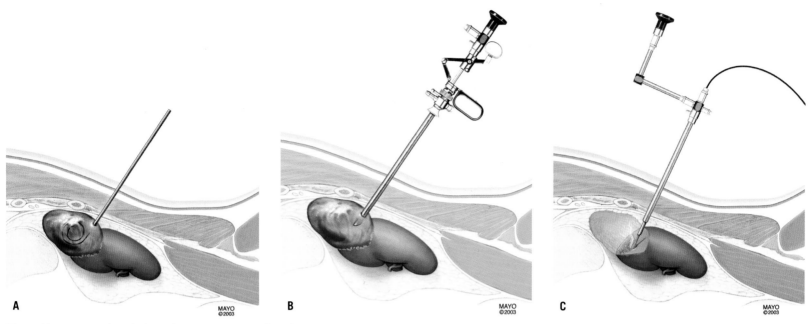

Figure 23-1 Transcystic technique of percutaneous resection of a renal cyst using a resectoscope. *A*, After guidewire placement into the renal cyst, the percutaneous access tract is dilated. *B*, A standard resectoscope is then used to resect the exophytic portion of the cyst wall. *C*, Electrocautery is then used to cauterize the parenchymal portion of the cyst with the assistance of a standard rigid nephroscope.

select patients with ADPKD that require native kidney removal, but laparoscopic treatment is quickly becoming the procedure of choice.[71] Open surgery also remains indicated as the treatment of choice for patients with complex renal cysts (Bosniak categories IIF and III). For patients with Bosniak IV lesions, a role continues to exist for open surgical techniques, especially when nephron-sparing techniques are considered.[11,14]

ARTERIAL EMBOLIZATION   Arterial embolization was recently reported as a minimally invasive nonsurgical management option for treatment of symptomatic anuric ADPKD patients on hemodialysis. Between 1996 and 2000, Ubara and colleagues treated 64 patients with renal artery embolization using intravascular coils.[99] Patients were followed at 3-month intervals after surgery and were noted to have a significant reduction in renal size, abdominal circumference, and dry weight. Serious complications were not encountered, but the authors did report minor complaints of fever and flank pain in the first week after the procedure. While the authors stated that embolization was effective for all patients, the procedure would be contraindicated for patients with an infectious indication for treatment.

CONCLUSION

A multitude of cystic lesions can arise in the kidney. Given the broad spectrum of renal cystic diseases and the variety of treatment options, efficacious treatment rests on an accurate clinical diagnosis. The overwhelming majority of cystic renal lesions are just benign asymptomatic cysts, and no additional treatment is required. When cystic renal lesions are uncovered or do become symptomatic, modern imaging techniques can classify renal cysts into clearly benign cysts and

cysts with possible malignant features. Benign symptomatic cysts can be treated with a variety of techniques, yet most investigators recommend percutaneous needle aspiration and sclerotherapy (unless the cyst is peripelvic) as the initial procedure of choice. The cyst fluid is routinely aspirated and sent for cytologic examination. If a benign cyst should recur and again cause the patient symptoms, then other minimally invasive procedures, such as endoscopic marsupialization procedures, percutaneous cyst resection, or laparoscopic cyst decortication, should be considered. Because of the significantly reduced morbidity and hospitalization time associated with minimally invasive surgical procedures as compared with open renal cyst unroofing, the latter should be reserved only for cases refractory to other minimally invasive therapies.

Oftentimes, regardless of symptomatology, patients with complex cystic lesions require more aggressive evaluation and treatment. At the present time, minimally invasive approaches do not appear indicated for the evaluation of most complex renal cysts (Bosniak category IIF, III, and IV). While minimally invasive laparoscopic treatments have been reported, traditional open renal exploration and treatment remains the procedure of choice. For patients with Bosniak category IV lesions, open surgery continues to have an important role in treatment, but utilization and efficacy of laparoscopic treatment is increasing, especially for lesions requiring complete nephrectomy.

REFERENCES

 1. Laucks SP, McLachlan SF. Aging and simple cysts of the kidney. Br J Radiol 1981;54:12.
 2. Tada S, Yamagishi J, Kobayashi H, et al. The incidence of simple renal cyst by computed tomography. Clin Radiol 1983;34:437.
 3. Terada N, Ichioka K, Matsuta Y, et al. The natural history of simple renal cysts. J Urol 2002;167:21.
 4. Nascimento AB, Mitchell DG, Zhang XM, et al. Rapid MR imaging detection of renal cysts: Age-based standards. Radiology 2001;221:628.
 5. Ishikawa I, Saito Y, Nakamura M, et al. Fifteen-year follow-up of acquired renal cystic disease - a gender difference. Nephron 1997;75:315.
 6. Kissane JM. The morphology of renal cystic disease. In: Gardner KD Jr, editor. Cystic diseases of the kidney. New York: John Wiley & Sons; 1976.
 7. Holmberg G, Hietala SO. Treatment of simple renal cysts by percutaneous puncture and instillation of bismuth-phosphate. Scand J Urol Nephrol 1989;23:207.
 8. Dalton D, Neiman H, Grayhack JT. The natural history of simple renal cysts: a preliminary study. J Urol 1986;135:905.
 9. Bosniak MA. The current radiological approach to renal cysts. Radiology 1986;158:1.
10. Lang EK. Renal cyst puncture studies. Urol Clin North Am 1987;14:91.
11. Kausik S, Segura JW, King BF Jr. Classification and management of simple and complex renal cysts. AUA Update Series 2002;21:82.
12. Bosniak MA. The small (3.0 cm) renal parenchymal tumor: detection, diagnosis, and controversies. Radiology 1991; 179:307.
13. Bielsa O, Lloreta J, Gelabert-Mas A. Cystic renal cell carcinoma: pathological features, survival and implications for treatment. Br J Urol 1998;82:16.
14. Corica FA, Iczkowski KA, Cheng L, et al. Cystic renal cell carcinoma is cured by resection.: a study of 24 cases with long-term followup. J Urol 1999;161:408.
15. Nassir A, Jollimore J, Gupta R, et al. Multilocular cystic renal cell carcinoma: a series of 12 cases and review of the literature. Urology 2002;60:421.
16. Aronson S, Frazier HA, Baluch JD, et al. Cystic renal masses: Usefulness of the Bosniak classification. Urol Radiol 1991;13:83.
17. Curry NS, Cochran ST, Bissada NK. Cystic renal masses: accurate Bosniak classification requires adequate renal CT. AJR 2000;175:339.
18. Wilson TE, Doelle EA, Cohan RH, et al. Cystic renal masses: a reevaluation of the usefulness of the Bosniak classification system. Acad Radiol 1996;3:564.
19. Cloix P, Martin X, Pangaud C, et al. Surgical management of complex renal cysts: a series of 32 cases. J Urol 1996;156:28.
20. Koga S, Nishikido M, Inuzuka S, et al. An evaluation of Bosniak's radiological classification of cystic renal masses. BJU Int 2000;86:607.
21. Siegal CL, McFarland EG, Brink JA, et al. CT of cystic renal masses: analysis of diagnostic performance and interobserver variation. AJR 1997;169:813.
22. Siegal CL, Fisher AJ, Bennett HF. Interobserver variability in determining enhancement of renal masses on helical CT. AJR 1999;172:1207.

23. Heneghan JP, Spielmann AL, Sheafor DH, et al. Pseudoenhancement of simple renal cysts: a comparison of single and multidetector helical CT. J Comput Assist Tomogr 2002;26:90.

24. Bae KT, Heiken JP, Siegel CL, Bennett HF. Renal cysts: is attenuation artifactually increased on contrast-enhanced CT images? Radiology 2000;216:792.

25. Macari M, Bosniak MA. Delayed CT to evaluate renal masses incidentally discovered at contrast-enhanced CT: demonstration of vascularity with deenhancement. Radiology 1999;213:674.

26. Israel GM, Bosniak MA. Calcification in cystic renal masses: is it important in diagnosis? Radiology 2003;226:47.

27. Ho VB, Allen SF, Hood MN, Choyke PL. Renal masses: quantitative assessment of enhancement with dynamic MR imaging. Radiology 2002;224:695.

28. Chicoskie C, Chaoui A, Kuligowska E, et al. MRI isolation of infected renal cyst in autosomal dominant polycystic kidney disease. Clin Imaging 2001;25:114.

29. Balci NC, Semelka RC, Patt RH, et al. Complex renal cysts: findings on MR imaging. AJR 1999;172:1495.

30. Kim AY, Kim SH, Kim YJ, Lee IH. Contrast-enhanced power Doppler sonography for the differentiation of cystic renal lesions: preliminary study. J Ultrasound Med 1999;18:581.

31. Holmberg G, Hietala SO, Ljungberg B. A comparison of radiologic methods in the diagnosis of renal mass lesions. Scand J Urol Nephrol 1988;22:187.

32. Lang EK, Macchia RJ, Gayle B, et al. CT-guided biopsy of indeterminate renal cystic masses (Bosniak 3 and 2F): accuracy and impact on clinical management. Eur Radiol 2002;12:2518.

33. Dechet CB, Sebo T, Farrow G, et al. Prospective analysis of intraoperative frozen needle biopsy of solid renal masses in adults. J Urol 1999;162:1282.

34. Rovsing T. Treatment of multiloculated renal cysts with multiple punctures. Hospitalstid 1911;4:105.

35. Buck FN, Bunts RC, Dodson AI. Preservation of renal function in polycystic disease. J Urol 1951;66:46.

36. Bricker NS, Patton JF. Renal-function studies in polycystic disease of the kidneys with observations on the effects of surgical decompression. N Engl J Med 1957;256:212.

37. Milam JH, Magee JH, Bunts CR. Evaluation of surgical decompression operation in polycystic kidneys by differential renal clearances. J Urol 1963;90:144.

38. Prat V, Kocvara S. Evaluation of results after surgical treatment of polycystic kidneys by separate glomerular filtration tests. Rozhl Chir 1961;40:383.

39. Elzinga LW, Barry JM, Torres VE, et al. Cyst decompression surgery for autosomal dominant polycystic kidney disease. J Am Soc Nephrol 1992;2:1219.

40. Holmberg G, Hietala SO, Karp K, Ohberg L. Significance of simple renal cysts and percutaneous cyst puncture on renal function. Scand J Urol Nephrol 1994;28:35.

41. Gabow PA, Ikle DW, Holmes JH. Polycystic kidney disease: prospective analysis of nonazotemic patients and family members. Ann Intern Med 1984;101:238.

42. Elzinga LW, Barry JM, Torres VE, Bennett WM. Surgical management of painful polycystic kidneys. Am J Kidney Dis 1993;22:532.

43. Kinder PW, Rous SN. Infected renal cyst from hematogenous seeding: a case report and review of the literature. J Urol 1978;120:239.

44. Veerman JT, Cate HW. Case report: infected solitary renal cyst. Neth J Surg 1980;32:59.

45. Sklar AH, Caruana RJ, Lammers JE. Renal infections in autosomal dominant polycystic kidney disease. Am J Kidney Dis 1987;10:81.

46. Fuse H, Ohkawa M, Asamoto T. Infected renal cystic mass associated with bacterial meningitis: a case report. Int J Urol 1996;3:301.

47. Ueno Y, Hosaka K, Hosaka K, Takezaki T. A case of infected renal cyst extending to leg abscess. Hinyokika Kiyo 2000;46:105.

48. Muther RS, Bennett WM. Cyst fluid antibiotic concentrations in polycystic kidney disease: differences between proximal and distal cysts. Kidney Int 1981;20:519.

49. Chapman AB, Thickman D, Gabow PA. Percutaneous cyst puncture in the treatment of cyst infection in autosomal dominant polycystic kidney disease. Am J Kidney Dis 1990;16:252.

50. Hemal AK, Gupta NP, Rajeev TP, et al. Retroperitoneoscopic management of infected cysts in adult polycystic kidney disease. Urol Int 1999;62:40.

51. Nadu A, Hoznek A, Salomon L, et al. Laparoscopic retroperitoneal nephrectomy for aspergillus-infected polycystic kidney. J Endourol 2002;16:237.

52. Ameur A, Lezrek M, Boumdin H, et al. Hydatid cyst of the kidney based on a series of 34 cases. Prog Urol 2002;12:409.

53. Horchani A, Nouira Y, Kbaier I, et al. Hydatid cyst of the kidney. A report of 147 controlled cases. Eur Urol 2000;38:461.

54. Zmerli S, Ayed M, Horchani A, et al. Hydatid cyst of the kidney: diagnosis and treatment. World J Surg 2001;25:68.

55. Pedersen JF, Emamian SA, Nielsen MB. Significant association between simple renal cysts and arterial blood pressure. Br J Urol 1997;79:691.

56. Schwarz A, Lenz T, Klaen R, et al. Hygroma renale: pararenal lymphatic cysts associated with renin-dependent hypertension (Page kidney). Case report on bilateral cysts and successful therapy by marsupialization. J Urol 1993;150:953.

57. Ekici S, Ziraman I, Ozen H, Erkan I. Marsupialization for bilateral pararenal lymphatic cysts. Scand J Urol Nephrol 2000;34:77.

58. Bongu S, Faubert PF, Porush JG, Gulmi F. Uncontrolled hypertension and hyperreninemia after hemorrhage in a patient with end-stage renal disease and acquired renal cysts. J Am Soc Nephrol 1994;5:22.

59. Lezrek M, Fassi-Fehri H, Badet L, et al. Remission of erythrocytosis and hypertension after treatment of a giant renal cyst. Urology 2002;60:164.

60. Uemasu J, Fujiwara M, Munemura C, et al. Effects of topical instillation on cyst size and renal function in polycystic kidney disease. Clin Nephrol 1993;39:140.

61. Gettman MT, Unni KK, Segura JW. Unusual case of multilocular cystic nephroma with prominent renal pelvis involvement treated with nephron-sparing techniques. J Urol 1999;162:482.

62. Fujimoto K, Samma S, Fukui Y, et al. Spontaneously ruptured multilocular cystic nephroma. Int J Urol 2002;9:183.

63. Hinman F Jr. Obstructive renal cysts. J Urol 1978;119:681.

64. Zeliak NV, Seniv IN. Intestinal obstruction, caused by kidney cyst. Klin Khir 1993;6:53.

65. Amar AD, Das S. Surgical management of benign renal cysts causing obstruction of renal pelvis. Urology 1984;24:429.

66. Brown JA, Segura JW, Blute ML. A giant left renal cyst presenting as obesity: a unique presentation. Arch Esp Urol 1998;51:105.

67. Welch TR. Current management of selected childhood renal diseases. Curr Probl Pediatr 1992;22:432.

68. Middleton AW, Melzer RB. Neonatal multicystic kidney with associated respiratory distress, obstruction of contralateral ureter, and gastric compromise. Urology 1989;34:36.

69. Johanson K-E, Plaine L, Farcon E, Morales P. Management of intrarenal peripelvic cysts. Urology 1974;4:514.

70. Kropp KA, Grayhack JT, Wendel RM, Dahl DS. Morbidity and mortality of renal exploration for cyst. Surg Gynecol Obstet 1967;125:803.

71. Flemming TW, Barry JM. Bilateral open transperitoneal cyst reduction surgery for autosomal dominant polycystic kidney disease. J Urol 1998;159:44.

72. Wahlqvist L, Grumstedt B. Therapeutic effect of percutaneous puncture of simple renal cyst. Follow-up investigation of 50 patients. Acta Chir Scand 1966;132:340.

73. Ohkawa M, Tokunaga S, Orito M, et al. Percutaneous injection sclerotherapy with minocycline hydrochloride for simple renal cysts. Int Urol Nephrol 1993;25:37.

74. Phelan M, Zajko A, Hrebinko RL. Preliminary results of percutaneous treatment of renal cysts with povidone-iodine sclerosis. Urology 1999;53:816.

75. Liatsikos EN, Siablis D, Karnabatidis D, et al. Percutaneous treatment of large symptomatic renal cysts. J Endourol 2000;14:257.

76. Peyromaure M, Debre B, Flam TA. Sclerotherapy of a giant renal cyst with povidone-iodine. J Urol 2002;168:2525.

77. Kim SH, Moon MW, Lee HJ, et al. Renal cyst ablation with n-butyl cyanoacrylate and iodized oil in symptomatic patients with autosomal dominant polycystic kidney disease: Preliminary report. Radiology 2003;226:573.

78. Ohta S, Fujishiro Y, Fuse H. Polidocanol sclerotherapy for simple renal cysts. Urol Int 1997;58:145.

79. Gelet A, Snaseverino R, Martin X, et al. Percutaneous treatment of benign renal cysts. Eur Urol 1990;18:248.

80. De Dominicis C, Ciccariello M, Peris F, et al. Percutaneous sclerotization of simple renal cysts with 95% ethanol followed by 24-48 h drainage with nephrostomy tube. Urol Int 2001;66:18.

81. Delakas D, Karyotis I, Loumbakis P, et al. Long-term results after percutaneous minimally invasive procedure treatment of symptomatic simple renal cysts. Int Urol Nephrol 2001;32:321.

82. Bozkurt FB, Boyvat F, Tekin I, et al. Percutaneous sclerotherapy of a giant benign renal cyst with alcohol. Eur J Radiol 2001;40:64.

83. Chung BH, Kim JH, Hong CH, et al. Comparison of single and multiple sessions of percutaneous sclerotherapy for simple renal cyst. BJU Int 2000;85:626.

84. Hanna RM, Dahniya MH. Aspiration and sclerotherapy of symptomatic simple renal cysts: value of two injections of a sclerosing agent. AJR 1996;167:781.

85. Fontana D, Porpiglia F, Morra I, Destefanis P. Treatment of simple renal cysts by percutaneous drainage with three repeated alcohol injection. Urology 1999;53:904.

86. Paananen I, Hellstrom P, Leinonen S, et al. Treatment of renal cysts with single-session percutaneous drainage and ethanol sclerotherapy: long-term outcome. Urology 2001;57:30.

87. Bean WJ. Renal cysts: treatment with alcohol. Radiology 1981;138:329.

88. Camancho MF, Bondhus MJ, Carrion HM, et al. Ureteropelvic junction obstruction resulting from percutaneous cyst puncture and intracystic iophendylate injection: an unusual complication. J Urol 1980;124:713.

89. Lang EK. Renal cyst puncture and aspiration: a survey of complication. AJR 1977;128:723.

90. Beyer D, Fiedler V. Is renal cyst puncture an available diagnostic procedure for differentiation of avascular, space-occupying renal lesions? Urologe 1977;16A:339.

91. Rubenstein SC, Hulbert JC, Pharand D, et al. Laparoscopic ablation of symptomatic renal cysts. J Urol 1993;150:1103.

92. Guazzoni G, Montorsi F, Bergamaschi F, et al. Laparoscopic unroofing of simple renal cysts. Urology 1994;43:154.

93. Hulbert JC, Hunter D, Young AT, Castañeda-Zúñiga W. Percutaneous intrarenal marsupialization of a perirenal cystic collection-Endocystolysis. J Urol 1988;139:1039.

94. Kavoussi LR, Clayman RV, Mikkelsen DJ, Meretyk S. Ureteronephroscopic marsupialization of obstructing peripelvic renal cyst. J Urol 1991;146:411.

95. Liaconis H, Pautler SE, Razvi HA. Ureteroscopic decompression of an unusual uroepithelial cyst using the holmium:YAG laser. J Endourol 2001;15:295.

96. Kavoussi LR, Clayman RV, Basler J. Flexible, actively deflectable fiberoptic ureteronephroscopy. J Urol 1989;142:949.

97. Kang Y, Noble C, Gupta M. Percutaneous resection of renal cysts. J Endourol 2001;15:738.

98. Plas EG, Hübner WA. Percutaneous resection of renal cysts: a long-term followup. J Urol 1993;149:703.

99. Ubara Y, Tagami T, Sawa N, et al. Renal contraction therapy for enlarged polycystic kidneys by transcatheter arterial embolization in hemodialysis patients. Am J Kidney Dis 2002;39:571.

Part III

Ureteroscopy

Rigid Ureteroscopes

Jim M. Adshead, MA, MD, FRCS (Urol.)
Anup Patel, MS, FRCS (Urol.)

In 1912 the first endoscopic visualization of the upper urinary tract was performed by Hugh Hampton Young. He achieved this by passing a 9.5 French (F) cystoscope directly to the renal pelvis of a child with megaureters.[1] Could our distinguished forefathers have predicted the technological advances in optics and instrumentation that have occurred thus far? The improvements in retrograde endoscopy of the upper urinary tract in recent times have been so fast and revolutionary that it is almost too difficult to imagine the ureteroscope of tomorrow.

The ultimate aim for patients is to diagnose and treat upper tract disease without the need for intervention, but although molecular diagnosis has made some inroads into reducing the need for endoscopy of the lower urinary tract, such applications are still very unreliable in the upper urinary tract. With improvements in the quality of radiologic imaging up to the point of virtual time of flight sequences with surface rendering (Figure 24A-1), development of quantitative urinary molecular markers of malignancy, extracorporeal and percutaneous treatments of upper tract pathology, ureteroscopic indications should have diminished by now, but in reality, the exact opposite has been true. The indications for ureteroscopy have been heavily scrutinized in some quarters, where it has been suggested that extracorporeal shock wave lithotripsy (ESWL) can be so successful at stone fragmentation that the ureteroscope could be "thrown away."[2] Provocative though this view-point may be, it is undeniable that ureteroscopy is currently going through an unprecedented renaissance and remains an invaluable diagnostic and interventional modality in the management of pathology as diverse as ureteric stones, strictures from urethro-vesical anastomosis—through ejaculatory duct to ureter and beyond (ureteropelvic junction [UPJ], intrarenal, and calyceal)—not to mention upper tract urothelial malignancy. It has allowed the possibility of precise targeting of energy sources under direct vision as well as providing a means of obtaining biopsy material from visibly abnormal or suspicious urothelium, and it is the final arbiter of diagnosis and therapy, where other less invasive modalities have failed. Nevertheless, controversy and debate continue as to whether ureteric stones are best treated ureteroscopically or with ESWL, particularly with reference to cost-benefit analysis. The advantages for ureteroscopy for stones in the distal ureter are undeniable, while upper and midureteral stone locations still remain controversial.

This chapter covers the historical evolution of ureteroscopy and ureterorenoscopy as well as the technical advances so far encompassed in modern ureteroscope design.

It would seem sensible to address these advances under the following categories.

- History
- Optical system and eyepiece design
- Sheath and tip design for atraumatic insertion
- Working channels
- Current designs
- Rigid versus flexible ureteroscopes.

HISTORY

Routine rigid ureteroscopy was first reported over a quarter of a century ago, in 1977, by Goodman[3] and by Lyon and colleagues.[4] Advances in fiberoptics had precociously led to the development and use of flexible ureteroscopes over a decade earlier, but their use did not achieve widespread acceptance at this time because of their limited capabilities. These early pioneering ureteroscopists did, however, demonstrate that excursion into the ureter was feasible.

Goodman reported using a pediatric cystoscope (11F) to inspect the distal ureters in 3 adults. In one of these patients, a distal ureteral tumor was fulgurated, marking the first ureteroscopically treated tumor. Lyon and colleagues[4] reported ureteroscopy in 5 adults using Jewett sounds for ureteral dilation before passing an 11F pediatric cystoscope. Most of these early ureteroscopy patients were women. Lyon and colleagues[5] reported in 1979 the use of specially designed ureteral dilators attached to the tip of a flexible probe. They were able to dilate the orifice to 16F, permitting insertion of a standard length 13F cystoscope for distal ureteroscopy in men. These early investigators demonstrated the ease and safety of rigid ureteroscopy for the distal ureter in both sexes.

The innovative work of Harold Hopkins made possible the further development of smaller rigid ureteroscopes. He revolutionized endoscope design when he developed the rod-lens system for rigid endoscopes in 1960.[6] Until then, endoscopic telescopes consisted of a hollow tube with a distal objective lens, an ocular lens, and a series of relay lenses through the length of the tube. These lenses had to remain in precise alignment. Any displacement of the lens resulted in loss of image transmission. There was also a significant loss of light transmission with this system, even under normal circumstances. The rod-lens system replaced the air spaces in the old design with glass rods. The air spaces between these rods functioned as the relay lenses. The telescope system was now made primarily of glass, which has a higher refractive index than air. The light and image transmission through this telescope was much more efficient. This made it possible for smaller outer diameter endoscopes to be more easily developed for use as ureteroscopes.

Richard Wolf Medical Instruments designed an endoscope specifically for ureteroscopy. Its use was reported in 1979 by Lyon and colleagues.[5] Modeled after the pediatric cystoscope, this 13F instrument had a working length of 23 cm. Sheath sizes of 14.5 and 16F, and a 16F resectoscope sheath were also available. The 13F sheath was used only for inspection, but the larger sheaths allowed simultaneous passage of a ureteral catheter or basket for stone manipulation and removal. For the first time, ureteral calculi were visualized, engaged in a basket, and removed.[5,7] A longer ureteroscope that could reach all the way to the renal pelvis was developed by Enriqué Pérez-Castro in collaboration with Karl Storz Endoscopy, and its use was reported in 1980.[8] Its 39 cm length allowed inspection of the renal pelvis for the first time. The other endoscope manufacturers quickly followed suit with rigid ureteroscopes in lengths

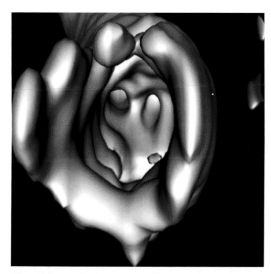

Figure 24A-1 Magnetic resonance image ureteroscopy with surface rendering.

ranging from 25 to 54 cm, sheath sizes of 9 to 16F, and working channels of 5F. Most of these designs used interchangeable lenses with 0- and 70-degree angles of view.

Ureteroscopy is most often performed for the treatment of urolithiasis. A major advancement in this field occurred with the introduction of ureteroscopic ultrasonic lithotripsy techniques. The early ultrasound probes were hollow, which allowed simultaneous destruction and removal of ureteral and renal calculi.[9] Unfortunately, the initial probes were 8F in diameter and not small enough to pass through the working channel of the ureteroscope. With these early devices, the stone was reached with the ureteroscope, visualized, and the telescope removed to allow placement of the ultrasound probe on the stone for treatment. The obvious disadvantage of this blind system was the potential for ureteral injury. Smaller solid probes (1.5–2.0 mm) were developed that could pass through the working channels but were too rigid to negotiate the angled instrument working ports.[10] The solution to this problem was the introduction of the offset eyepiece telescopes. These telescopes enabled the urologist to pass the ultrasound probe through a straight working channel of the ureteroscope to treat the stone under direct visual control. Rigid ureteroscopes were later designed with an interchangeable offset eyepiece and standard telescope. The ureteroscope could be more easily passed up the ureter using the standard telescope. This telescope could then be exchanged for one with an offset eyepiece for ultrasonic lithotripsy. A modification of this ureteroscope system came with the development of the Rigiflex ureteroscope by ACMI (Stamford, CT). This ureteroscope used flexible fiberoptics to produce a flexible "gooseneck" eyepiece. The eyepiece could be straightened for introduction into the ureteroscope and later deflected out of the way (or offset) for ultrasonic lithotripsy. The ACMI HTO-5 instrument was introduced in 1985 and was the first ureteroscope with a fiberoptic imaging system. It had a 5F single channel in a fairly rigid 12.7F shaft, while comparable rod-lens ureteroscopes of the time with a 5F work channel were 14.5 to 15F in size. These basic principles of ureteroscope design incorporating a straight working channel are still in use today. These types of ureteroscopes are used not only for ultrasonic lithotripsy, but also to accommodate use of larger sturdy reusable rigid working instruments 4 to 5F in size.

Improvements in the rod lens and fiberoptic lens systems, and the availability of smaller working instruments, permitted the development of smaller rigid ureteroscopes. Problems with the insertion of the larger ureteroscopes also made it apparent that smaller ureteroscopes were needed. In 1989, Huffman described a compact ureteroscope that was 8.5F in diameter and had a working channel of 3.5F.[11] The rod-lens telescope was integrated into the ureteroscope, which helped decrease the outer diameter while maintaining a good-sized working channel.

Laser lithotripsy, using the Candela laser company's pulsed-dye laser, reported in the late 1980s,[12] became a popular technique and prompted the use of other laser energy sources for lithotripsy in later years. The Candela laser company's thin, semirigid ureteroscope was the first to incorporate two independent channels, one for an accessory and one for flow, each of 2.1F size. It was the success of this 41 cm instrument with a 7.3F distal section that established it as the benchmark instrument of its time and prompted other U.S. manufacturers to develop competitive instruments of similar design, such as the MR-6 ureteroscope from ACMI. The MR-6 proved to be much more durable than the Candela scope and quickly gained supremacy. It had a sub-7F distal section with larger throughput capacity of one 2F and one 3F device in separate channels. The final distal shape was determined by enclosing the smallest size optical system the engineers could conceive at the time, along with the two separate throughput channels in a triangular-shaped outer tube, giving a 6.9F distal section. For the image system, by designing a conventional glass objective coupled to a 0.5 mm diameter fused quartz fiber bundle, more individual pixels of optical information were provided than the etched glass fiber bundle in either the Candela or the HTO-5 scopes. It came in a short 33 cm length version to allow access to the distal ureter and up to the UPJ of females. The MR-6L was 41 cm long and was intended for use in males and obese patients.

The recent introduction of holmium laser lithotripsy for the treatment of upper urinary tract stone disease in 1996[13] has been a huge step forward in endoscopic stone treatment, and is now the bedrock of contact lithotripsy in most departments with a tertiary referral practice. Its precision, minimal penetration into tissue (0.4 mm), and low potential for collateral damage has allowed safe use within ureter and renal pelvis. With regard to ureteroscope design, a further advantage of holmium laser lithotripsy is the ability to use very small fibers (200 and 365 micron) to deliver the laser energy to the stone, allowing deployment through yet smaller working channels and therefore smaller outer diameter ureteroscopes, or much improved flow and therefore better vision.

OPTICAL SYSTEM AND EYEPIECE DESIGN

Rigid ureteroscopes can be made with either flexible fiberoptic or rod-lens optical systems. The rod-lens systems provide excellent optical quality, but have larger diameters and do not allow angulation of the rigid ureteroscope. With angulation of a rigid ureteroscope using a rod-lens telescope, a dark crescent-shaped area will impinge on the image. These rod-lens telescopes can be interchangeable (from 0- to 70-degree angle of view) or integrated within the ureteroscope itself. The 70-degree lens is primarily used to inspect the

renal pelvis and calices with the rigid ureteroscope. With the development of high-quality flexible ureterorenoscopes that can be used to inspect the entire upper urinary system, these 70-degree lenses are now virtually obsolete. The interchangeable telescopes permitted some flexibility in the past, however, because a single telescope could be used with different sheath sizes. Most current rigid rod-lens ureteroscopes have integrated telescopes because of their smaller size advantage. The angle of view of these telescopes is usually 0 to 5 degrees. The advantage of a slight angulation of view is easier and quicker visualization of working instruments being passed out of the tip, reducing the potential for inadvertent iatrogenic injury to the normal urothelium.

The advantages of using flexible fiberoptics for image transmission are the lack of image distortion with angulation of the instrument, and a smaller diameter image transmission system that permits larger working channels within the same size scopes. Flexible fiberoptic image bundles are used in all of the new semirigid or miniureteroscopes and those ureteroscopes using a movable or flexible eyepiece.[14] Light transmission through the ureteroscope is provided by fiberoptic bundles in most current designs (Figure 24A-2).

The disadvantage of fiberoptic image bundles is the graining effect seen. The pixel density in most current semirigid ureteroscopes has now increased beyond 30,000, such that the images are much closer in quality and size to those of the traditional rod-lens system (Figure 24A-3).

Several different eyepiece designs are also available currently for rigid ureteroscopes. There has been a recent move away from the ocular focusing capability of ureteroscopes, which is now thought to be redundant for two reasons. Firstly, manufacturer resources have concentrated on improving camera quality, and secondly, the focusing mechanisms compromise the intent to design truly autoclavable scopes. The standard ureteroscope eyepiece was straight and in line with the scope axis, just like rigid cystoscopes. This design allowed easy introduction of the ureteroscope through the lower urinary tract and into the ureter. As discussed earlier, offset eyepieces became necessary when rigid ultrasound probes were developed for ureteroscopic lithotripsy. These probes, as well as larger more rigid working instruments, required a straight working channel for passage through the scope. These offset eyepieces could be either fixed or movable. Fixed offset eyepieces can be either angled or offset, but straight and parallel to the ureteroscope shaft, such as the Wolf designs based on the Marberger and Bichler models (Figure 24A-4).

SHEATH AND TIP DESIGN FOR ATRAUMATIC INSERTION

Early ureteroscopes were designed with sheath tips much like cystoscopes. These beaked tips caused problems with the introduction of the tip into the ureteral orifice and advancement of the ureteroscope. This tip design could result in ploughing of the ureteral epithelium. Most current tips are beveled for easier advancement into the ureter. The working channels are triangular or oval in cross-section to allow irrigation to continue around the sides of any deployed instrument within. Ureteroresectoscopes incorporate manually operated working elements much like standard transurethral resectoscopes. The tips of these scopes can also be insulated to permit use with electrocautery. Working elements, including resecting loops, cold and hot knife blades, and fulguration electrodes, can all be used with these ureteroresectoscopes. The range of tip designs of currently available ureteroscopes are shown in Figure 24A-5.

WORKING CHANNELS

To miniaturize ureteroscopes, the manufacturers combined smaller working channels and fiberop-

tics and incorporated them into a metal sheath. The optical system was much smaller using fiberoptics and could also be "bent" without distortion of the image. Dretler and Cho[15] first described this type of scope, which was developed with Candela, in 1989. The tip of the scope was 7.2F in diameter and it had two 2.1F working channels. Passing the smaller scope up the ureter often did not require active pre-dilation of the orifice. Smaller (6.9F) outer diameter scopes with larger working channels (3.4 and 2.3F) have been subsequently developed.[14] Having two separate channels meant that the operator could work through one channel without impeding irrigation flow through the other. It also allowed the simultaneous use of laser fiber and a basket or other such accessory while maintaining some flow. Most ureteroscopes are designed with oval-shaped accessory channels to allow irrigation to continue despite placement of an accessory. These twin-channel ureteroscopes incorporate a straight channel for more rigid accessories as well as a smaller channel for irrigation or a second accessory as shown in Figure 24A-6A. However, there are concerns about damaging the angled working channels by deployment of laser fibers. The repetitive angulation strain on the brittle quartz laser fiber can cause microfractures, and subsequent use may inadvertently release laser energy inside the working channel.

Furthermore, it is not practical to use even small diameter pneumatic lithotripsy probes through these angled channels owing to the frictional forces caused by the angulation. Miniureteroscopes or semirigid ureteroscopes, as these have come to be known, are probably still the most popular rigid ureteroscopes today.

A larger single channel permits the use of larger instruments and possible removal of small stone fragments or biopsy specimens through the sheath. The larger single channels can also permit dual instrumentation and the manufacturer labels are a useful reminder on size of accessory permitted via each channel port (Figure 24A-6B). The choice of design depends on the preference of the individual surgeon. The use of this design has facilitated the reduction in sheath diameter without compromising the working channel diameter.

CURRENT DESIGNS

Rigid ureteroscopes are available today in many of the designs previously described. Both inte-

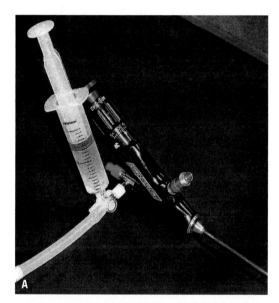

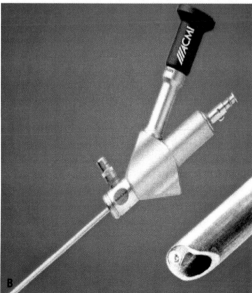

Figure 24A-2 Fiberoptic bundle for light transmission in modern ureteroscope design.

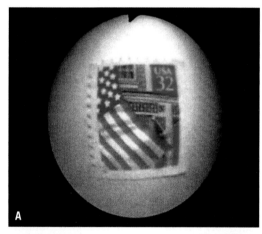

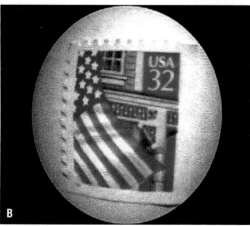

Figure 24A-3 With the latest improvements in image bundle density the image size can be increased without compromising the quality.

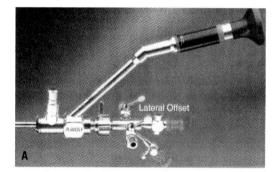

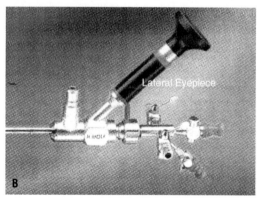

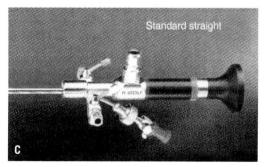

Figure 24A-4 The latest Wolf "E-line" series demonstrates the available eyepiece designs. These facilitate both easy insertion under direct vision with the standard design, as well as the ability to use straight rigid accessories in comfort with the offset designs.

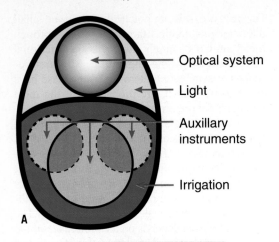

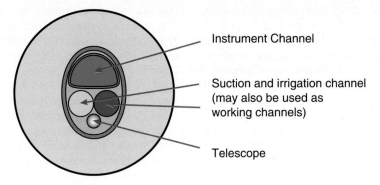

Figure 24A-7 Tip configuration of the Gelet ureteroscope.

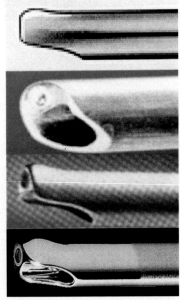

Figure 24A-5 *A*, The cross section depicts the possibilities available with single large- or twin-channel scopes with irrigation maintained. *B*, The tips from Storz, ACMI, Wolf, and Olympus are shown sequentially from top to bottom. The tips come beaked, beveled, and flat, as each manufacturer argues a case for easier atraumatic negotiation of the ureteric orifice.

grated and interchangeable rod-lens scopes are available. Ureteroresectoscopes are available in 9 to 12F sizes. The various offset eyepiece designs are available from most manufacturers, with the tips of the scopes ranging in size from 6.9 to 12.0F. Probably the most frequently used rigid ureteroscopes are the miniureteroscopes with fiberoptic imaging systems. Current designs have higher resolution, increased pixel density, and larger and brighter images.

Since the introduction of laser lithotripsy, particularly using the holmium laser, large working channels are less frequently needed for safe fragmentation itself. Likewise, many flexible acces-

sories and electrohydraulic lithotripsy can also now be used with probes as small as 1.6F. Most disposable working instruments are also available in sizes of 3F or less. Because of these advancements, many believe that a working channel of 3.4F may be adequate for most ureteroscopic work. The disadvantage of the 3.4F working channels is that many of the reusable rigid accessories will not pass because they are > 4F, with the obvious additional cost when expensive disposable accessories have to be used. These miniscopes can also be passed into the ureteral orifice without previous dilation in the majority of patients, and their fiberoptics permit a small amount of angulation, as described above. The Gelet scope from Storz incorporates an eyepiece and a light connection that are remote from the instrument itself to free up the working area. With this design, the operator can now use both hands to manipulate working instruments, while the optics are held remotely. In addition to two 3F channels for irrigation and suction or deployment of a disposable accessory, there is a larger ovoid central 4F work channel for interchangeable use of flexible and rigid accessories (Figure 24A-7). This does mean, however, that the instrument tip is not small at 10.5F, and the shaft gradually increases in a stepwise fashion to a base diameter of 13.5F.

Other instrument manufacturers (eg, ACMI and Olympus) have recently made attempts to reduce the trauma of insertion through modified shaft design and manufacture. The stepless dilation of the ureter using these new tapered shaft designs seems an attractive option, but it is yet to be conclusively shown that they are less traumatic than the traditional stepwise increase in sheath diameter. Previously, with the stepped shafts, bend stress was concentrated at solder points, leading ultimately to instrument failure at these sites. This possibility may be eliminated by the newer tapered shafts, which may ultimately be more durable as well as less traumatic.

The characteristics of the latest designs of currently available fiberoptic rigid ureteroscopes are given in Table 24A-1.

RIGID VERSUS FLEXIBLE URETEROSCOPES

Rigid and flexible ureteroscopes are used in a complementary fashion to access the entire upper urinary tract.[16] So complementary, in fact, that it is common practice to first use the semirigid ureteroscope (with its graduated increase in diameter) to optically dilate the lower ureter, both to ease passage of the flexible scope and increase the longevity of the delicate smaller caliber flexible ureterorenoscopes, as well as to maximally dilate the ureteral orifice to allow for atraumatic removal for larger stone fragments from the ureter at a later stage once fragmentation is completed. The rigid ureteroscopes are ideal for treating pathology in the lower ureter, particularly below the level of the iliac vessels, as this portion of the ureter can easily be accessed with this instrument in most patients. The advantages of rigid ureteroscopes include ease of introduction into the orifice under direct vision, excellent image transmission, and larger flow and working channels. Flexible ureteroscopes, on the other hand, are better suited for the upper ureter, renal pelvis, and calices. Flexible ureteroscopes are more difficult to use in the lower ureter because of their tendency to buckle into the bladder (though this can be overcome up to a point by passing them over a working guidewire to stiffen the shaft temporarily during insertion, before this working wire is sacrificed). The advantages of the flexible ureteroscopes are their ability to safely negotiate the angulations of the ureter, and they can access the entire upper collecting system in over 90% of patients with active and secondary passive deflection,[17] and now with secondary

Table 24A-1 Latest Data Summary of Semirigid Ureteroscope Characteristics

Model	Eyepiece	Tip Style	Mode of Ureteral Dilation	Diameter (F)	Working Length (cm)	No. of Channels	Size of Channel (F)	Field of View (degrees)	Angle of View (degrees)	Autoclavable	Focusing Ocular
ACMI (Stamford, CT)											
MRO-742A	Angle offset	Beveled Cutaway	Stepless	7 / 9.2 / 11.2	42	1	5.4	65	5	Yes	No
MRO-733 (742/715)	Angle offset	Beveled Cutaway	Stepwise	7.7 / 9.2 / 10.8	33 / 42 / 15	1	5.4	65	5	No*	Yes
MRO-633 (642)	Angle offset	Beveled	Stepwise	6.9 / 8.3 / 10.2	33 / 42	2	2.3 and 3.4	65	5	No*	Yes
MR-6 (6L/PC)	Standard	Beveled	Stepwise	6.9 / 8.3 / 10.2	33 / 42 / 15.5	2	2.3 and 3.4	65	5	No*	Yes
Olympus America (Lake Success, NY, and Tokyo, Japan)											
A2940/41A	Angle offset	Beaked	Stepless	6.4 / 7.8	43 / 33	1	4.2	90	7	Yes	No
A2942A	Angle offset	Beaked	Stepless	8.6 / 9.8	43	1	6.6	90	7	Yes	No
A2948/49A	Standard	Beaked	Stepless	6.4 / 7.8	43 / 33	1	4.2	90	7	Yes	No
A2943A	Angled	Flat	None	7.5	43	2	2.4 and 3.4	90	7	Yes	No
A2944/46A	Standard	Flat	None	7.5	43 / 33	2	2.4 and 3.4	90	7	Yes	No
Karl Storz Endoscopy (Culver City, CA, and Tuttlingen, Germany											
27410	Standard	Beaked	Stepwise	7.5 / 9 / 10.5	SL-34 / SK-43	2	2.5 and 4	60	8	Yes	No
27430	Angle offset	Beaked	Stepwise	8 / 9 / 10.5	K-34 / L-43	1	5	60	8	Yes	No
27023	Standard	Beaked	Stepwise	10 / 10.5 / 12 / 13	SA-34 / SB-43	1	5.5	60	8	Yes	No
27411	Angle offset	Beaked	Stepwise	10 / 10.5 / 12 / 13	K-34 / L-43	1	5.5	60	8	Yes	No
Richard Wolf Medical Instruments (Vernon Hills, IL, and Knittlinger, Germany)											
8702 (.523, .524)	Marberger Angle offset	Beaked	Stepless	6 / 7.5	.523–31.5 / .524–43	1 or 2	4 or 2×2.4F	–	5	Yes	No
8703 (.523, .524)	Marberger Angle offset	Beaked	Stepless	8 / 9.8	.523–31.5 / .524–43	1 or 2	5 or 2×3F	–	12	Yes	No
8702 (.533, .534)	Bichler Angle offset	Beaked	Stepless	6 / 7.5	.533–31.5 / .534–43	1 or 2	4 or 2×2.4F	–	5	Yes	No
8703 (.533, .534)	Bichler Angle offset	Beaked	Stepless	8 / 9.8	.523–31.5 / .524–43	1 or 2	5 or 2×3F	–	12	Yes	No

Information as available from manufacturers.
*Autoclavable from 2004.

active deflection.[18] Expertise with both rigid and flexible ureteroscopy allows the urologist to more safely diagnose and treat problems anywhere inside the upper urinary tract collecting system.

REFERENCES

1. Young HH, McKay RW. Congenital valvular obstruction of the prostatic urethra. Surg Gynecol Obstet 1929;48:509.
2. Olsburgh J, Ramsay J. Lithotripsy for ureteric stones: throw away the ureteroscope. BJU Int 2003;91:771–2.
3. Goodman TM. Ureteroscopy with paediatric cystoscope in adults. Urology 1977;9:394.
4. Lyon ES, Kyker JS, Schoenberg HW. Transurethral ureteroscopy in women: a ready addition to the urological armamentarium. J Urol 1978;119:35–6.
5. Lyon ES, Banno JJ, Schoenberg HW. Transurethral ureteroscopy in men using juvenile cystoscopy equipment. J Urol 1979;122:152–3.
6. Hopkins HH. British patent 954,629 and U.S. patent 3,257,902. 1960.
7. Huffman JL, Bagley DH, Lyon ES. Treatment of distal ureteral calculi using rigid ureteroscope. Urology 1982;20:574–7.
8. Pérez-Castro Ellendt E, Martinez-Piñeiro JA. [Transurethral ureteroscopy. A current urological procedure.] Arch Esp Urol 1980;33:445–60.
9. Huffman JL, Bagley DH, Schoenberg HW, Lyon ES. Transurethral removal of large ureteral and renal pelvis calculi using ureteroscopic ultrasonic lithotripsy. J Urol 1983;130:31–4.
10. Chaussy C, Fuchs G, Kahn R, et al. Transurethral ultrasonic ureterolithotripsy using a solid-wire probe. Urology 1987;29:531–2.
11. Huffman JL. Experience with the 8.5 French compact rigid ureteroscope. Semin Urol 1989;7:3–6.
12. Dretler SP, Watson G, Parrish JA, Murray S. Pulsed dye laser fragmentation of ureteral calculi: initial clinical experience. J Urol 1987;137:386–9.
13. Grasso M. Experience with the holmium laser as an endoscopic lithotrite. Urology 1996;48:199–206.
14. Abdel-Razzak OM, Bagley DH. The 6.9 F semi rigid ureteroscope in clinical use. Urology 1993;41:45–8.
15. Dretler SP, Cho G. Semirigid ureteroscopy: a new genre. J Urol 1989;141:1314–6.
16. Bagley DH. Ureteroscopy. AUA Update Series 1994;13:206.
17. Bagley DH. Intrarenal access with the flexible ureteropyeloscope: effects of active and passive tip deflection. J Endourol 1993;7:221–4.
18. Conlin M, Patel A, Schulam P, et al. Improved ureteroscopic access to the lower pole: results with a prototype flexible ureteroscope incorporating active secondary deflection. J Endourol 2002;16 Suppl 1:8–4, A29.

Flexible Ureterorenoscopes

Anup Patel, MS, FRCS (Urol.)

Jim M. Adshead, MA, MD, FRCS (Urol.)

Both flexible and rigid ureteroscopes are used in a complementary fashion to access, inspect, and treat pathology throughout the entire upper urinary tract collecting system.[1] The application of flexible ureteroscopy (9 French [F]) to visualize an impacted ureteral stone was first reported by Marshall in 1964.[2] Three years later, in 1966, Tagaki and colleagues[3] placed a similar instrument through an open ureterotomy to visualize the intrarenal anatomy. The subsequent development of a cystoscopically placed guide tube into the ureter (the original access sheath) allowed irrigant flow around the perimeter of the instrument for better visualization of the ureteral mucosa and pathology,[4] and by the 1980s, the irrigant channel and a working channel were combined and incorporated into the next generation of ureteroscopes at the University of Chicago by Bagley and colleagues.[5,6]

The upper ureter and particularly the intrarenal collecting system are both better suited to flexible ureteroscopes because of the angulations of the intrarenal collecting system, and therefore, perhaps they should really be called flexible ureterorenoscopes. Flexible ureterorenoscopes can be passed more safely beyond the iliac vessels, and then advanced all the way up to the calices under direct visual control, overcoming any undulations of the ureter around crossing vasculature. Often dilation of the ureteral orifice may not be required, especially now that disposable ureteral access sheaths are more widely available. The utility of flexible ureterorenoscopy has steadily increased as technological improvements have continued to be made in both instrument size and design. Advances in fiberoptic technology, improved deflecting mechanisms, and a greater diversity of working instrumentation, have all increased our ability to diagnose and treat a wider range of upper urinary tract disorders than was ever possible before.

All flexible ureterorenoscopes have similar essential basic components. These include a fiberoptic imaging bundle, a light transmission system, working channel, and deflection mechanism. The variations come in instrument size, the way that the light pillar is incorporated into the instrument, and whether the work channel is movable or fixed in position. We will review the characteristics of the latest designs of currently available flexible ureterorenoscopes.

OPTICAL SYSTEM

When light travels in a transparent medium such as glass, internal reflection of the light occurs at the interface between that medium and its surroundings. This was first demonstrated in 1854 by John Tyndall of London.[7] This physical property of internal reflection allows the "bending" of light within flexible glass. It was not until 1927 that the first patent for light transmission using glass fiber bundles was submitted. Current fiberoptic technology is based on this physical property of light demonstrated over a century ago.

Small-diameter flexible fibers can be fashioned out of molten glass. These fibers will uniformly transmit light from one end to the other, proportional to the light input. When they are bundled together with identical fiber orientation at each end (ie, coherent), these dots of light will coalesce to transmit images.[7–10] Improvements in fiberoptic technology have allowed bundling together of more fibers to produce sharper images. Newer techniques of cladding the fibers with a second layer of glass have improved their light transmission further. This second layer of glass has a different refractive index than the core glass. The interface between these two different glasses produces the internal reflection and is much more durable than previous uncladded designs.[7,9] This cladding does not transmit light and causes the meshlike ("chicken-wire") appearance of the image known as the Moiré effect. These advances in fiberoptics have improved imaging abilities, in turn allowing a reduction in size of the imaging part of the instrument, and allowing for both larger working channels and smaller outer diameters of the newer flexible ureterorenoscopes (Figure 24B-1).

The image transmission through the endoscope is dependent on a relatively clear, well-lit field. Light transmission to the tip of the scope begins with the source lamp. The most commonly used source lamps are halogen (150 watts) and xenon (300 watts).[9] A flexible light cord, which is also made up of fiberoptic bundles, transmits the light to the ureteroscope. This light cord can either plug onto a post on the ureteroscope (a separate cord) or be incorporated into the ureteroscope (an integrated cord). Further, one manufacturer (ACMI) of scopes with a separate cord has patented a rotatable light cord connection post so that it can be rotated into a convenient place for the operator, whilst accessing the work channel. The fiber bundles of an integrated light cord are continuous with the light fiber bundles traveling through the scope. A separate light cord will connect to a post on the scope to transmit light to the light fiber bundles. This connection invariably pro-

duces some loss of light power because of the inability to get perfect alignment of the fibers of the cord with those of the ureteroscope itself. This is usually not a significant problem because much more light is transmitted via the cord than is actually needed. The advantage of having a separate light cord is that only the cord must be replaced if it is damaged. In the instrument itself, the light is then transmitted through fiber bundles traveling along the full length of the shaft to the tip of the scope. Flexible ureterorenoscopes can carry either one or more of these light bundles (Figure 24B-2).

The light fibers in the cord and the scope don't need to be coherent because they are not responsible for image transmission.[7,9] This makes the manufacturing process easier and less costly than for the image fiber bundles. Only one manufacturer (Circon ACMI) has so far managed to incorporate a patented rotatable light post at right angles to the axis of the instrument, housed in the proximal portion of the handpiece of a flexible ureterorenoscope. This post has a 130-degree range of movement to improve the ergonomics of ease of access to the working portion of the instrument and can be fitted with a removable light cord. Using similar design, the work channel lower down the handpiece is also rotatable through 90 degrees.

The angle of view from the tip of the instrument can be modified by changing the axis of the optical system at the tip.[11] This is usually accomplished with a wedge lens system at the distal end of the imaging bundle. This modified angle of view can be up to 10 degrees in fluid and is help-

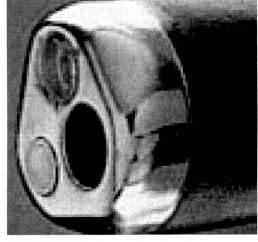

Figure 24B-1 Tip design of a flexible ureteroscope demonstrating the ends of the optical system, light transmission bundle, and working channel.

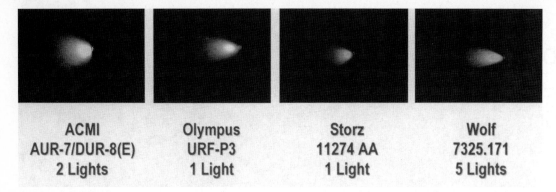

| ACMI
AUR-7/DUR-8(E)
2 Lights | Olympus
URF-P3
1 Light | Storz
11274 AA
1 Light | Wolf
7325.171
5 Lights |

Figure 24B-2 Lighting bundles and light patterns from the tips of different flexible ureterorenoscopes.

ful in visualizing working instruments as they emerge from the tip of the scope 29. This is particularly helpful when using the more translucent laser fibers, which, being made of quartz, can easily cause inadvertent damage to the urothelium if not carefully directed away. This is summarized in Figure 24B-3.

Flexible fiberoptics do have a drawback, as they provide a limited depth of field compared with the rod-lens optical system of the rigid endoscopes. To compensate for this relative deficiency, a focusing lens system is provided for flexible ureteroscopes. A virtual image is produced by the ocular lens at the eyepiece. The distance between the virtual image and the operator's eye is adjusted by the focusing control. Changing this distance compensates for any visual acuity differences between operators and allows for variation in the depth of field. Image magnification is also available (303–503) and will vary depending on the distance from the object being imaged to the tip of the scope. Greater magnification is produced the closer an object is to the distal tip.[7] The Wolf Viper flexible ureterorenoscope gives a large-screen image with up to a twofold better resolution[12] owing to its unique fused quartz bundle

design rather than using a glass bundle. The optical characteristics of each of the recently available flexible ureteroscopes are reviewed and summarized in Table 24B-1.

DEFLECTION MECHANISM

The early flexible ureterorenoscopes were only passively deflectable. There was no mechanism to actively control the tip deflection, and the ureterorenoscope was left to follow the course of the ureter or guidewire over which it traveled. This significantly reduced its usefulness, since only the most easily accessible portions of the upper urinary tract (ureter, renal pelvis, and possibly the upper calices) could be visualized.[13–16] Almost all current flexible ureterorenoscopes are equipped with a mechanism for primary active tip deflection in both directions in one plane,[17] while retaining the capability for passive secondary deflection. This active deflection is controlled by a manually operated thumb lever mechanism located on the hand-held portion of the ureterorenoscope, which places tension on control wires that run from here through movable metal rings within the ureterorenoscope shaft to

the distal tip where the wires are fixed.[7,16] The wires are effectively shortened by moving the control lever in order to get a range of deflection, which varies between scope models from different manufacturers. This results in tip deflection in the direction of that wire. Deflection in the opposite direction is accomplished by a wire on the opposite side of the ureteroscope. Deflection can be logical (an upward deflection on the handle deflects the scope tip upward, and vice versa), or it can be "reverse logic" (an upward deflection on the handle deflects the scope tip downward, as is the case with most European- and Japanese-designed instruments). Improvements in primary active deflection mechanisms now allow controlled deflection of the tip up to 180 degrees up or down in the same plane.

The optimal amount of tip deflection necessary to examine the entire intrarenal collecting system was determined to help with the design of flexible ureteroscopes. Bagley and Rittenberg measured the angle between the major axis of the ureter and the lower-pole infundibulum (the ureteroinfundibular angle) from the radiographs of 30 patients.[18] The average angle was 140 degrees with a maximum of 175 degrees. Primary active deflection of 175 degrees should allow ureteroscopic negotiation of this ureteroinfundibular angle in most patients.

The addition of secondary passive deflection allows lengthening of the deflected segment and permits inspection and treatment of the entire intrarenal collecting system.[19] Secondary passive deflection is made possible by a more flexible segment of the ureteroscope located just proximal to the point of active deflection (Figure 24B-4).

Passively bending the angled tip of the ureteroscope off the superior margin of the renal pelvis or the neck of a middle-pole calix when a baggy extrarenal pelvis is present moves the point of deflection proximally on the ureteroscope. This effectively extends the tip of the ureteroscope, allowing inspection of the lower-pole calices with greater ease. This portion of the collecting system can be visualized in over 90% of patients when passive deflection is possible.[19–21] The presence of either one- or two-way active deflection did not affect the ability to visualize the entire intrarenal collecting system.[19] Studies have shown that in flexible ureterorenoscopes smaller than 9 F, consecutive use leads to a deterioration in active deflection of up to 28%,[22] confirming that the active deflection unit is often the most fragile part of these instruments, and degradation in this unit or rough handling of the shaft leads to knock-on effects on the fiberoptic bundle.

The latest advances in active deflection have for the first time incorporated secondary active deflection into a flexible ureterorenoscope design, the first of a new generation of scopes. This unique design allows the operator to deflect the scope tip upward to 175 degrees and downward to 185 degrees by fully activating the primary deflection lever on the handpiece, and then by activating a second lever on the opposite side of the handle, a further 135 degrees of additional

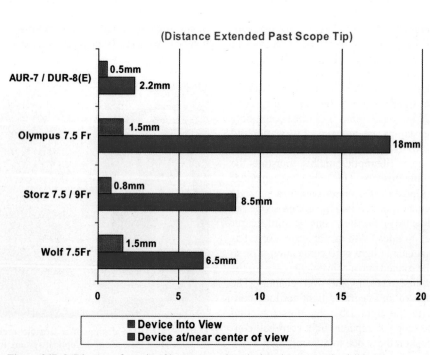

(Distance Extended Past Scope Tip)

AUR-7 / DUR-8(E): 0.5mm / 2.2mm
Olympus 7.5 Fr: 1.5mm / 18mm
Storz 7.5 / 9Fr: 0.8mm / 8.5mm
Wolf 7.5Fr: 1.5mm / 6.5mm

■ Device Into View
■ Device at/near center of view

Figure 24B-3 Distances from tip of instrument when deployed accessory is visible.

Table 24B-1 Latest Summary of Specifications of Flexible Ureterorenoscopes

Model	Tip Diameter (F)	Shaft Diameter (F)	Working Length (cm)	Channel Size (F)	Active Deflection Up (degrees)	Active Deflection Down (degrees)	Location of Passive Deflection (cm from tip)	Secondary Active Deflection (degrees)	Angle of View (degrees)	Field of View (degrees)
ACMI (Stamford, CT)										
AUR-7	7.2	7.4	65	3.6	120	160	5	N/A	12 in air, 9 in fluid	80
DUR8	6.75 Beveled Tip	8.6 Nitinol	65	3.6 super slippery	175	185	6	N/A	12 in air, 9 in fluid	80
DUR8-E	6.75 Beveled Tip	8.6 Nitinol	64	3.6 super slippery	170	180	6 (Active)	130	12 in air, 9 in fluid	80
Olympus (Lake Success, NY, and Tokyo, Japan)										
URF-P3	6.9	8.4	70	3.6	180	180	5	N/A	0	90
Karl Storz Endoscopy (Culver City, CA, and Tuttlingen, Germany										
11274 AA	7.5	8.0	70	3.6	120	170	5	N/A	0	90
11278 AU1 (Flex-X)	7.5	8.4	67.5	3.6	270	270	N/A	N/A	0	90
Richard Wolf Medical Instruments (Vernon Hills, IL, and Knittlinger, Germany)										
7330.072	–	9	70	4	130	160	–	N/A	0	–
7331.001	–	9	60	4.5	130	160	–	N/A	0	–
7325.172	6.8	7.5	70	3.6	130	160	6	N/A	0	65
Viper	6	8.8	68	3.6	270	270	–	N/A	0	86
Stryker Endoscopy (San José, CA)										
Flexvision	6.9	–	64	3.6	170	170	–	80	0	90

Information available from manufacturers.

downward deflection of the tip can be obtained, to give a total of 315 degrees downward deflection. The primary purpose of such a design is to improve access to the lower-pole calices, which are usually the hardest to reach and in which to treat pathology. Deflection can be up, down, or in both directions in one plane (Figure 24B-5). The first such scope was the DUR8 Elite from ACMI (now Gyrus-ACMI). With this instrument, when full primary deflection is achieved, a locking lever can be activated to make it easier to maintain the deflection, while the fingers are used on the opposite side of the barrel to activate the active secondary deflection cable. In addition, this instrument has incorporated unique features

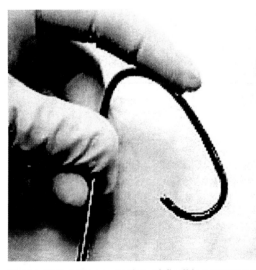

Figure 24B-4 Demonstration of flexible ureterorenoscopic, primary active followed by secondary passive deflection.

of a rotatable light post and irrigation/work channel (as with its predecessors), so that the operators can adjust these as necessary to optimize their working conditions, depending on the specific layout of the operating room.

A second scope called the Flex-X, has also been developed by Storz. This instrument has a greater range of primary deflection in each direction than any of its predecessors (Figure 24B-6), and the next generation from this manufacturer, the Flex-X2, has a special laser-resistant (Laserite) ceramic-coated distal tip of the work channel. This instrument also incorporates a shock absorbing mechanism at the scope's deflecting segment. The utility of these improvements in improving scope maneuverability and scope durability are not known. Other manufacturers have followed suit on both the concepts of increased primary active deflection and incorporation of primary and secondary active deflection, developing flexible ureterorenoscopes with some variations on a theme as is seen in Table 24B-2, but again, the durability of these newer instruments is also unknown at this time. The most durable instruments currently seem to be the DUR8 and the DUR8-Elite, according to the study by Monga and colleagues.[23]

However, when evaluating such instruments for use in real life, urologists must be aware that the wider the diameter of the turning circle of the deflectable tip, the greater the potential to damage the inside of the collecting system, particularly if the renal pelvis is not sufficiently capacious to accommodate the full turning circle of the instrument tip. This limitation can also lead to scope breakages if excessive deflection force is attempted by the operator. Further, if the point in the shaft where such active deflection is controlled

is too far proximal from the tip, it may be fixed in the upper ureter at or below the ureteropelvic junction (UPJ), and may negate any possibility to gain extra primary or secondary active deflection.

WORKING CHANNEL

The first flexible ureteroscopes were simply diagnostic tools, as they did not possess a working channel for irrigation or for the passage of accessory working instruments. It was not until the 1980s that their successors incorporated working channels for the first time, giving these instruments the ability to irrigate the field of view and pass small instruments for biopsy, fulguration, stone retrieval, and contact lithotripsy, depending on the size and design of the working channel. The working channel of a modern flexi-

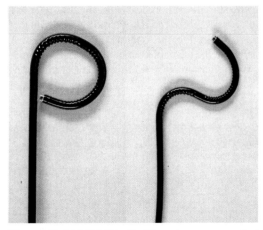

Figure 24B-5 DUR8-Elite flexible ureterorenoscope, first instrument that incorporates secondary active deflection.

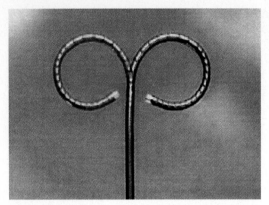

Figure 24B-6 Flex-X scope with large primary deflection.

ble ureterorenoscope is a smooth cylindrical plastic tube that travels through the length of the shaft from the lower part of the handle to the tip of the scope. It is usually located eccentrically or offset at the tip. This eccentricity is less accentuated in the smaller-diameter flexible ureteroscopes, because such a design causes less distortion of the working channel when the tip is deflected and allows for easier passage of working instruments.[17] Also, rotation of the ureteroscope may not be necessary when passing it through the ureteral orifice. Most available flexible ureterorenoscopes have working channels of up to 3.6F, though Wolf has recently produced an instrument that is 9F in size that has an offset eyepiece and a straight access work channel of 4.5F to specifically accommodate a pneumatic contact lithotripsy flexible probe. Many accessory instruments, including stone baskets, graspers, and biopsy forceps, are now available in sizes ranging from 3.2 to 1.5F, and electrohydraulic lithotripsy (EHL) probes even go down to 1.6F, while quartz laser fibers range from 150 to 1,000 microns in diameter. However, the stiffer the accessory, the less the deflection capacity of the scope tip (eg, deployment of a 200 micron laser fiber in the work channel of a DUR8 ureterorenoscope reduced primary active deflection from 143 degrees to 115 degrees, while a 500 micron laser fiber reduced it further to 47 degrees, but a nitinol accessory reduced it only to 123 degrees).[24] Hence, there is an increasing trend that the majority of modern stone retrieval accessories are made of nitinol, which is an alloy pliable enough not to restrict tip deflection nearly as much as its stainless steel counterpart. Working instruments passed through the channel will nevertheless decrease the available lumen for passage of standard irrigation.[14,25] Additional disassembly of the basket sheathing material may allow a greater

range of tip deflection with an occupied work channel, and a comparative 2- to 30-fold increase in irrigant flow, both of which are particularly important when access to pathology in the lower pole is required but cannot be achieved purely by activation of the available range of primary active deflection.[26] Poor irrigant flow through the restricted lumen of an occupied work channel can be overcome with the use of high-pressure irrigation.[14,25] Higher-pressure irrigation can be delivered by a pressurized irrigation bag, roller pump, hand-held syringe or bulb device (Bulbmaster), or foot-controlled device (Peditrol). Measurements of the flow rates available using these irrigation systems are given in Table 24B-2.

Clinical interpretation of this data suggests that flow rates of 20 mL/min provide adequate visualization in most circumstances. However, the downside of pressure irrigation is the potential for a higher incidence of septic systemic complications from pyelorenal reflux, and the possibility of seeding tumor cells from higher grades of transitional cell carcinoma, if present,[27] and as such, in our unit, there is seldom a need to use anything more than 1 to 1.5 m gravity head pressure irrigation. Bends in the shafts of flexible ureterorenoscopes may severely restrict subsequent active tip deflection by as much as 61 degrees.[28] In a study of scopes from all major manufacturers by Monga and Durfee, bending pressure was defined as the force required to deflect the tip of the ureterorenoscope by 15 degrees from a baseline horizontal position.[29] These authors found bending pressure to vary from 6 g for the Wolf 7325.172 ureterorenoscope (7.5F), to 10 g for the ACMI DUR8, to 12 g for the 9F Wolf 7330.072 instrument. Holding the instrument taut, placing a super-stiff guidewire in the shaft portion of the working channel, thus effectively stiffening it, or using an access sheath maximizes active deflection of the instrument tip. However, one must be careful that the instrument is not back-loaded onto the stiff rear end of the working wire, as this may punch a hole into the work channel lining, raising an invisible internal flap that may prevent the subsequent passage of any additional accessories during the rest of the case, leading to incompletely treated pathology and additional expensive repair bills. Furthermore, the wire inevitably reduces flow and vision, as well as hinders the possibility of injecting contrast down the work channel so that fluoroscopy can be used as an adjunctive means of monitoring progress in the upper tract, and most people prefer to use an access sheath when introducing small-diameter flexible ureterorenoscopes into the upper tract.[30]

The strength of tip deflection varies intrinsically from scope to scope[29] across a range from 46 g to 265 g (arbitrarily defined as the force that resulted in a loss of 10 degrees active deflection). It can also be limited by the additional rigidity of instruments within the working channel.[3,6] Moreover, passage of working instruments through the flexible ureterorenoscope may be difficult when the tip is deflected, and attempts to do so with either a stainless steel accessory or a quartz laser

fiber may easily damage the lining of the work channel and prevent further progress in the middle of a case, as well as lead to expensive repair bills. The maximization of flexible ureterorenoscope durability, especially with the small-caliber instruments, can be facilitated by straightening the tip before advancing the accessory through it, and the liberal use of jelly or silicone lubricant (eg, Glide) to reduce frictional forces, though some manufacturers have designed their instrument work channels to have a super slippery lining in the most recent models (eg, DUR8-E, Circon ACMI), and others have introduced ceramic linings at the tip of the work channel (though the practical impact of these is not yet known). The introduction of lasers for contact lithotripsy, tissue destruction, incision, and fulguration has significantly increased the usefulness of the flexible ureteroscopes, but can also potentially shorten their working lives. Lasers, specifically the holmium, neodymium:yttrium-aluminum-garnet (Nd:YAG), and pulsed-dye can be used with small fibers, improving irrigation and deflecting abilities with an occupied work channel. For lower-pole stones, the smallest laser fibers (150 and 200 micron) or EHL probes (1.6F) may be the better instruments if in situ fragmentation is called for. They are less rigid, and thus limit tip deflection to a smaller degree than the laser fibers.[26] The main risk of in situ fragmentation of stones with a maximally deflected scope tip is unseen damage to the inside of the work channel at the point of maximum deflection owing to energy released from microfractures of the stiff quartz core material. In most instances, this damage will not be discovered until after the scope has been sent for sterilization prior to next use, but may be suspected if there is no visible response of the target to energy discharge after foot-pedal activation. For this reason, in general it is better to relocate the target into a more favorable lie (upper or middle calix) within the kidney or into the ureter (for smaller stones), before it is treated, if the life of the delicate flexible ureterorenoscope is to be maximized.

Advances in fiberoptic technology have combined improved images, larger working channels, and smaller outer diameters. These factors and improvements in the working instruments expand the usefulness of these scopes. These working instruments will be discussed in greater detail in a later chapter.

COLUMN STRENGTH

Some small-caliber modern flexible ureterorenoscopes are built with a very rubbery shaft design. This means that they can buckle easily[28] and are very difficult to bare-pass and advance through the intramural portion of the ureter and up the remainder of the ureter. As a consequence, either an access sheath must be used, or the scope shaft must be stiffened temporarily by placing a 0.035- to 0.038-inch wire into the work channel (either antegradely or by backloading the instrument tip onto the rear end of a working wire—either a double floppy-tipped wire [which potentially prolongs

Table 24B-2 Irrigation Flow Rates for 3.6F Working Channels[31,41]

	Gravity (mL/min)	60 mL Syringe (mL/min)	Roller Pump (200 mm Hg) (mL/min)
Empty channel	32–35	110	104
2.5F instrument	5–7	24–55	26
0.038-inch wire	2	21	N/A

scope life] or a regular Bentson wire [which can potentially shorten scope life unless great care is taken to hold the scope straight so that the wire does not perforate the lining of the work channel at sites of bending]). The use of a wire to stiffen the instrument shaft inevitably means a 3- to 4-handed deployment requiring active involvement of both a primary surgeon and an assistant to deploy the instrument into the upper tract. Some manufacturers have increased column strength to facilitate passage of the instrument through the lower ureter by using proprietary polymers to construct the shaft for greater crush resistance as well as torque stability (Flex-X, Storz), while others have also used a Nitinol shaft design with a super slippery outer coating in a recent model (DUR8-Elite, ACMI), leading to stiffer but torque-stable durable shafts, in essence producing almost a semirigid instrument, but with a flexible deflectable tip.

CARE AND STERILIZATION

Flexible ureterorenoscopes are very delicate instruments and should be handled accordingly by a well-trained and knowledgeable team, and not by beginners! The endoscope should be coiled loosely and kept in a large, flat, well-padded rigid case when not in use. It should not be bent, but should be held by the handpiece with the tip in a dependent position, and care should be taken to avoid injury to the distal tip and the ocular piece. Because the glass optical fibers are contained in the body of the flexible endoscope, they can be easily damaged or broken if the instrument is kinked (Figure 24B-7) or dropped.

Inspecting an endoscope should include looking on the endoscope's exterior for dents or other signs of damage. Damaged fibers appear as small black dots within the image. If enough fibers are damaged, the flexible ureteroscope will be useless. Hence, before and after each use, the endoscope should be checked by the user for "peppering" from broken illumination fibers. In general, endoscopes should be sent for repair

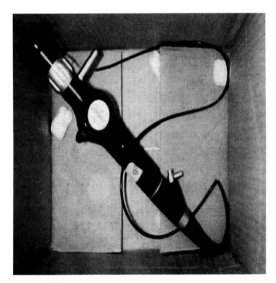

Figure 24B-7 Broken shaft of flexible ureteroscope due to rough handling.

when 18 to 20% of the fibers are broken, since adequate light can no longer be transmitted. A light meter is needed for exact measures. The optical fibers that transmit the image should also be checked both before and after each use. To check a flexible endoscope, hold it close to the object to be viewed. Should the image appear to be cloudy, the endoscope may need repair owing to moisture leaking into the optical fibers (Figure 24B-8) (usually from a hole in the work channel caused by a stiff guidewire or fractured brittle quartz laser fiber).

DEFLECTION CABLE TEST Before and after every use, ensure that all deflecting cables operate properly and deflect the tip to the recommended extent in each direction. If there is no deflection, the flexible endoscope should be sent for repair.

Ureteroscopes should be cleansed with warm water and a nonabrasive detergent to remove any debris following use. The working channel should be washed with a flow of water. This initial mechanical cleansing may be the most important step in the care and sterilization process.[31] Flexible endoscopes can be sterilized by gas (ethylene oxide) or disinfected by soaking in a glutaraldehyde solution.[7,31,32] Another option is the Steris system (Mentor, OH) (see Fig. 24B-2). This system provides automated washing and rinsing of the endoscopes with a peracetic acid solution, which will sterilize immersible instruments in 30 minutes.

The control bodies and light guide connectors of modern endoscopes are constructed with a water-impermeable seal to protect the optical systems and working mechanisms from fluid or moisture-seeping damage, and when these seals are damaged, expensive and lengthy repairs are bound to follow. They should be leak-tested before and after every procedure. Here, air pressure is applied to the mechanical channel of the endoscope insertion tube, and a leak is manifest either as a drop in the pressure gauge or by the appearance of air bubbles in the covering or channel wall. If external damage has already been spotted, further damage should not be risked by water immersion. During gas sterilization, changes in the temperature surrounding the endoscope can cause significant pressure changes within the sealed portion of the scope. Manufacturers have provided venting systems, usually a valve on the light post, to equalize the internal and external pressures during gas sterilization. Use of this venting mechanism is critical to prevent permanent damage to the endoscopes. Some flexible ureteroscopes have a more solid core with no internal air spaces. This permits gas sterilization without the need for an internal venting system. Recent engineering of flexible endoscopes has included automatic venting systems to avoid this costly problem with a patented Autoseal, which could potentially reduce repair costs by eliminating the need for gas, soak, or vent valves. An endoscope that is clearly damaged should be sent for repair immediately, for it

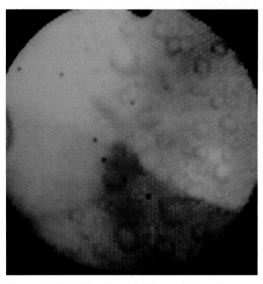

Figure 24B-8 Waterlogged fiberoptic bundle post-sterilization, indicative of work channel damage.

should be considered a contaminated medical device and is labeled for shipping following the Occupational Safety and Health Administration (OSHA) occupational exposure to blood-borne pathogens: final rule 29 CFR part 1910.1030, Federal Register (Dec. 6, 1991).

REFERENCES

1. Bagley DH. Ureteroscopy. AUA Update Series 1994;13:206–11.
2. Marshall VF. Fiber optics in urology. J Urol 1964;91:110–4.
3. Takagi T, Go T, Takayasu H, et al. A small-caliber fiberscope for the visualization of the urinary tract, biliary tract, and spinal canal. Surgery 1968;64:1033–8.
4. Takayasu H, Aso Y. Recent development for pyeloureteroscopy: guide tube method for its introduction into the ureter. J Urol 1974;112:176–8.
5. Bagley DH, Huffman JL, Lyon ES. Combined rigid and flexible ureteropyeloscopy. J Urol 1983;130:243–4.
6. Bagley DH, Huffman JL, Lyon ES. Flexible ureteropyeloscopy: diagnosis and treatment in the upper urinary tract. 1987;J Urol 138:280–5.
7. Barlow DE. Fiberoptic instrument technology. In: Tams TR, editor. Small animal endoscopy. St. Louis: CV Mosby; 1990.
8. Salmon PR. What is fibre-optics? In: Fibre-optic endoscopy. New York: Grune & Stratton; 1974.
9. Bordelon BM, Hunter JG. Endoscopic technology. In: Greene FL, Ponsky JL, editors. Endoscopic surgery. Philadelphia: WB Saunders; 1994. p. 6–17.
10. Wickham JEA. Basic physics and construction of fibre optic and solid lens endoscope. In: Percutaneous renal surgery. Edinburgh: Churchill Livingstone; 1983.
11. Higashihara E, Minowada S, Kameyama S, Aso Y. Angled optical axis for central viewing of endoscopic accessories. J Endourol 1990;4:361–4.
12. Abdelshehid C, Ahlering MT, Chou D, et al. Comparison of flexible ureteroscopes: deflection, irrigant flow and optical characteristics. J Urol 2005;173:2017–21.
13. Bagley DH. Active versus passive deflection in flexible ureteroscopy. J Endourol 1987;1:15–8.
14. Bagley DH. Flexible ureteroscopy. Semin Urol 1989;7:7–15.
15. Bagley DH. The use of flexible ureteropyeloscopy. Adv Urol 1992;5:95–105.
16. Bagley DH. Ureteropyeloscopy with flexible fiberoptic instruments. In: Huffman JL, Bagley DH, Lyon ES, editors. Ureteroscopy. Philadelphia: WB Saunders; 1988.
17. Grasso M, Bagley DH. A 7.5/8.2 F actively deflectable, flexible ureteroscope: a new device for both diagnostic and therapeutic upper urinary tract endoscopy. Urology 1994; 43:435–41.
18. Bagley DH, Rittenberg MH. Intrarenal dimensions. Guidelines for flexible ureteropyeloscopes. Surg Endosc 1987; 1:119–21.
19. Bagley DH. Intrarenal access with the flexible ureteropyeloscope: effects of active and passive tip deflection. J Endourol 1993;7:221–4.

20. Kavoussi L, Clayman RV, Basler J. Flexible actively deflectable fiberoptic ureteronephroscopy. J Urol 1989;142:949–54.

21. Abdel-Razzak OM, Bagley DH. Clinical experience with flexible ureteropyeloscopy. J Urol 1992;148:1788–92.

22. Afane JS, Olweny EO, Bercowsky, et al. Flexible ureteroscopes: a single center evaluation of the durability and function of the new endoscopes smaller than 9Fr. J Urol 2000;164:1164–8.

23. Monga M, Venkatesh R, Best S, et al. Durability of next generation flexible ureteroscopes: randomized prospective study [abstract 1477]. J Urol 2004;171(4 suppl):389.

24. Perry K, Shvarts O, Chin J, Schulam P. Improved functional deflection and access to lower pole renal calculi with new dual deflection flexible ureteroscope [abstract 29]. J Endourol 2002;16 Suppl 1:8–5.

25. Wilson WT, Eberhart RC, Preminger GM. Flow, pressure and deflection characteristics of flexible deflectable ureterorenoscopes. J Endourol 1990;4:283–9.

26. Landman J, Monga M, El-Gabry EA, et al. Bare naked baskets: ureteroscope deflection and flow characteristics with intact and disassembled ureteroscopic nitinol stone baskets. J Urol 2003;169:292–3.

27. Lim DJ, Shattuck MC, Cook WA. Pyelovenous lymphatic migration of transitional cell carcinoma following flexible ureterorenoscopy. J Urol 1993;149:109–11.

28. Monga M, Dretler SP, Landman J, et al. Maximizing ureteroscope deflection: "play it straight." Urology 2002;60:902–5.

29. Monga M, Durfee W. Evaluating flexible ureteroscope strength: buckling pressures and strength of deflection [abstract 28]. J Endourol 2002;16(Suppl 1):8–1.

30. Pietrow PK, Auge BK, Delvecchio FC, et al. Techniques to maximize flexible ureteroscope longevity. Urology 2002;60:784–8.

31. Gregory E, Simmons D, Weinburg JJ. Care and sterilization of endourologic instruments. Urol Clin North Am 1988; 15:541–6.

32. Bagley DH. Care and sterilization of ureteropyeloscopic instruments. In: Huffman JL, Bagley DH, Lyon ES, editors. Ureteroscopy. Philadelphia: WB Saunders; 1988.

Working Instruments

R. John D'A. Honey, MD, FRCSC

The introduction of smaller semirigid and double deflecting flexible ureteroscopes has created a challenging environment for the manufacturers of working instruments. However, the spectrum of instruments available has rapidly increased to meet the demands of the evolving field of endourology. It is therefore vital that the urologist has a thorough understanding of the different ureteroscopic instruments available and their unique characteristics.

GUIDEWIRES

Although guidewires were first introduced in the early 1960s, they did not become an important part of the urologist's armamentarium until the advent of endourology. Using a modification of the percutaneous entry technique, developed by Seldinger (1953),[1] access to the renal collecting system became possible without an open surgical procedure. Advances in technology and instrumentation, including the introduction of a variety of specialized guidewires, led to the development of a whole new field of percutaneous renal surgery. It was the guidewire that also allowed the urologist access to the ureter in a retrograde fashion for dilatation, stenting, and ureteroscopy.

Guidewires are available in a wide range of diameters, lengths, tip configuration, stiffness, and coatings. It is therefore important for the urologist to have an understanding of these various types, and be able to make the correct choice for the case at hand.

The basic construction of a guidewire involves a solid wire core, or mandrel, covered by a tightly coiled steel wire. A tapered mandrel allows transition from a stiffer shaft to a flexible tip, and the length and degree of tapering determines the flexibility of the tip. The outer coiled wire may be round or flat, the latter giving a smoother surface. Various coatings are used to decrease friction and facilitate introduction of the guidewire and the passage of instruments over it. These coatings include polytetrafluoroethylene (PTFE, Teflon) and various hydrophilic polymers. The Roadrunner (Cook, Spencer, IN) and the Glidewire (Terumo Corporation) use a solid nickel-titanium (nitinol) core and a polyurethane shell coated with a hydrophilic polymer. When wet, these hydrophilically coated wires become exceptionally slippery and, although difficult to handle, are particularly useful in negotiating tortuous segments of the ureter and bypassing impacted ureteral stones. An attachable handle is supplied with these that converts this to a torque wire

guide. A modification of this guidewire, the Sensor (Boston Scientific, Natick, MA) has a coiled wire covering to the shaft leaving the distal 5.5 cm bare, which makes it easier to handle, but loses some of the advantages of the uncovered hydrophilic guidewire.

Guidewires used in urologic procedures range in diameter from 0.021 inches (0.53 mm) to 0.038 inches (0.97 mm). They are available in lengths of 60 to 260 cm, although the 145 cm or 150 cm length is best suited for use during ureteroscopy. A double flexible tipped design permits safe passage into the ureter and guards against damage to the working channel of the flexible ureteroscope when it is advanced in a "monorail" fashion over the wire. A stiff proximal end can perforate the working channel and result in leakage of irrigant into the fiberoptic compartment of the endoscope. The Bentson and Newton Cerebral guidewires have a longer flexible tip of 10 to 15 cm, which is useful in negotiating strictures of the ureter with the least chance of perforation. The distal tip of the guidewire may be straight, J-shaped, angled, or deflecting up to 180 degrees. Movable core guidewires are available, where the length of the flexible portion of the tip can be adjusted by withdrawing or advancing the mandrel.

The stiffness of the guidewire depends on the diameter of the central mandrel. The Amplatz super- or extra-stiff wires are among the most rigid. These are useful in stent exchanges and as a working wire for percutaneous nephrostomy tract dilatation. By welding the outer coils to the inner mandrel, it is possible to transfer rotary motion, or torque, in a one-to-one ratio to the tip. The Lunderquist-Ring Torque Wire Guide is a torque wire with a malleable tip that can be refashioned into any shape or form to fit the particular situation.

INSTRUMENTS FOR STONE REMOVAL

Stone baskets were among the earliest devices introduced for endoscopic use in the upper urinary tract, and remain the most commonly used ureteroscopic working instrument. These are available in several different designs, constructed of steel or nickel/titanium and in a variety of French sizes (1.9–3.2F). Initially ureteroscopic stone baskets followed the classic helical Dormia design and were available with 3 or 4 wires, with or without a filiform tip projecting beyond the basket. The helical design makes it easier to rotate the basket as it is withdrawn, and facilitates engagement of the stone. A double-wire version is available that is designed to increase the lateral force and open the ureteral lumen (Figure 24C-1).

The Segura baskets have a nonhelical design, using flat steel wires that add stability and strength to the basket. They are designed to have a larger space between the wires to allow easier stone engagement. These baskets can also be used for caliceal stones, both percutaneously and ureteroscopically, but the protruding tip and the interference with deflection, especially with smaller flexible ureteroscopes, limits their use in these situations. Four- and six-wire designs are available from 2.5 to 3.2F diameter, with either 15 mm or 20 mm baskets. Filiform and spiral tipped baskets may on occasions help with manipulating the basket around an impacted stone. Laser baskets include a central channel to accommodate a laser fiber for simultaneous laser lithotripsy, but care must be taken not to cut the wire with the laser beam. The Segura basket can also be used to obtain large biopsy specimens prior to laser ablation of upper tract transitional cell carcinomas.

The more recently introduced tipless baskets are made of nitinol, a nickel/titanium alloy often referred to as the "memory metal," which has rev-

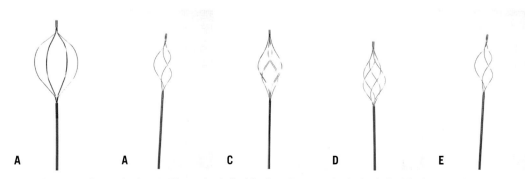

Figure 24C-1 *A,* Segura basket. *B,* Three-wire helical basket. *C,* Four-paired wire helical basket. *D,* Five-wire helical basket. *E,* Four-wire helical basket with filiform tip.

olutionized these instruments and overcome most of the shortcomings of the steel-wire baskets.[2] The increased flexibility allows an increased range of active deflection with flexible ureteroscopes, only limiting flexion by 10 degrees or less, rather than 70 to 80 degrees, seen with the 3.0F flat-wire basket (Figure 24C-2).[3]

The flexibility of the nitinol makes it possible to manipulate the wires carefully around a stone, in a controlled fashion, under direct vision. This can be done in the ureter or in a calix without fear of perforation or bleeding because of the tipless design and the soft "springy" nature of the wires. In addition, captured stones can easily be released by advancing the open basket beside the stone, which flips the wires back off the captured stone, after which the basket can be closed. Prior to the introduction of this technology, the inability to release a captured stone made many urologists reluctant to use baskets in the renal collecting system.[4]

The Holmium:YAG laser is capable of cutting through any of the endoscopic working instruments, including stone baskets. This was a concern with the stainless steel baskets, with the resulting "fish hook" configuration; however, fractured soft nitinol wires can be withdrawn without injury to the ureter.

The N-Circle stone extractor (Cook Urological, Spencer, IN) was the first basket introduced with this design,[5] but similar baskets are now available from a number of companies. These baskets are available in a variety of French sizes (2.2–3.2F) with basket diameters of 10 to 20 mm and a length of 115 to 120 cm for use with the flexible ureteroscope (Figure 24C-3). These can be used in the ureter and renal collecting system and are particularly effective in capturing and displacing stones from the lower pole into an upper-pole calix for more effective intracorporeal lithotripsy.[6]

An important safety feature of these baskets is that the handle can be removed and the basket disassembled within the ureteroscope. This will allow removal of the ureteroscope should a stone within the basket become entrapped. This will also allow the passage of a 200 µm laser fiber through the working channel beside the unsheathed basket for fragmentation of an entrapped stone with improved irrigation. This technique of using unsheathed nitinol baskets has been shown to increase the irrigant flow up to 30-fold and allow for additional deflection of the flexible ureteroscope.[7]

A number of modifications of the tipless design have been introduced, varying the number and configuration of the wires, but it is yet uncertain whether these will offer any advantage over the original four-wire design (Figure 24C-4).

Stone-grasping forceps are used in a similar manner to the nitinol tipless baskets rather than the helical baskets. Helical baskets are advanced beyond the stone, opened, and retracted back toward the ureteroscope which engages the stone. Grasping forceps, like nitinol baskets, are positioned close to the stone and opened. The opening motion advances the forceps, or the basket, onto the stone. As the forceps are closed, the tips retract away from the stone, making it necessary to simultaneously advance the instrument while closing. Grasping forceps are produced in two-, three-, and four-wire designs. Larger 5F three-pronged graspers are available for use through rigid ureteroscopes and smaller 3.0F and 2.4F graspers (Figure 24C-5) for use in the upper ureter and kidney through flexible ureteroscopes. Prior to the introduction of the nitinol baskets, graspers were frequently used in preference to stone baskets in the upper ureter and collecting system because of a concern about the inability to release entrapped stones.

The Graspit (Boston Scientific, Natick, MA) (Figure 24C-6) is an interesting modification of a grasping forceps. Its nitinol construction allows access into the mid- and some of the lower-pole calices, where stones can be grasped and released. This is available as a 2.6F instrument with an 8 mm tip opening and a 3.2F with a 10 mm opening. The forceps must protrude 8 mm before there is adequate separation of the jaws, which can be a disadvantage during flexible ureteroscopy.

Proximal migration of ureteral calculi during ureteroscopy and intracorporeal lithotripsy is more likely to occur with the pneumatic devices and during electrohydraulic lithotripsy than with the Holmium laser. The Stone Cone (Boston Scientific) (Figure 24C-7) is a modification of a nitinol guidewire housed within a sheath. When deployed above the level of the stone, the expanded cone-shaped coil fills the ureteral lumen to prevent proximal migration of stones and assist with removal of fragments after intracorporeal lithotripsy.[8] This is a 3.0F device and is available in 7 mm and 9 mm diameter coils.

INSTRUMENTS FOR INTRALUMINAL LITHOTRIPSY

Intraluminal lithotripsy is performed using ultrasound, electrohydraulic, electromechanical, pneumatic, or laser energy. These devices are discussed in detail in Chapter 5.

Ultrasound probes are available in hollow or solid designs. The hollow probes allow simultaneous suction of irrigation fluid and stone fragments. These are less frequently used now because the larger (4–6F) probes require rigid ureteroscopes of 9.5F or larger. The smaller 2.5F solid probes can be used with the small-caliber semirigid ureteroscopes and rely on lateral vibration alone.[9]

The Swiss Lithoclast is a safe and effective pneumatic intracorporeal lithotripter.[10] The rigid or semirigid probes, which are available in 2.4 and 3.0F, are suitable only for the treatment of ureteral calculi with semirigid ureteroscopes. Recently, a 0.6 mm Lithoclast flexible pneumatic probe has been introduced to be used via the smaller-caliber flexible ureteroscopes. Unfortunately, flexion of the probes results in a drop in the energy and a reduction in the efficiency of stone fragmentation.[11]

Electrohydraulic lithotripsy (EHL) remains an effective method of intracorporeal lithotripsy and 1.6F (Wolf) and 1.9F (Microvasive, ACMI) electrohydraulic probes are available for use with rigid and flexible ureteroscopes. However, the risk of perforation is higher than with the other energy sources, and bleeding within the collecting system tends to decrease visibility.

The Holmium:YAG laser is rapidly becoming the lithotripter of choice for ureteral and many renal calculi. Low water density quartz or silica fibers are available in various diameters from 200 to 1,000 µm. The 200 and 365 µm fibers are used for intracorporeal lithotripsy in the ureter and renal collecting system. Fragmentation rates using these two fibers are similar, but the 200 µm fibers are considerably more expensive. The effect on flexible ureterorenoscope deflection is larger for the 365 µm fiber, ranging from 18 to 37%, whereas the decrease in flexion when using the 200 µm fibers is from 7 to 16%.[12] The 365 µm fibers should therefore be used for the management of most ureteral stones and the 200 µm fibers for renal stones, where the increased flow of irrigant around the smaller

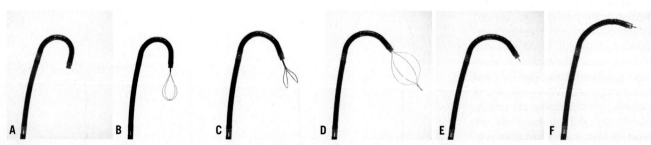

Figure 24C-2 Reduction in active deflection of a 7.5F Olympus flexible ureteroscope by various working instruments. *A*, Empty ureteroscope. *B*, N-Circle stone extractor (Cook). *C*, The Graspit (Boston Scientific). *D*, Segura Basket (Boston Scientific). *E*, 200 µm holmium laser fiber (Lumenis). *F*, 365 µm holmium laser fiber (Lumenis).

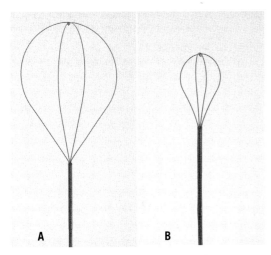

Figure 24C-3 Nitinol tipless baskets (Cook). *A,* 20 mm N-Circle (Megabasket). *B,* 10 mm N-Circle.

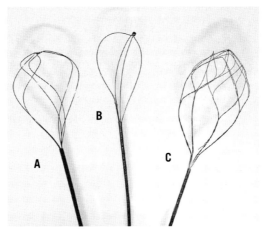

Figure 24C-4 New modifications of the nitinol tipless basket. *A,* Surcatch Tipless Basket (ACMI, Stamford, CT). *B,* Dimension Articulating Stone basket (Bard). *C,* Net Circle Basket (Cook).

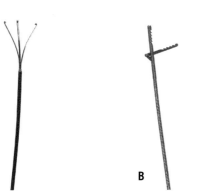

Figure 24C-5 *A,* Three-prolonged graspers. *B,* Alligator forceps.

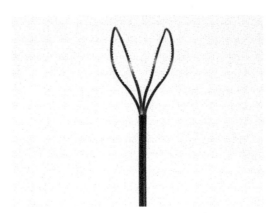

Figure 24C-6 The Graspit (Boston Scientific).

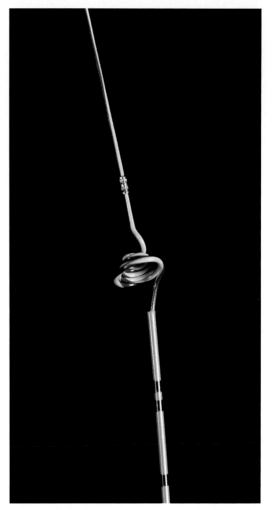

Figure 24C-7 The Stone Cone (Boston Scientific).

fiber is also an advantage. These fibers can also be used with the Holmium laser for tissue incision and destruction.[13]

ENDOLUMINAL ULTRASOUND

Endoluminal ultrasound imaging of the ureter is a useful modality for demonstrating ureteral and periureteral anatomy with a high degree of accuracy. Ultrasound probes are available in various sizes from 3.0 to 6.2F. These are usually passed over a guidewire, but may be passed directly through the working channel of a rigid ureteroscope. The transducers are 12.5 or 20 MHz, which give images with a penetration of 1.5 to 2 cm. A computer program is available to reconstruct these images into a three-dimensional (3D) format.[14] Endoluminal ultrasound is more sensitive than CT angiography[15] in demonstrating crossing vessels at the level of the ureteropelvic junction prior to endopyelotomy and has the added advantage of being able to demonstrate a septum between the ureter and the renal pelvis, seen when there is a high insertion of the ureter.[16] It has also been shown to be useful in the evaluation of various other conditions of the upper urinary tract including tumors, strictures, and embedded calculi.[17]

INSTRUMENTS FOR INCISION AND CAUTERIZATION

A variety of instruments are available for the endoscopic treatment of ureteropelvic junction obstruction and ureteral strictures, or for the ureteroscopic approach to upper tract transitional cell carcinoma and caliceal diverticula. Although the trend is toward the use of the Holmium laser,[18] a cold knife and electrocautery electrode are available for the larger 11.5F ureteroresectoscope, which can be used for retrograde endopyelotomy.[19] Small flexible electrodes with fine straight or hooked cutting tips, and ball coagulating tips, are available in 2.4F and 3.0F. These have control handles for precise work through either the semirigid or flexible ureteroscopes.

OTHER WORKING INSTRUMENTS

A variety of small cup biopsy forceps, ranging from 3.0 to 5.0F are available for use with both rigid and flexible ureteroscopes. Grasping forceps with various jaw and teeth designs (see Figure 24C-5) are produced in sizes 3.0F, 3.5F, and 5.0F for the removal of retained stents, foreign bodies, and embedded stones.

Small 3F dilating balloons with an inflated diameter of 4 mm and a maximum inflation pressure of 8.5 atm (Passport, Boston Scientific) are available in 2 cm and 4 cm lengths. These can be passed up the ureteroscope under direct vision for ureteral and infundibular dilatation, or to gain access to a caliceal diverticulum.

REFERENCES

1. Seldinger IS. Catheter replacement of the needle in percutaneous arteriography. Acta Radiol 1953;39:368–76.
2. el-Gabry EA, Bagley DH. Retrieval capabilities of different stone basket designs in vitro. J Endourol 1999;13:305–7.
3. Poon M, Beaghler M, Baldwin D. Flexible endoscope deflectability: changes using a variety of working instruments and laser fibers. J Endourol 1997;11:247–9.
4. Teichman JM, Kamerer AD. Use of the holium:YAG laser for the impacted stone basket. J Urol 2000;164:1602–3.
5. Honey RJ. Assessment of a new tipless nitinol stone basket and comparison with an existing flat-wire basket. J Endourol 1998;12:529–31.
6. Auge BK, Dahm P, Wu NZ, Preminger GM. Ureteroscopic management of lower-pole renal calculi: techniques of calculus displacement. J Endourol 2001;15:835–8.
7. Landman J, Monga M, El-Gabry EA, et al. Bare naked baskets: ureteroscope deflection and flow characteristics with intact and disassembled ureteroscopic nitinol stone baskets. J Urol 2002;167:2377–9.
8. Dretler SP. The stone cone: a new generation of basketry. J Urol 2001;165:1593–6.
9. Chaussy C, Fuchs G, Kahn R, et al. Transurethral ultrasonic ureterolithotripsy using a solid-wire probe. Urol 1987;29: 531–2.

10. Denstedt JD, Eberwein PM , Singh RR. The Swiss Lithoclast: a new device for intracorporeal lithotripsy. J Urol 1992; 148(3 Pt 2):1088–90.

11. Zhu S, Kourambas J, Munver R, et al. Quantification of the tip movement of lithotripsy flexible probes. J Urol 2000;164: 1735–9.

12. Kuo RL, Aslan P, Zhong P, Preminger GM. Impact of holmium laser settings and fiber diameter on stone fragmentation and endoscope deflection. J Endourol 1998;12:523–7.

13. Bagley DH, Erhard M. Use of the holmium laser in the upper urinary tract. Tech Urol 1995;1:25–30.

14. Bagley DH, Liu JB. Three-dimensional endoluminal ultrasonography of the ureter. J Endourol 1998;12:411–6.

15. Keeley FX Jr, Moussa SA, Miller J, Tolley DA. A prospective study of endoluminal ultrasound versus computerized tomography angiography for detecting crossing vessels at the ureteropelvic junction. J Urol 1999;162:1938–41.

16. Bagley DH, Liu JB, Goldberg B. Endoluminal sonographic imaging of the ureteropelvic junction. J Endourol 1996; 10:105–10.

17. Goldberg BB, Bagley DH, Liu J, et al. Endoluminal sonography of the urinary tract: preliminary observations. AJR Am J Roentgenol 1990;156:99–103.

18. Giddens JL, Grasso M. Retrograde ureteroscopic endopyelotomy using the holmium:YAG laser. J Urol 2000;164: 1509–12.

19. Thomas R. Endopyelotomy for ureteropelvic junction obstruction and ureteral stricture disease: a comparison of antegrade and retrograde techniques. Curr Opin Urol 1994;4:174.

25

Ureteral Anatomy

Omar M. Abdel Razzak, MBBCh, MSc, MD

The transition from open surgery to endoscopy has not diminished the urologist's need to be familiar with the anatomy of the urinary tract. A thorough understanding of the collecting system in its various permutations, from both a radiologic and an endoscopic point of view, is an invaluable aid to ureteropyeloscopy and is indispensable for orientation. Knowledge of the relationship of the ureter along its course enables one to predict the sites of curvature and narrowing, thus facilitating the manipulations of the ureteroscope up into the ureter.

SURFACE ANATOMY

The kidneys lie retroperitoneally on the posterior abdominal wall, on each side of the vertebral column between the twelfth thoracic and the third lumbar vertebrae. Because of the presence of the liver, the right kidney is slightly lower than the left. However, for all practical purposes, similar markings can be taken for either side.

Anteriorly, the upper pole of either kidney is found 5 cm from the midline at a level midway between the xiphisternal junction and the transpyloric plane. The lower poles are located 7 cm from the midline, midway between the transpyloric and intertubercular planes. The hilum lies along the transpyloric plane, 5 cm from the midline.

Posteriorly, the kidney is demarcated by two pairs of parallel lines: two horizontal lines, one at the level of the tip of the spinous process of the eleventh thoracic vertebra and the other at the lower border of the spinous process of the third lumbar vertebra; and two vertical lines located 2.5 and 9.5 cm, respectively, from the midline. The hilum is 5 cm from the midline at the level of the spinous process of the first lumbar vertebra.

The ureters extend vertically from the kidneys to the bladder. Anteriorly, their course can be traced from the hilum of the kidney to the pubic tubercle. Posteriorly, they can be said to run vertically from the renal hilum to pass across the posterior superior iliac spine.

GROSS ANATOMY

The ureter is the urinary conduit from the kidney to the bladder. As such, we might say it starts as a number of calices surrounding the renal papillae. There are usually 8 to 18 pyramids, but only 7 to 13 calices. A single calix may therefore enclose more than one papilla. In his classic study in 1964 Sykes[1] found the average number of calices to be 8.7 ± 0.30; the average number of papillae was 10.7 ± 0.33.

The upper pole usually contains three calices, less commonly, two; the hilar region, three to four calices; and the lower pole, two to three calices. These calices vary considerably in size and shape, since some receive a single papilla and others receive two or even three.[1] Compound papillae occur more commonly in the polar regions.[2]

The superior pole is usually drained by one unique midline caliceal infundibulum. The hilar zone is drained by paired calices arranged in anterior and posterior rows. The inferior pole is drained either by one unique midline calyceal infundibulum or by paired calices.[3]

The adult pelvicaliceal system is arranged in one of two basic types:

1. Divided pelvis or double caliceal type of arrangement: The pelvis is divided at the hilum into upper and lower portions. The lower portion is usually shorter but larger and often drains the hilar calices and the lower pole calices. The number of calices is usually higher than in the true pelvic arrangement.[4] This arrangement is significant during flexible endoscopy because there is no direct connection between the upper and lower calices.
2. True pelvis: This is the classic type of pelvis. The calices drain directly through elongated necks into an elongated pelvis.[1]

The pelvis may be completely within the renal sinus (intrarenal pelvis) or mostly outside it (extrarenal pelvis). In most kidneys, the pelvis has a capacity of 3 to 10 mL.[5] It is roughly pyramidal, with the base facing the parenchyma and the apex funneling down into the ureter. The ureter proper starts approximately at the level of the first lumbar vertebra.[6]

COURSE

The ureter proper is about 22 to 30 cm long, with the right side an average of 1 cm shorter than the left. It does not follow a straight course from the renal pelvis to the urinary bladder, but more an S-shaped course in both the sagittal and transverse planes (Figure 25-1).

The ureter usually displays three narrow sites at which calculi frequently become impacted. The most proximal is at the ureteropelvic junction, the second is at the crossing of the ureter over the iliac vessels, and the third or most distal site of narrowing is at the intramural part of the ureter. The latter is the narrowest region; thus, if this area is dilated, the rest of the ureter can usually be negotiated without difficulty.[7]

For anatomic purposes, the ureter can be conveniently divided into an abdominal portion above the iliac artery and a pelvic portion below it.

The abdominal part of the ureter starts imperceptibly from the renal pelvis at the ureteropelvic junction. It runs downward on the medial part of the psoas muscle, embedded in the subserous fascia and covered by the parietal peritoneum. It then reaches the bifurcation of the common iliac vessels to cross over their terminal part, or over the first part of the external iliac vessels, and to

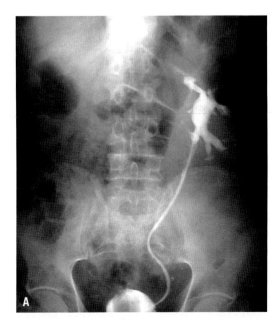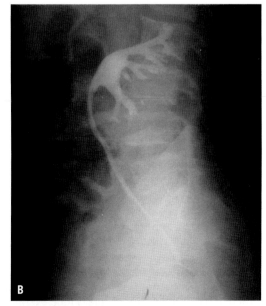

Figure 25-1 *A,* X-ray demonstrating exaggerated curves of ureter. *B,* Lateral view demonstrating S-shaped course.

begin its course in the pelvis. This part of the ureter can be further subdivided into a lumbar segment and an iliac segment, both of equal length—that is, about 8 cm.

As the ureters cross the iliac vessels, they are only 5 cm apart. In the case of hypertrophy of the psoas muscle, they may be even closer.[8] The ureters then diverge as they run downward and laterally on the lateral pelvic wall along the anterior border of the greater sciatic notch, still intimately related to the posterior parietal peritoneum. At the lower end of the greater sciatic notch the ureters curve again to be directed medially toward the lateral angle of the bladder. They then run obliquely for about 2 cm through the bladder wall to open at the angles of the trigone.

ANATOMIC RELATIONSHIPS

The origin of the right ureter from the ureteropelvic region is covered by the descending part of the duodenum. It then runs downward, lateral to the inferior vena cava, where it is crossed obliquely by the gonadal vessels. Further down, it is also crossed by the right colic and ileocolic vessels. Finally, it passes distal to the caudal part of the mesentery and the terminal ileum before entering the pelvis.

The beginning of the left ureter is covered by the initial part of the jejunum. On this side, the gonadal vessels cross the ureter after running parallel to it for a while. It is also crossed by the left colic vessels, and then, as it approaches the pelvis, it is crossed by the sigmoid colon and its mesocolon.

Posteriorly, both ureters lie anterior to the psoas major muscle at the site where it is crossed by the genitofemoral nerve. They then cross the ventral surface of transverse processes of the third to fifth lumbar vertebrae until they finally reach the bifurcation of the common iliac vessels to begin their course in the pelvis.

The upper part of the pelvic portion of the ureter is related to the sacral vertebrae, the lower part is related to the ischial spine, and finally, its termination into the bladder lies below the tip of the coccyx. On the right side, the appendix may overlie the ureter; on the left, the attachment of the sigmoid mesocolon usually lies anteriorly.

In males, the ureter enters the pelvis anterior to the internal iliac artery. Behind the artery are the internal iliac vein and the lumbosacral trunk. The ureter then crosses anterior and medial to the obturator vessels and nerve, the umbilical artery, and superior vesical artery. Opposite the ischial spine, the ureter makes a medial turn to descend in the endopelvic fascia with branches of the hypogastric nerves. Finally, before it enters the bladder, it is crossed anteriorly by the vas deferens. The ureter is then anterior and superior to the seminal vesicles as it reaches the posterolateral angle of the bladder within the lateral true ligament of the bladder. This ligament contains the nerves to the bladder, a plexus of veins, and the inferior vesical artery.

The ureter has a similar course in females, although of necessity the relations are somewhat different. Both ureters are medial to the ovarian vessels as they enter the suspensory ligaments.

Furthermore, each ureter is immediately behind the ovary to form the posterior boundary of the ovarian fossa. The ureter crosses over the uterine artery at its origin from the internal iliac artery; it then passes through the base of the broad ligament to cross below the uterine artery. These two structures are thus in close proximity or even in contact for 1.0 to 2.5 cm of their course. The ureter then runs lateral to the supravaginal part of the cervix as it enters the lateral true ligament of the bladder and inclines medially and downward, anterior to the vagina until it enters the bladder.

BLOOD SUPPLY

The blood supply to the ureters is both multiple and variable. In fact, the blood supply to the right and left ureters is usually asymmetric.[9] The upper part of the ureter is supplied by one or two branches of the renal artery. Supplementary branches are supplied by the gonadal, aortic, renal polar, capsular, or adrenal arteries. The pelvic portion of the ureter is supplied by branches from the common iliac artery, external iliac artery, gluteal arteries, deferential artery in the male, uterine artery in the female, and occasionally the obturator artery. Additional blood supply is also provided by the vaginal, superior vesical, and middle rectal arteries. The iliac region of the ureter thus has the fewest direct arterial branches.[10]

When planning an endoscopic incision in the ureter, it is useful to remember that the upper part of the ureter receives its vascular supply from its medial aspect, whereas the lower pelvic portion of the ureter receives its blood supply from its lateral aspect.[11] This takes the form of a variable number of long arteries that run close to the peritoneum and supply it with small twigs. These arteries divide into ascending and descending branches that travel in the adventitial cover of the ureter and anastomose with each other. The anastomosing arteries form a plexus on the surface of the ureter and send small branches into its substance to form a second more delicate plexus in the submucosa. The capillaries rejoin in a submucosal venous plexus that drains in an outer adventitial plexus. The veins then follow the arterial pathways.[6]

LYMPHATIC DRAINAGE

The lymphatics of the ureter start as plexuses within the ureter's muscular and adventitial layers. The lymphatics from the upper portion of the ureter end partly in the efferent vessels of the kidney and in part directly in the lateral aortic set of lumbar nodes. The middle portion above the pelvic brim drains into the common iliac nodes; the intrapelvic part of the ureter drains into the external and internal iliac nodes and more distally may also join efferent vessels from the bladder.[12]

NERVE SUPPLY

The ureter receives a rich autonomic nerve supply. Nerves to the ureter arise from the celiac, aorticorenal, and mesenteric ganglia and from the superior hypogastric and inferior hypogastric (pelvic) plexuses. The sympathetic supply arises from the preganglionic fibers of the eleventh and twelfth thoracic and first lumbar segments. The parasympathetic supply to the upper part of the ureter apparently arises from the vagal fibers via the celiac plexus. The lower portion of the ureter is supplied by the sacral segments S2, S3, and S4.

Similarly, afferent nerves from the upper portion of the ureter reach the spinal cord with the sympathetic fibers at T11, T12, and L1. Afferents from the lower ureter travel via the pelvic plexus to S2, S3, and S4.

The full significance of the various autonomic nerves to the ureters is not yet fully understood except for the fact that they conduct afferent sensory stimuli. The ultrastructural features of the human ureter seems to indicate that the autonomic nervous system has a minor role in the control of ureteral motility.[13] Furthermore, excised portions of the ureter continue to contract, and denervation of the lower portion of the ureter does not cause reflux to occur.[10]

MICROSCOPIC ANATOMY

As seen by light microscopy, the ureter consists of three distinct layers: the mucosa, muscularis, and adventitia. The mucosal lining consists of transitional epithelium, which has four to six layers of cells when the ureter is contracted. There are a large number of junctional complexes between these cells. This, together with the low but consistent level of keratin precursors within them, is probably responsible for the waterproof property of this layer.[13] This mucosal layer also contains many longitudinal folds, or rugae, that give the nondistended ureter a characteristic stellar outline.

The epithelium rests on a lamina propria of connective tissue that contains many blood vessels and unmyelinated nerve fibers. However, these nerve fibers seem to be absent from the inner third of the lamina propria.[6]

The muscular wall of the ureter is traditionally described as two longitudinal layers separated by a middle circular layer. However, a number of more recent studies seem to indicate that the muscle layers are actually arranged spirally. In the pelvic portion of the ureter, the inner spirals are steep and the outer spirals are horizontal, thus appearing in cross section as inner longitudinal and outer circular layers. In the abdominal portion of the ureter, the muscle bundles are arranged in loose helices, so that no actual layers can be discerned.[13]

The adventitia or outer layer of the ureter consists of a dense network of collagen and elastic fibers between which lie many blood vessels and unmyelinated nerve fibers. This layer is continuous proximally with the capsule at the renal pelvis. Distally, it is thickened by a specialized group of muscle fibers and fibrous tissue to form Waldeyer's sheath.

RADIOLOGIC ANATOMY

The first step in any endourologic procedure is examination of the excretory urogram. The right renal pelvis is usually opposite L2, with the left side 1 to 2 cm higher. In addition, the kidneys may move up to 4 cm with respiration, so that during inspiration the ureters may become kinked, mimicking adhesions or obstruction. Thus the urogram is best obtained in the expiratory phase.[14]

The kidney, as seen by radiography, is usually 11 to 14 cm in length, with the left side longer than the right by 0.5 cm. This is larger than the actual renal size because of the magnification obtained on the x-ray film and the diuresis associated with the contrast medium.

Although caliceal anatomy is usually demonstrated clearly, its interpretation is still a subject of controversy. In 1901 Brodel[4] published his classic article on renal vasculature and morphology in which he showed the anterior calices to be more medial than the peripherally situated posterior calices. This was challenged by Hodson,[2] who offered the view that the anterior row of calices is usually seen more peripherally from the side as cup-shaped structures, whereas the posterior papillae are seen more medially and from the end (ie, end on) as round concentrations of contrast.

Several elegant studies have since been conducted to settle this issue.[3,15] However, despite the use of such techniques as casts of cadaveric kidneys or CT scanning for differentiation, the only clear result of such studies seems to be that the pelvicaliceal anatomy is so varied as not to allow a simple rule of thumb for caliceal organization.

A new technique recently introduced allows the reprocessing of standard CT scans to produce three-dimensional reconstructed images of the pelvicaliceal system.[16] However, this seems to be of limited value in the presence of oblique and lateral x-ray views, ultrasound localization, or the injection of air into the pelvicaliceal system to identify posterior calices.

The renal pelvis may be completely intrarenal, completely extrarenal, or a combination of both. As the pelvis becomes more extrarenal, there is a tendency for the infundibula to insert directly into it and for the pelvis itself to dilate. This is not accompanied by caliceal dilatation and is a normal reflection of the decreased pressure around the pelvis. The pelvis may be box shaped with a distinct division between ureter and pelvis, or it may be funnel shaped, blending imperceptibly into the ureter.

The abdominal portion of the ureter usually descends vertically over the transverse processes of the lumbar vertebrae and lateral to their pedicles until it reaches the level of L5, where it becomes more medial. This course is very variable, and in fact the ureters may not be bilaterally symmetric. However, as a general rule, the ureter that is more than 1.5 cm lateral to the margin of the transverse process is suspect. Similarly, a ureter that crosses medial to a pedicle is usually abnormally displaced.[14] It should also be remembered that medial placement of one or both ureters may occur as a normal variant. This happens more frequently in young males, especially blacks, and is more common on the right side.[17]

Developmental variations in the cardinal vein system can cause displacement of the right ureter. If the subcardinal vein persisits to form the infrarenal portion of the inferior vena cava, the ureter will run medially behind it at the level of L3 and then return to its usual lateral position. The ureter may be distended above this level.[18]

Hypertrophy of the psoas muscles can also cause lateral displacement of the ureters below the renal pelvis. The ureters then turn medially to descend along the anteromedial surface of the psoas muscle. The ureters are often then displaced more medial than usual, especially from the level of L5 downward.[8]

CT scans have replaced lateral views of the kidneys and ureters in diagnosing displacement, but it is still useful to remember that in a standard crosstable lateral view, with a normal lumbar kidney, the renal collecting system should not project anteriorly beyond the spine. Similarly, the ureter stays behind the anterior margin of the vertebral bodies, then projects over the anterior margin at about the level of L4. At the level of L5, the ureter lies anterior to the vertebral body by approximately one-fourth of the width of the vertebral body.[19]

Between L3 and L5, the ureter is crossed and often indented anteriorly and obliquely by the gonadal vessels. The controversial ovarian vein syndrome is attributed to ureteral compression by a dilated ovarian vein and is more often diagnosed on the right side. Diagnosis is based on the clinical presentation in association with excretory urography showing partial obstruction of the ureter by extrinsic pressure at the pelvic inlet.[14]

During excretory urography, the entire length of the ureter is not usually seen in one film. Peristaltic activity or crossing vessels may simulate areas of narrowing or stricture. This can be overcome by ureteral compression, prone positioning, or the diuresis produced by infusion urography. In fact, contrast media may occasionally produce sufficient diuresis to simulate dilatation of the entire ureter.[14]

The diagnosis of a ureteral stricture should not be made without consistent evidence of localized narrowing on multiple films. Furthermore, dilatation should be demonstrated proximal to the site of narrowing and decreased filling below it. Conversely, if the entire ureter is completely filled, the possibility of obstruction or ureteral atony should be raised, especially if this persists on several films and is unilateral.[18]

It is useful to remember that evaluation of the ureter in the presence of a full bladder is often misleading because a distended urinary bladder may cause ureteral fullness. It is also important to have the patient empty his or her bladder because a contrast-filled bladder will obscure the distal ureter.[14]

Marked respiratory movements or moderate renal ptosis may produce ureteric kinks or angulations. Many kinks are also caused by ureteral peristalsis in a mobile ureter and last only a few seconds. These kinks are frequent in the ureteropelvic area and may be mistaken for true obstruction. They are amply demonstrated by oblique or multiple views.

The normal ureteral diameter is very variable, reaching 8 mm or even more (Table 25-1). The normal areas of narrowing are at the ureteropelvic junction, the pelvic brim, and the ureterovesical junction. The areas between them are called the abdominal and pelvic spindles, respectively. The narrowing at the pelvic brim is caused by the ureter crossing over the bifurcation of the iliac vessels. In some persons this may produce a posterior oblique indentation that may appear as an extrinsic filling defect, especially marked in older persons with atheromatous vessels. The dilatation above may mimic an obstruction, but there is no delay in emptying on a prone or erect film, and the renal pelvis and calices are not dilated.[14]

Below this area and anterior to the lower half of the sacroiliac joint, the ureter follows the inner margin of the iliac bone with a convex curve in a posterolateral arc. At the level of the ischial spine, the ureter turns anteriorly and medially to reach the bladder base, where the ureteric orifices are about 2 cm apart. Because of the x-ray beam divergence, a normal ureter may appear to insert abnormally low in the prone position.

If both pelvic portions of the ureters are straight (ie, no convexity or concavity) and are not displaced, they may be normal. However, if the ureter is concave laterally in the pelvic area, it is usually abnormal. Furthermore, a straight ureter with a convex mate is also suspect. Concavity and medial displacement of the pelvic segment of only one ureter are often caused by a bladder diverticulum, enlarged hypogastric nodes, or aneurismal dilatation of the hypogastric artery. Straightening or medial deviation of the pelvic part of the right ureter may also occur as a normal variant in adult females. The uterus is most often tilted to the left in these women. Medial displacement of the pelvic segments of both ureters might be caused by retroperitoneal fibrosis, pelvic lipomatosis, or following abdominoperineal surgery.[14]

In older males with prostatic hypertrophy, elevation of the bladder floor might be pronounced enough to cause the intramural section of the ureter to curve superiorly. This leads to angulation between the parietal and intramural parts of the pelvic portion of the ureter, which might constitute a narrowing in the ureter and might also present some difficulty during ureteroscopy. This is seen on excretory urography as the "hockey stick" or "fish hook" sign.[10]

A "jet" sign may be seen because of the ejection of dense contrast from the ureteral orifice into the bladder, which contains less dense contrast material. This should not be confused with ureteral ectopia, since the jet crosses the midline, whereas ectopic ureters do not.[14]

Table 25-1 The Normal Ureteral Diameter		
Level	Diam. (mm)	Size (F)
Intramural	1.5–3	5–9
Pelvis	4	12
Abdomen	5–6	15–18
UPJ	2–4	6–12

ENDOSCOPIC ANATOMY

Just inside the bladder neck is the trigone. It is a raised, smooth triangular area with its apex at the bladder neck and its base formed by the interureteric ridge extending between the two ureteral orifices. The trigone is the most vascular part of the bladder, and so it is more deeply colored than the rest of the bladder. It is formed by an extension of the longitudinal muscle fibers of the ureters superimposed over the detrusor muscle.

The elevation extending between the ureteral orifices is known as the interureteric ridge or Mercier's bar. It is more prominent in males than females; however, it can be identified in almost all bladders. The ureteral orifices are usually symmetrically located along this ridge, 1 to 2 cm from the midline.

The normal nonrefluxing orifice may have the configuration described as a volcano, a horseshoe, or some other variation. It might be prominent and obvious on endoscopy, or it might be an inconspicuous slit that can be identified only on close examination. A characteristic mucosal vascular pattern that surrounds the ureteral orifice might be helpful in these cases. Prominent mucosal vessels are often seen coursing in an arc medial, inferior, and lateral to the orifice unless they are obscured by an inflammation.[20] As the bladder fills, the ureteral orifices are pushed out laterally and the intravesical ureter is compressed, making ureteral access more difficult.

Alternatively, the ureteral orifice may be quite variable in position and appearance. In an attempt to establish a uniform classification of orifice characteristics, Lyon and colleagues[21] suggested categorizing the ureteral orifice according to these two criteria. They described the orifice as being in position A if it was in the normal medial aspect of the trigone. Position C was at the junction of the trigone and lateral bladder wall or on the lateral wall proper; position B was between A and C. Furthermore, they also graded the ureteral orifice according to its configuration: grade 0, the normal cone or volcano orifice; grade 1, the stadium orifice; grade 2, the horseshoe orifice; and grade 3, the golf-hole orifice. These configurations were associated with an increasing tendency to laterality and reflux as the grade progressed.

Starting from the ureteral orifice, the intravesical section of the ureter extends for about 1.5 cm. First, the submucosal part courses posterolaterally in the bladder for a distance of about 0.5 cm, then the intramural part runs obliquely through the bladder musculature at the detrusor hiatus for about 1 cm.[22] This represents the narrowest part of the ureter.

The normal ureter is easily distensible; however, there are three naturally narrow sites within the lumen. The narrowest portion is the ureterovesical junction, as previously mentioned. This requires dilation before introduction of large-caliber instruments. The other two narrow areas are at the pelvic brim and the ureteropelvic junction. These are relatively wider and are sufficiently dilated with irrigating fluid pressure to allow instrument passage.

These areas are identified endoscopically by a slightly stenotic appearance and relative nondistensibility. Furthermore, the pelvic brim constriction is at the area of the iliac vessels, which can be seen pulsating behind the ureter as this level is approached.

Following this is a relatively straight section where the middle of the ureter lies on the psoas muscle. It is here that the typical stellate appearance of the nondistended ureteral lumen can be discerned. This leads to the third constriction at the ureteropelvic junction, which is identified endoscopically as a narrowing in the ureter followed by the wide renal pelvis. A posterolateral lip of mucosa is sometimes seen in this region. It corresponds to the junction of the ureter with the more dependent part of the pelvis and is accentuated with the respiratory movements.

The kidney is a mobile structure that moves craniocaudally with respiration. This movement is readily apparent endoscopically, because the ureteropelvic region is approached from the relatively fixed ureter. The peristaltic contractions of the ureter, along with the opening and closing of the ureteropelvic junction, can also be observed endoscopically.

As the kidney lies posteriorly, the proximal aspect of the ureter passes posteriorly and laterally over the psoas muscle to enter the renal pelvis. The normal renal pelvis is usually conical on shape, with the apex of the cone leading to the ureteropelvic junction. It may also be more box shaped, with the ureteropelvic junction near the lower medial angle. The intrarenal pelvis is often small with short major calices. The extrarenal pelvis, on the other hand, is usually large, and because it lies outside the renal sinus, the major caliceal infundibula are by necessity long.

As the ureteroscope enters the renal pelvis, the first structures to be seen are the ostia of the major calices. These are circular openings with carinae separating the individual calices. A long tubular infundibulum connects each ostium to the apex of the major calix, which then branches into the minor calices. These are the next structures visible as the ureteroscope enters the infundibulum.

The ureteroinfundibular angle represents the angle of deflection necessary for a flexible ureteroscope to move from the axis of the upper section of the ureter to the axis of the lower infundibulum. This was found to be 140 degrees on average, although it may range from 104 to 175 degrees.[23]

The minor calices can be seen to contract periodically with obliteration of their lumen. This is due to a circular layer of muscle fibers that extends around the base of the papilla to help propel urine from the papillary ducts. An inner longitudinal layer of muscle fibers ends where the minor calix attaches to the renal papilla.

The papillae appear endoscopically as bulging discs covered with a pink friable epithelium and surrounded by the paler caliceal fornix. If more than one papilla projects into the calix, it is called a compound calix. The papillae are the apices of the renal pyramids, and as such they receive the papillary ducts of Bellini that drain the pyramids. These ducts can be seen as minute openings, which are dilated and more obvious in cases of obstruction.

REFERENCES

1. Sykes D. The morphology of renal lobulations and calices and their relationship to partial nephrectomy. Br J Surg 1964; 51:294–304.
2. Hodson J. The lobar structure of the kidney. Br J Urol 1972; 44:246–61.
3. Barcellos Sampaio FJ, Mandarim-de-Lacerda CA. 3-Dimensional and radiologic pelviocaliceal anatomy for endourology. J Urol 1988;140:1352–5.
4. Brodel M. The intrinsic blood vessels of the kidney and their significance in nephrotomy. Johns Hopkins Bull 1901;12: 10–3.
5. Kaye KW, Goldberg ME. Applied anatomy of the kidney and ureter. Urol Clin North Am 1982;9:3–13.
6. Davis JE, Hagedoorn JP, Bergman LL. Anatomy and ultrastructure of the ureter. In: Bergman H, editor. The ureter. New York: Springer-Verlag; 1981. p. 193–223.
7. Kabalin JN. Anatomy of the retroperitoneum and Kidney. In: Walsh PC, Retik AB, Stamey TA, Vaughan E Jr, editors. Campbell's urology. 6th ed. Philadelphia: WB Saunders; 1992. p. 3–39.
8. Bree RL, Green B, Keiler DL, Genet EF. Medial deviation of the ureters secondary to psoas muscle hypertrophy. Radiology 1976;118:691–5.
9. Daniel O, Shackman R. The blood supply of the human ureter in relation to ureterocolic anastomosis. Br J Urol 1952;24: 334–43.
10. Olsson CA. Anatomy of the upper urinary tract. In: Walsh PC, Gittes RF, Perlmutter AD, Stamey TA, editors. Campbell's urology. 5th ed. Philadelphia: WB Saunders; 1986. p. 12–46.
11. Racker DC, Braithwaite JL. The blood supply to the lower end of the ureter and its relation to Wertheim's hysterectomy. J Obstet Gynaecol Br Emp 1951;53:608–13.
12. Williams PL, Warwick R, Dyson M, Bannister LH, editors. Gray's anatomy. 37th ed. Edinburgh: Churchill Livingstone; 1989.
13. Hanna MK, Jeffs RD, Sturgess JM, Barkin M. Ureteral structure and ultrastructure, part 1. The normal human ureter. J Urol 1976;116:718–24.
14. Friedenberg RM. Excretory urography in the adult. In: Pollack HM, editor. Clinical urography. Philadelphia: WB Saunders; 1990. p. 101–207.
15. Kaye KW, Reinke DB. Detailed calyceal anatomy for endourology. J Urol 1984;132:1085–8.
16. Heyns CF, van Gelderen WFC. 3-Dimensional imaging of the pelviocaliceal system by computerized tomographic reconstruction. J Urol 1990;144:1335–8.
17. Adam EJ, Desai SC, Lawton G. Racial variations in normal ureteric course. Clin Radiol 1985;36:373–5.
18. Mellins HZ. Urography and cystourethrography. In: Walsh PC, Gittes RF, Perlmutter AD, Stamey TA, editors. Campbell's urology. 5th ed. Philadelphia: WB Saunders; 1986. p. 312–58.
19. Friedland GW, Filly R, Goris ML, et al. Anatomy. In: Friedland GW, Filly R, Goris ML, et al, editors. Uroradiology. An integrated approach. New York: Churchill Livingstone; 1983. p. 11–153.
20. Bagley DH, Huffman JL, Lyon ES. Normal anatomy of the urethra, prostate, and bladder. In: Bagley DH, Huffman JL, Lyon ES, editors. Urologic endoscopy. Boston: Little Brown; 1985. p. 3–12.
21. Lyon RP, Marshall S, Tanagho EA. The ureteric orifice: its configuration and competency. J Urol 1969;102:504–9.
22. Politano VA. Ureterovesical junction. J Urol 1972;107: 239–42.
23. Bagley DH, Rittenberg MH. Intrarenal dimensions. Guidelines for flexible ureteropyeloscopes. Surg Endosc 1987;1:119–21.

26

Indications for Ureteroscopy

Hiromi Kumon, MD, PhD

Fernando Abarzua MD

Yasutomo Nasu, MD, PhD

The trend in all surgical disciplines has been toward nonoperative or minimally invasive treatment. In urology, however, for more than a century these techniques have been used in cystoscopy. Cystoscopy is basically a noninvasive technique for diagnosing and treating diseases of the lower urinary tract and constitutes a major part of urologic practice. The field of ureteroscopy is an extension of cystoscopy, allowing urologists to inspect the entire urinary tract through the urethra.[1,2] The development of small accessory devices used in conjunction with endoscopes has transformed ureteroscopy into both a powerful therapeutic modality and an excellent diagnostic tool.

Ureteroscopy is generally performed in addition to other standard diagnostic techniques to establish more accurate diagnoses. It is also applied as a form of minimally invasive endoscopic surgery to replace more invasive standard procedures. With the development of increasingly miniaturized instruments, advanced optical and manipulation design and improved auxiliary devices, the field of ureteroscopy has expanded greatly during the last two decades.[3–11] In this chapter, four basic diagnostic indications for ureteroscopy will be described: differential diagnosis of filling defects, evaluation of lateralizing essential hematuria, evaluation of positive upper tract cytologic results, and surveillance of urothelial tumors. The second half of the chapter will deal with the main therapeutic indications for ureteroscopy: removal of calculi and foreign bodies, resection and fulguration of selected tumors and lesions, dilation and incision of strictures, and insertion of ureteral catheters for obstructions and fistulas. Therapeutic applications of ureteroscopy in the pediatric population are expanding, especially for the treatment of calculous disease.[12–14]

DIAGNOSTIC INDICATIONS

Ureteroscopy is a powerful tool for diagnosing upper urinary tract disorders when it is applied in appropriate circumstances with sufficient expertise. In this section, basic diagnostic techniques and applications of ureteroscopy will be discussed.

SYSTEMATIC APPROACH The first step is to determine which type of ureteroscopy to use. Basically, ureteroscopy is divided into rigid or flexible procedures, but now, one may choose from a wide variety of ureteroscopes with distinctive characteristics. For example, there is a semirigid fiberoptic miniature ureteroscope of 5 French to 7F,[3,15] a larger rigid multifunction ureteroscope with a size of 13.5F,[16,17] and small, actively deflectable flexible ureteroscopes of 7.4 to 9.8F.[11] The object is to select the best scopes to fit the individual patient and situation, and to vary the scopes, if necessary, so that a correct diagnosis can be made in a single diagnostic session. Care should also be taken to cover the entire collecting system with the small-range scopes and to avoid inducing any iatrogenic lesions.[18] A systematic approach recommended for diagnostic ureteroscopy follows.

First, the distal ureter should be directly evaluated with a semirigid fiberoptic miniature ureteroscope to avoid any iatrogenic mucosal damage caused by ureteral dilation. The ureter is observed as long as the insertion of the scope proceeds smoothly. At this point, a biopsy is performed, if necessary, and a guidewire is then placed below the portion of the ureter already examined. Next, an actively deflectable, flexible ureteroscope is inserted over the guidewire. Normally, no further dilation is needed because the miniature scope dilates the intramural ureter sufficiently.[5,11] The guidewire should be removed immediately after insertion of the flexible scope into the lower portion of the ureter to prevent an iatrogenic lesion. The scope is then advanced into the renal collecting system under direct endoscopic control with or without the aid of fluoroscopic monitoring. As reported by Kim and Gerber, performing flexible ureteroscopy through a cystoscope sheath prevents bucking of the ureteroscope and decreases the friction against the ureteroscope. This procedure is especially helpful in men with an enlarged prostate.[19] Routine use of the sheath, however, is not only cumbersome but risks damaging the ureteroscope. A detachable ureteroscope sheath[20] is recommended, if necessary.

Observations should be made in an orderly fashion, as demonstrated in Figure 26-1. To prevent iatrogenic traumatized bleeding, which could be mistaken for the source of bleeding, it is also important to maintain a low inflow pressure of irrigant (< 40 cm H_2O) during observation. Even though lack of visibility is present, manual

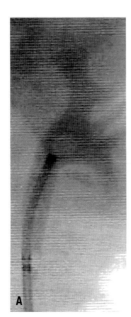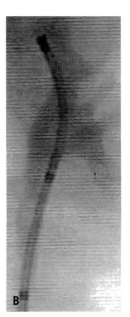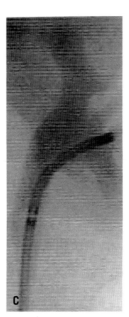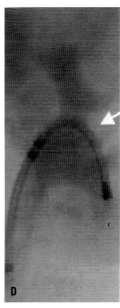

Figure 26-1 A systematic examination of the renal collecting system with an actively deflectable flexible ureteroscope. The evaluation starts in the renal pelvis (A). After observing the entire renal pelvis, including bases of major calices, all calices should be examined in an orderly fashion, proceeding from the upper-pole calices (B) to the middle calices (C) and finally to the lower-pole calices (D). Since a passively deflecting segment of the scope may injure the upper-pole infundibulum, as indicated by an *arrow* (D), the lower pole should be examined last.

flushing is not recommended; multiple, persevering replacement of irrigation fluid is the method of choice until specific lesions are detected. Usually a passive secondary (proximal) deflection is required for complete observation of lower calices,[7,11,21] which may induce indeterminate iatrogenic lesions at the upper infundibulum (see Figure 26-1). This is the reason the lower pole should be examined last. Similarly, any therapeutic maneuvers should be undertaken only after complete observation of the entire renal collecting system.

DIFFERENTIAL DIAGNOSIS OF FILLING DEFECTS

One of the most important and frequent diagnostic indications for ureteroscopy is the evaluation of ureteral or intrarenal filling defects in excretory urography. Filling defects in the upper urinary tract are common, but often no diagnosis can be made using standard methods. Ureteroscopy has been shown to facilitate the diagnosis in many of these cases. In 1986, Streem and colleagues, in a prospective study of 12 patients with upper tract filling defects, compared the diagnostic accuracy obtained by ureteroscopy with standard techniques.[22] They found that provisional diagnoses using standard techniques, including upper tract cytology and computed tomography (CT) with or without ultrasonography, were accurate in only seven cases, whereas the results of ureteroscopy proved to be correct in 10 cases. Of their two indeterminate cases, one involved a tumor in the lower infundibulum and the other an idiopathic renal pelvic hemorrhage (vasculitis). It should be noted that, in both cases, if a more recently developed, actively deflectable flexible ureteroscope had been used instead of a rigid ureteroscope, correct diagnoses would probably have been possible. In 1990, Bagley and Rivas, using the flexible scope, reported that definitive diagnoses were made in 62 patients with upper tract filling defects.[23] Therefore, with the combined use of rigid and flexible ureteroscopes, almost all filling defects in the upper urinary collecting system can be correctly diagnosed.[24,25]

The most common filling defect or lesion is a calculus.[24] It is usually identifiable by direct inspection, but in some cases, to make a diagnosis, the surface must be cleared by removing adherent blood clots, inflammatory debris, or even mucosa, with irrigant or instruments. Urothelial neoplasms are another common lesion, and they are often associated with macroscopic hematuria.[22–25] Through an endoscope, these tumors appear essentially identical to those of the bladder. Low-grade papillary tumors are easily identified (Figure 26-2), but sessile, solid, and non-papillary lesions, which are usually associated with high-grade tumors, are often difficult to differentiate from benign lesions such as inflammatory changes. In patients with positive upper-tract cytologic findings associated with a filling defect, a high-grade transitional cell carcinoma should be suspected[26] and ureteroscopy is neither necessary nor prudent.

In situations in which a lesion cannot be definitively diagnosed by visual inspection, both a biopsy specimen and a cytologic specimen should be obtained. To obtain larger samples, either remove the telescope first or remove the entire scope, including the forceps. In the latter instance, a ureteroscope access sheath may be helpful for repeated removal and insertion of flexible ureteroscopes into the upper urinary tract. Since ureteroscopic biopsy provides a very small sample in most cases, it is better to supplement it with cytologic specimens, particularly brushings taken under direct vision. Guarnizo and colleagues reported that a multi-biopsy approach provides the tissue diagnosis of upper urinary tract tumor in almost 90% of suspicious lesions.[27] Accurate histopathologic grading was achieved in 78% of cases, but concordance between ureteroscopic biopsy and surgical pathologic stage was 63% of

cases. Ureteroscopic biopsies do not necessarily provide sufficient information on tumor stage,[28] but the information on tumor grade is still helpful in choosing the subsequent treatment modality.

A variety of benign lesions can also be detected endoscopically.[22–25,29] These include pyelitis and ureteritis cystica, ureteral polyps, cholesteatoma, inverted papilloma, papillary necrosis, fungous balls, blood clots, peripelvic cysts, and ectopic papillae. Pyelitis and ureteritis cystica are usually easily identifiable on radiographs and from other test results. When doubt lingers, however, ureteroscopy is the best way to identify the lesion (see Figure 26-2). Occasionally it will become apparent that there are no true intraluminal filling defects. In some of these conditions, when an extrinsic pulsatile mass is visualized endoscopically in the area where the filling defect is present, an arterial impression or cross-

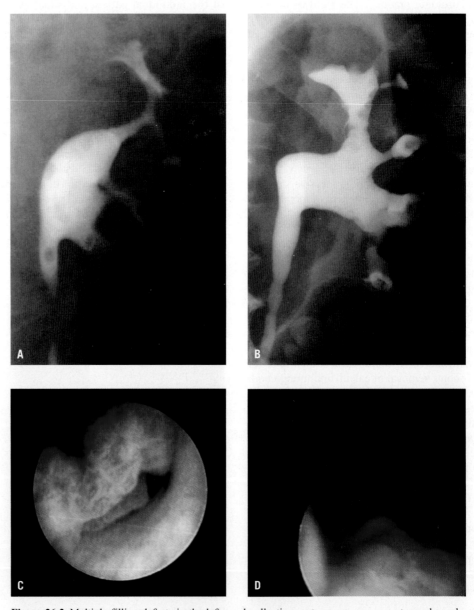

Figure 26-2 Multiple filling defects in the left renal collecting systems are seen on retrograde pyelograms in *A*, a 61-year-old man, and *B*, a 64-year-old man. These two patients had histories of transurethral resections of transitional cell carcinoma of the bladder. *C*, Ureteroscopy shows multiple papillary tumors consistent with low-grade transitional cell carcinoma in the 61-year-old man. *D*, Multiple cystic lesions are consistent with pyelitis cystica in the 64-year-old man.

ing vessels can be identified; intraluminal ultrasound is useful for its confirmation.[30–32]

Ureteral obstruction, another filling defect, may be considered a special case of occlusion of the lumen. This ureteral lesion can be intrinsic or extrinsic and is not usually detectable by ultrasonography or CT. To identify the lesion, direct inspection is normally sufficient, although a biopsy and cytologic studies may be needed to distinguish each intrinsic lesion. The major intrinsic lesions include post-inflammatory strictures, ureteral tumors, and calculi. On rare occasions, a benign ureteral polyp with a stalk (Figure 26-3) and primary non-Hodgkin lymphoma of the ureter is also present.[33]

EVALUATION OF LATERALIZING ESSENTIAL HEMATURIA   Lateralizing essential hematuria, which has also been called chronic unilateral hematuria or benign essential hematuria, is an uncommon syndrome characterized by intermittent or continuous gross hematuria that cannot be diagnosed by radiologic and hematologic tests. Only cystoscopic examination can positively establish that blood is coming from one of the upper collecting systems. Almost all lesions associated with this condition, including hemangiomas (Figure 26-4), minute venous rupture, and varix (Figure 26-5) are delicate vascular abnormalities that can be detected only by endoscopic examination.[18,24,34,35]

With hematuria, ureteroscopy should be performed when the patient is actively bleeding because a definitive diagnosis may be more difficult if the procedure is performed after the bleeding episode has ceased. Accordingly, our patients are asked to walk up and down several flights of stairs on the morning of the evaluation to sustain the bleeding.[18] For optimal detection of localized bleeding lesions, the ureter and renal collecting system must be inspected carefully and systematically, as described earlier in this chapter (see "Systematic Approach"). Every effort should be made to avoid causing iatrogenic traumatized bleeding throughout the ureteroscopic procedure. Usually traumatized bleeding induced by high irrigation pressure occurs at the fornical mucosa and not in the papillae. On the other hand, an iatrogenic guidewire lesion may occur at any site, including the papillae, in which the majority of lesions are found.

Prolonged studies in the United States and Japan have demonstrated the capacity of flexible ureteroscopy to facilitate diagnosis and treat patients suffering from hematuria.[18,34–37] In these studies, 70 of 111 patients were found to have localized lesions including hemangioma, minute venous rupture, and varix. Most of the lesions were in or around the papillae, although a few were found in the renal pelvis or infundibulum. In a small group (19 patients), the findings were nonspecific; in some (22 patients), there were no abnormal findings. Thus, it can be said that flexible ureteroscopy with actively deflectable endoscopes is an essential diagnostic and therapeutic procedure in patients with lateralizing hematuria (Table 26-1).

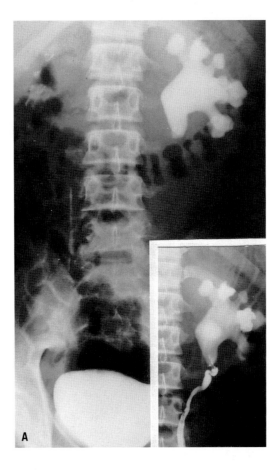

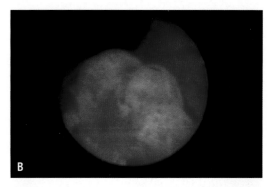

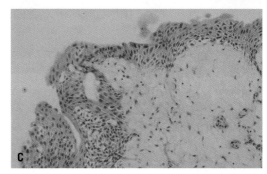

Figure 26-3 *A*, Radiograph of 16-year-old male patient. Left ureteropelvic junction obstruction caused by crossing vessels was suspected. *B*, A polypoid mass was detected and resected endoscopically. *C*, Histologic section reveals fibroepithelial polyp of the ureter.

OTHER APPLICATIONS   As described previously, a patient with positive cytologic results associated with a filling defect is not a candidate for ureteroscopy. But a patient with persistently positive cytologic findings in the presence of normal cystoscopic and intravenous and retrograde pyelographic findings presents a difficult problem. Unfortunately, there are no definitive data regarding ureteroscopic findings on carcinoma in situ of the upper urinary tract. From our own experience and that reported by others,[38] no specific lesions have been found in patients with positive cytologic findings but negative radiographic results, although low-grade tumors have been incidentally identified in patients with negative cytologic and radiographic results (see Table 26-1). Nevertheless, ureteroscopy should be performed after an upper tract localization study to detect concealed malignant lesions. If a suspicious lesion is not identifiable through systematic ureteroscopy, random cold cup biopsies with cytologic specimens may do the trick. Continued surveillance of this group of patients by radiography and cytology, with or without ureteroscopy, is probably the best way to ensure the earliest possible detection of any subsequent macroscopic tumors.

Another major diagnostic application of ureteroscopy is surveillance following conservative treatment of upper urinary tract tumors. It is often difficult to differentiate radiographically between the recurrence of malignancy and normal postoperative scarring. Ureteroscopy with or without biopsy provides an excellent method of checking previous segmental resection sites. In addition, a significant indication

for ureteroscopy is to follow up on a recent endourologic strategy[39–42] for treating low-grade and low-stage upper-tract transitional cell carcinoma. Concerning the surveillance after endoscopic surgery, urinalysis, urine cytology, and excretory or retrograde pyelography are not adequate, and ureteroscopic evaluation with upper trace biopsy is essential.[43,44] Although we need further studies, a reasonable surveillance regimen is ureteroscopy every 3 months until tumor-free, every 6 months for the next 2 years, and then annually thereafter.

In general, follow-up ureteroscopy is not difficult, and repeated ureteroscopy is often much easier to perform than the initial procedure. Andersen and Kristensen satisfactorily completed follow-up ureteroscopy in 42 units of 48 planned (87.5%).[42] Follow-up ureteroscopy, however, is stressful to the patient if it requires hospitalization and anesthesia. Kerbl and Clayman devised a routine office procedure for two patients that involved unroofing the ureteral orifice.[45] The widely patent refluxing ureteral orifice that resulted made possible repeated office-based flexible surveillance ureteroscopic procedures without fluoroscopy and without oral or parenteral analgesics. More recently, using small caliber flexible ureteroscopes and topical anesthesia, routine surveillance ureteroscopy is possible in the office setting without unroofing the ureteral orifice.[46,47]

THERAPEUTIC INDICATIONS

As suggested at the beginning of this chapter, ureteroscopic procedures have progressed from

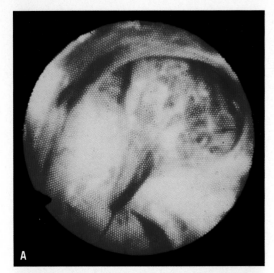

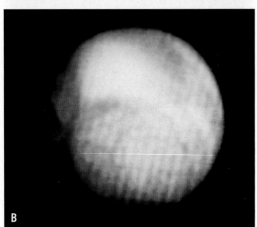

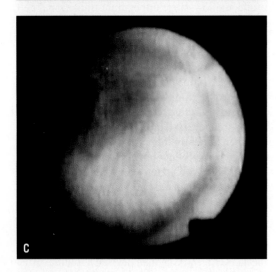

Figure 26-4 Endoscopic appearances of renal pelvic hemangiomas. *A*, Hemangiomas are frequently detected on the papillary tips as a dark-red granular mass. *B*, Small spherical mass with vascular-rich surface. *C*, Dark-red subtle mass.

basically a diagnostic tool to a powerful therapeutic option. In terms of therapeutic ureteroscopy, the advent of holmium:YAG laser has broadened its indications. In the following section, the primary indications for therapeutic ureteroscopy will be outlined.

CALCULI The treatment of calculi, or the removal of stones, from various regions remains

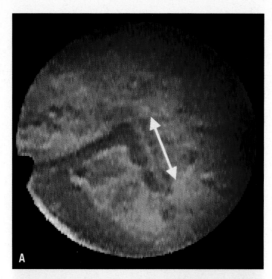

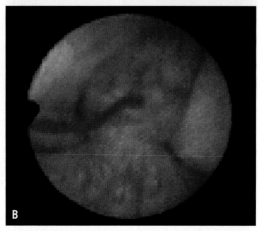

Figure 26-5 Endoscopic appearance of discrete lesion in chronic unilateral hematuria. *A*, Typical endoscopic appearance of minute venous rapture; a stream of blood from the tip of the papilla is clearly seen. *B*, Varix, a blood stream is arising from meandering, dilated vein (*white arrow*) in the papillae.

the most common application of ureteroscopy, even in the era of extracorporeal shock wave lithotripsy (ESWL). Ureteroscopy is particularly effective in the management of distal ureteral stones, and rigid ureteroscopy provides a stone removal rate of close to 100%.[48–50] A wide range of devices for intracorporeal lithotripsy, such as electrohydraulic lithotripsy, ultrasonic lithotripsy, ballistic lithotripsy, and laser lithotripsy are available. Among them, the holmium:YAG laser is capable of fragmenting any type of stone in 100% of cases and greatly decreases the possibility of ureteral injury during stone treatment. Although rigid ureteroscopy has a much lower success rate in removing stones from the middle and proximal ureter,[51] flexible ureteroscopy has been more successful for stones located in the middle and proximal ureter, with a success rate of more than 90%.[48] Lam and colleagues in their series achieved a stone-free rate of 100% for stones less than 1 cm in the proximal ureter, and a 93% stone-free rate in those bigger than 1 cm using holmium:YAG laser lithotripsy.[9] In the case of lower-pole stones, flexible ureteroscopy combined with holmium:YAG laser lithotripsy is safe

and reliable, with a success rate ranging between 82 and 89%.[52–54] In addition, displacement of the lower-pole stone into a more accessible calix before treatment by using a tipless nitinol basket is helpful.[55,56] Ureteroscopy for the treatment of urolithiasis in children has become easier and more common, with the development of the above-mentioned instruments and technique. Now, ureteroscopy is a safe and effective treatment, with results comparable to adult population. No long-term complications associated with ureteroscopic procedures have been reported.[12–14]

For the management of renal stones, there are several clinical situations in which ureteroscopic removal of renal stones is superior to ESWL—namely, residual stones after ESWL, stones associated with intrarenal stenosis, and stones that must be completely removed.

The removal of residual renal stones after ESWL, such as after insufficient fragmentation or delayed passage caused by anatomic alterations, is an excellent application of flexible ureteroscopy. In this situation, treatment time correlates directly with stone burden, and increasing stone size makes the retrograde approach cumbersome and potentially traumatic. Fuchs' guideline—size limits of 1.5 cm for solitary stones and < 5 mm for multiple stones (no more than five in number)—is reasonable for successful ureteroscopy.[57] Stones > 5 mm can be sufficiently fragmented using smaller electrohydraulic lithotripsy probes, high-power pulsed-dye lasers, or the holmium:YAG laser. In removing stones, it is often difficult to reach the lower infundibulum, particularly when there is an instrument in the channel of the flexible scope. In this situation, the stones in the lower infundibulum can be managed by dislodging with careful manipulation-for example, using manual flushing or a nitinol basket or grasper to redirect stones into the renal pelvis or upper infundibulum where they can be more easily removed. Alternatively, smaller-diameter 272 μm (the 200 micron fiber) holmium:YAG laser fiber can be successfully applied.

Renal stones associated with intrarenal stenosis, such as stones above infundibular strictures and in caliceal diverticula or stones associated

Table 26-1 Lateralizing Essential Hematuria: Endoscopic Findings

Discrete Lesions				
Hemangioma	11	11	5	7
Minute venous rupture	2	16	0	3
Papillary tumor	1	2	1	3
Varix	1	2	0	0
Calculus	1	1	1	2
Totals	16	32	7	15
Nonspecific Lesions				
Submucosal erythema	5	2	7	2
Abnormal papillary tip	1	0	0	1
Dilated collecting duct	1	0	0	0
Totals	7	2	7	3
No lesion seen	5	9	3	5

with ureteropelvic junction (UPJ) obstruction, are also indications for ureteroscopy. Although a percutaneous approach is the established method, the retrograde approach may afford a less invasive technique for the removal of such stones and treatment of the stenotic conditions.[7,58,59] In the case of a stenotic caliceal infundibulum balloon dilation, incision with a cutting electrode or holmium:YAG laser is performed to allow adequate access to the obscured area. The retained stones are then fragmented by intracorporeal lithotriptors and removed.

Flexible ureteroscopic removal of small renal stones appears to be particularly beneficial for patients in whom complete removal is indicated. Such patients include pilots, young women planning to become pregnant, and patients who intend to travel to countries with inferior medical infrastructures. For patients being prepared for organ transplantation, the complete removal of small fragments of renal stones, especially infection stones, is mandatory to prevent serious septic complications and simple stone attacks. It has been proven that bacterial biofilms are an essential component of primary and secondary infection stones, and significant bacteriuria and gradual enlargement of the fragments occur if the stones are not completely removed (Figure 26-6).[60] Therefore, in the face of residual fragments with positive stone cultures or positive urine cultures after ESWL, complete removal by flexible ureteroscopy is the method of choice to prevent stone recurrence (or enlargement) and to treat chronic, persistent urinary tract infections.

FOREIGN BODIES A foreign body in the upper urinary tract is not common, but normally can be diagnosed by clinical history and radiography. Most foreign bodies reported recently are migrated or fragmented double-pigtail catheters or broken parts of accessory devices such as portions of stone baskets. Ureteroscopy has been very successful in removing these foreign bodies,[61] although it is difficult when associated mucosal edema is prominent. Removal can be achieved using three-pronged grasping forceps, alligator forceps, or stone baskets.

UPPER-TRACT NEOPLASMS In selected cases, upper urinary tract transitional cell carcinoma has been successfully treated endoscopically without evidence of recurrence after long-term follow-up.[27,39–44,62] Initially, most authors recommended therapeutic ureteroscopy as an option for the following types of patients: (1) those who have a solitary kidney, bilateral upper-tract malignancy, or renal insufficiency and are not candidates for dialysis or a transplant, and (2) those who are poor risks for open surgery.[28,40,41] In these categories of patients, however, ureteroscopic procedures are regarded as a palliative option. Nevertheless, it has been reported that survival is not compromised by endoscopic treatment.[63] With the development of ureteroscopy and auxiliary devices, ureteroscopic treatment can be safely and effectively conducted as a first-

line therapy in properly selected patients with a normal contralateral kidney. Patients with small (< 2 cm) papillary and low-grade tumors, negative cytology, and no evidence of extended disease by conventional imaging studies, are sufficiently treated and followed by ureteroscopy.[44,64]

Concerning conservative management of upper urinary tract tumors, it has been demonstrated that, in low-grade and low-stage tumors of the upper tract, there is no difference in survival rates for patients treated with radical nephroureterectomy as compared with segmental resection.[62–65] It has also been reported that the occurrence of tumors in the contralateral or ipsilateral tract is small, although the occurrence of subsequent bladder tumors is high.[62] These results suggest that operations preserving the renal parenchyma can be considered as an alternative option for low-grade and low-stage tumors. On the other hand, the most common objection to ureteroscopy for neoplastic lesions concerns possible local and systemic seeding of tumor cells. The frequency of local recurrence after endoscopic treatment is no higher than after segmental resection. Reported recurrence rates within a follow-up period were 20 to 70% (mean: 36%, or 51 out of 140 patients),[39–42,62,65] and these recurrent tumors were successfully treated by ureteroscopy. In addition, no patient experienced retroperitoneal tumor seeding, although ureteral perforation and extravasation were observed in several patients.[40,62] Similar results have been obtained for bladder tumors following transurethral resection.[66] These rather low recurrence rates may be attributed to the weak malignant potential of low-grade transitional cell carcinoma. Nevertheless, pyelovenous lymphatic backflow is closely related to intrarenal pelvic pressure, and careful manipulation using low irrigation pressure is

mandatory since one case report indicated the migration of tumor cells from renal pelvic grade 2 transitional cell carcinoma to submucosal venous and lymphatic spaces during flexible ureterorenoscopy.[67]

The assessment of tumor stage by ureteroscopy can be unsatisfactory because of the small range of scopes and the restricted volume of biopsy specimens. Tumor grade and stage, however, are very closely related in transitional cell carcinoma of the upper urinary tract, and the presence of a low-grade tumor virtually guarantees mucosal confinement.[63,68] In addition, a multi-biopsy approach increases the accuracy range of histopathologic diagnosis.[27] Then the inspection and biopsy of both the tumor and the entire collecting system are sufficient to diagnose low-grade and low-stage tumors in the upper urinary tract. Therefore, in the era of ureteroscopy in which surveillance ureteroscopy following treatment can be performed as a routine procedure, ureteroscopic treatment can be considered a desirable option. Further longer-term, larger-sample studies are required to determine the final value of ureteroscopic treatment of upper-tract malignancy.

The technique for ureteroscopic treatment of upper urothelial tumors depends on the size and location of the lesion. In all cases, irrigation flow should be kept as low as possible. Small lesions can be removed completely with cold cup biopsy forceps, and the base of the tumor can be lightly fulgurated with a standard 2 or 3F electrode or a laser probe. Larger tumors in the ureter can be resected with a cutting loop fitted with a rigid ureteroscope. Because of the thinness of the ureteral and renal pelvic walls, which measure < 2 mm, a low-power setting is necessary to treat these tumors safely. In principle, laser energy is preferable to standard electrofulguration, because

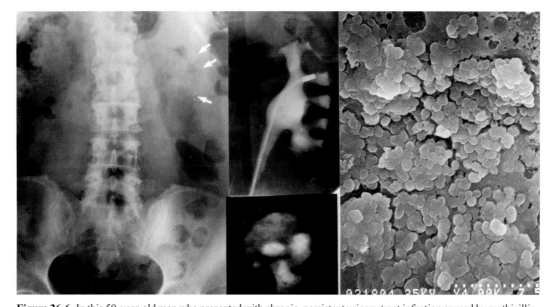

Figure 26-6 In this 59-year-old man who presented with chronic, persistent urinary tract infection caused by methicillin-resistant *Staphylococcus aureus* (MRSA), gradual enlargement of renal stone fragments was detected. At another institution the patient had undergone extracorporeal shock wave lithotripsy followed by percutaneous nephrolithotomy for multiple renal stones, leaving several small fragments. *A*, After the complete removal of multiple small stones (*arrows*) by flexible ureteroscopy, the intractable nosocomial infection was finally cured. *B*, Scanning electron microscopic study shows MRSA biofilms in these secondary infection stones.

penetration depth of laser energy is more controllable, resulting in less common occurrence of ureteral strictures.[39,41,65] The combination of the Nd:YAG, which penetrates tissue for 5 to 6 mm, and holmium:YAG, which is absorbed within 0.5 mm, can be used extremely effectively for treating urothelial tumors. Larger tumors located in the ureter and pelvis can be initially debulked and coagulated by using Nd:YAG without touching or altering the field of view, and the resulting coagulated tissue or tumor base is ablated with holmium:YAG.[69,70]

BENIGN LESIONS Benign lesions such as fibroepithelial polyps, inverted papilloma, and hemangioma are well suited to ureteroscopic resection or fulguration, although these lesions are rare. Figure 26-2 shows a fibroepithelial ureteral polyp that was resected successfully with a rigid ureteroresectoscope without any evidence of stricture or recurrence for 2 years. For renal hemangiomas, which are most often present on the papillary tips (see Figure 26-5) and are the most important cause of lateralizing essential hematuria, ureteroscopic fulguration is absolutely the first choice of treatment.[18,34–37]

STRICTURES Ureteral strictures can be treated by dilation or endoscopic incision through a retrograde, antegrade, or combined approach using rigid and/or flexible ureteroscopes.[71–73] Incision with a cold knife, cutting electrode, or laser fiber generally provides more promising results than simple balloon dilation. Overall success rates of about 60% are reported, but these rates are significantly influenced by the length of the stricture. Thomas performed a retrospective analysis of 36 ureteral strictures treated by ureteroscopic incision.[72] Among those with strictures 1.5 cm in length, 20 of 25 (80%) were successful. When the stricture was 1.5 cm in length, only 3 of 11 (27%) were successful. The density, nature, and cause of the stricture may also affect the success rate; a prior history of irradiation or a radical hysterectomy makes for a poor prognosis. Nevertheless, in most cases, ureteroscopic incision is an attractive option for short ureteral strictures of various kinds since the procedure is simple and noninvasive as compared with open surgery.

Normally, a cold knife incision with a rigid scope is the treatment of choice for ureteral strictures. Flexible ureteroscopes equipped with a small cutting electrode or laser fiber can be used to incise ureteroenteric or ureterovesical anastomotic strictures.[73,74] In cases involving completely strictured ureters a combined antegrade and retrograde approach may be necessary. After incision of the stricture, the area is splinted, usually with a 10 to 14F indwelling ureteral stent for 3 to 6 weeks. Follow-up periods of more than a year are necessary to establish the efficacy of, and the possible indications for, these procedures.

Holmium:YAG can be effectively applied to make the incision; a 200-micron fiber can easily pass through the working channel of a small-caliber rigid or flexible scope. These advantages significantly improve access to the UPJ and to pediatric patients. In the treatment of UPJ obstruction, retrograde techniques including ureteroscopic holmium laser incision are becoming preferred approaches, although percutaneous antegrade endopyelotomy for UPJ obstruction has been a well-established alternative to open pyeloplasty.[32,75]

FISTULAS Ureteroscopy is the treatment of choice for the resolution of fistulas such as a ureterovaginal fistula following hysterectomy. Even when catheters cannot be inserted by standard cystoscopic techniques, it is still possible to insert a rigid miniature ureteroscope beyond the fistula into the dilated proximal ureter under direct vision.[76] A guidewire is first inserted, and then a double-pigtail stent is positioned over the guidewire for 6 weeks. Although this procedure may not always be successful, it can remedy certain difficult problems and avoid re-operation.

CONCLUSION

The development of increasingly miniaturized ureteroscopes and accessory devices has dramatically expanded the indications for ureteroscopy. Miniaturization has also enhanced the safety margin of the procedure, resulting in fewer complications. Most of the diagnostic and therapeutic indications for ureteroscopy discussed in this chapter have been performed as a standard urologic procedure in most institutions. Although some of the therapeutic applications still need to be confirmed by longer-term follow-up and larger-sample studies, these applications will become more attractive to urologic surgeons, not only because they are minimally invasive but also because they will become simpler with advances in technology. Repeated innovations in associated technology will further broaden the applications of ureteroscopy and make them non invasive. The current revolution in medical engineering, nanotechnology, bio-imaging and information technology will be of major influence on ureteroscopy within the next decade.

REFERENCES

1. Pérez-Castro E, Martinez-Piñeiro JA. La ureterorrenoscopia transuretral. Un actual proceder urologico. Arch Esp Urol 1980;33:445–60.
2. Bagley DH, Huffman JL, Lyon ES. Flexible ureteropyeloscopy: diagnosis and treatment in the upper urinary tract. J Urol 1987;138:280–5.
3. Watson G, Murray S, Dretler SP, et al. An assessment of the pulsed dye laser for fragmenting calculi in the pig ureter. J Urol 1987;138:199–202.
4. Bagley DH. Active versus passive deflection in flexible ureteroscopy. J Endourol 1987;1:15.
5. Grasso M, Bagley DH. A 7.5/8.2 F actively deflectable, flexible ureteroscope: a new device for both diagnostic and therapeutic upper urinary tract endoscopy. Urology 1994;43:435–41.
6. Grasso M, Bagley DH. Small diameter actively delectable, flexible ureteropyeloscopy. J Urol 1998;160:1648–53.
7. Pearle MS. Renal urolithiasis: therapy for special circumstances. Part 1. AUA update series 2001. Vol XX: Lesson 30.
8. Parkin J, Keeley FX Jr, Timoney AG. Flexible ureteroscopes: a user's guide. BJU 2002;90:640–3.
9. Lam JS, Greene TD, Gupta M. Treatment of proximal ureteral calculi: holmium:YAG laser ureterolithotripsy versus extracorporeal shock wave lithotripsy. J Urol 2002;167:1972–6.
10. Pattaras JG. Ureteroscopic litthotripsy, AUA update series 2003. Vol. XXII: Lesson 19.
11. Bagley DH. Ureteroscopy: endoscopic techniques in the upper urinary tract. AUA course, May 2003.
12. Jayanthi VR, et al. Strategies for managing upper tract calculi in young children. J Urol 1999;162:1234–7.
13. Van Savage JG, Palanca LG, Andersen RD, et al. Treatment of distal ureteral stones in children similarities to the American Urological Association guidelines in adults. J Urol 2000;164:1089–93.
14. Schuster TG, Russell KY, Bloom DA, et al. Ureteroscopy for the treatment of urolithiasis in children. J Urol 2002;167:1813–6.
15. Abdel-Razzak OM, Bagley DH. The 6.9F semi-rigid ureteroscope in clinical use. Urology 1993;41:45–8.
16. Clayman R, Basler JW, Kavoussi L, et al. Uretero-nephroscopic endopyelotomy. J Urol 1990;144:246–52.
17. Kumon H, Ohmori H, Takei K. The "Universaltome," a new surgical endoscope for endourology. Jpn J Med Instru 1992;62:66–7.
18. Kumon H, Tsugawa M, Matsumura Y, et al. Endoscopic diagnosis and treatment of chronic unilateral hematuria of uncertain etiology. J Urol 1990;143:554–8.
19. Hyung LK, Glenn SG. Performing flexible ureteroscopy through a cystoscope introducer sheath. Urology 1999;54:557–8.
20. Abarzua F, Monden K, Nasu Y, et al. A detachable ureteroscope sheath for flexible ureteroscopy. Acta Medica Okayama, 2003.
21. Bagley DH. Intrarenal access with the flexible uretero-pyeloscope: effects of active and passive tip deflection. J Endourol 1993;7:221–4.
22. Streem SB, Pontes JE, Novic AC, et al. Uretero-pyeloscopy in the evaluation of upper tract filling defects. J Urol 1986;136:383–5.
23. Bagley DH, Rivas D. Upper urinary tract filling defects: flexible ureteroscopic diagnosis. J Urol 1990;143:1196–200.
24. Kavoussi L, Clayman RV, Basler J. Flexible actively deflectable fiberoptic ureteronephroscopy. J Urol 1989;142:949–54.
25. Kumon H, Uno S, Nishitani Y, et al. Flexible ureteroscopy: diagnosis and treatment of upper urinary tumors. Jpn J Endourol ESWL 1991;4:103–5.
26. Sarnacki CT, McCormack LJ, Kiser WS, et al. Urinary cytology and the clinical diagnosis of urinary tract malignancy: a clinicopathological study of 1400 patients. J Urol 1971;106:761–4.
27. Guarnizo E, Pavlovich CP, Seiba M, et al. Ureteroscopic biopsy of upper tract urothelial carcinoma: improved diagnostic accuracy and histopathological considerations using a multi biopsy approach. J Urol 2000;163:52–5.
28. Huffman JL, Bagley DH, Lyon ES, et al. Endoscopic diagnosis and treatment of upper tract urothelial tumors. A preliminary report. Cancer 1985;55:1422–8.
29. Kirschenbaum AM, Cohen EL, Goldman JH, et al. Ureteroscopic management of ureteral cholesteatoma. Urology 1986;28:397–8.
30. Bagley DH, Liu JB, Goldberg BB, et al. Endopyelotomy the importance of crossing vessels demonstrated by endoluminal ultrasound. J Endourol 1995;9:465.
31. Grasso M, et al. Examining the obstructed ureter with intraluminal sonography. J Urol 1999;162:1286–90.
32. Giddens JL, Grasso M. Retrograde ureteroscopic endopyelotomy using the holmium:YAG laser. J Urol 2000;164:1509–12.
33. Hashimoto H, Tsugawa M, Nasu Y, et al. Primary non-Hodgkin lymphoma of the ureter. BJU 1999;83:148–9.
34. Bagley DH, Allen J. Flexible ureteropyeloscopy in the diagnosis of benign essential hematuria. J Urol 1990;143:549–53.
35. Nakada SY, Elashry OM, Picus D, et al. Long term outcome of flexible ureterorenoscopy in the diagnosis and treatment of lateralizing essential hematuria. J Urol 1997;157:776–9.
36. Kumon H. Endoscopic management of renal hematuria of uncertain etiology. Nishinihon J Urol 1994;56:511–5.
37. Tawfiek ER, Bagley DH. Upper-tract transitional cell carcinoma. Urology 1997;50:321–9.
38. Huffman JL. Endoscopic management of upper urinary tract urothelial cancer. J Endourol 1990;4:S141.
39. Schmeller NT, Hofstetter AG. Laser treatment of ureteral tumors. J Urol 1989;141:840–3.
40. Blute ML, Segura JW, Patterson DE, et al. Impact of

endourology on diagnosis and management of upper urinary tract urothelial cancer. J Urol 1989;141:1298–301.

41. Kaufman RP, Carson CC. Ureteroscopic management of transitional cell carcinoma of the ureter using the neodymium:YAG laser. Lasers Surg Med 1993;13:625–8.

42. Andersen JR, Kristensen JK. Ureteroscopic management of transitional cell tumors. Scand J Urol Nephrol 1994;28:153–7.

43. Chen GL, El-Gabry EA, Bagley DH. Surveillance of upper urinary tract transitional cell carcinoma: the role of ureteroscopy, retrograde pyelography, cytology and urinalysis. J Urol 2000;164:1901–4.

44. Chen GL, Bagley DH. Ureteroscopic management of upper tract transitional cell carcinoma in patients with normal contralateral kidneys. J Urol 2000;164:1773–6.

45. Kerbl K, Clayman RV. Incision of the ureterovesical junction for endoscopic surveillance of transitional cell cancer of the upper urinary tract. J Urol 1993;150:1440–3.

46. Patel A, Fuchs GJ. New techniques for the administration of topical adjuvant therapy after endoscopic ablation of upper urinary tract transitional cell carcinoma. J Urol 1998;159:71–5.

47. Jones JS, Streem SB. Office based cystoureteroscopy for assessment of the upper urinary tract. J Endourol 2002;16:307–9.

48. Tawfiek ER, Bagley DH. Management of upper urinary tract calculi with ureteroscopic techniques. Urology 1999;53:25–31.

49. Turk TM, Jenkins AD. A comparison of ureteroscopy to in situ extracorporeal shock wave lithotripsy for the treatment of distal ureteral calculi. J Urol 1999;161:45–7.

50. Chow GK, Patterson DE, Blute ML, et al. Ureteroscopy: effect of technology and technique on clinical practice. J Urol 2003;170:99–102.

51. Kressel K, Hoffmann H, Butz M. Long-term experience with transurethral rigid ureteroscopy as a complementary method to extracorporeal shockwave lithotripsy. Urol Int 1992;48:76–80.

52. Bagley DH. Removal of upper urinary tract calculi with flexible ureteropyeloscopy. Urology 1990;35:412–6.

53. Behari F, Bagley DH. Ureteroscopic management of intrarenal calculi. J Urol 1998;159:1139.

54. Grasso M, Ficazzola M. Retrograde ureteropyeloscopy for lower pole caliceal calculi. J Urol 1999;162:1904–8.

55. Honey RJ. Assessment of a new tipless nitinol stone basket and comparison with an existing flat-wire basket. J Endourol 1998;12:529–31.

56. Schuster TG, Hollenbeck BK, Faerber GJ, et al. Ureteroscopic treatment of lower pole calculi: comparison of lithotripsy in situ and after displacement. J Urol 2002;168:43–5.

57. Fuchs GJ. Retrograde ureteroscopic intrarenal surgery. Probl Urol 1992;6:323–34.

58. Fuchs AM, Fuchs GJ. Retrograde intrarenal surgery for calculus disease: new minimally invasive treatment approach. J Endourol 1990;4:337–45.

59. Grasso M, Lang G, Loisides P, et al. Endoscopic management of the symptomatic caliceal diverticular calculus. J Urol 1995;153:1878–81.

60. Kumon H. Pathogenesis and management of bacterial biofilms in the urinary tract. J Infect Chemother 1996;2:18–28.

61. Bagley DH, Huffman JL. Ureteroscopic retrieval of proximally located ureteral stents. Urology 1991;37:446–8.

62. Elliott DS, Segura JW, Lightner D, et al. Is nephrectomy necessary in all cases of upper tract transitional cell carcinoma? Long term result of conservative endourological management of upper tract transitional cell carcinoma in individual with a normal contralateral kidney. Urology 2001;58:174–8.

63. Heney NM, Nocks BN, Daly JJ, et al. Prognostic factors in carcinoma of the ureter. J Urol 1981;125:632–6.

64. Elliott DS, Blute ML, Patterson DE, et al. Long term follow up of endoscopically treated upper transitional cell carcinoma. Urology 1996;47:819.

65. Murphy DM, Zincke H, Furlow W. Primary grade 1 transitional cell carcinoma of the renal pelvis and ureter. J Urol 1980;123:629–31.

66. Fitzpatrick JM, West AB, Butler MR, et al. Superficial bladder tumors (stage pTa, Grades 1 and 2): the importance of recurrence pattern following initial resection. J Urol 1986;135:920–2.

67. Lim DJ, Shattuck MC, Cook WA. Pyelovenous lymphatic migration of transitional cell carcinoma following flexible ureterorenoscopy. J Urol 1993;149:109–11.

68. Das AK, Carson CC, Bolick D, et al. Primary carcinoma of the upper urinary tract: effect of primary and secondary therapy on survival. Cancer 1990;66:1919–23.

69. Floratos DL, de la Rosette JJ. Lasers in urology. BJU 1999;84:204–11.

70. Wollin TA, Denstedt JD. The holmium laser in urology. J Clin Laser Med Surg 1998;16:13–20.

71. Netto NR, Ferreira U, Lemos GC, et al. Endourological management of ureteral strictures. J Urol 1990;144:631–4.

72. Thomas R. Choosing the ideal candidate for ureteroscopic endoureterotomy. J Urol 1993;149:314A.

73. Karamolowsky EV, Clayman RV, Weyman PJ. Endo-urological management of ureteroileal anastomotic strictures: Is it effective? J Urol 1987;137:390–4.

74. Ahmadzadeh M. Use of a prototype 3-Fr needle electrode with flexible ureteroscopy for antegrade management of stenosed ureteroileal anastomosis. Urol Int 1992;49:215–7.

75. Tawfiek ER, Liu JB, Bagley DH. Ureteroscopic treatment of ureteropelvic junction obstruction. J Urol 1998;160:1643–6.

76. Koonings PP, Huffman JL, Schlaerth JB. Ureteroscopy: a new assent in the management of postoperative ureterovaginal fistulas. Obstet Gynecol 1992;80:548–9.

27

Access to the Difficult Ureter

David E. Patterson, MD

INDICATIONS

With the advent of smaller rigid and flexible ureteroscopes, the difficulties with access of the ureter have decreased dramatically; there are, however, still select cases that require dilation of the ureteral orifice and ureter prior to introduction of the ureteroscope.[1–6]

PATIENT AND PREOPERATIVE PREPARATION

The ureteroscopic procedure begins with a frank discussion with the patient and family concerning realistic expectations of ureteroscopy. The procedure, hospitalization, necessity for ancillary procedures, and the possible open management of complications have to be discussed with the patient. The possibility of multiple procedures with prolonged hospitalization also must be clearly understood by the patient. Obtaining proper informed consent should minimize the risk of medical/legal litigation.

A complete history and physical examination needs to be performed. Previous history of pelvic surgery, radiation therapy, or trauma needs to be evaluated with preoperative cystoscopy and radiographic studies in order to define, precisely, the anatomy of the lower and upper urinary tract. Clearly, previous pelvic surgery, radiation or trauma may lead to grossly abnormal ureteral anatomy or leave the ureter fixed and fibrotic. Likewise, a urethral stricture or significant prostatic obstruction may make ureteroscopic access difficult or impossible unless these conditions can be corrected. Allergies to antibiotics and/or contrast media must be ascertained, thereby circumventing severe anaphylactic reactions. A review of current medications, including vitamin and herbal supplements, is mandatory to rule out the use of anticoagulants or other drugs, such as aspirin or nonsteroidal anti-inflammatory agents, that may predispose the patient to bleeding. Physical examination should be performed to determine overall prostatic size. All abdominal scars should be readily explained, as any prior pelvic or abdominal procedures may be associated with ureteral injury, fixation, or angulation, which may make access difficult or impossible.

Laboratory investigation should include a serum creatinine to assess renal function. The urinalysis and urine culture are necessary to rule out urinary tract infections. A coagulation battery including prothrombin time (PT), partial thromboplastin time (PTT), and platelet count should be performed.

All patients are given prophylactic antibiotics. These should be given one to two hours before the procedure and continued for two doses after the procedure. This will reduce the incidence of iatrogenically induced bacteria or sepsis.[7]

INSTRUMENTATION

The armamentarium necessary for successful access of the ureter is outlined below:

Fluoroscopy
Guidewires
    Sensor wire
    Floppy tips, 0.035 and 0.038 inch
    Bentson, Rosen, and Glidewire
Balloons
    Olbert, 4 to 10 cm, 12 to 18 atm
    Meatal
    Transureteroscopic
    Balloon injectors
Catheters
    Open-ended, 6 and 7 F
    Straight angiographic, 6 and 7 F
    Preformed tip angiographic, 5 and 6 F

FLUOROSCOPY Either fixed-table or C-arm fluoroscopes are necessary for successful access. Passage of guidewires, dilators, and catheters is facilitated by fluoroscopy. Visualization of a stone, its position and degree of obstruction, can only be accomplished with fluoroscopy. Any injuries or complications can also be detected quickly. Finally, placement of the post-procedure temporary ureteral catheter or Double-J stent can only be successfully accomplished using fluoroscopic control.

GUIDEWIRES A wide variety of guidewires are important in achieving access and for further manipulations in the upper urinary tract. Keeping an array of various types of guidewires will be very helpful in gaining access. The standard 0.035 or 0.038 Teflon- or non–Teflon-coated guidewires are being replaced by the new hybrid hydrophilic floppy tip with a traditional, stiffer wire. Other wires should include the Bentson "floppy tip" guidewire, Rosen guidewire, and the hydrophilic-coated "glide wire." (Figure 27-1 and Figure 27-2) These guidewires have many advantages. They help straighten the ureteral orifice in relation to the bladder neck, creating a straighter course for the introduction of the dilators and ureteroscope. They open the ureteral orifice and help elevate its upper lip, making introduction of the ureteroscope easier. By separating

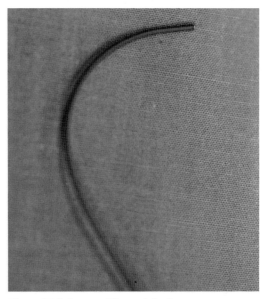

Figure 27-1 Bentson "floppy tip" wire.

the ureteral walls, they make introduction of the ureteroscope easier in areas above the ureteral orifice. Their intrinsic rigidity helps straighten minor angulations of the ureter. It can make identification of the orifice in difficult and complicated cases easier. It facilitates insertion of open-ended or double-J ureteral catheters. Be aware that, when using power transureteroscopic lithotriptors, damage can occur to the wire.[8]

BALLOONS The use of balloon dilators is the method of choice and the most popular way to

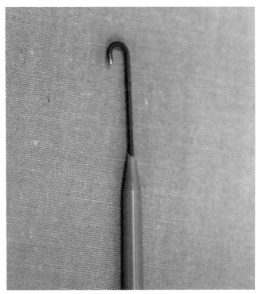

Figure 27-2 Rosen wire.

dilate the orifice and intramural ureter prior to ureteroscopy. There is a large variety of balloons available, ranging from 3 French to 30F in diameter, when inflated, and from 1 to 20 cm in length. As a rule, balloons that are used for dilation are not elastic, so that the outer diameter does not exceed the indicated size (Gruentzig type) (Figure 27-3). Dilation to 15F or 18F is more than adequate for the vast majority of ureteroscopic cases.[9,10] Other types of balloons that are used less frequently, but possibly critical to successful access, include the meatal balloons and transureteroscopic balloons. Meatal balloons are important particularly in cases of a Steinstrasse or an intramural ureteral stone where passage of the guidewire and traditional balloon dilation are impossible. Placing a meatal balloon through the cystoscope, just into the orifice and inflating it, can help with dilation of the orifice, which can then allow the introduction of a small ureteroscope and subsequent power lithotripsy (Figure 27-4). This may also permit direct visualization of the obstruction with subsequent passage of a guidewire. None of these maneuvers would be possible without the use of a meatal balloon. Occasionally, during passage of the ureteroscope, a poorly dilated segment becomes apparent. The use of a transureteroscopic balloon can be very helpful in dilating that segment (Figure 27-5).

When using balloons, a mechanical inflation device is mandatory. Using a simple 10 cc Luer-Lok syringe is inadequate due to the fact that it produces unequal and, often times, very high pressures within the balloon. Most importantly, it is very difficult for the operator to maintain constant pressure in the balloon. Various types of commercial inflation devices are available, ranging from the very expensive reusable devices used by angiographers for balloon angioplasty to the simple Leveen style inflation device shown in Figures 27-6 and 27-7. The LeVeen inflation device (Microvasive, Natick, MA) is a 10 mL syringe with a spiral piston that will advance or retract only when the shaft of the cylinder is screwed in clockwise or counterclockwise. The inflation is gradual and controlled. It does not require a lot of hand pressure to operate, and the pressure remains steady at the set point instead of at the pressure of the operator's thumb, which is constantly fluctuating if the simple 10 cc Luer-Lok syringe is used. The insertion of a pressure manometer gauge between the inflation device and the balloon will help more accurately measure the amount of pressure within these balloons (Fig-

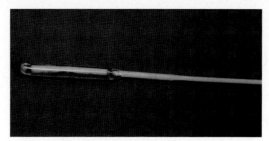

Figure 27-4 Meatal balloon.

ure 27-8). Overinflation of the balloon can lead to rupture and its attendant ureteral trauma.

OTHER DILATING DEVICES If necessary, balloon dilation of the ureter is the easiest and least traumatic to perform; in rare instances, however, balloon dilation will not be successful, and a back-up form of dilation should be available. A relatively new hydrophilic-coated, tapered, graduated 6/12 AQ dilator is quite cost-effective and has become the primary method for ureteral dilators in some practices.[11] A second line of attack, if the balloon does not work, includes Teflon and polyethylene dilators.

These devices, which are available from several manufacturers, are graduated, individual dilators with tips tapered to fit over a 0.038 inch guidewire smoothly and closely (Figure 27-9). These sets contain dilators sized from 6F to 18F increasing by an increment of 2F in the larger dilators. These dilators are used through a large cystoscope and, after passage of the 10F dilator, the lens of the cystoscope is removed for introduction of the larger dilators.

These devices are inferior to balloon techniques because their use requires multiple introductions of the dilator and the use of a large cystoscope. The introduction of these dilators can cause

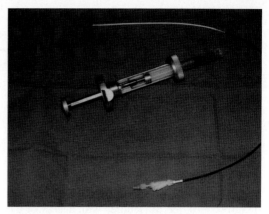

Figure 27-6 Angiographic balloon injector.

linear shearing of the ureteral mucosa, which can cause bleeding and, at times, injury to the muscular layer. Finally, these techniques cannot be used in the presence of distal stones or Steinstrasse.

ALTERNATIVE DILATION METHODS The following alternative methods are also available and suffer from the same drawbacks listed above, compared to the balloon dilation techniques: the one-step Nottingham ureteral dilator by Microvasive, metal bougies (Figure 27-10), and individual or multibead acorn metal dilators (Karl Storz Endoscopy - America, Culver City, CA). A telescoping, metal ureteral dilator is also manufactured by Storz. This principle is similar to the telescoping metal dilators used for fascial dilation of the nephrostomy tract for percutaneous renal procedures. Also available are ureteral access and peel-away inducer sets.[12] These sets consist of coaxial systems of either Teflon dilators or balloons that are placed over guidewires. Over these dilators and balloons are Teflon peel-away sheaths that can be advanced over the Teflon dilators or balloons on dilation. The inner dilators or balloons are removed, and the sheath is left in the ureter. The advantages of these systems, if properly placed, are that introduction of the ureteroscope, its retrieval and reintroduction can be performed very easily, allowing reduction in trauma to the ureteroscope, thus enhancing durability of the fragile, small ureteroscopes.[13,14] In addition, the large lumen of the sheath allows insertion and

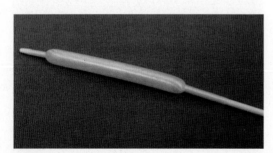

Figure 27-3 Olbert balloon.

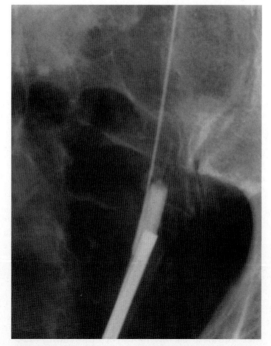

Figure 27-5 Transureteroscopic balloon.

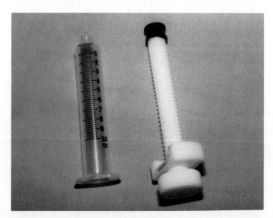

Figure 27-7 LeVeen inflation device.

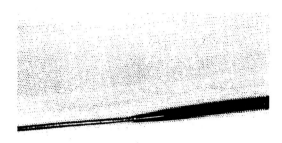

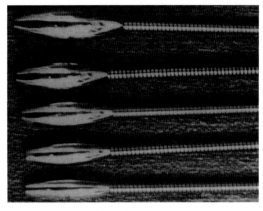

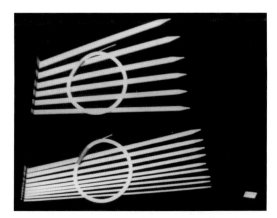

Figure 27-8 Inflation device connected to pressure gauge and balloon.

Figure 27-10 Metal bougies.

Figure 27-12 Angiographic straight catheter with tapered tip and side holes loaded over a guidewire.

placement of a Double-J stent at the completion of the procedure.[15] The drawbacks are that, if the guidewire cannot be advanced, neither can the dilators or the peel-away systems. They can cause injury to the wall of the ureter, particularly if the ureter is not distensible enough or if introduced forcibly. In male patients, the peel-away sheaths may get kinked in the bladder.[16] These sheaths are also not very useful in the presence of very distal pathology because there is not enough length to hold them in the ureter.

Finally, another system for ureteral dilation involves hydraulic dilation. This involves the hydraulic pump called the Ureteromat developed by Perez Castro and colleagues and manufactured by Storz.[17] This is a digital pump that creates a continuous pulsatile jet of irrigant at the tip of the ureteroscope. When the ureteroscope is introduced, the pulsatile stream of irrigant is aimed at the center of the ureteral orifice, which slowly dilates and stretches the ureteral wall. The major drawback with the Ureteromat is the continuous drainage of large volumes of irrigant into the bladder, necessitating periodic emptying of the bladder. Another option is to insert a small suprapubic catheter that can be removed at the end of the procedure. Some endourologists believe hydraulic dilation is the fastest and least traumatic method for ureteral dilation.[18]

CATHETERS   In addition to the usual assortment of open-ended straight urologic catheters, angio-graphic catheters should be included. These come in various sizes ranging from 5F to 7F. They are stiffer than the usual urologic catheters and are tapered at the end to slide smoothly over 0.035 or 0.038 guidewires. These work very well in straightening the ureter; (Figure 27-11 and Figure 27-12) and are manufactured by Cook Urological, Spencer, IN. Your local vascular radiologist can provide you with catheters with various preformed tips that are very useful in accessing the difficult ureter. (Figure 27-13) Use of these catheters will be discussed later in this chapter (see "Other Techniques").

URETEROSCOPES   These have been extensively discussed in a previous chapter (see Chapter 24A, "Instruments: Ureteroscopic"), but I want to emphasize the need for a small, rigid ureteroscope in the 4F to 6F range. This size ureteroscope is very important in accessing the difficult ureter. The use of this scope as an access tool will be discussed later in the chapter (see "Stone in the Intramural Tunnel").

METHODS OF DILATION

CHRONIC TECHNIQUE FOR URETERAL DILATION
It is well known that a ureteral catheter placed within the ureter over several days causes ureteral dilation.

This dilation procedure is usually easy to perform since standard techniques of ureteral catheterization are used. The largest catheter that will easily fit into the ureter is passed cystoscopically by standard techniques. The ureteral catheter is secured in position by placing a Foley

catheter in the bladder and tying the two catheters together attaching each to a drainage bag. In 48 to 72 hours, the ureter will be sufficiently dilated to accept the ureteroscope.

Self-retaining Double-J stents can be used to dilate the ureter by a mechanism similar to that of straight ureteral catheters. This allows the patient to remain ambulatory and be treated as an outpatient as the ureter is dilated with the stent in place. The self-retaining double-J catheter is excellent for long, narrowed areas or strictures within the ureter.

BALLOON DILATION OF THE URETER   Angio-graphic balloon catheters have been adapted for ureteral dilation. This technique is the treatment of choice for ureteral dilation prior to the introduction of the ureteroscope. As previously mentioned, these balloon catheters come in various lengths and diameters.

This technique is generally straightforward. First, the guidewire is placed through a standard cystoscope into the orifice and up into the renal pelvis (Figure 27-14A). The balloon catheter is placed over the guidewire into the orifice under cystoscopic visual control. The first dilation should be performed with the balloon protruding a few centimeters from the orifice to be certain that the orifice is dilated (Figure 27-14B). If a short, 4-cm balloon is used, it should be advanced after deflating and reinflated to dilate the ureter up to the point of disease (Figure 27-14C). As the balloon is inflated, it must never exceed the man-

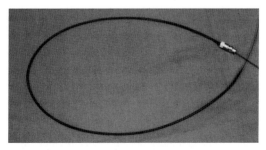

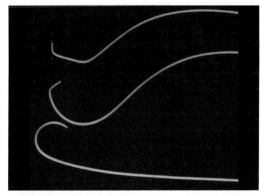

Figure 27-9 Teflon graduated tapered-tip dilators.

Figure 27-11 Angiographic straight catheter.

Figure 27-13 Angiographic catheters with various preformed tips.

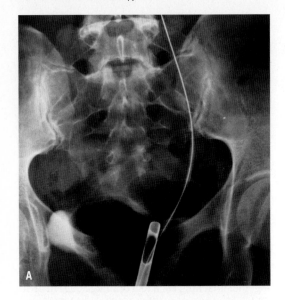

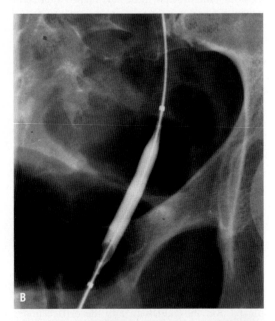

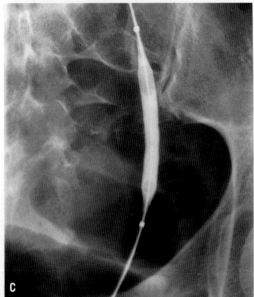

Figure 27-14 *A,* Guidewire placed into upper collecting system. *B,* Balloon inflated at level of ureteral orifice and intramural tunnel. *C,* Balloon deflated, advanced farther up the ureter and reinflated.

ufacturer's recommended pressure limits. A diluted solution of radiographic contrast medium is used for inflating the balloon so that the position and inflation can be followed fluoroscopically, thereby assuring full dilation without "waisting" (see "Waist" below) The majority of normal ureters will achieve adequate dilation with low pressures in the area of 4 to 6 atmospheres. Occasionally, higher pressures are needed, and up to 16 to 18 atmospheres can be safely used in the current high pressure balloons.

The major advantage of balloon dilation is the ease and speed of the dilating process as well as the capability of dilating the ureter at any level. The only disadvantage of balloon dilation is the cost of the catheters since they are recommended for one-time use only, whereas Teflon or hydrophilic-coated concentric coaxial dilators and metal bougies can be reused multiple times.

DILATING CHALLENGES

Most ureters can be readily dilated to accept any ureteroscope. There are, however, certain situations in which difficulty can be anticipated. A ureteral orifice that is inaccessible to the cystoscopic approach cannot be instrumented for dilation. Such situations occur rarely in patients with severe prostatic obstruction, ureteral reimplantation, or other surgical procedures with scarring of the orifice or ureterovesical junction. These conditions need to be rectified before ureteroscopic access can be accomplished.

The following special dilating problems can be overcome with the proper armamentaria, experience, and luck.

WAIST A waist occurs when a balloon is inflated and a segment of the ureter does not fully dilate to the outside diameter of the inflated balloon (Figure 27-15A). If a low-pressure balloon is used, it should be switched to a high-pressure balloon and reinflated across the narrowed segment, keeping the balloon inflated at the maximum pressure designated by the manufacturer. Usually, the waist will disappear in minutes. If this fails, a backup dilating technique can be applied using rigid coaxial Teflon dilators or metal bougies (Figure 27-15B and Figure 15C). Although more traumatic to the ureter than the balloon, these types of dilators can be effective in dilating waists. After using the rigid dilators, replace the balloon over the guidewire and reinflate. It is important to ascertain that the narrowed segment is fully distended. (Figure 27-15D). If these maneuvers fail to correct the waist, the final solution is to place a double-J catheter and let the ureter self-dilate over 48 to 72 hours and then return for the ureteroscopic procedure.

STONE IMPACTED AT ORIFICE If an impacted stone is present, passage of a guidewire is impossible (Figure 27-16). There are several options available to treat this situation. The easiest is to do a direct vision ureterotomy at the 12 o'clock posi-

tion incising over the stone for as much distance as is necessary to dislodge it from the distal trigonal portion of the ureter. Avoid using a Collings knife because thermal injury will occur when using this instrument. Certainly, reflux can occur, but this is low grade and of no clinical significance.[19]

Ultrasonic lithotripsy or the pulsed-dye laser will also work well for soft stones. Avoid electrohydraulic lithotripsy as it can create significant injury to the orifice and ureter if not used very carefully.

STONE IN THE INTRAMURAL TUNNEL One of the most difficult access problems occurs when a calculus is impacted in the intramural tunnel superior to the ureteral orifice. In these cases, often a guidewire cannot be passed. When this occurs, the meatal balloon is placed just inside the orifice and dilated. This will allow access with the ureteroscope up to a position below the stone, and under direct vision, a guidewire can usually be passed beyond the calculus into the upper collecting system. At this point, stone extraction can be successfully accomplished. (Figure 27-17) Alternatively, a small miniscope in the 4F to 6F range, can be carefully placed just inside the ureteral orifice where, under direct vision, a guidewire can be safely placed prior to manipulation of the stone.

PASSAGE OF THE URETEROSCOPE Once adequate dilation of the ureter has been performed, the next step is the introduction of the ureteroscope. Always keep the guidewire in the collecting system and secure it to the drapes in such a way that it will not be inadvertently removed. The ureteroscope is passed under direct vision through the urethra into the bladder. Because the lens system is offset from the center of the ureteroscope, attempts to pass the ureteroscope under direct vision in the usual orientation will cause the upper aspect of the end of the ureteroscope to impact into the superior lip of the orifice. Passing a guidewire through the working channel into the ureter for several centimeters and rotating the ureteroscope 180° will allow easier insertion of the ureteroscope through the orifice into the intramural tunnel (Figure 27-18). Once the ureteroscope is through the orifice, the guidewire is followed. The lumen should be open and directly in front of the scope, which should glide effortlessly along the ureter. The mucosa should be seen to slide directly underneath the ureteroscope without any bunching or telescoping in front of the ureteroscope (Figure 27-19). When telescoping of the mucosa or sudden resistance to passage of the scope occurs, stop immediately, pull the ureteroscope back, rotate the scope and try to reintroduce it through this segment. If this does not work, several options are available. One is to consider switching to a smaller caliber ureteroscope. Other options include using a transureteroscopic balloon or removing the ureteroscope and redilating the segment of the ureter with a high-pressure balloon. If

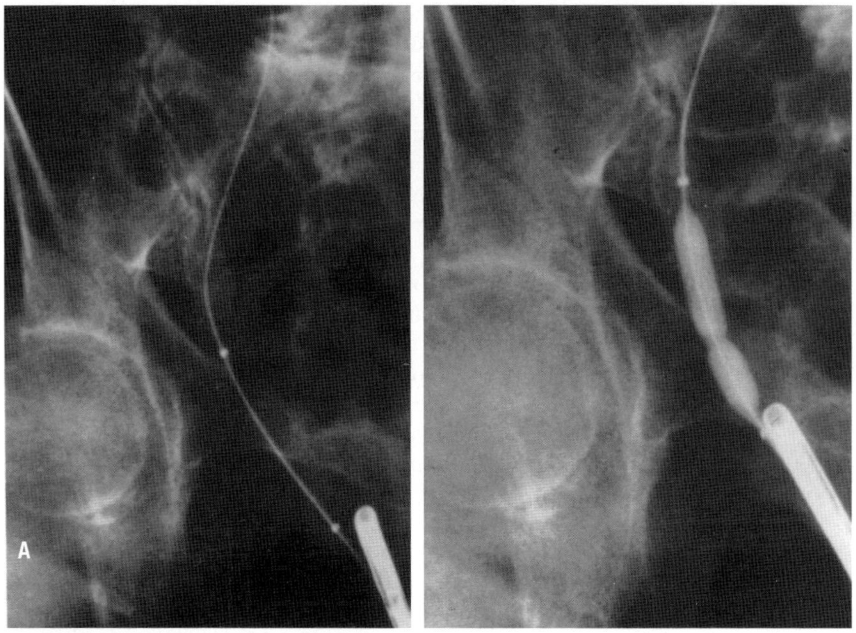

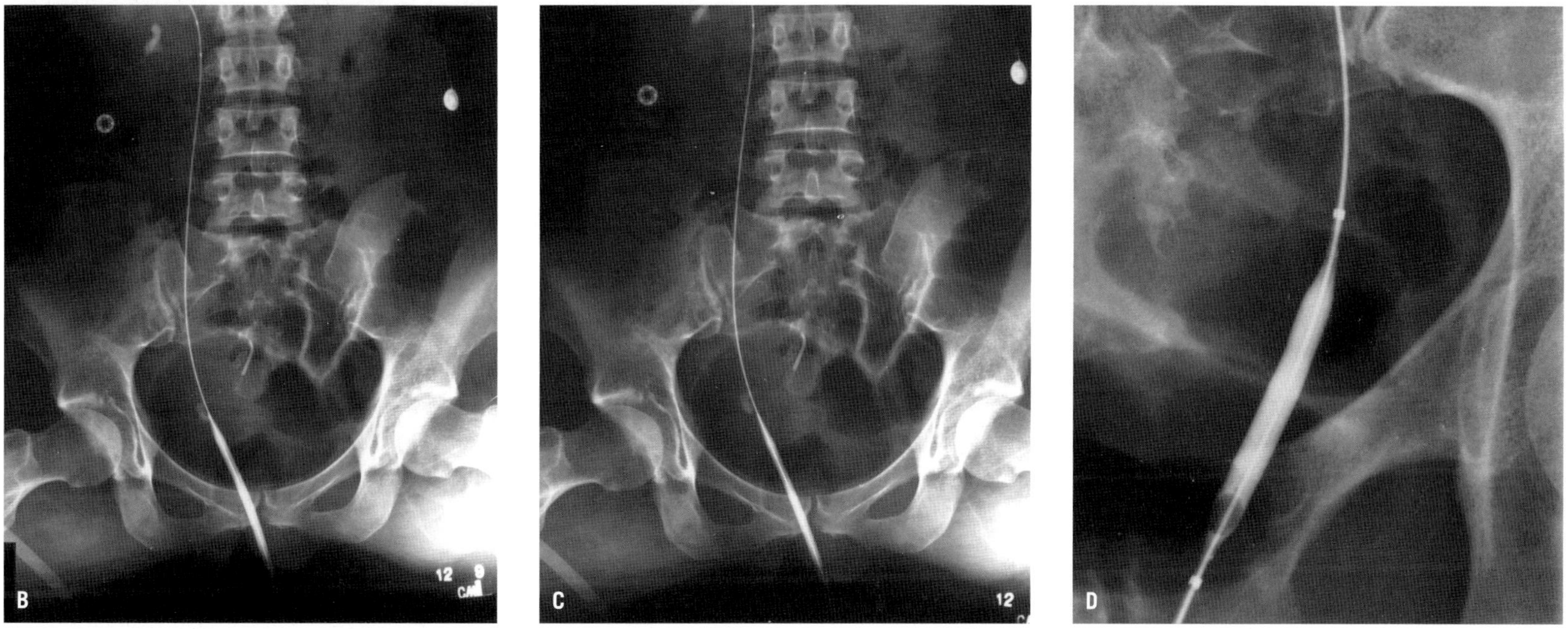

Figure 27-15 *A,* Example of a "waist" on the balloon at the level of the ureteral orifice. *B,* Teflon ureteral dilator passed through the orifice over the guidewire. *C,* Larger Teflon ureteral dilator passed through the orifice over the guidewire. *D,* Balloon confirmation of the elimination of the "waist" using the Teflon dilators.

these options fail or are not possible, consider placing a double-J catheter and allowing gradual ureteral dilation.

OTHER TECHNIQUES

Figures 27-20, 27-21, and 27-22 represent common problems in access encountered daily in our practices. Being able to access these collecting systems and deal therapeutically with these difficult access challenges can be made easier by using all or some of the various techniques that will subsequently be described.

Figure 27-20 shows an obvious impacted stone with significant ureteropyelocaliectasis proximal to the stone. In this case, shock wave lithotripsy would be the treatment of choice. Prior to that, it would be preferable to bypass the obstruction with a ureteral catheter or Double-J stent. The first step, under fluoroscopic control, is to pass the guidewire up to the stone, manipulate the wire by the calculus into the upper col-

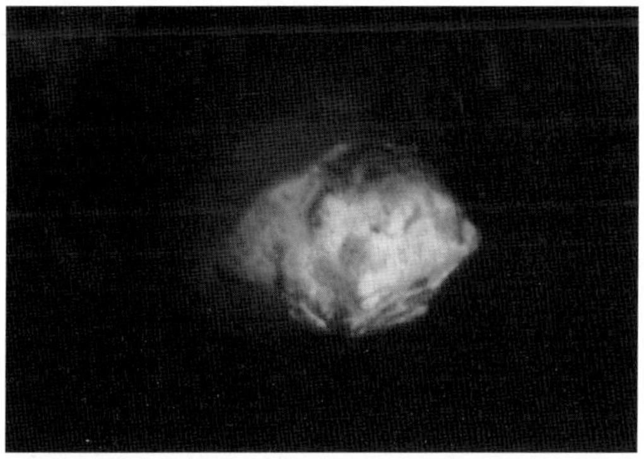

Figure 27-16 A large stone protruding from the ureteral orifice.

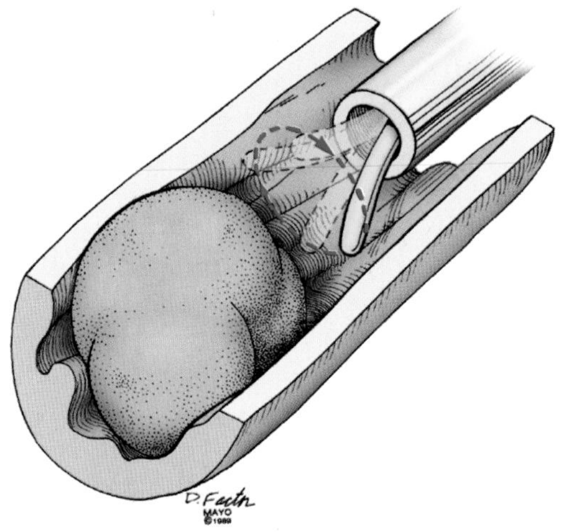

Figure 27-17 A small caliber ureteroscope just inside the intramural tunnel and attempted passage of a guidewire beyond an impacted stone.

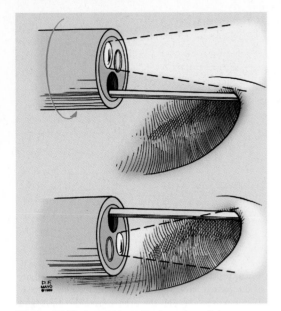

Figure 27-18 A technique for insertion of the ureteroscope into the orifice.

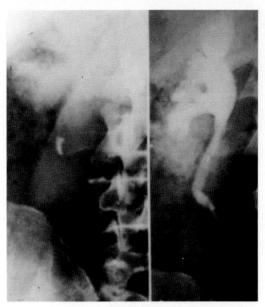

Figure 27-20 Impacted upper ureteral calculus.

tion of the ureter due to fibrosis or tumor, introduction of the angiographic catheter may not be satisfactory in straightening out the angulation. In these situations, the preformed tip angiographic catheters can be extremely helpful. After first placing the guidewire into the fixed portion of the ureter, a preformed tip catheter is passed over the wire. These catheters have memory enabling them to maintain a constant angle once they are introduced over the wire up to the point of obstruction, which facilitates manipulating various tortuosities within the ureter (Figure 27-24). Again, once the catheter is placed below the stone or obstruction, careful manipulation of a Glidewire or Sensor Wire will generally be successful in bypassing the obstruction. Orientation of the wire, as it exits the catheter below the

lecting system, and place a ureteral or Double-J stent over the guidewire. There is a risk involved: if manipulated too vigorously, a perforation may occur below the stone, necessitating a nephrostomy tube. If unable to bypass the stone, place the 6F angiographic catheter up to

the stone over the wire. This helps straighten the portion of the ureter below the stone, allowing the wire to project from the catheter in a different orientation than if the wire is simply passed without the aid of the straightening angiographic catheter (Figure 27-23). An attempt should then be made to manipulate the wire carefully beyond the calculus. At this point, extreme care should be taken to not perforate the ureter. In this particular situation, use a hydrophilic-coated wire, which easily slides through the angiographic catheter and will bypass the stone without causing trauma or perforation of the ureter. Once the Glidewire is in the proximal collecting system, the angiographic catheter is gently passed up into the renal pelvis. At this point, the Glidewire can be exchanged for a stiffer wire over which a Double-J stent or straight ureteral catheter can be placed. Use of the relatively new Sensor Wire obviates the need for multiple wire exchanges.

Figure 27-21 shows a ureter fixed by retroperitoneal fibrosis. In cases where there is fixa-

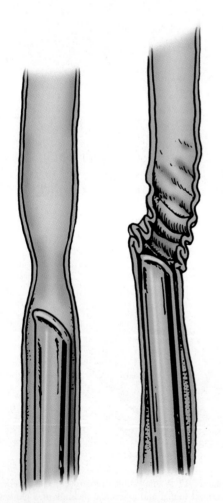

Figure 27-19 Telescoping of the ureter due to a poorly dilated segment.

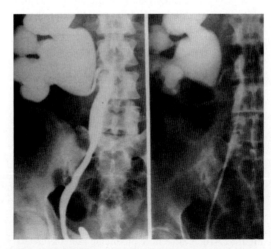

Figure 27-21 Retroperitoneal fibrosis with moderate pyelocaliectasis.

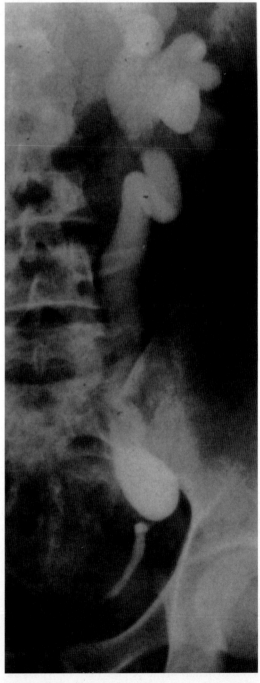

Figure 27-22 Post-hysterectomy ureteral stricture with massive hydroureteronephrosis

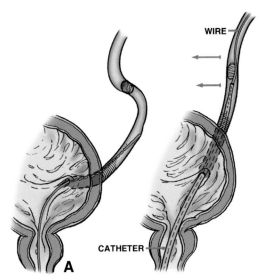

Figure 27-23 Realignment of ureter with passage of an angiographic straight catheter.

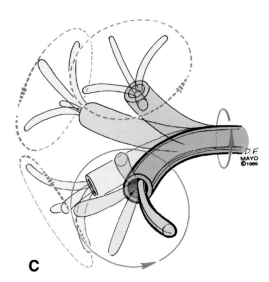

Figure 27-25 Use of a preformed tip catheter and guidewire creates an infinite number of potential chances for guidewire passage.

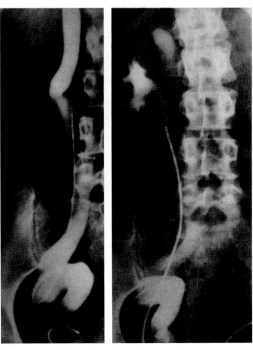

Figure 27-27 Accessing a difficult tortuous ureter.

obstruction, can occur in many different planes and angles, thereby allowing the wire to bypass the stone or obstruction. (Figure 27-25). Rotating the catheter can create an infinite number of exit points for the wire below the obstruction. By gently rotating the catheter and manipulating the wire carefully forward through the catheter, a space will ultimately be found through which the wire can pass beyond the obstruction into the upper collecting system. In cases in which there is tight obstruction, edema, or excessive friability, a soft, hydrophilic-coated wire can be used. Preformed tip angiographic catheters are also very helpful in negotiating multiple tortuosities

within the ureter as shown in Figure 27-26. By rotating the catheter and advancing the guidewire, multiple curves and bends within the ureter can be negotiated. Once the wire is beyond the curve or obstruction, careful manipulation of the catheter over the wire will allow gradual advancement up the tortuous ureter. For better orientation, the injection of contrast material will clearly outline the guidewire and catheter in the ureter. This also is helpful in detecting any perforations of the ureter.

In special situations, as demonstrated in Figure 27-22, use of the small caliber, short ureteroscope, with the passage of the guidewire under direct vision, will be less time-consuming and more successful. Particularly when dealing with

a pinpoint stricture or obstruction, sometimes the wire cannot be manipulated via the catheters as successfully as under direct vision. Also, if there is significant edema or friability of the mucosa, multiple attempts with catheters and guidewires may create more bleeding and false passages and ultimately lead to failure. By carefully passing the small ureteroscope to the point of obstruction and visually identifying the opening, passage of the guidewire will be less traumatic. (see Figure 27-17) Likewise, when dealing with a stone, with direct vision, a space can be identified between the ureteral mucosa and the stone, allowing careful manipulation of the wire into the upper collecting system.

CONCLUSION

In conclusion, with the use of various guidewires, catheters, small ureteroscopes, persistence, and a bit of luck, the vast majority of difficult retrograde ureteral access problems can be managed successfully (Figure 27-27).

REFERENCES

1. Lyon ES, Kyker JS, Schrenberg HW. Transuretheral ureteroscopy in women: a ready addition to the urological armamentarium. J Urol 1978;119:35.
2. Bagley DH, Huffman JL, Lyon ES. Flexible ureteropyeloscopy: diagnosis and treatment of the upper urinary tract. J Urol 1987;138:280.
3. Blute, ML, Segura, JW, Patterson, DE. Ureteroscopy. J Urol 1987;138:280.
4. Lyon SS, Huffman JL, Bagley DH. Ureteroscopy and ureteropyeloscopy. Urology 1984;23(Suppl 5):29.
5. Bagley DH, Huffman J, Lyon ES. Ureteroscopy for calculi in upper-tract neoplasms. In: Carson CC, Dunnick NR. Endourology. New York: Churchill Livingstone; 1985.
6. Perez-Castro, Ellendt E, Martinez-Prieiros JA. Transurethral ureteroscopy: a current urological procedure. Arch Esp Urol 1980;33:445.
7. Carson CC. Prophylactic antibiotics in urologic surgery. AUA Update Series 2:26, 1979.

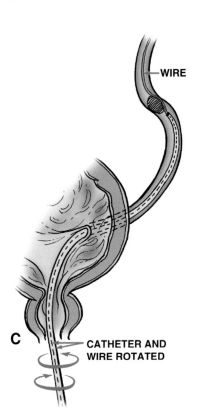

Figure 27-24 Use of a preformed tip angiographic catheter in the ureter.

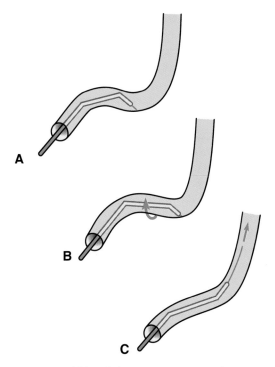

Figure 27-26 Negotiating a tortuous ureter using a preformed tip catheter and guidewire.

8. Freiha GS, King DHC, Teichman JMH. Holmium:YAG laser damage to ureteral guidewire. J. Endourol 1997;11:173–5.

9. Ford TF, Parkinson VM, Wickham JEA. Clinical and experimental evaluation of ureteric dilation. Br J Urol 1984; 56:460.

10. Clayman RV, Elbers J, Palmer JO, et al. Experimental extensive balloon dilation of the distal ureter. J Endourol 1987;1:19.

11. Gaylis, F, Bastuba, M, Bidair, M, Friedel, W. Ureteral dilation using a tapered dilator: A cost-effective approach. J Endourol 2000;14:447–9.

12. Newman RC, Hunter PT, Hawkins IF, Finlayson B. A general ureteral dilator sheathing system. Urology 1985;25:287.

13. Pietro PK, Auge BK, Delvecchio FC, et al. Techniques to maximize flexible ureteroscope longevity. Urology 2002; 60:784–6.

14. Monga M, Bhayani S, Landman J, et al. Ureteral access for upper urinary tract disease: the access sheath. J Endourol 2001;15:831–4.

15. Eiley DM, McDougall EM, Smith AD. Techniques for stenting the normal and obstructed ureter. J Endourol 1997; 11:419–29.

16. Lallas CD, Auge BK, Ganesh VR, et al. Laser doppler flowmetric determination of ureteral blood flow after ureteral access sheath placement. J Endourol 2002;16:583–90.

17. Perez-Castro, Ellendt E, Mancebo Gomes JM, Massara J. Dilatacion hidraulica con bomba impulsora de liquido irrigante: nueva aparataje en ureterorrenoscopic. Arch Esp Urol 1986;39(Suppl 1):3.

18. Eshghi M. Hydraulic dilation of the ureter for ureteroscopy [Abstract]. In: Proceedings of Fifth World Congress on Endourology and ESWL, Cairo, Egypt, November 1987. p. 23.

19. Patterson DE. Management of ureteral calculi. In: Stephen N. Rous, editor. Urology annual 1994, Vol. 8. New York: W. W. Norton and Company; 1994.

28

Techniques in Rigid Ureteroscopy

Damien M. Bolton, MD

When first introduced in the late 1970s, the utility of ureteroscopy appeared to be limited and confined mainly to the management of distal ureteric calculi. The initial experience at that time also indicated that its use would be associated with significant morbidity.[1,2] The large-diameter instruments used in the early experience with this procedure resulted in a significant incidence of ureteric injury, particularly mural perforation, and subsequent stricture formation. The delayed complications of these injuries occasionally were more significant than the problems caused by the original pathology that had been treated. Ureteroscopy has since evolved to become an essential and integral tool in the management of calculi and multiple other pathologies throughout the upper urinary tract. Its established place in the treatment of these conditions exemplifies the advances in ureteroscopy since its introduction, and renders historical the suboptimal results obtained with earlier and now superseded instrumentation.

The greatly expanded role of ureteroscopy is due to progress in fiberoptics and digital imaging, which affords better endoscopic vision with smaller-sized instrumentation, endoscopic baskets and laser power devices, and the development of improved ureteroscopic surgical techniques. The combination of these advances has made ureteroscopic treatment of upper, as well as lower and middle third ureteral calculi and mucosal lesions routine procedures with little resultant morbidity. Outpatient and bilateral ureteroscopic surgery for such indications has become standard practice in many centers.[3,4] Pathology in the upper third of the ureter and intrarenal collecting system is now also readily managed using ureteroscopic methods, reducing the need for both open and percutaneous renal surgery in such circumstances.[5,6] Ureteroscopy also has become standard of care in the management of urinary calculi in pregnancy.[7]

INSTRUMENTATION

Paramount to the success of any ureteroscopic procedure is the appropriate choice of instrumentation for the individual case. All necessary equipment should be selected, assembled, and tested before induction of anesthesia. It is important to ascertain at this time that the desired results of surgery will indeed be achievable with the equipment and consumables available. If stone fragmentation or tumor ablation is planned, the lithotrites and lasers in particular must be functional and calibrated to provide power precisely at the levels required.

The first generation of rigid ureteroscopic equipment had an external diameter of approximately 11.5 to 12.0 French (F). Such hardware was superseded by fiberoptic instruments of external diameter size 10.5 to 9.5F. The most recent class of instrumentation to be introduced has been the semirigid ureteroscopes of between 4.0 and 7.2F, which may graduate to a larger diameter along the shaft of the device. Such instruments range between 31.0 and 47.5 cm in length, and have working channels measuring between 1.8 and 5.5F. The type of ureteroscope used should be chosen with a view to most easily accessing and managing the particular stone, stricture, or tumor to be treated.

The larger ureteroscopes will permit passage of wider lithotrites that are able to fragment most urinary calculi, and have additional capabilities that may enhance the likelihood of immediate intraoperative stone clearance. Suction of irrigation fluid and stone fragments is possible through such ultrasonic lithotrite probes designed for use with the 10.5 to 12.0F ureteroscopes. Telescopes of this diameter, however, typically require dilation of the ureteral orifice and provide only limited access to the upper and middle thirds of the ureter. Smaller-diameter instruments pass more readily into the ureter without dilation and can be advanced into the upper third of the ureter without fear of mural perforation, but smaller lithotrites or laser fibers must be used. The availability of such smaller-diameter instrumentation has now become the accepted standard of care and has contributed in part to reducing the frequency of iatrogenic ureteral injury from historically high levels to being a rare event. The use of such smaller semirigid instrumentation is to be encouraged wherever possible.[8,9]

Most 6.0F and larger external diameter ureteroscope channels allow passage of the 1 mm diameter ultrasonic (without a suction channel) or lithoclast probes.[10] Only laser lithotripsy fibers and the small (1.6–1.9F) electrohydraulic lithotripsy probes can pass through the working channels of the smallest available 4.5F equipment (2.4F diameter working channel). A second working channel is available in some current-generation ureteroscopes. Such smaller-diameter equipment lenses also are more subject to the "crescent moon" effect—the limited visual field experienced when the telescope shaft is placed under pressure, causing it to bend out of a straight line. This effect is not seen with fiberoptic imaging bundles. Appropriate education of all levels of operating unit staff in regard to optimal methods of sterilization, storage, and presentation of ureteroscopes will help prolong the utility of such finely developed hardware.

The development of digital imaging systems has further extended the capability of ureteroscopic instrumentation. Current generation systems utilize either a halogen or xenon high-intensity light source that permits automatic light intensity adjustment, which may help compensate for technical difficulties during a procedure such as restriction to irrigation and ureteral dilation. Associated digital video cameras similarly allow for adjustment of camera aperture and exposure periods in order to try and achieve a constant balance of brightness and high clarity of the image. Such cameras may be single or more commonly three-chip systems that provide resolution of greater than 450,000 pixels, or more than 700 horizontal lines of image. More recently developed have been those ureteroscopes that have a digital chip in place at the distal end of the instrument instead of a camera, providing for a true digital image. Also available are magnifying and zoom endoscopes that provide for optimal imaging quality in occasional circumstances. Accessory equipment suitable for stone fragmentation, ureteral biopsy, and soft tissue ablation is available for use with practically all such variations of ureteroscope.

PREOPERATIVE PREPARATION

Access to all required ancillary equipment should be confirmed before the commencement of the procedure. Appropriate guidewires, stone baskets and grasping forceps, lithotrites, ureteral exchange catheters, and stents need to be on hand preoperatively to ensure the smooth progression of the case. Automated irrigation +/- suction systems may also be required to provide for optimal visualization in instances of difficult access to pathology such as a densely impacted calculus. X-ray facilities must be able to provide fluoroscopic and digital/hard-copy imaging that is of adequate quality for treatment, and that does not cause unnecessary scatter of radiation energy. An arrangement that delivers fluoroscopy from below the operating table is optimal and also provides the best protection for medical personnel against the risks of long-term radiation exposure (such as cataract formation). Digital enhancement settings for use at intervals during videoendoscopy has also been shown in a blinded study to significantly improve images from rigid and semirigid ureteroscopes, as has the use of a digital fiberscope filter during flexible ureteroscopy.[11] The importance of adequate preoperative imaging of the size, location, and number of urinary calculi also cannot be overstated prior to ureteroscopy. The use of newer 64-slice multidetector helical digital CT images, with the potential for reconstructions in coronal and saggital planes, as well as the plane of the length of the ureter and any stone within it, can be of great assistance in this regard (Figure 28-1).

TECHNIQUE

In most instances, insertion of a guidewire into the ureteral orifice and passage of the guidewire up into the renal pelvis are the initial steps in ureteroscopic surgery. Flexible-tip standard or hydrophilic guidewires each may be used to advantage depending on operator preference. Perforation of the ureteric wall is less likely with the more flexible hydrophilic guidewires, although these are somewhat more difficult to manipulate because of their lubricious coating. Ureteral perforation remains an uncommon event with standard guidewires, even in cases of complicated ureteral stone disease, provided such wires are placed with care. Hybrid wires that consist of a distal hydrophilic tip, a main body comprising a polytetrafluoroethylene (PTFE, Teflon) coating over a nitinol core, and a flexible proximal tip to permit retrograde passage through instrumentation are of particular use in occasional complicated surgery, but are more commonly used in flexible ureteroscopy.

A ureteral exchange catheter, usually 5F, is then passed over the wire. This permits a retrograde pyelogram to be obtained using dilute contrast medium injected under low pressure. This provides clear delineation of the anatomy of the upper urinary tract, and thereby reduces the likelihood of complications such as ureteral perforation, submucosal passage of guidewires and exchange catheters, and contrast extravasation. It is important for the endourologist to appreciate, however, that the images thus obtained provide only a two-dimensional picture of the ureteral course and do not delineate the variation in the anteroposterior dimension of the ureter throughout its normal course. The ureter naturally adopts a concave pelvic curve to the level of the iliac vessels and above this a less marked convexity over the psoas muscle (Figure 28-2). Special techniques are sometimes required later in the procedure to overcome surgical difficulties resulting from exaggerations of this normal anatomy.

If a guidewire will not pass beyond the ureteral calculus or lesion being treated, special techniques may be necessary to gain access to the renal pelvis. The injection of a small amount of dilute contrast agent from below the calculus may identify the nature of the obstruction and a potential passage around it. Similarly, the use of additional endoscopic guidewires may be advantageous. The length of the floppy tip of a coaxial guidewire may be increased to provide greater flexibility at the level of the calculus; a J-tipped wire also may permit more ready passage. More commonly, however, the use of hydrophilic guidewires allows the easiest access to the ureter beyond an obstructing stone. Once in place, the hydrophilic wire may be replaced by a standard PTFE-coated wire through a ureteral exchange catheter to permit a straighter ureteral lumen during endoscopic surgery, and to allow placement of a ureteral stent at the conclusion of the procedure. Occasionally the use of extra-stiff (Amplatz or Lunderquist-Cook) wires may be warranted to straighten a particularly tortuous ureter, and may be passed via a ureteral exchange catheter that has previously been advanced to the renal pelvis. Passage of such super-stiff guidewires directly via a cystoscope or partially inserted ureteroscope is to be discouraged owing to the potential for ureteral mural perforation.

In rare instances it will be impossible to place a wire retrogradely beyond an obstructing ureteral lesion. In such circumstances the urologist has two options. A percutaneous nephrostomy tube may be placed and attempts made to pass a guidewire down past the obstruction in an antegrade fashion, or alternatively, ureteroscopy may be undertaken to the level of the lesion and the wire passed beside the calculus under endoscopic vision. This latter technique is associated with a higher rate of ureteral perforation and should never be undertaken unless facilities for percutaneous nephrostomy are available should mural perforation result.

After the guidewire has been placed retrogradely into the renal pelvis, dilation of the ureteral orifice is undertaken, if necessary. The need for this ancillary technique has declined with the development of smaller-diameter ureteroscopes[12] and is rarely required if the ureter has been catheterized or stented previously. When dilation of the ureteral orifice is necessary, it is possible to use a balloon catheter placed over the guidewire and inserted into the ureteral orifice under endoscopic vision. The balloon catheter then is inflated to the pressure necessary to open the ureter on fluoroscopic monitoring. Alternatively, dilation may be performed using single- or serial-graduated Teflon sheaths, or less commonly, metal bougies, passed over the guidewire. The advent of the smaller-diameter ureteroscopes has meant that use of dilators of sizes greater than 10F in external diameter is now rarely required. Once dilation of the ureteral orifice has been completed, the cystoscope may be extracted from the bladder backward over the guidewire, which is kept secure in its positioning by light tension as the cystoscope is removed. The guidewire is then secured to the drapes with a clip to act as a guide during use of the ureteroscope.

The ureteroscope may now be introduced into the ureter. Previously, larger instruments may have required the use of a second guidewire and maneuvers such as rotating the telescope through 180 degrees so the port containing the wire was uppermost and the telescope was passed into the ureter through the widest possible aperture of the ureteral orifice. Smaller-caliber ureteroscopes can be passed directly without a second wire, although this option more often may be useful higher in the ureter where reduced luminal size, tortuous course, and prominent extramural anatomy may make passage toward the renal pelvis difficult. If the placement of two guidewires is warranted, it is preferable that the single, or both the twin working channels of the ureteroscope, can be left open to facilitate irriga-

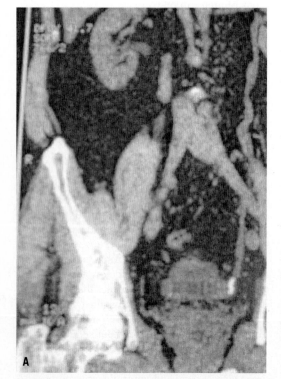

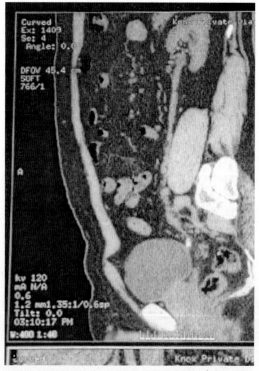

Figure 28-1 CT images of *A*, coronal and *B*, saggital reconstuctions of the kidney and ureter, demonstrating the presence of a 9 mm calculus situated 3 cm above the vesicoureteric junction, but below the iliac vessels, suitable for ureteroscopic fragmentation and extraction.

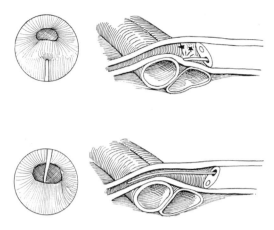

Figure 28-2 Schematic sagittal view of the ureteral course, demonstrating the curves normally followed within the pelvis and over the psoas muscle to reach the renal pelvis.

tion and endoscopic manipulation and retrieval. This can be achieved by backing the ureteroscope off the guidewire and reinserting the telescope if placement of the wire via the ureteroscope has been required. It is now rare that the ureteroscope needs to be inserted directly over a guidewire for purposes of gaining access to the upper ureter.

The ureteroscope should be advanced toward the stone or lesion under continuous endoscopic vision. The guidewire running to the renal pelvis provides an excellent reference point for orientation in an anteroposterior plane. Passive irrigation usually is adequate to allow sufficient proximal dilation of the ureter for the ureteroscope to pass without difficulty, and at the same time reduces the likelihood of proximal migration of any ureteric calculi back into the renal pelvis. The use of passive refilling and pressure irrigation devices (power irrigation) may occasionally be warranted to permit an adequate approach to a particular calculus or upper-tract tumour.[13] Such maneuvers will, however, increase the intraureteral pressure, and care must be taken not to flush the calculus being treated back to the renal pelvis. Even moving the ureteroscope within the collecting system without irrigant flow has been noted to elevate renal pelvic pressure approximately 25 mm Hg, which can be sufficient to dislodge a calculus.[14] The successful use of available automated irrigation/suction systems for controlling ureteral pressure and flow has, however, been associated with improved visibility and reduced operating time in ureteral stone surgery.[15]

Patient and methodical advancement of the telescope is the key to uncomplicated progression in a cephalad direction. Caution must be taken to avoid compression of the ureter into a "concertina," which occurs when excessive force is used in a narrowed segment (Figure 28-3). This can result in ureteral perforation or even avulsion.

A second wire passed through the instrument channel of the ureteroscope can facilitate proximal advancement through a narrow segment of ureter, for example, over the iliac vessels. Use of this technique, however, requires an appreciation of the potential complications if the wire is

placed extramurally. Every effort must be made to prevent this. Most useful in this regard is the technique of inverting the ureteroscope and taking advantage of the eccentrically placed manipulation channels within the instrument. This permits a second wire to pass more freely through the ureteral lumen and reduces the likelihood that the pressure of gentle advancement will perforate a weakened ureteral wall (Figure 28-4). The ureteroscope then can be restored to its usual orientation to facilitate proximal advancement in the normal fashion. This maneuver also may be used for positioning a ureteral exchange catheter beyond the tip of the ureteroscope to improve vision by permitting efflux of bloodstained irrigant if minor bleeding is a problem.

Once the urinary calculus or other pathology has been reached within the ureter, it must be dealt with in the most expeditious fashion possible, given the available resources. Several principles remain constant. Most importantly, care must be taken to avoid damaging the ureteral wall with the instrumentation. Tissue damage can be particularly severe with use of the electrohydraulic lithotrite, in which a cavitation bubble develops proportional in size to the energy applied. This can result in damage to the ureteral wall even when the probe is not in contact with the mucosa.[16] The selection of high-voltage and low-capacity settings reduces the size of this cavitation effect, resulting in short and steep pulses akin to those seen with laser lithotrites and limiting the extent of any ureteral injury. Avoiding direct pressure on the stone with the lithotrite also will reduce the likelihood of iatrogenic dislodgment into the renal pelvis or even the retroperitoneum. Although retroperitoneal dislodgment has a low rate of late complications, it can result in a confusing situation for both the patient and other physicians, and represents suboptimal management of urinary calculi.[17]

The use of laser lithotrites, predominantly those utilizing holmium:YAG laser energy, has been demonstrated to achieve higher stone-free rates than standard electrohydraulic lithotripsy and must now be regarded as the optimum stan-

dard of care in ureteroscopic stone management.[18] Such lasers provide light at a wavelength of 2,140 nm, which will produce a photothermal effect on the surface of the calculus at which it is directed, resulting in destabilization of the stone lattice and subsequent fragmentation.

Ideally, all calculi should be fragmented to a size where the greatest diameter of any residual debris is well below 5 mm and will pass spontaneously if not removed at the time of initial surgery. If the resulting fragments are larger, they must be retrieved using grasping forceps or stone baskets. Round-wire baskets can be torqued with some impunity to help entrap fragments, but flat-wire baskets should be used with greater caution because their sharper edges are more likely to cause ureteral injury. Sheathless baskets also may be used to optimize irrigant flow during ureteroscopy, and this technique also permits more substantial deflection of the flexible ureteroscope than when a standard sheathed basket is used.[19] Use of a stone-cone placed above a large calculus may avoid proximal migration of stone debris of significant dimensions. If multiple passages of a rigid instrument through the ureter will be required to remove a large bulk of fragmented calculus, consideration should be given to placing a Finlayson-type ureteral access sheath to reduce the trauma to the ureteral orifice, as is routine in flexible ureteroscopic surgery.

Care must be taken to avoid the complications specific to more complex procedures. In the pediatric population, increased attention must be given to avoiding trauma to the lower ureter and the ureterovesical junction during stone extraction.[20] Caution must be taken during ablation of superficial ureteral transitional cell carcinomas or other mucosal lesions to avoid damage to the deeper layers of the wall that could result in full-thickness ischemia with subsequent scarring of the ureter and possibly even retroperitoneal seeding of the tumor (Figure 28-5). Conversely, in retrograde management of ureteral and ureteropelvic junction strictures, efforts must be made to ensure that a full-thickness incision of the ureteral wall has been made and that the urologist is aware of

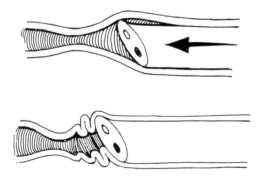

Figure 28-3 "Concertina" effect of the ureter that can result if the ureteroscope is advanced through a narrow segment of ureter without taking measures to maximize ureteral width. Ureteral perforation and even avulsion can result under such circumstances.

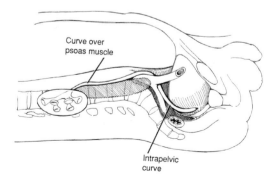

Figure 28-4 At points where the ureter does not follow a straight course (eg, over the iliac vessels), passage of the wire through the ureteroscope can result in it being pushed abruptly onto the ureteral wall. Inverting the ureteroscope permits the wire to pass more freely by taking advantage of the asymmetric placement of the instrument channel within the ureteroscope.

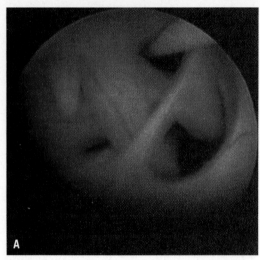

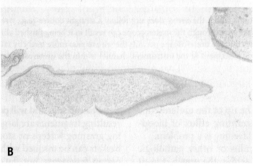

Figure 28-5 *A*, Endoscopic appearance of a fibroepithelial polyp of the upper urinary tract seen in the upper left corner. A guidewire can be seen passing into the upper pole calices. *B*, Histologic appearance of this benign tumor after it was endoscopically removed. The base of the lesion was fulgurated using ureteroscopic techniques.

the proximity of the planned incision to the large retroperitoneal vessels, which could easily be damaged during the procedure.[21,22] If treatment is being directed toward submucosal calculi, availability of endoluminal ultrasonographic equipment and familiarity with the appearance of the hyperechoic foci produced is mandatory to achieve optimal therapeutic results.[23]

POSTOPERATIVE CARE

The endourologist must individualize the operative plan so that the procedure can be accomplished in a single operation as far as is technically feasible. Occasionally, however, circumstances such as ureteral bleeding, large lesion size, or equipment failure make it necessary to discontinue a procedure and finish it a short time later. Under such circumstances, as at the completion of most routine rigid ureteroscopic cases, a Double-J stent should be placed, possibly along with a urethral catheter to monitor urine output and prevent urinary reflux in the early postoperative phase. The placement of a Double-J stent helps avoid the complications of pain and infection that can result from ureteral edema. Although the use

of stents with a long suture attached facilitates removal in the urologist's office, the strings often migrate proximally into the urethra, especially on penile erection. Removal then involves the flexible cystoscope and grasping forceps just as for stents without a suture attached. Stent placement has assisted greatly in permitting ureteroscopy to be performed on an outpatient basis. Recent data, however, suggest that with minaturization of ureteroscopes, ureteric stenting may not be required postoperatively as often as has traditionally been standard practice.[24]

In patients who have had prolonged renal drainage obstruction because of a ureteral lesion, the ureter above the site of the primary lesion may be distended and tortuous. This makes retrograde placement of stents difficult. Under such circumstances, the use of extra-stiff wires (Amplatz or Lunderquist) will assist in positioning the stent by straightening the varicose ureter. The urologist also must exercise caution in these cases to avoid placing the stent in the dilated upper ureter, rather than above the ureteropelvic junction in the renal pelvis as desired. Delineation of the anatomy of the collecting system by retrograde pyelography and the use of extra-long stents can be helpful in such cases.

If a nephrostomy tube was placed previously, it is often prudent to remove it under fluoroscopic guidance at the conclusion of the ureteroscopic procedure, when direct access to the Double-J stent can be obtained cystoscopically and the stent stabilized using grasping forceps, if necessary. Entwinement of the loop of a stent within that of a nephrostomy tube with subsequent percutaneous removal of both prostheses is a well-recognized pitfall that can complicate an otherwise technically perfect ureteroscopy.

CONCLUSION

Although the basic principles of endourology must be adhered to in ureteroscopy, there is no substitute for familiarity with the techniques that prevent the potential complications of these procedures. Caution, patience, and a thorough knowledge of endoscopic equipment and consumables ensure the optimum outcome for each procedure undertaken. The utilization of dedicated skill-center training modules has been demonstrated to improve technical outcomes in the process of learning to undertakes such procedures.[25] As the available equipment evolves and more techniques are added to the repertoire of the competent ureteroscopist, more complex and difficult procedures will continue to be proposed and undertaken. Most recently, such clinical instances have included pediatric urolithiasis,[26] ureteroscopy in pregnancy,[27] and in the evaluation and treatment of benign hematuria.[28] As endourologists, we look forward to further such challenges and the consequent evolution of this procedure.

REFERENCES

1. Lyon ES, Kyker JS, Schoenberg HW. Transurethral ureteroscopy in women: a ready addition to the urologic armamentarium. J Urol 1978;119:35–6.
2. Goodman TM. Ureteroscopy with the pediatric cystoscope in adults. Urology 1977;9:394.
3. Wills TE, Burns JR. Ureteroscopy: an outpatient procedure? J Urol 1994;151:1185–7.
4. Camilleri JC, Schwalb DM, Eshghi M. Bilateral same session ureteroscopy. J Urol 1994;152:49–52.
5. Grasso M, Loisides P, Beaghler M, Bagley D. The case for primary endoscopic management of upper urinary tract calculi. I. A critical review of 121 extracorporeal shock wave lithotripsy failures. Urology 1995;45:363–71.
6. Grasso M, Beaghler M, Loisides P. The case for primary endoscopic management of upper urinary tract calculi. II. Cost and outcome assessment of 112 primary ureteral calculi. Urology 1995;45:372–6.
7. Lifshitz DA, Lingeman JE. Ureteroscopy as a first-line intervention for ureteral calculi in pregnancy. J Endourol 2002;16:19–22.
8. Huffman JL. Ureteroscopic injuries to the upper urinary tract. Urol Clin North Am 1989;16:249–54.
9. Assimos DG, Patterson LC, Taylor CL. Changing incidence and etiology of iatrogenic ureteral injuries. J Urol 1994; 152(6 Pt 2):2240–6.
10. Ferraro RF, Abraham VE, Cohen TD, Preminger GM. A new generation of semirigid fiberoptic ureteroscopes. J Endourol 1999;13:35–40.
11. Aslan P, Kuo RL, Hazel K, et al. Advances in digital imaging during endoscopic surgery. J Endourol 1999;13:251–5.
12. Stoller ML, Wolf JS Jr, Hofmann R, Marc B. Ureteroscopy without routine balloon dilation: an outcome assessment. J Urol 1992;147:1238–42.
13. Menon A, Ather MH, Sulaiman MN. Three techniques for simpler, safer, and cost-effective rigid ureteroscopy. Tech Urol 2000;6:215–7.
14. Schwalb DM, Eshghi M, Davidian M, Franco I. Morphological and physiological changes in the urinary tract associated with ureteral dilation and ureteropyeloscopy: an experimental study. J Urol 1993;149:1576–85.
15. Lechevallier E, Luciani M, Nahon O, et al. Transurethral ureterorenolithotripsy using new automated irrigation/ suction system controlling pressure and flow compared with standard irrigation: a randomized pilot study. J Endourol 2002;17:97–101.
16. Vorreuther R, Corleis R, Klotz T, et al. Impact of shock wave pattern and cavitation bubble size on tissue damage during ureteroscopic electrohydraulic lithotripsy. J Urol 1995;153(3 Pt 1):849–53.
17. Evans CP, Stoller ML. The fate of the iatrogenic retroperitoneal stone. J Urol 1993;150:827–9.
18. Teichman JM, Rao RD, Rogenes VJ, Harris MJ. Ureteroscopic management of ureteral calculi: electrohydraulic versus holmium:YAG lithotripsy. J Urol 1997;158:1357–61.
19. Bhayani SB, Monga M, Landman J, Clayman RV. Bare naked baskets: optimizing ureteroscopic stone extraction. Urology 2002;60:147–8.
20. Thomas R, Ortenberg J, Lee BR, Harmon EP. Safety and efficacy of pediatric ureteroscopy for management of calculous disease. J Urol 1993;149:1082–4.
21. Yamada S, Ono Y, Ohshima S, Miyake K. Transurethral ureteroscopic ureterotomy assisted by a prior balloon dilation for relieving ureteral strictures. J Urol 1995;153:1418–21.
22. Clayman RV, Basler JW, Kavoussi L, Picus DD. Ureteronephroscopic endopyelotomy. J Urol 1990;144(2 Pt 1): 246–51.
23. Grasso M, Liu J, Goldberg B, Bagley D. Submucosal calculi: endoscopic and intraluminal sonographic diagnosis and treatment options. J Urol 1995;153:1384–9.
24. Chen YT, Chen J, Wong WY, et al. Is ureteral stenting necessary after uncomplicated ureteroscopic lithotripsy? A prospective, randomized controlled trial. J Urol 2002;167:1977–80.
25. Matsumoto ED, Hamstra SJ, Radomski SB, Cusimano MD. A novel approach to endourological training: training at the Surgical Skills Center. J Urol 2001;166:1261–6.
26. Satar N, Zeren S, Bayazit Y, et al. Rigid ureteroscopy for the treatment of ureteral calculi in children. J. Urol 2004;172:298–300.
27. Shokeir AA., Mutabagani H. Rigid ureteroscopy in pregnant women. Br J Urol 1998;81:678–81.
28. Dooley RE, Peitrow PK. Ureteroscopy for benign hematuria. Urol Clin North Am 2004;31:137–43.

29

Flexible Fiberoptic Ureteropyeloscopy

Danny M. Rabah, MD, FRCSC
Michael D. Fabrizio, MD, FACS

Hugh H. Young in 1912 described the first endoscopic view of the ureters when he passed a rigid cystoscope through a dilated ureter.[1] Fiberoptics have dramatically changed the therapeutic and diagnostic role of medical instruments in many medical specialties. The concept of light transmission through small-diameter glass fibers was first described in 1920.[2] The first clinical application was in 1956 when Hirshowitz and colleagues performed the first flexible esophagogastroduodenoscopy.[3] The first report of flexible ureteroscopy was by Marshall in 1964, who visualized a stone in the midureter using a 3 mm fiberscope.[4] This was followed in 1968 by Tagaki and colleagues who passed a similar scope through an open ureterotomy into the upper collecting system in a retrograde fashion.[5] Bagley and colleagues started their pioneering work in the early 1980s, developing improved flexible ureteroscopes that allowed better visualization, maneuverability, and working potential, allowing for therapeutic ureteroscopic techniques. The three major advances in design were as follows:

1. The addition of a working channel allowing irrigant, wires, and instruments to be passed through the flexible ureteroscopes.
2. Designing the mechanical system that allows for active deflection of the tip.
3. Softening and strengthening different parts of the ureteroscope shafts to allow for passive secondary deflection, and therefore improving access to the entire collecting system.[6–9]

INSTRUMENTATION

An understanding of the optical and mechanical design of the flexible ureteroscope allows a better appreciation of its potential as well as its limitations.

The basic concept of flexible scopes rests on fiberoptic technology. This relies on the physical property of light internal reflection, resulting in "bending" of light within flexible glass. Fiberoptics are fashioned out of molten glass that uniformly transmits light from one end to the other in proportion to the light input. These fibers are bundled together in the same orientation, which allows these dots of light to coalesce and transmit the resultant image. As the technology improves, more fibers are bundled together, resulting in better images.[10–13] A second layer of dissoluble glass is evenly dispersed between the fiberoptic quartz fibers and is known as cladding, which doesn't transmit light.[14] This even distribution is

known as pixel spacing and is what allows for softening and flexibility of the whole bundle. It is also responsible for the mesh-like appearance of the image or "insect-eye" pattern known as the morea. A distal and proximal optical lens transforms the fiberoptic bundle into a clinical telescope. A good light source is essential for adequate image transmission.

Current flexible scopes are capable of both active and passive tip deflection. The active deflection is lever controlled, which shortens or lengthens wires running to metal rings just proximal to the tip, which can cause the deflection in both directions in one plane.[15] Active deflection of the ureteroscope tip is essential to access the lateral and inferior infundibula.[16] The secondary passive deflection is a result of making the segment just proximal to the point of active deflection more flexible. Passive deflection of the ureteroscope off the wall of the renal pelvis moves the point of deflection proximally on the scope. This effectively extends the tip of the ureteroscope and allows inspection of the lower-pole calices with greater ease. When this maneuver is used, this portion of the collecting system is successfully visualized in over 90% of patients.[16–18] In order to access the lower-pole infundibulum, 104° to 175° (mean 140°) of deflection is required.[19] The passage of working instruments and laser fibers through the working chan-

nel of flexible ureteroscopes may decrease active deflection by up to 52%[20] (Figures 29-1, D and E, and 29-2, E and F). Deflection is inhibited when larger-diameter accessories are passed through the working channel. The flexible lithoclast, the non-nitinol baskets, and the 365-micron laser probes significantly inhibit the deflection of all scopes. The 200-micron laser fiber or the 1.6 to 1.9 French (F) is more flexible. Electrohydrolic lithotripsy (EHL) probes. Both the nitinol 1.9F basket as well as the 2.5F three-pronged grasper cause minimal inhibition and are ideal for use in lower-pole caliceal system.[21]

Flexible ureteroscopes have a single working channel. This allows fluid irrigation and passage of instruments for biopsy, fulguration, stone retrieval, and lithotripsy. This working channel is a smooth cylindrical plastic tube that travels trough the flexible ureteroscope. Most working channels are 3.6F in diameter and are eccentrically located. As newer, smaller-tip ureteroscopes become available, the eccentricity is less prominent. This allows for less distortion of the working channel while actively deflecting, and allows easier passage of working instruments.[16] Instruments that are 2.5F or smaller in size pass through the working channel more readily, improve irrigation, and cause less inhibition of the degree of active deflection of the scope.[16] Passage of working instruments may be difficult

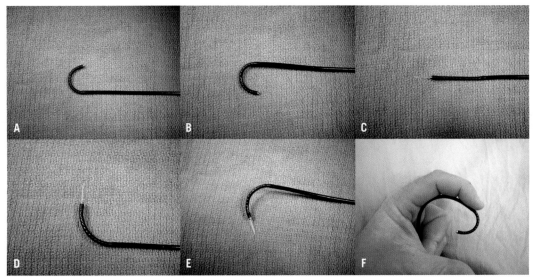

Figure 29-1 Flexible ureteroscope deflections. *A* and *B*, demonstrating 170° downward and 120° upward primary active deflection. *C*, 360-micron laser fiber passed beyond tip the ureteroscope. *D* and *E*, demonstrating loss of deflection angle obtained with the laser fiber in the working channel in both directions. *F*, Active primary and passive secondary deflection give a combined wider angle and easier access to the lower-pole calices.

when the scope is maximally deflected. In fact, the working channel may be damaged if passage is attempted while the scope is deflected. Therefore, passing instruments is best accomplished by passing the instrument with the scope straightened and adequately lubricating the instruments. High-pressure irrigation can increase the amount of flow around a working instrument. This may be accomplished by a pressurized irrigation bag, roller pump, or a hand-held syringe. Flow rates of 20 mL/min provide adequate visualization in most circumstances.[22]

Newer-developed flexible ureteroscopes have increasing angles of active deflection. This is seen in the ACMI DUR8-E flexible ureteroscope that allows two levers to control active deflection at two separate sites near the tip of the scope. The primary active deflection allows for up to 185° of downward deflection, while adding the secondary active deflection allows for a total of 270° in one direction. No passive deflection is available with this type of ureteroscope. Karl Storz has developed a different mechanism on their latest flexible ureteroscope. A single-lever mechanism that offers dual 270° of deflection. Figures 29-1 and 29-2, and Figure 29-3 demonstrate the range of motion of the new generation scopes and the amount of deflection lost by passing instruments in the working channels. Table 29-1 summarizes the characteristics of the flexible ureteroscopes available in the market today.

Failure to visualize the entire collecting system during diagnostic ureteroscopy or to access intrarenal calculi occurs in 10 to 14% of cases.[16,23]

Up to 61° of active deflection is lost if the proximal shaft of the ureteroscope is not kept in a straight alignment. The urologist must keep the shaft of the ureteroscope as straight as possible outside and inside the patient. Holding the ureteroscope taut by gentle manual back tension on the ureteroscope shaft provides additional

angulation at the tip. Using an access sheath also maximizes active deflection. The basic benefit of the sheath is in preventing buckling of the ureteroscope along the urethra or into the bladder, which is the major cause of decreased active tip deflection. Since tension on the midshaft of the ureteroscope results in improvements in upward and downward active deflection, placing a super-stiff guidewire in the working channel may maximize active deflection. This is accomplished by positioning the guidewire tip 2 cm proximal to the end of the ureteroscope. When positioned in this fashion, the 6 cm floppy tip of the wire will not interfere with its deflection mechanism. This may give up to 29° of improved maneuverability and is obviously of use only in diagnostic procedures.[24]

PREOPERATIVE AND PATIENT PREPARATION

In preparing for this procedure the urologist should assure the availability of the following:

1. Operating table suitable for cystoscopy and fluoroscopy. It must provide smooth and controlled positioning as well as a drainage device.
2. Video equipment, which allows the surgeon comfort as well as magnification. It also allows the staff in the operating room to work as team while following the procedure.
3. Flouroscopy unit.
4. The endoscope instruments, which include a cystoscope with all its axillaries, ureteroscope, rigid and flexible guidewires of various sizes and material composition, ureteral catheters and stents, dilators, syringes, and contrast material.
5. Anesthesia. Local anesthesia is adequate only when using smaller flexible endoscopes for surveillance ureteroscopy. General anesthesia is preferred over regional anesthesia because it

provides better pain control when working in the proximal ureters or collecting system. It also provides a relaxed patient, eliminating harmful sudden movements. One must remember to empty the bladder and prevent overfilling of the urinary tract, which may induce the anesthetized patient to move suddenly.

6. Positioning the patient in the standard lithotomy position. The leg contralateral to the side of interest is slightly extended and the hip abducted. This allows minimal angulation of the ureters. If necessary, flexible ureteroscopy may be done in the prone position as during percutanous nephrolithotomies. The legs are separated to allow access to the penis and urethra. Additional instruments may be required, including biopsy forceps, grasping forceps, ureteral brushes, ureteral resectoscopes, electrocautery, stone baskets pump syringe, lithotripsy energy sources, and ureteral catheters.
7. Sterile voided urine should be established prior to ureteroscopy. In a purely diagnostic setting, a single dose of prophylactic antibiotic (first generation cephalosporin) is administered just before starting the procedure. Broad-spectrum antibiotics may be given parenterally if a more vigorous therapeutic ureteroscopy is performed.

Informed consent should be obtained. This includes, but is not limited to, bleeding, infection, injury or loss of the ureter, injury or loss of the kidney, ureteral stricture, urinary extravasation, and anesthesia complications.

STEP-BY-STEP DESCRIPTION OF OPERATIVE PROCEDURE

RETROGRADE URETERAL ACCESS Use of a safety and a working guidewire is initially required for retrograde flexible ureteroscopy. This is done with cystoscopic and fluoroscopic guidance into the designated ureteral orifice. The wire should be passed in the intramural ureter beyond any ureteral lesion. The floppy tip should be coiled in the renal pelvis and caliceal system. The guidewire straightens the course of the ureter and secures the luminal path for low-friction passage of various instruments into the ureter. In the majority of cases a 0.038-inch (2.9F), 145 cm long, PTFE-coated (heavy duty) guidewire may be used. However, a combination of stents and guidewires with different properties may be used as the situation requires. For example, hydrophilic glidewires are readily used for access, but shouldn't be used as safety wires. Teflon-coated wires have less chance of migration during ureteroscopy.

A double lumen 10F catheter is passed over the *safety* guidewire into the distal ureters. A second *working* guidewire is passed up the ureters through the free lumen of the catheter. Passage of the double lumen catheter usually provides enough dilatation of the ureters for passage of the flexible ureteroscope. If the scope doesn't pass after this maneuver, a graduated dilating catheter

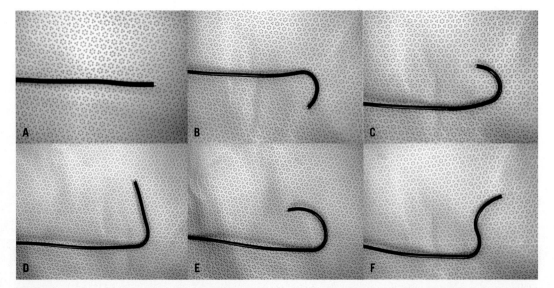

Figure 29-2 The new generation of scopes with wider deflection angles. Here are images of the Karl Storz Flex-X (11278AU1). *A*, straight. *B* and *C*, demonstrate 270° of deflection in both upward and downward directions using single lever active deflection mechanisms. *D*, acquiring an S-shaped configuration may allow access to difficult locations in the collecting system. *E* and *F*, loss of deflection angle with the 360-micron laser fiber in the working channel.

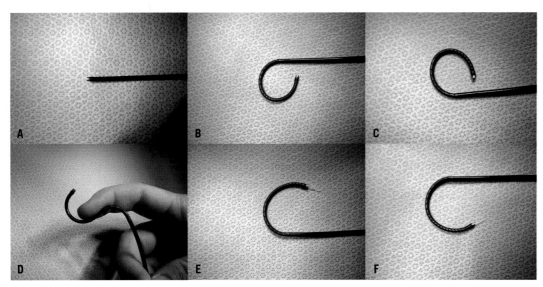

Figure 29-3 The new generation of scopes with primary and secondary active deflection mechanisms. Here are images of the ACMI DUR8-Elite. *A*, straight. *B* and *C*, primary active deflection downward 180° and upward 170°, respectively. *D*, secondary active deflection 130° in the downward direction. *E*, 270° of downward deflection using the combined primary and secondary deflection mechanism by a dual-lever system. *F*, acquiring an S-shaped configuration by moving both active deflection mechanisms spontaneously, but in the opposite direction.

RIGID VERSUS FLEXIBLE URETEROSCOPE

Semirigid ureterosopes efficiently address the distal ureteral lesions, while the flexible instrument is most efficient for the upper urinary tract above the iliac vessels. The use of the two should be complementary, according to the specifics of the case at hand. The newer semirigid instruments use the smaller fiberoptic technology to reduce the size of the tip to a range from 6.9 to 9.5F.[18,19] Starting the procedure by passing the semirigid scope dilates the intramural ureter and allows subsequent passage of the flexible instrument. If the flexible scope is used in the distal ureters, it has a tendency to migrate into the bladder, losing access.

INDICATIONS

DIAGNOSTIC APPLICATIONS Diagnostic indications for flexible ureteropyeloscopy include the following:

1. Evaluation and localization of hematuria.
2. Evaluation and localization of positive cytology.
3. Evaluation of filling defects seen on contrast studies.
4. Investigation of positive cultures localized to a specific urinary tract.
5. Surveillance ureteropyeloscopy for transitional cell carcinoma (TCC) cases of the upper tract managed endoscopically.

When evaluating for hematuria or possible malignancy, the initial exam should be done without a guidewire, using a semirigid ureteroscope to the highest point it can safely reach. It is important to evaluate the urothelium before passing the guidewire to minimize the risk of injury to the urothelial lining, which may mimic a mucosal lesion. After inspection and urine collection for cytology, the semirigid scope is removed and a guidewire is passed to the site last reached. The flexible ureteroscope is passed over as previously described, continuing the evaluation of the upper ureters, pelvis, and each calix. This is accomplished both under direct vision and with fluoroscopic guidance after injecting dilute contrast to delineate the upper collecting system. All suspi-

or balloon dilator is often used to establish safe access. The need for dilatation has decreased with improved design, modification, and downsizing of the scopes tip.[16] The Graduated dilator is 6F at the tip and will dilate the ureteral lumen to 12F. The balloon dilators are typically 150 cm long with a diameter ranging from 3 to 8F. Proximally, two ports are available; one for passage over the guidewire and the other is attached to a stopcock, which allows injection of half-strength contrast to inflate the balloon. This is done under fluoroscopic guidance with a Le Veen (Boston Scientific, Natick, MA) pressure gauge syringe. Constant monitoring of balloon pressure is imperative to avoid excessive inflation that could result in balloon rupture. The balloon is located at the distal end of the shaft with two radiopaque markers at both ends of the balloon. Inflated balloon lengths vary from 4 to 10 cm. The ureterovesical junction is the narrowest segment of the ureter, and is therefore the ideal location for placing the dilating balloon. This is rarely taken to a diameter more than 4 mm (12F). The dilators can be used at any narrow segment of the ureters encountered during the procedure. This not only allows smooth passage of the scope in and out of the ureter, but also allows easy stone extraction. Balloon dilators are never inflated over an obstructing calculus because of the risk of ureteral perforation. Once the dilatation is accomplished, the balloon is removed after adequate deflation, leaving the working guidewire intact.

Another means of ureteral dilatation is passive dilation. Passive dilation entails placement of either an open-ended or an indwelling Double-J stent for 24 or more hours before interval ureteroscopy or stone extraction.[25] This technique is commonly employed in situations in which a stone becomes impacted in a ureter. In this setting, a ureteral stent bypasses the obstruction, relieves symptoms of pain and colic, and can induce passive ureteral dila-

tion. Passive ureteral dilation provides safe and effective dilation of the entire ureter before ureteroscopy, but requires two separate procedures.

After emptying the bladder, the flexible ureteroscope is back loaded over the working guidewire in a monorail fashion under fluoroscopic guidance. It should be kept straight and in direct line with the wire. The scope is passed up like a catheter, free from any auxiliary attachments. Rotation of the shaft may be required to orient the working channel of the instrument to the 12-o'clock position. This depends on the ureteroscope tip design. When an eccentrically placed working channel is present, this step becomes necessary to prevent the ureteroscope lens from catching the roof of the ureteral orifice and telescoping the distal ureters during passage (Figure 29-4, A). The newer-designed tips have a more centrally located channel that obviates the need for rotation[16] (Figure 29-4, B).

After the tip of the flexible ureteroscope reaches the renal pelvis, the working wire is removed and the safety wire is secured to the drapes.

Table 29-1 Specifications of Available Flexible Ureteroscopes						
Specifications	ACMI DUR8-Elite	ACMI DUR8	Olympus URF-P3	Karl Storz 11278AU1	Karl Storz 11274AU	Wolf 7330.072
Diameter of distal tip (F)	6.75	6.75	8.1	6.7	6.7	7.4
Distal shaft diameter (F)	8.7	8.7	8.4	7.5	7.5	9
Shaft diameter (F)	9.4–10.1	9.4–10.1	8.4	8.4	8.4	9
Working channel size (F)	3.6	3.6	3.6	3.6	3.6	4.5
Working length (cm)	64	65	70	70	70	70
Primary active deflection	180° Down / 170° Up	185° Down / 175° Up	90° Down / 180° Up	270° Down / 270° Up	170° Down / 120° Up	160° Down / 130° Up
Secondary active deflection	130° Down	Non	Non	Non	Non	Non
Field of view	80° ± 5°	80° ± 5°	90°	90°	80°	65°
Direction of view	9°	9°	0°	6°	6°	0°
Ocular magnification	40×	40×	40×	60×	40×	50×

Specifications provided by the manufacturers.

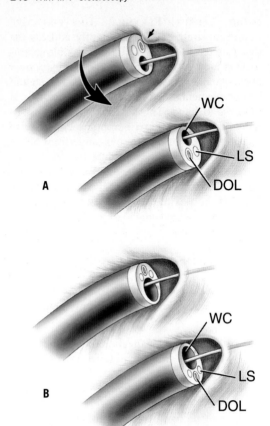

Figure 29-4 *A*, Intramural passage of the flexible ureteroscope varies with ureteroscope tip design. If the working channel is eccentrically placed, the ureteroscope must be rotated to position the working guidewire ventrally. *B*, The newer scopes with the smaller tips and centrally located working channel do not require rotation to be passed in the intramural ureter. WC = working channel; LS = light source; DOC = distal optical lens.

cious lesions are biopsied with the bases fulgurated, if necessary by Bugbee cautery or laser energy. Retrograde ureteropyelography should be done to assess for extravasation. The entire collecting system should be visualized as the scope is pulled out as a second review.

Brush biopsies may be used through a ureteroscope to exfoliate cellular material. This may be directed over suspicious areas. The scope and brush are removed as one unit and the cells retrieved are sent for cytologic assessment. Subsequently, a repeat washing using the ureteroscope or a stent may be done for collecting additional fluid for cytology.

When evaluating tumors of the upper tract, multiple biopsies using a cold-cup biopsy forceps should be performed. One should not evaluate the urinary tract above the lesion to avoid the risk of tumor avulsion until the first encountered lesion is thoroughly assessed. Therefore, biopsy is ideally done at the initial pass of the ureteroscope before increasing the risk of bleeding and poor visualization. A 3F flexible cold-cup endoscopy biopsy forceps is passed beyond the tip of the scope (Cook Urological, Spencer, IN). The jaws can be advanced into the lesion, or alternatively, the forceps and ureteroscope are advanced as one unit into the lesion to be biop-

sied. The forceps can be removed or the entire scope may be removed as a single unit to deliver the specimen. If multiple passes are to be done, a ureteral access sheath may be used. These sheaths range in size from 12 to 18F. The authors advocate a smaller sheath, if possible, to decrease the theoretical risk of ureteral stricture. The base of the lesion may be fulgurated with a Bugbee cautery or laser as needed.

Taking multiple biopsies has been found to provide a tissue diagnosis of transitional cell carcinoma in 89 to 94% of cases and has accurately assessed grade in 78 to 92%.[26,27]

THERAPEUTIC APPLICATIONS Endoscopic Lithotripsy

The success rate for treating proximal ureteral stones with small rigid and flexible ureteroscopes and the holmium laser is well over 90%. Lower-pole renal calculi can also be treated with a success rate of approximately 80%, which surpasses that of shock wave lithotripsy.[28] In a recent prospective cohort of 598 patients, the overall stone-free rate was 97%.[29]

Although more invasive than extracorporeal shock wave lithotripsy (ESWL), ureteroscopy with small, rigid, or flexible endoscopes is the most efficient technique for treatment and removal of ureteral stones.[30] Smaller ureteroscopes combined with holmium laser lithotripsy increased the single-procedure stone-free rate for ureteral stones to 97% in a large series of 492 consecutive patients.[30] When using a single-channel flexible ureteroscope, endoscopic graspers should be used to extract fragments. If the stone becomes impacted it can simply be released. A basket is ideally designed for a semirigid ureteroscope with two channels.

Electrohydrolic (EHL) probes and laser fibers (holmium or pulsed-dye) are passed through the working channels of most flexible ureteroscopes to fragment stones within the collecting system.

The EHL probe has the advantage of being very flexible and having a small diameter (as small as 1.6F), which allows it to pass through the flexible scope into the collecting system, including the lower-pole calices. All but the hardest calculi can be fragmented with this endoscopic lithotrite. However, it is more traumatic than the holmium:YAG laser.

The holmium lithotrite uses a low water density quartz laser fiber. It is available in 365 μm and 200 μm diameter for ureteroscopic use. This is a true thermal energy source, which can vaporize the hardest stone, including cystine.[31,32] Generally, pulse energies of 0.6 to 1.2 J and pulse rates of 5 to 15 Hz are used. Lowering the delivered energy setting and applying sufficient cooling saline irrigation can control the thermal effect and prevent damage to the surrounding tissue. When stones are fragmented, a "snowstorm" of dust develops. In order to acquire better visualization, power irrigation is frequently required. This is achieved by passing the pressurized irrigant beside the laser fiber in the working channel. The larger laser fiber is stiff, and it will inhibit the degree of active

deflection of the scope, making it difficult to reach stones deep in the collecting system, especially the lower-pole calices. Whereas EHL may cause injury to the ureter even when the probe is activated several millimeters away from the ureteral wall, the holmium laser may be safely activated at a distance of 0.5 to 1 mm from the ureteral wall.[33]

Because of the circumferential release of energy from either of the above described energy sources, care must be taken to fire at least 2 mm beyond the tip of the endoscope to avoid damaging the distal objective lens or causing a leak at the distal seal mechanism.

Mechanical or ballistic lithotripters that are very powerful are commonly used through rigid ureteroscopes but cannot be used with flexible ureteroscopes.

Complete fragmentation to a size less than that of the safety wire (0.035 inch) should allow passage of all fragments without sequelae. The larger fragments (2–3 mm) should be extracted if possible. The three-pronged grasper is the main instrument used for this purpose. The standard "retracting" three-pronged grasper should be advanced while closing in order to engage the stone. The other types of three-pronged graspers are "nonretracting" and are easier to engage the stone. However, owing to design, they are less efficient in extracting the stone. The stone fragments should be pulled out under direct vision in the lumen of the ureter. If resistance is met, one should avoid forceful traction as this may injure the ureter or break the instrument. Stone baskets are less frequently used with flexible ureteroscopes. This is due to higher risk of basket and stone entrapment. If this occurs, the ureteroscope should be removed after disassembling the basket handle and leaving the basket in place. The scope is then passed up along a guidewire next to the basket and an endoscopic lithotrite used. This can be avoided by simply using a grasper in a single channel ureteroscope.

Large stone burdens may require multiple passes of the flexible ureteroscope. In this setting, using a hydrophilic-coated ureteral access sheath may be beneficial in expediting the procedure. These sheaths not only dilate the ureters, but also reduce the potential for ureteral injury during repeat instrument exchange. Recently, a prospective, randomized study of 62 procedures focused on unaided ureteroscopy with no access sheath compared with ureteroscopy via a 12 to 14F ureteral access sheath. There was no significant difference in postoperative symptoms, complication rate, or stone-free status in the access sheath and nonaccess sheath groups. A significant increase in postoperative symptoms was noted when the balloon was used as a dilator compared with the access sheath. Operative time and costs in all patients who underwent access-sheath dilatation were less than in those in whom the access sheath was not used.[34]

Care must be taken during prolonged procedures to empty the bladder, as not doing so may inhibit ureteral access, reduce endoscopic view, and risk bladder rupture.

Routine ureteral stenting at the end of the procedure does not appear to be warranted in those patients who do not require ureteral dilation during ureteroscopic procedures. This was demonstrated in multiple recent prospective, randomized studies of patients undergoing ureteroscopic therapeutic procedures. Patients without stents had significantly less pain, fewer urinary symptoms, and decreased narcotic use postoperatively.[35–39]

TREATMENT OF UPPER URINARY TRACT UROTHELIAL MALIGNANCIES

Patients with TCC in a solitary kidney, renal insufficiency, synchronous bilateral tumors, high operative risk, and a predisposition to form multiple recurrences, such as endemic Balkan nephropathy, should be considered for nephron-sparing procedures. For patients with regionally extensive upper-tract urothelial neoplasms, use of endourologic techniques should be considered to control hemorrhage, relieve obstruction, and preserve as much functioning renal tissue as possible.[40] Patients must commit to a lifetime of follow-up with urine cytologies, radiographs, and endoscopy in order to be eligible for this mode of therapy. Endoscopic management is initiated after the diagnostic maneuvers mentioned earlier are completed, and only after the pathology shows that the patient is an acceptable candidate for continued minimally invasive endoscopic management. If the pathology is unresectable, high grade, or invasive, the patient should proceed immediately to nephroureterectomy. Staging the procedure may be considered for high-volume disease.

The urothelial lesions are treated with a combined use of rigid and flexible ureteroscope. The flexible instrument is usually reserved for proximal lesions. The tumor is addressed by debulking, using either grasping forceps or a flat wire basket engaged adjacent to the tumor and sending the specimen for pathologic evaluation.[41] The tumor may also be resected with a 3F Hulbert loop electrode.[42] Next, the tumor base is treated with either Bugbee electrocautery or laser energy sources. Both Nd:YAG and holmium:YAG lasers are used ureteroscopically to treat urothelial malignancies.[43] The holmium:YAG laser has the advantage of shallow tissue penetration (< 0.5 mm), which allows for tumor ablation with excellent hemostasis and minimal risk of full-thickness injury to the ureter and subsequent stricture formation.[44] It also removes coagulated tissue owing to its pulsed delivery mechanism. Settings most commonly used are energy of 0.6 to 1 joule with frequency of 10 hertz. The Nd:YAG may be used to coagulate the tumor at 30 watts followed by ablation with the holmium laser.

The overall recurrence rates for ureteral and renal pelvic lesions treated endoscopically were found to be 33% and 31.2%, respectively, in a retrospective literature review of 205 patients.[40]

A concern of potential tumor dissemination and metastatic spread secondary to ureteroscopic therapy has been raised. However, in a study by Kulp & Bagley on 13 patients who underwent multiple ureteroscopic treatments followed by nephroureterectomy, no unusual propagation of transitional cell carcinoma in the specimens was found.[45] This was further confirmed in a report of 96 patients that demonstrated no increased risk of metastatic disease in a group of patients who underwent ureteroscopy before nephroureterectomy when compared with a group undergoing nephroureterectomy alone.[46]

REMOVAL OF FOREIGN BODIES LOCATED WITHIN THE UPPER URINARY TRACT

Occasionally fragments of stents, laser fibers, guidewires, or stone baskets may be left in the upper urinary tracts postinstrumentation. Flexible ureteroscopy is used to inspect and grasp the foreign body using a three-pronged endoscopic grasper or a stone basket. Later, the urothelial surface is inspected for any injury and a ureteral stent may be left in the ureter for 2 to 3 days if necessary.

TREATMENT OF URETEROPELVIC JUNCTION (UPJ) OBSTRUCTION ENDOPYELOTOMY

The basic concept of retrograde endopyelotomy involves a full-thickness incision through the obstructing UPJ. The incision is stented and left to heal, based on the concept of an open, Davis intubated ureterotomy.[47] The advantage of performing ureteroscopic endopyelotomy over a fluoroscopically guided hot-wire balloon incision is that it allows direct visualization of the UPJ, assurance of a properly sited full-thickness incision, and visualization of pulsatile flow within vessels.[48]

After gaining ureteral access as explained earlier, the renal pelvis is drained to facilitate movement across the UPJ during the incision. The flexible ureteroscope is passed to the UPJ and positioned at the proximal extent of the UPJ. A 200- or 365-μ holmium fiber is placed through the working channel, and the UPJ is typically incised in a posterolateral direction while the ureteroscope is withdrawn back down across the UPJ. The position of the incision may vary from patient to patient. This procedure is repeated and the incision gradually deepened to extend into the peripelvic and periureteral fat. The incision is carried distally into normal ureteral tissue until the UPJ is widely patent. Injection of contrast material through the ureteroscope can demonstrate extravasation and confirm an adequate depth of incision. An endopyelotomy stent is left across the UPJ for 4 to 8 weeks. Alternatively, a 7 to 8F double-pigtail stent may be used.

Contemporary experiences with ureteroscopic endopyelotomy have reported success rates exceeding 82 to 87 %.[49–51]

POSTOPERATIVE CARE

Most ureteroscopies are performed as outpatient procedures. If mucosal edema or large blood clots and fragments are anticipated during the procedure, a Double-J ureteral stent may be left in place. Most diagnostic ureteroscopies in which the ureter is not dilated do not require a stent for drainage.

COMPLICATIONS

1. Ureteral perforation or false passage can occur during passage of a guidewire or ureteral stent, especially in cases in which there is ureteral obstruction. Ureteroscopic procedures, such as ureteral biopsy, resection, fulguration, stone fragmentation, or even overdistension of the collecting system with irrigant fluid may cause a ureteral leak. Longer duration of the ureteroscopic procedure is strongly associated with ureteral perforation. The likelihood of immediate postoperative complications is greater when renal calculi are treated and less when the surgeon is more experienced.[52]

2. When performing ureteroscopic lithotripsy, calculi may be iatrogenically driven into the wall of the ureter resulting in submucosal stones or lost stones. A submucosal stone removal is difficult, ureteral perforation with urinoma can occur, and intense fibrosis may result. If one is encountered, laser excision with prolonged stenting is recommended. A lost stone, however, is a stone that has been moved to a position outside the ureter, and it is usually harmless and requires no further treatment. But the perforation that placed the stone outside the ureter may induce stricture formation or a urinoma.

3. Ureteral strictures result after ureteral perforation, cauterization, or trauma. The incidence of both complications has steadily declined to 1.7% for perforations and 0.7% for strictures. This has been attributed to the advent of smaller ureteroscopes and better-controlled lithotripsy.[53,54]

4. Ureteral avulsion is the most serious complication of ureteroscopy. It most frequently occurs in the proximal ureters during basket extraction of a large stone without fragmentation. It has been reported to occur in as many as 0.6% of ureteroscopies.[55]

5. Urosepsis, which is best avoided by ensuring sterile urine before the procedure and adequate antibiotic coverage perioperativley.

6. Bleeding during manipulation of wires, scopes, or instruments on the mucosal wall of the collecting system may be encountered. Fortunately, this and most ureteroscopic complications respond favorably to simple drainage of urine with ureteral catheters or stents.

REFERENCES

1. Young HH, McKay RW. Congenital valvular obstruction of the prostatic urethra. Surg Gynecol Obstet 1929;48:509.
2. Baird JL. British patient specification. No. 20, 96927, 1927.
3. Curtis IE, Hirschowitz BI, Peters CW. A long fiberscope for internal medical examination. J Opt Soc Am 1956;46:1030.
4. Marshall VF. Fiberoptics in urology. J Urol 1964;91:110–4.
5. Tagaki T, Go T, Takayasu H, et al. A small caliber fiberscope for the visualization of the urinary tract, biliary tract and spinal canal. Surgery 1968;64:1033–8.
6. Berci G. Instrumentation: flexible fiber endoscopes. In: Berci G, editor. Endoscopy. New York: Appleton-Century-Crofts; 1976.
7. Bagley DH, Huffman JL, Lyon ES. Combined rigid and flexible ureteropyeloscopy. J Urol 1983;130:243–4.

8. Bagley DH, Huffman JL, Lyon ES. Flexible ureteropyeloscopy: diagnosis and treatment in the upper urinary tract. J Urol 1987;138:280–5.

9. Bagley DH. Intrarenal access with the flexible ureteropyeloscope: effects of active and passive tip deflection. J Endourol 1993;7:221–4.

10. Salmon PR. What is fiberoptics? In: Fiberoptic endoscopy. New York: Grune & Stratton; 1974.

11. Bordelon BM, Hunter JG. Endoscopic technology. In: Green FL, Ponsky JL, editors. Endoscopic surgery. Philadelphia: WB Saunders; 1994.

12. Wickham JE. Basic physics and construction of fiberoptic and solid lens endoscope. In: Wickman JE, Miller RA, editors. Percutaneous renal surgery. Edinburgh: Churchill Livingstone; 1983.

13. Siegmund WP. Fiberoptic imaging in medicine. Schott fiberoptics SPIE invited paper (1649–20), Bellingham, WA, August 1992.

14. Hicks JW. US Patent No. 3,004,368, 1961.

15. Grasso M, Bagley D. A 7.5/8.2 F actively deflectable, flexible ureteroscope: a new device for both diagnostic and therapeutic upper urinary tract endoscopy. Urology 1994;43: 435–41.

16. Bagley DH. Intrarenal access with the flexible ureteropyeloscope: effect of active and passive deflection. J Endourol 1993;7:221–4.

17. Kavoussi L, Clayman RV, Basler J. Flexible actively deflectable fiberoptic ureteronephroscopy. J Urol 1989;142: 949–54.

18. Abdel-Razzak OM, Bagley DH. Clinical experience with flexible ureteropyeloscopy. J Urol 1922;148:1788–92.

19. Bagley DH, Rittenberg MH. Intrarenal dimensions: guidelines for flexible ureteropyeloscopes. J Surg Endosc 1987;1:119–21.

20. Poon M, Beaghler M, Baldwin D. Flexible endoscope deflectability: changes using a variety of working instruments and laser fibers. J Endourol 1997;11:247–9.

21. Michel MS, Knoll T, Ptaschnyk T, et al. Flexible ureterorenoscopy for the treatment of lower pole calyx stones: influence of different lithotripsy probes and stone extraction tools on scope deflection and irrigation flow. Eur Urol 2002;41:312–7.

22. Conlin MJ, Bagley DH. Ureteroscopes and working instruments: flexible ureteroscopes. In: Smith A, Badlani G, Bagley D, et al, editors. Smith's textbook of endourology. 1st ed. St Louis: Quality Medical Publishing; 1996.

23. Menezes P, Dickinson A, Timoney AG. Flexible ureterorenoscopy for the treatment of refractory upper urinary tract stones. BJU Int 1999;84:257–60.

24. Monga M, Dretler SP, Landman J, et al. Maximizing ureteroscope deflection: "play it straight." Urology 2002;60:902–5.

25. Eshghi M. Dilatation of ureteral orifice for ureterorenoscopy. Urol Clin North Am 1988;15:301–14.

26. Guarnizo E, Pavlovich C, Seiba M, et al. Ureteroscopic biopsy of upper tract urothelial carcinoma: improved diagnostic accuracy and histopathologic considerations using a multi-biopsy approach. J Urol 2000;163:52–5.

27. Keeley FX Jr, Bibbo M, Bagley DM. Ureteroscopic treatment and and surveillance of upper urinary tract transitional cell carcinoma. J Urol 1997;157:1560–5.

28. Bagley DH. Expanding role of ureteroscopy and laser lithotripsy for treatment of proximal ureteral and intrarenal calculi. Curr Opin Urol 2002;12:277–80.

29. Sofer M. Holmium:YAG laser lithotripsy for upper urinary tract calculi in 598 patients. J Urol 2002;167:31–4.

30. Grasso M, Bagley D. Small diameter, actively deflectable, flexible ureteropyeloscopy. J Urol 1998;160:1648–53.

31. Dushinski JW, Lingeman JE. High-speed photographic evaluation of holmium laser. J Endourol 1998;12:177–81.

32. Wollin TA, Denstedt JD. The holmium laser in urology. J Clin Laser Med Surg 1998;16:13–20.

33. Santa-Cruz RW, Leveille RJ, Krongard A. Ex vivo comparison of four lithotriptors commonly used in the ureter: what does it take to perforate? J Endourol 1998;12:417–22.

34. Kourambas J. Does a ureteral access sheath facilitate ureteroscopy? J Urol 2001;165:789–93.

35. Byrne RR. Routine ureteral stenting is not necessary after ureteroscopy and ureteropyeloscopy: a randomized trial. J Endourol 2002;16:9–13.

36. Chen YT, Chen J, Wong WY, et al. Is ureteral stenting necessary after uncomplicated ureteroscopic lithotripsy? A prospective, randomized controlled trial. J Urol 2002;167:1977–80.

37. Borboroglu PG, Amling CL, Schenkman NS, et al. Ureteral stenting after ureteroscopy for distal ureteral calculi: a multi-institutional prospective randomized controlled study assessing pain, outcomes and complications. J Urol 2001;166:1651–7.

38. Netto NR Jr, Ikonomidis J, Zillo C. Routine ureteral stenting after ureteroscopy for ureteral lithiasis: is it really necessary? J Urol 2001;166:1252–4.

39. Denstedt JD, Wollin TA, Sofer M, et al. A prospective randomized controlled trial comparing nonstented versus stented ureteroscopic lithotripsy. J Urol 2001;165:1419–22.

40. Tawfiek ER, Bagley D. Upper-tract transitional cell carcinoma. Urology 1997;50:321–9.

41. Abdel-Razzak OM, Ehya H, Cubler-Goodman A, Bagley DH. Ureteroscopic biopsy in the upper urinary tract. Urology 1994;44:451–7.

42. Grasso M. Resecting upper-tract urothelial Ca by ureteroscope. Contemp Urol 1993;5:52–9.

43. Schmeller NT, Hofstetter AG. Laser treatment of ureteral tumors. J Urol 1989;141:840–3.

??. Bagley D, Erhard M. Use of the holmium laser in the upper urinary tract. Tech Urol 1995;1:25–30.

44. Johnson DE, Cromeens DM, Price RE. Use of the holmium:YAG laser in urology. Laser Surg Med 1992;12: 353–63.

45. Kulp DA, Bagley DH. Does flexible uretero-pyeloscopy promote local recurrence of transitional cell carcinoma? J Endourol 1994;8:111–3.

46. Hendin BN, Streem SB, Levin HS, et al. Impact of diagnostic ureteroscopy on long-term survival in patients with upper tract transitional cell carcinoma. J Urol 1999;161:783–5.

47. Davis DM. Intubated ureterotomy: a new operation for ureteral and ureteropelvic stricture. Surg Gynecol Obstet 1943;76:513.

48. Conlin MJ, Bagley DH. Ureteroscopic endopyelotomy at a single setting. J Urol 1998;159:727–31.

49. Tawfiek ER, Liu J, Bagley DH. Ureteroscopic treatment of ureteropelvic junction obstruction. J Urol 1998;160: 1643–6.

50. Gerber GS, Kim JC. Ureteroscopic endopyelotomy in the treatment of patients with ureteropelvic junction obstruction. Urology 2000;55:198–202.

51. Giddens JL, Grasso M. Retrograde ureteroscopic endopyelotomy using the holmium:YAG laser. J Urol 2000;164: 1509–12.

52. Schuster TG, Hollenbeck BK, Faerber GJ, Wolf JS Jr. Complications of ureteroscopy: analysis of predictive factors. J Urology 2001;166:538–40.

53. Abdel Razzak OM, Bagley DH. Clinical experience with flexible ureteropyeloscopy. J Urol 1992;148:1788–92.

54. Grasso M, Loisides P, Beaghler M. The case for primary endoscopic management of upper urinary tract calculi: cost and outcome assessment of 112 primary ureteral calculi. Urology 1995;45:372–6.

55. Blute ML, Segura JW, Patterson DE. Ureteroscopy. J Urol 1988;139:510–2.

30

Treatment of Ureteral Calculi

Jorge Gutierrez-Aceves, MD

Rodolfo Favela-Camacho, MD

Daniel Franco-Carrillo

Technological advances and improving skills with endourologic procedures have led to a continuous remarkable evolution in the treatment of ureteral calculi over the last 20 years. The removal of ureteral stones has been greatly facilitated by various endourologic treatment options, including extracorporeal shock wave lithotripsy (ESWL), retrograde ureteroscopy, antegrade percutaneous ureteroscopy, and recently, laparoscopic ureterolithotomy. ESWL has become an attractive option of treatment for ureteral stones; it has been accepted today as the first choice of treatment for proximal ureteral stones and as a valid option to treat distal ureteral stones. It is the least invasive treatment modality, and high success rates have been reported for calculi along the whole ureter.[1–4] Despite the high success rate reported for ESWL, other factors must be considered when selecting this modality of treatment: stones with limited prognosis for ESWL, time to clear stone fragments from the ureter, number of ancillary procedures, and rate of retreatments. Advances in instrumentation, smaller and more flexible ureteroscopes, and new lithotriptors have broadened the indications for endoscopic treatment, allowing stone fragmentation and removal of calculi along the whole course of the urinary tract, including the proximal ureter and intrarenal collecting system. A high success rate has been reported with the ureteroscopic treatment of distal ureteral calculi; recent series report close to 100% success rate with ureteroscopy in the distal ureter using smaller scopes with efficient instruments for stone fragmentation.[5–7] The success of ureteroscopy for proximal ureteral stones has dramatically increased; recent series report success rates above 90%,[8,9] and the invasiveness of the procedure has decreased, approaching that of ESWL. The majority of stones located in the ureter can be treated with ESWL or ureteroscopy when observation has failed. Antegrade percutaneous ureteroscopy may be used for the treatment of selective complex stones located in the proximal ureter, where the fragmentation capability with ESWL is limited and the retrograde ureteroscopic approach is difficult or challenging, or when ESWL or flexible retrograde ureteroscopy have failed. Although open ureterolithotomy is rarely performed today, it can always be considered an alternative in complex stone cases when a percutaneous approach cannot be recommended.

Whenever a patient might be considered for ureterolithotomy, retroperitoneal or transperitoneal laparoscopic ureterolithotomy is today a real, less-invasive alternative to open surgery.

The different options available to treat ureteral calculi are considered, and a discussion is presented on the alternatives to treat stones in the different locations of the ureter.

TREATMENT ALTERNATIVES

CONSERVATIVE TREATMENT   Although significant advances in minimally invasive procedures have led to increasing success in the treatment of ureteral stones, most patients pass calculi without interventions, and therefore, conservative treatment must still play a major role in the management of ureteral calculi.

Stone size, location, and impaction are the most important determinants for spontaneous stone passage. A large number of reported series in the literature sustain the contention that ureteral stones less than 5 mm in diameter may be expected to pass spontaneously in 71 to 98% of distal stones and 29 to 98% of proximal stones, whereas the spontaneous passage rate for stones between 5 and 10 mm ranges from 25 to 53% and from 10 to 53% for distal and proximal stones, respectively.[10] Coll and colleagues reported spontaneous stone passage rates, regardless of size, in 48%, 60%, 75%, and 79% for stones in the proximal, middle, distal, and intramural ureter, respectively.[11]

Allowing the patient the opportunity to pass the stone spontaneously may be an attractive alternative, but simple observation may be associated with recurrent pain and uncertainty of time to passage of the stone; it also risks urinary infection and deterioration in renal function. The rate of complications may increase to 20% when duration of symptoms reaches 4 weeks, versus 7% when the symptoms last less than 4 weeks.[12] Prediction of time for spontaneous stone passage is difficult. Overall, stone size of less than 5 mm, especially when located in the distal ureter, and downward stone progression are relative indicators for stone passage. Stones over 5 mm and prolonged stone impaction makes spontaneous passage unlikely. Other factors predicting stone passage for stones 10 mm or less include duration of pain less than 30 days, pyuria less than 100 white blood cells per high power field, lack of irregular stone surface and partial obstruction.[13] Miller and Kane

reported an average time to stone passage of 31 days for stones 2 mm or less, 40 days for stones 2 to 4 mm and 39 days for stones 4 to 6 mm in diameter; intervention was required in 50% of calculi greater than 5 mm.[14] Hubner and colleagues reported that spontaneous stone passage averaged 1.6 weeks for stones less than 4 mm and 2.8 weeks for stones between 4 to 6 mm. In their study, no calculus larger than 6 mm passed spontaneously.[12] Indications for intervention should be considered in patients with unremitting or recurrent disabling pain, urinary obstruction, persistent infection, solitary kidney, renal insufficiency or patients with specific occupations (eg, pilots).

Pharmacologic therapy has been used in an attempt to facilitate spontaneous stone passage. The use of α_1-adrenergic blocking agents appears to increase the rate of spontaneous passage of distal ureteral stones. In a recent randomized prospective study Dellabella and colleagues evaluated the efficacy of three drugs as medical expulsive therapy for distal ureteral calculi.[15] The expulsion rate was significantly higher using tamsulosin hydrochloride compared to phloroglucin and nifedipine, 97.1%, 64.3% and 77.1%, respectively, with less time to stone passage and decreased analgesic requirements. A similar study compared three different α_1-adrenergic blocking agents (tamsulosin hydrochloride, terazosin hydrochloride, and doxazosin mesylate) versus no medication. The calculi passed spontaneously in only 53.5% of the no-medication group, versus 79.3, 78.5, and 75.8% with the different agents, respectively. The expulsion time, the pain episodes, and the analgesic dosage were also found to be lower, and the α_1-adrenergic blocking agents were equally efficacious.[16]

ESWL   ESWL has become an attractive option for treatment of ureteral stones. It has been accepted as the first choice of treatment for proximal ureteral stones and as a valid option to treat distal ureteral stones. Several authors have proved the efficacy of ESWL with a success rate beyond 90% in the proximal ureter[1,2,17,18] and between 85 and 96% in the distal ureter.[3,4,6,19–23]

The physical environment surrounding a stone located in the ureter can have a significant effect on the efficacy of the shock wave action. The main limitation for success of ESWL in the ureter is observed in large impacted stones, because of the lack of a fluid-stone interface. It has been advocated that the existence of an expansion chamber in a non-impacted stone allows a better cavitation effect from the shock wave, helping the outer layer of stone to peel away and providing better penetration to the center of the stone.[24–26] Therefore, impacted ureteral stones represent a challenge, making in situ ESWL more difficult. The speed of stone elimination and symptom resolution is not always predictable. Initial fragmentation of the most proximal upper part of the stone may increase the amount of urine surrounding the stone and facilitate the stone fragmentation.

Manipulating the stone back to the kidney or bypassing the stone with a ureteral stent, in theory, provides the stone with an expansion chamber, increasing the likelihood of fragmentation. Initial reports demonstrated a clinical advantage with retrograde stone manipulation back to the kidney. Chaussy and Schmiedt reported a success rate of 50% with in situ lithotripsy versus more than 90% when the stones were manipulated.[27] Other authors have not found stone manipulation to be necessary. Several reports support the fact that in situ stone fragmentation may be achieved in 81% to more than 90%, mainly when treating stones less than 10 mm.[28] Second- and newer-generation lithotriptors using a decreased amount of energy made treatment with sedation or intravenous narcotics possible in most patients; therefore, to routinely perform a bothersome endoscopic manipulation is not indicated in most cases. Only selected stones (impacted or larger than 10 mm) can benefit from this approach.

ESWL represents a safe and effective method for approaching stones in different locations of the ureter; an adequate selection increases the success of the treatment. Stones with limited prognosis after ESWL are: stones more than 10 mm in length, badly impacted stones, hard stones (cistine, calcium-oxalate monohydrate), poorly visualized stones (uric acid), stones overlying bony structures, or stones associated with altered anatomy (ureteral kinking, ureteral strictures, previous ureteral surgery, radiation therapy).

URETEROSCOPY Rigid and flexible ureteroscopy has become a routine procedure in specialty endourology as well as in general urology. Advances in endoscopic technology combined with improvement in intracorporeal lithotriptors allow management of calculi along the course of the entire ureter with low risk and low morbidity.[29,30]

Instrumentation Urologists are no longer limited to large ureteroscopes that were often difficult to pass into the ureter and that presented a high incidence of ureteral injury. Today, newer semi-rigid, fiberoptic ureteroscopes can be passed with minimal ureteral trauma and, in the majority of cases, without ureteral dilatation.[30–33] At the same time, flexible ureteroscopes have facilitated access to the proximal ureter and intrarenal collecting system, allowing management of proximal ureter or renal stones in a retrograde fashion.[30]

The rigid ureteroscopes used today are semi-rigid scopes with fiberoptic bundles.[32] The currently available fiberoptic semi-rigid ureteroscopes produced by different manufacturers present an external diameter range from 6.9 French to 10.0F, with single or dual working channels up to 5.5F total. Some urologists prefer the use of 9.5 to 10F ureteroscopes with a straight 5F working channel. The use of large ureteroscopes improves visualization, and they have better consistency and a wide working channel that allows simultaneous use of the energy probe plus accessories. Using rigid reusable accessories (stone graspers) for stone fragmentation and removal can increase the chance of intact stone extraction. Some urologists advocate the use of smaller scopes (mini-scopes) with an external diameter between 6.9 and 8.5F. Small ureteroscopes pass easily into the ureter without dilatation, but may require several insertions into the ureter to remove fragments. They may bend easily to the point of instrument breakage. Some do not have a beveled tip and can cause problems with the introduction and advancement of the ureteroscope. The irrigation can be limited and compromised, and they may need costly flexible accessories because of a smaller working channel and, overall, potentially increased cost.

The recent advances of flexible endoscopy in the treatment of the upper urinary tract have been made possible by the development of actively deflecting fiberoptic endoscopes. Different manufacturers produce instruments with a small external diameter (7.5F), internal working channels up to 3.5F that accept instruments and allow adequate irrigation flow. They incorporate deflecting dual capabilities up to 270° or multiple deflection capabilities. These features have greatly improved the handling of the instruments and have increased the usefulness for diagnostic and therapeutic procedures in the ureter and kidney.

Ureteroscopy for stone fragmentation and removal is facilitated with the use of a wide variety of working accessories and instruments available in sizes 3F and less. Guidewires, introductory accessories, ureteral access sheaths, instruments for stone holding and stone removal (baskets, grasping forceps, loops and cones), instruments for intracorporeal lithotripsy, and stents are available. Urologists must be familiar with the design, advantages, and disadvantages of these different accessories to improve final results of ureteroscopy without unnecessarily increasing the overall cost of the procedure.

Rigid and flexible ureteroscopes are used in a complementary manner to access the entire upper urinary tract. The lower ureter can be accessed easily with a rigid ureteroscope. If the area of interest can be approached, even in the proximal ureter, it is suggested to use a rigid ureteroscope. Introduction of a rigid endoscope under direct vision is easier; they have a better image, a larger working channel, and provide excellent control of working instruments. Ureteral access sheaths may facilitate rigid ureteroscopy in the proximal ureter, but if a rigid endoscope cannot be used safely in the proximal ureter, or if the area of treatment is located in the intrarenal collecting system, a flexible endoscope should be used.

Surgical Technique Ureteroscopy has become a routine procedure for most urologists. Success rates can approximate 100% for fragmentation and stone removal in the distal ureter.[5,30–32,34] The procedure is minimally invasive, many patients can be treated under intravenous sedation,[35] and the vast majority of cases can be completed on an outpatient basis. Technical complications from instrumentation and the use of energy lithotriptors are avoidable, and complication rates approach 0%.

As in any other surgical procedure, it is important to adhere to some basic principles of ureteroscopy in order to accomplish optimal results and to reduce the risk of complications.

The basic principles of ureteroscopy can be summarized as follows:

1. Always observe a guideline (step-by-step approach).
   - As in any other surgery, ureteroscopy must be planned with a guideline that should be strictly followed.
2. Always have a safety guidewire bypassing the ureteral calculus up in the kidney.
   - After a cystoscopic evaluation of the bladder and the ureteral orifice, perform a retrograde ureterography and place a regular Teflon-coated guidewire. If the guidewire cannot bypass the obstacle, use a glide wire. A perforated tip catheter can be useful to create a fulcrum at the level of the obstacle. If it does not pass, use the ureteroscope but just to place the guidewire; once the guidewire has bypassed the stone, remove the scope and start the procedure over again, but now with a security guidewire in place. If the retrograde fashion fails, establish an antegrade percutaneous access to place the guide.
3. Never introduce and advance the ureteroscope with poor visualization.
   - Introduce the scope into the ureteral orifice alongside a safety guide wire. If not successful, try between two guidewires with a second wire running though the working channel of the ureteroscope, a tunnel is created between the two wires and the ureteroscope is advanced though the tunnel always under visual control. If not successful, consider dilation of the orifice. The dilation of the ureter used to be an essential part of ureteroscopy, but is now a very unusual requirement using fiberoptic instruments—even with 10F diameters.
4. Always visualize the field when advancing the ureteroscope.
   - While approaching the stone, continue advancing the scope alongside the safety wire keeping the ureteral lumen in full view. If the optical field is not satisfactory, use a second wire though the scope, improve irrigation, and advance the scope though the tunnel created between two wires. If not successful, consider stenting.

5. Never manipulate the stone with poor visualization.
   - Once the stone is approached, maintain good control of the optical field. When visualization is inadequate, improve irrigation, move backward, and reposition the scope on the stone, consider using a second guidewire through the scope (as described above) to improve exposure to the stone. Do not attempt to remove a stone or activate any energy source without full endoscopic control of the stone and the ureteral wall.
6. When unsure, or when encountering complications, consider stenting over the safety wire and consider scheduling a second session.

Following these basic principles of ureteroscopy, urologists have become more experienced, success rates have improved, and complication rates have dropped. Enhanced efficacy and decreased morbidity can be attributed to improvement in the technique of ureteroscopy.

Ureteroscopic Treatment of Stone: Removal versus Fragmentation When ureteroscopy is performed for management of ureteral stones, a decision needs to be made as to whether the stone can be removed intact or needs fragmentation prior to removal. Stones of 10 mm or less can be directly retrieved from the ureter.[36] The use of rigid reusable accessories (stone graspers) offers several advantages: if the stone is too large to be brought down the ureter, it can be released and fragmented; soft stones (even calcium-oxalate dihydrate and struvite) can be fragmented mechanically with the grasper. And they are reusable and cost-effective. The use of a basket has the disadvantage of extra cost for the procedure, but offers the advantage of trapping the stone prior to fragmentation and avoiding stone fragment migration, especially when using some energy sources such as pneumatic lithotripsy. After fragmentation, baskets allow removal of stone particles once they are reduced to less than 4 mm.

Ureteroscopic stone removal with or without fragmentation is a procedure that should never result in ureteral injury. Any maneuver performed with a stone retrieval instrument or any lithotriptor should not be activated without full endoscopic control of the stone and the ureteral wall. If this cannot be accomplished at the time of first access to the stone, placement of an indwelling stent for 2 weeks is a prudent decision.

If fragmentation is considered, the current options are electrohydraulic lithotripsy (EHL), ultrasound, pneumatic (Lithoclast) and holmium: yttrium-aluminum-garnet (holmium:YAG) laser. Because ureteroscope calibers have become smaller, ultrasonic probes may no longer fit in a small working channel, decreasing the applicability of this technology for the ureter. Electrohydraulic lithotripsy has been widely used with success; it is a low-cost and easily available technology, and usable with small, rigid or flexible instruments. Nevertheless, this technology uses disposable electrodes, cannot fragment stones of all composition (eg, monohydrated calcium oxalate and cistine), and has a lower safety margin for the ureteral wall.[37,38] Ballistic lithotripsy (Lithoclast) is a highly effective technology for fragmentation, has the highest safety margin for the ureter, has a reasonable cost, and uses nondisposable probes. The main disadvantages are retrograde stone propulsion and is restricted to use with rigid instruments.[39,40] Holmium:YAG laser technology can fragment all types of calculi, regardless of composition, by delivering energy through small-diameter quartz fibers. At the same time, it has the ability to fragment stones with an ablative effect, converting the stone to dust particles during the procedure and reducing the need for fragment removal. The smaller fibers can be used in any thin flexible instrument with only minimal interference with the acting deflection mechanism, allowing access to any part of the upper urinary tract. The main disadvantage is the higher cost compared with other energy sources.[41–43]

Even when all lithotriptors are not equal in terms of efficiency and safety margins, present options for intracorporeal lithotripsy have facilitated ureteral stone fragmentation while decreasing the possibility of ureteral injury during stone removal. The endpoint of a ureteroscopic procedure with stone removal or fragmentation is the stone-free ureter in one session, leaving only minute particles less than 1 mm, or the size of the safety wire.

Complications As instrumentation to endoscopically access the ureter has improved with the addition of small caliber rigid endoscopes, flexible ureteroscopes, and newer methods of intracorporeal lithotripsy with superior flexibility, the safety margins for endoscopic surgery in the ureter and kidney have improved.[5,30,32] Technical complications from instrumentation and the use of lithotriptors are avoidable, and complication rates, especially in the distal ureter, have decreased to less than 5%.[44,45]

Intraoperative complications are mostly associated with increased operative time and stone location, with a higher incidence from stones located in the kidney and lack of experience in the surgeon.[44] Most common complications related to ureteroscopy, however, can be recognized immediately, and most ureteral injuries can be managed conservatively. The most frequent intraoperative complication is ureteral perforation. Once false passage or perforation is recognized, stenting of the ureter most likely allows complete resolution of the injury. If a stent cannot be placed, or if the size of the perforation is more than 1 cm in length, it becomes necessary in most instances to place a nephrostomy tube. The length of stenting varies depending on the injury; an acceptable approach is to delay between 2 and 6 weeks before a contrast study is performed to document complete healing.

The most serious complication identified during the procedure is ureteral avulsion. In this case, the treatment depends on the extent and location of the avulsion. A distal avulsion may be repaired with ureteral reimplant with or without a psoas hitch or Boari flap, but avulsion in the middle or proximal ureter may require ureteral substitution or even nephrectomy.

A late complication of ureteroscopy is formation of a stricture. Ureteral strictures may be related to a mechanical or thermal injury with secondary devascularization and necrosis, or they can be produced due to ureteral wall fibrosis after a mucosal or complete wall perforation and secondary urine extravasation. Strictures are again encountered less frequently with the new, smaller fiberoptic instruments available, and most cases can be resolved using endourologic techniques to incise the narrow segment. Overall success rates are about 75%, depending mainly on the length and location of the stricture.[44,46,47]

PERCUTANEOUS ANTEGRADE URETEROSCOPY
Even with the high success rate of ESWL in the treatment of proximal ureteral stones, and the technological improvement of flexible ureteroscopy, percutaneous antegrade ureteroscopy can be considered a valid treatment alternative for proximal ureteral stones in select clinical conditions.

Large stones (> 2.0 cm) represent a relative contraindication to ESWL. The success rate with shock waves in this situation is reduced owing to the stone size and the poor expansion chamber usually present. Because these stones are, in general, chronically impacted, the manipulation required to position the stone back in the kidney is usually difficult. Also, large stones impacted in the proximal ureter are frequently positioned in ureteral kinkings, where access with the flexible ureteroscope may be difficult to obtain, and stone manipulation risky owing to the poor visualization produced by severe edema frequently associated with these stones.[48]

Another clinical condition that may indicate an antegrade approach is the patient with a reconstructed urinary tract secondary to bladder diversion. Reduced ureteral motility limits fragment passage after ESWL, and retrograde access to the ureter can be a challenge.[49] A stone positioned in the ureter just proximal to a ureteral stricture is better approached through percutaneous access and removed before a standard endoureterotomy is performed. Antegrade ureteroscopy can be considered an option to treat proximal ureteral stones with associated renal stones in the same renal unit, especially when the total stone burden is larger than 2.0 cm. Finally, percutaneous ureteroscopy must be considered the choice of treatment for complex ureteral stones where ESWL or flexible ureteroscopy have failed.

Stones in the upper ureter can usually be approached via middle-pole calix although, for stones located more distal in the ureter, an upper-pole access may be required. Most of the stones can be manipulated with a rigid scope. If the stone is 10 mm in diameter or smaller, it can be removed without intracorporeal lithotripsy. Rigid forceps can loosen the stone from the ureter and allow an atraumatic removal. If the stone is larger than 10 mm, various forms of mechanical lithotripsy can be used. Usually, there is minimal need for stone fragmentation, with the possibility of large stone fragment removal through a 30F Amplatz sheath. The use of flexible nephroscopes greatly facilitates the fragmentation and removal of stones located more distal in the ureter or for stones positioned in ureteral kinking. Holmium:YAG laser can be safely used to break impacted stones. EHL is still a valid alternative to holmium:YAG laser lithotripsy in these cases, although with higher potential risk of damage to the ureter. The new nitinol tipless basket may facilitate stone fragment removal through flexible scopes with reduced risk of ureteral damage. For stones located distal in the ureter, a flexible ureteroscope, or in selected cases, even a rigid small-caliber ureteroscope, can be advanced further into the ureter from an upper-pole access using the same technical principles considered for retrograde ureteroscopy.

LAPAROSCOPIC AND OPEN URETEROLITHOTOMY

The vast majority of ureteral calculi are treated with ESWL, ureteroscopy or antegrade percutaneous ureteroscopy in selected stones located in the proximal ureter. Although open ureterolithotomy is rarely performed today, it can always be considered an alternative in complex stones if endoscopic surgery fails. At the present time, there are very few conditions to indicate ureterolithotomy as the first option in the treatment of ureteral stones: stones larger than 2.0 cm, impacted stones located in ureteral kinking, impacted stones associated with severe edema, and stones in patients with reconstructed urinary tract secondary to bladder diversion. Under these conditions, the fragmentation capability with ESWL is limited, the retrograde or antegrade ureteroscopic approaches can be difficult or challenging, and stone manipulation risky due to poor visualization.

Whenever a patient might be considered for ureterolithotomy, retroperitoneal or transperitoneal laparoscopic ureterolithotomy is a less-invasive alternative to open surgery. Access to the ureter can be gained through transperitoneal or retroperitoneal approaches. The retroperitoneal approach, first described by Wickham offers advantages over the transperitoneal approach.[50] It avoids intra-abdominal manipulation and intra-abdominal organ mobilization, reduces the risk of visceral injury, and reduces the risk of intra-abdominal urine leakage. The retroperitoneum space can be easily prepared for laparoscopy using the technique described by Gaur[51] in combination with digital dissection. Once the laparoscope is introduced, further endoscopic dissection of the fibrofatty tissue over the retroperitoneum can be achieved. Using this approach, stones located in the proximal or distal ureter can be removed with laparoscopy. Once the ureter is located and dissected, ureterolithotomy is performed imitating with laparoscopy the same surgical technique as with open surgery: the ureter is incised in a longitudinal manner, the stone is extracted, and the ureterotomy closed with interrupted adventitial sutures. It is always recommended, especially for the surgeon with less experience, to place a guidewire into the collecting system and bypass the stone. During the procedure or at the end, a ureteral stent can easily

be placed in cases when a large incision is required or whenever any difficulty is found during the surgery.

Laparoscopic ureterolithotomy is an important advance in the management of ureteral stones. It is, in the beginning, a challenging procedure, but in experienced hands, is a safe and effective procedure with success rates approaching 100%. Gaur reported the largest series of laparoscopic ureterolithotomy, with a 93% success rate, and with the 8 failures mostly at the beginning of his experience.[52] As in many other conditions, laparoscopic ureterolithotomy is proven to have the same success as open surgery, with significant advantages for analgesia, hospital stay, recuperation time, and cosmesis.[53] Despite the increased experience of laparoscopic surgery for different pathologies in the retroperitoneal space, its role in the treatment of ureteral stones should still be considered as a salvage procedure for failed extracorporeal lithotripsy, ureteroscopy, or percutaneous antegrade ureteroscopy in proximal ureteral stones or in select complex cases as described above.

DECIDING THE BEST WAY TO TREAT URETERAL STONES

The main goal in the treatment of ureteral lithiasis must be to achieve the maximum success in terms of being stone-free after one treatment session with minimal invasiveness. Therefore, for every case, the urologist must select the best treatment alternative for a predictable, immediate high-success rate with the lowest morbidity. The only definition acceptable for success in the treatment of ureteral lithiasis must be total elimination of all stone fragments from the ureter, with complete resolution of symptoms.

ESWL is initially less invasive, with less anesthesia requirement and minimal or no instrumentation. Nevertheless, this alternative needs frequently repeated treatments and ancillary endoscopic procedures with an unpredictable outcome. When ESWL is performed for stones located in the ureter, the patient needs to be closely monitored until proven stone-free and with resolution of ureteral obstruction. On the other hand, endoscopic surgery offers immediate

results with a more predictable final outcome (Table 30-1), although it's more invasive and requires anesthesia.

For discussion of the different alternatives to treat ureteral stones, a two-part division of the ureter will be used, the upper or proximal ureter (above the segment of the ureter over the iliac vessels) and the lower or distal ureter (below this anatomic mark).

TREATMENT OF PROXIMAL URETERAL CALCULI

ESWL has been recommended as the primary treatment for proximal ureteral stones less than 1 cm in diameter. It is the least invasive treatment modality for management of proximal ureteral stones, although the success rate of shock wave lithotripsy varies according to stone size with less predictable results for large stones than for smaller stones. The meta-analysis by the American Urological Association (AUA) Ureteral Stones Clinical Guideline Panel reported an overall success rate of 84% for stones 1 cm or less treated with ESWL versus 72% for stones larger than 1 cm.[10]

Manipulating the stone back to the kidney or bypassing the stone with a ureteral stent, was initially advocated to improve stone fragmentation.[17] In theory, moving the stone back provides the stone with an expansion chamber and increases the likelihood of fragmentation. Nevertheless, several clinical trials have not demonstrated that stones that have been bypassed or manipulated into the renal pelvis get better fragmentation. In the same report, the AUA panel analysis showed, in 8,052 patients with stones 1 cm or less, a success rate of 87% for stones treated in situ, 77% for stones manipulated back in the kidney, and 83% for stones bypassed with a stent. Similar results were encountered in 2,708 patients with stones larger than 1 cm; success rates were 76%, 65%, and 76% for patients treated in situ, with stone manipulation, and bypassing the stone, respectively.[10] The differences in the way in which the results are reported in the literature make direct comparisons difficult; nevertheless, several comparative prospective studies failed to prove the advantage of stone manipulation and have not considered it necessary to bypass the stone before ESWL. Cass showed a 79% success rate in 815 patients treated

Table 30-1 Differences Between Endoscopic Surgery and ESWL		
Treatment	Advantages	Disadvantages
Endoscopic surgery	Immediate symptoms resolution High success rate for stone free Short predictable recovery Low morbidity after treatment Reduced long term complications Less cost	Invasive Anesthesia Indwelling stent Higher risk of complications
ESWL	Noninvasive No/minimal anesthesia No/minimal instrumentation	Uncertain immediate results Higher rate of re-treatment Ancillary procedures Prolonged stone clearance Potential morbidity during follow-up

ESWL = extracorporeal shock wave lithotripsy.

with in situ versus 73% in 903 patients with stone manipulation before shock wave lithotripsy.[54] In a similar study, Chang and colleagues reported stone fragmentation in 76.9% of patients treated in situ versus 59.3 in patients bypassed with a stent and 62.5% in patients treated under continuous irrigation with a ureteral stent.[55]

Routine placement of a ureteral stent to increase efficacy of fragmentation is not recommended as part of shock wave lithotripsy.[10] Mobley and colleagues, in a large retrospective series showed that placement of a ureteral stent had no effect on stone-free rates for stones at any ureteral location.[56] The use of a stent has potential complications and morbidity; stents may produce infection, bleeding, irritative voiding symptoms, and pain. At the same time, ureteral stents impair ureteral mobility with a subsequent delay in the transit time of fragments.[57] The major benefit of stents is to prevent ureteral obstruction and Steinstrasse as stone fragments pass further down in the ureter. Their use may result in fewer hospital readmissions and emergency room visits.[58] The use of stents during shock wave lithotripsy may be reserved for stones larger than 1 cm in diameter in order to prevent temporary urinary obstruction.

It seems that proximal ureteral stones may be treated in situ with similar results to stones manipulated back into the kidney. Stone clearance after ESWL, however, can vary and is influenced by stone size, degree of impaction, and chemical composition. Stones larger than 1 cm, impacted stones or hard stones (eg, monohydrated calcium oxalate, cystine) are often involved with treatment failures. The success rate of impacted stones has been reported to decrease to 35% versus 93% of non-impacted stones.[59] Overall, 15% of patients require secondary interventions after shock wave lithotripsy for proximal ureteral stones,[10] and the rate of auxiliary intervention may be more than 10%.[60] Moreover, ureteral stones that fail to clear after initial shock wave lithotripsy are less likely to clear after subsequent re-treatment. Pace and colleagues reported a significant reduction in the success rate (from 68% after the initial treatment to 46% after one, and to 31% after two re-treatments, with a stone-free rate significantly better for stones 10 mm or less than for stones 11 to 20 mm: 64% versus 43%, initially, and 49% versus 37% after re-treatment).[61] Because the re-treatment rate and the number of auxiliary procedures necessary to render a patient stone-free of ureteral calculi may be higher for ESWL, their report suggests that ureteroscopic management should be considered the first line of therapy for ureteral calculi in which shock wave lithotripsy failed after the initial treatment, particularly for large stones.

Ureteroscopy for the distal ureter has become a routine procedure for most urologists. Success rates can approach 100% for fragmentation and stone removal in the distal ureter,[5,30–32,34] technical complications from instrumentation and use of energy sources are avoidable, and complication rates approach 0%. Advances in instrumentation, smaller and more flexible ureteroscopes, and lithotriptors have broadened the indications for endoscopic treatment, allowing stone fragmentation and removal of calculi along the whole course of the urinary tract (including the proximal ureter and intrarenal collecting system). Rigid and flexible ureteroscopes are used in a complementary manner to access the entire upper urinary tract. The lower ureter can be accessed easily with a rigid ureteroscope. If the area of interest can be approached—even in the proximal ureter—it is suggested to use a rigid ureteroscope. Introduction of rigid endoscopes under direct vision is easier; they provide a better image, a larger working channel, and excellent control of working instruments.

Despite the use of rigid or semi-rigid scopes in the proximal ureter, some authors report that success rate for stone fragmentation and extraction decreases markedly—up to 50%.[62] If a rigid scope cannot be used safely in the proximal ureter, or if the area of treatment is located in the intrarenal collecting system, a flexible endoscope should be used. Flexible ureteroscopes and working instruments have undergone significant design advances within the last 10 years. A number of ureteroscopes available from different manufacturers incorporate an active deflecting mechanism and an internal working channel that accepts instruments as well as adequate irrigation flow. Thanks to small-caliber instruments, ureteroscopy can be performed without ureteral dilatation in most patients,[33,63] which avoids unnecessary trauma to the orifice. At the same time, stone fragmentation with flexible lithotriptors further minimizes ureteral wall trauma. Thus, routine ureteral stenting after ureteroscopy and intracorporeal lithotripsy may not be necessary in all cases, decreasing even more the morbidity of the procedure.[64,65] Flexible ureteroscopy allows a shorter total operative time, decreases the incidence of postoperative complications, and has the patient in ambulating status in a shorter period of time.[66] Overall, the success of treatment outcomes after flexible ureteroscopy has increased and the incidence of complications has declined.

Advances in technology have driven the evolution in ureteroscopy. Besides the advances in fiberoptic engineering, advancements in intracorporeal lithotripsy, as well as in the development of working instruments, have paralleled the improvements in ureteroscopic technology. The introduction of the holmium:YAG laser is largely responsible for the improvement and success of ureteroscopic stone management and the decreased risk of complications. This modality of lithotripsy can fragment all types of calculi, regardless of their composition, by delivering energy through small-diameter quartz fibers. It has the ability to fragment stones with an ablative effect, converting the stone to dust particles during the procedure and reducing the need for fragment removal. The smaller-diameter fibers can be used in any thin flexible instrument, with only minimal interference with the acting deflection mechanism and allowing access to any part of the upper urinary tract. Several authors have probed the safety and efficacy of holmium:YAG laser in endoscopic lithotripsy.[63,67,68]

The success rate of ureteroscopy for the treatment of proximal ureteral calculi has dramatically increased, and the invasiveness of the procedure approaches that of ESWL. Using flexible endoscopes and holmium:YAG laser lithotripsy, stone-free rates in the proximal ureter approach 100%. Dividing the ureter into proximal and middle segments, Sofer and colleagues reported (in a large series of patients) stone-free rates of 97 and 100%, respectively. Secondary intervention was required in 6%, and complications were observed in 4%, with a rate only 0.35% for major complications (ureteral strictures).[8] A number of authors have confirmed the evolution of ureteroscopy in the treatment of proximal ureteral stones in terms of efficacy and invasiveness of the procedure (Table 30-2).

Despite the fact that ESWL is currently the standard therapy for stones located in the upper ureter, the high success rate of ureteroscopy and the decrease in the invasiveness of the procedure suggest that the indications for the initial treatment for proximal ureteral stones may be revisited. ESWL is recommended as first-line treatment for single stones less than 1 cm. It has, however, provided poor and unpredictable results in several situations: stones larger than 1 cm, hard stones, impacted stones, stones in obese patients or with difficult body habitus, and after one failure of shock wave treatment.[61] Under these conditions, flexible ureteroscopy may be considered the initial treatment option. Lam and colleagues conducted a comparative study for treatment of proximal ureteral stones between in situ ESWL and ureteroscopy in combination with holmium:YAG laser.[9]

Table 30-2	Treatment of Proximal Ureteral Stones with Ureteroscopy		
Author	Ureteroscope	Stone –free rate (%)	Complication (%)
Blute, 1988	10–13.5F	51/77 (66)	20
Bagley, 1990	6.0–10.8F	27/34 (79)	—
Harmon, 1997	6.0–11.5F	13/17 (76)	12
Deravajan, 1998	7.5F	88/132 (77)	—
Tawfiek, 1999	6.9–9.8F	47/48 (98)	3
Soichi, 2000	6.9–7.8F	83 (96.2)	0
Hollenbeck, 2001	6.9–7.5F	60/68 (88)	9
Sofer, 2002	Flexible (7.5 y 9.8F) and rigid (6.9-11.5F)	194 (97)	4
Wu, 2004	Semirigid	36/39 (92%)	0 (major)

Initial stone-free rate for stones 1 cm or greater was 93% for ureteroscopic lithotripsy and 50% for in situ ESWL; for stones less than 1 cm, the success rate was 100% for ureteroscopy and 80% for ESWL. No major complications were found in either group. Wu and colleagues reported a similar study comparing ESWL and ureteroscopy in the treatment of large proximal stones. The stone-free rate achieved with ureteroscopy was 92% after a single surgery versus 61% with in situ ESWL, no major complications were observed in both groups.[69] Park and colleagues, in a comparative study between ESWL and ureteroscopic manipulation for stones in all ureteral locations (including the proximal ureter), reported that stone-free rate after ESWL is significantly affected by stone size.[70] Success was 84% for stones less than 1 cm and 42% for stones larger than 1 cm. The overall success rate for ureteroscopic treatment was 88% regardless of the size of the stones. In a recent review of several series treating proximal ureteral stones, Getttman and Segura reported an overall stone-free rate of 75% after ESWL, with a re-treatment rate of 30% and auxiliary procedures rate of 9.4%. Meanwhile, the overall stone-free rate with proximal ureteroscopy was 82%, the secondary procedure rate was 10% and the complication rate 6.6%.[71]

Another important factor in the decision of how to manage ureteral calculi is the cost of treatment. As discussed earlier, many ureteral calculi can be observed with a reasonable expectation of stone passage. Observation is usually the least costly modality of treatment, but when observation fails, ureteroscopy is the most cost-effective treatment alternative for ureteral stones at all locations of the ureter. Lotan and colleagues published an interesting study comparing the cost of management of ureteral calculi using a decision tree model. Observation was the least costly treatment modality when no financial cost was incurred due to failed observation.[72] Because the cost of observation can increase due to several factors, such as emergency or office visits, repeated radiographic

images, and other factors, stones that are unlikely to pass should be treated earlier with surgical intervention. Ureteroscopy was less costly than ESWL in treating stones at all sites in the ureter, with a cost difference of approximately $1,440, $1,670 and $1,750 (US) for proximal, mid-, and distal ureteral stones, respectively.

The majority of stones located in the proximal ureter can be treated with ESWL or ureteroscopy when observation has failed. Antegrade percutaneous ureteroscopy may be used for the treatment of select complex stones where the fragmentation capability with ESWL is limited, the retrograde ureteroscopic approach is difficult or challenging, and stone manipulation is risky due to poor visualization. The chances of patient complications increase when stones are larger than 2.0 cm; when impacted stones are located in ureteral kinking or associated with severe edema; with stones in patients with reconstructed urinary tracts secondary to bladder diversion; and with stones positioned in the proximal ureter just proximal to a ureteral stricture.[48,49] Antegrade ureteroscopy can be considered an option to treat proximal ureteral stones with associated renal stones in the same renal unit, especially when the total stone burden is larger than 2.0 cm, and it must be considered the treatment of choice for ureteral stones where ESWL or flexible ureteroscopy have failed.

Large complex stones located in the proximal ureter may be a treatment challenge. An endourologic combined approach may be required in selective complex cases. Initially, ureteroscopic retrograde stone manipulation allows the placement of a guidewire and perforated stent bypassing the stone, and subsequently, a percutaneous antegrade approach, usually using flexible endoscopes, completes the stone fragmentation and removal (Figure 30-1).

Although open ureterolithotomy is rarely performed today, it can always be considered an alternative in the complex stone cases mentioned above when a percutaneous approach cannot be

recommended due to patient condition, lack of expertise, or after failed percutaneous surgery. Whenever a patient might be considered for ureterolithotomy, retroperitoneal or transperitoneal laparoscopic ureterolithotomy is a less-invasive alternative to open surgery.[52,53] Despite the increased experience in laparoscopic surgery for different pathologies in the retroperitoneal space, there are still few conditions under which to recommend the laparoscopic approach as the first choice in the treatment of ureteral stones.

To summarize, for the treatment of proximal ureteral stones, ESWL is recommended as first-line treatment for single, non-impacted stones less than 1 cm, but ESWL has provided poor and unpredictable results in several situations: stones larger than 1 cm, hard stones, impacted stones, stones in obese patients, or patients with difficult body habitus and after one failure of shock wave treatment. In these circumstances, semi-rigid or flexible ureteroscopy is indicated as the initial treatment option. The high success rate of ureteroscopy and the decrease in the invasiveness of the procedure, suggest that this treatment modality may be a more frequent indication for the management of proximal ureteral stones in the future.

TREATMENT OF DISTAL URETERAL CALCULI

The optimal treatment alternative for ureteral stones located between the sacroiliac joint and the ureterovesical junction remains controversial. The two most frequently used options for the treatment of stones in the distal ureter are extracorporeal shock wave lithotripsy with either stent manipulation or in situ management, as well as ureteroscopy with either extraction of the stone or intracorporeal lithotripsy. Other treatment options, as discussed earlier, include open surgery, retroperitoneal or transperitoneal laparoscopic ureterolithotomy (indicated only in rare cases involving unusually large or complex stones), and blind or fluoroscopically guided basket extraction, which can no longer be encouraged as a treatment choice in the current era of ureteroscopy.

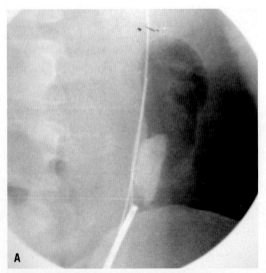 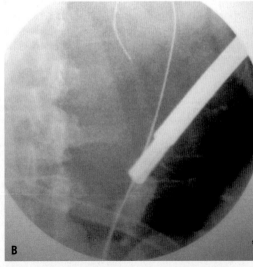 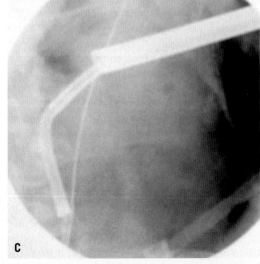

Figure 30-1 *A*, Large complex proximal stone, initial ureteroscopic retrograde manipulation by passing a guidewire into the collecting system. *B*, Antegrade percutaneous approach complete stone fragmentation. *C*, Flexible antegrade ureteroscopy allows complete evaluation and residual stone removal.

Ureteroscopy and ESWL are currently accepted treatment modalities for distal ureteral calculi. Each has advantages and disadvantages. Overall, ESWL is minimally invasive and can be performed without anesthesia or under intravenous sedation, but it may require multiple treatments for adequate fragmentation and is more likely to require ancillary treatments. Ureteroscopy has a higher success rate, with the least risk of multiple treatments and the least risk of ancillary procedures, but it is more invasive than ESWL.

The choice between ureteroscopy and ESWL for treatment for distal ureteral calculi is one of the most controversial issues in endourology. When deciding the most appropriate approach to treat distal ureteral stones, multiple factors must be considered. The following discussion tries to illustrate the advantages and disadvantages of each treatment method to select the best treatment alternative.

Stone-free Rate Comparative retrospective studies using different ureteroscopes and intracorporeal lithotriptors show higher success rates with ureteroscopy compared to ESWL. A meta-analysis presented by Wolf and colleagues showed a greater success rate for ureteroscopy over ESWL: 92.1% (range 89.7 to 95.7%) versus 74.3% (range 69.7 to 78.9%) after a single treatment.[73] Advances in endoscopic technology in combination with improvement in intracorporeal lithotripsy technology reduce the risk of complications and increase the success rate of ureteroscopy. Recent series report close to 100% success rates with ureteroscopy in the distal ureter using smaller scopes with efficient instruments for stone fragmentation.[5–7] A review of published series from 1990 to 2001 on the treatment of distal ureteral stones revealed success rates of 94.9% (range 90.4 to 100%) stone-free with ureteroscopy versus 87.2% (range 85.6 to 89.2%) after ESWL. When separately analyzing the first and second five-year periods, the success rate for ureteroscopy in the series reported between 1990 and 1995 was 91.2% versus 96.4% in the series reported between 1996 and 2001, supporting the fact that improvement of endoscopic technology increases the chances of treatment success.[74]

Most data in the literature come from retrospective reports from single-institution experiences where a variety of lithotriptors were used. Two series assessed the efficacy of ESWL with the unmodified HM3 lithotriptor for distal ureteral stones. Pearle and colleagues in a multicenter prospective randomized trial compare shock wave lithotripsy with the HM3 versus ureteroscopy.[75] At 21 and 24 days follow-up, the success rate for both treatments was 91%, but procedural time was shorter, and minor complications were less frequent with ESWL. Hochreiter and colleagues, in a large series of patients, reported 91% successful treatment with one ESWL session using the unmodified HM3 lithotriptor.[76] These data suggest that ESWL for distal ureteral stones with the powerful unmodified HM3 lithotriptor has superior results, in terms of stone-free rate and re-treatment rate, compared to those

obtained with any other second- or third-generation lithotriptor.

As is the case in proximal ureteral stones, the success rate of ESWL is related to size and number of stones. Parandalis and colleagues reported, in stones 1 cm or less, there was 100% success for ESWL versus 97% with ureteroscopy, but for stones larger than 1 cm, stone-free rate decreased to 85% with ESWL and 91% with ureteroscopy.[77] Eden and colleagues reported a single-treatment stone-free rate for ESWL and ureterolithotripsy of 75% and 90%, respectively, for single stones, whereas the success in treatment of multiple stones larger than 1 cm decreased after ESWL to 50% with virtually no modification in the success rate after ureteroscopy (89%).[78] These data suggest that ESWL provides effective treatment for small single stones, while larger and multiple stones must be managed with ureteroscopy.

Stone Clearance There are considerable differences between ESWL and ureteroscopy with regard to stone clearance after treatment. During ureteroscopy, the calculi are fragmented and the ureter is cleared of the fragments at the time of intervention. The endpoint of a ureteroscopic procedure with stone fragmentation is the stone-free ureter, leaving only minute particles less than 1 mm (or the size of the safety wire). Therefore, patients who desire a quick route to a stone-free state must be treated with ureteroscopy. Because fragments are left to clear spontaneously after ESWL, patients must accept a longer time interval to achieve a stone-free state, and they risk pain recurrence during this period. Bierkens and colleagues reported significant differences of stone clearance (28 days after ESWL vs. 1.3 days after ureteroscopy) with a considerably higher number of patients bothered by recurrent pain.[34]

Re-treatment Rate and Ancillary Procedures In terms of re-treatment, ureteroscopy has proven to be clearly superior to ESWL. Reported re-treatment rates for ureteroscopy range from 0 to 10%, whereas the re-treatment rates after ESWL for distal calculi range from 14 to 45%.[7,79] The number of treatments also varies with respect to size and number of stones; multiple and larger stones require a higher number of treatments with ESWL with no increase in the treatment rates with ureteroscopy. Eden and colleagues reported a mean treatment rate of 2.0 and 1.0 for ESWL and ureteroscopy, respectively, for single stones, but for multiple stones, the number of treatments increased to 2.8 after ESWL and stayed at 1.0 after ureteroscopy.[78] When analyzing the treatment rate with ESWL according to stone size, stones less than 8 mm required 1.6 treatments, while the number of treatments increased to 2.4 in stones larger than 8 mm. In patients treated with ureteroscopy, the number of treatments averaged 1.2 for stones less than 8 mm and 1.3 for stones larger than 8 mm. A review of published series from 1990 to 2001 showed a re-treatment rate of 17.3% (range 9.6 to 24.3%) for ESWL versus 5.56% (4.8 to 9.4%) for ureteroscopy.[74] The same review also found a significant increase in ancillary procedures after ESWL. Patients treated with ESWL required com-

plementary procedures in 10.3% of cases versus 1.4% for patients treated with ureteroscopy.

Complications The risk of significant complications in the treatment of distal ureteral stones after ESWL is estimated at 3.0%, and the estimated risk of ESWL plus ancillary procedures during treatment (bypass or push-back techniques) is 4.0%, whereas the estimated risk for ureteroscopy is 9%.[10] As discussed previously, with the development of newer smaller fiberoptic ureteroscopes and refined intracorporeal lithotriptors and working instruments with superior flexibility, the safety margins for endoscopic surgery in the ureter have improved and the incidence of complications during ureteroscopy has decreased. Using small-caliber instruments, complications following ureteroscopy are rare, and complication rates may be less than 5%.[5,6,30,32] When reviewing the literature separately, we encountered a higher complication rate for ureteroscopy in series published between 1990 and 1995: 5.3%, compared to 3.1% in the series published between 1995 and 2001.[74]

Anesthesia Ureteroscopy has been perceived as a more invasive procedure than ESWL. Again, with the availability of smaller ureteroscopes, ureteroscopy is less invasive than it used to be, and today's invasiveness of ureteroscopy can be questioned. Even though ureteroscopy is commonly performed with spinal, epidural, or general anesthesia, there are some reports on local anesthesia plus intravenous sedation.[35,80] This can be especially well tolerated if performing ureteroscopy for the distal ureter in women. ESWL frequently requires anesthesia. The need for anesthesia during ESWL depends largely on the energy source. Spark gap lithotriptors, while more effective, are more painful for patients, and anesthesia or intravenous sedation must be used. Although piezoelectric lithotripsy is associated with the least pain and anesthesia is not required, it has low efficacy.

Ureteral Stent Indwelling stents are seldom required for ESWL. Patients with distal ureteral stones can be treated without a ureteral catheter with the same success rate. Routine placement of a ureteral stent to increase efficacy of fragmentation is not recommended as part of shock wave lithotripsy.[10] Several authors have shown that placement of a ureteral stent had no effect on stone-free rates after ESWL at any ureteral location.[56] During ESWL, the presence of a stent may be of value only to facilitate location of sparse radiopaque stones and in patients with difficult body habitus. The major benefit of stents is to prevent ureteral obstruction and Steinstrasse as stone fragments pass further down in the ureter, but their use may result in fewer hospital readmissions and emergency rooms visits.[58] The use of a stent during shock wave lithotripsy may be reserved for stones larger than 1 cm in diameter in order to prevent temporary urinary obstruction.

Ureteral stent placement after ureteroscopy is still a common practice, and the prevalence of ureteral stenting after ureteroscopy ranges from 83 to 100%.[45,63,75] The use of a stent after ureteroscopy is thought to reduce or prevent the incidence of postoperative pain secondary to postoperative edema, to reduce the incidence of ureteral stricture, and possibly to aid with the passage of small fragments.[81] Their use, however, has potential complications and morbidity; they may produce infection, bleeding, irritative voiding symptoms, and bladder and flank pain. Moreover, stent placement usually requires longer operating room time, and their removal requires a re-instrumentation with a subsequent increase the overall cost of the procedure.

Several reports suggest that routine stenting after ureteroscopy for a distal ureteral stone is unnecessary. These studies consistently found that patients without stents have significantly fewer urinary symptoms, less bladder and flank pain, and the requirements for analgesic and narcotics were significantly less in the non-stented patients, especially one week after the procedure. None of these series reported ureteral strictures in the non-stented patients,[64,82–87] but they still risked persistent flank pain or fever and had a higher risk for readmittance. Reviewing the data from other series, 6% of patients without stents required an emergency room visit or rehospitalization versus less than 1% of the stented patients. Overall, there is a six-fold increase in the need for subsequent hospital management for pain if no stent is used after ureteroscopy.[88] Careful selection of patients may reduce the incidence of routine stent placement. The criteria for selective internal stenting are severe preoperative obstruction, tight stone impaction, significant residual obstruction, prolonged ureteroscopy, and complications during the procedure.[64] Uncomplicated ureteroscopy for distal ureteral calculi without ureteral dilatation can safely be performed without placement of a ureteral stent.

Limitations Although few, there are some recognized limitations when proposing treatment with ESWL. It is frequently difficult to image the distal calculi because of numerous calcifications within the bony pelvis, with the subsequent need of ureteral catheterization. Depending on the body characteristics and the lithotriptor used, positioning of the patient may cause some difficulties and reduce the success expectancy. In child-bearing women, the adverse effects on female fertility remain somewhat controversial.[28] In addition to potential damage to the ovaries from the shock wave, there is possible scarring of the fallopian tubes and the effects of radiation exposure. On the other hand, ureteroscopic removal of stones may be performed without incidence or limitations under any circumstances.

Cost Ureteroscopy seems to be a less expensive procedure than ESWL in the management of distal ureteral stones.[73] Observation is usually the least costly modality of treatment, but when observation fails, ureteroscopy is the most cost-effective treatment alternative for ureteral stones at all locations of the ureter. When the overall cost is calculated, factoring the need of re-treatments, ancillary procedures, office visits due to subsequent pain, and re-admission to emergency rooms, the mean cost of ESWL is significantly higher than ureteroscopy. The meta-analysis by Wolf and colleagues reported 21% higher costs for ESWL (overall cost, $6,745 for ESWL vs. $5,555 for ureteroscopy).[73] Lotan and colleagues recently published an interesting study comparing the cost of management of ureteral calculi using a decision tree model. Observation was the least costly treatment modality when no financial cost was incurred due to failed observation. Because cost of observation can increase due to several factors, such as emergency or office visits, repeated radiographic images and other factors, stones that are unlikely to pass should be treated earlier with surgical intervention. Ureteroscopy was less costly than ESWL for treating stones at all sites in the ureter with a cost difference of approximately $1,750 (US) for distal ureteral stones.[72] The numbers may vary depending on the site where the report is generated, but after reviewing the data reported in North America, it seems that ureteroscopy is a more cost-effective treatment compared to ESWL.

To summarize, for the treatment of stones in the distal ureter, ESWL and ureteroscopy are both efficacious procedures with low morbidity. Stone-free rates with ureteroscopy are higher than ESWL, with success rates close to 100%. With the development of new technology, complication rates have been reduced to nearly 0%. Ureteroscopy is now performed in an outpatient setting, and most urologists are able to perform this procedure, whereas access to ESWL for some urologists may be limited.

CONCLUSIONS

There are alternatives available to treat ureteral stones. The selection of a treatment option for the management of ureteral calculi depends on a number of factors: stone size, stone location, severity of impaction, composition, treatment cost, patient conditions and preference, and surgeon skill. Although ESWL is the standard therapy for stones located in the upper ureter, the high success rate of ureteroscopy and the decrease in the invasiveness of the procedure suggest that indications for initial treatment of proximal ureter stones may be revisited. ESWL is recommended as first-line treatment for single stones less than 1 cm, but ESWL has provided poor and unpredictable results in several cases: stones larger than 1 cm, hard stones, impacted stones, stones in obese patients or with difficult body habitus, and after 1 failure of shock wave treatment. Particularly in these circumstances, semi-rigid or flexible ureteroscopy may be considered as the initial treatment option in proximal stones. For distal ureteral stones, ESWL and ureteroscopy are reasonable choices, but several factors, such as stone-free rate, stone clearance, re-treatment rate, ancillary procedures, and cost favor ureteroscopy as the first treatment option for most distal stones. Percutaneous antegrade ureteroscopy must be reserved for complex stones located in the proximal ureter. The role of laparoscopy in the treatment of ureteral stones should still be considered as a salvage procedure for failed extracorporeal lithotripsy, ureteroscopy, or percutaneous antegrade ureteroscopy in proximal ureteral stones or in select complex cases.

REFERENCES

1. Liong ML, et al. Treatment options for proximal ureteral urolithiasis: review and recommendations. J Urol 1989;141:504–9.
2. Riehle RA Jr, Naslund EB. Treatment of calculi in the upper ureter with extracorporeal shock wave lithotripsy. Surg Gynecol Obstet 1987;164:1–8.
3. Erturk E, Herrman E, Cockett AT. Extracorporeal shock wave lithotripsy for distal ureteral stones. J Urol 1993;149:1425–6.
4. Jenkins AD. ESWL: distal ureteral stone management—1993. Urology 1993;42:353–5.
5. Peschel R, Janetschek G, Bartsch G. Extracorporeal shock wave lithotripsy versus ureteroscopy for distal ureteral calculi: a prospective randomized study. J Urol 1999;162:1909–12.
6. Turk TM, Jenkins AD. A comparison of ureteroscopy to in situ extracorporeal shock wave lithotripsy for the treatment of distal ureteral calculi. J Urol 1999;161:45–7.
7. Chang CP, et al. Optimal treatment for distal ureteral calculi: extracorporeal shockwave lithotripsy versus ureteroscopy. J Endourol 2001;15:563–6.
8. Sofer M, et al. Holmium:YAG laser lithotripsy for upper urinary tract calculi in 598 patients. J Urol 2002;167:31–4.
9. Lam JS, Greene TD, Gupta M. Treatment of proximal ureteral calculi: holmium:YAG laser ureterolithotripsy versus extracorporeal shock wave lithotripsy. J Urol 2002;167:1972–6.
10. Segura JW, et al. Ureteral Stones Clinical Guidelines Panel summary report on the management of ureteral calculi. The American Urological Association. J Urol 1997;158:1915–21.
11. Coll DM, Varanelli MJ, Smith RC. Relationship of spontaneous passage of ureteral calculi to stone size and location as revealed by unenhanced helical CT. AJR Am J Roentgenol 2002;178:101–3.
12. Hubner WA, Irby P, Stoller ML. Natural history and current concepts for the treatment of small ureteral calculi. Eur Urol 1993;24:172–6.
13. Ibrahim AI, et al. Prognostic factors in the conservative treatment of ureteric stones. Br J Urol 1991;67:358–61.
14. Miller OF, Kane CJ. Time to stone passage for observed ureteral calculi: a guide for patient education. J Urol 1999;162(3 Pt 1):688–91.
15. Dellabella M, Milanese G, Muzzonigro G. Randomized trial of the efficacy of tamsulosin, nifedipine and phloroglucinol in medical expulsive therapy for distal ureteral calculi. J Urol 2005;174:167–72.
16. Yilmaz E, et al. The comparison and efficacy of 3 different alpha1-adrenergic blockers for distal ureteral stones. J Urol 2005;173:2010–2.
17. Graff J, et al. Extracorporeal shock wave lithotripsy for ureteral stones: a retrospective analysis of 417 cases. J Urol 1988;139:513–6.
18. Netto NR Jr, et al. Treatment options for ureteral calculi: endourology or extracorporeal shock wave lithotripsy. J Urol 1991;146:5–7.
19. Rodrigues Netto N Jr, Lemos GC, Claro JF. Extracorporeal shock-wave lithotripsy with Lithostar lithotriptor. Urology 1992;40:430–4.
20. Becht E, et al. Treatment of prevesical ureteral calculi by extracorporeal shock wave lithotripsy. J Urol 1988;139:916–8.
21. Selli C, Carini M. Treatment of lower ureteral calculi with extracorporeal shock wave lithotripsy. J Urol 1988;140:280–2.
22. Thomas R, et al. An innovative approach to management of lower third ureteral calculi. J Urol 1993;149:1427–30.
23. Mattelaer P, et al. In situ extracorporeal shockwave lithotripsy of distal ureteral stones: parameters for therapeutic success. Urol Int 1994;53:87–91.
24. Paterson RF, et al. Shock wave lithotripsy of stones implanted in the proximal ureter of the pig. J Urol 2005;173:1391–4.
25. Mueller SC, et al. Extracorporeal shock wave lithotripsy of ureteral stones: clinical experience and experimental findings. J Urol 1986;135:831–4.
26. Parr NJ, et al. Mechanisms responsible for diminished fragmentation of ureteral calculi: an experimental and clinical study. J Urol 1992;148(3 Pt 2):1079–83.
27. Chaussy C, Schmiedt E. Shock wave treatment for stones in the upper urinary tract. Urol Clin North Am 1983;10:743–50.

28. Singal RK, Denstedt JD. Contemporary management of ureteral stones. Urol Clin North Am 1997;24:59–70.

29. Segura JW. Ureteroscopy for lower ureteral stones. Urology 1993;42:356–7.

30. Conlin MJ, Marberger M, Bagley DH. Ureteroscopy. Development and instrumentation. Urol Clin North Am 1997; 24:25–42.

31. Preminger GM. Technique versus technology: what is the most appropriate method for the removal of ureteral calculi. J Urol 1994;152:66–7.

32. Ferraro RF, et al. A new generation of semirigid fiberoptic ureteroscopes. J Endourol 1999;13:35–40.

33. Stoller ML, et al. Ureteroscopy without routine balloon dilation: an outcome assessment. J Urol 1992;147:1238–42.

34. Bierkens AF, et al. Treatment of mid- and lower ureteric calculi: extracorporeal shock-wave lithotripsy vs laser ureteroscopy. A comparison of costs, morbidity and effectiveness. Br J Urol 1998;81:31–5.

35. Hosking DH, Bard RJ. Ureteroscopy with intravenous sedation for treatment of distal ureteral calculi: a safe and effective alternative to shock wave lithotripsy. J Urol 1996;156:899–902.

36. Netto NR Jr, et al. Ureteroscopic stone removal in the distal ureter. Why change? J Urol 1997;157:2081–3.

37. Piergiovanni M, et al. Ureteral and bladder lesions after ballistic, ultrasonic, electrohydraulic, or laser lithotripsy. J Endourol 1994;8:293–9.

38. Zheng W, Denstedt JD. Intracorporeal lithotripsy. Update on technology. Urol Clin North Am 2000;27:301–13.

39. Denstedt JD, Eberwein PM, Singh RR. The Swiss Lithoclast: a new device for intracorporeal lithotripsy. J Urol 1992; 148(3 Pt 2):1088–90.

40. Menezes P, Kumar PV, Timoney AG. A randomized trial comparing lithoclast with an electrokinetic lithotripter in the management of ureteric stones. BJU Int 2000;85:22–5.

41. Grasso M. Experience with the holmium laser as an endoscopic lithotrite. Urology 1996;48:199–206.

42. Teichman JM, et al. Ureteroscopic management of ureteral calculi: electrohydraulic versus holmium:YAG lithotripsy. J Urol 1997;158:1357–61.

43. Cheung MC, et al. Outpatient holmium laser lithotripsy using semirigid ureteroscope. Is the treatment outcome affected by stone load? Eur Urol 2001;39:702–8.

44. Schuster TG, et al. Complications of ureteroscopy: analysis of predictive factors. J Urol 2001;166:538–40.

45. Harmon WJ, et al. Ureteroscopy: current practice and long-term complications. J Urol 1997;157:28–32.

46. Knowles DR, Staiman VR, Gupta M. Long-term results of the treatment of complete distal ureteral stenosis using a cutting balloon catheter device. J Urol 2001;166: 2087–90.

47. Matsuoka K, et al. Endoscopic antegrade laser incision in the treatment of urethral stricture. Urology 2002;60:968–72.

48. Kahn RI. Percutaneous approach for ureteral stones. Probl Urol 1993;7:1–9.

49. Wolf JS Jr, Stoller ML. Management of upper tract calculi in patients with tubularized urinary diversions. J Urol 1991;145:266–9.

50. Wickham JE. The surgical treatment of renal lithiasis. In: Livingstone C, editor. Urinary calculous disease; 1979. New York. p. 183–6.

51. Gaur DD. Laparoscopic operative retroperitoneoscopy: use of a new device. J Urol 1992;148:1137–9.

52. Gaur DD, et al. Laparoscopic ureterolithotomy: technical considerations and long-term follow-up. BJU Int 2002;89: 339–43.

53. Goel A, Hemal AK. Upper and mid-ureteric stones: a prospective unrandomized comparison of retroperitoneoscopic and open ureterolithotomy. BJU Int 2001;88:679–82.

54. Cass AS. Nonstent or noncatheter extracorporeal shock-wave lithotripsy for ureteral stones. Urology 1994;43:178–81.

55. Chang SC, Kuo HC, Hsu T. Extracorporeal shock wave lithotripsy for obstructed proximal ureteral stones. A prospective randomized study comparing in situ, stent bypass and below stone catheter with irrigation strategies. Eur Urol 1993;24:177–84.

56. Mobley TB, et al. Effects of stents on lithotripsy of ureteral calculi: treatment results with 18,825 calculi using the Lithostar lithotriptor. J Urol 1994;152:53–6.

57. Ryan PC, et al. The effects of acute and chronic JJ stent placement on upper urinary tract motility and calculus transit. Br J Urol 1994;74:434–9.

58. Chandhoke PS, et al. A randomized outcomes trial of ureteral stents for extracorporeal shock wave lithotripsy of solitary kidney or proximal ureteral stones. J Urol 2002; 167:1981–3.

59. Srivastava A, et al. Management of impacted upper ureteric calculi: results of lithotripsy and percutaneous litholapaxy. Br J Urol 1992;70:252–7.

60. Singh I, et al. Impact of power index, hydroureteronephrosis, stone size, and composition on the efficacy of in situ boosted ESWL for primary proximal ureteral calculi. Urology 2001;58:16–22.

61. Pace KT, et al. Low success rate of repeat shock wave lithotripsy for ureteral stones after failed initial treatment. J Urol 2000;164:1905–7.

62. Bagley DH. Ureteroscopic stone retrieval: rigid versus flexible endoscopes. Semin Urol 1994;12:32–8.

63. Tawfiek ER, Bagley DH. Management of upper urinary tract calculi with ureteroscopic techniques. Urology 1999;53: 25–31.

64. Denstedt JD, et al. A prospective randomized controlled trial comparing nonstented versus stented ureteroscopic lithotripsy. J Urol 2001;165:1419–22.

65. Hollenbeck BK, et al. Routine placement of ureteral stents is unnecessary after ureteroscopy for urinary calculi. Urology 2001;57:639–43.

66. Abdel-Razzak OM, Bagley DH. Clinical experience with flexible ureteropyeloscopy. J Urol 1992;148:1788–92.

67. Scarpa RM, et al. Holmium:YAG laser ureterolithotripsy. Eur Urol 1999;35:233–8.

68. Devarajan R, et al. Holmium:YAG lasertripsy for ureteric calculi: an experience of 300 procedures. Br J Urol 1998;82: 342–7.

69. Wu CF, et al. Comparison between extracorporeal shock wave lithotripsy and semirigid ureterorenoscope with holmium:YAG laser lithotripsy for treating large proximal ureteral stones. J Urol 2004;172(5 Pt 1):1899–902.

70. Park H, Park M, Park T. Two-year experience with ureteral stones: extracorporeal shockwave lithotripsy v ureteroscopic manipulation. J Endourol 1998;12:501–4.

71. Gettman MT, Segura JW. Management of ureteric stones: issues and controversies. BJU Int 2005;95 Suppl 2:85–93.

72. Lotan Y, et al. Management of ureteral calculi: a cost comparison and decision making analysis. J Urol 2002;167:1621–9.

73. Wolf JS Jr, Carroll PR, Stoller ML. Cost-effectiveness v patient preference in the choice of treatment for distal ureteral calculi: a literature-based decision analysis. J Endourol 1995;9:243–8.

74. Gutierrez-Aceves J. Ureteral calculi in stone disease. In: Segura J, Conort P, Khoury S, et al, editors. 1st International Consultation on Stones Diseases; 2003. Health Publications Ltd. p. 161–66.

75. Pearle MS, et al. Prospective randomized trial comparing shock wave lithotripsy and ureteroscopy for management of distal ureteral calculi. J Urol 2001;166:1255–60.

76. Hochreiter WW, et al. Extracorporeal shock wave lithotripsy for distal ureteral calculi: what a powerful machine can achieve. J Urol 2003;169:878–80.

77. Pardalidis NP, Kosmaoglou EV, Kapotis CG. Endoscopy vs. extracorporeal shockwave lithotripsy in the treatment of distal ureteral stones: ten years' experience. J Endourol 1999;13:161–4.

78. Eden CG, et al. Intracorporeal or extracorporeal lithotripsy for distal ureteral calculi? Effect of stone size and multiplicity on success rates. J Endourol 1998;12:307–12.

79. Hendrikx AJ, et al. Treatment for extended-mid and distal ureteral stones: SWL or ureteroscopy? Results of a multicenter study. J Endourol 1999;13:727–33.

80. Zisman A, Siegel YI, Lindner A. Ureteroscopy for ureterolithiasis with sedation only. Eur Urol 1995;27:151–3.

81. Pryor JL, Langley MJ, Jenkins AD. Comparison of symptom characteristics of indwelling ureteral catheters. J Urol 1991;145:719–22.

82. Hosking DH, McColm SE, Smith WE. Is stenting following ureteroscopy for removal of distal ureteral calculi necessary? J Urol 1999;161:48–50.

83. Netto NR Jr, Ikonomidis J, Zillo C. Routine ureteral stenting after ureteroscopy for ureteral lithiasis: is it really necessary? J Urol 2001;166:1252–4.

84. Rane A, et al. To stent or not to stent? That is still the question. J Endourol 2000;14:479–81.

85. Borboroglu PG, et al. Ureteral stenting after ureteroscopy for distal ureteral calculi: a multi-institutional prospective randomized controlled study assessing pain, outcomes and complications. J Urol 2001;166:1651–7.

86. Cheung MC, et al. A prospective randomized controlled trial on ureteral stenting after ureteroscopic holmium laser lithotripsy. J Urol 2003;169:1257–60.

87. Chen YT, et al. Is ureteral stenting necessary after uncomplicated ureteroscopic lithotripsy? A prospective, randomized controlled trial. J Urol 2002;167:1977–80.

88. Moon TD. Ureteral stenting—an obsolete procedure? J Urol 2002;167:1984.

31

Treatment of Upper Urinary Tract Calculi: Ureteropyeloscopic Lithotripsy

Michael Grasso III, MD

URETEROPYELOSCOPIC LITHOTRIPSY

In the ever changing world of minimally invasive surgical intervention, endoscopic lithotripsy has progressed with broader indications and improved instrumentation. Over two decades of refinements in surgical technique and the incorporation of a series of technological advancements have led to well-accepted therapies employed by the majority of clinical urologists.

In the early 1980s, endoscopic stone management commonly meant placing a rigid rod-lens ureteroscope into the distal ureter with stone extraction. Prior to the introduction of the ureteroscope, distal ureteral calculi were treated with blind basketing or with open surgery. Currently, open stone surgery is very rarely employed and makes up less than one-tenth of 1% of stone therapies at US centers. Blind basketing is a technique that today is felt to be unreasonably risky, with its use being restricted in the 1998 American Urological Association (AUA) Guidelines panel report.[1] Direct endoscopic visualization of a stone burden has thus become a universally accepted tenet of all endoscopic lithotripsy techniques. Clear visualization of the stone and endoscopic direction of an extraction accessory or an endoscopic lithotripsy device is routine.

Where first only distal ureteral stones were treated with ureteroscopic lithotripsy, the addition of flexible endoscopes and complementary lithotrites based on flexible probes allowed for treatment of stones in the more proximal collecting system. The introduction of fiberoptic endoscopes, electrohydraulic and laser lithotrites, and improved extractors based on new metal alloys allowed the endourologist to safely perform procedures of greater complexity. Based on technical advances, the twenty-first century has brought universal acceptance of retrograde endoscopic treatment of calculi throughout the upper urinary tract.[2,3] With contemporary instrumentation, the vast majority of upper urinary tract calculi can be successfully treated ureteroscopically, often irrespective of stone size, composition, and location.[4-8]

URETEROSCOPES: EVOLUTIONARY TO REVOLUTIONARY

Endoscopic telescopes began with sequential optical lens instruments that were large by today's standards and fragile. Illumination was the product of incandescent light at the distal end of the endoscope. Rod-lens endoscopes were pioneered by Hopkins, who first filed a patent application in 1959, and they were finally put into production by the Karl Storz Company in Tuttlingen, Germany, in 1967[9] (Figure 31-1). The rod-lens endoscopes were based on sequential cylindrical glass segments placed adjacent to each other with tight air interfaces. The Hopkins rod-lens system relies on the image being relayed through a series of rod lenses. The traditional system consisted of a tube of air with thin lenses of glass, but the new system consisted of a tube of glass within thin lenses of air.[10] This advancement revolutionized endoscopy for urologists and has remained a standard component of rigid cystoscopes and nephroscopes for some 30 years. These instruments were more durable, with excellent illumination and a crisp, clear image. In fact, the role of the rod-lens telescope in the development of standard therapies in the lower urinary tract (eg, transurethral treatment for prostatism, endoscopic resection of bladder lesions) was of great significance.

Rod-lens ureteroscopes were first employed in the late 1970s. In fact the first rigid ureteroscopes were pediatric cystoscopes placed into the ureter under direct vision.[11] The natural contours of the ureter and the frequent tortuosity associated with ureteral obstruction did pose limitations to the rod-lens ureteroscopes. These early 12 French (F) and larger instruments were designed to allow for only minimal passive bending of the shaft during placement into the ureter. In male patients, the prostatic urethra and distal ureter often required some, albeit minimal, passive deflection of the instrument shaft for access. This bending of the endoscope shaft caused buckling of the rod-lens optics, creating a crescent defect of the endoscopic image (Figure 31-2). The greater the deflection of the shaft, the larger the defect, and the more difficult the endoscopic therapy.

Fiberoptics was introduced in the 1920s.[12,13] It was not until 1956 that the first medical endoscope based on both fiberoptic imaging and illumination was described.[14,15] Gastroenterology was the first subspecialty, but urologic applications soon followed.[16] Marshall's description of the first fiberoptic ureteroscopy in 1964 was based on a 9F endoscope produced by American Cystoscope Makers (Pelham, NY).[17] This procedure represents the first flexible ureteroscopy for ureteral calculus disease. Of even greater significance was the application of fiberoptics in all rigid telescopes as a means of delivering bright light for illumination. All rigid endoscopes thus incorporated fiberoptics for illumination, even while maintaining rod-lens systems for visualization. This allowed for endoscope miniaturization while employing larger working channels (Figure 31-3).

Rod-lens ureteroscopes were abandoned in the late 1980s, as improved fiberoptics were developed and could be employed for visualization. Tightly packed bundles of glass fibers produced a clear image that was not distorted with

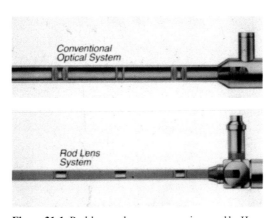

Figure 31-1 Rod-lens endoscopes were pioneered by Hopkins in 1959 and manufactured by the Karl Storz Company in 1967. They are based on sequential cylindrical glass segments placed adjacent to each other with tight air interfaces (Cockett and Cockett[9]). As compared with prior optical lens endoscopes, these instruments could be minimally bent or deflected during everyday usage without damage.

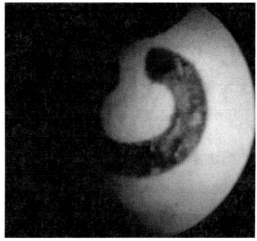

Figure 31-2 The early rigid ureteroscopes were 12F and allowed for only minimal passive bending of the shaft during placement into the ureter. This bending of the endoscope shaft caused buckling of the rod-lens optics and created a crescent defect of the endoscopic image.

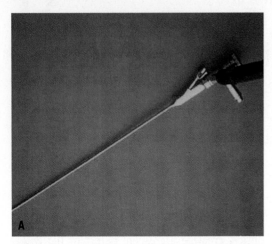

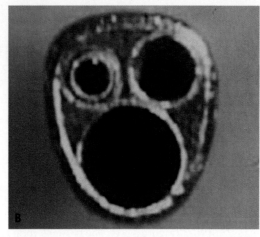

Figure 31-3 *A,* Rigid endoscopes incorporated fiberoptics for illumination, while maintaining the rod-lens system for visualization. *B,* This allowed endoscopic miniaturization, while maximizing the diameter of the working channels.

bending or deflection of the rigid instruments shaft (Figure 31-4). These instruments thus allowed the endoscopist to follow the contours of the prostate and distal ureter while maintaining a clear image. In addition, fiberoptics for visualization led to the development of even smaller diameter, now termed "semirigid" endoscopes.[18–20] This advancement in the later 1980s was associated with much enthusiasm for ureteroscopy in general. Now a small 6.9F, 2-channel endoscope could be placed into the distal ureter under direct vision, frequently without ureteral dilation, and with room to work in the ureter uninhibited by the bulk of the prior endoscopes. It is the semirigid, < 7F ureteroscopes (eg, ACMI MR6, American Cystoscope Manufacturers, Stamford, CT) that have been the most popular ureteroscopes among urologists for over 15 years, with only very minimal subsequent changes in design since their introduction in 1988.[21]

The limitations of the semirigid ureteroscope are based on the more proximal ureteral course and the intrarenal caliceal anatomy. Even though these instruments could be passed into the distal ureter under direct vision, in male patients they frequently could not be placed above the curve noted, as the ureter drapes over the iliac vessels. In addition, they had very minimal utility in the renal pelvis and intrarenal collecting system. Steerable, deflectable, flexible endoscopes were required. Marshall's initial report and Tagaki and colleagues' description of a flexible endoscope placed through a ureterotomy with visualization of papillae in 1966 reflect primitive maneuvers, based on today's standards, but which at the time were revolutionary.[17,22] These first flexible ureteroscopes were large in outer diameter, were not steerable, and did not have a working channel (Figure 31-5). Without the ability to direct the endoscope's tip or clear it of debris with irrigant, diagnostic endoscopy was often not fruitful, and no therapeutic endeavors could be performed. Passing the ureteroscope through a sheath or guide tube did facilitate concurrent irrigation and was one of many innovations employed early in the development of flexible ureteroscopic technique.

In the early 1980s, Aso in Tokyo, Japan, working with Olympus, and Bagley and colleagues working with ACMI began developing a new class of now steerable flexible ureteroscope with a dedicated working channel.[23–25] Endoscope outer diameter was set at 10F with a work-

ing channel diameter of 3.6F. Adjusting the stiffness of the endoscope along the shaft was found to be useful. Even with active tip deflection, the addition of a softer segment approximately 6 to 10 cm from the tip allowed for passive endoscope buckling. This was termed "secondary" deflection and became a standard in flexible endoscope design (Figure 31-6). It was the combination of active and passive tip deflection that facilitated lower-pole caliceal access. It was at this time that combination therapy based on distal ureter endoscopy with a semirigid endoscope and more proximal endoscopy with an actively deflectable, flexible instrument was first decribed.[24] This concept of complementary endoscopes continued as another tenet of ureteroscopy without challenge until recently.

In 1994 the next major advance in flexible ureteroscopy was led by Karl Storz Endoscopy and reflected significant endoscope miniaturization, while maintaining prior mechanical specifications that were essential for steerability throughout the caliceal system.[4,32] Smaller fiberoptics and mechanical improvement led to downsizing from 10 to 7.5F (Figure 31-7). Concepts including logical tip deflection (ie, thumb lever down causes tip

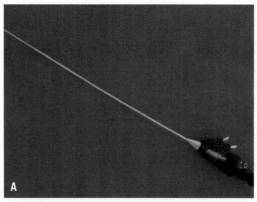

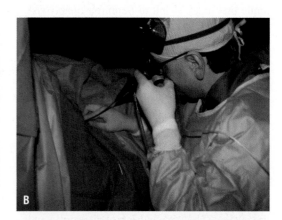

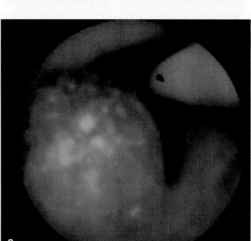

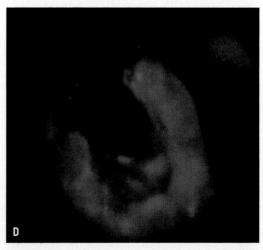

Figure 31-4 *A,* The MR-6 semirigid ureteroscope developed by ACMI permitted simultaneous application of two endoscopic accessories, such as laser fragmentation of a basketed ureteral stone, through its two dedicated working channels. *B,* A cystine stone in the middle-third ureter is visualized with a semirigid ureteroscope, and then *C,* a laser fiber is employed through the endoscope to pulverize the stone under direct vision. *D,* Tightly packed bundles of glass afford a clear optical image that is not distorted by bending or deflecting the rigid instruments.

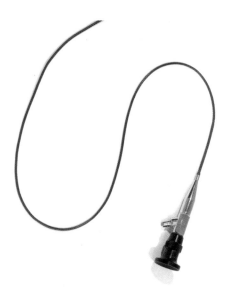

Figure 31-5 The first flexible ureteroscopes, developed in the 1960s, were revolutionary. They were large in outer diameter, were not steerable or deflectable, and did not have a working channel.

to go down and vice versa), passive secondary deflection, and maintaining a 3.6F working channel were now standard. These improvements led to growth in ureteroscopic procedures based in part on easier and less traumatic endoscope placement and greater directability in the intrarenal collecting system. A series of 1,000 consecutive procedures performed with this class of flexible ureteroscope underscores its versatility and usefulness in treating a variety of disorders.[2] Active intramural dilation for access with a balloon or graduated dilator was infrequently required. In addition, secondary deflection was useful in obtaining lower-pole intrarenal access in 57% of procedures performed.[2,4]

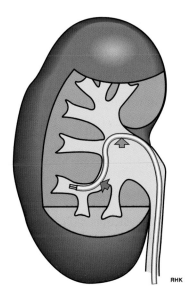

Figure 31-6 In the early 1980s steerable flexible ureteroscopes were introduced. These instruments incorporated both an active distal tip deflection and a passive "secondary" deflecting segment of the distal shaft approximately 6–10 cm from the tip, which facilitated intrarenal lower-pole caliceal access.

The next and most recent major advancement in flexible ureteroscope design was the mechanical addition of "exaggerated" or "active" secondary deflection in 2003 (Figure 31-8).[5] These instruments could now be directed more easily into the lower-pole calices with depression of a lever, and accessories, including the relatively stiff laser fibers that in the past had inhibited endoscope deflection, could now be more precisely placed in the lower pole and throughout the collecting system (Figure 31-9; Table 31-1).

Since the recent introduction of the actively deflectable, flexible ureteroscope with active secondary deflection, endoscopic technique has changed[5] (Table 31-2). Flexible ureteroscope access to the ureter is now commonly performed under direct vision without a guidewire. With the introduction of these instruments, for the first time the usefulness and necessity of the semirigid ureteroscope in treating distal ureteral lesions has now come into question. The trend currently is to flexible atraumatic ureteroscopy, employed throughout the upper urinary tract. When these endoscopes are combined with powerful and precise lithotrites, the clinical results can be extraordinary.

ENDOSCOPIC LITHOTRITES: SOUND, SPARKS, LIGHT, AND PERCUSSION

Ureteroscopic treatment of upper urinary tract calculi is based on either stone extraction or endoscopic lithotripsy. Blind basketing of ureteral calculi without the aid of a ureteroscope is prohibited.[1] Small calculi can, however, be safely extracted with either a helical round wire or spherical flat wire stainless steel basket (Figure 31-10). In addition, nitinol baskets represent a nonkinking, sturdy, and relatively atraumatic alternative that may completely replace the stainless steel accessories for stone fragment extraction.

Lithotripsy refers to stone fragmentation. Endoscopic lithotripsy is based on an endoscopic tool passed through the working channel of the ureteroscope employed to fragment calculi. The first endoscopic lithotrites were ultra-

sound based and were employed with rigid rodlens endoscopes.[26] The probes employed were either solid (eg, more powerful) or hollow and able to evacuate some debris. With the introduction of semirigid and flexible ureteroscopes, the usefulness of ultrasonic lithotripsy diminished appreciably. With even small deflection of the probes, power loss was dramatic with a corresponding drop in successful outcomes. Flexible lithotripsy probes were thus required to complement the changes in endoscopes.

Raney with Northgate presented a new endoscopic lithotripter in 1975.[27–29] The device employed an electrical spark on the end of a flexible cable that produced a shock wave strong enough to fragment a calculus (Figure 31-11). Electrohydraulic lithotripsy naturally meshed with the new endoscopes and became a standard lithotrite during the 1980s. Probes were downsized from 6 to 1.4F with the 3F and 1.9F being the most popular.[30] Cooling irrigant was essential to prevent urothelial thermal injury. Isotonic saline irrigant could be employed with the device to clear the optical field and cool the probe. Energy delivery was not only forward toward a calculus, but actually surrounded the probe tip as well. This was useful if the tip could only be placed adjacent to a stone, but did frequently cause urothelial and endoscope tip trauma. Attempts at directing energy exclusively forward with shielding were hampered by an inability to downsize to the working channel diameter of contemporary endoscopes.[31] Overall miniaturization (< 2F) produced a safer probe, which was unfortunately more fragile with a shorter working intraoperative lifespan.

A later addition was the pneumatic lithotripter based on a guidewire-like probe placed through the endoscope's working channel and driven back and forth like a mini-jackhammer. A bullet-like piston and a rotary engine design, which created sufficient kinetic energy delivered onto the probe for mechanical fragmentation, were both employed. The Lithoclast and Browne pneumatic impactor were two designs, with the Lithoclast being the only commercially available design[33,34] Figure 31-12. This device was reusable and cost

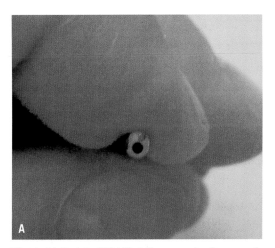

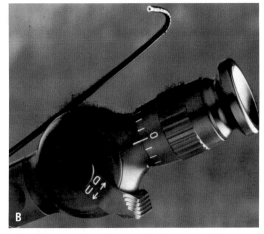

Figure 31-7 *A,* In 1994 Karl Storz was the first manufacturer to miniaturize the actively deflectable, flexible ureteroscope from 10 to 7.5F. *B,* Logical tip deflection and a 3.6F working channel became standard features henceforth.

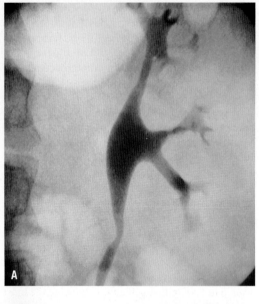
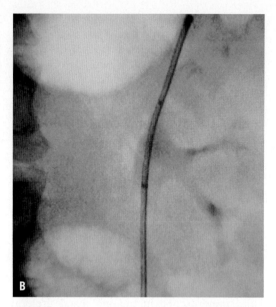
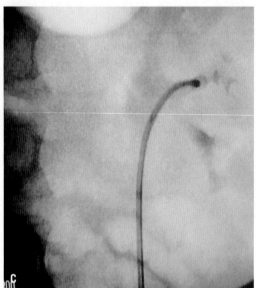
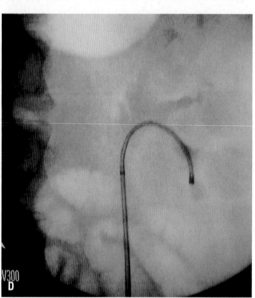

Figure 31-8 *A,* A retrograde pyelogram and subsequent diagnostic ureteroscopy with a 7.5F actively deflectable, flexible ureteroscope inspecting the *B,* upper-pole, *C,* midpole, and *D,* lower-pole calices.

effective. Limitations included retrograde stone migration, especially in dilated collecting systems, probe rigidity, and incompatibility with ureteroscopes as smaller and more flexible endoscopes became available. Flexible nitinol probes were initially an attractive addition, but were rarely, if ever, clinically employed, in part because of the simultaneous introduction of other devices that were superior in fragmentation.[33,34]

Laser lithotripsy was also introduced in the late 1980s with the coumarin-based pulsed-dye laser being the first clinically accepted device.[21] Now fiberoptics delivered a specific wavelength of light (504 nm), which, when applied in irrigant, created a plasma between a stone and the fiber tip. When delivered in a pulsatile manner, a photoacoustic effect was produced, converting light energy to audible sound and pressure waves that fragmented stones along fracture plains. The fiberoptic glass fibers were complementary with the small diameter and flexible ureteroscopes, and the device was thermal free and safe. Limitations

included limits of available energy based in part on fiber diameter, where, as an example, a 200 micron fiber could only deliver 80 mJ of energy. Frequently, more energy was required to fragment calcium oxalate monohydrate stones. Additionally, this laser energy had no effect on cystine calculi. This laser was unidimensional and could not be employed for other endoscopic therapies. Lastly, the liquid dye employed within the laser had a short half-life, was toxic, and had to be changed regularly, requiring special disposal.

The holmium laser was introduced in the early 1990s as a solid-state alternative to the pulsed-dye laser. As with the pulsed-dye laser, pulsatile light energy was delivered through flexible, low water density quartz fibers that could be passed easily through the working channels of the ureteroscopes. Holmium:YAG garnets were solid state and never required replacement. When excited with a flashlamp, they produced light energy of 2,150 nm, which created a vaporization bubble at the tip of the fiber when placed in

water-soluble irrigant or saline. This thermally produced bubble of water vapor would ablate stone, tissue, and urothelial lesions, if so desired. The combination of thermal effect and pulsatile delivery would disrupt stone structure, creating fine dust and small fragments. When employed in cooling irrigant, the thermal energy dissipates rapidly with minimal thermal effect a few millimeters from the fiber tip. In addition, even the smallest fibers can deliver sufficiently high energy to fragment all calculi irrespective of composition. The ablative effect converting stone and tissue to dust-like particles in a particularly controlled manner, the small fiber diameter delivery system, and the safety profile when employed in cooling irrigant, all have made this lithotrite a standard device employed universally (Figure 31-13).[35]

THE TECHNICAL ART OF URETEROSCOPIC LITHOTRIPSY

Ureteroscopic technique has progressed with technological advancements and the ever-broadening clinical experience of the endoscopist. The urologist has become first and foremost a primary endoscopist. In the office, flexible cystoscopy is a routine modality in diagnosing urothelial lesions. In the operating theatre, the flexible ureteroscope is the natural diagnostic extension when upper-tract diagnostic mapping of the urothelium is required. The natural progression from diagnostic to therapeutic endoscopy has led to therapies initially to treat distal ureteral lesions, with progression to the proximal ureter and intrarenal collecting system. With improvements in endoscopic instrumentation, technique is constantly being refined. Current endoscopic treatments for three common clinical presentations will be presented to frame current clinical technique. As with all presentations, the reader must place this work into proper perspective, for it is expected that with future advances in instrumentation, the technique will continue to change—all in an attempt to minimize tissue trauma and expedite complete stone clearance.

1. THE IMPACTED URETERAL CALCULUS

Ureteral stones treated ureteroscopically were for many years addressed differently based on their location in the ureter. Cystoscopic placement of a guidewire under fluoroscopic guidance with subsequent placement of a semirigid ureteroscope beside the safety wire is a commonly employed technique for distal ureteral calculi. Direct visualization of the calculus with placement of an endoscopic lithotrite passed through the working channel allowed for prompt stone fragmentation. Often, the stone would be disimpacted by the cooling irrigant employed to clear the optical field of view or by the endoscopic lithotrite during stone fragmentation. To prevent this, the use of a basket or coiled-wire backstop (Stone Cone, Boston Scientific, Natick, MA) was employed. Semirigid ureteroscopes were designed with two working channels, which allowed for simultane-

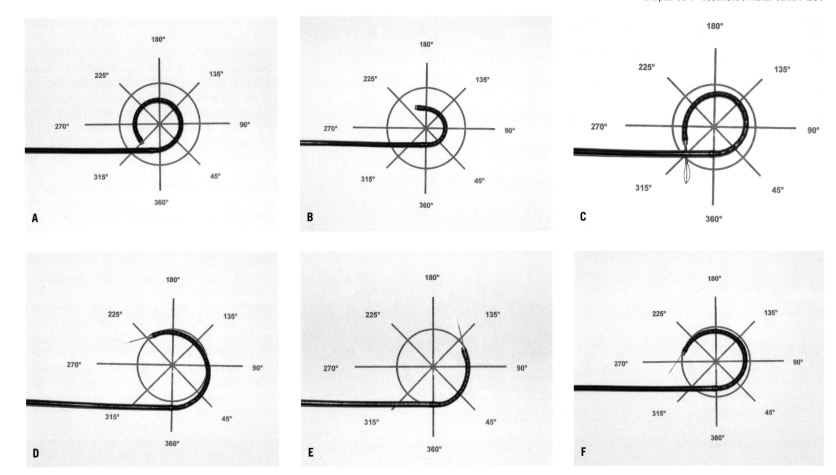

Figure 31-9 *A,* A new flexible ureteroscope released in 2003 (Flex-X, Karl Storz Endoscopy, Tuttlingen, Germany) with > 315 degrees of primary active tip deflection, and a longer radius of deflection—termed exaggerated deflection.[15] *B,* A standard 7.5F flexible ureteroscope with 180° of primary tip deflection employed for comparison.[17] *C,* Maximum active tip deflection with a 365 micron holmium laser fiber passed through the working channel of the Flex-X flexible ureteroscope (194°),[31] and for comparison, *D,* the prior standard 7.5F ureteroscope (103°).[33] *E,* Maximum active tip deflection with a 200 micron holmium laser fiber (238°),[35] *F,* A 2.5F nitinol basket (315°) passed through the working channel of the Flex-X flexible ureteroscope.[27] From Johnson GB and Grasso M.[5]

ous administration of a basket backstop and a laser fiber for fragmentation. A side-armed irrigation port cap was essential in this setting to allow for simultaneous irrigation while two accessories were employed (Figure 31-14).

The proximal ureter and the intrarenal collection system is the domain of the actively deflectable, flexible ureteroscope. When addressing an impacted proximal ureteral calculus, for example, guidewire placement proximal to the stone before endoscopic lithotripsy was suggested prior to the clinical introduction of the newest flexible ureteroscopes. These endoscopes with exaggerated active tip deflection allow for relatively easier access to the ureter and calculus, and are sufficiently stiff functioning as a safety wire

in and of themselves. Common practice in this setting would be to position the patient into mild Trendelenburg with the ipsilateral side raised. Direct flexible ureteroscopic access to the calculus and endoscopic lithotripsy with the holmium laser would be performed to fragment the stone into dust and small pieces. During the procedure, the remaining central stone mass would become mobile and would move proximally. With the patient in this position, the fragments can be easily followed into an upper- and middle-pole location where they can be treated completely. In most patients, the end result is tiny fragments and debris that do not require extraction and will subsequently pass. In patients with dilated ureters, fragments can be extracted with a minimally trau-

matic nitinol basket or grasper. The single working channel of the flexible ureteroscope will prohibit the simultaneous use of two accessories, so in most cases, total conversion of the stone burden to tiny material is the end point of lithotripsy.

A series of ureteroscopically treated ureteral stones performed at two institutions with contemporary technique is presented in Table 31-3. Since the publication of that manuscript, there have been additional advancements in instrumentation with concurrent refinement in technique.[3,5] Advances in flexible ureteroscope design, for example, and specifically the increased active tip deflectability combined with a more rigid shaft durometer has allowed for direct endoscopic inspection and treatment of all ureteral lesions

Table 31-1 Comparison of Active Deflection Prototype versus Standard Ureteroscope

		Baseline Deflection	Piranha 3F Biopsy Forceps	2.2F Nitinol Basket	3F Nitinol Basket	200 μm Laser Fiber	365 μm Laser Fiber
Flex-x	Down	318°	194°	315°	272°	238°	194°
Standard 7.5F	Down	180°	90°	162°	153°	125°	103°
% Increased Deflection of Prototype	Down	77%	116%	94%	78%	90%	88%
From Johnson GB and Grasso M.[5]							

Table 31-2 Comparison of Prototype versus Standard Ureteroscope

Indications for Flexible Ureteroscopy	Prototype	%	Standard	%
Endoscopic lithotripsy	51	44	491	49
Diagnostic ureteroscopy	26	23	215	21
Biopsy/treat upper tract TCCs	27	23	148	15
Retrograde endopyelotomy	3	3	45	4
Essential hematuria	0	–	31	3
Assisted perc. access	1	< 1	26	3
Incise obstructed infundibulum and caliceal diverticulum	3	3	19	2
Incise ureteral stricture	–	–	16	2
Remove foreign body	0	–	5	< 1
Incise and drain renal cysts	1	< 1	3	< 1
Resect fibroepithelia polyp	0	–	1	< 1
Total	115	–	1,000	–
Flexible Ureteroscopic Access Technique				
No wire	31	27	0	–
No active intramural dilation required (dual lumen catheter only)	54	46	347	35
Initial rigid ureteroscopy	12	10	290	29
Previous ureteral stents	45	39	245	25
Balloon dilation	0	–	63	6
Nottingham graduated dilators	4	3	55	5
Flexible Ureterscopic Access to the Lower-Pole Calix				
Passive secondary deflection	–	–	575	58
Active secondary deflection	99	86	N/A	–
Primary active deflection only	16	14	358	36
Unable to access lower pole	0	–	67	7

TCC = transitional cell carcinoma.
From Johnson GB and Grasso M.[5]

(including the distal ureter), thus minimizing the role of the semirigid endoscope. With distal ureteral stones, if the ureteral orifice is capacious, a technique based on direct flexible ureteroscope access without a guidewire can commonly be employed. If intramural ureteral dilation with either a balloon or graduated dilator is required for access, prior placement of a safety guidewire is important as a means of ultimately placing an internal ureteral stent. Ureteral stents are not absolutely required after endoscopic lithotripsy.[36] Ureteral trauma during the endoscopic lithotripsy, significant ureteral wall edema, or a sizeable volume of stone debris at the end of the treatment session are all relative indications. Even though uncomfortable while in place, ureteral stents help ensure renal drainage, facilitate passive ureteral dilation, and will ultimately make future passage of stone fragments and debris easier.

2. INTRARENAL CALCULUS Ureteroscopic lithotripsy of intrarenal calculi is based on flexible ureteroscopic application of a flexible lithotrite passed onto a calculus, under direct vision, through the working channel of the endoscope. Stone fragment extraction in this setting is most commonly performed with a nitinol grasper or basket. A series of retrograde ureteroscopic lithotripsy procedures performed at two institutions is presented in Table 31-4. Lower-pole stones are often the most challenging of retrograde endoscopic lithotripsy procedures. Parameters including the degree of hydronephrosis,

the length of the lower-pole infundibulum, and the infundibulopelvic angle have all been studied as potential parameters that could prohibit a successful outcome.[37] In one series of 90 consecutive flexible ureteroscopic lithotripsies, only the length of the lower-pole infundibulum in excess of 3 cm was a statistically significant variable associated with procedural failure (Table 31-5). With the addition of active secondary endoscope deflection, this limitation may be actually less significant. Other parameters, including severe hydronephrosis, did not prohibit a successful outcome in this series.

Technical issues when performing retrograde ureteroscopic treatment of intrarenal calculi include proper patient positioning and purposeful stone migration during endoscopic therapy. As with proximal ureteral calculi, positioning the patient in Trendelenburg and raising the ipsilateral side is useful. During treatment of lower-pole calculi, for example, initial fragmentation into large but mobile pieces with subsequent relocation to an upper- or middle-pole calix with a basket or grasper is frequently beneficial. As the intrarenal collecting system distends from the cooling irrigant applied during therapy, the ability to replace the endoscope and laser fiber into the lower pole will decrease. Prompt fragmentation and relocation to a more accessible cephalad calix will often facilitate complete treatment. It is important to note that very little can be gained from pursuing stone fragmentation when endoscopic visibility is poor. This often occurs during

vigorous ureteroscopic lithotripsy when either the bladder is full of irrigant or the intrarenal collecting system is coated with fine dust and fragments. Placement of a small-diameter Foley catheter into the bladder beside the flexible ureteroscope will frequently help clear the optical field and lower the overall pressure in the collecting system. If decreased visibility is secondary to buildup of stone debris, discontinuance and proceeding with staged therapy is essential. All patients with particularly large calculi where ureteroscopic therapy is planned are counseled that staged therapy will most likely be required to completely treat their stone burden.

3. LARGE INTRARENAL CALCULI Ureteroscopic treatment of large and branching intrarenal calculi is a relatively new application of retrograde endoscopic lithotripsy techniques.[35] The data from the largest clinical series on this subject are presented in Table 31-6. It must be clearly understood from the outset that this treatment was chosen for patients who were at higher risk of treatment with percutaneous endoscopic lithotripsy, or who had a prior complicated percutaneous nephrostolithotomy and sought out this form of treatment. It should also be clear that infectious calculi should not be treated in this fashion, especially if percutaneous endoscopic treatment can be performed safely as an alternative. In cases of uncorrectable bleeding diathesis or renal ectopy, where a nephrostomy cannot be placed safely because of the proximity of adjacent structures, these techniques could be employed for infectious stone burdens, even with higher risk.

All patients should have preoperative urine cultures performed, and those with positive cultures should be directed as previously described. Appropriate broad-spectrum antibiotic coverage is essential at the outset of the procedure. Regional anesthetic is preferred because these procedures can be lengthy, with a maximum of up to 3 hours in the published series.[37] Placement of a small diameter Foley catheter after positioning the flexible endoscope into the intrarenal collecting system will help keep the optical field clear and the intrarenal pressures as low as possible. All patients are counseled that serial, staged therapy will be required if their stone burden is in excess of 2.5 cm. If staged therapy is required, then patients are given the option of inpatient care with short breaks between endoscopic sessions of 24 to 36 hours, during which intrarenal irrigation is performed to clear dust and debris, or outpatient staged therapy with placement of a large 8F or 10F ureteral stent and subsequent a second outpatient sitting 1 or 2 weeks later.

In those patients with the largest calculi, multiple stages are required with intrarenal irrigation between sessions being particularly helpful. In this setting, a 5F Cobra catheter is positioned with its tip in the lower pole and a larger open-ended catheter is positioned in the upper pole (Figure 31-15). Irrigant is instilled via the Cobra

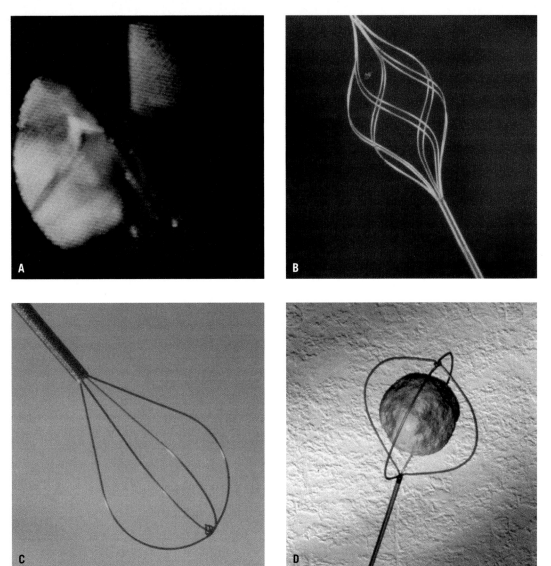

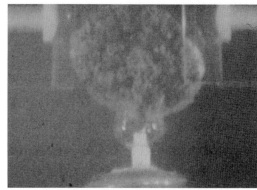

Figure 31-11 High-speed photography demonstrating the cavitation bubble formed by electrohydraulic lithotripsy.

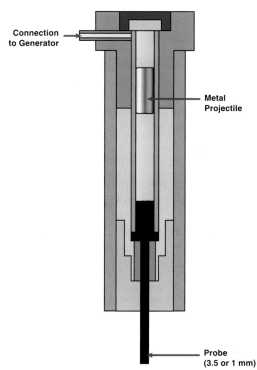

Figure 31-10 *A,* The Segura 2.5 and 3F flat wire stainless steel baskets are excellent tools for stabilizing calculi during semirigid ureteroscopic lithotripsy and/or extracting stones from a dilated ureter. *B,* The Gemini helical round wire stainless steel basket (Boston Scientific, Natick, MA) is useful in a tight, narrow-caliber ureter. *C, D,* The spherical nitinol baskets have many advantages, the most important of which is the fact that the wires are more kink resistant than the corresponding stainless steel variety. Nitinol baskets can also be manufactured to a specified outer diameter of < 2F. Clinically, these baskets are more flexible than stainless steel, minimally inhibiting the deflection of the flexible ureteroscope. If clinically warranted, nitinol baskets can also disengage a calculus that is found ureteroscopically to be too large to extract.

Figure 31-12 The ballistic, or jackhammer, mechanical lithotriptor (Lithoclast, Luzanne, Switzerland) is a pneumatically driven mechanical lithotrite. *A,* Compressed air drives a metallic projectile against a stainless steel probe, transforming kinetic energy into mechanical energy for fragmentation. *B,* The stainless steel probes are commonly placed through the working channels of both rigid and semirigid endoscopes. (Courtesy of John Denstedt, MD.)

catheter and either drains around both into the bladder or exits through the open-ended catheter. Instillation rates start at 50 cc per hour and are gradually increased to 100 cc per hour. Fever, flank pain, or nausea all can reflect obstruction with increased intrarenal pressures. If these symptoms occur, the continuous irrigation should be halted and the catheters manually irrigated and adjusted to clear debris. Irrigation solutions are based on stone composition. Patients with calcium-based stones are irrigated with sterile saline solution with 80 mg of gentamycin placed per liter of irrigant. Those with uric acid composition are treated with one-quarter normal sodium chloride solution with 1 or 2 amps of $NaHCO_3$ per liter. Cystine stone dust clears nicely with 0.4 M Mucomyst solution in THAM. Few cystine stone fragments larger than 2 to

3 mm clear with these irrigations, but the tremendous stone dust that prohibits endoscopic visibility will clear, thus facilitating the next endoscopic stage.

Operative success of retrograde endoscopic lithotripsy of large intrarenal calculi often is reflected in a post-procedural radiograph defining a smudge over the collecting system and no discrete radiopaque calculus. Other patients will have very small fragments throughout the caliceal system. Over time the majority of this debris will clear.[3,35] In those patients with longer than 6-month follow-up in the presented study, greater than 60% were completely stone free, while the remainder had a very small residual that frequently cleared over time (Table 31-7). In only those patients with uncontrollable metabolic disorder was new stone growth noted in follow-up.

LIMITATIONS AND COMPLICATIONS

As the indications for retrograde endoscopic lithotripsy broaden, the frequency and variety of intraoperative and post-operative problems should increase. Actually, the incidence of major complications associated with ureteroscopic lithotripsy has significantly decreased. This is felt to be secondary to smaller and sturdier endoscopes, improved and more universal training of ureteroscopic technique, and powerful yet precise endoscopic lithotrites like the holmium laser.

In Table 31-8 the effect on surgical complications of over a decade of advances in urteroscopic

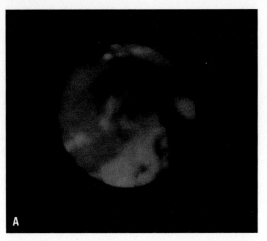
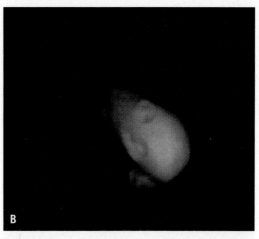
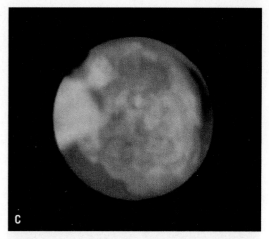

Figure 31-13 *A, B, C, D,* A staghorn calculus composed of calcium oxalate is visualized on plain radiography and then endoscopically. The holmium laser is then employed in a retrograde fashion through the actively deflectable, flexible ureteroscope to sequentially pulverize the stone into dust and small fragments.

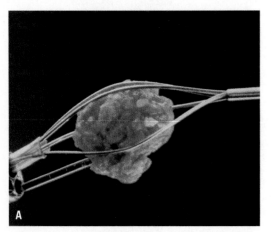
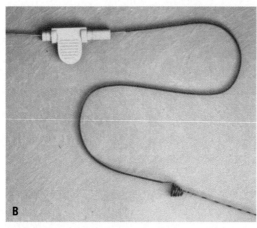
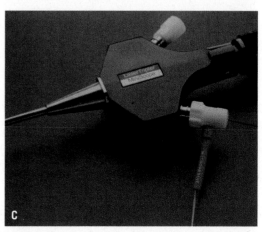

Figure 31-14 *A, B,* Semirigid ureteroscope with two working channels, which allows for simultaneous administration of a basket backstop and a laser fiber for stone fragmentation. *C,* A side-armed irrigation port cap is essential in this setting to allow for concomitant irrigation while two accessories are employed.

instruments and technique at three medical centers is presented. The Mayo Clinic, Jefferson Medical College, and the New York University experience changed significantly with the more liberal use of the flexible ureteroscope, with now a universally accepted major complication rate of less than 1%. Milestones, including endoscope miniaturization to 7.5F, the recent addition of active secondary deflection, and the universal use of the holmium laser as an endoscopic lithotrite, all have broadened indications while limiting major problems.

Minor complications are self limiting, requiring minimal or supportive care and include postoperative fever associated with a urinary tract infection, gross but transient and self-limiting hematuria, and voiding symptoms commonly associated with recent instrumentation or an internal ureteral stent. Minor ureteral wall abrasions associated with either access or vigorous endoscopic lithotripsy and small guidewire perforations 1 to 2 mm in diameter also fall into this category and are best treated with a short interval (few days to a week) of ureteral stenting (Figure 31-16).

Major intraoperative complications are infrequent, but without prompt and decisive care can lead to disastrous outcomes. Major complications include large ureteral wall perforations and avulsions (Figure 31-17). Once recognized, proximal drainage is required. Placement of a diverting nephrostomy, or, if technically feasible, ureteral stenting if the perforation can be managed in this fashion, is essential. In the rare case of an avulsion, placement of a nephrostomy should be performed promptly to prevent urinoma formation. Subsequent imaging after a period of healing will define the length of involved ureter and help direct the subsequent repair.

A significant postoperative complication occurring subsequent to ureteroscopic lithotripsy is ureteral stricture disease. This is an infrequent outcome and can be associated with prior stone impaction, vigorous endoscopic lithotripsy, and ureteral wall trauma. A good model is that of submucosal calculi that have found their way into the wall of the ureter either iatrogenically or because of long-standing impaction.[38,39] In a series of submucosal calculi evaluated with intraluminal sonography, the depth of the stone or fragments from the ureteral lumen correlated with subsequent stricture (Figure 31-18). Calculi

within 4 mm of the lumen were associated with obstruction and led to subsequent stricture and stone granuloma formation unless the fragments were promptly removed. Clearance of these fragments, if technically feasible, was performed with ureteroscopic unroofing and standard lithotripsy techniques emphasizing meticulous localization and extraction. Fragments deeper than 4 mm were felt to be outside the ureteral wall where treatment had little effect on the ultimate outcome. In another multi-institutional series lead by the group from Johns Hopkins, the rate of ureteral stricture disease after endoscopic lithotripsy of long-standing impacted calculi was 19%,[40] much higher than the less than 1% noted in the general population of calculi treated ureteroscopically.

Treatment of ureteral strictures is based in part on the stricture length, depth of fibrosis, and tissue viability. Short strictures (< 1.5 cm) can commonly be treated with either balloon dilation or endoscopic incision and transient stenting. Longer strictures and absent ureteral segments secondary to an avulsion require a more complex repair. Distal strictures or an absent distal ureter

Table 31-3 Grasso, The New York University Experience with Ureteroscopic Treatment of Ureteral Calculi Employing the Holmium:YAG Laser

Location	Number	Mean Diameter (range mm)	Success after Primary/ Secondary Treatment (%)*
Proximal third	75	11.3 (30–5)	95/96
Middle third	45	10.7 (60–5)	98/100
Distal third	91	10.3 (50–4)	99/100
Total	211	–	97/99

*Second stage required for stone diameter > 2.5 cm.[2]

Table 31-4 Grasso, The New York University Experience with Ureteropyeloscopic Treatment of Intrarenal Calculi Employ8ing the Holmium:YAG Laser

Location	Number	Mean Diameter (range mm)	Success after Primary/ Secondary Treatment (%)*
Upper pole	58	10.6 (35–4)	90/97
Middle pole	30	11.1 (23–4)	90/93
Lower pole	103	14.8 (40–3)	79/85
Renal pelvic	37	20.5 (60–6)	78/95
Total	228	–	81/90
Sofer et al.[3]			
Kidney	56	13.5 (5–30)	84**

*Second stage required for stone diameter > 2.5 cm.
**Staged therapy in eight patients.

Table 31-5 Prevalence of Collecting System Variants and Predictive Values for Surgical Failure

Collecting System Variants	No. Prevalence (%)	No. Failures with Variants (%)	Odds Ration (CI)
Long lower-pole infundibulum (> 3 cm)*	21 (23)	8 (38)	7.9 (5 ± 12.2)
Acute infundibulopelvic angle	29 (32)	5 (17)	1.3 (0.9 ± 2.1)
Dilated collecting system	23 (26)	4 (17)	1.3 (0.8 ± 2.1)
Infundibular stricture*	3 (3)	2 (67)	13.8 (10.9 ± 17.4)

*Statistically significant.
From Grasso M and Ficazzola M.[37]

Table 31-6a Surgical Indications for Retrograde Ureteroscopic Treatment of Large Upper Urinary Tract Calculi

Indication	No. Pts.
Complex comorbid medical conditions	12
Refused or failed prior percutaneous nephrostlithotomy	11
Failed prior ESWL	9
Failed medical therapy of radiolucent calculi	9
Bleeding diathesis:	
Chronic renal insufficiency	8
Anticoagulant therapy	1
Portal hypertension	1
Morbid obesity	4
Severe kyphoscoliosis, renal ectopia, solitary kidney	3

ESWL = extracorporeal shock wave lithotripsy.

sessions become routine throughout the upper urinary tract. The future of endoscopic lithotripsy mirrors the minimal to atraumatic ureteroscopy performed diagnostically to define upper urinary tract urothelial tumors. With greater tip control and a relatively stiff shaft, the newest flexible ureteroscopes allow for access and therapeutic maneuvers without a guidewire. In addition, the increase in active tip deflectability allows for the use of larger diameter accessories, including the larger, more efficient laser fibers.

Finally, an endoscopic lithotrite that would actually remove stone rather than converting into dust and small fragments, like the holmium:YAG laser, would be the next logical development. Experimental work with the erbium laser, for example, has shown some promise, but the delivery system is still either cost prohibitive and/or toxic. On a more positive note, there are many garnets that can be employed in this setting, all delivering a specific wavelength of light when stimulated, with unique mechanical properties when employed in a fluid medium. As with all recent advances, collaboration with industrial sources that are currently developing lasers for nonmedical applications may ultimately lead to the next endoscopic lithotrite.

are best repaired with a psoas hitch ureteroneocystostomy. The Boari flap technique is useful is gaining additional length to the middle third of the ureter. Proximal strictures are addressed in a similar fashion to secondary ureteropelvic junction obstructions with various flap repairs to gain length, and in the case of a small intrarenal pelvis, a ureterocalicostomy can be employed to bridge the segment. If the majority or ureter is absent, then either a bowel interposition employing ileum (ie, ileal ureter) or autotransplant are employed. There is a relative contraindication to employing transureterostomy in stone formers in this setting.

FUTURE DIRECTIONS

Advances in instrumentation continue to lead surgeons to new therapies. Where once only small ureteral calculi could be extracted with a fluoroscopically placed basket, today endoscopically directed treatment of large branching intrarenal stone burdens is performed. Endoscope advances, specifically improved imaging, illumination, instrument longevity, and mechanical parameters, including controlled tip deflection, will improve treatment efficiency and outcomes.

The more controlled the treatment the better the outcome. With the newest endoscopes allowing easier access and precise placement of endoscopic tools or lithotrites, endoscopic lithotripsy

Table 31-6b Stone Size and Locations

	No. Stone Burdens by Location	Smaller Secondary Component (mm)	Max. mm Stone Diameter	(Mean)
Renal calculi (45)				
Upper pole	5	8	30	(19.0)
Middle pole	6	20	35	(26.7)
Lower pole	11	6	40	(26.0)
Renal pelvic	23	10	60	(25.2)
Ureteral calculi (21)				
Proximal	9	8	30	(22.4)
Middle third	5	10	50	(22.0)
Distal	7	6	45	(24.6)

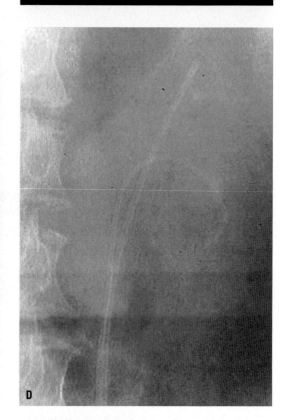

Figure 31-15 *A, B,* Lower-pole partial staghorn calculus is noted on computed tomographic imaging and retrograde pyelography. *C, D,* After the first session of endoscopic lithotripsy, the majority of the stone burden is fragmented. A 5F Cobra catheter is positioned with its tip in the lower pole and a larger open-ended catheter is positioned in the upper pole for continuous intrarenal irrigation. Retrograde intrarenal irrigation is employed for a variable period from one to a few days to clear dust and debris prior to the second staged endoscopic lithotripsy session.

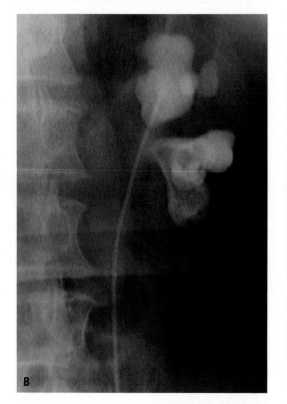

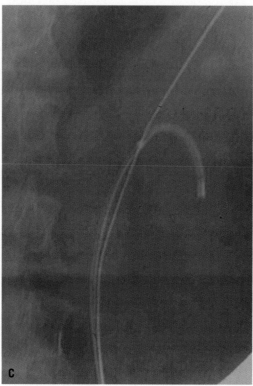

Table 31-7 Success of Ureteroscopic Treatment of Large Upper Urinary Tract Calculi		
	No./Total No. (%)	
	Renal Calculi	Ureteral Calculi
Immediate post-op success:		
Pulverized entire stone burden with consistent immediate imaging	27/45 (60)	18/21 (86)
Suspected significant residual fragments requiring second look endoscopy	15/45 (33)	3/21 (14)
Failure in access and/or visualization with conversion to percutaneous nephrostolithotomy	3/45 (7)	–
Second look endoscopy + multiple staged procedures:		
Fine dust and small debris noted on second look endoscopy	7/15	2/3
Stage 2 endoscopic therapy performed successfully	7/15	1/3
Stage 3 treatment required for largest stone burden	1/15	–
Success with multiple sessions:		
Overall initial success including normal second look endoscopy	34/45 (76)	20/21 (95)
Success after stage 2 lithotripsy	41/45 (91)	21/21 (100)
Additional stage 3 lithotripsy (1 case)	42/45 (93)	–

Table 31-8 Comparison of Ureteroscopic Complications

	Blute et al.[7]	Abdel-Razzak and Bagley[1]	Harmon et al.[20]	Current Study
Year	1988	1992	1997	2000
Procedure	346	290	209	1,000
Minor Complications	(%)	(%)	(%)	(%)
Colic/pain	–	9.0	3.5	4.2
Fever	6.2	6.9	2.0	1.3
False passage	0.9	–	–	0.4
Hematuria				
Minor	0.5	2.1	0	0.8
Prolonged	0.3	1.0	0	0.2
Extravasation	0.6	1.0	–	–
UTI	–	1.0	–	1.7
Pyelonephritis	–	–	–	1.0
Major Complications	(%)	(%)	(%)	(%)
Major perforation	4.6	1.7	1.0	0
Stricture	1.4	0.7	0.5	0.4
Avulsion	0.6	0	0	0
Urinoma	0.6	–	0	0
Urosepsis	0.3	0	0	0
CVA	–	–	0.5	0.1
DVT	–	–	–	0.1
MI	–	–	–	0.1

CVA = cerebral accident; DVT = deep vein thrombosis; MI = myocardial infarction; UTI = urinary tract infection.

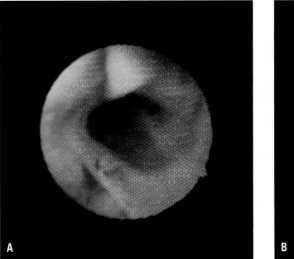 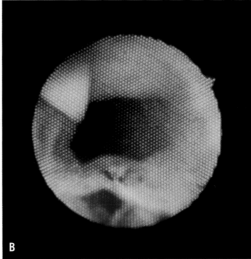

Figure 31-16 *A, B,* A guidewire perforation of the ureteral wall with a false passage will heal with minimal, if any, long-term sequelae so long as the small defect is not expanded with dilation or vigorous endoscopic manipulation and the defect is transiently bridged with a ureteral stent. (From Tenaja, Complications of Urologic Surgery.)

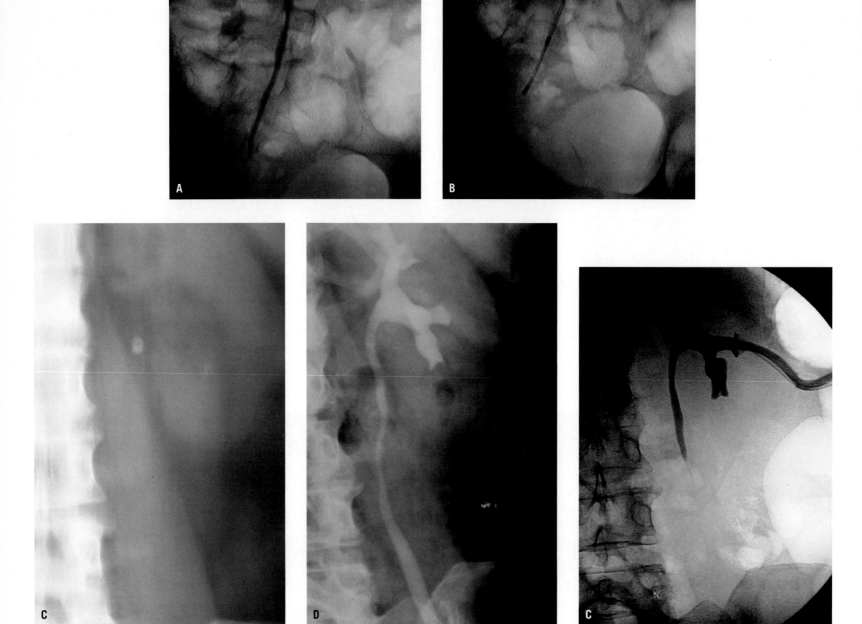

Figure 31-17 Distal ureteral avulsion. A distal ureteral calculus was engaged in an endoscopically placed basket, and during extraction the distal ureter was traumatized. Poor postoperative drainage required percutaneous nephrostomy placement. *A,* After transfer to another institution, an antegrade nephrostogram defined a blind-ending ureteral stump, which actually turns cephalad, representing a "snapping-off" effect. *B,* Simultaneous antegrade and retrograde endoscopy defined complete absence of the distal one-third of the ureter. This was repaired with an ureteroneocystostomy. *C,* Subtotal ureteral avulsion. This patient underwent extracorporeal shock wave lithotripsy to treat a lower-pole renal calculus. Poor fragmentation and migration of the stone burden led to severe colic and hospital admission. Plain radiography (C) and contrast imaging (D) define a nonobstructing proximal ureteral calculus. Ureteroscopic treatment was based on semirigid endoscopic access and attempted laser lithotripsy. When the laser lithotripter malfunctioned, an attempt at basket extraction produced an almost complete ureteral avulsion, whereby most of the ureter was brought down into the bladder with the endoscope. *E,* Antegrade nephrostogram performed at transfer to a tertiary referral center defines a ureteral cutoff just below the ureteropelvic junction, consistent with most of the now devascularized ureter being located in the bladder. Subsequent surgical repair is based on ileal substitution or renal autotransplantion. (From Tenaja's Complications of Urologic Surgery.)

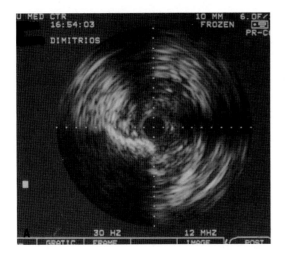

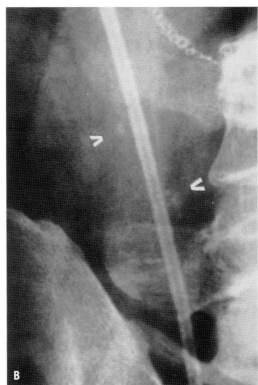

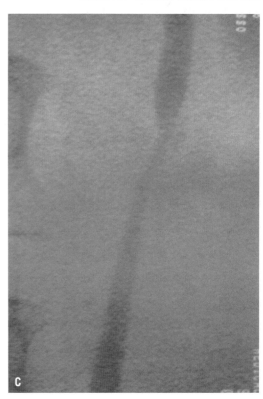

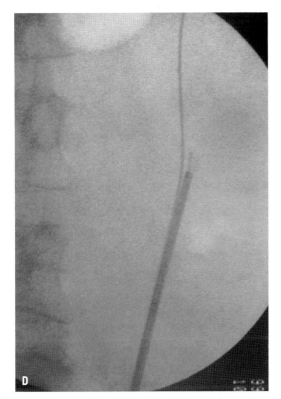

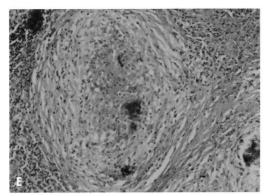

Figure 31-18 *A,* An introluminal ultrasonographic image of the ureteral wall defining a submucosal stone fragment, which was the product of prior vigorous electrohydraulic lithotripsy. *B, C, D, E,* Stone fragments such as these can be associated with granulomatous changes and subsequent stricture disease. If these fragments are located within the ureteral wall they should be removed promptly, if possible, to minimize foreign body reaction and subsequent fibrosis. (From Tenaja's Complications of Urologic Surgery)

REFERENCES

1. Segura JW, Preminger GM, Assimos DG, et al. Ureteral Stones Clinical Gudelines Panel summary report on the management of ureteral calculi. The American Urological Association. J Urol 1997;158:1915–21.

2. Grasso M. Ureteropyeloscopic treatment of ureteral and intrarenal calculi. Urol Clin North Am 2000;27:623–31.

3. Sofer M, Waterson J, Wollin T, et al. Holmium:YAG laser lithotripsy for upper urinary tract calculi in 598 patients. J Urol 2002;167:31–4.

4. Grasso M, Bagley DH. A 7.5/8.2 F actively deflectable, flexible ureteroscope: a new device for both diagnostic and therapeutic upper urinary tract endoscopy. Urology 1994; 43:435–41.

5. Johnson GB, Grasso M. Exaggerated primary endoscope deflection: initial clinical experience with prototypic flexible ureteroscopes. BJU Int 2004;93:109–14.

6. Lam JS, Greene, TD, Gupta, M. Treatment of proximal ureteral calculi: holmium:YAG laser ureterolithotripsy versus extracorporeal shock wave lithotripsy. J Urol 2002;167:1972–6.

7. Erhard M, Salwen J, Bagley DH. Ureteroscopic removal of mid and proximal ureteral calculi. J Urol 1996;155: 38–42.

8. Graff J, Pastor J, Funke PJ, et al. Extracorporeal shock wave lithotripsy for ureteral stones: a retrospective analysis of 417 cases. J Urol 1988;139:513–6.

9. Cockett WS, Cockett AT. The Hopkins rod-lens system and the Storz cold light illumination system. Urology 1998;51 Suppl 5A:1–2.

10. Gow JG. Harold Hopkins and optical systems for urology—an appreciation. Urology 1998;52:152–7.

11. Bagley DH, Huffman JL, Lyon ES. Flexible fiberoptic ureteropyeloscopy. In: Urologic endoscopy: a manual and atlas. Boston: Little, Brown; 1985. p. 207–17.

12. Baird JL. British Patent Specification No. 20, 96927. 1927.

13. Hansell CW. U.S. Patent No. 1,751,584. 1930, filed 1927.

14. Curtiss IE, Hirschowitz BI, Peters CW. A long fiberscope for internal medical examination. J Opt Soc Am 1956;46:1030.

15. Gow JG. Harold Hopkins and optical systems for urology–an appreciation. Urology 1998;52:152–7.

16. Hirchowitz BI, Curtiss IE, Peters CW, Pollard HM. Demonstration of a new gastroscope, the "fiberscope." Gastroenterology 1958;35:50.

17. Marshall VF. Fiberoptics in urology. J Urol 1964;91:100–4.

18. Stoller ML, Wolf JS Jr, Hofmann R, Marc B. Ureteroscopy without routine balloon dilation: an outcome assessment. J Urol 1992;147:1238–42.

19. Abdel-Razzak OM, Bagley DH. The 6.9F semirigid ureteroscope in clinical use. Urology 1993;41:45–8.

20. Bagley DH. Ureteroscopic stone retrieval: rigid versus flexible endoscopes. Semin Urol 1994;12:31–8.

21. Grasso M. Intracorporeal lithotripsy: ultrasonic, electrohydraulic, laser, and electromechanical. In: Marshall FF, editor. Textbook of operative urology. Philadelphia: WB Saunders; 1996. p. 77–90.

22. Tagaki T, Go T, Takayasu H, Aso Y. A small-caliber fiberscope for the visualization of the urinary tract, biliary tract, and spinal canal. Surgery 1968;64:1033–8.

23. Berci G. Instrumentation: flexible fiber endoscopes. In: Berci G, editor. Endoscopy. New York: Appleton-Century-Crofts; 1976.

24. Bagley DH, Huffman JL, Lyon ES. Combined rigid and flexible ureteropyeloscopy. J Urol 1983;130:243–4.

25. Bagley DH, Huffman JL, Lyon ES. Flexible ureteropyeloscopy: diagnosis and treatment in the upper urinary tract. J Urol 1987;138:280–5.

26. Goodfriend R. Disintegration of ureteral calculi by ultrasound. Urology 1973;1:260–3.

27. Raney AM. Electrohydraulic lithotripsy: experimental study and case reports with the stone disintegrator. J Urol 1975;113:345–7.

28. Raney AM. Electrohydraulic cystolithotripsy. Urology 1976;7:379–81.

29. Purohit GS, Pham D, Raney AM, Bogaev JH. Electrohydraulic ureterolithotripsy. An experimental study. Invest Urol 1980;17:462–4.

30. Denstedt JD, Clayman RV. Electrohydraulic lithotripsy of renal and ureteral calculi. J Urol 1990;143:13–7.

31. Bhatta KM, Rosen DI, Flotte TJ, et al. Effects of shielded and unshielded laser and electrohydraulic lithotripsy on rabbit bladder. J Urol 1990;143:857–60.

32. Bagley DH. Intrarenal access with flexible ureteropyeloscope: effects of active and passive tip deflection. J Endourol 1993;7:221–4.

33. Denstedt JD, Eberwein PM, Singh RR. The Swiss lithoclast: a new device for intracorporeal lithotripsy. J Urol 1992; 148(3 Pt 2):1088–90.

34. Grasso M, Loisides P, Beaghler M, Bagley DH. Treatment of urinary calculi in a porcine and canine model using the Browne Pneumatic Impactor. Urology 1994;44: 937–41.

35. Grasso M, Conlin M, Bagley DH. Retrograde ureteropyeloscopic treatment of 2 cm or greater upper urinary tract and minor staghorn calculi. J Urol 1998;160:346–51.

36. Denstedt JD, Wollin TA, Sofer M, et al. A prospective randomized controlled trial comparing stented versus non-stented ureteroscopic lithotripsy. J Urol 2001;165: 1419–22.

37. Grasso M, Ficazzola M. Retrograde ureteropyeloscopy for lower pole caliceal calculi. J Urol 1999;162:1904–8.

38. Giddens JL, Grotas AB, Grasso M. Stone granuloma causes UPJ obstruction after percutaneous nephrolithotomy and antegrade endopyelotomy.

39. Grasso M, Goldberg BB, Liu JB, et al. Submucosal calculi: endoscopic and endoluminal ultrasonographic diagnosis and treatment options. J Urol 1995;153:1384–9.

40. Roberts WW, Caddedu JA, Fabrizio MD, et al. Ureteral stricture formation following removal of impacted calculi: a multiinstitutional study [abstract]. J Urol 1999;1456:376.

32

Diagnostic Ureteroscopy

Kim Davenport, MBChB, MRCS (Glasgow)

Francis X. Keeley Jr, MD, FRCS (Edinburgh), FRCS (Urology)

Young reported the first endoscopic visualization of the ureter in 1912. Since then, technology has advanced from large, rigid ureteroscopes to smaller-diameter, semirigid instruments and the introduction of flexible steerable ureteroscopes. The first flexible instruments were dependent on passive deflection to allow adequate visualization of the upper tracts, which required considerable expertise. As newer, smaller instruments have become available, ureteroscopy has become a widely accepted method for both diagnosis and management of upper-tract pathology. Since the development of endoscopes with actively deflectable tips and channels adequate for working instruments, both the diagnostic and therapeutic roles have rapidly expanded.

This chapter aims to cover the technique of ureteroscopy when used for diagnostic purposes and discuss the potential indications.

GENERAL TECHNIQUE

The combined use of rigid ureteroscopy and flexible ureteroscopy allows access for full inspection of the upper tracts.[1] Flexible ureteroscopes have an actively deflectable tip, enabling deflection of up to 170 degrees within the collecting system. Most flexible fiberoptic ureteroscopes have an additional passively deflectable segment proximal to the actively deflectable segment, which allows further mobility and access into previously inaccessible areas of the collecting system. The latest generation of flexible ureteroscopes has taken deflection even further; one model incorporates an active secondary deflection mechanism, while another can deflect up to 270 degrees.

When using ureteroscopy for diagnostic purposes, it is important to take care to minimize trauma and artefact to prevent difficulty with interpretation of the endoscopic findings. Access sheaths and dilatation should be avoided because of the risk of associated trauma to the distal ureter. Guidewires should not be used until the distal ureter has been thoroughly inspected by rigid ureteroscopy.

The smallest ureteroscope possible should be used, again to minimize trauma. A rigid ureteroscope is used initially to inspect the distal ureter. Those currently available range in size from 6.9 to 12 French (F). Rigid ureteroscopy is carried out as far up the ureter as safely possible. A guidewire should be used only following the initial inspection of the distal ureter and should be inserted no further than has been visualized directly with the

ureteroscope. The guidewire is essential for the introduction of the flexible ureteroscope in an undilated ureter. The level inspected by the rigid ureteroscope can be confirmed using fluoroscopy, and the guidewire should be inserted under fluoroscopic guidance to ensure similar levels.

Flexible ureteroscopes range in size from 7.4 to 10.5F. The flexible ureteroscope is back loaded over the guidewire with no attachments, keeping the ureteroscope straight and in direct line with the guidewire. Fluoroscopy should be used to monitor the progress of the ureteroscope. The most common point of difficulty in passing the instrument is at the level of the ureteral orifice. If it does not pass, ensure that the guidewire is kept taught. Rotating the ureteroscope can also help. With smaller diameter (< 9F) ureteroscopes, dilation of the orifice is usually unnecessary. In cases needing dilatation, we recommend using a single pass of a dual-lumen catheter, which dilates the ureter to 10F, while keeping the tip of the catheter below the level examined by rigid ureteroscopy.

Once the flexible ureteroscope reaches the level inspected by rigid ureteroscopy, the guidewire is removed and the ureteroscope is advanced along the remaining length of the ureter under direct vision while irrigating with saline. A full 360-degree view must be maintained to ensure adequate visualization of the ureteral mucosa. Once within the intrarenal collecting system, the renal pelvis, upper, mid, and lower calices must be systematically inspected in order to minimize trauma to the mucosa.

Cytologic sampling and biopsies of any suspicious lesions should be performed during the initial pass of the instrument. Attempts at examining the entire upper tract prior to biopsy may lead to trauma or avulsion of the lesion during instrument passage. Following inspection and sampling, the working channel of the ureteroscope may be used to insert a further safety guidewire prior to any therapeutic procedure.

VISUAL RECOGNITION

The major advantage of ureteroscopy over other imaging techniques of the upper tracts is the ability to visually inspect the ureter and collecting system. This allows visual recognition of calculi, neoplasms, and other mucosal lesions. Benign ureteral strictures can often be distinguished from malignant strictures.

Extrinsic compression can be indicated by the presence of a narrowing in the absence of any

mucosal lesion. A visible pulsation or a compressible filling defect may indicate crossing vessels.

However, not all lesions are obvious. Some inflammatory lesions can be indistinguishable from malignant lesions.[2] Malignant lesions with surface calcification may be mistaken for calculi with a surrounding inflammatory reaction.

Fluid and tissue sampling should be used in conjunction with direct visualization to increase the diagnostic accuracy of ureteroscopy.

SAMPLING TECHNIQUES

The working channel of the endoscope provides access for several sampling instruments and techniques. The size of the channel ranges from 2.1 to 5.4F in the rigid instruments and 2.5 to 5F in the flexible ureteroscopes, depending on the instrument used. Following insertion of an instrument into the working channel of the flexible ureteroscope, the tip deflection may change slightly and, therefore, fluoroscopy and constant visual monitoring are essential to maintain the position at the lesion. The degree of instrument deflection is also limited to approximately 120 degrees when the working channel is in use, depending on the rigidity of the working instrument and the strength of the ureteroscope's deflecting mechanism.

A syringe may be connected to the working channel at the distal end of the endoscope to allow aspiration of irrigant fluid or urine from the area surrounding a suspicious lesion. This can then be sent for microscopy, culture, or cytology.

Brushing instruments may be used to exfoliate cellular material from suspicious lesions to enhance cytologic assessment. After multiple passes of the brush over the lesion, the ureteroscope and brush are removed. The cells are retrieved from the brush and sent to pathology for cytologic evaluation. Irrigation of the lesion with normal saline and aspiration of the fluid should follow this. This is sent along with the brushings to increase the accuracy of evaluation.

Tissue samples may be obtained using cold-cup biopsy forceps, graspers, baskets, and small-bore resectoscope loops (for distal ureteral lesions close to the vesicoureteral junction), depending on the nature of the lesion. The sample can be removed within the instrument leaving the ureteroscope in place, or both the instrument and the ureteroscope may be removed as a single unit. It is often safer to remove the entire unit to prevent losing the biopsy sample as the instrument is pulled through the working channel.

Tissue samples allow histologic examination and are more accurate than brushing techniques.[3] Obtaining these samples under direct vision improves the diagnostic accuracy. The size of the sample obtained is limited by the size of the working channel and the instruments used; for example, a 3F cup biopsy forceps provides a sample < 1 mm in diameter. Since the samples obtained are so small, techniques for handling and processing are crucial. These samples are often unable to survive the routine processing used for histologic specimens in the pathology department. A higher diagnostic yield, with a better estimate of tumor grade, can be determined by preparing a cell block. All retrieved urine, washes, and biopsy tissue are centrifuged together to make a cell block. An experienced cytopathologist is required to review the material.[4]

DIAGNOSTIC INDICATIONS

1. EVALUATION OF FILLING DEFECTS Upper-tract filling defects identified on intravenous urogram or retrograde ureteropyelography represent the most common diagnostic application of ureteroscopy. Ultrasound and computer tomography (CT) have both been used in an attempt to make a diagnosis. Ultrasound can be particularly useful for diagnosing renal calculi,[5] but it is poor at visualizing the ureteropelvic junction and ureter. CT can also be used to distinguish calculi from soft tissue filling defects owing to their high density. Small lesions may be missed because of the spacing of the slices, and definition can be poor. CT has been shown to be inaccurate for detecting muscle invasion of malignant lesions.[6]

Ureteroscopy can be used to directly inspect and sample the filling defect and obtain urine samples for cytology to aid diagnosis. The ureteroscope is passed to the site of the filling defect while inspecting the rest of the ureter and collecting system and minimizing trauma to the mucosa. The position and nature of the filling defect should be confirmed using contrast and fluoroscopy to prevent misidentification. In the majority of cases, direct visualization should provide a diagnosis. A calculus will be readily distinguishable from a low-grade papillary tumor. An extrinsic mass can be determined. Venous lesions are compressible, and so are less prominent as the pelvis fills with irrigant. Arterial lesions may have a visible pulsation.

Epithelial neoplasms can have a variety of appearances. Low-grade transitional cell carcinoma has a typical papillary appearance, similar to that found in the bladder. High-grade tumors tend to have a more sessile, less papillary appearance, often with necrotic or inflammatory debris on the surface.

Fibroepithelial polyps may be seen arising from the mucosa. They have an intact epithelial surface and, at the ureteropelvic junction, tend to be long, narrow, and worm-like and can be diagnosed on the basis of their gross appearance.

Where there is any suspicion as to the nature of the lesion, further intervention is necessary to obtain an accurate diagnosis. Ureteroscopic inspection and biopsy combined with cytologic techniques have been shown to provide accurate information regarding grade and stage of upper-tract transitional cell carcinoma.[7,8] The prognosis and behaviour of upper-tract transitional cell carcinoma is closely related to grade and stage,[9,10] and therefore accurate pathologic assessment is essential to guide further management.

Cytology of upper-tract urine aspirates has been shown to be approximately 60% accurate.[3] Low-grade lesions typically have fairly normal cytologic features, and so may be missed on cytology alone. High-grade lesions, especially carcinoma in situ, demonstrate a greater loss of cohesiveness and greater morphologic cell changes; for example, prominent nucleoli and high nuclear to cytoplasmic cell ratios.[11] They have a higher rate of desquamation, making the diagnosis more accurate.

Direct biopsy of an upper-tract lesion is more accurate for diagnostic purposes than brushing techniques.[3] In some cases, the brush serves only to move the tissue and fails to remove any fragments. Endoscopic biopsies have a reported sensitivity of up to 93%.[12] The formation of a cell block from all samples obtained has been shown to provide a diagnosis of transitional cell carcinoma in up to 94% of cases.[7] A multibiopsy technique is a suitable alternative, with an 89% diagnostic accuracy.[4] Seventy-eight percent of these specimens were correctly graded. A combination of these techniques has been advocated to provide the highest diagnostic accuracy.

Skolarikos and colleagues showed that, for patients with grade 2 biopsies, combining exfoliated upper-tract cytology with endoscopic biopsy improved the sensitivity and specificity of high-grade tumor detection from 43 to 55% and 23 to 85%, respectively.[8]

In summary, the following technique has been proposed to evaluate the nature of an upper-tract filling defect[7,13]:

- Voided urinary cytology
- Bladder lavage for cytology
- Place ureteric catheter to obtain urine prior to any further instrumentation or contrast
- Retrograde ureteropyelography
- Semirigid ureteroscopy of the distal ureter prior to guidewire insertion
- Flexible ureteroscopy of the proximal ureter and collecting system
- With the ureteroscope positioned near the area of interest, obtain samples
- Aspirate urine at the lesion
- Wash with saline solution and aspirate
- Sample with a basket or cup forceps
- Repeat saline wash and aspirate
- Send all samples (fresh) for cytopathologic study

2. SURVEILLANCE OF UPPER-TRACT TUMORS Ureteroscopy is proving to be a highly effective method for the treatment and surveillance of low-grade upper-tract tumors following endoscopic treatment in highly selected patients.[14–16] Since the alternative is nephroureterectomy, it is also useful in those patients with solitary kidneys, bilateral disease, renal insufficiency, or who are considered unfit for surgery.

Following successful treatment, the methods available for surveillance currently include urinalysis, urine cytology, intravenous urography, retrograde pyelography, and ureteroscopy. Chen and colleagues compared the effectiveness of these methods for surveillance.[12] Urinalysis to detect microscopic hematuria has the advantage of being inexpensive, easy to perform, and possible in the outpatient setting. Both urinalysis and urine cytology in the absence of any bladder tumors are highly specific for recurrent disease, but their sensitivity is low. Bladder drainage cytology obtained cystoscopically increased the specificity and sensitivity of urine cytology, but the sensitivity was still low. Retrograde pyelography read by the urologist at the time of the procedure and ureteroscopic biopsy or cytology were found to be more sensitive methods of detecting upper-tract recurrence, but these methods were less specific. The higher false-positive rate for upper-tract biopsies was felt to be due to artefactual changes in cell morphology as a result of instrumentation. Table 32-1 summarizes these results.

These results indicate that non-invasive methods for surveillance are inadequate in isolation as they yield a high number of false-negatives. Ureteroscopic evaluation with upper-tract biopsy is essential in these patients to detect early recurrence and prevent false-negative results. Ureteroscopic surveillance also allows treatment of the lesion during the same procedure. A combination of these methods provides the most information. Non-invasive methods of surveillance can be used between procedures along with regular cystoscopy to exclude bladder tumors. The threshold for ureteroscopic evaluation should be low. Some recommend periodic ureteroscopy as part of routine surveillance for upper-tract tumors and suggest this should be continued long term, even lifelong, in a similar way to surveillance for bladder cancer.[17]

The technique of ureteroscopy for tumor surveillance is no different to that for the investigation of upper-tract filling defects. The distal to midureter is inspected using a rigid ureteroscope and cytology is obtained by aspiration. A guidewire is inserted to the same level and the flexible ureteroscope is passed over the guidewire and used to inspect the proximal ureter and renal pelvis. Fur-

Table 32-1 Sensitivity and Specificity of Methods Available for Upper-Tract Transitional Cell Carcinoma Surveillance

Methods of Surveillance	Sensitivity	Specificity
Urinalysis	36	91
Urine cytology	38	91
Bladder drainage cytology	50	100
Retrograde pyelography	72	85
Ureteroscopic cytology/biopsy	93	65

ther aspirates are obtained for cytology and labeled appropriately. Contrast material is injected into the collecting system to guide a thorough examination of the calices. Any ureteral lesion identified should be biopsied at first view using either a flat wire basket or cup forceps. Once multiple specimens have been obtained for pathology, the remaining lesion should be treated with laser ablation or diathermy. All pathology specimens are sent directly to the cytopathology department for preparation.

3. Evaluation of Unilateral Hematuria

Macroscopic hematuria is a common problem. In the majority of patients, urine cytology and culture, routine upper-tract imaging, and cystoscopy are adequate to establish the presence or absence of a sinister abnormality. In a small minority of patients, gross hematuria can be localized to one upper tract at the time of cystoscopy. In some of these patients, routine investigations prove to be normal, as do second-line investigations, which may include selective upper-tract culture and/or cytology, clotting studies, percutaneous renal biopsy, renal angiography, renography, CT, or magnetic resonance imaging (MRI). This group of patients can be diagnosed as having benign lateralizing hematuria.

The traditional management of recurrent, prolonged, or life-threatening hematuria has been partial or complete nephrectomy. Conservative measures have included bed rest, blood transfusion, instillation of silver nitrate into the renal pelvis, oral administration of ε-aminocaproic acid, radiotherapy, and tamponade of the pelvicaliceal system with varying degrees of success. Flexible ureteroscopy has allowed the discovery of previously undiagnosed lesions in many of these patients.

Rigid ureteroscopy and then flexible ureteroscopy are used as previously described to visualize the distal to proximal ureter and collecting system in turn. Although the procedure can be performed more easily after the bleeding has settled, continuous irrigation via the working channel can be used during inspection to clear the field of view if bleeding continues. Contrast material can be added to the irrigant or used alone to delineate the caliceal anatomy and ensure complete inspection of all calices. Overfilling of the collecting system should be avoided as this may cause submucosal bleeding and further confusion.

According to the literature, the most common findings in these patients are hemangiomas. These are predominantly located at the tip or base of a papilla.[18] Other benign lesions reported include minute venous ruptures, peripapillary varices, abnormal configuration of a papillary tip, dilated collecting ducts, petechiae, focal and diffuse erythema, and inflammation. The working channel allows either diathermy fulgaration (using a 2–3F probe) or laser ablation using holmium:yttrium-aluminum-garnet (YAG) (Ho:YAG) or neodymium:YAG (Nd:YAG) of suitable lesions. We prefer using Nd:YAG because of its superior deep coagulative effects.

Rowbotham and Anson advocate the use of ureteroscopy earlier in the investigation of benign lateralizing hematuria than previously suggested.[18] They have suggested an algorithm to follow for the investigation of these patients (Figure 32-1).

Although benign lateralizing hematuria is an uncommon problem, it can cause life-threatening hemorrhage and considerable anxiety. Ureteroscopy has revolutionized the management of these patients and prevents many unnecessary, often repeated, investigations.

4. Calculi

Occasionally, a patient presents with symptoms typical of ureteral colic, but no stone or sign of obstruction can be visualized on radiography or ultrasound. This may be accompanied by microscopic hematuria. If symptoms persist, these patients require further evaluation. CT can be helpful but may still miss small calculi owing to the size of the slices. The next step is often cystoscopy and retrograde pyelography. If this fails to demonstrate any abnormality, then ureteroscopy can be diagnostic in the presence of small, radiolucent or poorly opaque calculi. The technique for ureteroscopy in these cases is similar to that for hematuria. The smallest ureteroscope should be used and trauma must be minimized to prevent bleeding. This prevents flushing small calculi from view. Any calculus viewed should be removed, regardless of size, as it may be responsible for the symptoms.

Submucosal calculi are rare. In many patients, they appear to be related to previous endoscopic lithotripsy or extracorporeal shock wave lithotripsy. A clinical history of retained fragments and the presence of a radiopaque lesion on radiography, plus or minus ureteral obstruction, can indicate submucosal calculi. In patients with stents in situ, submucosal calculi may be indicated by a visible gap between the stent and the opacity. The diagnosis can be confirmed by ureteroscopy and endoluminal ultrasound. Ureteroscopy reveals an intact mucosa and an open lumen. Fluoroscopy can be used to identify the position of the opacity, but endoluminal ultrasound is far more accurate and allows decisions to be made regarding management based on the stone size, number, and depth.[20]

Oral dissolution therapy can be used to treat uric acid calculi.[21] As these stones are radiolucent, it can be difficult to assess the adequacy of treatment. Ultrasound can be used to follow the progress of a renal calculus, but those within the ureter or at the ureteropelvic junction are often not visible. CT is more effective than intravenous urography to identify ureteral calculi,[22] but can still miss small stones between cuts.

Ureteroscopy may be indicated to assess the residual stone load in patients where assessment of the stone status proves impossible by any other method.

ENDOLUMINAL ULTRASOUND AS AN AUXILIARY DIAGNOSTIC TECHNIQUE

Endoluminal ultrasound has become possible as small catheter-based ultrasound probes have been developed. Catheters range in size from 3.0 to 7.2F and contain ultrasound transducers with frequencies of 12.5 or 20.0 MHz. The smaller catheters can be used within the working channel and guided endoscopically to the site of the lesion under direct vision. The larger catheters are passed over a guidewire and fluoroscopy is used to locate the required area. The transducer rotates at approximately 30 rps and provides an image with a penetration depth of 1.5 to 2 cm. This allows visualization deep to the lumen of the ureter or collecting system. Crossing vessels, fluid collections, scar tissue, and calculi can be distinguished as they all have typical appearances.

Endoluminal ultrasound has been used in many clinical situations. In the presence of submucosal calculi, it can be used to locate the calculus and identify the number of fragments and the depth from the mucosa to allow decisions to be made regarding further management.[20]

Endoluminal ultrasound is proving to be useful in ureteropelvic junction obstruction for identifying the presence or absence of crossing vessels or septae prior to endopyelotomy. Many studies suggest that the most important risk factor of failure of an endopyelotomy is the presence of a crossing vessel.[23–27] Endoluminal ultrasound can be used to direct the site of incision when crossing vessels are present, but even then, the results of endopyelotomy are disappointing.[27] It is therefore important to identify their presence prior to surgery. Conventional arteriography, CT angiography, MRI, Doppler ultrasound, and endoluminal ultrasound have all been used to identify crossing vessels in ureteropelvic junction obstruction. Keeley and colleagues showed that endoluminal ultrasound can be more sensi-

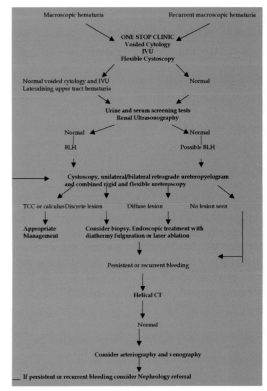

Figure 32-1 An algorithm for managing patients with benign lateralizing hematuria.

tive than CT angiography for detecting crossing vessels.[28] Endoluminal ultrasound detected vessels in 70% and septae in 35% of patients involved, whereas CT detected vessels in only 35% and no septae. Endoluminal ultrasound actually altered the choice of treatment or the direction of incision in 40% of these patients.

Endoluminal ultrasound can be useful in patients with evidence of ureteral obstruction where the cause is not identified by conventional imaging methods, for example, intravenous urography, CT, MRI, or retrograde urography. Extrinsic and intrinsic lesions may be differentiated. Extrinsic lesions diagnosed in this way included segmental retroperitoneal fibrosis, crossing vessels, periureteral fibrosis, adjacent fluid collections, and endometriosis.[29] Intrinsic lesions include mucosal edema, normal narrow ureter, and submucosal calculi. Endoluminal ultrasound can help to select those patients who would benefit from minimally invasive therapies and direct the endoscopic treatment.

STAGING

Accurate staging of upper-tract transitional cell carcinoma is impossible with ureteroscopy alone.[30] Although abdominal CT is still used to identify metastases, the resolution is inadequate for accurate staging. Endoscopic biopsy cannot provide a full thickness sample of the ureter or renal pelvis; therefore, microscopic examination of the muscle for invasion is rarely possible. However, there does appear to be good correlation between the grade of the tumor at ureteroscopic biopsy and the final pathologic stage in nephroureterectomy specimens.[7,8] Endoluminal ultrasound may also be used to estimate the depth of invasion at the time of ureteroscopy. The information obtained can be used to guide further management.

DISSEMINATION OF TUMOR

Diagnostic ureteroscopy for transitional cell carcinoma has been found to be safe and effective.[7,31] However, there has been concern that biopsy of an upper-tract neoplasm can disseminate tumor cells locally or possibly even systemically via pyelovenous or pyelolymphatic backflow. Lim and colleagues report a case where tumor cells were found outside the kidney in a nephroureterectomy specimen after ureteroscopic biopsy.[32] Despite this, ureteroscopy does not appear to negatively affect patient survival. Hendin and colleagues evaluated the surgical pathology of 96 patients who had undergone radical nephroureterectomy with or without preoperative ureteroscopy and found that long-term survival was unaffected.[33]

Careful attention to technique minimizes the risk factors of tumor dissemination. Tumor cells may migrate via ureteral perforations or secondary to high pelvic pressures generated by irrigation fluid. Irrigation pressure should be kept as low as possible.[34] Contrast within the irrigant fluid plus fluoroscopic monitoring can be used to indicate any extravasation. Dilatation of the ureteropelvic junction should be avoided when there is an intraluminal neoplasm, since extraluminal leakage of contrast has frequently been observed at this level.

CONCLUSION

Ureteroscopy has revolutionized the diagnosis and management of upper urinary tract lesions. It is particularly useful in conditions where all other currently available investigations are deficient, predominately, filling defects and upper-tract tumors, radiolucent and submucosal calculi, and benign lateralizing hematuria. Accurate information using a combination of urine cytology, washes, brushings, and biopsies can be obtained at ureteroscopy to allow diagnosis and plans for further management, especially with regard to transitional cell carcinoma. Previous concern regarding tumor seeding at diagnostic ureteroscopy appears to be unfounded.

The use of ureteroscopy is rapidly expanding. Further refinements of sampling methods will continue to improve the diagnostic accuracy of ureteroscopy. As small-diameter ureteroscopes become more durable and easier to use, the role of diagnostic ureteroscopy can only increase further.

REFERENCES

1. Kumar PVS, Keeley F, Timoney A. Safe flexible ureterorenoscopy with a dual-lumen access catheter and a safety guidewire. BJU Int 2001;88:638–9.
2. Aso Y, Ohtawara Y, Suzuki K, et al. Usefulness of fiberoptic pyeloureteroscopy in the diagnosis of upper urinary tract lesions. Urol Int 1984;39:355–7.
3. Gittes RF. Retrograde brushing and nephroscopy in the diagnosis of upper-tract urothelial cancer. Urol Clin North Am 1984;11:617–22.
4. Abdel-Razzack OM, Ehya H, Cubler-Goodman A, Bagley DH. Ureteroscopic biopsy in the upper urinary tract. Urology 1994;44:451–7.
5. Mulholland SG, Arger PH, Goldberg BB, Pollack HM. Ultrasonic differentiation of renal pelvic filling defects. J Urol 1979;122:14–6.
6. Badalament RA, Bennett WF, Bova JG, et al. Computed tomography of primary transitional cell carcinoma of the upper urinary tracts. Urology 1992;40:71–5.
7. Keeley FX, Kulp DA, Bibbo M, et al. Diagnostic accuracy of ureteroscopic biopsy in upper tract transitional cell carcinoma. J Urol 1997;157:33–7.
8. Skolarikos A, Griffiths TRL, Powell PH, et al. Cytologic analysis of ureteral washings is informative in patients with grade 2 upper tract TCC considering endoscopic treatment. Urology 2003;61:1146–50.
9. Murphy DM, Zincke H, Furlow WL. Primary grade 1 transitional cell carcinoma of the renal pelvis and ureter. J Urol 1980;123:629–31.
10. Murphy DM, Zincke H, Furlow WL. Management of high-grade transitional cell cancer of the upper urinary tract. J Urol 1981;125:25–9.
11. Kannan V. Papillary transitional-cell carcinoma of the upper urinary tract: a cytologic review. Diagn Cytolpath 1990; 6:204–9.
12. Chen GL, El-Gabry EA, Bagley DH. Surveillance of upper tract transitional cell carcinoma: the role of ureteroscopy, retrograde pyelography, cytology and urinalysis. J Urol 2000;164:1901–4.
13. Bian Y, Ehya H, Bagley DH. Cytologic diagnosis of upper urinary tract neoplasms by ureteroscopic sampling. Acta Cytol 1995;39:733–40.
14. Elliot DS, Segura JW, Lightner DJ, et al. Is nephroureterectomy necessary in all cases of upper tract transitional cell carcinoma? Long-term results of conservative endourologic management of upper tract transitional cell carcinoma in individuals with a normal contralateral kidney. Urology 2001;58:174–8.
15. Liatsikos EN, Dinlec CZ, Kapoor R, Smith AD. Transitional cell carcinoma of the renal pelvis: ureteroscopic and percutaneous approach. J Endourol 2001;15:377–83.
16. Chen GL, Bagley DH. Ureteroscopic management of upper tract transitional cell carcinoma in patients with normal contralateral kidneys. J Urol 2000;164:1173–6.
17. Keeley FX Jr, Bibbo M, Bagley DH. Ureteroscopic treatment and surveillance of upper urinary tract transitional cell carcinoma. J Urol 1997;157:1560–5.
18. Rowbotham C, Anson K. Benign lateralizing haematuria and upper tract endoscopy. BJU Int 2001;88:841–9.
19. McMurty JM, Clayman RV, Preminger GM. Endourologic diagnosis and treatment of essential hematuria. J Endourol 1987;1:145–51.
20. Grasso M, Liu JB, Goldberg B, Bagley D. Submucosal calculi: endoscopic and intraluminal sonographic diagnosis and treatment options. J Urol 1995;153:1384–9.
21. Moran ME, Abrahams HM, Burday DE, Greene TD. Utility of oral dissolution therapy in the management of referred patients with secondarily treated uric acid stones. Urology 2002;59:206–10.
22. Smith RC, Rosenfield AT, Choe KA, et al. Acute flank pain: comparison of non-contrast-enhanced CT and intravenous urography. Radiology 1995;194:789–94.
23. Danuser H, Ackermann DK, Bohlen D, Studer UE. Endopyelotomy for primary ureteropelvic junction obstruction: risk factors determine the success rate. J Urol 1998;159:56–61.
24. Van Cangh PJ, Wilmart JF, Opsomer RJ, et al. Long-term results and late recurrence after endopyelotomy: a critical analysis of prognostic factors. J Urol 1994;151:934–7.
25. Conlin MJ, Bagley DH. Ureteroscopic endopyelotomy at a single setting. J Urol 1998;159:727–31.
26. Van Cangh PJ, Nesa S, Galeon M, et al. Vessels around the ureteropelvic junction. Significance and imaging by conventional radiology. J Endourol 1996;10:111–9.
27. Parkin J, Evans S, Kumar PVS, et al. Endoluminal ultrasonography before retrograde endopyelotomy: can the results match laparoscopic pyeloplasty? BJU Int 2003;91:389–91.
28. Keeley FX Jr, Moussa SA, Miller J, Tolley DA. A prospective study of endoluminal ultrasound versus computerized tomography angiography for detecting crossing vessels at the ureteropelvic junction. J Urol 1999;162:1938–41.
29. Grasso M, Li S, Liu JB, et al. Examining the obstructed ureter with intraluminal sonography. J Urol 1999;162:1286–90.
30. Elashry OM, Elbahnasy AM, Rao GS, et al. Flexible ureteroscopy: Washington University experience with the 9.3F and 7.5F flexible ureteroscopes. J Urol 1997;157: 2074–80.
31. Huffman JL, Bagley DH, Lyon ES, et al. Endoscopic diagnosis and treatment of upper-tract urothelial tumours: a preliminary report. Cancer 1985;55:1422–8.
32. Lim DJ, Shattuck MO, Cook WA. Pyelovenous lymphatic migration of transitional cell carcinoma following flexible ureterorenoscopy. J Urol 1993;149:109–11.
33. Hendin BN, Streem SB, Levin HN, et al. Impact of diagnostic ureteroscopy on long-term survival in patients with upper tract transitional cell carcinoma. J Urol 1999;161:783–5.
34. Wilson WT, Preminger G. Intrarenal pressures generated during flexible deflectable ureterorenoscopy. J Endourol 1990;4:135–41.

33

Ureteroscopic Diagnosis and Treatment of Upper Urinary Tract Neoplasms

Demetrius H. Bagley, MD
Nathan Lewis Hatfield

Ureteroscopy has assumed a major role in the diagnosis and treatment of upper-tract neoplasms. Endoscopic techniques to visualize and sample neoplasms in the upper urinary tract have made accurate diagnosis possible. The same techniques combined with devices for tissue ablation have made treatment possible. Although both of these concepts have been widely accepted, there remains controversy over the selection of patients and the appropriate application of treatment and surveillance. Other diagnostic studies including radiologic, cytologic, and molecular techniques can provide initial or supportive diagnostic innovation, yet remain secondary to endoscopy as the definitive study.

Upper-tract neoplasms are relatively rare. Transitional cell carcinomas (TCCs) in the ureter and intrarenal collecting system account for only approximately 5% of all transitional cell carcinomas.[1] However, they are more common in patients with a previous history of carcinoma of the bladder.[2,3] The presentation may be different in these two groups of patients. In those with no history of bladder cancer, the most common presentation is with hematuria, either gross or microscopic. Hematuria is seen in approximately 80% of patients.[1,4,5] Flank pain can be seen in up to 30% of patients, while a lesion may be an incidental finding in 10 to 15% of patients. Physical findings are rarely present unless the patient has unusual masses or metastatic tumor or has hydronephrosis secondary to obstruction.

NONINVASIVE DIAGNOSIS

Noninvasive evaluation with radiologic studies usually includes intravenous contrast studies to outline the collecting system with excretory urography or computer tomographic urography. A filling defect is the most common radiologic finding, indicating urothelial neoplasm in the upper tract. The differential diagnosis includes blood clot, lucent calculus, air bubble, fungus ball, slough papilla, external compression with a crossing vessel, or benign inflammatory lesion. The diagnosis may be indicated by other diagnostic studies, yet can be confirmed by endoscopic inspection and biopsy.

Retrograde ureteropyelography may be indicated in the patient with severe contrast allergy with nonvisualization of the collecting system. It

has been reported to be accurate in up to 75% of cases of initial TCC of the upper urinary tract.[4]

Renal ultrasound can accurately define an intrarenal calculus or hydronephrosis. Renal masses are also well seen, but it is less useful to detect small intraluminal soft tissue masses.

Computed tomography (CT) can be more helpful. It can easily and accurately distinguish calculi from soft tissue masses. Larger renal masses are also easily detected, but smaller lesions are more controversial. An abdominal radiograph taken after the administration of contrast to provide an A-P ureteropyelogram can be extremely helpful in demonstrating these lesions. The cross sectional CT images are definitely of value in demonstrating masses extending beyond the collecting system or enlarged lymph nodes.[6,7]

Magnetic resonance imaging has similar limitations in a cross-sectional mode.[8] The magnetic resonance urogram designed to image the fluid of a distended collecting system can be helpful in certain patients with nonfunctioning kidneys or severe contrast allergies.

Cytologic study of voided urinary samples is of limited value because of the frequent false-positive and false-negative findings. It is often useful in detecting high-grade tumors that shed malignant-appearing cells in the urine. The sensitivity of voided urine cytology increases with an increasing grade of a neoplasm, ranging from 11% for grade 1 to 83% for grade 4 lesions.[9] Ureteral catheterization for the collection of urine from a radiographic area is no longer indicated if ureteroscopy can be performed. Selective ureteral catheterization for a specific upper-tract urinary sample for cytologic study may be indicated in patients with positive cytology without radiographic findings and with normal cystoscopy and bladder biopsy. Gill and colleagues and others[10–12] demonstrated the superiority of fluoroscopically guided brush biopsy of filling defects over catheterization. However, cystoscopic brush biopsy of radiographically demonstrated lesions is no longer indicated if a ureteroscope can be placed.

ENDOSCOPIC TECHNIQUES

Endoscopic evaluation of an abnormality in the upper urinary tract suspicious for a neoplasm includes inspection of the entire bladder and

involved collecting system. Cystoscopic inspection of the bladder is an essential component in evaluation of the patient with hematuria and/or filling defects because of the high risk of associated bladder tumors. It also provides access to the ureter for retrograde pyelography and for ureteral endoscopic access. After complete inspection of the bladder with biopsy of any suspicious lesion, the upper tract is studied. A ureteropyelogram may give more information regarding the filling defect or suspicious lesion. The cone-tipped retrograde injection efficiently outlines the entire collecting system without traumatizing the ureter itself. Initial ureteral catheterization without contrast study should be avoided since it can traumatize the lesion of interest and the otherwise normal ureteral mucosa. It may be necessary to use multiple injections of different concentrations of contrast with multiple radiographic views to define the extent of the lesion fully. Care should be used to prevent overfilling of the collecting system or overly dense radio-opacity, which can obscure filling defects.

A "no-touch technique" should be employed to examine the involved upper collecting system. The distal ureter is first inspected with a small rigid endoscope, preferably one small enough to pass into the orifice without other dilation. Thus, the ureter can be inspected without prior instrument trauma. The endoscope should be passed as far as possible into the lumen, and then a guidewire left in place as the rigid endoscope is removed. In a young muscular male, the rigid endoscope can usually be placed throughout the distal third of the ureter, where in an older female it may pass easily to the level of the renal pelvis. After completion of the proximal excursion of the rigid endoscope, a guidewire is left in place in the ureter as the endoscope is removed. It should be passed only to the level of the ureter that has been inspected or at most to the mid- or proximal ureter. It should not be passed into the collecting system where the tip can traumatize the calix or the renal pelvis and obscure subsequent visual inspection.

The smallest flexible ureteroscope is then passed over the guidewire into the ureter. Again, dilation should be avoided if possible. The flexible ureteroscope inspects the more proximal portion of the ureter not previously seen and the intrarenal collecting system. There, inspection should be systematic from the renal pelvis to the upper infundibula and calices to the mid and then the lower pole. The intent is to avoid trauma to the mucosa from the endoscope.

Continuous irrigation with saline is maintained through the working channel of the ureteroscope to clear the field of view. Iodinated contrast medium can be used in the irrigant to outline the collecting system for fluoroscopic monitoring. In this way, one can be certain that the entire kidney is inspected. Care should be taken to avoid overfilling the collecting system, since this can induce submucosa hemorrhage and rupture of the fornices.

Alternatively, in a patient with an adequate ureteral lumen, a flexible ureteroscope may be used initially to inspect the entire ureter.[13] If there is resistance to passage of the flexible endoscope at the level of the ureteral orifice, then it is better to revert to the use of rigid and flexible endoscopes.

If there is a specific lesion to be examined, such as a filling defect or a point of obstruction, then the distal portion of the urinary tract should be inspected first, followed by the lesion itself, in order to inspect it within a clear visual field without other manipulation that may cause bleeding and obscure the field of view. In the majority of cases, visual inspection alone can provide a diagnosis.[14–17] The appearance of a calculus will readily distinguish it from a low-grade papillary tumor. An extrinsic mass can also be readily distinguished. For example, a vascular impression of the renal pelvis will become more prominent as the pelvis is emptied and less prominent as it fills. In addition, an arterial impression can be seen pulsating. In each case, irrigant with contrast should be used so that fluoroscopy can demonstrate the tip of the ureteroscope at the filling defect. In this way, correct visualization and identification of the lesion can be confirmed.

Epithelial neoplasms may have totally different appearances. Low-grade transitional cell carcinomas have a typical papillary appearance, similar to the same lesions in the bladder. High-grade transitional cell carcinomas may be more sessile and less papillary, often with necrotic or inflammatory debris on the surface. Fibroepithelial polyps located within the pelvis and inverted papillomas throughout the upper collecting system have been seen to have a smooth, rounded surface.[18] There is the impression of an intact epithelial layer in the appearance. These differences have not been prominent enough to allow visual identification, but they have been strongly suggestive. Both fibroepithelial polyps and inverted papillomas located at the ureteropelvic junction can be narrow, elongated, and worm-like.

In a few circumstances, visual inspection alone may not be adequate to diagnose a neoplasm. High-grade urothelial neoplasms can be confused with inflammatory lesions or may be obscured by tumor growing submucosally or proximal to obstructive edema. There may be calculus material on the surface of a neoplasm, and thus appear as a solid calculus. Other tumors with a necrotic surface can appear the same as a soft, infectious stone covered with inflammatory debris. In these and many other situations, visual inspection alone is not adequate for diagnosis, and other interventional endoscopic maneuvers are necessary to obtain an accurate diagnosis.

BIOPSY

Ureteroscopic biopsy is important to sample upper-tract neoplasms to give a tissue diagnosis. It is particularly important in the unusual circumstances noted above. It is also of value to try to determine the malignancy of a lesion and the grade of a transitional cell carcinoma. Ureteroscopic biopsy is limited because of the size of the working channel within the ureteroscope and the limitation in the size of biopsy instrument that can be used. For example, the piece of tissue obtained with a 3 French (F) cup biopsy forceps is less than 1 mm in diameter and is usually too small to be prepared for histologic study using standard techniques. In contrast, it is a relatively large fragment of tissue for cytologic techniques. It can be prepared as a cell block and stained and examined as a histologic preparation to give a diagnosis and information on the grading when necessary.

Several different biopsy instruments and techniques are available. Abdel-Razzak and colleagues[19] evaluated samples from 55 procedures in 44 patients with a possible diagnosis of transitional cell carcinoma of the upper tract. They compared the diagnostic yield, considering only those samples that were specifically positive or negative for malignancy. Those that were "suggestive" or equivocal were not considered diagnostic. The techniques compared aspiration of urine at the level of the lesion, wash and aspiration with saline solution at the area of the lesion, and direct tissue sampling with brush basket or biopsy forceps.

The tissue sampling techniques gave the best yield, particularly with a flat-wire basket for large friable tumors and the cup forceps for more sessile lesions. The brush was less effective, and under endoscopic vision, the brush was observed to move the more flexible tissue without removing fragments. It may be more useful with flat or sessile lesions. Aspiration and wash prove to be valuable in providing a diagnosis for some patients in whom the other sampling techniques were inconclusive.

A flat-wire basket is quite effective for removing large fragments of papillary tissue with a small-diameter ureteroscope. Under endoscopic vision, the basket is placed on the tumor and partially closed. The entire unit consisting of tumor sample, basket, and ureteroscope is then removed from the ureter and bladder. This can often remove a large sample up to 1 cm in diameter, which is adequate for cytologic or histologic study. The ureteroscope is then replaced to repeat the inspection and biopsy or treat the neoplastic lesion.

One of the most important steps in handling the tissue for pathologic diagnosis is to work closely with the cytopathologist.[20–23] Samples are examined with both a smear and cytospin preparation. In addition, if there is any macroscopically visible tissue, a cell block is also prepared. This sample often demonstrates both the architecture of the neoplasm and the individual cells. Sufficient histologic structure has been present to allow grading of transitional cell carcinoma in most of the samples adequate for cell block. Multiple samples of the lesion are taken. In addition, urine and saline wash samples at the lesion before and after biopsy and/or treatment should be obtained (Table 33-1).

GRADING

Grading of transitional cell carcinoma of the upper tract is important in determining prognosis and directing therapy. The grade obtained from ureteroscopic biopsy has been shown to reflect the grade of the overall tumor with considerable accuracy. In 42 patients, Keeley and colleagues[24] found that the grade seen on a ureteroscopic biopsy prior to surgical treatment matched that in the final pathologic specimen in 86% of cases. Danashmand and colleagues[25] showed an overall accuracy of 90% in patients who had surgery early after biopsy and in those who had surgery within 2 months after ureteroscopic diagnosis. Combined cytology and ureteroscopic biopsy have been particularly valuable in patients with grade 2 TCC to provide an accurate diagnosis.[26]

STAGING

Accurate staging of upper-tract transitional cell carcinoma has not been possible with endoscopic techniques alone. The search for metastases includes the usual abdominal CT scans or magnetic resonance images and chest radiographs. Determining the depth of invasion of the primary tumor or other simultaneous lesions remains difficult. One series advocated multiple deep biopsies with cup forceps in an attempt to determine the presence of tumor in the lamina propria.[27] Most series have not been able to determine depth of invasion with accuracy. The grade of the primary tumor has often been associated with a stage, but it cannot be considered truly accurate staging. In Keeley's series,[24] increasing stage was noted with increasing grade exhibited on ureteroscopic biopsy. Other series of surgically treated patients have demonstrated the relationship of increasing stage with increasing grade.[28] Endoluminal ultrasound has been used in one series in an attempt to determine the depth of invasion.[29] It has shown some value but is severely limited by the availability of the instruments.

There has been concern that the ureteroscopic biopsy of an upper urinary tract neoplasm can disseminate tumor cells locally or systemically. The possibility of pyelovenous or pyelolymphatic

TABLE 33-1 Specimens for Cytology
Bladder urine
Aspirate at tumor
Biopsy
Aspirate
Treat
Aspirate

backflow has been cited as a possible mechanism. In a single case report, tumor cells were found outside the kidney in a nephroureterectomy specimen after ureteroscopic biopsy.[30] However, in a review of 13 nephroureterectomy specimens following ureteroscopic biopsy, no unusual metastatic pattern was seen.[31] In a well-controlled study of 96 patients, Hendin and colleagues[32] found no difference in long-term or disease-specific patients with upper-tract TCC who had surgical treatment proceeded either with or without ureteroscopic biopsy (Table 33-2). Hara and colleagues[33] reported the usefulness of ureteroscopic biopsy and added 50 patients to those who have had ureteroscopic biopsy without development of metastatic disease. These series have concluded that ureteroscopic biopsy can be a safe and very valuable procedure without any documented evidence of tumor dissemination.

SELECTION OF PATIENTS FOR URETEROSCOPIC BIOPSY

Ureteroscopic biopsy appears to be of value in any patient with an upper-tract filling defect in whom the diagnosis is in question. Thus, patients with a filling defect and voided urinary cytology without an abnormality or any abnormal finding less than a definitive (positive) diagnosis for malignant cells. The presence of individually malignant-appearing cells (positive cytology) indicates either carcinoma in situ (CIS) or a high-grade neoplasm. Biopsy may be avoided in patients with cytology that is definitively positive for malignant cells and who have a large irregular upper-tract filling defect, which can be considered classic for TCC.

URETEROSCOPIC TREATMENT

The advent of ureteroscopic access to the entire upper urinary tract has also provided options for the treatment of upper-tract neoplasms. These procedures are based on the extension of diagnostic procedures. Many devices can be placed through the working channel of the ureteroscopes to treat neoplasms.[34] These include graspers, electrodes, and laser fibers. There has been considerable interest and wide acceptance of these techniques for the treatment of some upper-tract neoplasms. The techniques for treatment and selection of patients are evolving as the value of this approach is being defined in relatively small series of patients. The rationale for conservative endoscopic therapy for upper-tract neoplasms has been based initially on the success of other conservative treatment modalities for similar lesions.

These series have defined the role of conservative treatment in the high-risk patient and have extended such therapy to other specific lesions. Conservative surgical techniques have been used to treat upper-tract tumors with mixed results, depending on the nature of the tumor and its location. Endoscopic treatment is a natural extension of these nephron-sparing procedures, evolving only as the instruments have become available. Similarly, these techniques can be considered an extension of endoscopic procedures used at the bladder level for the treatment of transitional cell carcinoma of the bladder. Since these series have not discovered prohibitive risks, other series in progress will continue to define appropriate applications of endoscopic therapy.

NATURAL HISTORY AND PROGNOSIS AFTER SURGICAL THERAPY

The natural history of neoplasms in the upper urinary tract must be considered in order to define the optimal mode of therapy. Transitional cell carcinoma constitutes the vast majority of endoluminal tumors in the upper collecting system; there remain a few benign lesions that can be considered separately. Since ureteroscopic access will allow us to treat only endoluminal lesions, transitional cell carcinoma is, for practical purposes, the only malignant neoplasm to be considered for treatment.

The behavior and prognosis of transitional cell carcinoma of the upper urinary tract, in both the ureter and the intrarenal collecting system, has repeatedly been shown to be related to the grade and stage of the lesion. In a series by Charbit and colleagues,[28] the overall survival rates at 5 and 10 years after treatment were 67.3% and 64.9%, respectively. Only 19.5% of patients died of metastases from the upper-tract tumor, 86% died within 1 year postoperatively, and the remainder died within 2 years. Among those with tumor-related deaths, 90% had high-grade tumors (grade 2 or 3/4) and 86% had presented with muscle invasion. Nielsen and Ostri[35] reviewed 36 patients treated surgically for primary carcinoma of the renal pelvis and found that 6 of 22 patients (27%) with grade 2/4 transitional cell carcinoma, and 8 of 11 (80%) with grade 3/4 lesions died of their disease. Both of the patients with grade 4 transitional cell carcinoma also died of this disease. The prognosis was statistically significantly poorer for patients with grades 3 and 4 TCCa than those with grade 2. Survival of 49 patients with grade 1 TCCa of the ureter or renal pelvis collected at the Mayo Clinic over a 22-year period was identical to that of an age-matched control group.[36] In contrast, the survival with higher-grade TCCa correlated with tumor stage and grade and was consistently lower than a control group.[37]

The grade and stage are also closely related and are reflected in the prognosis. Mufti and colleagues[38] found that survival of patients with superficial well-differentiated tumors was greater than 90% in groups treated either by total nephroureterectomy or by more conservative

resection. In the series of Nielsen and Ostri,[35] only 3 patients (14%) with grade 2/4 lesions had invasion of connective tissue, while 10 (91%) with grade 3 lesions and both with grade 4 had invasion. In the series by Charbit and colleagues,[28] 79% of the grade 2/3 tumors had invaded into or beyond the muscle layer. Lymphadenectomy was negative in all patients with low-grade tumors in whom it was performed, whereas 39% of those in patients with higher-grade tumors were positive.

The grade of the primary lesion also indicates the extent of mucosal abnormality. McCarron and colleagues[39] systematically mapped nephroureterectomy specimens and found that the grade of the principle neoplasm paralleled the extent of epithelial disturbance in the otherwise normal-appearing urothelium. They found that high-grade carcinomas were associated with severe epithelial changes and low-grade cancers with hyperplasia only. Cytologic study of specimens collected either from the upper tract (17 of 30 cases) or of bladder urine (13 cases) accurately reflected the grade of the principle neoplasm. It also indicated the presence of both contiguous and remote abnormalities. Among 7 patients with grade 1/3 tumors, 6 had negative cytologic studies and one was suspicious for carcinoma. However, among those with grade 3 lesions, 10 were positive for malignant cells, 3 were suspicious, and only 1 was negative.

Mazeman[40] found that a multiplicity of tumors formed a negative prognostic factor. He found that only 20% of patients with multiple tumors survived for 5 years, while 37% with single tumors survived. Survival was the same whether the primary tumor was within the renal pelvis, intrarenal collecting system, or in the ureter.

Standard surgical treatment of transitional cell carcinoma of the upper urinary tract has been nephroureterectomy including a cuff of bladder. High recurrence rates have been noted when a less extensive operation has been performed, particularly with more proximally located lesions. Mazeman[40] noted that there was a recurrence rate of 19% after total nephroureterectomy. This increased to 24% after subtotal nephroureterectomy, 32% after partial nephroureterectomy, and 48% after nephrectomy alone. Recurrences were noted to be distal to the primary tumor in any part of the urinary tract. The majority of the recurrences were in the bladder around the orifice. There is a low rate of occurrence in the contralateral kidney. The risk of bladder cancer in patients presenting initially with an upper-tract urothelial tumor was approximately 9%, and that of a contralateral urothelial tumor was 1%. In those with a previous history of bladder tumors, the risk of another vesical lesion was 53%.[28] Among patients with grade 2 or 3/4 lesions in a Mayo Clinic series, there was an incidence of bladder tumor of 30%.[37] Based on these and similar findings, recommendations for follow-up have included cystoscopy at intervals of 3 to 4 months and imaging of the remaining upper tracts at the first year. Recommendations for continued evaluation of the upper tract vary after that period.

Table 33-2 Effect of Ureteroscopic Biopsy		
	Biopsy	None
No. patients	48	48
Metastases	12.6%	18.8% (NS)
Died with recurrence	10.4%	10.4% (NS)
From Hendin et al.[32]		

CONSERVATIVE SURGICAL THERAPY

Conservative, nephron-sparing surgery has been attempted in special circumstances for transitional cell carcinoma of the upper urinary tract. The initial efforts at conservative surgical treatment have been in patients with a solitary kidney who were not candidates or refused to become anephric. Others with a compromised contralateral kidney, including bilateral tumors, were similarly included. There is also evidence that low-grade and stage, distal ureteral tumors can be treated by distal ureterectomy alone.

Major series have reviewed the results with local surgical treatment of upper-tract tumors both in the renal pelvis and the ureter. Generally, there has been a higher recurrence rate after the treatment of renal pelvic tumors and a much lower rate for ureteral tumors. Mazeman[40] and Zincke and Neves[41] have reported recurrence rates of 45 to 65% after the local resection of renal pelvic transitional cell carcinoma. In contrast, recurrences after resection of ureteral lesions range from 15 to 16%. The lesions treated, however, included a wide range of grade and stage. These and other series[36,42–44] have found that distal ureterectomy for low-grade transitional cell carcinoma in the distal ureter is often curative. Based on these results, some have recommended distal ureterectomy as primary therapy for distal ureteral lesions.

In summary, recommendations for conservative surgical therapy for transitional cell carcinoma of the upper urinary tract includes high-risk patients: those with a solitary kidney; a compromised contralateral kidney, including bilateral tumors; or overall compromised renal function. Also included are those in whom nephroureterectomy would be an overwhelming medical risk. Low-grade and stage, distal ureteral tumors can be successfully treated with distal ureterectomy.[36,42–45]

DIAGNOSIS, STAGING, AND GRADING

Diagnosis of an upper-tract lesion suspicious for neoplasm is essential before considering any form of therapy. This has been considered in detail in the previous chapter. In brief, it is now usually possible to diagnosis upper-tract filling defects that have been detected by radiographic studies but await endoscopic evaluation and sampling for a final diagnosis.

Grading of transitional cell carcinoma has also been possible with endoscopic sampling combined with cytopathologic techniques.[46,47] Others have previously demonstrated that high-grade lesions more frequently shed cells, giving positive urinary cytologic findings.[36,39,48] Since low-grade tumors rarely shed papillary structures indicating the presence of malignancy, a distinction in grading can sometimes be made on the basis of cytologic findings from the urine alone. This has been extended to endoscopic sampling techniques.

Staging of transitional cell carcinoma in the upper tract has been important to direct treatment and indicate prognosis. A search for metastatic disease and massive renal parenchymal invasion by transitional cell carcinoma is the same whether the treatment to be considered is surgical or endoscopic. Only when there is a decision to be made regarding radical or conservative (including endoscopic) therapy, does it become important to determine the stage preoperatively by learning whether there is local invasion by the neoplasm. The techniques available have generally failed in any attempt to sort out low-stage lesions.

ENDOSCOPIC THERAPY

Endoscopic therapy of transitional cell carcinoma is familiar and well accepted for lesions in the urinary bladder. The concept is new only when applied to lesions in the upper urinary tract. The instruments and techniques for endoscopic access for both diagnosis and treatment as well as for follow-up are now available. The size of the endoscopes employed and the ablative devices available as well as the access with rigid or flexible ureteroscopes must be considered in any endoscopic approach to upper-tract tumors. The neoplasm itself, including its diagnosis, grade, location, and size must also be considered in any decision for endoscopic treatment in an individual patient (Table 33-3). Ureteroscopy has become the major endoscopic technique for the diagnosis of upper-tract neoplasms. It also is the major technique for the treatment of upper-tract neoplasms. However, it is used with the complementary techniques of percutaneous nephroscopy with resection of larger neoplasms and laparoscopic nephroureterectomy or distal ureterectomy.

There are several techniques available that can be applied for the treatment of upper-tract neoplasms ureteroscopically. These techniques, which can remove or ablate tissue within the upper tract by a rigid or flexible ureteroscopes, include mechanical removal, electrosurgical resection, fulguration, and laser therapy. These are considered in specific detail because of their importance in treating neoplasms within the upper urinary tract.

The techniques used for the ureteroscopic biopsy of tumors result in the removal of tissue volume. A flat-wire basket can remove several millimeters of papillary tumor with each application. Although the cup biopsy forceps removes a small volume with each bite repetitive sampling, the base of the tumor can then be coagulated with one of the other instruments.

Electrosurgical techniques similar to those used in the bladder have been applied for small distal ureteral neoplasms. Historically, resection was the first use for treatment of upper-tract neoplasms.[49,50] Rigid ureteral resectoscopes, similar to a long version of a pediatric resectoscope can be used in a similar fashion to other resection procedures for tumors in the distal ureter. The resectoscopes are relatively large, approaching 12 to 13F. The loop takes a small bite of tissue, and it may become necessary to clean the look before proceeding to remove the second piece of tissue. This is often a slow procedure. After resection, the base of the tumor can be lightly fulgurated.

Table 33-3 Selection of Patients for Ureteroscopic Treatment		
Tumor Factors	For	Against
Size	Small	Large
Configuration	Papillary	Sessile
Number	Solitary	Multiple
Distribution	Single	Circumferential or extensive
Grade	Low	High
Cytology	Negative	Positive

Extreme care should be taken to avoid resecting through the full thickness of the ureteral or renal pelvic wall, and also to avoid fulgurating a large area of the ureter, which can result in scarring and stricture formation.[51] Electroresection has been superseded by other more efficient techniques.

The other major electrosurgical technique is simple fulguration with an electrocautery probe. This technique is suitable for very small lesions for the base of a tumor after removal of the bulk of the volume of the lesion. Small probes of 2 to 3F size are available and can be passed through the channels of small-diameter rigid flexible ureteroscopes. Again, care should be maintained to avoid fulgurating large areas of the ureter, which can result in stricture formation (Figure 33-1). Laser techniques have been applied widely for the treatment of upper-tract neoplasms ureteroscopically and have proven to be the most efficient. Small laser fibers of either 200 or approximately 400 micron core diameter can be passed through the working channel of small rigid or flexible ureteroscopes. The two major lasers presently available for urologic application can effectively treat upper-tract tumors with coagulation, ablation, and resection. The neodymium:YAG laser is the first laser used both for treatment of bladder tumors and for ablation of renal pelvic and ureteral neoplasms. This laser was first used with open surgical techniques to ablate TCC in the renal pelvis and intrarenal collecting system.[52] Long-term cures to that recurrence have been achieved with this technique. The Nd:YAG laser was subsequently used ureteroscopically to ablate TCC of the ureter.[53] In a comparative series, Schmeller and Hoffstetter[54] demonstrated the success of laser ablation of upper-tract tumors with the development of fewer ureteral strictures than after electrocoagulation.

The Nd:YAG laser can penetrate several millimeters into tissue after several seconds of exposure. This can be controlled by positioning the fiber onto the tumor without directly aiming it toward the wall of the ureter and by moving the fiber across the surface of the tissue to avoid prolonged exposure.[55] Ureteral damage can be limited since the laser fiber and beam are usually aimed at the tumor parallel to the surface of the ureter. Within the kidney, especially the renal pelvis, where there is a greater surface area and less risk of scarring and stricturing, the neoplasm can be coagulated safely with the Nd:YAG laser.[56] The laser is activated at 20 to 30 watts on contin-

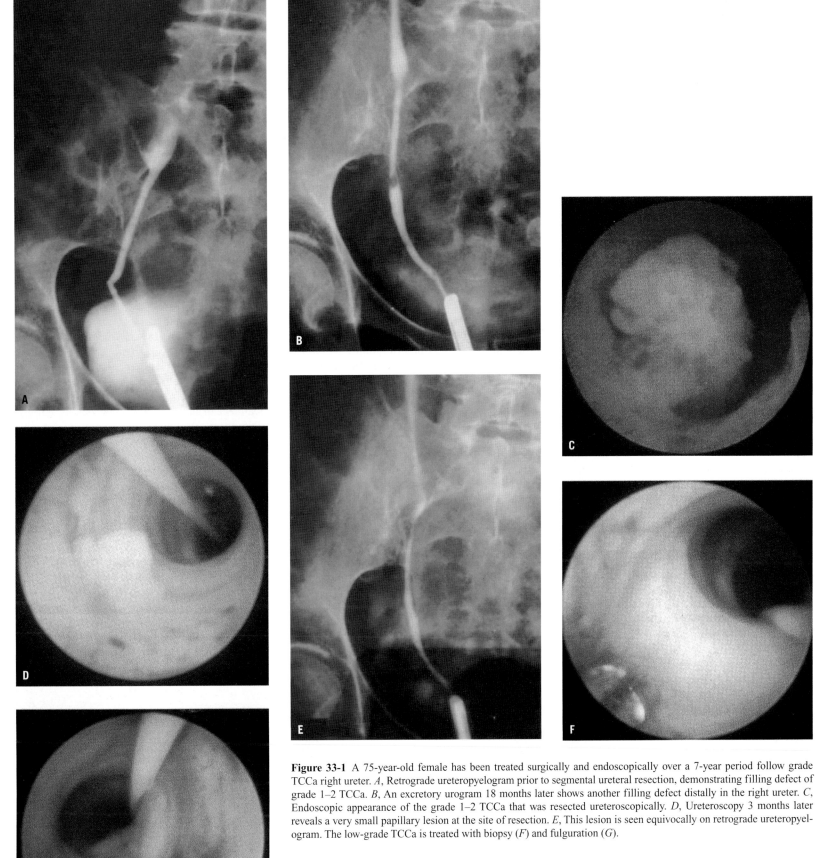

Figure 33-1 A 75-year-old female has been treated surgically and endoscopically over a 7-year period follow grade TCCa right ureter. *A*, Retrograde ureteropyelogram prior to segmental ureteral resection, demonstrating filling defect of grade 1–2 TCCa. *B*, An excretory urogram 18 months later shows another filling defect distally in the right ureter. *C*, Endoscopic appearance of the grade 1–2 TCCa that was resected ureteroscopically. *D*, Ureteroscopy 3 months later reveals a very small papillary lesion at the site of resection. *E*, This lesion is seen equivocally on retrograde ureteropyelogram. The low-grade TCCa is treated with biopsy (*F*) and fulguration (*G*).

uous mode and moved over the surface to coagulate the tissue. This can be seen as the color of the tissue changes to white. The laser fiber should not touch the tissue when it is activated because the tip will then char. For a relatively large lesion obstructing the ureter or an infundibulum, it may be necessary to remove some of the coagulated tissue to determine whether viable tumor remains after a single application. Since the laser can penetrate to a depth of approximately 5 to 6 mm, it may not affect the entire depth of the tumor. Coagulated tissue is removed with a grasper or basket to expose portions of the tumor otherwise not visible ureteroscopically. The remainder of the tumor is then treated similarly. There have been no reports of major renal or vascular injury or damage to associated organs from forward scatter of the Nd:YAG laser that has been used in the renal pelvis.

The holmium:YAG laser is widely applied for urologic applications. It is a solid-state pulsed laser that can fragment calculi and can coagulate and ablate tissue. This laser produces light at a wavelength of 2,100 nanometers that can be carried along long water-content fiber. The laser energy is absorbed within less than 0.5 mm of tissue and has essentially no risk of forward scatter. The effect observed is the only tissue effect achieved (Figure 33-2). The holmium:YAG can both coagulate and actually ablate and remove tissue. It is particularly useful for ureteral lesions, since it can ablate and remove a visually occlusive neoplasm to open the lumen for inspection more proximally.[57,58]

In use, the laser fiber must be placed in contact with or very close to the tissue to be treated. The laser is then activated at energies from 0.5 to 1 joule at a frequency of 6 to 10 or even 15 hertz. Irrigation is maintained to clear the visual field of tissue debris. It is often necessary to discontinue treatment to allow the field to clear, since considerable debris is formed during treatment. Bleeding occurs occasionally and can be controlled better at lower energies or by moving the fiber slightly away from the tissue to diffuse the laser beam and improve coagulation. The very limited penetration allows precise control, and the laser, thus, can be used for lesions located at the level of the iliac vessels and the renal pelvis near the renal vessels. Great care is employed to avoid ablation and resection through the wall of the ureter or renal pelvis itself.

The argon laser has major theoretical advantages for endoscopic treatment as well. Wavelengths of 488 to 514 nanometers have been used to treat superficial bladder cancer and also ureteral neoplasms. The penetration is limited to 1 mm and the laser light can be delivered with a fiber of 300 or 600 micron diameter. Johnson[59] reported treating tumors with continuous-wave argon laser energy with a quartz fiber utilizing a contact mode with the power set at 5 watts. There was satisfactory ablation of tumors in all 3 patients, but other confirmatory reports are still not available.

These lasers can also be used in combination. The effects of the Nd:YAG and Ho:YAG lasers are complimentary. The Nd:YAG laser can be used to coagulate the major volume of tumor since it penetrates several millimeters and can achieve this effect within the depth of the tissue. The coagulated tissue can then be removed mechanically or even more effectively with the Ho:YAG laser. The Ho:YAG can then be used to resect the tissue to the level of the wall of the ureter or renal pelvis. Thus, the benefits of each device can be used to the best advantage.

RESULTS OF TREATMENT

The results of ureteroscopic treatment of upper-tract TCC have been reported in several relatively small series. The techniques used for treatment, the location and characteristics of the tumors, and follow-up techniques and duration have varied widely. In the early report of Huffman and colleagues[49] on the treatment of upper-tract urothelial tumors, 8 patients with low-grade tumors were treated by ureteroscopic fulguration or resection. Surveillance was continued every 3 months with an average follow-up of 21 months. There were asynchronous recurrences in 3 patients, which remained low-grade, and no patient required surgical treatment during the study period. Grossman and colleagues[60] reported a higher recurrence rate, all treated endoscopically. Among their 8 patients, 2 were eventually treated surgically. One required a nephroureterectomy after the ureter could not be negotiated with the ureteroscope for treatment of a recurrence.

Several other larger series since these earlier reports have expanded the acceptable limits of treatment, including larger proximal lesions, and some have included higher-grade tumors. Over-all, this has resulted in a relatively high recurrence rate with a wide variation and an increasing need for nephroureterectomy, but stable development of new bladder tumors.[61-72]

RECURRENCES

Transitional cell carcinoma of the upper urinary tract recurs at significant rates just as locally treated bladder tumors do. There, too, it is impossible to determine whether the new neoplasms are the result of implantation of cells from the original tumor or if it is related to a field change in the urothelium. Successful treatment depends on thorough treatment of the primary neoplasm without irreversible damage to the organ system, coupled with the lack of local recurrence of the neoplasm as well as a lack of metastases. Several factors come into play in the adequacy of treatment.

Conservative surgical treatment with open excision of solitary upper-tract lesions also results in significant local recurrence. As noted above, the recurrence for ureteral lesions is approximately 12 to 18%, and higher when more proximal lesions were removed. Renal pelvic lesions treated surgically recur at an even higher rate of 48 to 66%.[40,41,70]

In collected series reporting ureteroscopic treatment of upper-tract tumors initially through 1995, there was a higher recurrence rate for renal pelvic lesions (Table 33-4). However, in reports through the following 5 years, there was an increase in the recurrence of ureteral tumor. This difference may be related to the ureteroscopic treatment of larger and more proximal ureteral lesions in the later years. These would be expected to be at higher risk of recurrence. A similar trend is seen in the increase of nephroureterectomies required in patients initially treated ureteroscopically. A similar shift in the selection of primary tumors treated would result in this higher failure rate.

It is more difficult to compare more recent studies since they have included larger tumors and higher-grade lesions. Recurrences have been seen

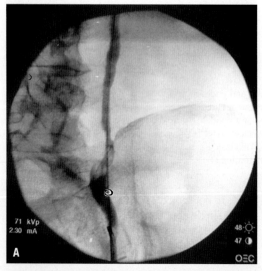
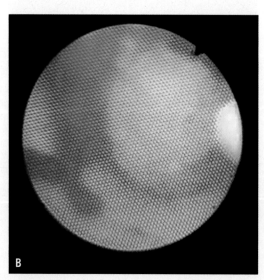
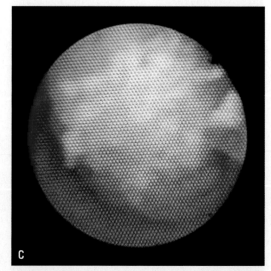

Figure 33-2 *A*, A retrograde pyelogram demonstrates the large filling defect nearly occluding the ureter. *B*, On endoscopy, a papillary tumor is evident. *C*, After biopsy of the lesion, it is treated with the holmium:YAG laser (0.6 J, 10 Hz at 700 microseconds). The entire tumor can be ablated with this technique.

Table 33-4 Tumor Recurrence after Ureteroscopic Treatment of Upper-Tract TCCa[53,54,60–67,77–79]		
	To 1995 (%)	To 2000 (%)
RP	6/15 (40)	22/60 (37)
Ureter	22/87 (25)	33/77 (43)
New BT	11/28 (39)	41/101 (41)
NU	4/102 (4)	19/137 (14)
BT = bladder tumor; NU = nephroureterectomy; RP = renal pelvis.		

in up to 80%+ of patients in some series. Most of the recurrent lesions are small and can be treated endoscopically. Only when there are extensive and rapid recurrences does nephroureterectomy become necessary.

There are several characteristics of primary upper-tract transitional cell carcinoma that appear to be related to the risk of recurrence (Table 33-5). Several of these characteristics are similar for risk and recurrence of bladder tumors. Recurrent disease is more likely for tumors over 1.5 cm in diameter than smaller lesions. There is also a higher risk of recurrence for high-grade tumors treated either ureteroscopically or by open surgery. There is evidence that positive urinary cytology at the time of treatment is a poor prognostic sign. The effect of the location of the primary tumor, whether in the intrarenal collecting system or ureter, has been inconsistent with some series reporting a higher rate for intrarenal neoplasms and others finding no difference or more frequent recurrence after ureteral primaries. However, multifocal lesions have consistently been seen to be associated with more frequent recurrences, both in the upper tract and in the bladder.

NEW BLADDER TUMORS

There is a higher risk of new bladder tumors forming in patients with upper-tract neoplasms. After surgical treatment with nephroureterectomy, nephrectomy, or segmental ureteral resection of upper-tract tumors, the risk of a new bladder tumor developing has ranged from 9 to 47% (Table 33-6). Some series note that the bladder tumor rate is related to the grade of the primary tumor, while the effect of grade was not considered in others. One report noted that the rate of new bladder neoplasm was related to a previous history of bladder cancer, where a 53% bladder tumor rate was noted.[28] A review of 89 patients[75] with total nephroureterectomy for localized TCC of the upper tract showed a direct effect of tumor multiplicity and surgical modality (laparoscopic vs open), and an inverse relationship of tumor

Table 33-5 Factors Related to Increase Risk of Tumor Recurrence
Multifocality
Tumor grade
Tumor size
Abnormal cytology
Previous bladder tumor
Tumor location

size and pathologic stage on subsequent development of bladder cancer. An overall rate of intravesical recurrence was 41.6%. Therefore, the patients most likely to be considered for endoscopic treatment, those with smaller low-stage tumors, may be more likely to develop bladder tumors. After ureteroscopic treatment, new bladder tumors occur in 28% of patients. This range may be expected since this group represents a mix of several grades and TCC history. Thus, ureteroscopic treatment does not appear to induce new bladder tumors.

LARGE TUMORS

Large neoplasms can be treated successfully ureteroscopically by staging treatment at intervals of approximately 8 weeks. At this time, the inflammatory changes following treatment are minimal, and significant new tumor growth should not be expected. Initially, the lesion is treated preferentially with the Nd:YAG laser or electrocoagulation to maximize coagulation of the tumor mass. This treated tissue is then resected with the holmium laser and the procedure is repeated as long as vesselicity permits. It may become impossible to distinguish the margin of the tumor that will become more distinct at a later interval. Tumors that regrow too rapidly or are too large to be treated ureteroscopically may require a percutaneous nephroscopic treatment or even nephroureterectomy.

HIGH-GRADE TUMORS

In general, high-grade tumors have not been considered good candidates for ureteroscopic treatment. However, in some instances, ureteroscopy may be the preferable option for a patient with a high-grade upper-tract neoplasm. Some ureteroscopic techniques are employed. There is some evidence that higher-grade lesions will recur more frequently, but long-term recurrences have also been reported.[68] Considerable care should be taken in the resection and subsequent surveillance of high-grade upper-tract tumors.

NORMAL CONTRALATERAL KIDNEYS

Ureteroscopic treatment of upper-tract TCC has also been extended to patients with a normal contralateral kidney. The results of endoscopic treatment in patients with a solitary kidney and compromised contralateral kidney can be extended to selected patients with an upper-tract tumor on one side and a normal contralateral kidney. Two series have demonstrated the feasibility of this treatment. Elliott and colleagues[77] reviewed 21 patients with 2 kidneys and found that 37% developed local recurrence averaging 7 months after treatment. There was a 46% recurrence rate among 13 ureteral tumors, and only 12% (1 of 8) for renal pelvic tumors. There was, however, a high mortality rate of 11 of 20 patients dying of unrelated causes, with 1 dying from invasive bladder cancer. There were no deaths

Table 33-6 New Bladder Tumor after Treatment of Upper-Tract TCCa	
Risk Group	New Bladder Tumors (%)
Gr 1 TCCa (NU, N, or segmental)[36,72,100]	20, 23, 33
Gr 2 or 3/4 (NU, N, or segmental)[37]	30
Any upper TCCa[28,53,99,101]	9, 31, 31, 34, 36, 36, 36, 42, 48
Previous history of bladder cancer[28]	53
Ureteroscopic treatment of upper TCCa[25,53,59,60,69]	28

related to the endoscopic tumor treatment or the upper-tract neoplasm. Only 4 patients (19%) required nephroureterectomy.

In the second series by Chen and Bagley,[78] 23 patients with 2 functional kidneys were treated ureteroscopically. The patients had several recurrences, but there was no significant grade increase and no patient developed metastatic disease. At the time of their follow-up, 17% had an ipsilateral recurrence, and 5% (1 patient) had developed a new contralateral neoplasm. However, 61% of patients were free of disease. Four (17%) had required nephroureterectomy.

Matsuoka and colleagues[69] reviewed their experience with ureteroscopic treatment of upper-tract tumors and found that there was a higher recurrence rate (86%) among patients treated for a strong indication such as a solitary kidney, while it was only 20% in those treated electively. Thus, again the results appear to be related to patient selection.

In summary, ureteroscopic treatment of upper urinary tract TCC can be performed safely and effectively with preservation of renal units, even in patients with a normal contralateral kidney.

SURVEILLANCE

Surveillance after ureteroscopic treatment of upper-tract neoplasms is essential because of the high recurrence rate. Cystoscopy has been well established as the standard technique to evaluate new bladder neoplasms after surgical treatment of upper-tract neoplasms. After endoscopic treatment, surveillance of the bladder must also be maintained with cystoscopy. Evaluation of the upper tracts for new or recurrent tumors must be maintained with other techniques (Figure 33-3).

Ureteroscopy is the most sensitive technique to evaluate the upper tract. It should be used routinely in follow-up surveillance. Grossman and colleagues[60] reported 1 patient with diffuse TCCa detected by ureteroscopy and confirmed on nephroureterectomy, who had a normal excretory urogram. Keeley and colleagues found that the sensitivity of retrograde pyelography for detecting recurrent upper-tract tumors was only 25%.[79] In another later series,[80] urinalysis, voided cytology, retrograde ureteropyelography, and ureteroscopic

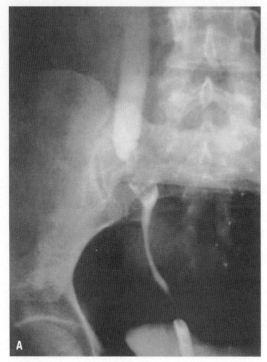 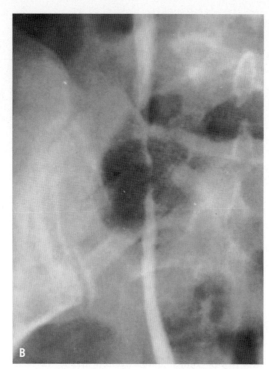 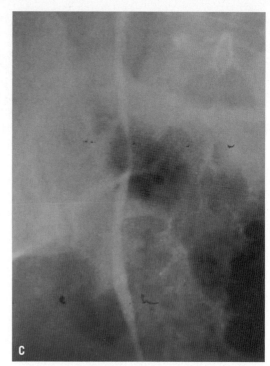

Figure 33-3 A 45-year-old female was previously treated with endoscopic resection and bacille Calmette-Guérin therapy for a large bladder tumor and with left distal ureterectomy and ureteroneocystostomy for a distal ureteral tumor. Both lesions were low-grade transtional cell carcinoma (TCCa). Follow-up studies show the filling defect of a grade 1 TCCa in the right ureter *A*, The tumor was treated with ureteroscopic Nd:YAG laser ablation and retrieval. At 3 months, *B*, and 6 months, *C*, after endoscopic treatment, there is drainage through the right ureter with small areas of residual tumor, again treated endoscopically.

biopsy were compared in patients with ureteroscopically visualized and treated tumors. None of those tests could accurately and routinely detect tumors. There was a high specificity of bladder urine cytology and urinalysis, which do support their use. If they are abnormal, the earlier endoscopy should be undertaken. Some authors have advocated excretory urography or retrograde ureteropyelography at intervals of 3 to 6 months, with ureteroscopy reserved only when specifically indicated. The author prefers to use the accuracy of ureteroscopy for surveillance. Ureteroscopy is continued at intervals of 3 months until the upper tract is clear, at which time the patient is examined ureteroscopically at 6-month intervals. Cystoscopy and cytology with urinalysis are continued at intervals of 3 months (Table 33-7).

COMPLICATIONS

Complications can occur with any ureteroscopic procedure, but there are some that appear to be specific to ureteroscopic tumor treatment. Many of the problems related to dilation of the ureterovesical junction can be avoided by the use of small-diameter rigid and flexible ureteroscopes. Electroresection is rarely used, and therefore the complications inherent in that procedure are avoided. With any of the techniques commonly used, electrocoagulation, laser coagulation, or resection with a neodymium:YAG or holmium:YAG laser, there remains a risk of stricture from scarring of the ureter. A review of complications from published series of ureteroscopic treatment of upper-tract tumors indicates a stricture rate of 13%, which is considerably higher than the less than 1% seen for stone treatment.[81] This may be an inherent risk of ureteroscopic tumor treatment, since the ureter itself is specifically traumatized with the treatment of the neoplasm, whereas such an effect on the ureteral wall is diligently avoided in stone treatment.

Perforation remains a strong theoretical risk. However, reported series have not shown any strong propensity toward intraluminal tumor dissemination, implantation, or extraluminal tumor or tumor extension. As noted above, there is no increased risk of tumor recurrence with ureteroscopic biopsy.[32]

ADJUVANT THERAPY

Adjuvant chemotherapy or immunotherapy is an attractive option in the treatment of upper-tract TCC, particularly because of the high recurrence rate. The safety and potential advantages of adjuvant therapy have been demonstrated in several short series, but this treatment has no proven role.

Bacille Calmette-Guérin (BCG) has been used as topical therapy in the upper tract with positive cytology. Sharpe and colleagues[82] administered BCG through retrograde ureteral catheters in patients with abnormal lateralizing cytology. Seventeen renal units were treated in 11 patients, and the urinary cytologic specimen normalized in 8 of the 11 patients with a median follow-up of 36 months. One patient experienced fever and required antituberculosis therapy without other complications in the group. Schoenberg and colleagues[83] also reported percutaneous instillation of BCG. One of 9 patients developed fever. Belman and colleagues[84] reported that 4 of 32 patients treated with BCG developed asymptomatic renal granulomatosis and 3 had fever that required treatment.

Mitomycin has also been used in the upper tract and has been found to be tolerated by patients. Eastham and Huffman[85] reported 7 patients with mitomycin C instilled in the intrarenal collecting system through a simple J ureteral catheter or a percutaneous nephrostomy tube after endoscopic resection of upper-tract tumors. No systemic side effects were noted, and there was no evidence of disease progression in 6 patients. Keeley and colleagues[86] similarly found that mitomycin could be administered without serious sequelae. They found that higher-risk grade 2 tumors, which were either larger or multifocal, treated with adjuvant mitomycin recurred at the same rate as the smaller, solitary grade 2 lesions without mitomycin after ureteroscopic treatment.

Thus, adjuvant therapy with either BCG or mitomycin has been seen to be feasible, but efficacy has not been demonstrated.

Table 33-7 Surveillance
3-Month Intervals
Cystoscopy
Cytology
6-Month Intervals (After Tumor-Free)
Ureteroscopy
12-Month Intervals
Imaging of contralateral kidney (IVP or retrograde)

TOTAL ENDOSCOPIC MANAGEMENT OF UPPER-TRACT TCC

Ureteroscopy constitutes an important facet in the totally endoscopic management of upper urinary tract TCC. Suspicious lesions are visualized and biopsied ureteroscopically, and many lesions can be treated ureteroscopically. Larger lesions, which cannot be treated ureteroscopically, may be treated more efficiently by percutaneous nephroscopy with laser or electrosurgical resection. Those that are too large or too extensive or higher grade, or those found through surveillance to be uncontrolled endoscopically, require nephroureterectomy, usually with hand-assisted laparoscopic nephroureterectomy. Surveillance is maintained with cystoscopy and ureteroscopy.[87,88] Upper urinary tract TCC, therefore, can be managed almost entirely endoscopically in the majority of patients (Table 33-8).

FAMILIAL NEOPLASM OF THE UPPER URINARY TRACT

Hereditary nonpolyposis colorectal cancer (HNPCC) syndrome is an autosomal dominant disorder that is characterized by germline mutations in DNA mismatch repair genes. It is a relatively common disorder, estimated to occur in 6 attempts out of colorectal cancers. The syndrome is associated with multiple colorectal neoplasms and extracolonic tumors, especially the endometrium, but also including the breast, the ovary, and the upper urinary tract. Bladder cancer does not appear to be increased in affected family members.[89]

The mutations found in HNPCC can be detected as microsatellite instability (MSI) in some DNA sequences, or alternatively, as the loss of immunostaining for the specific proteins. In one series, analysis showed MSI in 31.3% of consecutive upper urothelial tract carcinomas, which was noted to be the highest frequency reported in any type of tumor,[90] there is an increased risk of developing transitional cell carcinoma of the renal pelvis or ureter in patients with HNPCC. However, there is no increased risk of bladder cancer or renal cell carcinoma. Therefore, there is interest in screening these patients for upper-tract urothelial lesions. Excretory urography has been suggested as one option, and voided cytology and urinalysis are other options. The studies[91] on screening for recurrences after endoscopic treatment support the value of these same studies, but also note the lack of sensitivity.

In affected members, upper-tract neoplasms tend to occur at an earlier age and can be bilateral. These lesions can be treated as other upper-tract tumors have been. A conservative, endoscopic approach, even in patients with 2 functioning kidneys, should be considered because of the increased risk of developing additional lesions. Successful ureteroscopic treatment of bilateral ureteral tumors, renal pelvic neoplasms, and ureteral lesions in affected patients as young as 42 years have been reported. Screening in those patients has been by the routine endoscopic surveillance protocol noted above.[92] The presence of upper urinary tract tumors with a history of colon cancer, especially with other associated primary neoplasms at the sites, especially breast and ovaries, should be considered for screening for HNPCC. Conservative treatment options should be considered as first-line therapy.

BENIGN NEOPLASMS

Benign urothelial neoplasms are rare in the renal pelvis and ureter. Many individual cases or short series have been reported and include fibroepithelial polyps, inverted papillomas, and hemangiomas, as well as the more commonly noted ureteritis cystica.

Fibroepithelial polyps typically appear in young patients as a smooth pedunculated mass in the upper urinary tract, often occurring at the ureteropelvic junction. Historically, these lesions have been treated by open surgical resection. However, the availability of small ureteroscopes and appropriate biopsy or section devices, such as used for the transitional cell carcinomas, have permitted ureteroscopic diagnosis and treatment.[93–95] Follow-up after treatment is required only to confirm healing without significant stricture.

Inverted papillomas have also been considered a benign lesion, although there has been concern because of the association with transitional cell carcinoma in the difficult histopathologic diagnosis. Free erythrocyte protoporphyrin (FEP) is more common in the bladder than the upper urinary tract.[96] The most common presentation has been with hematuria. However, they also can cause obstruction with hydronephrosis. Endoscopically, these lesions as a smooth mucosal-based neoplasm. They lack the papillary configuration of low-grade transitional cell carcinoma, but can be confused with a higher-grade lesion. Endoscopic biopsy is a crucial diagnostic study.[97,98] Follow-up should be maintained both to confirm the patency of the urinary tract and because of the possible association with new transitional cell carcinoma. These neoplasms can be treated adequately ureteroscopically.

REFERENCES

1. Batata M, Grabstald H. Upper urinary tract urothelial tumors. Urol Clin North Am 1976;3:79–86.
2. Shinka T, Uekado Y, Aoshi H, et al. Occurrence of uroepithelial tumors of the upper urinary tract after the initial diagnosis of bladder cancer. J Urol 1988;140:745–8.
3. Rabbani F, Perrotti M, Russo P, Herr HW. Upper-tract tumors after an initial diagnosis of bladder cancer: argument for long-term surveillance. J Clin Oncol 2001;19:94–100.
4. Murphy DM, Zincke H, Furlow WL. Management of high grade transitional cell cancer of the upper urinary tract. J Urol 1981;125:25–9.
5. Bloom NA, Vidone RA, Lytton B. Primary carcinoma of the ureter. A report of 102 cases. J Urol 1970;103:590–8.
6. Lantz EJ, Hattery RR. Diagnostic imaging of urothelial cancer. Urol Clin North Am 1984;11:567–83.
7. McCoy JG, Honda H, Reznicek M, Williams RD. Computerized tomography for detection and staging of localized and pathologically defined upper tract urothelial tumors. J Urol 1991;146:1500–3.
8. Milestone B, Friedman AC, Seidmon EJ, et al. Staging of ureteral transitional cell carcinoma by CT and MRI. Urology 1990;36:346–9.
9. Zincke H, Aguillo JJ, Farrow GM, et al. Significance of urinary cytology in the early detection of transitional cell cancer of the upper urinary tract. J Urol 1976;116:781–3.
10. Gill WB, Lu CT, Thomsen S. Retrograde brushing: a new technique for obtaining histologic and cytologic material from ureteral, renal pelvic and calyceal lesions. J Urol 1973;109:573–8.
11. Sheline M, Amendola MA, Pollack HM, et al. Fluoroscopically guided retrograde brush biopsy in the diagnosis of transitional cell carcinoma of the upper urinary tract results in 45 patients. AJR Am J Roentgenol 1989;153:313–6.
12. Blute RD Jr, Gittes RR, Gittes RF. Renal brush biopsy: survey of indications, techniques and results. J Urol 1981;126:146–9.
13. Johnson GB, Grasso M. Exaggerated primary endoscope deflection: initial clinical experience with prototype flexible ureteroscopes. BJU Int 2004;93:109–14.
14. Streem SB, Pontes JE, Novick AC, Montie JE. Ureteropyeloscopy in the evaluation of upper tract filling defects. J Urol 1986;136:383–5.
15. Bagley DH, Rivas D. Upper urinary tract filling defects: flexible ureteroscopic diagnosis. J Urol 1990;143:1196–200.
16. Kavoussi L, Clayman RV, Basler J. Flexible, actively deflectable fibreoptic ureterorenoscopy. J Urol 1989;142:949–54.
17. Blute ML, Segura JW, Patterson DE, et al. Impact of endourology on diagnosis and management of upper urinary tract urothelial cancer. J Urol 1989;141:1298–301.
18. Bagley DH, McCue P, Blackstone AS. Inverted papilloma of the renal pelvis: flexible ureteroscopic diagnosis and treatment. Urology 1990;36:336–8.
19. Abdel-Razzak OM, Ehya H, Cubler-Goodman A, Bagley DH. Ureteroscopic biopsy in the upper urinary tract. Urology 1994;44:451–7.
20. Bian Y, Ehya H, Bagley DH. Cytologic diagnosis of upper urinary tract neoplasms by ureteroscopic sampling. Acta Cytol 1995;39:733–40.
21. Bagley DH, Kulp DA, Bibbo M. Ureteroscopic biopsy optimized by cytopathologic techniques. J Urol 1994;151:387A.
22. Low RK, Moran ME, Anderson KR. Ureteroscopic cytologic diagnosis of upper tract lesions. J Endourol 1993;7:311–4.
23. Tawfiek ER, Bibbo M, Bagley DH. Ureteroscopic biopsy: technique and specimen preparation. Urology 1997;50:117–9.
24. Keeley FX, Kulp DA, Bibbo M, et al. Diagnostic accuracy of ureteroscopic biopsy in upper tract transitional cell carcinoma. J Urol 1997;157:33–7.
25. Daneshmand S, Quek MD, Huffman JL. Endoscopic management of upper urinary tract transitional cell carcinoma: long-term experience. Cancer 2003;98:55–60.
26. Skolarikos A, Griffiths TRC, Powell PH, et al. Cytologic analysis of ureteral washings is informative in patients with grade 2 upper tract TCC considering endoscopic treatment. Urology 2003;61:1146–50.
27. Guarnizo E, Pavlovich CP, Seiba M, et al. Ureteroscopic biopsy of upper tract urothelial carcinoma: improved diagnostic accuracy and histopathological considerations using a multi-biopsy approach. J Urol 2000;163:52–5.
28. Charbit L, Gendreau MC, Mee S, Cukier J. Tumors of the upper urinary tract: 10 years of experience. J Urol 1991;146:1243–6.
29. Liu JB, Bagley DH, Conlin MJ, et al. Endoluminal sonographic evaluation of ureteral and renal pelvic neoplasms. J Ultrasound Med 1997;16:515–21.
30. Lim DJ, Shattuck MO, Cook WA. Pyelovenous lymphatic migration of transitional cell carcinoma following flexible ureterorenoscopy. J Urol 1993;149:109–11.
31. Kulp DA, Bagley DH. Does flexible ureteropyeloscopy promote local recurrence of transitional cell carcinoma? J Endourol 1994;8:111–3.
32. Hendin BN, Streem SB, Levin HS, et al. Impact of diagnostic ureteroscopy on long-term survival in patients with upper tract transitional cell carcinoma. J Urol 1999;161:783–5.
33. Hara I, Hara S, Miyake H, et al. Usefulness of ureteropyeloscopy for diagnosis of upper urinary tract tumors. J Endourol 2001;15:601–5.
34. Conlin MJ, Marberger M, Bagley DH. Ureteroscopy. Instrumentation and development. Urol Clin North Am 1997;24:25–42.

Table 33-8 Totally Endoscopic Management of Upper Urinary Tract Transitional Cell Carcinoma

Diagnosis – ureteroscopic
Treatment – ureteroscopic or PCN
Nephroureterectomy – laparoscopic
Surveillance – ureteroscopic

35. Nielsen K, Ostri P. Primary tumors of the renal pelvis: evaluation of clinical and pathological features in a consecutive series of 10 years. J Urol 1988;140:19–21.

36. Murphy DM, Zincke H, Furlow WL. Primary grade 1 transitional cell carcinoma of the renal pelvis and ureter. J Urol 1980;123:629–31.

37. Murphy DM, Zincke H, Furlow WL. Management of high grade transitional cell cancer of the upper urinary tract. J Urol 1981;125:25–9.

38. Mufti GT, Gove JRW, Badenoch DF, et al. Transitional cell carcinoma of the renal pelvis and ureter. Br J Urol 1989; 63:135–40.

39. McCarron JP Jr, Chasko SB, Gray GF Jr. Systemic mapping of nephroureterectomy specimens removed for urothelial cancer: pathological findings and clinical correlations. J Urol 1982;128:243–6.

40. Mazeman E. Tumours of the upper urinary tract calyces, renal pelvis and ureter. Eur Urol 1976;2:120–6.

41. Zincke H, Neves RJ. Feasibility of conservative surgery for transitional cell cancer of the upper urinary tract. Urol Clin North Am 1984;11:717–24.

42. Mills C, Vaughan ED Jr. Carcinoma of the ureter: natural history, management and 5-year survival. J Urol 1983;129: 275–7.

43. Heney NM, Nocks BN, Daly JJ, et al. Prognostic factors in carcinoma of the ureter. J Urol 1981;125:632–6.

44. Johnson DE, Babaian RJ. Conservative surgical management for noninvasive distal ureteral carcinoma. Urology 1979; 13:365–7.

45. Vest SA. Conservative surgery in certain benign tumors of the ureter. J Urol 1945;53:97–120.

46. Bian Y, Ehya H, Bagley DH. Cytologic diagnosis of upper urinary tract neoplasms by ureteroscopic sampling. Acta Cytol 1995;39:733–40.

47. Chaubal A, McCue PA, Bagley DH, Bibbo M. Multimodal cytologic evaluation of upper urinary tract urothelial lesions. J Surg Path 1995;1:31–5.

48. Zincke H, Aguilo JJ, Farrow GM, et al. Significance of urinary cytology in the early detection of transitional cell cancer of the upper urinary tract. J Urol 1976;116:781–3.

49. Huffman JL, Bagley DH, Lyon ES, et al. Endoscopic diagnosis and treatment of upper-tract urothelial tumors. Cancer 1985;55:1422–8.

50. Lyon E. The birth of modern ureteroscopy: the Albona Jaybis story. J Endourol 2004;18:525–6.

51. Huffman JL. Diagnostic and therapeutic approaches to upper tract urothelial tumors. In: Huffman JL, Bagley DH, Lyon ES, editors. Ureteroscopy. Philadelphia: W.B. Saunders; 1988. p. 107–23.

52. Malloy TR. Laser treatment of ureter and upper collecting system. In: Smith JA, editor. Lasers in urologic surgery. Chicago: YearBook Medical Publishers; 1985. p. 82–93.

53. Blute ML, Segura JW, Patterson DE, et al. Impact of endourology on diagnosis and management of upper urinary tract urothelial cancer. J Urol 1989;141:1298–301.

54. Schmeller NT, Hofstetter AG. Laser treatment of ureteral tumors. J Urol 1989;141:840–3.

55. Johnson DE. Use of the holmium:YAG (Ho:YAG) laser for treatment of superficial bladder carcinoma. Lasers Surg Med 1994;14:213–8.

56. Bagley DH. Ureteroscopic laser treatment of upper urinary tract tumors. J Clin Lasers Surg Med 1998;16:55–9.

57. Razvi HA, Chun SS, Denstedt JD, Sales JL. Soft-tissue applications of the holmium:YAG laser in urology. J Endourol 1995;9:387–90.

58. Bagley DH, Erhard M. Use of the holmium laser in the upper urinary tract. Tech Urol 1995;1:25–30.

59. Johnson DE. Treatment of distal ureteral tumors using endoscopic argon photoirradiation. Lasers Surg Med 1992; 12:490–3.

60. Grossman HB, Schwartz SL, Konnak JW. Ureteroscopic treatment of urothelial carcinoma of the ureter and renal pelvis. J Urol 1992;148(2 Pt 1):275–7.

61. Papadopoulos I, Wirth B, Bertermann H, Wand H. Diagnosis and treatment of urothelial tumors by ureteropyeloscopy. J Endourol 1990;4:55–60.

62. Tasca A, Zattoni F, Garbeglio A, et al. Endourologic treatment of transitional cell carcinoma of the upper urinary tract. J Endourol 1992;6:253–6.

63. Kaufman RP Jr, Carson CC. Ureteroscopic management of transitional cell carcinoma of the ureter using the neodymium:YAG laser. Lasers Surg Med 1993;13:625–8.

64. Gaboardi F, Bozzola A, Dotti E, Galli L. Conservative treatment of upper urinary tract tumors with Nd:YAG laser. J Endourol 1994;8:37–41.

65. Bales GT, Lyon ES, Gerber GS. Conservative management of transitional cell carcinoma of the kidney and ureter. Diagn Ther Endosc 1995;1:121–3.

66. Elliott DS, Blute ML, Patterson DE, et al. Long-term followup of endoscopically treated upper urinary tract transitional cell carcinoma. Urology 1996;47:819–25.

67. Grasso M, Fraiman M, Levine M. Ureteropyeloscopic diagnosis and treatment of upper urinary tract urothelial malignancies. Urology 1999;54:240–6.

68. Suh RS, Faerber GJ, Wolf JS Jr. Predictive factors for applicability and success with endoscopic treatment of upper tract urothelial carcinoma. J Urol 2003;170(6 Pt 1):2209–16.

69. Matsuoka K, Iida S, Tomiyasu K, et al. Transurethral endoscopic treatment of upper urinary tract tumors using a holmium:YAG laser. Lasers Surg Med 2003;32:336–40.

70. Iborra I, Solsona J, Casanova J, et al. Conservative elective treatment of upper urinary tract tumors: a multivariable analysis of prognostic factors for recurrence and progression. J Urol 2003;169:82–5.

71. Johnson G, Fraiman M, Grasso M. Broadening experience with the retrograde endoscopic management of upper urinary tract urothelial malignancies. BJU Int 2005;95 Suppl 2:110–3.

72. Sakamoto N, Naito S, Kotoh S, et al. Recurrence of bladder tumors following surgery for transitional cell carcinoma of the upper urinary tract. Eur Urol 1991;20:136–9.

73. Hisataki T, Miyao N, Masumori N, et al. Risk factors for the development of bladder cancer after upper tract urothelial cancer. Urology 2000;55:663–7.

74. Kang CH, Yu TJ, Hsieh HH, et al. The development of bladder tumors and contralateral upper urinary tract tumors after primary transitional cell carcinoma of the upper urinary tract. Cancer 2003;98:1620–6.

75. Matsui Y, Utsunomiya N, Ichioka K, et al. Risk factors for subsequent development of bladder cancer after primary transitional cell carcinoma of the upper urinary tract. Urology 2005;65:279–83.

76. Lim DJ, Shattuck MO, Cook WA. Pyelovenous lymphatic migration of transitional cell carcinoma following flexible ureterorenoscopy. J Urol 1993;149:109–11.

77. Elliott DS, Segura JW, Lightner D, et al. Is nephroureterectomy necessary in all cases of upper tract transitional cell carcinoma? Long-term results of conservative endourologic management of upper tract transitional cell carcinoma in individuals with a normal contralateral kidney. Urology 2001;58:174–8.

78. Chen GL, Bagley DH. Ureteroscopic management of upper tract transitional cell carcinoma in patients with normal contralateral kidneys. J Urol 2000;164:1173–6.

79. Keeley FX Jr, Bibbo M, Bagley DH. Ureteroscopic treatment and surveillance of upper tract transitional cell carcinoma. J Urol 1997;157:1560–5.

80. Chen GL, El-Gabry EA, Bagley DH. Surveillance of upper urinary tract transitional cell carcinoma: the role of ureteroscopy, retrograde pyelography, cytology and urinalysis. J Urol 2000;165:1901–4.

81. Chen GL, Bagley DH. Ureteroscopic surgery for upper tract transitional-cell carcinoma: complications and management. J Endourol 2001;15:399–404.

82. Sharpe JR, Duffy G, Chin JL. Intrarenal bacillus Calmette-Guérin therapy for upper urinary tract carcinoma in situ. J Urol 1993;149:457–60.

83. Schoenberg MP, VanArsdalen KN, Wein AJ. The management of transitional cell carcinoma in solitary renal units. J Urol 1991;146:700–3.

84. Bellman GC, Sweetser P, Smith AD. Complications of intracavitary bacillus Calmette-Guérin after percutaneous resection of upper tract transitional cell carcinoma. J Urol 1994;151:13–5.

85. Eastham JA, Huffman JL. Technique of mitomycin C instillation in the treatment of upper urinary tract urothelial tumors. J Urol 1993;150(2 Pt 1):324–5.

86. Keeley FX Jr, Bagley DH. Adjuvant mitomycin C following endoscopic treatment of upper tract transitional cell carcinoma. J Urol 1997;158:2074–7.

87. Lee D, Trabulsi E, McGinnis D, et al. Totally endoscopic management of upper tract transitional cell carcinoma. J Endourol 2002;16:37–41.

88. Keeley FX Jr, Tolley DA. Laparoscopic nephroureterectomy: making management of upper tract transitional cell carcinoma entirely minimally invasive. J Endourol 1998; 12:139–41.

89. Watson P, Lynch HT. The tumor spectrum in HNPCC. Anticancer Res 1994;14:1635–9.

90. Hartmann A, Cheville JC, Dietmaier W, et al. Hereditary nonpolyposis colorectal cancer syndrome in a patient with urothelial carcinoma of the upper urothelial tract. Arch Pathol Lab Med 2003;127:E60–3.

91. Sijmons RH, Kiemeney LA, Witjes JA, Vasen HF. Urinary tract cancer and hereditary nonpolyposis colorectal cancer: risks and screening options. J Urol 1998;160:466–70.

92. Bagley DH, Harlan M, Boman B. Management of upper urinary tract neoplasms in patients with HNPCC [Poster MP11/10]. J Endourol 2004;18:A71.

93. Bahnson RR, Blum MD, Carter MF. Fibroepithelial polyps of the ureter. J Urol 1984;132:343–4.

94. Bolton D, Stoller ML, Irby P III. Fibroepithelial ureteral polyps and urolithiasis. Urology 1994;44:582–7.

95. Lam JS, Bingham JB, Gupta M. Endoscopic treatment of fibroepithelial polyps of the renal pelvis and ureter. Urology 2003;62:810–3.

96. Witjes JA, van Balken MR, van de Kaa CA. The prognostic value of a primary inverted papilloma of the urinary tract. J Urol 1997;158:1500–5.

97. Bagley DH, McCue P, Blackstone AS. Inverted papilloma of the renal pelvis: flexible ureteroscopic diagnosis and treatment. Urology 1990;36:336–8.

98. Grasso M, Bagley DH. Inverted papilloma of the renal pelvis presenting as a filling defect on intravenous pyelogram: a case report. Surg Rounds 1991;14:711–3.

99. Koga F, Nagamatsu H, Ishimaru H, et al. Risk factors for the development of bladder transitional cell carcinoma following surgery for transitional cell carcinoma of the upper urinary tract. Urol Int 2001;67:135–41.

100. Mukamel E, Simon D, Edelman A, et al. Metachronous bladder tumors in patients with upper urinary tract transitional cell carcinoma. J Surg Oncol 1994;57:187–90.

101. Kulp DA, Bagley DH. Does flexible ureteropyeloscopy promote local recurrence of transitional cell carcinoma? J Endourol 1994;8:111–3.

Retrograde Ureteroscopic Endopyelotomy for Ureteropelvic Junction Obstruction

Freddy R. Mendez-Torres, MD

Raju Thomas, MD

Advances in technology and instrumentation have changed the practice of urology, especially over the past decade. One of the areas of major impact has been the treatment of ureteropelvic junction obstruction (UPJO), which is defined as an anatomic or functional impedance of urine flow from the renal pelvis into the ureter[1] (Figure 34A-1). This condition can be congenital or acquired in etiology, the congenital form being the more common. UPJO, although relatively uncommon, warrants prompt attention to alleviate symptoms and prevent deterioration of renal function. Several factors can play roles in the development of UPJO, including intrinsic aperistalsis of involved ureteral segment, crossing aberrant vessels causing direct compression to the ureter, renal stone disease, and previous surgical or endourologic manipulation.

The advent of smaller-caliber endoscopes, development of laparoscopic reconstructive techniques, the availability of laser technology, and robotics have diversified the treatment options for this condition.

Although the efficacy, decreased morbidity, decreased hospital stay, and decreased need for analgesia with endopyelotomy have been clearly demonstrated, several issues have still not been completely resolved. Should patients be managed initially by ureteroscopy? What are the exclusion criteria for these endoscopic procedures? What are the relative merits of antegrade versus retrograde approaches? In the era of minimally invasive laparoscopy and robotic-assisted surgery, is there still a role for endopyelotomy?

In this chapter we discuss the technique and results at our institution for retrograde ureteroscopic endopyelotomy for the treatment of ureteropelvic junction obstruction.

HISTORY

Several reconstructive procedures have been described for management of UPJO since Trendelenburg's first description of such a procedure in 1886. Open surgical management was the only mode of treatment for this condition before the introduction of endoscopic and laparoscopic techniques. Open surgical correction of the obstruction at the UPJ remains the gold standard of treatment for this condition, with success rates over 90%.[2] However, associated morbidity is not unusual with open surgery; specifically, there is fistula formation in 2.6% of patients, stricture of the UPJ in 2.4%, and the need for nephrectomy in 3.2%.[3]

The present-day endourologic approach to the management of UPJO can be traced back to the original descriptions of Albarran, Keyes, and Davis. Albarran did the first endosurgical repair of the UPJO in 1903, which actually described an *ureterotome externe*.[4] Keyes performed a similar procedure successfully in 1915.[5] Both the antegrade and retrograde endopyelotomy follow the concept of Davis's intubated ureterotomy, first described by Davis in 1943. In 1985, Bagley and colleagues reported a combined percutaneous and flexible ureteroscopic procedure approach for the management of an obliterated UPJ.[6] Wickham and Kellet described the first ureteroscopic pyelolysis of the UPJ in 1983.[7] Inglis and Tolley did the same in 1986.[8] Thomas and colleagues described their experience of ureteroscopic endopyelotomy in which pre-stenting was performed to facilitate ureteroscopy in 1996.[9] Single-setting, one-stage procedure was subsequently described by Soroush and Bagley in 1998.[10]

There are now multiple different options for the treatment of an obstructed UPJ, including antegrade nephroscopic endopyelotomy, retrograde ureteroscopic endopyelotomy, and Acucise (Applied Urology, Laguna Hills, CA), and laparoscopic- and robot-assisted pyeloplasty, as well as the traditional open surgical pyeloplasty. Open surgical dismembered pyeloplasty has been considered the gold standard for the treatment of UPJO, with success rates of over 90%. But many institutions now consider endopyelotomy a possible first-line therapy option for the treatment of this condition.[11–14]

Currently, a retrograde endopyelotomy can be performed in three ways: first, using a rigid ureteroscope and a cold-knife, electrocautery, or holmium laser incision; second, using a flexible ureteroscope and electrocautery or laser incision; and last, using a balloon with a cutting wire (Acucise, Applied Urology).[11]

Different series have reported success rates for retrograde ureteroscopic endopyelotomy to be in the range of 73 to 90%.[1,9,10,15–18] As compared with other treatment options, the ureteroscopic retrograde endopyelotomy is less invasive, requires less OR time, enables performing the procedure on an outpatient basis or with a very short hospital stay, and is associated with a shorter convalescence period.[1,12,20–24] Also, the initial report of ureteral stricture formation because of thermal injury from transmission of the electrocautery current has been eliminated with the use of insulated ureteroresectoscopes and with the use of holmium laser fibers.[19]

PATIENT SELECTION AND PREOPERATIVE PREPARATION

The presumptive clinical diagnosis of UPJO can be evaluated and/or confirmed with a renal ultrasound, intravenous pyelogram, diuretic renal scan, retrograde pyelogram, Whitaker test, or with a combination of them. The renal scan, beside aiding in the diagnosis of a UPJO, gives a quantitative differential renal function, which can be used to choose the best treatment option and, further, to allow for follow-up evaluation of the renal function.

Either a spiral-CT angiography or an endoluminal ultrasound is highly recommended to assess for the presence of an aberrant crossing vessel. The UPJ area can also be evaluated ureteroscopically for the presence of pulsations before performing the endopyelotomy incision.

Although ureteroscopic retrograde endopy-

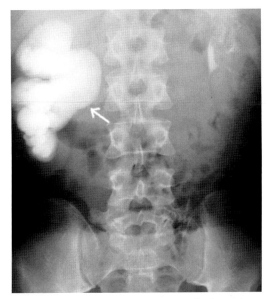

Figure 34A-1 Intravenous pyelogram of a Rt. ureteropelvic junction obstruction (*arrow*).

elotomy is applicable to most patients with UPJO, there exist some absolute and relative exclusion criteria. Among the absolute contraindications are patients with active infection and bleeding diathesis.

Patients with concurrent renal stone and UPJO, and patients with a nephrostomy tube in place, should be treated with an antegrade approach so that both the renal stone and the UPJO can be managed in a one-stage procedure.

Patients with relative long length of obstruction, usually > 2 cm, are best managed either open surgically, laparoscopically, or robotic assisted.

Patients with ipsilateral differential renal function of < 20% and severely decreased parenchymal thickness can be given a trial of drainage and reevaluation[11] or should be offered a laparoscopic simple nephrectomy for a poorly functioning or nonfunctioning kidney.

Patients with massive hydronephrosis should be treated with dismembered pyeloplasty, either open surgically, laparoscopically, or robot assisted because of the need for trimming and reduction of the redundant renal pelvis.

Controversy exists with patients with high insertion of the UPJ and crossing vessels. Although once considered a contraindication because of poor results, there are published series reporting that the type of ureteral insertion had no significant impact on the outcome of endopyelotomy,[25] and also that patients with crossing vessels had long-term success with retrograde endopyelotomy.[13] We routinely perform laparoscopic robotic-assisted pyeloplasty in either case of high insertion UPJO or a known crossing vessel.

Lastly, patients with known intractable stent intolerance should be considered candidates, either for an antegrade endopyelotomy or an open pyeloplasty with a nephrostomy tube and not for the ureteroscopic endopyelotomy.

Once the surgeon and patient have decided on the retrograde approach for management of an obstructed UPJ, an indwelling ureteral stent is usually placed to drain the obstructed renal unit for 1 to 2 weeks. This procedure not only drains the obstructed renal unit, but also stabilizes its renal function, dilates and straightens the UPJ, and facilitates subsequent passage of the ureteroscope into the renal pelvis. Above all, preoperative placement of the stent allows evaluation of any degree of stent intolerance and to identify improvement of renal function after drainage.

INFORMED CONSENT

On the day of the scheduled endopyelotomy, any final questions are answered and an informed consent is obtained after explaining and discussing with the patient the expected outcomes and benefits of the procedure (eg, improved renal drainage, preservation of renal function, diminished risk of calculus and infection, minimally invasive procedure), its associated risks or complications (bleeding, infection, possibility of conversion to open surgery, recurrence, etc), and the other minimally invasive treatment options avail-

able. Patients are informed that postoperative evaluations may show some residual caliectasis, especially in those with long-standing UPJO.

REQUIRED INSTRUMENTATION

A. HOLMIUM LASER URETEROSCOPIC ENDOPYELOTOMY

- 7.5 French (F) Rigid and/or flexible ureteroscope
- 200- or 365-Micron holmium laser fiber at the following settings:
  - 1.5 to 2.5 J
  - 10 to 15 Hz
- Superstiff guidewire (0.038-inch)
- Single-action pump system (Microvasive, Watertown, MA)
- 5F Open-ended catheter when used with the flexible ureteroscope
- Endopyelotomy stent (Microvasive or Applied Urology)
- Routine cystoscopy and fluoroscopy setup

B. URETEROSCOPIC ENDOPYELOTOMY WITH ELECTROCAUTERY

- 11.5F Ureteroresectoscope (Karl Storz, Culver City, CA, Richard Wolf, Rosemont, IL) (Figure 34A-2)
  - Insulated electrocautery knife
  - Cold knife and
  - Electrocautery attachments
- Superstiff guidewire (0.038-inch)
- Single-action pumping system (Microvasive)
- 5F Open-ended catheter
- Endopyelotomy stent (Microvasive or Applied Urology)
- Routine cystoscopy and fluoroscopy setup

STEP-BY-STEP OPERATIVE TECHNIQUE

After either a general or a spinal anesthesia, the patient is placed in the lithotomy position. Caution is taken so that all pressure points are well cushioned, and antiembolic stockings are used in high-risk patients.

With the use of a cystoscope, and under fluoroscopic guidance, a retrograde pyelogram is performed and subsequently a superstiff guidewire is passed and coiled into the renal pelvis. If the patient had a previously placed indwelling ureteral stent, it is removed and used to pass the guidewire prior to removing the stent. A retrograde pyelogram can assess any resolution of hydronephrosis and can be used as a prognostic indicator.

The next step varies depending on whether the endopyelotomy is done with electrocautery through a ureteroresectoscope or whether holmium laser is used through a rigid, semirigid, or flexible ureteroscope.

A. HOLMIUM:YTTRIUM-ALUMINUM-GARNET (YAG) LASER URETEROSCOPIC ENDOPYELOTOMY A 7.5F self-dilating rigid, semirigid, or flexible ureteroscope is passed alongside the superstiff guidewire. A balloon dilator can be

passed over the guidewire and the ureteral orifice dilated in case of difficulty advancing the ureteroscope within the ureter. If necessary, another guidewire can be passed through the ureteroscope and the narrow area subsequently balloon dilated.

Once at the UPJ, it is first inspected for the presence of any transmitted pulsations. A 365 µm holmium laser fiber, when using a rigid or semirigid ureteroscope, or a 200 µm, in the case of a flexible ureteroscope, is passed through the working channel of the ureteroscope. At a setting of 1.5 to 2.5 J and a frequency of 10 to 15 Hz, the UPJ is incised under direct vision either laterally or posterolaterally to avoid the risk of injuring any crossing vessel. The incision is carried on until periureteral fat is seen and the UPJ is wide enough to permit easy passage of the ureteroscope into the renal pelvis (Figure 34A-3).

After hemostasis of any venous bleeding is performed, the laser fiber and the ureteroscope are removed. The UPJ areas is dilated up to 24F using a balloon dilator under fluoroscopic guidance. The concept of balloon dilation of the UPJ is based on Davis's intubated ureterotomy, in which the incised and dilated ureteral fibers regenerate around the ureteral stent over a 6-week period[5] (Figure 34A-4).

The balloon dilator is then removed. An endopyelotomy stent is placed under fluoroscopic control, leaving the 14F or 10F end at the UPJ (depending on stent used) and the 7F end coiled in the bladder (Figure 34A-5). Alternatively, an 8F Double-J ureteral stent can be left in place. The authors recommend using a ureteral stent one size longer than anticipated to prevent downward migration of the renal coil into the incised UPJ.

An indwelling Foley catheter is placed to drain the bladder for 48 hours. This helps to maintain a low pressure in the urinary system and to prevent urinary reflux through the ureteral stent into the incised UPJ.

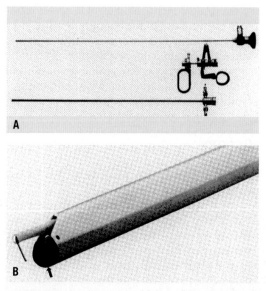

Figure 34A-2 11.5F Ureteroresectoscope with insulated tip.

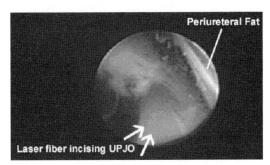

Figure 34A-3 Periureteral fat seen after the ureteropelvic junction was incised with holmium laser.

B. Ureteroscopic Endopyelotomy with Electrocautery

A 5F open-ended catheter is passed over the superstiff wire. The open-ended catheter works as an insulator, preventing contact with the electrocautery element, and avoiding transmission of current along the length of the guidewire. Also, the open-ended catheter may serve to continuously drain the renal pelvis of the irrigation fluid used during the procedure, once the wire is removed.

The ureteroresectoscope is passed directly alongside the insulated guidewire with the cold knife in place. The electrocautery element is right angled and would impede vision if placed during the insertion of the ureteroresectoscope.[1] If there is difficulty accessing the ureteral orifice or the intramural ureter, a balloon dilator can be passed over the guidewire to dilate the area. If there is resistance advancing the ureteroresectoscope along the ureter proximal to the UPJO, a smaller self-dilating ureteroscope can be passed to passively dilate the ureter and to inspect for the cause of the narrow area. If necessary, another guidewire can be passed through the self-dilating ureteroscope and the narrow area is balloon dilated.

Once at the UPJ, the cold knife and the working element are exchanged for the electrocautery element. Either water or 1.5% glycine solution are used as the irrigant during the incision.

The UPJ is first inspected for the presence of any transmitted pulsations, and then incised laterally, between 8 and 9 o'clock on the right and between 3 and 4 o'clock on the left. Short and shallow strokes should be performed and aggressive and deep incisions avoided. Any bleeding site is controlled by means of spot electrocoagulation. The incision is carried down until periureteral fat is seen and the ureteroresectoscope enters the renal pelvis with ease.

The ureteroresectoscope and the open-ended catheter are removed. The rest of the subsequent steps, balloon dilation, stenting, and Foley catheter drainage are the same as described above for the holmium:YAG laser endopyelotomy.

POSTOPERATIVE CARE

The vast majority of patients are discharged either the same day or within the first 24 hours following the procedure. Oral antibiotics, usually quinolones, are given for 3 to 5 days; oral antispasmodics and/or oral anticholinergics are given

as needed in case of irritative bladder symptoms. The Foley catheter is removed, often by the patient, after 48 hours. The ureteral stent is removed cystoscopically in 6 weeks.

Diuretic renal scans or intravenous pyelography are performed 4 weeks after the ureteral stent removal. Patients are followed-up with renal ultrasound or renal scan every 4 to 6 months during the first year and yearly thereafter or as needed.

Success following endopyelotomy is measured by evaluating improvement of the function and drainage of the involved kidney and alleviation of symptoms. After correction of the obstruction at the UPJ, postoperative radiographic images from an intravenous pyelogram (IVP) or CT scan often show caliectasis resulting from long-standing obstruction and dilatation that may not completely resolve.

RESULTS

We analyzed the outcome of 139 consecutive patients who underwent retrograde ureteroscopic endopyelotomy at Tulane University Health Sciences Center between 1989 and 2002. These patients included 7 pediatric patients, 4 solitary kidneys, 2 horseshoe kidneys, and 1 ptotic kidney.

The average postoperative hospital stay was less than 24 hours. Seventy-nine percent of the patients were discharged home on the same day, and 97% of them were discharged within 24 hours.

Of the 139 patients 32 (23%) required subsequent procedures to treat recurrence of obstruction, showing an overall long-term success rate for retrograde ureteroscopic endopyelotomy of

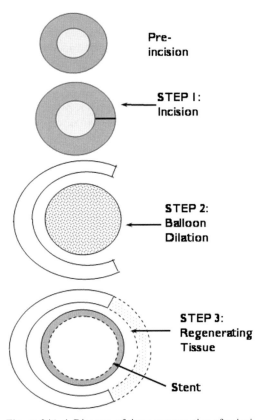

Figure 34A-4 Diagram of tissue regeneration after incision and balloon dilation.

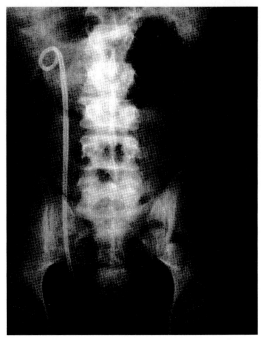

Figure 34A-5 Endopyelotomy indwelling stent in place after ureteropelvic junction obstruction incision.

77%. Fourteen of these patients (10%) required major open or laparoscopic surgical intervention, including nephrectomies for severe hydronephrosis and nonimprovement in renal function in 3 (2%) cases, emergent nephrectomy for severe bleeding in 1 (0.7%) case, dismembered pyeloplasties in 8 (5.7%) cases, and spiral flap pyeloplasties in 2 (1.4%) cases.

Eighteen (12.9%) patients required minor procedures, which included cystoscopy and balloon dilation of the ureteropelvic junction in 13 (9.3%), repeated retrograde endopyelotomy in 4 (2.8%), and 1 (0.7%) required long-term indwelling stent exchange. There were no ureteral strictures secondary to manipulation in our series.

After analyzing the failures of treatment in this series, two factors were obviously associated with poor results: (1) a long-standing obstruction with a decrease in ipsilateral renal function of less than 20% of the total renal function, and (2) a severely dilated renal pelvis, which did not improve drainage with an indwelling ureteral stent, resulted in nonimprovement of symptoms, drainage, and function after endopyelotomy.

After evaluation of these results, we conclude that patients with patulous redundant renal pelvis and borderline salvageable renal function should be considered candidates for treatment modalities such as open or laparoscopic pyeloplasty or nephrectomy, rather than endopyelotomy.

COMPLICATIONS

Since its initial description by Young in 1912, retrograde ureteroscopy has come a long way and has gained widespread acceptance as an option for the treatment of multiple pyeloureteric conditions. Further advances in technology have lead to the introduction of smaller-caliber ureteroscopes with the capacity to accommodate accessory instruments necessary to perform diagnostic and therapeutic upper urinary tract procedures.

As with ureteroscopy, the complications and adverse events associated with retrograde ureteroscopic manipulation of the ureter have decreased dramatically in the past 2 decades. Smaller-caliber ureteroscopes, the advent of laser technology, improved paraphernalia and, above all, experience in the procedures should be given credit. Although these advances have decreased the need for open ureteral surgery, iatrogenic injury can still occur with the endoscopic technique. Possible iatrogenic complications of ureteroscopy include ureteral perforation, stricture, false passage, ureteral avulsion, bleeding from the ureteral mucosa or adjacent structures, infection, and sepsis. Multiple studies have reported the overall complication rate of ureteroscopy fluctuates between 1 and 15%.[26–28]

The reported incidence of pain, fever, false passage, and urinary tract infection are 5.5%, 1.4%, 0.4%, and 1.6%, respectively, in one large ureteroscopy series.[29]

Other complications associated with incision of the UPJ can include bleeding from adjacent aberrant vessels, stent migration through the UPJ incision, and UPJO recurrence. Significant bleeding requiring emergent nephrectomy is another possible complication that justifies the need for vascular or three-dimensional radiographic studies to identify aberrant vessels. The use of a complete lateral incision at the UPJ helps to prevent injuries to those vessels.

Minor complications of retrograde ureteroscopic endopyelotomy could include proximal stent migration, stent intolerance, minor bleeding, and urinary tract infection after manipulation. Most of these complications are alleviated after removal of indwelling ureteral stents. The routine use of antispasmodic and anesthetic drugs after surgery improves tolerance to the stent and decreases complaints from the patient.

COMPARISON OF TREATMENT APPROACHES AND CONCLUSIONS

Multiple endourological and open surgical techniques are now available for the treatment of ureteropelvic junction obstruction. The choice of technique relies primarily on the urologist's experience with each procedure, available equipment, and the need to perform another concomitant procedure.

Antegrade endopyelotomy requires expertise in percutaneous renal surgery, with detailed knowledge of the intrarenal anatomy and adequate experience in "real time," two-dimensional fluoroscopic imaging. This is the preferred technique when treating concomitant intrarenal calculi, but it is also associated with a larger potential for complications and morbidity. The occurrence of pneumothorax, adjacent organ trauma (ie, bowel, spleen, liver), and hydrothorax are possibilities that need to be explained to the patient prior to the surgery. Antegrade and retrograde endopyelotomy share the potential for hemorrhage from injury to aberrant crossing vessels; however, antegrade access may also be associated with hemorrhage from the percutaneous renal tract and with a higher risk of infection owing to external urinary drainage through the percutaneous nephrostomy tube.

Acucise retrograde endopyelotomy relies on fluoroscopic imaging and not on direct visualization during cutting of the ureteropelvic junction. High-quality fluoroscopic imaging is critical for optimal electrode placement. Success rates of this procedure have been comparable to those obtained with retrograde ureteroscopic endopyelotomy and ranged from 66 to 84%.[30] Extreme cautions should be exercised when using this technique in the presence of aberrant crossing vessels. Preoperative CT scan with angiographic phase and three-dimensional reconstruction has been shown to be adequate to collect information regarding periureteral vasculature at the level of the obstruction.[31] Incision at the lateral position of the UPJ should minimize the risk of vascular injury while performing this procedure.

Multiple different indwelling stents can be used to maintain patency of the UPJ after an endopyelotomy. At our institution we use an 8F Double-J ureteral stent with postoperative results similar to those obtained with endopyelotomy stents. It is always important to use an indwelling stent one size longer than anticipated in order to avoid downward migration of the stent that could compromise endopyelotomy healing.

It is our belief that retrograde ureteroscopic endopyelotomy provides a safe and adequate first line of treatment for patients suffering from UPJO. With the advent of smaller scopes and devices, this technique has evolved to include larger children as possible patients. Adherence to strict endourologic principles and direct visualization makes retrograde ureteroscopic endopyelotomy a safe and effective treatment modality. Furthermore, this procedure has a short learning curve and can be performed in almost all general hospitals where ureteroscopy is performed.

REFERENCES

1. Thomas R, Monga M. Endopyelotomy. Retrograde ureteroscopic approach. Urol Clin North Am 1998;25:305–10.
2. Murphy LJT. The kidney. In: Murphy LJT, editor. The history of urology. Springfield, IL: Charles C Thomas; 1972. p. 197.
3. Scardino PT, Scardino PL. Obstruction at the ureteropelvic junction. In: Bergman H, editor. The ureter. 2nd ed. New York: Springer-Verlag; 1981. p. 697.
4. Albarran J. Operations plastiques et anastomoses dans le traitment des retentions de veim. These Paris, 1903.
5. Davis DM, Strong GH, Drake WM. Intubated ureterotomy: experimental work and clinical results. J Urol 1948;59:851–62.
6. Bagley DH, Huffman J, Lyon E, McNamara T. Endoscopic ureteropyelostomy: opening the obliterated ureteropelvic junction with nephroscopy and flexible ureteropyeloscopy. J Urol 1985;133:462–4.
7. Wickham JEA, Kellet MJ. Percutaneous pyelolysis. Eur Urol 1983;9:122–4.
8. Inglis JA, Tolley DA. Ureteroscopic pyelolysis for pelviureteric junction obstruction. Br J Urol 1986;58:250–2.
9. Thomas R, Monga M, Klein EW. Ureteroscopic retrograde endopyelotomy for management of ureteropelvic junction obstruction. J Endourol 1996;10:141–5.
10. Soroush M, Bagley DH. Ureteroscopic retrograde endopyelotomy. Tech Urol 1998;4:77–82.
11. Nakada SY, Johnson M. Ureteropelvic junction obstruction. Retrograde endopyelotomy. Urol Clin North Am 2000;27:677–84.
12. Danuser H, Ackermann DK, Bohlen D, Studer UE. Endopyelotomy for primary ureteropelvic junction obstruction: risk factors determine the success rate. J Urol 1998;159:56–61.
13. Ferraro RF, Abraham VE, Cohen TD, Preminger GM. A new generation of semirigid fiberoptic ureteroscopes. J Endourol 1999;13:35–40.
14. Van Cangh PJ, Nesa S, Tombal B. The role of endourology in ureteropelvic junction obstruction. Curr Urol Rep 2001;2:149–53.
15. Badlani GH, Karlin G, Smith AD. Complications of endopyelotomy: analysis in series of 64 patients. J Urol 1998;140:473–5.
16. Conlin MJ, Bagley DH. Ureteroscopic endopyelotomy at a single setting. J Urol 1998;159:727–31.
17. Meretyk I, Meretyk S, Clayman RV. Endopyelotomy: comparison of ureteroscopic retrograde and antegrade percutaneous techniques. J Urol 1992;148:775–83.
18. Hibi H, Yamada Y, Mizumoto H, et al. Retrograde ureteroscopic endopyelotomy using the holmium:YAG laser. Int J Urol 2002;9:77–81.
19. Thomas R. Endopyelotomy for ureteropelvic junction obstruction and ureteral stricture disease: a comparison of antegrade and retrograde techniques. Curr Opin Urol 1994;4:174–9.
20. Gerber GS, Kim JC. Ureteroscopic endopyelotomy in the treatment of patients with ureteropelvic junction obstruction. J Urol 2000;55:198–202.
21. Brooks JD, Kavoussi LR, Preminger GM, et al. Comparison of open and endourological approaches to the obstructed ureteropelvic junction. Urology 1995;46:791–5.
22. Shalhav AL, Giusti G, Elbahnasy AM, et al. Adult endopyelotomy: impact of etiology and antegrade versus retrograde approach on outcome. J Urol 1998;160(3 Pt 1):685–9.
23. Giddens JL, Grasso M. Retrograde ureteroscopic endopyelotomy using the holmium:YAG laser. J Urol 2000;164:1509–12.
24. Delvecchio FC, Preminger GM. Endourologic management of upper urinary tract strictures. AUA Update Series 2000;19:250–5.
25. Thomas R. Retrograde endopyelotomy for ureteropelvic junction obstruction. In: Smith AD, Badlani GH, Bagley DH, et al, editors. Smith's textbook of endourology. St Louis, MO: Quality Medical Publishing; 1996. p. 488–96.
26. Blute ML, Segura JW, Patterson DE, et al. Impact of endourology on diagnosis and management of upper urinary tract urothelial cancer. J Urol 1989;141:1298–301.
27. Low RK, Moran ME, Anderdion R. Ureteroscopic cytologic diagnosis of upper tract lesions. J Endourol 1993;7:311–4.
28. Fasihuddin Q, Hasan AT. Ureteroscopy (URS): an effective interventional and diagnostic modality. J Pak Med Assoc 2002;52:510–2.
29. Grasso M, Bagley D. Small diameter, actively deflectable, flexible ureteroscopy. J Urol 1998;160:1648–53.
30. Nakada SY, Pearle MS, Clayman RV. Acucise endopyelotomy: evolution of a less invasive technology. J Endourol 1996;10:133–9.
31. Quillin SP, Brink JA, Heiken JP, et al. Helical (spiral) CT angiography for identification of crossing vessels at the ureteropelvic junction. AJR Am J Roentgenol 1996;166:1125–30.

Ureteroscopic Management of Ureteral Stricture Disease

Daniel Janoff, MD

Michael Conlin, MD

Advances in ureteroscopic techniques, ureteroscope design, and working instrumentation have made endoscopic management of ureteral strictures a reasonable alternative to open surgery. Ureteral strictures can occur at any location along the ureter. There are many different causes of ureteral strictures, and the etiology can affect the success of incisional treatment. We will review these causes and treatment options, focusing on the endoscopic incisional treatment of benign intrinsic strictures, which are the most amenable to this treatment approach.

HISTORICAL PERSPECTIVE

Ureteral strictures were traditionally treated by open operative repair. Endoscopic management was first described by Hunner in 1924, with his review of 100 cases of retrograde catheter dilation.[1] In 1926, Illievitz and Dourmashkin reported the use of balloon dilation of the ureter for the endoscopic removal of ureteral calculi.[2,3] A "rubber bag" was fitted onto the end of a ureteral catheter and then inflated to dilate the segment just distal to an obstructing calculus. This would lay the groundwork for future balloon dilation of ureteral strictures.

Angiographic balloon dilators, initially developed for the dilation of arteriosclerotic vascular lesions, were later applied to the urinary tract. These 4-mm balloon catheters were first used to dilate ureteral strictures from an antegrade percutaneous approach.[4–13] In 1984, Finnerty and colleagues reported six patients with ureteral strictures treated with Grüntzig balloon catheters in a retrograde fashion.[14] They were successful in treating 83% of these strictures. Balloon dilation continues to be a reasonable treatment option today.[15]

Davis, in 1943 reported the intubated ureterotomy technique for the treatment of ureteropelvic junction (UPJ) obstruction and upper ureteral strictures.[16] This was first performed in an animal model and later successfully used in humans.[17] Since Davis's initial reports, several authors have studied the histologic changes following 4 to 8 weeks of stenting an incised ureteral stricture. They confirmed Davis's observation that ureteral musculature regenerates around the ureterotomy defect.[18–21] This new approach for stricture management became the foundation for the future endourologic treatment of ureteral obstruction.

Endoscopic incisional treatment of ureteral strictures grew out of experience with the management of UPJ obstruction. Wickham reported his technique of percutaneous pyelolysis (endopyelotomy) in 1983.[22] Extensive work by Smith and colleagues has shown excellent results using their endopyelotomy technique.[23–27] Although cold-knife incision was initially used for endopyelotomy, electrocautery and holmium:yttrium-aluminum-garnet (holmium:YAG) laser incision have also been used with good results. Retrograde endopyelotomy using a ureteroscopic approach was reported by Clayman and Picus in 1988.[28] These techniques were easily translated to the management of ureteral strictures.[29]

Use of the Acucise device (Applied Medical Resources, Laguna Hills, CA) was reported by Chandhoke and colleagues in 1993 for the treatment of UPJ obstruction and ureteral strictures.[30] This catheter was developed to simplify endopyelotomy and address the concern of ureteral stricture formation following retrograde endopyelotomy when larger diameter rigid ureteroscopes were used.[31] The Acucise devise permits treatment of UPJ obstruction and ureteral strictures from a retrograde approach under fluoroscopic control. The catheter design and treatment results are discussed later.

Over the past several years, new technology has permitted the creation of ureteroscopes of smaller caliber. Endoureterotomy could now be performed under direct visualization while minimizing the risk of stricture formation due to trauma from the scope.

Endoluminal ultrasound during endoureterotomy was reported in 1991 by Goldberg and colleagues.[32] This minimized the risk of bleeding by allowing the surgeon to obtain real-time images of surrounding periureteral vasculature prior to incision.

ETIOLOGY

Ureteral strictures can be classified by location and cause.[33] Operative trauma has traditionally been the most common source, but the incidence may be decreasing with improved ureteroscopic instrumentation.[34] Contemporary large ureteroscopic series now report the incidence of stricture following ureteroscopy to be as low as 0.5%.[34] Ureteral stones impacted for over 2 months in duration, however, have been associated with a 24% incidence of stricture formation following ureteroscopic treatment.[35] Inflammatory lesions can also result in ureteral strictures. Tuberculosis and bilharzial strictures remain common causes of ureteral obstruction in many parts of the world.[36–38] Malignancy should always be suspected in idiopathic strictures. Transitional cell carcinoma, adenocarcinoma of the prostate, and non-urologic malignancies causing extrinsic obstruction may be found. Other less common causes of ureteral obstruction include radiation injury, retroperitoneal fibrosis, compression by aneurismal arterial enlargement, arteriosclerotic periarterial inflammation, and ureteral ischemia following renal transplantation. Congenital strictures occur primarily at the UPJ and are reviewed in a separate chapter. We will focus our discussion on benign intrinsic ureteral strictures.

EVALUATION

The patient's history alone often reveals the diagnosis and cause of the ureteral obstruction. Most patients will present with flank pain; others may have hematuria, urinary tract infection, or a combination of these findings. As many as 25% of patients remain asymptomatic, despite high-grade obstruction.[33] Patients with a solitary kidney, underlying renal insufficiency, or bilateral involvement can present with renal failure. Any history of recent travel to countries with known schistosomiasis disease or concomitant tuberculosis should alert the urologist to possible infectious causes.

The first imaging evaluation of the urinary tract selected is often abdominal ultrasound. Although this can reveal hydronephrosis, excretory urography or retrograde ureteropyelography will be necessary to delineate the level and extent of obstruction (Figure 34B-1). Multi-detector computed tomography (CT) urogram may find an increasing role in evaluating ureteral strictures because it provides additional anatomic information about nearby vasculature compared to standard ureteropyelography.[39] If the presence of an obstruction is equivocal, renal scintigraphy with diuretic "washout" is usually diagnostic.[40] Difficult cases may require a pressure-flow study (the Whitaker test) for definitive diagnosis. A CT scan should be obtained if extrinsic or malignant causes are suspected.

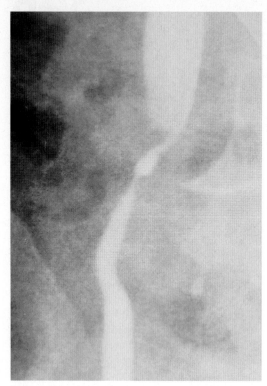

Figure 34B-1 Retrograde ureteropyelogram demonstrating a mid-ureteral stricture.

PREOPERATIVE PREPARATION

Preoperative imaging of the involved segment is critically important. The location and length of the stricture must be determined to plan the appropriate operative approach. An excretory urogram may be sufficient in some cases. A nephrostogram via percutaneous nephrostomy tube (when present) usually provides excellent imaging of the strictured segment. Combined antegrade and retrograde ureteropyelography can be performed preoperatively or at the time of surgery.

When pyelonephritis or diminished function of the obstructed kidney is present, management should begin with adequate drainage either by percutaneous nephrostomy or ureteral stent placement. This will optimize renal function and drain infected urine. Mild obstruction often does not require preoperative drainage. Urinary tract infections should be treated with antibiotics before surgical intervention.

Some surgeons advocate preoperative stenting across the strictured segment to passively dilate the ureter facilitating endoscopic access.[33] With a completely obliterated ureter, this may not be possible. When preoperative drainage is adequate, we prefer a one-stage approach, stenting preoperatively only if necessary for the other reasons listed above.

Informed consent should be obtained, and all options, including open operative repair, must be thoroughly discussed with the patient.

TREATMENT OPTIONS

The classic method of treating clinically significant ureteral strictures is by open surgical repair. The type of repair will depend on the location and length of the stricture. Open surgical options include ureteroureterostomy, ureteroneocystostomy (with or without Boari flap bladder reconstruction), ureteral replacement with ileum, urinary diversion, autotransplantation, or nephrectomy.

Ureteral dilation is usually the least traumatic endoscopic approach and a reasonable initial option. Slow, gentle dilation can be performed by placing progressively larger ureteral stents. This is rarely necessary, and it is usually more practical to dilate the ureter at one setting, using graduated dilating catheters or balloon dilating catheters.

The Acucise device can be used for treatment of ureteral strictures as well as UPJ obstruction. The incision, however, is made under fluoroscopic control only, and does not allow simultaneous imaging of the ureteral lumen or the periureteral tissues. Significant hemorrhage has been reported in at least seven patients.[30,41,42]

Ureteroscopic endoureterotomy may be performed with a cold knife, electrocautery, or holmium:YAG laser. A ureteroresectoscope or rigid ureteroscope can be used in the distal ureter, while a flexible ureteroscope is used for the proximal ureter. This combination of instruments permits access to strictures at any level. Injury to periureteral vasculature during endoureterotomy is a rare but significant complication.[43] Endoluminal ultrasonography at the time of surgery provides imaging of periureteral vessels, allowing them to be avoided during the incision.[44] Endoureterotomy can also be performed by an antegrade ureteroscopic approach. Combined antegrade and retrograde ureteroscopy is used when necessary for complete obliteration of the ureter.

INSTRUMENTATION

A variety of equipment has been used for endoscopic management of ureteral strictures. High-pressure ureteral dilation balloon catheters are available in inflated diameters of 4 to 8 mm and lengths of 5 to 10 cm. Many of these balloons are designed to withstand pressures from 12 to 20 atmospheres (atm), which is more than adequate for most ureteral strictures.

The Acucise RP35 device is a low-pressure (1 atm) balloon catheter. The balloon is 10 French in diameter and will inflate to 24F. It has a 6F catheter body and does not require preoperative stenting. A 150 μm electrocautery fiber, 3 cm in length, is exposed along the balloon's surface. This allows simultaneous balloon dilation and incision.

Cold-knife incision of the stricture requires the use of a rigid ureteroresectoscope (11 to 13F) (Figure 34B-2A). Knife blades are available in straight, half-moon, and hook configurations (Figure 34B-2B). Blades that pass over a guidewire are also available, adding to further control when passing the knife beyond the stricture. These over-the-wire blades are often only effective in partially opening the stricture, permitting passage of the resectoscope for further incision.[45]

Electrocautery incision is accomplished with either 2 to 3F ball-tip electrodes, Hulbert electrodes (Cook Urological, Spencer, IN), or the Rite cut device (Circon-ACMI, Stamford, CT) We prefer the Rite cut device for use through the flexible ureteroscope because it is small in caliber (3F), has an angled tip that can be rotated, and permits excellent control of the incision (Figure 34B-3). The holmium:YAG laser has also been used effectively for incision of ureteral strictures.[46] Energy can be delivered by 200 to 365 μm diameter fibers through both the rigid and flexible ureteroscopes. Low-power (25-watt) laser energy has been reported to be sufficient to successfully incise strictures.[47]

URETEROSCOPIC TECHNIQUE

The patient is placed in a lithotomy position for a standard retrograde approach. If simultaneous antegrade and retrograde access is needed, as in patients with strictures of significant length or total obliteration of the ureteral lumen, we recommend the split-leg prone position.[48] Alternatively, the patient can be placed in the dorsolithotomy position and the appropriate flank elevated with a roll to permit access to the nephrostomy site.

The first intraoperative step is to obtain imaging studies of the involved segment. Retrograde ureteropyelography will help guide the procedure. Before any manipulation, a guidewire should be passed across the strictured segment. This can be the most difficult portion of the procedure. Angled and straight hydrophilic-coated guidewires are helpful in passing beyond the stricture. (Access for completely obliterated lumens will be discussed later.) Once control is

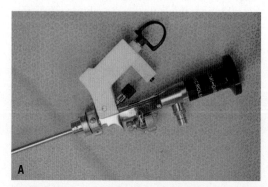
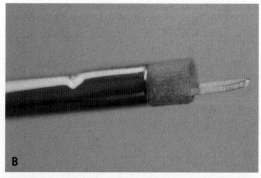

Figure 34B-2 *A*, 13F ureteroresectoscope often used for ureteroscopic incision. Because of its size, use is usually limited to the distal ureter. *B*, Tip of ureteroresectoscope with straight knife blade extended.

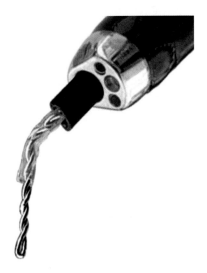

Figure 34B-3 3F Rite cut device permits excellent control of incision through a flexible ureteroscope.

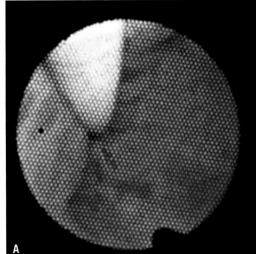

Figure 34B-4 *A,* Ureteroscopic view of mid-ureteral stricture. *B,* Same ureteral segment widely patent following endoureterotomy

obtained with a guidewire, the treatment can begin. The involved segment is now inspected under direct vision to rule out other causes of ureteral obstruction that may not have been evident by radiographic evaluation such as tumors and calculi. Before incision, if there is any question regarding the etiology of the stricture, biopsy and cytology samples can be obtained through the ureteroscope.

Knowledge of the ureteral surface anatomy and the surrounding vessels is critical to determine the safest location for incision of the ureter.[45] This safe zone is located posterolateral in the proximal ureter to the level of the iliac vessels. As the ureter crosses into the pelvis, the safest incision is made anteriorly to avoid injuring the iliac vessels. From the iliac vessels distally to the bladder, the incision should be made posteriorly. Again, intraoperative endoluminal ultrasonography offers the advantage of periureteral imaging to help choose the safest location for the incision.[49] If electrocautery is to be used, the safety wire must either be insulated with a ureteral catheter or replaced with an insulated wire, such as a polyurethane-coated nitinol wire. This will prevent transmission of the electrocautery energy to other parts of the ureter, which may result in damage and scarring. The incision can then be safely made using the cold knife, electrocautery probe, or holmium:YAG laser. The cold knife may be preferable because of theoretically less tissue injury and fibrosis. When using the flexible ureteroscope, we usually select the Rite cut electrode. Incisions should be made through the entire thickness of the ureter until fat is visible (Figure 34B-4), but in cases where there is significant periureteral fibrosis, this may be difficult or impossible to achieve. In these cases, the incision is made deep enough to restore an adequate luminal diameter. Following ureteroscopic incision, balloon dilation can then be performed to check for any "waisting" or persistent stricture. This will also gently open the ureterotomy to a larger diameter.

Stenting of the ureter is recommended. As with endopyelotomy patients, controversy exists regarding the appropriate size and duration of the stent.[50–52] We prefer using the gently tapered endoureterotomy stents (6/10F) unless the size of the ureter will not permit it. The 10F end can be positioned appropriately within a distal ureterotomy segment by inserting the stent upside down. Alternatively, two separate 6 or 7F stents can be placed simultaneously. Stenting with a regular 7 or 8F double-pigtail stent may be as effective, but definitive comparisons are lacking. Davis showed, in his animal studies of the intubated ureterotomy technique, that muscle had regenerated over 90% of the ureteral diameter by 6 weeks.[16] For this reason, we advocate stenting for a minimum of 6 weeks.

Postoperative follow-up should consist of imaging to detect recurrent obstruction—renal ultrasonography, excretory urography, retrograde ureteropyelography, or renal scintigraphy with diuretic washout can be used. Renal ultrasonography can demonstrate the presence of normal parenchyma and the absence of hydronephrosis, which makes the study adequate. It is also cost-effective and easier to tolerate than contrast studies. We routinely perform renal ultrasonography at 3 to 6 months postoperatively and annually if the patient's condition remains stable. Any change in the sonogram findings can be further evaluated with renal scintigraphy or contrast studies.

SPECIAL CONSIDERATIONS

Strictures that cause complete obstruction (the totally obliterated ureter) pose a more difficult problem (Figure 34B-5). Obtaining guidewire control across the strictured segment of the ureter constitutes the major portion of the procedure. If the segment is very short and the proximal and distal ends of the ureter are well aligned, the stiff end of a guidewire may be used to puncture the stricture under endoscopic and fluoroscopic guidance. Stabilization of the wire through a

ureteral catheter can facilitate puncture through the membrane. Longer strictures require ureteroscopically controlled incision from one end of the obliterated segment to the other. This usually requires simultaneous retrograde and antegrade ureteroscopy by a "cut to the light" technique. With both ureteroscope tips in their respective ureteral ends, the ends of the ureteroscopes are first aligned fluoroscopically in two planes. The light source for the operating ureteroscope is then turned off and the end of the opposing ureter is visualized by locating the light from that ureteroscope. Electrocautery can then be used to incise the end of each obliterated segment to establish continuity and obtain guidewire control of the ureter. The use of holmium:YAG laser for this purpose has also been described.[53] This process may require retroperitoneoscopy to properly align the ureteral segments. Once a guidewire is securely across this segment, one can proceed with treatment of the stricture.

Ureteroenteral anastomotic strictures following urinary diversion occur at rates up to 19%.[54] They can be difficult to manage because of extensive periureteral postoperative fibrosis, and complicated retrograde access from the enteral segment.

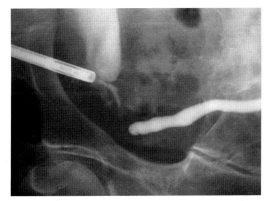

Figure 34B-5 Combined retrograde and antegrade contrast study demonstrating obliteration of a segment of distal ureter.

Also, because of the previous cancer history in these patients, local recurrence must be evaluated. The cause of ureteroenteral strictures is usually due to ischemia of the distal ureter or a technical problem in creating the anastomosis.[55,56] This is likely the reason why treatment is less successful when compared to other ureteral strictures.

Complete ureterovesical obstruction represents a similar problem, and identification of the ureter at the obliterated ureteral orifice can be difficult. Ureterovesical strictures occur most commonly following renal transplantation when ischemia to the distal segment and possible allograft rejection complicate the treatment (Figure 34B-6).[57,58] This problem can also occur after transurethral biopsy involving the ureteral orifice. Techniques for obtaining control across the scarred orifice include perforation of the proximal segment with a stiff guidewire and endoluminal ultrasound identification of the obstructed proximal segment at the ureterovesical junction, followed by perforation from below. The ureteral orifice can then be incised using any of the techniques and tools described above.[59]

RESULTS

There are few reported large series pertaining to endoscopic incisional treatment of ureteral strictures. Most incisional data are combined with results using other treatment modalities making the interpretation difficult. Comparisons of studies using different techniques can be misleading since the patient populations and stricture types often differ.

Balloon dilation alone has moderate success in resolving ureteral strictures and often requires repeat dilations. Long-term success has been reported to be 16 to 89% with average follow-up of 9 to 75 months.[4–13,30,60–63] Richter and colleagues showed that higher success was seen in patients with non-ischemic strictures with length < 2 cm (89.2% vs. 37.5%).[63] Patients with longer strictures that had compromised vascular supply did poorly, with a patency rate of 16.7%.

Preminger and colleagues conducted a multicenter trial evaluating the Acucise cutting balloon device.[41] They performed endoureterotomy on 49 patients and reported a 55% patency rate with a

follow-up of 8.7 months (range, 1.2 to 17 months).

Ureteroscopic endoureterotomy is performed with cold knife, cautery, or holmium:YAG laser. Reported results for ureteroscopic endoureterotomy are summarized in Table 34B-1. Eshghi and Lifson reported results of cold-knife endoureterotomy for 100 strictures in 89 patients.[33] Overall success was 95% for first-time treatment and 98% for repeat procedures. No complications were encountered using this technique. Franco and colleagues reported a 100% success rate at a follow-up of 3 to 8 months using cold-knife endoureterotomy to treat six patients with ureteral strictures.[64] Yamada and colleagues treated 19 patients with a mean follow-up of 18 months (range, 4 to 55 months) and found an 85% success rate.[43]

Thomas reviewed 36 ureteral strictures treated with endoureterotomy using electrocautery.[65] This was successful in 23 patients (64%). He also noted better results in patients with strictures less then 1.5 cm in length (success in 80%) compared with longer strictures (27% successful). Patients who had previously undergone radiation treatment also did worse, with only 33% success. Ghoneim and colleagues reviewed their experience with electrocautery incisional treatment of ureteral strictures.[37] Most of these strictures were bilharzial in origin. They were successful in 4 of 12 patients.

Singal and colleagues reported a success rate of 76% using holmium:YAG laser for endoureterotomy.[66] Five of their 21 patients failed. Thirteen ureteroileal strictures, one ureterovesical stricture following renal transplantation, and one strictured Boari flap were included in this data set.

In a multivariate analysis using a variety of techniques, including balloon dilation, Acucise, cold knife, or cautery endoureterotomy, Wolf and colleagues found their overall success in treating 38 benign ureteral strictures was 80% for 3 years.[67] The different modalities used did not significantly affect outcome, although these data are retrospective. All recurrences occurred within 1 year, and repeat endoureterotomy performed in 2 of these patients was successful. The authors also noted that all patients in whom the affected kidney provided < 25% of overall renal function had failed endoscopic management for their benign ureteral strictures. This may be because good urine flow through the cut section is important to keep the area patent. In addition, the group advocated the use of steroid injection to the stricture bed to decrease scar formation, although the efficacy of this treatment has not been clinically proven.

Incision of ureteroenteric strictures is less successful, likely due to their ischemic nature. Among 30 ureteroenteric stricture treatments,

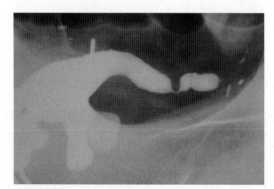

Figure 34B-6 Antegrade contrast study of renal allograft ureter with two strictures: a 1-cm mid-ureteral stricture and a ureterovesical anastomotic stricture.

Table 34B-1	Results with Endoureterotomy for Ureteral Strictures				
Series	Location	#Patients	Success (%)	Avg. Follow-up in Months (range)	
Acucise					
Preminger et al[41]	Proximal	4	50	8.7 (1.2–17)	
	Mid	10	50		
	Distal	26	58		
	Total	40	55		
Chandhoke et al[30]		8	75	3.8	
Cohen et al[74]		6	67	21.6 (14–29)	
Cold Knife					
Lopatkin et al[75]	Proximal	3	67	22 (6–48)	
	Distal	4	100		
	Total	7	85.8		
Yamada et al[43]		19	47	18 (4–55)	
Eshghi et al[45]		89	95		
Franco et al[64]	Distal	6	100	(3–20)	
Schneider et al[76]	Distal	12	67	15 (7–45)	
	Transplant	7	71		
	Ureterosig	2	100		
Strup et al[59]	UVJ (obliterated)	7	86	(14–64)	
Cautery					
Thomas[65]		36	64		
Ghoneim et al[37]		12	33		
Laser					
Singal et al[66]	Ureteral	10	80	(3–12)	
	Ureteroileal	9	89		
	Transplant	1	0		
Combined					
Conlin et al[72]	(obliterated)	8	75	87 (4–126)	
Wolf et al[67]	Proximal	4	75	28 (2–74)	
	Mid	5	100		
	Distal	29	78		
	Total	38	82		

Wolf and colleagues[67] reported success rates as low as 73, 51, and 32% at 1, 2, and 3 years, respectively. All endoscopic re-treatments failed. With the use of holmium:YAG laser, Watterson and colleagues had a 56% patency in 3 years, while Poulakis and colleagues reported a 3-year patency rate of 60.5% with cold knife endoureterotomy.[68,69] The Acucise cutting balloon catheter has also been used with a success rate at 30% for a median follow-up of 48 months.[70]

Ureterovesical obstruction is most often seen after renal transplantation. Bosma and colleagues reported 20 patients who failed conservative management with ureteral stenting.[71] Thirteen patients were treated endoscopically. Nine patients undergoing endoureterotomy resolved their obstruction, while all four patients treated with balloon dilation alone recurred. Mean follow up was 58 months. Strup and Bagley reported seven patients treated for complete obstruction of the ureterovesical junction by the method previously described.[59] Success was achieved in six patients, at a follow-up of 13 to 52 months. The sole failure resulted from recurrent transitional cell carcinoma.

Ureteroscopic management of completely obliterated ureteral segments is best performed on non-ischemic strictures < 2 cm in length. We have treated eight patients with obliterated segments of the ureter. Long-term patency with this technique was successful in 75% of our patients, with median follow up of 87 months.[72] One stricture > 6 cm recurred and was subsequently managed with nephrectomy. The other patient who was a treatment failure is now stent-dependent, refusing further treatment. Tsai and colleagues reported their results of 10 obliterated ureteral segments, three associated with ureterovaginal fistula.[73] Ureteral continuity was established across all strictures. Four patients required subsequent balloon dilation; one of these ultimately needed an open reimplantation. All 3 patients with vaginal fistulas were dry.

REFERENCES

1. Hunner GL. End results in one hundred cases of ureteral stricture. J Urol 1924;12:295–315.
2. Illievitz AB. A new method for the removal of stone in the ureter. Surg Gynecol Obset 1925;40:575–6.
3. Doumashkin RL. Dilation of ureter with rubber bags in the treatment of ureteral calculi. J Urol 1926;59:851–62.
4. Pingoud EG, Bagley DH, Zeman RK, et al. Percutaneous antegrade bilateral dilation and stent placement for internal drainage. Radiology 1980;134:780.
5. Reimer DE, Oswalt GC Jr. Iatrogenic ureteral obstruction treated with balloon dilation. J Urol 1981;126:689–90.
6. Kadir S, White RI, Engle R. Balloon dilation of a ureteropelvic junction obstruction. Radiology 1982;147:427–33.
7. Waller RM 3rd, Finnerty DP, Casarella WJ. Transluminal balloon dilation of a tuberculous ureteral stricture. J Urol 1983;129:1225–6.
8. Glanz S, Gordon DH, Butt K, et al. Percutaneous transrenal balloon dilatation of the ureter. Radiology 1983;149:101–4.
9. Banner MP, Pollack HM. Dilation of ureteral stenoses: techniques and experience in 44 patients. AJR 1984;143: 789–93.
10. Lang EK. Antegrade ureteral stenting for dehiscence, strictures, and fistulae. AJR Am J Roentgenol 1984;143:795–801.
11. Lang EK, Glorioso LW 3rd. Antegrade transluminal dilatation of benign ureteral strictures: long-term results. AJR Am J Roentgenol 1988;150:131–4.
12. Chang R, Marshall FF, Mitchell S. Percutaneous management of benign ureteral strictures and fistulas. J Urol 1987;137: 1126–31.
13. Shapiro MJ, Banner MP, Amendola MA, et al. Balloon catheter dilation of ureteroenteric strictures: long-term results. Radiology 1988;168:385–7.
14. Finnerty DP, Trulock TS, Berkman W, Walton KN. Transluminal balloon dilation of ureteral strictures. J Urol 1984; 131:1056–60.
15. O'Brien WM, Maxted WC, Pahira JJ. Ureteral stricture: experience with 31 cases. J Urol 1988;140:737–40.
16. Davis DM. Intubated ureterotomy. Surg Gynecol Obset 1943;76.
17. Davis DM, Strong GH, Drake WM. Intubated ureterotomy: experimental work and clinical results. J Urol 1948;74: 476–84.
18. Oppenheimer R, Hinman FJ. Ureteral regeneration: contraction vs. hyperplasia of smooth muscle. J Urol 1955;74:476–84.
19. McDonald JH, Calamas JA. Experimental ureteral stricture: ureteral regrowth following ureterotomy with and without intubation. J Urol 1960;84:52–9.
20. Figenshau RS, Clayman RV, Wick MR, Stone AM. Acute histologic changes associated with endoureterotomy in the normal pig ureter. J Endourol 1991;5:357–61.
21. Schmeller N, Leitl F, Arnholdt H. Histology of ureter after unsuccessful endoscopic intubated incision. J Urol 1992; 147:450–2.
22. Wickham JE. Percutaneous pyelolysis. In: Wickham JE, Miller RA, editors. Percutaneous renal surgery. New York: Churchill Livingstone; 1983. p. 150.
23. Badlani G, Eshghi M, Smith AD. Percutaneous surgery for ureteropelvic junction obstruction (endopyelotomy): technique and early results. J Urol 1986;135:26–8.
24. Badlani G, Karlin G, Smith AD. Complications of endopyelotomy: analysis in series of 64 patients. J Urol 1988;140: 473–5.
25. Karlin GS, Badlani GH, Smith AD. Endopyelotomy versus open pyeloplasty: comparison in 88 patients. J Urol 1988; 140:476–8.
26. Smith AD. Management of iatrogenic ureteral strictures after urological procedures. J Urol 1988;140:1372–4.
27. Motola JA, Badlani GH, Smith AD. Results of 212 consecutive endopyelotomies: an 8-year followup. J Urol 1993; 149:453–6.
28. Clayman RV, Picus DD. Ureterorenoscopic endopyelotomy. Preliminary report. Urol Clin North Am 1988;15:433–8.
29. Hulbert JC, Hunter D, Castaneda-Zuniga W. Classification of and techniques for the reconstitution of acquired strictures in the region of the ureteropelvic junction. J Urol 1988;140:468–72.
30. Chandhoke PS, Clayman RV, Stone AM, et al. Endopyelotomy and endoureterotomy with the acucise ureteral cutting balloon device: preliminary experience. J Endourol 1993; 7:45–51.
31. Meretyk I, Meretyk S, Clayman RV. Endopyelotomy: comparison of ureteroscopic retrograde and antegrade percutaneous techniques. J Urol 1992;148:775–83.
32. Goldberg BB, Bagley D, Liu JB, et al. Endoluminal sonography of the urinary tract: preliminary observations. AJR Am J Roentgenol 1991;156:99–103.
33. Eshghi M, Lifson B. Cold knife endoureterotomy. In: Smith AD, editor. Controversies in endourology. Philadelphia: WB Saunders; 1995.
34. Harmon WJ, Sershon PD, Blute ML, et al. Ureteroscopy: current practice and long-term complications. J Urol 1997; 157:28–32.
35. Roberts WW, Cadeddu JA, Micali S, et al. Ureteral stricture formation after removal of impacted calculi. J Urol 1998; 159:723–6.
36. Ramanathan R, Kumar A, Kapoor R, Bhandari M. Relief of urinary tract obstruction in tuberculosis to improve renal function. Analysis of predictive factors. Br J Urol 1998; 81:199–205.
37. Ghoneim MA, Nebeeh A, El-Kappany H. Endourologic treatment of ureteral strictures. J Endourol 1988;2:263–70.
38. ElAbd SA, ElShaer AF, ElMahrouky AS, et al. Long-term results of endourologic and percutaneous management of ureteral strictures in bilharzial patients. J Endourol 1996; 10:35–43.
39. Caoili EM, Cohan RH, Korobkin M, et al. Urinary tract abnormalities: initial experience with multi-detector row CT urography. Radiology 2002;222:353–60.
40. Krueger RP, Ash JM, Silver MM, et al. Primary hydronephrosis. Assessment of diuretic renography, pelvis perfusion pressure, operative findings, and renal and ureteral histology. Urol Clin North Am 1980;7:231–42.
41. Preminger GM, Clayman RV, Nakada SY, et al. A multicenter clinical trial investigating the use of a fluoroscopically controlled cutting balloon catheter for the management of ureteral and ureteropelvic junction obstruction. J Urol 1997;157:1625–9.
42. Walz J, Lecamus C, Lechevallier E, et al. [Complications of "Acucise" balloon endopyelotomy]. Prog Urol 2003;13: 39–45.
43. Yamada S, Ono Y, Ohshima S, Miyake K. Transurethral ureteroscopic ureterotomy assisted by a prior balloon dilation for relieving ureteral strictures. J Urol 1995;153:1418–21.
44. Grasso M, Loisides P, Rouse G, Bagley D. Intraluminal ultrasound: a new technique for assessing the upper urinary tract. J Urol 1994;151:336.
45. Eshghi M. Endoscopic incisions of the urinary tract. Part II. AUA Update Series 1989;37:298–303.
46. Bagley D, Erhard M. Use of the holmium laser in the upper urinary tract. Tech Urol 1995;1:25–30.
47. Kourambas J, Delvecchio FC, Preminger GM. Low-power holmium laser for the management of urinary tract calculi, strictures, and tumors. J Endourol 2001;15:529–32.
48. Nord RG, Cubler-Goodman A, Bagley D. Prone split-leg position for simultaneous retrograde ureteroscopic and percutaneous nephroscopic procedures. J Endourol 1991;5:13–5.
49. Bagley DH, Liu JB, Grasso M, Goldberg BB. Endoluminal sonography in evaluation of the obstructed ureteropelvic junction. J Endourol 1994;8:287–92.
50. Hwang TK, Yoon JY, Ahn JH, Park YH. Percutaneous endoscopic management of upper ureteral stricture size of stent. J Urol 1996;155:882–4.
51. Moon YT, Kerbl K, Pearle MS, et al. Evaluation of optimal stent size after endourologic incision of ureteral strictures. J Endourol 1995;9:15–22.
52. Kerbl K, Chandhoke PS, Figenshau RS, et al. Effect of stent duration on ureteral healing following endoureterotomy in an animal model. J Urol 1993;150:1302–5.
53. Thomas MA, Ong AM, Pinto PA, et al. Management of obliterated urinary segments using a laser fiber for access. J Urol 2003;169:2284–6.
54. Sullivan JW, Grabstald H, Whitmore WF Jr. Complications of ureteroileal conduit with radical cystectomy: review of 336 cases. J Urol 1980;124:797–801.
55. Kramolowsky EV, Clayman RV, Weyman PJ. Endourological management of ureteroileal anastomotic strictures: is it effective? J Urol 1987;137:390–4.
56. Vandenbroucke F, Van Poppel H, Vandeursen H, et al. Surgical versus endoscopic treatment of non-malignant ureteroileal anastomotic strictures. Br J Urol 1993;71:408–12.
57. Streem SB, Novick AC, Steinmuller DR, et al. Long-term efficacy of ureteral dilation for transplant ureteral stenosis. J Urol 1988;140:32–5.
58. Bhayani SB, Landman J, Slotoroff C, Figenshau RS. Transplant ureter stricture: Acucise endoureterotomy and balloon dilation are effective. J Endourol 2003;17:19–22.
59. Strup SE, Bagley DH. Endoscopic ureteroneocystostomy for complete obstruction at the ureterovesical junction. J Urol 1996;156:360–2.
60. Hall SJ, Babayan RK. Treatment of ureteral strictures and UPJ obstruction with the Acucise catheter: two-year followup. J Urol 1994;151:280.
61. Ravery V, de la Taille A, Hoffmann P, et al. Balloon catheter dilatation in the treatment of ureteral and ureteroenteric stricture. J Endourol 1998;12:335–40.
62. Kwak S, Leef JA, Rosenblum JD. Percutaneous balloon catheter dilatation of benign ureteral strictures: effect of multiple dilatation procedures on long-term patency. AJR Am J Roentgenol 1995;165:97–100.
63. Richter F, Irwin RJ, Watson RA, Lang EK. Endourologic management of benign ureteral strictures with and without compromised vascular supply. Urology 2000;55:652–7.
64. Franco I, Eshghi M, Bruder J, et al. Endourological management of 40 ureteral strictures. J Urol 1994;151:201.
65. Thomas R. Choosing the ideal candidate for ureteroscopic endoureterotomy. J Urol 1993;149:314.
66. Singal RK, Denstedt JD, Razvi HA, Chun SS. Holmium:YAG laser endoureterotomy for treatment of ureteral stricture. Urology 1997;50:875–80.
67. Wolf JS Jr, Elashry OM, Clayman RV. Long-term results of endoureterotomy for benign ureteral and ureteroenteric strictures. J Urol 1997;158:759–64.
68. Watterson JD, Sofer M, Wollin TA, et al. Holmium:YAG laser endoureterotomy for ureterointestinal strictures. J Urol 2002;167:1692–5.
69. Poulakis V, Witzsch U, De Vries R, Becht E. Cold-knife endoureterotomy for nonmalignant ureterointestinal anastomotic strictures. Urology 2003;61:512–7.

70. Lin DW, Bush WH, Mayo ME. Endourological treatment of ureteroenteric strictures: efficacy of Acucise endoureterotomy. J Urol 1999;162:696–8.

71. Bosma RJ, van Driel MF, van Son WJ, et al. Endourological management of ureteral obstruction after renal transplantation. J Urol 1996;156:1099–100.

72. Conlin MJ, Gomella LG, Bagley DH. Endoscopic ureteroureterostomy for obliterated ureteral segments. J Urol 1996;156:1394–9.

73. Tsai CK, Taylor FC, Beaghler MA. Endoscopic ureteroureterostomy: long-term followup using a new technique. J Urol 2000;164:332–5.

74. Cohen TD, Gross MB, Preminger GM. Long-term follow-up of Acucise incision of ureteropelvic junction obstruction and ureteral strictures. Urology 1996;47:317–23.

75. Lopatkin NA, Martov AG, Gushchin BL. An endourologic approach to complete ureteropelvic junction and ureteral strictures. J Endourol 2000;14:721–6.

76. Schneider AW, Conrad S, Busch R, Otto U. The cold-knife technique for endourological management of stenoses in the upper urinary tract. J Urol 1991;146:961–5.

35

Postoperative Care Following Ureteroscopic Procedures

Ramsay L. Kuo, MD

Advances in endoscopic technology have greatly reduced the caliber of today's ureteroscopes. This trend toward miniaturization has decreased procedural morbidity, as illustrated by a study comparing ureteroscopic complications at a single institution during the early 1980s to those in the early 1990s. Over this period, significant complications such as ureteral avulsion, stricture formation, and perforations decreased from 6.6% to 1.5%.[1]

Other factors have greatly expanded the range of applications for ureteroscopy. First, current flexible ureteroscopes provide significantly improved deflection capabilities, with some models possessing secondary active deflection and others enhanced primary active deflection.[2,3] This alone facilitates access to all portions of the collecting system. Refinements in adjunctive instruments have also been critical in facilitating the ureteroscopic treatment of upper tract pathology. For example, the holmium laser has proven itself to be a versatile lithotrite that is capable of fragmenting calculi of any composition.[4] As a result, more urologists are now employing ureteroscopic lithotripsy to successfully treat complex proximal stone burdens.[5] Holmium energy also produces precise soft tissue incisions in a hemostatic fashion, with a limited penetration depth of 0.4 mm.[6,7] This has made it a preferred modality for ureteroscopic endoureterotomies[8,9] and endopyelotomies.[10,11] Finally, improvements in instruments such as retrieval baskets and biopsy forceps as well as the neodymium:yttrium-aluminum-garnet (Nd:YAG) laser have led to effective ureteroscopic diagnosis and treatment of localized upper tract transitional cell carcinoma (TCC).

This chapter will provide a general overview of postoperative care following ureteroscopic procedures, with particular attention to care modifications needed after specific applications.

DIET AND ACTIVITY

Following the majority of ureteroscopic procedures, patients may be advanced as tolerated to a regular diet and are encouraged to ambulate once recovered from anesthesia. Increased oral fluid intake is often beneficial to help promote urine production and prevent clot formation. Most patients undergoing ureteroscopic lithotripsy are treated on an outpatient basis,[12] whereas overnight stays are suggested for those undergoing more invasive ureteroscopic interventions such as upper tract tumor ablation, endoureterotomy, or endopyelo-

tomy to ensure the absence of postprocedural complications such as hemorrhage. Other indications for hospital admission are listed in Table 35-1.

Patients with indwelling ureteral stents should avoid heavy lifting to prevent urine reflux into the stented kidney and associated flank discomfort. This also applies to patients who have undergone a full thickness ureteral incision to minimize the possibility of urine leak. These patients should also be counseled to perform timed voiding every 3 to 4 hours to prevent bladder overdistention and subsequent reflux.

POSTOPERATIVE MEDICATIONS

PAIN MEDICATIONS Postoperative discomfort is typically treated with oral narcotics. Patients with normal renal function may benefit from an adjunctive immediate dose of intravenous ketorolac postoperatively or in the recovery room. For those patients requiring indwelling ureteral stents, a course of a urinary analgesic such as phenazopyridine or Urised may be useful for relief of irritative voiding symptoms. A low-dose anticholinergic regimen may also be prescribed to decrease the severity of urgency and frequency symptoms associated with stenting.

ANTIBIOTIC COVERAGE A urinalysis and urine culture should have been obtained preoperatively in all patients, and active infections treated appropriately prior to ureteroscopic instrumentation. Postoperative bacteriuria has been documented following endoscopic procedures such as transurethral resection of the prostate and transurethral resection of bladder tumors. A prophylactic course of antibiotics can reduce the incidence of urinary tract infection.[13]

Table 35-1 Indications for Postoperative Admission following Ureteroscopy

Physical
Fever/sepsis
Intractable pain
Ureteral perforation or collecting system extravasation
Intractable nausea or emesis
Instillation of upper tract chemotherapy or immunotherapy

Social
Inability to arrange transportation
Lack of caretaker

Concern for the development of antibiotic resistance has led to efforts to clearly define both the most effective antibiotic type and the optimal duration of antibiotic prophylaxis following an endourologic procedure. A recent double-blinded, randomized trial examined the efficacy of a single 500 mg dose of oral ciprofloxacin compared to a gram of intravenous cefazolin given two hours preoperatively in 100 patients undergoing outpatient endourologic procedures, which included diagnostic and therapeutic ureteroscopy.[14] Because the incidence of postoperative UTI was not significantly different between the ciprofloxacin and cefazolin groups (8.1 vs 10.0%) and the cost of oral ciprofloxacin was substantially less, the authors concluded that administration of ciprofloxacin was preferable.

When stents are placed following ureteroscopy, the risk of urinary tract infection increases substantially with longer indwelling times.[15] This phenomenon is secondary to biofilm formation on the surface of stents, which leads to bacterial colonization.[16,17] To prevent infection, a 3- to 7-day course of prophylactic antibiotics is typically given after ureteroscopic procedures requiring an extended period of stenting.[16,18] In particular, fluoroquinolones have been shown to prevent adherence of organisms to stent surfaces and also absorb into stent materials.[17] For this reason, it has been suggested that the optimal stent prophylaxis regimen should consist of an immediate 3 days of fluoroquinolones postoperatively, followed by a 3-day course every 2 weeks while the stent remains in place.[16]

POSTOPERATIVE STENTING

Indwelling ureteral stents serve a number of purposes postoperatively, with specific situations requiring stenting described below. Following ureteroscopic lithotripsy, stents can not only bypass transient ureteral edema, but also passively dilate the ureter to assist in fragment passage. Following ureteroscopic endoureterotomy or endopyelotomy, a stent facilitates urine flow into the bladder and prevents stricture formation in the incised portion of the ureter. An indwelling stent should be placed following any ureteroscopic procedure with associated urinary extravasation (ie, collecting system or ureteral perforation) and left for 10 to 14 days.

It is important to counsel patients preoperatively that the stent itself can cause significant post-procedural irritative symptoms, including dysuria, urinary frequency and urgency, as well as hematuria and flank discomfort.[19–22] Stented patients who develop severe pain must be evaluated for stent migration, as this has been shown to occur in up to 3.7% of patients.[15] For those patients requiring extended stenting periods, the surgeon must emphasize the importance of follow-up for stent removal and keep diligent records of these patients to prevent severe complications associated with forgotten devices such as obstruction, sepsis, and stent calcification.

FOLLOWING URETERAL ORIFICE/INTRAMURAL URETER DILATION

The need for active dilation of the ureteral orifice and intramural ureter to facilitate ureteroscopic insertion has decreased dramatically as scopes have miniaturized. A study looking specifically at use of the 6.9 French (6.9F) semi-rigid ureteroscope found that ureteral dilation was required in only 6% of cases.[23] In general, a stent should be left for 4 to 5 days if the ureteral orifice has undergone either balloon or sequential dilation to facilitate ureteroscopic access. This management is based on minipig studies where dilation of the distal third of the ureter to 10F using graded Teflon dilators or pressure balloons resulted in obstruction for up to 96 hours postoperatively, as measured by DTPA renograms.[24]

With appropriate stenting after ureteral dilation, the incidence of stricture formation is low. In 122 patients who had had postoperative stents placed after dilation of the ureteral orifice and intramural ureter to 5 or 6 mm to facilitate ureteroscopic access, 45 had available intravenous pyelogram or retrograde pyelogram studies performed at a median of 12 months postoperatively showing no evidence of stricture.[25]

More recently, the ureteral access sheath has gained popularity as a method to facilitate insertion of flexible ureteroscopes. All access sheath devices gradually increase in caliber further proximally, such that the ureteral orifice undergoes gradual dilation upon insertion of the device. Because of the large caliber of these devices compared to those of the ureteroscopes themselves, concerns about potential ureteral ischemia and subsequent stricture formation have been raised. A swine model was used to examine proximal ureteral blood flow in a control group and in animals following insertion of 10/12F, 12/14F, and 14/16F access sheaths.[26] Laser Doppler flowmetry readings over 70-minute periods showed that blood flow was initially decreased over 50% from baseline in the 12/14F and 14/16F groups. Although ureteral blood flow gradually returned to normal during the evaluation period in all sheathed groups, the resumption of normal flow was slowest in the animals where the largest caliber sheaths were used.

Another study retrospectively examined the incidence of postoperative strictures following ureteral access sheath usage for ureteroscopic lithotripsy.[27] Of the 71 ureteroscopic procedures in which an access sheath was used, the mean follow-up for this patient cohort was 332 days, and the 12/14F sheath accounted for 78.9% of the devices employed. Notably, only one stricture (1.4%) was detected on postoperative imaging in a patient requiring multiple ureteroscopies for stone burden clearance. However, the majority of patients in this series (87.3%) were stented for 3 to 5 days postoperatively.

Although the incidence of complications associated with the use of ureteral access sheaths appears to be low, further long-term follow-up to accurately assess the incidence of stricture formation is needed. In the interim, it appears prudent to use smaller caliber sheaths and to place an indwelling stent for at least 3 days postoperatively.

STENTING AFTER UNCOMPLICATED URETEROSCOPIC LITHOTRIPSY

An area of continued debate is the need for postoperative stenting following uncomplicated ureteroscopic lithotripsy when the ureteral orifice has not been dilated. Traditionally, indwelling ureteral stents are placed for 48 to 72 hours, even if no significant stone fragments remain in the upper tract, in order to prevent transient renal obstruction. But the patient often suffers significantly decreased quality of life from the presence of the stent.[21] Others have also shown that stent placement can raise costs (eg, increased operating room time; costs associated with device removal).

Because of the negative aspects of ureteral stenting, the need for stent placement following uncomplicated ureteroscopic lithotripsy has been questioned. Many investigators have already shown that unstented patients have minimal complications following the ureteroscopic treatment of distal ureteral calculi.[28–30] More recently, a randomized, prospective clinical trial examined the outcomes of stented and unstented patients undergoing ureteroscopic lithotripsy of proximal, mid, and distal ureteral calculi.[31] The outcomes and complications in these two groups were not different; the stented patients, however, had significantly more urinary symptoms ($p < .005$). For these reasons, the authors concluded that routine placement of stents is not necessary.

The advent of biodegradable stents may eventually eliminate the debate on indwelling stent placement after uncomplicated ureteroscopic lithotripsy. The concept of a self-degrading stent is attractive because it would prevent immediate postoperative obstruction as well as the need for an additional procedure to remove the device. Recently, phase I and II clinical trials of a new biodegradable stent, termed a temporary ureteral drainage stent (TUDS), have been completed.[32,33] During the multicenter TUDS phase II trial, the devices were placed retrogradely following completion of uncomplicated ureteroscopy. Stent effectiveness was defined as adequate, intervention-free drainage for 48 hours with maintenance of ureteral position. In this trial, the overall stent effectiveness rate was 78.2%, with a median time of complete passage from the body of 15 days. Further refinements to these dissolvable stents, particularly an improvement in the predictability of short-term dissolution, may result in widespread use of these devices after ureteroscopic lithotripsy.

At present, the option of leaving the ureter unstented following routine ureteroscopic lithotripsy is left to the surgeon's discretion. Patients should be counseled that absence of a stent will greatly reduce the possibility of irritative voiding symptoms. The risk of readmission, however, tends to be higher in unstented patients (4.3 vs 1.5%),[34] and development of symptoms such as intractable pain, nausea, emesis, or fever in an unstented patient requires immediate evaluation.

URETEROSCOPIC ENDOPYELOTOMY AND ENDOURETEROTOMY

Conservatively, an indwelling stent should be left in place for 6 weeks to allow for complete urothelial regeneration and to prevent stenosis of the ureteropelvic junction or incised ureteral segment. This time period is based on the observed time period for ureteral regeneration following the Davis intubated ureterotomy.[35] The type of stent used can vary. In the past, the 7/14F endopyelotomy stent was typically used. More recently, smaller 7/10F stents and 7F double pigtail stents have become more popular.

IMMEDIATE FOLLOW-UP

URETEROSCOPIC LITHOTRIPSY

In cases of uncomplicated ureteroscopic lithotripsy, no postoperative labs are generally required. Patients with possible infection-related calculi should be very closely monitored for the development of sepsis (ie, hypotension, fever, pulmonary distress, increasing leukocytosis).

UPPER TRACT TCC

In general, an indwelling ureteral stent should remain for 2 to 7 days following an uncomplicated case of ureteroscopic surgery for upper tract TCC. In situations where patients have more aggressive pathology (Grade 2) or have a solitary renal unit, retrograde installation of agents through an open-ended ureteral catheter may be considered. Infusion of bacille Calmette-Guérin through ureteral catheters has been associated with the development of ureteral stricture formation[36] and should not be performed immediately post-treatment because of the risk of systemic infection through treated areas of the collecting system.

Use of mitomycin has been advocated immediately following ureteroscopic treatment of upper tract TCC because of its low–side-effect profile. Forty milligrams of mitomycin are diluted in 30 cc of saline and then administered through the open-ended ureteral catheter in 10 cc increments.[37] Additional prospective, randomized long-term studies are required to firmly define the efficacy of adjuvant agents used in the treatment of upper tract TCC.

URETEROSCOPIC ENDOPYELOTOMY AND ENDOURETEROTOMY

Serum chemistries and a complete blood count should be obtained in the recovery room postoperatively and on postoperative day 1. A foley catheter is left for at least 24 hours to prevent urinary extravasation through the endoscopic incision.

The safety of ureteroscopic endopyelotomy has been greatly improved through the use of preoperative imaging modalities such as computed tomography (CT) angiogram and the endoluminal ultrasonography. One series of 46 holmium laser ureteroscopic endopyelotomies had only one postoperative case of bleeding consisting of a subcapsular hematoma,[38] whereas another series of 28 cases imaged preoperatively with endoluminal ultrasonography had no incidents of intraoperative or postoperative hemorrhage.[39] Nevertheless, bleeding is the most potentially serious short-term complication in these patients, and therefore, postoperative hemoglobin levels and vital signs must be closely monitored to detect early evidence of hemorrhage.

LONG-TERM FOLLOW-UP

Ureteroscopic Lithotripsy   Imaging is generally obtained within 6 weeks postoperatively to document the presence and location of residual stone burden. The need for additional routine imaging (either intravenous pyelography or ultrasonography) to assess for the possibility of obstruction after ureteroscopic lithotripsy is a subject of debate. One retrospective review found that only patients with at least one of the following preoperative risk factors, including ureteral trauma, decreased renal function, chronic stone impaction, endoscopic evidence of stricture, postoperative flank pain, or postoperative fever, developed an obstruction; hence, the authors recommended that only patients with one of these risk factors should be assessed for post-procedural obstruction.[40] But another recent retrospective review of ureteroscopic lithotripsy procedures revealed asymptomatic obstruction in 7 patients, or 2.9% of the total cohort of 241 patients.[41] This lends support to obtaining routine postoperative upper tract studies that can assess patients for evidence of obstructive uropathy as well as calculi (renal ultrasonography with plain abdominal film, intravenous pyelogram with tomography images, or non-contrast CT scan).

Upper Tract TCC   Strict surveillance protocols combining cystoscopy, retrograde pyelograms and ureteroscopic evaluation of the upper tracts are necessary for the early detection of tumor recurrence. Chen and Bagley suggest that all three modalities should be performed every 3 months until the patient has been tumor free for 6 months.[42] Subsequently, a cystoscopy is performed every 3 months for 2 years, every 6 months for another 2 years, and then annually in conjunction with a retrograde pyelogram and ureteroscopic evaluation every 6 months. Ureteroscopy is essential for the early detection of recurrent tumors, as non-invasive tests such as urinalysis, urine cytology and retrogrades alone have inferior sensitivities as low as 25%.[43,44]

In the future, CT can be expected to play a larger role in the routine surveillance of upper tract TCC. For an initial evaluation of the upper urinary tract, CT offers superior sensitivity in the detection of renal masses and calculi as well as the ability to identify other abdominal pathology.[45] Unfortunately, assessment of intraluminal pathology has been suboptimal in the past and has necessitated the use of adjunctive intravenous pyelography. But current multi-detector row CT urography has successfully detected tumors as small as 5 mm.[46,47] As resolution improves in the future, CT will likely supplant other radiologic studies in the evaluation of the upper urinary tract.

Ureteroscopic Endoureterotomy   Overall, long term results of ureteroscopic endoureterotomy have shown success rates ranging from 62 to 80%.[8,48,49] Patency rates vary depending on the etiology of the ureteral stricture, with those resulting from ischemia and the setting of ureteroenteric anastomoses having very poor success rates. Follow-up should include an intravenous pyelogram or diuretic renal scan within 4 to 6 weeks of stent removal to document clinical improvement. For patients felt to be at high risk for stricture recurrence, radiographic surveillance should be diligently performed (ie, every 3 months during the first year postoperatively).

Ureteroscopic Endopyelotomy   An upper tract study consisting of either an intravenous pyelogram or diuretic renogram should be performed within 4 to 6 weeks after stent removal to document improvement in drainage. Long-term success rates of ureteroscopic endopyelotomies have ranged from 79 to 87.5%.[10,11,39,50,51] A recent manuscript found no significant differences among the restenosis rates of the hot-wire balloon, percutaneous antegrade and ureteroscopic endopyelotomy approaches.[52] Importantly, restenosis occurred at a mean of 10.3 months after surgery, with some failures presenting up to 3 years later. As a result, the authors recommend follow-up radiographic imaging through this time period to detect these late complications.

CONCLUSIONS

With advances in both ureteroscopes and adjunctive equipment, the range of upper tract pathology treatable with the ureteroscopic approach has become quite broad. Once skillful treatment of the patient has been accomplished, appropriate follow-up evaluations are required to ensure an optimal outcome. In the future, further technological developments are certain to further minimize complications and improve the results of ureteroscopic procedures.

REFERENCES

1. Harmon WJ, Sershon PD, Blute ML, et al. Ureteroscopy: current practice and long-term complications. J Urol 1997;157:28–32.
2. Lobik L, Lopez-Pujals A, Leveillee RJ. Variables affecting deflection of a new third-generation flexible ureteropyeloscope (DUR-8 elite). J Endourol 2003;17:733–6.
3. Johnson GB, Grasso M. Exaggerated primary endoscope deflection: initial clinical experience with prototype flexible ureteroscopes. BJU Int 2004;93:109–14.
4. Grasso M. Experience with the holmium laser as an endoscopic lithotrite. Urology 1996;48:199–206.
5. Chow GK, Patterson DE, Blute ML, Segura JW. Ureteroscopy: effect of technology and technique on clinical practice. J Urol 2003;170:99–102.
6. Kuo RL, Paterson RF, Siqueira TM Jr, et al. Holmium laser enucleation of the prostate: morbidity in a series of 206 patients. Urology 2003;62:59–63.
7. Razvi HA, Chun SS, Denstedt JD, Sales JL. Soft-tissue applications of the holmium:YAG laser in urology. J Endourol 1995;9:387–90.
8. Singal RK, Denstedt JD, Razvi HA, Chun SS. Holmium:YAG laser endoureterotomy for treatment of ureteral stricture. Urology 1997;50:875–80.
9. Gerber GS, Alsikafi NF. Retrograde ureteroscopic incision for the treatment of nonureteroenteric ureteral strictures. Tech Urol 2000;6:12–4.
10. Conlin MJ, Bagley DH. Ureteroscopic endopyelotomy at a single setting. J Urol 1998;59:727–31.
11. Gerber GS, Kim JC. Ureteroscopic endopyelotomy in the treatment of patients with ureteropelvic junction obstruction. Urology 2000;55:198–202; discussion 202–3.
12. Tawfiek ER, Bagley DH: Management of upper urinary tract calculi with ureteroscopic techniques. Urology 1999; 53:25–31.
13. Charton M, Mombet A, Gattegno B: Urinary tract infection prophylaxis in transurethral surgery: oral lomefloxacin versus parenteral cefuroxime. Am J Med 1992;92 (Suppl): 118–120.
14. Christiano AP, Hollowell CM, Kim H, et al. Double-blind randomized comparison of single-dose ciprofloxacin versus intravenous cefazolin in patients undergoing outpatient endourologic surgery. Urology 2000;55:182–5.
15. el-Faqih SR, Shamsuddin AB, Chakrabarti A, et al. Polyurethane internal ureteral stents in treatment of stone patients: morbidity related to indwelling times. J Urol 1991;146:1487–91.
16. Denstedt JD, Wollin TA, Reid G. Biomaterials used in urology: current issues of biocompatibility, infection, and encrustation. J Endourol 1998;12:493–500.
17. Wollin TA, Tieszer C, Riddell JV, et al. Bacterial biofilm formation, encrustation, and antibiotic adsorption to ureteral stents indwelling in humans. J Endourol 1998;12:101–11.
18. Mendez-Torres FR, Urena R, Thomas R. Retrograde ureteroscopic endopyelotomy. Urol Clin North Am 2004;31: 99–106.
19. Pollard SG, Macfarlane R. Symptoms arising from Double-J ureteral stents. J Urol 1988;139:37–8.
20. Pryor JL, Langley MJ, Jenkins AD. Comparison of symptom characteristics of indwelling ureteral catheters. J Urol 1991;145:719–22.
21. Joshi HB, Stainthorpe A, MacDonagh RP, et al. Indwelling ureteral stents: evaluation of symptoms, quality of life and utility. J Urol 2003;169:1065–9; discussion 1069.
22. Rane A, Saleemi A, Cahill D, et al. Have stent-related symptoms anything to do with placement technique? J Endourol 2001;15:741–5.
23. Abdel-Razzak O, Bagley DH. The 6.9 F semirigid ureteroscope in clinical use. Urology 1993;41:45–8.
24. Boddy SA, Nimmon CC, Jones S, et al. Acute ureteric dilatation for ureteroscopy. An experimental study. Br J Urol 1988;61:27–31.
25. Huffman JL, Bagley DH. Balloon dilation of the ureter for ureteroscopy. J Urol 1988;140:954–6.
26. Lallas CD, Auge BK, Raj GV, et al. Laser Doppler flowmetric determination of ureteral blood flow after ureteral access sheath placement. J Endourol 2002;16:583–90.
27. Delvecchio FC, Auge BK, Brizuela RM, et al. Assessment of stricture formation with the ureteral access sheath. Urology 2003;61:518–22; discussion 522.
28. Rane A, Cahill D, Larner T, et al. To stent or not to stent? That is still the question. J Endourol 2000;14:479–81.
29. Hosking DH, McColm SE, Smith WE. Is stenting following ureteroscopy for removal of distal ureteral calculi necessary? J Urol 1999;161:48–50.
30. Borboroglu PG, Amling CL, Schenkman NS, et al. Ureteral stenting after ureteroscopy for distal ureteral calculi: a multi-institutional prospective randomized controlled study assessing pain, outcomes and complications. J Urol 2001;166:1651–7.
31. Denstedt JD, Wollin TA, Sofer M, et al. A prospective randomized controlled trial comparing nonstented versus stented ureteroscopic lithotripsy. J Urol 2001;165:1419–22.
32. Lingeman JE, Schulsinger DA, Kuo RL. Phase I trial of a temporary ureteral drainage stent. J Endourol 2003;17:169–71.
33. Lingeman JE, Preminger GM, Berger Y, et al. Use of a temporary ureteral drainage stent after uncomplicated

ureteroscopy: results from a phase II clinical trial. J Urol 2003;169:1682–8.

34. Knudsen BE, Beiko DT, Denstedt JD. Stenting after ureteroscopy: pros and cons. Urol Clin North Am 2004;31:173–80.

35. Davis D, Strong G, Drake W. Intubated ureterotomy: experimental work and clinical results. J Urol 1948;59:851–862.

36. Yokogi H, Wada Y, Mizutani M, et al. Bacillus Calmette-Guerin perfusion therapy for carcinoma in situ of the upper urinary tract. Br J Urol 1996;77:676–9.

37. Keeley FX Jr, Bagley DH. Adjuvant mitomycin C following endoscopic treatment of upper tract transitional cell carcinoma. J Urol 1997;158:2074–7.

38. Matin SF, Yost A, Streem SB. Ureteroscopic laser endopyelotomy: a single-center experience. J Endourol 2003;17:401–4.

39. Giddens JL, Grasso M. Retrograde ureteroscopic endopyelotomy using the holmium:YAG laser. J Urol 2000;164:1509–12.

40. Beiko DT, Beasley KA, Koka PK, et al. Upper tract imaging after ureteroscopic holmium:YAG laser lithotripsy: when is it necessary? Can J Urol 2003;10:2062–7.

41. Weizer AZ, Auge BK, Silverstein AD, et al. Routine postoperative imaging is important after ureteroscopic stone manipulation. J Urol 2002;168:46–50.

42. Chen GL, Bagley DH. Ureteroscopic surgery for upper tract transitional-cell carcinoma: complications and management. J Endourol 2001;15:399–404; discussion 409.

43. Keeley FX Jr, Bibbo M, Bagley DH. Ureteroscopic treatment and surveillance of upper urinary tract transitional cell carcinoma. J Urol 1997;157:1560–5.

44. Chen GL, El-Gabry EA, Bagley DH. Surveillance of upper urinary tract transitional cell carcinoma: the role of ureteroscopy, retrograde pyelography, cytology and urinalysis. J Urol 2000;164:1901–4.

45. Joffe SA, Servaes S, Okon S, Horowitz M. Multi-detector row CT urography in the evaluation of hematuria. Radiographics 2003;23:1441–55; discussion 1455–6.

46. Caoili EM. Imaging of the urinary tract using multidetector computed tomography urography. Semin Urol Oncol 2002;20:174–9.

47. Caoili EM, Cohan RH, Korobkin M, et al. Urinary tract abnormalities: initial experience with multi-detector row CT urography. Radiology 2002;222:353–60.

48. Meretyk S, Albala DM, Clayman RV, et al. Endoureterotomy for treatment of ureteral strictures. J Urol 1992;147:1502–6.

49. Wolf JS Jr, Elashry OM, Clayman RV. Long-term results of endoureterotomy for benign ureteral and ureteroenteric strictures. J Urol 1997;158:759–64.

50. Meretyk I, Meretyk S, Clayman RV. Endopyelotomy: comparison of ureteroscopic retrograde and antegrade percutaneous techniques. J Urol 1992;148:775–82; discussion 782–3.

51. Tawfiek ER, Liu JB, Bagley DH.Ureteroscopic treatment of ureteropelvic junction obstruction. J Urol 1998;160:1643–6; discussion 1646–7.

52. Albani JM, Yost AJ, Streem SB. Ureteropelvic junction obstruction: determining durability of endourological intervention. J Urol 2004;171:579–82.

36

Ureteroscopy: Complications

Filiberto Zattoni, MD

Progression from urethrocystoscopy to the endoscopic examination of the ureter and pyelocaliceal cavities must be considered a natural continuum since ureteroscopy has become a routine examination for all urologists. The introduction of ureteroscopy modified the diagnostic approach to the ureter and renal cavities as well the treatment of urinary stones and other upper tract urinary diseases.

Both the miniaturization of the instruments (rigid ureteroscopes and ancillary devices) and the spreading use of flexible endoscopes will increase, more and more in the near future, the indications for the direct visual examination of the upper urinary tract. The continuous refinement of the instruments, combined with improved endourologic techniques, significantly shortened the learning curves, and at the same time, reduced the complication rate.[1] On these bases, ureteroscopy has been proposed as an outpatient procedure because of its inherent nature as a purely endoscopic examination with minimal bleeding and relatively short operative time.[2,3] This chapter, besides some notes on the pertinent anatomy and discussion of some technical aspects related to the endoscopic procedures, will offer a comprehensive summary of ureteroscopy as it pertains to intraoperative, early, and late complications. Suggestions on how to reduce undesirable events, and solutions to manage the different situations that may arise, will be offered based on the daily experience.

URETERAL ANATOMY RELEVANT TO THE ENDOSCOPIST

The ureter is a hollow muscular tube that measures approximately 25 to 30 cm in length; it connects the renal pelvis to the urinary bladder. It runs downward, closely adherent to the peritoneum throughout most of its course (Figure 36-1). The ureter has a relatively straight course in the abdominal cavity; after crossing the iliac vessels, it follows a broad lateral convex shape. The ureter is comprised of three layers: mucosal (lined by transitional epithelium), muscular, and fibrous. The ureteral diameter is different at the various segments (Table 36-1). The varying thickness of the layers in the ureteral wall, at different sites, explains the different types of complications that may occur during endoscopic instrumentation. Submucosal tunneling and false passage are more likely distally, where the transitional layer is more redundant and bulkier, and a thick muscular backing is present. On the other hand, perforation and avulsion occur more commonly in the proximal ureter where the muscular wall is less well-defined. The arteries supplying the ureter are branches from the aorta, renal, and gonadal arteries in the abdominal portion along with branches from the common and internal iliac, vesical, and uterine arteries in the pelvic portion. The close relationship with the gonadal vein in the upper part, with the iliac vessels in the mid-part, and with the internal iliac vessels in the lower part, must be kept in mind when a ureteral stricture is treated endoscopically. The site of the incision during ureterotomy should be carefully chosen, depending on the exact location of the stricture.[4]

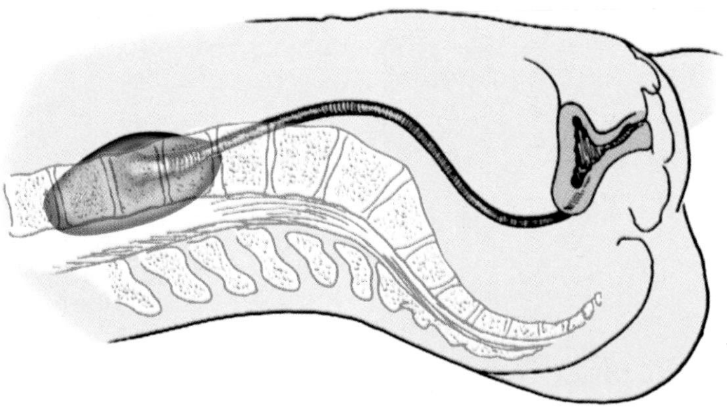

APPROACH TO THE URETER

The ureter is usually approached in a retrograde fashion. In case that retrograde approach is not feasible, an antegrade access to the upper urinary tract has to be performed. Such an approach may be considered for a stone located in the upper part of the ureter with dilation of the above ureter and renal cavities when the ureter, below the stone, is very tight and does not allow for instrument introduction, or the ureteral orifice is not found or reachable for any reason. Through the nephrostomic access, a flexible instrument can be used in order to reach the ureter (Figure 36-2). Otherwise, a rigid instrument is used in case the access to the kidney was created in a straight line with the ureter (Figure 36-3).

CONTROVERSIAL ISSUES

DILATION OF URETERAL ORIFICE Balloon dilation of the ureteral orifice allows for a more rapid and less forceful access into the ureter; an easier extraction of larger or irregularly shaped calculi is even permitted, often obviating the need for mechanical fragmentation.[5] Balloons of 4 to 10 cm in length are commercially available and inflate to 4 to 10 mm in diameter (12 French to 30 F). Four centimeters in length, with inflation simply obtained using a luer-lock syringe, is sufficient in most instances. Techniques for rigid ureteroscope access without dilation also have been described, especially using smaller ureteroscopes.[6] Flexible ureteroscopy usually requires ureteral orifice dilatation secondary to the flexibility and the low flow of irrigation of the instrument.[7] A peel-away introducer sheath can be suggested in the case of flexible ureteroscopy. Complications that can occur with such a dilatation include balloon rupture from overinflation; mucosal tearing, bleeding, and extravasation are possible if inflation is performed too rapidly. Stone impaction or extrusion can occur if the balloon straddles the stone prior to inflation.[8] Distal ureteral strictures, following orifice dilation, were usually associated with fascial dilators or metal bougies and not with balloon dilators.[9,10] On the other hand and under the economic point of view, a substantial decrease in operative costs should be expected by not using expensive balloon dilating catheters.

Figure 36-1 Lateral view of the serpentine course of the ureter.

Table 36-1 Ureteral Diameter at Various Locations		
Level of Ureter	Approximate Non-dilated Diameter (mm)	Size (F)
Intramural	1–2	3–5
Lesser pelvis	4	12
Intra-abdominal	15–18	5–6
Ureteropelvic junction	2–4	6–12

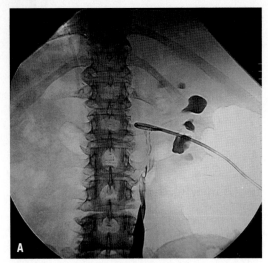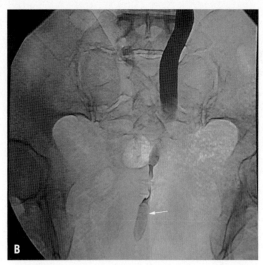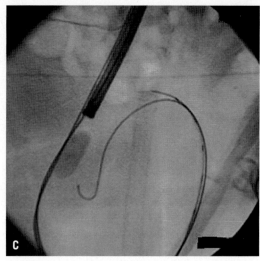

Figure 36-2 *A* and *B*, Antegrade nephrostogram showing a ureteral stone (*arrow*) in a female patient with ureterosigmoidostomy after cistectomy. *C*, Through a nephrostomic access a flexible instrument is used to reach the stone.

POSTOPERATIVE STENTING The routine placement of ureteral stents after ureteroscopic stone fragmentation is still considered the standard of care at most institutions, but it does not appear necessary when ureteroscopy is performed as a diagnostic procedure[2] or following uncomplicated ureteroscopy for distal ureteral stones.[11] This is especially true when ureteral dilation is not performed, when an atraumatic lithotripsy device such as the holmium laser is used for intracorporeal lithotripsy,[12] and when there is no ureteral injury or pronounced ureteral edema. In most of the patients undergoing uncomplicated ureteroscopy with removal of distal ureteral calculi, postoperative discomfort is modest, of short duration, and easily controlled with oral analgesics.[11,13] Operative time, surgical costs and

patient morbidity are consequently reduced.[14] An internal ureteral stent has been routinely advocated after the relief of ureteral obstruction that is secondary to soft tissue pathologic findings, including ureteral stricture dilation, ureterotomy, upper urinary tract transitional cell tumor removal or polipectomy.[2] The main advantages of stenting could be the prevention of ureteral stricture,[2,15] even promoting ureteral healing,[12] and of renal colic that may develop as a result of ureteral edema from balloon dilation or stone manipulation during ureteroscopy.[16] Ureteral stents may also aid the passage of stone fragments secondary to the passive ureteral dilation that occurs with indwelling ureteral stenting.[12] On the other side, the ureteral stent itself has been demonstrated to cause morbidity, including blad-

der irritation, loin pain, hematuria, encrustations, infection, and even possible migration.

In a prospective randomized controlled trial comparing non-stented versus stented ureteroscopic lithotripsy with the holmium laser, patients without any stent presented significantly fewer early symptoms postoperatively, in terms of abdominal and/or flank pain, dysuria, and frequency. No difference was demonstrated in non-stented versus stented ureteroscopy with respect to complications or stone-free status.[12] Neither the severity of preoperative obstruction and tight stone impaction nor intraoperative trauma would be determining factors for leaving a stent after ureteroscopic laser lithotripsy.[17] A decision on whether or not a ureteral stent placement is needed probably must be based on the complete-

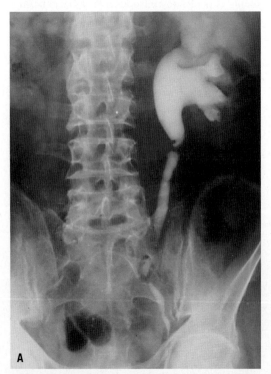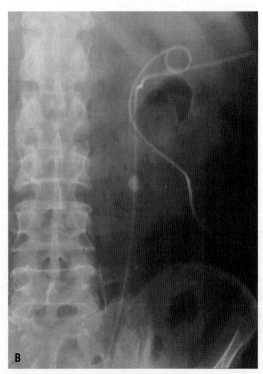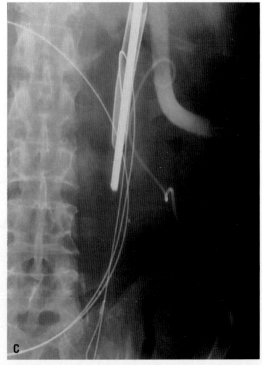

Figure 36-3 *A*, Intravenous pyelogram shows the presence of ureteral stenosis just below the ureteral pelvic junction, on the left side, in a patient with one functioning kidney. *B*, A stone is present above the stenosis; initial renal drainage was left in situ. *C*, A nephrostomic access, straight in line with the ureter was created and a rigid instrument inserted in the ureter.

ness of stone fragmentation.[17] Indications for stent positioning may be represented by failed ureteroscopy for which further procedures are planned[2,18] or in case the stone is flushed back to renal cavities and extracorporeal shock wave lithotripsy (ESWL) is indicated (Table 36-2).

ANESTHESIA Patients may receive general, spinal or epidural anesthesia at the beginning of the procedure, based on patient or anesthesiologist preference. General anesthesia, with muscle paralysis, may avoid potential ureteral injuries resulting from sudden and unexpected patient movement while the ureteroscope is within the ureter.[5] Kramolowsky reported ureteral perforation occurred when a patient coughed while under epidural anesthesia.[19] When peripheral anesthesia is used, patients must be informed about the procedure and the risks coming from sudden unintentional movements and they must be especially warned against unexpected cough shots. There are several reports of successful upper urinary tract procedures using local anesthesia and/or intravenous sedation.[14,20] Candidates for an outpatient ureteroscopy are to be classified as American Society of Anesthesiologist (ASA) class I or II with no previous history of any major anesthetic problems.[2]

INDICATIONS AND CONTRAINDICATIONS FOR URETEROSCOPY

Indications for flexible and rigid ureteroscopy are outlined elsewhere (see Chapter 28, "Techniques in Rigid Ureteroscopy" and Chapter 29, "Techniques in Flexible Ureteroscopy"). Generally, the choice for rigid or flexible ureteroscopes has to take into account the age of the patient, sex, site that has to be reached (which portion of the ureter and renal cavity), anatomy of both the lower urinary tract (presence of prostatic enlargement) and the upper urinary tract, indications for the procedure to be performed, availability of different instruments, and the surgeon's preference and training. Ureteroscopy can be performed for diagnostic and therapeutic purposes. The most common indication for therapeutic ureteroscopy is still ureteroscopic lithotripsy. It represented 66.5% of the cases for Harmon and colleagues.[5] According to these authors, indications differed

slightly from those of the 1980s, when 84% of all ureteroscopies were performed for calculus extraction, and 16% for diagnosis in their series.[5] Looking at the Harmon and colleagues series, as far as stone manipulation is concerned, an overall success, defined as removal of the stone, was achieved in 95% of the cases in a 1992 series, compared to 89% of stones successfully extracted in an earlier series. Stone removal was successful in 97% and 77% of stones in the distal ureter (below the pelvic brim) and upper ureter (above the pelvic brim), respectively.[5] Moving from these reproducible results, calculus extraction has been shown to be feasible even as an outpatient procedure.[2,18,21] In such cases, the proper selection of the patients, the preoperative preparation and the postoperative care play an important role in reaching the best results. There are some absolute contraindications to ureteroscopy, provided that the urethra is patent and the instrument can endoscopically get into the bladder. One such contraindication occurs when the ureteral lumen does not allow for the introduction of the instrument, owing to a discrepancy between the diameter of the lumen and that of the instrument. Ureteral kinking or angulation due to anatomic conditions, previous pelvic or retroperitoneal surgery, or radiation are better managed using a flexible instrument.

Urinary infection must be treated before ureteroscopy, unless it is due to urinary obstruction, which may be resolved by the endoscopic procedure itself. In case of upper urinary tract dilatation and simultaneous urinary infection, percutaneous urinary drainage should be considered prior to any retrograde ureteral maneuver. Prophylactic intravenous broad-spectrum antibiotics are routinely given in view of ureteroscopy, and antibiotics are eventually continued according to individual cases and preoperative urine cultures.

COMPLICATIONS FROM URETEROSCOPY

GENERAL CONSIDERATIONS Generally speaking, the best way to manage complications is to avoid complications. When the upper urinary tract is endoscopically approached, every effort must be made to minimize the risks of potential complications. Experience is very helpful, provided that it does not bypass the basic principles of proceeding in a correct way. In the light of that, only gentle maneuvers are advised and allowed. In case of retrograde approach, a guidewire must be placed into the renal collecting system under fluoroscopic guidance ("safety" guidewire) and eventual dilation of the ureteral orifice using a balloon dilation catheter may be considered to introduce the endoscope more easily. Sometimes it is advisable to insert the instrument along a second wire ("working" guidewire). If a stone is present, stone fragmentation must reduce the fragments as small as possible using the least invasive fragmentation system available on the market. A stent is eventually left in place, postoperatively, according to the surgeon's judgment. Preexisting anatomic situations, congenital or

acquired (eg, from previous surgery), may predispose the patient to possible complications and/or make the procedure impracticable. Complications include:

- so-called pre-ureteroscopic maneuvers, related to the insertion of the initial guidewire or to the dilation of the ureter orifice with whatever system;
- ureteroscopy itself: insertion of the instrument and its progression along the ureter to the renal cavities;
- application of different energy sources or use of the various accessories introduced into the endoscope, according to different situations;
- post-ureteroscopic maneuvers, stenting versus no stenting.

Stone disease, impacted stones and severity of impaction (Figure 36-4), large stones, the presence of ureteral dilatation above the stone, and the site of the stone (theoretically, the higher it is, the more difficult the extraction is, even if this is not always true) all represent negative prognostic factors that foretell possible complications during and after surgery.

Experience and availability of all (and the most sophisticated) instruments and accessories increase the possibility of success, reduce the incidence of complications, and allow for their resolution when they occur. Complications associated with ureteroscopy can be classified in different ways according to the following:

- time when complications occur: intraoperatively, early postoperatively, or late postoperatively (Table 36-3);
- severity of the injury: major or minor;
- frequency: some complications may be relatively frequent, some others purely anecdotal.

In the past, complications were reported to have an incidence of 9 to 20%, including fever and pain[8]; approximately 2 to 4% were listed as major.[22–24] Harmon and colleagues reviewed the

---

Table 36-2 Indications for Positioning an Internal Stent after Ureteroscopy

Severe obstruction at preoperative intravenous urogram
Endoscopic assessment of significant tissue trauma and edema at the impaction site
Significant holdup by on-table retrograde pyelogram despite stone clearance
Heavy renal stone load for which extracorporeal shock wave lithotripsy must be planned
Stone fragments flushed back to the pelvicaliceal system requiring additional intervention
Failed ureteroscopic lithotripsy requiring staged or further procedures

---

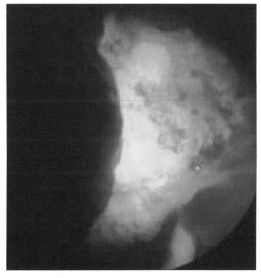

Figure 36-4 A stone impacted into the ureteral wall: on the right side, the stone is partially covered by the ureteral mucosa.

Table 36-3 Summary and Classification of Complications

Intraoperative complications	
Major	Minor
Ureteral perforation Ureteral avulsion Extravasation	Difficult access (introduction or progression of ureteroscope) Mucosal abrasion False passage Intussusception Bleeding Bladder overdistension Stone migration/extrusion Equipment malfunctions/ instrument breakage Thermal injury

Early postoperative complications	
Major	Minor
Infection/ fever	Severe pain Distal or proximal stent migration Bleeding /clot retention Steinstrasse Urinary retention Edema Vesicoureteral reflux

Late postoperative complications	
Major	Minor
Avascular ureteral necrosis Ureteral stricture	Vesicoureteral reflux Persistence of stone fragments

change in the complication rate with time at a single institution, and a decrease was observed in overall complications, to 12% from 20% in a 10-year interval. Significant complications, including ureteral perforation, avulsion, and stricture, likewise decreased to 1.5% from 6.6% in the same interval of time.[5] This reduced incidence was attributed to the use of smaller ureteroscopes and to an increase in surgeon experience. In terms of experience, from an analysis at 28 medical centers, Weinberg and colleagues had observed a decrease to 3.35% from 4.9% in the number of intraoperative injuries with an increase in surgeon experience.[25] Likewise, decreased surgeon experience may be significantly associated with an increased rate of immediate postoperative complications.[26] Age, sex, stone size, preoperative indwelling ureteral stent, need for ureteral orifice dilation, ureteral stent placement, and type of anesthesia were not apparently associated with significant postoperative complications.[26]

The diffuse and routine use of video monitoring during ureteroscopic procedures has led not only to improved teaching but also to a more comfortable, less fatiguing operation in an upright posture with finer dexterity and less jerky movements. Because the ureteral lumen can be observed on the monitor during the entire procedure, introduction of baskets, wires and other ancillary accessories can be accomplished with less risk of torquing or advancement of the telescope. This leads to a decrease in the likelihood of ureteral perforation or mucosal injury.[8]

INTRAOPERATIVE COMPLICATIONS *Difficult access* (the impossibility of introducing the ureteroscope or even the guidewire into the ureteral orifice in a male) is usually related to a prostatic enlargement, especially when a prominent median lobe exists modifying the alignment between urethra and ureter. In the female, a large cystocele may create some difficulty that can be overcome by using a finger to push the vagina upward. Difficulties are eventually encountered when dealing with a reimplanted ureteral orifice, a ureterocele, or in the case of reduced mobility of a contralateral hip.[27] When prostatic enlargement is present, it could be useful to introduce the guidewire into the ureteral orifice using curved angiographic catheters, available on the market with different designs, in order to better follow the course of the lower ureter and avoid perforations of the ureteral wall, which may occur when straight catheters or relatively rigid wires are used.

Progression of the ureteroscope could be difficult with the presence of ureteral stenosis, angulations or fixation (eg, from previous surgery), or ureteral spasm. A retrograde ureteropyelogram is helpful in demonstrating these particular situations, and must be suggested in all cases when the wire has some problems reaching the renal cavities with the simplest and basic maneuvers. Modifications of the Trendelenburg position may sometimes be of some aid. Usually the ureteral spasm recedes spontaneously after a few attempts; the injection of saline solution and lidocaine gel into the ureter has been suggested to facilitate the resolution of this spasm.[27] For other situations, ureteral balloon dilation under fluoroscopic control or ureteral incision using laser or cold blade has to be individually considered. Balloon dilation under visual control may be useful: a balloon catheter is passed through the ureteroscope and balloon inflation is performed just at the site where the ureteral lumen is reduced. Commercially available balloons are 2 to 4 cm in length and inflate to 4 to 5 mm in diameter (12F to 15F), are usable both for rigid and flexible endoscopes (Passport, Microvasive, Natick, MA; Bagley ureteroscopic balloon catheter, Cook Urological Inc., Spencer, IN). Instrument progression can be performed on the guide of the balloon catheter itself. Generally, it does not appear reasonable to attempt to push the ureteroscope into a non-receptive ureter owing to the risk of tearing the ureteral wall (Figure 36-5). It is safer and wiser to leave a catheter of adequate calibre (8F to 9F) in the ureter for a few days with modeling purposes. Postponing the endoscopic maneuvers is often successful. The risk of *ureteral perforation* is increased in the case of impacted stones or difficult ureteral access. Given this aspect, a significant association was pointed out between ureteral perforation and operative time.[26] When an impacted stone completely obstructs the ureteral lumen, a soft and flexible-at-the-tip guidewire must be used. Otherwise, if it does not find any room between the stone and the ureteral wall, it may perforate the wall of the ureter (Figure 36-6). Under these circumstances, it is convenient and safe to use hydrophilic "slippery" wires (Roadrunner, Cook Urological; Glidewire, Boston Scientific Corp., Natick, MA) since they are often able to bypass an impacted stone with ease and even offer less risk of submucosal passage. Otherwise, instead of forcing the guidewire, it is better to leave it just below the obstruction and try to advance it only with visual aid once the ureteroscope is introduced. That is in the case of an impacted, obstructive stone, when the stone must be partially fragmented before passing the wire over the obstacle while watching. When ureteral kinking or bending is found, especially if unrecognized, the passage of the guidewire, catheter, or instrument trying to go upward is sometimes difficult, predisposing the ureteral wall to perforation (Figure 36-7). When dilating the ureteral orifice,

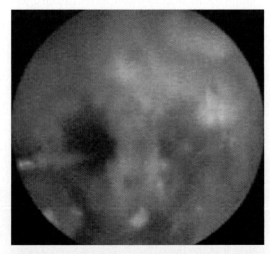

Figure 36-5 A guidewire is in the ureteral lumen (on the left side). A large mucosal tear (of whitish, pearly color) is evident on the right side of the ureteral wall as a consequence of an attempt to push a ureteroscope upward.

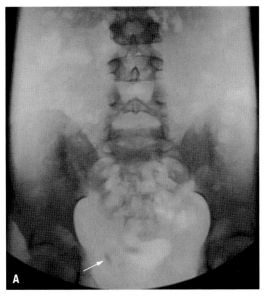

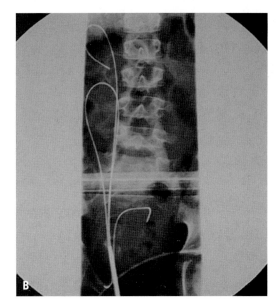

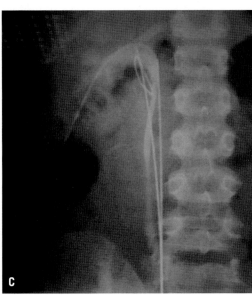

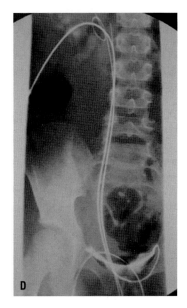

Figure 36-6 *A*, Plain film of the abdomen showing a stone in the right pelvic ureter. *B*, The stone was not bypassed by a wire, even under visual guidance; three wires were introduced perforating the ureteral wall below the impacted stone. *C*, Antegrade nephrostogram shows the wrong position of two retrogradely inserted wires. *D*, The ureter was later canalized through a nephrostomic access.

using graduated as well as balloon dilators, perforation is more likely in the distal part of the ureter. Dilation must never be performed over an impacted stone. This is especially true when the stone is localized in the distal part of the ureter. Any brutal manipulation of the endoscope in the attempt to make the instrument progress into the ureter must be avoided. Any tract of the ureter may be involved in perforation, and this is mostly dependent on the individual cases and it is often related to anatomic or pathologic situations. When enough force for stone or tumor destruction is applied, ureteral damage is possible. In stone fragmentation, electrohydraulic lithotripsy (EHL) represents the most dangerous, even if the most effective source of energy. Perforation is easily recognized by simply observing the breach in the ureteral wall or the periureteral fat lobules[28] (Figure 36-8). Ureteral perforation by itself does not represent an absolute indication to stop the procedure. It depends on the single case and on other concomitant factors (eg, presence of bleeding, the patient's situation, time of occurrence during the procedure). When a guidewire is safely in the ureter, complications from ureteral perforation are minimized and simpler, safer, and more conservative solutions can be adopted. External urinary drainage through a nephrostomy tube is rarely required if a ureteral catheter is correctly inserted. A stent, well-positioned and draining, has to be left in situ for a sufficient time, according to the severity of the injury.

Ureteral perforation can be associated with severe bleeding and/or urine extravasation.

Ureteral avulsion is a rare occurrence, with a reported incidence of 0.5% of all the ureteral procedures.[25,27] Attempts at ureteroscopic removal of calculi in the upper third of the ureter increase the risk of both perforation and avulsion[29] (Figure 36-9). This is probably the most catastrophic injury caused by ureteroscopy (Figure 36-10) and it is related to the difficulty of removing an impacted stone entrapped in a basket or the extraction of a stone still too large with excessive

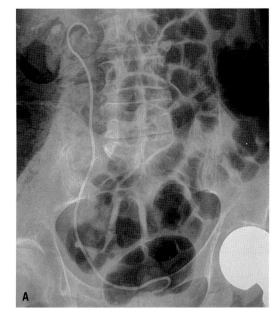

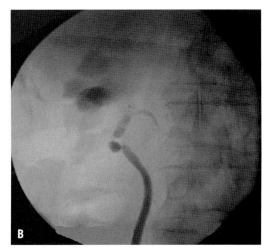

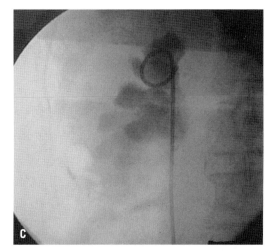

Figure 36-7 *A*, Plain film of the abdomen (A) and, *B*,retrograde ureteropyelogram showing the proximal end of a DJ stent out of the ureter. A bend in the upper ureter, below the ureteropyelic junction, was not bypassed by the wire, which perforated the ureteral wall leaving the stent in the wrong position. *C*, The stent was well-positioned as demonstrated by the final Rx-control.

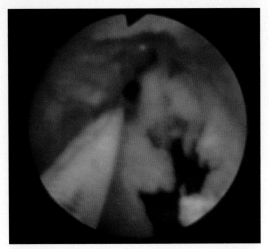

Figure 36-8 The ureteral wall is perforated (on the right side), while a guidewire is inserted into the ureteral lumen (on the left side).

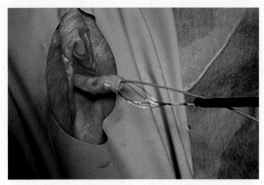

Figure 36-10 Ureteral avulsion: an impacted stone is entrapped into a basket. A long tract of ureter comes out of the external urethral meatus. A guidewire is still in the renal cavities.

and uncontrolled forces (Figure 36-11). Avulsion or intussusception can also occur during the endoscope advancement; this complication can be avoided by keeping the ureteral lumen in view, choosing an appropriately small endoscope, and balloon-dilating the ureteral orifice and fragmenting larger calculi before engagement into the stone basket.[8] The injury must be recognized and quite inevitably repaired in an open fashion. Immediate reconstruction was suggested in order to minimize the patient's discomfort. In our experience, there is no need to proceed with an immediate open surgery if a guidewire is safely positioned in the ureter and the most appropriate urinary drainage is guaranteed, most of the time through a ureteral stent or otherwise through a nephrostomic tube. Later on, the best surgical solution will be planned according to the length of the involved ureter. Nephrectomy should be

considered as the last solution and offered only in complicated cases.

Intraoperative bleeding may occur as a consequence of simple mucosal tear, submucosal trauma, or more severe injuries to the ureteral wall. Bleeding usually obscures the view and may create difficulties in moving the endoscope. If the view is not perfect, it is preferable to stop and postpone the procedure, leaving a stent in situ.

To avoid *bladder overdistention*, it could be advisable to introduce a small catheter into the bladder in the beginning of the procedure, or even during the procedure when it appears to last too long, especially if a forced washing is used and no access sheath was inserted.

If a stone is not fixed in the ureteral wall, *migration of the stone* into the renal cavities is possible (Figure 36-12). Probabilities of stone migration are inevitably higher when the stone is initially localized in the upper third of the ureter and the renal cavities are dilatated. Prevention of this complication includes some tricks (Table 36-4). In case of stone migration, it is possible to run after the stone, eventually into the renal cavities using a flexible endoscope. Otherwise it is preferable to leave a stent in situ (possibly a stent with withdrawal string) in order to avoid a possible remigration of the stone into the ureter. ESWL must be considered as a second treatment.

In some cases during fragmentation, *extrusion of the entire stone* or some fragments into the periureteral space may be found secondary to ureteral perforation. Stone hardness and a "weak" ureteral wall, as is found in case of impacted stones, are often associated with ureteral perforation and stone extrusion. It occurs infrequently, and aggressive attempts to retrieve extruded fragments may result in an increased incidence of ureteral injury and are frequently unnecessary. That is especially true if the stone or the stony fragments are far from the ureteral wall: the ureteral breach closes over the stone, usually without any residual (Figure 36-13). Observation is recommended in order to evaluate the risk of infection or abscess formation. Patients have to be informed in order to avoid future misunderstanding and mismanagement by other physicians.

As to *breakage of instruments, disruption of the burr tip of the ultrasonic lithotripter* during stone fragmentation may occur. It is a rare complication, initially described by Dalton and Brutscher.[30] Their two cases required open removal of both the stony fragments and the metallic tips. Conservative management of this complication should always be attempted because it is often successful, being possible to grasp and remove the broken tip using the ureteroscope and some forceps.

Likewise, the *breakage of the tip of the EHL probe or of the laser fiber* has also occurred. It is quite easy to become aware of this complication, which must be resolved immediately in a conservative, endoscopic way with the removal of the broken parts. When a stone, entrapped in a steel wire basket, is fragmented using the holmium laser, the wires may break or melt due to the high temperatures at the level of the fiber tip (Figure 36-14).[31] In such a case (Figure 36-15), the extraction of the basket may be difficult, especially if one of the wires penetrated the ureteral wall. To avoid this complication, every effort must be made to not entrap the stone in the basket until it is reduced to small fragments or, if the stone is in the basket, to shoot it directly, keeping the tip of the fibre away from the basket wires and from the ureteral wall, which can be damaged in the same

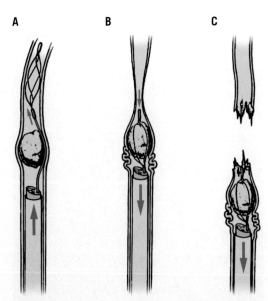

Figure 36-9 *A*, Antegrade passage of helical stone basket. Stone engaged and retrograde extraction attempted. *B*, Note proximal thinning of ureteral wall (*small arrow*) prior to avulsion. *C*, Complete avulsion (when excessive force is used).

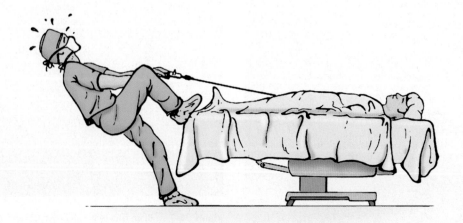

Figure 36-11 The golden rule: *Don't pull too hard!*

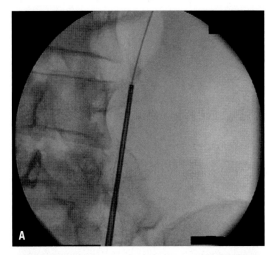

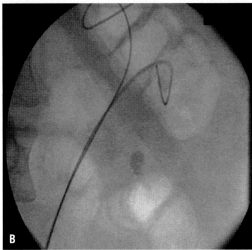

Figure 36-12 *A*, Plain film of the abdomen shows a ureteral stone located in the upper third of the ureter. Rigid ureteroscope is inserted into the ureter and laser fragmentation is performed. *B*, The stone was pushed back in the lower renal calices. Two wires are left in the renal cavities: one will be used for the insertion of a flexible ureteroscope.

way. A recently designed device (Stone Cone, Microvasive, Natick, MA) is inserted above the stone to prevent the fragments from migrating upward.[32] The material that coats the stainless steel wire was undamaged during pneumatic and electrohydraulic lithotripsy, but does not protect against the thermal effect of the holmium laser.[32]

As far as the endoscopes are concerned, with fiberoptics compact operating ureteroscopes, a *bending of the instrument* may occur during the procedure while still maintaining acceptable viewing conditions without the "half-moon" distortion of the normal circular field of vision typ-

Table 36-4 Prevention of Stone Migration
Insertion of a gentle guidewire completely under fluoroscopic control
Low pressure fluid irrigation during the ureteroscopy
Immediate introduction of a basket opened just above the stone as the stone is viewed
Meticulous disruption of the stone using the least explosive means (the holmium laser appears to be the most appropriate fragmentation system, under this point of view)

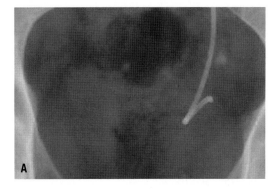

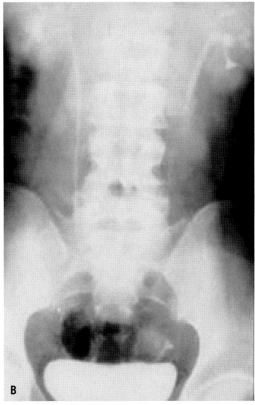

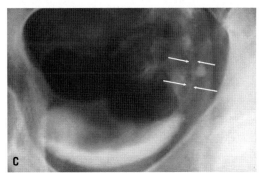

Figure 36-13 *A*, Plain film of the abdomen (pelvic particular) shows a stone far from a ureteral stent, inserted in left ureter, after ureteral wall perforation and stone extrusion. *B*, Intravenous pyelogram confirms the presence of the stone out of the ureter in its pelvic portion, *C*, with no interference with the ureteral course (see the *arrows*).

ical of the old rod lens telescopes (Figure 36-16). Excessive force can lead to further damage and impair the function until the fiberoptics are broken, totally compromising the viewing. This situation may be the consequence of undue bending as the rigid endoscope passes over the prostate or large psoas muscle.

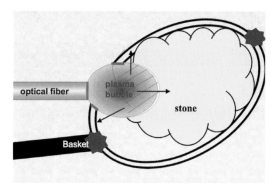

Figure 36-14 Schematic representation: at the tip of the Holmium laser fiber, plasma bubble is formed; that destroys both the stone and, eventually, the basket wires.

Major problems are encountered with the flexible instruments that appear to be prompter to the *rupture*, especially at the level of the actively deflecting portion. It is strongly recommended not to insert any accessory instrument when the flexible endoscope is bent, but to straighten it and then to insert the accessory instrument, which must be sufficiently pliable.

When EHL is used and the tip of the probe is too close to the tip of the instrument, *breakage of the objective lens* of the endoscope may occur with an immediate loss of view or the appearance of the typical black-dots that, in every case, lower the vision. It is advisable to keep the extremity of the probe far from the tip of the instrument and always in the field of view (Figure 36-17). The damages are usually quite expensive and often require replacement of the instrument. On the other hand, it should be accepted that the lower incidence of complications and the greater clinical applicability associated with the extended use of the small-diameter, rigid (and even more flexible) endoscopes must be weighed against their greater fragility.[1]

EARLY POSTOPERATIVE COMPLICATIONS *Bleeding* secondary to ureteral trauma after ureteroscopy is not a common finding and only rarely becomes severe. It may cause *clot ureteral obstruction* or *bladder retention*. The incidence of severe bleeding was less than 0.5% of all complications in Sosa and colleagues' initial series of

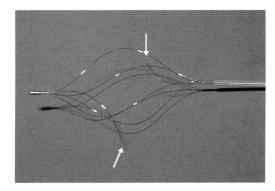

Figure 36-15 One of the basket wires is disrupted after using holmium laser for fragmentation of an entrapped stone.

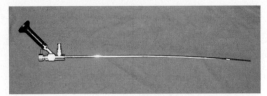

Figure 36-16 Ureteroscope appears curved along its axis.

ureteroscopies.[33] A wait-and-see approach is usually sufficient to obtain spontaneous resolution of this complication, only occasionally requiring blood transfusion. The case of life-threatening bleeding may be managed with angiographic techniques using embolization[34] or with open surgery. *Periureteral hematoma* may develop, where bleeding spreads into the periureteral space as well as into the retroperitoneum (Figure 36-18).

In the early postoperative period, *pain* is mainly related to the procedure itself, and on the first day, is associated with a longer operating time.[2] Drugs such as oral dextropropoxyphene have been suggested to manage the early postoperative pain.[2] An alternative is the combination of paracetamol (acetaminophen) and codeine, administered orally. Due to their complementary characteristics and pharmacokinetic properties, effective results are obtained without any increase in side effects.[35] Late postoperative pain is related to the ureteral stent. According to El Faqih and colleagues, dysuria and loin pain were associated with ureteral stenting in 79% and 29% of the patients, respectively.[36] Adequate hydration is advised and must be maintained, especially if a ureteral stent has been left in situ.

Stent migration can contribute to postoperative complications, and a stent that is too short might migrate at a higher rate[37] (Figure 36-19). The use of ureteral stents with a withdrawal string avoids the need for postoperative cystoscopy to remove it and prevents the complication itself.

Urinary infection secondary to ureteroscopy has been reported with an incidence of 1.3% in a

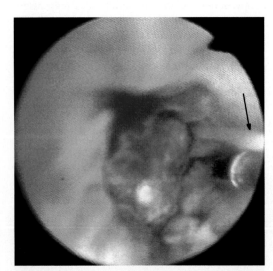

Figure 36-17 Impacted stone in the ureteral lumen. An insulating guidewire bypasses the stone (on the right side, *arrow*). The electrohydraulic lithotripsy probe is completely in the vision field.

large series.[33] When fever appears, antibiotics are continued at the appropriate dosage and time.

LATE POSTOPERATIVE COMPLICATIONS The only long-term complication following ureteroscopy in Harmon and colleagues' review was *ureteral stricture formation*[5] (Figure 36-20).

All the endourologic procedures are potentially associated with mucosal injuries or even ureteral perforation, which may result in stricture formation.[38] Ureteral strictures are the possible final result of different events[8,38–42] (Table 36-5).

With the earlier ureteroscopic experiences, stricture rates were reported ranging from 0 to 10%.[6,10,21,29,43–45] In the Harmon and colleagues series, with 67% radiologic follow-up and 100% clinical follow-up data, only one postoperative stricture was identified (0.5%). The improvement in stricture rate was associated with the routine use of smaller ureteroscopes through dilated ureteral orifices with postoperative stenting.[5] In the light of all that, it appears that the exact role of the ureteroscope as the only determining factor in causing stricture is far from being definitely defined.[21]

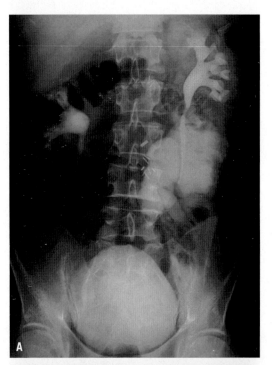

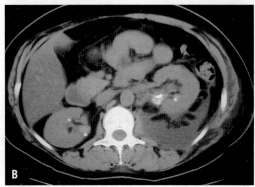

Figure 36-18 *A*, Intravenous pyelogram and, *B*, abdominal computed tomography scan show urine extravasation associated with retroperitoneal hematoma, following left ureteroscopy.

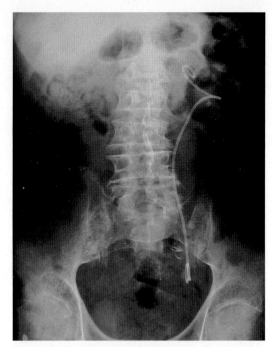

Figure 36-19 Upward stent migration.

Conservative endoscopic treatment can be attempted in case of ureteral stricture. Three techniques can be used: catheter dilation, balloon dilation and endoincision.[46]

Following Richter and colleagues, balloon dilation was successful in short ureteral strictures with intact vascular supply in 89.2% of the cases, but only in 37.5% of long strictures.[47] When vascular supply was considered compromised, the

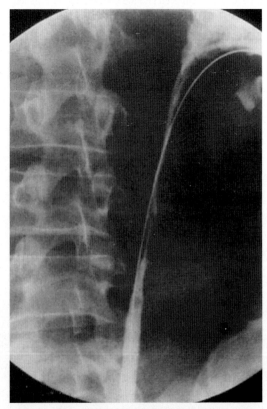

Figure 36-20 A long stricture developed after a ureteroscopic stone extraction in which there was a perforation leading to extensive extravasation.

Table 36-5 Possible Causes of Ureteral Strictures
Ureteral perforation at the site of stone with irrigation fluid extravasation
Ischemia of the ureteral wall due to stone impaction
Compressive effects due to ureteral stents causing ischemia
Stony fragments embedded in the periureteral wall with granuloma formation and subsequent tissue reaction
Thermal injury of the ureteral wall with delayed fibrosis, in relation with electrohydraulic, ultrasound, and holmium laser lithotripsy
Iatrogenic perforation of the ureter and calculi pushed into periureteral space

results were far less favorable: 40% for short ureteral strictures and 16.7% for long strictures.[47]

For benign ureteral strictures, endoureterotomy is best applied to strictures at the terminal segments of the ureter, proximal and distal, that are nonischemic in origin, that are short and of short duration. In the experience of Wolf and colleagues, the success rate of endoureterotomy for benign strictures was 80% at 1 year of follow-up and beyond.[48] In case of failure with conservative treatment, open surgical intervention is required and different procedures, such as ureteroureterostomy, transureteroureterostomy, autotransplantation, psoas hitch, Boari flap, ileal ureter and nephrectomy have been suggested according to the level, extension and severity of the ureteral lesion.

Ureteral necrosis is an extremely rare complication. Kaufman related the reported distal ureteral necrosis to a ureteral injury after stone manipulation: a mucosal tear led to urinary extravasation and eventually to severe stricture formation.[49] Lytton reported a similar result, which he believed was caused by submucosal passage of the ureteroscope with a devascularization of the longitudinal vascular plexus of the ureter due to irrigating fluid.[23] Submucosal passage of wires and stents may also result in similar injuries.[8]

Vesicoureteral reflux in uninfected adults is generally considered of little clinical significance. Convincing evidence for the safety of orifice dilation was reported by Garvin and Clayman, who demonstrated with intravenous pyelography and voiding cystography no clinical significant long-term sequelae from routine 24F ureteral orifice dilation.[43] Studies evaluating patients with voiding cystography following balloon dilation and ureteroscopy reported an incidence of 0 to 20% of postoperative low-grade reflux,[6,22,43,50,51] but there are no known reports of recurrent pyelonephritis or progressive renal insufficiency secondary to this reflux.[5]

The eventual *persistence of stone fragments* will be treated in accordance with their site and characteristics.

CONCLUSION

Ureteroscopy overcame the initial difficulties and, thanks to technical improvements and expanded experience, entered into the common practice of every urologist at least as far as the basic and simpler procedures are concerned. The extension of both the diagnostic and the surgical ureterorenoscopic maneuvers associated with the spreading use of the flexible instruments, has increased our knowledge of the complications and risks related to the procedure. But at the same time, we became aware of the great potential of this endoscopic procedure as a mini-invasive surgery. There are some "golden rules" that make ureteroscopy realizable and safe. From daily practice, it emerged that the rules must be followed, we would say, in a very routine way, ensuring that they are not bypassed by the experienced practitioner.

REFERENCES

1. Grasso M, Bagley D. Small diameter actively deflectable, flexible ureteropyeloscopy. J Urol 1998;160:1648–54.
2. Cheung MC, Lee F, Leung YL, et al. Outpatient ureteroscopy: predictive factors for postoperative events. Urology 2001;58:914–8.
3. Wills TE, Burns JR. Ureteroscopy: an outpatient procedure? J Urol 1994;151:1185–7.
4. Eshghi M. AUA Update Series 1989; Vol. 8, Lesson 38.
5. Harmon WJ, Sershon PD, Blute ML, et al. Ureteroscopy: current practice and long-term complications. J Urol 1997; 157:28–32.
6. Stoller ML, Wolf JS Jr, Hofmann R, Marc B. Ureteroscopy without routine balloon dilatation: an outcome assessment. J Urol 1992;147:1238–42.
7. Pang KK, Fuchs GJ. Ureteral stents and flexible ureterorenoscopy. J Endourol 1993;7:145–9.
8. Leveillee RJ, Hulbert JC. Complications. In: Smith AB, Badlani GH, Clayman RV, et al., editors. Smith's text book of endourology. St. Louis: Quality Medical Publishing; 1996.p. 513–25.
9. Netto NR Jr, Lemos GC, D'Ancona CAI, et al. Is routine dilatation of the ureter necessary for ureteroscopy? Eur Urol 1990;17:269–72.
10. Lytton B, Weiss RM, Green DF. Complications of ureteral endoscopy. J Urol 1987;137:649–53.
11. Hosking DH, McColm SE, Smith WE. Is stenting following ureteroscopy for removal of distal ureteral calculi necessary? J Urol 1999;161:48–50.
12. Denstedt JD, Wollin TA, Sofer M, et al. A prospective randomized controlled trial comparing nonstented versus stented ureteroscopic lithotripsy. J Urol 2001;165:1419–22.
13. Teichman JMH, Rao RD, Rogenes VJ, Harris JM. Ureteroscopic management of ureteral calculi: electrohydraulic versus holmium: YAG lithotripsy. J Urol 1997;158:1357–61.
14. Byrne RR, Auge BK, Kourambas J, et al. Routine ureteral stenting is not necessary after ureteroscopy and ureteropyeloscopy: a randomized trial. J Endourol 2002;16:9–13.
15. Boddy SM, Nimmon CC, Jones S, et al. Acute ureteric dilatation for ureteroscopy- an experimental study. Br J Urol 1988;61:27–31.
16. Weinberg JJ, Snyder JA, Smith AD. Mechanical extraction of stones with rigid ureteroscopes. Urol Clin North Am 1988;15:339–46.
17. Cheung MC, Lee F, Leung YL, et al. A prospective randomized controlled trial on ureteral stenting after ureteroscopic holmium laser lithotripsy. J Urol 2003;169:1257–60.
18. Cheung MC, Yip SK, Lee F, Tam PC. Outpatient ureteroscopic lithotripsy: selective internal stenting and factors enhancing success. J Endourol 2000;14:559–64.
19. Kramolowsky E. Ureteral perforation during ureterorenoscopy: treatment and management. J Urol 1987;138:36–8.
20. Hosking DH, Bard RJ. Ureteroscopy under intravenous sedation for treatment of distal ureteral calculi: a safe and effective alternative to shock wave lithotripsy. J Urol 1996;156:899–901.
21. Tawfiek ER, Bagley DH. Management of upper urinary tract calculi with ureteroscopic techniques. Urology 1999;53:25–31.
22. Stackl W, Marberger M. Late sequelae of the management of ureteral calculi with ureterorenoscope. J Urol 1986;136:386–9.
23. Lytton B. Complications of ureteroscopy. Semin Urol 1986; 4:183–90.
24. Schultz A, Kristensen JK, Bilde T, Eldrup J. Ureteroscopy: results and complications. J Urol 1987;137:865–6.
25. Weinberg JJ, Ansong K, Smith AD. Complications of ureteroscopy in relation to experience: report of survey and author experience. J Urol 1987;137:386–9.
26. Schuster TG, Hollenbeck BK, Faerber GJ, Wolf JS Jr. Complications of ureteroscopy: analysis of predictive factors. J Urol 2001;166:538–40.
27. Roumeguere T, Simon J, Schulman CC. Complications de l'ureteroscopie. Acta Urol Belgica 1997;65:31–4.
28. Morgentaler A, Bridge SS, Dretler SP. Management of the impacted ureteral calculus. J Urol 1990;143:263–6.
29. Sosa RE, Vaughan ED Jr. Complications of ureteroscopy. AUA Update Series 1988;7:274–8.
30. Dalton JR, Brutscher SP. Two cases of ureteroscopy and attempted stone disintegration complicated by disruption of the burr tip of the ultrasonic probe. J Urol 1986;135:778–9.
31. Cecchetti W, Tasca A, Zattoni F. Holmium laser in endourology: the phenomena related to plasma bubble formation [Abstract]. Eur Urol 2003;2: No. 687.
32. Dretler SP. The stone cone: a new generation of basketry. J Urol 2000;165:1593–6.
33. Sosa RE, Bagley DH, Huffman JL. Complications of ureteroscopy. In: Hufman JL, Bagley DH, Lyon ES, editors. Ureteroscopy. Philadelphia: WB Saunders; 1988. p. 159–68.
34. Kase DJ, Crystal KS, Naidich JB, et al. Embolization to control iatrogenic ureteral hemorrhage: a case report. J Urol 1994;151:420–1.
35. Moore A, Collins S, Carroll D, McQuay H. Paracetamol with and without codeine in acute pain: a quantitative systematic review. Pain 1997;70:193–201.
36. El Faqih SR, Shamsuddin AB, Chakrabarti A, et al. Polyurethane internal stents in treatment of stone patients: morbidity related to indwelling times. J Urol 1991;146:1487–91.
37. Slaton JW, Kropp KA. Proximal ureteral stent migration: an avoidable complication? J Urol 1996;155:58–61.
38. Grasso M, Liu JB, Goldberg B, Bagley DH. Submucosal calculi: endoscopic and intraluminal sonographic diagnosis and treatment. J Urol 1995;153:1384–9.
39. Roberts WW, Cadeddu JA, Micali S, et al. Ureteral stricture formation after removal of impacted calculi. J Urol 1998; 159:723–6.
40. Biester R, Gillenwater JY. Complications following ureteroscopy. J Urol 1986;136:380–2.
41. Kreigmair M, Schmeller N. Paraureteral calculi caused by ureteroscopic perforation. Urology 1995;45:578–81.
42. Doddamani D, Kumar R, Hemal AK. Stone granuloma—not to be forgotten as a delayed complication of ureteroscopy. Urol Int 2002;68:129–31.
43. Garvin TJ, Clayman RV. Balloon dilation of the distal ureter to 24F: an effective method for ureteroscopic stone retrieval. J Urol 1991;146:742–5.
44. Lyon ES, Kyker JS, Schoenberg HW. Transurethral ureteroscopy in woman: a ready addition to the urological armamentarium. J Urol 1978;119:35–6.
45. Esuvaranathan E, Tan EC, Tan PK, Tung KH. Does transurethral laser ureterolithotripsy justify its cost? J Urol 1992;148:1091–4.
46. Clayman RV, Kavoussi LR. Endosurgical techniques for non-calculous disease. In: Walsh PC, Retik AB, Stamey TA, Darracott Vaughan E Jr, editors. Campbell's urology, 6th ed. Philadelphia, WB Saunders; 1992. p. 2231–311.
47. Richter F, Irwin RJ Jr, Watson RA, Lang EK. Endourological management of benign ureteral strictures with and without compromised vascular supply. Urology 2000;55:652–7.
48. Wolf JS Jr, Elashry OM, Clayman RV. Long-term results of endoureterotomy for benign ureteral and ureteroenteric strictures. J Urol 1997;158:759–64.
49. Kaufman JJ. Ureteral injury from ureteroscopic stone manipulation. Urology 1984;23:267–9.
50. Kostakopoulos A, Sofras F, Karayiannis A, et al. Ureterolithotripsy: Report of 1000 cases. Br J Urol 1989;63:243–4.
51. Ford TF, Parkinson MC, Wickham JEA. Clinical and experimental evaluation of ureteric dilation. Br J Urol 1984;56:460–3.

37

Pediatric Ureteroscopy

Michael Erhard, MD

Ureteroscopy has benefited significantly from many technologic innovations in the field of endourology. There are well-documented beginnings of endourologic procedures, and numerous physicians, scientists and lay people can be credited with its evolution.

Many agree that cystoscopy originated with Max Nitze who, in 1894, introduced the refined operative cystoscope.[1] It is apparent that his ideas were based on Philip Bozzini who had previously published his use of the "lichtleiter" in 1806.[2] These early endoscopes had problems with optical magnification, and lacked a reliable or controllable light source which, therefore, limited their use. The first reported endourologic operation was performed by De'Sormeaux who in 1853 removed a tumor from the urethra of a male.[3]

It wasn't until the twentieth century that significant advances were made for the inherent problems of the early endoscopes. In the 1950s, Dr. James G. Gow of Liverpool consulted with Professor Harold H. Hopkins at the University College in London to help conquer some of these problems.[4] Professor Hopkins had developed a rod lens system for rigid endoscopes. Prior to this, endoscopic instruments consisted of a hollow tube with a distal objective lens, an ocular lens, and a series of relay lenses throughout the length of the tube. The revolutionary Hopkins rod lens system replaced the hollow air spaces with glass rods, thereby allowing a much higher refractive index, which provided more efficient transmission of both light and operative images.

Fiberoptic technology has early beginnings too. In the 1840s both Colladon and Babinet introduced novel ideas on light traveling through glass rods.[5,6] John Tyndall in 1854 has been widely credited with the first important demonstration of this principle, and its potential usefulness.[7] It was not until 1954, that Professor Hopkins as well as Dr. N. S. Kapany of London and Dr. Van Heel of the Netherlands each independently reported the transmission of images along tiny fibers of glass.[8] This work was based upon the principles of image bundling previously introduced by Hansel.[9] Hopkins and Kapany went on to refine this fiberoptic technology, leading to the production of the first endoscopes with rod lenses and fiberoptic lighting. This allowed for conduction of light without heat, and it was the American Cystoscope Makers Incorporated (ACMI) that produced the first "cold light" cystoscopes in 1963.

Pediatric cystoscopes were actually the first rigid rod lens ureteroscopes. Hugh Hampton Young reported in 1929 a ureteroscopic procedure that he had performed in 1912 on a 2-month-old boy with massively dilated ureters secondary to posterior urethral valves.[10] He utilized a 9.5 French pediatric cystoscope, which enabled visualization of the ureter as well as the intrarenal collecting system. Amazingly, it wasn't until the late 1970s that Goodman and Lyon each independently reported the use of an 11F pediatric cystoscope for ureteroscopy.[11,12] The first rigid endoscope specifically designed for ureteroscopy was produced by the Richard Wolf Instrument Company in 1979.[13] Essentially, it had a similar design to a pediatric cystoscope but was longer in length, and was available in two diameters: 13F and 16F. One problem with these early rigid ureteroscopes was that they used an interchangeable rod lens, and this was the most significant limitation to creating a smaller diameter scope. Fiberoptic technology not only enabled the miniaturization of these endoscopes, but also eliminated image distortion with flexing/bending of the endoscope, and allowed for a larger-diameter working channel.

Interestingly, even though rigid ureteroscopy had earlier beginnings, it is flexible ureteroscopy that was first reported in routine clinical use. In 1962, Dr. V. F. Marshall of New York succeeded in the diagnostic examination of the ureter as well the intrarenal collecting system using a 9F fiberoptic scope.[14] Early flexible endoscopes were modified bronchoscopes and gastroscopes, and problems with irrigation and deflection limited their acceptance. In 1968, the first flexible pyeloureteroscope with a working channel was introduced by Dr. H. Takayashu and was produced by the Olympus Company.[15] It wasn't until the 1980s that there was a renewed interest in flexible endoscopy owing to improvements in miniaturization as well as the addition of active deflection with adequate working channels and small-diameter working instruments. Current flexible ureteroscopes have at least two-way, active tip deflection and secondary, passive deflection, which effectively lengthens the deflected segment allowing inspection of the entire intrarenal collecting system.[16] Some flexible ureteroscopes have multidimensional active deflection similar to colonoscopes.

Finally, advancements in video technology now provide a clear magnified operative image and improved recording capabilities. Cameras can automatically adjust to varying light conditions, which produces a stable video image during any procedure, and filters have greatly improved the honeycombed appearance produced by fiberoptic bundles. Camera chips are now incorporated into the tip of some endoscopes, although their large size is currently a limiting factor. Clearer digital video images permit immediate chart documentation plus enhanced speaker presentation and resident/family education.[17]

INSTRUMENTS

URETEROSCOPES Two distinct types of ureteroscopes exist: (1) mini rigid (ie, semi-rigid) fiberoptic, and (2) flexible fiberoptic. There are no endoscopes produced specifically for use in children—only the length has been modified. The mini rigid fiberoptic ureteroscope has a metal outer casing, which is malleable enough to allow for limited bending without image distortion. Mini rigid endoscopes are particularly useful in the distal ureter, but may be difficult to pass proximal to the bony pelvis. One advantage of these endoscopes is two working channels—one for irrigation and the other for delivery of surgical instruments. They are more durable than flexible ureteroscopes due to their outer metal sheath, and some can be safely autoclaved for sterilization. The distal tip is as small as 4.7F, but all shafts gradually increase in diameter as you move more proximally towards the eyepiece. Constant vigilance is necessary in order not to injure a narrow male urethral meatus as the ureteroscope is advanced, particularly when a safety wire is present. They are produced in varying lengths; and I currently use a 15 cm and 33 cm ureteroscope with a 6.9F diameter (Figure 37-1).

Flexible ureteroscopes are particularly useful within the proximal and intrarenal collecting systems due to their active and passive deflection. Rarely is secondary passive tip deflection necessary for the complete inspection of the intrarenal pediatric collecting system because the arc of deflection alone is adequate to access the lower pole in most pediatric kidneys. The working channel of a flexible ureteroscope consists of a smooth cylindrical plastic tube located eccentrically at the tip. Most flexible ureteroscopes have a working channel of approximately 3.6F, which is adequate for a variety of instruments while still maintaining space for irrigation. Unfortunately, nearly all instruments will decrease the amount of active tip deflection.[18,19] In order to prevent damage, the ureteroscope should be straightened prior to passage of any working instrument. Silicone lubricant may aid in decreasing the resistance encountered during deployment.

Because of their flexible design, these ureteroscopes are more likely to be damaged and

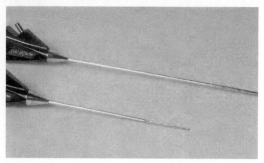

Figure 37-1 Semirigid ureteroscopes are useful for distal and mid-ureteral procedures. They can be used for proximal ureteral access if the patient's anatomy allows. It is helpful to have two separate channels, one for irrigation and one for working instruments. Different endoscope lengths provide easier surgeon control during pediatric ureteroscopy.

need to be handled with care. Technologic improvements to both the outer sheathing and deflecting mechanisms have increased their durability, but if enough fiberoptic bundles break, the image becomes distorted and repairs are required. Flexible endoscopes cannot be autoclaved, but can be safely soaked in cold solution, or gas-sterilized. The distal tip of the scope is generally the smallest diameter and usually under 8F. The shaft is tapered gradually, which strengthens the sheath and helps to protect the inner-bundle fibers. I have found that a variety of lengths (35, 50, and 65 cm) are necessary for use in children to decrease the amount of redundant shaft outside of the body, which helps to prevent damage during use (Figure 37-2).

GUIDEWIRES Guidewires are the most commonly used working instrument in endourology. They not only aid in access to the ureter, but help to prevent intraoperative complications, and are necessary for postoperative stenting. There are varying diameters, but I mainly use a 150 cm, .035-inch Teflon-coated guidewire with a 3 cm distal floppy tip as my working and safety wire. The basic design is an inner solid core wire, which is wrapped tightly by a coiled spring wire. Nitinol (nickel titanium) wires are resistant to kinking, and because of this, are the most durable small diameter wires. The distal tip of any wire may be straight or angled, and the length of the floppy flexible tip varies. A dual floppy tip wire is safest for passage of a flexible ureteroscope

because it minimizes potential damage to the working channel. The most common coating is Teflon although hydrophilic polymer coatings are helpful for negotiating tortuous or narrowed ureters, and also for placement of a wire proximal to an impacted ureteral calculus.

The full-length hydrophilic-coated guidewires should not be used as safety wires because they can easily dislodge. It is helpful to handle these slippery wires with a moistened gauze sponge. Extra-stiff wires help with straightening tortuous or reimplanted ureters and also make it easier to perform dilation (Figure 37-3). They are firm and should not be used as working wires for flexible endoscopes due to the risk of damaging the delicate working channel.

BASKETS AND GRASPERS Baskets and graspers are useful for the extraction of stone debris or any other foreign body within the collecting system.[20,21] They vary in diameter from 1.9 to 4.5F. Most often they are contained within a hydrophilic sheath to facilitate passage through endoscopes. Baskets traditionally either come as a flat wire (Segura) or helical design (Figure 37-4A,B). They can be made of three or four wires, and some are designed to increase the radial expansion of the ureter. There is a triangulated wire basket, which has significant radial expansion capabilities. The helical baskets are deployed proximally to the stone and are then drawn back to engage the calculus. The flat wire baskets should be positioned alongside the stone prior to deployment. The most significant improvement in basket design is the tipless nitinol basket. When deployed through a flexible endoscope it allows for near complete active deflection of the ureteroscope[22] (Figure 37-5). The tipless design and increased flexibility of the nitinol wires make it particularly safe and useful for extraction of calculi contained within calices. Some baskets have an inner central channel, which allows simultaneous placement of an electrohydraulic or laser lithotripsy device. Newer nitinol baskets allow controlled active angulation of the wires, and others form a canopy to engage multiple small fragments.

GRASPERS Grasping forceps are quite helpful during endoscopic stone extraction. They generally contain two, three or four wires, and some are made of nitinol. The most significant advan-

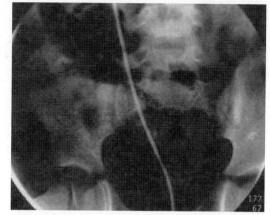

Figure 37-3 Access to the collecting system was made possible through the use of a stiff guidewire, which enabled the straightening of the previously reimplanted (cross-trigonal) ureter. At the conclusion of ureteroscopy, the course of the ureter will retain its preoperative appearance. Postoperative reflux is uncommon after ureteroscopy has been performed in a previously reimplanted ureter.

tage is that a grasper will disengage from a stone if it becomes lodged within a relatively narrow ureteral segment. This helps prevent trauma to the ureteral wall and also eliminates entrapment during stone removal. Grasper technique involves opening the forceps only as far as needed to engage the stone (Figure 37-6). Upon opening the forceps, the individual wires are advanced away from the operator; therefore, slight retraction is necessary to avoid pushing the stone more proximal. It is important to maintain contact with the stone while closing the graspers, and therefore, slight advancement of the sheath is needed while grasping the stone.

INTRACORPOREAL LITHOTRIPSY

There are four modes of intracorporeal lithotripsy available; electrohydraulic, ultrasonic, ballistic and laser. All have been extensively studied, and each has pros and cons.

Ultrasonic lithotripsy has been around since 1953.[23] The ultrasound probe is a metal probe, which transmits vibrational energy to the tip. When in contact with the stone, this results in disintegration due to cleavage of the crystal matrix. Solid probes as small as 2.5F have been used for stone fracture followed by fragment removal using endoscopic forceps or baskets. The disadvantages of use during ureteroscopy are proximal migration due to vibration, and the fact that any degree of bending of the probe decreases the delivery of energy. Although there is minimal tissue damage with the use of this energy, it is not the best modality for ureteroscopic stone disintegration.

Ballistic lithotripsy involves the mechanical impaction of stones by solid probes. This modality is effective in fragmenting all types of stones. There are flexible probes available, but loss of lithotripsy power with significant deflection, as well as retrograde migration due to pneumatic impaction, are two significant shortcomings.[24–27]

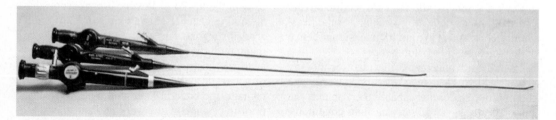

Figure 37-2 Flexible ureteroscopes provide the safest access to the proximal collecting system. These instruments are more delicate than semirigid ureteroscopes. In order to help prolong the working life of a flexible ureteroscope it is important to decrease the redundancy of the shaft located outside of the patient's body. Endoscopes of different lengths help to accomplish this in pediatric ureteroscopy since there is significant variability in patients.

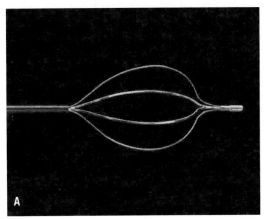
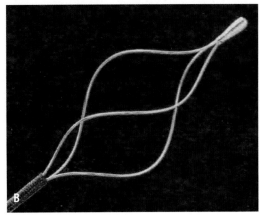

Figure 37-4 *A*, Basket design historically was either flat wire or, *B*, helical, and their primary material was metal. This not only limited active deflection of flexible endoscopes, but their protruding tips increased the risk of injury to the delicate collecting system.

Electrohydraulic lithotripsy (EHL) was discovered by Yutkin in 1955 and involves the generation of an electrical spark, which produces a cavitation bubble from heat.[28] With initial expansion and subsequent collapse of this bubble, there is energy significant enough to produce lithotripsy. The energy is maximized at a distance of approximately 1 mm from the stone; therefore, the tip of the probe should be kept just off the surface of the stone. This form of energy may not be able to fragment all stone compositions. One advantage is that deflection of a flexible scope does not decrease the energy transmitted. Probes come as small as 1.9F, they are relatively inexpensive to purchase and maintain, and they permit near complete deflection of ureteroscopes. One significant risk of EHL is lateral disbursement of energy, which can increase injury to the surrounding tissues, particularly within the small pediatric ureter.

Laser lithotripsy is the most effective, and, when used properly, the safest form of lithotripsy.[29]

Holmium laser lithotripsy has been shown in adults and children to be safe and effective in fragmenting all types of urinary calculi (Figure 37-7).[30,31] Holmium lithotripsy involves direct stone absorption of laser energy with subsequent disintegration. The holmium laser can also ablate tissue and, therefore, acts as a cutting instrument. Fibers as small as 200 μ, enable near complete deflection of the ureteroscope when working in the lower pole of the kidney. In order to prevent injury or endoscope damage from laser energy, you must always be aware as to the position of the tip of the probe. The fiber should be several millimeters outside of the end of the endoscope, and be placed near the stone or in direct contact for tissue ablation.

ELECTROSURGICAL PROBES

Cutting and fulgurating electrodes are available in sizes as small as 2F. Some of these probes are reusable, but most are disposable. Angled-tip 3F electrodes are quite helpful as cutting bipolar electrodes. When using these instruments, it is important to remember that there will be conduc-

tion of electrical current over non-coated guidewires, and therefore, the guidewire must either be insulated with a nonconductive coating (ie, hydrophilic) or be placed within an open-ended catheter.

URETEROSCOPY TECHNIQUE

Ureteroscopy in children requires general anesthesia. After the child is placed in the dorsal lithotomy position, he or she is padded well in order to prevent excessive limb abduction or pressure on nerves and limbs. In a male child, the urethral meatus is carefully inspected and gently dilated if necessary. Modern endoscopes are sufficiently small enough to prevent the need for routine dilatation. Cystoscopy is performed and the bladder is inspected and the ureteral orifices visualized. A mental picture of the intravesical anatomy is retained and a urine sample is collected.

First, gauge the caliber of the ureteral orifice using a 0.035-inch guidewire. If there appears to be sufficient room, a small-caliber, rigid mini-ureteroscope is guided over the wire under direct vision into the orifice (Figure 37-8). Persistence of congenital ureteral folds can make ureteroscopy in infants and young children challenging, but they are not an absolute contraindication (Figure 37-9). The ureter has three physiologic areas of narrowing, with the narrowest portion usually being the bladder orifice. There are known anatomic differences between adults and children regarding the diameter and size of the ureter. These anatomic differences are age-dependent

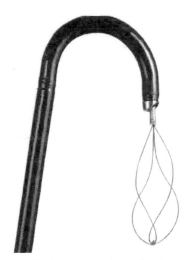

Figure 37-5 Nitinol (nickel-titanium) alloy is very flexible and has significant tensile strength. Because of these characteristics, utilization of baskets and graspers made by this material does not significantly affect the active deflection of flexible ureteroscopes. There are several basket designs, some of which are able to be actively manipulated, allowing for a more precise entrapment of a calculus.

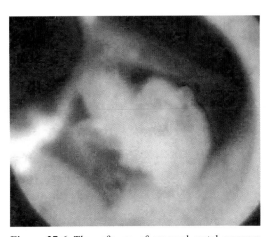

Figure 37-6 The safe use of pronged metal graspers requires opening the device only as large as needed to engage the outer rim of the calculus. This will help prevent inadvertent perforation or grasping of the ureteral mucosa. Metal-pronged forceps are particularly useful for the extraction of papillary tip calculi when they are embedded in the renal parenchyma.

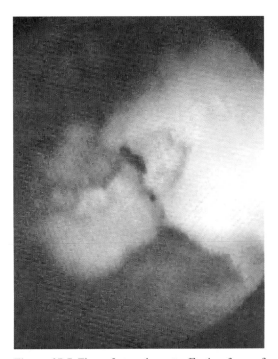

Figure 37-7 The safest and most effective form of lithotripsy is holmium laser energy. Unlike other modalities, this laser is capable of the disintegration of all types of urinary calculi. At increased energy levels, it can also perform tissue ablation, making it useful for incisional procedures. Small-caliber fibers allow near complete deflection of flexible endoscopes making it easier to treat conditions within the lower pole of the intrarenal collecting system.

and based on work by Cussen in 1971.[32] Access to the pediatric ureter is facilitated by using two guidewires (Figure 37-10): one inside the working channel and the other already independently placed in the ureter as a safety wire. This helps to not only increase the diameter, but also allows for a more controlled access. If the orifice appears "volcanic" and barely accepts a 0.035-inch guidewire, then either active dilatation or pre-stenting is performed.

Balloon dilatation of the ureteral orifice has been demonstrated to be effective and safe in children,[33,34] but clearly produces more dilatation than is actually necessary. If active dilatation is required, use a soft, graduated single shaft dilator that ranges from 6 to 10F (Figure 37-11). It is sometimes necessary to perform this technique through a 13F cystoscopic sheath to help decrease buckling of the dilator within the bladder. This type of active dilatation is best performed by using a stiff guidewire. If dilatation cannot be safely accomplished using one of these techniques, a ureteral stent should be placed passively dilating the ureter rather than performing active

balloon dilation. Any form of active dilation may be required in approximately 30% of children undergoing ureteroscopy, and age does not seem to be a predictive factor.[35]

When therapeutic maneuvers are anticipated, it is important to maintain a safety guidewire within the ureter. It is also important to either insulate the guidewire with an open-ended catheter, or to use a hydrophilic-coated guidewire if an electrosurgical procedure is planned. A hydrophilic wire should not be used as a routine safety wire due to the ease with which it may become dislodged. A semirigid ureteroscope can be inserted under direct vision alongside the guidewire or between two guidewires as previously stated. A flexible ureteropyeloscope requires either the use of an access sheath or a second working guidewire for placement of the ureteroscope into the proximal collecting system in a monorail fashion (ie, over the wire) (Figure 37-12). If it is difficult to traverse the ureteral orifice when accessing over a wire, rotating the flexible ureteroscope sequentially in 90° intervals may prove successful. If there is continued difficulty after turning the

scope 360°, then dilatation may be necessary in order to gain access to the ureter.

The safe use of access sheaths in children will most often require pre-stenting of the ureter to facilitate easier placement. I have found an access sheath to be most helpful when treating large renal or proximal ureteral stones, or when performing incisional procedures (ie, endopyelotomy). When retrieving stone fragments through an access sheath, ureteral injury can be avoided by preventing entrapment of the ureteral wall between the stone and the lip of the sheath. A 9.5F internal diameter (11.5F outer diameter) sheath is the smallest that permits passage of a 7.4F flexible ureteroscope and provides room for continuous flow irritation (Figure 37-13). Fluoroscopic guidance is absolutely necessary for proper positioning.

Once you are within the ureter it is important to maintain a three-dimensional image of your position within the collecting system. You should always keep in mind important surrounding structures prevalent throughout the course of the ureter. As you proceed proximally, you will appreciate caudal movement with inspiration and cephalad movement with expiration. When working within the intrarenal collecting system, contrast should be used to confirm complete inspection of all of the calices. Postoperative stenting is not always required, but should be performed after procedures requiring either extensive manipulation or significant active dilatation. It is also necessary if there is any injury or edema of the ureter, and after any incisional procedure. I prefer to leave a dangler string attached to facilitate removal without anesthesia if the stent will only remain for several days. Early, inadvertent removal has not been a problem.

Previous urologic surgery involving either the bladder neck, ureter, urethra, or ureteropelvic

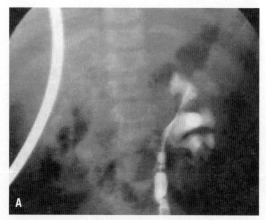

Figure 37-8 *A,* If there is sufficient room around the .035 inch guidewire when inserted into the ureteral orifice, direct access is usually able to be achieved through *B,* tenting up the mucosa and guiding the semirigid ureteroscope directly into the distal ureter. If the ureteral orifice is of small caliber and barely accepts the guidewire, it is usually most prudent to place an indwelling ureteral stent and continue the procedure under a separate anesthetic when there has been adequate time for passive dilatation.

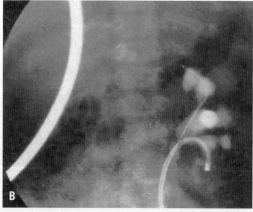

Figure 37-9 There are a variety of challenges encountered during pediatric ureteroscopy, which can make access to the collecting system more difficult. *A,* Congenital ureteral folds can be seen in infants and younger children. Their presence is not an absolute contraindication for pediatric ureteroscopy. *B,* Access to the intrarenal collecting system is accomplished through standard dilatation and guidewire access techniques. Postoperative stenting for this condition is recommended.

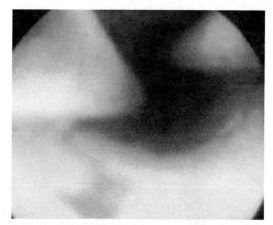

Figure 37-10 Sometimes it is necessary to access the distal ureter using a two-wire technique. The first guidewire is used to gauge the ureteral orifice. Primary access should be attempted if an adequate space is identified. When this attempt is unsuccessful, placing the semirigid ureteroscope between two guidewires can facilitate access by providing controlled dilatation. One wire is placed independently within the ureter and used as a safety wire, while the other is placed through the working channel. The ureteroscope can then be maneuvered to enter the ureter between the two wires.

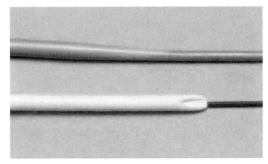

Figure 37-11 Controlled access using a soft graduated dilator is usually successful when active dilatation is needed. This is best performed over a stiff guidewire with a 6/10 French dilator (above). A second useful instrument is a dual lumen catheter (below). This permits simultaneous infusion of contrast material for opacification of the collecting system, and also for placement of a second guidewire when proximal ureteroscopy is planned.

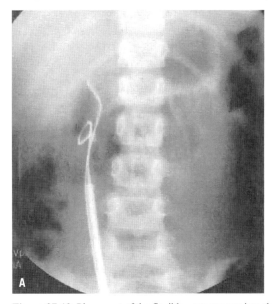 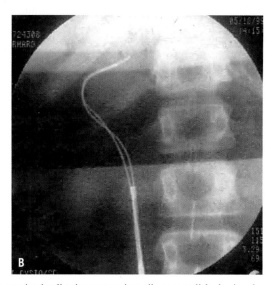

Figure 37-12 Placement of the flexible ureteroscope into the proximal collecting system is easily accomplished using the monorail technique. This involves advancing the ureteroscope over a previously placed guidewire. *A*, If no therapeutic intervention is planned, then only one guidewire is necessary. *B*, A second safety wire is appropriate when therapeutic maneuvers are being performed. The safety wire maintains continuity with the entire collecting system to allow access when needed during the procedure.

junction is not a contraindication for ureteroscopy. In the child who has had prior bladder neck reconstruction, it is important to use small-d iameter endoscopes to avoid disruption of the area. Many times, these children have had ureteral reimplantation at the time of their primary bladder neck repair and care must be taken not to over-torque the bladder neck when accessing the previously reimplanted ureter. For children who have undergone prior reimplantation, access to the ureter is dependent on the type of surgery previously performed. When either an advancement or extravesical procedure was performed, access is similar to the un-operated child because the orifice maintains its original position. When a cross trigonal reimplantation has been performed, access is more difficult, but usually the orifice can be cannulated with an angled guidewire. If this is unsuccessful, an activity deflecting guidewire can be used. Once access has been gained, the initial wire should be exchanged through an open-ended catheter with a stiff guidewire. This will straighten the intramural portion of the ureter allowing access for ureteroscopy. If dilatation is necessary, this should be performed with a soft graduated dilator and is usually necessary only at the ureteral orifice. When the procedure is completed, the ureter will return to its preoperative position. Significant recurrent reflux has not been demonstrated after ureteroscopy in the previously reimplanted ureter.

Intrarenal access after ureteropelvic junction (UPJ) repair does not usually require dilatation, provided there has been adequate healing and success of the previous surgery. Fortunately, the ureter remains supple, usually at the site of the previous repair, and is at no greater risk of injury due to fixation from scarring.

CALCULI

The minimally invasive treatment of urinary tract calculi in children has all but replaced open stone surgery. Debate continues regarding the most efficacious modality, and each case needs to be individualized in order to choose the best

form of treatment. Extracorporeal shock wave lithotripsy (ESWL) of the renal stones is the least invasive form of therapy and offers reasonable stone free rates of greater than 80% with minimal complications.[36–42]

The best rates of stone clearance are with the most powerful, first-generation HM3 lithotriptors. Subsequent second- and third-generation lithotriptors, while associated with less potential complications, certainly are less efficacious in stone treatment. Because of high re-treatment rates and the potential need for ancillary procedures in order to achieve maximum stone clearance, I have pursued retrograde ureteroscopic treatment of stones less than one centimeter contained within the entire urinary collecting system.

The most common presenting symptoms for stones in children include abdominal pain (40 to 75%), gross or microscopic hematuria (25 to 40%), and symptoms attributable to urinary tract infections (10 to 30%).[43–47] Although it has long been thought that the pediatric ureter is more forgiving than adults, recent data suggest that stones as small as 3 mm in size are likely to become trapped at the ureterovesical junction.[48] Some adult studies have suggested that the rate of spontaneous passage is different depending upon the stone's position within the ureter. In any event, neither the stone's position within the ureter or

overall size/configuration can be completely predictive of spontaneous passage. Conservative therapy for ureteral stones should be undertaken unless there are clinical signs of uncontrolled pain or vomiting, or any signs of urosepsis or significant obstruction. Proactive SWL should be considered for renal calculi > 5 mm due to the increased risk of non-spontaneous passage.

As technology has improved, the retrograde ureteroscopic treatment of stones becomes more popular in the pediatric population. Safety and efficacy in prepubertal children as young as 6 months of age has been documented.[31,35,50–61] It has also been suggested that the treatment of distal ureteral stones in children should mimic the American Urological Association guidelines for adults, and therefore a primary endoscopic procedure is recommended.[58]

Advantages of ureteroscopy for stone removal include negligible re-treatment rates with minimal complications. When performed on an outpatient basis, it has been demonstrated in adults that ureteroscopy is more cost-effective than SWL for stones within the ureter.[62,63] In children, both ESWL and ureteroscopy require general anesthesia offering no specific advantage for either therapy. Routine postoperative evaluation for iatrogenic vesicoureteral reflux is not necessary after ureteroscopy since clinically significant reflux

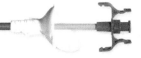

Figure 37-13 Access sheaths can be used in pediatric ureteroscopy. They are particularly useful when retrieving large stone burdens within the proximal collecting system. The smallest practical internal diameter that allows for adequate irrigation is 9.5 French. This has an outer diameter of 11.5F, therefore, making it difficult to be placed in a non-stented pediatric ureter.

has not been demonstrated even with dilatation to 15F. Currently, the primary ureteroscopic removal of stones less than or equal to 1 cm throughout the entire collecting system should be considered.

When performing ureteroscopy for stones within the urinary collecting system, access to the ureter is gained as previously mentioned. Previous urologic reconstructive surgery is not a contraindication to retrograde ureteropyeloscopy. If a Cohen cross-trigonal ureteral reimplantation has been performed, access is aided through the use of specifically designed deflecting wires. Once access is gained, a stiff guidewire will help straighten the ureter so that a mini rigid ureteroscope may be placed. Prior to any ureteroscopic endeavor, the bladder is drained to prevent filling during the procedure, and this is most critical for those previously augmented. A second safety wire is always left in place when there is a planned ureteral therapeutic procedure. Saline irrigation should be used and can be attached to a single spring-loaded syringe pumping system, which helps to control intraluminal pressures. Irrigation should be used sparingly in order to prevent proximal migration of calculi within a dilated collecting system.

A mini rigid ureteroscope should be used for distal and mid-ureteral calculi (Figure 37-14). It may be used for more proximal stones if it can be successfully passed above the pelvic brim. It is sometimes necessary to use a flexible ureteroscope for proximal ureteral calculi, and one should always be used for stones contained within the intrarenal collecting system. If the stone is impacted within the ureter, then either perform in situ holmium laser lithotripsy or attempt to dislodge the stone into the proximal dilated portion. The holmium laser produces dust particles and fragments of less than 2 mm, which are small enough to pass spontaneously. After gauging the size of the stone versus the diameter of the ureter, you can either "paint" the surface of the stone with the laser to smooth out rough edges or cleave the stone into distinct fragments for subsequent removal. Remember that the tip of the laser probe needs to be outside of the endoscope and directly visualized during the procedure in order to prevent local tissue injury or endoscope damage. Use graspers to remove calculus debris from the ureter and kidney due to the ease with which a stone fragment can be disengaged if it becomes lodged within a narrowed portion of the ureter. If a stone fragment becomes displaced outside the ureteral wall due to perforation, it is recommended to abandon further attempts at extraction of the migrated calculus. It is important to retrieve at least one stone fragment for crystallographic analysis, but once this is achieved, it is more efficient to deposit subsequent small fragments within the bladder to be removed through spontaneous voiding. Placement of a ureteral stent after ureteroscopy for stone removal is not always necessary.[55] It is difficult to know which patient will benefit from postoperative stenting, and there are no absolute predictive factors. A stent should be placed if there is any significant perforation or trauma to the ureteral wall, and if there was significant active dilation (balloon) or use of an access sheath in a non-dilated/pre-stented ureter. If stenting is performed, then leave a dangler string attached to facilitate removal in the office no sooner than 72 hours post-procedure.

UPJ OBSTRUCTION AND URETERAL STRICTURES

Traditionally, UPJ obstruction in the pediatric population has been corrected by open pyeloplasty, with success rates greater than 95%. The endourologic/laparoscopic management of this condition in adults is now considered by many to be the first option for treatment. When compared to an open surgical procedure, there is decreased morbidity and a comparable degree of success in adults. These benefits have not been demonstrated in any conclusive form in the pediatric population. At present, it is this authors' opinion that, in infants and toddlers, open surgical repair should still be considered the "gold standard" for children with primary UPJ obstruction.

Dr. Arthur Smith is credited for coining the phrase "endopyelotomy" when discussing the endourologic incision of the ureteropelvic junction. The procedure is a modification of the "ureterotomie externe" which was originally described in 1903 by Albarran.[64] The technique was later popularized by Dr. D.M. Davis in 1943 in his descriptive analysis of the intubated ureterotomy.[65] These techniques involved a longitudinal incision made outside the ureter extending into the internal ureteral lumen. A stent was placed for several weeks during ureteral regeneration. Early studies had demonstrated that a period of approximately 6 weeks is required for complete ureteral smooth muscle formation with return of active peristalsis.[66,67] The duration of postoperative indwelling stent placement is based upon these studies, and therefore, is suggested for 4 to 6 weeks, although more recent data suggests no significant difference in healing at 1, 3, or 6 weeks.[68]

Success for endopyelotomy in both adults and children appears to be related to several preoperative factors. Many agree that, in a kidney demonstrating severe (Grade IV) hydronephrosis or split renal function less than 25%, the outcome for endopyelotomy is significantly reduced.[69–74] More controversial in the failure of endopyelotomy is the role of crossing vessels in the area of the UPJ (Figure 37-15).[71,75] It has been suggested by some that the presence of such vessels is associated with a poor outcome. This has yet to be confirmed in prospective clinical trials.

Any cutting modality (ie, cold knife, electrosurgical, laser) can be used, provided it accomplishes through-and-through longitudinal incision extending to healthy urothelium both proximally and distally. It is important to maintain a solitary incisional groove in order to minimize subsequent scarring. Initially, it was felt that a posterior lateral incision would be safest, although a direct lateral incision may, in fact, be

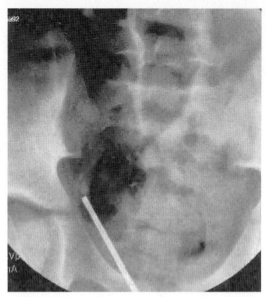

Figure 37-14 The mini rigid ureteroscope is best suited for mid and distal ureteroscopy. It can also be utilized for proximal ureteroscopy if the child's anatomy allows. In instances when there is an impacted ureteral calculus (shown here) the ureteroscope can be guided up to the stone under direct visualization allowing for a more precise placement of a guidewire in order to complete the endoscopic procedure.

associated with a lesser risk of intraoperative bleeding. Preoperative vascular radiologic assessment of the UPJ through either endoluminal ultrasound or computed tomography (CT) angiography is recommended prior to incision to avoid vascular damage.[72]

A postoperative ureteral stent remains indwelling for a period of 4 to 6 weeks. Stent size should be at least 7F although, if the ureter is of sufficient caliber, a 10F stent may be more beneficial. Optimum stent size and duration postoperatively continue to be debated. Several tapered endopyelotomy stents are manufactured, although necrosis has been reported after placement of a 14F tapered stent into an undilated ureter through an antegrade approach after endopyelotomy. Therefore, only leave tapered stents in pre-stented ureters.

After the diagnosis of UPJ obstruction has been made, a tailored treatment strategy needs to be discussed. It is important to mention to parents that the gold standard for repair of UPJ obstruction is an open pyeloplasty. Laparoscopy and robotic surgery are also becoming more accepted in young children and infants, which offers another surgical option.[77,111] From all published data on the endourologic incisional management of UPJ obstruction in children, there is an overall success rate of 81% for primary and 87% for secondary UPJ obstructions.[78–90] It is important to remember that most of these cases were performed in an antegrade fashion. Discussion of the risks for any procedure is mandatory when obtaining informed consent. These risks include bleeding, the possibility of open surgical correction, and the potential for loss of renal function. Prior to any endourologic

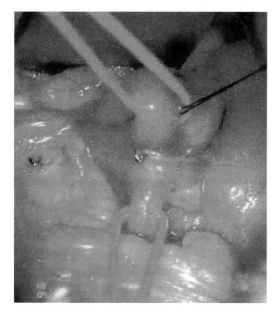

Figure 37-15 The role of primary endopyelotomy in children is limited because other minimally invasive techniques (ie, laparoscopy) have been found to have similar success rates when compared to standard open pyeloplasty. A lower–pole-crossing vessel (above) as pictured here during an open pyeloplasty, may alter the success of primary endopyelotomy. Their presence will also increase the risk for significant intraoperative bleeding if the vessels are inadvertently incised. Preoperative or intraoperative imaging is critical for assessment in order to help prevent such complications.

procedure, there should be documentation of sterile urine, and perioperative intravenous antibiotics should be administered.

After induction of general anesthesia, the patient is placed in the dorsal lithotomy position. Routine cystoscopic examination is performed, and a retrograde ureteropyelogram is obtained. Use of a 5F open-ended catheter is helpful to gauge the caliber of the ureteral orifice. A guidewire is then advanced into the renal pelvis and is confirmed using fluoroscopy. The bladder is emptied prior to removal of the cystoscope.

There are two distinctly different techniques for performing retrograde endopyelotomy or endoureterotomy. The first involves a balloon-cutting device and is performed under fluoroscopy. The second utilizes direct endoscopic visualization with either flexible or rigid ureteroscopy and surgical incision.

The direct retrograde ureteroscopic treatment of UPJ obstruction has been described for adults and is this author's preferred approach for endopyelotomy. This technique utilizes either flexible or rigid instrumentation as well as electrosurgical or holmium laser incision. Advantages to this approach include direct visualization of the area as well as confirmation of a transmural incision to expose retroperitoneal adipose tissue. After incision, active balloon dilation using either a 15 or 18F balloon catheter is performed to disrupt any remaining fibrous bands. Contrast extravasation is confirmed and a ureteral stent is placed and left indwelling for 4 to 6 weeks. A postoperative bladder catheter is removed the fol-

lowing day if the urine is clear. This technique is also applicable to ureteral strictures, keeping in mind the varying location of blood supply from medial to lateral as the ureter travels from the renal pelvis to the bladder (Figure 37-16).

CALICEAL DIVERTICULA

Caliceal diverticula are non-secreting, urothelial lined cavities which communicate with the collecting system through a narrow fornical channel. It was first described by Rayer in 1841 and he felt that this abnormality represented either a cyst or localized hydronephrosis. Their reported incidence is from 2.1 to 4.5 per 1,000 intravenous pyelograms. It is felt to be congenital in origin, but some have proposed vesicoureteral reflux as a main cause. There are two types that have been described. Type I are more common and are usually adjacent to a minor calix and are less likely to produce symptoms. Type II diverticula communicate directly with the renal pelvis or adjacent major calix. While Type I are usually less than 1 cm in size, Type II are usually larger, and therefore, are more likely to have associated symptoms. The incidence is similar for both children and adults, and there appears to be no predilection for either sex. They are bilateral in about 3% of cases.[91–94]

Approximately 50% of caliceal diverticula contain stones, and approximately 30% are symptomatic.[93] The most common complaint is pain, but they are also associated with infection and hematuria. Intervention is considered for chronic pain, gross hematuria, urolithiasis, recurrent infections, or progressive renal damage. While often times visualized on intravenous pyelogram, CT scan with delayed contrast images are quite helpful in demonstrating caliceal diverticula. Retrograde ureteropyelogram is also effective for demonstrating diverticula, but this is more invasive and generally not necessary as a primary diagnostic tool.

Open surgical techniques have been supplanted by lesser invasive forms of therapy. ESWL has been advocated as primary therapy, but overall symptom-free and stone-free percentages are 60% and 23%, respectively.[95,96] ESWL seems most appropriate for diverticula containing stones less than 1 cm and that have a patent neck, which would allow for post-lithotripsy drainage.[97]

Endourologic approaches for the treatment of caliceal diverticula include direct or indirect percutaneous puncture, retrograde ureteroscopic access, and laparoscopic unroofing. There is minimal data on the treatment of children, so most outcomes are based upon adult patient experience.

Percutaneous treatment is the most widely used and the most successful of the three modalities, with a stone-free rate of approximately 94% and a symptom-free rate of 93%.[98,99] In patients treated ureteroscopically, there were 80% stone-free and 85% symptom-free rates.[100–102] There was a successful report of the laparoscopic unroofing of peripheral diverticula with thinned parenchyma.[103] The ureteroscopic approach is well-suited for diverticula containing stones less than 1 cm within the upper and mid portions of the kidney (Figure 37-17). Diverticula within the lower pole may be more difficult to access and treat, therefore, a different treatment modality is suggested.

Debate regarding optimal treatment of the diverticular wall and neck continues. Some suggest that fulguration of the diverticular cavity, as well as incision of the diverticular neck versus dilatation, may result in better outcome for complete obliteration. Depth of incision should be minimal to avoid the deeper pericaliceal vessels, which are typically found in the anteroposterior plane. After balloon dilation of the neck, a drainage catheter is placed across the neck of the diverticulum. This is generally left indwelling for several weeks to permit caliceal decompression with subsequent obliteration.

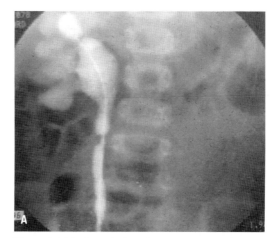
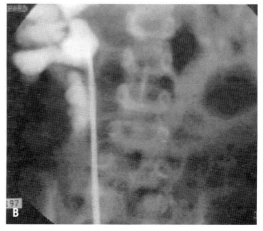

Figure 37-16 The technique for incisional procedures to correct urinary tract obstruction is similar, whether it is within the ureter or at the level of the ureteropelvic junction. *A,* A single incisional trough is made, and a complete incision is demonstrated by contrast extravasation, confirming a through-and-through incision. *A* and *B,* In cases of ureteral strictures, the direction of the incision should correspond to an area where the primary blood supply is less likely to be present. For this 3-year-old child with a proximal ureteral stricture, the incision was performed on the lateral margin of the ureter in hopes that this would prevent injury to the suspected medial blood supply.

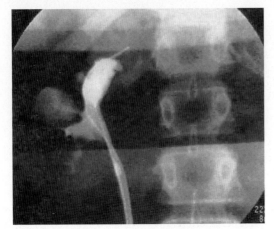

Figure 37-17 Caliceal diverticula can be treated in a variety of ways, which is mostly dependent upon their position within the collecting system and also any associated stone burden. An ureteroscopic approach can be performed if they are present within the mid- and upper-pole regions and have a stone burden that is small. It is important to avoid guidewire trauma, which could prevent adequate visualization of the tiny diverticular neck. A percutaneous or laparoscopic approach is probably better suited for large diverticula present within the lower pole of the collecting system or which are peripheral and contain a large amount of stones or are of large size.

HEMATURIA

Macroscopic (ie, gross) hematuria in children is most often benign and self-limiting. It is alarming to patients, family, and treating physicians, and occurs in approximately 1.3 per 1,000 children presenting to a pediatric emergency clinic. The origin of the hematuria is typically benign and of glomerular origin (eg, glomerulonephritis). Hematuria in children can result from lesions involving the glomerulus, interstitium, vascular or urothelium. Medical rather than surgical treatment is generally successful.[104,105]

Children presenting with gross hematuria should be evaluated through a careful history and physical examination accompanied by urinalysis, culture, as well as appropriate laboratory tests, or evaluation of medical diseases of the kidney.[106] Gross hematuria accompanied by lateralizing symptomatology may also represent renal or ureteral calculi. If the history and physical examination is consistent with this diagnosis, then upper tract imaging such as ultrasonography, excretory urography, or non-contrast CT scanning may reveal a urinary calculus. Persistent hematuria, with or without lateralizing symptoms, and a negative laboratory and a radiographic evaluation will often necessitate a pediatric urologic consultation.

Several papers demonstrate the successful ureteroscopic treatment of persistent gross hematuria in adults with lateralizing symptoms and negative upper-tract imaging.[107,108] Resolution of the hematuria tends to be durable over long-term follow-up, unless the upper-tract lesions were noted to be diffuse on the ureteroscopic examination. There have been few reports describing the ureteroscopic evaluation and treat-

ment of persistent lateralizing hematuria in children.[109,110] Discrete lesions were treated with fulguration, and none of these children had developed recurrent hematuria.

Sickle cell disease or trait can be associated with gross hematuria. This is thought to be secondary to microinfarcts of the renal papilla with subsequent spilling of blood into the urine. The character of the bleeding is generally dark blood rather than bright red blood. It is most often associated with the left kidney and collecting system. Conservative treatment is indicated as a first step and should include hydration, alkalinization and possibly oral/intravenous coagulating agents. The endoscopic installation of silver nitrate has also been effective in some instances. Ureteroscopy should be considered in children who have persistent flank pain secondary to obstruction due to blood clot formation, or any significant drop in their serum blood count. Most often, diffuse papillary bleeding will be present, but there are some reports of discrete lesions which responded well to electrocautery.

The technique for the evaluation of gross hematuria in children is similar to that previously described in adults. Care should be undertaken during the entire procedure to help prevent any iatrogenic trauma with subsequent hematuria. If no lateralizing symptomatology was demonstrated prior to endoscopic evaluation, then upon cystoscopy each ureteral orifice is individually examined and the side responsible for the hematuria is identified (Figure 37-18). Retrograde urography is then undertaken, making certain not to over-distend the collecting system.

The distal ureter as well as the ureteral orifice should be examined using a mini rigid endoscope. If a guidewire is necessary for traversing the ureteral orifice, then it should only be placed into the distal ureter to prevent proximal trauma. The mini rigid ureteroscope is advanced as far as possible without creating any harm. Fluoroscopy should confirm placement within the ureter at the

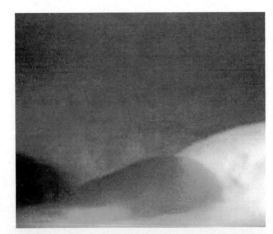

Figure 37-18 For patients with hematuria, it is sometimes necessary to perform your endoscopic evaluation at the time of active bleeding in order to localize the symptoms. As shown here, once the side of bleeding is identified, you can proceed with site-specific urography as well as ureteroscopy. Commonly, a specific source of bleeding will be identified, which can be properly treated by electrocauterization.

most proximal point of endoscopic evaluation. At this point, a guidewire should be placed, and the endoscope should be backed off this guidewire making certain not to inadvertently push the guidewire more proximally. A flexible ureteroscope is then placed over the guidewire in a monorail fashion under fluoroscopy to the area of previous examination. It is then carefully guided into the proximal collecting system and each individual infundibulum as well as calix should be examined. If electrocautery is indicated, then a 2F electrosurgical probe can be utilized. Postoperative stenting is not always necessary and should be avoided to help prevent postoperative trauma.

REFERENCES

1. Nitze M. Das Operation Skystoskop... Vorlaufige Mitteilund, Centr.bl. CHIR 1891;18:993.
2. Bozzini P, Lichtleiter J, der pract. Arzneykunde UND Wundarzneykunst. C.W. Hufeland 1806;24:107.
3. Desormeux AJ. De l'endoscope et de ses application an diagnostic et an traitment des affections de l'urethre et de la vessie. Paris 1865.
4. Gow JG. Harold Hopkins and optical systems for urology: an appreciation. Urol 1998;1:152–7.
5. Colladon D. On the reflections of a ray of light inside a parabolic liquid stream ,Comptes Rendus 1842;15:800.
6. Hecht J. City of lights: the story of fiberoptics. New York: Oxford University Press; 1999. p. 13–27.
7. Barlow DE. Fiberoptic instrument technology. TR, editors. Small animal endoscopy. St. Louis: C. Vosby Co, 1990.
8. Gow JG. Harold Hopkins and optical systems for urology, an appreciation. Urol 1998; 1:152-157.
9. Hansell CW. US Patent No 1751; 584, 1930.
10. Young HH, McKay RW. Congenital valvular obstruction of the prostatic urethra. Surg Gynecology Obstet 1929; 48:509–11.
11. Goodman TM. Ureteroscopy with a pediatric cystoscope in adults. Urol 1977;9:394.
12. Lyon ES, Kyker JS, Schoenbergh W. Transurethral ureteroscopy in women: a ready addition to urologic armamentarium. J Urol 1978;119:35–6.
13. Lyon ES, Banno JJ, Schoenberg HW. Transurethral ureteroscopy in men using juvenile pediatric cystoscopy equipment. J Urol 1979;122:152–3.
14. Marshall VG. Fiberoptics in urology. J Urol 1964;9:110–1.
15. Takagi T, Takayasu H, Aso Y. A small-caliber fiberscope for the visualization of the urinary tract, biliary tract, and spinal canal. Surgery 1968;64:1033–8.
16. Bagley DH. Intrarenal access with the flexible ureteropyeloscope. Effects of active and passive tip deflection. J Endourol 1993;7:221–4.
17. Tan YH, Preminger GM. Advances in video and imaging in ureteroscopy; Urol Clin North Am 2004;31:33–42.
18. Grasso M, Bagley DH. A 7.5/8.2 F actively deflectable, flexible ureteroscope: a new device for both diagnostic and therapeutic upper urinary tract endoscopy. Urol 1994;43:435–41.
19. Poon M, Beaghler M, Baldwin D. Flexible endoscopic defectability: changes using a variety of working instruments and laser fibers. J Urol 1997;11:247–9.
20. Ptsahnyk T, Cueva-Martinez A, Michel MS, et al. Comparative investigations on the retrieval capabilities of various baskets and graspers in four ex vivo models. Eur Urol 2002;41:406–10.
21. El-Gabry EA, Bagley DH. Retrieval capabilities of different stone basket designs in vitro. J Endourol 1999;13:305–7.
22. Kourambus J, Delvecchio FC, Munver R, et al. Nitinol stone retrieval-assisted ureteroscopic management of lower pole renal calculi. Urol 2000;56:935–9.
23. Mulvaney W. Attempted disintegration of calculi by ultrasonic vibration. J Urol 1953;70:704–6.
24. Schulze H, Haupt G, Piergiovanni M, et al. The Swiss lithoclast: a new device for endoscopic stone disintegration. J Urol 1993;149:15–8.
25. Haupt G, Pannek J, Herde T, et al. The Lithovac: new suction device for the Swiss lithocast. J Endourol 1995;9:375–7.
26. Ten CL, Fhong P, Preminger GM. Laboratory and clinical assessment of pneumatically driven intracorporeal lithotripsy. J Endourol 1998;12:163–9.
27. Loisides P, Grasso M, Bagley DW. Mechanical impactor employing nitinol probes to fragment human calculi:

fragmentation efficiency with flexible endoscope deflection. J Endourol 1995;9:371–4.

28. Yutkin L. Electrohydraulic lithotripsy. English translation for US Department of Commerce, Office of Technical Services; 1955. Dic 62-15184 MDL 1207/1-2.

29. Grasso M. Experience with the holmium laser as an endoscope lithotrite. Urology 1996;48:199–203.

30. Wollin TA, Teichman JM, Rogenes VJ, et al. Holmium:YAG lithotripsy in children. J Urol 1999;162:1717–20.

31. Reddy PP, Barrieras DJ, Bagli DJ, et al., Initial experience with endoscopic holmium laser lithotripsy for pediatric urolithiasis. J Urol 1999;162:1714–6.

32. Cussen LJ. The morphology of congenital dilatation of the ureter: intrinsic ureteral lesions. Austral and New Zeal J of Surg 1971;41:185–94.

33. Shepherd P, Thomas R, Harmon EP. Urolithiasis in children: innovations in management. J Urol 1988;140:790–2.

34. Thomas R, Ortenberg J, Lee BR, et al. Safety and efficacy of pediatric ureteroscopy for management of calculus disease. J Urol 1993;149:1082–4.

35. Minevich E, DeFoor W, Reddy P, et al. Ureteroscopy is safe and effective in prepubertal children. J Urol 2005;174:276–9.

36. Kroovand RL. Pediatric urolithiasis. Urol Clin North Am 1997;12:173.

37. Marberger M, Turk C, Steikogler. Piezoelectric extracorporeal shockwave lithotripsy in children. J Urol 1989;142:349–52.

38. Thornhill JA, Moran K, Moomey EE, et al. Extracorporeal shockwave lithotripsy monotherapy for paediatric urinary tract calculi. BJU Int 1990;65:348–50.

39. Picramenos D, Deliveliotis C, Alexopoulou K, et al. Extracorporeal shockwave lithotripsy for renal stones in children. Urol Int 1996;56:86–9.

40. Van Horn AC, Hollander JB, Kass EJ. First and second generation lithotripsy in children: results, comparison and follow-up. J Urol 1995;153:1969–71.

41. Rizvi S, Naqvi SA, Hussain Z, et al. Management of pediatric urolithiasis in pakistan: experience with 1,440 children. J Urol 2003;169:634–7.

42. Tan AH, Al-Omar M, Watterson JD, et al. Results of shockwave lithotripsy for pediatric urolithiasis. J Endourol 2004;18:527–30.

43. Choi H, Snyder HM III, Duckett JW. Urolithiasis in childhood: a current management. J Ped Surg 1987;22:158–64.

44. Polinsky MS, Kaiser BA, Baluarte HJ. Urolithiasis in children. Pediatr Clin North Am 1987;34:683–710.

45. Shepherd P, Thomas R, Harmon EP. Urolithiasis in children: innovations in management. J Urol 1988;140:790–2.

46. Milliner DS, Murphy ME. Urolithiasis in pediatric patients. Mayo Clinic Proceedings 1993;68:241–8.

47. Cohen TD, Ehreth J, King LR, Preminger GM. Pediatric urolithiasis: medical and surgical management. Urology 1996;47:292–303.

48. VanSavage JG, Palanca LG, Anderson RD, et al. Treatment of distal ureteral stones in children: similarities to the American Urological Association guidelines in adults. J Urol 2000;194 (3 pt 2):1089–93.

49. Morse R, Resnick M. Ureteral calculi: natural history and treatment in an era of advanced technology. J Urol 1991;145:263–5.

50. Caione P, DeGennaro M, Capozza N, et al. Endoscopic manipulation of ureteral calculi in children by rigid operative ureteroendoscopy. J Urol 1990;144:492–493.

51. Thomas R, Ortenberg J, Lee BR, et al. Safety and efficacy of pediatric ureteroscopy for management of calculous disease. J Urol 1993;149:1082–4.

52. Shroff S, Watson GM. Experience with ureteroscopy in children. Br J Urol 1995;75:395–400.

53. Scarpa RM, DeLisa A, Porru D, et al. Ureterolithotripsy in children. Urology 1995;46:859–62.

54. Smith DP, Jerkins GR, Noe HN. Urethroscopy in small neonates with posterior urethral valves and ureteroscopy in children with ureteral calculi. Urology 1996;47:908–10.

55. Kurzrock EA, Huffman JL, Hardy BE, et al. Endoscopic treatment of pediatric urolithiasis. J Ped Surg 1996;31:1413–6.

56. Minevich E, Rousseau MB, Wacksman J, et al. Pediatric ureteroscopy: technique and preliminary results. J Ped Surg 1977;32:571–4.

57. Wollin TA, Teichman JM, Rogenes VJ, et al. Holmium:YAG lithotripsy in children. J Urol 1999;162:1717–20.

58. Van Savage JG, Palanca LG, Anderson RD, et al. Treatment of distal ureteral stones in children: similarities to the American Urological Association guidelines in adults. J Urol 2000;164:1089–93.

59. Schuster TG, Russell KY, Bloom DA, et al. Ureteroscopy for the treatment of urolithiasis in children. J Urol 2002;167:1813–5.

60. Bassiri A, Ahmadnia H, Darabi MR, et al. Transureteral lithotripsy in pediatric practice. J Endourol 2002;16:257–60.

61. Satar N, Zeren S, Bayazit, et al. Rigid ureteroscopy for the treatment of ureteral calculi in children. J Urol 2004;172:298–300.

62. Kapoor DA, Leech JE, Yap WT, et al. Cost and efficacy of extracorporeal shock wave lithotripsy versus ureteroscopy in the treatment of lower ureteral calculi. J Urol 1992;48:1095–6.

63. Grasso M. Beaghler M, Loisides P. The case for primary endoscopic management of upper urinary tract calculi: II. Cost and outcome assessment of 112 primary ureteral calculi. J Urol 1995;45:372–6.

64. Albarran J. Operations plastiques et anastomoses dan la traitment des retentions de viem. These Paris 1903.

65. Davis DM. Intubated ureterotomy, new operation for ureteral and ureteropelvic stricture. Surg Gyn Obstet 1943;76:513–23.

66. Davis DM, Strong GH, Drake Wm. Intubated ureterotomy: experimental work and clinical results. J Urol 1948;59:851–62.

67. Davis DM. The process of ureteral repair: a recapitulation of the splinting question. J Urol 1958;79:215–23.

68. Kerbl K, Chandhoke PS, Figenshau RS, et al. Effect of stent duration on ureteral healing following endoureterotomy in an animal model. J Urol 1993;150:1302–5.

69. Thomas R, Cherry R, VandenBerg T. Long term efficacy of retrograde ureteroscopic endopyelotomy. J Urol 1993;149:276A.

70. Gupta M, Yuncay OL, Smith AD. Open surgical exploration after failed endopyelotomy: a 12-year perspective. J Urol 1997;157:1613–9.

71. Van Gangh PJ, Wilmart JF, Opsomer RJ, et al. Long term results and late recurrence after endoureteropyelotomy: a critical analysis of prognostic factors. J Urol 1994;151:934–7.

72. Figenshau RS, Clayman RV. Endourologic options for management of ureteropelvic unction obstruction in the pediatric patient. Urol Clin NA 1998;25:199–209.

73. Docimo SG, Kavovissi LR. The role of endourological techniques in the treatment of the pediatric ureteropelvic junction. J Urol 1997;158:1538.

74. Lam JS, Cooper KL, Greene TD, et al. Impact of hydronephrosis and renal function on treatment outcome: antegrade versus retrograde endopyelotomy. Urology 2003;61:1107–11.

75. Van Cangh PJ, Neea S. Galeon M, et al. Vessels around the ureteropelvic junction: significance and imaging by conventional radiology. J Endourol 1996;10:111–9.

76. Sutherland RS, Pfister RR, Koyle MA. Endopyelotomy associated ureteral necrosis: complete ureteral replacement using the Boari Flap. J Urol 1992;148:1490–2.

77. Peters CA. Robotically assisted surgery in pediatric urology. Urol Clin NA 2004;31:743–52.

78. King LR, Coughlin PW, Ford KK, et al. Initial experiences with percutaneous and transureteric ablation of postoperative ureteral strictures in children. J Urol 1984;131:1167–70.

79. Kavoussi LR, Meretyk S, Dierks SM, et al. Endopyelotomy for secondary ureteropelvic junction obstruction in children. J Urol 1991;145:345–349.

80. Tan HL, Najmaldin A, Webb DR. Endopyelotomy for pelviureteric junction obstruction in children. Eur Urol 1993;24:84–8.

81. Bolton DM, Bogaert GA, Mevorach RA, et al. Pediatric ureteropelvic junction obstruction treated with retrograde endopyelotomy. Urol 1994;44:609–13.

82. Faerber G, Ritchey M, Bloom DA. Percutaneous endopyelotomy in infants and young children after failed open pyeloplasty. J Urol 1995;154:1495–7.

83. Bogaert GA, Kogan BA, Mevorach RA, et al. Efficacy of retrograde endopyelotomy in children. J Urol 1996;156:734–7.

84. Towbin RB, Wacksman J, Ball WS. Percutaneous pyeloplasty in children: experience in three patients. Radiology 1987;163:381–4.

85. Netto NR, Ikari O, Esteves SC, et al. Antegrade endopyelotomy for pelviureteric junction obstruction in children. Br J Urol 1996;78:607–12.

86. Capolicchio G, Homsy YL, Houle AM, et al. Long-term results of percutaneous endopyelotomy in the treatment of children with failed open pyeloplasty. J Urol 1997;158:1534–7.

87. Schenkman EM, Tarry WF. Comparison of percutaneous endopyelotomy with open pyeloplasty for pediatric UPJ obstruction. J Urol 1998;159:1013–5.

88. Duschinsky J, Plaire J, Lingeman JE. Antegrade endopyelotomy in the pediatric population. World Congress of Endo Urol, Edinburgh Scotland, 1997.

89. Young JD, Gigenshau RS, Coplen DE, Clayman RV. Pediatric endopyelotomy: the Washington University experience. Society of Pediatric Urol, Dallas, Texas, 1999.

90. Tallai B, Toth C. Endopyelotomy in the child: our experience with 37 patients. J Urol 2003;17:A204.

91. Johnson DE. Calyceal diverticulum: report of 31 cases with reference to associated anomalies. South Med Journal 1969;62:220–2.

92. Middleton AW Jr, Pfister RC. Stone-containing pyelocalical diverticulum: embryogenic, anatomic, radiologic and clinical characteristics. J Urol 1974;111:2–6.

93. Timmons JW Jr, Malek RS, Hattery RR, Deweerd JH. Caliceal diverticulum. J Urol 1975;114:6–9.

94. Siegel MJ, McAlister WH. Calyceal diverticula in children: unusual features and complications. Radiology 1979;131:79–82.

95. Psihramis KE, Dretler SP. Extracorporeal shock wave lithotripsy of caliceal diverticula calculi. J Urol 1987;138:707–11.

96. Ritchie AWS, Parr MJ, Moussa SA, Tolley DA. Lithotripsy for calculi in caliceal diverticula? Br J Urol 1990;66:6–8.

97. Streem SB, Yost A. Treatment of caliceal diverticular calculi with extracorporeal shock wave lithotripsy: patient selection and extended follow-up. J Urol 1992;148:1043–6.

98. Jones JA, Lingeman JE, Steidle CP. The rules of extracorporeal shock wave lithotripsy and percutaneous nephrostolithotomy in the management of pyelocaliceal diverticula. J Urol 1991;146:724–7.

99. Shalhave AL, Soble JJ, Nakada SY, et al. Long-term outcome of caliceal diverticula following percutaneous endosurgical management. J Urol 1998;160:1635–9.

100. Grasso M, Lang G, Loisides P, et al. Endoscopic management of the symptomatic caliceal diverticular calculus. J Urol 1995;153:1878–81.

101. Batter SJ, Dretler SP. Ureterorenoscopic approach to the symptomatic caliceal diverticulum. J Urol 1997;158:709–11.

102. Baldwin DD, Beaghler MA, Ruckle HC, et al. Ureteroscopic treatment of symptomatic caliceal diverticular calculi. Tech Urol 1998;4:92–8.

103. Casale P. Grady RW, Joyner BW, et al. Transperitoneal laparoscopic pyelolithotomy after failed percutaneous access in the pediatric patient. J Urol 2004;172:680–3.

104. Patel HP, Bissler JJ. Hematuria in children. Pediatr Clin North Am 2001;48:1519–37.

105. Ingelfinger JR, Davis AE, Grupe WE. Frequency and etiology of gross hematuria in a general pediatric setting. Pediatrics 1977;59:557–61.

106. Tawfiek ER, Bagley DH. Ureteroscopic evaluation and treatment of chronic unilateral hematuria. J Urol 1998;160:700–2.

107. Bagley DH, Allen J. Flexible ureteroscopy in the diagnosis of benign essential hematuria. J Urol 1990;143:549–53.

108. Malada SY, Elashry OM, Picus D, Clayman RV. Long-term outcome of flexible ureterorenoscopy in the diagnosis and treatment of lateralizing essential hematuria. J Urol 1997;157:776–9.

109. Sloughenhoupt BL, Von Savage J. The evaluation and treatment of prolonged hematuria in adolescents. J Ky Med Assoc 1997;93:315–7.

110. Thiel D, Erhard MJ. The use of ureteropyeloscopy in the evaluation and treatment of adolescent hematuria. J Urol 2004;171:A573.

111. Lee RS, Retik AB, Borer JG, et al. Pediatric robot assisted laparoscopic dismembered pyeloplasty: comparison with a cohort of open surgery. J Urol 2006;175:683–7.

Part IV

Extracorporeal Shock Wave Lithotripsy

Part IV

Extracorporeal Shock Wave Lithotripsy

38

The Physics of Shock Wave Lithotripsy

Robin O. Cleveland, PhD

James A. McAteer, PhD

Shock wave lithotripsy (SWL) was introduced in the 1980s for the treatment of urinary stones and earned near-instantaneous acceptance as a first-line treatment option.[1] Since then SWL has revolutionized treatment in nephrolithiasis worldwide, and in the United States, it has been estimated that approximately 70% of kidney stones are treated using SWL.[2] Over the years, lithotripsy has undergone several waves of technological advancement, but with little change in the fundamentals of shock wave generation and delivery. That is, lithotriptors have changed in form and mode of operation from a user perspective—and in certain respects the changes have been dramatic—but the lithotriptor pressure pulse is still essentially the same. Lithotriptors produce a signature waveform, an acoustic shock wave. This pressure pulse, or shock wave, is responsible for breaking stones. However, it is also responsible for collateral tissue damage that in some cases can be significant.[3–6]

Lithotriptors produce a powerful acoustic field that results in two mechanical forces on stones and tissue: (1) direct stress associated with the high amplitude shock wave and (2) stresses and microjets associated with the growth and violent collapse of cavitation bubbles. Recent research has made significant advances in determining the mechanisms of shock wave action, but the story is by no means complete. What fuels this effort is the realization that a totally safe, yet effective lithotriptor has yet to be developed. Indeed, there is compelling evidence to suggest that a recent trend toward the development of lithotriptors that produce very high amplitude and tightly focused shock waves has led to increased adverse effects and higher re-treatment rates.[2,7–9]

A major objective within the lithotripsy community is to find ways to make SWL safer and more efficacious. The perfect lithotriptor may not exist, so urologists are left to determine how best to use the machines at hand. One step toward improving outcomes in SWL is to have a better understanding of how current machines work. Thus, the goal of this chapter is to introduce the basic physical concepts that underlie the mechanisms of shock wave action in SWL. Our aim is to give the background necessary to appreciate how the design features of a lithotriptor can affect its function. We also present a synopsis of current theories of shock wave action in stone breakage and tissue damage, and we summarize recent developments in lithotriptor technology. The main topics to be covered are as follows:

- Characteristics of a lithotriptor shock wave
- The acoustics of SWL
  - Acoustics primer
  - Acoustic cavitation
- The physics of clinical lithotriptors
  - Shock generation and shock focusing
  - Coupling the shock wave to the body
  - The focal zone of high acoustic pressure
- Mechanisms of shock wave action
  - How shock wave break stones
  - Mechanisms of tissue damage
- The evolution of the lithotriptor
- Future directions in lithotripsy

CHARACTERISTICS OF A LITHOTRIPTOR SHOCK WAVE

A typical shock wave measured at the focus of a lithotriptor is shown in Figure 38-1A. The wave is a short pulse of about 5 μs duration.* In this example, the wave begins with a near instantaneous jump to a peak positive pressure of about 40 MPa.† This fast transition in the waveform is referred to as a "shock." The transition is faster than can be measured and is less than 5 ns in duration.‡ The pressure then falls to zero about 1 μs later. There is then a region of negative pressure that lasts around 3 μs and has a peak negative

---

*1 microsecond (μs) is 1 millionth of a second.
†1 megapascal (MPa) is about 10 atmospheres of pressure.
‡1 nanosecond (ns) is 1 billionth of a second.

pressure around –10 MPa. The amplitude of the negative pressure is always much less than the peak positive pressure, and the negative phase of the waveform generally does not have a shock in it—that is, there is no abrupt transition. The entire 5 μs pulse is generally referred to as a shock wave, shock pulse or pressure pulse—technically, however, it is only the sharp leading transition that is formally a shock.

Figure 38-1B shows the amplitude spectrum of the shock pulse (that is, it displays the different frequency components in the pulse). We see that a lithotriptor shock wave does not have a dominant frequency or tone, but rather its energy is spread over a very large frequency range—this is a characteristic feature of a short pulse. It can be seen that most of the energy in the shock wave is between 100 kHz and 1 MHz. This means that it is unlikely that a lithotriptor breaks kidney stones by exciting its resonance—as an opera singer might shatter a crystal glass.

The waveform shown in Figure 38-1A was measured in an electrohydraulic lithotriptor. A description of different types of shock wave generators is given below (see "The Physics of Clinical Lithotripsy"). Most lithotriptors produce a similarly shaped shock wave, but depending on the machine and the setting, the peak positive pressure typically varies between 30 and 110 MPa and the negative pressure between –5 and –15 MPa. In Figure 38-2A, we compare waveforms measured in an electrohydraulic lithotriptor and

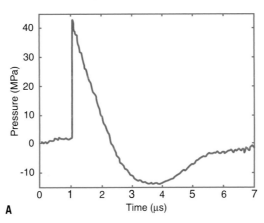
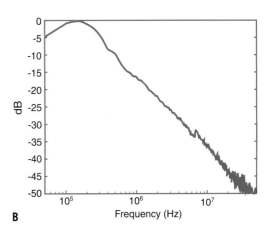

Figure 38-1 *A*, A pressure waveform measured at the focus of an electrohydraulic lithotriptor (Dornier HM3). *B*, The Fourier transform of the waveform in *A* showing how the energy is distributed as a function of frequency. (Both axes are shown on a log scale.) The peak of the amplitude response is around 300 kHz, which corresponds to the 4 μs duration. The energy between 1 MHz and 20 MHz can be attributed to the shock in the waveform. The steeper drop-off of energy for frequencies above 20 MHz is because that was the limit of the hydrophone for measuring the rise-time of the shock wave.

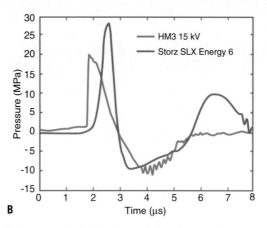

Figure 38-2 *A*, Focal waveforms measured in the Dornier HM3 at 24 kV and the Storz SLX at energy level 9. *B*, Comparison at lower settings—in this case the amplitudes are about the same, but the SLX waveform has not formed a shock.

an electromagnetic lithotriptor. It can be seen that the basic shape of both waveforms is very similar, consisting of a shock front, compressive phase, and tensile tail. For the settings chosen here, the main difference is the amplitude. Figure 38-2B shows waveforms measured at lower power settings of both machines, and again, the waveforms are similar, but the amplitudes are different.

Thus, lithotriptor shock waves show a unique form that contains a high amplitude, compressive phase of extremely rapid transition and short duration followed by a trailing tensile phase. The features of this waveform are similar regardless of the type of lithotriptor, but there are considerable differences in the amplitude and spatial extent of the acoustic output. It is likely that the amplitude and size of the focal zone of different lithotriptors affects their performance.

AN ACOUSTICS PRIMER FOR SWL

What is an Acoustic Wave?

An acoustic wave, or sound wave, is created whenever an object moves within a fluid (a fluid can be either a gas or liquid). In Figure 38-3, we show that, as an object moves, it locally compresses the fluid that surrounds it—that is, the molecules are forced closer together. The compressed mole-

cules in that region, in turn, push against the molecules next to them. This relieves the compression in the first region but leads to a new compressed region. The molecules in the second region then start to compress the next adjacent region, and so on; it is thus that a "wave" of compression travels through the fluid. This is an "acoustic wave," and the speed of wave propagation (called the sound-speed) is a material property of the medium. Note that individual molecules do not travel with the acoustic wave; rather, they just jostle their adjacent neighbors. Therefore, for an acoustic wave to propagate, there must be a medium present that can support the vibrations. This is an important physical difference between classical waves (eg, acoustic waves, seismic waves, water waves) and electromagnetic waves (eg, light, radio waves, x-rays). For electromagnetic waves, energy is carried by photons, which may be thought of as particles that physically travel through space; thus a medium is not needed for the signal to be transferred. Therefore, light can travel through a vacuum, but sound cannot.

Sound Waves Have Compressive and Tensile Phases

The explanation above describes the compressive phase of a sound wave (that is, where

the molecules are compressed). For the case where the object moves away from the fluid, there is a resulting rarefaction of the molecules (that is, the moving object leaves a partial vacuum). In this case, the neighboring molecules will move to fill the void, leaving a new region of rarefaction. This continues one region to the next, and the rarefactional disturbance propagates through the medium as a tensile acoustic wave. In most cases, a tensile wave propagates just like a compressive wave and with the same sound speed.

Typical acoustic sources, such as audio speakers, vibrate backwards and forwards. This produces alternating compression and rarefaction waves that are referred to as the compressive phase and tensile phase of the acoustic wave. Often the waveform is sinusoidal in nature. Note, however, that the majority of acoustic waves, including the acoustic pulses generated in lithotripsy, are not sinusoidal in form. For small-amplitude waves (linear acoustics), every point of the waveform moves at the same speed: the sound speed c_0. This is a material property, and for water and tissue, it is about 1,500 m/s. We will see later for large amplitude (nonlinear) acoustic waves, such as shock waves, that the sound speed is slightly changed by the presence of the wave.

The waveform shown in Figure 38-1 displays the pressure pulse as a function of time at a given point in space. This is typically how acoustic waves are measured; for example, a microphone will record how pressure varies in time at one point in space. Acoustic waves, however, also vary in space and it is often useful to think of the wave in terms of its spatial extent. The relationship between the temporal separation of points on an acoustic wave (Δt) and the spatial separation of the points (Δx) is related by:

$$\Delta x = \Delta t \, c_0 \qquad \text{(Equation 38-1)}$$

Recall that, in water or tissue, the sound speed is $c_0 = 1,500$ m/s = 1.5 mm/µs and therefore, for the shock wave shown in Figure 38-1, the positive part of the wave—a portion 1 µs long in time—will have a spatial extent in water of 1.5 mm. For a sinusoidal wave the spatial extent of one cycle of the wave is called the *wavelength*.

Sound Waves are not just Pressure Waves

When a sound wave propagates, it affects the density, pressure, and particle velocity of the fluid particles. The impact on the density occurs because, as molecules are compressed together, the local density (ρ) will increase and in regions of rarefraction the density will decrease. For an acoustic wave it is convenient to write the total density as:

$$\rho = \rho_0 + \rho_a \qquad \text{(Equation 38-2)}$$

where ρ_0 is the ambient density of the medium (in the absence of sound) and ρ_a is the variation in the density due to the acoustic wave.

The pressure in the fluid can similarly be written as the sum of two terms:

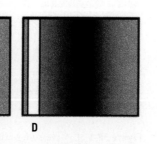

Figure 38-3 Illustration showing a molecular view point of a sound wave. *A*, Medium is at rest. *B*, A piston pushes all the molecules out of the left side, resulting in a localized region of compression at the face of the piston (dark region). *C*, The neighboring molecules are compressed and the compression region moves away from the piston. *D*, The wave continues to moved away from the piston. The molecules at the piston return to their ambient state.

$$p = p_0 + p_a \qquad \text{(Equation 38-3)}$$

where p_0 is the ambient pressure (in the absence of sound) and p_a, the *acoustic pressure*, is the fluctuation due to the sound wave. For most fluids, acoustic pressure and density are directly related by an "equation of state" which takes the form:

$$p_a = \rho_a\, c_0^2 \qquad \text{(Equation 38-4)}$$

That is, where the wave is compressed, the pressure will be positive, and where the fluid is rarefied, the pressure will be negative. Physically, pressure represents a force per unit area and has units of pascals (Pa). One pascal is quite a small pressure, and atmospheric pressure at sea level is approximately 100,000 Pa. In biomedical ultrasound, acoustic pressure is normally measured in megapascals (MPa).[§]

By way of example, the amplitude of the pressure from a diagnostic ultrasound scanner is about 2 MPa at the focus. Typically, values for ambient density and sound speed in tissue are $\rho_0 = 1{,}000$ kg/m^3 and $c_0 = 1{,}540$ m/s, and so this corresponds to a relative density perturbation of $\rho_a / \rho_0 = 0.0009$. For lithotripsy, peak pressures can be upwards of 100 MPa, which results in $\rho_a / \rho_0 = 0.04$. Therefore, the density disturbances associated with acoustic waves in medical devices—even the very strong waves that are produced in lithotripsy, actually result in very weak (less than 5%) compression of the fluid.

PROGRESSIVE WAVES AND PARTICLE VELOCITY
The case shown in Figure 38-3, where the compression wave moves in one direction, is referred to as a *progressive wave*. In contrast, when there are sound waves traveling in different directions, this is referred to as a *compound wave*, which will not be considered here. For a progressive wave, the molecules in the compressed region also have a small net velocity away from the source. The net velocity of the molecules in a region of space is referred to as the *particle velocity* (u_a) and for a progressive acoustic wave it can be expressed as:

$$u_a = p_a/\rho_0\, c_0 \qquad \text{(Equation 38-5)}$$

Using the example of a 100 MPa shock wave, the instantaneous particle velocity at the peak is about 67 m/s. We will see below that the particle velocity is needed in order to determine the energy in an acoustic wave. It has also been suggested that the particle velocity within a biological target may produce sufficient strain to damage the cells.

ACOUSTIC IMPEDANCE The density and sound speed of a material (Equation 38-4) determine its *specific acoustic impedance* ($Z_0 = \rho_0\, c_0$). This term is often shortened to *acoustic impedance* or just *impedance*. The impedance of tissue and water is about 1.5×10^6 kg m^{-2} s^{-1}. The units are

often referred to as Rayls—after the eminent nineteeth century acoustician Lord Rayleigh—although the Rayl is not an international standard.

Therefore, for a progressive acoustic wave, the pressure, density and particle velocity are not independent, but are linearly related to each other:

$$p_a = u_a\, Z_0 = \rho_a\, c_0^2 \qquad \text{(Equation 38-6)}$$

where the coefficients are material properties. It follows that regions of high pressure are also compressed, and high particle velocity (away from source) and regions of low pressure are rarefied and have a negative particle velocity (towards the source). As the acoustic wave travels, the fluctuations in density, pressure, and particle velocity all move together (ie, "in phase"). Therefore, in a fluid with known material properties, if one property of an acoustic wave (such as the acoustic pressure) is measured, then Equation 38-5 can be used to determine the other acoustic properties.

WAVE INTENSITY OR ENERGY A propagating acoustic wave carries energy. The amount of acoustic energy per unit area is called the *energy flux, energy density, energy flux density*, or the *pulse intensity integral*. The IEC standard[10][‖] calls this the "pulse intensity integral (energy density)" and it can be calculated by the following integral:

$$PII = \int p_a u_a dt \qquad \text{(Equation 38-7)}$$

where the integration is done over the duration of the pulse. This is the acoustic equivalent to the expression from physics "work equals force times distance," where acoustic pressure is the force per unit area and the time integral of the velocity gives the distance.

The units for the pulse intensity integral (*PII*) are joules per square meter (J/m^2). For a progressive wave, we know that the particle velocity is related to the acoustic pressure $u_a = p_a/Z_0$ and therefore:

$$PII = \int \frac{p_a^2}{Z_0} dt \qquad \text{(Equation 38-8)}$$

in which case, one only need measure the pressure of the wave to determine *PII*. Note that to calculate the integral, one needs to be able to accurately measure the entire pressure-versus-time waveform so that the integration can be done. The duration of a lithotripter pulse, for which this integral needs to be evaluated, is defined as the time from when the absolute value of the pressure first exceeds 10% of the peak pressure until the last time is exceeds 10% of the peak pressure.

To determine the energy in an acoustic wave, a specific area, A, has to be chosen, and the

energy that passes through that area can then be calculated as:

$$E = \iint PII\, dA \qquad \text{(Equation 38-9)}$$

where the double integral indicates a surface integral over the area A. The unit for energy is joules (J). The energy, E, will depend on both the size of the area A and how the intensity varies across the area. The *focal acoustic pulse energy* is calculated using the area in the focal plane, where the pressure is greater than half the maximum pressure (this is equivalent to the focal zone, see below). Energy can also be calculated over different areas, for example, the projected area of a stone or the area where the peak pressure is above 5 MPa.[11]

Another acoustic property used in the literature is the power per unit area, or the *intensity I*. Power is energy per unit time, and so the intensity is the energy density divided by the time over which the integration was done (Equation 38-8), which is normally the pulse length T_p:

$$I = \frac{PII}{T_p} \qquad \text{(Equation 38-10)}$$

Intensity has units of watts per square meter (W/m^2) but it is more common in biomedical ultrasound to use centimeters (W/cm^2).

For a sinusoidal pressure wave the integral can be calculated exactly and the intensity is:

$$I = \frac{\hat{p}^2}{2Z_0} \qquad \text{(Equation 38-11)}$$

where $\hat{p}$ is the peak pressure of the sinusoidal wave. If one substitutes the impedance for water or tissue ($Z_0 = 1.5$ MRayls) the relationship can be expressed as $\hat{p} = \sqrt{3I}$ where $\hat{p}$ is in atmospheres of pressure and I is in W/cm^2. For pulsed pressure waves, such as in lithotripsy, a simple expression does not exist for the intensity, as even small changes in the pulse shape can have a significant effect on the integration used to calculate *PII*.

REFLECTION AND TRANSMISSION OF SOUND WAVES When an acoustic wave encounters a medium with a different impedance, then part of the wave will continue to propagate into the new medium (the transmitted wave) and part of the wave will be reflected back into the original medium (the reflected wave). In the case of *normal incidence*, where the propagation direction of the shock wave is perpendicular to the surface, the amplitude of the transmitted and reflected waves depend only on the change in impedance between the two media, what is referred to as the *impedance mismatch*. In terms of acoustic pressure the transmission and reflection coefficients are:

$$R_p = \frac{Z_2 - Z_1}{Z_2 + Z_1} \qquad \text{(Equation 38-12)}$$

$$T_p = \frac{2Z_2}{Z_2 + Z_1} \qquad \text{(Equation 38-13)}$$

There is a different set of coefficients for the intensity or energy, called the intensity transmission and reflection coefficients:

$$R_I = \frac{(Z_2 - Z_1)^2}{(Z_2 + Z_1)^2} = R_p^2$$

$$\text{(Equation 38-14)}$$

$$T_I = \frac{4Z_1 Z_2}{(Z_2 + Z_1)^2} = 1 - R_I$$

$$\text{(Equation 38-15)}$$

In Figure 38-4, we show the intensity transmission coefficient for an acoustic wave going from water to another medium with different impedance. We indicate typical values for tissue, kidney stones, bone, and air. One can see that the transmission from water to tissue is very efficient. The water-to-stone transmission is also relatively high, with 75 to 95% of the energy transmitted into the kidney stones. But a water-air interface has an extremely small coefficient, and less than 0.1% of the energy of an acoustic wave in water will pass into air—that is, 99.9% is reflected. This is why shock wave generators in lithotripsy are water-filled, why immersion of the patient in water gives the most efficient coupling of shock waves to the body, and why in dry lithotriptors, great care must be taken to eliminate air pockets between the shock head and the body. This is also one reason why stones are not targeted for treatment through lung or segments of gas-filled bowel. Indeed the best *acoustic window*, which allows the shock wave a pure tissue path to the kidney, is on the flank of the patient (delineated by the ribs, spine and pelvic bone).

FOCUSING AND DIFFRACTION OF SOUND In lithotripsy, focusing of the shock waves is used to concentrate the acoustic energy onto the stone while reducing the impact on the surrounding tissue as much as possible. Lithotriptors achieve focusing by various means, including the use of reflectors, acoustic lenses, and spherically curved sources. Regardless of the method used, the physics that describes the focusing of the waves is similar for all these cases. An ideal focus would be the case where all energy is localized to an infinitesimally small region in space. However, the physics of wave propagation does not allow the energy to be focused to an arbitrarily small volume due to a process called *diffraction*. This means that, even though the acoustic pressure may be greatest at one point in space, there is a finite region or volume of surrounding space that is also at high amplitude. This is called the *focal zone*. For a theoretically optimal focusing arrangement, where sound can come in from all angles, diffraction puts a bound on the size of the focal zone of about one wavelength. For the realistic focusing arrangements used in lithotripsy, where the sound only comes from one direction, the focal zone can be from a few millimeters to tens of millimeters in size.

FOCAL ZONE The *focal zone* of a lithotriptor (equivalent terms include *focal region, hot spot, focal spot, focal volume, zone of high pressure*) is normally ellipsoidal in shape with its longest dimension along the axis of the shock wave. To demonstrate this, Figure 38-5 shows the predicted peak pressure of the focal zone in an unmodified Dornier HM3 lithotriptor.[12] The length and diameter of the focal zone depends on the diameter of the source, the focal length of the source, and the frequency content of the waveform. The dimension of the focal zone is thus one characteristic of any given lithotriptor that is determined by design features. Different lithotriptors have different focal zones and, as is discussed below, some lithotriptors generate extreme acoustic pressures delivered to a very narrow focal zone.

For a focused acoustic source that generates a sinusoidal waveform, such as an ultrasound transducer, there are analytical expressions for the size of the focal zone. The critical parameters are the wavelength of the sound wave (λ) and the half angle of the aperture:

$$\alpha = \arcsin(D/2F) \qquad \text{(Equation 38-16)}$$

where D is the diameter of the source and F the focal length. The formulae for the length (L_{FZ}) and the diameter (D_{FZ}) of the focal zone are:

$$L_{FZ} = \frac{0.6\lambda}{\sin^2(\alpha/2)} \qquad \text{(Equation 38-17)}$$

and

$$D_{FZ} = \frac{0.7\lambda}{\sin \alpha} \qquad \text{(Equation 38-18)}$$

Note that the focal length F is the distance from the mouth of the therapy head to the focus (where the stone should be placed). The focal length should not be confused with the length of the focal zone L_{FZ} which is the region around the focus where the pressure is high.

For a pulsed waveform, as is generated in lithotripsy, there are no explicit formulae for the size of the focal volume because the size depends on the waveform shape. But the focal region of a lithotriptor can be estimated using the formulae for the focal region of a sine wave. Figure 38-6A shows how the focal zone gets shorter and narrower as the diameter of the source aperture is increased. Figure 38-6B shows how the focal zone gets shorter and narrower as the focal length of the source (source-to-target distance) is decreased. Therefore, to make a small focal zone, a shock source with a large diameter aperture and short focal length would be desired. However, the size of the acoustic window in the flank and the need to be able to target stones deep in the body mean that, in most lithotriptors, both the focal

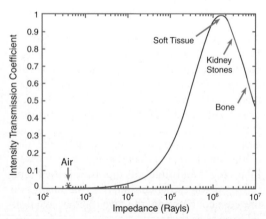

Figure 38-4 The intensity transmission coefficient (TI) from water ($Z = 1.5 \times 10^6$ Rayls) to a second medium, as a function of the impedance of the second medium. Typical values are indicated for soft tissue, kidney stones, bone and air. The transmission to soft tissue is very efficient. Coupling to air is very poor.

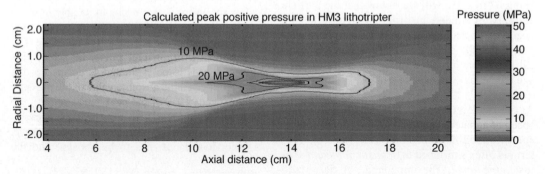

Figure 38-5 Predicted peak positive pressure in a Dornier HM3 lithotriptor. The pressure is not focused to a point but extends over a finite volume.

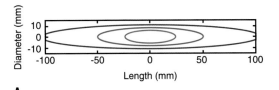

A

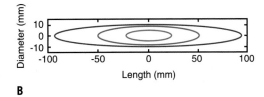

B

Figure 38-6 Predicted focal zone size as a function of the diameter of the source and the focal length of the source for a 500 kHz source. *A*, Contours show size of the focal zone for a source that has a focal length of 14 cm and with an aperture of 25 cm (red), 15 cm (green) and 10 cm (blue). The focal zone gets longer and wider as the aperture size decreases. *B*, Contours show the size of the focal zone for a source with fixed aperture diameter (15 cm) and varying focal length: 8 cm (red), 14 cm (green) and 20 cm (blue). The focal zone gets broader and longer as the focal length increases. For reference, the Dornier HM3 has focal length of 13 cm and an aperture diameter of 15 cm.

length and the diameter of the aperture are around 15 cm.

NONLINEAR ACOUSTICS When an acoustic wave has very large amplitude, for example a lithotriptor shock wave, the speed of the wave is no longer constant but depends on the local compression of the fluid. For "weak" shock waves (recall even at the focus of the highest power lithotriptor, the water is compressed by less than 5%) the speed of propagation ("phase speed") of an acoustic wave is:

$$c_{phase} = c_0 + \beta \, p_a / \rho_o \, c_0 \qquad \text{(Equation 38-19)}$$

where β is the *coefficient of nonlinearity* of the fluid and is a material property of the medium. For water, β is about 3.5, and for tissue, it varies from about 4 to 9. Normally, tissue of more complex structure has a greater coefficient of nonlinearity. A reasonable value for healthy soft tissue is β = 5.

Nonlinearity arises because of two physical processes; first, in regions of high pressure, the local sound speed is increased above the usual value; and second, the molecules in regions of high pressure have a higher particle velocity and are convected in the direction of acoustic propagation. For sound traveling through tissue, it is the first process that dominates the nonlinearity.

The difference between a nonlinear wave and a linear wave is that, for a nonlinear wave, different parts of the wave travel at different speeds as described by Equation 38-19. Figure 38-7 shows what happens to a sinusoidal wave as it propagates with nonlinearity present. The waveform becomes distorted in shape. In the absence of absorption, the wave obtains an infinite slope and then folds over and becomes multivalued. Ocean waves fanning up the beach are such waves, but this waveform is not physically realizable in acoustics—that is, it is not possible to have more than one pressure at any one point in space.

SHOCK FORMATION The point at which the waveform first attains an infinite slope is called the shock formation distance. For a sinusoidal waveform the *shock formation distance* is:

$$\bar{x} = \frac{\rho_0 c_0^3}{\beta \hat{p} 2\pi f} \qquad \text{(Equation 38-20)}$$

Any acoustic wave can result in a shock wave if it can propagate for a long enough distance. For most sound waves encountered in everyday life, however, the shock formation distance is so long that the wave has been absorbed before it can form a shock. In lithotripsy the sound waves are intense enough that the wave typically does form a shock in the approximately 10 cm propagation path to the kidney.

RISE TIME In acoustics, waveforms are prevented from folding over (or breaking) by the presence of acoustic loss mechanisms. All acoustic waves will leave behind a small fraction of their energy as they propagate through a fluid—this loss of energy is referred to as absorption. The absorption of sound is greater from waveforms with steep gradients. In the case of a shock wave where the slope tends towards infinity, the absorption will also tend towards infinity. The shock will, therefore, never attain an infinite slope, but instead, a balance between nonlinear distortion and absorption will result in a shock front where the pressure jumps in a very short time. This time is referred to as the *rise time* of the shock (or the Taylor shock thickness). For a shock wave in water, the expression for the Taylor shock thickness is:

$$T_{rt} = \frac{5}{\Delta P} \text{ns} \cdot \text{MPa} \qquad \text{(Equation 38-21)}$$

where ΔP is the pressure jump in MPa and the rise time (in ns) is defined as the time to go from 10% to 90% of ΔP. From this expression one finds that a 1 MPa shock should have a rise time of 5 ns and a 10 MPa shock a rise time of 0.5 ns. As a shock becomes stronger, the rise time shortens. Using Equation 38-1, one finds that the corresponding spatial extent of the rise time of the 1 MPa and 10 MPa shock waves is 7.5 μm and 0.75 μm, respectively.

Nonlinear acoustics phenomena are also important in other areas of biomedical ultrasound. In diagnostic ultrasound, nonlinear effects can create problems such as excess heating of tissue[13,14] but can also be beneficial by enhancing image quality in tissue harmonic imaging.[15–17] Nonlinear effects are also important in high intensity focused ultrasound surgery (HIFU or FUS), where ultrasonic heating of tissue is exploited to destroy specific regions of tissue or

to coagulate blood (see ter Haar G,[18] Hynynen K,[19] Arefiev A,[20] and Bailey MR, et al[21]).

ABSORPTION OF SOUND BY TISSUE As mentioned above, when a sound wave passes through a medium, most of the energy remains in the sound wave, but a small amount of it is absorbed by the medium. The amplitude of an acoustic wave will therefore slowly decay, or *attenuate*, as it propagates through a medium. The absorption in water is very low, and aside from controlling the rise time of the shock front, has little effect on lithotriptor waveforms. The absorption in tissue, however, is about 1,000 times larger than that in water and has a measurable effect on lithotriptor shock waves as they pass through the body and into the kidney. Typical values for absorption in muscle, fat and kidney are shown in Figure 38-8 as a function of frequency. One can see that the

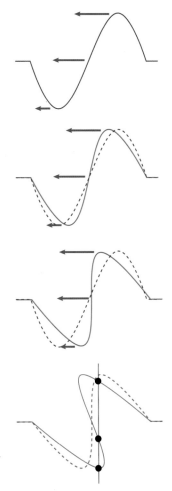

Figure 38-7 Nonlinear distortion of a sine wave based on Equation 38-19. *A*, Initial waveform; the length of the arrows shows the local phase speed of different points to the waveform. The peak will move the most quickly and the trough the least quickly. *B*, Waveform after a short amount of propagation (dashed line is waveform in *A*) showing how the shape has distorted. *C*, Shock formation distance where the slope of the waveform first becomes infinite (dashed line is waveform in *A*). *D*, Predicted multivalued waveform—the vertical line indicates that there are three different pressures predicted at one point in time (dashed line is from *C*). This shape is non-physical because absorption will prevent the wave from folding over.

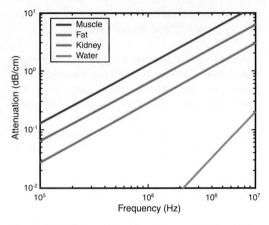

Figure 38-8 Attenuation of sound as a function of frequency for muscle, fat, and kidney tissue (listed in decreasing order of loss). Also shown is the attenuation in water, which is much less (1,000 times less at 1 MHz) than the attenuation of tissue.

absorption increases (almost linearly) with frequency. This means that energy is removed more effectively from the higher frequencies of the sound wave. In lithotripsy waveforms, the high frequency components are associated with the shock front. The primary action of tissue absorption is to increase the rise time of the shock front, and this will also result in the peak amplitude being reduced. The main energy components of the wave (which are around 500 kHz) will not be significantly impacted by tissue attenuation, and therefore, the basic shape of the pulse should not be affected by propagation through tissue, and the peak negative pressure, in particular, will not be sensitive to tissue absorption.

HOW SHOCK WAVES ARE MEASURED

Hydrophones Measure Shock Waves The main physical property of a lithotriptor is the spatial and temporal distribution of its acoustic pressure field. The acoustic field is typically measured in water using a hydrophone, which converts pressure into an electrical signal. Lithotriptors generate short (wide frequency band) high amplitude acoustic pulses, which are focused to a small volume in space. These physical parameters require that the hydrophone needs to (1) be very wide bandwidth (60 kHz to > 20 MHz), (2) be robust, to withstand the high pressures of the shock waves, and (3) possess a small active area ≈ 0.5 mm. The first reliable measurements of lithotripsy shock waves were performed with a hydrophone made of PVDF—a piezoelectric plastic.[22] PVDF has very wide bandwidth, is capable of measuring high amplitude acoustic pressures, and can be manufactured so that only a small region is active. Both membrane hydrophones and needle hydrophones have been used, however membrane hydrophones are considered to yield the best measurement of the shock wave.[23] One problem with PVDF is that the adhesion between water and PVDF is not strong and the tensile phase of the lithotripsy pulse can result

in cavitation at the surface of the PVDF. This is a significant limitation that has two main consequences. First, it limits the ability of the hydrophone to measure the tensile phase of the shock wave because, once the bubble forms, the negative pressure is relieved and the hydrophone registers a pressure close to zero. Second, when the cavitation bubbles collapse, they can irreversibly damage the hydrophone.

Recently, a new hydrophone was developed—the fiber optic probe hydrophone (FOPH).[24] This is now considered to be the state-of-the-art for measuring lithotripsy shock waves and is the recommended device in the international measurement standard.[10] The FOPH consists of a laser that injects light into one end of an optical fiber; the other end of the fiber is placed in the lithotriptor field. The FOPH measures the light that is reflected from the end of the fiber and exploits the fact that the amplitude of the reflection depends on the pressure in the fluid. Several features make the FOPH superior to the PVDF membrane. Similar to PVDF, the FOPH has wide bandwidth and is capable of measuring very high pressure amplitudes. The diameter of the active area of the FOPH (100 μm) is smaller than most PVDF hydrophones (500 μm). Also, the FOPH is made of an optical fiber (silica), and the adhesion between water and silica is very high. This means that cavitation is much less likely to occur at the surface of the FOPH, and therefore, it can more accurately capture the tensile phase of the shock wave. This also means that the FOPH is less susceptible to damage from cavitation. The main drawback with the FOPH is that the signal it generates is weak and therefore not good for measuring low pressures (≈2 MPa and less).

Measuring Shock Waves in the Body All published measures of dimensions of the focal zone come from in vitro experiments, and there have been few attempts to collect any shock wave pressure data within animals. Both the high attenuation and inhomogeneous nature of tissue will affect shock waves as they propagate through the body. Figure 38-9 shows representative pressure waveforms for a Dornier HM3 measured in water and for a PVDF membrane hydrophone implanted in a pig.[25] The in vivo waveform is very similar in basic shape to the in vitro waveform. The main difference is that the in vivo waveform has a 30% decrease in peak positive pressure and a greatly increased shock rise time (70 ns). Both of these effects are consistent with the higher attenuation associated with tissue.

What is Acoustic Cavitation? A second mechanical force generated by lithotriptor shock waves is *acoustic cavitation*. This refers to the generation of cavities in a fluid (ie, bubbles) when the tensile phase (negative pressure) of the acoustic wave is sufficiently strong to rip the fluid apart. In lithotripsy, the tensile phase of the shock wave is large enough (≈10 MPa) to generate violent cavitation events. Cavitation is believed to play a significant role in tissue damage during SWL and to contribute to stone comminution.[26–28]

Typically, cavitation is initiated at micron size motes in the fluid or at sites of small gas pockets trapped on rough surfaces.[29] There are a number of different theories available[30,31] that can describe how acoustic cavitation proceeds once the cavity has been formed—at this point, the cavity is normally referred to as a bubble. In Figure 38-10, we show the predicted radius of a spherical bubble as a function of time in response to a lithotriptor shock wave. The bubble is first compressed by the positive phase of the shock wave. Then the tensile phase of the shock wave causes the bubble to grow from 1 μm radius to about 1 mm radius over a period of 150 μs. Note that the bubble continues to grow long after the shock wave has passed (5 μs time frame), and this is referred to as inertial cavitation as the dynamics of the bubble are no longer driven by acoustics, but instead, by the inertia of the fluid surrounding the bubble. While the bubble is large, some amount of gas and vapor from the fluid will diffuse into the bubble. The bubble will then collapse by virtue of the near vacuum inside the bubble and the roughly 1 atmosphere of ambient pressure in the surrounding fluid. It takes a further 150 μs for the bubble to collapse. The collapse is very violent, and the gas that diffused inside is heated and compressed to such an extent that it can produce light.[32] The main collapse is followed by rebounds, after which the gas that had diffused into the bubble will slowly diffuse back out into the fluid. Also shown in Figure 38-10, is the acoustic emission radiated by the bubble; a lithotripsy-induced cavitation bubble

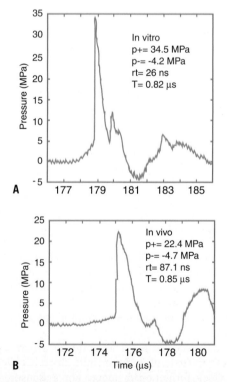

Figure 38-9 *A*, Waveform measured in water with a miniature PVDF hydrophone in a Dornier HM3 at 18 kV. *B*, Waveform measured in vivo in a pig for the same settings. The peak amplitude in vivo was about 30% less than that in water, and the rise time in vivo (87 ns) was much longer than that measured in water (26 ns).

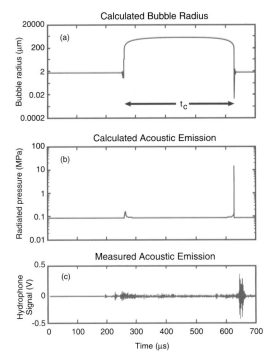

Figure 38-10 *A,* Calculated radius versus time curve of a spherical bubble subject to a lithotriptor pulse (as in Figure 38-1). In this time scale, the shock wave arrives at the focus at 250 μs, and the bubble is initially crushed by the leading compressive phase. The bubble grows to a millimeter-size bubble at about 450 μs. It then starts to collapse, with a violent collapse occurring at 650 μs. The time between the two collapse signals is the characteristic time t_C. *B,* The predicted acoustic emissions that the bubble calculated in *A* will radiate. There are two emissions due to the two collapses. *C,* Measured acoustic emissions in a Dornier HM3 using a PCD (see Figure 38-11). The measured emissions agree with the calculations.

generates two acoustic emissions, one when it is hit by the compressive wave, and one when it collapses hundreds of microseconds later. This unique "double-bang" signature can be used to detect the cavitation events.[32]

There are numerous techniques by which cavitation can be measured.

High-Speed Photography Bubble behavior can be observed using a high-speed camera in an in vitro setting.[33–36] In principle, this allows the entire dynamics of a bubble to be tracked from genesis to extinction. In practice, this is not feasible. During the growth phase, the bubble needs to be imaged at millimeter-length scales and tens of microseconds time scales. At the nadir of the collapse, the bubble radius is less then a 1 μm, and the dynamics of the collapse is at nanosecond time scales. The remnant bubble left after the rebounds, is on order of 10 μm and slowly dissolves over hundreds of milliseconds. Thus, the range of temporal and spatial scales makes it virtually impossible to capture all the bubble dynamics photographically. Therefore, investigators have found it necessary to study cavitation in segments. A further limitation of imaging is that cameras have a limited depth of field and cannot give an adequate record of bubble dynamics throughout the substantial volume of the cavitation field.

Laser Scattering of Single Bubbles The dynamics of a single spherical bubble can be measured very precisely by laser scattering.[37] In this case, a laser beam is used to illuminate a bubble, and a photodetector is used to collect the light scattered by the bubble. For a spherical bubble, the amplitude of the scattered light varies in a known way as the bubble radius changes. This method is able to capture most of the temporal and spatial scales associated with the dynamics of a lithotripsy-excited cavitation bubble. But laser scattering has several restrictions: the sample volume is very small, the method requires unrestricted visual access at high magnification, and the theory that is used to recover the actual bubble size is based on a single spherical bubble. This means the technique will only yield qualitative information about bubble clouds or nonspherical bubbles, both of which are very common in lithotripsy induced cavitation.

Acoustic Detection Can Be Used In Vivo Acoustic detection of bubbles is very powerful, in part, because it can be used to characterize bubble dynamics within living subjects. Acoustic detection normally works in one of two modes: active cavitation detection (ACD) and passive cavitation detection (PCD).[38–40] In ACD, one transducer is used to send an acoustic wave toward the cavitation field, while a second transducer picks up sound reflections from the bubbles—this is the acoustic analogue to laser scattering. In PCD, one or more receiving transducers listen for the "double-bang" acoustic emissions from cavitation bubbles. In the case where two receiving transducers (dual PCD) are used, it is possible to take advantage of coincidence detection to sample a small, discrete volume of the cavitation field where the transducers intersect.[41] The timing and amplitude of the two emissions is influenced by various factors, such as the size of the initial bubble and the amplitude of the lithotriptor pulse. Thus, although acoustic detection does not image bubbles (that is, it cannot provide information on bubble number and size) it gives valuable data that can be used to help

characterize the acoustic output of a lithotriptor and assess the environment and dynamics of the cavitation field.[35,41,42]

Other techniques have also been developed for measuring cavitation (Figure 38-11). It has been observed that cavitation leads to pitting on metal foils, and the number and depth of pits can be used to assess the violence of cavitation.[26,43,44] An electromagnetic probe device has been used to measure the mechanical force exerted on a steel ball by both the incident shock wave and the cavitation activity.[45] The high pressures and temperatures in the interior of the bubble provide an environment that can produce light emissions (sonoluminescence) and also result in enhanced chemical reaction rates (sonochemistry). Production of light and byproducts from chemical reactions have both been used to quantify cavitation activity.[37,42] These are secondary measurements of the cavitation field, and interpreting the results in terms of physical processes can be complicated.

THE PHYSICS OF CLINICAL LITHOTRIPSY

SHOCK GENERATION AND FOCUSING Three shock wave generating principles have been used in clinical lithotriptors.

Electrohydraulic Lithotriptors The electrohydraulic lithotriptor (EHL) has a spark source, which generates a shock wave that is focused by an ellipsoidal reflector (Figure 38-12). In an EHL, the pressure pulse originates as a shock wave and remains a shock wave at all times during its propagation from the spark source to the reflector, and then as it focuses to the target. As we will see below, this is not the case for other types of shock wave sources. In an EHL, focusing of the shock wave is critically dependent on the placement of the spark at the first focus of the ellipse. Misalignment by just a few millimeters can lead to a significant loss in focusing and a lengthening and broadening of the focal zone. Thus, EHLs are designed so that the

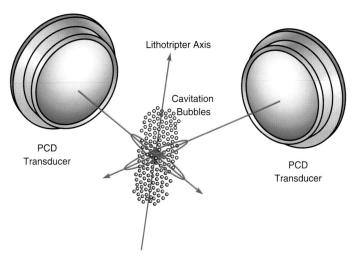

Figure 38-11 Schematic showing the dual passive cavitation detection system. Two focused transducers are placed so that their ellipsoidal focal zones intersect. Acoustic emissions that occur in the shaded region of intersection can be localized by searching for simultaneous events on both transducers.

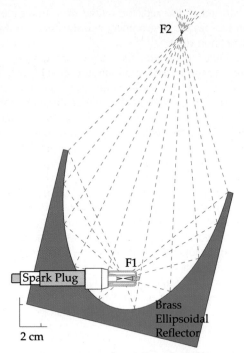

Figure 38-12 The focusing design of a Dornier HM3 electrohydraulic lithotriptor. A spark plug is located at the focus (F1) of an ellipsoidal reflector. Energy from the spark plug is reflected and focused to the second focus of the ellipsoidal reflector (F2).

tion in measured pressure waves is less than 10%. Thus, the shock waves generated by electromagnetic lithotriptors are inherently more consistent than in EHL. An additional advantage is that there are no electrodes to replace.

One difference between the acoustics of an EML and an EHL is that the acoustic pulse generated by an EML does not start as a shock wave; the displacement of the plate generates a high-intensity ultrasonic wave, which has a smooth waveform with no discontinuities. The amplitude of the wave at clinically relevant power settings is normally high enough that nonlinear distortion occurs during propagation, and a shock is produced before the wave reaches the focus. A second difference is that the EML waveforms have a relatively small trailing positive pressure after the negative phase. This peak likely has little impact on the stress inside the stone but may affect the cavitation dynamics.

Piezoelectric Lithotriptor The piezoelectric lithotriptor (PEL) uses piezoelectric crystals to form an ultrasonic wave. When a voltage is applied to a piezoelectric crystal it deforms and creates an acoustic wave. The crystals are placed on the inside of a spherical cap

and the acoustic wave focuses at the centre of the curvature of the sphere, (Figure 38-14A). This focus is highly reproducible, and very small variations in the focal waveforms are reported. Similar to the EML, the acoustic waveform in the PEL starts as an acoustic pulse, and a shock wave is created by nonlinear propagation distortion. For most clinical settings, a shock is produced before the wave reaches the focus. Figure 38-14B shows a representative waveform from a piezoelectric lithotriptor.[46] Also similar to the EML is the presence of a tail, or coda, at the end of the pulse. The coda is much more pronounced for a PEL. This is because the piezoelectric crystals "ring" for a couple of cycles after they are excited—a phenomenon not present in an EHL or EML. As with the EML, the PEL coda should not affect the stress in the stone but may affect the cavitation.

COUPLING OF THE SHOCK SOURCE TO THE BODY
Efficient transfer of acoustic energy from one medium to another only occurs when the acoustic impedances are very close. A water/tissue interface results in very good coupling, and theoretically, it should be possible to transfer more than

alignment of the electrode is consistent. Still, there is variability of the precise location of the spark discharge across the spark gap that is not easy to control. Therefore, from shot-to-shot, there can be significant variation (upwards of 50%) in the amplitude of the shock wave, and there can be some shift in the position of the focal zone at the target. A unique "feature" of EHLs is that the target is insonified by two pulses. The main focused pulse is preceded by the so-called "direct wave," which travels directly from the spark to the target without bouncing off the reflector. The direct wave arrives about 30 μs earlier and because it undergoes spherical spreading it is low in amplitude. However, it has been shown that this direct wave can influence the cavitation generated by the focussed wave.

In EHL, the electrodes wear out and must be replaced. Some lithotriptor manufacturers have found ways to enhance the lifetime of their electrodes, such as by encapsulating them and filling the casing with an appropriate electrolyte. Still, electrodes eventually show wear and this can affect their acoustic output.

Electromagnetic Lithotriptors The electromagnetic lithotriptor (EML) uses an electrical coil in close proximity to a metal plate as an acoustic source. When the coil is excited by a short electrical pulse, the plate experiences a repulsive force and this is used to generate an acoustic wave. If the metal plate is flat, the resulting acoustic wave is a plane wave that can be focused by an acoustic lens (Figure 38-13A). If the plate is in the shape of a tube, the resulting cylindrical wave can be focused by a parabolic reflector (Figure 38-13B). In both cases, focusing is very reproducible, and the varia-

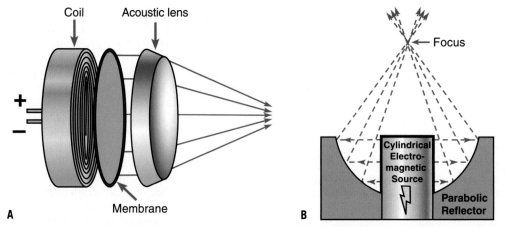

Figure 38-13 The two focusing mechanisms employed in electromagnetic lithotriptors. *A*, In a Siemens or Dornier lithotriptor, a membrane is driven by a coil to produce a plane wave, which is then focused by an acoustic lens. *B*, In a Storz lithotriptor, a coil excites a cylindrical membrane, which generates a wave that is focused by a parabolic reflector.

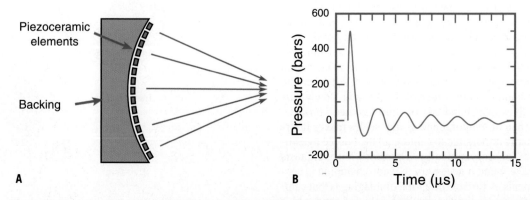

Figure 38-14 *A*, Fundamental principles for a piezoelectric lithotriptor. Piezoceramic elements are placed onto the surface of a sphere. The wave will focus to the center of the radius of curvature of that sphere. *B*, A typical waveform measured at the focus of a piezoelectric lithotriptor—notice the long ring-down for time greater than 3 μs.

99% of the energy of the shock wave into the body. But the presence of even a small pocket of air at the skin surface will result in a dramatic reduction in energy transfer to the patient (see Figure 38-4). Thus, the manner in which the shock wave is coupled to the body is critical.

Water-Bath Lithotriptors The "first-generation" lithotriptors (eg, the Dornier HM3) were electrohydraulic lithotriptors and used an open water bath in which the patient was immersed. Thus, there was nothing but water between the shock source and the patient. This is ideal except that the bubbles that drift up from the spark-gap, or the cavitation bubbles that form along the path of the shock wave, have the potential to collect against the skin of the patient and interfere with the propagation of subsequent shock waves. To help prevent this, the ellipsoidal reflector of the shock source is fixed off vertical—in the Dornier HM3 the angle is 14 degrees—and the water in the bath is continuously degassed.

Dry Lithotriptors Most current lithotriptors have the shock wave source mounted in a "therapy head," which is filled with water. The therapy head is capped by a thin rubber membrane pressed against the patient and through which the shock wave passes. A coupling agent such as gel or oil is smoothed on the rubber membrane and the patient's skin to ensure good coupling by reducing air pockets. The water in the therapy head of most lithotriptors is continuously recirculated and degassed to remove any bubbles that might interfere with the shock wave propagation. Although this design is more convenient in the clinic than a water–bath-type of lithotriptor, it is inherently less effective at allowing shock waves to pass because the presence of the rubber (although well-matched to water and tissue) adds additional reflecting interfaces. Further, even with the application of a couplant, the presence of small air bubbles between the skin and membrane is almost impossible to avoid. In vitro experiments have shown that the type of couplant can have a significant effect on stone breakage.[47] At present, the convenience of a dry therapy head appears to outweigh performance issues.

The Focal Zone of the Lithotriptor

In lithotripsy, acoustic energy is focused to a relatively small zone surrounding the *focal point* of the lithotriptor. The focal point is a geometric point in space (eg, in an EHL, this point is the second focal point [F2] of the ellipsoidal reflector) and is usually the location of the stone for treatment. All extracorporeal lithotriptors have a focal point, but lithotriptors differ in the dimensions of the zone of high pressure (*focal zone*) that surrounds this point. The dimensions and the pressure characteristics of the focal zone are the most important features that distinguish one lithotriptor from another.

There are many definitions of the focal zone that may be appropriate for lithotripsy. The IEC standard for measuring lithotriptor pulses[10] defines it as the volume within which the measured peak acoustic pressure is at least half the maximum peak positive pressure. The peak posi-

tive pressure (p+) of a waveform (see Figure 38-1) is the highest positive pressure in that waveform. The maximum peak positive pressure is the highest value of p+ in the field of the lithotriptor, and the location of the maximum peak positive pressure is defined as the focus.[10] The maximum peak pressure will vary with the power of the machine. The resulting focal zone is normally an elongated, elliptical "cigar-shaped" volume. It is worth noting that maximum peak pressure does not necessarily occur at the location the manufacturer will indicate a stone should be placed, and the location of the focus and the dimensions of the focal zone may change as the power setting is changed.

The Dornier HM3 has been used clinically more than any other lithotriptor and has been studied and characterized more extensively than any other lithotriptor. As such, data for the Dornier HM3 prove to be a useful standard for reference. Because different lithotriptors, even the same type of lithotriptor, may perform somewhat differently, and because investigators have used different means to map the acoustic field of their lithotriptors, published values for peak pressures and dimensions of the focal zone of a given type of lithotriptor may not coincide perfectly. Representative focal zones of selected lithotriptors are shown in Figure 38-15. Typical published values for the Dornier HM3 electrohydraulic lithotriptor report the maximum peak positive pressure to be 40 MPa at 20 kV and the focal zone to be about 60 mm long by 12 mm in diameter. In contrast. the Storz Modulith electromagnetic lithotriptor has a maximum peak positive pressure around 100 MPa at energy level 8 and a focal zone that is about 35 mm long and only 4 mm in diameter. Reported values for piezoelectric lithotriptors indicate a maximum peak positive pressure of 80 MPa and a focal zone 20 mm long and 3 mm in diameter.[48,49] Thus, there is a considerable difference in the dimensions of the focal zone between lithotriptors, and typically lithotriptors with narrower focal zones have higher peak pressures.

The half-maximum focal zone (also known as –6 dB focal zone because the contour corresponds to the pressure being 6 decibels less than at the maximum) is recommended in the IEC standard, but this may not necessarily be the best descriptor of the focal zone of a lithotriptor. For example, in a Storz lithotriptor, with a peak pressure of 110 MPa at energy level 9, the focal zone will correspond to a surface where the peak pressure is 55 MPa. For an Dornier HM3, which only has a peak pressure of 40 MPa, the focal zone will correspond to a surface where the pressure is just 20 MPa. Therefore, when comparing the focal zones of these machines, the absolute pressure levels are very different—indeed the focal zone of a Dornier HM3 would be zero if the 55 MPa level of the Storz focal zone were used. Other suggestions for the focal zone include: (1) half the peak negative pressure, (2) half the energy density, (3) the surface where the peak pressure is 5 MPa, or (4) even using the energy that passes through a volume with diameter 10 mm (about

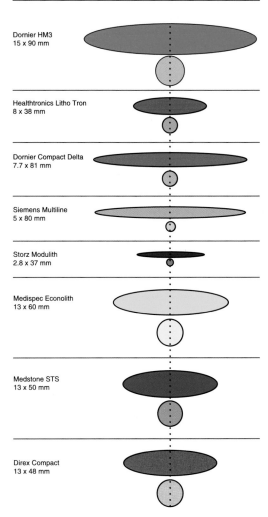

F2 Size Comparisons

Figure 38-15 Comparison of the focal zones of selected clinical lithotriptors showing their dimensions along the axis of the lithotriptor (ellipses) and in the focal plane at the focus (circles). Image courtesy of P. Blomgren.

the size of a typical stone). Until there is a better understanding of how shock waves fragment stones, it is unlikely that an alternative metric will be agreed upon within the literature.

The smaller, tighter, focal spot of an electromagnetic or piezoelectric lithotriptor would at first glance appear to be advantageous because it should allow for more accurate targeting on the stone, and thus, less damage to the surrounding tissue. But in vitro experiments (where stones are stationary) indicate that the electromagnetic or piezoelectric lithotriptors, with their very high pressures, are no better at breaking stones that an electrohydraulic lithotriptor and often are not as effective.[50,51] High peak positive pressure does not appear to correlate with enhanced stone fragmentation in the clinic.[2]

Further, stone motion due to respiration means that, with a tight focal zone, fewer shock waves actually hit the stone, and more shock wave energy is deposited directly into tissue.[52] When one considers that some tight focal zone lithotriptors have peak pressures in excess of

100 MPa, this suggests that tissue is being subjected to a very high dose of acoustic energy. This may help explain the increased incidence of adverse effects, such as subcapsular hematomas observed with these machines.[3,8]

DEVICE EQUIVALENCY/EQUATING LITHOTRIPTOR PERFORMANCE

At present, there are no agreed metrics by which the acoustic output of different lithotriptors can be compared, and there is no straightforward means to operate any given lithotriptor so that it is equivalent to another. This is partly due to the fact that, although all lithotriptors produce shock waves that have similar waveforms, the amplitude and focal zone of different lithotriptors is not the same, and measurements of the properties of the acoustic field can yield very different values. This is illustrated in Table 38-1, where we show a number of physical measurements made on an electrohydraulic and an electromagnetic lithotriptor.[53] For the settings chosen, the only parameter that was roughly equivalent was the energy incident on a 6.5 mm diameter stone (0.484 mJ versus 0.528 mJ). Other physical measurements, however, varied tremendously; for example, the peak positive pressure in the electromagnetic lithotriptor was three times that of the electrohydraulic lithotriptor.

Therefore, although it is possible to find settings on two given machines that give equivalency on one physical property, it is unlikely that there will be equivalency on other properties, and indeed, there are likely to be significant differences. For example, if the power setting were to be reduced on the electromagnetic lithotriptor to yield the same pressure as the electrohydraulic lithotriptor, then the energy measurements would drop by almost a factor of 10.

A further confounding issue is the number of shock waves to be used. The clinical literature suggests that typically fewer shock waves are required to break stones with an electrohydraulic device than with an electromagnetic device. In addition, the rate at which shock waves are delivered has also been reported to affect fragmentation efficiency.[54] Therefore, at the current time, there is no clear way in which the three main parameters of shock wave delivery for a lithotriptor (power, number of shock waves and rate of shock wave delivery) can be adjusted to ensure equivalency between different machines.

MECHANISMS OF SHOCK WAVE ACTION

WAVES IN STONES The acoustic field in stones is more complex than the acoustic theory described above. Kidney stones are elastic solids and support two types of waves: a longitudinal or compression wave (which is akin to an acoustic wave) and transverse of shear waves, where the motion of the vibration is transverse to the direction of propagation. In a shear wave, the transverse vibration does not result in the molecules being compressed and rarefied, but rather they oscillate in a manner analogous to the wave motion of a rope excited by a snap of the wrist. Longitudinal waves and shear

Table 38-1 Comparison of Physical Properties Measured in an Electrohydraulic Lithotriptor (EHL) and an Electromagnetic Lithotriptor (EML)

	L_{FZ}	W_{FZ}	p+	p-	E_{FZ}	E_{STONE}	t_c
EHL	54 mm	9 mm	37.5 MPa	-7.8 MPa	4.25 mJ	0.484 mJ	250 μs
EML	32 mm	3.5 mm	115 MPa	-14.6 MPa	3.35 mJ	0.528 mJ	350 μs
Ratio EH/EM	1.69	2.57	0.33	0.53	1.27	0.92	0.71

The columns show measurements of the length (L_{FZ}) and width (W_{FZ}) of the focal zone, the peak pressures (p+ and p-), the energy in the focal zone (EFZ) (Equation 38-9 using the area given by the width of the focal zone), the energy incident on a stone (E_{STONE}) (Equation 38-9 using the area given by the 6.5 mm diameter of the stone), and the characteristic time of cavitation (tc), which is a measure of the strength of cavitation. The bottom row shows the ratio of the values in the EHL to the EML. For the settings used here, the energy delivered to the stone was the one quantitative parameter that was approximately equivalent. Adapted from Chitnis PV.[53]

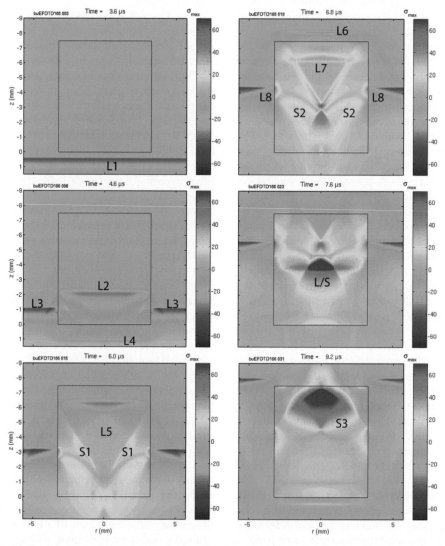

Figure 38-16 Snap-shots of the tensile stress generated by the propagation of a lithotripsy shock wave through a model kidney stone surrounded by fluid. The cylindrical stone (6.5 mm wide by 7.5 mm high) has the following properties p=1700 kg/m3, c_T=3000 m/s c_S=1500 m/s. The shock wave is incident from below and colour scale depicts the tensile stress (in MPa) where yellow through red indicate regions of tensile stress and blue regions of compression. In the first frame (3.6 μs) the leading compressional phase of the shock wave in the fluid (L1) is almost incident on the proximal surface of the stone. At 4.6 μs the shock wave has entered the stone as a longitudinal wave (L2), note because the propagation axis is normal to the surface no shear waves are generated at this interface. Because the speed in the stone is higher than in the fluid, the wave in the stone advances ahead of the wave in the fluid (L3). The reflection of the shock wave by the proximal surface can be seen leaving the bottom of the image (L4). At 6.0 μs the tensile tail of the incident shock wave can be seen in the stone (L5) following the leading compressive phase. The interaction of the longitudinal wave in the stone with the lateral walls of the stone results in the production of shear waves (S1)that propagate towards the axis of the stone. At 6.8 μs the leading compressive phase has been partially transmitted (L6) and reflected (L7) at the distal surface. The reflection coefficient is approximately -0.5 and results in a tensile phase (L7) that generates significant tensile stress (red region) near the distal surface—this is spall. The wave on the outside of the stone (L8) is inducing further shear waves (S2) inside the stone. At 7.6 μs the reflected longitudinal wave and the shear waves interact to produce a large region of tensile stress in the centre of the stone (L/S). At 9.2 μs the shear waves interact near the distal surface to generate another region of high tensile stress (S3).

waves travel at different speed and the longitudinal wave speed (cL) is always faster than the transverse wave speed (cT).

When a shock wave passes from urine or tissue into a stone the transmitted energy is divided between the longitudinal and transverse waves in the stone. The proportion of the energy that each wave gets depends on the material properties of the stone and the angle of incidence. If the wave is normally incident on the stone surface then all the energy is converted into a longitudinal wave in the stone and no energy is available for transverse waves. As the angle of incidence increases less energy is converted into a longitudinal wave and more is converted into transverse waves. The complex shape of many natural stones results in a non-trivial partition of energy between the two types of wave.

The basic features of the interaction of shock waves with a stone can be illustrated by means of a computer simulation. The computer simulation solves the equations of motion for particles in an elastic solid.[55] Figure 38-16 shows a series of snap-shots of the interaction of an lithotripter shock wave with a cylindrical shaped stone. The snap-shots show the distribution of the maximum tensile stress inside the stone at each instant of time. In the first two frames the shock wave can be seen to enter the stone as compressional waves. The third and fourth frames show that the longitudinal wave inside the stone and the acoustic wave outside the stone result in the generation of shear waves from the lateral walls. Further, between the third and fourth frames the shock wave reflects from the rear wall. Because the impedance of the surrounding fluid is less than that of the stone the reflected pressure wave is inverted and the leading compressive wave is reflected as a tensile wave. This is because the pressure reflection coefficient R_P given in Eq. 38-19 is negative if $Z_2 < Z_1$. The last two frames show the shear and longitudinal waves interfere to produce the high tensile stresses in the stone.

Acoustic Properties of Stones The most important material properties of kidney stones from the point of view of wave propagation are (1) density ρ_0, (2) longitudinal sound-speed c_L, and (3) transverse wave velocity c_T. Figure 38-17 shows reported measurements from human stones.[56–58] There is a large variation in the reported properties for uric acid, calcium oxalate monohydrate and cystine stones, for example, the sound speed in calcium oxylate monohydrate varies between 3,000 m/s and 4,500 m/s. This variation is likely due to the natural variation in the properties of the stones but may also be related to the preparation of the stones (eg, the amount of hydration).

How Shock Waves Break Stones Numerous mechanisms by which shock waves may fragment stones have been described in the literature. Here, we give a synopsis of some of the most likely mechanisms (Figure 38-18).

Spall Fracture *Spallation* occurs after the shock wave enters the stone and subsequently reflects from the rear of the stone (see Figure

38-16). The stone/urine interface inverts the large positive pressure pulse, resulting in a large tensile stress. This stress is added to the tensile stress of the still-incoming negative pressure tail, resulting in a very large tensile stress near the back wall.[59–62] Most solids are much weaker in tension than in compression, and so the large tensile stress near the rear of the stone can be expected to make the material fail.

Shear Stress *Shear* stresses will be generated by a combination of both shear waves and compressive waves that develop as the shock wave passes into the stone (Figure 38-19).[55,63] Many materials are weak in shear, particularly like kidney stones if they consist of layers, as the bonding strength of the matrix between layers often has a low ultimate shear stress.[59,60,64,65] Furthermore, the organic binder of kidney stones is much softer than the crystalline phase, and as the shock front

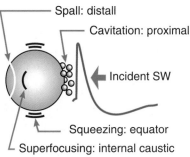

Figure 38-18 Schematic showing regions where different stone fracture mechanisms will act.

passes through the stone, it will induce very large shear stresses at the binder/crystal interfaces, which likely contribute to the fracture of the kidney stone.[55,66] Shear waves in the stone can also result in large tensile stresses that exceed the tensile stress induced by spallation.[55] In Fig 38-16 it was shown that shear waves interfere with the reflected longitudinal wall to produce the largest tensile stress in the cylindrical stone.

Superfocusing *Superfocusing* is the amplification of stresses inside the stone due to the geometry of the stone. The shock wave that is reflected at the distal surface of the stone can be focused either by refraction (associated with the high sound-speed and geometry of the stone) or by diffraction from the corners of the stone. It has been shown that these reflected waves can be focused to caustics (regions of high stress) in the interior of the stone and that this can lead to failure.[65,67] The regions of high stress (both tensile and shear) can be determined from the geometry of the stone and its elastic properties (eg, density, longitudinal wave speed, and shear wave speed).

Squeezing *Squeezing/splitting* occurs because of the difference in sound speed between

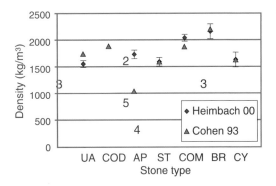

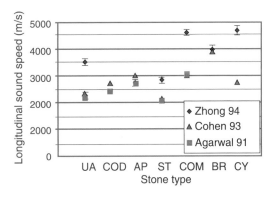

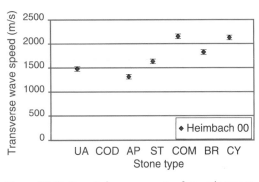

Figure 38-17 Reported measurements of acoustic properties in human stones. Top: density; Middle: sound speed; Bottom: shear wave speed. (UA = uric acid; COD = calcium oxylate dihydrate; AP = Apatite; ST = Struvite; COM = calcium oxylate monohydrate; BR = brushite; CY = cystine). Adapted from Agarwal R, Singh VR,[56] Cohen NP, Whitfield HN,[57] and Zhong P, Preminger GM.[58]

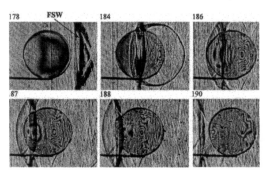

Figure 38-19 Images of the stress waves in a cylindrical stone (14 mm diameter), which was subject to a shock wave from a Dornier HM3. At 178 μs, the shock wave is almost incident on the stone. At 184 μs, the shock wave has entered the stone and has also reflected. At 186 μs, the compressive phase of the shock wave has just made it to the distal surface of the stone, and a shear wave can be seen at the midpoint of the stone. At 187 μs, the compressive wave has exited the stone, and the shear wave is focused along the axis of the stone. At 188 μs, the shear wave reaches the distal surface of the stone. At 190 μs, the shock wave has passed by the stone but stress waves are still reverberating inside the stone. (Images courtesy of Dr. P. Zhong—Figure 9a of [65].)

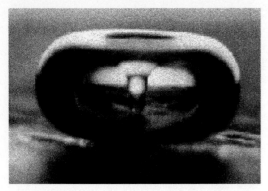

Figure 38-20 Image of a cavitation bubble collapsing on a metal surface. A jet of fluid can be seen punching through the center of the bubble toward the metal surface. Reproduced with permission from Crum LA.[27]

the stone (greater than 2,500 m/s) and the surrounding fluid ($\approx$1,500 m/s). The shock wave inside the stone "runs away" from the shock wave propagating through the fluid outside of the stone (see Figure 38-16C and Figure 38-16D). The shock wave that propagates in the fluid outside the stone results in a circumferential force on the stone (known as a hoop stress). This results in a maximum tensile stress at proximal and distal ends of the stone and leads to an axial "splitting" failure. It has been theorized that squeezing should be enhanced when the entire stone falls within the diameter of the focal zone, and a lithotriptor based on this principal has recently been built and described in the literature.[68,69]

Cavitation *Cavitation* refers to small bubbles (or cavities) that grow in the urine surrounding the stone in response to the large negative pressure tail of the acoustic pulse. When a cavitation bubble collapses near a solid surface (eg, a kidney stone) a microjet of fluid is formed that pierces the bubble and impacts the surface (Figure 38-20) with speeds upwards of 100 m/s.[27] This jet likely plays a role in cavitation-induced damage to kidney stones.[27,28] The collapse of the cavitation bubble also results in the emissions of secondary shock waves that are radiated into the bubble. These secondary shock waves have an amplitude comparable to that of the focused shock wave. In vitro experiments where cavitation is suppressed show significant reduction in stone fragmentation.[43,70,71] Cavitation is principally a surface-acting mechanism, and experiments indicate that it acts most strongly on the proximal (shock wave incident) surface of the stone.[28,61,72] It has also been suggested that the stresses imparted by cavitation can act by a spall mechanism.[67,73] Recent work has recognized that the cavitation generated by lithotriptors acts as a cluster of bubbles (Figure 38-21) rather than individual bubbles, and that the coherent collapse of the cluster may enhance the destructive power of cavitation.[36,74,75]

Fatigue *Fatigue* is a process that may occur anywhere in the stone. Its hallmark is the progressive development of cracks.[76,77] The cracks are nucleated at sites of small imperfections that occur in almost all materials—these nucleation sites will be present in all kidney stones. The imperfections are sites of "stress concentrations" which, when a shock wave passes, can lead to local stresses far in excess of the average stress induced by the shock wave. With the impact of repetitive shock waves, the imperfections frow into microcracks. With subsequent shock waves, the microcracks grow into macrocracks, and eventually produce cracks large enough to induce failure. The cracks can be grown either by large tensile stresses or by large shear stresses. Therefore, fatigue will be enhanced wherever regions of high stress coincide with weak points in the stone. This means that there could be a synergistic effect between fatigue and some of the other mechanisms that result in localized regions of high tensile or shear stress. There are two pieces of evidence that strongly support the argument that stone comminution is a fatigue process. First, the internal structure of stones has been shown to affect how they fragment in lithotripsy.[55,78–80] Second, normally more than 1,000 shock waves are required to progressively fragment stones into sufficiently small pieces; the use of multiple stress cycles to fracture a material is a classic hallmark of fatigue.[76,77]

Although, present understanding of shock wave lithotripsy indicates that the stones fail through a fatigue process, it is not clear which mechanism drives the fatigue. The two most commonly cited mechanisms are direct stresses (spall and shear) and cavitation or some combination of them.[81] Part of the problem in determining which mechanism is that only limited data on the material strength of kidney stones have been reported (eg, ultimate strength in compression, fracture toughness, Knoop hardness, and Vickers microhardness.[56–58,82–85]) Of note is the paucity of data for the tensile and shear strength of kidney stones. This is most likely because determining these properties in brittle materials is fraught with technical difficulties. Further, most of the data have been measured in quasi-static tests, with the stress applied over many minutes, and the results may not be representative of the material properties when subject to shock waves, where the stress is applied and removed in microseconds.[66] At present, the data on material strength of kidney stones is not sufficient for the fracture process to be described.

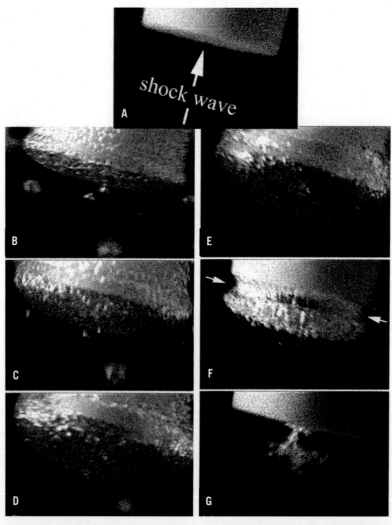

Figure 38-21 Images of cavitation bubble cluster collapse on a model stone 6.5 mm in diameter and 7.5 mm long. *A*, Orientation of shock wave to stone. *B*, 100 μs after shock wave arrival, a bubble cluster has formed on the proximal surface and a few bubbles have formed in the surrounding fluid. *C to E*, (200, 300 and 400 μs after shock wave arrival) the cluster continues to grow. *F*, The cluster begins to collapse in a mushroom like shape. *G*, The final collapse of the cluster at the center of the stone. Reproduced with permission from Pishchalnikov YA, et al.[36]

MECHANISMS OF TISSUE DAMAGE It is now well recognized that SWL results in trauma to the kidney and that, in some cases, the injury can be severe.[6] The clinical implications of such adverse effects are still under investigation (see Chapter 41, "Complications").

The notion that lithotriptor shock waves can pass harmlessly through the body is simply not true. It is likely that all patients who receive at least an average dose of shock waves (2,000 shock waves at midrange power or higher) experience some form of tissue trauma. Lithotripsy has been very beneficial for a large number of patients but has also led to severe, even catastrophic, adverse effects for others.[86] To better understand how shock waves have the potential to cause tissue trauma, consider the physics of the problem.

As discussed above lithotriptors produce a focused acoustic pulse. The acoustic field is broad at the source and narrow at the focus. The focal zone, the area of highest acoustic pressure, is elongated and of dimensions that cannot be localized exclusively to a stone. Although shock waves are targeted onto the stone, the surrounding tissue is also subject to significant mechanical forces. We have seen that the length of the focal zone of most lithotriptors is about 50 mm (see Figure 38-15), and this means that the entire thickness of the kidney is subject to high amplitude shock waves. In addition, patient motion, due to respiration or discomfort, likely results in the stone spending a good portion of the treatment time out of the focal region, and thus, many of the shock waves will interact solely with tissue.

Fortunately, tissue has physical properties that make it far less susceptible to damage by shock waves than kidney stones. For example, the fact that the acoustic impedance of tissue is close to that of water means that shock waves can pass through a tissue-to-water interface without significant reflection. Thus, tissue is not subjected to the extreme tensile forces that cause stones to fail by spallation. Further, the sound speed in tissue is almost constant, and so tissue will not be under a differential squeezing stress that could result in splitting. Tissue is, however, subject to shear forces induced by the pressure wave and to cavitation induced by the tensile phase of the shock wave. We will briefly describe the mechanisms that may contribute to tissue injury.

Mechanical Stress The positive pressure of a lithotriptor pulse leads to significant compression of tissue. Although tissue is usually robust to isotropic compression, the leading shock front has a rise time of the order of 70 ns in tissue which corresponds to a spatial scale of 100 μm. Therefore, tissue structures in the range of 10 μm to 1 mm will experience a significant variation in stress across them as the shock wave passes. The short rise time associated with the shock will lead to non-uniform straining of the tissue, resulting in shear forces. It is generally recognized that tissue structures are sensitive to shear stress, and the distortion of the tissue by the shock wave could induce enough shear to cause damage.[87,88]

Shear Induced by Inhomogeneities Tissue is an inhomogeneous medium at multiple length scales. Spatial variation in the sound speed on the millimeter length scale can have a dramatic effect on the focusing of ultrasonic pulses in tissue.[89] As the shock wave focuses, parts of the wavefront that passed through tissue with high sound speed will be advanced, and the parts that passed though low sound speed tissue will fall back. This distortion in the wavefront will lead directly to shear stresses in the tissue. Again these shear stresses could be strong enough to induce mechanical damage of the tissue.[87]

Cavitation Cavitation is known to occur in tissue during lithotripsy.[35,90,91] Measurements using passive cavitation detection in both humans and pigs have detected the unique acoustic signature associated with cavitation. Measurements have indicated the presence of cavitation in the perirenal fat, the collecting system, the parenchyma, and in subcapsular hematomas. Cavitation has been well documented to have a significant biological effect in many in vitro settings (see Carstensen EL, et al,[92] Miller DL and Thomas RM,[93] Miller M, et al,[94] Dalecki D, et al,[95] Delius M, et al,[96] and Williams JC, et al[97]). Experiments in lithotripsy indicate that damage to in vitro cells and in vivo tissue is dramatically reduced when cavitation is reduced or eliminated.[97–99] Cavitation is most likely the dominant cause of damage in tissue.

Cavitation is more likely to result in injury within blood vessels than within the surrounding tissue. This is because a bubble surrounded by tissue will be constrained and will not be able to go through a violent growth-and-collapse cycle. In a blood vessel, there is a fluid environment for the bubbles to grow and collapse. There are at least two mechanisms by which bubbles could produce mechanical damage to organs such as the kidney:

Collapsing Bubbles When cavitation bubbles collapse asymmetrically, they form high-velocity microjets of fluid focused to a small spot. These liquid microjets, forceful enough to pit foils or etch metal surfaces, seem easily capable of puncturing the fragile wall of a capillary or other blood vessel. Thus, just as cavitation bubble cluster collapse is believed to contribute to the breakage of stones, bubble collapse may play a role in the rupture of vessels. The weakness of this argument is that the blood vessels that are injured during lithotripsy typically are not large enough to allow cavitation bubbles to undergo a complete growth-collapse cycle.

Bubble Expansion Bubbles may rupture vessel walls during the expansion phase of the bubble cycle. That is, as the negative pressure of the shock wave passes through the vessel, it causes the bubble to undergo explosive growth (see Figure 38-10) pushing outward on the vessel and rupturing it. This is consistent with the observation that damage occurs first in the capillaries, which, due to their small size, will be subject to greater stresses during the most explosive part of the growth cycle. Experiments using capillary phantoms in an in vitro setting support the explosive bubble hypothe-

sis.[100,101] This mechanism may also allow for other tissue to be damaged, for, if bubble growth is capable of rupturing vessels, it may be able to rip apart other tissue structures in the vicinity as well.

Once blood vessels have been ruptured and blood has collected in pools, in a hematoma for example, there is a greater potential for cavitation to occur. The pooling of blood provides a large fluid-filled space for cavitation bubbles to grow and collapse. Also, existing bubbles, which can act as nuclei for subsequent cavitation events, will not be swept away by blood flow, but will remain in the pooled region. This explains the intense PCD cavitation signals and B-scan ultrasound echogenicity collected from hematomas during SWL.[90,91,102] The violent cavitation in such a region could lead to further disruption of cells in the area.

Research continues in this area, with the goal of confirming whether the physical processes outlined here, or some other processes, are responsible for tissue damage in shock wave lithotripsy. This is partly due to the fact that the mechanical response of the tissue, at least at strain rates relevant in shock wave lithotripsy, is not well understood and so damage criteria are also not well defined. Further, there are few experimental systems that can be used to test and validate different hypotheses. Although the general consensus among researchers is that cavitation is the primary mechanism for tissue injury, this field still requires much study.

THE EVOLUTION OF THE LITHOTRIPTOR How Lithotriptors Have Changed Over the Years It is more than 25 years since the introduction of lithotripsy to clinical practice, and there have been a number of noteworthy changes in equipment design, but none that have involved a fundamental change in the acoustics of the lithotriptor. That is, lithotriptors have changed—they are now compact, modular, use dry shock heads, have improved imaging—but the acoustic signature of the lithotriptor pressure pulse remains remarkably similar. The focal waveform generated by a Dornier HM3 is virtually the same as the waveform produced by any of the numerous lithotriptors available on the market today. This is not to imply that the lithotriptor industry has been static. Indeed, there has been a very active effort on the part of manufacturers to produce machines that are easier and more practical to use. In this regard, lithotripsy has seen numerous refinements. At the same time, however, it is essential to note that success rates in lithotripsy have declined. The use of newer lithotriptors, specifically those that produce a tight focal zone of extreme peak positive pressure, has led to decreased efficiency of stone breakage and to an increase in collateral damage.[2] Thus, progress in lithotripsy has taken a step back—improved convenience has been gained, but at a cost.

The first lithotriptors were electrohydraulic devices in which the shock wave was generated by underwater spark discharge, and shock wave coupling was achieved by immersion of the patient in a water bath. The Dornier HM3 was a very popular lithotriptor of this era, and at some centers is still in use today. By today's standards, the Dornier HM3 produces moderate peak positive pressures ($\approx$ 40 MPa) delivered to a generous focal zone ($\approx$ 15 by 60 mm). The Dornier HM3 was a very successful machine, and it is probably safe to say that the early success and rapid acceptance of lithotripsy was built on the back of this particular lithotriptor.

Even though the Dornier HM3 was a very effective lithotriptor, it was perceived by some to have several significant drawbacks. It used an open water bath to couple shock waves to the body, treatment was painful, requiring the patient to be sedated (or even anaesthetized), and the lithotriptor was a large, stationary piece of equipment that required a dedicated water treatment plant. What physicians (and patients) really wanted was lithotripsy that was painless and convenient, with minimal to no anesthesia—a fully ambulatory walk-in/walk-out therapy. Lithotriptor manufacturers responded with a number of modifications. Problems related to the overall physical design of the lithotriptor were challenging but solvable. For example, the issue of the open water bath was addressed by enclosing the shock head and by using a rubber membrane to couple the shock wave to the body. This was not a perfect solution, as there is no better way to achieve acoustic coupling than through a water-tissue interface. Elimination of the water bath, however, meant that medical staff had much easier access to the patient, the lithotriptor did not necessarily have to be tied down to a dedicated facility, and that lithotriptors could be designed as modular systems. Many modern lithotriptors have indeed been designed to be portable and are used in mobile lithotripsy units.

Another perceived disadvantage of the Dornier HM3 was the limited life span of the electrodes. It is necessary to replace the electrode one or more times during a treatment. Electromagnetic and piezoelectric lithotriptors do not use electrodes, which is an advantage in terms of cost, time, and convenience. In addition to the need to periodically change electrodes, electrode wear is an issue with electrohydraulic lithotriptors. As the spark gap widens with use, there is increased variability in the path of the arc discharge. Several manufacturers of current electrohydraulic machines have found various ways to improve electrode life, and some use designs such as encapsulation in an electrolyte-filled housing to extend the life of the electrode.[103,104]

The attempt to design a lithotriptor so that it can be operated "anesthesia-free," on the other hand, has proven to be a much more difficult problem. Discomfort during shock wave treatment is due primarily to the sensation of cutaneous pain over the area of shock wave entry at the surface of the body. One attempted solution was to widen the aperture at the shock source in order to spread the energy over a broader area. A wider aperture broadens the acoustic field along the shock wave axis, but it narrows the focal zone of the pressure pulse. Many current lithotriptors have a very narrow focal zone (on the order of 5 mm or less). Some of these lithotriptors also generate huge peak positive pressures (in excess of 100 MPa). Use of a tight focal zone might prove to be an advantage if it could be kept directly on target, but it cannot. Because of respiratory motion, shooting at a stone using a narrow focal zone proves to be harder than when using a broad focal zone. Further, regardless of which lithotriptor is used, lithotripsy is uncomfortable for the patient. If the patient is not sedated he or she will move to try to get more comfortable. Thus, attempts to build a totally anesthesia-free device have not yet been successful.

Future Directions in Lithotriptor Design
There have been recent developments in lithotripsy that could herald a positive change for the future of SWL. That is, there has been an effort to introduce novel approaches in lithotriptor design that build upon well-tested theory—and positive experimental results—targeting ways to improve stone breakage and reduce tissue injury. One approach is a response to the recent trend toward tight–focal-zone, high–acoustic-pressure machines. The Xi Xin-Eisenmenger lithotriptor[69] is a wide-focus and low-pressure lithotriptor that generates the largest focal zone (18 by 180 mm) and lowest range of acoustic pressures (10 to 25 MPa) currently in use in clinical practice. This machine was developed to test the hypothesis that a very broad focal zone could be used to enhance stone breakage by circumferential squeezing.[68] It was reported in an early trial that this machine delivered a high stone-free rate (86%) and can be used anesthesia-free.[69]

Cavitation control may be a means to improve lithotripsy. The cavitation bubble cycle—the time for a bubble to grow and then collapse—lasts on the order of 300 μs in the free field and $\approx$ 600 μs at the surface of a stone.[105] Recent studies have shown that cavitation bubbles generated by one lithotriptor pulse can be manipulated by a second pulse.[106,107] If the second pulse arrives while bubbles are in their early growth phase, further expansion is stopped and the bubbles collapse with minimal damage. If, however, the second pulse arrives later in the cycle, bubble collapse is accelerated and damage is enhanced. Thus, the timing of the two pulses is critical. Bailey originated dual pulse lithotripsy, and in his studies used twin shock sources oriented coaxially facing one another.[108] Others have built upon this concept and developed lithotriptors that fire multiple pulses along the same axis[109-111] or machines that use dual treatment heads offset at an angle to accommodate the constraints imposed by the anatomy of a patient.[112-114] At the time of writing, dual pulse lithotripsy is under development and testing. The concept holds promise, as this may be a means to tailor acoustic forces within the focal zone for better breakage of stones, hopefully with reduced collateral damage. But it is too early to endorse such machines as there are, as yet, no data that assess these lithotriptors for efficacy and safety compared to conventional lithotriptors.

The safety of lithotripsy is a very important issue. Shock waves cause trauma, and any strategy that results in lowering the dose of shock waves needed to treat a patient should be welcomed. One way to reduce unnecessary shock wave impact on tissue is to track the stone during treatment and only fire when the shock wave will hit the stone. Devices have been proposed that would monitor stone location and only allow shock waves to be fired when the stone is at the focus of the lithotriptor.[115-118] A device has also been proposed to exploit acoustic time-reversal to dynamically change the focus of the lithotriptor and so hit the stone even as it moves.[119,120] Such concepts have the potential to dramatically reduce the number of shock waves required to break a stone. However, clinical devices do not currently employ real-time tracking.

SUMMARY

Shock wave lithotripsy is a superb example of the successful transition of engineering technology into the clinical area. We have outlined the underlying acoustic principles that describe (1) the generation of the shock pulse, (2) focusing, (3) nonlinear distortion, (4) coupling of the shock source to the body, and (5) absorption of sound by the body. The exact mechanisms by which shock waves can damage stones and tissue are still not fully understood, although it is likely that direct stresses and cavitation are dominant in stone fragmentation, and that cavitation is dominant in tissue injury. Improvements in lithotripsy, whether through improved use of existing lithotriptors or through the development of new technologies, are likely to come only from an improved understanding of the acoustics and the physics of this problem.

In this chapter we have attempted to make the following main points.

- Most lithotriptors produce a similar type of shock wave, which consists of a leading positive pressure shock front (compressive wave) lasting about 1 μs followed by a negative pressure trough (tensile wave), which lasts about 3 μs. There is a large range in the amplitude of the shock waves used, with peak positive pressures of 30 to 110 MPa depending on the type of shock source and the power setting.
- The intense compressive wave induces mechanical forces inside the stone that may lead to fragmentation, most likely by a spall mechanism. The tensile component of the shock wave is lower amplitude (about −8 to −15 MPa). This negative pressure drives cavitation bubble activity that is critical to stone comminution, but also causes vascular trauma to the kidney.
- Various types of shock wave sources and focusing mechanisms have been exploited in lithotripsy. Electromagnetic and electrohydraulic lithotriptors dominate the lithotripsy market today.
- The size and dimensions of the focal zone are controlled by diffraction. Typically, electro-

magnetic lithotriptors have a smaller focal zone than electrohydraulic devices and generate substantially higher peak positive pressures. A smaller focal zone is not necessarily an advantage because patient motion means that the stone can easily spend a significant amount of time outside the focal region. Currently, there is no good metric to determine equivalent action of different types of machines.

- Shock waves are coupled into the body using a water path that, ideally, is devoid of bubbles. Most current lithotriptors use an enclosed water path in which the shock head is capped by a rubber membrane of low acoustic impedance. Such dry lithotriptors tend not to be as efficient as the older water-bath lithotriptors in which the patient is immersed in water during treatment—and this reduced efficiency could be due, at least in part, to poorer coupling.

- The acoustic waveforms measured in vitro and in vivo are very similar, despite the presence of absorption and heterogeneity in tissue. This is a significant finding for it validates in vitro experimentation as being representative of the in vivo condition.

- Numerous mechanisms have been proposed to explain how shock waves break urinary stones. No single mechanism gives an adequate explanation, and it appears that multiple mechanisms involving cavitation and spallation are at play. For tissue injury on the other hand it appears that cavitation, and shock wave/bubble interaction, are the most likely cause of trauma.

- Since its inception, lithotripsy has undergone a fascinating evolution. Water bath-type, electrohydraulic devices have given way to modular, highly portable lithotriptors, many of which employ electromagnetic shock wave generators. Most lithotripsies are now performed using mobile units delivered by truck to subscribing hospitals. This improved convenience has come at a price as stone re-treatment rates have increased and reports of collateral damage are on the rise. One explanation is that the newer lithotriptors are not as efficacious and have the potential to cause more collateral damage.

- New technologies of shock wave delivery are now being applied to patient treatment. Dual-pulse lithotripsy uses two shock heads to fire separate pulses. In theory, it should be possible to treat patients faster, and the potential for control over the properties of the acoustic field could lead to improved efficacy and safety. Likewise, initial success with a new lithotriptor that produces a very broad focal zone and is operated at low peak positive pressures suggests that a return to some of the features of the original lithotriptor could also be a step toward improved lithotripsy.

ACKNOWLEDGEMENTS

We would like to thank Drs. Michael Bailey, Andrew Evan, James Lingeman, Yura Pishchalnikov, David Wang and James Williams Jr for their comments on this chapter. This research was supported in part by grants from the National Institutes of Health (NIH DK43881, DK55674) and the Whitaker Foundation (RG-01-0084).

REFERENCES

1. Holmes S, Whitfield HN. The current status of lithotripsy. Br J Urol 1991;68:337–44.
2. Kerbl K, Rehman J, Landman J, et al. Current management of urolithisasis: progress or regress? J Endourol 2002;16: 281–8.
3. Kohrmann KU, Rassweiler JJ, Manning M, et al. The clinical introduction of a 3rd generation lithotriptor - Modulith Sl-20. J Urol 1995;153:1379–83.
4. Lingeman JE, Newmark J. Adverse bioeffects of shock-wave lithotripsy. In: Coe FL, et al, editors. Kidney stones: medical and surgical management,. Philadelphia: Lippincott-Raven; 1996. p. 605–14.
5. Janetschek G, Frauscher F, Knapp R, et al. New onset hypertension after extracorporeal shock wave lithotripsy: age related incidence and prediction by intrarenal resistive index [see comments]. J Urol 1997;158:346–51.
6. Evan AP, Willis LR, Lingeman JE, McAteer JA. Renal trauma and the risk of long-term complications in shock wave lithotripsy. Nephron 1998;78:1–8.
7. Tan EC, Tung KH, Foo KT. Comparative studies of extracorporeal shock wave lithotripsy by Dornier HM3, EDAP LT 01 and Sonolith 2000 devices. J Urol 1991;148: 294–97.
8. Ueda S, Matsuko K, Yamashita T, et al., Perirenal hematomas caused by SWL with EDAP LT-01 lithotriptor. J Endourol 1993;7:11–15.
9. Fuselier HA, Prats L, Fontenot C, Gauthier A. Comparison of mobile lithotriptors at one institution: Healthtronics Lithotron, Dornier MFL-5000, and Dornier Doli. J Endourol 1999;13: 539–42.
10. IEC61846, Ultrasonics - Pressure pulse lithotriptors - Characteristics of fields, T.-. Ultrasonics, Editor. 1998.
11. Dreyer T, Riedlinger RE, Steiger E. Experiments on the relation of shock wave parameters to stone disintegration. 16th International Congress on Acoustics 1998. Seattle, WA, USA: Acoustical Society of America.
12. Averkiou MA, Cleveland RO. Modeling of an electrohydraulic lithotriptor with the KZK equation. J Acoust Soc Am 1999;106:102–12.
13. Fry FJ, Dins KA, R. C.R., G. S.A. Losses in tissue associated with finite amplitude ultrasound transmission. Ultrasound Med Biol 1989;15:481–97.
14. Hynynen K. The role of nonlinear ultrasound propagation during hyperthermia treatments. Med Phys 1991;18: 1156–63.
15. Averkiou MA, Hamilton MF. Nonlinear distortion of short pulses radiated by plane and focused circular pistons. J Acoust Soc Am 1997;102:2539–48.
16. Ward B, Baker AC, Humphrey VF. Nonlinear propagation applied to the improvement of resolution in diagnostic medical ultrasound. J Acoust Soc Am 1997;101:143–54.
17. Christopher T. Finite amplitude distortion-based inhomogeneous pulse echo ultrasonic imaging. IEEE Trans Ultrason Ferroelectr Freq Control 1997;44:125–39.
18. ter Haar G. Ultrasound focal beam surgery. Ultrasound Med Biol 1995;21:1089–100.
19. Hynynen K. Review of ultrasound therapy. In: 1997 IEEE Ultrasonics Symposium Proceedings: An International Symposium; 1997; Toronto, Canada. New York: IEEE.
20. Arefiev A, Prat F, Chapelon JY, et al. Ultrasound-induced tissue ablation: studies on isolated, perfused porcine liver. Ultrasound Med Biol 1998;24:1033–43.
21. Bailey MR, Khokhlova VA, Sapozhnikov OA, et al. Physical mechanisms of the therapeutic effect of ultrasound (a review). Acoustical Physics 2003;49:369–88.
22. Coleman AJ, Saunders JE, Preston RC, Bacon DR. Pressure waveforms generated by a Dornier extracorporeal shock-wave lithotriptor. Ultrasound Med Biol 1987;13: 651–57.
23. Campbell DS, Flynn HG, Blackstock DT, et al. The acoustic fields of the Wolf electrohydraulic lithotriptor. J Lithotr Stone Dis 1991;3:147–56.
24. Staudenraus J, Eisenmenger W. Fibre-optic probe hydrophone for ultrasonic and shock-wave measurements in water. Ultrasonics 1993; 31:267–73.
25. Cleveland RO, Lifshitz DA, Connors BA, et al. In vivo pressure measurements of lithotripsy shock waves in pigs. Ultrasound Med Biol 1998;24:293–306.
26. Coleman AJ, Saunders JE, Crum LA, Dyson M. Acoustic cav-

27. Crum LA. Cavitation microjets as a contributory mechanism for renal calculi disintegration in ESWL. J Urol 1988; 140:1587–90.
28. Delius M, Brendel W, Heine G. A mechanism of gallstone destruction by extracorporeal shock waves. Naturwissenschaften 1988;75:200–1.
29. Atchley AA, Prosperetti A. The crevice model of bubble nucleation. J Acoust Soc Am 1989;86(3):1065–84.
30. Church C. A theoretical study of cavitation generated by an extracorporeal shock wave lithotriptor. J Acoust Soc Am 1989;86:215–27.
31. Matula TJ, Hilmo PR, Storey BD, Szeri AJ. Radial response of individual bubbles subjected to shock wave lithotripsy pulses in vitro. Phys Fluids 2002;14(3):913–21.
32. Coleman AJ, Choi MJ, Saunders JE, Leighton TG. Acoustic emission and sonoluminescence due to cavitation at the beam focus of an electrohydraulic shock wave lithotriptor. Ultrasound Med Biol 1992;18:267–81.
33. Philipp A, Delius M, Scheffczyk C, et al. Interaction of lithotriptor-generated shock waves with air bubbles. J Acoust Soc Am 1993;93:2496–509.
34. Sass W, Matura E, Dreyer HP, et al. Lithotripsy-mechanisms of the fragmentation process with focussed shock waves. Electromedica 1993;61:2–12.
35. Zhong P, Cioanta I, Cocks FH, Preminger GM. Inertial cavitation and associated acoustic emission produced during electrohydraulic shock wave lithotripsy. J Acoust Soc Am 1997;101:2940–50.
36. Pishchalnikov YA, Sapozhnikov OA, Bailey MR, et al. Cavitation bubble cluster activity in the breakage of kidney stones by lithotriptor shockwaves. J Endourol 2003;17:435–46.
37. Matula TJ, Hilmo PR, Bailey MR, Crum LA. In vitro sonoluminescence and sonochemistry studies with an electrohydraulic shock-wave lithotriptor. Ultrasound Med Biol 2002;28:1199–207.
38. Coakley W. Acoustical detection of single cavitation events in a focused field in water at 1 MHz. J Acoust Soc Am 1971; 49:792–801.
39. Roy RA, Madanshetty SI, Apfel RE. An acoustic backscattering technique for the detection of transient cavitation produced by microsecond pulses of ultrasound. J Acoust Soc Am 1990;87:2451–8.
40. Madanshetty SI, Roy RA, Apfel RE. Acoustic microcavitation: its active and passive acoustic detection. J Acoust Soc Am 1991;90:1515–26.
41. Cleveland RO, Sapozhnikov OA, Bailey MR, Crum LA. A dual passive cavitation detector for localized detection of lithotripsy-induced cavitation in vitro. J Acoust Soc Am 2000;107:1745–58.
42. Coleman AJ, Whitlock M, Leighton T, Saunders JE. The spatial distribution of cavitation induced acoustic emission, sonoluminescence and cell lysis in the field of a shock wave lithotriptor. Phys Med Biol 1993;38:1545–60.
43. Bailey MR, Blackstock DT, Cleveland RO, Crum LA. Comparison of electrohydraulic lithotriptors with rigid and pressure-release ellipsoidal reflectors. II. Cavitation fields. J Acoust Soc Am 1999;106:1149–60.
44. Lifshitz DA, Williams JC Jr, Sturtevant B, et al. Quantitation of shock wave cavitation damage in vitro. Ultrasound Med Biol 2001;23:461–71.
45. Pye SD, Dineley JA. Characterization of cavitational activity in lithotripsy fields using a robust electromagnetic probe. Ultrasound Med Biol 1999;25:451–71.
46. Church CC, Crum LA. A theoretical study of cavitation generated by four commercially available extracorporeal shock wave lithotriptors. In: Frontiers of Nonlinear Acoustics: Proceedings of 12th ISNA; 1990; Austin (TX). New York: Elsevier.
47. Cartledge JJ, Cross WR, Lloyd SN, Joyce AD. The efficacy of a range of contact media as coupling agents in extracorporeal shockwave lithotripsy. BJU Int 2001;88:321–4.
48. Coleman AJ, Saunders JE. A survey of the acoustic output of commercial extracorporeal shock wave lithotriptors. Ultrasound Med Biol 1989;15:213–27.
49. Buizza A, Dell'Aquila T, Giribona P, Spagno C. The performance of different pressure pulse generators for extracorporeal lithotripsy: a comparison based on commercial lithotriptors for kidney stones. Ultrasound Med Biol 1995;21:259–72.
50. Chuong CJ, Zhong P, Preminger GM. A comparison of stone damage caused by different modes of shock wave generation. J Urol 1992;148:200–5.
51. Teichman JMH, Portis AJ, Cecconi PP, et al. In vitro comparison of shock wave lithotripsy machines. J Urol 2000;164: 1259–64.

52. Cleveland RO, Anglade R, Babayan RK. Effect of stone motion in vitro comminution efficiency of a Storx Modulith SLX. J Endourol 2004;18:629–33.

53. Chitnis PV. Characterization and comparative analysis of extracorporeal shock wave devices. In: Aerospace and mechanical engineering. Boston: Boston University; 2002. p. 108.

54. Paterson RF, Lifshitz DA, Lingeman JE, et al. Stone fragmentation during shock wave lithotripsy is improved by slowing the shock wave rate: studies with a new animal model. J Urol 2002;168:2211–15.

55. R.O Cleveland and O.A. Sapozhnikov. Modeling elastic wave propagation in kidney stones with application to shock wave lithotripsy. J Acoust Soc Am 2005;118:2667–76.

56. Agarwal R, Singh VR. A comparative study of fracture strength, ultrasonic properties and chemical constituents of kidney stones. Ultrasonics 1991;29:89–90.

57. Cohen NP, Whitfield HN. Mechanical testing of urinary calculi. World J Urol 1993;11:13–8.

58. Zhong P, Preminger GM. Mechanisms of differing stone fragility in extracorporeal shockwave lithotripsy. J Endourol 1994;8:263–68.

59. Chaussy C, Brendel W, Schmiedt E. Extracorporeally induced destruction of kidney stones by shock waves. Lancet 1980;2:1265–8.

60. Chaussy C. Extracorporeal shock wave lithotripsy: new aspects in the treatment of kidney stone disease. 1982. Basel, Switzerland: S Karager.

61. Sass W, Braunlich M, Dreyer H-P, et al. The mechanisms of stone disintegration by shock waves. Ultrasound Med Biol 1991;17:239–43.

62. Ding Z,. Gracewski SM. Response of constrained and unconstrained bubbles to lithotriptor shock wave pulses. J Acoust Soc Am 1994;96:3636–44.

63. Sapozhnikov OA, Cleveland RO, Bailey MR, Crum LA. Modeling of stresses generated by lithotriptor shock wave in cylindrical kidney stone. In: 3rd International Symposium of Therapeutic Ultrasound. 2004. Lyon, France.

64. Dahake G, Gracewski SM. Finite difference predictions of P-SV wave propagation inside submerged solids. II. Effect of geometry. J Acoust Soc Am 1997;102:2138–45.

65. Xi X, Zhong P. Dynamic photoelastic study of the transient stress field in solids during shock wave lithotripsy. J Acoust Soc Am 2001;109:1226–39.

66. Sylven ET, Agarwal S, Cleveland RO, Briant CL. High strain rate testing of kidney stones. J Mater Sci Mater Med 2004;15:613–17.

67. Gracewski SM, Dahake G, Ding Z, et al. Internal stress wave measurements in solids subjected to lithotriptor pulses. J Acoust Soc Am 1993;94:652–61.

68. Eisenmenger W. The mechanisms of stone fragmentation in ESWL. Ultrasound Med Biol 2001;27:683–93.

69. Eisenmenger W, Du XX, Tang C, et al. The first clinical results of "wide focus and low pressure" ESWL. Ultrasound Med Biol 2002;28:769–74.

70. Holmer NG, Almquist LO, Hertz TG, et al. On the mechanism of kidney-stone disintegration by acoustic shock-waves. Ultrasound Med Biol 1991;17:479–89.

71. Sapozhnikov OA, Khokhlova VA, Bailey MR, et al. Effect of overpressure and pulse repetition frequency on cavitation in shock wave lithotripsy. J Acoust Soc Am 2002; 112(3).

72. Delacretaz G, Rink K, Pittomvils G, et al. Importance of the implosion of ESWL-induced cavitation bubbles. Ultrasound Med Biol 1995; 21:97–103.

73. Zhong P, Chuong CJ, Preminger GM. Propagation of shock waves in elastic solids caused by cavitation microjet impact. II: Application in extracorporeal shock wave lithotripsy. J Acoust Soc Am 1993;94:29–36.

74. Pittomvils G, Lafaut JP, Vandeursen H, et al. Macroscopic ESWL-induced cavitation: in vitro studies. Ultrasound Med Biol 1995;21:393–8.

75. Tanguay M, Colonius T. Numerical investigation of bubble cloud dynamics in shock wave lithotripsy. In: 2002 ASME Fluids Engineering Division Summer Meeting. 2002.

76. Sturtevant B. Shock wave physics of lithotriptors. In: Smith AD, editor. Smith's textbook of endourology. St. Louis: Quality Medical Publishing, Inc.; 1996. p. 529–52.

77. Lokhandwalla M, Sturtevant B. Fracture mechanics model of stone comminution in ESWL and implications for tissue damage. Phys Med Biol 2000;45:1923–40.

78. Pittomvils G, Vandeursen H, Wevers M, et al. The influence of internal stone structure upon the fracture behaviour of urinary calculi. Ultrasound Med Biol 1994;20:803–810.

79. Cleveland RO, McAteer JA, and Muller R. Time-lapse nondestructive assessment of shock wave damage to kidney stones in vitro using micro-computed tomography. J Acoust Soc Am 2001;110:1733–6.

80. Williams JC Jr, Saw KC, Paterson RF, et al. Variability of renal stone fragility in shock wave lithotripsy. Urology 2003;61:1092–6.

81. Zhu S, Cocks FH, Preminger GM, Zhong P. The role of stress waves and cavitation in stone comminution in shock wave lithotripsy. Ultrasound Med Biol 2002;28:661–71.

82. Burns JR, Shoemaker BE, Gauthier JF, Finlayson B. Hardness testing of urinary calculi. In: Schwille PO, Others ETC, editors. Urolithiasis and related clinical research. New York: Plenum Press; 1985. p. 703–6.

83. Ebrahimi F, Wang F. Fracture behavior of urinary stones under compression. J Biomed Mater Res 1989;23:507–21.

84. Singh VR, Dhawan JB. Ultrasonic velocity and attenuation measurement in kidney stones: correlation to constituents and hardness. Biomed Mater Eng 1992;2:79–82.

85. Zhong P, Chuong CJ, Preminger GM. Characterization of fracture toughness of renal calculi using a microindentation technique. (Extracorporeal shock wave lithotripsy). J Mater Sci Lett 1993;12:1460–2.

86. Tuteja AK, Pulliam JP, Lehman TH, Elzinga LW. Anuric renal failure from massive bilateral renal hematoma following extracorporeal shock wave lithotripsy. Urology 1997;50: 606–8.

87. Lokhandwalla M, Sturtevant B. Mechanical haemolysis in shock wave lithotripsy (SWL). I. Analysis of cell deformation due to SWL flow-fields. Phys Med Biology 2001; 46:413–37.

88. Lokhandwalla H, McAteer JA, Williams JC Jr, Stuftevant B. Mechanical haemolysis in shock wave lithotripsy (SWL): II. In vitro cell lysis due to shear. Phys Med Bio 2001;46:1245–64.

89. Mast TD, Hinkelman LM, Metlay LA, et al. Simulation of ultrasonic pulse propagation, distortion, and attenuation in the human chest wall. J Acoust Soc Am 1999;106:3665–77.

90. Coleman AJ, Choi MJ, Saunders JE. Detection of acoustic emission from cavitation in tissue during clinical extracorporeal lithotripsy. Ultrasound Med Biol 1996;22: 1079–87.

91. Sapozhnikov OA, Bailey MR, Crum LA, et al. Ultrasound-guided localized detection of cavitation during lithotripsy in pig kidney in vivo. IEEE Ultrasonics Symposium 2001. p. 1347–50.

92. Carstensen EL, Child SZ, Crane C, et al. Lysis of cells in Elodea leaves by pulsed and continuous wave ultrasound. Ultrasound Med Biol 1990;16:167–73.

93. Miller DL, Thomas RM. Contrast-agent gas bodies enhance hemolysis induced by lithotriptor shock waves and high-intensity focused ultrasound in whole blood. Ultrasound Med Biol 1996;22:1089–95.

94. Miller M, Miller D, Brayman A. A review of in vitro bioeffects of intertial ultrasonic cavitation from a mechanistic perspective. Ultrasound Med Biol 1996;22:1131–54.

95. Dalecki D, Raeman CH, Child SZ, Carstensen EL. A test for cavitation as a mechanism for intestinal hemorrhage in mice exposed to a piezoelectric lithotripter. Ultrasound Med Biol 1996;22:493–6.

96. Delius M, Denk R, Berding C, et al. Biological effects of shock waves: cavitation by shock waves in piglet liver. Ultrasound Med Biol 1990;16:467–72.

97. Williams JC Jr, Woodward JF, Stonehill MA, et al. Cell damage by lithotriptor shock waves at high pressure to preclude cavitation. Ultrasound Med Biol 1999;25:1445–9.

98. Delius M. Minimal static excess pressure minimises the effect of extracorporeal shock waves on cells and reduces it on gallstones. Ultrasound Med Biol 1997;23:611–7.

99. Evan AP, Willis LR, McAteer JA, et al. Kidney damage and renal functional changes are minimized by waveform control that suppresses cavitation in shock wave lithotripsy. J Urol 2002;168:1556–62.

100. Zhong P, Cioanta J, Zhu S, et al. Effects of tissue constraint on shock wave-induced bubble expansion in vivo. J Acoust Soc Am 1998;104:3126–9.

101. Zhong P, Zhou Y, Zhu S. Dynamics of bubble oscillation in constrained media and mechanisms of vessel rupture in SWL. Ultrasound Med Biol 2001;27:119–34.

102. Kuwahara M, Ioritani N, Kambe K, et al. Hyperechoic region induced by focused shock waves in vitro and in vivo: possibility of acoustic cavitation bubbles. J Lithotr Stone Dis 1989;1:282–8.

103. Bourlion M, Dancer P, Lacoste F, et al. Design and characterization of a shock wave generator using canalized electrical discharge: application to lithotripsy. Rev Sci Instrum 1994;65:2356–63.

104. Cleveland R, Chitnis P, Gerbus B, McAteer J. An in vitro comparison of open-cage and encapsulated electrodes in shock wave lithotripsy (SWL). European Association of Urology. 2004.

105. Bailey MR, Cleveland RO, Williams JC Jr, et al. Effect of increased ambient pressure on lithotripsy-induced cavitation in bulk fluid and at solid surfaces. In: Joint Meeting of the Acoustical Society of America, European Acoustics Association and German Acoustics DAGA Conference. 1999. Berlin, Germany: Deutsche Gesellschaft fur Akustik (DEGA).

106. Sokolov DL, Bailey MR, Crum LA. Use of a dual-pulse lithotriptor to generate a localized and intensified cavitation field. J Acoust Soc Am 2001;110(3 Pt 1):1685–95.

107. Sokolov DL, Bailey MR, Crum LA. Dual-pulse lithotriptor accelerates stone fragmentation and reduces cell lysis in vitro. Ultrasound Med Biol 2003;29:1045–52.

108. Bailey MR. Control of acoustic cavitation with application to lithotripsy. J Acoust Soc Am 1997;102:1250–1250.

109. Prieto FE, Loske AM. Bifocal reflector for electrohydraulic lithotriptors. J Endourol 1999;13:65–75.

110. Huber P, Debus J, Jöchle K, et al. Control of cavitation activity by different shockwave pulsing regimes. Phys Med Biol 1999;44:1427–37.

111. Zhong P, Zhou YF. Suppression of large intraluminal bubble expansion in shock wave lithotripsy without compromising stone comminution: methodology and in vitro experiments. J Acoust Soc Am 2001;110:3283–91.

112. Zhong P, Cocks FH, Cionta I, Preminger GM. Controlled, forced collapse of cavitation bubbles for improved stone fragmentation during shock wave lithotripsy. J Urol 1997;158:2323–8.

113. Xi X, Zhong P. Improvement of stone fragmentation during shock-wave lithotripsy using a combined EH/PEAA shock-wave generator-in vitro experiments. Ultrasound Med Biol 2000;26:457–67.

114. Sheir KZ, El-Sheikh AM, Ghoneim MA. Synchronous twin-pulse technique to improve efficacy of SWL: Preliminary results of an experimental study. J Endourol 2001; 15:965–74.

115. Kuwahara MA, Kambe K, Taguchi K, et al. Initial experience using a new type extracorporeal lithotriptor with an anti-misshot control device. J Lithotr Stone Dis 1991;3:141–6.

116. Orkisz M, Farchtchian T, Saighi D, et al. Image based renal stone tracking to improve efficacy in extracorporeal lithotripsy. J Urol 1998;160:1237–40.

117. Chang CC, Liang SM, Pu YR, et al. In vitro study of ultrasound based real-time tracking of renal stones for shock wave lithotripsy: part I. J Urol 2001;166:28–32.

118. Chang CC, Manousakas I, Pu YR, et al. In vitro study of ultrasound based real-time tracking for renal stones in shock wave lithotripsy: Part II - A simulated animal experiment. J Urol 2002;167:2594–97.

119. Thomas J-L, Wu F, Fink M. Time reversal focusing applied to lithotripsy. Ultrason Imaging 1996;18:106–21.

120. Montaldo G, Roux P, Derode A, et al. Ultrasound shock wave generator with one-bit time reversal in a dispersive medium, application to lithotripsy. Appl Phys Lett 2002;80:897–9.

39

Lithotripsy Systems

James E. Lingeman, MD

The concept that extracorporeally generated shock waves could be used to successfully fragment urinary calculi in a non-invasive manner has revolutionized the management of urolithiasis.[1–3] Open surgical lithotomy is now rarely performed. Extracorporeal shock wave lithotripsy (ESWL) has become a well established and routine urologic technique, and the majority of patients with symptomatic urolithiasis can be managed initially with ESWL.[4,5] The success of ESWL has resulted in its rapid acceptance worldwide[6,7] and has spawned the development of a variety of extracorporeal lithotripsy devices by numerous manufacturers. A variety of methods for extracorporeal destruction of kidney stones with shock waves have been introduced in the past decade.[8–10] In this chapter, as much information as could be garnered from industry sources and the published literature regarding the many devices currently available will be presented. The various components required for any lithotripsy system will be reviewed. Technical information regarding the plethora of lithotriptors currently marketed will be presented in tabular format. Perhaps as important as the lithotriptor itself is the recent appreciation that attention to the technique of shock wave administration that may enhance the effectiveness of ESWL. Anesthesia techniques appropriate to ESWL will be reviewed. An attempt has been made to review the available clinical data to allow meaningful comparison of machine efficiency. Treatment of renal and ureteral stones is addressed separately (see Chapter 40, "Helical Computed Tomography and Shock Wave Lithotripsy Treatment of Renal and Ureteral Calculi").

LITHOTRIPTOR BASICS

Certain features are common to all ESWL devices. Even the most basic lithotriptor will require an energy source, a focusing mechanism for the shock wave, a coupling medium, and a stone localization system. In the most fundamental sense, all that is required of a lithotriptor is that it transform urinary calculi into particles small enough for spontaneous discharge by the patient. In the 1990s, there was a trend towards development of lithotripsy devices that were multifunctional and could be utilized for diagnostic radiologic procedures and endourologic procedures as well as ESWL. Over the last decade, there has been a trend away from such designs. Furthermore, there has been a strong trend away from large, fixed-site systems towards smaller, modular, easily transportable lithotripsy devices.

SHOCK WAVE GENERATION AND FOCUSING

A variety of energy sources capable of generating shock waves sufficient for stone fragmentation have been developed or investigated, including electrohydraulic, electromagnetic, piezoelectric, microexplosion, and focused laser.[11–15] Currently, the most commonly utilized energy source for lithotripsy is electromagnetic, but electrohydraulic lithotriptors remain in common use. Piezoelectric lithotriptors are significantly less common than electromagnetic and electrohydraulic devices. A detailed discussion of the physics of the various lithotripsy energy sources is presented elsewhere (see Chapter 38, "The Physics of Shock Wave Lithotripsy") and will not be repeated here.

IMAGING FOR STONE LOCALIZATION

The original Dornier lithotriptors used fluoroscopy for stone localization, an imaging technology with which urologists are familiar and comfortable. Many renal calculi, however, can be imaged with ultrasonography. In the late 1980s and early 1990s, interest in the potential for lithotripsy to treat radiolucent biliary calculi stimulated the introduction of many lithotripsy systems that used ultrasonography exclusively for stone targeting. Biliary lithotripsy proved unsuccessful, and the inability to image many ureteral calculi with ultrasonography has resulted in the de-emphasizing of ultrasonography for kidney stone lithotripsy. At the present time, fluoroscopic stone localization, often using portable C-arm technology, is the accepted standard for lithotriptors. Since the decision by the United States Food and Drug Administration (FDA) in 1989 to not approve biliary lithotripsy, interest in this treatment approach for cholelithiasis has greatly decreased.[16–18] Currently, biliary lithotripsy is rarely, if ever, considered as a treatment option for cholelithiasis, and thus, the utility of a lithotriptor capable of biliary lithotripsy (ie, one with ultrasonography) is questionable .

Ultrasonography does have some potential advantages for lithotripsy in that radiation exposure is minimized and real-time (ie, continuous) imaging to monitor stone targeting is possible during treatment.[19] In lithotripsy systems with dual localization (meaning both fluoroscopy and ultrasonography), some operators will localize the stone initially with fluoroscopy and then monitor the treatment with ultrasonography. Ultrasonography is problematic in obese patients, a problem of epidemic proportions among urolithiasis patients in the United States. Currently, all manufacturers of lithotripsy systems provide either fluoroscopic or fluoroscopic plus ultrasonography. There would appear to be little, if any, reason to consider for urologic purposes a lithotriptor that has only an ultrasound capability.

SHOCK WAVE COUPLING

The original ESWL device, the Dornier HM-3 (Dornier MedTech), had a large water bath for coupling the shock wave to the patient during lithotripsy. Body tissue has an acoustical impedance very close to that of water, and therefore, a shock wave generated in water will pass into the body with minimal reflection or absorption of energy at the water/skin interface. Although the water bath is the theoretical ideal for shock wave coupling, it is bulky and inconvenient. Shock waves sufficient for stone fragmentation can be transmitted through membranes of similar acoustic density, thereby eliminating the inconvenience of the water bath. The acoustics of shock wave coupling are reviewed elsewhere (see Chapter 38, "The Physics of Shock Wave Lithotripsy"). The incorporation of "dry" shock wave energy sources in lithotriptor design provides several advantages. A flat table can be incorporated into such a system, which facilitates patient positioning, particularly when treating stones in the mid- and lower ureter.[20,21] Prone positioning, which may be advantageous when treating patients in the middle ureter, horseshoe kidneys, or pelvic kidneys, is straightforward with lithotriptors that have a water cushion energy source, although the HM-3 is also adaptable for such positions.[22–25]

The water bath may be the reason that ESWL with the Dornier HM-3 lithotriptor has been associated with cardiac arrhythmias. When a water bath is used, the initial unfocused shock wave (which precedes the more powerful focused shock wave) expands spherically upon emanating from the ellipsoid reflector, and some shock wave energy likely passes through the heart, requiring that shock waves with this device be released during the refractory period of the ventricle to prevent extrasystoles.[11] Although arrhythmias have been reported with water cushion lithotriptors using electrohydraulic, electromagnetic, and piezoelectric energy sources, rhythm disturbances are significantly less common with these devices than with the HM-3. Current lithotriptors do not routinely require coordination of shock wave administration to the cardiac cycle.[26,27] One consequence of non-electrocardiogram gating of the lithotriptor has been an industry-wide trend towards administration of shock waves at higher rates (100 to120 Hz) thereby shortening the ESWL treatment time. The practice of administration of shock waves at higher rates may not be a positive development. The influence of shock wave administration rate on the effectiveness of stone fragmentation is reviewed later in this chapter and elsewhere (see Chapter 40, "Helical Computed Tomography and Shock Wave Lithotripsy Treatment of Renal and Ureteral Calculi").

MODULAR SYSTEMS

Early lithotriptors such as the Dornier HM-3 and the Siemens Lithostar (Siemens AG, Munich, Germany) were large, bulky, expensive devices (Figure 39-1 and 39-2). Some early lithotriptor systems utilized water baths (HM-3, Technomed 2000) and many had two x-ray systems (HM-3 and HM-4, THS International Inc.; Lithostar, Siemens AG). With the evolution towards "dry" lithotriptor energy sources and the adoption of portable C-arms into lithotriptor designs, substantial downsizing of these devices and lowering of costs was made possible (Figure 39-3). In addition, lithotriptors could be broken down into their modular components (treatment table, treatment head, portable C-arm) allowing the

machines to be easily moved around the treatment facility as needed, or even transported from one facility to another. Currently, all lithotriptor manufacturers provide modular designs. There remain a few manufacturers who produce traditional, large, fixed-site lithotriptor designs, but such devices represent a distinct minority of machines currently utilized worldwide .

ANESTHESIA

The approach to anesthesia for lithotripsy has changed considerably since the first clinical application of ESWL in 1980. At the beginning of ESWL, regional or general anesthesia was used in all instances as treatment at recommended kilovolt levels with the HM-3 device produced intolerable pain. Subsequently, urologists and lithotriptor manufacturers realized that the recommended kilovolt settings for the HM-3 were greater than generally necessary for the fragmentation of most renal calculi, an observation that spawned interest in less powerful lithotriptors and lithotriptors with decreased anesthesia requirements.[8–10] Anesthesia requirements were noted to be decreased with the original HM-3 lithotriptor by utilizing lower kilovolt settings which still resulted in excellent treatment results.[28–31] The discomfort experienced during ESWL is directly related to the energy density of the shock waves that pass through the skin and

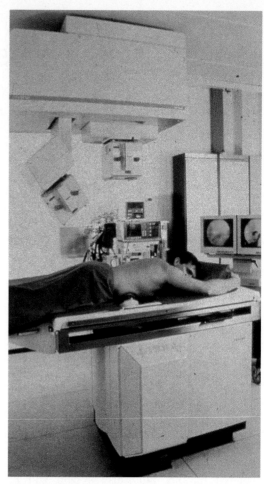

Figure 39-2 The Siemens Lithostar was the most successful of the second-generation lithotriptors. The combination of a flat table with multiplane fluoroscopic imaging greatly facilitates the treatment of ureteral stones.

also the size of the focal point. The large aperture of the piezoelectric lithotriptors combined with their extremely small focal point make them the least painful.[32]

Recent development of new anesthetic techniques adaptable to ESWL have greatly influenced the way that lithotripsy sessions are conducted.[33–35] Short-acting agents such as the narcotic alfentanil hydrochloride and the sedative-hypnotics midazolam and propofol have been used in various combinations to allow most ESWL treatments with any lithotriptor (including the unmodified Dornier HM-3) to be accomplished comfortably for the patient without the need for general or regional anesthesia if the patient so desires. For this reason, anesthetic considerations have not been included in the technical data on lithotriptors presented in Tables 39-1 to 39-4.

Monk and colleagues compared two sedative-analgesic techniques (midazolam/alfentanil vs fentanyl citrate/propofol) and found both techniques provided anesthesia comparable to epidural anesthesia for ESWL.[36] Anesthesia and recovery times, however, were significantly shorter than with epidural anesthesia techniques. Arroyo and colleages noted that a continuous alfentanil infusion supplemented with midazolam as needed provided satisfactory anesthesia

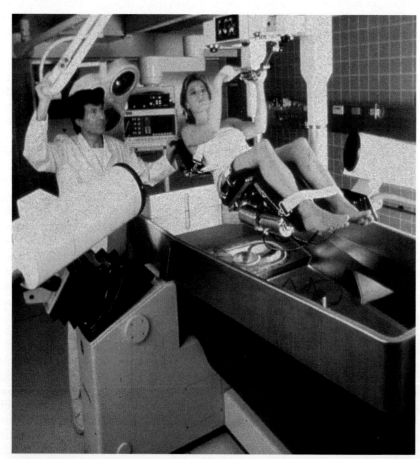

Figure 39-1 The success of the Dornier HM-3 revolutionized the treatment of urolithiasis patients.

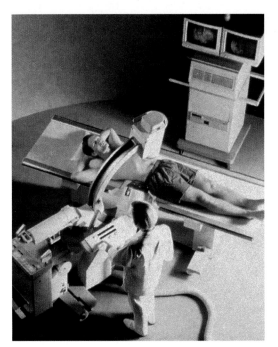

Figure 39-3 The LithoDiamond uses an electrohydraulic shock wave integrated into a portable C-arm. The system is typical of the modular designs now in common use for ESWL. Modular systems facilitate moving ESWL devices from one room or facility to another.

for 88 of 90 patients treated with a Medstone STS lithotriptor, another powerful device.[37]

Another approach to minimize anesthesia requirements during ESWL has been the use of topical agents. Fair and Malhotra first reported that ESWL could be accomplished successfully in some patients by infiltrating the skin over the area of shock wave entry with lidocaine.[38] This technique, however, was cumbersome and time-consuming. More recently, the use of EMLA cream, a eutectic mixture of lidocaine and prilocaine hydrochloride, has been demonstrated to significantly reduce anesthesia requirements during ESWL.[30,31,39,40] EMLA cream, a topical agent, should be applied at least 45 minutes prior to ESWL. The combination of topical agents and short-acting intravenous agents would likely minimize the amount of these agents required and lead to shortened recovery times.[36]

A variety of factors need to be considered when choosing the preferred anesthetic technique for ESWL. Calculi composed of cystine, calcium oxalate monohydrate (whellelite), and brushite are known to be resistant to fragmentation,[41,42] and if their presence is anticipated or known, the delivery of higher levels of shock wave energy that are required means that anesthetic requirements will also be greater. Thin patients will have more pain during ESWL because the converging shock wave will be more concentrated at the point of skin penetration. Children and extremely anxious individuals may be best served by general anesthesia. If a lengthy treatment session is anticipated (ie, bilateral ESWL or treatment of ureteral and renal stones), the larger amounts of topical and intravenous agents that will be required lessens their appeal.

TECHNIQUE OF SHOCK WAVE ADMINISTRATION

Over the past 20 years, changes in lithotriptor technology have been incremental. The shock waves produced by current-generation lithotriptors are fundamentally the same as that produced by the original Dornier HM-3 device. At the time of the introduction of ESWL, understanding of the basic science of how shock waves interacted with stone and tissue was minimal. As new knowledge has been gained regarding the basic science of shock wave lithotripsy, a number of new approaches to the technique of shock wave administration are being investigated. In ESWL treatment, the urologist has control over just a few parameters of shock wave delivery: voltage/power, number of shock waves, the sequence of shock wave administration, and the rate at which shock waves are fired. Each of these parameters has the potential to influence lithotripsy outcomes.

A number of studies have shown that increased doses of shock waves (ie, higher number, higher voltage/power) result in increased renal tissue injury.[43,44] An extensive review of the biologic effects of shock waves on renal tissue may be found elsewhere (see Chapter 41, "Complications"). Given the progressive effects of increasing shock wave dosage on renal tissue, the safety of ESWL is enhanced by limiting the treatment dose to as low as is necessary for stone comminution.

The influence of shock wave rate on the effectiveness of ESWL is a recent observation and is

Table 39-1 Mechanical Aspects — Electrohydraulic Lithotriptors								
Company	Machine	Method of Focusing SW	Aperture (cm)	Focal Distance (cm)	Peak Pressure at Focal Point (PVDF)	Focal zone (W × L mm)	Electrode life span (SW)	SW Coupling
Dornier Medical Systems	HM-3*	Ellipsoid reflector	15.6, 17.2	13	220–360, 320–390	15 × 90, 10 × 40	2000	Water bath
Medispec Ltd.	Econolith	Ellipsoid reflector	17.6*	13.5	760	13 × 60	3000	Water cushion
Medispec Ltd.	E-2000	Ellipsoid reflector	17.6	13.5, 15.0	760	13 × 60	3000	Water cushion
Medispec Ltd.	E-3000	Ellipsoid reflector	17.6	13.5, 15.5	910	13 × 60	3000	Water cushion
Healthtronics	Litho Tron	Ellipsoid reflector	20	15	530	8 × 38	8000	Water cushion
Healthtronics	Litho Tron Ultra	Ellipsoid reflector	20	15	530	8 × 38	8000	Water cushion
HMT-USA	LithoDiamond	Ellipsoid reflector	20	15	580	11 × 96	20,000	Coupling water cushion
Comair Professor H. Wiksell AB	Lithocut C-3000S**	Ellipsoid reflector	23	15	820	5 × 16	Approx. 5 sessions	Water cushion
Comair Professor H. Wiksell AB	Lithocut C-3000A**	Ellipsoid reflector	23	15	200–820	3.5 × 12	Approx. 5 sessions	Water cushion
Direx Systems Corp.	Tripter X-1 Compact	Ellipsoid reflector	18.1	13.5	240-440	13 × 48	3000	Water cushion
Direx Systems Corp.	Duet	Dual ellipsoid reflectors	18.1	14.2	240–480	13 × 48	3–12,000	Dual water cushion
Direx Systems Corp.	Nova Ultima**	Rotating ellipsoid reflector	18.1	13.5	240–440	13 × 48	3–12,000	Water cushion
Medstone International	STS	Ellipsoid reflector	15	15	481	12 × 90	3600	Water cushion
Medstone International	STS-TC	Ellipsoid reflector	15	15	481	12 × 90	3600	Water cushion
ELMED Lithotripsy Systems	Multimed Classic**	Ellipsoid reflector	17.6	13.5	N/A	7.5 × 22	4500	Water cushion
ELMED Lithotripsy Systems	Complit**	Isocentric moveable ellipsoid reflector	17.6	13.5	N/A	7.5 × 22	4,500	Water cushion
EDAP Technomed	Sonolith Praktis	Ellipsoid reflector	21.9	13	106	25 × 3.6	27,000 at 100%	Water cushion
EDAP Technomed	Sonolith Vision	Ellipsoid reflector	21.9	13	106	25 × 3.6	27,000 at 20 KV	Water cushion
FMD, LLC	Twinheads TH101	Ellipsoid reflector	14.7	12.7	1100	15.4 × 15.6	3,000	Two water cushions
FMD, LLC	Twinheads TH103	Ellipsoid reflector	14.7	12.7	1100	15.4 × 15.6	3,000	Two water cushions

*No longer manufactured.

**Not FDA approved.

*Not interchangeable w/Econolith 2000 ellipsoids.

Table 39-2   Imaging/Financial Aspects—Electrohydraulic Lithotriptors

Company	Machine	ECG Gaiting	Endourology Capability	Stone Localization	Portability	Purchase Price	Service Contract	Upgrade Possibility	Upgrade Cost
Dornier Medical Systems	HM-3*	Yes	No	X-ray	Semi-trailer	$25 K used*	$45K	Digital X-ray	$60K
Medispec Ltd.	Econolith	Optional	Yes	X-ray, Portable C-arm, Optional US	Yes	$350K	$15-21K	ECG monitor, Endo., C-arm upgrades, comp. Console	N/A
Medispec Ltd.	E-2000	Optional	Yes	X-ray, Portable C-arm, Optional US	Yes	$380K	$15-26K	ECG monitor, Endo., C-arm upgrades	N/A
Medispec Ltd.	E-3000	Optional	Yes	X-ray, Portable C-arm, Optional US	Yes	$399K	$15-26K	ECG monitor, 4 or 5 axis Endourology Table, Console, C-arm upgrades	N/A
Healthtronics	Litho Tron	Optional	Yes	X-ray, Portable C-arm, Optional US	Yes	$350-400K	$48K	No	N/A
Healthtronics	Litho Tron Ultra	Optional	Yes	X-ray, Optional US	No	$700K	$65K	N/A	N/A
HMT-USA	LithoDiamond	Optional	Yes	X-ray, Optional US	Yes	$400K	N/A	N/A	N/A
Comair Professor H. Wiksell AB	Lithocut C-3000S**	Yes/No	Yes	X-ray, Optional US	Yes	$250K	Sub-unit exch. sys	N/A	N/A
Comair Professor H. Wiksell AB	Lithocut C-3000A**	Yes/No	Yes	X-ray, Optional US	Yes	$200K	Sub-unit exch. sys	N/A	N/A
Direx Systems Corp.	Tripter X-1 Compact	Yes	Yes	X-ray, Portable C-arm	Yes	$395K	$28-35K	Triple generator, non ECG gaiting	N/A
Direx Systems Corp.	Duet	Yes	Yes	X-ray, Portable C-arm, Optional US	Yes	$435K	$35K	Ultrasound	N/A
Direx Systems Corp.	Nova Ultima**	Yes	Yes	X-ray, Portable C-arm, Optional US	Yes	N/A	N/A	Triple generator	N/A
Medstone	STS	Yes	Yes	Digital X-ray, US	No	$500K	$25-80K	Yes	variable
Medstone	STS-TC	Yes	Yes	Digital X-ray, US	Yes	$433,350	$20-55K	Yes	$49.5-54K
ELMED Lithotripsy Sys.	Multimed Classic**	Yes	Yes	X-ray, Ultrasound	Yes	$55-135K	$25K	Comp. controlled US localization	$15K
ELMED Lithotripsy Sys.	Complit**	Yes	Yes	X-ray, Ultrasound	Yes	$65-145K	$25K	Comp. controlled US localization	$15K
EDAP Technomed	Sonolith Praktis	Optional	Yes	X-ray and U/S	Yes	$400K	$35K	Yes	N/A
EDAP Technomed	Sonolith Vision	Optional	Yes	X-ray and U/S	Yes	$500K	$50K	Yes	N/A
FMD, LLC	Twinheads TH101	Yes	Yes	Flouroscopy, Integrated U-Arm	Semi-Portable	$540K	$50K	US, Laser Printer, DICOM 3	$9.8-56K
FMD, LLC	Twinheads TH103	Yes	Yes	Works with stand-alone C-arm	Semi-Portable	$495K	$40K	US, Laser Printer, DICOM 3	$9.8-56K

*No longer manufactured.

**Not FDA approved.

*Disassembly/reinstallation—add $55K.

generally a counter to trends in the clinical practice of ESWL over the last two decades. Early lithotriptors were associated with a risk of extrasystoles and were, therefore, tethered to the heart rate with the shock wave pulse being released during the refractory period of the ventricle, thus minimizing the risk of arrhythmias.[11] Newer "dry" lithotriptors are much less likely to produce arrhythmias, and, in order to increase the speed of the ESWL session, most newer lithotriptors are designed to treat at 100 to 120 Hz. Given our recent increased understanding about the physics of shock wave lithotripsy, the trend towards more rapid shock wave administration may have been a counterproductive strategy as recent experimental and clinical studies have suggested that stones break better at slower shock wave administration rates. Wiksell and Kinn first suggested an inverse relationship between rate and stone fragmentation in an in vitro model in 1995.[45] Similar in vitro findings supporting a

relationship between rate and stone fragmentation were reported by Greenstein and Matsken, as well as Lifshitz and colleagues and Weir and colleagues.[46–48] These in vitro studies were followed by an in vivo study done by Paterson and colleagues utilizing a porcine model. A model stone was implanted percutaneously via an upper pole access with positioning of the stone into a lower pole calyx.[49] Stones treated at 30 shock waves per minute broke more completely than stones treated at 120 shock waves per minute, findings that were very similar to those reported in an in vitro study from the same institution (Figure 39-4).[12] In a recent randomized, controlled trial reported by Pace and colleagues, treatment of patients with ESWL at 1 Hz resulted in a significantly better success rate than those patients receiving treatment at 2 Hz (Table 39-5).[50] The mechanism responsible for this rate effect is not known but likely involves the role of cavitation in stone breakage. Shock waves initiate cavitation,

and bubbles can persist well beyond the passage of the shock pulse. At higher shock wave rates, persistent or residual bubble activity at the surface or in the vicinity of the stone may act as a barrier to subsequent shock waves.[51] A detailed discussion of cavitation during ESWL was presented earlier (see Chapter 39, "Shock Wave Lithotripsy Devices and Techniques").

Recent in vitro experiments suggest that stone breakage can also be improved by changing voltage/power during treatment. When ESWL is performed with sedation, shock wave delivery is often initiated at a low power setting to acclimate the patient to treatment. This may actually be a good strategy for stone breakage, as well. In experiments using an electrohydraulic lithotriptor, groups of gypsum model stones were exposed to shock waves in various stepwise regimens (15 to 20 kV) of increasing or decreasing charge potential.[52] When the same total shock wave energy was delivered, stones treated with

Table 39-3 Mechanical Aspects

Electromagnetic Lithotriptors

Company	Machine	Method of Focusing SW	Aperture (cm)	Focal Distance (cm)	Peak Pressure at Focal Point (PVDF)	Focal Zone (W × L mm)	Generator Life Span (SW)	SW Coupling
Siemens Medical Systems	Lithostar Multiline	Acoustic lens	17	12	800	5 × 80	1 million	Water cushion
Siemens Medical Systems	Lithostar Modularis Vario† (with C-plus)	Acoustic lens	12.5	14	570	12 × 130 to 13 × 146	1.5 million	Water cushion
Siemens Medical Systems	Lithostar Modularis (with C-plus†)	Acoustic lens	12.5	14	570	12 × 130 to 13 × 146	1.5 million	Water cushion
Karl Storz Lithotripsy	Modulith SL20*	Parabolic reflector	30	16.5	189–1056	4.6 × 34 to 2.8 × 37	6 million	Water cushion
Karl Storz Lithotripsy	Modulith SLX-MX	Parabolic reflector	30	16.5	189–1056	4.6 × 34 to 2.8 × 37	8 million	Water cushion
Karl Storz Lithotripsy	Modulith SLX-T	Parabolic reflector	30	16.5	189–1056	4.6 × 34 to 2.8 × 37	8 million	Water cushion
Karl Storz Lithotripsy	Modulith SLX-F2	Parabolic reflector	30	16.5	90–160	2.0 × 22 to 3.5 × 50	N/A	Water cushion
Dornier MedTech	Compact Delta	Acoustic lens	14	15	315–550	4.7 × 57	1 million	Water cushion
Dornier MedTech	Compact Sigma	Acoustic lens	14	15	315–550	4.7 × 57	1 million	Water cushion
Dornier MedTech	DoLi S 140	Acoustic lens	14	15	160–550	4.7 × 57	1 million	Water cushion
Dornier MedTech	DoLi S 220	Acoustic lens	22	15	288–991	2.5 × 41	1 million	Water cushion
Dornier MedTech	DoLi S 220-XP*	Acoustic lens	22	15	200–900	3.4 × 46	1 million	Water cushion
Dornier MedTech	DoLi S 220-XXP*	Acoustic lens	22	15	490–900	4.1 × 60.5	1 million	Water cushion
Dornier MedTech	DoLi S II 140	Acoustic lens	14	15	160–550	4.7 × 57	1 million	Water cushion
Dornier MedTech	DoLi S II 220	Acoustic lens	22	15	288–991	2.5 × 41	1 million	Water cushion
Dornier MedTech	DoLi S II 220-XP*	Acoustic lens	22	15	200–900	3.4 × 46	1 million	Water cushion
Dornier MedTech	DoLi S II 220-XXP*	Acoustic lens	22	15	490–900	4.1 × 60.5	1 million	Water cushion

Piezoelectric Lithotriptors

Wolf	P3000†	Concave Dish	26	15	1320	3 × 16	>5 mil	Water cushion

*Not sold in the US.
†Not FDA approved.

increasing voltage/power broke significantly better. Similar results have been reported using different stone models.[53] These reports suggest that the application of low energy shock waves condition stones for improved fragmentation by high-energy pulses. Thus, stone comminution is dependent not only on the total energy delivered but on how the energy is delivered.

Perhaps one of the most interesting and significant new findings to come from animal studies in ESWL is the observation that treatment of the kidney with a preconditioning dose of low-voltage/low-power shock waves protects the kidney from damage when a subsequent clinical dose of higher-energy shock waves is delivered. In one study reported by Willis and colleagues, groups of pigs received either 100 or 500 shock waves at 12 kV followed by 2,000 shock waves at 24 kV delivered to the same pole.[54] The animals were then sacrificed and processed for quantitative determination of the volume of the hemorrhagic lesion in the renal parenchyma secondary to shock wave exposure. When compared to animals that received only high-energy shock waves, the low-kV pretreatment animals had a significantly reduced lesion size (less than 0.5% vs 6.1% for all of the 24-kV animals) (Figure 39-5). This means that pretreatment with a small number of shock waves (less than 100) at low power may protect the kidney from subsequent injury. The protective effect noted is thought to be mediated by vasoconstriction, as shown by lack of protection when vasoconstriction was blocked by infusion of dopamine prior to shock wave administration.

Based on the new findings reviewed above, attention to the technique of ESWL may have as much, or more, to do with the success of lithotripsy treatment as the choice of lithotriptor technology.

CURRENT LITHOTRIPTORS

Information regarding 38 extracorporeal shock wave lithotriptors marketed by 14 manufacturers is presented in Tables 39-1 to 39-4.

COMPARISON OF LITHOTRIPTORS

Although there was a surge in publications in the urologic literature in the 1980s addressing lithotripsy, few (if any) appropriately designed comparative trials of lithotriptors have been published to date. Although there is a general consensus that re-treatment rates are an appropriate indicator of lithotriptor effectiveness, the lack of clinical agreement about the appropriate outcome of lithotripsy (ie, stone-free vs residual fragments of various sizes) hampers appropriate comparison of various lithotriptors.[55] Only a tiny fraction of the literature published to date on ESWL results contains data stratified sufficiently to allow any comparative analysis.[56] Currently, extracorporeal shock wave lithotriptors have been designated as Class 2 devices by the FDA, meaning that very little animal or clinical data is required for approval. Therefore, few studies with meaningful data on the newer lithotripsy systems are available.

A substantial amount of well-stratified data have been published for two early lithotriptors: the unmodified Dornier HM-3 and the Siemens Lithostar.[57–63] The overall results from these publications have been compared by integrating stone free rates stratified by size into a regression model (Figure 39-6). The stone-free rates achieved with the unmodified HM-3 lithotriptor are significantly better than those with the less powerful Lithostar. To date, despite the proliferation of lithotriptors and the variety of solutions devised for stone targeting and shock wave delivery, no lithotripsy system has convincingly equaled or surpassed the results produced by the unmodified Dornier HM-3 device. That the most effective lithotriptor was invented first is a remarkable achievement for Dornier, particularly considering the incomplete understanding of the physics of shock wave lithotripsy at the time of the introduction of this device. Despite claims to the contrary, the unmodified HM-3 remains the gold standard for ESWL.

A small amount of partially stratified data has been published for a variety of different lithotriptors other than the Dornier HM-3 and the Siemens Lithostar (Table 39-6). In general, the less powerful lithotriptors with smaller focal points result in lower stone-free rates and/or higher re-treatment rates.

There have been several comparative trials of lithotriptors reported, most of which involve studies of second-generation machines (the modified HM-3 is considered a second-generation device). Tan and colleagues from Singapore reported that a small non-randomized series comparing the unmodified Dornier HM-3 with an EDAP LT.01 and a Sonolith 2000 (an earlier version of the Sonolith 4000) in which they found 3-month stone free rates of 66%, 67%, and 58%, respectively, with re-treatment rates of 4%, 42%, and 26%, respectively.[64] This is the only direct (albeit non-randomized) trial reported in the literature noting equivalent stone-free rates between the unmodi-

Table 39-4   Imaging/Financial Aspects

Electromagnetic Lithotriptors

Company	Machine	ECG Gaiting	Endourology Capability	Stone Localization	Portability	Purchase Price	Service Contract	Upgrade Possibility	Upgrade Cost
Siemens Medical Systems	Lithostar Multiline	Yes	Yes	X-ray, Inline US	No	$650K	N/A	N/A	N/A
Siemens Medical Systems	Lithostar Modularis (with Cplus)	Yes	Yes	X-ray, Co-axial US	Yes	$495K	N/A	N/A	N/A
Siemens Medical Systems	Lithostar Modularis Vario (with Cplus)	Yes	Yes	X-ray, Co-axial US	Yes	$455K	N/A	N/A	NA
Karl Storz Lithotripsy	Modulith SL20	No	Yes	Inline X-ray and US	No	$295K used‡	$69K	No	N/A
Karl Storz Lithotripsy	Modulith SLX-MX	No	Yes	Inline X-ray and US	No	$695K	$80K	No	N/A
Karl Storz Lithotripsy	Modulith SLX-T	No	Yes	Inline X-ray and US	Yes	$525K	$62.5K	No	N/A
Karl Storz Lithotripsy	Modulith- SLX-F2	No	Yes	Inline X-ray and US	N/A	N/A	N/A	N/A	N/A
Dornier MedTech	Compact Delta	Optional	Yes	X-ray, US optional, isocentric fluoro	Yes	$430k	$52k	US, laser printer, DICOM 3	$50K, $10K, $25K
Dornier MedTech	Compact Sigma	Optional	Yes	X-ray, US optional, mobile C-arm	Yes	$440k	$52k	US, laser printer, DICOM 3	$50K, $10K, $7K
Dornier MedTech	DoLi S 140	Optional	Yes	X-ray, US optional, isocentric fluoro	No	$695K	$73.5k	US, laser printer, DICOM 3	$50K, $10K, $25K
Dornier MedTech	DoLi S 220	Optional	Yes	X-ray, US optional, isocentric fluoro	No	$695K	$73.5k	US, laser printer, DICOM 3	$50K, $10K, $25K
Dornier MedTech	DoLi S, 220-XP*	Optional	Yes	X-ray, US optional, isocentric fluoro	No	N/A	N/A	US, laser printer, DICOM 3	N/A
Dornier MedTech	DoLi S, 220-XXP*	Optional	Yes	X-ray, US optional, isocentric fluoro	No	N/A	N/A	US, laser printer, DICOM 3	N/A
Dornier MedTech	DoLi S II, 140	Optional	Yes	X-ray, US optional, isocentric fluoro	No	$695K	$73.5k	US, DICOM 3 included	$50k
Dornier MedTech	DoLi S II, 220	Optional	Yes	X-ray, US optional, isocentric fluoro	No	$695K	$73.5k	US, DICOM 3 included	$50k
Dornier MedTech	DoLi S II, 220-XP*	Optional	Yes	X-ray, US optional, isocentric fluoro	No	N/A	N/A	US, DICOM 3 included	N/A
Dornier MedTech	DoLi S II, 220-XXP*	Optional	Yes	X-ray, US optional, isocentric fluoro	No	N/A	N/A	US, DICOM 3 included	N/A

Piezoelectric Lithotriptors

Company	Machine	ECG Gaiting	Endourology Capability	Stone Localization	Portability	Purchase Price	Service Contract	Upgrade Possibility	Upgrade Cost
Wolf	P3000‡	No	Yes	Coaxial x-ray & US	Yes	N/A	N/A	Yes	N/A

*Not sold in the U.S.
†disassembly/reinstallation - add 53K.
‡disassembly/reinstallation - add 20K.

fied Dornier HM-3 and second-generation lithotriptors. In another study comparing first- and second-generation lithotriptors, Sofras et al[65] found that the unmodified Dornier HM-3 achieves significantly higher stone-free rates overall than the EDAP LT.01. For small renal calculi (less than 1 cm), however, the machines achieved equivalent stone-free rates. More recently, a matched pairs analysis was reported by Portis and colleagues comparing the unmodified Dornier HM-3 and the Healthtronics Lithotron.[66] Only patients with solitary renal calculi were included in this study. The stone-free rate for the unmodified Dornier HM-3 was 79% vs. 58% for the Lithotron. Factors trending for failure of lithotripsy with the Lithotron included stone location in the lower pole, stone size > 10 mm, or a body mass index > 30.

Rassweiler and colleagues compared a modified (low-pressure generator and smaller F2) Dornier HM-3 and a Wolf Piezolith 2200 (predecessor of the Wolf P3000).[67] Stone-free rates were not reported, but stone fragmentation rates were equivalent. Re-treatment was necessary in 12% of the modified Dornier HM-3 patients and in 54%

of the Wolf Piezolith cases. Additionally, this was one of the first reports to note problems with ultrasound stone location/localization of ureteral calculi, with 58% of the cases of ureteral stone

failing ultrasound stone localization. The current version of the Wolf Piezoelectric lithotriptor, the Piezolith 3000, was studied in a matched pairs analysis and compared to the previous generation

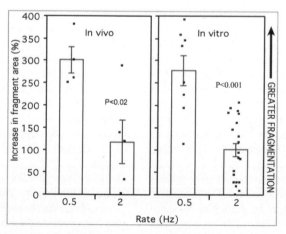

Figure 39-4 Stone fragmentation efficiency in vitro and in vivo (in a porcine model) is inversely proportional to shock wave administration rate.

Table 39-5	Clinical Evidence for a Shock Wave Rate		
	60 SW/min (N = 78)	120 SW/min (N = 71)	*p*-Value
Overall success rate (3 months)	82%	63%	−.039
Success stone area ≥ 100 mm	88%	31%	−0.002
Ancillary procedure rate within 3 months	10%	32%	−0.003
Number of SWs administered	2480	2884	< 0.001
Treatment time (minutes)	41	24	< 0.001

device, the Piezolith 2300. The stone-free rate at 3 months for the Piezolith 3000 and Piezolith 2300 were 36% and 48%, respectively.[68] The Piezolith 3000 produced significantly more discomfort than the Piezolith 2300. Sebold and colleagues also compared a modified Dornier HM-3 with another Dornier device, the MPL9000, once again noting problems with ultrasonography for stone localization and for assessing stone fragmentation.[69] Fragmentation results were lower for the MPL9000 than for the modified HM-3 (73% vs 95%). Additionally, 18% of patients initially starting therapy with the MPL9000 eventually crossed over to complete their lithotripsy therapy in the modified HM-3 device, whereas only 3% of patients being treated with the modified HM-3 subsequently crossed over to the MPL9000. The Dornier HM-4 lithotriptor with a low-pressure generator was compared with the Dornier MPL9000 in a study by Tailly.[70] He noted that the MPL9000 appeared to be a more efficient machine with a slightly lower re-treatment rate than the modified Dornier HM-4 (1.11 vs 1.17) but also noted prob-

lems with ultrasound stone localization for ureteral stones and in obese patients. It should be noted that Dornier no longer produces electrohydraulic lithotriptors (HM-3, HM-4, MPL9000, MFL5000) although these devices are often available on secondary markets.

Bierkens and colleagues examined five second-generation lithotriptors (Siemens Lithostar, Dornier HM-4, Wolf Piezolith 2300, Direx Tripter X-1, and Breakstone) in a multicenter trial involv-

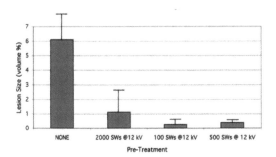

Figure 39-5 Lesion size produced by high-energy shock waves after pre-treatment with low-energy shock waves

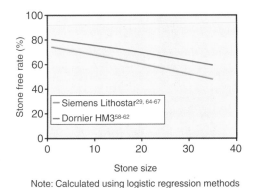

Note: Calculated using logistic regression methods

Figure 39-6 Comparison of stone-free rates for the Lithostar and the unmodified Dornier HM-3 lithotriptors.

Table 39-6	Lithotriptor Comparisons: Clinical Results					
Lithotriptor & Series	No. of Patients	% Retreatment*	Avg. Stone Size Data Stratified (yes/no)	3-month Stone-Free Rates (Data Stratified by Size, Yes/No)		% Auxiliary Procedures Pre-Post-ESWL†
Medstone STS						
Thomas and Cass‡[81]	81	11§	Y	72	Y	3
Lipson et al[82]	50	8§	Y	46§	N	8
Cass[83]	1212	5.4	Y	68	Y	2.7
Modultih SL20						
Liston et al[84]	500	31.8	Y	78§	N	2.8
Sonolith 2000						
Benson et al[85]	142	10.4§	N	59§	N	NA
Martin et al[86]	245	14.2	N	62	N	27
Tan et al[64]	104	54	N	42	N	9
MFL 5000						
Lingeman et al[26]	46	NA	Y	64§	Y	NA
Ehreth et al[87]	658	NA	Y	66	Y	13
Direx Tripter X-1						
Frang et al[88]	169	11§	Y	NA		14.1
Servadio et al[89]	37	7.5§	N	54§	N	8.1
Bierkens et al[71]	355	8.5	N	46	N	40
EDAP LT.01						
Tan et al[90]	180	40§	N	64	Y	15
Vallancien et al[91]	374	11.2§	Y	NA		7
Kiely et al[92]	872	NA	Y	64§	Y	15
Miller et al[93]	461	24	Y	51	N	NA
Kim et al[94]	398	30	N	NA		4.5
MPL 9000						
Talati et al[95]	464	42.1	Y	72.8§	N	9.1
Oshima et al[97]	336	16.4	N	64.9	N	
Wolf 2200						
Bowsher et al[97]	367	62	N	53§‖	N	11,4
Marberger et al[98]	426	35	N	81	Y	26
Wolf 2300						
Cope et al[99]	220	43#	N	82#	N	28
Bierkens et al[71]	438	34	N	50	N	29
Fegan et al[100]	100	21	Y	43**	N	NA

NA = not available.

*All stones overall average retreatment.

†Auxiliary procedures, both pre- and post-ESWL, include (1) stone manipulation (push back), (2) stent placement, (3) ureteroscopy, (4) PCNL, (5) nephrostomy drainage, (6) ureterolithotomy, pyelolithotomy, and open surgery.

‡All patients morbidly obese (mean wt 326 lb; range 300–402 lb).

§Ureteral and large stones included.

‖2-month follow-up.

#Stones < 2cm.

**2-week follow-up.

ing over 1800 patients.[71] The overall stone-free rate was only 45% with a re-treatment rate of 20%. There were no significant differences in the stone-free rates among the various machines. But re-treatment rates were higher with the Wolf Piezolith than the other lithotriptors.

A prospective randomized trial comparing the modified Dornier HM-3 with the Dornier MFL5000 was reported by Chan and colleagues.[72] Although more patients with large stones were treated with the HM-3, overall stone-free results were equivalent with the two machines. The authors noted that the stone-free rates achieved in the lower pole for the modified HM-3 were significantly better than those achieved by the MFL5000 (80% vs 56%, $p = .05$). Since these two lithotriptors used the same ellipsoid and shock wave generator, this study supports the observation that a water bath is the ideal mechanism for transmitting shock wave energy into the body (see Chapter 38, "Shock Wave Lithotripsy Devices and Techniques"). Chan and colleagues also noted that treatment times were significantly shorter with the unmodified HM-3 device and concluded that the MFL5000 lithotriptor offered no significant clinical advantage over the modified HM-3 in terms of lithotriptor efficiency, although the multifunctional table did provide more versatility for stone treatment (ie, ureteral stones).

Treatment outcomes with newer Dornier electromagnetic lithotriptors have yielded mixed results in the United States. Johnson and colleagues reported a stone-free rate of 73% in 176 patients treated with a Doli-S device.[73] Mean stone size, however, was only 9.7 mm. Sorenson and colleagues reported poor results with a Doli-U50 lithotriptor in patients whose lithotripsy sessions were performed with sedation. When patients were completely anesthetized, treatment outcomes improved significantly, presumably due to decreased motion and improved stone targeting.[74] At 3 months, the stone-free rates for those treated under intravenous sedation and those treated under general anesthesia were 55% vs 87%, respectively ($p < .001$). Similar findings were reported by Eichel and colleagues.[75] Matin and colleagues reported a comparison of results with the MFL5000 (mean stone size 103 mm^2: stone-free rate 77%) to the Storz Modulith SLX (mean stone size 71 mm^2: stone-free rate 67%).[76]

ESWL is now recognized as a form of trauma similar to renal contusions, occasionally resulting in adverse clinical sequela, a topic reviewed in detail later (see Chapter 41, "Complications"). Fortunately, while further study is necessary regarding the bioeffects of ESWL, early concerns about a major adverse long-term effect of lithotripsy have not materialized.[77,78] Nonetheless, there are certain patients such as the pediatric patient, patients with preexisting renal disease, or elderly or hypertensive patients who may be at increased risk of adverse effects with ESWL (see Chapter 41, "Complications"). The amount of lithotripsy that can be safely tolerated by a kidney during a single session of ESWL remains to be determined for current lithotriptors.

FUTURE CONSIDERATIONS

Until very recently, lithotriptors have not changed fundamentally since the introduction of the first lithotriptor, the HM-1, in 1980 in that all lithotripsy devices use basically the same shock wave. With recent developments in increasing our understanding of shock wave physics (see Chapter 38, "The Physics of Shock Wave Lithotripsy"), some novel approaches to ESWL are being explored. These new approaches to lithotripsy attempt to make use of the realization that cavitation plays a fundamental role in both stone comminution and tissue injury during ESWL (a principle unknown at the time of the introduction of Dornier lithotriptors in the early 1980s). To date, two fundamentally different approaches to manipulating cavitation events during ESWL have been investigated. Zhong and Preminger from Duke University have modified the ellipsoidal reflector of a Dornier HM-3 lithotriptor with an insert that produces a secondary shock pulse arriving at F2 just after the normal lithotriptor pulse (Figure 39-7).[79] The purpose of this weak secondary shock wave is to limit the size of the cavitation bubbles produced by the lithotriptor pulse. This group has presented evidence that the intravascular growth of cavitation bubbles in the small capillaries and venules during lithotripsy may be the explanation for rupture of these blood vessels and subsequent hemorrhage. By controlling the size of bubble growth, they have been able to document (Figure 39-8) that there is reduced trauma to tissue in a porcine

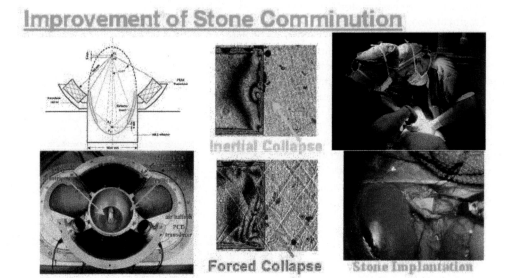

Figure 39-7 Manipulations of cavitation during ESWL. *A*, An HM-3 ellipsoid has been modified by adding an insert and a piezoelectric array, modifications which limit the diameter of bubble growth and enhance bubble collapse (middle panel). *B*, Artificial stones are implanted surgically for in vivo testing (see Figure 39-8).

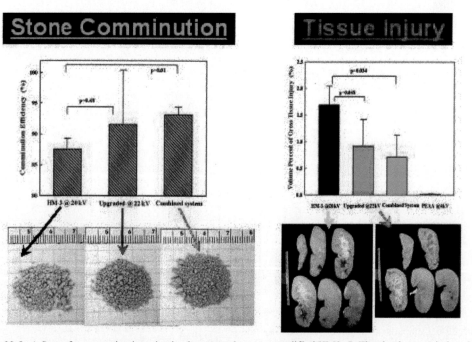

Figure 39-8 *A*, Stone fragmentation is maintained compared to an unmodified HM3. *B*, The shock–wave-induced renal parenchymal lesion is less with the modified than with the unmodified system.

model. Cavitation bubble collapse is believed to be an important contributor to stone comminution. Therefore, a third pulse generated by a piezoelectric array mounted on top of the ellipsoid is timed to coincide with cavitation bubble collapse, enhancing this aspect of stone fragmentation. At least in an experimental system, Preminger and Zhong's approach seems to maintain the highly desirable stone comminution properties of the HM-3 lithotriptor while at the same time minimizing adverse tissue effects. This innovative approach to lithotriptor shock wave design has yet to be subjected to clinical trials.

A different approach to the manipulation of cavitation is to use two lithotriptor pulses, released simultaneously, both focused at the same F2. This concept of dual pulse lithotripsy was first reported by Bailey and colleagues utilizing a coaxial system (Figure 39-9), a configuration that causes the lithotriptor pulse to be additive within F2 where the pulses arrive simultaneously.[80] Outside of F2, however, the asynchronous interaction of the pulses inhibits cavitation. In Bailey and colleagues' in vitro studies, stone fragmentation was enhanced and tissue effects minimized.

Two dual-source ESWL devices are currently in clinical use. In these devices (Direx Duet and FMD Twinheads), the shock wave sources are not coaxial as in the work by Bailey and colleagues but are rather offset at 70 to 90 degrees. The significance and effect of these new lithotriptor designs on stone comminution and tissue effects have not been well studied. Evan and colleagues in a porcine study of tissue effects of the Direx Duet found significantly greater tissue effects than with the Dornier HM-3 under similar study conditions. Although the potential advantages of dual source lithotriptors is intriguing from a physics standpoint, these devices require significantly more testing before they are put in widespread clinical use.

DISCLOSURE

Dr. Lingeman has no current or previous financial relationships with any lithotriptor manufacturer. This work was supported in part by NIH grant PO1 DK43881.

REFERENCES

1. Chaussy C, Brendel W, Schmidt E. Extracorporeal induced destruction of kidney stones by shock waves. Lancet 1980;2:1265.
2. Chaussy C, Schmidt E, Jocham D, et al. First clinical experience with extracorporeal induced destruction of kidney stones by shock waves. J Urol 1982;127:417.
3. Chaussy C, Schmidt E, Jocham D, et al. Extracorporeal shock wave lithotripsy (ESWL) for treatment of urolithiasis. Urology 1984;23:59.
4. Lingeman JE, Woods JR, Toth PD, et al. Role of lithotripsy and its side effects. J Urol 1989;141:793.
5. Prevention and treatment of kidney stones. NIH Consensus Conference Statement. JAMA 1988;260:978.
6. Power EJ. The adoption and use of extracorporeal shock wave lithotripsy by hospitals in the United States. Int J Technol Assess Health Care 1987;3:397.
7. Bloom BS, Hillman AL, Schwartz JS. Abruptly changing patterns of diffusion and use of extracorporeal shock wave renal lithotripsy. Am J Kidney Dis 1991;18:103.
8. Wilbert DM, Reichenberger H, Noske E, et al. New general shock wave lithotripsy. J Urol 1987;138:563.
9. Marberger M, Turk C, Steinkogler I. Painless piezoelectric extracorporeal lithotripsy. J Urol 1988;139:695.
10. Marberger M, Turk C, Steinkogler I. Painless piezoelectric extracorporeal lithotripsy by ultrashort waves with the EDAP LT.01 device. J Urol 1988;139:689.
11. Chaussy C. Extracorporeal shock wave lithotripsy: new aspects in the treatment of kidney stone disease. Munich, Germany: Karger; 1982.
12. Cathignol D, Mestas JL, Gomez F, et al. Influence of water conductivity on the efficiency and the reproducibility of electrohydraulic shock wave generation. Ultrasound Med Biol 1991;17:819.
13. Kuwahara M, Kambe K, Kurosu S, et al. Clinical application of extracorporeal shock wave lithotripsy using microexplosions. J Urol 1987;137:837.
14. Mayo ME, Chapman WH, Ansell JS. Progress report on the Lasertripter. J Urol 1986;135:160A.
15. Coleman AJ, Saunders JE. Comparison of extracorporeal shock wave lithotriptors. In: Coptcoat MJ, Miller RA, Wickham JEA, editors. Lithotripsy II. London: BDI Publishing; 1987.
16. Schoenfield LJ, Maglinte DDT, Berci G, et al. The effect of Ursodiol on the efficacy and safety of extracorporeal shock wave lithotripsy of gallstones. The Dornier National Billiary Lithotripsy Study. N Engl J Med 1990; 323:1239.
17. Maglinte DDT, Graffis R, Jordan L, et al. Extracorporeal lithotripsy of gallbladder stones: a pessimistic view. Radiology 1991;178:29.
18. United States Food and Drug Administration. FDA Medical Devices Advisory Committee Meeting, October 19–20, 1989. Rockville, MD: FDA.
19. Preminger GP. Sonographic piezoelectric lithotripsy: more bang for your buck. J Endourol 1989;3:321.
20. Mobley TB, Myers DA, Grine WB, et al. Low energy lithotripsy with Lithostar: treatment results with 19,962 renal and ureteral calculi. J Urol 1993;149:1419.
21. Cass AS. Extracorporeal shock wave lithotripsy for stones in middle third of ureter (overlying pelvic bone). Urology 1994;43:182.
22. Jenkins AD, Gillenwater JY. Extracorporeal shock wave lithotripsy in the prone position: treatment of stones in the distal ureter or anomalous kidney. J Urol 1988; 139:911.
23. Wiatrak M, Ohl DA, Sonda LP. Stryker frame gantry modification of extracorporeal shock wave lithotripsy to circumvent positioning problems. J Urol 1991;146:283.
24. Eisenberger F, Rassweiler J. ESWL: technique in evolution. In: Lingeman JE, Smith LH, Woods JR, et al, editors. Urinary calculi: ESWL, endourology, and medical therapy. Philadelphia: Lea & Febiger; 1989. p. 415–32.
25. Scott JW, Lingeman JE, Newman DM. Successful extracorporeal shock wave lithotripsy of stones in ectopic pelvic kidney. J Endourol 1987;1:201.
26. Lingeman JE, Newman DM, Siegel YI, et al. Shock wave lithotripsy with the Dornier MFL 5000 lithotriptor using an external fixed rate signal. J Urol 1995;154:951.
27. Kataoka H. Cardiac dysrhythmias related to extracorporeal shock wave lithotripsy using a piezoelectric lithotriptor in patients with kidney stones. J Urol 1995;153:1390.
28. Newman DM, Lingeman JE, Mosbaugh PM, et al. Extracorporeal shock wave lithotripsy using only intravenous analgesia with an unmodified Dornier HM3 lithotriptor. In: Lingeman JE, Newman DM, editors. Shock wave lithotripsy 2: urinary and biliary lithotripsy. New York: Plenum Press; 1989. p. 411–5.
29. Tiselius HG. Treatment of large staghorn stones and ureteral stones without anesthesia. Scand J Urol Nephrol 1989; 122 Suppl:25.
30. Tiselius HG. Anesthesia-free in situ extracorporeal shock wave lithotripsy of ureteral stones. J Urol 1991;146:8.
31. Pettersson B, Tiselius HG, Andersson A, et al. Evaluation of extracorporeal shock wave lithotripsy without anesthesia using a Dornier HM3 lithotriptor without technical modifications. J Urol 1989;142:1189.
32. Rassweiler J, Westhauser A, Bub P, et al. Second generation lithotriptors: a comparative study. J Endourol 1988;2:193.
33. Richards MJ, Skues MA, Jarvis AP, et al. Total IV anesthesia with propofol and alfentanil: dose requirements for propofol and the effect of premedication with clonidine. Br J Anaesth 1990;65:157.
34. Reves Gl, Glass PSA, Lubarsky DA. Nonbarbiturate intravenous anesthetics. In: Miller RD, editor. Anesthesia. New York: Churchill Livingstone; 1994. p. 247–90.
35. Bailey PL, Stanley TH. Intravenous opioid anesthetics. In: Miller RD, editor. Anesthesia. New York: Churchill Livingstone; 1994. p. 291–388.
36. Monk TG, Bouré B, White PF, et al. Comparison of intravenous sedative-analgesic techniques for outpatient immersion lithotripsy. Anesth Analg 1991;72:616.
37. Arroyo CS, Michaels EK, Laurito CE, et al. Use of continuous infusion alfentanil for spark-gap lithotripsy. J Endourol 1995;9:41.
38. Fair WR, Malhotra V. Extracorporeal shock wave lithotripsy (ESWL) using local infiltration anesthesia. J Urol 1986; 135:181A.
39. Tiselius HG. The treatment of large staghorn stones and ureteral stones without anesthesia. Scand J Urol Nephrol 1989;122 Suppl:25.
40. Bierkens AF, Maes RM, Hendrikx JM, et al. The use of local anesthesia in second generation extracorporeal shock wave lithotripsy: eutectic mixture of local anesthetics. J Urol 1991;146:287.
41. Dretler SP. Stone fragility: a new therapeutic distinction. J Urol 1998;139:1124.
42. Klee LW, Brito CG, Lingeman JE. The clinical implications of brushite calculi. J Urol 1991;145:715.
43. Willis LR, Evan AP, Connors BA, et al. Shock wave lithotripsy: dose related effects on renal structure, hemodynamics, and tubular function. J Endourol 2005;19:90.
44. Delius M, Enders G, Xuan ZIR, et al. Biological effects of shock waves: kidney damage by shock waves in dogs: dose dependence. Ultrasound Med Biol 1988;14:117.
45. Wiksell H, Kinn AC. Implications of cavitation phenomena

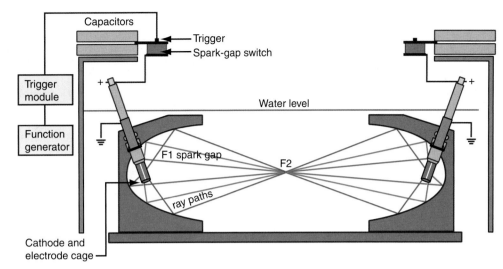

Figure 39-9 Dual pulse lithotripsy. Coaxially aligned electrohydraulic shock wave sources with a common F2. If released simultaneously, the shock wave pulses are additive in F2, but to either side of F2, they minimize cavitation.

for shot intervals in extracorporeal shock wave lithotripsy. Br J Urol 1995;75:720.

46. Greenstein A, Matzkin H. Does the rate of extracorporeal shock wave delivery affect stone fragmentation? Urology 1999;54:430.

47. Lifshitz DA, Williams JC Jr, Lingeman JE, et al. Efficiency of SWL stone fragmentation in vitro is improved by slowing the SW delivery rate [Abstract 1501]. J Urol 2000;163 Suppl:338.

48. Weir MJ, Tariq N, Honey RJ. Shockwave frequency affects fragmentation in a kidney stone model. J Endourol 2000;14:547.

49. Paterson RF, Lifshitz DA, Lingeman JE, et al. Stone fragmentation during shock wave lithotripsy is improved by slowing the shock wave rate: studies with a new animal model. J Urol 2002;168:2211.

50. Pace KT, Harju M, Dyer S, et al. Shock wave lithotripsy at 60 or 120 shocks per minute: a randomized, single-blinded trial [Abstract]. J Urol 2003;169 Suppl:487.

51. Zeman RK, Davros WJ, Garra BS, et al. Cavitation effects during lithotripsy. Part I. Results of an in vitro experiment. Radiology 1990;177:157.

52. McAteer JA, Baird T, Williams J, et al. Voltage-stepping during SWL influences stone breakage independent of total energy delivered: in vitro studies with model stones. J Urol 2003;169 Suppl:487.

53. Zhou Y, Cocks FH, Preminger GM, et al. The effect of treatment strategy on stone comminution efficiency in shock wave lithotripsy. J Urol 2004;172:349.

54. Willis LR, Evan AP, Connors BA, et al. Same-pole application of low- and high-energy shock waves protects kidney from SWL-induced tissue injury [Abstract]. J Urol 2004; 171 Suppl:294.

55. Tolley DA, Wallace DMA, Tiptaft RC. First UK consensus conference on lithotriptor terminology—1989. Br J Urol 1991;67:9.

56. Lingeman JE, Siegel YI, Steele B, et al. Management of lower pole nephrolithiasis: a critical analysis. J Urol 1994;151:663.

57. Drach GW, Dretler SP, Fair WR, et al. Report of the United States Cooperative Study of extracorporeal shock wave lithotripsy. J Urol 1986;135:1127.

58. Graff J, Diederichs W, Schulze H. Long-term follow up in 1003 extracorporeal shock wave lithotripsy patients. J Urol 1988;140:479.

59. Politis G, Griffith DP. ESWL: stone-free efficacy based upon stone size and location. World J Urol 1987;5:255.

60. El-Damanhoury H, Schärfe T, Ruth J, et al. Extracorporeal shock wave lithotripsy of urinary calculi: experience in treatment of 3,278 patients using the Siemens Lithostar and Lithostar Plus. J Urol 1991;145:484.

61. Psihramis KE, Jewett MAS, Bombardier C, et al. Lithostar extracorporeal shock wave lithotripsy: the first 1000 patients. J Urol 1992;147:1006.

62. Netto NR, Lemos GC, Claro JFA. Extracorporeal shock wave lithotripsy with Lithostar lithotriptor. Urology 1992;40:430.

63. Clayman RV, McClennan BL, Garvin TJ, et al. Lithostar: an electromagnetic acoustic shock wave unit for extracorporeal lithotripsy. J Endourol 1989;3:307.

64. Tan EC, Tung KH, Foo KT. Comparative studies of extracorporeal shock wave lithotripsy by Dornier HM3, EDAP LT01 and Sonolith 2000 devices. J Urol 1991;146:294.

65. Sofras F, Karayannis A, Kastriotis J, et al. Extracorporeal shock-wave lithotripsy or extracorporeal piezoelectric lithotripsy? Comparison of costs and results. Br J Urol 1991;68:15.

66. Portis AJ, Yan Y, Pattaras JG, et al. Matched pair analysis of shock wave lithotripsy effectiveness for comparison of lithotriptors. J Urol 2003;169:58.

67. Rassweiler J, Gumpinger R, Mayer R, et al. Extracorporeal piezoelectric lithotripsy using the Wolf lithotriptor versus low energy lithotripsy with the modified Dornier HM3: a cooperative study. World J Urol 1987;5:218.

68. Ng CF, McLornan L, Thompson TJ, et al. Comparison of 2 generations of piezoelectric lithotriptors using matched pair analysis. J Urol 2004;172:1887.

69. Siebold J, Rassweiler J, Schmidt A, et al. Advanced technology in extracorporeal shock wave lithotripsy: the Dornier MPL 90000 versus the upgraded Dornier HM3. J Endourol 1988;2:173.

70. Tailly GG. Experience with the Dornier HM3 and MPL 9000 lithotriptors in urinary stone treatment. J Urol 1990;144: 622.

71. Bierkens AF, Hendrikx AJM, DeKort WJW, et al. Efficacy of second generation lithotriptors: a multicenter comparative study of 2206 extracorporeal shock wave lithotripsy treatments with the Siemens Lithostar, Dornier HM4, Wolf Piezolith 2300, Direx Tripter X1, and Breakstone lithotriptors. J Urol 1992;148:1052.

72. Chan SL, Stothers L, Rowley A, et al. A prospective trial comparing the efficacy and complications of the modified Dornier HM3 and MFL 5000 lithotriptors for solitary renal calculi. J Urol 1995;153:1794.

73. Johnson DB, Lowry PS, Schluckebier JA, et al. University of Wisconsin experience using the Doli S lithotriptor. Urology 2003;62:410.

74. Sorensen C, Chandhoke P, Moore M, et al. Comparison of intravenous sedation versus general anesthesia on the efficacy of the Doli 50 lithotriptor. J Urol 2002;168:35.

75. Eichel L, Batzold P, Erturk E. Operator experience and adequate anesthesia improve treatment outcome with third generation lithotriptors. J Endourol 2001;15:671.

76. Matin SF, Yost A, Streem SB. Extracorporeal shockwave lithotripsy: a comparative study of electrohydraulic and electromagnetic units. J Urol 2001;166:2053.

77. Lingeman JE, Kulb TB, Newman DM, et al. Hypertension following ESWL. J Urol 1987;137:142A.

78. William CM, Kaude JV, Newman RC, et al. Extracorporeal shock wave lithotripsy: long-term complications. AJR 1998;150:311

79. Zhou Y, Cocks FH, Preminger GM, et al. Innovations in shock wave lithotripsy technology: updates in experimental studies. J Urol 2004;172:1892.

80. Bailey MR. Control of acoustic cavitation with application of lithotripsy. PhD dissertation. Austin, TX: University of Texas at Austin; 1997.

81. Thomas R, Cass AS. Extracorporeal shock wave lithotripsy in morbidly obese patients. J Urol 1993;150:30.

82. Lipson SB, Ross LS, Sonda LP. Initial clinical trials with a tubeless lithotriptor. J Urol 1990;143:10.

83. Cass AS. Equivalence of mobile and fixed lithotriptors for upper tract stones. J Urol 1991;146:290.

84. Liston TG, Montgomery BSI, Bultitude MJ, et al. Extracorporeal shock wave lithotripsy with the Storz Modulith SL20: the first 500 patients. Br J Urol 1992;69:465.

85. Benson RC, Bagley DH, Kandel LB, et al. Results of the United States trial of the Technomed Sonolith 2000 lithotriptor: preliminary report. J Endourol 1988;2:189.

86. Martin X, Kata J, Daware M, et al. Second generation extracorporeal lithotriptor using ultrasound stone localization. J Litho Stone Dis 1989;1:133.

87. Ehreth JT, Drach GW, Arnett ML, et al. Extracorporeal shock wave lithotripsy: multicenter study of kidney and upper ureter versus middle and lower ureter treatments. J Urol 1994;152:1379.

88. Frang D, Hamvas A, Kámán J, et al. Experience with the Direx Tripter X1 shock wave lithotriptor. Int Urol Nephrol 1992;24:481.

89. Servadio C, Livne P, Winkler H. Extracorporeal shock wave lithotripsy using a new, compact and portable unit. J Urol 1988;139:685.

90. Tan EC, Tung KH, Foo KT. Piezoelectric extracorporeal shock wave lithotripsy by EDAP LT01: the Singapore experience. J Litho Stone Dis 1990;2:19.

91. Vallancien G, Aviles J, Munoz R, et al. Piezoelectric extracorporeal lithotripsy by ultrashort waves with the EDAP LT01 device. J Urol 1988;139:689.

92. Kiely EA, Madigan D, Ryan PC, et al. Ultrasonic imaging for extracorporeal shockwave lithotripsy: analysis of factors in successful treatment. Br J Urol 1990;67:127.

93. Miller HC, Collins LA, Turbow AM, et al. EDAP LT01 lithotripsy group experience in the United States. J Urol 1989;142:1412.

94. Kim SC, Moon YT, Kim KD. Extracorporeal shock wave lithotripsy monotherapy: experience with piezoelectric second generation lithotriptor in 642 patients. J Urol 1989;142:674.

95. Talati J, Shah T, Memon A, et al. Extracorporeal shock wave lithotripsy for urinary tract stones using MPL 9000 spark gap technology and ultrasound monitoring. J Urol 1991;146:1482.

96. Oshima S, Yoshinari O, Masafumi S, et al. Extracorporeal shock wave lithotripsy using the Dornier MPL 9000 lithotriptor. Urol Int 1994;52:17.

97. Bowsher WG, Carter S, Phillip T, et al. Clinical experience using the Wolf Piezolith device at two British stone centers. J Urol 1988;139:695.

98. Marberger M, Türk C, Steinkogler I. Painless extracorporeal lithotripsy. J Urol 1988;139:695.

99. Cope RM, Middleton RG, Smith JA. A 2-year experience with the Wolf piezoelectric lithotriptor: impact of repeat treatment on results and complications. J Urol 1991;145: 1141.

100. Fegan J, Camp LA, Wilson WT, et al. Treatment philosophy and retreatment rates following piezoelectric lithotripsy. J Urol 1993;149:12.

40

Helical CT Imaging and SWL Treatment of Renal and Ureteral Calculi

Ryan F. Paterson, MD

Samuel C. Kim, MD

James C. William Jr, PhD

The basic techniques for treatment of urinary calculi with shock wave lithotripsy (SWL) have changed little since the introduction of SWL in the 1980s. As detailed in the previous chapter, dry-head lithotriptors have largely replaced the original HM3 lithotriptor (which immersed the patient in a water bath for treatment), but the mechanics of the treatment process are quite similar to that described in the earliest days of SWL. In itself, this is not negative, because SWL continues to be an excellent mode of treatment for urinary stones and is clearly the best choice for many patients. But there is considerable evidence to suggest that the overall effectiveness of SWL has been declining over the years.[1] This is an unfortunate trend, and the explanation for this apparent reduction in SWL effectiveness is not obvious. Part of the problem could be related to machine design, as there is evidence that no lithotriptor has been able to match the effectiveness of the Dornier HM3,[2,3] but the mechanistic reasons for this lessening of effectiveness are not clear. That is, no one can point to any one aspect of machine design and identify this as universally problematic in breaking stones. Moreover, some of the decline in SWL effectiveness could be due to changes in practice, such as an increase in the use of a rapid shock wave (SW) rate.

This concern about a decline in the effectiveness of SWL is heightened by our present awareness of the damaging effects of lithotriptor SWs on the kidney. All surgical procedures are accompanied by risk to the patient, but SWL was considered by many—for most of its first two decades of use—to be completely benign. It was thought that SWs passed through human tissue without effect, bringing their great energy to bear only upon hard objects, like stones. We know now that lithotriptor SWs cause damage to kidneys,[4] which includes the breaking of blood vessels and which leaves scarring.[5] SWL treatment may induce new-onset hypertension in some patients,[6,7] and may even lead to the production of difficult-to-treat (brushite) stones.[8] Additional concern has been raised about the documented tendency of tight-focus, high-pressure lithotriptors to cause perirenal hematomas,[9–12] and indeed, as of this writing, the major lithotriptor manufacturers are already addressing this specific problem in their newer designs.[13]

Thus, one must think of SWL treatments as carrying significant risk to the patient, though this risk may still be considerably less than more invasive procedures. If SWL were always successful, this risk might be of small significance; but SWL is not always successful. Thus, possible injury to the patient with SWL could be lessened if the success rate of SWL could be improved, or if the success of SWL on a particular patient case could be predicted, so that SWL could be used (or bypassed) as appropriate.

This chapter describes recent work that helps the urologist use helical computed tomography (CT) to learn about the stones identified in the patient, such that more rational decisions can be made about mode of treatment. It also describes recent work on SW rate—the effect of the frequency of firing of a lithotriptor on stone comminution—as an example of how SWL effectiveness may be improved, even using presently available technology. Finally, the chapter summarizes advisable practice in treating urinary calculi using SWL, based on the anatomic location of the stones.

HELICAL CT IMAGING OF URINARY STONES

The role of helical CT in the evaluation of stone patients has greatly expanded in the last decade, and helical CT has become the radiologic tool of choice in the assessment and treatment of patients with urinary tract calculi, with up to a 95% sensitivity, 98% specificity, and 97% accuracy for the detection of urolithiasis.[14–27]

As a single imaging study, non-contrast CT can provide important stone details, such as the shape, number, size, and location of urinary calculi. But the full potential of helical CT to differentiate between stone types, and thus predict SWL outcome for a patient, has yet to be realized. As early as 1988, Dretler pointed to radiologic methods for predicting the SW fragility of a patient's stone, so that the physician could plan treatment accordingly,[28] and he and his colleagues have continued to develop this concept over the years since.[29–33] Renewed interest in this topic is demonstrated by recent reports describing work to identify the composition of stones

using CT, and work that relates SWL success to stone attenuation values as measured on CT.[34–41] The rationale for all of these studies is that, if patient CT images of urinary stones could provide information about stone fragility or stone composition, then stones that are resistant to SWL could be identified at diagnosis.

It is important to understand that studies seeking to explore imaging of urinary stones can stumble over two potential errors inherent in CT: (1) they can fail to appreciate the interaction of stone size with CT axial resolution (ie, beam collimation, or slice width), and/or (2) they can fail to exploit the ability of CT to resolve structural detail inside stones. Thus, some studies have sought to link SWL success to stone composition when really they are "measuring" stone size with CT attenuation (as described below in Error 1). Other studies have not fully utilized existing technology to gain information about the stones that is relevant to their clinical aims (as described below in Error 2). It is worthwhile elaborating on these errors, as they are due primarily to the rapid advancement of CT technology.

CT ERROR 1: FAILURE TO APPRECIATE THE INTERACTION BETWEEN STONE SIZE AND APPARENT CT ATTENUATION VALUES Helical CT is performed using an x-ray source and a detector head that rotates around the patient while obtaining images; these images are processed by a computer and representative slices of the patient's body are produced. At the edges of any object, the CT will average the x-ray attenuation of the object with that of the surroundings—a phenomenon known as "volume averaging." In the case of urinary stones, the surrounding urine and tissue has a much lower x-ray attenuation value (measured in Hounsfield units) as compared to the stone. In a larger stone, this error is small, but as stone size decreases to about twice the slice width of the scan, the attenuation measured on the CT image will be significantly lower than the true value for the stone, and for smaller stones, this error is further magnified. Typical CT scans performed for suspected urolithiasis are performed using a "slice width" (or collimation) of 3 to 5 mm. With this resolution of CT scan, the Hounsfield unit measurements for stones less than 1 cm in diameter will be lower than the true value for CT attenuation of the stones.[42] Moreover, this error becomes increasingly large as the size of the stone decreases,[43] as shown in Figure 40-1. As clinically significant urinary stones range in size from about 4 mm to about 2 cm, the potential for volume averaging to artifactually affect CT attenuation values is quite real, especially at the smaller stone sizes.

With slice widths commonly used clinically, the CT attenuation of the stone will be a product of both the stone composition and the stone size. Some studies have considered attenuation values to be affected only by the stone composition, and thus the researchers possibly misinterpreted their data. Others have recognized the effect of stone size on apparent CT attenuation and sought to correct for this by using smaller collimation.[44–47] In the long run, the size artifact for stone attenuation values will disappear with increasing scanner resolution and decreasing collimation, as scanner technology continues to improve.[48–51] Urologists wishing to use CT imaging to determine stone composition must be cognizant of the size of the stone and the collimation of the CT scan. Further, most stones are heterogeneous,[52] and properly restricted regions-of-interest (ROI) areas must be drawn for accurate determination of stone composition using attenuation values, as described under CT Error 2.

CT ERROR 2: UNDERUTILIZATION OF PRESENTLY AVAILABLE CT TECHNOLOGY TO VIEW STONE HETEROGENEITY Helical CT is capable of showing much more information on urinary calculi than merely their size and location, but this capability may not be widely recognized. When viewing helical CT scans for the diagnosis of nephrolithiasis, images are almost always viewed using 'abdominal windows' (350W/40L) that allow distinction of different soft tissues within the abdominal cavity. Viewing windows are not part of the settings used to collect the patient images, but rather are the settings with which the images are viewed afterward. Using abdominal windows, one can distinguish abdominal organs, and identify foreign bodies and tumors. With abdominal windows, calculi are visualized as bright white, enabling them to be easily recognized against the darker surrounding tissue. Abdominal windows, although useful for the identification of urinary stones, obscure the internal structure within the stone.[41,53,54]

Stone structure, however, *can* be seen in helical CT images. This is evident even from older CT studies, which describe inhomogeneities observed inside many stones.[55,56] If one uses bone windows (2500W/480L) when viewing CT images, then internal structure is visible within the stones.[53] Visualizing compositional heterogeneity in stones can also allow one to use ROIs to measure the attenuation values of just part of a stone.[41] The value of this approach is illustrated in Figure 40-2, which compares determinations of CT attenuation values for four types of stone in two studies that used different protocols for drawing the ROIs on the CT image. For the data shown in the blue bars, stones were viewed using traditional abdominal windows, with ROIs drawn within the stone image.[57] Note that the blue bars show considerable overlap in CT attenuation measured for stones of different composition, as has been observed in many studies.[15,35,44,46,47,55,56,58–60] For the data shown in the red bars, stones were viewed using bone windows, with ROIs drawn in regions of relative homogeneity (which had additionally been confirmed to be of a single mineral using laboratory micro-CT).[41] Note that the CT attenuation values of ROIs obtained using bone windows (red bars) do not overlap between types of stone mineral.

The differences between the two sets of data shown in Figure 40-2 can be explained by the inclusion of more than one material in the portion of the stones measured using ROIs drawn with traditional viewing windows. For example, calcium phosphate—represented here by apatite—has the highest x-ray attenuation of any stone mineral, but apatite stones may have other mineral or organic material mixed within them. These lower attenuation regions cannot be seen when CT images are viewed using abdominal windows, and could easily be included in the ROI, thereby lowering the average attenuation value measured in apatite stones. In the case of struvite or uric acid stones, regions of calcium mineral are often present, thus accounting for the higher attenuation values seen in some of these stones.

All of these examples of viewing stone structure and attenuation values come from in vitro studies. But reports are beginning to emerge that describe the use of CT to examine stones in patients,[39,61] and it appears that a great deal of stone structure can be seen inside the patient. Again, more work remains to be done in this area, but the field shows promise that patient CT scans may be used both for diagnosis and for planning treatment as more data on stone composition and structure and their relationship to stone comminution in SWL are reported. It seems likely that these data will be part of the larger set of patient data—including patient age, stone location, and renal anatomy—that have been described as important for predicting SWL outcome.[62–64] Specifics of several of these criteria are covered further below.

THE EFFECT OF SW RATE ON THE EFFICIENCY OF SWL

The original clinical lithotriptor, the Dornier HM-3, was synchronized with the patient's electrocardiogram (ECG), and thus, the SW rate did not exceed 60 to 80 SW/minute in most cases. Experience with second and third generation machines, however, revealed that un-gating the SW treatment from the patient's ECG (nonsynchronous SWL) resulted in few cardiac abnormalities,[65–67] and today, administration of SWL at rates of 100 to 120 SW/minute is commonplace. No study has conclusively demonstrated that treating stones at fast rates provides a significant advantage in SWL success, and multiple in vitro studies have reported that slowing the SW rate improves stone fragmentation.[68–72] In a recent animal study, Paterson and colleagues implanted matched, artificial stones percutaneously into the lower pole calyx of both kidneys of pigs, exposed the stones to SWL at either 30 or 120 SW/minute, and recovered the stone fragments to quantitate breakage.[73,74] They found significantly better stone comminution with the slower rate of SW delivery.

A recent randomized, single-blind clinical study of SW rate has been reported that corroborates the results of in vitro and in vivo animal studies.[75] The group randomized 218 patients with radiopaque renal calculi > 5 mm diameter (stratified by location and size) to SWL at either 60 or 120 SW/minute. Success was defined as stone-free, asymptomatic fragments < 5 mm, or sand (fragments ≤ 2 mm). An increased success rate was demonstrated in the 60 SW/min group at 3 months of follow-up. As seen in Table 40-1, the rate effect was particularly evident for larger stones. A reduction in the need for follow-up

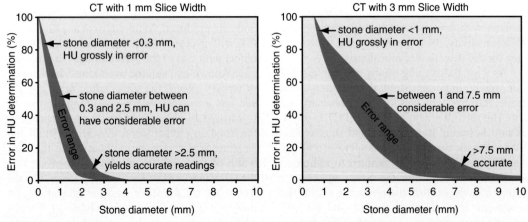

Figure 40-1 Predicted error in measuring computed tomography (CT) attenuation value in a spherical stone of given diameter, at two helical CT slice widths (or beam collimation widths). Vertical range of error is due to location of CT slice on stone, with least error when slice falls across center of stone. Adapted from Hu H, Fox SH,[42] as described in Williams JC Jr, et al.[43]

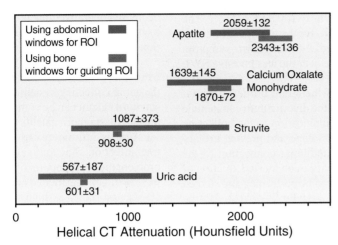

Figure 40-2 Computed tomography (CT) attenuation values measured in four types of stone, using high-resolution (1 mm or thinner) helical CT. Ranges are illustrated by bars, with mean values ± standard deviations shown next to bars. Data for blue bars are stones that were not examined for heterogeneity of content with abdominal viewing windows. Data from red bars use bone windows to draw restricted regions of interest (ROIs). Adapted from Saw KC, et al,[57] and Zarse CA, et al.[41]

treatment in the first 3 months was also reported, reflecting improved stone fragmentation during SWL sessions at a slower rate. There was no additional morbidity to SWL at a slower rate with a reduction in the total number of SWs delivered and an average increase in treatment time of only 17 minutes.

The optimal rate for SW delivery has not yet been determined, so guidelines for SW delivery currently cannot be given. Indeed, the optimal SW delivery rate may be machine-specific and also may be affected by the size and location of stones. The rate effect may differ depending on the energy source (electrohydraulic vs. electromagnetic) of the lithotriptor used and further work is warranted. Nevertheless, in vitro studies, animal experiments, and initial clinical data are remarkably consistent: SW administration at fast rates can reduce the effectiveness of SWL. The urologist should consider slowing down SW rate in lithotripsy to improve stone breakage and clinical outcome.

SWL OF RENAL CALCULI

Stone burden is often the most important factor to consider when selecting the appropriate treatment for an individual with a renal stone.[76] Regardless of the measure used to characterize a patient's stone burden—such as stone area, size and number, maximal stone diameter, aggregate stone diameter, or even stone volume—the greater the amount of stone material to be treated, the harder a stone-free status is to achieve.[77–83]

Stone composition also has a significant effect on treatment outcome. Stones differ in fragility by composition, and although in vitro studies have shown tremendous variability in fragility for any given mineral type,[30,84–86] it is widely appreciated that calcium oxalate monohydrate, brushite, and cystine stones can be very difficult to break using SWL.[87,88] Cystine and calcium oxalate monohydrate stones also produce larger size fragments that may be less apt to clear from the urinary tract.[87,89]

SWL is most effective on stones located in the renal pelvis. In early work by Chaussy's group, a 90% success rate was reported for calculi in the renal pelvis.[90,91] Success rate for SWL of renal stones is less if located in the lower pole calyx, in caliceal diverticula, and when the collecting system is filled with stone material (staghorn). In addition, unusual renal conformations, such as ectopic and horseshoe kidneys, complicate SWL treatment of stones. These cases will be considered later in this section.

Treatment of renal stones that are not staghorn calculi is commonly stratified by size. Mean stone-free rates of SWL for solitary renal calculi 10 mm or less, 11 to 20 mm, and greater than 20 mm are 80% (range 63 to 90%), 64% (range 50 to 83%) and 54% (range 33 to 81%).[82,83,92,93] SWL of stones less than 10 mm is generally successful regardless of stone location or composition as indicated previously by a mean stone-free rate of approximately 80%.

The majority of urinary calculi between 10 and 20 mm are still managed initially with SWL.[94] For stones this size, composition and location influence the results of SWL and should be taken into consideration when choosing treatment options.

Lower pole caliceal stones and harder stones such as brushite or cystine may result in less successful outcomes when treated with SWL.

When reviewing the NIH Consensus Conference recommendation for stones > 20 mm, the percutaneous approach was favored as the initial treatment option.[95] Lingeman and colleagues demonstrated that multiple treatments increased from 10 to 33% for SWL of stones from 10 to 20 mm and 20 to 30 mm respectively.[96] In addition, the stone-free rate for SWL was only 34%, while percutaneous nephrostolithotomy (PNL) resulted in a 90% stone-free rate.[97] Psihramis and colleagues treated 94 renal stones > 20 mm with SWL and only rendered 33% stone free.[92] Higher re-treatment rates after SWL for stones > 20 mm have led the NIH Consensus Panel to recommend the more invasive percutaneous approach for calculi of this size. SWL, however, is the mainstay of treatment for calculi 20 mm or less in size.

LOWER POLE CALICEAL CALCULI SWL, when compared to PNL, results in significantly less clearance of lower pole caliceal stones.[93,99] When comparing treatment of lower pole renal calculi greater than 10 mm with PNL and SWL, the Lower Pole Study Group showed much improved stone-free rates of 91% for PNL when compared to 21% for SWL.[99] Retreatment rates (16% vs. 9%) and ancillary treatment rates (14% vs. 2%) were also higher for SWL. When the same study group prospectively examined ureteroscopy versus SWL for lower-pole stones 10 mm or less, the stone-free rate of 50% for ureteroscopy was comparable to 35% for SWL ($p = .92$).[100] For lower-pole calculi 11 to 25 mm in size, PNL achieved better stone-free rates than ureteroscopy (74% vs. 40%).[100]

Several groups have suggested that the variable anatomy of the lower pole calyx can explain why SWL is successful in some cases with stones in this region and not in others. Sabnis and colleagues initially concluded that an infundibular angle (IA) > 90°, an infundibular width (IW) < 4 mm, and a complex caliceal pattern, individually affected stone clearance after SWL.[101] Every patient with all three of the aforementioned characteristics had residual stones in follow-up. Elbahnasy and colleagues popularized the concept that an IA less than 70°, an IW ≤ 5 mm, or an infundibular length (IL) > 3 cm can limit lower pole clearance after SWL.[102] If all three of the criteria were met, the chance of being stone-free after the SWL was less than 50%.

Table 40-1 Summary of Results Showing Increased Success Rate			
	60 SW/min ($n = 110$)	120 SW/min ($n = 108$)	p value
Overall success rate (3 mo)	75%	61%	$p = .027$
Success rate on stones ≥ 100 mm²	71%	32%	$p = .002$
SWL retreatment (≤ 3 mo)	18%	32%	$p = .018$
Number of SWs administered	2423	2906	$P < .001$
Treatment time (min)	41	24	$P < .001$

SW = shock wave
Adapted from Pace KT et al.[75]

Following these studies, others have also assessed the ability of differing aspects of lower-pole anatomy to predict clearance of fragments after SWL, but only one study was prospective in design. This report, from the Lower Pole Study Group, concluded that lower-pole calyx anatomy has no correlation with stone-free status after SWL. One of the difficulties of assessing the effect of lower-pole anatomy is the fact that there are numerous factors to evaluate (eg, width, angle, length, and height), and there is little agreement on how each of these factors should be measured. For example, a study by Knoll and colleagues demonstrated that the value found for IA is dependent on the method of measurement used and interobserver variability is high.[103] Thus, although it seems intuitive that some aspect of the anatomy of the lower calyx should correlate with success in SWL for stones in this region, no method for predicting SWL success in the lower pole calyx is widely accepted, and the difficulty of standardizing measurements in the various studies makes interpreting them problematic. A comprehensive prospective study examining all of the reported factors using carefully standardized measurements may help elucidate what factors indeed may be significant.

CALCULI IN CALICEAL DIVERTICULA   Minimally invasive treatment options for stones in caliceal diverticula include SWL, ureteroscopy, laparoscopy, and PNL. SWL is initially an attractive option but it provides relief of pain in only 36 to 70% of patients, and stone-free rates are low, ranging from 4 to 20%.[104,105] Only one study series has reported stone-free rates as high as 58% for SWL monotherapy.[106]

Ureteroscopic approaches for the treatment of caliceal diverticular stones are possible with actively deflectable flexible endoscopes. Stone-free rates for ureteroscopy range from only 19 to 58%, and diverticular obliteration is as low as 18%.[107,108] These success rates are low, reflecting several major disadvantages of ureteroscopy with stones in a diverticulum. First, the normal retrograde approach for ureteroscopy is most appropriate only for upper and interpolar regions because lower pole diverticula can be difficult to enter.[107,108] Second, larger stone burdens in a diverticulum are not efficiently treated with ureteroscopy alone and may require a combined retrograde ureteroscopic and antegrade percutaneous procedure.[109] Finally, the operative times for retrograde techniques are longer, lasting from 1.25 to 4 hours.[107,109]

Laparoscopy for stones in caliceal diverticula is also an option, but the indications for such an approach are limited. It has been suggested that anterior diverticula, especially if there is a thin layer of parenchyma overlying a large anterior cavity, are well suited for laparoscopy.[110,111] Operative times are long (up to 2.5 hours) even in expert hands.[110]

Percutaneous treatment of caliceal diverticular calculi achieves excellent stone-free rates (87.5 to 100%) and successful obliteration of the diverticular cavity (76 to 100%).[104,112–114] The superior results of PNL for the treatment of diverticular stones coupled with long-term symptom relief[113] justify its use over the less invasive SWL or ureteroscopy.

After removal of the stone burden percutaneously, treatment of the diverticulum can include creating a large communication to the collecting system to promote drainage and prevent urinary stasis. When the infundibular connection to the renal collecting system can be located, dilation of this communication can be performed and stented with a nephrostomy tube.[104,113,114] If the infundibular connection cannot be found or traversed with a wire, some authors have created a neoinfundibulum to the calix or the renal pelvis.[115,116] Both techniques require the placement of a nephrostomy tube for many days to ensure that the channel will remain open. Neoinfundibulotomy cannot be performed when the diverticulum is located anteriorly and normal parenchyma is traversed and dilated in order to form a connection to the collecting system.[116]

Another treatment strategy is to fulgurate the diverticular lining and allow the cavity to collapse. Monga and colleagues performed a direct percutaneous puncture in conjunction with fulguration of the diverticular lining without any attempt at cannulating the infundibular communication.[117] As all patients had a ureteral catheter placed initially, the catheter was exchanged for a ureteral stent that was left in place for 2 to 4 weeks. The success rate for complete diverticular ablation in this cohort was 100%, and all patients were symptom-free at 38 months follow-up.

At our institution, we use a modified minimally invasive technique in which percutaneous access is placed via an infracostal approach directly into the diverticular cavity without the aid of a retrograde catheter.[118] The lining of the cavity is fulgurated using a rollerball electrode, and the infundibular communication is neither cannulated nor identified. In our cohort, 95% were discharged tubeless on postoperative day one. On follow-up intravenous pyelography, all diverticula decreased in size, and 87.5% had complete resolution.

Our approach offers a number of advantages over the standard PNL for diverticular calculi. As a retrograde ureteral catheter is not placed, there is no risk of ureteral obstruction and no need for an indwelling stent. The mean operative time of 58.5 minutes is short when compared to other percutaneous approaches (Table 40-2). The decreased operative time is due to the elimination of both the retrograde catheter and the localization/dilation of the infundibular communication.

STAGHORN CALCULI   Staghorn stones can fill the entire collecting system of a kidney. Although staghorn calculi can be composed of any mineral, the classic staghorn calculus is composed of struvite and is intimately associated with urinary tract infection. Staghorn calculi tend to be highly problematic, with reports of chronic renal failure in 36% of patients treated conservatively[119] and a 10-year mortality as high as 28% for untreated staghorn stone patients.[120]

The strategy for management of staghorn stones is threefold. First, complete removal of the stone must be achieved, as only then can the kidney be sterilized of urea-splitting organisms. Second, any metabolic abnormalities need to be identified and addressed. Finally, any anatomic abnormalities contributing to stasis should be addressed.

Staghorn calculi have long been treated by open surgery, and anatrophic nephrolithotomy as described by Smith and Boyce was an effective technique in removing any size renal calculi.[121] The stone-free rate for open stone surgery as reported by Griffith and colleagues was about 85%, with a 30% recurrence rate over the following 6 months.[122,123] When comparing PNL combined with SWL to anatrophic nephrolithotomy, Kahnoski and associates reported a similar stone-free rate of 85%; convalescence and hospital stay for PNL were shorter, and blood loss was reduced.[124] Further, when PNL was compared to SWL monotherapy for staghorn stones, the stone-free rate for PNL (with or without SWL) was 84%, but for SWL alone was only 51%.[125] Almost a third (30.5%) of the SWL group also required auxiliary procedures, whereas only 3.4% of the PNL group needed additional interventions. SWL monotherapy was successful in a subgroup of patients with 500 mm^2 or smaller stone burden in non-dilated collecting systems, a subgroup encompassing only 3% of all staghorn patients.[125] Meretyk and colleagues compared staghorn patients undergoing SWL to those treated with PNL (with or without SWL) and reported stone-free rates of 22% and 74%, respectively.[125a] The significantly higher complication rate and number of ancillary procedures for the SWL group also led these authors to conclude that PNL was superior to SWL alone for staghorn treatment. The reliance of SWL on residual fragments being cleared by patients with

Table 40-2 Comparison of Percutaneous Approaches to Caliceal Diverticular Calculi							
Patient Cohort	Age (yr)	Operative Time (min)	Stone Area (mm^2)	Hospital Stay (d)	Stone-Free Rate	Percent Diverticulum Obliterated	Ureteral Catheter?	Neoinfundibulotomy or Dilation of Diverticular Neck?
Kim et al. 2005[118]	42.6	56.1	135.3	1.0	85.7%	87.5%	No	No
Monga et al. 2000[117]	33.4	162.0	10.2*	2.3	100%	100%	Yes	No
Auge et al. 2002[115]	37.4	N/A	140.4	2.8	80%	63%	Yes	Yes
Shalhav et al. 1998[113]	36	171	N/A	4.1	93%	76%	Yes	Yes

*Maximum stone diameter only reported.

infected stones can prevent sterilization of the urinary tract and increase the risk of recurrent stones and infection. A combination of multiple endourologic techniques described by Streem and coworkers as "sandwich" therapy (which consisted of primary percutaneous debulking, followed by SWL of the residual stone burden, then secondary PNL) gave results similar to PNL and open surgery when treatments were separated by 1 to 2 days.[126,127] Currently, the management of staghorn calculi is primarily a percutaneous approach—which with the liberal use of flexible nephroscopy and judicious use of additional accesses make essentially all calyces accessible. The use of flexible equipment and the holmium laser allows for the fragmentation and removal of previously difficult-to-access stones, and decreases or eliminates the additional use of SWL.[128]

The American Urological Association (AUA) Nephrolithiasis Committee published recommendations for the treatment of staghorn calculi based on a meta-analysis of peer-reviewed published articles.[95] As a guideline, PNL should be the recommended primary therapy for large-volume staghorn calculi, and SWL and PNL are equal options for small-volume staghorn stones when the renal collecting system is not hydronephrotic. Open surgery may be appropriate in unusual circumstances where a staghorn stone may not be removed with a reasonable number of PNL and/or SWL treatments. Nephrectomy is an option for a poorly functioning kidney containing a staghorn stone.

ECTOPIC KIDNEY   An ectopic kidney can be found in a pelvic, iliac, abdominal, thoracic, or crossed position. Pelvic kidneys are the most common, and although the retroperitoneal location of these can create positioning problems during SWL, calculi in pelvic kidneys should be approached initially with SWL when feasible.[129,130] If the stone is shielded by the bony pelvis, a prone position may be used. When SWL fails or if a larger stone burden is present, alternative approaches should be selected. Flexible ureteroscopy is an excellent treatment modality if the stone burden can be managed with this approach. Laparoscopic-assisted PNL or even laparoscopic pyelolithotomy can offer alternative techniques for this challenging problem.

HORSESHOE KIDNEY   Horseshoe kidney is the most common congenital renal anomaly complicated by urinary stones.[131] The ureteropelvic junction can be abnormal due to the high insertion of the ureter, resulting in impaired drainage. Although SWL can be used to treat stones in horseshoe kidneys, localization of the stones can be difficult because the calyces are anomalous. The prone position[132] or a "blast path" technique using high pressures produced some distance from F2[133] have been used successfully. The stone-free rate for SWL in horseshoe kidneys varies from 28 to 78%.[134–137] Renal calculi in horseshoe kidneys require a higher number of SWs and a greater number of re-treatments (30% vs. 10%) compared to similarly sized stones in

normal kidneys.[138,139,140,141] SWL can achieve satisfactory results in properly selected patients (stones < 1.5 cm and normal urinary drainage). Larger stones or kidneys with compromised urinary drainage should undergo PNL as primary surgical therapy. The results for PNL are better than that for SWL, with a mean stone-free rate of 84% (range 74 to 100%).[134,142,143]

SWL OF PROXIMAL URETERAL CALCULI   Common treatment options for proximal ureteral stones include SWL in situ, SWL after "push back," SWL after stent insertion, PNL, ureteroscopy, and open stone surgery. The AUA Ureteral Stones Clinical Guidelines Panel,[144] which performed a meta-analysis of 320 suitable articles on ureteral calculi published from 1966 to 1996, reported that for stones < 1 cm, the stone-free rates for SWL and ureteroscopy were 84% and 56%, respectively, and for stones > 1 cm, 72% and 44%, respectively. A surprisingly high risk of significant complications following SWL and ureteroscopy (4% and 11%, respectively) was also reported. Due to the greater efficacy and lower morbidity of SWL, the panel suggested that SWL should be the primary approach for stones less than 1 cm in the proximal ureter. In contrast, for stones larger than 1 cm in diameter, SWL, PNL, and ureteroscopy are all acceptable choices.[144] The results of a study by Park and colleagues provided additional support of using a size cut-off of 1 cm when choosing treatment for ureteral calculi.[145] The authors compared the results of in situ SWL and ureteroscopy for ureteral stones (proximal and distal) and showed that while the efficacy of SWL dropped significantly for stones larger than 1 cm (84% vs. 42%), the stone-free rate with ureteroscopic manipulation was not affected by stone size (89% vs. 86%).

Since publication of the AUA guidelines in 1997, great progress has been made in the development of small flexible ureteroscopes, with a significant improvement in results for proximal ureteral stones from ureteroscopic lithotripsy and stone-free rates equivalent or superior to the results achieved by SWL, with minimal complications.[146–150] Despite these excellent results from ureteroscopic lithotripsy, many urologists choose SWL as the initial approach for typical proximal ureteral stones < 1 cm and use flexible ureteroscopy for stones presumed to be hard (eg brushite, cystine), stones that fail SWL, distal obstruction, impacted calculi, and patients who are obese or who have bleeding diatheses.[148] In addition, several recent reports suggest that ureteroscopy should be the primary approach for impacted ureteral stones. Mugiya and colleagues demonstrated the efficiency of small flexible ureteroscopes (6.9 French to 7.5F) combined with holmium laser lithotripsy in 104 patients with impacted ureteral stones, including 83 stones in the proximal ureter.[151] Of the 104 stones, 100 (96.2%) were completely fragmented by a single endoscopic procedure. At one month, the stone-free rate was 100%, and there were no significant complications. Similarly,

Yagisawa and colleagues reported a stone-free rate at 1 month of 91% for patients treated with ureteroscopic pneumatic lithotripsy.[152]

Years of clinical experience with SWL have revealed that treatment of stones impacted in the ureter is often unsuccessful.[153–157] The experience of urologists during the early years of SWL resulted in multiple studies reporting improved stone fragmentation when the stone was first relocated into the pelvicaliceal system ("push-back" technique).[158–165] Push-back is rarely performed today, and most proximal ureteral stones are treated with either SWL in situ or with more invasive endourologic procedures.[147–148] A study by Gross and colleagues, however, provided additional support for stone manipulation in the treatment of proximal ureteral stones.[165] The authors compared 105 patients who underwent pre-SWL stone manipulation to 93 patients receiving SWL in situ. Stone manipulation into the renal pelvis was successful in 91.4% of the patients with a reduction in the mean number of SWL treatments in the push-back group versus in situ SWL (1.4 and 2.1 treatments, respectively).

The reduced effectiveness of SWL in the treatment of impacted ureteral calculi may be due to the lack of a fluid interspace between the stone and the wall of the urinary tract, possibly leading to decreased cavitation.[155,157] Mueller and colleagues reported a novel in vitro model system for SWL research consisting of a Penrose drain filled with water (or gelatin) connected to a spring balance with a balloon catheter inside the drain to allow for pressure recordings.[158] The authors treated standardized artificial stones (primarily composed of calcium hydrogen phosphate) with SWL at 16 kV and reported that increasing tension on the Penrose drain (mimicking increased impaction of the stone) resulted in impaired stone comminution. Interestingly, impaired fragmentation was also seen when the stone was surrounded by gelatin, a medium that prevented stone fragments from easily falling away from the stone edge. The authors postulated that close apposition between the stone and the ureteral wall resulted in a shell of small fragments on the outside of the stone that reflected or absorbed the incoming SWs, resulting in reduced effectiveness of subsequent SWs. Along similar lines, Parr and colleagues also investigated the local environment of a stone treated with SWL in vitro.[155] The authors treated a total of 24 artificial stones of the same composition (9 mm by 9 mm cylinders) placed within a latex tube and surrounded by saline (a medium known to support cavitation). Four treatment groups (free, confined, confined and impacted, and impacted and stented) were then subjected to piezoelectric SWL (400 SW; 70 SW/minute; power level 3). The authors reported significantly improved stone fragmentation when stones were "free" compared to the other three groups with no significant difference in stone fragmentation between the confined, confined and impacted, and impacted and stented groups. Interestingly, the only erosions seen in the confined and impacted group were on the end faces of the stone cylinders that were exposed to saline. In addition, in the impacted and stented group, erosions were seen on the end faces of the cylinders, and along the course of the stent, further supporting the argument that a fluid interspace surrounding a stone is important for stone comminution.

An in vivo model has recently been developed to investigate SWL of proximal ureteral stones.[166] Artificial stones were inserted into the pig kidney by a reverse-percutaneous protocol,[73] and then guided into the proximal ureter. The stones were treated using a Dornier HM-3 (0.5 Hz; 20 kV; 400 SW); the urinary tract was harvested en bloc, and the stone fragments were collected and quantitated. Breakage of stones implanted in the proximal ureter was significantly less than that for stones located in the renal calyx treated with the same dose of SWs (134% vs. 327%, $p < .001$). Interestingly, when the artificial stones were located at the ureteropelvic junction, the portion of the stone protruding into the renal pelvis (with a large amount of fluid surrounding the stone) had significant fragmentation in contrast to the portion of the stone impacted in the ureter.

Some authors have reported improved fragmentation of ureteral stones with SWL when saline is injected via catheter below the stone in an attempt to create a larger stone-fluid interspace.[154] But attempts to bypass impacted stones with a ureteral stent or catheter prior to SWL—which creates an increased fluid interspace surrounding the stone—do not result in a significant improvement in stone fragmentation over in situ SWL.[144,155,167–170] Although the placement of a ureteral catheter appears promising, Ryan and colleagues reported that ureteral stents can impair ureteral motility, potentially delaying transit time of ureteral stones or fragments.[171] Ureteral stenting is not routinely performed prior to SWL of ureteral stones, however, stenting is appropriate for the relief of obstruction/infection, injection of radiographic contrast for stones difficult to visualize, and in the setting of a solitary obstructed kidney.

A variety of medications have been evaluated to reduce ureteral colic post-SWL.[172,173,176,177] Recently, the use of a combination of nifedipine and deflazacort after SWL of ureteral calculi has been reported to show promise.[177] This prospective randomized study of 80 patients reported a 75% complete fragment expulsion in the treated group compared to 50% in the placebo group ($p = .02$) with a reduced need for diclofenac sodium post-SWL. Over a decade ago, indomethacin was reported to show promise[176,178] but little interest has been evident recently. Ketorolac tromethamine, another nonsteroidal anti-inflammatory has been commonly employed for pain control emergently for acute ureteral colic[179,180] as well as pain relief post-ureteroscopy and post-PNL. But little has been written about its use after SWL,[181] and many urologists are reluctant to use this medication owing to potential risks of delayed renal bleeding. Other medications, such as glucagons,[172] have

shown no significant benefit in ameliorating post-SWL ureteral colic.

A few additional points on the treatment of proximal ureteral calculi deserve mention. First, the stone-free rate for the re-treatment of ureteral calculi with SWL after an initial failed SWL session is not significantly better than that of a single session alone, such that proceeding with ureteroscopic lithotripsy after failed SWL is justified.[182] Second, multiple clinical series of patients treated with SWL have reported that patients with proximal ureteral stones are often treated at a higher energy level and with an increased number of SWs than comparable stones located within the kidney without a corresponding improvement in stone-free status.[159,161,162,167,174,175,183–187] As tissue injury is known to increase with higher energy levels and shock wave number,[5,188,189] the treatment of ureteral stones at higher energy settings and at increased total number of SWs appears to pose an unnecessary risk to the patient without offsetting benefit.

Finally, the reader should be aware that a significant percentage of proximal ureteral stones will pass spontaneously: 29 to 98% of patients pass proximal ureteral stones < 5 mm, and 10 to 53% with stones 5 to 10 mm in diameter.[144,190] Thus, appropriate analgesic treatment is recommended as a first step for patients with proximal ureteral stones < 1 cm in diameter. Inability to pass the stone in several weeks or recurrent symptoms may prompt surgical intervention.

DISTAL URETERAL STONES

As noted in the proximal ureter, many distal ureteral stones can pass spontaneously. Stones presenting in the distal ureter are even more likely to pass than those in the proximal ureter: 71 to 98% of stones < 5 mm and 25 to 53% of stones with a diameter of 5 to 10 mm have been reported to pass spontaneously from the distal ureter.[144,190] Conservative management is certainly a reasonable option for patients willing to attempt to pass smaller distal ureteral stones, with intervention only when unable to pass the stone or when symptoms recur.

Multiple surgical options are available for the treatment of distal ureteral calculi, including SWL with or without a stent, ureteroscopy with stone basket extraction or intracorporeal lithotripsy, and open and laparoscopic stone surgery. Direction for treatment is again provided by the meta-analysis published by the AUA Ureteral Stones Guideline Panel, which reported that for stones < 1 cm, the median stone-free rates for SWL and ureteroscopy were 85% and 89%, respectively, and for stones > 1 cm, 74% and 73%, respectively. Given these equivalent efficacies, SWL and ureteroscopy were both considered acceptable treatment options.[144] Again, these results must be balanced against the significant improvements in ureteroscopes and intracorporeal lithotriptors that have allowed the stone-free rates for the treatment of distal ureteral stones—both stones < 1 cm and > 1 cm—to

approach 100%. But SWL has many advantages, including short procedure times, a reduced need for anesthesia, short recovery times, avoidance of ureteral dilation or postoperative ureteral stenting, and minimal complications.[191]

Multiple limitations of SWL in the treatment of distal ureteral calculi exist. These include a higher re-treatment rate and a longer time required to achieve a stone-free state with SWL than that seen with ureteroscopic management. In addition, smaller stones may be obscured and poorly visible, and successful treatment may still require ancillary steps in the form of placement of a ureteral catheter to allow for adequate targeting, or intravenous administration of radiographic contrast to target the bottom of the contrast column (and presumed stone location). Occasionally, stones will be located in the ureter overlying the bony pelvis or pre-sacral area with the pelvic bones blocking the path of the SWs. In this setting, prone positioning has been shown to eliminate the interference of the pelvis, and allow successful lithotripsy.[192–194]

Concern has been raised as to the safety of SWL for the treatment of stones in the distal ureter in women of childbearing age, but these concerns have not been substantiated clinically. Vieweg and colleagues assessed 10 childless women who attempted pregnancy after SWL of distal ureteral stones and reported 7 normal children from 6 of the subjects.[195] Three miscarriages occurred, all more than one-year after SWL. Similarly, Erturk and colleagues treated 10 women of childbearing age with distal ureteral stones with the Dornier HM-3, using an average of 2,079 SW at 21 kV, and reported 11 pregnancies, no spontaneous abortions and no malformations.[196] Appropriate counseling of the female patient as to the risk versus benefits of SWL compared with ureteroscopy should be undertaken, but untoward effects of SWL have not been demonstrated to date in women of childbearing age. In contrast, SWL is contraindicated for all pregnant women. Animal studies on the effects of SWs on fetal development show mixed results, but conventional wisdom argues that SWL not be performed during pregnancy. Ureteroscopy is the frontline surgical therapy for the treatment of urolithiasis in pregnancy.[197,198]

Significant progress has been made in ureteroscopic lithotripsy since the AUA guidelines were published, with improved efficiency and lower morbidity using the latest generation ureteroscopes and intracorporeal lithotrites (especially the holmium laser). At the same time, second- and third-generation SWL devices, which have smaller focal points and higher positive peak pressures, have become popular.[81] A review of the current literature reported the mean stone-free rates for SWL versus ureteroscopy were 81% (50 to 99%) and 94% (86 to 100%), respectively, while re-treatment rates were 27% (7 to 50%) and 8% (1 to 20%), respectively.[145,199–204] Two recent randomized studies intended to help clarify the optimal treatment of distal ureteral calculi have reported conflicting results, and the debate of SWL versus ureteroscopy for distal ureteral calculi will continue into the foreseeable future. Pearle and colleagues reported 64 patients with distal ureteral stones (less than 15 mm) that were randomized to SWL or ureteroscopy.[205] At 3 weeks follow-up, 91% of patients in each group imaged with plain film showed resolution of the target stone. A significantly shorter procedural and operating room time was reported with SWL versus ureteroscopy (34 and 72 minutes vs. 65 and 97 minutes, respectively) with a larger percentage of patients in the SWL group able to be sent home the same day (94% vs. 75%). In contrast, Peschel and colleagues reported 80 patients with distal ureteral stones stratified randomized to SWL or ureteroscopy.[203] Ureteroscopy was found to be significantly better in terms of operative time, fluoroscopy time, and time to achieve stone-free status. All patients were subsequently stone free. But the re-treatment rate in the SWL group was 15% for stones greater than 5 mm and 10% for stones less than 5 mm. Re-treatment was not required in the ureteroscopic group. Smaller stones (less than 5 mm) that had not passed spontaneously by 3 weeks were more efficiently treated with ureteroscopy, as they are the most difficult to visualize and focus with SWL and may also be associated with relative narrowing of the intramural ureter.[206]

Excellent results for SWL of distal ureteral stones have been reported with the Dornier HM-3.[205,207] Unfortunately, many urologists who have experienced the gratifying results with the HM-3 have been disappointed when their HM-3 has been replaced with a newer generation lithotriptor. Review of the literature supports this anecdotal experience (Table 40-3).[200,208–214] In contrast to the large focal zone of the HM-3 with excellent shock wave transmission through a water bath, the newer generation lithotriptors are all limited by small focal zones and suboptimal coupling to the patient as SWs pass through the membrane of the water cushion and coupling jelly.

As randomized studies do not clearly determine the optimal treatment for distal ureteral calculi, patients should be offered an educated choice between SWL and ureteroscopy based on current data. Furthermore, issues of cost-effectiveness, physician expertise, equipment availability, and patient occupation also need to be considered. Although SWL may result in a successful outcome, ureteroscopy is favored in settings where the lithotriptor is not on-site or immediately available, or if a patient prefers to be stone free without dependence on passage of stone fragments. Airline pilots may be a classic example in which an endoscopic approach would be best for a distal ureteral stone.[215]

CONCLUSION

SWL remains an excellent method for the successful treatment of many urinary calculi. Recent work suggests that SWL results can be improved by simple adjustments in the treatment proto-col—such as the use of a slower SW rate. Further, helical CT may emerge as a technology that not only is useful for patient diagnosis, but which can also provide important information on stones for planning treatment. Studies that compare SWL with other modalities consistently show greater patient satisfaction with SWL—as long as SWL is successful. Thus, being able to predict the success of SWL in a given patient is essential, and there is promise that the ability to make such predictions is improving over time.

Table 40-3 Shock Wave Lithotripsy for Distal Ureteral Stones: Newer Lithotriptors

Author/Machine	Patients	% Stone Free	Procedures/patient	MPa at F2
Bendhack/Multiline[209]	25	72	2.04	80
Eden/Modulith[200]	313	74.8 (after 1st session)	2.25	105.6
Strohmaier/Modulith Compact[210]	37	59	1.60	105.6
Goethuys/Multiline[208]	157	85	1.90 (No. of SWL sessions only)	80
Nabi/Dornier Compact Delta[212]	26	79	1.80	
Johnson/Dornier Doli S[211]	12	79		
Sheir/MFL 5000[214]	48	93.7	1.54	35–80
Sheir/Doli S[214]	31	93.6	1.58	28–84

REFERENCES

1. Kerbl K, Rehman J, Landman J, et al. Current management of urolithiasis: Progress or regress? J Endourol 2002;16:281.
2. Bierkens AF, Hendrikx AJ, de Kort VJ, et al. Efficacy of second generation lithotriptors: a multicenter comparative study of 2,206 extracorporeal shock wave lithotripsy treatments with the Siemens Lithostar, Dornier HM4, Wolf Piezolith 2300, Direx Tripter X-1 and Breakstone lithotriptors. J Urol 1992;148:1052.
3. Tan EC, Tung KH, Foo KT. Comparative studies of extracorporeal shock wave lithotripsy by Dornier HM3, EDAP LT 01 and Sonolith 2000 devices. J Urol 1991;146:294.
4. McAteer JA, Williams JC Jr, Evan AP, et al. Mechanisms of cell and tissue damage in shock wave lithotripsy. In: Andrew MA, Crum LA, Vaezy S, editors. Proceedings of the International Symposium on Therapeutic Ultrasound. Seattle: University of Washington; 2003. p. 491.
5. Evan AP, Willis LR, Lingeman JE, McAteer JA. Renal trauma and the risk of long-term complications in shock wave lithotripsy. Nephron 1998;78:1.
6. Knapp R, Frauscher F, Helweg G, et al. Age-related changes in resistive index following extracorporeal shock wave lithotripsy. J Urol 1995;154:955.
7. Janetschek G, Frauscher F, Knapp R, et al. New onset hypertension after extracorporeal shock wave lithotripsy: age related incidence and prediction by intrarenal resistive index. J Urol 1997;158:346.
8. Parks JH, Worcester EM, Coe FL, et al. Clinical implications of abundant calcium phosphate in routinely analyzed kidney stones. Kidney Int 2004;66:777.
9. Ueda S, Matsuoka K, Yamashita T, et al. Perirenal hematomas caused by SWL with EDAP LT-01 lithotripter. J Endourol 1993;7:11.
10. Fuselier HA, Prats L, Fontenot C, Gauthier A Jr. Comparison of mobile lithotripters at one institution: healthtronics lithotron, Dornier MFL-5000, and Dornier Doli. J Endourol 1999;13:539.
11. Piper NY, Dalrymple N, Bishoff JT. Incidence of renal hematoma formation after ESWL using the new Dornier Doli-S lithotriptor [Abstract]. J Urol 2001;165:377.
12. Dhar N, Yost A, Streem SB. The incidence of and a multivariate analysis of risk factors associated with subcapsular hematoma formation following electromagnetic lithotripsy [Abstract]. J Urol 2004;171:495.
13. McAteer JA, Bailey MR, Williams JC, et al. Strategies for improved shock wave lithotripsy. Minerva Urologica e Nefrologica 2005;57:271.
14. Federle MP, McAninch JW, Kaiser JA, et al. Computed tomography of urinary calculi. AJR 1981;136:255.
15. Hillman BJ, Drach GW, Tracey P, Gaines JA. Computed tomo-graphic analysis of renal calculi. AJR Am J Roentgenol 1984;142:549.
16. Van Arsdalen KN, Banner MP, Pollack HM. Radiographic imaging and urologic decision making in the management of renal and ureteral calculi. Urol Clin North Am 1990;17:171.
17. Sommer FG, Jeffrey RBJ, Rubin GD, et al. Detection of ureteral calculi in patients with suspected renal colic: value of reformatted noncontrast helical CT. AJR 1995;165:509.
18. Smith RC, Verga M, McCarthy S, Rosenfield AT. Diagnosis of acute flank pain: value of unenhanced helical CT. AJR Am J Roentgenol 1996;166:97.
19. Fielding JR, Steele G, Fox LA, et al. Spiral computerized tomography in the evaluation of acute flank pain: a replacement for excretory urography. J Urol 1997;157:2071.
20. Hubert J, Blum A, Cormier L, et al. Three-dimensional CT-scan reconstruction of renal caluli. A new tool for mapping-out staghorn calculi and follow-up of radiolucent stones. Eur Urol 1997;31:297.
21. Dalrymple NC, Verga M, Anderson KR, et al. The value of unenhanced helical computerized tomography in the management of acute flank pain. J Urol 1998;159:735.
22. Preminger GM, Vieweg J, Leder RA, Nelson RC. Urolithiasis: Detection and management with unenhanced spiral CT—a urologic perspective. Radiology 1998;207:308.
23. Vieweg J, Teh C, Freed K, et al. Unenhanced helical computerized tomography for the evaluation of patients with acute flank pain. J Urol 1998;160:679.
24. Boulay I, Holtz P, Foley WD, et al. Ureteral calculi: diagnostic efficacy of helical CT and implications for treatment of patients. AJR Am J Roentgenol 1999;172:1485.
25. Fielding JR, Silverman SG, Rubin GD. Helical CT of the urinary tract. AJR Am J Roentgenol 1999;172:1199.
26. Katz DS, Hines J, Rausch DR, et al. Unenhanced helical CT for suspected renal colic. AJR Am J Roentgenol 1999;173:425.
27. Smith RC, Levine J, Rosenfeld AT. Helical CT of urinary tract stones. Epidemiology, origin, pathophysiology, diagnosis, and management. Radiol Clin North Am 1999;37:911.
28. Dretler SP. Stone fragility—a new therapeutic distinction. J Urol 1988;139:1124.
29. Dretler SP. The clinical significance of variations in urinary stone fragility. J Lithotr Stone Dis 1989;1:192.
30. Bhatta KM, Prien EL Jr, Dretler SP. Cystine calculi—rough and smooth: a new clinical distinction. J Urol 1989;142:937.
31. Dretler SP. Special article: calculus breakability—fragility and durility. J Endourol 1994;8:1.
32. Dretler SP, Polykoff G. Calcium oxalate stone morphology: fine tuning our therapeutic distinctions. J Urol 1996;155:828.
33. Dretler SP, Spencer BA. CT and stone fragility. J Endourol 2001;15:31.
34. Joseph P, Mandal AK, Singh SK, et al. Computerized tomography attenuation value of renal calculus: can it predict successful fragmentation of the calculus by extracorporeal shock wave lithotripsy? A preliminary study. J Urol 2002;167:1968–71.
35. Pareek G, Armenakas NA, Fracchia JA. Hounsfield units on computerized tomography predict stone-free rates after extracorporeal shock wave lithotripsy. J Urol 2003;169:1679.
36. Stern JA, Kimm SY, Chang C-H, et al. Computerized tomography density accurately predicts success of shockwave lithotripsy [Abstract]. J Urol 2003;169:460.
37. Lowry PS, Pozniak M, Leverson GE, Nakada SY. Ratio of peak attenuation to stone size predicts uric acid stones using spiral computerized tomography [Abstract]. J Urol 2003;169:464.
38. Sacco DE, Cay O, Mueller PR, Dretler SP. Combining com-

puterized tomography attenuation values with stone diameter predicts the success of extracorporeal shock wave lithotripsy on ureteral stone clearance [Abstract]. J Urol 2003;169:487.
39. Jacobsen N, Ng D, Varma V, Wollin T. Does internal structure of renal calculi on high resolution CT predict SWL treatment outcome? J Endourol 2003 17(Suppl 1):A36.
40. Gupta NP, Kumar P, Aron M, et al. Role of NCCT in predicting the outcome of shockwave lithotripsy. J Endourol 2003;17(Suppl 1):A263.
41. Zarse CA, McAteer JA, Tann M, et al. Helical CT accurately reports urinary stone composition using attenuation values: In vitro verification using high resolution micro CT calibrated to FT-IR microspectroscopy. Urology 2004;63:828.
42. Hu H, Fox SH. The effect of helical pitch and beam collimation on the lesion contrast and slice profile in helical CT imaging. Med Phys 1996;23:1943.
43. Williams JC Jr, Saw KC, Monga AG, et al. Correction of helical CT attenuation values with wide beam collimation. Acad Radiol 2001;8:478.
44. Nakada SY, Hoff DG, Attai S, et al. Determination of stone composition by noncontrast spiral computed tomography in the clinical setting. Urology 2000;55:816.
45. Saw KC, McAteer JA, Fineberg NS, et al. Calcium stone fragility is predicted by helical CT attenuation values. J Endourol 2000;14:471.
46. Motley G, Dalrymple N, Keesling C, et al. Hounsfield unit density in the determination of urinary stone composition. Urology 2001;58:170.
47. Mostafavi MR, Ernst RD, Saltzman B. Accurate determination of chemical composition of urinary calculi by spiral computerized tomography. J Urol 1998;159:673.
48. Hu H, He HD, Foley WD, Fox SH. Four multidetector-row helical CT: Image quality and volume coverage speed. Radiology 2000;215:55.
49. Mueller-Lisse UG, Mueller-Lisse UL, Oberneder R. Multidetector CT of the kidney. In: Reiser MF, Takahashi M, Modic M, Bruening R, editors. Multislice CT. Berlin: Springer Verlag; 2001. p. 23.
50. Dawson P, Lees WR. Multi-slice technology in computed tomography. Clin Radiol 2001;56:302.
51. Boiselle PM, Dippolito G, Copeland J, et al. Multiplanar and 3D imaging of the central airways: comparison of image quality and radiation dose of single–detector row CT and multi–detector row CT at differing tube currents in dogs. Radiology 2003;228:107.
52. Daudon M, Donsimoni R, Hennequin C, et al. Sex and age-related composition of 10617 calculi analyzed by infrared-spectroscopy. Urol Res 1995;23:319.
53. Williams JC Jr, Paterson RF, Kopecky KK, et al. High resolution detection of internal structure in renal calculi by helical computerized tomography. J Urol 2002;167:322–326.
54. Tanrikut C, Sahani D, Dretler SP. Distinguishing stent from stone: Use of bone windows. Urology 2004;63:823.
55. Mitcheson HD, Zamenhof RG, Bankoff MS, Prien EL. Determination of the chemical composition of urinary calculi by computerized tomography. J Urol 1983;130:814.
56. Newhouse JH, Prien EL, Amis ES, et al. Computed tomographic analysis of urinary calculi. AJR Am J Roentgenol 1984;142:545.
57. Saw KC, McAteer JA, Monga AG, et al. Helical CT of urinary calculi: effect of stone composition, stone size, and scan collimation. AJR Am J Roentgenol 2000;175:329.
58. Kuwahara M, Kageyama S, Kurosu S, Orikasa S. Computed tomography and composition of renal calculi. Urol Res 1984;12:111.
59. Herremans D, Vandeursen H, Pittomvils G, et al. In vitro analysis of urinary calculi: type differentiation using computed tomography and bone densitometry. Br J Urol 1993;72:544.
60. Hubert J, Descotes JL, Bellin MF. Imaging and urinary stones. Progres En Urologie 2003;13:993.
61. Kim SC, Zarse CA, McAteer JA, et al. Stone internal structure is visible in patients by helical CT [Abstract]. J Urol 2004;171(4 Suppl):509.
62. Bon D, Dore B, Irani J, et al. Radiographic prognostic criteria for extracorporeal shock-wave lithotripsy: a study of 485 patients. Urology 1996;48:556.
63. Hamid A, Dwivedi US, Singh TN, et al. Artificial neural networks in predicting optimum renal stone fragmentation by extracorporeal shock wave lithotripsy: a preliminary study. BJU Int 2003;91:821.
64. Abdel-Khalek M, Sheir KZ, Moktar AA, et al. Prediction of success rate after extracorporeal shock-wave lithotripsy of renal stones. Scand J Urol Nephrol 2004;38:161.
65. Lingeman JE, Newman DM, Siegel YI, et al. Shock wave lithotripsy with the Dornier MFL 5000 lithotriptor using an external fixed rate signal. J Urol 1995;154:951.
66. Winters JC, Macaluso JN Jr. Ungated Medstone outpatient lithotripsy. J Urol 1995;153:593.
67. Cass AS. The use of ungating with the Medstone lithotriptor. J Urol 1996;156:896.
68. Vallancien G, Munoz R, Borghi M, et al. Relationship between the frequency of piezoelectric shock waves and the quality of renal stone fragmentation. In vitro study and clinical implications. Eur Urol 1989;16:41.
69. Greenstein A, Matzkin H. Does the rate of extracorporeal shock wave delivery affect stone fragmentation? Urology 1999;54:430.
70. Lifshitz DA, Williams JC Jr, Lingeman JE, et al. Efficiency of SWL stone fragmentation in vitro is improved by slowing the SW delivery rate (abstract). J Urol 2000;163:338.
71. Weir MJ, Tariq N, Honey RJ. Shockwave frequency affects fragmentation in a kidney stone model. J Endourol 2000; 14:547.
72. McAteer JA, Paterson RF, Lifshitz DA, et al. In vitro model of shock wave lithotripsy (SWL) produces stone breakage equivalent to that seen in vivo. Proceedings 17th International Congress on Acoustics VII:180, 2002.
73. Paterson RF, Lingeman JE, Evan AP, et al. Percutaneous stone implantation in the pig kidney: a new animal model for lithotripsy research. J Endourol 2002;16.
74. Paterson RF, Lifshitz DA, Lingeman JE, et al. Stone fragmentation during shock wave lithotripsy is improved by slowing the shock wave rate: Studies with a new animal model. J Urol 2002;168:2211.
75. Pace KT, Ghiculete O, Harju M and Honey RJD. Shock wave lithotripsy at 60 or 120 shocks per minute: a randomized, double-blinded study. J Urol 2005;174:595–99..
76. Motola JA, Smith AD. Therapeutic options for the management of upper tract calculi. Urol Clin North Am 1990;17:191.
77. Drach GW, Dretler S, Fair W, et al. Report of the United States cooperative study of extracorporeal shock wave lithotripsy. J Urol 1986;135:1127.
78. Lingeman JE, Newman D, Mertz JH, et al. Extracorporeal shock wave lithotripsy: the Methodist Hospital of Indiana experience. J Urol 1986;135:1134.
79. Politis G, Griffith DP. ESWL: stone free efficacy based upon stone size and location. World J Urol 1987;5:255.
80. El-Damanhoury H, Scharfe T, Ruth J, et al. Extracorporeal shock wave lithotripsy of urinary calculi: experience in treatment of 3,278 patients using the Siemens Lithostar and Lithostar Plus. J Urol 1991;145:484.
81. Mobley TB, Myers DA, Grine WB, et al. Low energy lithotripsy with the Lithostar: treatment results with 19,962 renal and ureteral calculi. J Urol 1993;149:1419.
82. Logarakis NF, Jewett MAS, Luymes J, Honey RJD. Variation in clinical outcome following shock wave lithotripsy. J Urol 2000;163:721.
83. Cass AS. Comparison of first generation (Dornier HM3) and second generation (Medstone STS) lithotriptors: treatment results with 13,864 renal and ureteral calculi. J Urol 1995;153:588.
84. Williams JC Jr, Saw KC, Paterson RF, et al. Variability of renal stone fragility in shock wave lithotripsy. Urology 2003;61:1092.
85. Sakamoto W, Kishimoto T, Takegaki Y, et al. Stone fragility—measurement of stone mineral content by dual photon absorptiometry. Eur Urol 1991;20:150.
86. Wang YH, Grenabo L, Hedelin H, et al. Analysis of stone fragility in vitro and in vivo with piezoelectric shock waves using the EDAP LT-01. J Urol 1993;149:699.
87. Pittomvils G, Vandeursen H, Wevers M, et al. The influence of internal stone structure upon the fracture behaviour of urinary calculi. Ultrasound Med Biol 1994;20:803.
88. Saw KC, Lingeman JE. Management of calyceal stones. AUA Update Series XVIII:154, 1999.
89. Rutchik SD, Resnick MI. Cystine calculi. Diagnosis and management. Urol Clin North Am 1997;24:163.
90. Chaussy C, Schmiedt E. Extracorporeal shock wave lithotripsy (ESWL) for kidney stones. An alternative to surgery? Urologic Radiology 1984;6:80.
91. Schmiedt E, Chaussy C. Extracorporeal shock-wave lithotripsy of kidney and ureteric stones. Urol Int 1984; 39:193.
92. Psihramis KE, Jewett MA, Bombardier C, et al. Lithostar extracorporeal shock wave lithotripsy: the first 1,000 patients. J Urol 1992;147:1006.
93. Lingeman JE, Siegel YI, Steele B, et al. Management of lower pole nephrolithiasis: a critical analysis. J Urol 1994;151:663.
94. Clayman RV, McDougall EM, Nakada SY: Percutaneous therapeutic procedures. In: Walsh PC, Retick AB, Vaughan ED, Wein AJ, editors. Campbell's urology, 7th ed. Philadelphia: WB Saunders; 1998. p. 2809–64.
95. Segura JW, Preminger GM, Assimos DG, et al. Nephrolithiasis Clinical Guidelines Panel summary report on the management of staghorn calculi. J Urol 1994;151:1648.
96. Lingeman JE, Coury TA, Newman DM, et al. Comparison of results and morbidity of percutaneous nephrostolithotomy and extracorporeal shock wave lithotripsy. J Urol 1987;138:485.
97. Lingeman JE, Smith LH, Woods JR. Staghorn calculi. In: Lingeman JE, Smith LH, Woods JR, Newman DM, editors. Urinary calculi. Philadelphia: Lea and Febiger; 1989. p. 163.
98. This reference is missing. See comments at citation of #99 and near #125 and 126 for possible source of the problem.
99. Albala DM, Assimos DG, Clayman RV, et al. Lower pole I: a prospective randomized trial of extracorporeal shock wave lithotripsy and percutaneous nephrostolithotomy for lower pole nephrolithiasis—initial results. J Urol 2001;166:2072–80.
100. Pearle MS, Lingeman JE, Leveillee RJ, et al. Prospective, randomized trial comparing shock wave lithotripsy and ureteroscopy for lower pole calyceal calculi 1 cm or less in size. J Urol 2005. [In press]
101. Sabnis RB, Naik K, Patel SH, et al. Extracorporeal shock wave lithotripsy for lower calyceal stones: can clearance be predicted? Br J Urol 1997;80:853.
102. Elbahnasy AM, Shalhav AL, Hoenig DM, et al. Lower caliceal stone clearance after shock wave lithotripsy or ureteroscopy: the impact of lower pole radiographic anatomy. J Urol 1998;159:676.
103. Knoll T, Musial A, Trojan L, et al. Measurement of renal anatomy for prediction of lower-pole caliceal stone clearance: reproducibility of different parameters. J Endourol 2003;17:447.
104. Jones JA, Lingeman JE, Steidle CP. The roles of extracorporeal shock wave lithotripsy and percutaneous nephrostolithotomy in the management of pyelocaliceal diverticula. J Urol 1991;146:724.
105. Psihramis KE, Dretler SP. Extracorporeal shock-wave lithotripsy of caliceal diverticula calculi. J Urol 1987; 138:707.
106. Streem SB, Yost A. Treatment of caliceal diverticular calculi with extracorporeal shock wave lithotripsy: patient selection and extended followup. J Urol 1992;148:1043.
107. Batter SJ, Dretler SP. Ureterorenoscopic approach to the symptomatic caliceal diverticulum. J Urol 1997;158:709.
108. Auge BK, Munver R, Kourambas J, et al. Endoscopic management of symptomatic caliceal diverticula: a retrospective comparison of percutaneous nephrolithotripsy and ureteroscopy. J Endourol 2002;16:557.
109. Grasso M, Lang G, Loisides P, et al. Endoscopic management of the symptomatic caliceal diverticular calculus. J Urol 1995;153:1878.
110. Miller SD, Ng CS, Streem SB, Gill IS. Laparoscopic management of caliceal diverticular calculi. J Urol 2002;167: 1248.
111. Ruckle HC, Segura JW. Laparoscopic treatment of a stone-filled, caliceal diverticulum: a definitive, minimally invasive therapeutic option. J Urol 1994;151:122.
112. Hulbert JC, Reddy PK, Hunter DW, et al. Percutaneous techniques for the management of caliceal diverticula containing calculi. J Urol 1986;135:225.
113. Shalhav AL, Soble JJ, Nakada SY, et al. Long-term outcome of caliceal diverticula following percutaneous endosurgical management. J Urol 1998;160:1635.
114. Bellman GC, Silverstein JI, Blickensderfer S, Smith AD. Technique and follow-up of percutaneous management of caliceal diverticula. Urology 1993;42:21.
115. Auge BK, Munver R, Kourambas J, et al. Neoinfundibulotomy for the management of symptomatic caliceal diverticula. J Urol 2002;167:1616.
116. Al-Basam S, Bennett JD, Layton ZA, et al. Treatment of caliceal diverticular stones: transdiverticular percutaneous nephrolithotomy with creation of a neoinfundibulum. J Vasc Interv Radiol 2000;11:885.
117. Monga M, Smith R, Ferral H, Thomas R. Percutaneous ablation of caliceal diverticulum: long-term followup. J Urol 2000;163:28.
118. Kim SC, Kuo RL, Paterson RF, Lingeman JE. Percutaneous nephrolithotomy for caliceal diverticular calculi: a novel single stage approach. J Urol 2005. [In press]
119. Koga S, Arakaki Y, Matsuoka M, Ohyama C. Staghorn calculi—long-term results of management. Br J Urol 1991; 68:122.

120. Blandy JP, Singh M. The case for a more aggressive approach to staghorn stones. J Urol 1976;115:505.
121. Smith MJ, Boyce WH. Anatrophic nephrotomy and plastic calyrhaphy. Trans Am Assoc Genitourin Surg 1967;59:18.
122. Griffith DP, Gibson JR, Clinton CW, Musher DM. Acetohydroxamic acid: clinical studies of a urease inhibitor in patients with staghorn renal calculi. J Urol 1978;119:9.
123. Griffith DP. Struvite stones. Kidney Int 1978;13:372.
124. Kahnoski RJ, Lingeman JE, Coury TA, et al. Combined percutaneous and extracorporeal shock wave lithotripsy for staghorn calculi: an alternative to anatrophic nephrolithotomy. J Urol 1986;135:679.
125. Lam HS, Lingeman JE, Barron M, et al. Staghorn calculi: analysis of treatment results between initial percutaneous nephrostolithotomy and extracorporeal shock wave lithotripsy monotherapy with reference to surface area. J Urol 1992;147:1219.
125a. Meretyk S, Gofrit ON, Gafni O, Complete Staghorn calculi: random prospective comparison between extracorporeal shock wave lithotripsy monotherapy and combined with percutaneous nephrostolithotomy. J Urol 1997;157:780.
126. Streem SB, Lammert G. Long-term efficacy of combination therapy for struvite staghorn calculi. J Urol 1992;147:563.
127. Streem SB, Yost A, Dolmatch B. Combination "sandwich" therapy for extensive renal calculi in 100 consecutive patients: immediate, long-term and stratified results from a 10-year experience. J Urol 1997;158:342.
128. Lam HS, Lingeman JE, Mosbaugh PG, et al. Evolution of the technique of combination therapy for staghorn calculi: a decreasing role for extracorporeal shock wave lithotripsy. J Urol 1992;148:1058.
129. Harmon WJ, Kleer E, Segura JW. Laparoscopic pyelolithotomy for calculus removal in a pelvic kidney. J Urol 1996;155:2019.
130. Zafar FS, Lingeman JE. Value of laparoscopy in the management of calculi complicating renal malformations. J Endourol 1996;10:379.
131. Evans WP, Resnick MI. Horseshoe kidney and urolithiasis. J Urol 1981;125:620.
132. Jenkins AD, Gillenwater JY. Extracorporeal shock wave lithotripsy in the prone position: treatment of stones in the distal ureter or anomalous kidney. J Urol 1988; 139:911.
133. Locke DR, Newman RC, Steinbock GS, Finlayson B. Extracorporeal shock-wave lithotripsy in horseshoe kidneys. Urology 1990;35:407.
134. Esuvaranathan K, Tan EC, Tung KH, Foo KT. Stones in horseshoe kidneys: results of treatment by extracorporeal shock wave lithotripsy and endourology. J Urol 1991; 146:1213.
135. Vandeursen H, Baert L. Electromagnetic extracorporeal shock wave lithotripsy for calculi in horseshoe kidneys. J Urol 1992;148:1120.
136. Theiss M, Wirth MP, Frohmuller HG. Extracorporeal shock wave lithotripsy in patients with renal malformations. Br J Urol 1993;72:534.
137. Kirkali Z, Esen AA, Mungan MU. Effectiveness of extracorporeal shockwave lithotripsy in the management of stone-bearing horseshoe kidneys. J Endourol 1996;10:13.
138. Lampel A, Hohenfellner M, Schultz-Lampel D, et al. Urolithiasis in horseshoe kidneys: therapeutic management. Urology 1996;47:182.
139. Kupeli B, Isen K, Biri H, et al. Extracorporeal shockwave lithotripsy in anomalous kidneys. J Endourol 1999;13:349.
140. Drach GW, Dretler S, Fair W, et al. Report of the United States cooperative study of extracorporeal shock wave lithotripsy. J Urol 1986;135:1127.
141. Lingeman JE, Newman D, Mertz JH, et al. Extracorporeal shock wave lithotripsy: the Methodist Hospital of Indiana experience. J Urol 1986;135:1134.
142. Jones DJ, Wickham JE, Kellett MJ. Percutaneous nephrolithotomy for calculi in horseshoe kidneys. J Urol 1991; 145:481.
143. Al-Otaibi K, Hosking DH. Percutaneous stone removal in horseshoe kidneys. J Urol 1999;162:674.
144. Segura JW, Preminger GM, Assimos DG, et al. Ureteral Stones Clinical Guidelines Panel summary report on the management of ureteral calculi. J Urol 1997;158:1915.
145. Park H, Park M, Park T. Two-year experience with ureteral stones: extracorporeal shockwave lithotripsy v ureteroscopic manipulation. J Endourol 1998;12:501.
146. Netto NR, Claro JF, Lemos GC, Cortado PL. Treatment options for ureteral calculi: endourology or extracorporeal shock wave lithotripsy. J Urol 1991;146:5.
147. Grasso M, Loisides P, Beaghler M, Bagley DH. The case for primary endoscopic management of upper urinary tract calculi: I. A critical review of 121 extracorporeal shock-wave lithotripsy failures. Urology 1995;45:363.
148. Grasso M, Beaghler M, Loisides P. The case for primary endoscopic management of upper urinary tract calculi: II. Cost and outcome assessment of 112 primary ureteral calculi. Urology 1995;45:372.
149. Grasso M. Ureteroscopic lithotripsy. Curr Opin Urol 1999; 9:329.
150. Tawfiek ER, Bagley DH. Management of upper urinary tract calculi with ureteroscopic techniques. Urology 1999;53:25.
151. Mugiya S, Nagata M, Un-No T, et al. Endoscopic management of impacted ureteral stones using a small caliber ureteroscope and a laser lithotriptor. J Urol 2000;164:329.
152. Yagisawa T, Kobayashi C, Ishikawa N, et al. Benefits of ureteroscopic pneumatic lithotripsy for the treatment of impacted ureteral stones. J Endourol 2001;15:697.
153. Green DF, Lytton B. Early experience with direct vision electrohydraulic lithotripsy of ureteral calculi. J Urol 1985; 133:767.
154. Morgentaler A, Bridge SS, Dretler SP. Management of the impacted ureteral calculus. J Urol 1990;143:263.
155. Parr NJ, Pye SD, Ritchie AWS, Tolley DA. Mechanisms responsible for diminished fragmentation of ureteral calculi—an experimental and clinical study. J Urol 1992; 148:1079.
156. Farsi HMA, Mosli HA, Alzimaity M, et al. In-situ extracorporeal shock-wave lithotripsy for primary ureteral calculi. Urology 1994;43:776.
157. Roberts WW, Cadeddu JA, Micali S, et al. Ureteral stricture formation after removal of impacted calculi. J Urol 1998;159:723.
158. Mueller SC, Wilbert D, Thueroff JW, Alken P. Extracorporeal shock wave lithotripsy of ureteral stones: clinical experience and experimental findings. J Urol 1986;135:831.
159. Lingeman JE, Shirrell WL, Newman DM, et al. Management of upper ureteral calculi with extracorporeal shock wave lithotripsy. J Urol 1987;138:720.
160. Riehle RA, Naslund EB. Treatment of calculi in the upper ureter with extracorporeal shock wave lithotripsy. Surg Gynecol Obstet 1987;164:1.
161. Evans RJ, Wingfield DD, Morollo BA, Jenkins AD. Ureteral stone manipulation before extracorporeal shock wave lithotripsy. J Urol 1988;139:33.
162. Fetner CD, Preminger GM, Seger J, Lea TA. Treatment of ureteral calculi by extracorporeal shock-wave lithotripsy at a multi-use center. J Urol 1988;139:1192.
163. Lingeman JE. Ureteral calculi. In: Lingeman JE, Smith LH, Woods JR,Newman DM, editors. Urinary calculi: ESWL, endourology, and medical therapy. Philadelphia: Lea & Febiger; 1989. p. 192.
164. Bolton DM, Costello AJ, Lenaghan D. Comparative study of the role of endo-urological manipulation in the treatment of ureteric calculi using extracorporeal shock wave lithotripsy. Aust N Z J Surg, 1991;61:654.
165. Gross AJ, Kugler A, Seseke F, Ringert RH. Push and smash increases success rates in treatment of ureteric calculi by ESWL. Int Urol Nephrol, 1998;30:417.
166. Paterson RF, Kim SC, Kuo RL, et al. Shock wave lithotripsy of stones implanted in the proximal ureter of the pig. J Urol 2005;173:1391.
167. Rassweiler J, Lutz K, Gumpinger R, Eisenberger F. Efficacy of in situ extracorporeal shock wave lithotripsy for upper ureteral calculi. Eur Urol 1986;12:377.
168. Holden D, Rao PN. Ureteral stones—the results of primary in situ extracorporeal shock-wave lithotripsy. J Urol 1989;142:37.
169. Cass AS. Nonstent or noncatheter extracorporeal shock-wave lithotripsy for ureteral stones. Urology 1994;43:178.
170. Mobley TB, Myers DA, Jenkins JM, et al. Effects of stents on lithotripsy of ureteral calculi: treatment results with 18,825 calculi using the Lithostar lithotripter. J Urol 1994;152:53.
171. Ryan PC, Lennon GM, McLean PA, Fitzpatrick JM. The effects of acute and chronic JJ stent placement on upper urinary tract motility and calculus transit. Br J Urol 1994;74:434.
172. Kahnoski RJ, Lingeman JE, Woods JR, et al. Efficacy of glucagon in the relief of ureteral colic following treatment by extracorporeal shock wave lithotripsy: a randomized double-blind trial. J Urol 1987;137:1124.
173. Cole RS, Palfrey EL, Smith SE, Shuttleworth KE. Indomethacin as prophylaxis against ureteral colic following extracorporeal shock wave lithotripsy. J Urol 1989;141:9.
174. Hendrikx A, Bierkens A, Oosterhof G, Debruyne F. Treatment of proximal and midureteral calculi: a randomized trial of in situ and pushback extracorporeal lithotripsy. J Endourol 1990;4:353.
175. Schmidt A, Rassweiler J, Gumpinger R, et al. Minimally invasive treatment of ureteric calculi using modern techniques. Br J Urol 1990;65:242.
176. Ou YC, Hwang TI, Yang CR, et al. Use of indomethacin in the prophylaxis of ureteral colic following extracorporeal shock wave lithotripsy. Scand J Urol Nephrol 1992;26:351.
177. Porpiglia F, Destefanis P, Fiori C, et al. Role of adjunctive medical therapy with nifedipine and deflazacort after extracorporeal shock wave lithotripsy of ureteral stones. Urology 2002;59:835.
178. Cole RS, Palfrey EL, Smith SE, Shuttleworth KE. Indomethacin as prophylaxis against ureteral colic following extracorporeal shock wave lithotripsy. J Urol 1989;141:9.
179. Ergene U, Pekdemir M, Canda E, et al. Ondansetron versus diclofenac sodium in the treatment of acute ureteral colic: a double blind controlled trial. Int Urol Nephrol 2001; 33:315.
180. Jones JB, Giles BK, Brizendine EJ, Cordell WH. Sublingual hyoscyamine sulfate in combination with ketorolac tromethamine for ureteral colic: a randomized, double-blind, controlled trial. Ann Emerg Med 2001;37:141.
181. Fredman B, Jedeikin R, Olsfanger D, Aronheim M. The opioid-sparing effect of diclofenac sodium in outpatient extracorporeal shock wave lithotripsy (ESWL). J Clin Anesth 1993;5:141.
182. Pace KT, Weir MJ, Tariq N, Honey RJ. Low success rate of repeat shock wave lithotripsy for ureteral stones after failed initial treatment. J Urol 2000;164:1905.
183. Cass AS. Do upper ureteral stones need to be manipulated (push back) into the kidneys before extracorporeal shock wave lithotripsy? J Urol 1992;147:349.
184. Cass AS. In situ extracorporeal shock wave lithotripsy for obstructing ureteral stones with acute renal colic. J Urol 1992;148:1786.
185. Parr NJ, Pye SD, Ritchie AWS, Tolley DA. Mechanisms responsible for diminished fragmentation of ureteral calculi—an experimental and clinical study. J Urol 1992; 148:1079.
186. Danuser H, Ackermann DK, Marth DC, et al. Extracorporeal shock wave lithotripsy in situ or after push-up for upper ureteral calculi: a prospective randomized trial. J Urol 1993;150:824.
187. Mobley TB, Myers DA, Grine WB, et al. Low energy lithotripsy with the Lithostar: treatment results with 19,962 renal and ureteral calculi. J Urol 1993;149:1419.
188. Willis LR, Evan AP, Connors BA, et al. Relationship between kidney size, renal injury, and renal impairment induced by shock wave lithotripsy. J Am Soc Nephrol 1999;10: 1753.
189. Connors BA, Evan AP, Willis LR, et al. The effect of discharge voltage on renal injury and impairment caused by lithotripsy in the pig. J Am Soc Nephrol 2000;11:310.
190. Whitfield HN. The management of ureteric stones. Part II: therapy. BJU Int 1999;84:916.
191. Deliveliotis C, Stavropoulos NI, Koutsokalis G, et al. Distal ureteral calculi: ureteroscopy vs. ESWL. A prospective analysis. Int Urol Nephrol 1996;28:627.
192. Jenkins AD, Gillenwater JY. Extracorporeal shock wave lithotripsy in the prone position: treatment of stones in the distal ureter or anomalous kidney. J Urol 1988;139:911.
193. Puppo P, Bottino P, Germinale F, et al. Extracorporeal shock-wave lithotripsy in the prone position for stones situated anteriorly. Eur Urol 1988;15:113.
194. Tiselius HG, Pettersson B, Andersson A. Extracorporeal shock-wave lithotripsy of stones in the mid ureter. J Urol 1989;141:280.
195. Vieweg J, Weber HM, Miller K, Hautmann R. Female fertility following extracorporeal shock wave lithotripsy of distal ureteral calculi. J Urol 1992;148:1007.
196. Erturk E, Ptak AM, Monaghan J. Fertility measures in women after extracorporeal shockwave lithotripsy of distal ureteral stones. J Endourol 1997;11:315.
197. Lifshitz DA, Lingeman JE. Ureteroscopy as a first-line intervention for ureteral calculi in pregnancy. J Endourol 2002;16:19.
198. Watterson JD, Girvan AR, Beiko DT, et al. Ureteroscopy and holmium:YAG laser lithotripsy: an emerging definitive management strategy for symptomatic ureteral calculi in pregnancy. Urology 2002;60:383.
199. Bierkens AF, Hendrikx AJ, De La Rosette JJ, et al. Treatment of mid- and lower ureteric calculi: extracorporeal shock-wave lithotripsy vs laser ureteroscopy. A comparison of costs, morbidity and effectiveness. Br J Urol 1998;81:31.

200. Eden CG, Mark IR, Gupta RR, et al. Intracorporeal or extracorporeal lithotripsy for distal ureteral calculi? Effect of stone size and multiplicity on success rates. J Endourol 1998;12:307.

201. Kupeli B, Biri H, Isen K, et al. Treatment of ureteral stones: comparison of extracorporeal shock wave lithotripsy and endourologic alternatives. Eur Urol 1998;34:474.

202. Pardalidis NP, Kosmaoglou EV, Kapotis CG. Endoscopy vs. extracorporeal shockwave lithotripsy in the treatment of distal ureteral stones: ten year's experience. J Endourol 1999;13:161.

203. Peschel R, Janetschek G, Bartsch G. Extracorporeal shock wave lithotripsy versus ureteroscopy for distal ureteral calculi: a prospective randomized study. J Urol 1999; 162:1909.

204. Turk TM, Jenkins AD. A comparison of ureteroscopy to in situ extracorporeal shock wave lithotripsy for the treatment of distal ureteral calculi. J Urol 1999;161:45.

205. Pearle MS, Nadler R, Bercowsky E, et al. Prospective randomized trial comparing shock wave lithotripsy and ureteroscopy for management of distal ureteral calculi. J Urol 2001;166:1255.

206. Van Cangh PJ. Upper tract urinary calculi-the comeback of the friendly endourologist [Editorial]. J Urol 1999;162:1920.

207. Hochreiter WW, Danuser H, Perrig M, Studer UE. Extracorporeal shock wave lithotripsy for distal ureteral calculi: what a powerful machine can achieve. J Urol 2003;169:878.

208. Goethuys H, Winnepenninckx B, Van Poppel H, Baert L. The new generation Siemens Multiline lithotripter tube "M": early results in ureteral calculi. J Endourol 1996;10:403.

209. Bendhack ML, Grimm MO, Ackermann R, Vogeli T. Primary treatment of ureteral stones by new multiline lithotripter. J Endourol 1999;13:339.

210. Strohmaier WL, Schubert G, Rosenkranz T, Weigl A. Comparison of extracorporeal shock wave lithotripsy and ureteroscopy in the treatment of ureteral calculi: a prospective study. Eur Urol 1999;36:376.

211. Johnson DB, Lowry PS, Schluckebier JA, et al. University of Wisconsin experience using the Doli S lithotriptor. Urology 2003;62:410.

212. Nabi G, Baldo O, Cartledge J, et al. The impact of the Dornier Compact Delta lithotriptor on the management of primary ureteric calculi. Eur Urol 2003;44:482.

213. Portis AJ, Yan Y, Pattaras JG, et al. Matched pair analysis of shock wave lithotripsy effectiveness for comparison of lithotriptors. J Urol 2003;169:58.

214. Sheir KZ, Madbouly K, Elsobky E. Prospective randomized comparative study of the effectiveness and safety of electrohydraulic and electromagnetic extracorporeal shock wave lithotriptors. J Urol 2003;170:389.

215. Zheng W, Beiko DT, Segura JW, et al. Urinary calculi in aviation pilots: what is the best therapeutic approach? J Urol 2002;168:1341.

41

Extracorporeal Shock Wave Lithotripsy: Complications

Andrew P. Evan, PhD

Lynn R. Willis, PhD

Extracorporeal shock wave lithotripsy (ESWL) for the treatment of urinary stones was introduced to clinical practice in the early 1980s. Today, even with the refinement of endourologic methods for stone removal, such as ureteroscopy and percutaneous nephrolithotomy, ESWL remains an important treatment for uncomplicated upper urinary tract calculi.[1,2] Although considered to be highly successful, lithotripsy is not a benign procedure, in that it is plagued by the occurrence of adverse effects and increased rates of significant injury linked to the use of high acoustic output machines. Clinical experience and studies with experimental animals treated with the first lithotriptor (the Dornier HM3) have shown that a dose of shock waves sufficient to comminute a stone invariably causes trauma to the kidney.[3-5] This injury can be severe and can lead to long-term complications such as new-new-onset hypertension,[6-7] diabetes mellitus,[7] and potentially brushite stone disease.[7a] Moreover, morbidity may occur following a technically successful procedure as a result of the stone fragments produced. Complications following ESWL treatment result from stone-related problems, infection, effects of treatment on tissue and renal function, and a possible increased risk of stone recurrence.

In addition, recent studies now show that the present generation of "high-pressure" lithotriptors produce low stone-free rates, high re-treatment rates and an increased incidence of adverse effects.[8-24] Thus, a technology that should provide the best treatment option has become more problematic, and the lithotriptor has become a risk factor itself.

ACUTE AND CHRONIC RENAL INJURY IN ESWL

ACUTE EXTRARENAL DAMAGE: CLINICAL OBSERVATIONS ESWL can induce acute injury to all extrarenal tissues that are within the boundaries of the focused shockwave front.[3,25-27] Patients treated with an unmodified HM3 at 18 to 24 kV commonly complain of pain localized to the posterior body wall (flank) near the site of shock wave entry and renal colic.[28] Lithotripsy manufacturers have attempted to reduce the amount of flank pain by increasing the diameter of the entering shock front and have had some suc-

cess. ESWL has been associated with significant trauma to such organs as the liver and skeletal muscle as detected by elevated levels for total bilirubin, cholecystokinin, lactic dehydrogenase, serum glutamic transaminase and creatinine phosphokinase within 24 hours of treatment.[28-31] These parameters begin to fall within 3 to 7 days post-ESWL and are normal at 3 months. It should be noted that most of these findings were associated with the use of an unmodified HM3. This does not mean the unmodified HM3 is more prone to injury. The problem is that current clinical studies reporting on the use of second- and third-generation machines have inadequately reported side effects.

Gastric or duodenal erosion with hematoma formation are thought to represent one of the most common extrarenal complications of ESWL therapy[32-36] with the potential of spillage of enteric contents[37-41] and hematochezia.[33] The incidence of bowel perforation is not known, but if one uses the data from the largest series ever reported (19,960 patients), only one small bowel perforation was noted.[23] Treatment in prone position might be an additional risk factor and should be used with caution.[37,41]

ESWL-induced injury to other extrarenal organ systems has an incidence of 1% or less. The lung parenchyma is injured if exposed directly to shock waves.[42] Acute pancreatitis associated with a marked rise in serum amylase and lipase levels has been observed or an increase in amylase levels in the absence of manifest pancreatitis[28,29,43,44] as well as other forms of tissue injury.[45] Patients having a previous history of pancreatitis may be at a greater risk.[46] ESWL-induced splenic rupture may require a splenectomy.[47-50] This complication may actually have a higher incidence for the third-generation machines characterized by tight focal zone and high-energy. Other ESWL-induced complications include, aortic aneurysms,[51-54] iliac vein thrombosis,[55] portal vein thrombosis,[56] scrotal bruising,[57-59] and stimulation of the obturator nerve.[60,61] In the early years of ESWL, it was recognized that shock waves could induce extrasystoles, thus, requiring electrocardiographic synchronization with R-wave triggering on the Dornier HM3 device.[42] More recent clinical studies, however, have concluded that ungating was safe and effective in allowing patients with an

abnormal cardiac rhythm to be treated with the same shock time as gated cases (normal cardiac rhythm).[62,63] This was probably a mistake, in that increasing the rate of ESWL delivery reduces the efficiency of stone breakage (see "Chapter 38, "The Physics of Shock Wave Physics Lithotripsy" and Chapter 40, "Treatment of Renal and Ureteral Calculi").

ACUTE RENAL INJURY: CLINICAL OBSERVATIONS
A clinical dose of shock waves induces a consistent and predicable pattern of acute structural changes in the treated kidney characterized primarily as a vascular insult with an acute inflammatory response. Gross hematuria always occurs (within the initial 200 to 300 shock waves, for the Dornier HM3), generally resolving within 12 hours[42,64] and occurs regardless of the type of lithotriptor employed. In fact, a lack of hematuria indicates a problem with shock wave delivery. The source of hematuria is direct injury to the renal parenchyma within the region of the focused shock wave.[65] Morphologic studies using both magnetic resonance imaging (MRI) and quantitative radionuclide renography or computed tomography (CT) have suggested that 63 to 85% of all ESWL patients exhibit one or more forms of renal injury within 24 hours of treatment,[19,30,64,66-71] values much larger than that reported by Chaussy and Schmidt.[21] These changes are not specific to any particular lithotriptor, in that numerous reports have now documented identical renal bioeffects induced by the second- and third-generation lithotriptors.[14-17,72,73]

Hemorrhage and edema within or around the kidney are the two most common renal side effects seen immediately after ESWL, causing the kidney to be enlarged (approximately 84%) and show a loss of corticomedullary demarcation (Figure 41-1).[19,64,68,74-77] Clinically significant perirenal and subcapsular fluid (blood and/or urine) (Figure 41-2) accumulation was initially determined to occur in less than 1% of lithotripsy treatments[19-23] except for the report by Ueda and colleagues,[17] where they detected a 4.1% hematoma rate. But these values rise to 32% of patients when screened by CT or MRI.[19,64,68,73] In addition, the newer generation lithotriptors that have very small focal areas and extremely high peak positive pressures are reporting higher clinically significant hematoma rates of 3 to

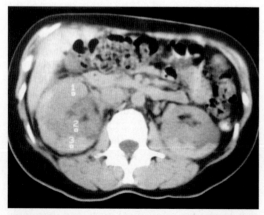

Figure 41-1 Magnetic resonance image of stone patient treated with extracorporeal shock wave lithotripsy demonstrating loss of corticomedullary junction demarcation in right kidney.

12%,[14–17,24] a trend that is worrisome. Dhar and colleagues reported new clinical results with a Storz Modulith showing that the probability of developing a subcapsular hematoma increased 2.2 times for every 10-year increase in patient age.[24] All of these new data suggest that the lithotriptor itself is now a risk factor for increased tissue injury. Hemorrhagic changes can range in severity from mild contusions localized within the renal parenchyma to large hematomas, which can be associated with severe bleeding requiring blood transfusions, arteriographic embolization, or percutaneous draining.[78] Such hemorrhage may produce a Page kidney with hypertension,[79–81] a state of acute renal failure,[82–87] may require a partial or total nephrectomy,[88–91] and may result in death if the condition is not identified early.[23] Rubin and associates, using CT scans, noted changes in the perirenal soft tissues consisting of an increase in the number of septal strands and a thickening of Gerota's fascia suggesting focal regions of edema.[68] Usually, the perirenal fluid disappears within a few days, while

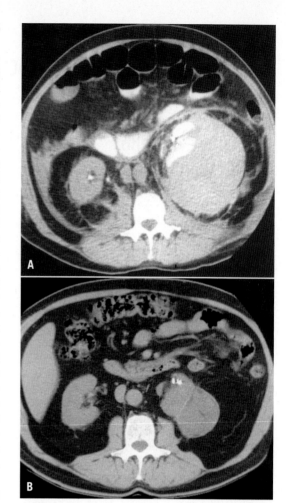

Figure 41-2 Computed tomography scan showing bilateral perinephric hematomas following bilateral simultaneous extracorporeal shock wave lithotripsy of a stone patient.

the subcapsular fluid or blood may take 6 weeks to 6 months (or more) to resolve (Figure 41-3).[19]

Acute histopathologic changes in the ESWL-treated kidney and surrounding tissues include dilation of veins with endothelial damage and thrombus formation, disruption of most renal corpuscles at F2, as well as milder degenerative changes in the nephron accompanied by hemosiderin granules and cast material.[92] Seitz and colleagues studied the kidneys from four patients treated with a piezoelectric lithotriptor and detected sites of intraparenchymal hemorrhage at the corticomedullary junction that increased in severity with increasing numbers of shocks (4,000 to 20,000).[93] They commented on how the gross and histologic appearance of these four ESWL-treated kidneys mirrored exactly the results published in animal studies. Human cadaver kidneys treated with a clinical dose always induced injury to nephrons and small to medium-sized blood vessels within F2.[94–96] Again, as the number of shock waves was increased so was the amount of damage detected. In addition, Roessler and colleagues determined the size of lesion induced by an electromagnetic versus an electrohydraulic lithotriptor and found a much larger lesion with the electrohydraulic machines.[96] This ex vivo model has numerous drawbacks, which prevents an investigator from drawing valid conclusions on the real extent of ESWL-induced damage and, therefore, should not be used.

ESWL-induced nephron injury has been assessed by detecting the spillage of tubular enzymes into the urine immediately after treatment.[31,72,97–103] The list of tubular enzymes found elevated after ESWL includes: N-acetyl-β-D-glucosaminidase (NAG), alkaline phosphatase and β-galactosidase as proximal tubular lysosomal enzymes, γ-glutamyltransaminase (GGT) and angiotensin-converting enzymes for brush border of proximal tubular cells, calbindin-D for distal tubular cells and β2-microglobulin as a small circulating protein that is freely filtered but almost completely reabsorbed in the proximal tubules. There appears to be great variation in the levels of these markers in stone patients when pre- and post-ESWL levels were compared,[104] and no attempt has been made to document the presence or absence of bilateral stone disease. Significant proteinuria has been documented immediately after ESWL, which resolved 3 to 6 months post-treatment without detectable changes in whole kidney glomerular filtration rate.[105] Others have reported transient microalbuminuria.[103,106] Transient increases in both prostaglandin E2 and thromboxane B2 levels have been noted in the urine and serum but they quickly return to baseline values.[107] Sarica and colleagues determined the plasma and urine levels of nitrite and adrenomedullin as markers of tubular and glomerular cell injury in stone formers and controls treated with lithotripsy.[108] Both markers were elevated in the plasma and urine of only the stone formers 24 hours post-ESWL and returned to normal at one week. Generally, in ESWL-treated adult patients, the enzyme

Figure 41-3 *A,* Computed tomography (CT) scan of a stone patient 48 hours after left extracorporeal shock wave lithotripsy (ESWL) for a 1 cm non-obstructive stone in the left renal pelvis. The patient received 1,000 shocks at 22 kV with an unmodified HM3 lithotriptor. *B,* Abdominal CT 8 years after ESWL demonstrating persistence of a smaller hematoma around the left kidney.

changes return to baseline in a week; in children, however, the functional regeneration time increases to two weeks.[109] Clearly, there are conflicting reports on this topic that can be explained, in part, by the great variation in the parameters of ESWL delivery and the lack of appropriate control groups. Despite these issues, the majority of observations on human stone formers suggest that all portions of the kidney and surrounding tissues are vulnerable to shock waves, with the microvasculature being the most susceptible, and that the amount of injury increases with shock number.

Acute changes in renal function have also been found immediately after ESWL treatment, as documented by specialized imaging techniques such as radionuclide studies using orthoiodohippurate to measure effective renal plasma flow (ERPF), creatinine clearance for glomerular filtration rate (GFR) and color Doppler ultrasound for a measure of change in the vasoconstriction of intrarenal blood vessels. While these techniques are relatively imprecise, there are reports of a significant reduction in ERPF and GFR between 24 and 48 hours post-ESWL. Kaude and colleagues, the first group to report ESWL-induced changes in renal function, found an immediate decrease in effective plasma flow, measured by renal scans, in 30% of kidneys treated with a clinical dose of ESWL (1,800 shock waves).[64] Several investigators have confirmed the decrease in ERPF[110-112] and/or a delay in—to complete loss of—contrast excretion in unobstructed ESWL-treated kidneys.[64,74] These studies are supported by the observations that there is an apparent transient reduction of intrarenal blood flow at F2.[113-116] While there are clearly studies that have not found functional changes,[110] these different observations appear to be linked to the number of shocks administered. Thomas and associates found that a treatment regimen of approximately 1,500 shocks was safe, but higher levels induced a fall in renal plasma flow.[117] Orestano and colleagues noted that fewer than 2,500 shocks produced changes in renal function that totally regressed by 30 days post-ESWL.[118] However, a dose of greater than 2,500 shocks induced more extensive changes in renal function (reduction in clearance, prolonged 131 I-Hippuran transit) in the treated kidney as well as in the contralateral kidney. Other investigators have also detected functional changes in both the treated and untreated kidneys.[111,119] Similar observations have been reported in the pig.[120,121] As stated earlier, acute renal failure has been reported in a few ESWL patients; in most instances, however, this condition has been reversible. The majority of the studies just described indicate that renal function is acutely affected by a clinical dose of shock waves. There are reports that ESWL can result in a significant improvement in renal function in some patients.[42] Many such patients, however, show evidence of ureteral obstruction prior to treatment, thereby biasing the functional changes (ie, increased clearance) in the direction of improvement.

In view of the adverse effects the ESWL treatment may have acutely on renal function, several investigators have attempted to protect the kidney from ESWL-induced injury. The protective effects of nifedipine and allopurinol on high-energy shock–wave-induced acute changes of renal function have been studied in 40 patients in a prospective randomized study, and the results indicated that nifedipine and/or allopurinol exhibits a protective effect on high-energy shock–wave-induced renal damage. [122] In their original two studies Strohmaier and colleagues aimed to outline the limitation of shock–wave-induced renal tubular dysfunction by nifedipine and verapamil in 24 patients with renal pelvic or caliceal stones undergoing anesthesia-free ESWL.[123,124] To assess renal tubular function, the urinary excretion of α_1-microglobulin (A1M), N-acetyl-β-glucosaminidase (NAG) and Tamm-Horsfall protein (THP) were measured before, immediately, 12 hours and 24 hours after ESWL. Their results indicated that nifedipine and verapamil exhibit a protective effect on shock–wave-induced tubular damage similar to verapamil. Chan and colleagues and Benyi and colleagues have shown that pretreatment with aminophylline, nifedipine or allopurinol also blocks the fall in renal blood flow induced by ESWL.[125,126]

The underlying mechanism(s) on how these drugs produce this effect is unclear; they may have a direct action on tubular cells or alter the effect that shockwaves have on the renal vasculature. A new study on pigs has shown that a pretreatment set of 100 to 500 shock waves administered at a low kilovolt level can greatly reduce a predicted lesion induced from a subsequent delivery of a clinical dose of shock waves.[127] These findings and the application to a clinical setting are discussed later in this chapter.

CHRONIC RENAL INJURY: CLINICAL OBSERVATIONS Although little information exists to date on the possible chronic renal changes after ESWL,[3,7,25,26,128] potential long-term adverse effects are still emerging but include an accelerated rise in systemic blood pressure, a decrease in renal function, onset of hypertension, an increase in the rate of stone recurrence, diabetes mellitus and the development of brushite stone disease. All of these effects appear to be linked to the observation that the acute injury usually progresses to scar formation with time and is accompanied by a loss of functional tissue and blood vessels. Lechevallier and colleagues performed pre- and post-ESWL (30 days) single photon emission computed tomography (SPECT) studies in 12 patients treated with a piezoelectric lithotriptor.[129] All ESWL-treated kidneys showed some loss of renal function, with 4 of the 12 kidneys showing a loss of local tracer uptake of greater than 4%. In addition, there were sevem scars in the region of F2. Umekawa and colleagues examined a kidney of a patient in acute renal failure that occurred 90 days post-ESWL treatment and found evidence of anti-glomerular basement membrane production in glomeruli at F2.[130]

The possibility that ESWL treatment might be associated with a long-term reduction in renal function has been suggested by several investigators. Williams and Thomas found a significant decrease in the percentage of effective renal plasma flow 17 to 21 months after ESWL for patients with two kidneys.[131] Orestano and colleagues noted that patients receiving more than 2,500 shocks had a reduction in clearance and a prolongation of 131 I-Hippuran transit time at 30 days post-ESWL in the treated kidney and occasionally in the contralateral kidney.[118] Brito and colleagues reported that patients with a solitary kidney showed elevated serum creatinine levels five years post-ESWL.[132] These observations stand in contrast to the early reports by Chaussy, suggesting a significant increase in renal function three months to one year following ESWL.[42] In addition, a longer-term follow-up study of patients treated in Munich failed to confirm this increase in renal function[133] as did other studies that looked at patients who received bilateral treatment[134] and those who received unilateral treatment.[135]

There has been increasing concern and controversy over the association between ESWL and the development of hypertension. Peterson and Finlayson were the first investigators to suggest the possibility that ESWL might be associated

with significant changes in systemic blood pressure.[136] Subsequently, Lingeman and colleagues reported that 8.2% of 243 patients who were normotensive at the time of ESWL developed blood pressure changes requiring antihypertensive medication.[137] Mean follow-up in this group of patients was 1.5 years, giving an annualized incidence of hypertension of 5.5%. Similar data have been reported by Williams and Thomas.[131]

While this initial association between hypertension and ESWL may be alarming, not all data support the connection,[133,138-141] and it has been suggested that stone patients have a higher incidence of hypertension to start with.[142,143] Montgomery and associates retrospectively reviewed patients following ESWL on the HM3 and determined the rate of hypertension to be 8.1%; but the hypertension developed de novo in only 2.9%.[139] Yokoyama and associates retrospectively reviewed patients treated with the HM3 for either renal or ureteral calculi and determined an annualized incidence of new-onset hypertension to be 0.65%.[144] There was, however, a statistically significant annualized increase in diastolic blood pressure (DBP) (0.78 mm Hg). They suggested that a dose-response relationship might exist between blood pressure changes and shockwave energy administered. Claro and associates retrospectively reviewed blood pressure data from patients treated on a Lithostar lithotriptor and found that DBP was statistically higher after treatment, but the incidence of hypertension was not significant.[140] All of these studies suffer from being retrospective in nature. Interestingly, in a small prospective study by Zanetti and colleagues following blood pressure changes in patients treated with an HM3, no significant increase in DBP was noted, although the incidence of new-onset hypertension was 6%.[141]

In an attempt to further elucidate the long-term association between ESWL and hypertension, Lingeman and associates retrospectively surveyed 961 stone patients treated at Methodist Hospital of Indiana for stone disease.[145] Eighty percent of the study group received therapy that exposed them to ESWL. The remainder of the patients were treated with percutaneous surgery or ureteroscopy and consequently were not exposed to shock waves and served as controls. Follow-up blood pressures were measured with random-zero devices at least one year following treatment. In patients treated with ESWL, the annualized incidence of hypertension (2.4%) did not differ significantly from that in control patients (4.0%). Moreover, in those patients exposed to ESWL, there was no correlation between the incidence of hypertension and the laterality of treatments, the number of shock waves administered, the voltage applied, or the power index. There was, however, a statistically significant rise in DBP after treatment with ESWL (0.78 mm Hg) that was not present in the control group (–0.88 mm Hg). These data were remarkably similar to findings reported by Yokoyama and colleagues.[144] As an extension of this survey, a second set of follow-up blood pressure measurements was conducted approximately 4 years after treatment in 749 patients (77.9%). The annualized incidence of new onset hypertension in ESWL patients was 2.1% compared to 1.6% in non-ESWL patients (not significant). A statistically significant difference in the annualized mean DBP was identified and was notably higher in the ESWL-treated patients compared to the non-ESWL patients at all time intervals following treatment. This change in blood pressure remains statistically significant even after controlling for other statistically significant risk factors such as pretreatment blood pressure, patient gender and patient age, as well as various treatment factors such as years since treatment, direct shock wave exposure to the kidney, and multiple shock wave sessions. Although exposure to shock waves was associated with a small but statistically significant rise in DBP up to 4 years following treatment, there was a trend of DBP back toward baseline during later follow-up.

A recent study from the Mayo Clinic reported on a retrospective chart review of 687 SWL treatments in 630 kidney stone patients over a 19-year period.[7] The pthe SWL and control groups with the SWL groups more likely to have hypertension. The new-onset hypertension was not related to the total number of shock waves, average intensity or total intensity but with bilateral treatment.

A prospective study has addressed the issue of hypertension as a possible long-term complication of ESWL therapy.[6,115,146] A group of investigators from the University of Innsbruck, Austria, calculated the intrarenal resistive index in 76 patients treated with a Dornier MFL 5000 lithotriptor. In 15 of 20 patients over 60 years of age, the resistive index was higher than the upper limit of normal immediately following ESWL in the treated kidney but not in the untreated kidney. At 26 months of follow-up in these patients, the resistive index continued to increase in all nine patients who developed hypertension and a strong positive correlation (0.903) between the pathological resistive index levels and blood pressure was found. With one exception, an elevated resistive index and hypertension were observed exclusively in patients older than 60 years. No significant change in plasma rennin activity was observed in the four patients with new-onset arterial hypertension whose values were available because their blood pressures were not normalized with diuretics or angiotensin-converting enzyme inhibitors. Moreover, their rennin levels were not different from the values observed in five normotensive patients. Because in the condition of hypertension mediated by vascular disturbances originating in the kidney one would expect rennin values to be high, this result is surprising and raises speculations about the importance of local tissue activation of the rennin-angiotensin system or the release of another vasoactive peptide such as endothelin.

Therefore, age is probably a risk factor of new-onset hypertension due to ESWL. Resistive index has never been taken into account in previous studies, which may explain the lack of clear evidence that hypertension in elderly patients can

be a chronic complication of ESWL therapy. What is not known at this time is the future health risk for these patients or who is at risk. Clearly there are studies that have found no change in blood pressure after ESWL.[26,138] The long-term effects of hypertension, if it is occurring, include an increased risk of stroke, myocardial infarction, and renal failure. Therefore, any therapy that might increase the incidence of hypertension should be rigorously examined.

Other groups have focused on determining if kidney stone patients have a greater risk for a loss of renal function, as detected by a change in creatinine clearance,[147] or GFR.[148] Such a change in renal function would suggest that stone patients have a kidney disease as the result of specific alterations in their kidneys. These data indicate that there is a significant interaction between the GFR value and the body mass index (BMI) level. In other words, if a stone patient had a BMI level greater than 27 kg/m^2, there was a significant association between a history of renal stones and a lower GFR value. If these data hold up, one must be concerned with any stone removal technique that would cause additional loss of renal mass in this subset of stone patients.

The recent Mayo Clinic study also detected the development of diabetes mellitus in 16.8% of the SWL-treated stone patients. The diabetes mellitus was related to the number of administered shock waves and treatment intensity. The authors suggested that the diabetes mellitus could be a result of damage to pancreatic islet cells, because a portion of the pancreas was probably located within the blast path of the HM3 machine.

An additional concern has been raised suggesting that stone recurrence rates may be higher following ESWL because of residual stone debris forced into the lining of the renal pelvis.[149] A recent study by Carr and colleagues documented all new stone formation in 298 consecutive patients who initially were determined to be stone-free after ESWL and compared those findings to 62 patients treated with percutaneous nephrolithotomy.[150] Their data showed a significant increase ($p = .004$) in the rate of new stone formation within one year of ESWL treatment compared to percutaneous nephrolithotomy. Furthermore, the location of the new stones changed from their original treatment site to the calices. The authors suggested that fine sand debris generated from ESWL treatment remained in the kidney, and gravity acted to position them as a nidus of the caliceal system.

Lastly, our group has determined that there has been a significant rise in the number of calcium phosphate (CaP) stone formers over the last three decades,[151] an observation supported by others.[152] An intriguing finding (noted when all kidney stone formers were analyzed for the number of ESWL procedures) was that the CaP stone formers had received a significantly higher number of procedures than the idiopathic calcium oxalate stone formers when adjusted for number of stones and duration of stone disease. Furthermore, the brushite stone formers had received a

significantly higher number of ESWL treatments than the apatite stone formers. The histopathology of the brushite stone formers revealed advanced levels of tissue changes in the renal cortex and papilla that included interstitial fibrosis, tubular atrophy, glomerular obsolescence, and deposition of large amounts of hydroxyapatite in the lumens of inner medullary collection ducts.[153] While these data do not establish a cause-and-effect relationship, clearly there is an association between brushite stone disease and high levels of ESWL treatment sessions. Because we believe that apatite stone disease is primarily related to higher urinary pH levels in these patients, the animal studies showing the initial site of ESWL injury to be localized to the microvessels and collecting duct of the renal papilla might explain a loss of control over normal urinary fluid pH at this level.

RISK FACTORS Risk factors may predispose ESWL patients to increased acute renal injury. Knapp and associates found stone patients with existing hypertension to be at increased risk for the development of perinephric hematomas as a consequence of ESWL.[19] In particular, those patients having unsatisfactory control of their hypertension at the time of ESWL had the highest incidence of hematomas. Dhar and colleagues reported new clinical results with a Storz Modulith showing that the probability of developing a subcapsular hematoma increased 2.2 times for every 10-year increase in patient age.[24] Additional risk factors included increased thromboplastin time and the use of aspirin[154] (even when discontinued up to two weeks prior to treatment), again not agreed on by all groups.[155] When the power setting and number of shock waves administered were evaluated as potential risk factors, no correlation was found with the occurrence of hematomas. Newman and Saltzman confirmed these observations.[22] They noted that patients with coagulopathies and thrombocytopenia were at greater risk of developing a subcapsular hematoma. Additional risk factors identified for increased incidence of hemorrhage were diabetes mellitus, coronary artery disease, and obesity, all suggesting a link to a vascular disorder. In relation to risk factors, an interesting observation is that some patients with preexisting hypertension require higher doses of their blood pressure medication following ESWL therapy.[64] This suggests that preexisting hypertension is a potential risk factor for adverse acute effects of ESWL. In a study of solitary kidneys, Karlsen and Berg reported a significant reduction in GFR three months following ESWL.[110]

Age is a factor on both ends of the scale; children and the elderly appear to be at a greater risk for structural and functional changes following exposure to ESWL.[6,156] The concern for children is that the smaller size of their growing kidneys to the fixed size of the focal area will always damage a greater proportion of their functional renal mass compared to the large adult kidney and the fixed size of the focal area. Although pediatric

ESWL is thought to be clinically well-tolerated and is reported to be associated with few adverse effects, there are only a few studies with a small number of patients that have addressed the issue of possible long-term complications.[157–166] Adams and colleagues reported the results of ESWL in a group of 44 pediatric patients and noted normal renal growth in 14 treated renal units after a mean follow-up time of 23 months.[157] That initial study was followed up by a longer-term study (mean 9 years) on 29 patients where actual and predicted renal growth rates were compared.[156] The treated kidneys were stratified into normal and abnormal groups based on a history of renal surgery, evidence of recurrent infections and obvious anatomic abnormalities. Fifty-six upper urinary tract calculi were treated in 34 renal units. Twenty-two renal units were rendered stone-free and 65% of the patients continued to be stone-free. At follow-up, one patient was classified as having new-onset hypertension, and the mean serum creatinine was 0.93 ± 0.08 mg/dL. At treatment, the abnormal group of kidneys seemed to be smaller than expected (mean $Z -1.30 \pm 1.10$), whereas the group of normal kidneys was very close (mean $Z\ 0.18 \pm 0.54$) to the predicted mean. At follow-up, the deviations between actual and predicted renal length were significantly more negative. Although there was a trend toward the abnormal group having smaller kidneys than the normal group, both groups showed the same trend toward an age-adjusted reduction in renal growth at follow-up. The alterations in renal growth patterns observed in this population are unsettling and could be secondary to treatment effect (ie, ESWL) or, more likely, to some underlying pathology intrinsic to pediatric kidneys with urolithiasis. The results of this clinical study and the observations from several studies on immature and juvenile animals[59,167,168] must still caution us about the potential for long-term complications in children treated by ESWL. Until further data are available, ESWL in the pediatric population should be applied with caution and at the lowest dosage sufficient to achieve stone breakage.

In addition to the list of risk factors described above that relate to conditions the patient brings to ESWL treatment, another set of factors is linked to the parameters of treatment. These factors include the discharge voltage, number of total shock waves administered, rate of shock wave delivery, and type of lithotripsy. Most of these data have been collected in animals so will be discussed below. The issues of increased side effects induced by the third-generation machines have already been cited above.

Acute renal injury may be an important consequence of ESWL, but a number of questions still need to be addressed that will require continual investigation. It is not known if renal function is altered in all ESWL patients, or if only a subset of patients is at risk. It is not known if patients with two kidneys tolerate ESWL therapy better than those with one kidney. Importantly, numerous data suggest that risk factors may predispose

the ESWL patient to acute renal injury, although such factors have yet to be fully defined.

ACUTE RENAL INJURY: EXPERIMENTAL STUDIES

In contrast to the early misperception within the medical/scientific community that ESWL does not produce injury[42] subsequent animal studies have clearly demonstrated structural and functional changes in various organs,[3,25,26,120,121,127,169–189] particularly the kidney, after shock wave administration, and that these changes correlate well with side effects observed in ESWL patients. Investigators have used a variety of animals that include the rat,[42,188,189] the rabbit,[185–187] the dog,[169–171,173,175–178] and the pig.[3,25,26,65,120,121,127,175,180–182,184] Clearly, the pig is the most appropriate animal model for these studies (Figure 41-4).[3,26,65]

Macroscopically, the acute changes noted in dog and pig kidneys treated with a clinical dose of shock waves are strikingly similar to those described for ESWL patients. The lesion is predictable in size, focal in location, and unique in the types of injuries (primarily vascular insult) induced. These changes include hematuria, contusion-like lesions, subcapsular hematomas, hemorrhage, and kidney enlargement. Hemorrhage has been found in three general locations: perirenal, subcapsular, and intraparenchymal (but always at or near F2). The perirenal fat is a common site of extensive hemorrhage. Subcapsular hemorrhage is found to spread diffusely along the length of the capsule and/or form discrete hematomas (Figure 41-5). Sites of intraparenchymal hemorrhage are generally wedged-shaped being most severe at the corticomedullary junction, and extend from the papillary tip to the capsule. It has been our observation that the initial sites of damage always occur in the renal papilla involving injury to the wall of vasa recta and

nearby collecting ducts.[180] Hematomas localized within the renal parenchyma or subcapsular zone range in size, from very small to 0.5 cm in diameter,[171–177] and in number, from 1 to 10 per kidney. Our group has quantitated the hemorrhagic lesion and found it to be about 2% of the functional mass in an adult pig treated with an unmodified HM3, 2,000 shocks at 24 kV.[120,121] Larger hematomas appear to compress the adjacent tissue. Interstitial edema is also common. The diffuse nature of this change would appear to account for enlargement of the kidney.

Histologic analysis has shown that the regions of hemorrhage are always near the site of F2 (Figure 41-6).[3,26,65,167–170,180,187] These regions of damage reveal rupture of nearby thin-walled veins, walls of small arteries, glomerular and peritubular capillaries, which correlate with the vasoconstriction measured in both the treated and untreated kidneys.[120,121] Venous thrombi are frequently associated with interlobular and arcuate veins located at the sites of hemorrhage. Evidence of extensive endothelial damage in these veins is noted by a loss of endothelial cells and the immediate attachment of numerous polymorphonuclear (PMN) cells and activated platelets to the luminal surface of these vessels depicting a vasculitis (Figure 41-7).[3,180] Nephrons located near areas of massive hemorrhage show evidence of damage. These alterations consist of vacuolar changes in individual cells, tubular dilation, cast formation (hyaline-like, RBCs) and mild tubular necrosis.[3,4,169,171,172,182] These observations show that both the microvasculature and nephron are susceptible to shock wave damage; the primary injury, however, appears to be a vascular insult.

Of great interest are those experimental animal studies that have determined factors of ESWL administration that appear to influence the degree of renal trauma induced by shock

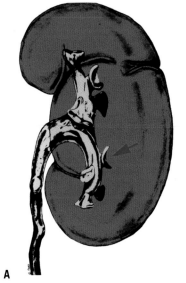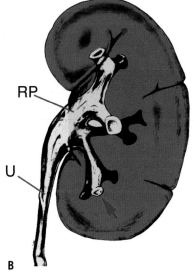

Figure 41-4 *A*, Drawing of the collection system of a human kidney. *B*, Drawing of the collection system of a pig kidney. Both the human and pig kidney are multi-papillary and may show considerable variability in the form of the collecting system. Generally, the human kidney has a greater number of minor calyces (*arrows*) than the pig, with longer calyceal stems and a larger renal pelvis (RP). U = ureter.

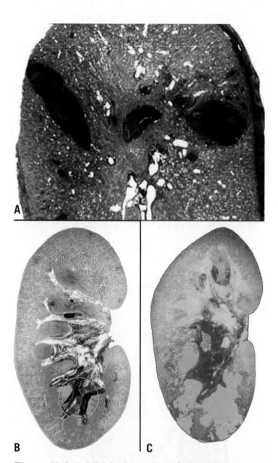

Figure 41-5 Magnetic resonance image of a pig kidney treated with 2,000 shocks at 24 kV with an unmodified HM3 lithotriptor demonstrating a large subcapsular hematoma much like that seen in Figure 41-3A.

Figure 41-6 *A*, Histologic section of pig kidney treated with 2,000 shocks at 24 kV with unmodified HM3. This kidney shows sites of parenchymal hemorrhage extending from the renal papilla to the capsule. *B*, Digitized image of a pig kidney treated with 2,000 shocks at 24 kV or *C*, with 8,000 shocks at 24 kV and then processed, sectioned and captured by digital camera. The hemorrhagic lesion (colored light blue in *B* and *C*) seen in both the 2,000 and 8,000 shocked kidney was selectively segmented by a color range identifier for blood so that the area of the lesion could be determined for all serial sections. The site of F2 is signified by an *open circle*.

waves.[120,121,171–174,180,181,185] Delius and colleagues[171] and Willis and colleagues[121,183] have noted that, as shock number is increased (1,000 to 8,000 shocks), a greater number of hematomas are formed, and lesion size increases, but not as a direct correlation with shock number (Figure 41-8). The higher shock number was also associated with larger hematomas. This is related to the fact that larger arteries are injured at high shock numbers.[3] Delius and colleagues have also shown that more massive hemorrhage and tubular damage are induced by increasing the rate (1 shock/second to 100 shocks/second) at which the shocks are administered and by administering the shock waves in pairs.[171–174] Kidney size is clearly a risk factor for increased intraparenchymal hemorrhage, in that lesion size is 6% in a juvenile pig versus 2% in an adult pig (Figure 41-9).[4,120,121,183,184] In addition, Evan and colleagues noted that the degree of injury induced by a clinical dose of ESWL is potentiated by a preexisting condition like acute pyelonephritis.[181] Under such conditions, a 2,000-shock dose acts as an 8,000-shock dose. Lastly, the degree of renal injury has been linked to the type of shock wave generator used.[176,185] But these data are difficult to compare in that the parameters for shock wave delivery are so varied between instruments. Hypertension has been noted as a risk factor in animals treated with ESWL. A significant increase in post-ESWL arterial blood pressure was found in immature white rabbits.[167] Weber and colleagues tested the hypothesis that ESWL treatment induces hypertension.[188] They treated F1-hybrids of spontaneously hypertensive rats (rats with borderline hypertension) and normal Wistar rats with a clinical dose of shock wave and determined their blood pressure post-ESWL therapy. ESWL-induced hypertension in only the F1-hybrids indicated a potential risk factor for shock–wave-induced hypertension in genetically predisposed patients.

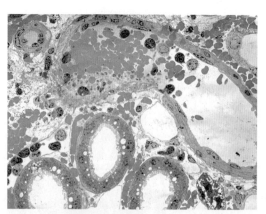

Figure 41-7 Transmission electron micrograph showing extracorporeal shock wave lithotripsy-induced vascular injury. This low-magnification image shows a damaged intermediate-sized artery from a pig kidney 1 hour after treatment with 2,000 shocks at 24 kV with an unmodified HM3 lithotriptor. The left side of the vessel shows extensive injury to the endothelium and smooth muscle cells of the vessel wall permitting the extravasation of blood into the underlying interstitial space. Numerous polymorphonuclear neutrophils and other leukocytes have migrated to the site of injury.

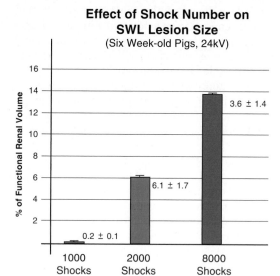

Effect of Shock Number on SWL Lesion Size
(Six Week-old Pigs, 24kV)

Figure 41-8 Effects of 1,000, 2,000 and 8,000 shocks at 24 kV with an unmodified HM3 lithotriptor on lesion size. Data are expressed as mean ± SEM. *N* indicates the number of individual kidneys sectioned and quantified in each group. *$p < .05$.

An obvious void in the experimental ESWL literature has been studies that documented changes in renal function after shock wave administration. Two early studies were done in dogs.[190,191] Jaeger and Constantinides reported a significant decrease in creatinine clearance and an elevation of glucose excretion one-hour post-ESWL in dogs treated with 3,000 shocks (1,500 shocks per pole of kidney).[191] Both values returned to normal by 24 hours post-ESWL. They also noted an increase in serum glutamic-oxaloacetic transaminase and glutamic-pyruvic transaminase levels at one-hour post-ESWL. The study by Karlsen and colleagues found an increase in urinary osmolality and urine flow while renal plasma flow was reduced about one-third at 2 hours post-ESWL in dogs treated with 1,500 at 18 kV.[190] These authors found no change in glomerular filtration rate or urinary electrolyte excretion. A series of experiments by Willis and colleagues[120,121,183,184] expanded these observations to include bilateral kidney function in the pig. These studies show that the application of 2,000 shocks at 24 kV with an unmodified Dornier HM3 lithotriptor to one kidney consistently reduces renal blood flow (RBF) and GFR in that kidney (Figure 41-10). At 1 hour post-ESWL, the fall in RBF was 27% for the young adult animals and 50% in the juvenile pigs. By 4 hours post-ESWL, RBF returned to baseline in the young adult pigs but was still significantly reduced in the juvenile pigs. GFR followed a similar course but was reduced to a lesser extent than RBF measurements. In addition, these studies found a significant reduction in RBF in the untreated kidney at the 1-hour post-ESWL time point. These investigators also measured tubular function using *p*-aminohippurate extraction and found a significant reduction in the treated kidney but no fall in the untreated kidney. Again, the greatest reduction occurred in the juvenile pig

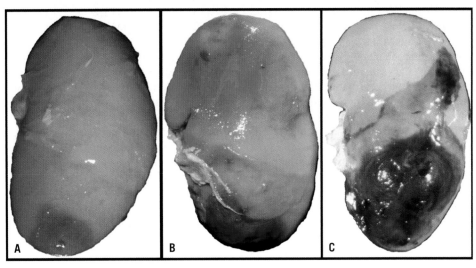

Figure 41-9 Gross appearance of pig kidneys treated with 2,000 shocks at 12 (A), 18 (B), and 24 (C) kV with an unmodified HM3. Note that the size of the subcapsular hematoma increases with increasing kV level.

found a direct correlation between the number of shock waves and the size of the resulting scar.[198] As the number of shocks was increased from 1,000 to 2,000, the size of the scar increased from 1.37% to 12.76%. In addition, Banner and colleagues have noted mesangioproliferative glomerulopathy in pigs treated with either the HM3 or the EDAP lithotriptor.[199] With time, deposits of complement C3 and traces of immunoglobulin G (IgG) were found to increase in amount in the mesangium. Interestingly, these changes were noted to occur in both the treated and the untreated (contralateral) kidney to about the same degree, suggesting the induction of a systemic factor or bilateral injury induced by ESWL. Delius and associates reported that most of these renal alterations were reversible in sev-

compared to the young adult pig. These results show that the major change in renal function is vasoconstriction, and kidney size is indeed a risk factor for increased side effects. Willis and colleagues[120,121,183] have found that high shock numbers (8,000 shocks) do not generate a greater decrease in RBF at 1 hour post-ESWL, but induce a sustained reduction noted at 24 hours post-treatment. Connors and colleagues evaluated the effect of kilovolt level of both RBF and lesion size and found lesion size to clearly increase as the kilovolt level was increased from 12 to 24 kV.[180] But the maximal vasoconstrictive response was already induced at the 12 kV level and remained there regardless of the kilovolt level used. These studies point out the sensitivity of the renal vasculature to shock wave lithotripsy. Elegant studies by Brendel and colleagues have shown, by video microscopy, that when shock waves are directed at a simple microvascular bed, acute spasms of arterioles and hemorrhage of venules are induced.[168] Vasoconstriction begins within and reaches its maximum after 20 to 30 seconds, lasting between 4 to 10 minutes. Dilation follows the constrictive event. Along with the sites of microhemorrhage in the small veins are areas showing leakage of macromolecules, and platelet aggregation. These authors also suggested that vasoconstriction was most pronounced in the region of peak pressure generated by the shock wave. Studies are needed that would directly correlate the physical characteristics of the shock wave with tissue damage.

Our group has uncovered a practical way to protect the treated kidney from the predicted lesion induced by a clinical dose of shock waves.[127] Prior to giving a clinical dose of 2,000 shocks at 2 kV with an unmodified HM3 to the lower pole of a kidney, a pre-treatment dose of 100 to 500 shock waves at 12 kV is administered, followed by the full clinical dose to the same site. Under those conditions, the normal lesion of about 6% is reduced to about 0.3%, a highly significant change (Figure 41-11). Our present thinking about the possible

mechanism of this outcome is that the pre-dose of shock waves induces a significant vasoconstrictive event that could prevent an incoming stress from shearing the vessel wall or perhaps prevent/reduce the number of cavitation events. A reduction in cavitation would potentially protect the parenchyma from cavitation-induced injury. A clinical trial is needed to test this result in stone patients.

Investigators have suggested that the vascular injury might induce an ischemic injury to the already damaged tissue.[3,26,182,187] Thus, Cohen and colleagues[192] and Brown and colleagues[193] determined in the pig that a clinical dose of shock-waves induces lipid peroxidation and free radical formation in the treated kidney. The concern for ischemic changes is for both the treated and untreated kidney, in that ESWL induces a vasoconstrictive response in both kidneys.[4,120,121] Delvecchio and colleagues recently determined a dose-related increase in conjugated diene ratio levels from the pole of the treated kidney[194] and, to a lesser degree, from the untreated kidney—a result consistent with the data from Willis and colleagues.[120] Animal models have also been used to investigate protective agents against shock–wave-induced renal injury. Verapamil[184,195–197] and antioxidant vitamins (E plus C)[58] can significantly reduce shock–wave-induced renal injury.

CHRONIC RENAL INJURY: EXPERIMENTAL OBSERVATIONS Chronic changes in renal structure after shock wave treatment have received minimal investigation. At two weeks post-ESWL, Jaeger and Constantinides noted calcium deposits, streaky fibrosis, and encapsulation of sites of acute hemorrhage.[191] Newman and coworkers identified permanent morphological changes in the dog kidney 30 days after ESWL treatment.[175] These alterations consisted of diffuse interstitial fibrosis, focal areas of calcification, nephron loss, dilated veins, and hyalinized to acellular scars running from the cortex to the medulla (Figure 41-12). Morris and colleagues

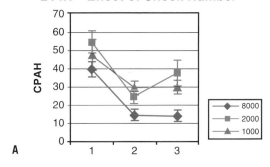

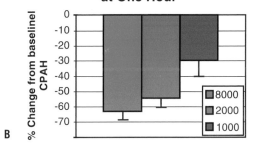

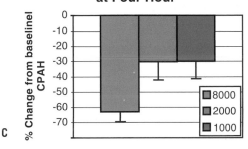

Figure 41-10 *p*-Aminohippurate clearance in treated pig kidney after 1 and 4 hours post-extracorporeal shock wave lithotripsy (ESWL) treatment with 2,000 shocks at 24kV. *A*, All three dosage levels induce a significant fall in *p*-aminohippurate clearance at one hours post-ESWL. *B*, The 8,000 shock treatment induced a greater fall in *p*-aminohippurate clearance compared to the 1,000 shock dose. *C*, At four hours post-ESWL, the 1,000 and 2,000 shock dose show similar changes while the 8,000 shock dose shows a persistent reduction in *p*-aminohippurate clearance.

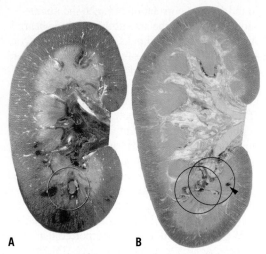

A   **B**

Figure 41-11 *A*, Digitized image of a pig kidney treated with 2,000 shocks at 24 kV. *B*, Digitized image of a pig kidney treated with 500 shocks at 12 kV followed immediately with 2,000 shocks at 24 kV to the same pole. This pre-treatment protocol protects the kidney from the predicted lesion induced by 2,000 shocks at 24 kV. *Arrowhead* shows the only site of hemorrhage in the kidney that received the pretreatment protocol. The sites of F2 are signified by an *open circle*.

eral weeks except for some of the large hematomas.[171] These observations suggest that the acute changes induced in the kidney can be classified as either reversible or irreversible; but a clinical dose of ESWL always induces irreversible injury that ends as a region of scar. In contrast to these studies, Chaussy reported no

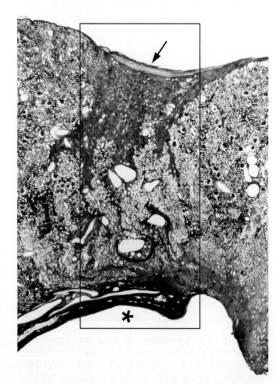

Figure 41-12 Histologic section from a pig kidney treated with 2,000 shocks at 24 kV in an unmodified HM3. The acute injury induced at the site of F2 (seen within *rectangle*) resulted in a scar that extends from the renal capsule (*arrow*) to the renal medulla. The renal papilla is no longer present, being reduced to scar tissue (*asterisk*).

histologic abnormalities in the dog kidney up to 1 year post-ESWL.[42]

Only a few studies have attempted to determine the chronic changes in renal function induced by ESWL. Neal and colleagues treated infant adult rhesus monkeys with 1,500 shocks at 15 kV or 2,000 shocks at 18 kV to each kidney, while adult animals were treated with 2,000 shocks at 18 kV to each kidney.[168] A highly significant decrease in effective renal plasma flow was noted in the infant group 6 months post-treatment when those values were indexed to body surface area. In another study, immature rabbits receiving 1,000 to 2,000 shocks developed a significant rise in mean arterial blood pressure at 4 and 8 weeks post-ESWL compared to controls.[200] Pre-treatment of these animals with either allopurinol or mannitol prevented the development of hypertension. Both of these studies suggest strongly that there can be long-term functional consequences to a clinical dose of ESWL and that the young or immature are a great risk for such complications.

The mechanism for the traumatic effects of ESWL is not known; Delius and colleagues, however, have speculated that cavitation bubbles generated by the shock waves are primarily responsible for the cellular changes.[171] This idea is based on data showing the presence of cavitation bubbles in the liver during shock wave application, and that lithotriptor shock wave can cavitate water and blood in vitro.[201,202] Crum[203] documented that ESWL does produce acoustic cavitation, possibly as the result of the high intensity of the shock wave amplitude. He noted that cavitation microjets are sufficiently forceful to pit or deform metal test foils. But acoustic cavitation has only been detected in the parenchyma of the treated kidney after 1,000 shock waves and at a time when pooling of fluid within the tissue or at the capsule was noted.[204] Of interest are the animal studies that employed a Styrofoam insert into the brass reflector of an unmodified HM3 lithotriptor.[205] Neither lesion nor renal functional changes were seen in these kidneys, compared to our usual result with a clinical dose using the unmodified HM3.[120] This insert had been shown to reverse the normal pressure wave so that the negative tail precedes the positive portion of the wave.[206] Cavitation activity is greatly reduced and so is the renal parenchymal lesion. It is tempting to link the reduction in cavitation activity with the smaller lesion. But there is still another potential mechanism for tissue injury: shear stress. Lokhandwalla and Sturtevant showed by computation that shock waves are capable of causing cell rupture by inducing unsteady flows (shear waves) in the surrounding media.[207] Subsequent experimental studies using overpressure to eliminate cavitation and a parabolic reflector to refocus the wave field within the sample vial showed that, even in the absence of cavitation, shock waves could deform foils, and that cell lysis was significantly enhanced by shock wave focusing.[208] This gives validation to shear as a damage mechanism.

PROBLEMS RELATED TO STONE FRAGMENTS

Much of the morbidity associated with ESWL results when stone fragments fail to pass out of the ureter after lithotripsy. This may be caused by poor fragmentation, so that larger stone pieces pass and obstruct the ureter, or a stone that is finely disintegrated may pass down the ureter, resulting in a column of sand—Steinstrasse ("street of stone")—that may obstruct the kidney (Figure 41-13). This occurs in less than 10% of patients.[209] Several factors are responsible for the degree of fragmentation after lithotripsy. The nature of the stone burden treated may affect how successfully a stone is fragmented by ESWL. The risk of Steinstrasse increases with larger stone burdens—in one study of 885 patients, it occurred in 0.3% of stones less than 10 mm, 7% of stones between 10 and 20 mm, and 11.5% of stones between 20 and 30 mm.[210] In a series of 4,634 patients, multivariable analysis showed stone size > 20 mm to be an independent predictor of Steinstrasse, with a 3.7-fold increase in risk compared to smaller stones.[211] Larger calculi fracture less completely, and more often require additional treatment. The stone composition will also affect the degree of fragmentation. Struvite, uric acid, and calcium oxalate dihydrate calculi fracture into small particles that can pass relatively easily. On the other hand, calculi of calcium phosphate dihydrate (brushite) and calcium oxalate monohydrate tend to break up into larger pieces that are more difficult to pass.[212] Cystine calculi are especially difficult to treat with lithotripsy since, as an organic compound, cystine has acoustic properties that do not differ greatly from those of the surrounding tissues.[213] Recognition that stone size and composition can affect the degree of fragmentation, and, therefore, treatment outcome can help urologists determine which modality is best. Other important factors

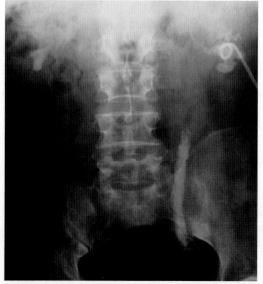

Figure 41-13 Complex Steinstrasse following treatment of a large staghorn calculus by extracorporeal shock wave lithotripsy.

include stone location, the type of lithotriptor used, and the power index (number of shocks and generator voltage). Lingeman noted that multiple ESWL treatments are more likely to be required when stones are located in the lower pole.[214]

Most Steinstrasse are short and will pass with only mild discomfort. Longer Steinstrasse are more troublesome (see Figure 41-13). Steinstrasse can produce a variety of symptoms or a patient may be completely asymptomatic. Renal colic will occur in almost a third of patients treated with the Dornier HM-3 lithotriptor[28] and occurs in almost all patients with Steinstrasse.[215] To identify silent obstruction, the urologist must follow up with plain abdominal films, ultrasound, and/or an intravenous pyelogram 4 to 6 weeks after ESWL.[216]

Steinstrasse is best managed by averting the problem if possible before ESWL is performed. Placement of an indwelling ureteral stent in kidneys with moderate stone burden (aggregate stone diameter 0.25 mm) before ESWL can significantly reduce the incidence of symptomatic Steinstrasse.[217] The theoretic advantage of using ureteral stents with ESWL is that they may allow continued passage of urine and gravel. Initially, small particles pass around the stent. With time, the ureter dilates, and after stent removal, larger fragments pass through the distended ureter.[218] Fine and colleagues noted that, during fluoroscopic examinations, ureteral stents allowed urine reflux from the bladder to the kidney.[219] They proposed that this initiates ureteral peristalsis, propelling urine and gravel into the bladder.

The use of ureteral stents is not without problems, however. Bregg and Riehle found that a third of lithotripsy patients with indwelling stents had moderate discomfort that was not associated with stent material, size, or location.[220] Of their patients, nearly half complained of severe to intolerable pain that was relieved after stent removal. They also noted obstruction caused by the stent itself. In another study of ureteral stents and ESWL, symptoms from the stents often led to the necessity for early stent removal.[221]

In general, stones 0.3 cm are best managed percutaneously; if ESWL is performed, however, the incidence of Steinstrasse is lowered if ureters are stented prior to treatment.[222] Overall, morbidity is reduced when stents are placed prior to ESWL therapy of larger stones.[217] Smaller calculi less frequently result in significant Steinstrasse.[223] Moreover, stents do not decrease the incidence of Steinstrasse following lithotripsy of small to moderately sized stones.[224] Consequently, small calculi rarely require ureteral stenting.

One must weigh the benefits, risks, and costs associated with ureteral stents that are placed before ESWL. The routine use of ureteral stents is generally not indicated because fragments from smaller stones will pass spontaneously with minimal discomfort and with little risk of obstruction. In general, stents should be reserved for a large stone burden (0.25 mm or 300 mm²), for patients with a solitary kidney, or to assist in stone localization.

Steinstrasse that is asymptomatic or minimally symptomatic can be followed conservatively as long as function of the affected kidney is not impaired. Management of symptomatic Steinstrasse is based on the symptoms and the degree of ureteral involvement. In one study, for symptomatic Steinstrasse with an average length of 2.6 cm, observation and symptomatic treatment resolved the obstruction in 64% of patients.[215] In the same study, one-third of patients were treated with ESWL in situ, and Steinstrasse resolved completely in 90% of patients. Similar results have been reported by Miller and Hautmann.[225] Sigman and colleagues managed distal Steinstrasse by performing a ureteral meatotomy.[226] Although one-third had a great reduction in the length of Steinstrasse, more than half demonstrated vesicoureteral reflux on cystograms 2 months later. Ureteroscopy and basket extraction are useful, especially if a large lead fragment is present. Several authors have described a variety of techniques to irrigate the sand from the ureter.[227,228] If retrograde methods are not successful, percutaneous nephrostomy will decompress the kidney and often allow gravel to pass spontaneously.[42]

At the Methodist Hospital of Indiana, management of Steinstrasse depends on the degree of ureteral involvement. Simple Steinstrasse are defined as columns of gravel 0.5 cm in length in a patient who has no evidence of urosepsis. If symptoms require intervention, simple Steinstrasse can be effectively managed by ureteroscopy if a guidewire can be passed beyond the obstruction. Bypassing the Steinstrasse is often facilitated with the use of hydrophilic guidewires. If a guidewire cannot be passed, ureteroscopic manipulation should be abandoned because the risk of ureteral perforation during manipulation is greatly increased. Alternatively, ESWL in situ to the obstructed region of the ureter can relieve the obstruction in many cases, especially if a large lead fragment can be identified. Complex Steinstrasse, in which columns of stone fragments 5 cm are present or there are signs of urosepsis, is a more serious problem. In this situation, the risk of ureteral injury with ureteroscopy increases significantly. In addition, the sequelae of urosepsis demand rapid resolution of the obstruction. Consequently, complicated Steinstrasse is best managed with a percutaneous nephrostomy to allow decompression of the kidney and alleviate symptoms. Ureteral peristalsis will aid spontaneous stone passage even without urine flow. A guidewire can be placed in an antegrade manner to facilitate future ureteroscopic manipulation if necessary.

INFECTION

Overall, the reported incidence of sepsis following ESWL is less than 1%,[2] although for staghorn calculi, the rate is 2.7%.[229] The risk of sepsis increases if a urine culture yields positive results before ESWL.[230] The renal trauma and vascular disruption associated with ESWL may allow bacteria in urine to enter the bloodstream. Moreover, with the destruction of infected calculi, bacteria are released from the stone into the urine and may be absorbed systemically. In the presence of urinary obstruction, the risk of urosepsis increases dramatically. The rate of bacteremia following ESWL has been reported to be as high as 14%.[231] Infectious complications of ESWL include perinephric[232,233] and psoas abscess,[234] miliary tuberculosis,[235] and endophthalmitis.[236–238] Although rare, death from sepsis following ESWL can occur.[239] In general, while routine administration of prophylactic antibiotics for ESWL is not necessary,[240–242] certain clinical and radiographic factors may indicate the need for antibiotic therapy. Prophylactic antibiotics do not prevent infectious complications[238] but should be considered in patients at high risk for them. Therefore, ESWL should be performed only in the presence of sterile urine and in the absence of distal obstruction.

SUMMARY: CAN LITHOTRIPSY BE IMPROVED?

We see at least two logical paths that can lead to significant improvements in ESWL: (1) reinvention of the lithotriptor, and (2) rediscovery of how to use it. Our look at the evolution of lithotripsy shows that patient outcomes were never better than during the era of the first-generation lithotriptor, the unmodified Dornier HM3. Subsequent technological advances did not produce a better instrument and did not yield better results. Instead, lithotriptors have progressively become too powerful. With the widespread adoption of these machines, stone-free rates have dropped, re-treatment rates are up, and reports of adverse effects are on the rise.

There is an important lesson to be learned from the history of lithotripsy. We cannot expect to solve the problems associated with shock wave therapy solely from what we have learned about the physics of lithotriptors. We need to pay attention to the clinical findings as well. When manufacturers saw that their second-generation machines did not perform to expectations, they found a solution based on laboratory results. Boosting the power of the lithotriptor broke stones better in vitro. For example, the Storz Modulith breaks stationary artificial stones better than the Dornier HM3.[243] This result does not take into account that, in a living breathing patient, it is more difficult to keep the third-generation machine on target, and that excessively powerful shock waves lead to increased trauma to the kidney.

There is recent evidence for a move back to the basics. As mentioned above, a new lithotriptor has been introduced that, like the first-generation Dornier HM3, produces low-to-moderate acoustic pressures focused to a relatively broad focal zone. Initial clinical findings with the Xi Xin-Eisenmenger machine are encouraging.[244] This lithotriptor may not prove to be a solution to the problems that currently face ESWL—independent assessment of the device is needed—but it appears to be a step in the right direction. To be sure, this machine is a departure from the trend in ESWL toward high–acoustic-pressure devices. If this machine continues to deliver good results, it may set a new trend. We may see the development of other low- to moderate-power devices—a reinvention of the first-generation lithotriptor.

On the other hand, how lithotripsy is performed may be more important than which lithotriptor is used. Our endorsement of the HM3 is a matter of siding with the "lesser of two evils." We are well aware that adverse effects occur with the HM3. It is safe to say that any lithotriptor can be used to overtreat a patient. Likewise, it seems reasonable to suggest that, with the proper treatment protocol, most any lithotriptor can be used more effectively and with improved safety.

There are several basic conditions of shock wave treatment that will give better outcomes. All physicians should: (1) use lower power, (2) treat at a slow shock-wave rate, (3) sedate the patient and (4) keep the dose (number of shock waves) low.

As for power, there are no good published studies to show the effect of power setting on stone comminution. In our experience using the Dornier HM3 (at the Methodist Hospital) we have found that most classes of stones respond well to treatment at 12 to 15 kV. Use of low power has been recognized to be effective in the treatment of pediatric patients. Also, initial results with the Xi Xin-Eisenmenger lithotriptor report using this machine at very low power. We recommend starting treatment at low power and increasing the power only if the stone does not break up.

As for shock wave rate, there are several reports to show that slowing the rate of shock wave administration improves the effectiveness of treatment.[245,246] This concept was first tested in vitro and then demonstrated using model stones implanted in pig kidneys.[245] Preliminary results from the first prospective randomized clinical trial of shock wave rate show that treatment at 1 SW/sec is more effective than treatment at 2 SW/sec.[246] Also, the initial report of favorable results with the Xi Xin-Eisenmenger lithotriptor describes treatment at a very slow rate (0.3 Hz, 20 SW/min).

The issue of sedation is controversial. Many patients would rather not be sedated. Many urologists would rather not sedate their patients. Many lithotriptors are intended to be used as "anesthesia-free" machines. Still, there is very good evidence to show that outcomes are much better when the patient is under sedation.[11] This may be simply a matter of targeting the lithotriptor. When the patient moves around, it is more difficult to hit the stone.

The severity of collateral damage to the kidney increases with the dose of shock waves. The fewer the number of shock waves delivered, the better. Some urologists take the position that it is better to overtreat than to re-treat. We contend that it is best to monitor treatment closely and to stop as early as possible. We realize that a major part of this issue is the poor quality of our present imaging equipment. What is needed is better imaging tools to help the physician know more precisely when

complete stone comminution has been achieved. Ongoing refinements in diagnostic ultrasound and radiologic imaging should lead to advancements that will improve this aspect of ESWL.

There may be other factors, other features of treatment that can and should be improved in ESWL. Shock wave coupling is one. In "dry table" lithotripsy, transmission of shock wave energy into the body is dependent on the gel interface between the shock head and the skin. This interface can be a site for attenuation of the shock wave and possibly scattering or refocusing of the pulse. We know of no systematic study that has assessed the quality of coupling on stone comminution or on tissue injury.

In some respects, lithotripsy has been an ongoing experiment. A lot of observations have been made but few improvements have been realized. We think there is reason to expect that lithotripsy is about to change for the better. For one, awareness has never been higher that ESWL can cause adverse effects. As a result, urologists are more keenly aware of the potential for collateral damage and are more likely to treat conservatively. We now know that some lithotriptors are more dangerous than others. We expect that urologists will begin to demand better instruments, and that this will lead to the development of safer, more effective lithotriptors. We are beginning to learn that how shock waves are delivered (how the urologist controls the parameters of shock wave delivery) can have a significant effect on the outcome of treatment. This is a positive development and will improve how ESWL is performed regardless of the lithotriptor that is used.

REFERENCES

1. Kerbl K, Rehman J, Landman J, et al. Current management of urolithiasis: progress or regress? J Endourol 2002;16:281–8.
2. Smith AD, Marcovich R. Renal pelvic stones: choosing shock wave lithotripsy or percutaneous nephrolithotomy. International Braz J Urol 2003;29:195–207.
3. Evan AP, McAteer JA. Q-Effects of shock wave lithotripsy. In: Coe FL, Favus MJ, Pak CYC, Preminger GM, editors. Kidney stones: medical and surgical management. Philadelphia: Lippincott-Raven; 1996. p. 549–70.
4. Evan AP, Willis LR, Lingeman J, McAteer JA. Renal trauma and the risk of long-term complications in shock wave lithotripsy. Nephron 1998;78:1–8.
5. Lingeman, JE, Newmark JR. Adverse bioeffects of shock-wave lithotripsy. In: Coe FL, Favus MJ, Pak CYC, Preminger GM, editors. Kidney stones: medical and surgical management. Philadelphia: Lippincott-Raven; 1996. p. 605–614.
6. Janetschek G, Frauscher F, Knapp R, et al. New onset hypertension after extracorporeal shock wave lithotripsy: age-related incidence and prediction by resistive index. J Urol 1997;158:346–51.
7. Krambeck AE, Gettman MT, Rohlinger AL, et al. Diabetes mellitus and hypertension associated with shock wave lithotripsy of renal and proximal ureteral stones. J Urol 2006;175:1742–47.
7a. Parks, JH, Worcester E, Coe FC, et al. Clinical implications of abundant calcium phosphate in routinely analyzed kidney stones. Kidney Intl 2004;66:777–85.
8. Lingeman JE, Safar FS. Lithotripsy systems. In: Smith AD, Badlani GH, Bagley DH, et al, editors. Smith's textbook of endourology. St. Louis: Quality Medical Publishers, Inc.; 1996. p. 553–89.
9. Lingeman JE. Extracorporeal shock wave lithotripsy devices: are we making progress? In: Lingeman JE, Preminger GM, editors. Topics in clinical urology. New York: Igaku-Shoin Medical Publishers; 1996. p. 79–96.
10. Grenabo L, Lindquist K, Adami HO, et al. Extracorporeal

11. Eichel L, Batzold P, Erturk E. Operator experience and adequate anesthesia improve treatment outcome with third-generation lithotripters. J Endourol 2001;15:671–3.
12. Tan EC, Tung KH, Foo KT. Comparative studies of extracorporeal shock wave lithotripsy by Dornier HM3, EDAP LT 01 and Sonolith 2000 devices. J Urol 1991;148:294–7.
13. Fuselier HA, Prats L, Fontenot C, Gauthier A. Comparison of mobile lithotripters at one institution: Healthtronics Lithotron, Dornier MFL-5000, and Dornier Doli. J Endourol 1999;13:539–42.
14. Kohrmann KU, Rassweiler JJ, Manning M. The clinical introduction of a third generation lithotripter Modulith SL 20. J Urol 1995;1379–83.
15. Piper NY, Dalrymple N, Bishoff JT. Incidence of renal hematoma formation after ESWL using the new Dornier Doli-S lithotripter [Abstract]. J Urol 2001;165:377.
16. Thuroff S, Thorsten B, Chaussy C. Anatomy related shockwave (SW) power using Siemens Lithostar multiline [Abstract]. J Urol 1998;159:34.
17. Ueda S, Matsuko K, Yamashita T, et al. Perirenal hematomas caused by SWL with EDAP LT-01 lithotripter. J Endourol 1993;7:11–5.
18. U.S. Food and Drug Administration, Center for Devices and Radiological Health. Manufacturer and User Facility Device Experience database (MAUDE).
19. Knapp PM, Kulb TB, Lingeman JE, et al. Extracorporeal shock wave lithotripsy induced perirenal hematomas. J Urol 1988;139:700–3.
20. Krishnamurthi V, Streem B. Long-term radiographic and functional outcome of ESWL induced perirenal hematomas. J Urol 1995;154:1673–5.
21. Chaussy C, Schmidt E. Extracorporeal shock wave lithotripsy (ESWL) for kidney stones: an alternative to surgery? Urol Radiol 1984;6:80–7.
22. Newman LH, Saltzman B. Identification of risk factors in the development of clinically significant subcapsular hematomas following shock wave lithotripsy. In: Lingeman JE, Newman DM, editors. Shock wave lithotripsy 11: urinary and biliary lithotripsy. New York: Plenum Press; 1989. p. 207–10.
23. Mobley TB, Myers DA, Grine WB, et al. Low energy lithotripsy with the Lithostar: treatment results with 19,962 renal and ureteral calculi. J Urol 1993;149:1419–24.
24. Dhar N, Yost A, Streem SB. The incidence of and a multivariate analysis of risk factors associated with subcapsular hematoma formation following electromagnetic shock-wave lithotripsy [Abstract]. J Urol 2004;171:495.
25. Evan AP, Willis LR, Connors B, et al. Shock wave lithotripsy induced renal injury. Am J Kidney Dis 1991;17:445–50.
26. Evan AP, McAteer JA. Current perspectives on shock wave adverse effects. Lingeman JE, Shock wave lithotripsy bioeffects: the yin and the yang of stone fragmentation and tissue injury. New York: Igaku-Shoin Medical Publishers; 1996. p. 3–20.
27. Lingeman JE, McAteer JA, Kempson SA, Evan AP. Bioeffects of extracorporeal shock wave lithotripsy. J Endourol 1987;1:89–97.
28. Lingeman JE, Newman D, Mertz JH, et al. Extracorporeal shock wave lithotripsy: The Methodist Hospital of Indiana experience. J Urol 1986;135:1134–7.
29. Drach GW, Dretler S, Fair W, et al. Report of the United States cooperative study of extracorporeal shock wave lithotripsy. J Urol 1986;135:1127–33.
30. Parr KL, Lingeman JE, Jordan M, Coury EA. Creatinine kinase concentrations and electrocardiographic changes in extracorporeal shock wave lithotripsy. Urology 1988;32:21–3.
31. Ruiz-Marcellan FJ, Ibarz-Servio L. Evaluation of renal damage in extracorporeal lithotripsy by shock waves. Eur Urol 1986;12:73–5.
32. Karawi MA, Mohamed AR, El-Etaibi KE. Extracorporeal shock wave lithotripsy (ESWL) induced erosions in upper gastrointestinal tract. Urology 1987;30:224–7.
33. Cass AS. Colonic injury with ESWL for an upper ureteral calculus. Proceedings of the 4th Symposium on Shock Wave Lithotripsy: State of the Art. Indianapolis; 1988. p. 2.
34. Ilyckyj A, Hosking DH, Pettigrew NM, et al. Extracorporeal shock wave lithotripsy causing colonic injury. Dig Dis Sci 1999;44:2485–7.
35. Etzkorn KP, Mihalov M, Brown RD, et al. Colonic injury after ESWL of renal calculi. Gastrointest Endosc 1996;44:511–2.
36. Hidalgo PF, Conte VA, Rebassa LM, et al. Rectorrhage as an unusual extrarenal complication after ESWL. Actas Urol Exp 1998;22:366–8.
37. Geh JL, Curley P, Mayfield MP. Small bowel perforation after

shock wave lithotripsy for the treatment of renal stones. Arch Surg 1997;132:20–6.

extracorporeal shock wave lithotripsy. Br J Urol 1997;79: 648–9.
38. Holmberg G, Spinnell S, Sjodin JG. Perfusion of the bowel during SWL in prone position. J Endourol 1997;11:313–4.
39. Kurtz V, Muller-Sorg M, Federmann G. Perforation of the small intestine after nephrouretero-lithotripsy by ESWL—a rare complication. Chirurg 1999;70:306–7.
40. Castillon I, Frieyro O, Gonzalez-Enguita C, et al. Colonic perforation after extracorporeal shock wave lithotripsy. BJU Int 1999;83:720–1.
41. Olsson LE, Anderson KR, Foster HE Jr. Small bowel perforation after extracorporeal shock wave lithotripsy. J Urol 2000;164:775.
42. Chaussy C. Extracorporeal shock wave lithotripsy: new aspects in the treatment of kidney stone disease. Basel, Switzerland: S Karger; 1982.
43. Abe H, Nisimura T, Osawa S, et al. Acute pancreatitis caused by extracorporeal shock wave lithotripsy for bilateral renal pelvic calculi. Int J Urol 2000;7:65–8.
44. Mullen KD, Hoofnagle JH, Jones EA. Shock wave induced pancreatic trauma. Am J Gastroenterol 1991;86:630–2.
45. Hung SY, Chen HM, Jan YY, et al. Common bile duct and pancreatic injury after extracorporeal shock wave lithotripsy for renal stone. Heptogastroenterology 2000;46:1162–3.
46. Deliveliotis C, Sofras F, Alivizatos G, et al. The effect of ESWL of renal calculi on pancreatic function. Int Urol Nephrol 1998;30:665–70.
47. Marcuzzi D, Gray R, Wesley-James T, et al. Symptomatic following extracorporeal shock wave lithotripsy. J Urol 1991;145:547–8.
48. Rashid P, Steele D, Hunt J. Splenic rupture after extracorporeal shock wave lithotripsy. J Urol 1996;156:1756–7.
49. Fugita OE, Trigo-Rocha F, Mitre AI, et al. Splenic rupture and abscess after extracorporeal shock wave lithotripsy. Urology 1998;52:322–3.
50. Fuselier HA, Prats L, Fontenot C, et al. Comparison of mobile lithotriptors at one institution: Healthtronics Lithotron, Dornier MFL-5000, and Dornier Doli. J Endourol 1999; 13:539–42.
51. Patel KL, Gross J. Extracorporeal shock wave lithotripsy induced abdominal aortic aneurysm rupture. J Am Geriatr Soc, 1991;39:318–9.
52. Taylor JD, McLoyghlin GA, Parsons KF. Extracorporeal shock wave lithotripsy induced rupture of abdominal aortic aneurysm. Br J Urol 1995;76:262–3.
53. Lazarides MK, Drista H, Arvanitis DP, et al. Aortic aneurysm rupture after extracorporeal shock wave lithotripsy. Surgery 1997;122:112–3.
54. Neri E, Capannini G, Diciolla F, et al. Localized dissection and delayed rupture of the abdominal aorta after extracorporeal shock wave lithotripsy. J Vascular Surgery 2000; 31:1052–5.
55. Desmet Y, Baett L, Vandeursen H, et al. Iliac-vein thrombosis after extracorporeal shock wave lithotripsy. N Engl J Med 321:907,189.
56. Abecassis JP, Delaitre B, Morel MP, et al. Portal vein thrombosis after extracorporeal shock wave lithotripsy. Lancet 1991;338:316–7.
57. Kaye MC, Streem SB, Yost A. Scrotal hematoma resulting from extracorporeal shock wave lithotripsy for a distal ureteral calculi. J Urol 1993;150:481–2.
58. Biri H, Sinik Z, Alkibay T, et al. Scrotal bruising as a sign of retroperitoneal hematoma following extracorporeal shock wave lithotripsy. Int Urol Nephrol 1997;29:287–90.
59. Blacklock AR. Painless scrotal bruising following extracorporeal shock wave lithotripsy for renal calculus. Br J Urol 1994 ;74:675–6.
60. Cass AS, Doce CD, Ugarte RR. Extracorporeal shock wave lithotripsy induced stimulation of the obturator nerve. J Urol 1994;151:144–5.
61. Deliveliotis C, Picramenos D, Kiriakakis C, et al. Stimulation of the obturator nerve during extracorporeal shock wave lithotripsy. Int Urol Nephrol 1995;27:515–9
62. Lingeman JE, Newman DM, Siegel YI, et al. Shock wave lithotripsy with the Dornier MFL 5000 lithotriptor using an external fixed rate signal. J Urol 1995;154:951–4.
63. Cass AS. The use of ungating with the Medstone lithotriptor. J Urol 1996;156:896–8.
64. Kaude JV, Williams MC, Millner MR, et al. Renal morphology and function immediately after extracorporeal shock wave lithotripsy. AJR 1985;145:305–14.
65. Evan AP, McAteer JA, Steidle CP, et al. The mini-pig: an ideal large animal model for studies of renal injury in extracorporeal shock wave lithotripsy research. In: Lingeman JE, Newman DM, editors. Shock wave lithotripsy 11: urinary and biliary lithotripsy. New York: Plenum Press; 1989. p. 35–40.
66. Knapp PM, Scott JW, Lingeman JE. Magnetic resonance imaging following extracorporeal shock wave lithotripsy with the Dornier HM3 lithotriptor. J Urol 1987;137:287.
67. Wilson WT, Miller GL, Morris JS, et al. Morphologic renal changes following piezoelectric lithotripsy or spark-gap lithotripsy. In: Lingeman JE, Newman DM, editors. Shock wave lithotripsy 11: urinary and biliary lithotripsy. New York: Plenum Press; 1989. p. 19–22.
68. Rubin JI, Arger PH, Pollack HM, et al. Kidney changes after extracorporeal shock wave lithotripsy: CT evaluation. Radiology 1987;162:21–4.
69. Grote R, Dohring W, Aeikens B. Computed tomographic and aonographic detection of renal and perirenal changes following extracorporeal shock wave lithotripsy. Rofo: Fortschr Geb Rontgenstr Nuklearmed 1986;144:434–9.
70. Baumgartner BR, Dickey KW, Ambrose SS, et al. Kidney changes after extracorporeal shock wave lithotripsy: appearance on MR imaging. Radiology 1987;163:531–4.
71. Krysiewicz S. Complications of renal extracorporeal shock wave lithotripsy reviewed. Urol Radiol 1992;13:139–45.
72. Karlin GS, Urivetsky M, Smith AD. Side effects of extracorporeal shock wave lithotripsy: assessment of urinary excretion of renal enzymes as evidence of tubular injury. In: Lingeman JE, Newman DM, editors. Shock wave lithotripsy 11: urinary and biliary lithotripsy. New York: Plenum Press; 1989. p. 3–6.
73. Preminger GM. Sonographic piezoelectric lithotripsy: more bang for your buck. In: Lingeman JE, Newman DM, editors. Shock wave lithotripsy ii: urinary and biliary lithotripsy. New York: Plenum Press; 1989. p. 437–43.
74. Grantham JR, Millner MR, Kaude JV, et al. Renal stone disease treated with extracorporeal shock wave lithotripsy: short-term observations in 100 patients. Radiology 1986; 158:203–6.
75. Dyer RB, Karstaedt N, McCullough DL, et al. Magnetic resonance imaging evaluation of immediate and intermediate changes in kidneys treated with extracorporeal shock wave lithotripsy. In: Lingeman JE, Newman DM, editors. Shock wave lithotripsy 11: urinary and biliary lithotripsy. New York: Plenum Press; 1989. p. 203–5.
76. Bex A, Goepel M, Mollhoff S. Extensive retroperitoneal hematoma following extracorporeal shock wave lithotripsy with second-generation lithotriptor. Urol Int 1992;48:11–4.
77. Maziak DE, Ralph EA, Detile M, et al. Massive perirenal and intra-abdominal bleeding after SWL: case report. Ca J Surg 1994;37:329–34.
78. Umekawa T, Yamate T, Amasaki N, et al. Continuous evaluation for retroperitoneal hematoma following ESWL. Urol Int 1993;51:114–6.
79. Lemann J Jr, Taylor AJ, Collier BD, et al. Kidney hematoma due to extracorporeal shock wave lithotripsy causing transient rennin mediated hypertension. J Urol 1991;145:1238–41.
80. Graham CW, Lynch SC, Muskat PC, et al. Laparascopic evacuation of a subcapsular renal hematoma causing symptomatic hypertension. J Endourol 1998;12:551–3.
81. Sasaguri M, Noda K, Matsumoto T, et al. A case of hyperreninemic hypertension after extracorporeal shock wave lithotripsy. Hypertens Res 2000;23:709–12.
82. Stoller ML, Litt L, Salazar RG. Severe hemorrhage after extracorporeal shock wave lithotripsy. Ann Inten Med 1989;111:612–3.
83. Littleton RH, Melser M, Kupin W. Acute renal failure following bilateral extracorporeal shock wave lithotripsy without ureteral obstruction. In: Lingeman JE, Newman DM, editors. Shock wave lithotripsy 11: urinary and biliary lithotripsy. New York: Plenum Press; 1989. p. 197–201.
84. Treglia A, Moscoloni M. Irreversible acute renal failure after extracorporeal shock wave lithotripsy. J Nephrol 1999; 12:190–2.
85. Tuteja AK, Pulliam JP, Lehman TH, et al. Anuric renal failure from massive bilateral renal hematoma following extracorporeal shock wave lithotripsy. Urology 1997;50: 606–8.
86. Diaz-Tejeiro R, Diaz EG, Fernandez G, et al. Irreversible acute renal failure after extracorporeal shock wave lithotripsy. Nephron 1993;63:242–3.
87. Kleinknecht D, Pallot JL, Chauveau P. Bilateral acute tubular necrosis after unilateral extracorporeal shockwave lithotripsy. Nephron 1994;66:360–1.
88. Donahue LA, Linke CA, Rowe JM. Renal loss following extracorporeal shock wave lithotripsy. J Urol 1989;142:809–11.
89. Antoniou NK, Karanastasis D, Stenos JL. Severe perinephric hemorrhage after shockwave lithotripsy. J Endourol 1995; 9:239–41.
90. Davidson T, Tung K, Constant O, et al. Kidney rupture and psoas abscess after ESWL. Br J Urol 1991;68:657–8.
91. Seddiki A, Thomas J, Tobelem G, et al. A rare complication of extracorporeal shock wave lithotripsy: rupture of the kidney. Apropos of a case. J Urol (Paris) 1991;97:224–7.
92. Colombo PR, Francesca F, DiGirolamo V, et al. Histological and ultrastructural evaluation of extracorporeal shock wave lithotriptor-induced acute renal lesions: preliminary report. Eur Urol 1989;16:207–11.
93. Seitz G, Pletzer K, Neisius D, et al. Pathologic-anatomic alterations in human kidneys after extracorporeal piezoelectric shock wave lithotripsy. J Endourol 1991;5:17.
94. Brewer SL, Atala AA, Ackerman DM, et al. Shock wave lithotripsy damage in human cadaver kidneys. J Endourol 1988;4:333–9.
95. Roessler W, Steinbach P, Nicolai H, et al. Effects of high-energy shock waves on the viable human kidney. Urol Res 1993;21:273–7.
96. Roessler W, Wieland WF, Steinbach P, et al. Side effects of high-energy shock waves in the human kidney: first experience with model comparing two shockwave sources. J Endourol 1996;10:507–11.
97. Assimos DG, Boyce WH, Furr EG, et al. Selective elevation of urinary enzyme levels after extracorporeal shock wave lithotripsy. J Urol 1989;142:687–90.
98. Krongrad A, Saltzman B, Tannenbaum M, et al. Enzymuria following extracorporeal shock wave lithotripsy. J Urol 1988;139:324.
99. Kishimoto T, Senju M, Sugimoto T, et al. Effects of high energy shock wave exposure on renal function during extracorporeal shock wave lithotripsy for kidney stones. Eur Urol 1990;18:290–8.
100. Kirkali Z, Kirlali G, Tahiri Y. The effects of extracorporeal electromagnetic shock waves on renal proximal tubular function. Int Urol Nephrol 1994;26:255–7.
101. Hasegawa S, Kato K, Takashi M, et al. Increased levels of calbindin-D in serum and urine from patients treated by extracorporeal shock wave lithotripsy. Urol Int 1998;48: 420–4.
102. Jung K, Kirschner P, Wille A, et al. Excretion of urinary enzymes after extracorporeal shock wave lithotripsy: a critical reevaluation. J Urol 1993;149:1409–13.
103. Akdas A, Turkeri LN, Ilker Y, et al. Short-term bioeffects of extracorporeal shock wave lithotripsy. J Endourol 1994; 8:187–90.
104. Krongrad A, Saltzman B, Tannenbaum M. Enzymuria after extracorporeal shock wave lithotripsy. J Endourol 1991; 5:209–11.
105. Gilbert BR, Richie RA, Vaughan ED. Extracorporeal shock wave lithotripsy and its effect on renal function. J Urol 1988;139:482.
106. Barak M, Ginesin Y, Hornstein L, et al. Excretion of urinary protein induced by extracorporeal piezo-electric lithotripsy. Br J Urol 1990;66:575–80.
107. Horgan PG, Hanley D, Burke J, et al. Extracorporeal shock wave lithotripsy induces the release of prostaglandins which increase ureteric peristalsis. Br J Urol 1993;71:648–52.
108. Sarica K, Balat A, Erbagei A, et al. Effects of shock wave lithotripsy on plasma and urinary levels of nitrite and adrenomedullin. Urol Res 2003;31:347–51.
109. Villanyi KK, Szekely JG, Farkas LM, et al. Short-term changes in renal function after extracorporeal shock wave lithotripsy in children. J Urol 2001;166:222–4.
110. Karlsen SJ, Berg K. Acute changes in renal function following extracorporeal shock wave lithotripsy in patients with a solitary kidney. J Urol 1991;145:253–6.
111. Bomanji J, Boddy SAM, Britton KE, et al. Radionuclide evaluation pre and post extracorporeal shock wave lithotripsy for renal calculi. J Nucl Med 1987;28:1284–9.
112. Saxby MF. Effects of percutaneous nephrolithotomy and extracorporeal shock wave lithotripsy. Scand J Urol and Nephrol 1997;31:141–4.
113. Mostafavi MR, Chavez DR, Cannilo J, et al. Redistribution of renal blood flow after SWL evaluated by Gd-DTPA-enhanced magnetic resonance imaging. J Endourol 1998; 12:9–12.
114. Kataoka T, Kasahara T, Kobashikawa K, et al. Changes in renal blood flow after treatment with ESWL in patients with renal stones: studies using ultrasound color Doppler method. J Urol 1993;84:851–6.
115. Knapp R, Frauscher F, Helweg G, et al. Age-related changes in resistive index following extracorporeal shock wave lithotripsy. J Urol 1995;154:955–8.
116. Nazaroglu H, Akay AF, Bukte Y, et al. Effects of extracorporeal shock-wave lithotripsy on intrarenal resistive index. Scand J Urol Nephrol 2003;37:408–12.
117. Thomas R, Roberts J, Sloane B, et al. Effects of extracorporeal shock wave lithotripsy on renal function. J Endourol 1988;140:141–4.
118. Orestona F, Caronia N, Gallo G, et al. Functional aspects of

the kidney after shock wave lithotripsy. In: Lingeman JE, Newman DM, editors. Shock wave lithotripsy 11: urinary and biliary lithotripsy. New York: Plenum Press; 1989. p. 15–17.
119. Eterovic D, Juretic-Kuscic L, Capkun V, et al. Pyeleolithotomy improves while extracorporeal shock wave lithotripsy impairs kidney function. J Urol 1999;161:39–44.
120. Willis LR, Evan AP, Connors BA, et al. Relationship between kidney size, renal injury, and renal impairment induced by shock wave lithotripsy. J Am Soc Nephrol 1999;10: 1753–62.
121. Willis LR, Evan AP, Lingeman JE. The impact of high-dose lithotripsy on renal function. Contemp Urol 1999;45–50.
122. Li B, Zhou W, Li P. Protective effects of nifedipine and allopurinol on high energy shock wave induced acute changes of renal function. J Urol 1995;153:596–8.
123. Strohmaier WL, Bichler KH, Koch J, et al. Protective effect of verapamil on shock wave induced renal tubular dysfunction. J Urol 1993;150:27–9.
124. Strohmaier WL, Koch J, Balk N. Limitation of shock-wave-induced renal tubular dysfunction by nifedipine. Eur Urol 1994;25:99–104.
125. Chan AL, Prasad PV, Priatna A, et al. Protective effect of aminophylline on renal perfusion changes induced by high-energy shockwaves identified by Gd-DTPA-enhanced first-pass perfusion MRI. J Endourol 2000;14: 117–21.
126. Benyi L, Weizheng Z, Puyun L. Protective effects of nifedipine and allopurinol on high-energy shock wave induced acute changes of renal function. J Urol 1995;153:596–8.
127. Willis LR, Evan AP, Connors BA, et al. Prevention of lithotripsy-induced renal injury by pretreating kidneys with low-energy shock waves. J Am Soc Nephrol 2006; 17:663–73.
128. Lingeman JE, Woods JR, Toth PD, et al. The role of lithotripsy and its side effects. J Urol 1989;141:793–7.
129. Lechevallier E, Siles S, Ortega JC, et al. Comparison by SPECT of renal scars after extracorporeal shock wave lithotripsy and percutaneous nephrolithotomy. J Endourol 1993;7:465–7.
130. Umekawa T, Kohri K, Yashioka K, et al. Production of antiglomerular basement membrane antibody after extracorporeal shock wave lithotripsy. Urol Int 1994;52:106–8.
131. Williams CM, Thomas WC. Permanently decreased renal blood flow and hypertension after lithotripsy. N Engl J Med 1989;321:1269–70.
132. Brito CG, Lingeman JE, Newman DM. Long-term follow-up of renal function in ESWL-treated patients with solitary kidney. J Urol 1990;143:299.
133. Liedl B, Joacham D, Lunz C, et al. Five-year follow-up of urinary stone patients treated with extracorporeal shock wave lithotripsy. J Endourol 1988;2:157–62.
134. Pienkny AJ, Streem SB. Simultaneous versus staged bilateral extracorporeal shock wave lithotripsy. J Urol 1999;162: 1591–3.
135. Chandhoke PS, Albana DM, Clayman RV. Long-term comparison of renal function in patients with solitary kidneys and/or moderate renal insufficiency undergoing extracorporeal shock wave lithotripsy or percutaneous nephrolithotomy. J Urol 1992;147:1226–30.
136. Peterson JC, Finlayson B. Effects of ESWL on blood pressure. In: Gravenstein JS, Peter K, editors. Extracorporeal shock wave lithotripsy for renal stone disease: technical and clinical aspects. Boston: Butterworths; 1986. p. 145–50.
137. Lingeman JE, Kulb TB, Newman DM, et al. Hypertension following ESWL. J Urol 1987;137:142.
138. Jewett MAS, Bombardier C, Logan AG et al. A randomized controlled trial to assess the incidence of new onset hypertension in patients after shock wave lithotripsy for symptomatic renal calculi. J Urol 1998;160:1241–3.
139. Montgomery B, Cole R, Palfrey E. Does extracorporeal shock wave lithotripsy cause hypertension? Br J Urol 1989;64;567–71.
140. Claro JA, Lima A, Ferreira U. Blood pressure changes after extracorporeal shock wave lithotripsy in normotensive patients. J Urol 1993;150;1765–7.
141. Zanetti GR, Montanari E, Guarneri A, et al. Long-term follow-up after extracorporeal shock wave lithotripsy treatment of kidney stones in solitary kidneys. J Urol 1992;148:1011–4.
142. Strohmaier WL, Schmidt J, Lahme S, et al. Arterial blood pressure following different types of urinary stone therapy. Eur Urol 2000;38:753–7.
143. Borghi L, Meschi T, Guerra A, et al. Essential arterial hypertension and stone disease. Kidney Intl 1999;55:2397–406.
144. Yokoyama M, Shoji F, Yanagizawa R. Blood pressure changes following extracorporeal shock wave lithotripsy for urolithiasis. J Urol 1992;147:553–8.
145. Lingeman JE, Woods JR, Toth PD. Blood pressure changes after extracorporeal shock wave lithotripsy and other forms of treatment for nephrolithiasis. JAMA 1990;63; 1789–94.
146. Knapp R. Frauscher F, Helweg G, et al. Blood pressure changes after extracorporeal shock wave nephrolithotripsy: prediction by intrarenal resistive index. Eur Radiol 1996; 6:665–9.
147. Worcester EM, Parks JH, Thisted R, et al. Causes and consequences of kidney loss in patients nephrolithiasis. Kidney Intl 2004;64:2204–13
148. Gillen, DL, Worcester, EM, Coe, FL. Decreased renal function among adults with a history of nephrolithiasis: a study of NHANES III (In Press: KI)
149. Pearle M, Watamull LM, Mullican MA. Sensitivity of noncontrast helical computerized tomography and plain film radiography copred to flexible nephroscopy for detecting residual fragments after percutaneous nephrolstolithotomy. J Urol 1999;162:23–6.
150. Carr LK, Honey JD'A, Jewett MAS, et al. New stone formation: A comparision of extracorporeal shock wave lithotripsy and percutaneous nephrolithotomy. J Urol 1996;155:1565–7.
151. Parks JH, Worcester E, Coe FL, et al. Clinical implications of abundant calcium phosphate in routinely analyzed kidney stones. Kidney Intl 2004;66:777–85.
152. Mandel N, Mandel I, Fryjoff K, et al. Conversion of calcium oxalate to calcium phosphate with recurrent stone episodes. J Urol 2003;169:2026–9.
153. Evan AP, Lingeman JE, Coe FL, et al. Crystal associated nephropathy in patients with brushite nephrolithiasis (In Press: KI)
154. Ruiz H, Saltman B. Asprin-induced bilateral renal hemorrhage after extracorporeal shock wave lithotripsy therapy: implications and conclusions. J Urol 1990;143: 791–2.
155. Zanetti GR, Kartalas-Goumas J, Montanari E, et al. Extracorporeal shockwave lithotripsy in patients treated with antithrombotic agents. J Endourol 2001;15:237–41.
156. Lifshitz DA, Lingeman JE, Zafar FS, et al. Alterations in predicted growth rates of pediatric kidneys treated with extracorporeal shock wave lithotripsy. J Endourol 1998; 12:469–75.
157. Adams MC, Newman DM, Lingeman JE. Pediatric ESWL: long-term results and effects on renal growth. J Endourol 1989;3:245.
158. Frick J, Sarica K, Kohle R, et al. Long-term follow-up after to extracorporeal shock wave lithotripsy in children. Eur Urol 1991;19:225–9.
159. Thomas R, Frentz JM, Harmon E, et al. Effect of extracorporeal shock wave lithotripsy on renal function and body height in pediatric patients. J Urol 1992;148:1064–6.
160. Corbally MT, Ryan J, FitzPatrick JR, et al. Renal function following extracorporeal lithotripsy in children. J Pediatr Surg 1991;26:539–40.
161. Goel MC, Baserge NS, Ramesh Babu RV, et al. Pediatric kidney: functional outcome after extracorporeal shock wave lithotripsy. J Urol 1996;155:2044–6.
162. Lottman H, Archambaud F, Helal B, et al. Extracorporeal shock wave lithotripsy in children: study of the effectiveness and renal consequences in a series of eighteen children. Ann Urol 1955;29:136.
163. Lottman HB, Traxer O, Archambaub F, et al. Monotherapy extracorporeal shock wave lithotripsy for the treatment of staghorn calculi in children. J Urol 2001;165:2324–7.
164. Sarica K, Kupei S, Sarica N, et al. Long-term follow-up of renal morphology and function in children after lithotripsy. Urol Int 1995;54:95–8.
165. Shukla AR, Hoover DL, Homsy YL, et al. Urolithiasis in the low birth weight infant: the role and efficacy of extracorporeal shockwave lithotripsy. J Urol 2001;165:2320–3.
166. Villanyi KK, Szekely JG, Lszlo M, et al. Short-term changes in renal function after extracorporeal shock wave lithotripsy in children. J Urol 2001;166:222–4.
167. Kaji DM, Xie HW, Hardy BE, et al. The effects of extracorporeal shock wave lithotripsy on renal growth function and arterial blood pressure in an animal model. J Urol 1991;146:544–7.
168. Neal DE, Harmon E, Hlavinka T, et al. Effects of multiple sequential extracorporeal shock wave treatments on renal function: a primate model. J Endourol 1991;5:217–21.
169. Brendel W. Effect of shock waves on canine kidney. In: Gravenstein JS, Peter K, editors. Extracorporeal shock wave lithotripsy of renal stone disease: technical and clinical aspects. Boston: Butterworths; 1986. p. 141–2.
170. Delius, M. Biomedical shock wave research: a brief update. In: Chaussy C, Eisenberger F, Jocham D, Wilbert D, editors. High energy shock waves in medicine. Stuttgart: Georg Thieme Verlag; 1997. p. 1–10.
171. Delius M, Enders G, Xuan Z, et al. Biological effects of shock waves: kidney damage by shock waves in dogs-dose dependence. Ultrasound Med Biol 1988;14:117–22.
172. Delius M, Jordan M, Eizenhoefer H, et al. Biological effects of shock waves: kidney hemorrhage by shock waves in dogs-administration rate dependence. Ultrasound Med Biol 1988;14:689–94.
173. Delius M, Denk R, Berding C, et al. Biological effects of shock waves: cavitation by shock waves in piglet liver. Ultrasound Med Biol 1990;16:467–73.
174. Delius M, Mueller W, Goetz A, et al. Biological effects of shock waves: kidney hemorrhage in dogs at a fast shock wave administration rate of fifteen Hertz. J Lithotripsy Stone Dis 1990;2:103–10.
175. Newman R, Hackett R, Senior D, et al. Pathologic effects of ESWL on canine renal tissue. Urology 1987;29:194–200.
176. Neisius D, Seitz G, Gebhardt T, et al. Dose-dependent influence on canine renal morphology after application of extracorporeal shock waves with Wolf Piezolith. J Endourol 1989;3:337–45.
177. Jaeger P, Redha, Uhlschmid G, et al. Morphological changes in canine kidneys following extra-corporeal shock wave treatment. Urol Res 1988;16:161–6.
178. Thibault P, Dory J, Cotard JP, et al. Lithotripsy by ultra short pulsation: experimental study in renal lithiasis in the dog. Ann Urol (Paris) 1986;20:20–5.
179. Connors BA, Evan AP, Willis LR, et al. Separation of SWL-induced cavitation and renal injury from impairment of hemodynamics. J Urol 1988;159 (Suppl):32.
180. Connors BA, Evan AP, Willis LR. The effect of discharge voltage on renal injury and impairment caused by lithotripsy in the pig. J Am Soc Nephrol 2000;11:310–8.
181. Evan AP, Connors BA, Pennington DJ, et al. Renal disease potentiates the injury caused by SWL. J Endourol 1999; 13:619–28.
182. Shao Y, Connors BA, Evan AP, et al. Morphological changes induced in the pig kidney by extracorporeal shock wave lithotripsy: nephron injury. Anat Rec 2003;75:979–89.
183. Willis LR, Evan AP, Connors BA, et al. Lingeman effect of high-dose lithotripsy on renal function and structure. (In Press: J Urol).
184. Willis LR, Evan AP, Connors BA, et al. Effects of extracorporeal shock wave lithotripsy to one kidney on bilateral glomerular filtration rate and PAH clearance in minipigs. J Urol 1996;156:1502–6.
185. Morris JS, Husmann DA, Wilson WT, et al. Piezoelectric v electrohydraulic lithotripsy: a comparison of morphologic alterations. In: Lingeman JE, Newman DM, editors. Shock wave lithotripsy 11: urinary and biliary lithotripsy. New York: Plenum Press; 1989. p. 29–33.
186. Sarica K, Soygur T, Yaman O, et al. Stone recurrence after shock wave lithotripsy: evaluation of possible enhanced crystal deposition in traumatized tissue in rabbit model. J Endourol 1996;10:513–7.
187. Sarica K, Kosar A, Yaman O, et al. Evaluation of ischemia after ESWL: detection of free oxygen radical scavenger enzymes in renal parenchyma subjected to high-energy shock waves. Urol Int 1996;57:221–3.
188. Weber C, Gluck U, Staehler G, et al. Extracorporeal shock wave treatment raises blood pressure in borderline hypertensive rats. J Urol 1995;154:232–6.
189. Weber C, Moran ME, Braun EJ, et al. Injury of rat vessels following extracorporeal shock wave treatment. J Urol 1992;147:476–8.
190. Karlsen SJ, Smevik B, Stenstrom J, et al. Acute physiological changes in canine kidneys following exposure to extracorporeal shock waves. J Urol 1990;143:1280–3.
191. Jaeger P, Constantinides C. Canine kidneys: changes in blood and urine chemistry after exposure to extracorporeal shock waves. In: Lingeman JE, Newman DM, editors. Shock wave lithotripsy 11: urinary and biliary lithotripsy. New York: Plenum Press; 1989. p. 7–10.
192. Cohen TD, Durrani AF, Brown SA, et al. Lipid peroxidation induced by shock wave lithotripsy. J Endourol 1998;12: 229–32.
193. Brown SA, Munver R, Delvecchio FC, et al. Microdialysis assessment of shock wave lithotripsy-induced renal injury. Urology 2000;56:364–486.
194. Delvecchio FC, Auge BK, Munver R, et al. Shock wave lithotripsy causes ipsilateral renal injury remote from the focal point: the role of regional vasoconstriction. J Urol 2003;169:1526–9.
195. Strohmaier WL, Abelius A, Billes I, et al. Verapamil limits shockwave-induced renal tubular damage in vivo. J Endourol 1994;8:269–73.

196. Yaman O, Sarica K, Ozer G, et al. Protective effect of verapamil on renal tissue during shockwave application in rabbit model. J Endourol 1996;10:329–33.

197. Sarica K, Bakir K, Yagci F, et al. Limitation of shockwave-induced enhanced crystal deposition in traumatized tissue by verapamil in rabbit model. J Endourol 1999;13:343–7.

198. Morris JS, Husmann DA, Wilson WT, et al. Temporal effects of shock wave lithotripsy. J Urol 1991;145:881–3.

199. Banner B, Ziesmer D, Collins LA. Proliferative glomerulopathy following extracorporeal shock wave lithotripsy in the pig. J Urol 1991;146:1425–8.

200. Feagins BA, Alexander M, Dollar M, et al. Prevention of lithotripsy-induced hypertension in a juvenile animal model. J Urol 1991;145:258.

201. Coleman AJ, Saunders JE, Crum LA, et al. Acoustic cavitation generated by an extracorporeal shockwave lithotriptor. Ultrasound Med Biol 1987;13:69–76.

202. Coleman AJ, Saunders JE, Preston RC, et al. Pressure waveforms generated by a Dornier extracorporeal shock wave lithotriptor. Ultrasound Med Biol 1987;13:651–7.

203. Crum L. Cavitation microjets as a contributory mechanism for renal calculi disintegration in ESWL. J Urol 1988;140:1587–90.

204. Bailey MR, Pishchalnikov YA, Sapozhnikov OA, et al. Cavitation detection during shock wave lithotripsy. (In Press: UMB).

205. Evan AP, Willis LR, McAteer JA, et al. Kidney damage and renal functional changes are minimized by waveform control that suppresses cavitation in shock wave lithotripsy.

206. Bailey MR, Blackstock DT, Cleveland RO, Crum LA. Comparison of electrohydraulic lithotripters with rigid and pressure-release ellipsoidal reflectors. I. Acoustic fields. J Acoust Soc Am 1999;106:1149–57.

207. Lokhandwalla M, Sturtevant B. Fracture mechanisms model of stone comminution in ESWL and implications for tissue damage. Phys Med Biol 2000;45:1923–40.

208. Lokhandwalla M, McAteer JA, Williams JC, Sturtevant B. Mechanical hemolysis in shock wave lithotripsy (SWL): II. In vitro cell lysis due to shear. Phys Med Biol 2001;46:1245–64.

209. Marcovich R, Smith AD. Renal pelvic stones: choosing shock wave lithotripsy or percutaneous nephrolithotomy. Intl Braz J Urol 2003;29:295–207.

210. Sayed MA, El-Taher AM, Aboul-ella HA, Shaker SE. Steinstrasse after extracorporeal shock wave lithotripsy: aetiology, prevention and management. BJU Intl 2001;88:675–8.

211. Madbouly K, Sheir KZ, Elsobky E, et al. Risk factors for the formation of a Steinstrasse after extracorporeal shock wave lithotripsy: A statistical model. J Urol 2002;167:1239–42.

212. Dretler SP. Stone fragility—a new therapeutic distinction. J Urol 1988;139:1124.

213. Dretler SP. Extracorporeal shock wave lithotripsy: a review of its first two years of operation in the United States. Urol Ann 1987;1:1.

214. Lingeman JE. Bioeffects and long-term results of ESWL. In: Lingeman JE, Smith LH, Woods JR, Newman DM, editors. Urinary calculi: ESWL, endourology and medical therapy. Philadelphia: Lea & Febiger; 1989. p. 273–92.

215. Kim SC, Oh CW, Moon YT, et al. Treatment of Steinstrasse with repeat extracorporeal shock wave lithotripsy: experience with piezoelectric lithotriptor. J Urol 1991;145:489–91.

216. Hardy MR, McLeod DG. Silent renal obstruction with severe functional loss after extracorporeal shock wave lithotripsy: a report of 2 cases. J Urol 1987;137:91.

217. Libby JM, Meacham RB, Griffith DP. The role of silicone ureteral stents in extracorporeal shock wave lithotripsy of large renal calculi. J Urol 1988;139:15.

218. Ramsay JWA, Crosker RP, Ball AJ, et al. Urothelial reaction to ureteric intubation: a clinical study. Br J Urol 1987;60:504.

219. Fine H, Gordon RL, Lebensart PD. Extracorporeal shock wave lithotripsy and stents: fluoroscopic observations and a hypothesis on the mechanisms of stent function. Urol Radiol 1989;11:37.

220. Bregg K, Riehle RA. Morbidity associated with indwelling internal ureteral stents after shock wave lithotripsy. J Urol 1989;141:510.

221. Pryor JL, Jenkins AD. Use of double-pigtail stents in extracorporeal shock wave lithotripsy. J Urol 1990;143:475.

222. Anderson PAM, Norman RW, Awad SA. Extracorporeal shock wave lithotripsy experience with large renal calculi. J Endourol 1989;3:31.

223. Preminger GM, Kettelhut MC, Elkins SL, et al. Ureteral stenting during extracorporeal shock wave lithotripsy: help or hindrance. J Urol 1989;142:32.

224. Bierkens AF, Hendrikx AJ, Lemmens WA, et al. Extracorporeal shock wave lithotripsy for large renal calculi: the role of ureteral stents. A randomized trial. J Urol 1991;145:699.

225. Miller K, Hautmann R. Treatment of distal ureteral calculi with ESWL: experience with more than 100 consecutive cases. World J Urol 1987;5:259.

226. Sigman M, Laudone V, Jenkins AD. Ureteral meatotomy as a treatment of Steinstrasse following extracorporeal shock wave lithotripsy. J Endourol 1988;2:41.

227. Dretler SP. Management of ureteral calculi. Presented at the Fifth World Congress on Endourology and ESWL, Cairo, Egypt, November 1-4, 1987.

228. Rubenstein MA, Norris DM. Variation on water-pik technique for treatment of Steinstrasse after ESWL. Urology 1988;32:429–30.

229. Lam HS, Lingeman JE, Barron M, et al. Staghorn calculi: analysis of treatment results between initial percutaneous nephrostolithotomy and extracorporeal shock wave lithotripsy monotherapy with reference to surface area. J Urol 1992;147:1219.

230. Zink RA, Frohmueller HG, Eberhardt JE, et al. Urosepsis following ESWL. J Urol 1988 139:265A.

231. Müller-Mattheis VGO, Schmale D, Seewald M, et al. Bacteremia during extracorporeal shock wave lithotripsy of renal calculi. J Urol 1991;146:733.

232. Karamalegos AZ, Diokno AC, Moylan DF. Formation of perinephric abscess following extracorporeal shock wave lithotripsy. Urology 1989;34:277.

233. Peiser J, Kaneti J, Lissmer L, et al. Perinephric inflammatory process following extracorporeal shock wave lithotripsy. Int Urol Nephrol 1991;23:107.

234. Davidson T, Tung K, Constant O, et al. Kidney rupture and psoas abscess after ESWL. Br J Urol 1991;68:657.

235. Federmann M, Kley HK. Miliary tuberculosis after extracorporeal shock wave lithotripsy [Letter]. N Engl J Med 1990;323:212.

236. Greenwald BD, Tunkel AR, Morgan KM, et al. Candidal endophthalmitis after lithotripsy of renal calculi. South Med J 1992;85:773.

237. Westh H, Mogensen P. Extracorporeal shock wave lithotripsy of a kidney stone complicated with *Candida albicans* septicaemia and endophthalmitis. Scand J Urol Nephrol 1990;24:81.

238. Kremer I, Gaton DD, Baniel J, et al. *Klebsiella* metastatic endophthalmitis—a complication of shock wave lithotripsy. Ophthalmic Surg 1990;21:206.

239. Silber N, Kremer I, Gaton DD, et al. Severe sepsis following extracorporeal shock wave lithotripsy. J Urol 1991;145:1045.

240. Kattan S, Husain I, El-Faqih SR, et al. Incidence of bacteremia and bacteriuria in patients with non-infection-related urinary stones undergoing extracorporeal shock wave lithotripsy. J Endourol 1993;7:449.

241. Dejeter SW, Abbruzzese MR, Reid BJ, et al. Prospective randomized evaluation of antimicrobial prophylaxis in patients undergoing extracorporeal shock wave lithotripsy. J Endourol 1989;3:43.

242. Pettersson B, Tiselius HG. Are prophylactic antibiotics necessary during extracorporeal shock wave lithotripsy. J Urol 1991;144:15.

243. Cleveland RO, Chitnis PV, Anglade R, Babayan RK. Measurements of the pressure field and in vitro stone fragmentation of a Stortz Modulith SLX lithotripter [Abstract]. J Acoust Soc Am 2001;109:2482.

244. Eisenmenger W, Du XX, Tang C, et al. The first clinical results of "wide-focus and low-pressure" ESWL. Ultrasound Med Biol 2002;28:769–74.

245. Paterson RF, Lifshitz DA, Lingeman JE, et al. Stone fragmentation during shock wave lithotripsy is improved by slowing the shock wave rate: studies with a new animal model. J Urol 2002;168:2211–5.

246. Pace K, Bilgasem S, Dyer S, Honey RJ. Shock wave lithotripsy: interim results for a randomized, double-blinded trial to compare shock wave frequencies of 60 and 120 hertz [Abstract]. J Endourol 2002;16:20.

Part V

Basic and Procedural Laparoscopy

42

Patient Preparation and Operating Room Setup

Andrew B. Joel, MD

Marshall L. Stoller, MD

A prepared patient and skilled surgeon are prerequisites for successful laparoscopic procedures. Laparoscopic surgical candidates must be fully informed and medically suitable. Surgeons should be cognizant of the physiologic changes characteristic of specific laparoscopic surgery and proficient in laparoscopic techniques. Expertise in open surgery does not fully prepare a surgeon for the specific demands of operating in the confines of a limited working space with specialized laparoscopic instrumentation. Acquiring surgical proficiency involves a steep learning curve, as evidenced by the relatively high incidence of early complication [1–3] (Figure 42-1). Despite the challenges that laparoscopy can present, the outcomes can be as good as, or more often better than, their open counterparts. Patients who have undergone laparoscopic procedures require fewer analgesics, leave the hospital sooner and return to work and daily activities more quickly. Such outcomes are the result of preparing your patient for the laparoscopic experience. This includes informing the patient and the family about postoperative expectations such as initiating oral intake of food the evening of surgery and even anticipating discharge the day following surgery.

THE LAPAROSCOPIC TEAM: AN INTEGRATED APPROACH

To perform laparoscopic surgery safely, the surgical, anesthesia, and nursing staff must be experienced with laparoscopic techniques and familiar with specialized instrumentation. Once in the operating suite, the responsible surgeon must assume the role as team leader, orchestrating anesthesia, operating assistants, and nursing staff. An open line of communication between personnel before, during, and after laparoscopic surgery is mandatory (Figure 42-2).

INFORMED CONSENT

Patients must be given adequate information to obtain an informed consent prior to any surgical procedure. Alternative treatment modalities and relative risks and benefits should be discussed prior to laparoscopic surgery. Proper patient preparation begins with a frank discussion of the advantages and limitations of a laparoscopic approach. This includes describing potential risks specific to laparoscopy (which could include carbon dioxide [CO_2] diaphragmatic irritation, subcutaneous emphysema, gas embolism, and Veress needle and trocar injuries). Laparoscopic techniques represent "minimal access" surgery not "minimally invasive" surgery. The potential risks of an open surgical approach also apply to laparoscopic techniques. Patients must understand that conversion to an open procedure may be necessary if laparoscopic injury requires laparotomy. Patient and physician must enter a laparoscopic procedure with realistic expectations.

ASSESSING ANESTHETIC AND SURGICAL RISKS

Patient evaluation begins by assessing the general risks associated with anesthesia and surgery. As in open procedures, most minimal access procedures require tolerance to general anesthesia, fluid shifts, and stress on the cardiopulmonary system. Patients should be nutritionally fit and in a medically optimal condition prior to undergoing elective surgery.

Anesthetic risks specific to laparoscopic surgery must be considered when assessing patients' tolerance and suitability for laparoscopy. Such specific risks relate to absorption of insufflating CO_2, head-down positioning, and transmitted pneumoperitoneal pressure. Patients with impaired pulmonary function and/or significant cardiovascular dysfunction may not tolerate hypercarbia and/or respiratory compromise from peritoneal CO_2 insufflation. Both Trendelenburg positioning and increased abdominal pressures decrease pulmonary vital capacity, increase ventilation/perfusion mismatch, and impair oxygenation.[4–6] consequently, significant underlying pulmonary and cardiovascular disease are risk factors that may preclude a laparoscopic approach; such patients may be managed more safely using an open procedure. Additionally, Trendelenburg positioning during laparoscopic pelvic and transperitoneal abdominal surgery can decrease cerebral vascular flow and increase intracranial and intraocular pressures.[7,8] Patients with cerebral disease, glaucoma, or known cerebral metastases

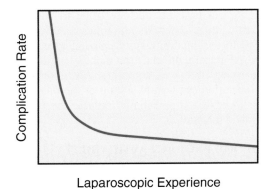

Figure 42-1 Correlation of initial learning curve and complications of laparoscopy.

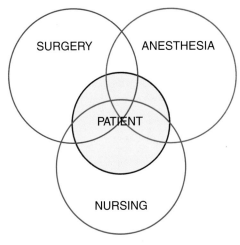

Figure 42-2 Optimal patient care requires integration of surgical, anesthetic, and nursing personnel.

are not ideal candidates for a laparoscopic approach. In reality, these are more theoretical issues than actual ones and rarely do we find our operative plans altered on their basis alone.

CONTRAINDICATIONS

The only absolute contraindication to laparoscopic surgery is improperly trained staff and lack of equipment. All other risks of surgery are determined by the surgeon's clinical judgment and weighed against alternative treatment options. Relative contraindications can be classified as infectious, anatomic, or systemic (Table 42-1) A history of either diffuse or prior severe peritonitis should be an indication for an open surgical approach. Bowel distention and abdominal adhesions associated with these forms of peritonitis greatly increase the risk of bowel injury and the difficulty of dissection. Performing laparoscopic surgery on morbidly obese patients should be considered only by the most experienced laparoscopists. The increased abdominal wall mass complicates trocar placement and necessitates increased pneumoperitoneal pressures to maintain an adequate working space.

Most risks related to anatomic deformities are associated with organ perforation or laceration during Veress needle or primary trocar insertion. These risks can be minimized by placing a Hasson cannula under direct vision to establish transperitoneal pneumoperitoneum or by using a retroperitoneal approach.[9] It should be noted, however, that open trocar placement does not guarantee having no injury to either visceral or vascular structures. Patients with abdominal wall hernias are at a theoretical risk for bowel herniation and strangulation during peritoneal insufflation. Similarly, patients with diaphragmatic or large hiatal hernias can extrude bowel into the chest cavity, impairing pulmonary function. As previously stated, patients with severe cardiac or pulmonary disease are not ideal candidates for laparoscopic surgery because of the possible side effects of CO_2 absorption and the physiologic

stress related to body position changes and establishing the pneumoperitoneum.

BOWEL PREPARATION

Initially, most patients undergoing transperitoneal laparoscopic procedures undergo full mechanical and antibiotic bowel preparation. As surgeons became more experienced and skilled at laparoscopic techniques, the need for bowel preparation has diminished. Today, bowel preparation for renal and adrenal laparoscopic surgery is generally not suggested. In addition, no bowel preparation is needed for laparoscopic varicocelectomy, pelvic lymph node dissection, diagnostic procedures, or procedures through a retroperitoneal approach. Laparoscopic procedures that involve a bowel anastomosis or that involve removal of the prostate typically require a bowel preparation. Mechanical bowel preparation can ease bowel dissection and mobilization and potentially minimize the interference from distended bowel. Furthermore, the addition of an antibiotic bowel preparation can reduce the morbidity from an actual bowel injury. One must keep in mind, however, that a full bowel may actually help with medial reflection of the colon during transperitoneal upper tract renal or adrenal surgery. Ultimately, the decision to administer a bowel preparation depends on the risk of bowel perforation. The risk of bowel perforation is multifactorial and depends on the individual patient, the surgeon, and the intended laparoscopic procedure. Patient risk factors relate to the presence of anterior abdominal wall adhesions, which are influenced by the number and type of previous abdominal surgical procedures. A prior uncomplicated open cholecystectomy, for example, may have little effect on adhesion formation and pelvic visualization for a laparoscopic pelvic lymph node dissection. In contrast, a history of previous bowel resection for an enteral fistula and inflammatory bowel disease may preclude a safe laparoscopic approach. Table 42-2 presents general guidelines for bowel preparation.

If a bowel preparation is indicated, we generally use either 4 L of GoLytely or two bottles of magnesium citrate solution given orally in conjunction with dietary clear liquids on the day prior to surgery. In addition, patients may undergo oral antibiotic preparation consisting of three oral doses of both erythromycin and neomycin base on the day prior to surgery. Lastly, broad-spectrum antibiotics are given on call to the operating suite. Having initiated a bowel preparation, one must make every attempt to ensure that it is complete. An incomplete preparation can lead to soiling of the operating room table and potentially increase the risk of wound infection.

BLOOD PRODUCT AVAILABILITY

All patients undergoing elective surgery should be given the opportunity to donate autologous blood preoperatively. Aortic and common iliac

vessel injury during Veress needle and primary trocar insertion can cause significant bleeding. Although the reported incidence of major vascular injury is low (0.03% to 0.09%), immediate laparotomy to obtain hemostasis is required.[10,11] The mean estimated blood loss in the larger reported series ranges from 172 to 219 cc for laparoscopic nephrectomy, and consequently, the risk of transfusion is less than 2%.[12–15] Infants, young children, and thin adults are at greatest risk for penetrating vascular injury, given the short distance between the anterior abdominal wall and great vessels, increasing the risk during Veress needle and trocar insertion.

Once a surgical team is proficient with laparoscopic techniques, blood availability requirements should be similar to those for an equivalent open surgical procedure (Table 42-3). Ideally, the patient should have a type and screen and "hold" prior to laparoscopic nephrectomy. Likewise, a serum type and screen is all that is required for pelvic operations including laparoscopic pelvic lymph node dissection. At least a type and "hold" is appropriate for laparoscopic prostatectomy. For challenging procedures involving major retroperitoneal dissections near the great vessels, two units of cross-matched blood, either autologous or not, should be considered.

AN ALGORITHM FOR A LAPAROSCOPIC SURGICAL APPROACH

After the decision is made to proceed with surgery, treatment options are presented to the patient in an objective fashion. If a laparoscopic approach is desirable and there are no contraindications, the patient is then medically optimized with appropriate medication as necessary. The operative staff is prepared and a team approach undertaken. Specialized equipment is made available and the operating suite is prepared. If necessary, the appropriate bowel preparation is initiated along with preoperative blood work and screening tests. A systematic decision tree for screening patients for a laparoscopic approach is presented in Figure 46-3.

Table 42-1 Relative Contraindications

Infectious States

Peritonitis
Abdominal wall infection
Sepsis

Anatomic Conditions

Mechanical or functional bowel obstruction
Multiple prior laparotomies
History of severe adhesions
Morbid obesity
Large intra-abdominal mass
Organomegaly
Ascites
Umbilical hernia
Large aneurysm of major blood vessel
Near-term pregnancy
Abdominal wall or diaphragmatic hernia

Systemic Factors

Severe cardiac or pulmonary disease
Shock
Uncorrected coagulopathy

Table 42-2 Bowel Preparation Guidelines

Diagnostic procedures	None
Procedures requiring improved visibility	Mechanical preparation
Procedures requiring improved visibility and minimalization of bowel injury	Mechanical and antibiotic preparation

Table 42-3 Blood Availability Guidelines

Diagnostic procedures	None
Pelvic procedures	Type and screen
Renal and major retroperitoneal procedures	Type and screen, "hold," or crossmatch

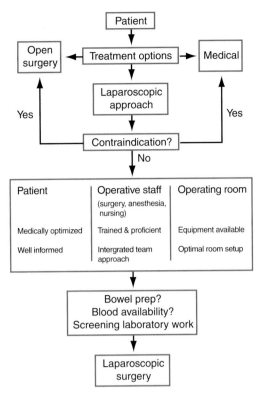

Figure 42-3 Preoperative algorithm for patients being considered for laparoscopic surgery.

ADJUNCTIVE ENDOSCOPIC PROCEDURES

Adjunctive endoscopic procedures performed either simultaneously or prior to peritoneal insufflation may facilitate laparoscopic surgery. Endoscopic placement of ureteral identification devices, cystoscopic light sources into bladder diverticula to aid in dissection, and bladder cuff incision prior to nephroureterectomy have all been described.[16–20] Ureteral identification is an important first step in laparoscopic ureteral surgery (including ureterolithotomy, ureterolysis, ureterectomy, and ileal loop urinary diversion) as well as in extirpative renal surgery and retroperitoneal lymph node dissections. In the early days of laparoscopy, ureteral identification was facilitated by preoperative placement of balloon occlusion catheters and ureteral catheters and stents to provide tactile and visual information about ureteral location.[16] Some even tried placement of ureteral illuminators to aid in ureter localization.[17] Currently, no such procedures or devices are necessary for extirpative renal surgery. The most important aid in ureteral localization is having a firm grasp on the anatomic relationship between the ureter and the gonadal vein. Almost always, the ureter will be found just anterior to the psoas muscle and lateral to the gonadal vein on both the right and left. Some laparoscopic procedures do require placement of ureteral stents or catheters. For example, a ureteral catheter during a partial nephrectomy allows instillation of methylene blue or indigo carmine into the renal pelvis to enable identification of a collecting system leak. Ureteral catheter placement during an ipsilateral ureteroureterostomy helps to discriminate between the upper and lower pole ureter. Furthermore, a Double-J stent placed immediately before laparoscopic pyeloplasty allows for postoperative drainage of the dilated system.

Transmitted cystoscopic light when cystoscopy is being performed simultaneously with laparoscopic bladder diverticulectomy can help localize diverticula and aid the dissection. Parra and colleagues initially described this technique using a rigid endoscope, but we have had equal success using a flexible cystoscope.[18] Traditionally, adjunctive transurethral endoscopic procedures have required either a change from the lithotomy position to the supine position or performing laparoscopic surgery in the dorsolithotomy position. Changing positions intraoperatively requires inordinate time, and the dorsolithotomy position can restrict surgeon mobility and visualization of video images. These problems can be resolved by preparing and draping the abdominal and genital areas with the patient supine and using flexible cystoscopy to perform adjunctive endoscopic procedures.

ADJUNCTIVE RADIOLOGIC PROCEDURES

Preoperative radiologic studies are imperative prior to laparoscopic surgery to provide vital anatomic information regarding genitourinary structures as well as adjacent organ orientation. Anatomic relationships become even more important when operating on dysmorphic patients or patients with anatomic variants. Computed tomography (CT) is the most widely used imaging modality. Angiography was once a useful adjunct for better delineating the vascular anatomy prior to partial nephrectomy or donor nephrectomy. Now, with the capabilities of CT angiography with 3D reconstruction and magnetic resonance imaging, traditional angiography has a limited role. We do not routinely perform additional imaging beyond a CT scan for the vast majority of adrenal and renal procedures. Even donor nephrectomy is performed without angiography. CT angiography with 3D reconstruction can be particularly helpful in identifying the presence or absence of a crossing lower pole vessel when planning ureteropelvic junction repair. Furthermore, this modality of imaging is excellent for delineating anomalous vascular anatomy such as a right-sided precaval renal artery. It cannot be stressed enough that no imaging can replace a very keen understanding of the anatomic relationships of one organ to the next, and of "safe" versus "unsafe" areas of dissection. For example, Chan et al described dividing the renal artery with minimal posterior dissection because no major structures lie behind the arter.[19] Placing a radiopaque marker on a known cutaneous landmark can help determine optimal trocar placement (Figure 46-4).

DEEP VENOUS THROMBOSIS PROPHYLAXIS

No studies are available to document an increased risk of lower extremity deep venous thrombosis or pulmonary embolism in patients undergoing laparoscopic surgery. A cumulative review of laparoscopic pelvic lymph node dissections performed at eight different medical centers revealed a 1.3% (5 of 372 patients) incidence of lower extremity deep vein thrombosis and no clinical pulmonary emboli.[21] Transmitted pneumoperitoneal pressures can collapse pelvic veins and compromise lower extremity venous return.[22] The placement of sequential pneumatic compression stockings has been shown to normalize pelvic venous flow during laparoscopic cholecystectomy.[23] In general, placement of lower extremity support stockings and sequential pneumatic compression devices are recommended for laparoscopic pelvic procedures and any intra-abdominal procedure lasting longer than 1 hour. The role of prophylactic subcutaneous heparin administration is controversial.

MEASURES TO PREVENT VISCERAL INJURY

Measures to prevent visceral injury include appropriate patient selection and intraoperative precautions. Laparoscopy should be avoided in patients with prohibitive risk factors for visceral injury.

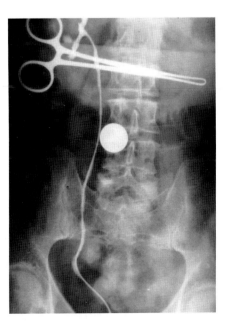

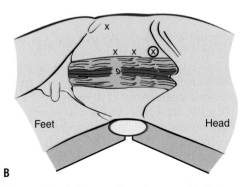

Figure 42-4 *A*, Retrograde pyelogram with sterile coin and Allis clamp placed as cutaneous markers to aid in optimal trocar placement. *B*, Patient positioning and trocar placement for laparoscopic nephrectomy.

Patients with bowel obstruction, inflammatory bowel disease, history of severe peritonitis, or history of extensive previous abdominal surgeries should not be considered ideal candidates for a laparoscopic approach. Despite precautionary measures, visceral injury remains a risk of laparoscopic surgery. An incidence of bowel injury of 0.01 to 0.03% is reported in the gynecologic laparoscopy literature.[10,24,25] Injury to the urinary tract is less common, with a 0.05% incidence in a cumulative series of laparoscopic pelvic lymph node dissection.[21] Most visceral injuries occur during blind passage of the Veress needle or primary trocar. A smaller percentage of injuries result from electrothermal burns that often are unrecognized at surgery and can result in a high morbidity.[26] Intraoperative placement of a nasogastric tube and indwelling urethral Foley catheter to decompress the bowel and bladder is recommended prior to establishing the pneumoperitoneum. Bladder drainage is vital in pediatric patients, because the bladder lies more intra-abdominally as compared to adults. A pediatric feeding tube can be used in place of a Foley catheter in infants and young children. The surgeon should also confer with the anesthesiologist to ensure that the patient is fully relaxed. This facilitates maximum pneumoperitoneum, and thus provides that additional distance between the anterior abdominal wall and the viscera. Veress needle placement at the umbilicus carries some risk for visceral perforation because of the potential for periumbilical adhesions or for a subclinical umbilical hernia. Changing Veress needle placement to Palmer's point has been shown to be both safe and effective.[27] This point is found just lateral to the lateral border of the rectus abdominis muscle and approximately two finger breadths below the costal margin. This site allows for obtaining safe pneumoperitoneum and for upper port placement for transperitoneal adrenal and renal procedures. One should always remember that the Veress needle may be placed into the contralateral side of the abdomen if one expects extensive adhesions at the intended site of surgery. Administration of nitrous oxide anesthesia has been associated with bowel distention and is discouraged, especially during long procedures.[28,29] Finally, a retroperitoneal approach to the genitourinary system further reduces the risk of bowel injury.

PATIENT POSITIONING

Intraoperative position changes and ancillary endoscopic or radiologic procedures must be taken into consideration. An operative table that enables intraoperative Trendelenburg and lateral side-to-side positioning is a necessity. Tables should allow attachment of lower extremity stirrup devices for dorsolithotomy positioning and fluoroscopic capability for adjunctive radiologic procedures. Once positioned, patients should be secured to the table using strap restraints and/or wide cloth tape at the level of the shoulders, pelvic girdle, and knees. A vacuum-activated beanbag device (Olympic Vac-Pac, Seattle, WA) to maintain patient position and pad pressure points can

be helpful during lateral decubitus positioning for retroperitoneal surgery on the adrenal glands, kidneys, and urinary collecting system. All pressure points should be padded prior to abdominal preparation and draping. In general, laparoscopic procedures may be longer than similar open procedures, making positioning and pressure point padding more critical. The table should be rotated into Trendelenburg, and lateral rotation and pressure points rechecked during the position changes. An axillary roll should be placed under the dependent axilla in patients in the lateral decubitus position. Shoulder restraints should be placed prior to pelvic procedures in which steep Trendelenburg positioning is anticipated. Conversely, a foot rest should be placed for procedures in which reverse Trendelenburg positioning is likely. Another effective way to prevent patients from slipping on the operating table is to apply benzoin and foam padding directly to the back of those who are likely to be positioned steeply. When using a robotic surgical system, the position of the patient and the table may not be changed after the patient and robot are coupled.

TRANSPERITONEAL PROCEDURES Transperitoneal access is preferred for approaching the adrenal glands, intra-abdominal and pelvic genitourinary organs, and their associated lymphatic drainage. It is considered the standard approach for laparoscopic varicocelectomy. Standard positioning begins with placing the patient in a lateral decubitus position. With the patient at approximately a 60° angle to the table, the table is then flexed. After placing an axillary roll, the down-arm is positioned and padded, with the elbow slightly flexed and the wrist slightly extended. The up-arm is draped over one or two folded pillows that are placed over the down-arm. It should appear as if the patient is hugging the pillows. Care must be taken not to hyperabduct the shoulders beyond 90 degrees to avoid brachial plexus injury.

RETROPERITONEAL APPROACH Patients undergoing retroperitoneal surgery on the adrenal glands, kidneys, or upper/middle ureters are placed in a similar lateral decubitus position. A vacuum-activated beanbag device can be used to stabilize patients placed in the lateral decubitus position. Percutaneous endoscopic retroperitoneal surgery was revolutionized when Gaur developed a balloon expansion device to create a retroperitoneal working space.[30] Advantages of a retroperitoneal versus transperitoneal approach to retroperitoneal structures are avoidance of hazards associated with establishing a pneumoperitoneum; lack of interfering mobile loops of bowel; a more direct approach to the renal hilum—particularly the renal artery—during extirpative renal surgery; and optimal visualization of the renal collecting system for reconstructive procedures. Exposure of the short right adrenal vein is improved through a retroperitoneal approach. Potential disadvantages of this approach are the relatively small working space and unfamiliar laparoscopic landmarks.

PELVIC PROCEDURES Laparoscopic pelvic lymph node dissection, bladder neck suspension, varicocelectomy, and prostatectomy are the most common pelvic urologic procedures. Patients are placed in either the supine or low lithotomy position. Access to the perineum and vaginal vault allows transvaginal elevation of the bladder neck while placing suspension sutures during incontinence procedures. Abducting and flexing the thighs allegedly opens the obturator space, facilitating pelvic lymph node dissection.[31] Patients are placed in a 10° to 15° Trendelenburg position for Veress needle insertion. Further Trendelenburg and lateral rotation may aid surgical exposure by displacing bowel. Positioning for an intraperitoneal or extraperitoneal approach to pelvic organs is similar. An extraperitoneal approach prevents visual obstruction from interfering loops of bowel and minimizes the amount of Trendelenburg rotation necessary to optimally visualize pelvic landmarks.

SURGICAL PREPARATION AND DRAPING

Once the patient and laparoscopic equipment have been properly positioned, the surgical area is cleansed and sterile drapes placed. Prior to draping, it should be verified that an electrical grounding pad for the electrosurgical unit has been connected. A Bair Hugger warming device (Augustine Medical, Eden Prairie, MN) is useful to maintain core body temperature for long laparoscopic procedures. Skin preparation should accommodate the need for conversion to an open operation. Emergency laparotomy rarely may be necessary to control bleeding, repair intra-abdominal injuries, or complete the planned procedure. The incidence of open laparotomy during laparoscopic pelvic lymph node dissection ranges from 2.6 to 4.3%.[21]

Surgical preparation for transperitoneal abdominal procedures extends from the nipple line to thighs and laterally to the posterior axillary line. Limiting skin preparation to the subcostal margin is adequate for pelvic procedures. Shaving of hair-bearing areas at planned trocar insertion sites is recommended. Preparation and exposure of the genitals during laparoscopic varicocelectomy allows traction of the ipsilateral testicle to aid cord structure identification and to manually decompress the pneumoscrotum (if present) prior to removal of trocars. Urethral access permits flexible cystoscopy for adjunctive endoscopic procedures.

LAPAROSCOPIC EQUIPMENT

Laparoscopic equipment and supplies vary according to the planned procedure and surgeon preferences (Table 42-4). Some laparoscopic equipment, however, is universally used in nearly all laparoscopic procedures. Abdominal adhesions and difficulty in establishing the pneumoperitoneum require that a Hasson cannula is available for peritoneal access. Sterile bags of

Table 42-4 Basic Laparoscopic Equipment
Main Instrument Table
Video monitoring
Rigid laparoscope: 0- and 30-degree lenses
Warming solution for laparoscope
Antifogging solution
Video camera
Fiberoptic light cord
Establishing pneumoperitoneum
Insufflation tubing
Veress needle or Hasson cannula
Laparoscopic portals
Trocars (number and size depend on procedure
and surgeon preference)
Reducer valves
Fascial threads
Suction/irrigation apparatus
Heparinized saline solution
Electrocautery instrument
Handpiece
Electrodes (hook, spatula)
Hand ports
Laparoscopic clamps
Satinsky clamps
Bulldog clamps
Atraumatic bowel clamp
Clips/Staplers
GIA/TA stapler
Weck clips
Special laparoscopic instruments
Needle drivers
Suture devices
Mechanical arm devices
Leonard arm
Laparoscopic Bookwalter
OMNI
Special Equipment
Tissue morcellator
Argon beam coagulator
Harmonic scalpel
Ligature
Intraoperative ultrasound
Fibrin products
Laparoscopic sponges
Robotic Systems
da Vinci
Zeus
Aesop
Secondary Instrument Table
Laparotomy set

premixed heparinized solution should be prepared for the irrigation setup. Standard solutions consist of 5,000 U of heparin in 1,000 mL of either normal saline or lactated Ringer's solution. Mechanical arm devices to stabilize and hold the laparoscope or retractors are available from a variety of manufacturers. These devices can substitute as a second surgical assistant and maximize the working space, comfort, and vision of the primary and first assisting surgeons. The need for specialized equipment must be conveyed well in advance to operating room personnel to ensure availability. Laparoscopic handports are readily available by a number of manufacturers. Ultimately, the surgeon must decide on the necessity

of such devices and on which particular brand best suits his or her laparoscopic needs. Laparoscopic staplers have become a very useful adjunct to procedures that require dividing significant vascular structures. Both GIA and TA staplers ought to be readily accessible. Many types and styles of laparoscopic instruments are available, and ultimately, the best instrument is the one that the surgeon is the most familiar with and feels the most comfortable with using. Depending on the particular procedure, the surgeon should have instruments that allow for intracorporeal sewing and knot tying. Laparoscopic Satinsky and "bulldog" clamps have facilitated performing nephrectomies with renal vein thrombus as well as partial nephrectomies. Laparoscopic bowel clamps are also available for procedures requiring bowel anastomoses. Electrocautery instruments are excellent for dividing tissue whether it is done with a hook or spatula. The Harmonic Scalpel (Ethicon Endosurgery, Cincinnati, OH) is useful for dissection and dividing small vessels. A handpiece to permit laparoscopic argon beam coagulation (ABC, Birtcher Medical Systems, Irvine, CA) to aid in hemostasis has proven useful during laparoscopic partial nephrectomy and fulguration of renal cysts and caliceal diverticula.[21,32,33] Care must be taken to vent the peritoneal cavity through accessory trocars during ABC operation to prevent excessive peritoneal pressures. Perhaps one of the most useful adjuncts to laparoscopic procedures is the availability of various fibrin tissue sealants that can be applied with the use of laparoscopic applicators.[34] Other useful equipment includes laparoscopic ultrasound and rolled sponges (Kittner Roll Gauze, Care Free Surgical Specialties, New Castle, CA) that can be placed through 10 mm ports.[35] The later can facilitate hemostasis and therefore improve visualization without using laparoscopic irrigators and suction which can compromise pneumoperitoneum when it is most needed.

IMAGING EQUIPMENT

Most hospitals do not have operating suites designed to accommodate the large amount of specialized equipment necessary for laparoscopic surgery. As a result, the organization and room setup for laparoscopic surgery often requires efficient use of room space and modification of existing operating rooms designed for traditional open surgery. Mobile equipment carts allow stacking units for housing video imaging and insufflation equipment (Figure 42-5). The main television monitor cart is positioned across from the primary surgeon and houses the insufflation unit and video monitoring equipment. This includes the camera console box, laparoscope light source, and videocassette recorder. The insufflator monitor should be positioned high on the equipment cart in clear view of the primary surgeon to allow monitoring of insufflation and intraperitoneal pressures. Video imaging has revolutionized laparoscopic surgery by facilitating coordination of surgeon and assistant

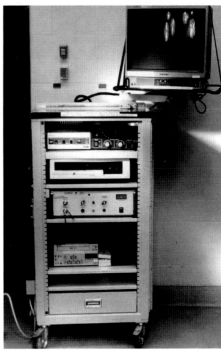

Figure 42-5 Mobile primary video monitor cart housing insufflator, light source, and video recording equipment.

movements. It is also an invaluable teaching aid. The electrocautery unit, camera, light source, video equipment, and specialized devices should be verified prior to patient positioning, preoperative testing and setting of the insufflator and reserve tank. A secondary equipment cart can house an accessory monitor, and if available, should be positioned across from the surgical assistant (Table 42-5).

POSITIONING OF EQUIPMENT AND SURGICAL TEAM RELATIVE TO PATIENT

In general, a coaxial alignment of surgeon, surgical area of interest, and video monitor optimizes vision and body positioning. The optimal configuration places the primary surgeon on the contralateral side of interest and the video monitor on the ipsilateral side. The availability of two video monitors allows a relaxed position for the operator(s) and maximizes the view. Optimal positioning of video monitor(s) also varies with the type of laparoscopic procedure (pelvic, abdominal, or retroperitoneal). Figure 42-6 depicts a typical

Table 42-5 Imaging Equipment
Main Television Monitor Cart
Video monitor on swivel arm extension
Insufflator
Camera console box
Light source
Videocassette recorder
Secondary Equipment Cart
Accessory monitor
Second insufflator if necessary

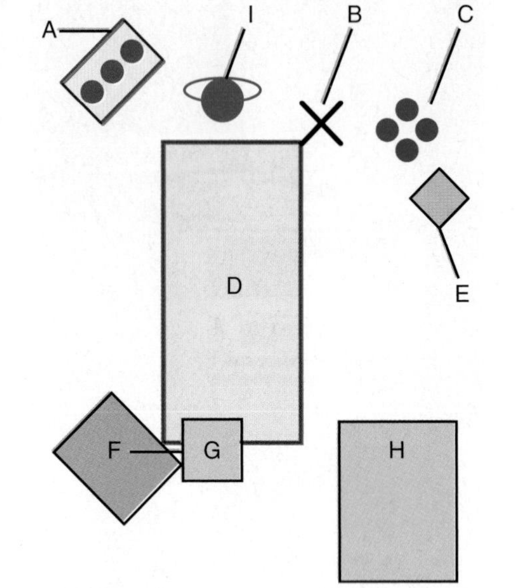

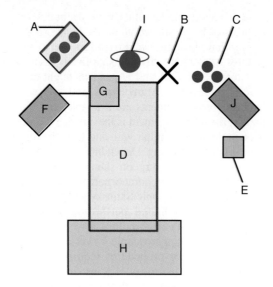

Figure 42-6 Diagram of general operating room setup for laparoscopic pelvic procedures. A = anesthesia monitor; B = intravenous pole; C = suction canisters; D = operating table; E = electrocautery unit; F = main equipment cart; G = primary video monitor; H = instrument table; I= anesthesiologist.

Figure 42-8 Diagram of general operating room setup for laparoscopic transperitoneal upper abdominal and retroperitoneal procedures. A = anesthesia monitor; B = IV pole; C = suction canisters; D = operating table; E = electrocautery unit; F= main equipment cart; G = primary video monitor; H= instrument table; I= anesthesiologist; J= secondary video cart and monitor.

room organization and setup for laparoscopic pelvic procedures. A single video monitor placed at the foot of the operating table permits unobstructed vision for the primary surgeon and assistants. Upper transperitoneal abdominal procedures do not afford this luxury given the space required for the anesthesiologist and monitoring equipment. Mounting the primary video monitor on a swivel arm allows for placement of the monitor over the patient's head (Figure 42-7). Figure 42-8 depicts a routing room organization for transperitoneal abdominal and/or retroperitoneal procedures. When a second video monitor is available, the instrument table is placed at the end of the operating table and video monitors positioned near the head opposite the primary and first assisting surgeons. Suction canisters and the electrocautery unit are positioned next to the secondary equipment cart. Ancillary equipment such as the Harmonic Scalpel or the argon beam coagulator can be positioned wherever room

space permits. The introduction of robotics demands even more space in an already crowded operating room. For example, the da Vinci Surgical System (Intuitive Surgical, Sunnyvale, CA) requires additional space for both the robotic element and the console. When using such a device, operating in large rooms can facilitate positioning and movement of this equipment. Others have used projectors to allow the assistant in robotic surgery to have 3D imaging during the operation.

CONCLUSION

Laparoscopic surgery is an extension of minimally invasive endoscopic techniques pioneered in urology. As with all urologic procedures, the safety and success of laparoscopic urologic procedures rely on proper patient selection and specific training of health care personnel. Preoperative patient preparation and open lines of communication between the patient and laparoscopic team members enhances the safety of the procedure and permits an objective evaluation of laparoscopic techniques. Technologic advances in laparoscopic instrumentation will continue to expand the use of minimally invasive techniques in urology.

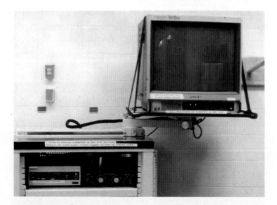

Figure 42-7 Video monitor mounted on swivel arm to optimize space.

REFERENCES

1. Kerbl K, Clayman RV, Petros JA, et al. Staging pelvic lymphadenectomy for prostate cancer: A comparison of laparoscopic and open techniques. J Urol 1993;150:396–9.
2. Hawasli A, Lloyd LR. Laparoscopic cholecystectomy. The learning curve: Report of 50 patients. Am Surg 1991; 57:542–4.
3. Wolfe BM, Gardiner BN, Leary BF, Frey CF. Endoscopic cholecystectomy: An analysis of complications. Arch Surg 1991;126:1192–6.
4. Altschule MD. The significance of changes in the lung vol-
5. ume and its subdivisions during and after abdominal operations. Anesthesiology 1943;4:385–91.
5. Wilcox S, Vandam LD. Alas, poor Trendelenburg and his position: a critique of its uses and effectiveness. Anesth Analg 1988;67:574–8.
6. Hodgson C, McClelland RMA, Newton JR. Some effects of the retroperitoneal insufflation of carbon dioxide at laparoscopy. Anaesthesia 1970;25:382–90.
7. Prentice JA, Martin JT. The Trendelenburg position. Anesthesiologic considerations. In: Martin JT, editor. Positioning in anesthesia and surgery. Philadelphia: WB Saunders; 1987. p. 127–45.
8. Gartner S, Beck W. Ocular tension in the Trendelenburg position. Am J Ophthalmol 1965;59:1040–3.
9. Hasson HM. Open laparoscopy: a report of 150 cases. J Reprod Med 1974;12:234–8.
10. Reidel HH, Lehmann-Willenbrock E, Conrad P, Semm K. German pelviscopic statistics for the years 1978-1982. Endoscopy 1978;18:219–22.
11. Mintz M. Risks and prophylaxis in laparoscopy: A survey of 100,000 cases. J Reprod Med 1977;18:269–72.
12. Portis AJ, Yan Y, Landman J, et al. Long–term followup after laparoscopic radical nephrectomy. J Urol 2002;167: 1257–62.
13. Gill IS, Merany AM, Schweizer DK, et al. Laparoscopic radical nephrectomy in 100 patients: a single center experience from the United States. Cancer 2001;92:1843–55.
14. Dunn MD, Portis AJ, Shalhav AL, et al. Laparoscopic versus open radical nephrectomy: a 9-year experience. J Urol 2000;164:1153–9.
15. Siqueira TM Jr, Kuo RL, Gardner TAAA, et al. Major complications in 213 laparoscopic nephrectomy cases: the Indianapolis experience. J Urol 2002; 168:1361–5.
16. Albala DM, Kavoussi LR, Clayman RV. Laparoscopic nephrectomy. Semin Urol 1992;10:146–51.
17. Low RK, Moran ME. Laparoscopic use of the ureteral illuminator. Urology 1993;42:455–7.
18. Parra RO, Hagood PG, Boullier JA. Endocavitary bladder surgery. Urology 1993;41:26–32.
19. Chan DY, Su LM, Kavoussi LR. Rapid ligation of renal hilum during transperitoneal laparoscopic nephrectomy. Urology 2001;57:360–2.
20. Chandhoke PJ, Clayman RV, Kerbl K, et al. Laparoscopic ureterectomy: initial clinical experience. J Urol 1993;149: 992–7.
21. Capelouto CC, Kavoussi LR. Complications of laparoscopic surgery. Urology 1993;42:2–12.
22. Jorgenson JO, Hanel K, Lalak NJ, et al. Thromboembolic complications of laparoscopic cholecystectomy [letter]. Br Med J 1993;306:518–9.
23. Millard JA, Hill BB, Cook PS, et al. Intermittent sequential pneumatic compression stockings in prevention of venous stasis associated with pneumoperitoneum during laparoscopic cholecystectomy. Arch Surg 1993;128:914–9.
24. Yuzpe AA. Pneumoperitoneum needle and trocar injuries in laparoscopy. A survey on possible contributing factors and prevention. J Reprod Med 1990;35:485–90.
25. Cunanan RG Jr, Courey NG, Lippes J. Complications of laparoscopic tubal sterilization. Obstet Gynecol 1980;55:501–6.
26. Wheeless CR. Thermal gastrointestinal injuries. In: Phillips JM, editor. Laparoscopy. Baltimore: Williams & Wilkins; 1977. p. 231–5.
27. Chung H, Meng MV, Abrahams HM, Stoller ML. Upper quadrant access for urologic laparoscopy. Urology. [In press]
28. Eger EI II, Saidman LJ. Hazards of nitrous oxide in bowel obstruction and pneumothorax. Anesthesiology 1965;26: 61–6.
29. Scheinin B, Lindgren L, Scheinin TM. Perioperative nitrous oxide delays bowel function after colonic surgery. Br J Anaesth 1990;64:154–8.
30. Gaur DD. Laparoscopic operative retroperitonoscopy: use of a new device. J Urol 1992;147:1137–9.
31. Guazzoni G, Montorsi F, Bergamaschi F, et al. Open surgical revision of laparoscopic pelvic lymphadenectomy for staging of prostate cancer: the impact of laparoscopic learning curve. J Urol 1994;151:930–3.
32. Stoller ML, Irby PB III, Osma M, Carroll PR. Laparoscopic marsupialization of a simple renal cyst. J Urol 1993;150: 1486–8.
33. Gluckman GR, Stoller M, Irby P. Laparoscopic pyelocaliceal diverticula ablation. J Endourol 1993;7:315–7.
34. Shekarriz B, Stoller ML. The use of fibrin sealant in urology. J Urol 2002;167:1218–25.
35. Gholami SS, Shekarriz B, Rudnick D, et al. The laparoscopic cigarette sponge. J Urol 2001;166:194.

43

Basic Laparoscopy: Instrumentation

Stephen V. Jackman, MD

Jay T. Bishoff, MD

Modern advances in laparoscopy are due, in large part, to the progress in the development of new laparoscopic instrumentation. Currently, only the surgeon's imagination and the willingness of the industry to produce innovative equipment limit the development of new devices. In this chapter, we describe the current state of the art in laparoscopic instrumentation with the goal of increasing the surgeon's knowledge of the devices available to assist them in their laparoscopic surgical procedures. Many of these instruments and techniques for their use are described in detail in subsequent chapters.

OPTICAL SYSTEM

A high-resolution magnified image of the operative site is a significant advantage of laparoscopy. Fine dissection, the ability to anticipate instrument needs, and teaching are enhanced by the equal availability of this image for the surgeon and other participants. The cost is a limited field of view and the occasional loss of visualization due to fogging, soiling, or equipment failure. Excellent visualization is essential for optimal completion of the procedure. A large and continually improving group of devices is available. The basic components are outlined in this section.

LAPAROSCOPES The laparoscope is a rod-lens, fiberoptic, or camera-on-a-chip endoscope. They are available with straight, angled (commonly 30° and 45°) and flexible lenses. Sizes range from "needleoscopes" that can pass through a Veress needle to 12 mm. Light transmission decreases as angle increases and size decreases.

LIGHT SOURCE Light is transmitted through the laparoscope via fiber optic cable from the light source. Halogen and xenon bulbs are the most common sources of high intensity light. Integrated light source and camera systems allow for automatic adjustment of light intensity. Damage to fiber optic cables will reduce light throughput and should be prevented.

CAMERA The camera system consists of the camera box and camera head. The head can be integrated into the laparoscope, either at the back or at the distal tip (camera-on-a-chip). Three-chip cameras provide better resolution and color but are heavier and more expensive. The camera box processes the image for output to the monitors. Adjustments commonly include white balance, gain, zoom, and shutter control.

VIDEO MONITOR Standard high-resolution CRT monitors are increasingly being replaced by the lighter flat-screen LCD monitors. This allows for easier and more ergonomic positioning using lightweight booms. Projection systems placing the image directly over the patient offer potentially the most intuitive images but suffer from lack of brightness and resolution. Advanced three-dimensional images are available with the da Vinci Surgical System (Intuitive Surgical, Mountain View, CA) described later.

RECORDING DEVICES Any type of video capture device can be adapted to document laparoscopic procedures. Still photos and VCRs are giving way to miniDV, direct-to-DVD, and flash memory recording devices.

ACCESS

Complications during laparoscopic surgery may occur at the time of initial access to the peritoneal cavity.[1] The traditional method of Veress needle insufflation followed by blind insertion of a cutting trocar is being replaced by new techniques including dilating-tip trocars, visual obturators, and variations on the open Hasson technique. Balloon dissection may be used to rapidly develop the retroperitoneal or retropubic spaces.

INSUFFLATION Pneumoperitoneum or pneumoretroperitoneum creates and maintains the working space for laparoscopic procedures. Carbon dioxide (CO_2) gas is currently used owing to its easy availability and lack of combustibility. The acidosis caused by CO_2 is countered by increased ventilation in all but the most severe pulmonary patients. These same patients are those for whom a flank incision would be most detrimental postoperatively, and thus, poor pulmonary status should not be an absolute contraindication to laparoscopy.

Insufflation pressures typically are kept between 8 and 20 mm Hg. Higher pressures improve working space and can be vital to completing procedures in heavier patients. The trade-off is higher gas resorption that is only a problem if not compensated for by increased ventilation. Higher pressure can increase postoperative pain in minor procedures but is not a factor in the majority of urologic laparoscopic procedures, where the type of procedure determines the pain.[2]

Insufflation pressure and gas flow is controlled with an insufflator. Current high-flow models can deliver 30 to 40 liters per minute, which can be useful when there is a port site leak or when using a hand-assist device. The use of two insufflators is also an option. Heated and humidified insufflation may reduce peritoneal irritation and pain.[3]

VERESS NEEDLE Initial access to, and insufflation of, the peritoneal space is still commonly performed using a Veress needle. It allows rapid and safe access in the virgin abdomen and can often be inserted in the right or left upper quadrant in patients with a history of prior surgery. This needle consists of an inner spring-loaded blunt tip and an outer sharp sheath (Figure 43-1). The blunt tip is compressed and exposed when pressed against firm structures such as fascia, but springs out to prevent injury to more compliant structures such as bowel.

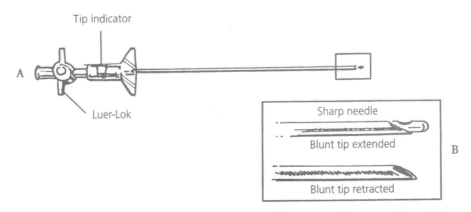

Figure 43-1 The Veress needle tip has an inner blunt core that retracts when encountering resistance from tissue but pops forward once the needle is in the peritoneal cavity.

TROCARS Cutting trocars offer rapid access to the peritoneal cavity, but their safety has been questioned for initial port placement, especially in the previously operated-upon abdomen. Even with secondary port placement under direct internal vision, the risk of laceration of body wall blood vessels and muscle exists. Transillumination of the abdominal wall is often useful for locating blood vessels in thin patients, but this is not possible in many cases. Finally, cutting trocars ≥ 10 mm make incisions in the fascia that require closure. For these reasons, dilating-tip or non-bladed trocars were developed. Many manufacturers offer versions of this style of trocar. The tips are typically cone-shaped, often with laterally placed fins to assist in the dilation. The fins can vary from sharp to dull. Advantages include smaller fascial openings after port removal, which do not require closure, and a higher likelihood of pushing aside rather than lacerating blood vessels and muscle.[4] This technology may be combined with direct visualization as described below. Disadvantages include a higher insertion force and increased difficulty penetrating compliant structures such as the peritoneum and bladder.[5]

VISUAL OBTURATORS Visual obturators, or direct-view trocars, are systems combining sheath, cutting or dilating element and laparoscope, allowing direct visualization of the layers and blood vessels of the body wall during entry. These devices are typically used after insufflation. Two disposable instruments in this category are the Visiport RPF Optical Trocar (U.S. Surgical, Norwalk, CT) and the Optiview Non-bladed Obturator (Ethicon Endo-Surgery, Cincinnati, OH) (Figures 43-2 and 43-3). The Visiport uses a trigger-activated cutting blade to enter the abdomen, whereas the Optiview has two dilating fins. The Optiview requires more pressure and rotation to enter the abdomen but retains the advantages of non-bladed instruments, including smaller fascial defects that may not require closure. The EndoTIP system (Karl Storz GmbH & Co. KG, Tuttlingen, Germany) is a reusable threaded screw-in trocar that allows visualization and also incorporates a dilating tip.

OPEN ACCESS DEVICES Open access using the Hasson technique is a viable option for entering

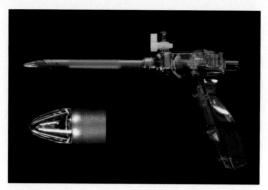

Figure 43-3 The Optiview (Ethicon Endo-Surgery, Cincinnati, OH) uses two sharpened plastic fins on the tip of the trocar.

the peritoneal cavity. This type of access is particularly important in children where standard-size laparoscopic trocars may be more likely to damage vital structures. Disadvantages of the Hasson technique include the need for a larger incision, more cumbersome trocar systems that may leak gas if not well secured, and increased difficulty in obese patients. The Step System (U.S. Surgical) is a modification of this method that solves some of these problems (Figure 43-4). Through a small skin incision, the fascia and peritoneum are opened 2 to 3 mm under direct visualization. The mesh sleeve is then inserted and dilated with a rigid cannula and dilator to the desired size (5 to 12 mm). The entire system can also be used over a Veress needle, but the advantages of open insertion are lost. The fascial defect left after removing a Step trocar has been shown to be 50% smaller than that of a conventional cutting trocar.[6] Overlying tissue and muscle planes

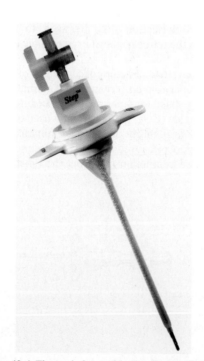

Figure 43-4 The mesh sleeve of the Step System (U.S. Surgical, Norwalk, CT) can be placed in an open fashion or used with a Veress needle as shown. The cannula and dilator is then passed through the sleeve. Photographs courtesy of United States Surgical, a division of Tyco Healthcare.

return to their preoperative location after removal and provide further closure of the wound.

A prospective randomized trial in 250 patients showed that the Step System results in significantly less intraoperative cannula site bleeding and postoperative wound complications than conventional cutting trocars.[7] Furthermore, no port site hernias were seen, despite not closing any of the Step port sites.

Another modification of the Hasson technique for access to non-peritoneal locations is use of a balloon to rapidly develop the space. This was initially done using a red-rubber catheter with a glove finger secured to the end. More convenient commercial products are now available, which perform the same task. A useful combination of balloon and visual obturator, the Preperitoneal Distention Balloon System (U.S. Surgical) or Spacemaker II Balloon Dissector (U.S. Surgical) are available to allow direct observation during space creation (Figure 43-5). They require use of a balloon-tipped or Hasson trocar to seal the initial incision. The Blunt-tipped Trocar (U.S. Surgical) is a significant advance over the standard Hasson trocar. It has a balloon at the distal end to hold it in place, and a sliding foam ring proximally to seal it to the abdomen. This allows full 360° motion without leakage in a small footprint device (Figure 43-6).

INSTRUMENTATION

Basic laparoscopic grasping, dissecting and cutting instruments are available from many manufacturers and are quite similar. They vary in size (2 to 10 mm), handle type, action (single or double), jaw curvature, ability to lock closed, rotate or roticulate, and presence of insulation for electrocautery use. Five millimeter scissor-handle, rotating, insulated, curved jaw instruments are most common. High-use basic instruments include the curved atraumatic grasper (Maryland-type), atraumatic locking bowel grasper, curved scissors and hook electrode. Surgeons will develop their own preferences with training and experience.

IRRIGATOR/ASPIRATOR The irrigator/aspirator is an essential tool for both cleaning up the operative site for optimal visualization as well as dis-

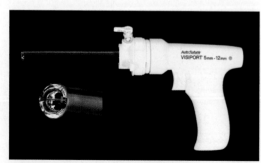

Figure 43-2 The Visiport (U.S. Surgical, Norwalk, CT) uses a recessed blade that extends out of the end of the obturator as the surgeon fires a trigger.

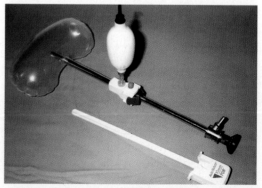

Figure 43-5 With the Preperitoneal Distention Balloon System (U.S. Surgical, Norwalk, CT), the retroperitoneal space can be balloon-developed under direct vision.

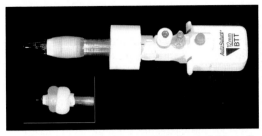

Figure 43-6 The blunt tip trocar (U.S. Surgical, Norwalk, CT) uses a balloon, inflated after insertion through the entry site, and a sliding foam collar to seal the trocar site at the fascia. Only a small amount of the trocar protrudes into the working space.

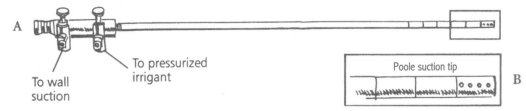

Figure 43-7 *A*, Combined irrigator/aspirator has a trumpet valve mechanism for separately activating irrigation and suction. *B*, Poole suction tip.

section. The Poole suction design and blunt tip of most devices minimizes impaction of tissue in the device and allows gentle bursts of suction to be used to tease apart tissue planes (Fig. 43-7).

RETRACTORS Safe retraction of organs, such as the liver and bowel, is often necessary for access to the operative site. When adequate gravity retraction is not possible, numerous instruments are available. They typically are variations on the design of a straight 5- or 10-mm instrument that transforms into a wider configuration once inserted.

An innovative reusable device is the Diamond Flex 80 mm Angled Triangular Liver Retractor (Genzyme Surgical Products Corp., Tucker, GA) (Figure 43-8). This long multi-jointed instrument passes through a 5-mm port and then transforms into a rigid triangular shape after its knob is tightened. Other sizes and configurations exist. Disadvantages include the initial expense and the metal construction that does not hold organs as securely as some disposable fabric devices.

The PEER retractor (Jarit Surgical Instruments, Hawthorne, NY) is another reusable device that opens to provide retraction in a variety of situations. It is available in 5 and 10 mm sizes (Figure 43-9).

Fan retractors are available from several manufacturers in either reusable or disposable form. They typically fit through a 10-mm port and "fan" open into a triangular shape. Other common variations include balloon or fabric that expands after insertion.

Retraction of some structures during laparoscopic surgery can be accomplished using a 2-0 or larger suture on a straight needle passed directly through the skin and anterior abdominal wall. Once in the surgical field, the needle is passed though or around the tissue to be retracted and then back through the abdominal wall with both strands of suture held in place at the skin surface with a hemostat.

INSTRUMENT HOLDERS Several mechanical instrument holders have been developed to take the place of the assistant. The instrument is then positioned and locked in place by one of several methods. The basic Martin Arm (Mick Radio-Nuclear Instruments, Inc., Mount Vernon, NY) is a multi-jointed stainless steel arm that requires

each joint to be positioned and hand-tightened. The Unitrac Retraction System (Aesculap, Center Valley, CA) is an advanced version of the Martin Arm that uses compressed air to allow pneumatic locking and unlocking with a single button (Figure 43-10). The Endoholder (Codman Inc., Cincinnati, OH) is an innovative device with a flexible gooseneck that can be quickly bent into position.[8] The TISKA Endoarm (Karl Storz, Endoskope, Tuttlingen, Germany) is a system developed to assist with trocar and instrument positioning. This device maintains the position of the trocar sheath at a fixed point at the trocar puncture site, while instruments or laparoscopes are changed or removed. Routine laparoscopic needs such as tissue retraction can easily be performed with this system. When combined with a robotic camera holder, these instrument holders permit many procedures to be done completely without assistance.

HEMOSTASIS Some of the most significant advances in laparoscopic instrumentation have been achieved in obtaining hemostasis. Excessive bleeding from even small venous vessels can quickly obscure the surgical field, making it difficult to find the correct planes of dissection. The availability of new delivery systems for electrocautery, ultrasound, clips, staples, clamps and fibrin products have allowed laparoscopy to approach open surgery in even the most challenging cases.

Electrocautery Monopolar electrocautery has been the mainstay for hemostasis of small

vessels during dissection. In the monopolar circuit, the active electrode is in the surgical site, and the return electrode is the grounding pad. Consequently, the current passes through the body of the patient to complete the circuit.

When using monopolar electrocautery, the current is not localized to the visible portion of the instrument. Since only 15% of the entire length of the electrocautery instrument is seen with the laparoscope at any given time, injuries from stray energy can occur out of the surgeon's field of view.[9] More than half of laparoscopic bowel injuries reported in the literature result from monopolar electrocautery.[10] Application of monopolar electricity to duct-like strands of tissue attached to bowel, even during a short burst of energy can result in tissue death at the bowel segment.[11] Unrecognized bowel injuries can also occur from the use of monopolar electrocautery when stray energy is released from unrecognized breaks in the integrity of the insulated coating or from capacitive coupling along the shaft of the monopolar instruments or trocar.

Cautery injury can be minimized through the use of active electrode monitoring (AEM) devices or insulation scanners for monopolar instruments and bipolar electrocautery. The Electroscope AEM system (Electroscope, Inc., Boulder, CO) includes a unique set of laparoscopic instruments that are simultaneously connected to a standard electrocautery machine and to a separate device that continuously searches for stray

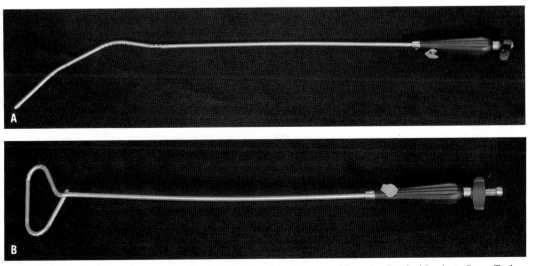

Figure 43-8 *A*, The Diamond Flex 80 mm Angled Triangular Liver Retractor (Genzyme Surgical Products Corp., Tucker, GA) fits through a 5-mm cannula. *B*, Twisting the handle converts the retractor to a rigid, angled triangular shape with large surface area.

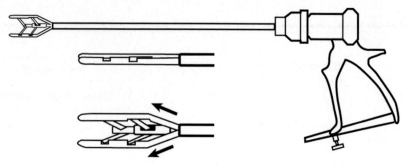

Figure 43-9 The reusable PEER retractor (Jarit Surgical Instruments, Hawthorne, New York) is available in 5-mm and 10-mm sizes, which expand to provide a 20-plus or 40-plus mm surface for retraction.

energy escaping along the shaft of the instrument. When stray energy is detected, the active electrode monitoring system deactivates the electrosurgical generator before injury can occur. The integrity of the insulated coating on the shaft of laparoscopic instruments can also be determined on the back table, prior to placing the instrument into the patient, by using the InsulScan (Medline Industries, Inc., Mundelein, IL). Both disposable and reusable instruments can be tested for visually undetectable holes in the insulation sheath.

In bipolar electrocautery, the active electrode and the return electrode functions are performed at the site of surgery between the tips of the instrument. The waveform is continuous, low current, and low voltage. Since the flow of current is restricted between the contact points of the instrument tip, only the tissue grasped is included in the electrical circuit, minimizing the risk of injury from stray surgical energy. Thermal injury can be prevented by vigilant surveillance of monopolar contact points during dissection.

The Ligasure (Valleylab, Boulder, CO) is a specialized electrosurgical generator/instrument system developed to reliably seal tissue and blood vessels up to 7 mm in diameter during laparoscopic or open surgery. The electrical generator delivers a continuous wave form of low-voltage, high-current flow and pulsed electrosurgical energy to tissue between the jaws of the instrument. The tissue is under a predetermined amount of pressure set by the unique locking jaws of the instrument. The vessel lumen is obliterated as collagen, and elastin in the vessel wall fuses to form a permanent seal. The seal zone is then divided with standard laparoscopic scissors. The

newest version (Ligasure Atlas, Valleylab) is a 10-mm instrument that incorporates a blade in the jaws of the instrument to safely divide the obliterated tissue.

Monopolar Radiofrequency For nephron-sparing surgery, the quest for hemostasis without the need for total renal ischemia led to the investigation of new delivery systems for electrical energy. The Floating Ball (Tissue Link Medical Inc, Dover, NH) has been shown to be of some assistance during partial nephrectomy. As a conductive fluid drips from the tip of the device, radiofrequency energy is transmitted through the fluid at the point of tissue contact. Collagen in tissues shrinks, stopping blood flow in treated tissues.[12]

Argon Gas Coagulation Argon–gas-enhanced coagulation is useful for the treatment of solid organ bleeding, including from the kidney, liver, and spleen. This system uses a stream of argon gas to improve the delivery of the electrosurgical current. Argon gas is noncombustible and inert, making it a safe gas to use in the presence of electrosurgical current. The argon gas is ionized by the electrical current, making it more conductive than air. The flow of argon gas also disperses blood, improving visualization during coagulation. During argon beam coagulation the pressure inside the abdomen can quickly rise above the preset level. Consequently, an insufflation port should be opened during coagulation and the intra-abdominal pressure carefully monitored.

Ultrasound A relatively new tool for laparoscopic dissection uses ultrasonic energy to achieve precise cutting and coagulation. Three devices are currently available (The UltraCision System, Ethicon Endo-Surgery; The AutoSonix System, U.S. Surgical; SonoSurg, Olympus America, Inc., Melville, NY). Energy is delivered using a laparoscopic 5-mm or 10-mm hand piece with a shaft tuned to conduct the ultrasonic vibration at the rate of approximately 55,000 cycles per second. The vibration causes heat, which is more precisely located at the vibrating tip and, at 50° to 100°C, is much lower than conventional electrocautery. Different tip configurations are available, including hooks, shears, and blunt probes. As the tissue is compressed between the jaws of the shears, blood vessels are occluded and the vibration causes intracellular water vaporization. Proteins are denatured in the tissue, and pro-

tein coagulum forms to seal the blood vessels while the tissue is divided. Hemostasis and division of tissue occurs at temperatures less than conventional cautery, without the wide dispersion of heat creating a small band of tissue necrosis. Water vapor is emitted in the abdomen instead of smoke. While the cords are reusable for all three systems, only the Olympus SonoSurg offers an autoclaveable, reusable hand piece.

Temporary Vessel Occlusion Laparoscopic partial nephrectomy is now possible owing to instruments that allow temporary occlusion of the renal hilar vessels. Two manufacturers offer bulldog clamps that are endoscopically applied through a 10-mm trocar. The jaws range in size from 17 to 45 mm and come in curved and straight configurations (Klein Surgical Systems, San Antonio, TX; Aesculap, Inc., Center Valley, PA;) (Figure 43-11). A 5-mm laparoscopic Satinsky clamp is also available but requires the placement of an additional trocar (Klein Surgical Systems).

Surgical Clips Occlusive clips are useful for small veins and arteries and have become standard equipment in many laparoscopic cases. Most endoscopic clips today are made of titanium, and vary in size from 5 to 12 mm. Nonabsorbable, polymer locking clips are also available and offer the advantage of being radiolucent (Weck Closure Systems, Research Triangle Park, NC) (Figure 43-12). There are absorbable clips, and some research shows no difference in adhesion formation between metallic and absorbable clips.[13]

Most laparoscopic clip appliers are single-use and multi-load, carrying between 15 and 30 clips per unit (Table 43-1). The ability to fire multiple clips without exiting the abdomen to reload can save significant time and decreases blood loss. In general, the diameter of the shaft depends on the size of the clips. The Endoclip (U.S. Surgical) 5-mm shaft, single-use clip applier can deliver a slightly larger clip than other 5 mm clippers: its hinged jaws are normally retracted within the shaft, but upon squeezing the handles they advance and expand, and a clip is automatically loaded. Most disposable clip appliers have 360° rotating shafts, allowing the handle of the instrument to rest comfortably in the hand while placing the tips around the target tissue at an ideal angle. Right-angle clip appliers (U.S. Surgical) are also available and can offer a visual advantage in situations where the tips of straight appliers are not well seen.

Tacking Staples The laparoscopic biting stapler was originally developed for laparoscopic hernia repair with mesh, but these devices are also useful in refashioning the peritoneum in laparoscopic ureterolysis and fixing mesenteric defects in bowel resections. Much like the staplers used for skin wound closure, laparoscopic staplers fire titanium staples with sharp ends that enter the tissue and then undergo deformation into a rectangular shape or deploy in cork-screw formation to secure tissue. Most contemporary devices are single-use and multi-load, with 15 to 30 staples per unit. A 360° rotating shaft allows accurate placement of the staple. Some devices

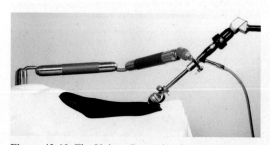

Figure 43-10 The Unitrac Retraction System (Aesculap, Center Valley, CA) is locked in place with compressed air. It can hold various instruments for retraction. Photograph courtesy of Aesculap.

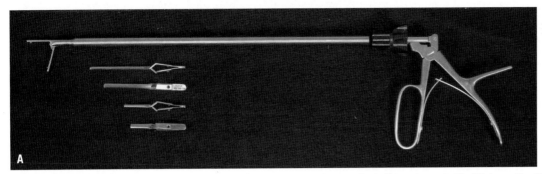
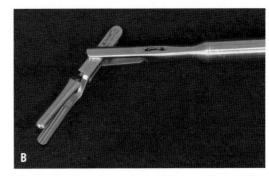

Figure 43-11 *A*, This 10-mm applier allows laparoscopic placement of a vascular bulldog clamp. *B*, The Klein applier (Klein Surgical Systems, San Antonio, TX) also allows rotation and angulation of the bulldog clamp.

also come with a 60° to 65° distal articulating head, which permits tacking hard-to-reach areas like the anterior abdominal wall and deep pelvis.

Linear Staplers Laparoscopic linear staplers are essential for rapid, safe intracorporeal tissue division and re-approximation of visceral structures. With a squeeze of a handle, these devices deploy multiple, closely spaced, parallel rows of titanium staples. Staples come in three different "loads": thin/vascular, medium, and large/thick, and are color-coded for easy recognition. Thin staples penetrate tissue to a depth of 2 to 2.5 mm, deform to an exaggerated b-shape, and form a reliably hemostatic staple line. These staples are ideal for rapid division of vascular pedicles. Medium to large staples are 3.0 to 4.8 mm thick in their closed form, and are useful in securing thicker tissues like bowel, bladder, and ureter. The larger staples do not fold to the same tight shape as small staples and should not be used for primarily hemostatic ligation. Staplers today allow the same instrument to fire between 8 and 25 separate loads before stapler disposal.

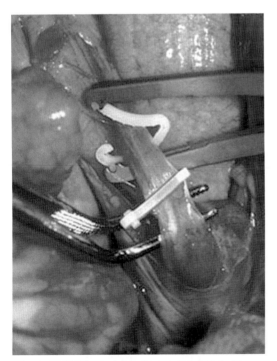

Figure 43-12 Hem-o-lok polymer clips (Weck Closure Systems, Research Triangle Park, NC). Photograph courtesy of Weck Closure Systems.

Linear staplers can be broadly classified into cutting and non-cutting. Cutting versions deploy loads with six intercalated parallel rows of staples. As the staples are fired, a knife follows closely behind and incises the tissue between the staples, leaving 3 rows of staples on each side. The staple line extends past the range of the cutting knife by one or two staples to avoid incising non-secured tissue. Once the staples are fired, a safety feature on all devices prevents accidental re-deployment of the cutting knife until a new load with staples is in place. Non-cutting staplers simply fire three to four parallel rows of staples, and are useful for closing enterotomies and repairing bladder injuries.

Laparoscopic linear cutting staplers are further distinguished by the length of their staple line (30/35 mm, 45 mm, and 60 mm), and whether their firing heads are articulated or not (Table 43-2). An articulating head gives a greater range of motion from a fixed trocar, but also adds to the price. All devices offer a rotating shaft, which allows proper visualization of the tips during firing. On most models, a replacement load consists of a fresh six rows of staples but uses the same knife and anvil inherent to the actual stapling device. The Endo GIA Universal linear cutting stapler (U.S. Surgical) is a universal firing device that accommodates both articulating and non-articulating loads of varying lengths (30 mm, 45 mm, and 60 mm). The stapler is unique in that the jaws, anvil and knife are inherent to the load and not part of the actual base unit (ie, each reload comes with a new knife). This system also allows the surgeon to use loads (articulating or fixed) of varying lengths without having to open a new stapler. The minimum-size limitation posed by the width of the staple load

requires use of a 10 mm or larger port for all currently available staplers.[14]

Loop ligation Loop ligatures are valuable in securing an already transected pedicle. A length of suture with a preformed sliding, locking knot is passed intracorporeally. The structure to be ligated is then retracted through the loop with a grasper, and the loop cinched down with a knot pusher. Two loop ligature systems are available with both 0 and 2-0 plain gut, chromic gut, polyester and synthetic absorbable varieties (Surgitie from U.S. Surgical; Endoloop from Ethicon). The plastic knot pusher is only available in one length, and may be too short to reach the target site if the wrong port is chosen. Two hands are needed to cinch the knot, requiring an assistant to grasp the tissue and hold it still.

Fibrin Products Fibrin tissue adhesive (FTA) has gained widespread acceptance in a variety of surgical procedures as an adhesive, sealant, hemostatic agent, carrier for growth factors or antibiotics. It has been used in many different urologic procedures to assist with hemostasis and tissue adhesion.[15,16] FTA can also be valuable in treating complications of laparoscopic surgery, including spleen and liver injury, urinary fistula formation, and wound dehiscence.[17] At present, FTA is made from autologous preparations using a patient's own blood or from homologous sources using a single donor or pooled samples.

Concentrates of coagulation factors are known for their adhesive and coagulation properties. In addition, fibrin in surgical wounds promotes healing by supplying a network for the growth of fibroblasts and activating macrophages.[18] Surgeons have prepared their own fibrin sealants for many years. These locally prepared products, however, are not standardized, and the sources of

Table 43-1 Clip Appliers (Multi-load, Single Use)					
	Ligaclip Allport	Ligaclip ERCA	Right Angle AccuClip	Endoclip 5 mm	Endoclip II
Company	Ethicon	Ethicon	U.S. Surgical	U.S. Surgical	U.S. Surgical
Port size	5 mm	10 and 12 mm	8 mm	5 mm	10 mm
Clips	20	20	20	12	20
Clip sizes	Medium, Medium/Large	Medium, Medium/Large, Large	Medium/Large	Medium/Large	Medium/Large, Large
Clip load	Automatic	Automatic	Automatic	Separate lever	Automatic
Cost	$146	$111	$245	$335	$236

Table 43-2 Linear Staplers

	Endopath ETS	Endopath ETS/ flex articulating	Endopath EZ45: cutter	Multifire Endo GIA 30	Multifire Endo TA	Endo GIA Universal
Company	Ethicon	Ethicon	Ethicon	U.S. Surgical	U.S. Surgical	U.S. Surgical
Port size	12 mm	12 mm	18 mm	12 mm	12 mm	12 mm, 15 mm
Staple size	2.5,3.5,4.1 mm	2.5, 3.5, 4.1 mm	3.8, 4.5 mm	2.0, 2.5 3.5 mm	2.5, 3.5 mm	2.0, 2.5, 3.5,4.8 mm
Staple length	35m, 45 mm	35 mm, 45 mm	45 mm	30 mm	30 mm	30, 45 & 60 mm
Rotating shaft	Yes	Yes	Yes	Yes	Yes	Yes
Articulating	No	Yes	No	No	No	Yes
Cost	$269	$311	$260	$375	$375	$451

fibrinogen are not virally inactivated. Blood-derived products are now commercially available for topical application to control bleeding and seal tissue. The basic principle is the same for these kits. Human thrombin and fibrinogen are applied separately to a bleeding site resulting in formation of a layer of fibrin that controls the bleeding and seals tissue.

Commercial preparations reproduce the final stage of coagulation resulting in their adhesive, hemostatic and healing effects through the polymerization of fibrin chains with collagen of adjacent or damaged tissue. These fibrin sealants are made from different combinations of fibrinogen and thrombin derived from human plasma and fibrinolysis inhibitor, a substance of bovine origin. As part of normal coagulation, fibrinogen undergoes proteolysis by the enzyme thrombin to form a fibrin monomer that polymerizes into fibrin strands, making up a major component of the actual clot. Thrombin also activates clotting factor XIII, promoting cross-linking of the fibrin monomer to stabilize the fibrin network. Thrombin is found in the plasma as an inactive precursor—prothrombin. After proteolysis, the active enzyme thrombin is formed. Proteolysis occurs as a result of tissue damage to cell membranes (extrinsic pathway) or trauma to the blood vessel walls, exposing collagen (intrinsic pathway) resulting in the activation of thrombin followed by fibrin clot formation. The clotting time of fibrin sealant is dependent on the concentration of thrombin in the sealant.

Commercial fibrin sealants are typically packaged as freeze-dried concentrates of human fibrinogen and thrombin in separate containers. The powders are reconstituted, and bovine fibrinolysis inhibitor (Aprotinin) is added to the liquid fibrinogen. When the fibrinogen and thrombin solutions are mixed, they become active, forming a clot or adhesive (Haemacure Corp, Sarasota, FL; Tisseel, Baxter Healthcare Corporation, Glendale, CA). Another product currently available uses the patient's own plasma mixed with bovine thrombin and bovine collagen (CoStasis, U.S. Surgical) but is FDA approved for hemostasis alone and not for tissue sealing or tissue adhesion.

The American Red Cross developed a lyophilized fibrinogen and thrombin product in powder formulation and as a 4-by-4 pressure bandage. The powder spray formulation has been shown to prevent bleeding and urine leak, in a laparoscopic porcine heminephrectomy model, without any suturing of the parenchyma or collecting system.[19] A similar product as a 4-by-4 bandage is designed to be applied directly to the wound in open cases.[20–23] When these products contact the surgical site or blood, they are activated and rapidly form a dense synthetic clot. The lyophilized formulation is currently under investigation and not FDA-approved for human use.

Since fibrin sealants commonly consist of human and bovine products, there is a theoretical risk of viral transmission, anaphylaxis, and coagulopathy. Viral transmission is of concern, because pooled human plasma is used to make the sealant. Donor screening, heat treatment of tissue, and solvent/detergent treatment seem to be effective in maintaining the safety of these products by preventing the transmission of HIV, Epstein-Barr virus, cytomegalovirus and hepatitis.[24] Four patients, however, are known to have been infected with parvovirus B19 following treatment with fibrin sealant.[25,26] Infection with parvovirus B19 is usually asymptomatic or may present with a minor febrile illness. Rarely, transient aplitic crisis with rapid red blood cell turnover can occur. There is an isolated report of a patient who developed rash, bronchospasm and circulatory collapse following use of fibrin sealant to close an enterocutaneous fistula. A complete investigation showed her to have aprotinin-specific antibodies, which were the most likely cause of the severe anaphylactic reaction.[27] Fibrin sealants are designed for topical use and are not designed for systemic injection. Intravenous injection could result in systemic activation of the coagulation cascade and fatal thrombosis. No systemic effects have been reported using sealants on surgical bleeding sites.

SUTURING Given the complexity of suturing in the laparoscopic environment, the majority of early laparoscopic urologic cases were extirpative and required little to no reconstruction. Unique demands to be overcome include a fixed center of motion, limited needle and suture handling ability, lack of three-dimensional perspective, and intracorporeal knot tying. Today, with the increasing interest in laparoscopic radical prostatectomy, more urologists are becoming proficient in free-hand suturing. This technique is applicable to most situations and offers the greatest flexibility with respect to suture and needle choices as well as the angle at which a needle may be held. Most popular needle drivers have single action and a Castro-Viejo–type inline locking mechanism. For special circumstances and for those less experienced in free-hand techniques, several instruments have been developed to facilitate laparoscopic suturing.

The EndoStitch (U.S. Surgical) is an innovative device that passes a small needle back and forth between jaws allowing both running and interrupted suturing techniques without the need to worry about reloading the needle. It also facilitates rapid intracorporeal knot tying. Limitations of the EndoStitch include its 10 mm width and short dull needle, which cannot be passed through thick tissue and is more traumatic than a similar-sized swedged-on suture. The needle can only be passed perpendicularly from jaw to jaw and may require excess tissue manipulation for proper suture placement. Finally, the device is disposable and reloads are costly adding to the expense of a case. Despite these disadvantages, the EndoStitch has been used very successfully, even in cases requiring delicate reconstruction, such as laparoscopic pyeloplasty.[28]

The Suture Assist (Ethicon Endo-Surgery, Cincinnati, OH) is a 5-mm instrument designed to quickly place a pre-tied knot after using either the device or a needle driver to place a single or figure-of-eight throw. Running sutures are not possible without using an alternative knot-tying method for the second knot. Like the EndoStitch, the Suture Assist is disposable and relies on reloads.

A newer 5-mm instrument, the Sew-Right SR5 (LSI Solutions, Rochester, NY), uses two built-in needles to place a simple suture precisely through even relatively thick tissue. Advantages include its 5-mm size and needle passage parallel to the device, which may be better for some applications. With tenacious tissue, if the needle deviates or does not fully penetrate the tissue, it may miss or not engage the suture at the distal jaw. Again, this is a disposable instrument, and only a single, simple suture can be placed per load.

A final device, the Quik-Stitch (Pare Surgical, Englewood, CO) is available in 3-mm, 5-mm, 10-mm and 12-mm versions. This system consists of a proprietary needle driver passed through a spool containing a pre-tied knot. A single or figure-of-eight suture is placed or passed followed by release, setting, and advancement of the knot. The device and needle driver are reusable, making it economical. Straight, curved, and blunt needles are available on absorbable and non-absorbable suture.

Early in the course of laparoscopy, knots were tied extracorporeally and transported to the site with a knot pusher. Intracorporeal knot tying is quicker and more versatile once practiced. Intracorporeal knot tying, especially the second knot of a running suture, can be complicated. This is due to the short suture length often available for tying, the need to tie a single strand to a loop, and difficulty maintaining constant tension on a knot. Two instruments are available to assist with this task. The Lapra-Ty (Ethicon Endo-Surgery) is a Vicryl clip delivered by a reusable 10-mm device.

The LapraTy can be placed on the tail of a suture as the first knot or at the end of a running or simple suture instead of tying. A concern is that a large number of clips may incite an inflammatory reaction or fistula. It is therefore most valuable for the final "knot" of running sutures.

A second "knot-tying" instrument is the Ti-Knot TK5 (LSI Solutions). This device is designed to replace extracorporeal knot tying. Once the two suture ends have been brought out through the trocar, they are snared and fed through a titanium cylinder at the end of the device. While holding the sutures under the proper tension, the instrument is advanced to the closure site and fired. This crimps the titanium knot onto the suture and trims the extra. Advantages promoted by the manufacturer include precise tensioning, one-step suture tying and cutting, and titanium's nonreactivity. Disadvantages are the need for extracorporeal loading of the suture into the device and the costs of a disposable instrument.

With experience, surgeons will find most suturing and knot tying is best done intracorporeally with two standard needle drivers. The above instruments, however, may be useful early in one's experience and in special circumstances.

TISSUE RETRIEVAL Anyone who has struggled to place an organ or tissue in a bag can immediately appreciate new advances in retrieval technology. Retrieval devices are available from two different manufacturers. The Endocatch (U.S. Surgical) is a self-opening bag that comes in several sizes, including 10 mm and 15 mm. The Endopath (Ethicon Endo-Surgery) is available in only the 10-mm size. Once the instrument is placed through a trocar or directly through the skin, the inner core handle slides forward advancing the bag. A metal band automatically opens the bag and can be used to scoop up the tissue to be removed. A separate string is pulled, closing the bag and tearing it away from the metal ring. The ring is pulled back into the handle, and the device removed, leaving the closed bag and string in the working space. The current bags are not strong enough to withstand automated tissue morcellation, but are useful when intact removal of specimens is required.

If the specimen is to be morcellated, a Lap Sac (Cook Urological, Inc., Spencer, IN) fabricated from a double layer of plastic and nondistensible nylon must be used. This device has been shown to withstand morcellation and remain impermeable to bacteria and tumor cells.[29] In the past, placing large specimens in the Lap Sac was often a consuming and frustrating experience. Using several simple tricks, the bag can now be modified to allow rapid entrapment of specimens. A stiff hydrophilic wire can be double-passed through the holes in the Lap Sac, creating a rigid opening. The bag and wire can be rolled up and inserted through an 11-mm trocar site with the trocar removed. Replacing the trocar alongside the protruding ends of the wire allows the pneumoperitoneum to be reestablished. The modified Lap Sac opens easily, and the rigid wire

maintains the mouth of the sac open. Once the specimen is entrapped, the wire can be pulled from the holes in the sac, and the mouth of the sac brought out through a trocar site.

MORCELLATION At the conclusion of any extirpative laparoscopic procedure, the organ must be removed from the patient. When malignancy is not involved and an incision is otherwise not required, morcellation and removal through the largest port site is ideal. This requires entrapment in a suitably sized pouch and mechanical reduction in size to allow passage through the port site. Morcellation of malignant lesions continues to be controversial.[30,31] There is clear cosmetic benefit and possibly a small decrease in postoperative morbidity with morcellation. Computed tomography (CT) has proven to be an effective tool for planning surgery and predicting pathologic findings.[32] To date, there have been no reports of peritoneal seeding or local tumor recurrence in the renal fossa following laparoscopic nephrectomy with specimen morcellation. There have been two reports of trocar site seeding after radical nephrectomy.[33,34] One study compared pain and hospital stay in patients after morcellation versus those requiring conversion to an open procedure by subcostal incision.[35] Not surprisingly, there was less narcotic analgesic use and a shorter stay in the morcellation group. A more equal comparison would be that of hand-assisted laparoscopic nephrectomy versus laparoscopic nephrectomy with morcellation. This has not shown a morbidity advantage for morcellation.[36]

Once the decision has been made to morcellate an organ, it must first be placed in an impermeable bag (Lap Sac, Cook Urological). Once closed, the strings of the bag are removed through the chosen port site, removing the trocar at the same time. The area is then carefully draped with towels to prevent tumor contamination. The simplest, cheapest, and quickest option is to extend the fascial incision to 20 mm to allow manual fragmentation and extraction of the tissue using a combination of ring forceps, Kocher clamps, etc. The laparoscope should be used throughout this process to visually confirm bag integrity from inside the abdomen. The advantage of this technique is that it creates relatively large pieces of tissue and, with the addition of India ink, may allow preservation of much staging and margin information.[37]

HAND-ASSIST DEVICES The merits of hand-assisted laparoscopy (HAL) versus pure laparoscopy in urology are a matter of significant current debate. Proponents point to the proven ability to decrease operative times, allow performance of complex procedures, and aid in resident teaching.[38] This is achieved with a slight increase in postoperative pain but no significant increase in recovery times.[36] The issue of cost can be balanced by shorter operating room times and decreased need for other disposables, such as trocars and entrapment bags. Furthermore, injuries related to Veress needle and initial trocar

access should be eliminated as all of the HAL devices except the Pneumo Sleeve (Weck Closure Systems) can be used for primary insufflation. The GelPort and Lap Disc also allow airtight passage of the laparoscope to visually direct subsequent port placement.

Opponents object to hand-assist techniques because they are not minimally invasive since HAL requires an incision large enough to allow placement of the surgeon's hand into the abdomen. The same complex cases are being done "purely laparoscopically" by experts often in shorter times than those reported in hand-assist series. These experts argue that use of the hand is a "crutch" rather than a "bridge" to improved surgical ability.[39] Other disadvantages of HAL include device failure, air leakage, hand pain and fatigue with extended dissection or tight incisions, decreased view and working room due to the intra-abdominal placement of the surgeon's hand, and cosmetic concerns created by the larger incision.

Currently, there are three FDA approved devices available for hand-assisted laparoscopic surgery (Table 43-3). They all incorporate two basic features: an airtight seal between the device and the incision, and a second seal between the device and the surgeon's arm (Figure 43-13). Little data exist comparing the different HAL devices. A prospective evaluation of three now-discontinued HAL devices (the HandPort, Intromit, and Pneumo Sleeve) showed highest overall satisfaction with the Intromit.[40] It was easier to exchange hands or lap pads with the Intromit or HandPort than the Pneumo Sleeve. The HandPort was the easiest to set up but also had the highest failure rate. Surgeons are encouraged to try several devices prior to selecting one for routine use. Regardless of the device chosen, some gas leakage can be expected, especially in longer cases. A high-flow or dual insufflation system is desirable.

CLOSURE Exiting the abdomen consists of visually controlled port removal and purging the carbon dioxide gas. Port sites 10 mm in size or larger have traditionally been closed to prevent port-site hernias. These have been reported to happen in up to 3% of cases.[41] Despite newer trocars that may not require fascial closure up to 12 mm, most surgeons continue to close ports $\geq$ 10 mm in adults and 5 mm sites in children.

Conventional open suture closure of port sites can be difficult, especially in obese patients. Multiple instruments have been developed to simplify and expedite this task. Most follow the same basic principle of suture passage through the fascia and into the peritoneal cavity under direct vision followed by suture retrieval with a second pass through the opposite side of the fascia. The Carter-Thomason Needle-Point Suture Passer (Inlet Medical Inc., Eden Prairie, MN) and Berci Fascial Closure Device (Karl Storz GmbH & Co. KG) are two commonly used non-disposable instruments based on this model (Figure 43-14). Both have a sharp beak, which punctures the fascia and then opens to capture or release the suture. The

Table 43-3 Hand-Assist Laparoscopic Devices

	Omniport	GelPort	Lap Disc
Company	Weck Closure Systems, Research Triangle Park, NC	Applied Medical, Rancho Santa Margarita, CA	Ethicon Endo-Surgery, Cincinnati, OH
Seal to incision	Inflation/wound retractor	Wound retractor	Wound retractor
Seal to arm	Inflation	Gel	Iris
Cost (Jan 2004)	$440	$575 (kit w/ 2 trocars & clip applier)	$490

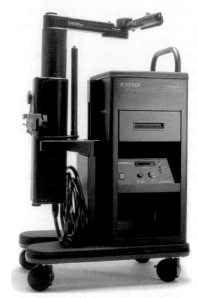

Figure 43-15 The AESOP robot (Intuitive Surgical, Mountain View, CA). Photograph courtesy of Intuitive Surgical.

Carter-Thomason is currently only available as the disposable Inlet CloseSure Procedure Kit (Inlet Medical Inc.). The EndoClose (U.S. Surgical) is a similar disposable device. Its rigidity is less and the suture capture opening smaller, making it somewhat more difficult to use.

MISCELLANEOUS Lasers can be applied laparoscopically. Experimentation has been carried out using the CO_2, holmium, and neodymium lasers, but no clear indication yet exists for their routine use.

Laparoscopic ultrasound probes are now available, which are steerable in three dimensions. These are essential for obtaining proper margins in procedures such as partial nephrectomy and cryoablation of renal lesions.

ROBOTICS

Once a mere fantasy, robotic-assisted surgery is now reality. Currently available robots vary in complexity and degree of involvement in the procedure. Simple robots are used for laparoscope holding and direction, while others are more directly involved in tissue manipulation at the surgeon's direction. The automated endoscopic system for optimal positioning or AESOP robotic device (Intuitive Surgical, Mountain View, CA, formerly Computer Motion Inc., Santa Barbara, CA) was the first FDA-cleared surgical robot. The AESOP system attaches to the side of the operating room table and incorporates a 7°-of-freedom robotic arm to hold and position the endoscope during laparoscopic surgery. The robot is voice-activated allowing control by the operating surgeon, eliminating unintentional movement, and ensuring a stable surgical image (Figure 43-15).

Currently, only one FDA-approved robot is being marketed for tissue manipulation during laparoscopic surgery. Since the surgeon actually performs the procedure with the assistance of the mechanic device, these systems are not purely robotic. The da Vinci Surgical System (Intuitive Surgical) is a master-slave system that uses robotic technology with three-dimensional visualization (Figure 43-16A). The surgeon operates while seated at a console, viewing the surgical field. At the patient side, three robot arms position and maneuver the Endowrist endoscopic instruments and laparoscope with a wide range of movements and 360° maneuverability through laparoscopic trocars (Figure 43-16B). The instruments are capable of delivering 7° of freedom, like the human wrist (Figure 43-17). The surgeon's movements are translated into movements of the instruments, allowing precise dissection, manipulation, and suturing.[42–44]

Robotic assistance has the potential to enhance the surgeon's capabilities. The machine translates the surgeon's movements into more steady and precise results at the end of laparoscopic instruments. With these new devices, there is the potential to decrease the learning curve associated with traditional laparoscopic surgery, where instrument movements and degrees for freedom are limited. Motion-scaling allows for more precise movements from the surgeon's hand. Intention and resting hand tremor is considerably diminished, compared to open surgery, but is virtually eliminated with robotics.

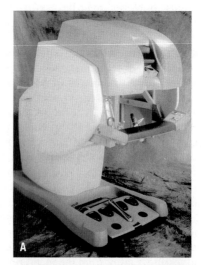

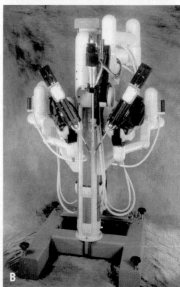

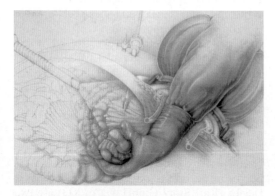

Figure 43-13 The Pneumo Sleeve (Weck Closure Systems, Research Triangle Park, NC) in cross-section showing the airtight seals between the device and abdominal wall, and the device and the surgeon's arm. Photograph courtesy of Weck Closure Systems.

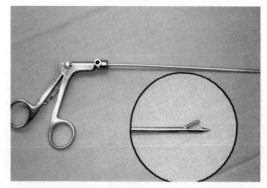

Figure 43-14 Berci fascial closure device (Karl Storz GmbH & Co. KG, Tuttlingen, Germany) with tip close-up.

Figure 43-16 *A*, The da Vinci Surgical System (Intuitive Surgical, Mountain View, CA) consists of the surgeon console, and *B*, the patient-side cart that provides the two robotic arms and one endoscope arm. Photographs courtesy of Intuitive Surgical.

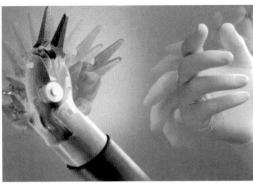

Figure 43-17 The 7°-of-freedom Endowrist (Intuitive Surgical, Mountain View, CA) end-effector of the da Vinci Surgical System. Photograph courtesy of Intuitive Surgical.

REFERENCES

1. Bhoyrul S, Vierra MA, Nezhat CR, et al. Trocar injuries in laparoscopic surgery. J Am Coll of Surg 2001;192:677–83.
2. Chow GK, Jackman SV, Chan DY, et al. Effect of gas insufflation pressure on post-operative pain in laparoscopic urologic surgery. J Urol 2000;163(Suppl):22.
3. Demco L. Effect of heating and humidifying gas on patients undergoing awake laparoscopy. J Am Assoc Gynecol Laparosc 2001;8:247–51.
4. Liu CD, McFadden DW. Laparoscopic port sites do not require fascial closure when non-bladed trocars are used. Am Surg 2000;66:853–4.
5. Bohm B, Knigge M, Kraft M, et al. Influence of different trocar tips on abdominal wall penetration during laparoscopy. Surg Endosc 1998;12:1434–8.
6. Bhoyrul S, Mori T, Way LW. Radially expanding dilatation. A superior method of laparoscopic trocar access. Surg Endosc 1996;110:775–8.
7. Bhoyrul S, Payne J, Steffes B, et al. A randomized prospective study of radially expanding trocars in laparoscopic surgery. J Gastrointest Surg 2000;4:392–7.
8. Dunn MD, McDougall EM, Clayman RV. Laparoscopic radical nephrectomy. J Endourol 2000;14:849–55.
9. Grosskinsky CM, Hulka JE. Unipolar electrosurgery in operative laparoscopy. Capacitance as a potential source of injury. J Reprod Med 1995;40:549–52.
10. Bishoff JT, Allaf ME, Kirkels W, et al. Laparoscopic bowel injury: incidence and clinical presentation. J Urol 1999; 161:887–90.
11. Saye WB, Miller W, Hertzman P. Electrosurgery thermal injury: myth or misconception. Surg Laparosc Endosc 1991;4:223–8.
12. Venkatesh R, Vanlangendonck SF, Figenshau AS, et al. Laparoscopic resection of renal tumor assisted by a water cooled high density monopolar radiofrequency device with out renal vascular clamping [Abstract]. J Endourology 2003;MP14.26, (Abstract) 105.
13. Ling FW, Stovall TG, Meyer NL, et al. Adhesion formation associated with the use of absorbable staples in comparison to other types of peritoneal injury. Int J Gynaecol Obstet 1989;30:361–6.
14. Tierney AC, Nakada SY. Laparoscopic stapling and reconstruction. In: Bishoff JT, Kavoussi LR, editors. Laparoscopic retroperitoneal surgery. Philadelphia: WB Saunders; 2000. p. 33–56.
15. Shekarriz B, Stoller ML. The use of fibrin sealant in urology. J Urol 2002;167:1218–25.
16. McDonough RC, Morey AF. Urologic applications of fibrin sealant bandage. In: Lewandrowski KU, Tantolo DJ, Gresser JD, et al, editors. Tissue engineering and biodegradable equivalents: Scientific and clinical applications. New York: Marcel Dekker; 2003.
17. Canby E, Morey AF, Jatoi I, et al. Fibrin sealant treatment of splenic injury during open and laparoscopic left radical nephrectomy. J Urol 2000;164:2004–5.
18. Leibovich SJ, Ross R. The role of macrophages in wound repair. Am J Pathol 1975;78:71–100.
19. Bishoff JT, Cornum RL, Perahia B, et al. Laparoscopic hemi-nephrectomy using a new fibrin sealant powder. Urology 2003;62.
20. Cornum RL, Morey AF, Harris R, et al. Does the absorbable fibrin adhesive bandage facilitate partial nephrectomy? J Urol 2000;164:864–7.
21. Morey AF, Anema JG, Harris R, et al. Treatment of grade 4 renal stab wounds with absorbable fibrin adhesive bandage in a porcine model. J Urol 2001;165:955–8.
22. Cornum RL, Bell J, Gresham V, et al. Intraoperative use of the absorbable fibrin adhesive bandage: long term effects. J Urol 1999;162:1817–20.
23. Perahia B, Bishoff JT, Cornum RL, et al. The laparoscopic hemi-nephrectomy: made easy by the new fibrin sealant powder [Abstract]. J Urol 2002;167(Suppl 2):167.
24. Greenhalgh DG, Gamelli RL, Lee M, et al. Multicenter trial to evaluate the safety and potential efficacy of pooled human fibrin sealant for the treatment of burn wounds. J Trauma 1999;46:433–40.
25. Morita Y, Nishii O, Kido M, Tsutsumi O. Parvovirus infection after laparoscopic hysterectomy using fibrin glue hemostasis. Obstet Gynecol 2000;95:1026.
26. Hino M, Ishiko O, Honda K, et al. Transmission of symptomatic parvovirus B19 infection by fibrin sealant used during surgery. Br J Haematol 2000;108:194–5.
27. Scheule AM, Beierlein W, Lorenz H, Ziemer G. Repeated anaphylactic reactions to aprotinin in fibrin sealant. Gastrointest Endosc 1998;48:83–5.
28. Bauer JJ, Bishoff JT, Moore RG, et al. Laparoscopic versus open pyeloplasty: assessment of objective and subjective outcome. J Urol 1999;162:692–5.
29. Urban DA, Kerbl K, McDougall EM, et al. Organ entrapment and renal morcellation: permeability studies. J Urol 1993; 150:1792–4.
30. Bishoff JT. Laparoscopic radical nephrectomy: morcellate or leave intact? Definitely morcellate! Reviews in Urology 2202;4:34–7.
31. Kaouk JH, Gill IS. Laparoscopic radical nephrectomy: morcellate or leave intact? Leave intact. Reviews in Urology 2002;4:38–42.
32. Shalhave AL, Leibovitch I, Lev R, et al. Is laparoscopic radical nephrectomy with specimen morcellation acceptable cancer surgery? J Endourol 1998;12:255–7.
33. Fentie DD, Barrett PH, Taranger LA. Metastatic renal cell cancer after laparoscopic radical nephrectomy: long-term follow up. J Endourol 2000;14:407–11.
34. Castilho LN, Fugita OE, Mitre AI, Arap S. Port site tumor recurrences of renal cell carcinoma after videolaparoscopic radical nephrectomy. J Urol 2001;165:519.
35. Walther MM, Lyne JC, Libutti SK, Linehan WM. Laparoscopic cytoreductive nephrectomy as preparation for administration of systemic interleukin-2 in the treatment of metastatic renal cell carcinoma: a pilot study. Urology 1999;53:496–501.
36. Wolf JS, Moon TD, Nakada SY. Hand assisted laparoscopic nephrectomy: Comparison to standard laparoscopic nephrectomy. J Urol 1998;160:22–7.
37. Meng MV, Koppie TM, Duh QY, Stoller ML. Novel method of assessing surgical margin status in laparoscopic specimens. Urology 2001;58:677–81.
38. Wolf JS. Hand-assisted laparoscopy: pro. Urology 2001;58: 310–2.
39. Gill, IS. Hand-assisted laparoscopy: con. Urology 2001;58: 313–7.
40. Stifelman M, Nieder AM. Prospective comparison of hand-assisted laparoscopic devices. Urology 2002;59:668–72.
41. Bowrey DJ, Blom D, Crookes PF, et al. Risk factors and the prevalence of trocar site herniation after laparoscopic fundoplication. Surg Endosc 2001;15:663–6.
42. Abbou CC, Hoznek A, Salomon L, et al. Laparoscopic radical prostatectomy with a remote controlled robot. J Urol 2001;165:1964–6.
43. Binder J, Kramer W. Robotically-assisted laparoscopic radical prostatectomy. BJU Int 2001; 87:408–10.
44. Sung GT, Gill IS. Robotic laparoscopic surgery: a comparison of the da Vinci and Zeus systems. Urology 2001;58: 893–8.

44

Anesthetic Considerations

Matthew D. Dunn, MD
Terri G. Monk, MD

With an increasing trend toward laparoscopic surgery in most surgical specialties, the unique physiologic changes created pose a new challenge for the anesthesiologist that differs from open surgery. As was mentioned in the last edition of this text, the teamwork approach between the surgeon and the anesthesiologist cannot be overemphasized. More so than in open surgery, communication between physicians is vital. Counterbalancing the advantages of laparoscopy is the potential for significant disaster as a result of unique hemodynamic alterations. Intraoperatively, a high level of clinical awareness and anticipation of potential cardiopulmonary disasters is required, which usually falls upon the responsibility of the anesthesiologist.

PHYSIOLOGIC CHANGES DURING LAPAROSCOPY

While a detailed account of the physiologic changes associated with laparoscopy are detailed in chapter 45, major effects as they pertain to anesthetic management during laparoscopy are worth mentioning.

CARDIOVASCULAR CHANGES Hemodynamic changes during laparoscopy have been extensively studied and though not all studies agree, the majority identify relatively consistent cardiac changes that stem from the increased intra-abdominal pressure. Such changes are also affected by the type of insufflant used, the cardiovascular status of the patient, and somewhat by patient positioning. Other important patient factors include body weight, preexisting cardiopulmonary disease, and preoperative volume status.

One has to remember that induction of general anesthesia by itself leads to hemodynamic changes independent of insufflation. General anesthesia can lead to a reduction of mean arterial pressure (MAP), cardiac output (CO) and cardiac index (CI) with elevation of pulmonary pressures and systemic vascular resistance (SVR).[1,2] Interestingly, these effects tend to normalize with time during open surgery but not during laparoscopy. Creation of a pneumoperitoneum causes additional hemodynamic changes such as increasing right and left sided cardiac filling pressures (CVP, MPAP, and PCWP), reducing CO and CI, and stroke volume (SV).[1,3,4] An increase in MAP, SVR, and $PaCO_2$ by 12% has been demonstrated.[5,6] Change in heart rate is variable and has been shown to increase or

remain stable.[2] In obese patients, insufflation has been shown to increase the mean heart rate, blood pressure, and cardiac output and index.[7] Fortunately these changes are rarely clinically significant and usually normalize after desufflation.[1]

Positive pressure pneumoperitoneum leads to compression of the abdominal contents, which affects the splanchnic vasculature. In animal models, a decrease in blood flow in the superior mesenteric artery and hepatic portal vein is demonstrated in pressures above 12 mm Hg.[8,9] In healthy humans, a decrease in splanchnic blood flow has been demonstrated, which worsens with insufflation time.[10,11] Hepatic arterial flow has been reported either to decrease or remain constant.[8,10–12] Increased peripheral vascular resistance is noted during insufflation with carbon dioxide. It is hypothesized that the increased intra-abdominal pressure causes an increase in the SVR, which thus redistributes the splanchnic blood flow leading to the above changes.[11,13,14]

Increased SVR and redistribution of flow may also result from an increase in catecholamine secretion, which is known to occur during laparoscopy. During development of the pneumoperitoneum, a catecholamine response is noted, with rise in both epinephrine and norepinephrine, although the secretion of each may have different etiologies. The release of epinephrine is centrally mediated, whereas the release of norepinephrine is more locally mediated. In a study of patients undergoing laparoscopic fundoplication, the use of opioids to suppress centrally mediated catecholamines had no effect on the stimulation of norepinephrine indicating local production and control.[15] The local release of norepinephrine, as well as the mechanical effect of the pneumoperitoneum, most likely explain the changes in SVR and redistribution of splanchnic blood flow.

Volume status has also been shown to affect the above hemodynamic parameters after establishment of a positive pressure pneumoperitoneum. In animal models, significant decreases in CO are seen in hypovolemic animals. In contrast, minimal changes are noted in normovolemic animals and beneficial effects are appreciated in hypervolemic animals, illustrating the benefits of preoperative volume loading.[11,16–18]

The type of gas used to create the pneumoperitoneum also plays a major role in hemodynamic changes. Carbon dioxide (CO_2), nitrous oxide (N_2O), helium, and argon have all been used for laparoscopic surgery. The most commonly used insufflant is CO_2, mainly because it is inex-

pensive, chemically stable, rapidly eliminated, non-combustable, and highly soluble compared to the other insufflants.[8] Absorption into the blood stream occurs through the peritoneal cavity, where CO_2 is converted to carbonic acid. High levels resulting in acidosis directly inhibit cardiac function. In contrast, moderate levels stimulate the sympathetic nervous system enough to improve cardiac output and counteract the inhibitory effect of the pneumoperitoneum.[11,19,20] The other gases mentioned do not affect the sympathetic nervous system and therefore result in a lower cardiac output when used for insufflation.

Compensatory increase in the minute ventilation rapidly excretes the excess CO_2 to avoid hypercarbia and its ill effects. For healthy patients without pulmonary disease, this is usually well tolerated and easily managed. Though the serum pH and $PaCO_2$ may change during insufflation they usually remain within the normal range. The pattern of change may not be the same for all patients. In those undergoing laparoscopic cholecystectomy, $PaCO_2$ levels did not rise until the middle of the case, with maximum levels at the end of the procedure. Other studies showed an increase in $PaCO_2$ at the beginning of the surgery. Yet other reports identify no difference in acid base balance with intra-abdominal pressures of 10 mm Hg or 15 mm Hg. Typically, the change in acid base balance is toward acidosis, with the majority of cases illustrating respiratory and mixed acidosis.[21–24]

The effect of position on the hemodynamic status during laparoscopy is controversial. The Trendelenburg, or head-down tilt, position has been associated with improved cardiac function in normovolemic and normotensive patients for pelvic laparoscopy.[11,25–27] In another study of patients undergoing laparoscopic hysterectomy, the head-down tilt position was found to increase pulmonary arterial pressures, central venous pressures, pulmonary capillary wedge pressures which increased further with CO_2 insufflation.[2] Conversely, the head-up tilt, or reverse Trendelenburg, position has been attributed to a decrease in cardiac output during laparoscopy.[29–30] The lateral position was noted to partially reverse some of the deleterious effects of the head-up tilt in one study.[11,30] Other reports indicate that the lateral position has few other effects except for a modest decrease in SVR and MAP, although extreme lateral flexion can obstruct the vena cava and decrease venous return.[11,31]

In contrast to the above, others have demonstrated that changes in position fail to show a constant change in hemodynamic parameters.[4] One study identified an increase in heart rate, blood pressure, and cardiac output with the pneumoperitoneum, but little effect was seen with patient positioning in both obese and non-obese patients.[32] Interpretation of the available data indicates that induction of general anesthesia and a positive pressure pneumoperitoneum induce greater hemodynamic changes than patient positioning. Ultimately the effects of positioning are probably negligible except for patients with significant cardiopulmonary compromise.[33]

PULMONARY CHANGES In a similar fashion to the above hemodynamic effects, pulmonary changes during laparoscopy result from the increased abdominal pressures, body habitus, preexisting pulmonary disease, and type of insufflant gas used. Introduction of gas into the peritoneum or retroperitoneum not only compresses the abdominal and retroperitoneal contents but transmits pressure to the thoracic cavity, adversely affecting pulmonary mechanics. The elevated pressure mechanically compresses and limits movement of the diaphragm, reducing pulmonary compliance, vital capacity, functional residual capacity, and total lung volume.[34] Pneumoperitoneum with an intra-abdominal pressure of 15 mm Hg led to a 27% decrease in respiratory system compliance and an increase of peak inspiratory pressures by 35% without any significant effect of patient positioning.[33] Oxygenation (PaO_2) is not adversely affected for most patients, except in those who are morbidly obese, where a decrease in PaO_2 has been documented.[35]

Aside from effects of the pneumoperitoneum, body habitus also appears to affect pulmonary mechanics. Obese patients demonstrate an increased inspiratory resistance compared to non-obese patients. Whereas increasing the respiratory rate and tidal volume improves ventilation and blows off CO_2, increasing the tidal volume or respiratory rate does not appear to affect oxygenation in morbidly obese patients.[36] Interestingly, other reports have failed to show any significant differences in respiratory mechanics when comparing laparoscopic to open bariatric surgery.[37]

An increase in ventilation-perfusion (V/Q) mismatch and dead space during laparoscopy has been reported but is controversial. This was addressed by Anderssen and colleagues, who evaluated patients intraoperatively during laparoscopic cholecystectomy. They demonstrated that at intraoperative pressures of 11 to 13 mm Hg, the pulmonary shunt actually decreased after development of the pneumoperitoneum, and then gradually rose to normal during the case.[5] They also noted that patient positioning had little effect on pulmonary dynamics. In contrast to this, others have reported that the head-down tilt position exacerbates the pulmonary effects.[11,38]

During insufflation, CO_2 is absorbed through the peritoneal surface and can only be excreted through the lungs. Because CO_2 is very soluble in blood, it leads to hypercarbia and respiratory acidosis.[8] Absorption is dependent on many factors, including physical properties of the gas, temperature, and vascularity of the exposed tissue.[11,39–45] The peritoneal cavity provides an excellent absorptive mesothelial surface that is well vascularized. CO_2 and N_2O are highly soluble and therefore rapidly absorbed during insufflation. The baseline production of CO_2 in adults is 150 to 200 mL/min.[11,46] The amount of CO_2 absorbed during transperitoneal laparoscopy has been estimated to range from 14 to 48 mL/min.[47–51] To manage this, minute-volume of ventilation must be increased during insufflation by approximately 30% to drive off the excessive CO_2.[8] It is important to realize that not all of the absorbed CO_2 can be excreted by ventilation during the course of surgery. In fact, up to 120 L can be stored in the body, the largest reservoir being the bones. This means that a significant amount of retained CO_2 is still being excreted during the recovery phase.[8] Respiratory acidosis and increased CO_2 output are reported to last at least up to 1 hour postoperatively, despite intraoperative normoventilation in ASA I-II patients.[8,52,53] During the recovery period extra ventilatory work is needed to remove the absorbed CO_2, which may be an issue in patients with COPD or pulmonary compromise.[8]

Position may affect placement of the endotracheal tube, usually leading to downward shifting of the endotracheal tube into the right mainstem bronchus. In a double-blinded, prospective, controlled study of 60 patients undergoing gastroplasty, patients in the laparoscopic group had a higher incidence of endotracheal tube (ETT) displacement than patients undergoing open gastroplasty. In most situations, the endotracheal tube moved down into the bronchus after positioning and placement in the head down or Trendelenburg position. This may have more to do with pushing contents upward rather than the ETT shifting downward.[54]

General anesthesia itself also affects pulmonary mechanics, usually leading to pulmonary atelectasis in patients postoperatively. For morbidly obese patients, one should be aware that they already have more atelectasis than non-obese patients, even before surgery. This also increases post induction of anesthesia, and remains so (even 24 hours later), placing morbidly obese patients at higher risk for pulmonary complications.[55]

Despite the pulmonary changes associated with the increased abdominal pressure, laparoscopy has been shown to reduce postoperative pulmonary complications after such procedures as cholecystectomy, fundoplication, bariatric surgery and nephroureterectomy, especially when compared to open surgery.[56–65]

ANESTHETIC TECHNIQUES

The goals of laparoscopic anesthesia are listed in Table 44-1. The anesthesiologist should evaluate the patient preoperatively to identify potential risk factors that may affect anesthetic management. Patients with a history of diabetes, obesity, hiatal hernia, or gastric outlet obstruction are at risk for gastroesophageal reflux, which may be exacerbated with pneumoperitoneum and the Trendelenburg position.[48,66–68] Despite the use of a cuffed endotracheal tube, which should protect against aspiration, prophylaxis is considered prudent. Metacloropromide, a dopamine antagonist with central and peripheral actions, stimulates gastric emptying and increased lower esophageal sphincter tone, and, with an H2 antagonist (eg, cimetidine, ranitidine, famotidine), can stimulate gastric emptying and decrease gastric secretions and volume.[11,69,70]

For longer and complicated laparoscopic procedures, preoperative preparation should include a blood specimen for type and screen. Intravenous access through a large-bore IV or central line is important due to the risk of sudden cardiovascular complications. An oro- or gastric tube, along with a urethral catheter, decompresses the stomach, small intestine, and bladder, limiting a viscous perforation during insufflation and trocar placement. An open laparotomy tray should be available at a moment's notice.

Positioning the patient is the responsibility of both the surgeon and anesthesiologist, with special attention to certain pressure points to prevent a neurologic or pressure-induced injury. Specifically, bony prominences such as ankles, knees, hips, and elbows should be well padded. Strapping with tape at the lower leg, hips, and shoulder prevents inadvertent movement if repositioning of the table is required during the procedure. The use of shoulder braces during extreme, head-down, tilt position for pelvic laparoscopy may place too much pressure on the shoulders if the rest of the body is poorly secured. This may result in brachial plexus injuries[40] unless the patient is adequately secured to the table. Likewise, excessive leg abduction and external hip rotation during dorsolithotomy may induce a femoral nerve injury.[71]

Insufflation is associated with a decrease in peripheral venous flow.[3,72] The use of intermittent, sequential pneumatic compression devices on the lower extremeties augments femoral venous flow velocity and provides protection against deep venous thrombosis.[73,74]

GENERAL ANESTHESIA

ANESTHETIC AGENTS The choice of anesthetic agent is rarely the problem for the surgeon but one of obvious importance for the anesthiologist. Nitrous oxide is frequently avoided because of bowel distention, which can intrude into the surgical field and potentially increases postoperative nausea and vomiting. This is, however, controversial. There are plenty of reports demonstrating no difference in the above parameters with nitrous oxide.[75] Taylor and colleagues, in a blinded study, noted no difference in bowel distention between groups receiving N_2O or air.[76] A more compelling argument against the use of N_2O is an animal study showing that it worsens the negative cardiovascular effects of venous CO_2 or helium gas emboli, thus increasing the risk of emboli-induced death when CO_2 or helium is used to create the pneumoperitoneum.[77]

Table 44-1 Goals of Laparoscopic Anesthesia

Provide amnesia
Induce analgesia
Minimize risk of anesthesia
Produce abdominal wall relaxation
Allow expedient conversion to laparotomy if necessary
Maintain hemodynamic and respiratory stability
Control diaphragmatic excursion in upper retroperitoneal procedures
Maintain hypercarbia at acceptable level (PETCO$_2$ usually < 45 mm Hg)
Allow rapid emergence and recovery
Minimize postoperative pain
Prevent postoperative nausea

As an alternative, halogenated, remifentanil-, and propofol-based general anesthetic regimens have been used. A comparison of remifentanil with propofol versus remifentanil with desflurane identified both to be suitable regimens with respect to rapid recovery. The use of propofol, however, led to decreased postoperative analgesic use and nausea.[78] Certain halogenated anesthetics, such as halothane, are associated with an increased incidence of cardiac arrhythmias. Respiratory acidosis (hypercapnea) with increased catecholamine levels in the presence of these anesthetics is thought to be the etiology. Enflurane and isoflurane have a lower incidence of catecholamine-induced arrhythmias than does halothane.[79] Other adverse effects have been reported. Enflurane may decrease cardiac output more than other inhalational agents, and isoflurane has been associated with a higher incidence of headache (44%) after laparoscopy.[11,80,81] Desflurane, a short-acting agent, causes a high incidence of airway irritation when used for induction.[82]

Anesthetic agents have been reported to affect the stress responses during laparoscopic surgery. In one study comparing remifentanil versus alfentanil for outpatient laparoscopic gynecologic surgery, remifentanil patients showed fewer stress responses to surgical stimuli, required fewer doses of drugs, and showed quicker recovery of psychomotor function. Patients receiving remifentanil, however, demonstrated a higher incidence of intraoperative bradycardia and required more pain medication than patients receiving alfentanil.[83] Likewise, the type of volatile anesthetic significantly affects the stress response. Specifically, the use of sevoflurane as opposed to isoflurane in women undergoing laparoscopic pelvic surgery demonstrated a more favorable metabolic and lower stress response.[84] In a prospective randomized blinded comparison of sevoflurane and isoflurane for laparoscopic bariatric surgery in morbidly obese patients, sevoflurane provided the advantage of a faster recovery and earlier discharge from the recovery unit over isoflurane. The extubation, emergence and response times were shorter with sevoflurane. No differences were seen in hemodynamic parameters or complications. Postoperative pain was similar in both groups.[85] One study looking at the effects of remifentanil in addition to sevoflurane for obese patients undergoing laparo-

scopic cholecystectomy demonstrated an advantage to remifentanil, which facilitated awakening from anesthesia and decreased the needed concentration of sevoflurane used.[86]

In establishing the correct balance between quality of anesthesia and recovery time, the dosing regimen for combination of remifentanil and sevoflurane was evaluated. The combination of 14 μg × kg(–1) × h(–1) remifentanil and 1.24% end-tidal sevoflurane achieved the optimal balance between quality and recovery from anesthesia.[87]

The use of neuromuscular relaxant during laparoscopy has been evaluated. Comparing short-acting (mivacurium chloride) versus intermediate-acting (rocuronium bromide) neuromuscular relaxants in a randomized fashion for patients undergoing gynecologic laparoscopy demonstrated that the intermediate-acting neuromuscular relaxant (rocuronium) better facilitated intubation more rapidly, improved hemodynamic stability, required less frequent used of maintenance doses and was not associated with erythema compared to the short-acting neuromuscular relaxants.[88]

INTUBATION VERSUS LARYNGEAL MASK Effective airway management during general anesthesia for laparoscopic surgery is important in order to control the adverse effects of the CO_2 pneumoperitoneum. Protection of the airway is more reliable with cuffed endotracheal intubation and is considered the standard of care for many reasons; the risk of aspiration is decreased, it allows for controlled ventilation to prevent hypercapnea, it allows for abdominal wall relaxation and muscle paralysis, and ensures adequate oxygenation. In general, endotracheal intubation better enables the anesthesiologist to maintain cardiovascular and pulmonary stability throughout the procedure and will certainly prepare the patient for a quick laparotomy at a moment's notice if necessary.

Despite the above, there are many successful reports of general anesthesia with laryngeal mask for gynecologic laparoscopic surgery. The use of laryngeal mask airway (LMA) for laparoscopy is controversial because of the lack of airway control. In one study, however, use of the LMA-ProSeal in patients undergoing laparoscopic cholecystectomy was just as effective in ventilating patients when compared to endotracheal intubation, except for obese patients. There was no difference in SpO$_2$ or the CO$_2$ in expired gas (PETCO$_2$), nor was there significant gastric distention in non-obese patients. Certainly, in obese patients, it is contraindicated due to high risk of airway obstruction, poor oxygenation, and aspiration.[89] In a series by Drummand and Duncan, LMA was used successfully for gynecologic pelvic laparoscopy.[90] The use of low doses of opioids in this setting, however, changes the mechanics of breathing by increasing rigidity of the abdominal wall and stimulating active expiratory activity, which normally is passive. The use of the LMA requires that the patient be spontaneously breathing. As such, the addition of even small doses of opioids, such as fentanyl citrate, can alter the dynamics of breathing and place the

patient at risk. Aspiration pneumonia has been reported in patients undergoing laparoscopic cholecystectomy with a laryngeal mask, illustrating the potential hazard of regurgitation without airway control.[91] In addition, patients managed with spontaneous (as opposed to assisted) ventilation during CO_2 laparoscopy demonstrate higher increases of PaCO$_2$.[48,49,92] Controlled ventilation avoids this. When used judiciously with positive end-expiratory pressure (PEEP), mechanical ventilation with a cuffed endotracheal tube allows for pulmonary expansion in the face of increased intra-abdominal pressure. PEEP should be used carefully because it may exacerbate the hemodynamic suppression of the pneumoperitoneum.[93–96]

For those patients with abnormal airways who cannot be intubated, it is possible to consider high-frequency jet ventilation, which allows for positive pressure ventilation without an endotracheal tube. Such a case was described in a patient with a vocal fold abnormality, who underwent a laparoscopic cholecystectomy with an abdominal lift technique. Clearly, insufflation was not performed, so whether this can correlate to positive pressure pneumoperitoneum is unknown.[97]

REGIONAL ANESTHESIA Most physicians agree that general anesthesia with endotracheal intubation remains the standard of care for abdominal and retroperitoneal laparoscopy. Epidural or spinal anesthesia, however has been described as a suitable alternative to general anesthesia for certain laparoscopic procedures. For short duration, pelvic or lower abdominal procedures, this has been shown to work well. Epidural anesthesia for gynecologic laparoscopy has been reported since the 1970s.[98] Small-dose selective spinal anesthesia for gynecologic laparoscopy has been successfully performed.[99] Good results were reported by Azurin and colleagues when they used epidural anesthesia for extraperitoneal herniorrhaphy.[100] The disadvantages of regional anesthesia include less protection against aspiration of gastric contents, less control of respiratory compensation, and potential loss of vascular resistance.[80] Using epidural anesthesia for transperitoneal abdominal laparoscopic surgery is more of a challenge since a higher spinal level of analgesia is required. Complete peritoneal anesthesia and abdominal relaxation requires a T4-level blockade, which may also impair respiratory function. Shoulder pain may not be relieved completely until a cervical-level blockade is achieved.[101] Nonetheless, Gramatica and colleagues reported their experience with epidural anesthesia in patients with COPD undergoing laparoscopic cholecystectomy, in which 48% of patients experienced intraoperative shoulder pain but all patients tolerated the procedure well with no conversions to general anesthesia required.[102] Complications were minimal and usually related to urinary retention. It was also cheaper than general anesthesia. A case report of successful epidural anesthesia for retroperitoneoscopic renal biopsy was reported with a T4-level of analgesia obtained.[103] Thoracic epidural anesthesia-analgesia has also been used for laparoscopic colectomy, giving a T8-9 or T9-10 level of anesthesia. In one report, this was successfully performed on five patients. When compared to five patients undergoing standard general laparoscopy, patients in the epidural group had a shorter hospital stay and were able to eat sooner.[104]

Despite the concerns of respiratory compromise, healthy patients without significant pulmonary disease may remain quite stable during regional anesthesia. Patients increase their minute ventilation by increasing the respiratory rate more so than tidal volume in order to maintain adequate ventilation.[105] The use of sedatives and narcotics, however, could decrease the sensitivity to CO_2 retention and may also lead to hypoxia. In a series of patients undergoing extraperitoneal hernia repair, regional anesthesia did not compromise respiratory compensation and showed no change with respect to stress parameters. Most patients who received regional anesthesia in this study showed severe agitation, often accompanied by chest pain. As such, these authors did not recommend regional anesthesia for laparoscopy.[106]

In summary, for the cooperative and healthy patient, regional anesthesia is a viable alternative for shorter procedures where minimal tissue manipulation is performed. This also requires the care of an expert anesthesiologist.

LOCAL ANESTHESIA The experience with local anesthesia with or without sedation for laparoscopic surgery has been limited to short procedures in young and healthy patients where minimal manipulation is required. It has been used for laparoscopic gynecologic procedures and extraperitoneal hernia repairs.[107] Clearly, the advantages are a rapid postoperative recovery, but the disadvantages include anxiety, dyspnea, and abdominal and shoulder pain.[108–110] The need for a higher level of analgesia and tight control of intraoperative cardiopulmonary parameters limits the effectiveness of local anesthesia for most abdominal laparoscopic procedures. Similar to regional anesthesia, this technique should be limited to short diagnostic procedures where minimal tissue manipulation is required.

INTRAOPERATIVE ANESTHETIC MANAGEMENT

MONITORING Intraoperative monitoring techniques during laparoscopy are no different than other procedures requiring general anesthesia and mechanical ventilation. Standard methods to measure intraoperative cardiac and pulmonary function include an electrocardiogram, blood pressure manometer, an in-line oxygen monitor, capnometer, and continuous monitoring of airway pressure and tidal volume. Monitoring the effectiveness of ventilation can be performed with serial blood gases measuring the $PaCO_2$ from an arterial line. In lieu of this, capnography (which measures the CO_2 in expired gas) may be used as a noninvasive substitute for $PaCO_2$ in evaluating the adequacy of ventilation. There is controversy about whether this is an adequate method of monitoring ventilation. Using the $PETCO_2$ as a guide to ventilation assumes a constant gradient between arterial CO_2 and end-tidal CO_2, which is generally valid in healthy patients and for shorter procedures. The $PETCO_2$ is roughly 3 to 4 mm Hg lower than $PaCO_2$ for healthy patients.[50,111–114] Controversy lies over the adequacy of $PETCO_2$ as a substitute for monitoring ventilation for longer procedures and in patients with preexisting cardiopulmonary disease. In a review of 28 healthy patients undergoing laparoscopic cholecystectomy, $PETCO_2$ was a reasonable approximation of $PaCO_2$ in patients free from cardiopulmonary disease. It was not a satisfactory index of $PaCO_2$ if it exceeded 41 mm Hg and if large volumes of CO_2 were insufflated.[115] In pregnant patients undergoing laparoscopy, $PETCO_2$ is only effective in preventing respiratory acidosis if it is maintained at 32 mm Hg.[116] In patients with preoperative cardiopulmonary disease, the $P(a-et)CO_2$ gradient increases. As such, increases in $PaCO_2$ are not reflected by comparable increases in $PETCO_2$ during insufflation, rendering the latter unreliable as a method to monitor ventilation.[117] $PaCO_2$ may also be underestimated by $PETCO_2$ if there is a reduction in cardiac output or an increase in alveolar dead space. Rarely, $PETCO_2$ may even overestimate $PaCO_2$.[118] For patients with significant cardiopulmonary disease, arterial blood gas monitoring of $PaCO_2$ should be measured to better assess ventilation and to avoid hypercarbia and the resulting acidosis. The arterial line will also allow for continuous blood pressure monitoring and detect adverse fluctuations earlier than an arm cuff manometer. Preoperative pulmonary function tests showing low forced expiratory volume (< 70% of predicted values), low diffusion constants (< 80% of predicted values), and vital capacity and a high ASA level can predict patients at risk for developing hypercarbia and acidosis during laparoscopic cholecystectomy. Age and duration do not seem to be strong influencing factors.[119] Invasive Swan-Ganz catheterization may be needed for high-risk ASA III-IV patients to monitor the hemodynamic response to insufflation. In this setting, the increased abdominal pressure from insufflation has shown a greater adverse affect on cardiac function.[120,121] Since patients with a low intravascular volume have the most marked decrease in cardiac output, invasive cardiac monitoring may help to direct fluid management. Overall, it gives the anesthesiologist better control in managing the patient.

RENAL EFFECTS AND FLUID MANAGEMENT Fluid management during laparoscopic surgery can be a challenge for the anesthesiologist owing to diminished urine output and lower insensible fluid loss, compared to open surgery.[122–123] Oliguria is a common finding during laparoscopy and results from mechanical compression of the renal parenchyma and vasculature by the pneumoperitoneum.[124–126] In a study comparing patients undergoing laparoscopic versus open gastric bypass surgery, there was a 64% decrease in the urine output, compared to the open surgery group at one hour post incision. This continued to remain lower than that of the open group by 31 to 50% throughout the operation. Postoperative blood urea nitrogen and creatinine levels, however, remained within the normal range. Antidiuretic hormone, aldosterone, and plasma renin activity peaked at 2 hours post-incision, although they were not significantly different from the open surgery group.[127] The creatinine clearance has been reported to decrease intraoperatively during laparoscopic cholecystectomy, although not consistently for all patients.[128] Despite expanding the blood volume, increasing the intra-abdominal pressure from 0 to 20 mm Hg increases renal vascular resistance and decreases the glomerular filtration rate. This effect may last for hours postoperatively, as well. Oliguria during laparoscopy is refractory to intravenous fluid hydration.[129] Likewise, ureteral obstruction is not a major factor because placement of ureteral stents preoperatively does not improve urine output during the procedure.[130] A comparable clinical situation would be an abdominal compartment syndrome due to hemorrhage leading to oliguria or anuria, which usually responds to laparotomy.[18,131,132] The etiology for low urine output is multifactorial and includes compression of the renal parenchyma, stimulation of the renin-angiotensin-aldosterone cycle, and compression of the renal vasculature, along with increased vascular resistance. Plasma renin activity and arginine vasopressin levels are significantly increased after insufflation.[133]

The combination of decreased fluid requirement and decreased urine output explains why volume overloading can easily occur. In the early nephrectomy series reported by Clayman and colleagues, two of the first 10 patients developed congestive heart failure; most likely due to aggressive fluid administration intraoperatively.[134] On the one hand hypovolemia predisposes patients to decreased cardiac output after insufflation, whereas overhydration in elderly patients may be just as compromising. A recommendation for minimizing fluid-related complications is to hydrate preoperatively and then limit fluid replacement intraoperatively to a maintenance rate of 5 to 10 mL/kg/hr.[11]

The concern about potential renal function impairment during laparoscopy is important for patients donating a kidney for renal transplantation, or for patients with preexisting renal insufficiency. In a rodent model looking for signs of chronic ischemia from prolonged pneumoperitoneum, no signs of chronic ischemic histologic changes were identified for a period of 3 months after up to a 5-hour period of insufflation at 15 mm Hg.[135] To date, there have been no reports of permanent renal failure from prolonged pneumoperitoneum. Even in animal studies where the renal mass has been surgically reduced to 22% of normal, acute renal dysfunction may occur initially, but by 1 week postoperatively, the glomerular filtration rate returns to preoperative levels. This indicates that there is no long-term impact, even in animals with pre-existing renal dysfunction.[136]

HYPOTHERMIA Heat loss is a concern during any prolonged surgical procedure and is usually a challenge for both the anesthesiologist and nursing staff. Induction of anesthesia has been shown to significantly decrease core body temperature ($< 36°C$) seen in 36% of patients.[137] The added risk of hypothermia with laparoscopy has been reported and is felt to correlate to the duration of surgery and the insufflation flow rate.[138] The incidence of hypothermia in patients undergoing laparoscopic gynecologic surgery has been reported as high as 94%. Despite reports that laparoscopic surgery leads to a higher incidence of hypothermia, compared to open surgery, many studies also fail to show any higher incidence.[139,140] In one study, after insufflation, the temperature decreased further, which did not differ from patients undergoing open surgery.[141] In another study evaluating laparoscopic versus open colon surgery, there was no higher incidence of perioperative hypothermia in the laparoscopic group.[142] Also reported in one study is a gender difference, in that men showed less variability in temperature change than women.[143] Intra-abdominal temperatures will decrease with insufflation of non-heated CO_2 gas, sometimes quite dramatically, as high as 27.7°C. Core temperature, however, may not change, despite this. In fact, one study comparing heated versus non-heated insufflated CO_2 demonstrated no significant change in core temperature with heated gas.[144] This is somewhat controversial since the converse has also been reported (see below).

Numerous methods of maintaining core temperature intraoperatively have been used. Warmed irrigation fluid has been shown to decrease, but not eliminate, the drop in core temperature.[145] Likewise the use of warmed intravenous fluids does not appear to affect maintenance of core body temperature during laparoscopic cholecystectomy.[146] Other techniques include resistive heating, forced air heating, circulating water mattresses. Of these, resistive heating and forced air heating units were superior to circulating water mattresses in maintaining core temperature while also offering the advantage of adjustable heating.[147] Warming the insufflated gas has been developed to prevent hypothermia sometimes associated with prolonged laparoscopic cases. In an animal study, heating and humidifying the insufflant gas decreased the drop in temperature, compared to insufflating with cool dry gas. Animal studies have pointed to water evaporation as the main source of heat loss during laparoscopy.[148] Humidifying and heating units have been shown to reduce intraoperative hypothermia, as well as reduce the length of recovery room stay, and reduce postoperative pain. In a randomized, prospective, blinded multicenter study, heating and humidifying the insufflant gas was superior to room temperature gas with less

hypothermia and even postoperative pain.[149] Another randomized trial demonstrated that, although the intra-abdominal temperature remained higher in the heated and humidified patients, it did not significantly alter core temperature nor reduce postoperative pain.[150] Regardless of effect on core temperature, there may be another beneficial effect from humidification that is not initially appreciated. In an animal study on thoracoscopy, electron microscopy indicated that insufflation with dry gas, when compared to humidified gas for insufflation, resulted in greater structural injury to the pleura.[151] Whether this can be extrapolated to similar effects on the peritoneum is unknown at this time.

ANESTHETIC AND PHYSIOLOGIC COMPLICATIONS In the last edition, this chapter mentioned that one-third of complications during laparoscopy were cardiopulmonary in nature.[11] Most will be diagnosed and managed by the anesthesiologist. Again, one must remember that general anesthesia has negative cardiovascular effects, such as a depressed baroreceptor response, decreased cardiac contractility, and basal autonomic tone.[11,152] These effects will be obvious after anesthetic induction and before insufflation. Acute hypotension, hypoxemia, and cardiovascular collapse after development of the pneumoperitoneum have been reported, and possible causes include tension pneumoperitoneum, pneumothorax, pneumopericardium, and pneumomediastinum, gas embolism, arrhythmias, and severe hypercapnea (Table 44-2).[11]

Excessive distention of the peritoneum may lead to numerous complications. When abdominal pressures exceed 20 mm Hg for prolonged periods of time, a tension pneumoperitoneum can occur, impairing cardiac and pulmonary function as mentioned earlier.[153] In this situation, desufflation may be all that is necessary to improve the patient's status and continue with the procedure. Rapid and excessive peritoneal distention in the face of elevated CO_2 may also stimulate vagal tone leading to significant bradycardia and even cardiac arrest.[19,154,155] Anticholinergic agents such as atropine may be needed to prevent excessive vagal stimulation during laparoscopy. Conversely, rapid exsufflation was reported to have caused cardiovascular collapse in a patient undergoing laparoscopic cholecystectomy.[156] Hypercarbia may lead to cardiac arrhythmia, which is noted in 17 to 22% of cases.[19,157,158] Careful monitoring of $PaCO_2$ levels should prevent this.

In a 1967 survey of 63,845 laparoscopic procedures, pneumomediastinum and pneumothorax were reported in 0.08% and 0.03% of cases.[159] Pathways through which insufflated gas may enter into the thorax are demonstrated in Figure 44-1. Such gas accumulations can inhibit cardiac filling and limit lung expansions with harmful effects.[160,161] Since peak airway pressures rise during insufflation, barotrauma may also occur, leading to pneumothoraces.[11,50,162] A limited pneumothorax will usually resolve if

CO_2 or N_2O is used as the insufflant, since both gases will be absorbed.[163,164] For a large or symptomatic pneumothorax, chest tube insertion should be performed.

The incidence of clinically significant venous gas emboli is estimated to be between 0.002 and 0.08%, although careful surveillance may increase the incidence to 0.59%.[159,165-169] Etiologic factors include open venous channels, high insufflating pressures (> 15 mm Hg), and even Veress needle insufflation directly into a vessel.[47] Small amounts of CO_2 that enter the vascular system are usually quickly absorbed and excreted by the lungs, but larger emboli may have catastrophic consequences. Unfortunately, there have been deaths due to this complication.[167,168,170-172] The greatest risk is during the initial insufflation. The anesthesiologist usually makes the diagnosis in the setting of profound hypotension, cyanosis, asystole, pulmonary edema, increased peak inspiratory pressures, jugular venous distention, and arrhythmias after development of the pneumoperitoneum. Initially, with smaller emboli, the $PETCO_2$ may increase. For larger emboli, a sudden decrease in $PETCO_2$ is noted, potentially associated with a mill wheel murmur, a widened QRS complex, and right heart strain patterns on electrocardiogram.[11,172] Treatment includes immediate desufflation, rapid ventilation with 100% oxygen, and placing the patient in a steep head-down tilt with the right side up.[173]

Deep venous thrombosis is another complication with potentially fatal consequences. The incidence after laparoscopic surgery is overall quite low, but variable. Bergqvist and Lowe reviewed the literature of prospective studies evaluating thromboembolism in patients undergoing laparoscopic cholecystectomy. The incidence varied between 0 and 55 % although some patients received prophylaxis, and overall patient numbers were small.[174] Lindberg and colleagues also reviewed the literature for the incidence of thromboembolic complications after laparoscopic cholecystectomy. They reviewed 60 studies, which included 153,832 patients.[175] Taking into consideration that some patients received prophylaxis, the overall average incidence of deep venous thrombosis was 0.03%, pulmonary embolism, 0.06%, and fatal pulmonary embolism, 0.02%. In contrast, a review of 587 patients

Table 44-2 Anesthetic and Physiologic Complications of Laparoscopy

Tension pneumoperitoneum
Thoracic gas collections
Pneumomediastinum
Pneumopericardium
Pneumothorax
Cardia dysrhythmias
Venous gas embolism
Hypercarbia
Hypoxemia
Hypertension
Hypothermia
Venous thrombosis

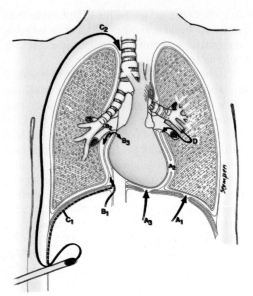

Figure 44-1 Possible routes of gas into thoracic spaces. Persistent fetal connections include the pleuroperitoneal membrane (A1), pleuropericardial membrane (A2), and pericardioperitoneal canal (A3). Gas may pass around great vessels in an extrafascial plane such as at the diaphragmatic hiatus (B1), pulmonary hiatus (B2), or the entry/exit of the great vessels at the heart (B3). Extraperitoneal or extrapleural gas can dissect in between fibers of the diaphragm (C1) and subcutaneous gas may extend directly from the anterior neck into the superior mediastinum (C2). Finally, barotraumas may allow ventilatory gas to enter the pleural cavity or mediastinum (D).

undergoing laparoscopic cholecystectomy failed to identify any clinical symptoms of DVT or pulmonary embolism, and questioned whether DVT prophylaxis is needed.[176] Older patients may be at higher risk of DVT since they appear to have a more significant reduction in lower extremity venous outflow during pneumoperitoneum.[177] Other risk factors for DVT formation include the pneumoperitoneum, long operative times (> 2 hours), and the reverse Trendelenberg position.[178] The use of sequential compression devices for the lower extremities does improve flow and is appropriate as a form of prophylaxis. Portal vein thrombosis has been reported as a complication of laparoscopic sigmoid colectomy for diverticulitis.[179]

Hypertension may occur during laparoscopy but usually results from other factors such as hypoxemia, hypercarbia, light anesthesia, or excessive stimulation of catecholamines, renin-angiotensin-aldosterone system, and vasopressin from an increased abdominal pressure.[11] Other complications reported include cardiac arrest during use of an argon beam coagulator in an elderly woman during laparoscopic cholecystectomy. The exact etiology was not definitive, but an argon gas embolism was suspected because a mill wheel murmur was heard on auscultation.[180] A case of fatal large bowel ischemia was reported in an elderly man following laparoscopic inguinal hernia repair. An infrarenal aortic aneurysm was noted on autopsy, which may be an added risk factor for laparoscopy.[181]

POSTOPERATIVE ANESTHETIC CONSIDERATIONS

POSTOPERATIVE PAIN CONTROL Numerous series have consistently demonstrated the advantage of laparoscopic surgery over open surgery with respect to a decrease in postoperative pain and analgesic requirement.[182] But postoperative pain and discomfort is still an issue for most patients. Common sources of pain include visceral and peritoneal irritation at the operative site, tissue manipulation at the trocar or hand-assist site, diaphragmatic irritation from retained gas, and release of inflammatory mediators.[183,184]

The use of preemptive analgesia has been extensively evaluated, although the timing of analgesic administration is controversial. The application of long-acting local anesthetics such as bupivacaine hydrochloride to the surgical area has been shown to improve postoperative pain when used in patients undergoing laparoscopic hernia repair.[185] Uzunkoy and colleagues determined that the use of bupivacaine (locally infiltrated into the trocar site) significantly decreased postoperative pain compared to placebo. But there was no difference if given before trocar placement or after trocar removal.[186] In contrast, if given before trocar insertion, Lee and colleagues reported less postoperative pain for the first 3 hours.[187] These authors also reported the benefits of intraperitoneal bupivacaine at the initiation of surgery. When bupivacaine is injected into the trocar and incision sites, it augments the analgesic effect of intraperitoneal lidocaine in patients undergoing gynecologic laparoscopy.[188] Certainly, the use of local anesthesia at the trocar site improves perioperative pain, but in one study, it was also found to decrease cost in patients undergoing laparoscopic cholecystectomy due to less medication usage.[189]

Regarding peritoneal irritation, N_2O has less of an irritating effect on the peritoneum than CO_2. The use of N_2O over CO_2, however, is controversial due to the former's combustible nature. Nonetheless, there are reports of its successful use.[190,191] In a prospective randomized trial comparing N_2O and CO_2 for laparoscopy, patients who had an N_2O pneumoperitoneum had less pain up to one day postoperatively, compared to patients who had CO_2 pneumoperitoneum. Pain medication use was not statistically different between the two groups. No adverse events were reported.[192]

The incidence of shoulder pain following laparoscopic surgery varies from 35 to 63%.[193] Intraoperative instillation of a local anesthetic significantly decreases shoulder pain following outpatient laparoscopy.[194] Likewise, placement of a cutaneous piroxicam patch on the skin of each shoulder prior to anesthetic induction showed decreased postoperative shoulder pain, and was significantly better than a bilateral suprascapular nerve block.[193] A rectus sheath block has been shown to decrease both pain and narcotic use after diagnostic laparoscopy.[195] To address visceral irritation as the source of pain, topical etidocaine has been shown to significantly reduce pain after laparoscopic tubal ligation.[196,197]

To reduce residual gas as a source of ongoing irritation, placing a drain through the umbilical trocar site for 6 hours postoperatively has been shown to reduce pain through the following 24-hour period.[11,198] Instillation of 1 to 2 L of fluid at the end of the procedure is a simple way to reduce subdiaphragmatic and shoulder pain postoperatively (from 76% down to 22%).[11,199] It has been suggested that a retroperitoneal approach to nephrectomy and pelvic surgery may be associated with less postoperative pain, perhaps due to less peritoneal irritation.[200,201] A comparison of retroperitoneal nephrectomy to hand-assisted transperitoneal laparoscopy demonstrated no significant difference in postoperative analgesic requirement.[202]

Postoperative administration of narcotic and nonsteroidal anti-inflammatory drug (NSAID) analgesics is commonly used for managing postoperative pain.[203–208] The specific anesthetic agent does not appear to have much influence on postoperative pain.[209] Nondepolarizing agents have not been shown to produce less pain than the depolarizing agent succinylcholine chloride during laparoscopy.[210,211]

Clonidine hydrochloride, which is used intraoperatively to maintain hemodynamic stability, has been shown to enhance analgesia. The use of clonidine in a prospective randomized setting for patients undergoing laparoscopic cholecystectomy showed it to improve heart rate variability and decrease the need for analgesics with the 24-hour postoperative period.[212]

POSTOPERATIVE NAUSEA Many patients cite the fear of postoperative nausea and vomiting as more prevalent than the fear of postoperative pain.[213] Postoperative nausea and vomiting is a common complaint after laparoscopic surgery and is especially noted after laparoscopic cholecystectomy. When prophylactic antiemetics are not used, the incidence ranges from 25 to 42%.[214] It is also common in patients who receive a general anesthetic.[215] Likewise, the type of anesthetic is important; nausea is more common after inhalational anesthesia than total intravenous anesthesia.[216]

Risk factors for manifesting postoperative nausea and vomiting are female gender, young age, a history of postoperative nausea and vomiting, non-smoking, long duration of anesthesia, and the use of opioids and volatile anesthetics.[217] Delayed gastric emptying does not appear to be a factor in postoperative nausea and vomiting in patients undergoing laparoscopic cholecystectomy.[218] The use of reversal drugs such as neostigmine for neuromuscular blockade is associated with an increase in postoperative nausea and antiemetic requirements.[219]

Prophylaxis of postoperative nausea and vomiting has been the focus of numerous studies. The use of selective serotonin (5-HT3) antagonist antiemetics in preventing postoperative nausea and vomiting is well documented. Ramosetron (a 5-hydroxytryptamine type 3 receptor antagonist) is effective at a minimum dose of 0.3 mg for preventing postoperative nausea and vomiting

48 hours postoperatively in patients undergoing laparoscopic cholecystectomy.[220] Ondansetron has demonstrated a decrease in nausea and vomiting by 50% or more.[215,221–223] A comparison of tropisetron and ondansetron both improve postoperative nausea and vomiting compared to placebo. Ondansetron appears to be more effective during the first 3 hours, but tropisetron has a longer duration of action.[224] Interestingly, postoperative nausea and vomiting is not related to an increase in the peripheral release of serotonin, suggesting a more central phenomenon.[225] The dosage may also be important in preventing nausea and vomiting. Prophylactic administration of ondansetron at a higher dose (8 mg) is more effective than 4 mg in patients undergoing laparoscopic cholecystectomy.[226]

The addition of steroids has demonstrated an antiemetic effect. The use of dexamethasone at or before the induction of anesthesia is effective as prophylaxis of postoperative nausea and vomiting and is as effective as other antiemetics, (ie, tropisetron) in patients undergoing laparoscopic cholecystectomy.[227] Because of this, the combination of an antiemetic plus dexamethasone has been evaluated. In a randomized, double-blinded study, granisetron plus dexamethasone was found to be superior to granisetron alone, without causing any adverse side effects.[228] In a similar fashion, a prospective, randomized, double-blinded study comparing the use of dolasetron plus dexamethasone versus dolasetron alone showed that, although the incidence of nausea and vomiting was no different, the dexamethasone group had a shorter stay and more rapid discharge.[229] Fujii and colleagues demonstrated that the addition of 8 mg of dexamethasone to granisetron reduced the incidence of nausea and vomiting from 17% to 2%.[230,231] In patients with a history of motion sickness, dexamethasone given before anesthetic induction is associated with a decreased incidence of postoperative nausea and vomiting.[232] Optimal timing of antiemetic administration is controversial, although one study indicates that dolasetron given before the induction of anesthesia is as effective as if given at the end of laparoscopy or at the end of anesthesia for outpatient laparoscopy.[233] Other combinations of antiemetics have been evaluated. Granisetron plus droperidol was more effective than granisetron alone in preventing postoperative nausea and vomiting after laparoscopic cholecystectomy.[234]

Due to the high costs of newer antiemetics, less expensive alternatives have been studied. In one study, dimenhydrinate (Dramamine) was found to be as effective as ondansetron in preventing postoperative nausea and vomiting in patients undergoing laparoscopic cholecystectomy.[235] In another study, cyclizine and ondansetron were equally effective at preventing nausea and vomiting postoperatively after gynecologic laparoscopy.[236] Metoclopramide hydrochloride has been reported to be equivalent to placebo, but less effective than dolasetron in patients undergoing laparoscopic cholecystectomy.[237] In contrast, a higher dose of metoclopramide (20 mg) given at the end of

laparoscopic cholecystectomy resulted in a similar incidence of postoperative nausea and vomiting as ondansetron (8 mg). Interestingly, patients receiving metoclopramide had less pain than patients receiving ondansetron.[238]

Regional anesthesia has a lower incidence of nausea and vomiting compared to general anesthesia.[11] Total intravenous anesthesia with propofol is associated with a 40 to 50% decrease in the incidence of nausea and vomiting, compared to inhalational techniques.[239–242] Avoiding opioids may limit emesis, while NSAIDs may give less nausea and vomiting for equivalent analgesia.[206] The addition of supplemental oxygen does not seem to prevent nausea and vomiting in women undergoing outpatient gynecologic laparoscopy.[243]

Pain is often associated with an increased frequency of nausea and vomiting, and the prevention of pain with local anesthetics may decrease the incidence.[196,197] Likewise, antiemetics have been associated with decreased postoperative pain. Preoperatively, metoclopramide can significantly decrease morphine requirement in the PACU but had no impact on pain intensity as rated by pain scale scores.[244]

When looking at alternative forms of prevention, non-pharmacologic approaches to treatment have focused mainly on acupuncture and acupressure. This method is based on the belief that a patient's well-being is related to the balance of energy in the body. It is thought that energy flows within the body through paths termed meridians, which can be manipulated to restore the balance of energy. Results have been variable when used for treating nausea and vomiting due to morning sickness, chemotherapy, general anesthesia, or narcotic use.[245] In one study, acupressure appears to have no effect in preventing nausea and vomiting compared to placebo.[246] Conversely, another study shows that acupressure is more effective than placebo and is as effective as ondansetron.[245] The use of acustimulation in the form of Relief-Band, which provides transcutaneous electrical P6 acupoint stimulation in combination with ondansetron, was more effective than either treatment alone.[247] Non-pharmacologic methods are controversial, and their responses variable and not definitively proven at this point.

CONCLUSION

Ensuring a successful outcome is the goal to any surgery. This begins with proper patient preparation and assessment of potential risk factors. It also relies on adequate communication between surgeon and anesthesiologist. The surgeon should inform the anesthesiologist about the anticipated length of the procedure, the needed position, the potential for blood loss, and possibility of open conversion. Conversely, the surgeon should be aware of the concerns of the anesthesiologist when planning the surgery.[11]

For most operative laparoscopy, general anesthesia with entotracheal intubation is the standard of care, and the physiologic responses to insufflation are usually well-tolerated with proper anes-

thetic management. Carbon dioxide is the most commonly used insufflant, which may lead to metabolic and respiratory alterations that are, fortunately, usually easy to manage. Intraoperative monitoring is dictated by the type and length of procedure as well as the patient's cardiopulmonary status. For longer procedures, an arterial line provides better monitoring of $PaCO_2$, and a central venous and/or Swan Ganz catheter may be needed for higher risk patients. Preventative measures such as antiemetics and preemptive analgesics may facilitate a smoother postoperative course. Knowledge of the potential pitfalls and complications unique to laparoscopic surgery will not only help prevent disasters but allow for proper management and secure a safe outcome.

REFERENCES

1. Galizia G, Prizio G, Lieto E, et al. Hemodynamic and pulmonary changes during open, carbon dioxide pneumoperitoneum and abdominal wall-lifting cholecystectomy. A prospective, randomized study. Surg Endosc 2001;15:477–83.
2. Hirvonen EA, Nuutinen LS, Kauko M. Hemodynamic changes due to Trendelenburg positioning and pneumoperitoneum during laparoscopic hysterectomy. Acta Anaesthesiol Scand 1995;39:949–55.
3. Alishahi S, Francis N, Crofts S, et al. Central and peripheral adverse hemodynamic changes during laparoscopic surgery and their reversal with a novel intermittent sequential pneumatic compression device. Ann Surg 2001;233:176–82.
4. Zuckerman R, Gold M, Jenkins P, et al. The effects of pneumoperitoneum and patient position on hemodynamics during laparoscopic cholecystectomy. Surg Endosc 2001;15:562–5.
5. Andersson J, Lagerstrand L, Thorne A, et al. Effect of CO2 pneumoperitoneum on ventilation-perfusion relationships during laparoscopic cholecystectomy. Acta Anaesthesiol Scand 2002;46:552–60.
6. Donati A, Munch C, Marini B, et al. Transesophageal Doppler ultrasonography evaluation of hemodynamic changes during videolaparoscopic cholecystectomy. Minerva Anesthesiol 2002;68:549–54.
7. el-Dawlatly AA, al-Dohayan A, Favretti F, Samarkani A. Anaesthesia for morbidly obese patients: a study of haemodynaci changes during bariatric surgery. Middle East J Anesthesiol 2002;16:411–7.
8. Koivusalo AM, Lindgren L. Effects of carbon dioxide pneumoperitoneum for laparoscopic cholecystectomy. Acta Anaesthesiol Scand 2000;44:834–41.
9. Ishizaki Y, Bandai Y, Shimomura K, et al. Safe intra-abdominal pressure of carbon dioxide pneumoperitoneum during laparoscopic surgery. Surgery 1993;114:549–54.
10. Schilling MK, Redaelli C, Krahenbuhl L, et al. Splanchnic microcirculatory changes during CO2 laparoscopy. J Am Coll Surg 1997;184:378–82.
11. Wolf JS, Monk TG. Anesthetic considerations. In: Smith AD, Badlani GH, Bagley DH, et al, editors. Smith's Textbook of Endourology. St. Louis: Quality Medical Publishing; 1996. p. 731–53.
12. Masey SA, Buck JR, Koehler RC, et al. Effects of increased intra-abdominal pressure on regional blood flow in newborn lambs. Anesthesiology 1983;59:A425.
13. Caldwell CB, Ricotta JJ. Changes in visceral blood flow with elevated intra-abdominal pressure. J Surg Res 1987;43:14020.
14. Kotzampassi K, Kapanidis N, Kazamias P, Eleftheriadis E. Hemodynamic events in the peritoneal environment during pneumoperitoneum in dogs. Surg Endosc 1993;7:494–9.
15. Myre K, Raeder J, Rostrup M, et al. Catecholamine release during laparoscopic fundoplication with high and low doses of remifentanil. Acta Anaesthesiol Scand 2003;47:267–73.
16. Ho HS, Saunders CJ, Corso FA, Wolfe BM. The effects of CO2 pneumoperitoneum on hemodynamics in hemorrhaged animals. Surgery 1993;114:381–7.
17. Toomasian JM, Glavinovich G, Johnson MN, Gazinga AB. Hemodynamic changes following pneumoperitoneum and graded hemorrhage in the dog. Surg Forum 1978;29:32–3.
18. Cullen DJ, Coyle JP, Teplick R, Long MC. Cardiovascular,

pulmonary, and renal effects of massively increased intra-abdominal pressure in critically ill patients. Crit Care Med 1989;17:118–21.
19. Price HL. Effects of carbon dioxide on the cardiovascular system. Anesthesiology 1960;21:652–63.
20. Richardson DW, Wasserman AJ, Patterson JL. General and regional circulatory responses to change in blood pH and carbon dioxide tension. J Clin Invest 1961;40:31–43.
21. Sefr R, Puszkailer K, Jagos F. Randomized trial of different intra-abdominal pressures and acid-base balance alterations during laparoscopic cholecystectomy. Surg. Endosc. 2003;17:947–50.
22. Iwasaka H, Miyakawa H, Yamamoto H, et al. Respiratory mechanics and arterial blood gases during and after laparoscopic cholecystectomy. Can J Anaesth 1996;43: 129–33.
23. Kantorova I, Svoboda P, Ochmann J, et al. Does insufflation of the abdomen affect acid-base and ventilatory parameters in laparoscopic surgery? Rozhl Chir 1998;78:332–6.
24. Shuto K, Kitano S, Yoshida T, et al. Hemodynamic and arterial blood gas changes during carbon dioxide and helium pneumoperitoneum in pigs. Surg Endosc 1995;9:1173–8.
25. Gentili DR, Benjamin E, Berger SR, Iberti TJ. Cardiopulmonary effects of the head-down tilt position in elderly postoperative patients: a prospective study. South Med J 1994;81:1258–60.
26. Taylor J, Weil MH. Failure of the Trendelenburg position to improve circulation during clinical shock. Surg Gynecol Obstet 1967;124:1005–10.
27. Sibbald WJ, Paterson NAM, Holliday RL, Baskerville J. The Trendelenburg position: hemodynamic effects in hypotensive and normotensive patients. Crit Care Med 1979;7:218–24.
28. Williams MD, Murr PC. Laparoscopic insufflation of the abdomen depresses cardiopulmonary function. Surg Endosc 1993;7:12–6.
29. Joris JL, Noirot DP, Legrand MJ, et al. Hemodynamic changes during laparoscopic cholecystectomy. Anesth Analg 1993;76:1067–71.
30. Cunningham AJ, Turner J, Rosenbaum S, Rafferty T. Transoesophageal echocardiographic assessment of the haemodynamic function during laparoscopic cholecystectomy. Br J Anesth 1993;70:621–5.
31. Lawson NW. The lateral decubitus position. In: Martin JT. Positioning in anesthesia and surgery. Philadelphia: WB Saunders; 1987. p. 155–79.
32. Fried M, Krska Z, Danzig V. Does the laparoscopic approach significantly affect cardiac functions in laparoscopic surgery? Pilot study in non-obese and morbidly obese patients. Obes Surg 2001;11:293–6.
33. Rauh R, Hemmerling TM, Rist M, Jacobi KE. Influence of pneumoperitoneum and patient positioning on respiratory system compliance. J Clin Anesth 2001;13:361–5.
34. Baroncini S, Gentili A, Pigna A, et al. Anaesthesia for laparoscopic surgery in paediatrics. Minerva Anestesiol 2002; 68:406–13.
35. Casati A, Comotti L, Tommasino C, et al. Effects of pneumoperitoneum and reverse Trendelenburg position on cardiopulmonary function in morbidly obese patients receiving laparoscopic gastric banding. Eur J Anaesthesiol 2000;17:786–7.
36. Sprung J, Whalley DG, Falcone T, et al. The effects of tidal volume and respiratory rate on oxygenation and respiratory mechanics during laparoscopy in morbidly obese patients. Anesth Analg 2003;97:268–74.
37. Demiroluk S, Salihoglu Z, Zengin K, et al. The effects of pneumoperitoneum on respiratory mechanics during bariatric surgery. Obes Surg 2002;12:376–9.
38. Prentice JA, Martin JT. The Trendelenburg position. Anesthesiologic considerations. In: Martin JT. Positioning in anesthesia and surgery. Philadelphia: WB Saunders; 1987. p. 127–45.
39. Kety SS. The theory and application of the exchange of inert gases at the lungs and tissues. Pharmacol Rev 1951;3:1–41.
40. Piiper J, Canfield RE, Rahn H. Absorption of various inert gases from subcutaneous gas pockets in rats. J Appl Physiol 1962;17:268–74.
41. Piiper J. Physiological equilibria of gas cavities in the body. In: Fenn WO, Rahn, editors. Handbook of physiology. Section 3: Respiration. Vol 2. Washington (DC): American Physiological Society; 1965. p. 1205–18.
42. Van Liew HD. Coupling of diffusion and perfusion in gas exit from subcutaneous pocket in rats. Am J Physiol 1968; 214:1176–85.
43. Collins JM. Inert gas exchange of subcutaneous and intraperitoneal gas pockets in piglets. Respir Physiol 1981;46: 391–404.
44. Loring SH, Butler JP. Gas exchange in body cavities. In: Fishman AP, editor. Handbook of physiology. Section 3: The respiratory system. Vol 4. Bethesda (MD): American Physiological Society; 1987. p. 283–95.
45. Nunn JF. The effects of changes in the carbon dioxide tension. In: Applied respiratory physiology. London: Butterworths; 1987. p. 460–70.
46. Nunn JF. Carbon dioxide. In: Applied respiratory physiology. London: Butterworths; 1987. p. 207–34.
47. Seed RF, Shakespeare TF, Muldoon MJ. Carbon dioxide homeostasis during anaesthesia for laparoscopy. Anaesthesia 1970;25:223–31.
48. Lewis DG, Ryder W, Burn N, et al. Laparoscopy—an investigation during spontaneous ventilation with halothane. Br J Anaesth 1972;44:685–91.
49. deSousa J, Tyler IL. Can abdorption of the insufflation gas during laparoscopy be hazardous? Anesthesiology 1987; 67:A476.
50. Puri GD, Singh H. Ventilatory effects of laparoscopy under general anaesthesia. Br J Anaesth 1992;68:211–3.
51. Tan PL, Lee Tl, Tweed WA. Carbon dioxide absorption and gas exchange during pelvic laparoscopy. Can J Anaesth 1992;39:677–81.
52. Critchley L, Critchley J, Gin T. Haemodynamic changes in patients undergoing laparoscopic cholecystectomy: measurement by transthoracic electrical bioimpedance. Br J Anaesth 1993;70:681–83.
53. Kazama T, Ikeda K, Kato T, Kikura M. Carbon dioxide output in laparoscopic cholecystectomy. Br J Anaesth 1996;76: 530–5.
54. Ezri T, Hazin V, Wartners D, et al. The endotracheal tube moves more often in obese patients undergoing laparoscopy compared with open abdominal surgery. Anesth Analg 2003;96:278–82.
55. Eichenberger A, Proietti S, Wicky S, et al. Morbid obesity and postoperative pulmonary atelectasis: an underestimated problem. Anesth. Analg 2002;95:1788–92.
56. Suter M, Martinet O. Postoperative pulmonary dysfunction after bilateral inguinal hernia repair: a prospective randomized study comparing the Stoppa procedure with laparoscopic total extraperitoneal repair (TEPP). Surg Laparosc Endosc Percutan Tech 2002;12:420–5.
57. Joris JL, Hinque PE, Laurent CJ, et al. Pulmonary function and pain after gastroplasty performed via laparotomy or laparoscopy in morbidly obese patients. Br J Anaesth 1998;80:283–8.
58. Olsen MF, Josefson K, Dalenback J, et al. Respiratory function after laparoscopic and open fundoplication. Eur J Surg 1997;163:667–72.
59. Rovina N, Bouros D, Tzanakis N, et al. Effects of laparoscopic cholecystectomy on global respiratory muscle strength. Am J Respir Crit Care Med 1996;153:458–61.
60. Karayannaki AJ, Makri GG, Mantzioka A, et al. Postoperative pulmonary function after laparoscopic and open cholecystectomy. Br J Anaesth 1996;77:448–52.
61. Frazee RC, Roberts JW, Okeson GC, et al. Open versus laparoscopic cholecystectomy. A comparison of postoperative pulmonary function. Ann Surg 1991;213:651–4.
62. Schauer PR, Luna J, Ghiatas AA, et al. Pulmonary function after laparoscopic cholecystectomy. Surgery 1993;144:389–99.
63. Joris J, Cigarini I, Legrand M, et al. Metabolic and respiratory changes performed via laparotomy or laparoscopy. Br J Anaesth 1992;69:341–5.
64. Poulin EC, Mamazza CJ, Breton G, et al. Evaluation of pulmonary function in laparoscopic cholecystectomy. Surg Laparosc Endosc 1992;2:292–6.
65. Shalhav AL, Dunn MD, Portis AJ, et al. Laparoscopic nephroureterectomy for upper tract transitional cell cancer: the Washington University experience. J Urol 2000; 163:1100–4.
66. Fishburne JI, Keith L. Anesthesia. In: Phillips JM, editor. Laparoscopy. Baltimore (MD): Williams & Wilkins; 1977. p. 69–85.
67. Duffy BL. Regurgitation during pelvic laparoscopy. Br J Anaesth 1979;51:1089–90.
68. Carlsson C, Islander G. Silent gastropharyngeal regurgitation during anesthesia. Anesth Analg 1981;60:655–7.
69. Gibbs CP, Modell JH. Management of aspiration pneumonitis. In: Miller RS, editor. Anesthesia. New York: Churchill Livingstone; 1990. p. 1193–319.
70. O' Sullivan G, Sear JW, Bullingham RES, Carrie LES. The effect of magnesium trisilicate mixture, metoclopramide, and randitidine on gastric pH, volume and serum gastrin. Anaesthesia 1985;40:246–53.
71. Hershlag A, Loy RA, Lavy G, DeCherney AH. Femoral neuropathy after laparoscopy. J Reprod Med 1990;35:575–6.
72. Ido K, Suzuki T, Kimura K, et al. Lower extremity venous stasis during laparoscopic cholecystectomy as assessed using color Doppler ultrasound. Surg Endosc 1995;9:310–3.
73. Millard JA, Hill BB, Cook PS, et al. Intermittent sequential pneumatic compression in prevention of venous stasis associated with pneumoperitoneum during laparoscopic cholecystectomy. Arch Surg 1993;128:914–9.
74. Schwenk W, Bohn B, Fugener A, et al. Intermittent pneumatic sequential compression (ISC) of the lower extremeties prevents venous stasis during laparoscopic cholecystectomy. Surg Endosc 1998;12:7–11.
75. Cunninghan AJ, Mcaleese JAM. Anesthesia for laparoscopic surgery. In: Barash P, Cullen B, Stoelting RK, editors. Clinical anesthesia. Philadelphia: Lippincott-Raven Publishers; 1996. p. 991–9.
76. Taylor E, Feinstein R, White PF, Soper N. Anesthesia for laparoscopic cholecystectomy. Is nitrous oxide contraindicated? Anesthesiology 1992;76:541–3.
77. Junghan T, Bohm B, Meyer E. Influence of nitrous oxide anesthesia on venous gas embolism with carbon dioxide and helium during pneumoperitoneum. Surg Endosc 2000;14: 1167–70.
78. Grundman U, Silomon M, Bach F, et al. Recovery profile and side effects of remifentanil-based anaesthesia with desflurane or propofol for laparoscopic cholecystectomy. Acta Anaesthesiol Scand 2001;45:320–6.
79. Harris MNE, Plantevin OM, Crowther A. Cardiac arrhythmia during anaesthesia. Br J Anaesth 1984;56:1213–6.
80. Schoeffler P, Henry C, Monteillard C. Anesthesia. In: Bruhat M, Mage G, Pouly JL, et al, editors. Operative laparoscopy. New York: McGraw-Hill; 1992. p. 33–8.
81. Tracey JA, Holland AJC, Unger L. Morbidity in minor gynecological surgery: a comparisoni of halothane, enflurane, and isoflurane. Br J Anaesth 1982;54:1213–5.
82. Van Hemelrijck J, Smith I, White PF. Use of desflurane for outpatient anesthesia. A comparison with propofol and nitrous oxide. Anesthesiology 1991;75:197–203.
83. Chinachoti T, Werawatganon T, Suksompong S, et al. A multicenter randomized double-blind comparison of remifentanil and alfentanil during total intravenous anaesthesia for out-patient laparoscopic gynecological procedures. J Med Assoc Thai 2000;83:1324–32.
84. Marana E, Annetta MG, Meo F, et al. Sevoflurane improves the neuroendocrine stress response during laparoscopic pelvic surgery. Can J Anaesth 2003;50:348–54.
85. Torri G, Casati A, Albertin A, et al. Randomized comparison of isoflurane and sevoflurane for laparoscopic gastric banding in morbidly obese patients. J Clin Anesth 2001;13:565–70.
86. Paventi S, Santevecchi A, Perilli V, et al. Effects of remifentanil infusion bis-titrated on early recovery for obese outpatients undergoing laparoscopic cholecystectomy. Miverva Anesth 2002;68:651–7.
87. van Delden PG, Houweling PL, Bencini AF, et al. Remifentanil-sevoflurane anaesthesia for laparoscopic cholecystectomy: comparison of three dose regimens. Anaesthesia 2002; 57:212–7.
88. Dahaba AA, Schweitzer E, Fitzgerald RD, Schwarz S. Equilasting doses of rocuronium, compared to mivacurium, result in improved neuromuscular blockade in patients undergoing gynecological laparoscopy. Can J Anaesth 2001;48:1084–90.
89. Maltby JR, Beriault MT, Watson NC, et al. The LMA-ProSeal™ is an effective alternative to tracheal intubation for laparoscopic cholecystectomy. Can J Anaesth 2002;49:857–62.
90. Drummond GB, Duncan MK. Abdominal pressure during laparoscopy: effects of fentanyl. Br J Anesth 2002;88: 384–348.
91. Griffin RM, Hatcher IS. Aspiration pneumonia and the laryngeal mask airway. Anaesthesia 1990;45:1039–40.
92. Kenefick JP, Leader A, Maltby JR, Taylor PJ. Laparoscopy: blood-gas values and minor sequelae associated with three techniques based on isoflurane. Br J Anaesth 1987; 59:189–94.
93. Ekman LG, Abrahamsson J, Biber B, et al. Hemodynamic changes during laparoscopy with positive end-expiratory pressure ventilation. Acta Anaesthesiol Scand 1988;32: 447–53.
94. Burchard KW, Ciombor DM, McLeod MK, et al. Positive end expiratory pressure with increased intra-abdominal pressure. Surg Gynecol Obstet 1985;161:313–8.
95. Moffa SM, Quinn JV, Sltohman GJ. Hemodynamic effects of carbon dioxide pneumoperitoneum during mechanical ventilation and positive end-expiratory pressure. J Trauma 1993;35:613–7.
96. Luz CM, Polarz H, Bohrer H, et al. Hemodynamic and respiratory effects of pneumoperitoneum and PEEP during laparoscopic pelvic lymphadenectomy in dogs. Surg Endosc 1994;8:25–7.

97. Barreca M, Maronian N, Bowdle TA, Sinanan MN. Combined use of high-frequency jet ventilation and abdominal lift for laparoscopic cholecystectomy in a patient with glottic impairment. Surg Endosc 2003;17:658.

98. Brindernbaugh LD, Soderstrom RM. Lumbar epidural block anesthesia for outpatient laparoscopy. J Reprod. Med 1979;23:8–12.

99. Stewart AV, Vaghadi H, Collins L, Mitchell GW. Small-does delective spinal anaesthesia for short-duration outpatient gynaecological laparoscopy: recovery characteristics compared with propofol anaesthesia. Br J Anaesth 2001; 86:570–2.

100. Azurin DJ, Go LS, Cwik JC, Schuricht AL. The efficacy of epidural anesthesia for endoscopic preperitoneal herniorrhaphy: a prospective study. J Laparoendosc Surg 1996;6: 369–73.

101. Borten M. Choice of anesthesia. In: Laparoscopic complications. Toronto: BC Decker Inc; 1986. p. 173–84.

102. Gramatica L, Brasesco OE, Mercado Luna A, et al. Laparoscopic cholecystectomy performed under regional anesthesia in patients with chronic obstructive pulmonary disease. Surg Endosc 2002;16:472–5.

103. Micali S, Jarrett TW, Pappa P, et al. Efficacy of epidural anesthesia for retroperitoneoscopic renal biopsy. Urology 2000;55:590xv–590xvi.

104. Senagore AJ, Whalley D, Delaney CP, et al. Epidural anesthesia-analgesia shortens length of stay after laparoscopic segmental colectomy for benign pathology. Surgery 2001;129:672–6.

105. Ciofolo MJ, Clergue R, Seebacher J, et al. Ventilatory effects of laparoscopy under epidural anesthesia. Anesth Analg 1990;70:357–61.

106. Hirschberg T, Olthoff D, Borner P. Comparative studies of total extraperitoneal hernioplasty in combined spinal epidural anesthesia versus balanced general anesthesia. Anaesthesiol Reanim 2002;27:144–51.

107. Alexander GD, Goldrath M, Brown EM, Smiler BG. Outpatient laparoscopic sterilization under local anesthesia. Am J Obstet Gynecol 1973;116:1065–8.

108. Sogge MR, Goldner FH, Butler ML. Pain response comparison between carbon dioxide and nitrous oxide in peritoneoscopy. Gastrointest Endosc 1980;26:78.

109. Sharp JR, Pierson WP, Brady CE III. Comparison of CO2 and N2O induced discomfort during peritoneoscopy under local anesthesia. Gastroenterology 1982;82:453–6.

110. Minoli G, Terruzzi V, Spinzi GC, et al. The influence of carbon dioxide and nitrous oxide on pain during laparoscopy: a double-blind controlled trial. Gastrointest Endosc 1982;28:173–5.

111. Liu SY, Leighton T, Davis I, et al. Prospective analysis of cardiopulmonary responses to laparoscopic cholecystectomy. J Laparoendosc Surg 1991;1:241–6.

112. Brown DR, Fishburne JI, Robertson VO, Hulka JF. Ventilatory and blood gas changes during laparscopy with local anesthesia. Am J Obstet Gynecol 1976;124:741–5.

113. Ciofolo MJ, Clergue F, Seebacher J, et al. Ventilatory effects of laparoscopy under epidural anesthesia. Anesth Analg 1990;70:357–61.

114. Pillalamorri ED, Bhangdia P, Rudin RS, et al. Effect of CO2 pneumoperitoneum during laparoscopy on A.B.G.'s, end-tidal CO2 and cardiovascular dynamics. Anesthesiology 1983;59:A424.

115. Wahba RWM, Mamazza J. Ventilatory requirements during laparoscopic cholecystectomy. Can J Anaesth 1993;40:206.

116. Bhavai-Shankar K, Steinbrook RA, Brooks DC, Datta S. Arterial to end-tidal carbon dioxide pressure difference during laparoscopic surgery in pregnancy. Anesthesiology 2000;93:370–3.

117. Wittgen CM, Andrus CH, Fitzgerald SD. Analysis of the hemodynamic and ventilatory effects of laparoscopic cholecystectomy. Arch Surg 1991;126:997–1000.

118. Bhavani-Shanker K, Moseley J, Jumar AY, Delph Y. Capnometry and anesthesia. Can J Anaesth 1991;39:617.

119. Wittgen CM, Naunhei KS, Andrus CH, Kaminski DL. Preoperative pulmonary evaluation for laparoscopic cholecystectomy. Arch Surg 1993;128:880.

120. Iwase K, Takenaka H, Yagura A, et al. Hemodynamic changes during laparoscopic cholecystectomy in patients with heart disease. Endoscopy 1992;24:771–3.

121. Safran D, Sgambati S, Orlando R III. Laparoscopy in high-risk cardiac patients. Surg Gynecol Obstet 1993;176:548–54.

122. Vukasin A, Lopez M, Shichman S, et al. Oliguria in laparoscopic surgery [Abstract]. J Urol 1994;151:343.

123. Wakizaka Y, Sano S, Koike Y, et al. Changes of arterial CO2 (PaCO2) and urine output by carbon dioxide insufflation of the peritoneal cavity during laparoscopic cholecystectomy. Nippon Geka Gakkai Zasshi 1994;95:336–42.

124. Kirsch AJ, Hensle TW, Chang DT, et al. Renal effects of CO2 insufflation: oliguria and acute renal dysfunction in a rat pneumoperitoneum model. Urology 1994;43:453–9.

125. McDougall EM, Monk TG, Hicks M, et al. Effect of pneumoperitoneum on renal function in an animal model [Abstract]. J Urol 1994;151:462.

126. Harman PK, Kron IL, McLachlan HD, et al. Elevated intra-abdominal pressure and renal function. Ann Surg 1982;196:594–7.

127. Nguyen NT, Perez RV, Fleming N, et al. Effect of prolonged pneumoperitoneum on intraoperative urine output during laparoscopic gastric bypass. J Am Coll Surg 2002;195: 476–83.

128. Kubota K, Kajiura N, Teruya M, et al. Alterations in respiratory function and hemodynamics during laparoscopic cholecystectomy under pneumoperitoneum. Surg Endosc 1993;7:500–4.

129. Chang DT, Kirsch AJ, Sawczuk IS. Oliguria during laproscopic surgery. J Endourol 1994;8:349–52.

130. Dunn MD, McDougall EM. Renal physiology; laparoscopic considerations. Urol Clin N Amer;27:609–14.

131. Richards WO, Scovill W, Shin B, Reed W. Acute renal failure associated with increased intra-abdominal pressure. Ann Surg 1983;197:183–7.

132. Fietsam R, Villalba M, Glover JL, Clark K. Intraabominal compartment syndrome as a complication of ruptured abdominal aortic aneurysm repair. Am Surg 1989;55:396–402.

133. Stone J, Dyke L, Fritz P, et al. Hemodynamic and hormonal changes during pneumoperitoneum and Trendelenburg positioning for operative gynecologic laparoscopic surgery. Primary Care Update Ob Gyns 1998;5:155.

134. Clayman RV, Kavoussi LR, Soper NJ, et al. Laparoscopic nephrectomy: review of the initial 10 cases. J Endourol 1992;6:127–32.

135. Cadeddu JA, Molnar-Nadasdy G, Enriquez D, et al. Chronic effect of pneumoperitoneum on renal histology. J Endourology 1999;13:279–82.

136. Cisek LJ, Gobet RM, Peters CA. Pneumoperitoneum produces reversible renal dysfunction in animals with normal and chronically reduced renal function. J Endourology 1998;12:95–100.

137. Nguyen NT, Fleming NW, Singh A, et al. Evaluation of core temperature during laparoscopic and open gastric bypass. Obes Surg 2001;11:570–5.

138. Barrat C, Capelluto E, Champault G. Intraperitoneal thermal variations during laparoscopic surgery. Surgical Endoscopy 1999;13:136–8. Bessel JR, Karatassas A. Hypothermia induced by laparoscopic insufflation. Surgical Endoscopy 1995;9:791–6.

139. Makinen MT. Comparison of body temperature changes during laparoscopic and open cholecystectomy. Acta Anaesthesiol. Scand 1997;41:736–40.

140. Berber E, String A, Garland A, et al. Intraoperative thermal regulation in patients undergoing laparoscopic vs. open surgical procedures. Surg. Endosc 2001;15:281–5.

141. Danelli G. Berti M, Perotti V, et al. Temperature control and recovery of bowel function after laparoscopic or laparotomic colorectal surgery in patients receiving combined epidural/general anesthesia and postoperative epidural analgesia. Anesth Analg 2002;95-467–71.

142. Nguyen NT, Fleming NW, Singh A, et al. Evaluation of core temperature during laparoscopic and open gastric bypass. Obes Surg 2001;11:570–5.

143. Stewart BT, Stitz RW, Tuch MM, Lumley JW. Hypothermia in open and laparoscopic colorectal surgery. Dis Colon Rectum 1999;42:1292–5.

144. Luck AJ, Moyes D, Maddern GJ, Hewett PJ. Core temperature changes during open and laparoscopic colorectal surgery. Surg Endosc 1999;13:480–3.

145. Jacobs VR, Morrison JE, Mettler L, et al. Measurement of CO2 hypothermia during laparoscopy and pelviscopy: how cold it gets and how to prevent it. J Am Assoc Gynecol Laparoscopy 1999;6:289–95.

146. Moore SS, Green CR, Wang FL, et al. The role of irrigation in the development of hypothermia during laparoscopic surgery. Am J Obstet Gynecol 1997;176:598–602.

147. Ekkis-Stoll CC, Anderson C, Cantu LG, et al. Effect of continuously warmed i.v. fluids on intraoperative hypothermia. AORN J 1996;63:599–606.

148. Matsuzaki Y, Matsukawa T, Ohki K, et al. Warming by resistive heating maintains perioperative normothermia as well as forced air heating. Br J Anaesth 2003;90:689–91.

149. Bessell, JR, Ludbrook G. Millard SH, et al. Humidified gas prevents hypothermia induced by laparoscopic insufflation: a randomized controlled study in a pig model. Surgical Endoscopy 1999;13:101–5.

150. Ott DE, Reich H, Love B, et al. Reduction of laparoscopic-induced hypothermia, postoperative pain and recovery roon length of stay by pre-conditioning gas with the Insuflow device: a prospective randomized controlled multi-center study. JSLS 1998;2:321–9.

151. Nguyen NT, Furdui G, Fleming NW, et al. Effect of heated and humidified carbon dioxide gas on core temperature and postoperative pain: a randomized trial. Surg. Endosc 2002;16:1050–4.

152. Mouton WG, Bessell JR, Pfitzner J, et al. A randomized controlled trial to determine the effects of humidified carbon dioxide insufflation during throacoscopy. Surg Endosc 1999;13:382–5.

153. Seagard JL, Bosnjak AJ, Hopp FA, et al. Cardiovascular effects of general anesthesia. In: Covino BG, Fozzard HA, Rahder K, Strichartz G, editors. Effects of anesthesia. Baltimore (MD): Williams & Wilkins; 1985. p. 149–77.

154. Lew JKL, Gin T, Oh TE. Anaesthetic problems during laparoscopic cholecystectomy. Anaesth Intensive Care 1992;20:91–2.

155. Myles PS. Bradyarrhythmias and laparoscopy: A prospective study of heart rate changes with laparoscopy. Aust NZ J Obstet Gynecol 1991;31:171–3.

156. Doyle DJ, Mark PWS. Laparoscopy and vagal arrest. Anaesthesia 1989;44:448.

157. Barake A. Cardiovascular collapse after carbon dioxide exsufflation in a patient undergoing laparoscopic cholecystectomy [Letter]. Anesth Analg 1994;78:603.

158. Scott DB. Some effects of peritoneal of carbon dioxide at laparoscopy. Anaesthesia 1970;25:590.

159. Scott DB, Julian DG. Observations on cardiac arrhythmias during laparoscopy. Br Med J 1972;1:411–3.

160. Bruhl W. [Complications of laparoscopy and liver biopsy under vision: the results of a surgery]. German Med Monthly 1967;12:31–2.

161. Horwitz ST. Laparoscopy in gynecology. Obstet Gynecol Survey 1972;27:1013.

162. Sivak BJ. Surgical emphysema: report of a case and review. Anesth Analg 1964;43:415–7.

163. Monk TG, Weldon BC, Lemon D. Alterations in pulmonary function during laparoscopic surgery. Anesth Analg 1993;76:S274.

164. Batra MS, Driscoll JJ, Coburn WA, Marks WM. Evanescent nitrous oxide pneumothorax after laparoscopy. Anesth Analg 1983;62:1121–3.

165. Murray DP, Rankin RA, Lackey C. Bilateral pneumothoraces complicating peritoneoscopy. Gastrointest Endosc 1984;30:45–6.

166. Loffer FD, Pent D. Indications, contraindications and complications of laparoscopy. Obstet Gynecol Survey 1975; 30:407–27.

167. Phillips J, Keith D, Hulka J, et al. Gynecologic laparoscopy in 1975. J Reprod Med 1976;16:105–17.

168. Brown JAC, Chamberlain GVP, Jordan JA, et al. Gynaecological laparoscopy: the report of the working party of the confidential enquiry into gynaecological laparoscopy. Br J Obstet Gynaecol 1978;85:401–3.

169. Mintz M. Risks and prophylaxis in laparoscopy: a survey of 100,000 cases. J Reprod Med 1977;18:269–72.

170. Hynes SR, Marshall RL. Venous gas embolism during gynaecological laparoscopy. Can J Anaesth 1992;39:748–9.

171. Jernstrom P. Air embolism during peritoneoscopy. Am J Clin Pathol 1951;21:573–5.

172. Root B, Levy MN, Pollack S, et al. Gas embolism death after laparoscopy delayed by "trapping" in portal circulation. Anesth Analg 1978;57:232–7.

173. Beck DH, McQuillan PJ. Fatal carbon dioxide embolism and severe haemorrhage during laparoscopic salpingectomy. Br J Anesth 1994;72:243–5.

174. Oppenheimer MJ, Durant TM, Lynch P. Body position in relation to venous air embolism and the associated cardio-respiratory changes. Am J Med Sci 1953;225:362–73.

175. Bergqvist D, Lowe G. Venous thromboembolism in patients undergoing laparoscopic and arthroscopic surgery and in leg casts. Arch Intern Med 2002;162:2173–6.

176. Lindberg F, Bergqvist D, Rasmussen I. Incidence of thromboembolic complications after laparoscopic cholecystectomy: review of the literature. Surg Laparoscopic Endosc 1997;7:324–31.

177. Blake AM, Toker SI, Dunn, E. Deep venous thrombosis prophylaxis is not indicated for laparoscopic cholecystectomy, JSLS 2001;5:215–9.

178. Maillo CL, Martin E, Lopez J, et al. Effect of pneumoperitoneum on venous hemodynamics during laparoscopic cholecystectomy. Influence of patients age and time of surgery. Med Clin Barcelona 2003;120:330–4.

179. Catheline JM, Gaillard JL, Rizk N, et al. Thrombolembolism prophylaxis and incidence of thromboembolic complica-

tions after laparoscopic surgery. Int J Surg Investig 2000;2:41–7.
180. Baixauli J, Delaney CP, Senagore AJ, et al. Portal vein thrombosis after laparoscopic sigmoid colectomy for diverticulitis: report of a case. Dis Colon Rectum 2003;46:550–3.
181. Kono M, Yahagi N, Kitahara M, et al. Cardiac arrest associated with use of an argon beam coagulator during laparoscopic cholecystectomy. Br J Anaesthesia 2001;4:644–6.
182. Bandyopadhyay D, Kapadia CR. Large bowel ischemia following laparoscopic inguinal hernioplasty. Surg. Endosc 2003;17:520–1.
183. Dunn MD, Portis AJ, Shalhav AL, et al. Laparoscopic versus open radical nephrectomy: a 9 year experience. J. Urology 2000;164:1153–9.
184. Yu HP, Hseu SS, Yien HW, et al. Oral clonidine premedication preserves heart rate variability for patients undergoing laparoscopic cholecystectomy. Acta Anaesth Scand 47:185–90.
185. Alexander JI. Pain after laparoscopy. Br J Anaesth 1997; 79:369–78.
186. Edelman DS, Misiakos EP, Moses K. Extraperitoneal laparoscopic hernia repair with local anesthesia. Surg Endosc 2001;15:976–80.
187. Uzunkoy A, Coskun A, Akinci OF. The value of pre-emptive analgesia in the treatment of postoperative pain after laparoscopic cholecystectomy. European Surgical Research 2001;33:39–41.
188. Lee IO, Kim SH, Kong MH, et al. Pain after laparoscopic cholecystectomy: the effect and timing of incisional and intraperitoneal bupivicaine. Can J. Anaesth 2001;48: 545–50.
189. Helvacioglu A, Weis R. Operative laparoscopy and postoperative pain relief. Fert Steril 1992;57:548–52.
190. Hasaniya NW, Zayed FF, Faiz H, Severino R. Preinsertion local anesthesia at the trocar site improves perioperative pain and decreases costs of laparoscopic cholecystectomy. Surg Endosc 2001;15:962–4.
191. Neuhaus SJ, Gupta A, Watson DI. Helium and other alternative insufflation gases for laparoscopy. Surg Endosc 2001; 15:553–60.
192. Spivak J, Nudelman I, Fuco V, et al. Laparoscopic extraperitoneal inguinal hernia repair with spinal anesthesia and nitrous oxide insufflation. Surg Endosc 1999;13:1026–9.
193. Tsereteli Z, Terry ML, Bowers SP, et al. Prospective randomized clinical trial comparing nitrous oxide and carbon dioxide pneumoperitoneum for laparoscopic surgery. J Am College Surg 2002;195:173–9.
194. Hong JY, Lee IH. Suprascapular nerve block or a piroxicam patch for shoulder tip pain after day case laparoscopic surgery. Eur J Anaesthesiol 2003;20:234–8.
195. Narchi P, Benhamou D, Fernandez H. Intraperitoneal local anaesthetic for shoulder pain after day-case laparoscopy. Lancet 1991;338:1569–70.
196. Smith BE, Suchak M, Siggins D, Challands J. Rectus sheath block for diagnostic laparoscopy. Anaesthesia 1988;43: 947–8.
197. McKenzie R, Phitayakorn P, Uy NT, et al. Topical etidocaine during laparoscopic tubal occlusion for postoperative pain relief. Obstet Gynecol 1986;67:447–9.
198. Baram D, Smith C, Stinson S. Intraoperative topical etidocaine for reducing postoperative pain after laparoscopic tubal ligation. J Reprod Med 1990;35:407–10.
199. Alexander JI, Hull MG. Abdominal pain after laparoscopy. The value of a gas drain. Br J Obstet Gynecol 1987;94: 267–9.
200. Perry CP, Tombrello R. Effect of fluid instillation on postlaparoscopy pain. J Reprod Med 1993;38:768–70.
201. McDougall EM, Clayman RV, Fadden PT. Retroperitoneoscopy: the Washington University Medical School experience. Urology 1994;43:446–52.
202. Kuenkel MRF, Schaller G, Korth K. Rationale for a retroperitoneoscopic approach in PLND [Abstract]. J Urol 1994;151:344.
203. Batler RA, Campbell SC, Funk JT, et al. Hand-assisted vs. retroperitoneal laparoscopic nephrectomy. J Endourol 2001;15:899–902.
204. Edwards ND, Barclay K, Catling SJ, et al. Day case laparoscopy: a survey of postoperative pain and an assessment of the value of diclofena [see comments]. Anaesthesia 1991;46:1077–80.
205. Hovorka J, Kallela H, Korttila K. Effect of intravenous diclofenac on pain and recovery profile after day-case laparoscopy. Eur J Anaesthesiol 1993;10:105–8.
206. Crocker S. Paech M. Preoperative rectal indomethacin for analgesia after laparoscopic sterilization. Anaesth Intensive Care 1992;20:337–40.
207. Ding Y, White PF. Comparative effects of ketorolac, dezocine, and fentanyl as adjuvants during outpatient anesthesia [see comments]. Anesth Analg 1992;75:566–71.
208. Gillberg LE, Harsten AS, Stahl LB. Preoperative diclofenac sodium reduces post-laparoscopy pain. Can J Anaesth 1993;40:406–8.
209. van EE R, Hemrika DJ, van der Linden CT. Pain relief following day-case diagnostic hysteroscopy-laparoscopy for infertility: a double-blind randomized trial with preoperative naproxen versus placebo. Obstet Gynecol 1993;82: 951–4.
210. Smith I, Ding Y, White PF. Muscle pain after outpatient laparoscopy—influence of propofol versus thiopental and enflurane. Anesth Analg 1993;76:1181–4.
211. Zahl K, Apfelbaum JL. Muscle pain occurs after outpatient laparoscopy despite the substitution of vecuronium for succinylcholine. Anesthesiology 1989;70:408–11.
212. Poler SM, Watcha MF, White PF. Mivacurium as an alternative to succinylcholine during outpatient laparoscopy. J Clin Anesth 1989;4:127–33.
213. Yu HP, Hseu SS, Yien HW, et al. Oral clonidine premedication preserves heart rate variability for patients undergoing laparoscopic cholecystectomy. Acta Anaesthesiol. Scand 2003;47:185–90.
214. van Wijk MGF, Smalhout B. A postoperative analysis of the patient's view of anaesthesia in a Netherlands' teaching hospital. Anaesthesia 1990;45:679–82.
215. Fujii Y, Saitoh Y, Tanaka H, Toyooka H. Granisetron/dexamethasone combination for the prevention of postoperative nausea and vomiting after laparoscopic cholecystectomy. European J of Anaesthesiol 2000;17:64–8.
216. Raphael JH, Norton AC. Antiemetic efficacy of prophylactic ondansetron in laparoscopic surgery: randomized, double-blind comparison with metroclopramide. Br J Anaesth 1993;71:845–8.
217. Paech MJ, Lee BH, Evan SF. The effect of anaesthetic on postoperative nausea and vomiting after day-case gynaecological laparoscopy. Anaesth Intensive Care 2002;30: 153–9.
218. Apfel CC, Roewer N. Risk factors for nausea and vomiting after general anesthesia: fiction and facts (German) Anaesthesist 2000;49:629–42.
219. Wattwil M, Thorn SE, Lovqvist A, et al. Perioperative gastric emptying is not a predictor of early postoperative nausea and vomiting in patients undergoing laparoscopic cholecystectomy. Anesth. Analg 2002;95:476–9.
220. Lovstad RZ, Thagaard KS, Berner NS, Raeder JC. Neostignime 50microg Kg(-1) with glycopyrrolate increases postoperative nausea in women after laparoscopic gynaecological surgery. Acta Anaesthesiol Scand 2001;45: 495–500.
221. Fujii Y, Uemura A, Tanaka H. Prophylaxis of nausea and vomiting after laparoscopic cholecystectomy with ramosetron: randomized controlled trial. Eur J Surg 2002;168:583–6.
222. Malins AF, Field JM, Nesling PM, Copper GM. Nausea and vomiting after gynaecological laparoscopy: comparison of premedication with oral ondansetron, metoclopramide and placebo. Br J Anaesth 1994;72:231–3.
223. Bodner M, White PF. Antiemetic efficacy of ondansetron after outpatient laparoscopy [see comments]. Anesth Analg 1991;73:250–4.
224. Kovac A, McKenzie R, O'Connor T, et al. Prophylactic intravenous ondansetron in female outpatients undergoing gynaecological surgery: a multicentre dose-comparison study. Eur J Anaesthesiol 1992;6:37–47.
225. Argiriadou H, Papaziogas B, Pavlidis T, et al. Tropisetron vs. ondanseetron for prevention of postoperative nausea and vomiting after laparoscopic cholecystectomy: a randomized double-blind, placebo-controlled study. Surg Endosc 2002;16:1087–90.
226. Nicole PC, Trepanier CA, Lessard MR. Nausea and vomiting after laparoscopic surgery are not associated with an increased peripheral release of serotonin. Can J Anaesth 2002;49:453–7.
227. Paventi S, Santevecchi A, Ranieri R. Efficacy of a single-dose ondansetron for preventing postoperative nausea and vomiting after laparoscopic cholecystectomy with sevoflurane and remifentanil infusion anaesthesia. Eur Rev Med Pharmacol Sci 2001;5:59–63.
228. Wang JJ, Ho ST, Uen YH, et al. Small-dose dexamethasome reduces nausea and vomiting after laparoscopic cholecystectomy: a comparison of tropisetron with saline. Anesth Analg 2002;95:229–32.
229. Biswas BN, Rudra A. Compariseon of granisetron plus dexamethasome for the prevention of postoperative nausea and vomiting after laparoscopic cholecystectomy. Acta Anaesthesiol Scand 2003;47:79–83.
230. Coloma M, White PF, Markowitz SD, et al. Dexamethasone in combination with dolasetron for prophylaxis in the ambulatory setting; effect on outcome after laparoscopic cholecystectomy. Anesthesiology 2002;96:1346–50.
231. Fujii Y, Saitoh Y, Tanaka H, Toyooka H. Granisetron/dexamethasone combination for the prevention of postoperative nausea and vomiting after laparoscopic cholecystectomy. European J Anaesthesiol 2000;17:64–8.
232. Fujii Y, Saitoh Y, Tanaka H, Toyooka H. Granisetron/dexamethasone combination for reducing nausea and vomiting during and after spinal anesthesia for cesarian section, Anesth. Analg 1999;88:1346–50.
233. Lee Yi, Lai HY, Lin PC, et al. Dexamethasone prevents postoperative nausea and vomiting more effectively in women with motion sickness. Can J Anesth 2003;50:232–7.
234. Chen X, Tang J, White PF, et al. The effect of timing of dolasetron administration on its efficacy as a prophylactic antiemetic in the ambulatory setting Anesth Analg 2001; 93:906–11.
235. Ozmen S, Yavuz L, Ceylan BG, et al. Comparison of granisetron with granisetron plus droperidol combination prophylaxis in post-operative nausea and vomiting after laparoscopic cholecystectomy, J Int Med Res 2002;30: 520–4.
236. Kothari SN, Boyd WC, Bottcher ML, Lambert PJ. Antiemetic efficacy of prophylactic dimenhydrinate (Dramamine) vs. ondantestron (Zofran): a randomized, prospective trial of inpatients undergoing laparoscopic cholecystectomy. Surg Endosc 2000;14:926–9.
237. Grimsehl K, Whiteside JB, Mackenzie N. Comparison of cyclizine and ondansetron for the prevention of postoperative nausea and vomiting in laparoscopic day-case gynecological surgery. Anaesthesia 2002;57:61–5.
238. Piper SN, Suttner SW, Rohm KD, et al. Dolasetron, but not metaclopramide prevents nausea and vomiting in patients undergoing laparoscopic cholecystectomy. Can J Anesth 2002;49:1021–8.
239. Quaynor H, Raeder JC. Incidence and severity of postoperative nausea and vomiting are similar after metoclopramide 20mg and ondansetron 8mg given by the end of laparoscopic cholecystectomies, Acta Anaesthesiol. Scand 2002;46:109–13.
240. Marshall CA, Jones RM, Bajorek PK, Cashman JN. Recovery characteristics using isoflurane or propofol for maintenance of anaesthesia: a double-blind controlled trial. Anaesthesia 1992;47:461–6.
241. Raftery S, Sherry E. Total intravenous anaesthesia with propofol and alfentanil protects against postoperative nausea and vomiting. Can J Anaesth 1992;39:37–40.
242. Randel GI, Levy L, Kothary SP, Pandit SK. Propofol versus thiamylal-enflurane anesthesia for outpatient laparoscopy. J Clin Anesth 1992;4:185–9.
243. Chanvej L, Kijsirikul S, Thongsuksai P, Naheem L. Postoperative nausea and vomiting in out-patient gynecologic laparoscopy: a comparison of thiopental-nitrous oxide, propofol-nitrous oxide and total intravenous anesthesia using propofol. J. Med Assoc Thai 2001;84:697–704.
244. Purhonen S, Turunen M, Ruohoaho UM, et al. Supplemental oxygen does not reduce the incidence of postoperative nausea and vomiting after ambulatory gynecologic laparoscopy. Anesth Analg 2003;96:91–6.
245. Gibbs RD, Movinsky BA, Pellegrini J, Vacchiano CA. The morphine-sparing effect of metoclopramide on postoperative laparoscopic tubal ligation patients. AANA J 2002; 70:27–32.
246. Agarwal A, Bose N, Gaur A, et al. Acupressure and ondansetron for postoperative nausea and vomiting after laparoscopic cholecystectomy. Can J Anesthesia 2002;49: 554–60.
247. Samad K, Afshan G, Kamal R. Effect of acupressure on postoperative nausea and vomiting in laparoscopic cholecystectomy. J Pak Med Assoc 2003;53:68–72.
248. Coloma M, White PF, Ogunnaike BO, et al. Comparison of acustimulation and ondansetron for the treatment of established postoperative nausea and vomiting, Anesthesiology 2002;97:1387–92.

45

Physiologic Effects of the Pneumoperitoneum

Margaret S. Pearle, MD
Jeffrey A. Cadeddu, MD

Until 1990, laparoscopy was used primarily as a diagnostic tool; occasionally, simple therapeutic procedures such as tubal ablation for sterilization were performed through the laparoscope. The procedures were generally brief in duration, associated with little morbidity, and most commonly performed on healthy young females. As the skill and instrumentation of the laparoscopic surgeon expanded, so did the complexity and duration of the procedures. With the introduction of laparoscopic cholecystectomy in 1990[1] and laparoscopic nephrectomy in 1991,[2] the removal of large solid organs became feasible, and laparoscopy moved from the realm of diagnostic procedure to therapeutic application. Current laparoscopic procedures address a variety of pathologic conditions in patients with varied states of health. As a result, the effect of prolonged pneumoperitoneum has become a pertinent issue. This chapter addresses the physiologic effects of pneumoperitoneum and the potential complications arising from it.

HISTORY

In 1902, Kelling in Germany coined the term "koelioskopie" for a procedure in which he examined the abdominal cavity of a dog using a cystoscope introduced through the anterior abdominal wall.[3] A pneumoperitoneum was first established by insufflating filtered air through a separate needle; a trocar was then used to establish a tract for the Nitze cystoscope.

Jacobaeus of Stockholm is credited with the first endoscopic abdominal inspection in a human patient.[4] Unaware of Kelling's work, he reported two cases in 1910, one abdominal and one thoracic, in which the pneumoperitoneum or pneumothorax, respectively, was established after introduction of the trocar. He subsequently published a series of 115 procedures (80 laparoscopies and 35 thoracoscopies) in which laparoscopy was primarily performed in patients with ascites[5]; after introduction of the trocar, the ascitic fluid was withdrawn and replaced with air.

In 1920, Orndoff, a radiologist in Chicago, devised a new instrument to facilitate peritoneoscopy.[6] He fashioned a pyramidal-tipped trocar that contained three faces, each with sharp edges. The cannula surrounding the trocar was fitted with a valve that prevented release of the insufflated gas. Using oxygen as an insufflant, Orndoff operated on 42 patients with pelvic and abdominal pathologic conditions with this new instrument.

Although most early laparoscopists used air to insufflate the peritoneum, Zollikofer of Switzerland in 1924 suggested that CO_2 was a more practical choice because it is more readily absorbed from the peritoneal cavity.[7] Although other gases have been used to insufflate the peritoneal cavity, CO_2 remains the medium of choice for establishing the pneumoperitoneum.

Overall, although laparoscopic instrumentation has become more sophisticated, enabling surgeons to perform a wide spectrum of reconstructive, extirpative, and diagnostic procedures, the basic principles of establishing the pneumoperitoneum have changed little since the time of Kelling. But our understanding of the physiologic consequences of the pneumoperitoneum continue to expand. The physiologic effects of the pneumoperitoneum can be attributed to the effect of two independent variables: increased intra-abdominal pressure and absorption of the gaseous medium used for insufflation.

PRESSURE-RELATED EFFECTS

CARDIOVASCULAR EFFECTS   The net cardiovascular effect of increased intra-abdominal pressure is determined by changes in cardiac function and venous return (Table 45-1). Animal studies suggest that elevated intra-abdominal pressure leads to an increase in total peripheral vascular resistance, which negatively influences cardiac function.[8–10] The effect of increased intra-abdominal pressure on venous return is determined by changes in venous resistance and mean systemic pressure. At low right atrial pressures, venous return is inhibited by increased intra-abdominal pressure, primarily due to compression of the vena cava. In contrast, at high right atrial pressures, the vena cava resists compression, and venous return is augmented by increased intra-abdominal pressure.[8–11] Likewise, as intra-abdominal pressure increases, mean systemic pressure increases as a result of compression of the small capacitance vessels and augmented venous return. Kashtan and colleagues demonstrated that increased mean systemic pressure enhanced venous return and right atrial pressure in hypervolemic animals[8]; consequently, cardiac output increased by the Starling mechanism. In normo- and hypovolemic animals, however, the increased mean systemic pressure was outweighed by the increased venous resistance caused by compression of the vena cava;

consequently, venous return and cardiac output dropped. In all cases the increase in total peripheral resistance depressed cardiac function, but its effect was more pronounced in hypovolemic animals because the arterioles were more readily compressed in the low-volume state.[8]

Clinically, the degree to which various vascular and cardiac parameters change during surgery (see Table 45-1) is a function of several factors, including intra-abdominal pressure, patient position, CO_2 absorption, intravascular volume status, preexisting cardiopulmonary status, and current medications. Pneumoperitoneum appears to uniformly induce phasic hemodynamic changes that are characterized by a decrease in cardiac index to approximately 50% of preoperative values within 5 minutes of insufflation, after which there is a gradual increase in cardiac index as systemic vascular resistance drops after 10 minutes of insufflation.[12] Wallace and colleagues randomized 40 healthy patients undergoing laparoscopic cholecystectomy to insufflation pressures of 7.5 or 15 mm Hg and demonstrated that the fall in cardiac index after insufflation lasted longer (7 versus 2 minutes) at a pressure of 15 mm Hg although both corrected to baseline.[13] Dexter and colleagues also randomized 20 laparoscopic cholecystectomy patients to either low (7 mm Hg) or high (15 mm Hg) pressure pneumoperitoneum.[14] Although heart rate and mean arterial pressure increased to a similar degree in both groups, stroke volume and cardiac output were depressed to a greater extent in the 15 mm Hg group. Despite these measurable changes, the European Association for Endoscopic Surgery practice guidelines consensus surmised that, at intra-abdominal pressures up to 15 mm Hg, the decrease in venous return and cardiac output is minimal and without consequence in healthy

Table 45-1 Cardiovascular and Renal Effects of Increased Intra-abdominal Pressure (10 to 20 mm Hg)	
Parameter	Change
Heart rate	Unchanged , up
Mean arterial pressure	Up
Systemic vascular resistance	Up
Venous return	Down
Central venous pressure	Up
Cardiac output/index	Unchanged , Down
Glomerular filtration rate	Down
Urine output	Down

patients.[15] At this pressure, adequate volume loading mitigates the cardiovascular effects of the pneumoperitoneum, which are most pronounced during its induction.[16] In patients with limited cardiac reserve, however, the increased work required to circulate the blood dictates that close attention be directed to the intra-abdominal pressure set point as well as to volume status and blood pressure in order to avoid potentially dangerous cardiovascular changes.[15,17]

RENAL EFFECTS Elevated intra-abdominal pressure has also been observed to affect renal hemodynamics (see Table 45-1). As early as 1923, Thorington and Schmidt noted that intra-abdominal pressures > 15 mm Hg were associated with oliguria in dogs[18]; pressures > 30 mm Hg resulted in anuria. Likewise, in 1947, in a study of 17 normal human volunteers, Bradley and Bradley observed a decrease in urine flow after pressurizing a pneumatic abdominal girdle to 80 mm Hg, which corresponds to an average intra-abdominal pressure of 20 mm Hg.[19] Inferior vena caval pressure rose from 5.8 to 18.3 mm Hg. In addition, they found a reduction in effective renal plasma flow and glomerular filtration rate (GFR).

Several mechanisms have been proposed to account for the renal dysfunction seen with increases in the intra-abdominal pressure. Thorington and Schmidt implicated increased renal vein pressure as the etiology of the observed renal functional changes.[18] Others speculated that direct renal compression accounts for the changes in renal blood flow (RBF) and functional impairment. Finally, changes in antidiuretic hormone (ADH) levels were suggested to play a role in the oliguria seen clinically in patients with increased intra-abdominal pressure. Decreased cardiac output, ureteral compression, and renal ischemia, however, have been shown not to play a role in laparoscopy-associated oliguria.[16,20–22]

The clinical experience with elevated intra-abdominal pressure due to bleeding or edema parallels that seen during laparoscopy. Richards and colleagues noted oliguria or anuria postoperatively in four patients who subsequently required reexploration for bleeding associated with abdominal distention.[23] In all four cases, urine output remained low despite vigorous fluid resuscitation and normal to high-normal arterial and central venous pressures. Operative decompression resulted in a prompt diuresis in each case. Likewise, Fietsam and colleagues described an "intra-abdominal compartment syndrome" in four patients with massive retroperitoneal interstitial edema after abdominal aortic aneurysm repair, who developed severe oliguria despite elevated central venous pressures.[24] With decompressive laparotomy, urine output increased significantly.

In a laboratory model, Harman and colleagues favored direct renal compression as the cause for decreased renal blood flow and GFR in seven anesthetized dogs.[16] Inflation of an intraperitoneal bag with air to a pressure of 20 mm Hg resulted in a 22% reduction in GFR; at 40 mm Hg, three dogs became anuric, and the

GFR in the remaining four dogs dropped to 7% of baseline. Likewise, renal blood flow decreased from a baseline of 160 mL/min at 0 mm Hg pressure to 36 and 9 mL/min at 20 and 40 mm Hg intra-abdominal pressure, respectively. Cardiac output was similarly affected by the increased intra-abdominal pressure, decreasing by 17% and 37% at 20 and 40 mm Hg, respectively. Intravascular expansion doubled the cardiac output but had no effect on GFR or RBF. Inferior vena cava and renal vein pressure correlated with intra-abdominal pressure; in contrast, renal artery pressure was relatively unaffected by changes in intra-abdominal pressure. With elevated intra-abdominal pressure, the increase in renal vascular resistance far exceeded the increase in systemic vascular resistance. These findings suggest that direct effects on the kidney, rather than changes in systemic hemodynamics, are responsible for the renal dysfunction seen with increased intra-abdominal pressure.

A number of investigators have correlated changes in renal hemodynamics with increased intra-abdominal pressure during laparoscopy. Chiu and colleagues studied the effects of increased intra-abdominal pressure in six pigs undergoing laparoscopy.[25] Using air as the insufflant, intra-abdominal pressure was gradually increased from 0 to 40 mm Hg; measurements of carotid artery blood flow (CABF, representing cardiac output), carotid artery blood pressure (CABP), inferior vena caval pressure (IVCP), and RBF were recorded at various intra-abdominal pressures. As noted in previous studies, IVCP correlated directly with intra-abdominal pressure. Although CABP remained constant with increasing intra-abdominal pressure, CABF decreased linearly. Interestingly, renal cortical blood flow (RCBF) decreased exponentially with increasing intra-abdominal pressure. In contrast, renal medullary blood flow increased up to an intra-abdominal pressure of 20 mm Hg and then dropped steadily as intra-abdominal pressure reached 40 mm Hg. The decrease in RCBF could not be accounted for solely by decreased cardiac output: CABF decreased linearly with rising intra-abdominal pressure, whereas RCBF decreased exponentially. McDougall and colleagues [21] used noninvasive magnetic resonance imaging to similarly evaluate renal vessel blood flow and also demonstrated reduced cardiac output, reduced flow velocity in the renal vessels, and decreased renal parenchymal perfusion associated with abdominal insufflation. They also demonstrated reduced renal cortical and medullary blood flow. It seems likely, then, that the direct compressive effect of increased intra-abdominal pressure on the renal parenchyma accounts for the profound effect on renal blood flow, although whether or not a shunting phenomenon occurs remains unclear.

Along this same line, McDougall and another group of colleagues[26] performed a series of experiments using anesthetized farm pigs showing that decreased renal vein blood flow is invariably associated with oliguria during laparoscopy. At intra-abdominal pressures ≥ 10 mm Hg, urine

output, creatinine clearance, and renal vein flow decreased significantly, despite minimal change in cardiac output. These effects were not gas-specific; similar findings were observed with CO_2 or argon as an insufflant. Administration of renal doses of dopamine (2 μg/kg/min) and the use of ureteral catheters failed to overcome the effects of elevated intra-abdominal pressure. ADH was also measured, and no significant change was observed in any group, despite increasing intra-abdominal pressure. Of note, 2 hours after desufflation, ADH fell by 50% in all groups. Overall, these data suggest that impaired renal vein flow may be one, but not the sole, mechanism accounting for the observed decrease in urine output.

A number of clinical investigators in the early 1990s noted that patients undergoing lengthy laparoscopic procedures had a marked decrease in urine output that resolved after desufflation.[27,28] This is now a well-known clinical phenomenon. The role of ADH (arginine vasopressin) in promoting the oliguria seen during laparoscopy is unclear. Several investigators have measured increased levels of ADH during insufflation.[29,30] Solis Herruzo and colleagues evaluated 47 patients undergoing laparoscopy for a variety of conditions and noted a significant increase in plasma arginine vasopressin (AVP) levels with nitrous oxide insufflation of 6 to 10 mm Hg compared to baseline.[30] The change in AVP levels was independent of underlying liver disease, blood pressure changes, heart rate, carbon dioxide partial pressure (P_{CO2}) or oxygen partial pressure (P_{O2}), or plasma osmolality; however, increases in central venous pressure correlated closely with AVP levels. The authors suggested that the stimulus to AVP release may be a decrease in the left atrial pressure gradient that occurs with increased intra-abdominal pressure during laparoscopy. Whether AVP release contributes to the oliguria observed during laparoscopy remains unproved.

The hemodynamic and renal effects of pneumoretroperitoneum are similar to conventional pneumoperitoneum. Unilateral pneumoretroperitoneum results in a similar reduction in renal vein flow[26] and also results in oliguria due to a gradual decrease in contralateral kidney perfusion and increase in intra-abdominal pressure.[31]

In summary, at abdominal pressures of 10 to 15 mm Hg, urine output decreases significantly and is associated with decreased renal blood flow. Other hemodynamic changes, ADH levels, and direct ureteral compression play no discernible role in the transient oliguric state.

NONRENAL VISCERAL EFFECTS Changes in blood flow observed with elevated intra-abdominal pressure are not limited to the kidney. Gastric mucosal perfusion, assessed by measuring gastric intramucosal pH and used as a surrogate measure of splanchnic perfusion, decreases significantly (a decrease in pH) during pneumoperitoneum and can persist into the postoperative period.[12,32] Caldwell and Ricotta assessed blood flow to a number of intra-abdominal organs in dogs subjected to varying intra-abdominal pressures with an intraperitoneal inflatable bag.[33] In all organs measured (stomach, small bowel, pancreas, colon, liver, spleen, and kidney), visceral blood flow decreased out of proportion to the decrease in cardiac output, with the exception of the adrenal gland, which demonstrated an increase in blood flow. Likewise, Hashikura and colleagues measured blood flow to the liver and kidney in seven pigs subjected to intra-abdominal pressures of 6, 12, 18, and 24 mm Hg during CO_2 insufflation[34]; at the higher pressures, blood flow to the liver was significantly decreased. Since splanchnic ischemia is a known risk factor for bacterial translocation across the gut wall, it is not surprising that pneumoperitoneum has been associated with increased bacterial translocation from the peritoneum into the blood.[35] This phenomenon, however, has not been recognized as a clinical cause of laparoscopic morbidity.

INTRACRANIAL PRESSURE   A number of experimental[36–40] and clinical[41] studies have demonstrated an increase in intracranial pressure (ICP) with induced CO_2 pneumoperitoneum during laparoscopy. Although two clinical studies showed a direct correlation between ICP and PCO_2,[42,43] Josephs and colleagues found in an animal model that the rise in ICP was independent of changes in arterial PCO_2, PO_2, pH or mean arterial pressure.[36] Likewise, Schob and colleagues showed that the rise in ICP with pneumoperitoneum also occurred with nitrous oxide and helium as insufflants although to a lesser degree than with the use of CO_2.[44]

Several theories have been proposed to account for the rise in ICP seen during laparoscopy. One hypothesis incorporates the modified Monroe-Kellie doctrine, by which a change in one intracranial compartment (among four compartments: vascular, cerebrospinal fluid (CSF), osseous and parenchymal) results in a compensatory change in the other non-osseous compartments. With rapid changes in one compartment, however, there may be insufficient time for compensation, and ICP rises. Este-McDonald and colleagues attributed the rise in ICP to obstruction of venous outflow from the spinal cord via the lumbar and pelvic plexuses as a consequence of increased intrathoracic pressure, thereby increasing the volume of the vascular compartment and inducing a rise in ICP.[38]

In another theory, impaired absorption of CSF is hypothesized to account for the increase in ICP. Halverson and colleagues showed a linear increase in ICP and inferior vena caval pressure with increasing intra-abdominal pressure in 10 anesthetized domestic pigs (from an ICP of 14 mm Hg before insufflation to an ICP of 30 mm Hg at 15 mm Hg abdominal pressure), suggesting that impaired venous drainage from the lumbar venous plexus contributes to the rise in ICP.[40] This theory is further supported by the finding of impaired CSF absorption in anesthetized pigs in which radioiodinated human serum albumin (RISA) was injected into the CSF. A reduced rate of CSF absorption (by 55%) was demonstrated by measuring RISA in the blood over a 4-hour period during CO_2 pneumoperitoneum to 15 mm Hg pressure.[45]

Rosenthal and colleagues, on the other hand, postulated that the rise in ICP is mediated by a two-phase mechanism, including an early, passive, venous effect and a late, active, arterial effect (Figure 45-1).[37,46] In the early, mechanical stage, increased intra-abdominal pressure results in compression of the inferior vena cava and an increase in central venous pressure (CVP), thereby impairing venous drainage from the lumbar plexus and raising ICP. In the late stage, hypercarbia, due to ventilation-perfusion mismatch and peritoneal absorption of CO_2, causes vasodilatation of the intracranial vessels and a rise in ICP. Furthermore, acute elevation in ICP elicits a central nervous system response (Cushing reflex) mediated by release of catecholamines and vasopressin, leading to an increase in mean arterial pressure and systemic vascular resistance to maintain cerebral perfusion, and reduced splanchnic and visceral blood flow to enhance central venous return. By this mechanism, the array of hemodynamic changes observed with increased intra-abdominal pressure may be accounted for by the rise in ICP. Although this theory is compelling, it requires further validation.

In a pig model of head injury in which a Foley balloon catheter is inserted intracranially to simulate a mass lesion, changes in ICP similar in magnitude and direction to the noninjured pig model (but from a higher baseline ICP) were observed with increasing intra-abdominal pressure.[36–38] In contrast, no significant changes in ICP were observed with use of an apneumic retractor[38] or with low pressure laparoscopy (5 mm Hg intra-abdominal pressure) in a pig model.[47]

The clinical significance of these findings in patients without existing intracranial lesions or head injury is unknown, but to date no cases of significant neurologic impairment thought to be related to pneumoperitoneum have been reported. In patients with a head injury or an intracranial lesion, however, the potential for increased ICP during CO_2 pneumoperitoneum could be dangerous. As such, laparoscopy may be contraindicated in these patients or should be undertaken only under conditions of low intra-abdominal pressure or by gasless laparoscopy to avoid potentially dangerous elevations in ICP. The use of intra-operative ICP monitoring in this situation is advisable.[37,38,40]

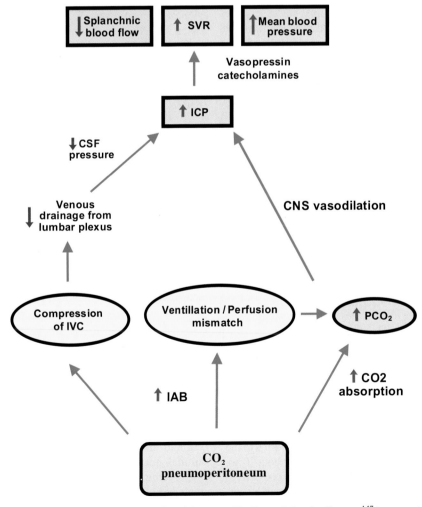

Figure 45–1 Schematic diagram of model proposed by Rosenthal and colleagues[147] to account for increased intracranial pressure and subsequent hemodynamic effects with CO_2 pneumoperitoneum. CVP=central venous pressure; IAP= intra-abdominal pressure; ICP= intracranial pressure; IVC= inferior vena cava; SVR= systemic vascular resistence.

Table 45-2 Pulmonary Effects of Increased Intra-abdominal Pressure (10 to 20 mm Hg)

Respiratory Parameter	Change
Peak inspiratory pressure	Up
Chest wall mechanical resistance	Up
Pulmonary compliance	Down
Pulmonary dead space	Unchanged
Functional reserve capacity	Down
Vital capacity	Down

RESPIRATORY EFFECTS Alterations in respiratory mechanics have also been noted with increased intra-abdominal pressure (Table 45-2). Numerous studies have documented that airway pressures increase, pulmonary compliance decreases (by nearly 50%), and functional reserve capacity decreases.[12,48,49] Motew and colleagues noted that the average peak airway pressure required to maintain a constant tidal volume in 10 women undergoing laparoscopy increased from 17.9 mm Hg at 0 mm Hg intra-abdominal pressure to 25.9 mm Hg at 20 mm Hg intra-abdominal pressure.[50] Likewise, Alexander and colleagues evaluated 24 patients undergoing laparoscopy and found that significantly increased airway pressure was required to maintain adequate ventilation during insufflation to 20 mm Hg intra-abdominal pressure.[51] The excess effort necessary to mechanically ventilate a healthy patient under general anesthesia is usually not clinically significant. In obese patients or those with lung disease, however, these perioperative changes can have deleterious effects, placing them at higher risk of pulmonary complications. Application of positive end expiratory pressure is generally necessary to adequately compensate in these patients.

ABSORPTION OF CARBON DIOXIDE

CARBON DIOXIDE HOMEOSTASIS Independent of the direct effect of increased intra-abdominal pressure, the pneumoperitoneum can alter hemodynamic and respiratory parameters as a result of the influence of absorbed CO_2. To understand the potential impact of infusing CO_2 under pressure into the abdomen, a review of basic CO_2 homeostasis is in order.

CO_2 is the predominant by-product of cellular metabolism. As such, an efficient mechanism for its elimination is required. The carbonic acid–bicarbonate buffer system provides a means of removal of CO_2; it also serves to prevent marked changes in arterial pH. Both components of the system can be regulated: bicarbonate in the kidney and CO_2 in the lungs. CO_2 in the tissues diffuses into capillaries. A small fraction of the CO_2 (about 7%) dissolves in the blood and is transported to the lungs. By far, the majority of the CO_2 (about 70%), however, combines with water in red blood cells to form carbonic acid in a reaction catalyzed by carbonic anhydrase. Almost as rapidly as it is formed, carbonic acid dissociates into hydrogen ions, which complex with hemoglobin, and bicarbonate ions, which diffuse into the plasma:

$$CO_2 + H_2O \leftrightarrows H_2CO_3 \leftrightarrows H^+ + HCO^-_3$$

The remaining minor fraction of CO_2 will complex with hemoglobin and plasma proteins for delivery to the lungs.[52] The carbonic acid–bicarbonate system therefore provides a powerful buffering system: the elimination of CO_2 drives the reaction to the left, thereby reducing the number of hydrogen ions and increasing pH. In addition, increases in CO_2 or hydrogen-ion concentration directly stimulate the chemosensitive area of the medulla, leading to respiratory stimulation, and consequently, to increased excretion of CO_2.[52,34]

Whether CO_2 is produced as a by-product of metabolism at the tissue level or is instilled into the peritoneum for laparoscopy, it is absorbed into the blood and ultimately equilibrates in the lungs. The movement of gas from one body compartment to another is controlled by the process of diffusion, which generally occurs from an area of high concentration to an area of low concentration. The rate at which a dissolved gas in liquid crosses an interface is determined by a number of factors, including the pressure differential across the interface, the solubility of the gas in the liquid, the distance the gas must traverse, the cross-sectional area of the fluid, the molecular weight of the gas, and the temperature of the gas and fluid. The *diffusion coefficient* defines the rate of diffusion of a specific gas for a given pressure differential and diffusion distance, thereby encompassing the solubility and molecular weight of the given gas. The diffusion coefficient is a relative number based on the diffusion coefficient of oxygen. The diffusion coefficients for several important respiratory gases are as follows:

Oxygen	1.00
Carbon dioxide	20.30
Carbon monoxide	0.81
Nitrogen	0.53
Helium	0.95

Indeed, CO_2 is highly soluble in water, and accordingly, has a high diffusion coefficient. CO_2 is more readily diffusible in body tissues than any of the other respiratory gases, a fact of some importance in its choice as insufflant for laparoscopy. With establishment of a CO_2 pneumoperitoneum, the CO_2 partially dissolves in the peritoneal fluid and subsequently reaches equilibrium with the tissues and blood as determined by the diffusion coefficient.

PHYSIOLOGIC CONSEQUENCES OF CARBON DIOXIDE ABSORPTION The hemodynamic consequences of hypercarbia have been well described (Table 45-3). Price divided the effects of hypercarbia into direct and indirect effects.[53] In isolated animal hearts, decreased pH, whether due to hypercarbia or otherwise, is associated with myocardial depression, which is manifest by decreased heart rate and force of contraction. Isolated blood vessels respond to a low pH by vasodilating. In contrast, CO_2 directly enhances sympathetic activity, which promotes cardiac contraction

and induces peripheral vasoconstriction. Cardiac output and myocardial oxygen consumption increase in response to hypercarbia and may reflect increased sympathetic activity. Peripherally, increases in mean arterial pressure are modest and suggest that local peripheral vasodilatory effects outweigh the central sympathomimetic effects. Cullen and Eger evaluated the circulatory response to increased inhaled CO_2 in 42 healthy volunteers.[54] Like Price, they found increases in heart rate, stroke index, myocardial contractility, and peripheral blood flow; in contrast, total peripheral resistance dropped significantly.

The CO_2 pneumoperitoneum has been implicated in a number of hemodynamic and respiratory alterations seen during laparoscopy. Early investigators noted that patients allowed to breathe spontaneously during laparoscopy began to hyperventilate[55–57]; likewise, in patients under controlled ventilation, significant hypercarbia and acidosis requiring ventilatory changes occurred in patients undergoing laparoscopy. Alexander and colleagues evaluated 24 healthy patients undergoing laparoscopy with a 20 mm Hg CO_2 pneumoperitoneum[51]; arterial blood gases were obtained before insufflation and during laparoscopy. A significant increase in P_{CO_2} by 8.6 mm Hg and a decrease in arterial pH by 0.082 pH units were measured after insufflation; P_{O_2} remained constant. Alexander and Brown subsequently showed that the effect occurred only with CO_2 insufflation and not nitrous oxide insufflation,[58] thereby implicating CO_2 absorption from the peritoneal cavity, rather than hypoventilation, as the etiology of the hypercarbia and acidosis. Seed and colleagues also measured a significant increase in end-tidal CO_2 concentration after insufflation, even in patients maintained on constant-volume ventilation during laparoscopy with a CO_2 pneumoperitoneum.[59] Likewise, Hodgson and colleagues and Montalva and Das showed that patients undergoing laparoscopy at intra-abdominal pressures of 15 to 20 mm Hg developed significant hypercarbia despite being maintained at a constant minute volume. Montalva and Das demonstrated an increase in P_{CO_2} of 5 mm Hg from pre- to post-insufflation P_{CO_2} in 10 female patients undergoing laparoscopy at a working pneumoperitoneum of 20 mm Hg.[60] Hodgson and colleagues found a difference of 8 mm Hg in the P_{CO_2} measured before and after insufflation to 15 to 20 mm Hg in patients breathing spontaneously during laparoscopy[55]; in 10 patients maintained at constant minute volumes, the mean change in P_{CO_2} was 10.1 mm Hg.

These data suggest that significant quantities of CO_2 are absorbed from the peritoneal cavity during laparoscopy with a 15 to 20 mm Hg CO_2 pneumoperitoneum. The absorption of CO_2 appears to reach a steady state between 15 and 30 minutes after the initiation of insufflation. Tan and colleagues measured CO_2 elimination in 12 patients undergoing pelvic laparoscopy (insufflation pressure was not mentioned) to estimate CO_2 absorption during insufflation.[61] CO_2 excretion increased from 146 mL/min before insufflation to 183 and 172 mL/min at 15 and 30 minutes

Table 45-3 Hemodynamic Effects of Hypercarbia

Hemodynamic Parameter	Experimental Effect		Clinical Effect
	Direct Effect*	Indirect Effect†	
Heart rate	Down	Up	Up
Cardiac contractility	Down	Up	CO up
Vascular resistance	Down	Up	SVR down
Mean arterial pressure	No data	Up	BP slightly up

BP = blood pressure; CO = cardiac output; SVR = systemic vascular resistance.
*Direct local effect of hypercarbia.
†Indirect effect of hypercarbia due to sympathetic stimulation.

after insufflation, respectively. This translated into a rate of CO_2 absorption from the peritoneal cavity of 42 and 39 mL/min, respectively. Likewise, Mullet and colleagues measured CO_2 excretion at 2-minute intervals after insufflation in 20 patients undergoing laparoscopic cholecystectomy (10 patients) or gynecologic laparoscopy (10 patients)[62]; in both groups, CO_2 excretion began to increase 8 to 10 minutes after the initiation of insufflation and reached a plateau by 15 to 20 minutes. The maximum increase in CO_2 excretion in the cholecystectomy group was 32 mL/min and, in the gynecologic laparoscopy group, was 18 mL/min, representing a 25% and 12% increase, respectively, from baseline.

Lister and colleagues also confirmed that significant CO_2 absorption occurs from the peritoneal cavity during laparoscopy[63] and further defined the relationship of CO_2 absorption and intra-abdominal pressure. Twelve anesthetized pigs maintained at constant ventilatory parameters underwent CO_2 or helium insufflation in 5 mm Hg increments from 0 to 25 mm Hg. At each insufflation pressure, measurements were taken of CO_2 excretion (Vco_2), dead space, and hemodynamic parameters. In the CO_2 pneumoperitoneum group, CO_2 excretion increased in a nonlinear fashion with increasing intraperitoneal pressure, reaching a plateau at a pressure of 10 mm Hg. In the helium pneumoperitoneum group, no increase in CO_2 excretion was noted. Pco_2 increased with rising intra-abdominal pressure in both groups, although the increase in Pco_2 was greater in the CO_2 group as compared to the helium group. Dead space ventilation increased by 24% in both groups with increased insufflation pressure. Hemodynamic parameters (heart rate, mean arterial pressure and cardiac output) were relatively stable at all pressures tested in both groups. The authors concluded that CO_2 absorption from the peritoneal cavity during insufflation reaches a maximum at a relatively low intra-abdominal pressure (ie, 10 mm Hg); up to that point there is a rapid increase in peritoneal surface area available for diffusion as intra-abdominal pressure increases. At higher pressures minimal additional surface area is recruited, further limiting CO_2 absorption. Pco_2, however, continues to rise as a result of increasing dead space ventilation, perhaps as a consequence of decreased delivered tidal volume. Use of a helium pneumoperitoneum avoids the delete-

rious effects of direct CO_2 absorption from the peritoneal cavity but produces the same ventilatory compromise resulting from increased intra-abdominal pressure.

The capacity of the lungs to excrete the excess absorbed CO_2 is limited; consequently, absorbed CO_2 is generally stored immediately in the body tissues until it can be eliminated by the lungs.[59] The capacity of individual tissues to store CO_2 is variable and depends on their perfusion and storage capacity. Although bone is the largest potential reservoir, muscle may play a larger role in immediate CO_2 storage because of its high perfusion rate.[64] For brief periods of increased CO_2 absorption, alveolar and blood stores primarily mediate homeostasis. For longer periods of CO_2 retention (ie, during laparoscopy), skeletal muscle and visceral stores come into play as well.[59] According to Fowle and Campbell, an immediate storage capacity of approximately 40 mL for each mm Hg rise in Pco_2 is available.[65] Therefore, if Pco_2 rises by 5 to 10 mm Hg with a 20 mm Hg CO_2 pneumoperitoneum, a corresponding 200 to 400 mL increase in CO_2 occurs. In the short term, this excess CO_2 is buffered in the alveolar-arterial and visceral stores, but potentially dangerous elevations in Pco_2 may result in serious hemodynamic alterations if compensatory changes in ventilation are not made. Furthermore, the need for elimination of excess CO_2 from visceral stores continues during the recovery phase after laparoscopy. With underlying pulmonary disease, elimination of CO_2 may be compromised, thereby necessitating prolonged mechanical ventilation in the postoperative period.[66,67]

Although hypercarbia associated with CO_2 pneumoperitoneum is well recognized, the choice of an appropriate monitoring technique is controversial. Liu and colleagues prospectively evaluated 16 healthy patients undergoing laparoscopy using CO_2 pneumoperitoneum.[68] Capnography was used to measure end-tidal CO_2 during insufflation; arterial blood gases were obtained intermittently to simultaneously assess arterial Pco_2. Good correlation was found between the two measurements: end-tidal CO_2 increased from 31 to 42 mm Hg and Pco_2 increased from 33 to 44 mm Hg, respectively, during the procedure. Based on end-tidal CO_2 measurements, minute ventilation was increased in 81% of patients to maintain normocarbia. Because of its noninva-

sive nature, capnography was recommended for monitoring healthy patients during laparoscopy. Wittgen and colleagues also found good agreement between capnography and arterial blood gas analysis in assessing Pco_2 in healthy patients undergoing cholecystectomy, but found capnography to be unreliable in estimating Pco_2 in patients with cardiopulmonary disease.[66] In 20 ASA class I patients, a small increase in Pco_2 and decrease in pH were noted after insufflation to between 12 and 15 mm Hg but the change did not reach statistical significance. In contrast, 10 ASA class II or III patients demonstrated a significant increase in arterial Pco_2 and a decrease in pH after insufflation. No significant difference in end-tidal CO_2 was found between the two groups after insufflation, suggesting that end-tidal CO_2 underestimated the arterial Pco_2 in the less healthy patients. Because of the poor correlation between end-tidal CO_2 and Pco_2 in patients with pulmonary disease, invasive monitoring with arterial blood gas analysis is necessary to reliably evaluate patients with cardiopulmonary disease during laparoscopy.

The cardiovascular effects of hypercarbia are difficult to distinguish from the effects of increased intra-abdominal pressure during laparoscopy. Some, but not all, of the hemodynamic effects occur regardless of the insufflant, whereas others appear to be gas-specific. In 10 healthy women undergoing laparoscopic tubal ablation, Motew and colleagues noted that CO_2 insufflation to 20 mm Hg was associated with increased central venous and arterial pressure, tachycardia, and hypercarbia[50]; cardiac output was unchanged. In contrast, at an intra-abdominal pressure of 30 mm Hg, central venous and arterial pressure and cardiac output dropped, although these changes were not statistically significant. Likewise, Liu and colleagues used transesophageal ultrasonography to measure cardiac output in 16 healthy patients undergoing laparoscopic cholecystectomy.[68] Although a significant rise in blood pressure was noted with insufflation (intra-abdominal pressure was not specified), no change in cardiac output was measured. Marshall and colleagues also found no change in cardiac output in seven young women undergoing laparoscopic tubal ablation,[69] but significant increases in central venous pressure, mean arterial pressure, and heart rate occurred with insufflation to between 15 and 21 mm Hg. At low intra-abdominal insufflation pressures (10 mm Hg), Kubota and colleagues also found no change in cardiac output or pulmonary arterial pressure compared to baseline.[70]

Lenz and colleagues used impedance cardiography to measure cardiac output in 24 women undergoing laparoscopy.[71] They found a modest reduction in stroke volume (by 23%) and cardiac output (by 17%) with CO_2 insufflation that was linearly related to the amount of CO_2 insufflated. Westerband and colleagues also used impedance cardiography to evaluate 16 patients undergoing laparoscopic cholecystectomy.[72] With CO_2 insufflation to 15 mm Hg, they noted a 30%

Table 45-4 Direct Effects of Patient Position Compared with Baseline Supine Position

Hemodynamic Parameter	Patient Position	
	Head Up	Head Down
Heart rate	Up	Down
Mean arterial pressure	Down	Up
Systemic vascular resistance	Up	Down
Cardiac output	Down	Up
Intracranial pressure	Down	Up

reduction in cardiac output compared to baseline: to 2.3 from 3.2 L/min/m^2. In addition, a significant increase in mean arterial pressure to 97 mm Hg from 84 occurred with a corresponding increase in total peripheral resistance (to 3,808 from 2,125 dyn 3 sec/m^5 3 m^2).

Several randomized trials compared the hemodynamic and respiratory consequences of high- and low-pressure CO_2 pneumoperitoneum during laparoscopic cholecystectomy. Wallace and colleagues randomized 40 patients to low-pressure (7.5 mm Hg) versus high-pressure (15 mm Hg) pneumoperitoneum and found no significant differences between the two groups with regard to PCO_2 or end-tidal CO_2, peak airway pressure, heart rate, cardiac index, stroke index or mean arterial pressure.[13] However, the decrease in cardiac index that was observed in both groups, was greater and lasted longer in the high pressure group. Dexter and colleagues, however, found that stroke volume increased from baseline in 10 patients undergoing low-pressure laparoscopy (7 mm Hg pressure) but decreased in 10 patients undergoing high-pressure (15 mm Hg pressure) laparoscopy.[14] Likewise, cardiac output remained at or below baseline levels in the high-pressure group but increased after an initial drop, to a level 20% above baseline in the low-pressure group. From these studies, there may be a slight hemodynamic advantage to low-pressure laparoscopy.

HEMODYNAMIC IMPACT OF PATIENT POSITION
Patient position influences hemodynamic parameters (Table 45-4) and alters the changes seen during laparoscopy. Williams and Murr evaluated the hemodynamic response of 10 dogs undergoing CO_2 insufflation in various positions.[73] In the horizontal position at a pressure of 15 mm Hg, cardiac output dropped to 79% of baseline; at 30 mm Hg pressure, cardiac output measured 77% of baseline. Positioning the animal head down resulted in a smaller reduction in cardiac output during insufflation to 15 mm Hg than was seen in the horizontal position (cardiac output 86% of baseline); at 30 mm Hg, cardiac output was 82% of baseline, similar to that seen in the horizontal position. The head-up position further reduced cardiac output at both 15 and 30 mm Hg pressure: 70% and 67% of baseline, respectively.

Joris and colleagues also found hemodynamic parameters to be position-dependent in 15 patients undergoing laparoscopic cholecystectomy at an intra-abdominal pressure of 14 mm Hg.[74] Hemo-

dynamic parameters were measured before and after induction of anesthesia, after positioning the patient head up, at various time intervals after insufflation, and after desufflation. Induction of anesthesia with the patient supine, before insufflation, resulted in a 9% decrease in a mean arterial pressure and a 25% decrease in cardiac index. Tilting the patient to the head-up position further reduced the mean arterial pressure by 17% and the cardiac index by 14%. With insufflation, the mean arterial pressure increased by 37% and the cardiac index decreased by 18% compared to the head-up position prior to insufflation. Systemic vascular resistance and pulmonary vascular resistance increased significantly with insufflation. Overall, mean arterial pressure was unchanged, and the cardiac index decreased by 50% from the preanesthestic value (from 3.6 to 1.8 L/min/m^2 at 5 minutes after insufflation). Systemic vascular resistance and pulmonary vascular resistance increased by 107% and 128%, respectively. The authors suggested that the reduction in cardiac index may have been caused by increased afterload (systemic vascular resistance) as well as decreased venous return. The increase in systemic vascular resistance was likely a consequence of increased venous and arteriole resistance arising from increased intra-abdominal pressure as well as from enhanced sympathetic activity resulting from elevated PCO_2. This study demonstrated the cumulative effects of anesthesia, patient positioning, and insufflation on the hemodynamic status of patients undergoing laparoscopy.

Kelman and colleagues compared hemodynamic parameters in 39 patients undergoing gynecologic laparoscopy in either the horizontal position (21 patients) or head-down position (18 patients).[75] In the horizontal position, cardiac output rose from 3.9 L/min before insufflation to 4.5 L/min after insufflation to between 10 and 20 cm H_2O. Baseline cardiac output was higher in the head-down position (4.8 L/min) compared to the horizontal position (3.9 L/min). After insufflation to between 10 and 20 cm H_2O, cardiac output increased to 5.3 L/min in the head-down group. At an intra-abdominal pressure of 30 to 40 cm H_2O, however, cardiac output fell in both groups to 4.4 L/min in the horizontal position and to 4.8 L/min in the head-down position. The changes in cardiac output reflected changes in central venous pressure; patients in the head-down position had higher central venous pressures than patients in the horizontal position, and the cardiac output was correspondingly higher.

Unlike Kelman and colleagues, Hirvonen and colleagues detected a decrease in cardiac index from baseline in 20 female patients undergoing laparoscopic hysterectomy in the head-down position at 13 to 16 mm Hg pneumoperitoneum.[76] In addition increases in pulmonary arterial pressure, central venous pressure and pulmonary capillary wedge pressure were noted. In a similar study examining the effects of the head-up position during laparoscopic cholecystectomy, Hirvonen and a different group of colleagues noted

decreases in central venous pressure and pulmonary capillary wedge pressure, and a gradual decrease in cardiac index during laproscopy.[77] Preoperative volume loading, and wrapping the lower extremities in elastic bandages reduced the magnitude of the drop in cardiac index usually seen with the head-up position.

The increase in intra-abdominal pressure along with the head-up position impairs venous return from the lower extremities. As such, the risk of deep venous thrombosis is theoretically enhanced. The use of intermittent sequential compression devices on the lower extremities has been shown to reduce venous stasis and partially compensate for the negative effects of position and intra-abdominal pressure.[78]

The effect of patient position on ICP is well known; the head-up position reduces ICP and the head-down position increases it. The combined effect of position and intra-abdominal pressure has been investigated in an animal model, in which increases in ICP were apparent with increasing intra-abdominal pressure in the supine, head-down and head-up positions.[40] ICP was correspondingly higher in the head-down position than any other position at each intra-abdominal pressure tested. Furthermore, head-up positioning failed to prevent the rise in ICP seen with insufflation.

In summary, three variables influence hemodynamic parameters during laparoscopy and contribute to the net hemodynamic effect (see Table 45-4): intra-abdominal pressure, choice of insufflant, and patient position. In patients undergoing laparoscopy in the supine position, cardiac output is unaffected or decreases with insufflation to low to moderate intra-abdominal pressure (10 to 15 mm Hg); mean arterial pressure and systemic vascular resistance increase. Higher intra-abdominal pressures (> 20 mm Hg) adversely affect cardiac output by decreasing venous return. Urine output falls precipitously, but returns to normal shortly after desufflation. The choice of insufflant contributes to the net hemodynamic effect; if CO_2 insufflation is used, hypercarbia generally has a stimulatory effect on the circulatory system, causing a further increase in heart rate, stroke volume, and myocardial contractility, while decreasing peripheral vascular resistance. Absorption of inert gases such as helium generally causes no additional hemodynamic changes. The head-down position results in favorable hemodynamic changes; cardiac output is higher than in the supine position but is still dependent on intra-abdominal pressure. However, ICP increases in the head-down position, which could be potentially dangerous in patients already at risk for increased ICP.

STRESS RESPONSE AND IMMUNOLOGIC FACTORS

The effect of pneumoperitoneum on immune and metabolic responses has been extensively studied, primarily based on alterations in cytokines and other immune response mediators, although correlation of these findings with actual immune function and clinical complications has not been forthcoming. Nonetheless, alterations in the stress and immune response to laparoscopic surgery may provide insight into the observed clinical outcomes.

Alterations in the stress and immune response correlate with the severity or extent of injury[79]; as such, the physiologic response to laparoscopic surgery may differ from that of open surgery. The primary mediators of the acute phase response are the inflammatory cytokines interleukin-1 (IL-1), interleukin-6 (IL-6) and tumor necrosis factor (TNF), which are released from peritoneal macrophages.[80] The hepatic component of the acute phase response is regulated by IL-6, which stimulates production of acute phase response proteins, including C-reactive protein, which is the primary marker.[79,81,82] TNF and IL-β1β mediate the non-hepatic manifestations of the acute phase response, such as fever and tachycardia.[81]

A number of investigators have compared IL-6 levels after laparoscopic and corresponding open operations, for which cholecystectomy is the best studied. Numerous series have demonstrated significantly higher levels of IL-6 with open as compared with laparoscopic cholecystectomy,[83–85] and some have also found a correlation between peak IL-6 and C-reactive protein concentrations.[86,87] The results for laparoscopic-assisted colon resection are less definitive. In a non-randomized trial comparing laparoscopic-assisted with open colon resection, Harmon and colleagues detected reduced IL-6 levels with the laparoscopic approach.[88] Likewise, Leung and colleagues randomized 34 patients with organ-confined rectosigmoid carcinoma to laparoscopic-assisted versus open colon resection and found significantly lower IL-6 and IL-1β levels after laparoscopic surgery.[89] On the other hand, Stage and colleagues measured higher levels of IL-6 and C-reactive protein in the laparoscopic group among a mixed group of patients randomized to laparoscopic-assisted or open colectomy.[90] Differences in patient and tumor characteristics in the study groups may account for the discrepancies in these studies. Differences are also evident between studies evaluating IL-6 levels after laparoscopic fundoplication[91,92] and hernia repair.[93] But the effect on the immune response of a small incision, as in laparoscopic-assisted surgery, either with or without pneumoperitoneum, is not known.

The effect of laparoscopic surgery on C-reactive protein has also been investigated. Although most studies demonstrated more modest increases in C-reactive protein with laparoscopic compared to open cholecystectomy,[84,86,89,92,94,95] a few demonstrated no difference in acute phase response proteins between the two groups.[96,97]

The influence of the specific gas used for insufflation on immune function has been addressed experimentally. Chekan and colleagues compared the immune competence of mice, as determined by their ability to clear an intraperitoneally administered intracellular pathogen, *Listeria monocytogenes*, after undergoing abdominal laparotomy or laparoscopy using either CO_2 or helium as an insufflant.[98] Although all interventions were associated with impaired cell-mediated immunity (decreased clearance of interperitoneal bacteria), CO_2 pneumoperitoneum resulted in a lower bacterial clearance rate than either laparotomy or helium pneumoperitoneum, with helium pneumoperitoneum demonstrating the best clearance rates. The mechanism of the immune defect was not addressed in this study. Sandoval and colleagues, however, found no impairment in natural killer cell activity in rats subjected to CO_2 pneumoperitoneum.[99] On the other hand, West and colleagues demonstrated significantly lower levels of TNF and IL-1 in response to bacterial lipopolysaccaride when macrophages were incubated in CO_2 compared with air or helium.[100] In a separate study, they and some other colleagues proposed that the impairment in macrophage cytokine production was due to intracellular acidification as a result of the CO_2 pneumoperitoneum.[101]

Other factors related to the pneumoperitoneum have also been investigated to assess their effect on immune function. In a randomized clinical trial of laparoscopic cholecystectomy, cytokine production was attenuated when using warmed, as opposed to room temperature, CO_2.[102]

Stress response with respect to neuroendocrine factors has also been compared between laparoscopic and open surgery. In a randomized trial comparing laparoscopic and open cholecystectomy, Karayiannakis and colleagues detected significantly higher levels of cortisol, epinephrine, and norepinephrine in the postoperative period after open cholecystectomy.[103] Likewise Le Blanc-Louvry and colleagues found reduced levels of corticotropin as well as urinary cortisol and catecholamine metabolites in patients randomized to laparoscopic versus open cholecystectomy.[104] In contrast, Hendolin and colleagues found no significant differences in plasma cortisol or catecholamines between patients undergoing laparoscopic versus open cholecystectomy in a randomized trial.[105]

Further correlation of the immune and stress response and immunologic outcome is required in order to determine their significance with regard to laparoscopic complications, postoperative recovery and tumor implantation or metastasis.

COMPLICATIONS

A variety of adverse effects have been attributed to establishment and maintenance of the pneumoperitoneum. Hemodynamic and ventilatory consequences of insufflation have been described, but a number of complications can occur due to misplacement of the Veress needle and/or trocar with subsequent insufflation.

Subcutaneous emphysema is the most common manifestation of a poorly positioned Veress needle or trocar. In this case, leakage of CO_2 around the trocar or direct insufflation of CO_2 into the subcutaneous or properitoneal tissues results in blunt dissection along extraperitoneal tissue planes. Generally, subcutaneous emphysema is harmless, but if severe, it may lead to hypercarbia.[106–109] Wolf and colleagues found that subcutaneous emphysema was one of several factors, along with increased duration of insufflation and an extraperitoneal approach, that correlated with increased CO_2 absorption (as measured by CO_2 excretion) during pelvic laparoscopy.[109] Likewise, Sosa and colleagues noted that, among patients undergoing laparoscopic pelvic lymph node dissection, those who developed significant hypercarbia ($P_{CO_2} \geq 50$ mm Hg) were more likely to have associated subcutaneous emphysema (7 of 8 patients) than patients who maintained normocarbia ($P_{CO_2} < 47$ mm Hg) (0 of 8 patients).[107]

Unlike intraperitoneal gas, retroperitoneal or properitoneal gas is not limited by the peritoneal membrane. As such, it may traverse a variety of tissue planes to enter the pleural or extrapleural space, mediastinum, or pericardium. Insufflation of gas along the great vessels or from the anterior neck allows entrance into the mediastinum.[110] From the mediastinum, gas may rupture into the pericardium or travel along the pulmonary vessels to the pleural space, resulting in pneumopericardium[111–114] or pneumothorax,[110,114,115] respectively. Direct seepage of gas between diaphragmatic fibers provides access to the extrapleural space and subsequently the mediastinum. Generally, in the absence of hemodynamic or respiratory compromise, small pneumothoraxes may be managed conservatively. Large or symptomatic pneumothoraxes are treated with needle aspiration or tube thoracostomy.

A dangerous and potentially fatal complication of pneumoperitoneum is gas embolism.[116–122] Typically, in this catastrophic complication, the Veress needle is inadvertently positioned in a vein, resulting in injection of gas directly into the venous system. The gas bubble travels to the right heart and lodges in the atrium or pulmonary arterial system; the gas lock may obstruct venous return to the atrium, leading to a dramatic fall in cardiac output, or it may block pulmonary blood flow, causing pulmonary hypertension and right heart failure. The diagnosis is suggested by dramatic, sudden cyanosis, hypoxia, hypercarbia, arrhythmia, or hypotension during insufflation; the classic mill wheel murmur is pathognomonic, but variably present. Capnography may be useful in the early diagnosis of gas embolism.[119,121] An abrupt decrease in end-tidal CO_2 may be the first sign of a gas embolism; the "air lock" completely obstructs pulmonary blood flow, leading to the decrease in CO_2 excretion.[120] The most sensitive means of detecting gas embolism is transesophageal echocardiography (TEE), which can detect a bolus of CO_2 as small as 0.02 cc.[123] Couture and colleagues compared the sensitivity of TEE, end tidal CO_2, pulmonary artery pressure and precordial auscultation for detecting CO_2 embolism in anesthetized pigs and found that TEE was superior to the other modalities, which were of comparable sensitivity, in detecting gas embolism.[124]

Although gas embolism occurs most commonly as a result of Veress needle misplacement and insufflation into a large vein, embolism as a result of venous injury during pneumoperitoneum is also a theoretical concern.[117,125,126] O'Sullivan and colleagues detected gas emboli after 20 of 22 venotomies created in anesthetized pigs undergoing laparoscopy with CO_2 pneumoperitoneum at 10 to 25 mm Hg pressure.[123] The degree of embolization correlated with the decrease in central venous pressure due to blood loss or distal venous compression, the duration and amount of manipulation of the venotomy and intraperitoneal pressure. As such, in the event of significant venous injury during laparoscopy, intravascular volume should be maintained and the site of bleeding should be occluded directly.

Treatment of gas embolism consists of immediate desufflation, initiation of 100% inspired oxygen, and resuscitative measures. In addition, the patient is turned laterally and placed head down with the right side up; in this position, further air is prevented from entering the pulmonary circulation, and the air bubble can theoretically be aspirated with a central venous catheter placed in the right atrium.

Cardiac dysrhythmias have also been associated with laparoscopy. Carmichael reported three cases of marked bradycardia that occurred shortly after initiation of CO_2 insufflation.[127] He suggested that reflex vagal stimulation from stretching of the peritoneum accounted for the bradycardia. Two further cases of cardiac dysrhythmia, both ventricular in nature, were also reported; in these cases, ventilatory insufficiency was theorized to be responsible for the cardiac response. Scott and Julian reviewed 100 consecutive patients undergoing laparoscopy using CO_2 insufflation and compared them to 45 patients undergoing laparoscopy with nitrous oxide insufflation.[128] Among the patients undergoing CO_2 insufflation, 17% experienced cardiac arrhythmias compared with 4% of the nitrous oxide patients. The arrhythmias were characterized primarily by extrasystolic ventricular beats. In addition, the post-insufflation P_{CO_2} was significantly higher in the CO_2 insufflation patients versus the nitrous oxide patients; the authors attributed the higher incidence of arrhythmias in the CO_2 group to the hypercarbia.

ALTERNATE GASES FOR ESTABLISHING PNEUMOPERITONEUM

The ideal gas for peritoneal insufflation should be colorless, inert, unable to support combustion, easily absorbed from the peritoneal cavity, inexpensive, and readily available. Early laparoscopists used air to establish the pneumoperitoneum, but reports of air embolism and prolonged postoperative distention from persistent intraperitoneal air led some investigators to search for a more suitable gas for insufflation.

In 1933, Fevers used oxygen to insufflate the peritoneum of a patient undergoing laparoscopy.[129] He reported a dramatic explosion that resulted from combustion of the intraperitoneal oxygen during electrocautery. This report effectively eliminated the use of oxygen to obtain a pneumoperitoneum.

CO_2 satisfies the need for a colorless, noncombustible, inexpensive gas, and its ready absorption from the abdomen prevents prolonged peritoneal irritation and postoperative abdominal distention. However, the adverse cardiorespiratory effects resulting from absorption of CO_2 from the peritoneum have detracted from its appeal in some patients, and in other patients it has been associated with postoperative diaphragmatic irritation and shoulder pain.

Nitrous oxide pneumoperitoneum was historically used as an alternative to CO_2 because it avoids the sequelae of hypercarbia and acidemia seen with CO_2 pneumoperitoneum. El-Minawi and colleagues compared patients undergoing diagnostic laparoscopy with either CO_2 or nitrous oxide and concluded that the acid-base and cardiovascular consequences were greater with CO_2 than nitrous oxide pneumoperitoneum.[130] After insufflation, the CO_2 group showed significant changes in pH (decreased by 0.11 pH units), P_{CO_2} (increased by 12.5 mm Hg), and P_{O_2} (decreased by 43.9 mm Hg); in contrast, the changes in pH, P_{CO_2}, and P_{O_2} in the nitrous oxide group were insignificant. In contradistinction to CO_2 insufflation, which had no effect on cardiac output,[69] nitrous oxide insufflation reduced cardiac output by an average of 25%.[131] The decreased cardiac output seen with nitrous oxide compared to CO_2 insufflation may reflect the absence of hypercarbia-induced stimulation; in CO_2 pneumoperitoneum, this effect offsets the reduction in cardiac output resulting from increased intra-abdominal pressure. In addition to fewer adverse cardiorespiratory effects resulting from nitrous oxide pneumoperitoneum compared with CO_2 pneumoperitoneum, nitrous oxide has been shown to be associated with less peritoneal irritation during insufflation.[132,133]

Despite the advantages of nitrous oxide pneumoperitoneum, nitrous oxide at high concentrations supports combustion, and thus, its use is limited to diagnostic laparoscopy in which cautery is not needed.[134] Moreover, Ooka and colleagues suggested that absorption of nitrous oxide from the peritoneum interferes with oxygen exchange in the lungs.[135] They evaluated 12 patients undergoing laparoscopic cholecystectomy with either CO_2 or nitrous oxide insufflation. Although P_{CO_2} increased after insufflation only in the CO_2 group, P_{O_2} decreased by 25 mm Hg in the nitrous oxide group compared to 13 mm Hg in the CO_2 group. This is in contradistinction to the work of El-Minawi and colleagues who showed a decrease in P_{O_2} after insufflation with both nitrous oxide and CO_2,[130] although the difference reached statistical significance only in the CO_2 group.

The preferred alternatives to CO_2 insufflation in high-risk pulmonary or cardiac patients are helium or argon. Both are inert, inexpensive, and noncombustible. Leighton and colleagues compared hemodynamic parameters in eight anesthetized, ventilated pigs undergoing sequential insufflation with helium and then with CO_2.[136] Significant hypercarbia occurred within 30 minutes of CO_2 insufflation; in contrast, helium insufflation was not associated with hypercarbia. Likewise, CO_2 pneumoperitoneum was associated with acidemia at all study points, whereas pH changes were not significant during helium pneumoperitoneum. Pulmonary hypertension developed as a result of hypercarbia in the CO_2 group; pulmonary artery pressures were unchanged in the helium group.

Further studies by Leighton and colleagues in a pig model showed that the use of helium insufflation prevented the physiologic consequences of hypercarbia.[137] Moreover, the volume of helium in exhaled gas was minimal (0.2%) and constituted no threat to alveolar oxygen exchange.

A clinical drawback to helium or argon as insufflant is that they are not as readily diffusible as CO_2, which can result in prolonged subcutaneous emphysema and gas retention in the peritoneum or pleural space. In addition, cost favors the use of CO_2 for insufflation.

EXTRAPERITONEOSCOPY

Absorption of CO_2 and subsequent hypercarbia appear to be greater when an extraperitoneal/retroperitoneal laparoscopic approach is used, as compared to an intraperitoneal approach. This is especially true in the presence of subcutaneous emphysema.[138] In a study by Mullet and colleagues, a group of patients undergoing pelvic laparoscopy via an extraperitoneal approach ($n = 10$) was compared to two groups of patients (10 each) undergoing transperitoneal laparoscopy (laparoscopic cholecystectomy and gynecologic laparoscopy).[62] In all groups, an increase in CO_2 excretion was observed during insufflation. The increase in CO_2 excretion was significantly greater in the extraperitoneal group (71%) than in either of the transperitoneal groups (12% for the gynecologic laparoscopy group and 25% for the laparoscopic cholecystectomy group) despite a duration of insufflation (45 minutes) that was comparable to the gynecologic laparoscopy group (43 minutes) and a third as long as the pelvic laparoscopy group (125 minutes). Wolf and colleagues also found an association between increased CO_2 excretion and the extraperitoneal approach.[139] They reviewed 59 patients undergoing laparoscopic renal surgery in whom CO_2 excretion was measured before and after insufflation; 32% of patients were approached extraperitoneally, whereas 68% underwent transperitoneal laparoscopy. The increase in CO_2 excretion (from baseline to maximum excretion after insufflation) was significantly greater in the extraperitoneal group (4.7 mL/min) compared to the transperitoneal group (2.4 mL/min). Nevertheless, any adverse sequelae of hypercarbia are routinely managed with an appropriate ventilatory strategy (hyperventilation).

The physiologic effects of pneumoretroperitoneum on the kidney and vascular system are similar to transperitoneal laparoscopy (see Table 45-1),[138] but the rapidity of renal vein flow reduction, oliguria, elevation of mean arterial pressure, and decrease in venous pressure are less pronounced than with pneumoperitoneum.

LOW-PRESSURE AND GASLESS LAPAROSCOPY

Regardless of the gas used, insufflation of the peritoneal cavity can be associated with significant adverse effects from increased intra-abdominal pressure and/or absorption of insufflant. To avoid these problems, a number of investigators have examined the use of low-pressure pneumoperitoneum and gasless laparoscopy. Banting and colleagues developed an abdominal lift device that suspends the abdominal wall, thereby reducing the intra-abdominal pressure needed to create a working space.[140] A 10 to 12 mm Hg pneumoperitoneum was established, and the lift device was employed under endoscopic vision. An external hook and chain assembly secured to the side of the table was used to provide traction to suspend the anterior abdominal wall. They used this device in eight patients with cardiopulmonary disease; with use of the abdominal wall lift, a working pneumoperitoneum of only 6 to 8 mm Hg was sufficient to perform cholecystectomy.

Araki and colleagues used a similar device in 151 patients undergoing laparoscopic cholecystectomy.[141] A low-pressure pneumoperitoneum (4 mm Hg) was established to allow placement of the abdominal wall retractor. In 121 patients, the abdomen was desufflated after the gallbladder was identified; in 30 obese patients, the pneumoperitoneum was maintained until the cystic duct and artery were secured. No adverse effects were attributable to the abdominal wall-lift device. End-tidal CO_2 was recorded before pneumoperitoneum, during pneumoperitoneum, and after desufflation; end-tidal CO_2 varied from 29, to 35, to 30 mm Hg, respectively, which is less than the 10 mm Hg increase reported by Hodgson and colleagues during CO_2 pneumoperitoneum at 15 to 20 mm Hg.[55]

Kitano and colleagues prospectively randomized 83 patients with symptomatic gallstones to laparoscopic cholecystectomy using either traditional CO_2 pneumoperitoneum or a U-shaped abdominal lift retractor.[142] The laparoscopic procedure was completed in 88% of patients in the pneumoperitoneum group and in 100% of patients in the abdominal wall retractor group. When the gallbladder was severely fibrotic, the success rate was higher in the retractor group (100% of six patients) compared with the pneumoperitoneum group (12% of six patients). The authors concluded that the abdominal lift device was safer and more efficacious than traditional pneumoperitoneum for laparoscopic cholecystectomy.

Gasless laparoscopy has become easier with the development of commercial abdominal retractors/elevators secured to the side of the operating table (eg, Laparolift, Origin Medsystems, Menlo Park, CA). As in the studies noted above, all abdominal lift devices mechanically elevate the anterior abdominal wall away from the intra-abdominal organs, thereby creating a working space and eliminating the need for insufflation. Such instruments have been used for a variety of laparoscopic procedures, including pelvic lymph node dissection,[143] repair of a traumatic gastric perforation,[144] herniorrhaphy,[145] cholecystectomy,[145] and appendectomy.[145] Smith and colleagues used the Laparolift device in 58 patients undergoing elective (31) or trauma-related (27) procedures.[146] Of the elective procedures (cholecystectomy, appendectomy, and diagnostic procedures), exposure was judged by the operating surgeon to be equivalent to the pneumoperitoneum in 97% of the cases. Among 26 attempted cholecystectomies, 21 were completed via the gasless technique; conversion to a pneumoperitoneum in four cases resulted in success in two, whereas two required open cholecystectomy. One patient underwent minilaparotomy for repair of a small bowel injury and completion of the cholecystectomy. Three complications occurred in the Laparolift elective surgery group: two superficial wound infections at the Laparolift insertion site and one enterotomy. Postoperative pain was not objectively quantified, but several Laparolift patients noted abdominal wall discomfort that was believed to be a result of abdominal wall retraction. Hospital stay was comparable among patients undergoing gasless and pneumoperitoneum laparoscopic cholecystectomy (2.0 vs. 2.1 days).

CONCLUSION

The vast majority of laparoscopic procedures can be safely performed with a CO_2 pneumoperitoneum. The physiologic consequences of increased intra-abdominal pressure and absorption of CO_2 from the peritoneum are generally well-tolerated in the healthy individual on controlled ventilation. During retroperitoneoscopy the risks associated with CO_2 absorption are comparable, if not higher, than the conventional transperitoneal approach. Because of the problems of hypercarbia with either approach, alternative gases such as helium should be considered in debilitated patients with cardiopulmonary compromise. Finally, as an alternative, especially in the high-risk patient or the patient at risk for increased intracranial pressure, gasless laparoscopy or low-pressure pneumoperitoneum may likewise provide comparable visibility and working space to the CO_2 pneumoperitoneum but without the associated adverse consequences.

REFERENCES

1. Dubois F, Icard P, Brethelot G, Levard H. Coelioscopic cholecystectomy: preliminary report of 36 cases. Ann Surg 1990;211:60–2.
2. Clayman RV, Kavoussi LR, Soper NJ, et al. Laparoscopic nephrectomy: initial case report. J Urol 1991;146:278–82.
3. Kelling G. Uber oesophagoskopie, gastroskopie und koelioskopie. Munch Med Wochenschr 1902;49:21–4.
4. Jacobaeus HC. Uber die moglichkeit die zystoskope bei untersuchung seroser hohlung anzuwenden. Munch Med Wochenschr 1910;57:2090–2.
5. Jacobaeus HC. Kurze ubersicht uber meine erfahrungen mit der laparo-thorakoskopie. Munch Med Wochenschr 1911;58:2017–9.
6. Orndoff RH. The peritoneoscope in diagnosis of diseases of the abdomen. J Radiol 1920;1:307–25.
7. Zollikofer R. Zur laparoskopie. Schweiz Med Wochenschr 1924;54:264–5.
8. Kashtan J, Green JF, Parsons EQ, Holcroft JW. Hemodynamic effects of increased abdominal pressure. J Surg Res 1981;30:249–55.
9. Ivankovich AD, Miletich DJ, Albrecht RF, et al. Cardiovascular effects of intraperitoneal insufflation with carbon dioxide and nitrous oxide in the dog. Anesthesiology 1975;42:281–7.
10. Diamant M, Benumof JL, Saidman LJ. Hemodynamics of increased intra-abdominal pressure: interaction with hypovolemia and halothane anesthesia. Anesthesiology 1978;48:23–7.
11. Richardson JD, Trinkle JK. Hemodynamic and respiratory alterations with increased intra-abdominal pressure. J Surg Res 1976;20:401–4.
12. O'Malley C, Cunningham AJ. Physiologic changes during laparoscopy. Anesthesiol Clin North America 2001;19:1–19.
13. Wallace DH, Serpell MG, Baxter JN, O'Dwyer PJ. Randomized trial of different insufflation pressures for laparoscopic cholecystectomy. Br J Surg 1997;84:455–8.
14. Dexter SP, Vucevic M, Gibson J, McMahon MJ. Hemodynamic consequences of high- and low-pressure capnoperitoneum during laparoscopic cholecystectomy. Surg Endosc 1999;13:376–81.
15. Neudecker J, Sauerland S, Neugebauer E, et al. The European Association for Endoscopic Surgery clinical practice guideline on the pneumoperitoneum for laparoscopic surgery. Surg Endosc 2002;16:1121–43.
16. Harman PK, Kron IL, McLachlan HD, et al. Elevated intra-abdominal pressure and renal function. Ann Surg 1982; 196:594–7.
17. Wolf JS Jr, Stoller ML. The physiology of laparoscopy: basic principles, complications and other considerations. J Urol 1994;152:294–302.
18. Thorington JM, Schmidt CF. A study of urinary output and blood-pressure changes resulting in experimental ascites. Am J Med Sci 1923;165:880–90.
19. Bradley SE, Bradley GP. The effect of increased intra-abdominal pressure on renal function in man. J Clin Invest 1947;26:1010–22.
20. Kirsch AJ, Hensle TW, Chang DT, et al. Renal effects of CO2 insufflation: oliguria and acute renal dysfunction in a rat pneumoperitoneum model. Urology 1994;43:453–9.
21. McDougall EM, Bennett HF, Monk TG, et al. Functional MR imaging of the porcine kidney: physiologic changes of prolonged pneumoperitoneum. JSLS 1997;1:29–35.
22. Micali S, Silver RI, Kaufman HS, et al. Measurement of urinary N-acetyl-beta-D-glucosaminidase to assess renal ischemia during laparoscopic operations. Surg Endosc 1999;13:503–6.
23. Richards WO, Scovill W, Shin B, Reed W. Acute renal failure associated with increased intra-abdominal pressure. Ann Surg 1983;197:183–7.
24. Fietsam R Jr, Villalba M, Glover JL, Clark K. Intra-abdominal compartment syndrome as a complication of ruptured abdominal aortic aneurysm repair. Am Surg 1989;55: 396–402.
25. Chiu AW, Azadzoi KM, Hatzichristou DG, et al. Effects of intra-abdominal pressure on renal tissue perfusion during laparoscopy. J Endourol 1994;8:99–103.
26. McDougall EM, Monk TG, Wolf JS Jr, et al. The effect of prolonged pneumoperitoneum on renal function in an animal model. J Am Coll Surg 1996;182:317–28.
27. Kerbl K, Clayman RV, McDougall EM, Kavoussi LR. Laparoscopic nephrectomy: the Washington University experience. Br J Urol 1994;73:231–6.
28. Chang DT, Kirsch AJ, Sawczuk IS. Oliguria during laparoscopic surgery. J Endourol 1994;8:349–52.
29. Melville RJ, Frizis HI, Forsling ML, LeQuesne LP. The stimulus for vasopressin release during laparoscopy. Surg Gynecol Obstet 1985;161:253–6.
30. Solis Herruzo JAJ, Castellano G, Larrodera L, et al. Plasma arginine vasopressin concentration during laparoscopy. Hepatogastroenterology 1989;36:499–503.
31. Chiu AW, Chang LS, Birkett DH, Babayan RK. The impact of pneumoperitoneum, pneumoretroperitoneum, and gasless laparoscopy on the systemic and renal hemodynamics. J Am Coll Surg 1995;181:397–406.
32. Koivusalo AM, Kellokumpu I, Ristkari S, Lindgren L. Splanchnic and renal deterioration during and after laparoscopic cholecystectomy: a comparison of the carbon dioxide pneumoperitoneum and the abdominal wall lift method. Anesth Analg 1997;85:886–91.

33. Caldwell CB, Ricotta JJ. Changes in visceral blood flow with elevated intraabdominal pressure. J Surg Res 1987;43: 14–20.
34. Hashikura Y, Kawasaki S, Munakata Y, et al. Effects of peritoneal insufflation on hepatic and renal blood flow. Surg Endosc 1994;8:759–61.
35. Evasovich MR, Clark TC, Horattas MC, et al. Does pneumoperitoneum during laparoscopy increase bacterial translocation? Surg Endosc 1996;10:1176–9.
36. Josephs LG, Este-McDonald JR, Birkett DH, Hirsch EF. Diagnostic laparoscopy increases intracranial pressure. J Trauma 1994;36:815–8.
37. Rosenthal RJ, Hiatt JR, Phillips EH, et al. Intracranial pressure. Effects of pneumoperitoneum in a large-animal model. Surg Endosc 1997;11:376–80.
38. Este-McDonald JR, Josephs LG, Birkett DH, Hirsch EF. Changes in intracranial pressure associated with apneumic retractors. Arch Surg 1995;130:362–5.
39. Moncure M, Salem R, Moncure K, et al. Central nervous system metabolic and physiologic effects of laparoscopy. Am Surg 1999;65:168–72.
40. Halverson A, Buchanan R, Jacobs L, et al. Evaluation of mechanism of increased intracranial pressure with insufflation. Surg Endosc 1998;12:266–9.
41. Irgau I, Koyfman Y, Tikellis JI. Elective intraoperative intracranial pressure monitoring during laparoscopic cholecystectomy. Arch Surg 1995;130:1011–3.
42. Fujii Y, Tanaka H, Tsuruoka S, et al. Middle cerebral arterial blood flow velocity increases during laparoscopic cholecystectomy. Anesth Analg 1994;78:80–3.
43. Abe K, Hashimoto N, Taniguchi A, Yoshiya I. Middle cerebral artery blood flow velocity during laparoscopic surgery in head-down position. Surg Laparosc Endosc 1998;8:1–4.
44. Schob OM, Allen DC, Benzel E, et al. A comparison of the pathophysiologic effects of carbon dioxide, nitrous oxide, and helium pneumoperitoneum on intracranial pressure. Am J Surg 1996;172:248–53.
45. Halverson AL, Barrett WL, Iglesias AR, et al. Decreased cerebrospinal fluid absorption during abdominal insufflation. Surg Endosc 1999;13:797–800.
46. Ben-Haim M, Rosenthal RJ. Causes of arterial hypertension and splachnic ischemia during acute elevations in intra-abdominal pressure with CO2 pneumoperitoneum: a complex central nervous system mediated response. Int J Colorectal Dis 1999;14:227–36.
47. Rosin D, Brasesco O, Varela J, et al. Low-pressure laparoscopy may ameliorate intracranial hypertension and renal hypoperfusion. J Laparoendosc Adv Surg Tech A 2002; 12:15–19.
48. Odeberg-Wernerman S. Laparoscopic surgery—effects on circulatory and respiratory physiology: an overview. Eur J Surg Suppl 2000;585:4–11.
49. Safran DB, Orlando R 3rd. Physiologic effects of pneumoperitoneum. Am J Surg 1994;167:281–6.
50. Motew M, Ivankovich AD, Bieniarz J, et al. Cardiovascular effects and acid-base and blood gas changes during laparoscopy. Am J Obstet Gynecol 1973;115:1002–12.
51. Alexander GD, Noe FD, Brown EM. Anesthesia for pelvic laparoscopy. Anesth Analg 1969;48:14–8.
52. Guyton AC, editor. Textbook of Medical Physiology. Philadelphia: W. B. Saunders Company; 1981.
53. Price HL. Effects of carbon dioxide on the cardiovascular system. Anesthesiology 1960;21:652–63.
54. Cullen DJ, Eger EI. Cardiovascular effects of carbon dioxide in man. Anesthesiology 1974;41:345–59.
55. Hodgson C, McClelland RMA, Newton JR. Some effects of the peritoneal insufflation of carbon dioxide at laparoscopy. Anaesthesia 1970;25:382–90.
56. Desmond J, Gordon RA. Ventilation in patients anaesthetized for laparoscopy. Can Anaesth Soc J 1970;17:378–87.
57. Baratz RA, Karis JH. Blood gas studies during laparoscopy under general anesthesia. Anesthesiology 1969;30:463–4.
58. Alexander GD, Brown EM. Physiologic alterations during pelvic laparoscopy. Am J Obstet Gynecol 1969;105: 1078–81.
59. Seed RF, Shakespeare TF, Muldoon MJ. Carbon dioxide homeostasis during anaesthesia for laparoscopy. Anaesthesia 1970;25:223–31.
60. Montalva M, Das B. Carbon dioxide homeostasis during laparoscopy. South Med J 1976;69:602–3.
61. Tan PL, Lee TL, Tweed WA. Carbon dioxide and gas exchange during pelvic laparoscopy. Can J Anaesth 1992;39:677–81.
62. Mullet CE, Viale JP, Sagnard PE, et al. Pulmonary CO2 elimination during surgical procedures using intra- or extraperitoneal CO2 insufflation. Anesth Analg 1993; 76:622–6.
63. Lister DR, Rudston-Brown B, Warriner CB, et al. Carbon dioxide absorption is not linearly related to intraperitoneal carbon dioxide insufflation pressure in pigs. Anesthesiology 1994;80:129–36.
64. Farhi LE, Rahn H. Dynamics of changes in carbon dioxide stores. Anesthesiology 1960;21:604–14.
65. Fowle ASE, Campbell EJM. The immediate carbon dioxide storage capacity of man. Clin Sci 1964;27:41.
66. Wittgen CM, Andrus CH, Fitzgerald SD, et al. Analysis of hemodynamic and ventilatory effects of laparoscopic cholecystectomy. Arch Surg 1991;126:997–1001.
67. Koivusalo AM, Lindgren L. Respiratory mechanics during laparoscopic cholecystectomy. Anesth Analg 1999;89:800.
68. Liu S, Leighton T, Davis I, et al. Prospective analysis of cardiopulmonary responses to laparoscopic cholecystectomy. J Laparoendosc Surg 1991;1:241–6.
69. Marshall RL, Jebson PJR, Davie IT, Scott DB. Circulatory effects of carbon dioxide insufflation of the peritoneal cavity for laparoscopy. Br J Anaesth 1972;44:680–4.
70. Kubota K, Kajiura N, Teruya M, et al. Alterations in respiratory function and hemodynamics during laparoscopic cholecystectomy under pneumoperitoneum. Surg Endosc 1993;7:500–4.
71. Lenz RJ, Thomas TA, Wilkins DG. Cardiovascular changes during laparoscopy. Anaesthesia 1976;31:4–12.
72. Westerband A, Van De Water JM, Amzallag M, et al. Cardiovascular changes during laparoscopic cholecystectomy. Surg Gynecol Obstet 1992;175:535–8.
73. Williams MD, Murr PC. Laparoscopic insufflation of the abdomen depresses cardiopulmonary function. Surg Endosc 1993;7:12–6.
74. Joris JL, Noirot DP, Legrand MJ, et al. Hemodynamic changes during laparoscopic cholecystectomy. Anesth Analg 1993;76:1067–71.
75. Kelman GR, Swapp GH, Smith I, et al. Cardiac output and arterial blood-gas tension during laparoscopy. Br J Anaesth 1972;44:1155–62.
76. Hirvonen EA, Nuutinen LS, Kauko M. Hemodynamic changes due to Trendelenburg positioning and pneumoperitoneum during laparoscopic hysterectomy. Acta Anaesthesiol Scand 1995;39:949–55.
77. Hirvonen EA, Poikolainen EO, Paakkonen ME, Nuutinen LS. The adverse hemodynamic effects of anesthesia, head-up tilt, and carbon dioxide pneumoperitoneum during laparoscopic cholecystectomy. Surg Endosc 2000;14:272–7.
78. Schwenk W, Bohm B, Fugener A, Muller JM. Intermittent pneumatic sequential compression (ISC) of the lower extremities prevents venous stasis during laparoscopic cholecystectomy. A prospective randomized study. Surg Endosc 1998;12:7–11.
79. Cruickshank AM, Fraser WD, Burns HJ, et al. Response of serum interleukin-6 in patients undergoing elective surgery of varying severity. Clin Sci (Lond) 1990;79:161–5.
80. Perlmutter DH, Dinarello CA, Punsal PI, Colten HR. Cachectin/tumor necrosis factor regulates hepatic acute-phase gene expression. J Clin Invest 1986;78:1349–54.
81. Pullicino EA , Carli F, Poole S, et al. The relationship between the circulating concentrations of interleukin 6 (IL-6), tumor necrosis factor (TNF) and the acute phase response to elective surgery and accidental injury. Lymphokine Res 1990;9:231–8.
82. Baumann H, Gauldie J. Regulation of hepatic acute phase plasma protein genes by hepatocyte stimulating factors and other mediators of inflammation. Mol Biol Med 1990;7:147–59.
83. Glaser F, Sannwald GA, Buhr HJ, et al. General stress response to conventional and laparoscopic cholecystectomy. Ann Surg 1995;221:372–80.
84. Cho JM, LaPorta AJ, Clark JR, et al. Response of serum cytokines in patients undergoing laparoscopic cholecystectomy. Surg Endosc 1994;8:1380–3.
85. Chaudhary D, Verma GR, Gupta R, et al. Comparative evaluation of the inflammatory mediators in patients undergoing laparoscopic versus conventional cholecystectomy. Aust N Z J Surg 1999;69:369–72.
86. Joris J, Cigarini I, Legrand M, et al. Metabolic and respiratory changes after cholecystectomy performed via laparotomy or laparoscopy. Br J Anaesth 1992;69:341–5.
87. Maruszynski M, Pojda Z. Interleukin 6 (IL-6) levels in the monitoring of surgical trauma. A comparison of serum IL-6 concentrations in patients treated by cholecystectomy via laparotomy or laparoscopy. Surg Endosc 1995; 9:882–5.
88. Harmon GD, Senagore AJ, Kilbride MJ, Warzynski MJ. Interleukin-6 response to laparoscopic and open colectomy. Dis Colon Rectum 1994;37:754–9.
89. Leung KL, Lai PB, Ho RL, et al. Systemic cytokine response after laparoscopic-assisted resection of rectosigmoid carcinoma: a prospective randomized trial. Ann Surg 2000; 231:506–11.
90. Stage JG, Schulze S, Moller P, et al. Prospective randomized study of laparoscopic versus open colonic resection for adenocarcinoma. Br J Surg 1997;84:391–6.
91. Zieren J, Jacobi CA, Wenger FA, et al. Fundoplication: a model for immunologic aspects of laparoscopic and conventional surgery. J Laparoendosc Adv Surg Tech A 2000;10:35–40.
92. Perttila J, Salo M, Ovaska J, et al. Immune response after laparoscopic and conventional Nissen fundoplication. Eur J Surg 1999;165:21–8.
93. Hill AD, Banwell PE, Darzi A, et al. Inflammatory markers following laparoscopic and open hernia repair. Surg Endosc 1995;9:695–8.
94. Roumen RM, van Meurs PA, Kuypers HH, et al. Serum interleukin-6 and C reactive protein responses in patients after laparoscopic or conventional cholecystectomy. Eur J Surg 1992;158:541–4.
95. Yoshida S, Ohta J, Yamasaki K, et al. Effect of surgical stress on endogenous morphine and cytokine levels in the plasma after laparoscopoic or open cholecystectomy. Surg Endosc 2000;14:137–40.
96. Watson RW, Redmond HP, McCarthy J, et al. Exposure of the peritoneal cavity to air regulates early inflammatory responses to surgery in a murine model. Br J Surg 1995; 82:1060–5.
97. McMahon AJ, O'Dwyer PJ, Cruikshank AM, et al. Comparison of metabolic responses to laparoscopic and minilaparotomy cholecystectomy. Br J Surg 1993;80:1255–8.
98. Chekan EG, Nataraj C, Clary EM, et al. Intraperitoneal immunity and pneumoperitoneum. Surg Endosc 1999;13:1135–8.
99. Sandoval BA, Robinson AV, Sulaiman TT, et al. Open versus laparoscopic surgery: a comparison of natural antitumoral cellular immunity in a small animal model. Am Surg 1996;62:625–30.
100. West MA, Baker J, Bellingham J. Kinetics of decreased LPS-stimulated cytokine release by macrophages exposed to CO2. J Surg Res 1996;63:269–74.
101. West MA, Hackam DJ, Baker J, et al. Mechanism of decreased in vitro murine macrophage cytokine release after exposure to carbon dioxide: relevance to laparoscopic surgery. Ann Surg 1997;226:179–90.
102. Puttick MI, Scott-Coombes DM, Dye J, et al. Comparison of immunologic and physiologic effects of CO2 pneumoperitoneum at room and body temperatures. Surg Endosc 1999;13:572–5.
103. Karayiannakis AJ, Makri GG, Mantzioka A, et al. Systemic stress response after laparoscopic or open cholecystectomy: a randomized trial. Br J Surg 1997;84:467–71.
104. Le Blanc-Louvry I, Coquerel A, Koning E, et al. Operative stress response is reduced after laparoscopic compared to open cholecystectomy: the relationship with postoperative pain and ileus. Dig Dis Sci 2000;45:1703–13.
105. Hendolin HI , Paakonen ME, Alhava EM, et al. Laparoscopic or open cholecystectomy: a prospective randomised trial to compare postoperative pain, pulmonary function, and stress response. Eur J Surg 2000;166:394–9.
106. Kent RB. Subcutaneous emphysema and hypercarbia following laparoscopic cholecystectomy. Arch Surg 1991; 126:1154–6.
107. Sosa RE, Weingram J, Stein B, et al. Hypercarbia in laparoscopic pelvic lymph node dissection. J Urol 1992;147: 246A.
108. Hall D, Goldstein A, Tynan E, Braunstein L. Profound hypercarbia late in the course of laparoscopic cholecystectomy: detection by continuous capnometry. Anesthesiology 1993;79:173–4.
109. Wolf JS Jr, Clayman RV, Monk TG, et al. Carbon dioxide absorption during laparoscopic pelvic surgery. J Am Coll Surg 1995;180:555–60.
110. Sivak BJ. Surgical emphysema: report of a case and review. Anesth Analg 1964;43:415–7.
111. Knos GB, Sung Y, Toledo A. J Clin Anesth 1991;3:56–9.
112. Nicholson RD, Berman ND. Chest 1979;76:605–7.
113. Herrerias JM, Ariza A, Garrido M. Endoscopy 1980;12: 254–5.
114. Pascual JB, Baranda MM, Tarrero MT, et al. Subcutaneous emphysema, pneumomediastinum, bilateral pneumothorax and pneumopericardium after laparoscopy. Endoscopy 1990;22:59.
115. Murray DP, Rankin RA, Lackey C. Bilateral pneumothoraces complicating peritoneoscopy. Gastrointest Endosc 1984;30:45–6.

116. Yacoub OF, Cardona I, Coveler LA, et al. Carbon dioxide embolism during laparoscopy. Anesthesiology 1982;57:533–5.

117. Root B, Levy MN, Pollack S, et al. Gas embolism death after laparoscopy delayed by "trapping" in portal circulation. Anesth Analg 1978;57:232–7.

118. Hynes SR, Marshall RL. Venous gas embolism during gynaecological laparoscopy. Can J Anaesth 1992;39:748–9.

119. Jernstrom P. Air embolism during peritoneoscopy. Am J Clin Pathol 1951;12:573–5.

120. Shulman B, Aronson HB. Capnography in the early diagnosis of carbon dioxide embolus during laparoscopy. Can Anaesth Soc J 1984;31:455–9.

121. Ostman PL, Pantle-Fisher FH, Faure EA, Glosten B. Circulatory collapse during laparoscopy. J Clin Anesth 1990;2:129–32.

122. Greville AC, Clements EA, Erwin DC. Pulmonary air embolism during laparoscopic laser cholecystectomy. Anesth Analg 1991;46:113–4.

123. O'Sullivan DC, Micali S, Averch TD, et al. Factors involved in gas embolism after laparoscopic injury to inferior vena cava. J Endourol 1998;12:149–54.

124. Couture P, Boudreault D, Derouin M, et al. Venous carbon dioxide embolism in pigs: an evaluation of end-tidal carbon dioxide, transesophageal echocardiography, pulmonary artery pressure, and precordial auscultation as monitoring modalities. Anesth Analg 1994;79:867–73.

125. Derouin M, Couture P, Boudreault D, et al. Detection of gas embolism by transesophageal echocardiography during laparoscopic cholecystectomy. Anesth Analg 1996;82:119–24.

126. Schmandra TC, Mierdl S, Bauer H, et al. Transoesophageal echocardiography shows high risk of gas embolism during laparoscopic hepatic resection under carbon dioxide pneumoperitoneum. Br J Surg 2002;89:870–6.

127. Carmichael DE. Laparoscopy—cardiac considerations. Fertil Steril 1971;22:69–70.

128. Scott DB, Julian DG. Observations on cardiac arrythmias during laparoscopy. BMJ 1972;1:411–3.

129. Fevers C. Laparoskopie mit dem cystoskop. Med Klin 1933;29:1042–5.

130. El-Minawi MF, Wahbi O, El-Bagouri IS, et al. Physiologic changes during CO2 and N2O pneumoperitoneum in diagnostic laparoscopy. J Reprod Med 1981;26:338–46.

131. Marshall RL, Jebson JR, Davie IT, Scott DB. Circulatory effects of peritoneal insufflation with nitrous oxide. Br J Anaesth 1972;44:1183–7.

132. Sharp JR, Pierson WP, Brady CEI. Comparison of CO2- and N2O induced discomfort during peritoneoscopy under local anesthesia. Gastroenterology 1982;82:453–6.

133. Minoli G, Terruzi V, Spinzi GC, et al. The influence of carbon dioxide and nitrous oxide on pain during laparoscopy: a double-blind, controlled trial. Gastrointest Endosc 1982;28:173–5.

134. El-Kady AA, Abd-El-Razek M. Intraperitoneal explosion during female sterilization by laparoscopic electrocoagulation. A case report. Int J Gynaecol Obstet 1976;14:487–8.

135. Ooka T, Kawano Y, Kosaka Y, Tanaka A. Blood gas changes during laparoscopic cholesystectomy-comparative study of N2O pneumoperitoneum and CO2 pneumoperitoneum. Japanese Journal Anesthesiology 1993;42:398–401.

136. Leighton TA, Bongard FS, Lie S-Y, et al. Comparative cardiopulmonary effects of helium and carbon dioxide pneumoperitoneum. Surg Forum 1991;42:485–7.

137. Leighton TA, Liu S-Y, Bongard FS. Comparative cardiopulmonary effects of carbon dioxide versus helium pneumoperitoneum. Surgery 1993;113:527–31.

138. Dunn MD, McDougall EM. Renal physiology. Laparoscopic considerations. Urol Clin North Am 2000;27:609–14.

139. Wolf JS Jr, Monk TG, McDougall EM, et al. The extraperitoneal approach and subcutaneous emphysema are associated with greater absorption of carbon dioxide during laparoscopic renal surgery. J Urol 1995;154:959–63.

140. Neuberger TJ, Andrus CH, Wittgen CM, et al. Prospective comparison of helium versus carbon dioxide pneumoperitoneum. Gastrointest Endosc 1994;40:P30.

141. Araki K, Namikawa K, Yamamoto H, et al. Abdominal wall retraction during laparoscopic cholecystectomy. World J Surg 1993;17:105–8.

142. Kitano S, Iso Y, Tomikawa M, et al. A prospective randomized trial comparing pneumoperitoneum and U-shaped retractor elevation for laparoscopic cholecystectomy. Surg Endosc 1993;7:311–4.

143. Etwaru D, Raboy A, Ferzli G, Albert P. Extraperitoneal endoscopic gasless pelvic lymph node dissection. J Laparoendosc Surg 1994;4:113–6.

144. Brams DM, Cardoza M, Smith RS. Laparoscopic repair of traumatic gastric perforation using a gasless technique. J Laparoendosc Surg 1993;3:587–91.

145. Newman LI, Ruben DM, Eubanks S. Laparoscopic herniorrhaphy without pneumoperitoneum. Surg Laparosc Endosc 1993;3:213–5.

146. Smith RS, Fry WR, Tsoi EK, et al. Gasless laparoscopy and conventional instruments. The next phase of minimally invasive surgery. Arch Surg 1993;128:1102–7.

147. Rosenthal RJ, Friedman RL, Kahn AM, et al. Reasons for intracranial hypertension and hemodynamic instability during acute elevations of intra-abdominal pressure: observations in a large animal model. J Gastrointest Surg 1998;2:415–25.

46

Obtaining Access: Pneumoperitoneum—Closed vs Open Techniques

Scott Troxel, MD

Sakti Das, MD

The invention of the incandescent light bulb was a significant building block in the development and advancement of laparoscopic instrumentation and techniques. In 1901, a Russian gynecologist by the name of Dimitri Ott was the first to report on ventroscopy, using a head mirror and speculum through a small anterior abdominal wall incision. Concurrently, Kelling described the use of a separate needle to establish pneumoperitoneum in the dog model. However, it was not until 1918 that the first automatic insufflation needle was developed by Goetze, only to be refined by Veress in 1938—still the most widely used device for creating pneumoperitoneum. As the optics, instrumentation, and automatic insufflation control systems improved through the 1970s and 1980s, the focus of laparoscopy changed from primarily a diagnostic tool to an interventional technique. Over the past 15 years, laparoscopic applications have exploded, from the first laparoscopic cholecystectomy to the current use of robotics and telemedicine. Currently, both hand-assisted and pure laparoscopy are standard elements of resident training, and with this, safe initial access is the key to success.

PNEUMOPERITONEUM: CLOSED TECHNIQUE

VERESS NEEDLE The basic Veress needle has remained unchanged since the initial invention in 1938. It consists of a blunt-tipped, spring-loaded, inner stylet surrounded by a sharp outer needle. During placement, the resistance of the abdominal wall pushes the inner stylet within the outer needle, allowing the sharp outer needle to work its way through the layers of the abdominal wall. Once the sharp needle has entered the peritoneal cavity, the loss of resistance on the inner stylet allows it to extend forward and protect the abdominal contents from the sharp needle. On the majority of prototypes, there is some form of color-coded system that instructs the surgeon as to whether the blunt-tipped inner stylet is extended or retracted, an important addition that helps both with safety and in determining proper placement within the peritoneal cavity.

The Veress needle comes in both disposable and reusable forms. Both are routinely used, although some surgeons prefer the reusable form as it assures a sharp needle for each use. The standard dimensions are 14 gauge by 120 mm or 150 mm in length. However, both 100 mm and 200 mm lengths are also available. At the distal end of the needle, a stopcock allows connection to the insufflation tubing. The proximal end of the inner stylet has a lateral hole that allows for insufflation. The space between the inner stylet and outer needle is minimal, preventing back leakage.

VERESS NEEDLE INSUFFLATION Following assessment of the abdomen for surgical scars and organomegaly, the site of initial trocar placement is chosen. Traditionally, this has been the umbilicus, both for aesthetic reasons as well as the technical advantage of access through the linea alba, where the parietal peritoneum is most adherent. Because of the presence of small bowel and the division of the great vessels at this level, the possibility of vascular or bowel injury is a concern. As an alternative, percutaneous access in the right or left subcostal midclavicular line or lateral to the rectus muscle on either side of the umbilicus are also widely used. Proponents of the subcostal midclavicular line approach feel that the rib cage acts as a fixation point for the fascia and underlying peritoneum, decreasing the risk of organ injury. Furthermore, the risk of bowel adhesions to the liver or spleen is low, and the risk of inadvertent needle puncture to either of these organs is insignificant, requiring no further intervention.[1] The authors feel that any of the above sites of initial entry are safe, and that the site selected should be chosen according to the planned trocar pattern for the selected case. More important than the initial site of access chosen, is having a thorough understanding of the underlying anatomy prior to percutaneous access.

A No. 15 or No. 11 scalpel blade is used to make a curvilinear 5 to 10 mm incision in the umbilical skin, depending on the port size to be placed. The location within the umbilicus (inferior, superior, lateral) is chosen according to procedure to be performed. Remember that there is less preperitoneal fat in this location, and an aggressive skin incision may result in unplanned entry into the peritoneum. Following the skin incision, a blunt-tipped clamp is helpful to clear away the subcutaneous fat and expose the linea alba. There is some dispute regarding the benefit, prior to needle placement, of outward traction on the abdominal wall, either by pinching the abdominal wall with the nondominant hand, placing towel clamps through the skin, or by using Kocher clamps in the fascia, etc. Some feel that this provides counter traction for the Veress needle as well as lifting the peritoneum away from the abdominal contents. Others feel that the peritoneum is independent of the abdominal wall, resulting in an increased distance between the linea alba and the peritoneum, making percutaneous access more difficult.[2] The authors prefer to use upward traction to aid in piercing the external oblique fascia, but then relaxing to enter the peritoneum.

The Veress needle should be held firmly in the dominant hand like a dart, making sure that the built in color-coded safety mechanism functions properly. Whether needle placement is done freehand or with the ulnar border of the hand resting on the patient is up to the surgeon's preference. The abdominal wall is retracted upward with the nondominant hand, and the needle is inserted with steady constant pressure with the tip aimed away from the great vessels. In general, the needle should be advanced at a 45° angle. Acute angulation of the needle often results in scything of the peritoneum and ultimate preperitoneal placement. One should feel two areas of resistance through the abdominal wall, one as the needle traverses the linea alba or the external fascia, and the second as it traverses the peritoneum. Depending on the direction of the needle placement, Trendelenburg or reverse Trendelenburg positioning may help minimize the risk of bowel injury.

Prior to initiating insufflation, there are several steps to help determine proper positioning of the needle within the peritoneal cavity. Initial return of blood, intestinal contents, or urine indicates improper positioning and appropriate measures should be taken. A 10 cc syringe partially filled with saline is then attached to the stopcock. The initial maneuver is to aspirate and should result in air return within the syringe. Next, the syringe is removed leaving a small water droplet on the stopcock. Lifting on the abdominal wall should generate negative pressure on the droplet, pulling it into the peritoneal cavity. Only when proper needle placement is established should the insufflation tubing be connected and low flow of carbon dioxide (CO_2) initiated. Initial intraabdominal pressures should be less than 10 mm Hg, and flow through the needle unobstructed. An obstructed gas flow pattern or high opening pressures indicate improper needle placement, most commonly encountered during preperitoneal or omental insufflation. After the instillation of 1 L with maintenance of low pressure, high flow can be established. Insufflation at 1 to 3 L/min is recommended, and the average adult patient requires 4 to 6 L to establish an intraperitoneal pressure of 12 to 15 mm Hg.

TROCAR INSERTION As with Veress needle insertion, the initial trocar placement is blind. A thorough understanding of the working mechanism of the trocar is therefore necessary to avoid injury to vasculature or bowel. The majority of trocar systems have an inner blade protected by an outer sheath. When properly loaded, the outer sheath will retract secondary to the resistance of the abdominal wall, then reposition over the blade once the trocar has entered the peritoneal cavity. Assuring proper function of this mechanism and proper loading prior to placement is imperative to avoid injury to the intra-abdominal contents.

For initial trocar placement, the intra-abdominal pressure should be set at a minimum of 16 mm Hg. This will maximally expand the peritoneal cavity to create the greatest distance between the abdominal wall and the peritoneal contents, as well as provide adequate outward pressure on the abdominal wall to facilitate percutaneous puncture. Reich and colleagues reported on 3,041 procedures in which the intraperitoneal pressure was set at 25 to 30 mm Hg for initial trocar insertion. They had no vascular injuries, two bowel injuries and no complications related to the elevated intra-abdominal pressure.[3] Prior to insertion of the trocar, make sure that the skin incision is of adequate length to accept passage of the trocar. The trocar should be held in the dominant hand with the butt end positioned within the palm, and the index finger extended. The extended finger will act as a stop-gap, preventing overzealous advancement of the trocar. The trocar is then advanced through the abdominal wall with steady constant pressure in a twisting motion until the peritoneal cavity is entered and the outer sheath locks forward into place. The inner sheath is then removed and immediate placement of the laparoscope evaluates for bowel or vascular injury. Following placement of the initial trocar, the remaining trocars are placed, viewed directly with the laparoscope. Once all trocars are in position, the intra-abdominal pressure is reduced to 12 to 14 mm Hg.

RADIALLY EXPANDING TROCAR SYSTEM An alternative closed access and trocar system is the radially expanding trocar system. It also requires use of the Veress needle to establish pneumoperitoneum, but when the needle is removed, it is back-loaded with an expandable mesh sleeve trocar (Step, Innerdyne, Sunnyvale, CA) and reinserted as before. The Veress needle is then removed, leaving the mesh sleeve in place. The mesh sleeve can then be dilated to the desired size by using the nondominant hand to support the sleeve and the dominant hand to advance a blunt-tipped fascial dilator back-loaded with a laparoscopic port. The mesh sleeve can be initially expanded to 5 mm, 10 mm, or 12 mm, and can also be converted to any size during the case. A modified open (or "drop-in" technique) is also described. After the appropriately sized skin incision, the subcutaneous fat is cleared down to the external oblique fascia, and a small opening large enough for the mesh sleeve is made in the fascia as well as the peritoneum. The mesh sleeve is placed, and the dilation process is the same as described above. The main advantage of this modified open technique is that the fascial incision remains the diameter of the trocar placed, preventing leakage of CO_2 during the case. Shekarriz and colleagues reported on 62 cases using the Step system, including 24 with previous abdominal surgery.[1] There were no complications secondary to placement or dilation of the mesh sleeve. The fascia was not closed at any port site, and they reported no port site hernias at 12-month follow-up. Galen and colleagues reported on 212 women who had a total of 541 radially expanding ports placed.[4] There were no significant vascular or intestinal injuries, abdominal wall hematomas or port site hernias. One patient developed a postoperative mesenteric hematoma felt to be related to initial Veress needle placement. The Step system has clearly been shown to be a safe alternative to the more conventional trocar systems. The main advantages are the ability to easily change trocar diameter during the case and the time saved in avoiding closure of the fascia. Autosuture also makes a radially expanding trocar system called the VersaStep Plus (Autosuture, Norwalk, CT), which combines the radially expanding sheath and the VersaSeal Plus universal seal. The VersaSeal Plus allows multiple instrument changes without losing the CO_2 tight seal and accepts 5 to 12 mm instruments.

VISUALIZING TROCAR SYSTEMS An alternative technique for safe peritoneal access is the visualizing trocar. Two such systems are the Optiview (Ethicon Endo-Surgery, Cincinnati, OH) and the Ternamian EndoTip system (Karl Storz Endoscopy, Tuttlingen, Germany). As the name implies, the first system allows the surgeon to visualize the tip of the trocar as it traverses the abdominal wall, providing a more controlled access. The Optiview is a hollow trocar with a clear plastic conical tip that has two external ridges. A 10 mm camera is placed within the trocar, and the whole assembly is passed through the abdominal wall to enter the peritoneal cavity under direct vision. Marcovich and colleagues retrospectively compared the Optiview visualizing trocar to Veress needle access.[5] They evaluated 100 consecutive transperitoneal cases in which the Veress needle was used as initial access in 96 cases and the Optiview used after Veress needle failure in 22 cases and as initial access in four cases. Optiview access was successful in 25 of 26 cases with no complications. Veress needle access was successful in 72 of 96 cases (75%) with four minor complications. Jirecek and colleagues evaluated 546 cases using the optical tro-

car with no complications,[6] and String and colleagues evaluated 650 cases with one bowel injury, including 25 cases in which the Optiview was placed through a previous trocar site.[7]

The Ternamian EndoTIP has an external spiral edge down the length of the trocar that engages and atraumatically spreads the tissue as it is advanced in a clockwise manner through the abdominal wall. A laparoscope lens is positioned within the trocar so that access can be accomplished under direct vision. Visualizing trocar systems are a safe and proven alternative to the Hasson open technique and avoid the problems with CO_2 leakage.

PNEUMOPERITONEUM: OPEN ACCESS

OPEN HASSON TECHNIQUE For patients that are obese, have had prior abdominal surgery, or have failed Veress needle access, the open technique is the preferred form of entry. The standard open approach is the Hasson cannula technique, first described in 1971.[8] After an initial 2 to 3 cm midline skin incision, the subcutaneous fat is cleared and stay sutures are placed in the fascia on either side of the midline. The fascia is then opened between the stay sutures, the preperitoneal fat cleared, and the peritoneum entered under direct vision. After palpating the peritoneal lining for the absence of adhesions, the Hasson trocar is positioned and the stay sutures secured to the port. An adjustable gasket acts as a seal to prevent CO_2 leak. There is no need to test for proper intraperitoneal placement so high-flow insufflation can begin immediately. There are both disposable and reusable versions of this system as well as various systems for anchoring and preventing CO_2 leakage.

The obvious advantage to the open Hasson technique is that access is obtained under direct vision, minimizing the risk of injury to vasculature or bowel. The potential disadvantages include poor esthetics, CO_2 leakage at the Hasson port site, and added time to obtain access. Several studies have attempted to evaluate the two forms of access with regard to safety. Mayol and colleagues retrospectively evaluated 203 patients undergoing Veress needle access vs 200 patients undergoing open Hasson cannula access.[9] They found that there were no injuries related to Veress needle placement, but that the closed technique did correlate with a higher complication rate. There was one aortic injury related to initial trocar placement, and six patients developed umbilical hernias compared to no vascular injuries or umbilical hernias in the open Hasson group. The Hasson technique, however, is not without risk, as several authors have reported both vascular and visceral injuries with this technique as well.[10] Furthermore, there have been numerous studies supporting the safety of closed access. Bonjer and colleagues retrospectively evaluated 489,335 closed access cases and found the incidence of visceral and vascular injuries to be 0.083 and 0.075%.[11] Arnott and Wilson reported no significant complications in over 1,400 Veress needle accesses,[12] and Florio and colleagues reported no vascular or bowel injuries during 2,126 Veress needle accesses.[13] While the risk of vascular injury does exist for closed access, the authors believe this risk to be minimal and it should not prevent one from using the Veress needle technique. The open Hasson technique is preferred for patients with prior laparoscopic or open surgery at the site of initial entry, but in standard cases, the route of access should be determined by the comfort level of the surgeon.

BLUNT TIP ACCESS   In order to maintain the theoretical advantages of open access, but avoid the issues of CO_2 leakage and added surgical time, modifications to the Hasson open technique have been developed. One such modification is the blunt-tipped trocar technique, of which there are two main descriptions. The TrocDoc trocar (Storz, Tuttlingen, Germany) was developed by removing the sharp tip of a 10/11 mm trocar and replacing it with a longer blunt tip (10 mm at the connection site, tapering to 5 mm at the tip). The balloon blunt-tip trocar (United States Surgical Corp., Norwalk CT) has a blunt tip with an inflatable balloon cuff that can be inflated and pulled up against the peritoneum for an airtight seal. A sponge collar on the extracorporeal side can then be tightened against the external abdominal wall to hold the intracorporeal balloon snug in place.

The procedure begins by making a 15- to 20-mm skin incision at the desired port location. After sweeping away the subcutaneous fat, the external oblique fascia is grasped with a pair of Kocher clamps. The abdominal wall is lifted anteriorly and a 6- to 8-mm vertical incision is made in the linea alba. Crile forceps are then used to bluntly puncture the peritoneum, and the peritoneal opening is probed for adhesions. The blunt-tipped trocar is then placed, and insufflation begun. The advantages over the Hasson technique are that there are no stay sutures to secure and the incision in the fascia and peritoneum is smaller, preventing CO_2 leakage. In a comparison to Veress needle and open Hasson techniques, Bemelman and colleagues and Bernik and colleagues both reported no CO_2 leakage and time to full insufflation to be statistically shorter for the blunt tip approach.[14,15] Bernik and colleagues have reported the largest series on blunt-tipped trocar insertion and had no vascular or bowel injuries and one port site hernia in their series of 118 patients. We have not used the blunt-tipped technique, but feel that it is a safe alternative to the open Hasson trocar.

ACCESS IN PEDIATRIC LAPAROSCOPY

The anteroposterior dimension of a child's abdomen is relatively narrow, raising the concern of potential injury during closed Veress needle and trocar insertion. We therefore routinely recommend open access technique during pediatric laparoscopy. Our initial access is at the umbilicus where a curvilinear skin incision is made inside the upper edge. There is a physiologic, hernia-like, small out-pouching of the parietal peritoneum at this position that can be held up with forceps and opened directly. A box stitch of 2-0 polyglycolic acid suture is loosely placed through the fascia and peritoneum. The trocar is inserted through the loop of the box stitch, which is then tied with a single knot to prevent CO_2 leakage. At the end of the procedure, the trocar is removed and the box stitch tied down, thereby allowing a rapid and efficient closure.

HAND-ASSISTED LAPAROSCOPY

The hand-port incision can be made either prior to or following insufflation of the peritoneal cavity. The advantage of making the hand-port incision initially is that one avoids the potential risk and added time of Veress needle placement. Urologists are comfortable with open entry to the abdominal cavity and can therefore accomplish peritoneal entry safely and relatively quickly. The advantage of prior insufflation with the Veress needle is the added safety and speed in which the hand-port incision can be made. The authors prefer to make the hand-port incision initially as we have found this to be more efficient. Once the peritoneal cavity is entered, the anterior abdominal wall and small bowel are checked for adhesions. Particular attention should be focused around the incision so that the hand-assist device can be seated safely. The authors then prefer to place the camera port prior to positioning of the hand-port and establishment of pneumoperitoneum. A folded lap pad is placed intracorporeally and positioned on top of the bowel underlying the chosen site for the trocar. After making the appropriately sized skin incision, the nondominant hand is placed intracorporeally to apply counter-traction on the abdominal wall while the dominant hand is used to place the trocar. Following proper positioning of this trocar, the hand-assist device is placed and pneumoperitoneum established. The remaining trocars are then placed under direct vision, again using an intracorporeal lap pad to protect the bowel.

CONCLUSION

For the majority of patients, initial Veress needle access is a safe and proven technique for the establishment of pneumoperitoneum with minimal risk of bowel or vascular injury. But in select patients, an open access is preferred, such as in patients with previous abdominal surgery, following failed closed access, and in the pediatric population. Critics of the routine use of open access will point to poor aesthetics, increased time to obtain access, and potential CO_2 leakage during the case. As a result, modifications to both the closed and open access instrumentation have been developed in an attempt to combine the advantages of both techniques, such as the radially expanding, and direct-vision, and blunt-tipped trocar systems. Currently there are numerous options for obtaining pneumoperitoneum, all of which have been shown to be safe and effective. It is truly the surgeon's preference as to which system is to be used.

REFERENCES

1. Shekarriz B, Gholami SS, Rudnick DM, et al. Radially expanding laparoscopic access for renal/adrenal surgery. Urology 2001;58:683–7.
2. Clayman RV, Griffith DP, Kavoussi LR. Laparoscopy: tips on technique. Contemp Urol 1991;3:23.
3. Reich H, Ribeiro SC, Rasmussen C, et al. High-pressure trocar insertion technique. JSLS 1999;3:45–8.
4. Galen DI, Jacobson A, Weckstein LN, et al. Reduction of cannula-related complications using a radially expanding access device. J Am Assoc Gynecol Laparosc 1999;6: 79–84.
5. Marcovich R, Del Terzo MA, Wolf JS Jr. Comparison of transperitoneal laparoscopic access techniques: Optiview visualizing trocar and Veress needle. J Endourol 2000;14:175–9.
6. Jirecek S, Drager M, Leitich H, et al. Direct visual or blind insertion of the primary trocar. Surg Endosc 2002;16:626–9.
7. String A, Berber E, Foroutani A, et al. Use of the optical access trocar for safe and rapid entry in various laparoscopic procedures. Surg Endosc 2001;15:570–3.
8. Hasson HM. A modified instrument and method for laparoscopy. Am J Obstet Gynecol 1971;110:886–7.
9. Mayol J, Garcia-Aguilar J, Ortiz-Oshiro E, et al. Risks of the minimal access approach for laparoscopic surgery: multivariate analysis of morbidity related to umbilical trocar insertion. World J Surg 1997;21:529–33.
10. Hanney RM, Carmalt HL, Merrett N, et al. Vascular injuries during laparoscopy associated with the Hasson technique. J Am Coll Surg 1999;188:337–8.
11. Bonjer HJ, Hazebrock EJ, Kazemier G, et al. Open versus closed establishment of pneumoperitoneum in laparoscopic surgery. Br J Surg 1997;84:599–602.
12. Arnot RS, Wilson T. Methods for achieving pneumoperitoneum at laparoscopy. J R Coll Surg Edinb 2001;46:68–9.
13. Florio G, Silvestro C, Polito DS. Periumbilical Veress needle pneumoperitoneum: technique and results in 2,126 cases. Chir Ital 2003;55:51–4.
14. Bemelman WA, Dunker MS, Busch ORC, et al. Efficacy of establishment of pneumoperitoneum with the Veress needle, Hasson trocar, and modified blunt trocar(TrocDoc): a randomized study. J Laparoendosc Adv Surg Tech A 2000;10:325–30.
15. Bernik TR, Trocciola SM, Mayer DA, et al. Balloon blunt-tip trocar for laparoscopic cholecystectomy: improvement over traditional Hasson and veress needle methods. J Laparoendosc Adv Surg Tech A 2001;11:73–8.

47

Pneumoretroperitoneum

Antonio Finelli, MD, MSc, FRCSC
Jihad H. Kaouk, MD

Unlike the peritoneal cavity, the retroperitoneum is a potential, rather than actual anatomic space. A retroperitoneal space needs to be created by mechanical means in order to provide adequate surgical exposure. Although Wickham[1] performed a ureterolithotomy using pneumoretroperitoneal insufflation and a standard laparoscope in 1979, it was not until Gaur[2] described an atraumatic balloon dilation technique to expand the retroperitoneum that retroperitoneoscopy became a viable laparoscopic approach. The retroperitoneal approach avoids the peritoneal cavity and minimizes handling of bowel during surgery. Although retroperitoneoscopy was described more than a decade ago and is now an accepted approach during laparoscopy, it is often avoided due to limited surgical space and subtle anatomical landmarks. However, the retroperitoneal approach is indispensable for morbidly obese patients or those with an extensive history of transperitoneal surgery.

SURGICAL ANATOMY

The lumbar retroperitoneal space is bounded anteromedially by the peritoneum, posterolaterally by the paraspinal and flank muscles, superiorly by the diaphragm, and joins the pelvic extraperitoneal space inferiorly.[3] Capelouto and coworkers showed that the anteroposterior dimension of the retroperitoneal space increases twofold when patients are repositioned from a supine to lateral decubitus position.[4] Moreover, the distance between the colon and the quadratus lumborum muscle increased by approximately threefold when changing from supine to the lateral decubitus position.[5] Likewise, the flank position results in anterior displacement of the lateral peritoneal reflection by the gravity-related traction exerted on the mesocolon.[3] Although the flank position results in increased retroperitoneal space, further development of the surgical field by mechanical means is necessary.

During retroperitoneoscopy, the posteroinferior aspect of Gerota's fascia and the lower pole of kidney are initially visualized and the orientation of the kidney is caudad to cephalad.[6] After retroperitoneal balloon dilation and port insertion, several surgical landmarks could be identified with the following frequencies: psoas muscle (100%), Gerota's fascia (100%), peritoneal reflection (83%), ureter (61%), renal artery pulsations (56%), aorta during left retroperitoneoscopy (50%), and inferior vena cava during right retroperitoneoscopy (25%).[7] The most important surgical landmark is the psoas muscle, which should be kept in a horizontal position to maintain orientation

PHYSIOLOGY

The physiologic consequences of laparoscopy are addressed in detail elsewhere in this text.[8]

RESPIRATORY The potential for developing hypercarbia exists during both transperitoneal and retroperitoneal CO_2 pneumo-insufflation. During retroperitoneoscopy, CO_2 is absorbed through preperitoneal adipose and connective tissue.[9] Although mild elevations in CO_2 are generally well-tolerated, patients with preexisting respiratory compromise should be monitored closely. Respiratory rate and tidal volume should be adjusted to rising end-tidal CO_2 values. If ventilatory maneuvers are insufficient, pneumoperitoneal pressures should be lowered while maintaining adequate working space to facilitate expeditious completion of the surgery. Although CO_2 absorption occurs with either transperitoneal or retroperitoneal laparoscopy, controversy exists as to which approach is associated with greater absorption.[10,11] A prospective comparison of CO_2 absorption during transperitoneal and retroperitoneal laparoscopic renal surgery concluded that there was no difference between the two approaches.[12] Regardless of the approach used, subcutaneous emphysema is a risk factor for hypercarbia. The risk of subcutaneous emphysema appears to be higher during retroperitoneal laparoscopy.[10,12] In order to minimize subcutaneous emphysema, the primary trocar should be airtight at the level of the lumbodorsal fascia before insufflation. The commercially available Bluntport (PDB, Origin Medsystems, Menlo Park, CA) is particularly advantageous in this regard. Regardless of the port used, the basic principles of a small port site incision and adequate port positioning to avoiding port displacement above the fascia should be adhered to. The minimal necessary insufflation pressure should be used. It was shown that a pressure ≤ 12 mm Hg was associated with significantly less episodes of subcutaneous emphysema as compared to pressures ≥ 15 mm Hg[13].

CARDIOVASCULAR AND RENAL Using a porcine model, Giebler and associates demonstrated that there were statistically significant differences in cardiovascular physiologic parameters when comparing transperitoneal to retroperitoneal CO_2 insufflation.[11] Specifically, there was a greater increase in cardiac output, pulmonary artery and central venous pressures during transperitoneal versus retroperitoneal laparoscopy for the same insufflation pressures.

Notably, intraperitoneal insufflation—in contrast to retroperitoneal insufflation—induced a marked inferior vena caval pressure gradient. Oliguria associated with laparoscopy however, is believed to be due to decreased renal blood flow and direct pressure on the renal parenchyma.[8] Although a limited area of aorta and inferior vena cava are exposed to pneumo-insufflation during retroperitoneoscopy, the renal effect of a pneumoretroperitoneum is similar to that seen with a pneumoperitoneum. An elevated retroperitoneal pressure may lead to oliguria, and when insufflation pressure is maintained for 2 hours, it can cause gradual decrease in contralateral kidney perfusion and a concomitant increase of the intra-abdominal pressure.[5] Oliguria is usually reversible with no renal pathologic consequences.

INDICATIONS/CONTRAINDICATIONS

Where laparoscopy is indicated, a retroperitoneal approach can be used for adrenalectomy, simple nephrectomy, radical nephrectomy, partial nephrectomy, donor nephrectomy, radical nephroureterectomy, renal cyst decortication, pyeloplasty, pyelolithotomy and ureterolithotomy. Morbid obesity, previously considered a relative contraindication because of the excessive fat and consequent inadequate surgical landmarks, has become an indication for this approach.[14,15] Retroperitoneoscopy provides direct access to the renal hilum and avoids the thick abdominal fat that is displaced medially away from the surgical field when the patient is placed in the flank position during retroperitoneoscopy. In addition, the retroperitoneal approach provides direct exposure of renal tumors located posteriorly or posterolaterally during laparoscopic nephron-sparing surgery.

General contraindications include previous ipsilateral retroperitoneal surgery, severe cardiopulmonary impairment, uncorrected coagulopathy, and abdominal sepsis. Relative contraindications include dense perirenal or retroperitoneal adhesions due to retroperitoneal pathology including renal tuberculosis, xanthogranulomatous pyelonephritis, and perirenal abscess.

PATIENT POSITIONIING

For most retroperitoneoscopic renal and adrenal surgery, the patient is placed in the standard 90-degree full flank (lateral decubitus) position (Figure 47-1). The patient is secured to the operative table in position with a safety belt and broad adhesive tape. All bony prominences are carefully padded to prevent pressure sores or adverse neuromuscular sequelae. The operative table is mildly flexed to maximize the space between the twelfth rib and iliac crest. Occasionally, the kidney rest is raised to achieve an adequate subcostal space for initial port placement. The relevant anatomic landmarks include the twelfth rib superiorly, iliac crest inferiorly, and paraspinal muscle posterolaterally. The surgeon and assistant stand facing the back of the patient.

SURGICAL TECHNIQUE

INITIAL RETROPERITONEAL ACCESS   The retroperitoneal space can be accessed using either closed or open techniques. The open approach (Hasson technique) is most commonly employed to develop the retroperitoneal working space and subsequent insertion of the primary port under direct vision. Initially, a horizontal 1.5 cm skin incision is made at the tip of the twelfth rib.[16] S-retractors are used to bluntly split the flank muscle fibers until the anterior thoracolumbar fascia is identified. The thoracolumbar fascia is then incised with an electrocautery and the retroperitoneal space is developed using blunt finger dissection (Figure 47-2). The proper plane is confirmed by finger-palpation of the psoas muscle posteriorly and Gerota's fascia anteriorly. To minimize air leak and consequent subcutaneous emphysema, the incision length should be limited to surgeon's finger admittance, and dissection above the fascia plane should be avoided.

Alternatively, the closed access technique involves placement of a Veress needle in Petit's triangle.[4,17] A horizontal 1-cm incision is made above the iliac crest, and muscle fibers are spread with a Kelly clamp until the lumbodorsal fascia is identified. A Veress needle is inserted and the space is developed with an insufflation pressure of 30 mm Hg. Standard methods of confirming Veress needle location for intraperitoneal access may be unreliable in this setting. Incorrect placement and insufflation may complicate the retroperitoneoscopic procedure and may necessitate conversion to a transperitoneal approach.[4] Thus, the open approach for initial retroperitoneal access provides a more reliable technique for subsequent balloon dilation.

DEVELOPMENT OF RETROPERITONEAL SPACE

A variety of techniques have been used to develop the retroperitoneal space. The most commonly employed method involves balloon (commercial or self-styled) dilation. Gaur's original technique involved securing a No. 7 latex glove over the end of a red-rubber catheter connected to a sphygmomanometer that was pumped to a pressure of 110 mm Hg.[2] An alternative medium is saline. In an ex vivo laboratory study, it was shown that a volume of 1,000 mL resulted in a mean retroperitoneal pressure of 15 mm Hg.[17] Clinically, volumes of 800 to 1,000 mL often suffice.[6] Self-fashioned latex balloons often rupture because of a relative lack of tensile strength. Given that silicone balloons have more tensile strength than latex, a 30-ml Foley catheter balloon can be used, but the potential space developed is limited to the size of the balloon.[18] An alternative approach is to develop the retroperitoneal space with a combination of digital blunt dissection through the initial incision at the tip of the twelfth rib followed by blunt dissection using the laparoscope during insufflation.[13] Although feasible, this technique often necessitates frequent cleaning of the laparoscope and must be performed cautiously due to initial lack of clear landmarks. It has also been suggested that this method may be more time-consuming and tedious compared to preliminary distension with a balloon device.[18]

We routinely develop the retroperitoneal working space with a commercially available trocar-mounted balloon device (PDB, Origin Medsystems, Menlo Park, CA) (Figure 47-3). The balloon is inflated with 800 mL of air for adults and 400 to 600 mL for children. The balloon is routinely placed outside of and posterior to Gerota's fascia, and anterior to the psoas muscle (Figure 47-4). Although previously described for simple nephrectomy, balloon placement inside of Gerota's fascia is no longer advocated because it was not routinely feasible and impaired access to the hilar vessels. The stiff shaft that the balloon is affixed to facilitates precisely directed placement of the balloon. Direct visualization of the developed space can be confirmed by introducing the laparoscope through the transparent shaft. Secondary balloon dilation is performed cephalad to the original site for retroperitoneoscopic adrenalectomy[7] and caudad for procedures requiring ureteral mobilization.[19]

PORT PLACEMENT   The primary port is inserted in place of the balloon dilator at the tip of the twelfth rib. We use a 30–cc–balloon-mounted port (PDB, Origin Medsystems) that contains an internal doughnut-shaped fascial retention balloon at the port tip and an external adjustable foam cuff that can be cinched together against the flank wall creating an airtight seal (see Figure 47-3).

After pneumoretroperitoneum is achieved, a 30° lens laparoscope is introduced through the primary port, and preliminary retroperitoneoscopic examination is performed. Secondary ports are then placed under direct laparoscopic vision. An anterior port is placed between the mid- and anterior axillary line, approximately 5 cm cephalad to the iliac crest, and a posterior port is placed at that junction of the twelfth rib with the paraspinal muscles. Either 5- or 12-mm ports are placed depending on the procedure. Rarely, an additional port may be necessary and is inserted at the tip of the eleventh rib to assist in counter traction. The ports should be placed as far apart as possible to avoid intraoperative clashing of instruments. Inadvertent peritoneal injury during port placement can occur when trocars are placed too medially. In order to maximize working space and diminish the likelihood of this adverse event, a technique of atraumatic peritoneal dissection from the abdominal wall with an Endo Peanut (United States Surgical, Norwalk, CT) has been described.[20] After completion of the procedure, the fascia of 10 to12 mm port incisions is closed.

SURGICAL CAVEATS

MORBIDLY OBESE PATIENTS   During initial access, it may be difficult to palpate the tip of the twelfth rib. A spinal needle (18 gauge, 15 cm) may be used to identify the twelfth rib by inserting the needle percutaneously to feel and confirm the rib position. Another caveat in these circumstances is to perform ultrasonography for clear identification of the bony landmarks before trocar insertion. Other considerations during retroperitoneoscopy for morbidly obese patients include the intraoperative use of two CO_2 insufflators to maintain adequate retroperitoneal working space.[14,15]

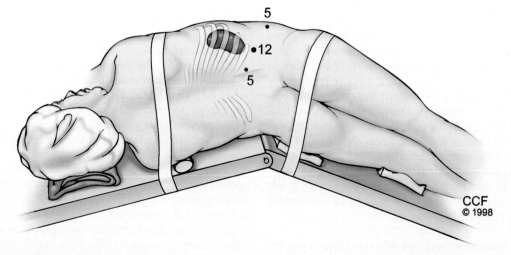

5

•12

5

CCF
© 1998

Figure 47-1 The patient is placed in the 90° flank position and the operative table is flexed. Three subcostal ports are inserted as shown. Adapted from Hsu TH et al.[27]

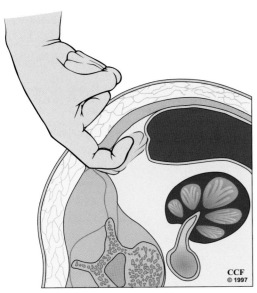

Figure 47-2 The surgeon's index finger is inserted through a 1 cm incision made at the tip of the twelfth rib. After the flank muscles are split and the thoracolumbar fascia sharply incised, a retroperitoneal space is created by gently mobilizing the lateral peritoneal reflection medially. Adapted from Gill IS.[6]

PREVIOUS PERCUTANEOUS RENAL SURGERY Contrary to previous open or laparoscopic retroperitoneal surgery, percutaneous procedures are not considered contraindications to retroperitoneoscopy. Adhesions may form, secondary to percutaneous procedures, but they are often localized. Initial balloon dilation may not initially develop an adequate working space, but secondary balloon dilation or blunt dissection of adhesions with the laparoscope usually results in an adequate space.

BLEEDING FROM INITIAL PORT ENTRY Bleeding from a port site is particularly troublesome during retroperitoneoscopy because of the proximity of the ports and smaller working space. An increase in insufflation pressure will diminish minor bleeding and facilitate insertion of the anterior port. Electrocautery is then introduced to cauterize and control bleeding.

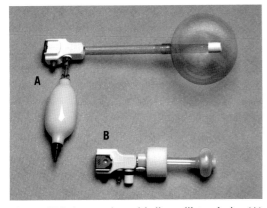

Figure 47-3 A preperitoneal balloon dilator device (A) and a 30–cc–balloon-mounted port with an internal doughnut-shaped fascial retention balloon at the port tip and an external adjustable foam cuff (B) (PDB, Origin Medsystems, Menlo Park, CA).

INADVERTENT PERITONEOTOMY This is not an infrequent occurrence, having been reported to occur in 5 to 20% of retroperitoneoscopic cases.[21–23] Peritoneotomy may occur during balloon dilation, anterior port placement or with dissection during the procedure. Although a peritoneotomy may increase the difficulty of surgery by reducing the retroperitoneal working space, gravity displaces the intraperitoneal organs away from the surgical field while the patient is in the flank position, making this less of an issue. Also increasing the insufflation pressure or inserting an additional port for additional retraction can help maintain the retroperitoneal working space.[23] Rarely, conversion to transperitoneal laparoscopy or open surgery is required

COMPLICATIONS

The potential adverse sequelae of pneumoretroperitoneum are most commonly related to subcutaneous emphysema. Subcutaneous emphysema occurs more frequently during retroperitoneal versus transperitoneal laparoscopy. Also, with routine postoperative chest x-rays, up to 7% of patients may have radiographic evidence of pneumothorax and/or pneumomediastinum.[10] Clinically significant absorption of CO_2, however, occurs in 7% of patients, and pneumothorax and/or pneumomediastinum in 0.6%.[24]

An international survey documented an overall major complication rate of 4.7% with retroperitoneal and extraperitoneoscopic surgery.[24] Vascular injuries constitute most major complications encountered during laparoscopic surgery.[25] Without discriminating between retroperitoneal or transperitoneal laparoscopy, a review of 2,407 patients found a 1.7% rate of vascular injuries.[25] This is identical to the rate of vascular injuries that occurred in a series of 404 patients undergoing retroperitoneoscopic procedures.[26]

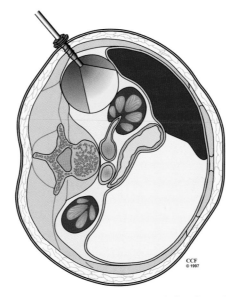

Figure 47-4 The balloon dissector is inflated anterior to the psoas muscle and a space is developed outside of Gerota's fascia. The kidney is mobilized medially and the renal hilum is exposed. Adapted from Gill IS.

By limiting the surgical field to the retroperitoneal space, the risk of injury to intraperitoneal organs should be diminished, but it should be kept in mind that, although the intraperitoneal viscera are not visualized, they are in close proximity. The rate of injury to intraperitoneal viscera was 0.7% in a multi-institutional review of retroperitoneal and extraperitoneal laparoscopic surgery.[24] In other series, 0.25% to 0.32% of patients undergoing retroperitoneoscopy suffered a bowel injury.[23,26] The risk of port site hernia is diminished, but nonetheless, documented cases have been reported.[23] Thus, although unique features and challenges of retroperitoneoscopy exist, the rate of complication is no different from that of transperitoneal laparoscopy.

CONCLUSIONS

Retroperitoneoscopy provides direct access to the extraperitoneally located urological organs. The aforementioned techniques for obtaining pneumoretroperitoneum and developing adequate retroperitoneal working space are reliable and reproducible. Pneumoretroperitoneum is safe and does not result in increased complications compared to the transperitoneal approach. Facility with both transperitoneal and retroperitoneal laparoscopy expands the surgical repertoire allowing optimal access for specific procedures.

REFERENCES

1. Wickham JEA. The surgical treatment of renal lithiasis. In: Urinary calculous disease. New York: Churchill Livingstone; 1979. p. 145–98.
2. Gaur DD. Laparoscopic operative retroperitoneoscopy: use of a new device. J Urol 1992;148:1137–9.
3. Gill IS, Kerbl K, Meraney AM, Clayman RV. Basic principles, techniques, and equipment of laparoscopic surgery. In: Walsh PC, et al., editors. Campbell's Urology. 8th ed. Vol. 4. Saunders; 2002.
4. Capelouto CC, Moore RG, Silverman SG, Kavoussi LR. Retro-peritoneoscopy: anatomical rationale for direct retroperitoneal access. J Urol 1994;152(6 Pt 1): 2008–10.
5. Chiu AW, Chang LS, Birkett DH, Babayan RK. The impact of pneumoperitoneum, pneumoretroperitoneum, and gasless laparoscopy on the systemic and renal hemodynamics. J Am Coll Surg 1995;181:397–406.
6. Gill IS. Retroperitoneal laparoscopic nephrectomy. Urol Clin North Am 1998;25:343–60.
7. Sung GT, Gill IS. Anatomic landmarks and time management during retroperitoneoscopic radical nephrectomy. J Endourol 2002;16:165–9.
8. Dunn MD, McDougall EM. Renal physiology. Laparoscopic considerations. Urol Clin North Am 2000;27:609–14.
9. Collins JM. Inert gas exchange of subcutaneous and intraperitoneal gas pockets in piglets. Respir Physiol 1981;46: 391–404.
10. Wolf JS Jr, Monk TG, McDougall EM, et al. The extraperitoneal approach and subcutaneous emphysema are associated with greater absorption of carbon dioxide during laparoscopic renal surgery. J Urol 1995;154:959–63.
11. Giebler RM, Kabatnik M, Stegen BH, et al. Retroperitoneal and intraperitoneal CO2 insufflation have markedly different cardiovascular effects. J Surg Res 1997;68:153–60.
12. Ng CS, Gill IS, Sung GT, et al. Retroperitoneoscopic surgery is not associated with increased carbon dioxide absorption. J Urol 1999;162:1268–72.
13. Rassweiler JJ, Seemann O, Frede T, et al. Retroperitoneoscopy: experience with 200 cases. J Urol 1998;160:1265–9.
14. Doublet J, Belair G. Retroperitoneal laparoscopic nephrectomy is safe and effective in obese patients: a comparative study of 55 procedures. Urology 2000;56:63–6.
15. Abreu SC, Kaouk JH, Steinberg AP, Gill IS. Retroperitoneoscopic radical nephrectomy in a super-obese patient (BMI 77 kg/m2). Urology 2004;63.

16. Gill IS, Grune MT, Munch LC. Access technique for retroperitoneoscopy. J Urol 1996;156:1120–4.

17. McDougall EM, Clayman RV, Fadden PT. Retroperitoneoscopy: the Washington University Medical School experience. Urology 1994;43:446–52.

18. Keeley FX Jr, Tolley DA. Retroperitoneal laparoscopy. BJU Int 1999;84:212–5.

19. Gill IS, Munch LC, Lucas BA, Das S. Initial experience with retroperitoneoscopic nephroureterectomy: use of a double-balloon technique. Urology 1995;46:747–50.

20. Wakabayashi Y, Kataoka A, Johnin K, et al. Simple techniques for atraumatic peritoneal dissection from the abdominal wall and for preventing peritoneal injury during trocar placement under retroperitoneoscopy. J Urol 2003;169:256–7.

21. Gasman D, Saint F, Barthelemy Y, et al. Retroperitoneoscopy: a laparoscopic approach for adrenal and renal surgery. Urology 1996;47:801–6.

22. Gaur DD, Rathi SS, Ravandale AV, Gopichand M. A single-centre experience of retroperitoneoscopy using the balloon technique. BJU Int 2001;87:602–6.

23. Kumar, M, R Kumar, AK Hemal, and NP Gupta, Complications of retroperitoneoscopic surgery at one centre. BJU Int, 2001. 87(7): p. 607–12.

24. Gill IS, Clayman RV, Albala DM, et al. Retroperitoneal and pelvic extraperitoneal laparoscopy: an international perspective. Urology 1998;52:566–71.

25. Fahlenkamp D, Rassweiler J, Fornara P, et al. Complications of laparoscopic procedures in urology: experience with 2,407 procedures at 4 German centers. J Urol 1999;162 (3 Pt 1):765–70; discussion 70-1.

26. Meraney AM, Samee AA, Gill IS. Vascular and bowel complications during retroperitoneal laparoscopic surgery. J Urol 2002;168:1941–4.

27. Hsu TH, Sung GT, Gill IS. Retroperitoneoscopic approach to nephrectomy. J Endourol 1999;13:713–8; discussion 18–20.

48

Basic Laparoscopy: Hand-Assisted Techniques

J. Stuart Wolf, Jr, MD

The introduction of hand-assisted laparoscopic surgery (HALS) has contributed greatly to the explosive growth in laparoscopic urology over the past few years. More urologists than ever are performing laparoscopy, specifically laparoscopic nephrectomy. Just a few years ago, this procedure was limited predominantly to academic medical centers, but now laparoscopic nephrectomy is performed by many urologists in practice—young and old, urban and rural, large group and solo practice. Why this dramatic increase, when laparoscopic nephrectomy, for close to a decade prior to this, languished in the view of the typical general urological practitioner somewhere along the continuum of "ridiculous" to "investigational" to "occasionally useful"? This history of laparoscopic nephrectomy contrasts starkly with that of other laparoscopic procedures introduced in the same time period (late 1980s to early 1990s). Laparoscopic cholecystectomy, laparoscopic pelvic lymph node dissection (until its utility was reduced by prostate-specific antigen risk-profiling), and laparoscopic hysterectomy all achieved widespread use soon after their introduction. Why was laparoscopic nephrectomy different? The primary reason proposed in the mid-1990s was that laparoscopic nephrectomy was too difficult for the average urologist to develop and maintain the necessary operative skills, given the relative infrequency of nephrectomy in a typical practice. There were other factors as well, including concern about oncologic efficacy, the inefficiency of increased operative time, safety of the procedure in case of vascular injury, and others.

Although there likely were many developments that spurred on the widespread acceptance of laparoscopic nephrectomy, HALS was one of the major factors. HALS addresses many of the perceived problems with laparoscopic nephrectomy: (1) it technically simplifies the procedure, which allows even urologists with a low-volume practice to develop and maintain skills; (2) it facilitates wide dissection and intact specimen removal, which may provide some reassurance as to the oncologic efficacy of the procedure (although there is no evidence that HALS provides any different outcome than standard laparoscopic nephrectomy in this regard); (3) it reduces operative time for most surgeons; and (4) it provides more rapid control of vascular injury. Combined with patient demand, once a critical mass of surgeons started performing laparoscopic nephrectomy, the (still increasing) popularity of laparoscopic nephrectomy was inevitable.

Following a brief history of hand-assistance, this chapter first describes the various HALS devices that are currently available in the United States along with their application, advantages, and disadvantages. Then, the results of HALS are provided, with emphasis on series that compare HALS to other laparoscopic techniques. Finally, an assessment of the role of HALS in urology is made.

HISTORY

By 1993, surgeons had reported the insertion of a gloved hand through a tight fascial incision to allow direct manual manipulation while maintaining pneumoperitoneum during laparoscopy.[1] Tierney and associates, and then Tschada and Rassweiler reported laparoscopic radical nephrectomy using this technique in 1994 and 1995, respectively.[2,3] Commercial devices to facilitate laparoscopic hand-assistance were under development by this time,[4] and in 1996, Bannenberg and colleagues[5] reported hand-assisted laparoscopic nephrectomy in a porcine model using a prototype of a commercial HALS device. Later that same year, Nakada and colleagues performed the first clinical laparoscopic nephrectomy with a commercial HALS device.[6] In 1997, Keeley and associates reported the first HALS nephroureterectomy,[7] and in 1998, Wolf and co-workers described the first HALS donor nephrectomy.[8] HALS was soon applied to a number of other urologic laparoscopic procedures. The introduction of second-generation HALS devices that do not require the use of a sleeve has further accelerated the acceptance of HALS in urology.

DEVICES FOR HAND-ASSISTED LAPAROSCOPY

The first commercial HALS devices were affixed to the abdomen with adhesive, the Pneumo Sleeve (Dexterity Surgical, Roswell, GA; Figure 48-1) and the Intromit (Medtech Ltd., Dublin, Ireland; Figure 48-2). The HandPort (Smith & Nephew, Andover, MA; Figure 48-3) also had a separate base and sleeve, with the base held on with inflatable compression rather than adhesion. None of these first-generation devices remains in production. Lessons learned through their use, however, prompted the development of the improved second-generation devices.

There are three commercial devices for HALS currently available. None require a separate sleeve, which was a limitation of the first-generation devices. The Gelport (Applied Med-

ical, Rancho Santa Margarita, CA; Figure 48-4) has three components that fit together on the abdomen, affixing by compression and providing gas occlusion with a gel that fits snugly around the surgeon's forearm. The Lap Disc (Ethicon Endo-Surgery, Cincinnati, OH; Figure 48-5) is a single-piece device that is held in place by compression and occludes gas with an iris valve that closes around the surgeon's forearm. The Omniport (Advanced Surgical Concepts, Bray, Co. Wicklow, Ireland), distributed in the United States by Weck Closure, Raleigh, NC, (Figure 48-6) is a cylinder that inflates to provide both abdominal fixation and gas occlusion.

GELPORT The Gelport kit contains a flexible skirt that fits into the abdominal cavity, a rigid base that is placed on the abdomen, and the seal gel cap that snaps onto the base. This device does not require a separate sleeve. The HALS incision is made initially, and the skirt is inserted into the abdomen, pulling up the free end to retract the inner ring of the skirt against the underside of the abdominal wall. There are two skirts in the kit, one for average and one for large body walls. The free end of the skirt is hooked over tabs on the base to open the incision and fix the base to the abdominal wall (Figure 48-7). The laparoscopic ports can be inserted now under manual guidance, or later after insufflation (Figure 48-8). Once the gel cap is snapped onto the base, the abdomen is gas-tight. The gel expands enough to allow insertion of a hand through its central slit, but will also occlude the incision with nothing passing through it (Figure 48-9). For this device, as for all of the devices that do not require a sleeve for gas occlusion, a dark second glove

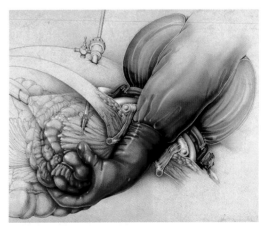

Figure 48-1 Pneumo Sleeve (discontinued).

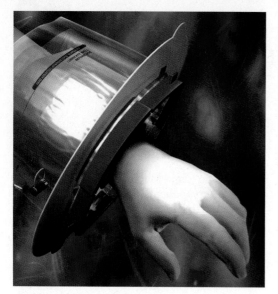

Figure 48-2 Intromit (discontinued).

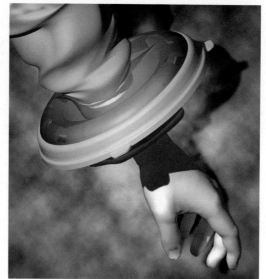

Figure 48-4 Gelport.

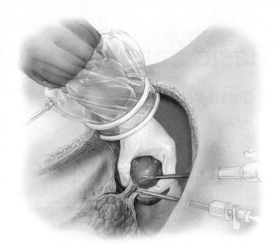

Figure 48-6 Omniport.

should nonetheless be worn, placed over a water-proof liner around the forearm, to prevent soak-through of body fluids. In addition, ports and bare instruments can be passed through the central slit in the gel, or through a separate stab incision in the gel. An instrument can be passed through the gel alone, or when the hand is in place. Two kits are available, described as 100 mm and 120 mm by the manufacturer (total circumferences are 13 and 16 cm, respectively). The former is preferred in most settings to reduce crowding of trocars. The new Gelport XE uses an integrated wound retractor that fits into the rigid base (Figure 48-10), replacing the skirt, and it is more resistant to gas leakage.

LAP DISC The Lap Disc is a one-piece device that consists of a pair of locking rings that close an iris valve, with an inner ring that holds the device in the abdomen. After making the incision, the ports can be inserted under manual guidance, or later after insufflation. The inner ring of the Lap Disc is inserted inside the

abdomen (Figure 48-11), and the tension from the elastic sheath connecting the inner ring to the outer locking rings holds the latter in place on the abdominal wall. There are two sizes of the device to accommodate varying thicknesses of the abdominal wall in different patients. To use a hand intra-abdominally, the hand is inserted to the desired depth and the iris valve is tightened around the forearm by turning the outermost ring clockwise and locking it onto the middle (stable) ring by way of ratcheted teeth (Figure 48-12). Slight inward movements of the forearm can be made, but large movements require the iris valve to be opened a bit. Similarly, pulling back or removing the forearm necessitates tightening the valve to prevent gas leak. The valve can be completely occluded, or it can be tightened around a port to allow use of a laparoscopic instrument. Since this port can be used for both insufflation and visualization, after initial insertion of the device, the insufflated abdomen can be inspected and subsequent ports can be inserted under direct visualization. This method of secondary port

placement can be used with any of the devices that allow placement of a port through the device.

OMNIPORT The Omniport is also a one-piece device. It is a cylindrical inflatable cuff fitted with two retention rings. A separate inflating bulb can be disconnected once the device is in place. After making the incision, the entire device is placed into the abdomen (Figure 48-13). The outer retention ring (the one on the side of the inflation port) is pulled out onto the abdominal surface while the inner ring is pulled up against the inner aspect of the abdominal wall. This fixes the cylindrical inflatable cuff in place. Inflating the cuff with the intra-abdominal hand in place provides gas occlusion (Figures 48-14 and 48-15). Minor in and out movements of the forearm can be made without deflating the cuff, but for extreme inward movements and removal of the hand, the cuff does need to be deflated first. In addition, the cuff cannot be occluded completely enough to allow pneumoperitoneum to be maintained without anything going through the device, although it can be inflated enough to hold in place a 12-mm laparoscopic port with only slight gas leakage.

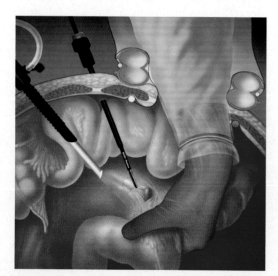

Figure 48-3 HandPort (discontinued).

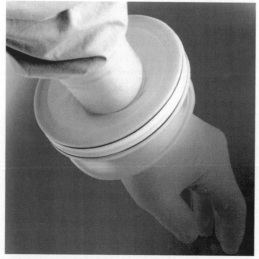

Figure 48-5 Lap Disc.

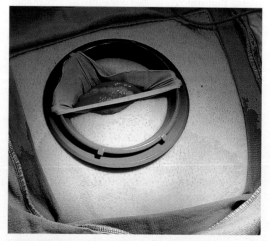

Figure 48-7 Gelport: The skirt, with the inner ring inside the abdomen, has been pulled up and partially hooked onto the tabs of the rigid base.

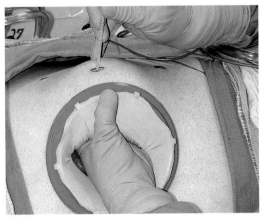

Figure 48-8 Gelport: The skirt has been completely attached and a non-bladed system is being used to insert ports under manual guidance.

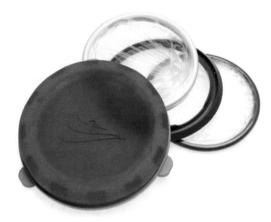

Figure 48-10 Gelport XE.

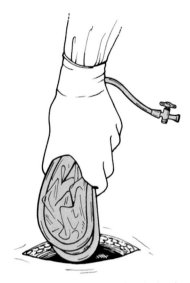

Figure 48-13 Omniport: The entire device is slipped inside the abdomen.

DIFFERENCES BETWEEN DEVICES Table 48-1 summarizes the important differences between the HALS devices. An important consideration is the device diameter. Especially in small patients, the size of the HALS device sometimes necessitates suboptimal port placement. This is less of a problem with the three current devices, all measuring 12 to 13 cm in diameter, than it was with the first-generation devices. Gas leakage or premature removal of the device is in most cases only an inconvenience, but sometimes the resulting loss of pneumoperitoneum can hinder the procedure considerably. The Gelport and Lap Disc leak infrequently, as long as the incision is not too large (≤ 8 cm), but even a slight enlarging of the incision, usually made in an attempt to allow deeper access for the intra-abdominal hand, can result in gas leakage with these two devices. The Omniport probably has the lowest tendency to leak gas, but it has the distinct disadvantage of loss of pneumoperitoneum when the hand is removed. The ability to use a laparoscopic instrument through the HALS device is possible with all three, but only the Gelport allows simultaneous insertion of the hand and an instrument.

ADJUNCTS FOR HALS Fluid can track up the intra-abdominal forearm and soak through the surgeon's gown above the glove. Double gloving

does not necessarily prevent this, and some additional barrier is recommended. We have found the simplest and most effective to be a Steri-Drape Small Towel Drape 1000 (3M Co., St. Paul, MN). The adhesive strip is wrapped around the wrist and the rest of the drape trails down over the forearm, covered by a second glove over the hand and adhesive strip. The second glove should be dark to minimize glare. Other surgeons have overcome the fluid problem by using a disposable impervious gown.

CHOICE OF POSITION FOR SURGEON, HALS DEVICE, AND PORTS Either the primary or the assistant surgeon can have the intra-abdominal hand. When the primary surgeon's hand is intra-

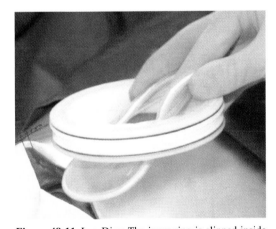

Figure 48-11 Lap Disc: The inner ring is slipped inside the abdomen and the outer locking rings are left outside.

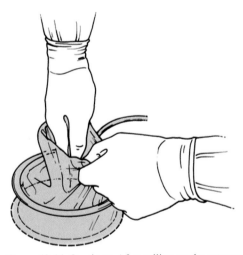

Figure 48-14 Omniport: After pulling out the outer retention ring, the cuff is held in place while the intra-abdominal hand is inserted to the desired depth.

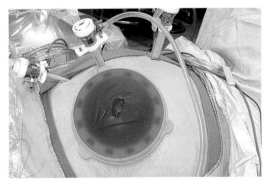

Figure 48-9 Gelport: Gel cap has been attached, and maintains pneumoperitoneum even without the hand through the device.

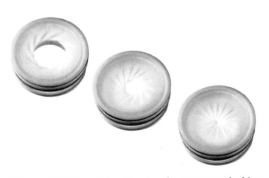

Figure 48-12 Lap Disc: Turning the outermost locking ring clockwise closes down the iris valve.

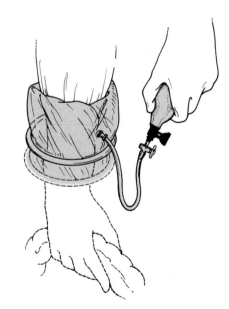

Figure 48-15 Omniport: With the cuff inflated around the intra-abdominal forearm (after which the hand pump can be removed), pneumoperitoneum is maintained.

Table 48-1 Differences between HALS devices

	Gelport (100mm and XE)	Lap Disc	Omniport
Abdominal fixation	Compression, variable elastic	Compression, fixed elastic	Compression, inflatable
Gas occlusion	Compression, fixed elastic	Compression, variable elastic	Compression, inflatable
Diameter	13 cm	12 cm	12 cm
Major advantages	Maintenance of pneumoperitoneum at all times, can insert ports or instruments alongside hand	Smallest and simplest device, can insert one port through the middle	Gas leakage rare, even if incision too large
Major disadvantages	Gas leakage if incision is too large, can feel tight	Gas leakage if incision is too large	Loss of pneumoperitoneum when remove hand

abdominal, direct manual dissection is possible, but the primary surgeon has only one hand free to manipulate a laparoscopic instrument. If the assistant's hand is in the abdomen, then the primary surgeon can use two laparoscopic instruments, but then the hand is used primarily only for retraction. This distinction is important, inasmuch as it can alter port placement. Figure 48-16 indicates the most common HALS device and port arrangements when the surgeon's hand is intra-abdominal. Figure 48-16A is the most typical arrangement for a left nephrectomy by a right-handed surgeon. The non-dominant (left) hand is placed through the HALS device in the periumbilical midline. This allows simultaneous retraction of bowel and finger dissection of the kidney. The assistant operates the videolaparoscope through a 10/12 mm port at the level of the umbilicus, 1 to 2 cm lateral to the edge of the HALS device (see #2 in Figure 48-16A), and an instrument placed through a lateral 5 mm assisting port (see #4 in Figure 48-16A). The surgeon's 10/12 mm working port is placed 1 to 2 cm below

the costal margin (see #3 in Figure 48-16A), on the line that extends from the videolaparoscope port to the patient's ipsilateral shoulder. There is more variation for right nephrectomies by a right-handed surgeon. Some, including this author, recommend an arrangement that is the mirror image of the left-sided procedure (Figure 48-16B). The right hand is used intra-abdominally, which allows retraction of the liver by the back of the hand while dissecting the kidney. The surgeon's left hand is used to manipulate laparoscopic instruments, which some right-handed surgeons find less effective. The ability to use either hand intra-abdominally is valuable, and if an "ambidextrous" approach is used when starting out with HALS, then it is quickly learned.

An alternative for right nephrectomy by a right-handed surgeon is depicted in Figure 48-16C. Here, the surgeon's left hand is placed through the HALS device and the right hand operates an instrument through the working port (see #3 in Figure 48-16C). The assistant operates the videolaparoscope (#2) and an assisting instrument (#4). Some

place the HALS device obliquely in the ipsilateral lower quadrant when using this approach. A number of HALS device placements have been described, including midline (supraumbilical, periumbilical, and infraumbilical), paramedian, subcostal, lower quadrant oblique ("muscle-splitting" Gibson incision), and transverse suprapubic (Pfannenstiel). Each will be associated with slightly different port placements, depending on whether the surgeon or assistant has the intra-abdominal hand. The general principles that guide device and port placement in HALS are maximization of effectiveness of the hand, minimization of videolaparoscope obstruction by the hand, and centering the videolaparoscope between instruments, rather than working with the hand and instruments all off to one side. Use of a 30° videolaparoscope is very useful during HALS to reduce obstruction of vision by the intra-abdominal hand.

RESULTS OF HALS

SERIES OF HALS In urology, HALS is most commonly applied to nephrectomy. The first reported use of HALS in urology was for radical nephrectomy,[2] as was the first use of a commercial HALS device in urology.[6] In a large series of HALS for radical nephrectomy, Stifelman and colleagues reported 95 HALS radical nephrectomies for large specimens.[9] The mean operative time was 158 minutes, and the major complication rate was only 4%, with a rate of conversion to open surgery of 3%. In a notable series of 96 HALS radical nephrectomies from Japan with appreciable follow-up, the 4-year actuarial survival free of renal cell carcinoma recurrence was 84%.[10]

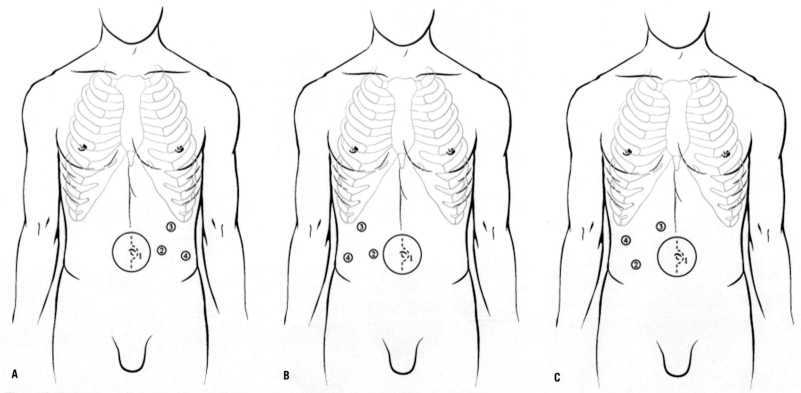

Figure 48-16 *A*, typical port placement for left HALS nephrectomy using the surgeon's left hand in the abdomen. *B*, Mirror image, for right HALS nephrectomy using the surgeon's right hand in the abdomen. *C*, One alternative for right HALS nephrectomy using the surgeon's left hand in the abdomen. 1 = HALS device; 2 = videolaparoscope port; 3 = working port for surgeon; 4 = assisting port.

There have been 11 published series (containing 10 or more patients) of HALS nephroureterectomy for urothelial neoplasm (not including series that have been updated by subsequent ones).[11–21] In the total of 368 patients described in these series, the operative time averaged 298 minutes, with 10% major and 17% minor complication rates overall. Conversion to open surgery was required in only 3.2% of cases. The non-vesical recurrence rate was 10% with 17-month mean follow-up.

Many of the recently reported series of donor nephrectomy have been with HALS.[22–40] Among these 19 series (reporting 848 patients in total), the mean operative time was 210 minutes, and the mean warm ischemia time, 2.7 minutes. The minor and major complication rates were 10.2% and 1.7%, respectively, with a conversion to open surgery in only 1.4% of patients. In the studies that reported convalescence, the mean return to non-strenuous activity levels was 10.1 days. Graft function has been excellent, with 97.3% functioning at a mean follow-up of 15 months. Delayed function of the allograft occurred in 3.6%, and ureteral complications occurred in 1.7%. Of the first 200 HALS donor nephrectomies performed by the author at the University of Michigan, the ureteral complication rate has been 4%.[41] The one-month, one-year, and three-year actuarial graft survival rates are 97%, 95%, and 94%, respectively.

Series of HALS for partial nephrectomy,[42,43] bilateral nephrectomy,[44,45] and multi-organ removal[46,47] have also been reported. The latter two procedures can be particularly challenging with standard laparoscopic techniques, and are perfectly suited to HALS. Other difficult maneuvers, such as radical nephrectomy with associated excision of vena caval thrombus,[48] are facilitated by HALS.

COMPARISONS TO OTHER TECHNIQUES Although HALS has been reported in the setting of retroperitoneoscopic surgery,[16,17,36,39] this is not yet a commonly accepted technique. As such, when assessing the role of HALS in urologic laparoscopy, this chapter considers it to be a transperitoneal approach. Transperitoneal HALS, standard transperitoneal laparoscopy, and standard retroperitoneoscopy all have advantages and disadvantages. In this section, comparisons between the techniques are presented.

Wolf and associates reported the initial comparison of hand-assisted and standard transperitoneal laparoscopic nephrectomy using the first hand-assisted ($n = 13$) and standard ($n = 8$) transperitoneal laparoscopic nephrectomies performed at the University of Michigan and the University of Wisconsin.[49] The mean operative time for hand-assistance was 90 minutes shorter than that for of standard laparoscopy, but without a significant difference in measures of convalescence. This study suggests that, early in a surgeon's experience, HALS "shortens the learning curve" for transperitoneal nephrectomy. A subsequent report from the University of Michigan made the same comparison after more experience had been gained.[50] Of 38 laparoscopic radical

nephrectomies, 16 were performed with standard transperitoneal laparoscopy and 22 with HALS. Tumor size, specimen weight, and body mass index tended to be greater in the hand-assisted group (Table 48-2; statistically significant only for tumor size). Despite these differences, HALS was over 60 minutes quicker than standard laparoscopy overall. With experience, however, the operative time for standard transperitoneal laparoscopy decreased (while that for HALS remained constant), such that HALS was 90 minutes faster during the first half of the series and 30 minutes faster in the second half. The benefit of HALS was still evident, but of less magnitude. The intensity and duration of convalescence was generally the same in the two groups, although there was a trend (not statistically significant) toward more pain specifically in the abdomen with hand-assistance (Table 48-3).

The six non-randomized, retrospective studies comparing standard transperitoneal laparoscopic and hand-assisted donor nephrectomies are summarized in Table 48-4.[27–30,32–33] The hand-assisted procedures tended to be faster, were associated with shorter warm ischemia time, had fewer complications, required conversion less frequently, and were associated with a shorter hospital stay. Although convalescence parameters were not consistently assessed, in two of the studies[27,30] there tended to be more postoperative narcotic use in the hand-assisted group.

Batler and associates compared their experience with retroperitoneoscopic and hand-assisted laparoscopic transperitoneal nephrectomy (all but one were radical nephrectomies).[51] Although this was the initial approach of the authors with these two techniques, they were already experienced in the technique of standard transperitoneal laparoscopic nephrectomy. In this setting, the authors found that HALS decreased operative time only slightly compared to retroperitoneoscopy (238

versus 256 minutes, $p = .54$). Similarly, Baldwin and associates reported a retrospective comparison of 13 standard transperitoneal laparoscopic radical nephrectomies and 8 HALS radical nephrectomies in patients at high anesthetic risk (American Society of Anesthesiologists score of 3 or 4), in which the primary surgeon already had more than 5 years experience with standard transperitoneal laparoscopic radical nephrectomy.[52] Given this prior experience, operative time was equivalent (2.8 hours) in both groups. These authors found that analgesic use and recovery time tended to be greater in the HALS group, although not significantly so.

Comparing 11 standard transperitoneal laparoscopic and 16 hand-assisted laparoscopic nephroureterectomies, Landman and associates found that hand-assistance reduced mean operative time by 72 minutes but did not significantly alter any measure of the intensity and duration of convalescence.[12] This difference was noted despite the authors' extensive prior experience with standard transperitoneal laparoscopic nephroureterectomy. Length of hospital stay did tend to be longer in the hand-assisted group, but the difference was not statistically significant (3.3 versus 4.5 days).

In the general surgery literature, two randomized clinical trials of standard transperitoneal versus hand-assisted laparoscopic colectomy both determined no differences in operative time (< 3 hours in both), complications, or recovery parameters.[53,54] Conversion to open surgery (or to HALS), however, was more frequent in the standard transperitoneal group (22% versus 14%,[53] and 22% versus 7%[54]), suggesting that hand-assistance enhances the ability of the surgeon to complete difficult laparoscopic procedures in a minimally invasive fashion.

Overall, then, published data suggests that HALS is generally faster than standard transperi-

Table 48-2 Laparoscopic Radical Nephrectomy at the University of Michigan

	Body Mass Index	Tumor Size (cm)	Specimen Weight (g)	Operating Time (min)*
Standard TP ($n = 16$)	26.7	4.1	386	270
Hand-assisted ($n = 22$)	29.1	6.3	658	205
p Value	$> .10$	.006	$> .10$	.008

Adapted from Nelson CP, Wolf JS Jr.[50]

TP = transperitoneal.

*Hand-assisted was 90 min faster in first half of series and 30 min faster in second half of series, owing to a decrease to 232 minutes from 293 minutes in mean operative time of standard transperitoneal laparoscopy.

Table 48-3 Postoperative Data from Laparoscopic Radical Nephrectomy at the University of Michigan

	Overall Pain at 2 Weeks	Abdominal Pain at 2 Weeks	Time to Normal, Non-strenuous Activity (min)	Change in PHS of SF-12 at 6 weeks
Standard TP ($n = 16$)	4.0	2.4	14	−7.1
Hand-assisted ($n = 22$)	3.5	4.1	14	−7.3
p Value	$> .10$	.07	$> .10$	$> .10$

Adapted from Nelson CP, Wolf JS Jr.[50]

TP = transperitoneal.

Table 48-4 Published Series Comparing Standard Transperitoneal Laparoscopic to Hand-Assisted Laparoscopic Donor Nephrectomy

Study	Number/Type of Procedure	OR time (min)	Warm Ischemia (min)	Minor/Major Complications	Conversions	Hospital Stay (days)
Ruiz-Deya et al[27]	11 standard	215	3.9	1/1	0	1.6
	23 hand-assisted	165	1.6	2/0	1	2.0
Lindstrom et al[28]	11 standard	270	5.0	3/0	0	6.5
	11 hand-assisted	197	3.6	0/0	0	6.2
Velidedeoglu et al[29]	40 standard	255	–	–	3	3.2
	60 hand-assisted	260	–	–	1	2.6
Gershbein and Fuchs[30]	15 standard	276	3.8	1/0	0	2.0
	29 hand-assisted	205	2.4	2/0	1	2.3
Mateo et al[32]	29 standard	311	3.7	5/2	4	4.1
	18 hand-assisted	269	3.4	2/1	1	4.1
El-Galley et al[33]	28 standard	306	3.0	0/0	0	2.0
	17 hand-assisted	249	2.0	1/0	0	2.0
Total	134 standard	278*	3.7*	11%/3.2%†	5.2%†	3.1*
	158 hand-assisted	232*	2.5*	7.1%/1.0%†	2.5%†	2.8*

*Weighted average.
†% occurrence of summed totals.

Table 48-6 General Situations in which Hand-Assistance is Most Useful

Intact specimen removal is required
Limited experience
  With laparoscopy in general
  With specific procedure
Difficult procedure
Large specimen
Reoperation
Perihilar mass that limits accept to vasculature
Other process (eg, inflammation, fibrosis) that renders dissection difficult
Medical comorbidities necessitate rapid procedure

toneal laparoscopy, but that the difference decreases with increasing surgeon experience. Although firm conclusions cannot be made from the limited data to date, the magnitude of the effect of HALS on operative time appears to vary with the alternative technique as well as the type of surgery. The study of Batler and associates suggests that the difference may be less marked when the comparison is made to retroperitoneoscopy (which tends to be a more rapid approach in experienced hands).[51] The report of Landman and associates suggests that this difference may be more dramatic when a complex procedure such as nephroureterectomy is considered, even if there is prior experience.[12] In general, the intensity and duration of post-surgical recovery is slightly increased by HALS, but the magnitude of the difference between HALS and standard laparoscopy is much less than that between HALS and open surgery. For advanced procedures, HALS appears to reduce the likelihood of conversion to open surgery.

SELECTIVE USE OF HALS

Table 48-5 lists the advantages and disadvantages of HALS. The relative impact of these considerations differs by surgeon and procedures. Table 48-6 lists the general situations in which HALS is most useful. HALS is an excellent choice when intact specimen removal is required because it takes advantage of the required incision throughout the entire procedure rather than just at the conclusion. Another major consideration is surgeon experience with both laparoscopy in general or with a new procedure. HALS is an excellent way for an inexperienced surgeon to start performing laparoscopy, or for an experienced surgeon to start performing a new procedure. Similarly, a difficult procedure is a good indication for the use of HALS. Large specimens, reoperation, a perihilar mass, or anytime the surgical planes or

tissue identification are indistinct, can result in a prolonged and complication-prone laparoscopic procedure. HALS can make the difference between conversion to open surgery and completion of a minimally invasive procedure. Finally, for a patient with severe chronic obstructive pulmonary disease or congestive heart failure, in whom a rapid procedure is necessary because of problems due to hypercapnia or elevated intra-abdominal pressure, HALS can be very useful.

With these considerations in mind, HALS is best selected when there is a clear advantage (eg, in terms of operative time, safety, or specimen manipulation) over standard laparoscopic techniques. The degree of advantage or disadvantage of HALS is determined for the individual surgeon. The best procedures for HALS are advanced extirpative renal procedures. For radical nephrectomy, HALS offers the most advantage when the specimen is large or the anatomy is difficult. For partial nephrectomy, HALS might

Table 48-5 Advantages versus Disadvantages of HALS

Typical Advantages of HALS over Standard Laparoscopy

Faster
Easier
More control in operating room by surgeon
Better control of vascular injury
Reduced need for conversion to open surgery
Enhanced teaching

Typical Disadvantages of HALS compared to Standard Laparoscopy

Larger incision
Sometimes leak gas
Sometimes necessitates suboptimal port placement
Hand can get in the way
Physical pain for surgeon
Small degree of increased postoperative pain relative to standard laparoscopy

facilitate accurate resection, collecting system repair, and/or hemostasis for tumors that are large or central in location . For straightforward radical nephrectomies and for partial nephrectomy for peripheral tumors, standard transperitoneal or retroperitoneal techniques are effective in the hands of many. During procedures where intact specimen removal is required, such as nephroureterectomy for urothelial carcinoma or live donor nephrectomy, HALS takes advantage of the required incision throughout the entire procedure rather than just at the conclusion.

For some procedures, HALS is less useful—or may even hinder the procedure. Laparoscopic simple nephrectomy can be performed in a straightforward manner with standard transperitoneal or retroperitoneal techniques unless the specimen is inflamed (ie, pyonephrosis or xanthogranulomatous pyelonephritis) or very large (ie, autosomal dominant polycystic kidney disease). Standard laparoscopic techniques are also adequate for renal cyst resection and adrenalectomy in most cases. For reconstructive procedures such as laparoscopic pyeloplasty or nephropexy, there is little advantage to HALS. Although there has been interest in the hand-assisted laparoscopic approach to radical cystoprostatectomy, the tight confines of the pelvis reduce the utility of HALS for pelvic laparoscopic procedures.

In summary, HALS is technically easier than standard laparoscopy, with a "shorter learning curve" for most procedures. The current devices are easily applied and effective. Although there is considerable variation in port-placement, especially with regard to right nephrectomy for right-handed surgeons, the general techniques are standardized. Evidence suggests that convalescence associated with HALS is similar to that of standard laparoscopy, with a minimal increase in the intensity and duration of postsurgical recovery. Unless there is extensive laparoscopic experience, HALS offers more rapid operating times and a tendency towards safer procedures than standard laparoscopy for most extirpative renal procedures. Given prior experience, HALS offers minimal if any improvement over standard laparoscopy for straightforward renal procedures, reconstructive procedures, and most pelvic procedures. HALS is most useful for difficult extirpative laparoscopic procedures, and when intact extraction is desired.

CONCLUSION

HALS is …

- …technically easier than standard laparoscopy, with a shorted learning curve;
- …associated with minimal increase in the intensity and duration of postsurgical recovery compared to standard laparoscopy;
- …an approach with definite advantages and disadvantages, and should be used selectively;
- …associated with more rapid operating times, unless there is extensive laparoscopic experience;
- …most useful for difficult extirpative laparoscopic procedures, and when intact extraction is desired.

REFERENCES

1. Boland JP, Kusminsky RE, Tiely EH. Laparoscopic mini-laparotomy with manipulation: the middle path. Minim Invas Ther 1993;2:63–7.
2. Tierney JP, Oliver SR, Kusminsky RE, et al. Laparoscopic radical nephrectomy with intra-abdominal manipulation. Min Inv Ther 1994;3:303–5.
3. Tschada RK, Rassweiler JJ. Laparoscopic tumornephrectomy—the German experiences [abstract]. J Urol 1995; 153 (Suppl):479.
4. Leahy P, Bannenberg J, Meijer D. Laparoscopic colon surgery-a difficult operation made easy [abstract]. Surg Endosc 1994;8:992.
5. Bannenberg JJG, Meijer DW, Bannenberg JH, Hodde KC. Hand-assisted laparoscopic nephrectomy in the pig: initial report. Minim Invasive Ther Allied Technol 1996;5:483–7.
6. Nakada SY, Moon TD, Gist M, Mahvi D. Use of the Pneumo Sleeve as an adjunct in laparoscopic nephrectomy. Urology 1997;49:612–3.
7. Keeley FX, Sharma NK, Tolley DA. Hand assisted laparoscopic nephroureterectomy [abstract]. J Urol 1997; 157 (Suppl):399.
8. Wolf JS Jr, Tchetgen MB, Merion RM. Hand-assisted laparoscopic live donor nephrectomy. Urology 1998;52:885–7.
9. Stifelman MD, Handler T, Nieder AM, et al. Hand-assisted laparoscopy for large renal specimens: a multiinstitutional study. Urology 2003;61:78–82.
10. Harano M, Eto M, Omoto K, et al. Long-term outcome of hand-assisted laparoscopic radical nephrectomy for localized stage T1/T2 renal-cell carcinoma. J Endourol 2005; 19:803–7.
11. Li C-C, Chou Y-H, Shen J-T, et al. Comparison of hand-assisted laparoscopic nephroureterectomy with open surgery for upper urinary tract tumor. Kaohsiung J Med Sci 2001;17:615–9.
12. Landman J, Lev R, Bhayani S, et al. Comparison of hand assisted and standard laparoscopic radical nephroureterectomy for the management of localized transitional cell carcinoma. J Urol 2002;167:2387–91.
13. Wong C, Leveillee RJ. Hand-assisted laparoscopic nephroureterectomy with cystoscopic en bloc excision of the distal ureter and bladder cuff. J Endourol 2002;16:329–32.
14. Uozumi J, Fujiyama C, KMeiri H, et al. Hand-assisted retroperitoneoscopic nephroureterectomy for upper urinary-tract urothelial tumors. J Endourol 2002;16:743–7.
15. Munver R, Del Pizzo JJ, Sosa RE. Hand-assisted laparoscopic nephroureterectomy for upper urinary-tract transitional-cell carcinoma. J Endourol 2004;18:351–8.
16. Kawauchi A, Fujito A, Soh J, et al. Hand-assisted retroperitoneoscopic radical nephrectomy and nephroureterectomy. J Endourol 2004;18:365–9.
17. Hsueh TY, Huang Y-H, Chiu AW, et al. A comparison of the clinical outcome between open and hand-assisted laparoscopic nephroureterectomy for upper urinary tract transitional cell carcinoma. BJU Int 2004;94:798–801.
18. Wolf JS Jr, Dash A, Hollenbeck BK, et al. Intermediate follow-up of hand-assisted laparoscopic nephroureterectomy for urothelial carcinoma: factors associated with outcomes. J Urol 2005;173:1102–7.
19. Chen C-H, Wu H-C, Chen W-C, et al. Outcomes of hand-assisted laparoscopic nephroureterectomy for managing upper urinary tract transitional cell carcinoma - China Medical University Hospital experience. Urology 2005; 65:687–91.
20. Gannon GM Jr, Averch T, Colen J, et al. Hand-assisted laparoscopic nephroureterectomy with open cystotomy for removal of the distal ureter and bladder cuff. J Endourol 2005;19:973–5.
21. Brown JA, Strup SE, Chenven E, et al. Hand-assisted laparoscopic nephroureterectomy: analysis of distal ureterectomy technique, margin status, and surgical outcomes. Urology 2005;66:1192–6.
22. Wolf JS Jr, Marcovich R, Merion RM, Konnak JW. Prospective, case-matched comparison of hand-assisted laparoscopic and open surgical live donor nephrectomy. J Urol 2000;163:1650–3.
23. Kercher K, Dahl D, Harland R, et al. Hand-assisted laparoscopic donor nephrectomy minimizes warm ischemia. Urology 2001;58:152–6.
24. Buell JF, Alverdy J, Newell K, et al. Hand-assisted laparoscopic live-donor nephrectomy. J Am Coll Surg 2001;192:132–6.
25. Wolf JS Jr, Merion RM, Leichtman AB, et al. Randomized controlled trial of hand-assisted laparoscopic versus open surgical live donor nephrectomy. Transplantation 2001; 72:284–90.
26. Stifelman MD, Hull D, Sosa RE, et al. Hand assisted laparoscopic donor nephrectomy: a comparison with the open approach. J Urol 2001;166:444–8.
27. Ruiz-Deya G, Cheng S, Palmer E, et al. Open donor, laparoscopic donor and hand assisted laparoscopic donor nephrectomy: a comparison of outcomes. J Urol 2001;166:1270–4.
28. Lindstrom P, Haggman M, Wadstrom J. Hand-assisted laparoscopic surgery (HALS) for live donor nephrectomy is more time- and cost-effective than standard laparoscopic nephrectomy. Surg Endosc 2002;16:422–5.
29. Velidedeoglu E, Williams N, Brayman KL, et al. Comparison of open, laparoscopic, and hand-assisted approaches to live-donor nephrectomy. Transplantation 2002;174:169–72.
30. Gershbein AB, Fuchs GJ. Hand-assisted and conventional laparoscopic live donor nephrectomy: a comparison of two contemporary techniques. J Endourol 2002;16:509–13.
31. Buell JF, Hanaway MJ, Potter SR, et al. Hand-assisted laparoscopic living-donor nephrectomy as an alternative to traditional laparoscopic living-donor nephrectomy. Am J Transplant 2002;2:983–8.
32. Mateo RB, Sher L, Jabbour N, et al. Comparison of outcomes in noncomplicated and in higher-risk donors after standard versus hand-assisted laparoscopic nephrectomy. Am Surg 2003;69:771–8.
33. El-Galley R, Hood N, Young CJ, et al. Donor nephrectomy: a comparison of techniques and results of open, hand assisted and full laparoscopic nephrectomy. J Urol 2004; 171:40–3.
34. Maartense S, Idu M, Bemelman FJ, et al. Hand-assisted laparoscopic live donor nephrectomy. Br J Surg 2004;91: 344–8.
35. Nakajima I, Tojimbara T, Sato S, et al. Hand-assisted laparoscopic live donor nephrectomy: report of 100 cases. Trans Proc 2004;36:1898–1900.
36. Tsuchiya N, Iinuma M, Habnuchi T, et al. Hand-assisted retroperitoneoscopic nephrectomy for living kidney transplantation: initial 44 cases. Urology 2004;64:250–4.
37. Baron PW, Baldwin DD, Hadley HR, et al. Hand-assisted laparoscopic donor nephrectomy is safe and results in increased kidney donation. Amer Surg 2004;70:901–5.
38. Seo SI, Kim JC, Hwangbo K, et al. Comparison of hand-assisted and open donor nephrectomy: a single center experience from South Korea. J Endourol 2005;19:58–62.
39. Wadstrom J. Hand-assisted retroperitoneoscopic live donor nephrectomy: experience from the first 75 consecutive cases. Transplantation 2005;80:1060–6.
40. Maciel RF, Deboni LM, Guterres JC, et al. Hand-assisted laparoscopic nephrectomy versus transperitoneal anterior approach in living donors for renal transplantation. Trans Proc 2005;37:2748–9.
41. Fisher PC, Montgomery JS, Johnston WK III, Wolf JS Jr. 200 consecutive hand-assisted laparoscopic donor nephrectomies: evolution of operative technique and outcomes. J Urol. [In press]
42. Wolf JS Jr, Seifman BD, Montie JE. Nephron-sparing surgery for suspected malignancy: open surgery compared to laparoscopy with selective use of hand-assistance. J Urol 2000;163:1659–64.
43. Stifelman MD, Sosa RE, Nakada SY, Schichman S. Hand-assisted laparoscopic partial nephrectomy. J Endourol 2001;15:161–4.
44. Rehman J, Landman J, Andreoni C, et al. Laparoscopic bilateral hand assisted partial nephrectomy for autosomal dominant polycystic kidney disease: initial experience. J Urol 2001;166:42–7.
45. Rubenstein JN, McVary KT, Nadler RB, Gonzalez CM. Patient positioning and port placement for bilateral hand-assisted laparoscopic nephrectomy. Urology 2002;59:441–3.
46. Troxel S, Das S. Hand-assisted laparoscopic approach to multiple-organ removal. J Endourol 2001;15:895–7.
47. Landman J, Figenshau RS, Bhayani S, et al. Dual-organ ablative surgery using a hand-assisted laparoscopic technique. A report of four cases. J Urol 2002;16:215–6.
48. Sundaram CP, Rehman J, Landman J, Oh J. Hand assisted laparoscopic radical nephrectomy for renal cell carcinoma with inferior vena caval thrombus. J Urol 2002;168: 176–9.
49. Wolf JS Jr, Moon TD, Nakada SY. Hand-assisted laparoscopic nephrectomy: comparison to standard laparoscopic nephrectomy. J Urol 1998;160:22–7.
50. Nelson CP, Wolf JS Jr. Comparison of hand-assisted versus standard laparoscopic radical nephrectomy for suspected renal cell carcinoma. J Urol 2002;167:1989–94.
51. Batler RA, Campbell SC, Funk JT, et al. Hand-assisted vs. retroperitoneal laparoscopic nephrectomy. J Endourol 2001;15:899–902.
52. Baldwin DD, Dunbar JA, Parekh DJ, et al. Single-center comparison of purely laparoscopic, hand-assisted laparoscopic, and open radical nephrectomy in patients at high anesthetic risk. J Endourol 2003;17:161–7.
53. HALS Study Group. Hand-assisted laparoscopic surgery vs standard laparoscopic surgery for colorectal disease: a prospective randomized trial. Surg Endosc 2000;14: 896–901.
54. Targarona EM, Gracia E, Garriga J, et al. Prospective randomized trial comparing conventional laparoscopic colectomy with hand-assisted laparoscopic colectomy: applicability, immediate clinical outcome, inflammatory response, and cost. Surg Endosc 2002;16:234–9.

49

Secondary Trocar Placement

Debora K. Moore, MD
Robert G. Moore, MD

Trocars provide access for performing laparoscopy. Interventional laparoscopy requires one or more trocars to act as conduits for working instruments. Number, size, and arrangement of secondary trocars depend on the type of procedure and the surgeon's individual preference. This chapter will address anterior abdominal wall, general considerations, technique, and rationale for secondary trocar configuration.

ANTERIOR ABDOMINAL WALL ANATOMY

A thorough knowledge of the anterior abdominal wall anatomy is essential for secondary trocar placement. This will decrease the possibility of vascular injury, hernia formation, or loss of access. The abdominal wall muscles are organized into two separate groups: anterolateral and posterior. The quadratus lumborum is the sole muscle in the posterior group.[1] The anterolateral group of abdominal muscles is divided into two subgroups based on the orientation of muscle fibers. The rectus abdominis and pyramidalis are the two vertical muscles of the anterolateral abdominal group. The external abdominal oblique, internal abdominal oblique, and transversus abdominis muscles are three, thin, muscular layers that alternate in their fiber direction. The linea alba is a midline fusion of the aponeurosis of both the external and internal oblique that runs from the xiphoid process to the symphysis pubis. The linea alba is devoid of muscle and is ideal for placement of the primary and secondary trocars.

Blood vessels of the anterolateral abdominal wall that can affect laparoscopic port placement are divided into two groups: superficial (or cutaneous) and deep.[1] Superficial vessels include the superficial epigastric vessels (Figure 49-1). The superficial epigastric artery originates from the femoral artery just below the inguinal ligament. This artery traverses the femoral sheath to course toward the umbilicus in the subcutaneous tissue. Avoidance of these vessels and their branches is possible by transilluminating the abdominal wall.

The deep anterolateral abdominal wall vessels that influence laparoscopic port placement include: superior and inferior epigastric vessels, intercostal vessels, subcostal vessels, and the ascending branch of the deep circumflex iliac vessels (Figure 49-2).[1] The superior epigastric artery is the termination of the internal thoracic artery, and courses downward posterior to the rectus abdominis muscle in the rectus sheath. The inferior epigastric artery originates from the external iliac artery just medial to the deep inguinal ring (lateral to the medial umbilical ligament). The inferior epigastric vessel courses toward the umbilicus and traverses the transversalis fascia at the arcuate line to ascend in the rectus sheath posterior to the rectus muscle. Both the superior and inferior epigastric vessels anastomose near the umbilicus. Both vessels supply numerous branches to the rectus muscle and umbilicus. These vessels are often not seen on transillumination of the abdominal wall with a laparoscope. For this reason, trocar placement through the rectus abdominis muscle should be avoided.

Intercostal vessels (X and XI) and the subcostal vessels traverse the lateral abdominal muscles, coursing in an oblique diagonal fashion from lateral to medial (midline) (Figure 49-2).[1] The ascending branch of the deep circumflex iliac artery originates near the anterior superior spine and ascends toward the costal margin. These vessels are generally not visualized during transillumination of the abdominal wall.

GENERAL CONSIDERATIONS

While ablative laparoscopic urological procedures have led the way in the development of minimally invasive urological procedures, reconstructive urologic procedures are becoming more mainstream. Most reconstructive procedures, while feasible, are technically difficult compared to open or laparoscopic ablative procedures. The most difficult aspect of reconstructive procedures is the necessity for laparoscopic suturing for the anatomizing portion of the procedure. While few studies exist on standardization of laparoscopic intracorporeal suturing and knotting techniques, one thing that is known is that the positioning or placement of the access ports plays a crucial role.

Trocar configuration and placement should be well thought out ahead of time to maximize the utility of each individual cannula. Several basic tenets for trocar placement are useful to the laparoscopist.

Trocars should be placed within the operative field so that the sheath is pointing toward the operative field.[2] Placing the ports in such a manner minimizes resistance when manipulating instruments. Placement of cannulas pointing away from the area of dissection can result in decreased maneuverability and tactile feedback transmitted through the instruments. The force needed to redirect the sheath can cause a tear in the peritonotomy and result in subcutaneous air. Seasoned laparoscopists know that this leads to

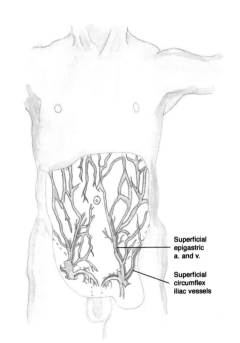

Figure 49-1 Superficial (cutaneous) vessels of the anterolateral abdominal wall.

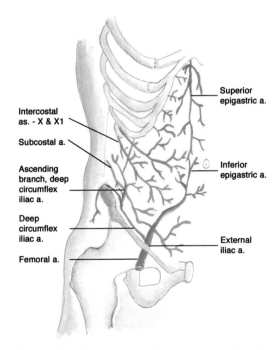

Figure 49-2 Deep arteries of the anterolateral abdominal wall.

leakage of gas at the port site, difficulty keeping the trocar in place, and increases gas absorption. The former events turn even a simple laparoscopic case into a major struggle.

Another known fact is that secondary trocars must be adequately spaced so that external interlocking and internal overlapping of cannulas will not hamper maneuverability. For the novice, prior to secondary trocar placement, individual trocar sites can be mapped with a surgical marking pen to ensure adequate working distance between the trocars. Eventually this can be carried out mentally without actually marking the field.

If one is to use anterior abdominal trocars, they should be placed in the midline or lateral to the rectus muscle to avoid the epigastric vessels and branches. In addition, trocars should be placed away from bony structures because this limits mobility. When the planned procedure requires a dorsal lithotomy or split frog-leg position, lower, laterally placed trocars may pose difficulties. Placement of a secondary trocar at the midline suprapubic area will allow greater trocar movement in these specific cases.

Frede and colleagues described other special considerations given to secondary trocar configurations for laparoscopic reconstructive procedures in which laparoscopic suturing is needed.[3] They discussed three general rules to optimize laparoscopic suturing. First and foremost, they state that "an isosceles triangle trocar instrument arrangement is needed for optimal suturing." Rule two dictates that the angle between laparoscopic instruments be adjusted between the angles of 25° to 45°. Rule three states that the angle between the horizontal plane and instruments should be kept at an angle of less than 55°. According to the authors by using the above general principles they decreased their suturing time by 75%.

Choice of trocar size will vary depending on the size of instruments needed to perform the desired procedure. Trocars routinely used vary in width from 5 to 12 mm. Larger trocars are available for insertion of larger instruments (ie, specialized bowel staplers) and passage of suture material. In most instances one of the secondary trocars should be a 10/12 mm cannula to accommodate larger instruments (eg, clip applicators, tissue removal forceps). The standard trocar length is 10 cm; extra-long trocars (15 cm) are often used in obese patients.

Table 49-1 provides a simple outline for the beginning laparoscopist for specific port and instrument placement for several laparoscopic procedures. This guideline is only a starting point that will be modified with experience and over time by the individual.

TECHNIQUE

After successful creation of the pneumoperitoneum and placement of the initial trocar, secondary trocars are placed under videoendoscopic vision. Prior to trocar placement the intra-abdominal pressure is increased to ≥ 20 mm Hg. This increases the rigidity of the anterior

Table 49-1 Optimal Trocar/Instrument Position for Retroperitoneoscopic Laparoscopic Procedures			
Procedure	Video Endoscope	Suturing	Dissector
Nondismembered Pyeloplasty			
R	Petit's triangle	Above iliac crest	Subcostal
L	Petit's triangle	Subcostal	Above iliac crest
Dismembered Pyeloplasty			
R	Petit's triangle	Anterior axillary Medial trocar	Above iliac crest
L	Subcostal	Petit's Triangle	Above iliac crest
Nephropexy			
R	Petit's triangle	Above iliac crest	Subcostal
L	Petit's triangle	Subcostal	Above iliac crest
Radical Prostatectomy			
	Umbilical	R lower Medial	L upper Lateral
Bladder Neck Suspension			
	Umbilical	R lower Medial	L upper Lateral

R = right; L = left.
Adapted from Frede T, et al.[3]

wall providing a stronger platform, which facilitates the downward trocar placement. The room is darkened and the laparoscope is used to transilluminate the anterior abdominal wall. This helps visualize the superficial anterior abdominal wall vessels, which aids in avoiding these structures. After the appropriate trocar site is selected, preemptive analgesics are injected into the area, and a skin incision just large enough to admit the trocar is made along Langer's lines. The subcutaneous tissue is spread with a clamp to push the superficial vessels away from the trocar entry site. The secondary trocar site is checked by pushing downward at the site on the abdominal wall. While watching the interior structures via the camera, the appropriate entry site is recognized by the deformity of the peritoneal surface and is deemed safe or another site is chosen. Again, epigastric or abdominal wall vessels should be avoided.

For the traditional cutting trocar, the technique for placement is as follows. The trocar is held in the palm of the dominant hand with the middle finger extended to act as a brake.[4] If a shielded trocar (a trocar with a safety shield) is used, the shield should be in the set position. The side port stopcock is closed prior to placement. The cannula is placed in the direction of the dissection. But if two separate operative fields are required, as in a nephrourerterectomy, the trocars are placed perpendicular to the abdominal wall.

All secondary cannulas are placed under laparoscopic monitoring. The trocar is checked so that it fits into the incision site. An insufficient skin opening can result in excess force required to enter the peritoneal cavity. Forward pressure is applied using a slow continuous right-to-left twisting motion. The trocar tip is visualized as it enters the abdominal cavity by the deformity of the peritoneum (Figure 49-3). As the trocar tip

comes close to the underlying viscera, it is redirected up and away from the viscera. Once the trocar tip is in the abdominal cavity, the safety shield springs forward. The trocar is advanced further into the abdominal cavity until the sheath is within the peritoneal cavity. The inner obturator is then removed, and the sheath is advanced 1 to 2 cm within the peritoneal cavity.

Once the trocar is placed, it should be fixed in place to prevent accidental removal during dissection. Several manufacturers have integrated retentive grooves built into the sheath or make detachable retentive grooves to prevent movement of the trocar sheath (Figure 49-4). In contrast to inte-

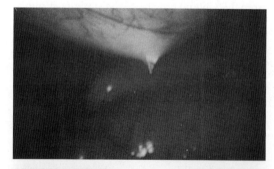

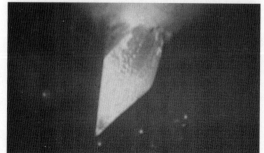

Figure 49-3 Direct visual placement of a secondary trocar.

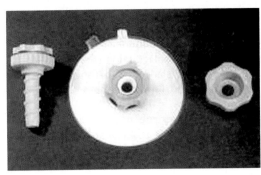

Figure 49-4 Detachable retentive grooves allow for the intra-abdominal portion of the cannula to be adjusted and they prevent inadvertent removal of the trocar from the abdominal wall.

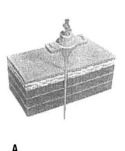 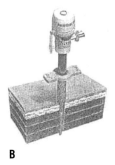 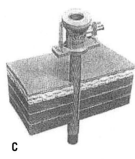

A **B** **C**

Figure 49-6 The mesh-like expandable sleeve of the Step Access System (Weck Closure Systems, Research Triangle Park, NC) is back-loaded over a Veress insufflation needle and introduced in the peritoneal cavity in standard fashion (A). After removal of the Veress needle the mesh-sleeve is expanded to the desired diameter (5-12 mm) by a blunt tipped obturator and cannula under direct laparoscopic vision (B). The obturator is removed and the cannula/mesh is adjusted until 2 cm of cannula is placed in the peritoneal cavity (C). Adapted from Moore et al.[19,20]

grated grooves, detachable grooves allow adjustment of the depth of placement without changing the trocar. Other retentive devices include "Malecot" or balloon-tipped sheaths. Trocars can also be secured by placing a suture through the skin and tying the suture to the sidearm port (Figure 49-5). This suture prevents the trocar from being pulled out of the abdominal cavity while allowing the operator to advance the trocar further into the peritoneal cavity. Suturing the port in place is useful when operating deep within the pelvis.

New to the laparoscopic lineup are radial dilating trocars (Figure 49-6). The advantages of these trocars over cutting trocars in randomized comparison studies are numerous. Radial dilating trocars have fewer entry complications, plus less gas leakage, trocar site bleeding, and hernia formation. In addition, the studies have demonstrated less postoperative pain at the trocar site with the radial dilating trocars versus the traditional cutting trocars.[5–7]

Radial dilating secondary trocars are placed under direct vision. A skin incision is made to admit the desired trocar size. The expandable mesh sleeve is back-loaded onto a 14-gauge Veress needle. With no dissection of the subcutaneous tissue, this apparatus is passed through the

abdominal wall under direct vision. The inner Veress needle is removed, and a blunt-tipped fascial dilator is back-loaded with its corresponding cannula through a sleeve. It is critical to hold countertraction with the nondominant hand while passing the dilator/cannula with the dominant hand. This step is facilitated by using a constant right-to-left twisting downward pressure. Care is taken to prevent inadvertant injury to intra-abdominal organs. Once the canula has been passed through the abdominal wall, the obturator is removed and the canula depth is adjusted. No stay suture is needed to secure the radial dilating trocars. The fascial defect is reported to be one-half of that of the traditional cutting trocar.

Ultrasonically activated trocar systems are the latest addition to the trocar armamentarium (SonoSurg G2, Olympus, Tokyo, Japan).[8–9] The 5-mm pyramidal tip is activated with a frequency of 23.5 kHz and amplitude of 150 μm (Figure 49-7 and Figure 49-8). The trocar fits a 5-mm plastic sheath that is introduced inside a 10-mm dilator with a conical tip. The plastic sheath isolates the abdominal muscles from the lateral spread of ultrasonic energy once the tip has passed the tissue.

After making a skin incision at the desired port site, the tip is applied to the abdominal wall and the generator is activated via a foot pedal. The power of the ultrasonic generator (which is the same generator used for the Olympus harmonic scalpel) is set at 100%, the power necessary for a cutting effect. The trocar tip penetrates the abdominal wall by a combination of ultrasonic vibration and gravity without force applied to the trocar. Once the trocar tip has passed the peritoneum, the plastic sleeve is pushed in, the trocar is withdrawn, and the 10-mm dilator/cannula is inserted using the plastic sleeve as a guide. The dilator is then removed and only the cannula remains in place.

The ultrasonic trocar is available in only a 5-mm diameter since insertion of a 5-, 10-, or 12-mm cannula is then made by expansion of the port site. In a basic science comparison study, Gossot and colleagues compared the conventional cutting (pyramidal tip) trocar to the ultrasonic trocar. Peak force ranged from 4.8 kg-Force (KgF) to 9.2 KgF (mean of 6.8 KgF) using conventional trocars, versus 0.2 to 0.6 KgF (mean of 0.4) for the

ultrasonic trocar. The reported average time needed for trocar insertion was lower with ultrasonic trocars at 4.5 s (range 1.5 to 8.5 s) versus 12.8 s (range 4.0 to 21 s) using ultrasonic versus conventional trocars, respectively. Lastly, there was little to no increase in abdominal pressure during trocar insertion with the ultrasonic trocar (range, 0 to 2 mm Hg; average, 0.85 mm Hg) while the insertion of the conventional trocar resulted in a significant increase in abdominal pressure (range, 4 to 11 mm Hg; average, 7.6 mm Hg).[8]

Risk factors for trocar injuries include; lack of experience, peritoneal adhesions, patient conformation and trocar tip shape. However, the main factor is the need to exert force on the trocar. The more force that needs to be applied, the more hazardous the insertion because the trocar may escape and hit any organ. The ultrasonic trocar system offers theoretical advantages compared to the conventional trocars. The ultrasonic system should reduce bleeding, incisional hernia rate, and postoperative pain. Advantages to the ultrasonic trocar system include ease of insertion with minimal force and expected decrease in cost because it can be sterilized with an autoclave, which makes it reusable. Clinical trials are currently underway to verify these claims.

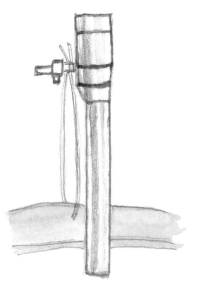

Figure 49-5 A retentive suture can also be used to prevent accidental removal of a trocar. Reproduced with permission from Clayman RV.[2]

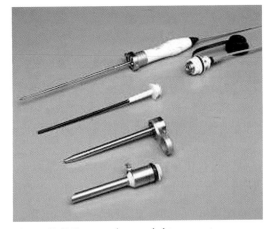

Figure 49-7 Sonosurg intergraded trocar system components. From top to bottom: cutting Sonosurg end-effector, insulation sleeve, fascial dilating sleeve, and nondisposable trocar cannula.

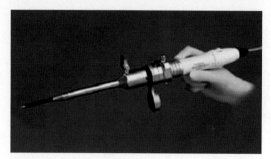

Figure 49-8 Proper grip for completely assembled Sonosurg ultrasonic trocar system.

PRIMARY TROCAR SITE INSPECTION After the initial secondary trocar has been placed, a laparoscope is passed through this cannula. The primary trocar site is inspected at its entry point into the peritoneal cavity.[2] If any abdominal viscera (eg, omentum, bowel) have been traversed, appropriate reparative actions must be initiated. This is also the optimal time to secure the primary trocar to the abdominal wall. Additional secondary trocars are placed as outlined above.

EXCHANGING TROCARS Occasionally, trocars must be exchanged to increase the size of the trocar (ie, 5 to 10/12 mm sheath) or to correct a trocar defect (ie, gas leak).[2,10] Exchanging a cannula for the same size sheath can be accomplished by passing an appropriately sized solid metal bar or Amplatz dilator (5 mm sheath = 16F; 10 mm sheath = 30F). When using the Amplatz dilators to interchange trocars, an 8F Amplatz catheter should be passed first, followed by the appropriate dilator. Interchanging a smaller sheath (5 mm) for a larger sheath (10/12 mm) can be performed by first placing an 8F Amplatz catheter. A 16F Amplatz dilator is placed over the 8F catheter and the 5 mm trocar sheath is removed. Sequential Amplatz dilators are used until the 30F dilator is reached. The 10 mm sheath is then placed over the 30F dilator. Exchange of a radial dilating trocar from a smaller size to larger size simply entails increasing the skin incision and removing the smaller cannula and placing the larger cannula obturator through the sleeve.[5]

SECONDARY TROCAR CONFIGURATION

Selection of trocar size and secondary trocar arrangement depends on the type of procedure and the surgeon's individual preference. Individual surgeons may choose different trocar configurations based on the patient's body habitus, surgical approach (transperitoneal versus extraperitoneal), and availability of specialized instruments. This section will give some basic startup secondary trocar arrangements for specific urologic procedures.

PELVIC PROCEDURES Laparoscopic urologic pelvic procedures are performed with two different types of trocar arrangements: a fan or diamond array.[3,10–12] Procedures using the fan or diamond configurations include pelvic lym-

phadenectomy, bladder neck suspension, and radical prostatectomy.

In both of these trocar configurations, at least two 10/12 mm trocars are needed. One 10/12 mm port is used for the camera, and the other port is used for passage of suture material or to remove tissue. The fan configuration is advantageous because this allows use of both hands (Figure 49-9) and has been advocated for use in obese patients. A modified fan configuration (Figure 49-10) was designed for laparoscopic radical prostatectomies. In this configuration, the lower trocars are moved from lateral to a medial or paramedian position. The upper trocars are moved slightly lateral to the midclavicular line. This rearrangement allows specialized suturing instruments to reach deep into the pelvis where one may need to perform a vesicourethral anastomosis or it may be useful in laparoscopic bladder neck suspension. Using this trocar configuration, Frede and colleagues recommended specific tasks for each trocar when performing a radical prostatectomy or a bladder neck suspension (see Table 49-1).[3]

For pelvic procedures, the patient is often positioned in a dorsal lithotomy position. In this position, the diamond trocar (Figure 49-11) array gives the surgeon maximal freedom in moving the suprapubic trocar. One also needs to be aware that the medial umbilical ligament can interfere with instruments passed through the lower midline trocar of the diamond configuration. The diamond configuration is also used when a pelvic lymphadenectomy is being performed in conjunction with a laparoscopic-assisted perineal prostatectomy.

Bladder Neck Suspension When using a diamond trocar array (see Figure 49-11) in performing a Burch bladder neck suspension, secondary trocar size depends on the reconstructive instrumentation used.[13,14] For example, if an Endostitch suturing device is used, all trocars placed will be 10/12 mm. If conventional suturing is used for

securing the anterior vaginal wall to Cooper's ligament, then 5 mm trocars can be substituted. Alternatively, Frede and colleagues recommended a modified fan configuration (see Figure 49-10) for laparoscopic bladder neck suspension.[3]

Varix Ligation/Orchiopexy When performing a varix ligation (unilateral or bilateral), three trocars are usually needed (Figure 49-12).[15] They are arranged in a triangular configuration. In addition to the primary umbilical 10/12 mm trocar or a 5 mm trocar for the camera, two secondary trocars are placed in the midclavicular line at the level of the anterior superior iliac spine. One of these midclavicular trocars is used for clipping the spermatic veins. This trocar arrangement also can be used when clipping the spermatic vessels in a staged orchiopexy.

Several 5 mm secondary trocars are needed to perform a laparoscopic primary orchiopexy for the treatment of intra-abdominal testes (Figure 49-13).[16] A 5 mm umbilical primary trocar is needed for the camera. Two 5 mm trocars are placed in the midclavicular line at the level of the anterior superior spine for dissection of the spermatic vessels. A final 5 mm trocar is placed through the scrotum into the peritoneal cavity for transfer of the intra-abdominal testes into the scrotum. This is accomplished by back-feeding a 5 mm trocar over a 5 mm straight grasper that has been passed through the midclavicular trocar (ipsilateral to the intra-abdominal testes) over the pubic ramus and through the scrotal incision.

Ureter Port placement to access the abdominal ureter includes a port placed just lateral to the umbilicus. Another port is placed below the costal margin in the midclavicular line, and the third trocar is positioned in the lower ipsilateral quadrant in the midclavicular line (Figure 49-14). Trocar placement for the lower pelvic ureter includes a trocar at the umbilicus and one to two ports in each lower quadrant, 2 cm medial to the corresponding anterior iliac spine. This

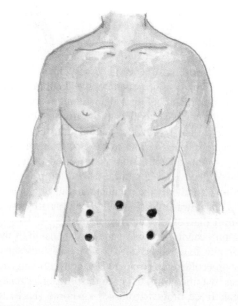

Figure 49-9 Fan configuration has been commonly used for performing pelvic lymph node dissection.

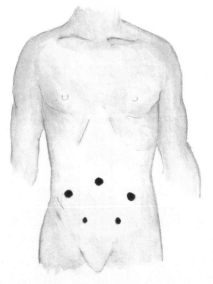

Figure 49-10 Modified fan configuration has been commonly used for laparoscopic radical prostatectomy and retropubic bladder neck suspension.

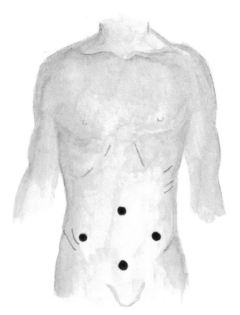

Figure 49-11 The diamond trocar configuration is used for either pelvic lymphadenectomy or bladder neck suspension.

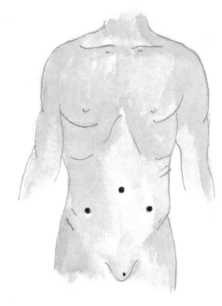

Figure 49-13 This trocar configuration is used for a primary orchiopexy. A 5-mm scrotal trocar is used to deliver the testicle into the scrotum.

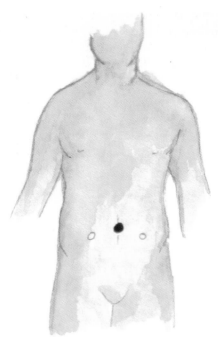

Figure 49-15 Trocar arrangement for access to the pelvic ureter. A triangular arrangement is advocated with a 10/12-mm port at the umbilicus and two 5-mm ports as shown.

configuration provides optimal access to the pelvic ureter from the iliac vessels to the ureterovesical junction (Figure 49-15). When access to the entire ureter is a concern, a combination port placement is necessary (Figure 49-16). Three to four trocars are required to perform a transperitoneal laparoscopic procedure on the upper ureter.[17] A periumbilical 12 mm primary trocar is used for the videoendoscope. A 10/12 mm trocar is placed in the midclavicular line at the level of the umbilicus. Two 5 mm trocars are used, one in the epigastric area and one in the anterior axillary line between the iliac crest and the twelfth rib. Suture passage is via the midclavicular trocar, while suturing is performed via both the mid-clavicular and epigastric trocars

(port placement for pyeloplasty or ureterolysis is seen in Figures 49-17 and 49-18). Ureterolithotomy port placement is dependent on whether the upper or lower ureter is involved. A stone located in the upper ureter can be approached similar to a pyeloplasty procedure, while for lower ureteral stones, the 10 mm port is placed contralateral to the side to be addressed (Figure 49-19).

RENAL PROCEDURES Nephrectomy Three to five trocars are needed to carry out a transperitoneal laparoscopic nephrectomy and other laparoscopic renal surgeries (Figure 49-20).[18] A 10/12 mm periumbilical cannula is used for the

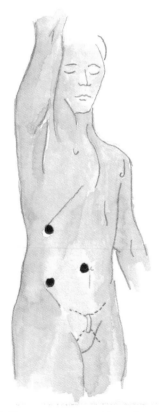

Figure 49-14 Three trocars are used to perform a reconstructive upper ureteral procedure. An optional 5-mm trocar can be placed in the anterior axillary line for refraction of a large redundant renal pelvis and the exit point for a retroperitoneal drain.

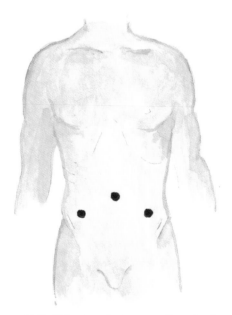

Figure 49-12 This triangular trocar configuration is used for varix ligation (unilateral or bilateral).

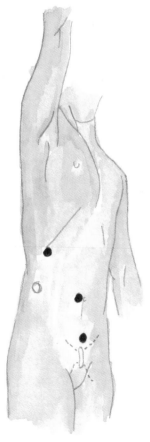

Figure 49-16 Combination port placement for access to the entire ureter.

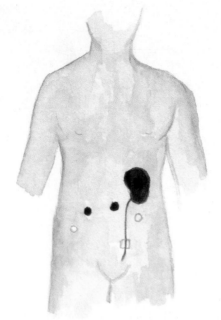

Figure 49-19 Trocar configuration for a left lower laparoscopic ureterolithotomy. Place the 10/12-mm port contralateral to the side in question.

Figure 49-17 Port placement for laparoscopic pyeloplasty is similar to the abdominal ureter port placement. However, an additional 5-mm trocar may be placed in the anterior axillary line midway between the costal margin and iliac crest.

camera. The dissection ports are placed at the epigastric and midclavicular position similar to the positioning used for performing a laparoscopic procedure on the upper ureter. If an endovascular

stapler or vascular bulldog clamp is to be used for vascular control, one or both of these trocars needs to be a 10/12 mm trocar(s). Additional laterally placed trocars are used for retraction of the renal helium, lateral dissection or suture repair as well as treatment probe insertion for nephron-sparing procedures. In all cases, the lateral trocars are either 5 or 8 mm in size; the exception is during cytoreductive nephrectomy when an endovascular stapler is needed to control the parasitic vessels. In this case, 10/12 mm lateral trocars are used.

Retroperitoneoscopic Nephrectomy Retroperitoneoscopic nephrectomy and renal surgery require an entirely different trocar arrangement. These trocar configurations are often "tighter" with less distance between the cannulas, which is reflective of the much smaller working space of the retroperitoneum compared to the peritoneal cavity. A triangular/diamond configuration is used (Figure 49-21). The initial trocar (10/12 mm) is placed off the tip of the twelfth rib and between the iliac crest. Additional trocars are placed in Petit's triangle (10/12mm) and the anterior axillary line. A fourth and fifth port is optional. The camera site is usually the most dependent cannula. However, the videoendoscope is often moved to other trocars to facilitate the procedure.

Nephroureterectomy Trocar configuration for laparoscopic nephroureterectomy is identical to the configuration for the laparoscopic nephrectomy. An additional suprapubic port is used to secure the bladder cuff. (Figure 49-22) Some surgeons use a vascular GIA stapler to complete this task. When using the GIA stapler, a 10/12 mm suprapubic trocar is needed. Other surgeons perform primary resection with subsequent conventional suturing reconstruction of the bladder. This requires a 5 mm trocar.

Donor Nephrectomy Laparoscopic transperitoneal donor nephrectomy requires the same three primary trocars used for laparoscopic simple nephrectomy, with additional retraction trocars. For left laparoscopic donor nephrectomy. a 15-mm suprapubic trocar is used for medial retraction of the bowel (Figure 49-23). For right-sided procedures, this trocar is moved upward to the epigastric region (Figure 49-23B). Trocar configuration for left-sided, hand-assist, donor

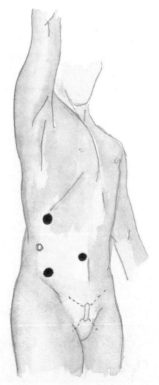

Figure 49-18 Port placement for laparoscopic ureterolysis is similar to the laparoscopic pyeloplasty. In this case the 5-mm port is used for retraction.

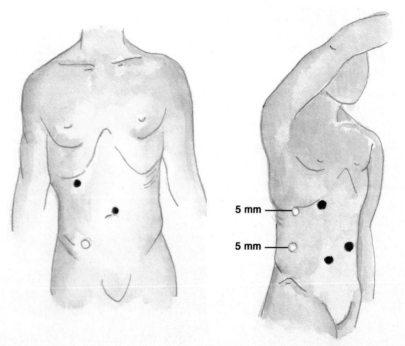

5 mm

5 mm

Figure 49-20 Two 12-mm ports are placed initially at the umbilicus and upper midclavicular line. Three other ports may be 5-mm ports and are placed at the lower midclavicular line, lower anterior axillary line, and upper anterior axillary line. At times the upper axillary line port may be changed out for a 12 mm port.

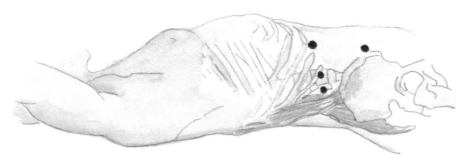

Figure 49-21 Trocar configuration for a retroperitoneoscopic nephrectomy. One may start with all 10/12-mm ports and with time and experience convert some ports to 5-mm ports.

nephrectomy starts with an epigastric-placed hand-assist device. In addition, two 12 mm ports are placed at the umbilicus and mid-clavicular area with an optional (if retraction is needed) lateral 5 mm port placed at the anterior axillary line.

Partial Nephrectomy/Calyceal Diverticulectomy During laparoscopic partial nephrectomy or caliceal diverticulum resection, laterally placed trocars are used for renal resection, renal reconstruction, or drain placement. In the morbidly obese patient, it is important to remember to move all trocars laterally and place the midline trocars in the paramedian line.[19]

Hand-assist Nephrectomy The trocar configuration for hand-assist laparoscopic nephrectomy (HALN) is very different from both transperitoneal and retroperitoneal laparoscopic nephrectomy. Secondary trocar arrange-

ment is dependant on placement of the hand-assist device and is arranged to optimize visualization with the camera port and dissection with the two working instruments. As with traditional laparoscopic procedures, these three ports are arranged in triangular configurations. For left-sided HALN, the hand-assist device is placed within the periumbilical area, with the working port and camera ports placed in the midclavicular line and anterior axillary line, respectively (Figure 49-24A). For right-sided HALN, the hand-assist device is placed in the right lower quadrant, with the working and camera ports placed in the periumbilical area and epigastric area, respectively (Figure 49-24 B).

Adrenal Laparoscopic adrenalectomy has multiple trocar placement configurations depending on approach, transperitoneal versus retroperitoneal versus thoracic and side of interest right or

left-sided. For right sided transperitoneal adrenalectomy, the trocars are arranged in a circular configuration. The camera port (10/12 mm) is placed in the periumbilical region. The dissection trocars are positioned in the anterior axillary and midaxillary line. A fourth port is placed between the two above-mentioned trocars and is used for retraction of the liver (Figure 49-25). An optional fifth port can be placed in the posterior axillary line to retract the upper pole of the kidney. Trocars are placed in a similar fashion for performing a left transperitoneal adrenalectomy.

For the retroperitoneoscopic adrenalectomy, the access ports are positioned later over the retroperitoneal space. The camera port is placed below the tip of the twelfth rib for both the left and right retroperitoneal approach. A posterior trocar is placed directly below the camera port in the angle between the twelfth rib and the paraspinous muscle. An anterior port is placed directly medial to the camera port in the anterior axillary line. Occasionally, additional retraction trocars are placed superior to the iliac crest to assist in retraction of the liver and inferior vena cava for right retroperitoneoscopic adrenalectomy. Lastly, Gill and colleagues have reported thorascopic transdiaphrag-

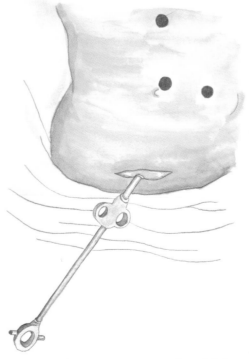

Figure 49-23 Trocar arrangement for a left laparoscopic donor nephrectomy. A suprapubic "thoracoport" and Endo-catch II entrapment device may be useful at the extraction site.

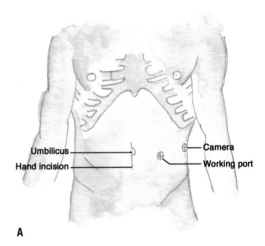

A

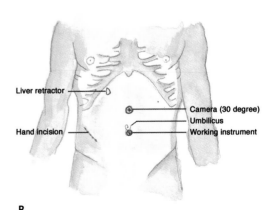

B

Figure 49-24 *A,* Hand-assist device and trocar configuration for left-sided hand-assist nephrectomy. *B,* Hand-assist device and trocar configuration for right-sided hand-assist nephrectomy.

Figure 49-22 Trocar arrangement for laparoscopic nephroureterectomy. The 12-mm port is used for passing the GIA stapler across the bladder cuff. Again placing a 5-mm port for retraction is optional.

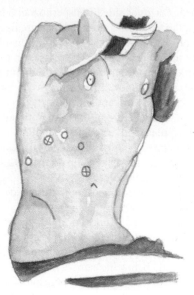

Figure 49-25 Four ports are typically used for a transperitoneal laparoscopic adrenalectomy. The first trocar is usually placed in the anterior axillary line. The next two are placed under direct vision at the subcostal midclavicular and midline. After the kidney has been identified, a fourth trocar may be placed subcostally in the posterior axillary line.

matic adrenalectomy with four-port configuration depicted in Figure 49-26.

Retroperitoneal Lymph Node Dissection
Four to five ports are usually used. Some surgeons recommend only 10/12 mm ports to allow maximal flexibility, and it enables use of larger

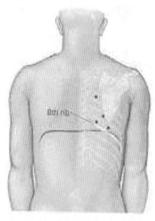

Figure 49-26 Trocar configuration using Gill's right transthoracoscopic approach to an adrenalectomy.

grasping forceps for specimen retrieval. Port positioning for laparoscopic retroperitoneal lymph node dissection for testicular cancer is a diamond-shaped configuration with the camera port at the umbilicus. Two 12 mm working ports are placed in the mid-clavicular line, one at the costal margin and one at the level of the anterior superior spine. A lateral retraction port is placed in the anterior axillary line at the level of the umbilicus (Figure 49-27).

CONCLUSION

With careful planning, secondary trocars can be placed safely and effectively under videoendoscopic vision. For surgeons who are early on in the learning curve, we recommend using an established trocar placement for a given procedure and suggest modifying them as one gains

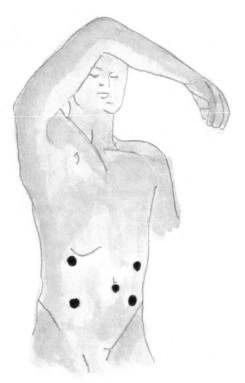

Figure 49-27 Trocar positioning is in an "X" arrangement for a right retroperitoneal lymphadenectomy for testicular cancer. Usually the surgeon will use laparoscopic scissors at the infraumbilical port and grasping forceps at the lower quadrant port. The contralateral port is optional and may be used by an assistant. The upper right quadrant port is the camera site.

experience to fit personal preferences and one's own experience with established trocar arrangements. As the experienced laparoscopic surgeon well knows, the prudent arrangement of the laparoscopic trocars can mean the difference between an effortlessly orchestrated procedure versus a tiresome melee.

REFERENCES

1. Woodburne RT. The abdomen. In: Essentials of human anatomy. 7th ed. New York: Oxford University Press; 1983. p. 367–88.
2. Clayman RV. Secondary trocar placement. In: Clayman RV, McDougall EM, editors. Laparoscopic urology. St. Louis: Quality Medical Publishing; 1993. p. 66–85.
3. Frede T, Stock C, Rassweiler JJ, Alken P. Retroperitoneoscopic suturing: tips and strategies for improving efficiency. J Endourol 2000;14:905–14.
4. Hulka JB. Abdominal entry. In: Hulka JF, editor. Textbook of laparoscopy. Orlando: Grune & Stratton; 1985. p. 61–73.
5. Rubenstein JN, Blunt LW, Lin WW, et al. Safety and efficacy of 12-mm radial dilating ports for laparoscopic access. BJU Int 2003; 92:327–9.
6. Bhouryl S, Payne J, Steffes B, et al. A randomized prospective study of radial expanding trocars in laparoscopic surgery. J Gastrointest Surg 2000;4:392–7.
7. Feste JR, Bojahr B, Turner DJ. Randomized trial comparing a radial expandable needle system with cutting trocars. JSLS 2000;4:11–5.
8. Gossot D, Validire P, Matsumoto S, et al. Development of an ultrasonically activated trocar system: preliminary experimental evaluation. Surg Endosc 2002;16:210–4.
9. Yamakawa T, Kitano S, Kimura T, Matsumoto S. New integrated ultrasonic surgical system 'Sonosurg'. Digestive Endoscopy 2002;14:163–6.
10. Clayman RV. Secondary trocar placement. In: Soper NJ, Odem RR, Clayman RV, McDougall EM, editors. Essentials of laparoscopy. St. Louis: Quality Medical Publishing; 1993. p. 82–103.
11. Moore RG, Kavoussi LR. Laparoscopic lymphadenectomy in genitourinary malignancies. Surg Oncol 1993;2 (Suppl 1):51.
12. Loughlin KR, Kavoussi LR. Laparoscopic lymphadenectomy in the staging of prostate cancer. Contemp Urol 1992; 4:69.
13. Vancaille TG, Schuessler W. Laparoscopic bladder neck suspension. Laparoendosc Surg 1991;1:169.
14. Polascik TJ, Moore RG, Rosenburg MT, Kavoussi LR. Comparison of laparoscopic and open retropubic urethropexy for treatment of stress urinary incontinence. Urology 1995;45:647.
15. Donovan JF, Winfield HN. Laparoscopic varix ligation. J Urol 1992;142:77.
16. Docimo S, Moore RG, Kavoussi LR. Laparoscopic orchiopexy for the palpable true undescended testicle: Preliminary experience [Abstract]. J Endourol 1994;8 (Suppl 1):95.
17. Kavoussi LR, Peters CA. Laparoscopic pyeloplasty. J Urol 1993;150:1811.
18. Kavoussi LR, Kerbl K, Capelouto CC, et al. Laparoscopic nephrectomy for renal neoplasms. Urology 1993;42:603.
19. Textbook of minimially invasive urology. Moore, Bishoff, Loening, Docimo, editors. London: Martin-Dentiz Publishing; Chapters 16 & 34, 2005.

Minimally Invasive Urologic Reconstructive Techniques: Suture, Staple, and Clip Technology

Michael E. Moran, MD

INTRODUCTION

In the overall emergence of endourology, there has been a rapid diaspora of such technologies and philosophy into all areas of urology; so much so, in fact, that there is no area in the whole spectrum of genitourinary surgery that has remained untouched by advancements that were once the "staple" (pun intended) of this specialty. Now, faced with the pervasiveness of minimally invasive modalities in every aspect of genitourinary surgery, it is now a monumental effort to broadly characterize current trends of just one aspect of endourology-reconstructive techniques. Sakti Das has quipped recently that laparoscopic urology has passed through four phases of progress. First was the phase of initial exposure, where diagnostic laparoscopy was used to identify undescended testes. Second was the phase of initial exploration heralded by Howard Winfield's research work from Washington University and presented at the 1988 American Urologic Association meeting and followed by Ralph Clayman's first laparoscopic nephrectomy. The third phase was the decline in laparoscopic urologic surgery, thought by many to be secondary to limited benefits of certain "high-volume" procedures such as pelvic lymph node dissection and varicocelectomy. The fourth, or current phase, is the re-emergence of more complex laparoscopic urologic procedures.[1] Technology is the driving force behind this re-emergence and possibly represents the inherent appeal of minimally invasive surgery to patients, and nowhere is this more evident than with the recent and burgeoning robotic urologic realm.[2] Yet, as rapid as this evolution has occurred, there is ongoing the incursion of the next newest technology, telerobotics, into the urologic armamentarium. Technology has been a fundamental characteristic of humanity since we first evolved from our homo cousins. Tekne⁻ comes from the Greek root that means "art" or "craft," and logia means "the study of."

Proceeding with advances in laparoscopic urologic reconstructive techniques, the technology is rapidly progressing, especially in surgical robotics. In addition, as with the previous edition of this textbook, series remain small in some areas, but are rapidly expanding in others. One must fight the tendency to view such series with skepticism. However, the exact opposite extreme is likewise not necessarily true. Technologic surgery in its infancy arouses justifiable concerns,

but some simple facts remain. First, patients who are given an option of a less invasive alternative will in many instances opt for it, regardless of sufficient evidence to support that decision. Next is the continual availability of newer technologies (ie, telerobotic surgical systems) that potentially can make even the most arduous reconstructive techniques widely available. Third is the fact that a new genre of surgeons are now available who have been exposed to these technologies and the laparoscopic environment for their entire careers. I have interviewed a young fourth-year resident recently at an epicenter program of advanced technologic laparoscopic teaching who has never seen an open radical prostatectomy! It is little wonder that this field is exploding. Finally, there is growing basic scientific evidence that the patients are really benefiting from being less cut upon. The nay-saying philosophy of "why work through a keyhole when you can just walk through the door" is being eroded. There are growing numbers of studies indicating that minimally invasive laparoscopic surgeries cause less catecholamine response, less catabolic insult, fewer intra-abdominal adhesions, etc. There are real reasons that this type of surgery will continue to advance and expand. But do not expect complacency from our current reconstructive methods, no matter how sophisticated they might now appear. Evolving already are even less invasive "natural-orifice" surgeries that are just beginning to emerge as the next great era in surgical evolution. The laparoscopic methods that are so diligently sought in this chapter, that we the practicing urologists have sought to master for the past decade, are about to be wiped out or at best redefined by the boundaries of this next level of less invasive surgery.[3]

Having stated in a somewhat circuitous way that things are about to change in rapid fashion, one could just throw out all the previous concepts about reconstructive techniques presented in the past edition of *Smith's Endourology*. Doing so, though, would not provide the rich historical context that is classically considered necessary to master a complex skill such as the reconstruction of a human viscus. The argument that an intelligent machine-driven database could synthesize and provide the exact same experience in a fraction of the time, and being linked to a surgical end effector would probably make this herculean effort laughable. But, like Sisyphus, the author feels compelled to be as complete and current as

possible, so once again into the breach of reconstructive surgery we will plod.

RECONSTRUCTION TIMELINE

The early history of laparoscopic surgery is dominated by diagnostic endeavors of those interested in hepatobiliary and gynecologic pathology. The instruments and procedures were necessarily limited. With the advent of more complex operative tasks, the gynecologists became increasingly interested in the capability of reproducing what were previously open surgical interventions as laparoscopic procedures. The need to suture was clear as long ago as 1972, when Clarke described a series of instruments and techniques applicable to gynecologic surgery.[4] Extracorporeal knots and the search for methods of placing ligatures followed.[5] The adaptation of an otolaryngologist's suture ligature for tonsillectomies was incorporated into the routine practices of innovative laparoscopic gynecologic surgeons.[6] The Roeder knot was probably the first of a series of extracorporeally tied knots that could be slipped tightly so as to achieve hemostasis or tissue realignment (Figure 50-1). Weston described several other variations, which are derived from fishing and sailing knots (Figure 50-2).[7] All of the extracorporeal knots do not improve the endoscopic surgeon's ability to place sutures or perform an entire anastomosis intracorporeally. Specifically designed laparoscopic suturing instruments have been available only for the last 2 years. The problems of instruments designed to both gently reapproximate tissues and firmly grasp laparoscopic needles has been a difficult manufacturing goal. Endoscopic suturing devices

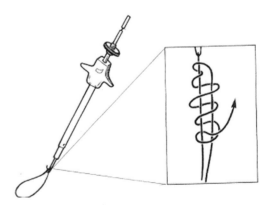

Figure 50-1 Roeder loop knot.

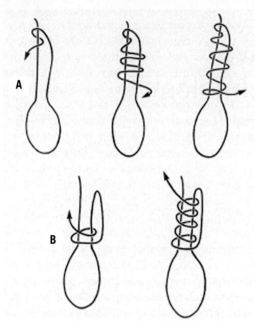

Figure 50-2 Other types of extracorporeally tied slipknot configurations. A, Roeder vs B, Duncan vs C, jamming loop knot.

will be discussed in detail later, but recently, a one-handed automatic suturing instrument utilizing the principles of a loom is being marketed. Such instruments are allowing endoscopic surgeons to rapidly reproduce even the most arduous urologic reconstructive procedures.

Surgical stapling has its foundations in the large, cumbersome prototypes investigated and utilized by the Russians during the 1950s.[8] In the United States, these instruments were investigated and rapidly achieved widespread surgical utilization in the 1970s.[9] A large number of metallic stapling devices have since been developed, and it should be no surprise that these mechanical systems should be rapidly incorporated into the newer laparoscopic techniques. Limitations imposed by a closed laparoscopic environment would favor a quick mechanical system to achieve hemostasis or reconstruct an organ. Laparoscopic utilization of a linear stapler was initially utilized for intracorporeal bowel resections and reconstruction utilizing a functional end-to-end technique.[10,11] Urologic adaptation for controlled hemostatic renal pedicle division during nephrectomy and for the distal portion of a nephroureterectomy have been reported.[12–14] The device has also been used to aid in the formation of a laparoscopic ileal conduit.[15] As with all such technologies, advantages and disadvantages have become apparent, and modifications of the endoscopic staplers have occurred, in fact, the staples themselves have been recently modified. Despite these advances, metallic staples within the urinary tract provide a foreign body nidus with well-recognized risks of encrustation and stone formation. To overcome this problem, absorbable staples have been developed for investigational purposes.[16–18] Biofragmentable rings have been developed for sutureless intestinal anastomoses.[19,20] Clip technology

has advanced since the last edition of this textbook. Now available from four different manufactures are endoscopic clip applicators that are in the 5 mm category. Each of the laparoscopic clip appliers has had changes, and review of the recent literature is vital to understanding the nuances between these devices.

In the early 1990s, urologists at centers committed to advancing laparoscopic procedures persisted despite the "national decline" in urologic laparoscopy. Scheussler and Raboy pioneered reconstructive work on pyeloplasty and vesicourethral anastomoses, which laid the foundations for others to methodically begin investigations to improve instruments and methods. In 1991, our labs at U.C. Davis began to systematically reevaluate all aspects of laparoscopic suturing, including needle design, suture types, suture colors, suturing techniques, knotting techniques, and instrument design. By 1993, we published on the outcomes of some of these investigations in laparoscopic radical prostatectomy in a canine model.[21] Rassweiller and colleagues have further augmented our knowledge of intracorporeal suturing and knotting and continued to stress the need for "skill" development.[22] Perhaps some of the most exciting areas in all surgical research currently are focusing on methods of surgical skill acquisition.[23]

Clinical series with advanced reconstructions include Lou Kavoussi's pyeloplasty and Gilleneau and Vallencein's work on radical prostatectomy with sutured vesicourethral reanastomosis. These techniques have had rapid proliferation into the urologic community with a large number of secondary centers beginning to report on their own respective results. No longer are advanced laparoscopic techniques within the sole domain of the endourologists, urologic oncologists are rightly reclaiming some of these techniques as their own and fostering further clinical applications.[24] Advancing technology, especially telerobotic surgical systems are now poised to further diffuse these complex laparoscopic reconstructive methods into widespread application.[25] Detailed discussion of this specific reconstructive capacity will follow later in this chapter as a newly added section since the first publication. In a recent review of the past decades' experience with laparoscopic surgical procedures from a single "cutting-edge" institution, Costi and colleagues have noted that the quality of laparoscopic surgery has improved. They reviewed 3,022 consecutive patients undergoing 99 different laparoscopic procedures at the Institut Mutualiste Montsouris in Paris over the past decade. A complex database included the types of laparoscopic procedures, conversion of access, duration of the surgery, complications, further hospitalizations and reoperations, and duration of the hospital stay. General trends confirm more difficult laparoscopic surgery peformed in the latter half of the decade and fewer easier procedures. In addition, evolution of the surgery itself was demonstrated by the development of new procedures. All of this was noted without a significant

increase in the number of complications.[26] Complex robotic series are burgeoning, yet just as this technologic incursion is profoundly reshaping urologic practice, another even less invasive methodology is just beginning. The current robotic instruments are large, costly, cumbersome, and lack significant haptic feedback. As natural orifice surgical incursions become more sophisticated, a new genre of robots should be expected. Look for more degrees of freedom, dexterity enhancements on a microscale, image guidance outside of human vision, and fusion-image guidance, all capable of being delivered per orally or transrectally.

ESSENTIALS OF MINIMALLY INVASIVE RECONSTRUCTION

BASICS Surgical knot tying is one of the first skills every medical student delights in mastering. One- and two-handed throws are next developed throughout the surgical residency for controlling hemorrhage or reapproximating tissues. Typically, surgical application of stapling devices follows mastery of basic suturing skills. Laparoscopic urologic surgery is accomplishing the same fundamental operation as would an open incision, except with electronic imaging and small, fixed portals of access to the closed environment. The laparoscopic environment makes suturing and knotting a most difficult task.[21,27] It is for this reason that urologic reconstructive surgeries have been only sporadically reported and usually rely on automated stapling technologies.

It is doubtful that a urologist would perform any of the operations we do if told from the outset that suturing or knot tying could not be accomplished. It has been stated that laparoscopic urologic reconstruction can be facilitated only if there are stapling devices that can rapidly reapproximate tissue margins. These statements are made despite our continuing experience with metallic staples and the accompanying litany of complications when used within the genitourinary tract.[28,29]

HEMOSTASIS Hemostasis in the closed environment imposed by minimal access surgery is one obstacle blocking progression to more complex intracorporeal techniques. The ability to maintain a clear surgical field allows complex tasks such as suturing to be performed.[29] Some of the instruments discussed in this chapter are essential components to the surgeon's hemostatic armamentaria. There are five basic modalities at the surgeon's disposal for the augmentation of local hemostasis (Table 50-1). These are in addition to the methods of systemically altering the physiologic clotting parameters that might facilitate hemostasis. Of those particularly germane for this discussion are stapling and clip application.

Vascular pedicles have been safely ligated and divided by autostaplers for 2 decades.[31,32] The concern for arteriovenous fistula development is certainly worth consideration, especially if both structures are taken en bloc.[33] The vascular autostapling devices are theoretically designed to

Table 50-1 Methods of Laparoscopic Hemostasis Excluding Augmenting Peripheral Clotting Parameters
Parameters
Mechanical
pressure
clamping
Thermal
radiofrenquency electrocautery
monopolar
bipolar
endothermal
argon beam coagulator
Lasers
cryoprobes
radiofrenquency energy
microwave energy
Chemical
fibrin glue, calcium-impregnated swabs EndoAvitene
Suture/Ligation
Stapling/Clipping

separate the artery and the vein prior to fixing into the staple delivery mode. The laparoscopic autostaplers have little clinical data yet to support their widespread applicability. Laboratory studies indicate that it is crucial to anticipate the trajectory necessary for delivering the 12 mm device to the targeted pedicle vasculature. The wrong approach results in untoward tension on the vessels during the engagement process. During transperitoneal laparoscopic nephrectomies, anterior axillary line portals, both cranially or caudad to the laparoscope portal, were effective to autostaple the renal artery and vein.[34]

Clip application during pedicle dissection has been addressed in the general surgical literature.[35,36] There are proponents for loop ligation and for titanium clipping. Urologically, the laparoscopic nephrectomy animal model indicated that clips were associated with more blood loss than autostapling techniques.[34] One investigation of the two major manufacturers of laparoscopic clip appliers studied the pressures necessary to dislodge each type of clip in vitro and in vivo.[37] In detailed measurements on both axial and horizontal displacement, the Ethicon clips held more effectively than the U.S. Surgical clips. Both types had an unusually high rate of distractibility during the in vivo studies.[37] A second study quantifying the force to dislodge the newer generation of U.S. Surgical clips, found EndoClip II to be much more difficult to dislodge.[38] Each study was respectively funded by the manufacturer whose clip was felt to be better, so conclusions must be weighed carefully. The surgeon should be aware that these clips can become dislodged during the course of subsequent dissecting if either radial or horizontal traction is applied near or at the clip.

Metallic clips, and automated staplers have been described to secure the renal pedicle during laparoscopic nephrectomy and nephroureterectomy.[33] Comparing these two modalities with open suture ligation of the renal pedicle in a porcine animal model, all three methods were equally efficacious at preventing arterial leakage at physiological pressures. At superphysiologic pressures (avg 1,364 mm Hg), 5 of 6 pigs leaked from renal arteries secured with an EndoGIA 30.[33] This multifire vascular stapler cuts between 2 triple-staggered rows of 2.5 mm staples. Application of three 9 mm titanium clips and suture ligation with a 2-0 silk stick and 0-silk free tie both prevented leakage, even at renal artery burst pressures (avg 1,821 mm Hg). Moran similarly found renal artery branch vessel ligation with 3 clips transversely placed in opposing directions and linear stapling equally efficacious in a porcine animal model.[34] En masse occlusion of the renal pedicle without separating the artery and vein, using a 12 mm vascular stapler, has also been examined in animals. One of 3 animals followed for 6 months demonstrated an arteriovenous fistula on aortography.[33] The true risk of arteriovenous fistula formation from en masse renal pedicle ligation may be even higher given previous studies documenting their formation 5 months to 40 years after surgery.[39–41] Current practice recommendations are to use 9 mm titanium clips to secure renal vessels. A total of 5 clips, 3 placed proximally and 2 on the specimen side, placed transversely in opposing directions prior to vessel division is recommended. Finally, a case where a partial nephrectomy was performed utilizing a linear cutting stapler has been described.[42]

TISSUE REAPPROXIMATION AND HEALING The ability of the laparoscopic surgeon to reconstruct the genitourinary tract is fundamentally the same in the closed versus the open abdomen. The five techniques available for tissue reapproximation are listed in Table 50-2. More than one modality can be combined as in Dr. Avant's end-to-end anastomotic device and tissue laser welding techniques that will be mentioned later.[43] The surgical literature is replete with arguments for and against suturing versus stapling for gastrointestinal reconstruction.[44–47] Much research has been fostered into the mechanisms of tissue healing following various reconstruction techniques.[45] Suffice it to say that the integrity of the intrinsic blood supply is paramount to the ability of mucosa-to-mucosa sealing.[45] In fact, the newest rapidly proliferating method of robot-assisted surgical reconstruction utilizes a single-knot method, which although in theory is easier to perform, has its own potential theoretical disadvantages that need to be seriously discussed (more on this later).

Anastomosis and complex enteric-uroepithelial composite appositions are the rule for urologic reconstruction. A number of synthetic, autograft, and xenograft materials have been sought to further diminish the trauma of urologic reconstruction.[48] Methods to reapproximate these and native bowel segments to the bladder laparoscopically are being investigated. Stapled and sutured bladder resections and closures have been described.[12,49–51] Bladder diverticula have been removed and partial cystectomies with and without nephroureterectomy have been described.[13,16,52] Both clinical study and animal work on the use of metallic autostapling instruments suggest that this technique is successful.[14] Delayed complications, specifically incrustation on the foreign body nidus have not been observed to date. This probably reflects the investigator's careful apposition methods, trying to keep the staple line from direct contact with the urine. Upper-tract reconstructions have also been reported. Dismembered pyeloplasties,[53] anterior pyelocaliceal diverticulectomy with omental patch,[54] and partial nephrectomies[55,56] have all been performed. The reconstructions to date have been hampered by constraints of limited instrument technology; lack of stereoscopic imaging; and closed, fixed, operative access to the urologic areas of interest.

SKILL DEVELOPMENT AND ASSESSMENT The field of laparoscopic urologic surgery has experienced a period of rapid regrowth in the past 4 years.[1] Despite the initial skepticism that should generally be expected by such technologically demanding surgical procedures, this resurgence of interest has made popular demands on training courses at the national meetings, local academic centers, and at international courses. The urologist must initially have an interest in laparoscopic surgery. The nuances associated with all the instrumentation are significant. If one is not exposed early to laparoscopic instrumentation, the breadth of information necessary can seem staggering. Once the instrumentation has been mastered, the physiologic consequences of operating on patients must next be addressed. Safe utilization of electronic, high-speed insufflators and specific problems associated with pneumoperitoneum must always be understood during these cases. On top of all of this background material, the surgeon must become adept at utilizing complex instruments in the laparoscopic environment. The laparoscopic environment consists of limited fixed portals of access, longer than normal surgical instruments, and angles of access that at times must cross over one another to work within a brightly illuminated but small focal area within a live patient. Next, consider that the reliance on the electronic image is complete. That is to say, the movements within the operative field are within the surgeon's control, but there are activities often occurring outside the surgeon's view, such as retraction. Finally, add to this a lack of "true" stereotactic, three-dimensional vision and little ability to utilize the sense of touch (in the laparoscopic environment, the surgeon cannot palpate an organ or feel for the pulsations of a nearby artery), and you have summed up the potential limitations of working laparoscopically. But there are advantages as well, or dedicated laparoscopic

Table 50-2 The Five Methods of Tissue Reapproximation. Each Can Be Applied Alone or in Combination with the Others
Suturing
Stapling
Crimping
Thermal welding (Laser)
Gluing

urologic centers would not have evolved. The brightly illuminated, magnified surgical field is an enticing environment in which to perform surgery, rather akin to microsurgery. The precision capable in such an environment is unparalleled. In addition, following the greatest traditions in urology, the technology fostered by laparoscopic surgery is itself attractive.

Research currently focuses on methods of learning, measuring, teaching, and modifying the mental and motor abilities to accomplish complex laparoscopic surgery.[57] This is one of the most exciting areas of research in *all* of surgery currently. How do surgeons learn? What makes one person recognize pathways to practical motor problems quickly where others need to be shown? Should we be able to pick those potential urologic residents that will be able to master complex laparoscopic procedures by testing certain aptitudes? Are all urologic surgeons capable of adapting to the laparoscopic environment and mastering the techniques necessary to safely apply these in their practice? What skills are essential, and can they be modeled and practiced to increase proficiency? These are some of the basic questions and clinical research currently being investigated on psychomotor skill necessary to perform complex laparoscopic surgery.

Psychomotor Skills Surgical education to date has relied on the formal apprenticeship model exemplified by the doctrine, "see one, do one, teach one."[58] Laparoscopic surgery has been defined by degrees of difficulty, with increasingly complex procedures resulting in "steep learning curves." These curves are usually but not always exemplified by the amount of time taken to accomplish the laparoscopic procedure, often comparing this with the open surgical equivalent.[59] In addition, there are relatively few centers where advanced techniques are occurring with regularity. On top of this, hospitals and regulatory agencies (particularly in the United States) are struggling with credentialing issues that surround "surgical proficiency." It is no wonder that the number of laparoscopic, urologic, intracorporeal sutured reconstructions have not proliferated to any great extent. But the envelope continually expands, and small groups of investigators such as Clayman, Janeschtek, Kavoussi, Gill, Gilleneou, Rassweiler, and others push us into rethinking the possibilities of this technology.

Paralleling the growing amount of research on laparoscopic suturing are investigations in the acquisition and development of psychomotor skills and skill evaluation. Derossis and colleagues from the McGill University evaluated 42 subjects to better understand how structured, objectively measured tasks could be utilized to improve performance during laparoscopic surgery. They demonstrated that the ability to develop suturing skills correlated with overall improvement in a wide variety of laparoscopic activities.[60] Hanna and colleagues at the University of Dundee have investigated the differing abilities of right- and left-handed individuals to develop psychomotor skills for complex endo-

scopic manipulations. Utilizing a complex in vitro system, 10 right-handed and 10 left-handed individuals were evaluated for psychomotor aptitude using both the dominant and nondominant hands. They demonstrated that the right-handed surgeons performed fewer errors and exhibited better first-time accuracy than the left-handed individuals. In addition, accuracy definitely favored the dominant hand in both groups.[61] This same center reported on the improvement of skill performance by optical axis manipulation. They noted that even small decreases in the viewing angle were attended by significant degradation in performance.[62] Others have demonstrated this same phenomenon, such as Holden's group from The Hadassah Hebrew University Medical Center. They demonstrated that changes in either the camera's or the surgeon's position profoundly disrupted the surgeon's performance.[63]

However, when the surgeon and camera positions were altered together, these detrimental effects could be altered and skilled performance could be regained. More specific to our topic at hand, endoscopic skills have been extensively evaluated by our group and others. Hanna, again from Dundee, evaluated the influence of direction of view, target-to-endoscope distance, and manipulation angles on the efficiency of intracorporeal knot tying. These authors confirmed our observations that the closer the endoscope is to the targeted reconstruction site, the more magnified the field of view and the more difficult will be the performance of the suturing task. They specifically evaluated distances of 50, 75, 100, 125, and 150 mm from the targeted task. The 50 mm distance uniformly resulted in the longest times. In addition, the 60-degree manipulation angle had the shortest execution times compared with 30 and 90 degrees. Finally, some recent investigations have sought how to minimize these problems utilizing a 90-degree laparoscope to achieve movement parallax. In this investigation, the authors report on the theoretical advantages of manipulating the endoscopic image to the surgeon's advantage, essentially recapitulating all the problems alluded to previously. By synchronizing a flexible laparoscope to the movement of a surgeon's head, movement parallax or compensated visual enhanced-movement is achieved.[64] They note that a head-controlled flexible 90-degree laparoscope improves the surgeon's depth perception and hand-eye coordination. This has not been significantly reported for expensive 3-D imaging systems.[65,66]

The primary problem with these types of investigations is that the small study groups do not reflect the community of surgeons that will be attempting these procedures. In addition, the *ability* of a surgeon to perform a given task is a complex issue involving adaptive capacity, traits, and aptitudes that a person brings to any given situation. This is quite different from the *skill* of a surgeon. Skill is referred to when specific combinations of techniques are deftly employed to accomplish a given task.[66,67] Numerous investigators have begun to focus the attention of their

investigations on how surgical residents develop laparoscopic skills and how we can best foster this skill transfer? Reznick, at the University of Toronto, has written extensively regarding this issue. He summarizes the crucial nature of these research endeavors by stating that the teaching of technical skills is one of the most important tasks of surgical educators. He concludes by calling for adherence to simple principles: treat pupils as adult learners; set specific objectives; realize that operative skills are multidimensional; and be there to observe, to be patient, to provide feedback, to be positive, and to seriously structure the assessment process.[68] Many struggle with the notion that there are individuals who have an aptitude for innately performing difficult laparoscopic maneuvers deftly. This has found little documented validity and many cling to the notion that all interested surgeons who seek to be trained should avail themselves of advanced courses. In practice, however, there is increasing pressure on our specialty societies, hospitals, and governmental watchdogs that more scrutiny is warranted.[69] Macmillan and Cuschieri, also from the Dundee group, recently reported on a method of identifying individuals who appear to have innate aptitude to perform complex dexterous laparoscopic tasks. They propose that if larger studies confirm these initial observations, that selection of candidates for advanced laparoscopic training might be possible.[70]

Skills Training *Theory* Surgical education has struggled with methods to objectively scrutinize surgical performance of housestaff for many years. The methods of formal education have had some limited application, but as the complexity of modern laparoscopic surgery has manifested itself, departments across the country and around the world have begun to evaluate how to assess competency, skill development, teaching methodologies, and communications skills.[71] The complexity of this task has resulted in a surprising number of papers in the surgical literature on trends in education. Extensive lists are beginning to be generated on measurable psychomotor skills, but the ability of young surgeons to communicate is significantly important, especially for advanced laparoscopic procedures. Important aspects that deserve attention are psychomotor skills, congnitive decision making, incorporation of video-enhanced motor coordination, two-handed surgical maneuvering, and rhetorical ability. Students of advanced laparoscopic surgery are themselves independent learners. There are various approaches each will take to gaining laparoscopic skills. A whole host of research endeavors have begun to focus on the surgeon's ability to learn.[72] At least four factors can be attributed to learning orientation: concrete experiences, abstract conceptualization, active experimentation, and reflective observation. D.A. Kolb is widely quoted in research regarding learning orientation. It is these orientations that help research investigators study learning. They identify four dominant learning styles: convergence, divergence, assimilation, and accommodation.

The convergence learner stresses abstract conceptualization and active experimentation. These learners stress hypothetical-deductive reasoning to analyze their problems. Divergers rely on contrasting orientations of concrete experience and reflective observation. Their information processing can thus be protracted and often they do not feel impelled to act. Assimilators tend to use inductive development of concepts such as unifying theories to explain their observations. They tend to focus on the soundness or fitness of ideas, and thus, are less concerned about the practical value of observations. Last are the accommodators who emphasize orientations of active experimentation and concrete experience.[73] Kolb's learning styles have been used successfully to evaluate medical students and the educational environment for medical learning. In addition, this theory has also recently been applied to third-year medical students rotating on their general surgery clerkships at the University of Nebraska. They identified that the bulk of third-year students were convergers (45%), assimilators (26%), accommodators (21%), divergers (8%). They were primarily interested in how best to evaluate the performance of the students and not to predict methods to better teach psychomotor skills. But applications of modern learning theory are evident. They stated that clinical performance requires additional cognitive skills and abilities that need to be further quantified.[73]

The ability to measure and impart laparoscopic psychomotor skill is another area undergoing intense scrutiny. The ability to ascertain those individuals who have innate ability should also be possible. Components recognized as crucial for laparoscopic surgery include muscle strength, speed, precision, dexterity, balance, spatial resolution, as well as poise and endurance. Kaufman and colleagues at the University of West Virginia have begun an active program interested in three aspects of surgical education. First, can prospective surgeons be screened with regards to their psychomotor skills? Second, can the application of modern educational psychomotor concepts help in the development of advanced skills? Third, can evaluation methods of psychomotor skill proficiency adequately guage the acquisition and performance of complex surgical tasks? Their methodology is complex, but applies a wide battery of psychomotor tests at the initiation of, during, and following training to better evaluate skill acquisition. Their tests include the following: McCarron Assessment of Neuromuscular Development (MAND), to measure motor function and fatigue; Purdue Pegboard, to assess fine motor control; Minnesota Rate of Manipulation Test (MRMT), to measure speed and precision; Minnesota Paper Form Board (MPFB), to measure spatial perception; Haptic Visual Discrimination Test (HVDT), to measure spatial perception; and California Psychological Inventory (CPI), to measure poise, confidence, and relaxation. During preliminary evaluations, they have developed an equation that balances psychomotor ability with the acquisition of motor skill, factoring in time of training.

$$\text{Psychomotor ability} \times \text{amount of practice} = \text{motor skill proficiency}^{74}$$

The United States Army represents another wealth of information regarding the ability to perform tasks and the ability to measure skill. Again, they have reported two major determinates for performance: length of time spent doing a given task and aptitude. Using isoperformance curves, relationships between experience and aptitude are possible mathematically. Now changing the relationships can be measured and the effect of training can be calculated on isoperformance curves.[75] As these studies continue, one can hope that directed methods of training will be possible for those interested in advanced laparoscopic surgery that will bring performance to a peak level and maintain it there.[76–92]

Flight Simulators   The premise that the skill of the surgeon can be equated to the outcomes of the operations over time is a fundamental concept in modern surgery. Those surgeons who perform the most complex operations and have the lowest morbidity are encouraged. This concept is fundamental to other more intensively scrutinized professions as well, most notably commercial aviation. Flight simulation has a long and interesting history.[93] Simulators have been attempted with surgical procedures such as laparoscopic cholecystectomy, laparoscopic-assisted vaginal hysterectomy, and laparoscopic inguinal hernia repair (Figure 50-3).[77,81] But to date, they lack ability to function in the manner in which the aeronautics profession is capable. Current simulators are available in anesthesia, interventional radiology, and emergency medicine, but these are far from clinical reality. Fidelity in haptic feedback has been an ongoing problem with surgical simulators. In addition, the ability for the computer to add nuances of human anatomical variability has not been easy to achieve. Yet, simulation is making rapid advances as the brain behind this machine, the computer, likewise rapidly advances in speed, performance, and processing power.

Computerized Education   The explosion in computer performance, hardware, and software has had profound effects on education, data management, communication, and entertainment. The ability for this modality to impact on surgical education is just beginning to be felt.[94] The "information age" has quietly crept into the surgical training programs throughout the country.[95] It is no surprise to see that the housestaff, raised with familiarity with computer technologies gladly accept these methodologies. One recent study investigated the use of multimedia interactive computer programs to familiarize residents in laparoscopic skills. The comparative scale for most effective method to familiarize and raise their knowledge regarding new laparoscopic procedures was as follows: textbook (4.7), lectures

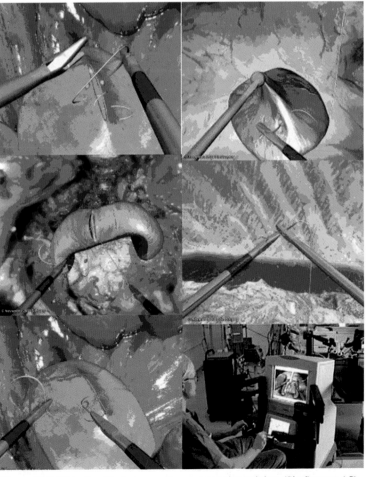

Figure 50-3 Virtual reality laparoscopic reconstructive training. (SimSurgery AS)

(5.1), videos (6.0), animal labs (7.3), and multimedia interactive computer programs (8.8). There are lots of problems with the more standard methods of surgical education when applied to laparoscopic surgery.[95] First, with printed material such as this syllabus, there is no method of questioning the information unless those truly interested seek out references, read those, and synthesize their own opinions. Lectures provide the student with the possibility of real-time interaction through questioning and answering. The limitation of this modality is that it is entirely dependent on the skill and knowledge of the lecturer. Couple with this the inherent problems of inhibitions of students in a large group, which can stifle potential educational interaction. Videos can be a very good reference, but again, like textbooks lack the ability to interact with questions and answers. Animal labs allow the student to experience live surgery; make mistakes and have to correct them; and provide animate experience with such issues as tissue handling, bleeding, and visual imaging problems. These experiences are costly, limited in availability, and lack true educational value unless a skilled proctor is present continuously to provide feedback.[96] Multimedia interactive computer programs can provide all the aforementioned qualities necessary, and also provide interactive references to specific questions via HELP commands. In addition, computer programs have been shown to increase retention of important facts and decrease the learning curves, can be scaled to individual performance abilities, are inexpensive compared with animal labs, and are mobile. The computer method of training can be self-directed, self-paced, as well as interactive. Rosser and colleagues at Yale University's Minimally Invasive Surgery group has developed a CD-ROM tutorial to aid in transferring cognitive knowledge thought to be essential for establishing laparoscopic skills. The tutorial was designed to provide surgeons with the knowledge base thought to be essential for acquiring basic laparoscopy skills originally designed for an intense 2-day course (Yale Laparoscopic Boot Camp). The main menu consisted of 8 main menus that could be taken in any sequence. They were as follows: dexterity drills, laparoscopic equipment, strategy of positioning, operating procedures, troubleshooting, clinical applications, post-test, and statistical analysis. The tutorial requires almost no reading with audio prompts to a layered, regimented program with abundant illustrations and embedded videos. Using the embedded post-test and statistics package, they were able to show no difference in post-test scores for students taking the 2-day course versus the multimedia computerized tutorial.[95]

Virtual Reality Jaron Lanier introduced the term "virtual reality" in 1989, but the concept that computers would have enough power to interface with a human's sensory perceptions formed the basis of Ivan Sutherland's doctoral thesis from MIT in 1963. As with most things in the computer world, the first head-mounted display became a reality, and a young entrepreneur, Morton Heilig, tried to sell "Sensorama," a simulated computerized motorcycle ride through a virtual city. Computational capacity has been the only limiting factor in the advance of these technologies. Gordon Moore, Intel Corporation's cofounder is now best known for Moore's law, stating that a computer's power would double every 18 to 24 months. He has made this statement from observing trends for the past 35 years. In addition, the cost of that technology has almost halved in the same period. In other words, the supercomputer of 1990 that cost $100,000 (US) is today available in a $150 (US) Nintendo system. Randall Tobias, former vice-president of ATT is widely quoted as saying, "if we had similar progress in the automotive industry, a Lexus would cost $2 (US), it would travel at the speed of sound, and go 600 miles on a thimbleful of gas."[97]

One of the first major advances in the development of VR surgical systems came with the Visible Human Project. Sponsored by the National Library of Medicine, 1 mm cross-sectional anatomy was stored on a computer for 3-D reconstructive purposes. This database became the first available human subset for computer VR programs.[98]

Virtual reality surgery overcomes several of the limitations of education in an operating room (see Figure 50-3). First, the teaching session in the OR cannot always be well designed or orchestrated. The prime focus remains on the patient. The scheduled case may not be well suited for the resident at that given time. The corollary to this is that the technical nuances of the particular case may be above or below the skills of the student, making the educational potential limiting. The execution of the surgical procedure may not be altered to satisfy an educational goal. Likewise, the dissection and exposure cannot always proceed in a fashion best structured for educational potential. Finally, the steps of the surgical procedure cannot be repeated. Errors that occur can be corrected, but they cannot be repeated.[99] All these shortcomings are nonexistent in the virtual operating room. In addition, there is more evidence that learning complex tasks is significantly impaired by increasing the amount of stress in the environment.[100] An operating room is inherently filled with stress. Factors contributing to the high-stress environment of the OR include time constraints, technical difficulties, concern for the patient, equipment failures, interpersonal issues, handling telephone calls, and lack of rest. Investigators now are sure that the greatest learning and performance occurs in environments with moderate stress. The psychomotor tasks are learned in three ways, all facilitated in the virtual environment. In the cognitive phase of learning, the student attains a degree of understanding of the task. The second phase is the associative process. During the associative phase, the student practices the task and compares performance with an expert. The differences are considered errors and mastery is achieved by minimizing these errors. Finally comes the autonomous phase, where skill is performed without cognitive awareness.[101–103]

Telementoring and Remote Surgery Several factors are associated with altering the rules of surgical education. The hospital inpatient population is becoming more complicated and surgical therapy is potentially becoming more technologically complex. Insurance payers and, in particular, government watchdogs, are requiring more supervision and less autonomy of the residents. The residents are being asked to learn the same or more material in fewer working hours. Practicing urologists are facing the same phenomena, which is increasingly taxing the endurance to stay current. This is the scenario that is poised for *all* of the just-discussed technologies to merge with telecommunications and allow guided preceptorships remotely. If you throw in robotic surgery, then telementoring is not even necessary. The expert at one location can perform the surgery at another without physically being present.[104]

Telementoring has already been performed for multiple surgeries as well as urologic laparoscopic cases. Dr. Kavoussi's group at Johns Hopkins has gained significant notoriety for their pioneering efforts. In their initial studies, the surgeon mentor was located in a control room > 1,000 feet from the operating room. Fourteen advanced and 9 basic laparoscopic procedures were performed. Telementoring was accomplished using real-time computer video images, two-way audio communication links, and a robotic arm to control the videoendoscope. Success was achieved in 22 of 23 cases without increased operative times or complications. They then extended their investigations and distances between the Johns Hopkins Bayview Medical Center and the Johns Hopkins Hospital (distance = 3.5 miles) for 27 more telementoring laparoscopic procedures utilizing public phone lines. Finally, they have extended their novel surgical instruction capabilities to the international arena with 1 case in Innsbruck, Austria, and 2 cases in Bangkok, Thailand.[105] Others have reported on the technology necessary for successful telementoring. The U.S. Navy recently studied the feasibility of laparoscopic hernia repairs aboard the *USS Abraham Lincoln* while cruising the Pacific Ocean. Telementoring was possible from remote locations in Maryland and California.[106] In a recent research investigation, Broderick and colleagues at the Virginia Commonwealth University reported that decreasing transmission bandwidth does not significantly affect laparoscopic image clarity or color fidelity as long as the laparoscopes are positioned and maintained at their optimal working distance.[107]

Now for the ultimate in technophilia, a recent Internet study on the attitudes and practices of general surgeons was performed. Over 2 months, 459 surgeons were enrolled in a study on the World Wide Web (WWW). Those polled stated that the Internet was used to expand their knowledge of surgery in 74.5%, more than half of them stated that they favored more advances in technology such as robotics in the operating room (53%), and most (78%) favored the technology necessary for telementoring to learn new laparoscopic procedures.[108]

Technology and advances in urologic surgery are being paralleled by research interests in the methods of acquiring skills and teaching. There is no doubt that computer-assisted methods of education will proliferate, that the classic methods for keeping current will be transitioned into a high-tech data stream of information. Telementoring is already a reality at those institutions that have been on the forefront of laparoscopic surgery. It is only a matter of time when an "off-the-shelf" package will be added to an operating room in your locale for furthering training of interested surgeons. There are centers cropping up around the globe interested in expanding the envelope of technology on laparoscopic surgical education. Most of these centers currently come with a high price tag. But as seen so clearly with computerized systems, this too should become an integral part of surgical education at any institution interested in less invasive surgical technology. One such center (Center for Minimal Access Surgery [CMAS] in London, Ontario) has recently published its first paper on the establishment of a "state-of-the-art" multidisciplinary technological education and research center for minimally invasive surgical techniques. Among the technologies available for skill acquisition include high fidelity Minimal Access trainers, Body Form Simulator, a VR system, a computerized laparoscopic skills workstation, and a multimedia library of laparoscopic procedures. In addition, the CMAS has started a videoconferencing system to be integrated with its various components to enhance education via telementoring.[109]

EXTRACORPOREAL KNOTTING

Extracorporeal knotting techniques have evolved for a diverse variety of laparoscopic purposes. First, they can be utilized to secure hemostasis of the anterior abdominal wall.[110] Best described as a "sling-suture" technique, the utility in stopping active hemorrhage from trocar sites has been demonstrated by several authors. The technique of sling suturing extracorporeally includes both straight and curved needles of various sizes.[111] For control of anterior abdominal wall hemorrhage, a transverse ligature is necessary to encompass the area of the vessel. The first stitch should be below the vessel if the culprit is from a lower abdominal trocar injury and above if upper abdominal. The trocar should be removed only after control of hemorrhage. Alternative maneuvers may be necessary to control trocar site bleeding, including but not limited to percutaneous fulguration (resectoscope), transportal placement of a Foley catheter for direct pressure application, and others. This extracorporeal knot can also facilitate intra-abdominal visualization by "slinging" obstructing structures out of the visual pathway. Nathanson and Cushierie utilized just such an extracorporeal knot as a "falciform lift" and the same can be done with the urachus. Recently, several extracorporeal assist mechanisms for passing these sling sutures have been marketed (Figure 50-4). These instruments are primarily being marketed for visually assisted fascial closures (Figure 50-5).

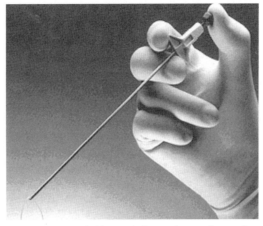

Figure 50-4 EndoClose needle carrier can be used to sling or lift structures out of the field of view, for close fascial defects, or to stop bleeding from anterior abdominal wall vessels. (U.S. Surgical, Norwalk, CT)

Extracorporeal knotting has had its most common application with loop ligation techniques. A variety of loop knots are utilized and the laparoscopic surgeon can use pretied ligatures or tie one with standard sutures. Several knot configurations are also available, and the surgeon can utilize fly-fishing knot variants or sailor's knots for the same purpose.[5] Clinically, the most commonly utilized loop ligature still employs the Roeder knot.[112] The Roeder knot can be applied pretied as a loop ligature or can be tied after needle ligature intracorporeal placement and then synched (Figure 50-6).[36,54] The only investigation on the safety of vessel occlusion reported that dry-gut Roeder knots provide vascular occlusion for up to 3 mm arteries.[111]

The other knot configurations that have also been successfully employed include the Duncan knot (with or without a half hitch), Fisherman's clinch knot, jamming loop knot, and Weston's configurations (Figure 50-7).[7,115,116] Loop ligatures by design can incorporate any of these aforementioned slipknot modalities. Several manufacturers offer prepackaged, slipknot loop ligatures. Common features include a variable-length pusher (usually 80 cm) over monofilament or braided

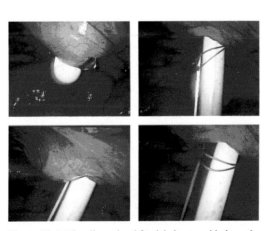

Figure 50-5 Visually-assisted fascial closure with through-and-through stitches. eXit puncture closure device shown here. (Advanced Surgical, Princeton, NJ)

sutures. Application of pretied slipknot loop ligatures has been simplified by disposable applicators. Chromic gut, plain gut, polydioxanone (PDS and PDSII), silk, polyglactin (Vicryl, Dexon, or Polysorb), and Dacron (Surgidac) are all clinically available laparoscopic suture materials.

The endoscopic loop ligature is passed backward through a reducer sleeve (3 mm) and then into the appropriate trocar (Figure 50-8). The pushrod is then advanced until the loop is fully opened within the abdomen. A grasping instrument is passed through the loop and the targeted tissue is grasped. The back end of the plastic pushrod is snapped and the rod advanced to tighten the slipknot. The synching suture is cut at least 2 cm from the knot.

Finally, extracorporeal knotting can be utilized with intracorporeal suturing when knot pushers are available.[116] Various reports indicate that with practice, these knots can be applied fairly quickly (below 5 minutes).[113] Any available suture material can be utilized for these extracorporeal techniques providing that adequate length is available to traverse the trocar (usually 80 cm). Various braided sutures do not slide as well as others if standard square knots are utilized and should be avoided. Prepackaged endoscopic ligatures with variable needle configurations are available for this purpose from most manufacturers. One unique approach to this technique employs a specifically designed knotting instrument. Oko and Rosin report the ability to suture and place knots with almost any material and then adjust tension and knot position with his device (Figure 50-9).[117] The same type of knotting technique was described by Puttick and colleagues utilizing a laparoscopic Babcock clamp.[118] A multitude of manufacturers tout their knot pushers for ease of cinching. The primary problem with all techniques of extracorporeal knotting includes the need to maintain long suture tails, multiple passages via trocars, no

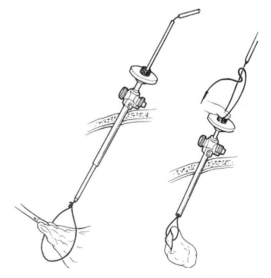

Figure 50-6 Application of Roeder slipknot loops. Technique of applying pretied loop ligatures, left. Technique of tying Roeder slipknot extracorporeally, right. Completion of the extracorporeally tied Roeder knot.

ment represents the primary hindrance to mastering these techniques. Fixed portals of entrance limit the "approach" to the targeted suture site. The intra-abdominal viscera are rarely stationary and the ability to move a needle driver's approach is limited by these fixed entrance portals. Specifically designed assisting instruments (Figure 50-10, bottom flamingos) (Karl Storz, Culver City, CA) can manipulate nonfixed tissues for correct alignment and overcome the problem of fixed portal positioning. In addition, the camera site and the surgeon's right and left hands also remain fixed. Adding an additional trocar is always possible, but it defeats the philosophical goal of minimal access surgery. The camera position of choice when first attempting intracorporeal reconstructions should lie between the surgeon's right and left hands. For maximum efficiency the right and left hand portals should not be over an acute angle with each other. The optimal angle to work is 80 to 110 degrees, and each trocar should be greater than 8 cm, separated at the surface skin sites to allow the maximal ability for the tips to interact.

Figure 50-7 Other types of extracorporeal knots, left is the Weston II, and right is the fisherman's clinch. The fisherman's clinch has also been utilized for throwing intracorporeal knots using straight needles or pin vise needle drivers.

direct control of the sutures at the tissue while knots are being thrown, and the need to suture intracorporeally. Kennedy has shown that multiple extracorporeally tied knots can be sequentially thrown with the aid of a pusher, thus simplifying the reentry problems.[119] Complex urinary reconstructions typically require end-to-end or layered closures, which are nearly impossible using extracorporeal techniques.

Prior to addressing intracorporeal suturing and knotting techniques, mention should be made to those who advocate clips to secure the intracorporeal suture or suture line. Although not an extracorporeal technique, the primary claims of those exploring this method of suture anchoring are avoiding the potential loosening of slipknot ties or the cumbersome multiple trocar passages required by extracorporeal knotting. Metallic and absorbable clips have been successfully used to secure intracorporeal sutures.[120] Metallic sphere clips have likewise been devised to more securely maintain suture tension. There exists only one study evaluating the security of these differing modalities to secure a suture. Utilizing a ten-

siometer, distraction forces were measured following a standard three-throw knot versus titanium clips versus locking polyglactin clips versus malleable collars. No technique approximated the security of the standard three-throw knot. By doubly throwing the suture through the collar, the distraction force approached that of the knot (knot 4.9 kg [SD = 3.22] vs doubly thrown collar 5.4 kg [SD = 3.22]).[120]

INTRACORPOREAL SUTURING AND KNOTTING

INTRACORPOREAL SUTURING DIFFICULTIES Laparoscopic urologic reconstruction requires intracorporeal suturing skills at present. The fact that more work on urinary diversion or bladder reconstruction has not been done reflects the difficulties inherent in this task. Intracorporeal suturing and knotting represent the most difficult surgical techniques the advanced laparoscopic surgeon can acquire. Reasons for the difficulty in performing intracorporeal suturing are multifactorial (Table 50-3). The closed operating environ-

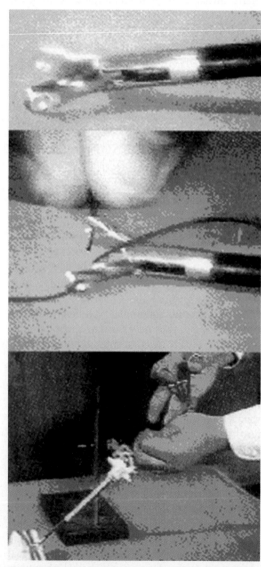

Figure 50-9 Oko's OR laparoscopic ligator. Allows extracorporeal knotting and nonderailing of sutures during trocar passage. (Photo courtesy of Dr. Oko and G.U. Manufacturing Co., London, Eng.)

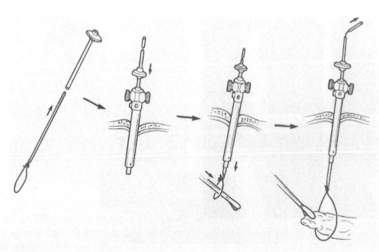

Figure 50-8 Steps in successfully passing and applying endoscopic loop ligatures.

Table 50-3 The Barriers Limiting Rapid Mastery of Intracorporeal Suturing Skills

Environmental
1. fixed access portals
2. rigid access portals
3. limited visual field by rigid laparoscopes
4. lack of stereoscopic image
5. bloodless field

Instrumentation

Skills (needle driving, suturing, knotting)
1. control
2. coordination
3. choreography

Another important factor to control in this closed, fixed environment is image stability.[121] A stable image is readily obtainable by replacing the human camera assistant with a robotic arm. A wide variety of choices are available, ranging in price and complexity from simple mechanical devices to computer-controlled, servo-assisted systems (Figure 50-11). These instruments allow for maximally stable images even with close zooming with the laparoscope. An added bonus of these robotic arms is the free lateral space at the side of the operating room table allowed by the low profile of some of these assist-systems.

Rigid portals are another hindrance to rapidly adapting suturing skills. Surgeons are used to suturing with fluid wrist movements that accentuate needle driving forces, forming loops in suture to facilitate knotting, and keeping tension on swaged-end portion for secure running stitches. Rigid portals eliminate these finesse skills and magnify the perceived difficulties of intracorporeal suturing. Flexible trocar portals have been recently marketed (Figure 50-12) (Karl Storz, Tubingen, Germany) that may permit some degree of fine movement assistance currently lacking in endoscopic suturing. More appropriate and well known to microsurgeons are the utility of curved needle graspers. Primarily employed because the curved instrument allows continuous visualization of the needle and driver's tip during all aspects of suturing in microsurgery, the curved needle driver also has advantages to overcome problems of fixed portals in intracorporeal suturing. By changing the orientation and position of the needle along the curved needle driver, the same fine alignments can be achieved for entrance and exit bites during needle driving without reliance on flexibility at the trocar site. It

takes hours of practice with handling the needle under videolaparoscopic conditions to master these new skills, but mastery facilitates fluid intracorporeal suturing. Another way around fixed trocars is to have access to the region of interest with part or all of the surgeon's hand.[122] Conventional suturing instruments could be utilized if requirements for pneumoperitoneum are abandoned, such as with gasless laparoscopy.[123] The surgeon's hand need not be introduced at all if mechanical systems that provide the degrees of freedom necessary to overcome fixed portal insertion site limitations can be developed.[124,125]

Another limiting factor preventing rapid acquisition of endoscopic suturing skills is the limited visual field. Open surgeons take for granted the ability to lift tissues so as to allow visualization during all phases of suturing. Although the concept of atraumatic tissue handling during suturing is a fundamental skill, the tissue handling represents the key to visually controlled needle placement. The laparoscope brightly illuminates the visual field but does not allow unlimited circumferential views without repositioning or changing to a different angle. A flexible or semiflexible laparoscope would make these angled adjustments, but the degree of interaction with the surgeon would have to be such that anticipated needle path trajectories could be followed. The only current method of overcoming this problem is to have an assistant tissue grasper manipulate the targeted suture site for correct visual alignment toward the laparoscope.

Next on the list of environmental limitations to intracorporeal suturing is the lack of stereoscopic vision. This is a result of current imaging technology. Videolaparoscopic images are magnified and 2-dimensional. With time and practice, the feedback from both surgeon's hands and the interaction with hand-eye coordination make even the most difficult intracorporeal maneuvers possible. In a study of videolaparoscopic suturing over standard suturing, the degree of difficulty was approximated to be 8 times greater. Developing a memorized systematic method of tying with both hands cooperating to minimize the movements necessary to tie can overcome this problem (Figure 50-13).[21] This results in "economy of motion." The right and left hand develop orchestrated interactions very much like in microsurgery.[21] Small motions result in faster, more fluid magnified suturing skills. Of course stereoscopic videolaparoscopes could decrease the dif-

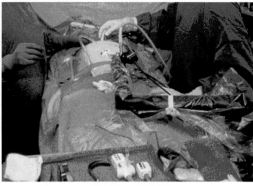

Figure 50-11 Robotic arm assisted laparoscopic surgery. Aesop system. (Computer Motion, Inc., now a part of Intuitive Surgical, Mountain View, CA)

ficulty of intracorporeal suturing. Such systems are in prototypic application.[126] Clinical cases of laparoscopic gastrojejunostomy, bowel anastomoses, and even colonoscopic suturing have already been accomplished with these scopes. The major anticipated drawback of these systems initially will be purchase prices (estimates approximate $100,000 [US]).[126] As with any type of magnified, endoscopic-assisted surgery, it is the surgeon who is highly trained and dexterous who performs flawlessly even in difficult conditions. It may be expected, but is not proven, that the stereoscopic systems will benefit most those who have already mastered the difficulties of intracorporeal suturing.

Finally, one last environmental limitation must be mentioned as a hindrance of intracorporeal suturing—hemorrhage. The closed environment of laparoscopic surgery imposes a formidable barrier to the safe maintenance of hemostasis. During intracorporeal suturing, bleeding, even in small amounts, can make identification of correct tissue planes an arduous or impossible task. Complex intracorporeal suturing requires a bloodless field in order to expedite the already difficult maneuvers mentioned previously. During the division of the viscera it is crucial to be able to achieve hemostasis without compromising the viability of the tissue to be reconstructed. In preliminary

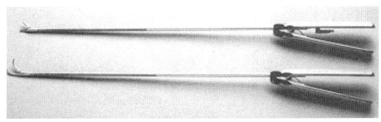

Figure 50-10 Szabo-Berci flamingo tissue grasper and the parrot-jawed needle driver. These represent the first set of intracorporeal instruments specifically designed to overcome many of the difficulties outlined in this chapter. (Karl Storz, Culver City, CA)

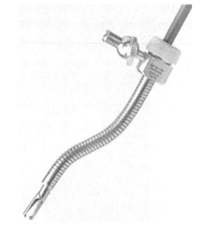

Figure 50-12 Flexible trocars may allow instruments with more degrees of freedom to be passed intracorporeally to facilitate reconstructions. (Karl Storz, Culver City, CA)

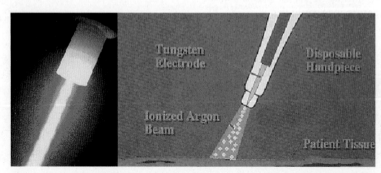

Figure 50-13 Two-handed intracorporeal suturing facilitating bilateral vesicopsoas hitches. Note that when the left hand moves, the right hand follows in choreographed control; this facilitates intracorporeal knotting.

investigations, the argon beam coagulator (Con-Med, Utica, NY) demonstrated unique abilities for this specific purpose (Figure 50-14).[30] A plasma from flowing argon gas molecules allows precise cauterization with very limited depth of penetration. The flowing gas also clears the targeted field, allowing the cautery to be more effective on the bleeding vessels and decrease the time of thermal exposure. There are still risks of thermal necrosis from overzealous exposure from argon beam coagulators. This instrument probably has its greatest utility in its unique hemostatic effects for the reconstructive laparoscopist.

INSTRUMENTATION AND SKILLS   Closed environmental constraints aside, there are two other significant barriers limiting rapid mastery of intracorporeal suturing skills: instrumentation and skills. Instrumentation initially relied on adaptation of grasping instruments for the purpose of laparoscopic suturing. Limitations of general purpose graspers are their inability to grasp and maintain the torque needed for driving needles through tissue. To overcome this problem, several manufacturers developed pin vise-like needle drivers that would rapidly facilitate needle driving (Figure 50-15) (WISAP, Tomball, TX, and Cook Urological, Cook OB/GYN, Spencer, IN). The torque problem was eliminated but all the other problems discussed previously have not been addressed. The result is a perfectly good needle driver but not a good intracorporeal suturing instrument. There is no other function that the driver can accomplish and the second hand of the surgeon must multitask to facilitate just the needle driving.

Brute force by the needle driver does not necessarily create an improved sutured reconstruction. By forcing the needle along an inappropriate trajectory through the tissues, irregularly spaced intervals, bunching of tissues, and inability to catch mucosa are all possible. Forceful needle drivers should not be allowed to replace surgical finesse. In a study of 7 different needle drivers, the ergonomics of laparoscopic suturing was recently studied.[127] Wide variability in the torque and flexion forces are obtainable. Specifically designed intracorporeal suturing instruments have been developed addressing many of the problems outlined previously (Figure 50-16). The shorter the needle driver, the less magnification of small movements at the tip from the surgeon's hands. By removing finger rings, the surgeon's

hands are no longer entrapped. Fine movements with the palm or with thumb and index finger can be accomplished (Figure 50-17). In addition, because of the complexity of intracorporeal suturing, removal of the finger rings greatly eases the cramping and paresthesias that develop when the fingers and thumb are fixed within an instrument for hours. Finally, the needle driver's jaws are another essential feature affecting performance. Although most instruments rely on the standard open diamond jaw configuration to firmly grasp the needle, other variations are just beginning to emerge as effective alternatives (Figure 50-18). The only intracorporeal suturing sets that provide an assistant tissue grasper and a dedicated needle driver are the Szabo-Berci flamingo and parrot-jawed instruments (Figure 50-19) (Karl Storz, Culver City, CA). Many individuals painfully aware of the limitations of current suturing instruments are beginning to develop "prototypic" devices. Agarwal and colleagues describe a simple 10 mm instrument with a fixed needle at the tip of the driver to facilitate intracorporeal suturing.[128]

The last barrier for accomplishing intracorporeal suturing is skill. Defined as the ability to do something well, intracorporeal suturing skill requires remastery of tasks surgeons use daily, but with much more attention to detail. This was referenced during the discussion of lack of stereoscopic vision. Intracorporeal suturing can be divided into three distinct tasks that can be practiced and mastered separately. These are needle driving, suturing, and knotting.

Needle Driving   Laparoscopic intracorporeal needle driving requires successful, safe introduction of the needle and suture material through a trocar or through the anterior abdominal wall. This requires the knowledge of which needles will pass through a specific-sized trocar. The safest method to avoid inadvertent injury to the trocar's flapper valve mechanism and the patient's underlying viscera is to grasp the suture 2 to 3 mm behind the swage, open the valve, and begin passing the needle driver and suture simultaneously (Figure 50-20).[129] Second, the needle and suture must be grasped by the needle driver and correctly aligned prior to beginning. Here, the assisting instrument grasps either the suture close to the needle or the needle itself, and then

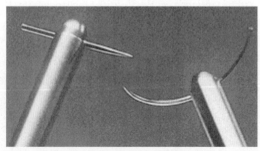

Figure 50-14 Argon beam coagulation may allow more effective hemostasis with less tissue necrosis. Both are essential features for advancing intracorporeal reconstruction. (ConMed Utica, NY)

Figure 50-15 Pin vise laparoscopic suturing instruments. The design limits utilization of these needle drivers for few other purposes. (WISAP U.S.A., Tomball, TX, or Cook Urologic, Cook OB/Gyn, Spencer, IN)

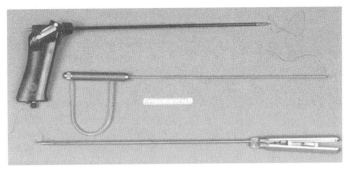

Figure 50-16 Various types of intracorporeal needle drivers. Each represents a unique design modification. What is common to all is the lack of finger rings that limit laparoscopic surgical dexterity.

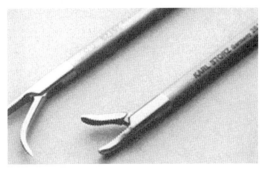

Figure 50-19 The Szabo-Berci parrot-jaw needle driver and flamingo tissue grasper close-up. (Karl Storz, Culver City, CA)

the needle is turned by both instruments close to the laparoscope until proper alignment is achieved. Needles are best held perpendicular to the jaws of the driver and in line with the proposed suture line. A curved needle is best grasped halfway along its circumference, whereas the ski-types can be grasped along the straight shaft. An assisting instrument is utilized for tissue alignment and countertraction. Correct alignment and needle handling is crucial to preventing deflection of the needle within the driver's jaws as the needle point enters the tissue for the entrance bite. The most common problems encountered during initial experiences with intracorporeal suturing are frustrating deflections during the entrance bite, needle advancement, or the exit bite. It is recommended that while mastering this skill, the surgeon slows the motions down to the point of control and thinks

about each step while maintaining alignment of needle, driver, countertraction, and tissues (Figure 50-21). At the exit bite, the assistant instrument provides countertraction, the needle is released by the driver and regrasped further back toward the swage and pushed through the tissues. It can at this point be regrasped by the driver.[128]

Suturing   Suturing is the next skill to be relearned for intracorporeal reconstruction. Simple stitches require only one pass through the tissues and one knot to be synched. The goal of the laparoscopic surgeon should be to achieve a perfect stitch, equally apposed entrance and exit bite sizes to avoid tension on one side of the anastomosis or the other.[130] Suture length should be kept to the absolute minimum required for this purpose. During microsurgical laparoscopic suturing, 8 cm is adequate for simple stitches. This allows ample room for the loops necessary for knotting even in thick, muscular bladder reconstructions. Urologic reconstruction can require the utilization of simple running, or running locking sutures on the bladder. These stitches require more length of intracorporeal suture material and careful attention to tension along the repair. A good rule of thumb is that twice the length of a linear incision in suture material is required. Here, as the needle is driven through the tissues at each exit bite, the assistant grasper is utilized to aid in pulling the running stitch through for the given length and creating the desired tension while the needle driver with the reloaded needle is utilized to provide counter

pressure. Since the intracorporeal suturing is arduous, it behooves the surgeon to make sure the suture line is perfect the first time, if this takes time, it is still better than redoing it. Attention to the detail of an ideal suture is paramount. The running suture should start 2 to 3 mm proximal to the incision and run to 2 to 3 mm beyond prior to tying the end knot.[129] Locking is not particularly difficult but should also be carefully orchestrated and not started until the suture line's tension has been rechecked. It is far easier to tighten a running line of suture before rather than after it has been locked intracorporeally. The suture should run at least one needle-driven point beyond the end of the incision. Knotting a running intracorporeal stitch can be more difficult than a simple suture. This will be discussed in the next section.

Knotting   Knot tying represents the final hurdle for proficiency of intracorporeal suturing. Were suturing and needle driving not difficult in themselves, one might say that extracorporeal knotting would certainly be the method of choice. But because the skills necessary for complex endosurgical reconstruction are all linked, knotting represents the last, most difficult task. In addition, once mastered, intracorporeal knots can be manipulated to the endoscopic surgeon's advantage for complex anastomoses very much as in microsurgery (more on this later).[131] The key to successfully mastering intracorporeal knotting has been careful, small, orchestrated movements of the instruments in both of the surgeon's hands.

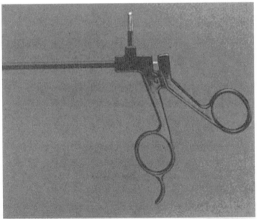

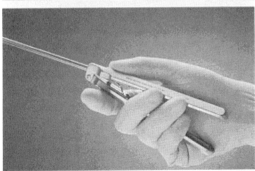

Figure 50-17 Classic finger-ringed instruments entrap the surgeon's hands, right. Left, newer instruments allow fine manipulation of the instrument's tip without encumbering the hands.

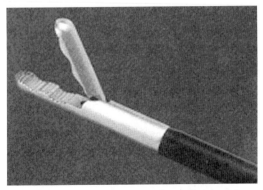

Figure 50-18 A unique laparoscopic needle driver's jaws, close-up. (EndoLap Inc., contour tip with Rack & Pinion power drive.)

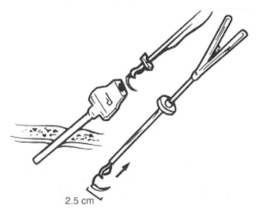

2.5 cm

Figure 50-20 Intracorporeal passage of needles.

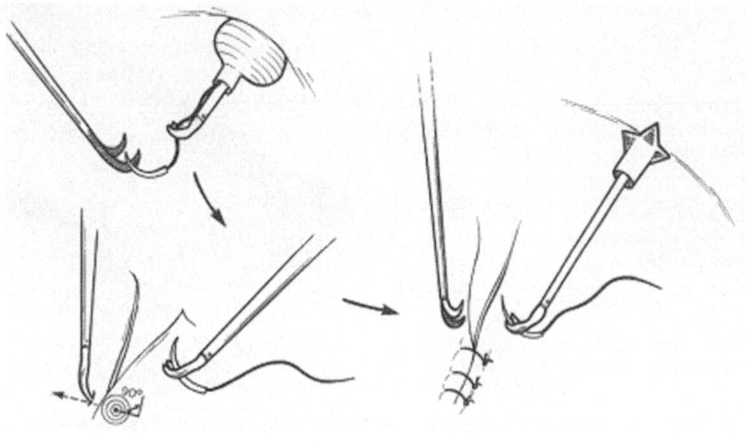

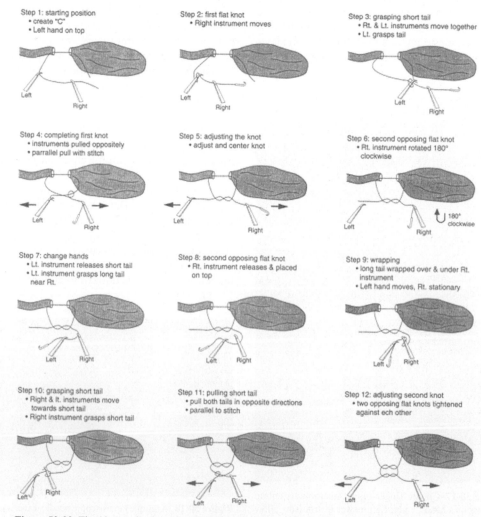

Figure 50-21 The principles of intracorporeal needle driving. Movements should be slowed to the point of control and an understanding of the forces at the entrance and exit bites can prevent frustrating needle deflections.

The intracorporeal knot of most utility is the simple square knot. A square knot is two apposed half hitches, one atop the other. To orchestrate the movements necessary to tie such a knot and eliminate wasted motions, each key movement must be identified and the entire sequence practiced. Reported previously, we discussed the 12 steps in tying an intracorporeal square knot (Figure 50-22).[132] Step 1 is the starting position. A C-shape is made in the suture with the right hand grasping the swaged end of the suture and the left stabilizing the tail. Step 2, the right hand only moves to create a loop around the tip of the left instrument. Step 3, the right and left hands move together as the left instrument grasps the tail of the suture. Step 4, the instruments are pulled in opposite directions paralleling the pull with the suture. Step 5, the knot is adjusted to center the first half hitch directly above the laceration by placing more tension on the right or left hand grasp of suture. Step 6, sets up throwing the second half hitch. The right grasps the swaged end and is rotated 180 degrees clockwise. Step 7, the left instrument releases the short tail and grasps the swaged end near the right grasper. Step 8, the right instrument releases the suture and is placed on top, directly in front of the left grasper. Step 9, the left hand moves to create a loop around the right, which remains stationary. Step 10, the right and left instruments move together toward the short tail, which the right then grasps. Step 11, both instruments are pulled in opposite directions parallel to the stitch. Step 12, the two opposing half hitches are tightened against each other. This concludes the exercises necessary to orchestrate fluid interaction and minimize wasted motions, thus limiting the surgical frustration.

Methods other than that described above can be utilized for laparoscopic intracorporeal knotting. By prefacing these techniques with the reminder that intracorporeal suturing is difficult, but with time, patience, and practice it can be mastered. Utilizing microsurgical principles adapted for the laparoscopic environment, knots and sutures can be manipulated to the surgeon's advantage. This should be kept in mind when considering intracorporeal suturing techniques and taking shortcuts.[133]

Depending on the intracorporeal instruments utilized, a variety of intracorporeal knotting strategies can be performed. If a pin vise needle driver is chosen, an intracorporeal "twist" technique can be performed (Figure 50-23). Utilized by H.C. Topel in Park Ridge, IL, and L. Sharpe in Minneapolis, MN, a sequence of twists (usually 2–3) on the needle wrap the suture around the assistant grasper, keeping the needle curve parallel to the introducer. The free grasper helps release the needle and swage from the jaws, carefully maintaining the loops. Then the looped grasper can grasp the tail and the instruments move in opposite directions to tighten the half hitch. This "twisting" technique can be utilized for both curved and straight needles. Straight needles can be utilized with conventional laparoscopic instruments. Here, the needle is used to wrap the swaged end about the assistant grasper, as long as the instrument is oriented toward the assistant. The tail can then be grasped from the now "looped" grasper. Another technique reported to simplify intracorporeal knotting describes grasping both ends, forming a loop above the repair.[134] The needle driver can then loop through either side to facilitate formation of each half hitch (Figure 50-24). This technique hopes to eliminate "complicated, dextrous, simultaneous two-handed motions." The "smiley-face" technique is another method of promoting the intracorporeal formation of knots (Figure 50-25). During intracorporeal suturing with this technique, emphasis is placed on manipulating both swage and tail segments with the needle.

Figure 50-22 The 12 steps in choreographing the right and left hands for accomplishing fluid intracorporeal suturing and knotting. (Reprinted with permission of W.B. Saunders).

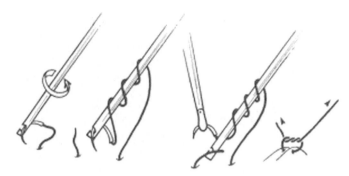

Figure 50-23 Pin vise suturing technique.

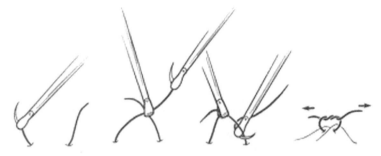

Figure 50-24 Pietrafitta's technique of stabilizing each half hitch.

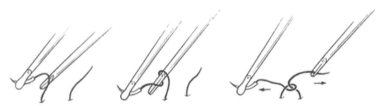

Figure 50-25 Smiley face technique of intracorporeal knotting.

The needle is grasped midshaft with each end pointed upward forming a "smiley face." Each half hitch is then facilitated by wrapping the needle around the assisting instrument to form loops. This technique results in fixed orientation and a stable continuing starting place. Kozminski and colleagues have recently described a fly-casting technique to aid with intracorporeal knotting with interrupted sutures.[135] The tail is grasped and held up in space, next the swage is passed over the tail and allowed to drop by gravity. The swage is retrieved from the underside for the first half hitch (Figure 50-26). Mirror image repeat of

this sequence results in a square knot. Finally, a prelooped needle and suture are available for intracorporeal stitching (Laparomed, Irvine, CA). Once introduced to the area of reconstruction, the needle is advanced and grasped by the driver. The needle is then passed through the preformed double loops and pulled in opposite directions. The applicator plunger is next pushed, pulling the tail and tightening the slipknot. A surgeon's knot can be incorporated by placing 2 loops around the left grasper during the first half hitch. A surgeon's knot adds to the security against slipping, especially with monofilament

sutures such as polypropylene. If further modifications of the knot are required, then the surgeon's knot should not be deployed.

Running sutures may require special intracorporeal knotting techniques. Depending on the type of suture material utilized, there is the need to maintain the tension on the trailing segment of the stitch. Because of the fixed point of exit from the incision, the tail's end must be looped, causing a double-tailed segment that must be manipulated with the free swaged end. This double-stranded loop can result in increased demands on the needle driver and assistant instrument to maintain tension on the suture line while performing intracorporeal knotting. Some monofilament sutures can fracture because of pressures applied by the instruments during knotting. Because of these problems, alternatives have been sought for running intracorporeal knotting. The jamming loop knot (Dundee jamming loop knot) can be thrown extra- or intracorporeally (Figure 50-27). The running suture line can be initiated with the knot outside the abdomen. The suture is then grasped along the swage and passed intracorporeally, usually with the aid of a reducing sleeve. The needle is then passed through the tissues and pulled until the loop approximates the tissues. The needle is then passed back through the loop, and swage and tail ends are pulled in opposite directions, jamming the knot.[136] J.W. Rollero describes the use of a noose-like knot to start running intracorporeal suture lines (Figure 50-28). First, 2 loops are made in a counterclockwise fashion. The tail crosses over the loop and is passed through the center. A third loop is formed by passing back through the center. The first running stitch is passed back through this third noose, anchoring it into place as the tension is applied. The Aberdeen (crochet) knot allows the intracorporeal completion of the running suture line (Figure 50-29). Its major advantage over simple square knots is the avoidance of unequal lengths being manipulated intracorporeally and excessive force being applied to monofilament suture materials. Here the suture is first passed beneath the last running stitch before it is tightened to form a loop. A second loop through the first is fashioned, then the swage with needle is passed through, tightening the loop and synching the knot.[137]

Recently, the interest in running sutured anastomosis has prompted resurgent interest in this technique, particularly as it applies to the vesi-

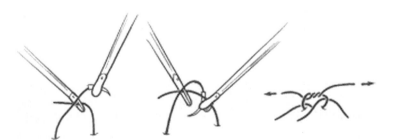

Figure 50-26 Fly-casting method for intracorporeal knotting.

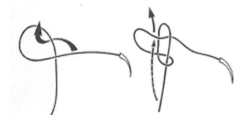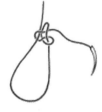

Figure 50-27 Jamming loop knot (Dundee) shown previously can be used for extracorporeal knotting or starting a running stitch.

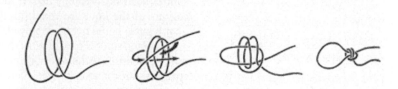

Figure 50-28 Rollero's method of starting a running suture line.

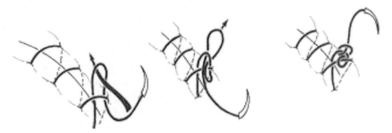

Figure 50-29 The Aberdeen knot (crochet) can be used to securely synch a running intracorporeal suture line if concern exists about crimping a monofilament suture.

courethral repair following laparoscopic radical prostatectomy and during the repair phase of robotic pyeloplasty. This running technique, as mentioned in the introduction to this section, has attracted some significant research attention lately and will be addressed more completely in the section "Running Suturing" below.

INTRACORPOREAL NEEDLES Laparoscopic intracorporeal needle configuration has received limited attention by manufacturers to date. Because of the limitations of the closed working environment and difficulty of intracorporeal suturing, it might be expected that needle configurations should approximate those of microsurgery. Needles should be high-quality stainless steel or carbon steel. Carbon steel needles are harder but are more brittle, and "on-table" adjustments could result in weakening or breaking of the shaft. Homogenous stainless steel is preferred but more costly. The needle profile of choice has not been rigorously investigated.[130] In our study of intracorporeal bladder neck reconstructions, we identified three configurations that facilitated intracorporeal suturing.[132] A curved 3/8 needle, a ski configuration and an S-shaped profile were most helpful (Figure 50-30). Needle points can be taper point, cutting, spatulated, or taper cut, depending on the tissue and resistance expected in suturing.

The spatial constraints limit the needle size, shape, and suture lengths needed to most expeditiously accomplish intracorporeal suturing. For urologic pelvic work on the urethra or bladder neck, the deep recesses of the retropubic space permit only a small 1/2 or 3/8 (RB-1 or TF) taper-point–configured needle to allow eversion of knots when reconstruction is performed. Some investigators have advocated straight needles (SC-1 Ethicon, TS-20 Davis & Geck, EndoSuture WISAP, or ELW U.S. Surgical). These have primary advantage on surface structures or when intracorporeal suturing with straight needle graspers.

INTRACORPOREAL SUTURES Suturing under laparoscopic conditions also produces other influences on the choice of suture materials. Surgical knots must hold and the choice of a woven or monofilament, absorbable versus nonabsorbable must be carefully chosen with this constraint foremost. For urological applications, intracorporeal suturing with plain or chromic gut and polydiox-

anone has advantages for the security of the half-hitch throws. Unfortunately the coloring of each of these suture materials is such that if blood is present at the laceration site, specified ends, crucial for the orchestrated movements already discussed, become impossible. Blood has a tendency to adhere to these suture materials and strict attention to hemostasis is warranted. In addition, the coloration absorbs the light in all these materials except for the blue PDS.[138] As multiple untied sutures are placed but not tied as is required for complex end-to-end anastomoses, swage and tail ends become indistinct (Figure 50-31, left). Brightly colored, optically fluorescent colors are required to overcome this problem. Currently, dye materials that have been investigated to enhance visibility when exposed to xenon light have also demonstrated carcinogenic properties. Despite this, colors most efficacious for laparoscopic suturing include pink, yellow, green, and purple (see Figure 50-31, right).[132]

The next problem for intracorporeal suturing is introducing the correct length of suture material. Available endoscopic suture materials that come prepackaged have no conception as to the requirements of the surgeon for the given task. Therefore, the sutures are often long (> 80 cm). For a simple stitch the length required should be no more than 8 cm for a surface knot or 10 cm for deep stitches.[139] Running sutures are more difficult to approximate, but as previously mentioned, a rule of thumb is to utilize approximately twice the length of the incision.[140] Keeping the length to the minimum required results in less surgical frustration in manipulating long tail segments.

OTHER INTRACORPOREAL SUTURING TECHNIQUES An enormous effort has been placed on developing innovative methods of intracorporeal suturing to obviate the difficulties we have spent so much time outlining above.[16,141] Sheath systems that allow the needles and graspers to be positioned simultaneously have been described (Laparomed Suture Applier, Irvine, CA). Metal clips for replacing intracorporeal knots have been designed and marketed specifically for this pur-

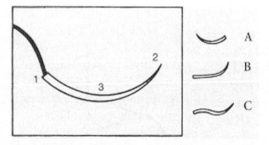

Figure 50-30 Useful needle configurations for intracorporeal urologic reconstruction. 1. swage, 2. point, 3. body. A, 3/8 curve, B, ski configuration, C, S-shaped needle.

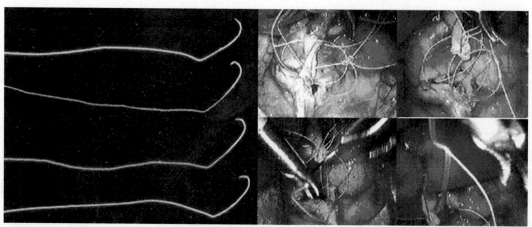

Figure 50-31 Brightly colored sutures that fluoresce in xenon lighting. Left, shows each color identifies swage and tail segments necessary for complex end-to-end anastomoses. Right, close-up of sutures, shows multiple square knot simple sutures ready for conversion to suspension stitches. (Studies from Ethicon indicate a potential carcinogenic property of certain dyes that fluoresce under xenon lighting.)

pose (Ehticon, Cincinnati, OH).[31] Special techniques of tying that produce knots with straight pin vise-type needle drivers have been reported.[50] Mechanical devices are the latest devices that are attempting to reduce the difficulty of intracorporeal suturing and knotting. Stoller has described a simple device that will throw an intracorporeal knot automatically. A suture scope has also been invented with a mechanism for aligning tissues and driving a long needle through two opposing tubular structures (Figure 50-32).[142] Utilizing this device, an endoscopic ureteroneocystostomy has already been performed. The ultimate mechanical suturing device would be an automatic endoscopic sewing machine. Current work with such a device has been investigated and utilized clinically via a large colonoscope by Saclarides and colleagues.[143] The Auto Suture Company has recently introduced its automated, single-handed, 10 mm suturing instrument, EndoStitch, for clinical application (Figure 50-33). This device utilizes a loom-like mechanism to pass a straight needle back and forth through tissues from either end of its jaws. Controllable with a single hand, the needle can simply be reversed and regrasped with a flick of the switch. Intended to be a single-patient use item, the EndoStitch device can be reloaded with the same or different suture materials. Suture materials are available currently in Polysorb (coated, braided, synthetic, polyglactin), Bralon (coated, braided nylon), Sofsilk (coated, braided silk), and Surgidac (coated, braided polyester). The lengths of these preloaded sutures are 18 and 120 cm, with size being dependent on the suture material but ranging from 4-0 to 0 (USP sizing).

Another approach to intracorporeal suturing would be to take advantage of the brightly illuminated, magnified image from the video systems and apply the reconstructive advantages of microsurgery.[21,116,143] This of course requires bringing the laparoscope in close proximity to the

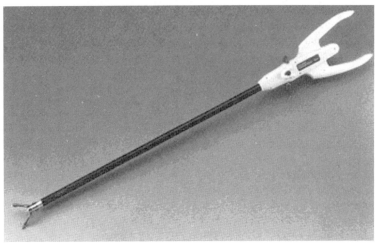

Figure 50-33 EndoStitch is an automatic, loom-like, 10 mm intracorporeal suturing device. With practice, knotting can also be facilitated with this instrument for simple and running sutures. (U.S. Surgical, Norwalk, CT)

area of interest. Each move of the laparoscopic instrument's tips speeds up in equal magnitude to the degree of magnification.[21] All of the intracorporeal skills discussed earlier must be precisely applied or this becomes an impossible task. Hemostasis is even more crucial during laparoscopic microsurgical suturing.[141] The ability to observe small movements of the suture material through tissues is fundamental to smoothly facilitate needle driving, suturing, and knotting. Complex urologic anastomoses have been accomplished utilizing microsurgical techniques, including vesicourethral reanastomosis, augmenta-

tion cystoplasties, and others.[132] The degree of difficulty of microsurgical intracorporeal suturing is twice again as difficult as regular laparoscopic suturing.[132] The advantages of microsurgical reconstruction in urology include less need for long-term urinary diversion or drainage, less infiltration with scar tissue, and visually secure suture placement.[132] In addition, because of the magnification, special suturing techniques can be performed that make end-to-end anastomoses nearly foolproof.[131] Suspension suturing is the technique of converting a square knot into a slipknot and back again on demand (Figure 50-34). This can only be

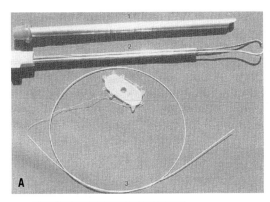

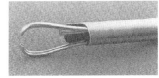

Figure 50-32 A suturoscope from Gomes da Silva. A, Shows the 8 mm outer sleeve (1), the suturing device (2), and the suture material (3). B, Shows a close-up of the suturing devices tip.

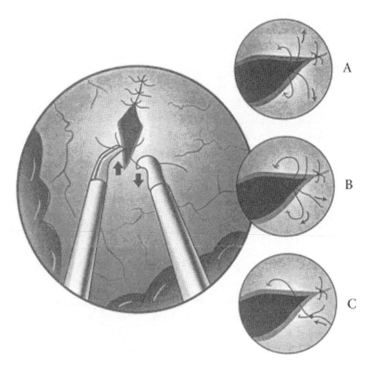

Figure 50-34 Suspension stitch technique for converting square knots to slipknots. Primary utility for end-to-end laparoscopic anastomoses (modified from microsurgery, Dr. Z. Szabo). Top right, square knot opposing pulls to set. Middle right, apposing tension to same side threads converts square knot to slipknot configuration. Bottom right, advancement of slip configuration. Finally, reconversion to square knot by apposing pulls as in top right. (Reprinted with permission of W.B. Saunders).

accomplished if magnification allows careful suture manipulation. With these techniques, spatial constraints and limited visual fields do not prevent the surgeon from even small anastomoses.

RUNNING SUTURING Despite considerable attention just given to suturing techniques, it is felt that one recent suturing method requires separate consideration. Initially Hoznek and colleagues described a simplified urethrovesical anastomosis using two hemicircle sutures with three intracorporeal knots.[144] Van Velthoven further simplified this technique by pretying two 6-inch, 3-0 polyglycolic acid sutures (one dyed and one undyed). Both needles are passed through the posterior bladder neck at the 6 o'clock position where the knot rests (Figure 50-35). Sewing upward on either side of this results in a water-tight closure. If a bladder discrepancy exists, the suture line can be run onto the anterior bladder neck, forming a tennis-racket closure. Van Velthoven and colleagues report utilization in 122 laparoscopic and 8 robotic-assisted radical prostatectomies, with an average anastomotic time of 35 minutes. They have had no postoperative anastomotic leaks and at short follow-up have reported no symptomatic bladder neck contractures.[145] Menon's group has taken this technique and rapidly expanded its clinical application in the robotic-assisted VIP

series at Henry Ford Hospital. Now with over 1,000 consecutive cases presented, the mean operating time has dwindled to 150 minutes.[146]

This technique is easily transposable to other urinary reconstructive procedures, such as Anderson-Hynes dismembered pyeloplasty, ureteroureterostomy, ureteroneocystostomy, and ureteroenterostomy. Preliminary reports of this suturing methodology are beginning to accrue. Much has yet to be learned about this technique. But questions are numerous. Would a monofilament absorbable suture be better than the braided polyglcolic acid suture? Are two colors necessary? Are the two 6-inch lengths ideal? This sutured reconstruction technique appears to facilitate both free-hand as well as robotic-assisted repairs and may well be a true advance in the technique of laparoscopic reconstructive urology. Basic research may yet solve some of the dilemmas, such as the ideal length of a running suture.[147]

But from the beginning there has always existed a conundrum on purely theoretical grounds regarding running sutures. Advantages of interrupted, single suturing methods include the following: nonreliance on a single suture; safer; slower, which allows for more precision; less ischemia potential; and less scarring. Advances for running sutures include the following: quicker, even distribution of tension in a circle,

water-tight closure, more hemostatic, and less scarring. Note that some advantages claimed by both are feasible. Disadvantages of single interrupted suturing include the following: slower than running, more knots need to be placed and tied, more knots yield more inflammatory response, and greater potential for leakage. Finally, disadvantages for running anastomoses are as follows: potiential for ischemia is greater, radial force distortion can be caused by two dissimilar areas approximated, and disruption of entire anastomoses by failure at any point in the single suture. A review of the literature for the past 30 years using PubMed failed to substantiate any of these theoretical claims to suturing. However, a clear renaissance of interest has occurred in the urologic literature particularly in regards to the vesicourethral anastomoses.[148] There are now 101 citations rising exponentially in the past decade prompted by minimally invasive methods. Sutured anastomoses still predominate; however, there has been a spattering of hybrid methodologies, making for more sophisticated repairs. Underscoring the significance of this resurgent research effort are reports by Bariol and colleagues that simply how the suture material is handled effects its integrity.[149] Perhaps seen as no real risk, there are rising numbers of case reports of complete anastomotic separation distantly from the time of the robotic surgery, suggesting that, in fact, the running techniques do contain an Achilles' heal.[150] Finally, the actual problem that may yet come from the technology focusing on this key issue in reconstructive surgery may be the scientific basis whereby *all* the questions that have never formally been answered might now be capable of resolution. We recently completed a series of experiments utilizing the da Vinci Surgical System and micorfiber phantoms to evaluate the number of running suture bites to best perform a simulated vesicourethral anastomosis. Twelve suture bites seemed to be the minimal number that improved measurable variables in this in vitro model (Figure 50-36).[151] Is any of this important you might ask. One complete disruption of a urinary anastomosis is a catastrophic complication, and this era where risk directly correlates with complications, any effort to minimize complications should be sought. This brings us to a potential solution to the Achilles' heel, or running suture lines, that is, hybrid techniques such as suturing and gluing. Could a suture glue be devised that could combine the security of gluing with the unparalleled advantages of absorbable sutures in the urinary tract? We have been investigating just such a material that has no real glue, but an innovative bidirectional barbed suture that acts like glue but can be used like standard suture. Using the same fiduciary model that was used to optimize the number of suture bites, we have been investigating Quill (Quill Sutures, Research Triangle Park, NC) barbed, bidirectional sutures versus the standard Van Velthoven method. The Quill sutures were faster to deploy, were very accurately placed, and most significantly, were very fault tolerant. Cutting every fourth suture resulted in no

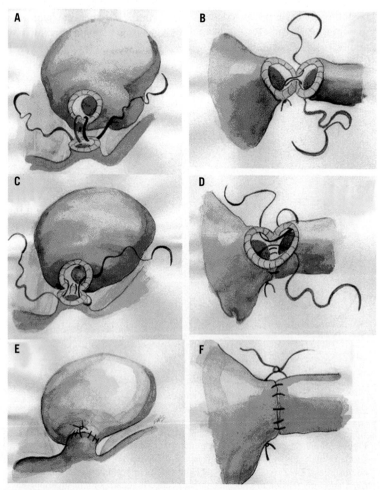

Figure 50-35 Van Velthoven's method of running vesicourethral anastomosis with a single intracorporeal knot. Two 6-inch lengths are tied together extracorporeally with 2 different colored absorbable sutures.

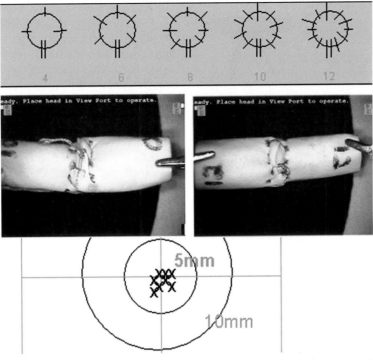

Figure 50-36 Running suture technique for investigations into robotic-assisted anastomoses.

loss of the anastomosis, cutting every other suture resulted in some separation of edges, but again, the suture line held against disruption.[152]

EXTRACORPOREAL STAPLING

The first utilization of surgical stapling technology in laparoscopic surgery was for the resection of bowel. The development of large abdominal trocars allowed the surgeon to deliver the isolated bowel segment extracorporeally for the stapled resection using classic "open" techniques. These trocars were specially designed with sizes approaching 30 and 40 mm. In experimental models, the bowel could be easily mobilized on its vascular mesentery, opening a window for the resected segment intracorporeally. The segment could then be grasped with endoscopic, Babcock-type clamps and delivered via the large working trocar (Figure 50-37). Standard functional end-to-end anastomoses utilizing linear cutting staplers and TA staplers have been performed. Urologically, this technique was first utilized by Kozminski's group to perform an ileal conduit urinary diversion.[15] End-to-end anastomoses have been accomplished with a variety of techniques using extracorporeally assisted circular staplers (Figure 50-38). The esophagus and colon have been the prime organs resected in this fashion. Following colon resection, a purse-string suture is placed to secure both luminal ends, two to secure the open stapler and one to fix the anvil. An alternative to EEA staplers is the biodegradable anastomotic ring (BAR) device (see Figure 50-38). This instrument (Valtrac, Davis and Geck, Stamford, CT) (bottom of Figure 50-47) has been utilized for laparoscopic-assisted colon anastomoses via small celiotomies. Purse-string sutures are again

necessary prior to applying this anastomotic ring; however, special applicators for the purse-string application are being devised.[143] These devices have compared favorably with standard stapler reconstruction in comparative clinical trials.[19] Laparoscopic application has been described by Sackier and colleagues.[144] This may yet be of significance, especially with increasing concerns regarding the devascularizing effects of triple-stapled, functional side-to-side anastomoses resulting in long-term luminal narrowing.[44]

INTRACORPOREAL CLIPPING AND STAPLING

The primary applications of intracorporeal stapling and clipping have been discussed during the

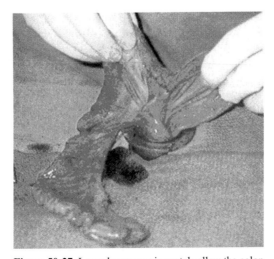

Figure 50-37 Large laparoscopic portals allow the colon to be delivered to the anterior abdominal wall. Extracorporeal suturing techniques can then be performed.

theory of laparoscopic hemostasis and tissue reapproximation. Now attention will be focused on the use of these devices. As with almost every laparoscopic instrument, there are the considerations of reusable versus disposable devices. Clip appliers come in both forms, but as of this writing the automatic staplers are single-patient–use items. One primary problem with these devices is the lack of research data regarding their reliability, problems commonly encountered during utilization, tissue reactivity, and ease of use. Because of the extensive utilization of their open counterparts, they have become instantly popular amongst laparoscopic surgeons. Because of the many barriers to intracorporeal suturing, clip appliers and automatic staplers have become routine instruments on many operating room tables.

CLIP APPLIERS Clip appliers are primarily available from a variety of manufacturers: Ethicon EndoSurgery (Cincinnati, OH), Tyco Healthcare (U.S. Surgical, Norwalk, CT), Weck Closure Systems, North Carolina (Figures 50-39 and 50-40) and Surgicon (Stratford, CT). Clip appliers have several crucial features warranting careful scrutiny by the surgical consumer (Table 50-4). The size, shape, and security of the applied metallic clips should be initially discussed. Titanium clip sizes range from 6.0 to 11.0 mm. Each company's clip has a characteristic "footprint." Investigations imply that all laparoscopic clips are capable of being distracted.[36] Dislodgement should be a feature recognized by all laparoscopists. Once applied, further dissection around the clip is capable of transversely dislodging them from their occluded target. Nondisposable clip appliers require multiple passages through the entrance trocar for multifiring. There is only the initial purchase price of the instrument and the reloadable cartridges versus each disposable clip applier. The disposable clip appliers have additional features that are currently not available on the reusable instruments. Disposable devices are multifire capable (20 or 30 clips) with rotatable shafts. The pistol grip can comfortably rest in the surgeons palm, as the angle of application can be adjusted 360 degrees. At present, small and medium clip appliers are designed for placement through 10 mm portals. Larger clip appliers can be placed via 12 mm portals. When a clip is

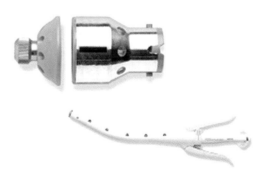

Figure 50-38 End-to-end anastomotic stapler. (Premium Plus CEEA single-use stapler, U.S. Surgical, Tyco Healthcare, Norwalk, CT)

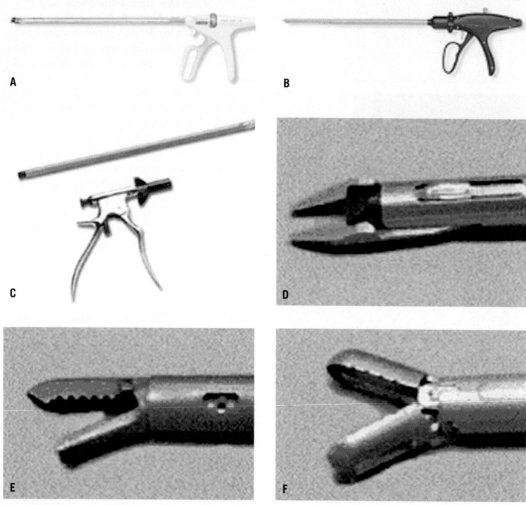

Figure 50-39 Three manufacturers' disposable clip appliers, top row is 10 mm U.S. Surgical appliers (left is single use and right is reusable, middle is the Applied Urology TiGold (Applied Medical), and below are three companies' (5 mm) clip appliers.

reusable applicator coupled with the cost of the polymer clips (approximately $60 [US]) certainly puts them at a fiscal advantage. In addition, centers such as the Cleveland Clinic have now begun to use the 5 mm clip during the dissection of the vascular pedicle during the laparoscopic radical prostatectomy. A clip placed during the lateral dissection of the prostatic base off the bladder neck results in less risk of thermal injury to the neurovascular bundles. In addition, the nonabsorbable polymer clip has no image artifact on subsequent CT or MR scanning, and it won the Gold Award for Medical Design in Manufacturing (MDEA 2000).

Research work has also been performed on the tissue reactivity of various types of clips.[26] All clips can potentially cause adhesion formation.[83] In studies of metallic versus absorbable types of clips, no significant difference could be made for one type versus the other. Others have been concerned about the reliability of these clips for maintaining hemostasis.[9] We have already discussed the distractibility of these laparoscopic clips.[13] The technique of vascular pedicle application deserves further discussion. Most investigators mention that more than 1 clip is necessary on major vascular structures. In addition, the clips are probably most secure if placed in an oppositely opposed fashion such that the open jaws are not facing the same direction. Electrocautery should not be used when dividing clipped vessels because conductance should occur with these metallic structures. Necrosis could result in sloughing of the vessels within the occluding clips. Finally, studies have been performed on the ability to perform CT and MR imaging following titanium clip application. Although they produce artifacts, they do so less than other steel clips, yet more than absorbable ones.

BITING CLIP APPLIERS Clip appliers were specifically designed to occlude and control vascular structures. The need to reapproximate and hold tissues together in fixed positions prompted the development of biting clip appliers. The surgeon's interest in laparoscopic herniorrhaphy was the primary driving force for the availability of both reusable and disposable instruments.[84] These must be applied carefully to take full advantage of the biting ends (Table 50-5). Initially, the surgeon should have the two opposing tissue edges approximated with graspers. Next, the clip applier's trig-

deployed, the vessels should be carefully positioned by assisting graspers for alignment perpendicular to the jaws. Using multifire, disposable clip appliers, the clip should be loaded intracorporeally to avoid inadvertent dislodgement during passage through the flapper valves of the trocar. By gently squeezing the trigger, the clip applier more firmly grasps the clip so that the exact deployment site can be selected. The trigger is then firmly squeezed. If too much force is used, or too much tissue is taken, then the delicate autoloading mechanisms can malfunction, precluding further use of an approximately $150 (US) disposable device.

The most recent addition to the market of metallic clips is the Surgicon 5 mm closed-biased device (Figure 50-41). It delivers a spring design and not a crushing clip applier as do all the rest presented here. This new clip design generates force between spring arms even in the closed position, thus in theory creating higher distracting forces to dislodge the clip. Also, the manufacturers suggest that because of the closed-spring–biased design, there cannot develop during deployment "clip scissoring." Riskin and Schwaitzberg recently published a comparitive evaluation of this clip on in vitro tubings of vari-

ous diameters. They noted that the Surgicon clip was the most reliable clip in terms of distraction forces (see Figure 50-41). They noted that 10 mm clips are more predictable than 5 mm devices in general. They noted that all the 5 mm devices had the widest range of holding strength, except for the Surgicon device. In fact, the Surgicon 5 mm clip applier has the highest holding force on all tested substrates and ranged from 18% to as much as 225% stronger than all the competition.[153] Notably lacking for comparison in this study is the Weck Hem-o-lok clips.

The Weck clips are available for use in either a 5 mm or 10 mm reusable applier. The clip cartridges have 6 clips per cart and come in 14 cartridges per box. The 10 mm clip applier can securely close a vessel as large as 13 mm, but can close larger, deformable vessels such as the renal vein. The 5 mm, Endo5 can be applied to a vessel as large as 10 mm. The Weck also has a 32 cm endoscopic clip removal device for both the 10 mm and 5 mm clip appliers. These clips have been utilized extensively in laparoscopic urologic surgery for control of the renal hilar vasculature (Figure 50-42). Problems with the clip application has anecdotally been reported, but most of the feedback is positive. The cost effectiveness of the

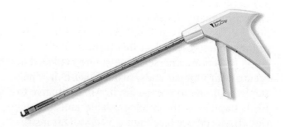

Figure 50-40 The AcuClip disposable clip applier for right-angle application. It has 20 clips and a 28 cm shaft, clip sizes are 3.8 to 8 mm long. (U.S. Surgical, Tyco Healthcare, Norwalk, CT)

Table 50-4 Laparoscopic Clip Appliers

Manufacturer	Clip Applier Name	Diameter	Length	Clip Size	Clips/Unit
Aesculap	SLS	5.5 mm	30 mm	Small/Medium	NA – single fire
		6.5 mm	30 mm	Medium	NA – single fire
		10 mm	33 mm	Medium or Large	NA – single fire
	Sovereign	10 mm	26 mm	Medium/Large	8
	Multifire	10 mm	37 mm	Medium/Large	8
Applied Med	TiGold	10 mm	?	Medium/Large	14
CONMED	Reflex	5 mm	?	Medium/Large	15
	Reflex ELC	10 mm	?	Medium/Large	20
	PermaClip Multi	10 mm	?	Medium/Large	10
Ethicon	LigaClip	10 mm	2.8 mm	Medium	20
	ERCA			Medium/Large	20
				Large	20
	ALLPORT LLS	5 mm	33.8 mm	Medium	30
		5 mm	30.2 mm	Large	20
Microline	Microline Multifire	10 mm	?	Medium/Large	19
SOLOS Endo	Clip Applying Forceps	10 mm	?	Small	NA – single fire
				Medium	NA – single fire
				Large	NA – single fire
U.S. Surgical	AcuClip	10 mm	?	Medium	20
	EndoClip	5 mm	28 mm	Medium	12
	EndoClip ML	10 mm	33 mm	Medium/Large	20
	EndoClip M	10 mm	33 mm	Medium	20
	EndoClip L	10 mm	33 mm	Large	15
	EndoClip II ML	10 mm	29 mm	Medium/Large	20
	EndoClip MultApplier	10 mm	32.5 mm	Medium	8
Wisap	Clip-	10 mm	28 mm	Large	NA – single fire
	Applicator Titan Clip LT 300	10 mm	33 mm	Large	NA – single fire
Wolf	Clip Applier	10 mm	34 mm	Large	NA – single fire

ger is pulled so as to just expose the biting ends. Each tip is carefully positioned to centrally locate the clip across the tissue edges. Finally, further tension on the trigger produces the "B" configuration in an ideal location of the tissues to be approximated. Utilization of these devices has been in reperitonealization following transabdominal bilateral pelvic lymphadenectomy, fixation of mesh for hernia repairs,[84] retracting viscera from the pelvis for high-dose radiation therapy with mesh,[85] fixation of vesicourethral slings,[86,87] and closure of mesenteric defects after bowel resection.[44] Another refinement of the biting clip applicator is the addition of a distal articulating segment. This additional degree of motion allows angulation upward to 40 degrees. The surgeon can thus fixate materials such as mesh to the anterior abdominal wall or deep pelvic recess (ie, Cooper's ligament) from a fixed access trocar.

The U.S. Surgical clip applier incorporates an articulating head so as to angle the clip applier toward the stapler's head, maximizing the angle of entrance upward to the anterior abdominal wall. These instruments have been described for the reperitonealization following transabdominal laparoscopic pelvic lymphadenectomies and for the securing of pubo-bladder neck slings in research studies. A new biting, nonperforating clip applier (VCS clip applier, U.S. Surgical) is a 5 mm applier that has been used by the Washington University group to experimentally perform pyeloplasties and ureterostomies without difficulty and with no encrustation in the porcine model. A newer prototype, the EndoTriceps (U.S. Surgical) is being evaluated for eversion of edges during tissue reapproximation using the same VCS technology.[154]

Both Ethicon and U.S. Surgical produce disposable multifire biting clip appliers with either 10 or 20 clips per instrument. Both devices have a 360-degree rotatable shaft and a distal articulating feature. There exists one investigation comparing sutures with each of these company's clips for security following placement. Prolene sutures resulted in higher burst pressures, thus more security followed by the Ethicon EMS staple, followed by the U.S. Surgical Endohernia staple in decreasing order of strength.[88]

TACKERS OR ANCHORS The biting clips discussed previously were the forerunners of more sophisticated methods of tissue reapproximation that now include tackers and anchoring devices. Not long ago, the market for these devices was limited to fixation of mesh for repair of hernias. Now a wide range of applications is beginning to be appreciated for these sophisticated devices and novel methods of tissue approximation. The Ethicon EndoAnchor is a 5 mm device that penetrates the tissue for fixation of mesh during hernia repairs (Figure 50-43, top). The anchoring system deploys nitinol harpoon-like fixators through the applied mesh to keep it from moving and is approximately 6.7 mm across and 5.9 mm in depth. The AutoSuture device is likewise a 5 mm instrument called the ProTack.[155] This is a helical tacking system that literally is screwed through the mesh and anchored into the adjacent tissues (see Figure 50-43 bottom). It is 4.0 mm in diameter and 3.8 mm in depth. Two fixation devices are available from ONUX Medical (Hampton, NH), the Touché, which is a 5 mm titanium suturing device, and the Salute a single stroke fixation device (Figure 50-44). The final device that can be placed within this category is the U-Clip device from anastomotic device (Coalescent Surgical, Sunnyvale, CA). This is an extrudable nitinol device with a unique retainer end that allows it to function similarly to an anastomotic suture (Figure 50-45).[156]

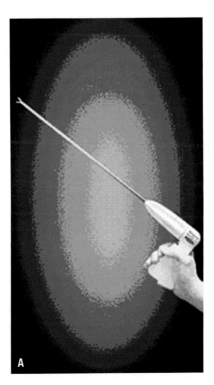

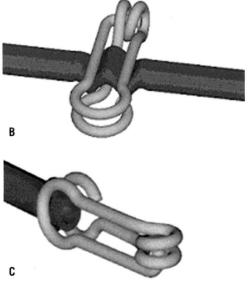

Figure 50-41 Surgicon's unique spring-biased laparoscopic clip. (Surgicon's SpringLock Ligation System, Stratford, CT)

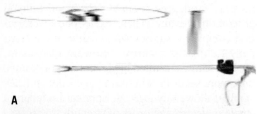

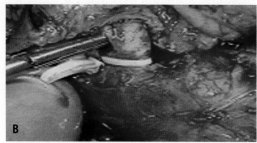

Figure 50-42 Weck Hem-o-lok clip applier with the clinical application of the larger and smaller clips on the renal artery and renal vein. Five mm applier is above, and 10 mm applier is below. (Weck Teleflex Medical, Research Triangle Park, NC)

Table 50-5 Laparoscopic Biting Clip Appliers (also Referred to as Tackers)							
Manufacturer	Device Name	Type	Diameter	Length	Clip Diameter	Clip Length	Tack per Unit
Davol/Bard	Salute Fixation System	Tacking	5 mm	380 mm	4.1 mm	NA	10
	Salute Fixation System	Tacking	5 mm	38 mm	4.1 mm	NA	50
Ethicon	EndoAnchor	Tacking	5 mm	360 mm	6.7 mm	5.9 mm	20
U.S. Surgical	TACKER	Tacking	5 mm	–	–	–	30
	Mesh Fixation System ProTack 5 mm	Tacking	5 mm	180 mm	4.1 mm	NA	30

AUTOMATIC STAPLERS Endoscopic stapling technology probably has advanced the least of all of the reconstructive methods that have been discussed to this point, but there are notable exceptions that deserve attention. In addition, some newer modifications are likely to have an impact on these most useful laparoscopic devices. Also, the utilization of laparoscopic staplers has had widespread applicability, and large series are available to better understand the efficacy of these devices and their clinical hazards.[157]

Automated stapling devices allow the rapid deployment of multiple, metallic staples to facilitate division and reapproximation of visceral structures (Figure 50-46). These devices are available for laparoscopic, intracorporeal utilization with a variety of features. There are linear cutting manual, linear cutting powered, linear noncutting manual, and linear noncutting powered multifire disposable staplers currently marketed (Table 50-6). Each stapler has a specific size trocar limitation. The EndoGIA 30 (Tyco Healthcare, U.S. Surgical, Norwalk, CT) is the original mechanical linear cutting device. It requires a 12 mm laparoscopic portal for placement. The EndoGIA 60 requires a 15 mm trocar. Ethicon's EndoPath 30 and EndoPath 60 (Ethicon EndoSurgery, Cincinnati, OH) require a 12 mm and 18 mm trocar, respectively. All automatic staplers have a 360-degree rotatable shaft and many are reticulated.

The EndoGIA 30 and EndoPath 30 each deploy 2 triple rows of staples from the 30 mm blades. The staples are available in reloadable, color-coded cartridges: white 2.5 mm, blue 3.8 mm, and green 4.8 mm. Staple size depends on the thickness of tissues being reapproximated or divided. The white 2.5 mm staples are usually used on vascular structures because of their compressibility. The larger blue 3.8 mm and green 4.8 mm staples are ideal more for thicker visceral structures such as thickened ureter, small bowel,

large bowel, or the bladder. An endoscopic sizer is available for tissue compression that will indicate which size staples will produce the best anastomosis or occlusion (EndoGauge, U.S. Surgical).

Linear cutting staplers usually deploy 3 rows of staples on either side of the cutting blade. The one exception is the EndoPath 60, which fires double rows. An important consideration in utilizing automated staplers is that the knife cuts short of the end of the staple line. Also, the staples are not loaded to the ends of the cartridges, making deployment length shorter than the 30 or 60 mm of the instrument. For this reason, when applying a linear cutting stapler, the ends should be seen protruding beyond the distal side of tissue prior to engaging the firing mechanisms. The actual placement and firing of an endoscopic stapler is similar to their open cousins. Once in an intracorporeal cavity, the release mechanism allows the jaws to be opened. Graspers are utilized to guide the targeted visceral structure into the opened jaws. The graspers then align the tissues so as to provide a straight, smooth staple line without tissue bunching. The safety is disengaged and the trigger is pulled, which fires the staples and moves the knife that separates the tissues. The manufacturers have utilized a safety lockout mechanism that will prevent the knife from cutting tissue if the staple cartridge is empty or if a misfire should occur. In addition, these disposable staplers can multifire reloaded cartridges up to 3 additional firings (a total of 4).

Linear noncutting staplers are available in both 30 and 60 mm lengths. Theoretically, these staplers reapproximate tissues with less incorporation of tissue mass. The Ethicon EndoPath 30

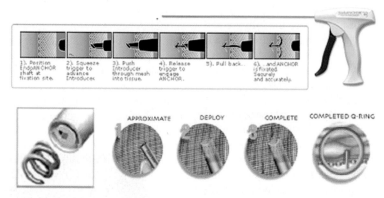

Figure 50-43 Ethicon's EndoSurgery's EndoAnchor on top. U.S. Surgical's spiral tacking device is below (Protack), and ONUX Medical's Salute (ONUX Medical, Hamptom, NY).

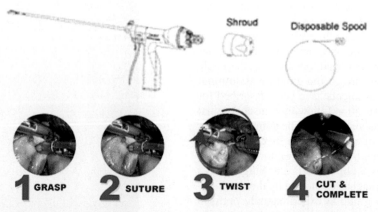

Figure 50-44 The ONUX Medical Touche suturing system (top) and Salute single stroke endoscopic fixation system. (ONUX Medical, Hampton, NH)

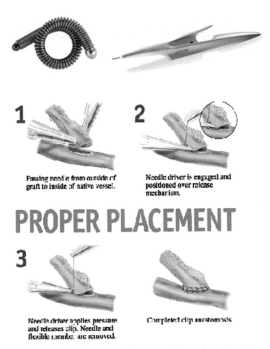

PROPER PLACEMENT

1 Passing needle from outside of graft to inside of native vessel.

2 Needle driver is engaged and positioned over release mechanism.

3 Needle driver applies pressure and releases clip. Needle and flexible member are removed.

Completed clip anastomosis.

Figure 50-45 The U-clip Anastomotic Device from Coalescent Surgical (Sunnyvale, CA)

really is a major advance for laparoscopic urologic reconstruction.

As mentioned in the opening paragraph of this section, stapler and staple designs are beginning to be investigated for modifications that could improve efficiency. The leg and crown design of the staple itself has recently been altered by U.S. Surgical (Tyco Healthcare, Norwalk, CT). Coupled with changes in the anvil of the stapler, the B-mode configuration of the staples can be more reliably formed and deployed.

Another method of stapling is the rapid application in general surgical series of EEA staplers. A whole host of surgical bypass procedures have been performed laparoscopically with the aid of these end-to-end, circular intestinal stapling devices. Novel methods of deploying the anvil of the circular stapler have been developed and used on literally thousands of patients. Gastric bypass for morbid obesity, Roux-en-Y procedures, and low anterior resections have all been performed with laparoscopic techniques utilizing this stapling methodology.[158] The technology has advanced to the point that "intelligent" computer-assisted stapling devices are beginning to be uti-

lized, such as the SurgASSIST laparoscopic stapling device. This instrument consists of an in situ autocalibration computer to aid in precision staple application. It is capable of being used for open and laparoscopic procedures with a flexible shaft that rotates 360 degrees. The distal jaw closure ensures that 55 mm of tissue can be resected and sealed with the stapler. Essentially, this computer-mediated transection device (CMTD) can replace all the other staplers that currently occupy operating room space with one device. The flexible shaft of this unit allows the surgeon to reach and repair viscera that have been inaccessible with conventional, fixed stapling devices (Figure 50-47).[159] As with most of this cutting-edge technology, the price tag speaks for itself. The Digital Loading Unit (DLU) costs approximately $50,000 (US). The disposable portions, ie, the stapling parts, each cost $360 (US), which is the approximate cost of current circular staplers.

Laparoscopic stapling devices are complex mechanical systems and the utilizing urologist should be intimately aware of their mechanisms of action and also their potential for misfiring. Several recent reports have clearly delineated the risks

and EndoPath 60 deploy 4 staple rows. The Tyco Surgical EndoTA is a pneumatically powered noncutting linear stapler that deploys 3 rows. The staples on all the noncutting instruments are identical to their cutting relatives.

Linear cutting staplers have been utilized for a wide variety of general surgical, thoracic, gynecologic, and urologic applications. As previously mentioned, the 30 mm length, 2.5 mm stapler has been utilized to divide vascular pedicles. The availability of larger linear cutting staplers is responsible for intracorporeal gastrointestinal resections and reconstructions. Small bowel resections, partial colectomies, laparoscopic-assisted low anterior resections, gastric resections, gastrojejunostomies, esophageal resections, pulmonary wedge resections, lobectomies, and pneumonectomies have all been facilitated with linear cutting staplers. Solid viscera have also been removed with the aid of these devices, including the spleen, kidney, and uterus. Urologic reconstructions, including ileal conduit formation and distal ureterectomy and partial cystectomy, have been accomplished intracorporeally with the aid of these staplers. The noncutting staplers were originally developed for thoracoscopic purposes but are useful for closing enterotomies.

The major drawback other than the nonabsorbable foreign body within the urinary tract is cost for these automated staplers. Estimates for linear cutting staplers run from $250 to $350 (US) per instrument. Reloadable cartridges can currently be placed for no more than four applications. Each cartridge costs from $100 to $130 (US). To date there are no circumferential end-to-end anastomotic, intracorporeal staplers. There are no currently available absorbable automated, intracorporeal staplers. Despite these drawbacks, the ability to rapidly, hemostatically, and reliably separate viscera and reapproximate them intracorpo-

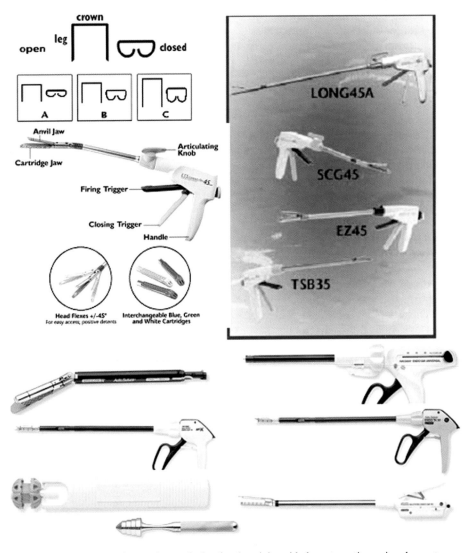

Figure 50-46 Linear cutting staplers, reticulated and straight, with the pneumatic version shown, top are Ethicon's and below are U.S. Surgical's. Bottom left is U.S. Surgical's Valtrac Biofragmetable anastomotic ring device (with purse string suture device).

Table 50-6 Laparoscopic Linear Cutting Staplers*

Name	EndoPath ETS	EndoPath ETS Flex Articulating	EndoPath EZ45 cutter	EndoPath EZ45 no cutting	Multifire EndoTA 30	Multifire EndoTA 30	EndoGIA Universal
Manufacturer	Ethicon	Ethicon	Ethicon	Ethicon	US Surg	US Surg	
Port Size	12	12	12	12	12	12	12
Staple Size (mm)	vasc thin	vasc thin	reg	reg	2/2.5/3.5	2.5/3.5	2/2.5/3.5/4.8
Staple Length (mm)	35	35	45	45	30	30	30/45/60
All have rotating shafts 360°							
Reticulating	no	yes	no	no	no	no	yes
Price (est) (USD)	$1,174 (3)	$1,467 (3)	$1,456 (3)	$1.456 (3)	$969 (3)	$900 (3)	$594 (3)

Note: Staple loads cost between $150 and $225 for each reload.
*Data from 1998 lists.

of EndoGIA staplers misfiring during crucial vascular division in laparoscopic nephrectomy cases.[160] During a 6-year period, 353 patients underwent laparoscopic donor nephrectomy at Johns Hopkins Medical Institutions, and there were only 2 endovascular GIA misfires.[161] A larger survey by Meng and colleagues also points out how disastrous this complication can be, arguing for being always instantly prepared for this rare complication. This same group has essentially given up using the cutting linear staplers for control of the renal vasculature, opting instead for the endoscopic TA staplers.[162] There is much to be said for this cautious approach.

One other rare but definite risk of endoscopic staplers has been recently noted, the ability of loose metallic foreign bodies to migrate and cause insidious complications, such as mechanical small-bowel obstruction and staple erosion into the urinary tract and the subsequent identification of microtacks in the urinary bladder. Finally, there are anecdotal cases of major vascular ligation and division utilizing these staplers. The infrarenal aorta and vena cava have both been reported to be inadvertently stapled and divided during advanced laparoscopic surgery.[163]

LAPAROSCOPIC UROLOGIC RECONSTRUCTION

In the first edition of this textbook, series were small in the urologic reconstructive realm of laparoscopy. This is no longer the case. Well over 3,000 laparoscopic radical prostatectomies have been performed worldwide with reconstructed, sutured vesicourethral anastomosis. Over 500 laparoscopic pyeloplasties have been reported with sutured repair. Now emerging with larger series is laparoscopic radical cystectomy with either orthotopic or heterotopic sutured/stapled urinary diversion. The implications and abilities for the urologist to intervene and reconstruct the urinary tract are now widely being applied. In this section, each urinary organ will be isolated and discussed with review of the relavent literature. Every aspect of urologic reconstruction has been attempted on the kidney, ureter, bladder, bladder neck, urethra, and genitalia. Recently, the inferior epigastric artery was isolated and harvested for reconstruction of the penile vasculature for impotence.[164] Laparoscopic ileal vaginal reconstruc-

tion has been accomplished in a young woman with Mayer-Rokitansky-Küster-Hauser syndrome.[165] Virtually every intersexual condition has now been reported to be successfully treated with the aid of laparoscopic reconstructive measures.[166] The following will be a discussion of the most recent series of laparoscopic urologic reconstructive surgery with historical references when relavent.

RENAL RECONSTRUCTION Literally every open procedure performed on the kidney has now been done laparoscopically. Procedures include the following: pyeloplasty, parital nephrectomy for malignancy, partial nephrectomy for duplication anomalies, partial nephrectomy for fusion anomalies, lower-pole partial nephrectomy for stones, ureterocalicostomy, pyelolithotomy, anatrophic nephrolithotomy, pyelocaliceal diverticulectomy, renovascular surgery, autotransplant, donor transplantation, and nephropexy. Here, the literature will be viewed from the standpoint of the laparoscopic reconstruction efforts. Attention will be particularly paid to those methods that the investigators are utilizing to repair the genitourinary tract, and their postoperative management and outcomes.

Laparoscopic Pyeloplasty Of all the renal procedures currently being done, the most commonly performed ,short of nephrectomy, is reconstruction for primary or secondary ureteropelvic junction obstructions (Figure 50-48). The laparoscopic approach to the repair of this condition is so successful at some institutions that it has become the "method of choice" for repairing all patients presenting with UPJ obstruction. Oth-

ers argue that less invasive endopyelotomy approaches remain viable alternatives in selected patients with a high probability of success. Marcovich and colleagues recently reported on trends from 37 endourologists in North America. They found that 41% were still performing endopyelotomy, that 51% were performing laparoscopic pyeloplasty, and about 50% were still performing open pyeloplasty. Of note, about 20% of thosed polled would now choose a laparoscopic pyeloplasty as first-line therapy.[167] A single institution's comparison of laparoscopic pyeloplasty, Acucise endopyelotomy, and open pyeloplasty showed success rates of 94%, 54%, and 86%, respectively.[168] It is easy to understand that the trend among endourologists is to consider laparoscopic pyeloplasty as first-line therapy.

Schuessler and colleagues have reported their first 6 cases of laparoscopic dismembered pyeloplasty.[53] All were performed with running 4-0 polyglactin sutures, 2 had reduction pyeloplasties, and all were drained postoperatively. He has subsequently reported on 6 additional cases with operative times ranging from 180 to 420 minutes.[169] Two additional laparoscopic pyeloplasties are reported using a 4-0 absorbable suture material. The largest single series has come from Johns Hopkins with 100 reported cases. Seventy-one of these 100 cases were Anderson-Hynes dismembered pyeloplasties with sutured reconstruction. Their average operative time was 252 minutes (range 120–480 minutes). The success rate is reported to be 96% at a mean follow-up of 32.4 months.[170] Gaur and colleagues described 8 patients who underwent laparoscopic pyelolithotomy without closure of the pyelotomy inci-

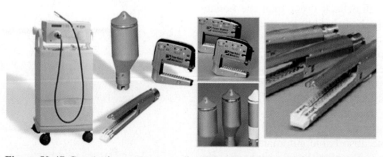

Figure 50-47 SurgAssist computer-mediated flexible endoscopic surgical stapler. Comes with circular, right angle linear, and linear stapling capability. (Power Medical Interventions, New Hope, PA)

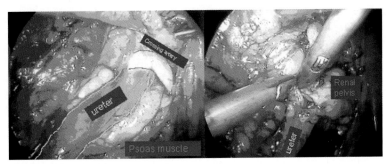

Figure 50-48 Laparoscopic pyeloplasty.

sion.[171] They have subsequently described a homemade intracorporeal suturing instrument to solve the problem of open drainage in order to reconstruct the pyelotomy.[128] Laparoscopic pyeloplasty has also been utilized to synchronously extract calculi and repair the obstructed ureteropelvic junction. In the single largest cohort, 19 patients with 20 renal units underwent simulateous interventions. Varying methods of laparoscopic reconstruction were used, including the Anderson-Hynes (11), Y-V plasty (8), and Heinecke Mickulicz (1). Stone-free status was 90% (17 of 19) and 90% had no obstruction at 3 months follow-up. Two of these patients have recurrent stones at follow-up for an 80% stone-free rate (16 of 20).[172] Laparoscopic pyeloplasty has been evaluated for the treatment of secondary UPJ obstructions. In a multi-institutional evaluation of 36 patients with an average of 1.3 prior procedures (range 1–4), the reported patency rate for a laparoscopic pyeloplasty is 89% and the reasonable objective response was 94%.[173] In addition to salvage for secondary UPJs, other reconstructive urologic procedures may be necessary in patients who have had previous surgery and long segmental defects affecting the UPJ. Kaouk and colleagues reported the use of a dismembered tabularized flap repair in a 73-year-old with a solitary kidney who had failed multiple prior procedures.[174] In addition, a laparoscopic ileal ureter reconstruction was described by the same group from the Cleveland Clinic. An 87-year-old with a solitary left kidney had a solitary proximal ureteral tumor and underwent a total ureterectomy and an ileal ureteral interposition.[175]

One recent review used a decision tree analysis to compare the costs of each method of UPJ repair at a single institution. A retrograde ureteroscopic endopyelotomy was the least costly ($3,842 [US]). The Acucise endopyelotomy was next ($4,427 [US]), followed by antegrade endopyelotomy ($5,297 [US]), laparoscopic pyeloplasty ($7,026 [US]) and open pyeloplasty ($7,119 [US]).[176] The authors are quick to point out that the financial data are arbitrary to the decision, but in the current health care environment the failure to consider this is likewise unacceptable. In conclusion, patients with UPJ obstructions, especially with crossing vessels, are increasingly being considered for laparoscopic pyeloplasty. The success of this operation is very good, rivaling that of its open alternative. The

method of choice for the repair has yet to be answered; however, for patients with crossing vessels, the Anderson-Hynes dismembered pyeloplasty appears to be the most reliable method with intracorporeally sutured anastamosis.

Partial Nephrectomy Reconstruction As every other aspect of open renal surgery has been reproduced laparoscopically, it is important to consider the reconstructive aspects of partial nephrectomy. Partial nephrectomies in the earlier edition of this textbook were anecdotal, now a MedLine search shows greater than 56 published articles on this primarily. Most partial nephrectomies are performed for malignancy. The largest series was reported at the 2003 American Urologic Association Meeting by Gill and colleagues. They compared laparoscopic and open partial nephrectomies in 200 consecutive patients. Pyelocaliceal repair was performed in 63.9% of the laparoscopic cases versus 73.4% of the open cases ($p = 0.20$). Pyelocaliceal repair was performed utilizing suture ligation of intrarenal vessels and renal parenchymal reconstruction.[177] Another recent investigation of pure laparoscopic versus laparoscopic-assisted partial nephrectomy in a porcine animal model noted that surgeons rated suture placement and tying much easier in the pure laparoscopic technique over the assisted alternative.[178] Most investigators have taken to covering their sutured repair with fibrin glue or modification with a Surgicel patch (fibrin glue-impregnated patch). A flap of extrarenal fat can likewise be swung and sutured for a layered covering. In addition, many papers reviewed also utilized stenting judiciously in order to decrease the risk of urinary leakage.[179,180]

Laparoscopic Ureterocalicostomy Two small series of investigations utilizing this technique have been reported, both in swine models. Cherullo and colleagues performed a laparoscopic lower-pole nephrectomy by transverse amputation in 10 pigs. Next, a sutured ureterocalicostomy was carried out with interrupted absorbable sutures. All anastomoses were stented and the mean operative time was 165.3 minutes (range 105–240).[181] The group at U.C. Irvine is likewise investigating this complex reconstruction utilizing a similar porcine model but with a unique reconstructive twist. A novel nitinol tacker has been used for vascular anastomoses. Since previous reports by this same group have revealed little lithogenic potential for titanium

during the use of an EndoGIA for reduction of the renal pelvis during laparoscopic pyeloplasty, this device deserves further attention.[182] The U-Clip device from anastomotic device (Coalescent Surgical, Sunnyvale, CA).[183]

Laparoscopic Calicorrhaphy and Calicoplasty Anatrophic nephrolithotomy has been the last bastion of open renal stone surgery.[184] This has now been modeled in the procine surgical research lab and brought into clinical practice at the Cleveland Clinic. Laparoscopic anatrophic nephrolithotomy was performed in 10 pigs and 11 kidneys using vascular pedicle clamping, contact surface kidney cooling, renal parenchymal incision laterally along the avascular plane, and sutured reconstruction. This group has reported on the clinical application of this technique in 2 patients.[185] Coupled with the methods of laparoscopic, intraoperative ultrasonography, it might be expected to expand to other applications such as the radial nephrotomy for obstructed calices.

Laparoscopic Renal Vascular Surgery Renal vascular surgery can be performed for nascient renovascular disease or during the reconstruction phase of renal transplantation and auto-transplantation. In the former category, nascient renovascular disease, laparoscopic repair would of course have to compete with the less invasive alternative of percutaneous transluminal balloon catheter angioplasty with renal artery stenting.[186] The Cleveland group has also evaluated laparoscopic renovascular reconstruction. In their preliminary animal series, 5 female swine underwent a 7-step renal artery repair.[187] This group followed with a case report of a laparoscopic repair of a 3 cm sacular left renal artery aneurysm in a 57-year-old woman. A 4-port transabdominal technique was utilized allowing circumferential mobilization, Rummel tourniqueting of the main renal artery, bivalving of the aneurysm with excision, followed by 4-0 polypropylene sutured repair using an RB-1 needle. Total repair time was 31 minutes with an approximate 100 cc blood loss.[188] Splenorenal bypass is another method for managing renal artery stenosis. This has been investigated in a canine model of 6 animals. In this laboratory model, a spatulated, end-to-end anastomosis of the renal to the splenic artery was accomplished using 6-0 polypropylene sutures on an RB-2 needle. Mean anastomotic time was 71 minutes (SD = 8).[189] More distal vascular aneurysms are also approachable laparoscopically. This same group recently reported a 51-year-old male with a multilobulated intrarenal aneurysm from the upper-pole branch of the renal artery. Laparoscopic Statinsky clamping controlled the renal hilum en bloc, the aneurysm was circumferentially mobilized, clipped, and divided. They completed this using 4 ports with a total warm ischemia time of 39 minutes.[190] Ming and colleagues have performed laparoscopic-assisted autotransplantation in patients with devastating ureteral and UPJ injuries. The kidney is mobilized in much the same manner for a donor nephrectomy, only a small separate lower-quadrant incision is made for the autotransplant. Finally, the ultimate vascular reconstruction has been a robotic-assisted kidney transplantation where all anastomoses, both vascular and ureterovesical, have been performed with the aid of the da Vinci robot.[191]

Pyelocaliceal Diverticulectomy Gluckman first reported a laparoscopic ablation of a pyelocaliceal diverticulum by unroofing and ablation, but little was mentioned in the way of reconstruction.[192] Two separate reports of pyelocaliceal diverticula ablations have been reported.[54,193] In both cases the anterior diverticula were incised and the linings marsupialized and fulgurated. Omentum was used in the first case and the colon in the second to isolate and cover the exposed raw surfaces. Since then, there have continued anecdotal reports of a case and one published small series representing 5 cases with detailed description of technique. In this series, a vertical incision was made over the thinnest avascular plane over the diverticulum. All stones or stone debris is removed into an endoscopic sack. Figure-of-eight 3-0 polyglactin sutures were used to obliterate the ostium. An argon beam coagulator was used to obliterate the epithelial lining after thorough inspection to ensure no inadvertent malignancies. Adjacent perirenal fat is mobilized and sutured into the diverticular defect. A Jackson-Pratt drain is placed prior to exiting. Stents were utilized routinely.[194] A final series of 4 cases has been recently described on the management of type II pyelocaliceal diverticula (Figure 50-49). Two of these 4 patients underwent laparoscopic repair in a similar fashion to that reported by Miller with excellent outcomes and functional recovery of the kidneys.[195]

Nephropexy Nephroptosis, or the "floating kidney," is most commonly identified in thin, young females and preferentially involves the right side. It has an uncertain incidence in the modern era, but the correction of this condition resulted in large series published in the early modern surgical literature.[196] With the advent of laparoscopic techniques, it is certainly possible to provide surgical fixation to these floating kidneys. Urban and colleagues first reported a laparoscopic nephropexy in 1993 using clip fixation techniques.[197] Elashry and colleagues presented a group of 6 patients who underwent 2 methods of laparoscopic nephropexy: transperitoneal (4) and retroperitoneal (2). The nephropexy was performed using a vertical and horizontal row of 1-0 silk sutures through the renal capsule into the quadratus lumborum fascia. Mean operative time was 4 hours (range 2.5–7 hours).[198] Larger series with longer follow-up is now available. Plas and colleagues presented 30 patients who have had a transabdominal laparoscopic nephropexy since 1992. Seventeen of 30 have been followed for greater than 5 years and all are asymptomatic. In 10 completely evaluated patients, 8 have no nephroptosis, but 2 (20%) have greater than 5 cm displacement. Their technique is decidedly different from the Washington University series. They describe fixation using a polypropylene mesh shaped like an ellipse to cover the sagittal

aspect of the kidney during active cephalad displacement. Fascial staples are used to fix the mesh to the abdominal wall from the upper pole to the lower. The average operating time was 154 minutes (range 90–300).[199] A final series comes from Lubeck, reporting transperitoneal laparoscopic nephropexy in 22 women and 1 man. A round-bodied double-stranded No.2 nonabsorbable polyester suture was passed via the abdominal wall and used to fixate the upper pole to the psoas or quadratus lumborum with a single simple stitch. A second suture is made to fix the convexity of the kidney laterally. They compared this procedure with 12 open nephropexies performed at their hospital showing previously. The mean operative time was 61 minutes (40–85) laparoscopic versus 49 minutes (28–70) for open nephropexy. Narcotic use, complications, hospital stay, and mean days to return to work all favored the laparoscopic approach. All patients in this series had correction of the nephroptosis by IVP at 6 weeks. There appears no definite method that reliably fixes the kidneys from these series, but the historical literature is replete with methods of renal fixation, well over 170 operative techniques. Szekely recently reported in a letter to the editor of the *Journal of Urology* that the same thing could be accomplished by placing a circle (U) nephrostomy tube for 2 weeks.[200]

URETERAL RECONSTRUCTION The ureter has been opened, repaired, or reconstructed predominately utilizing sutured techniques.[201] Nezhat and colleagues probably were the first to report a clinical application of intracorporeal sutured reconstruction of a ureter obstructed by endometriosis. Excision of the involved segment and ureteroureterostomy was performed over 7 French (F) catheter with 4 interrupted 4-0 absorbable sutures (PDS). A CO_2 laser was utilized for the bloodless dissection prior to reconstruction with an estimated surgical time of 117 minutes.[202] Wickham explored and performed a laparoscopic ureterolithotomy without repair of the ureter in 1978.[203] Closure of the ureteral wall following ureterolithotomy was described utilizing a running 4-0 PDS anchored on each end with absorbable clips (Ethi EndoClip, Ethicon, Cincinnati, OH).[204] The procedure lasted approximately 180 minutes. We have recently resected a stenotic segment of ureter with an eroded proximal calculus and performed a Heinike-Mikulitz type of ureteroureterostomy with interrupted 4-0 chromic gut sutures intracorporeally tied over a stent. A case of a right circumcaval ureter requiring transposition has also been reported.[205] Retrograde dissection of the right ureter from the iliac vessels identified the postcaval segment. Next, the middle third of the ureter was dissected until it passed behind the cava to the renal hilum. The renal pelvis was identified and dissected to the area of obstruction and divided, and the distal ureter was spatulated and anastomosed with 5 4-0 polyglactin interrupted sutures over a guidewire. This procedure was accomplished in 560 minutes and stented following the repair. Others have repeated the

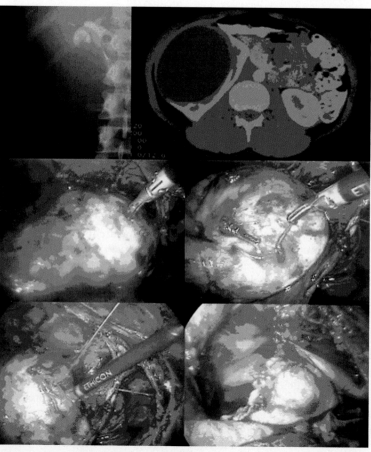

Figure 50-49 Laparoscopic type II pyelocaliceal diverticulum.

procedure of ureteral repair for retrocaval ureter, most now support a complete intracorporeal sutured repair.[206] The laparoscopic approach and treatment of benign retroperitoneal fibrosis has been described.[207] After mobilizing the ureter in a 15-year-old female, the ureter was secured within the abdomen with a biting clip applier. The correction of vesicoureteral reflux using laparoscopic biting clips to reapproximate the muscularis over the distal ureter and create a nonrefluxing tunnel has been described in the porcine model.[49,208] There are now several series in which retroperitoneal fibrosis has been explored, biopsied, and peritonealization of the ureter has been accomplished. In fact, Puppo and colleagues have even reported on the classic method of bilateral ureterolysis because of the risk of bilateral involvement.[209] Finally, the ureter has been taken apart and reconstructed laparoscopically with intracorporeal suturing techniques for severe endometriosis in 9 patients. Long-term follow-up for these laparoscopic ureteroureterostomies is available between 2 months and 7 years. Only 1 patient developed a mild ureteric stricture that required balloon dilation.[210]

BLADDER RECONSTRUCTION Most laparoscopic bladder reconstructions to date have been performed with linear cutting staplers. A growing number of sutured reconstructions include diverticulectomy, closure of traumatic cystorrhaphies, ureteroneocystostomy, ureterocystoplasty, augmentation cystoplasty, seromyotomy (autoaugmentation), and partial cystectomy.[211] The bladder neck has been suspended and bladder neck slings have been placed with the aid of laparoscopic sutures. Das reported resecting a large bladder diverticulum and suturing the ostium with 3-0 polyglycolic acid in a continuous, double-layered fashion.[50] Intracorporeal knotting was utilized and the procedure took 288 minutes. Most bladder diverticuli are posterior and tend to be eccentrically located at or near a ureteral orifice. We have used simultaneous flexible cystoscopy and ureteral illumination to aid in the dissection and sutured reconstruction (Figure 50-54).[212] Laparoscopic sutured cystorrhaphy following an iatrogenic intraperitoneal bladder laceration has been reported.[213] A 75-year-old male with a large intraperitoneal bladder perforation required laparoscopic 2-layered running suture repair. Using 3-0 polyglycolic acid suture (first layer mucosa and muscularis and second muscularis and parietal peritoneum), all knots were tied intracorporeally. The entire procedure of laparoscopic cystorrhaphy lasted 27 minutes. Two cases of vesicoureteroplasty have been reported.[214] A 2-year-old boy and a 5-year-old girl with grades III and IV, respectively, vesicoureteral reflux underwent laparoscopic mobilization of the distal ureter for 3 to 4 cm. A 3 cm straight horizontal myotomy was then created as a tunnel with the ureter sutured in situ by 4 3-0 polyglactin, interrupted sutures. Extracorporeal knotting was used in the first case and intracorporeal knotting in the latter. The mean time for

vesicoureteroplasty was 182.5 minutes (range 170–195). Seromyotomy or bladder autoaugmentation has been performed laparoscopically at several centers.[215,216] Very little reconstruction is necessary following excising a portion of the detrusor muscle. Detrusor flaps were sutured to the pelvic side wall at Cooper's ligament utilizing 1-0 polyglactin secured intracorporeally with clips. The time of surgery ranged from 70 to 330 minutes. Augmentation cystoplasty utilizing xenograft human lyophilized dura mater and collagen-impregnated polyglactin mesh were accomplished laparoscopically in beagles.[217] The bladders of 4 animals were opened after the fashion of Blaivas, and bilateral vesicopsoas hitches were performed utilizing 3-0 polyglactin sutures with intracorporeal knotting. This type of bladder opening allowed onlay of the xenograft such that two simple suture lines could accomplish the cystoplasty. Running 4-0 polyglactin sutures, synched with intracorporeal knots allowed the cystoplasties to be water tight with an average time of surgery of 134 minutes. One case of laparoscopically assisted continent catheterizable cutaneous appendicovesicostomy has been accomplished.[218] A 15-year-old female with an obliterated bladder neck from multiple previous surgeries underwent mobilization of her appendix laparoscopically utilizing a 12 mm linear cutting stapler. The cecum was reattached to the side wall with PDS sutures tied intracorporeally. The appendix was anastomosed isoperistaltically to the bladder via a trocar passed transvesically. The base of the appendix was delivered through a predetermined stoma site via a 10 to 11 mm trocar and the appendicovesicostomy was finished using the Mitrofanoff principle with a 4 cm subepithelial tunnel through a small open cystotomy. The total operating time was 360 minutes. Finally, Anderson and colleagues described an animal model for laparoscopic continent urinary diversion in swine.[219] In 9 male swine, in situ ureterosigmoidostomy in a 5 to 6 cm detubularized rectosigmoid pouch was performed. A Boari flap for reconstruction of the distal ureter has been described by several investigators. The first case was done because of distal ureteral involvement by endometriosis.[220] A series has been presented by the Johns Hopkins group. There were 2 left- and 1 right-sided distal ureteral obstructions with 6 to 8 cm of distal ureteral involvement. An anterior bladder flap was harvested from the bladder after dividing the the superior and middle vesical arteries with the EndoGIA. The ureter was anastomosed to the flap using interrupted 4-0 polyglactin suture.[221]

Visually-guided transvaginal techniques have been employed in 7 women with types I and II genuine stress incontinence (GSI).[222] A formal intracorporeal Burch and Marshall-Marchetti-Krantz suspension has been performed in over 92 incontinent patients with a mean operative time of 65 minutes. One to 2 2-0 nylon sutures are placed on either side of the bladder neck and then into Cooper's ligament or the pubic periosteum.[223,224] Bladder neck suspensions for genuine stress uri-

nary incontinence were being widely performed, but long-term follow-up investigations have failed to adequately demonstrate that laparoscopic colposuspension maintains continence.[225,226] Some centers continue to persist in evaluating the potential for laparoscopy to treat stress urinary incontinence.[227] Laparoscopic mesh fixations have been performed for severe pelvic prolapse sysndromes in women. The "gold standard" sacrocolpopexy has now been performed laparoscopically. Of the vaginal restorative procedures, uteroscacral lligament vault suspension, iliococcygeous, and sacrospinous fixation each have their proponents. There is marked utilization of mesh materials to reconstruct these prolapse syndromes, requiring suturing to these anatomic structures. All types of prosthetic mesh materials are being investigated and utilized.[228]

The urachus is an unusual site for urologic disease, but it too has been successfully approached by laparoscopic maneuvers. Most commonly, urachal sinuses and cysts have been laparoscopically resected and ligated. More common in children, these occasionally present in adulthood. A case of a 34-year-old male underwent a laparoscopic resection of a 4 cm cyst from the urachus using a voice-controlled laparoscope.[229] One series of pediatric management of urachal anomalies has been published. Four children ranging in age from 4 to 10 underwent laparoscopic radical excision of the urachus.[230] Four adults have also been managed laparoscopically in a report by Cadeddu and colleagues. In these cases the urachus, and medial umbilical ligaments were detached just caudal to the umbilicus and dissected caudad to the bladder dome. In 75% of cases a bladder cuff was taken with the specimen because of fibrotic attachments. The bladder defect in these cases was sewn in 2 layers with 2-0 polysorbate loaded on an EndoStitch device.[231]

Laparoscopic cystectomy represents the ultimate surgical site for laparoscopic urologic reconstruction. For purposes here, the radical prostatectomy portion that requires reanastomosis to the urethra will be considered separately and discussed later. Now, attention will focus on methods of laparoscopic cystectomy and urinary diversion. Brief mention will also be placed on laparoscopic efforts at urinary undiversion. Initially, however, the first attempts at laparoscopic bladder reconstructive surgery focused on bladder diverticula resection and repair. Automated staplers have a wide application for laparoscopic procedures involving the bladder. The multifire linear cutting stapler has been used to divide the vascular pedicles and urethra during a laparoscopic cystectomy in a 27-year-old female with recurrent pyocystis and previous urinary diversion.[51] The endostapler has also been used to close bladder defects following diverticulectomy and distal ureterectomy for upper-tract transitional cell carcinomas.[12,13] Parra and colleagues reported the first laparoscopic bladder diverticulectomy in an 87-year-old man with a superiorly positioned, narrow-necked diverticulum and chronic urinary tract infections. Adequate healing without urinary extravasation was documented by cystography 8 days after surgery.[51] In addition to expediting surgery, automated staplers may have an added benefit during excision of bladder diverticula containing urothelial malignancies by preventing potential spillage of tumor cells into the peritoneum. Neoplastic changes in the lining of diverticula occur in approximately 0 to 13.5% of cases.[232–235] Laparoscopic division of a bladder cuff during nephroureterectomy and ureterectomy in porcine experiments and humans has been described by Kerbl and colleagues.[14] After cystoscopically incising the ureteral orifice and submucosal tunnel, a 2 cm juxtaureteral bladder cuff is dissected laparoscopically. A linear cutting, multifire stapler is then utilized to close and excise the cuff of bladder.[14]

Parra was the first to perform a laparoscopic cystectomy in a patient with pyocystis. Porcine animal studies have been performed to evaluate methods of cystectomy and urinary diversion. Anderson and Clayman described a method of ureterosigmoidostomy.[236] Kaouk and colleagues presented an animal model of orthotopic ileal neobladder.[237] Baldwin and colleagues described an attempt to simplify the laparoscopic reconstructive effort by using the "dunk" technique for ureteroileal anastomoses. In addition, they used Lapra-Ty suture clips (Ethicon EndoSurgery, Cincinnati, OH) to facilitate intracorporeal knotting. Two of 3 of the "dunked" ureters were partially or completely strictured. In addition, the shortcut method of knot substitution resulted in Lapra-Ty migration and subsequent urinary obstruction by the foreign body in 2 animals.[238] Now, laparoscopic radical cystoprostatectomy is becoming increasingly performed. Large series are beginning to accrue patients into the laparoscopic group. Simonato and colleagues recently reported their technique in 10 patients using a 5-port technique. The urinary reconstructive aspects included the orthotopic ileal neobladder in 6, sigmoid ureterostomies in 2, and cutaneous ureterostomy in 2. The mean operating room time was 166 minutes (range 150–180). Two patients have diffuse metastatic disease, with 8 free of disease at a mean 12.3 months (range 5–18).[239] Another method has been utilized by Abdel-Hakim and colleagues. Laparoscopic radical cystoprostatectomy was performed in 9 patients. Here the authors removed the laparoscopic specimen through a 3 to 5 cm right iliac fossa incision through which a detubularized modified Camey II orthotopic neobladder was performed.[240] Matin and Gill from Cleveland have detailed their method of complete intracorporeal urinary diversion following laparoscopic radical cystectomy. Here the authors performed a completely hand-sewn anastomosis of the orthotopic neobladder and the ureteroileal anastomoses.[241] They have summarized the application of this technique in 2 patients using 6-ports with an average time of 9.5 hours.[242] This same group previously published a series of 5 patients who had undergone a laparoscopic radical cystectomy with ileal conduit urinary diversion using a 6-port technique.[243]

Another group has performed 11 laparoscopic radical cystectomies with intracorporeal construction of a continent urinary diversion (Mainz pouch II). Their average operating time was 6.7 hours.[244]

Segmental bowel excision and reconstruction using automated staplers has been practiced during open surgery for many years. Bohm and colleagues described the technique of laparoscopic intestinal resection and intraperitoneal reanastomosis.[245] After mobilization of the selected intestinal segment and isolation of the vascular pedicle, the linear cutting stapler is inserted into enterotomies on the antimesenteric border of afferent and efferent limbs of the future anastomosis. Two consecutive firings of the 3 or 6 cm stapler create a 5 to 11 cm anastomosis. A cotton umbilical tape encircling the bowel close to the anastomosis provides countertraction and prevents spillage of intestinal contents into the peritoneum. Firing the linear stapler across both loops of bowel near the corner of the anastomosis transects the specimen and completes the anastomosis. Kozminski and Partamian reported the first urologic application of automated stapling for laparoscopic bowel resection and intracorporeal ileal conduit formation.[15] Their initial clinical case involved performing the palliative supravesical diversion in an 83-year-old male for unresectable fibrosarcoma of the prostate. Intracorporeal ureteral and bowel mobilization was accomplished through six 10 to 12 mm trocars. Bowel resection and reanastomosis were performed extracorporeally with linear stapling devices after evacuating the pneumoperitoneum and pulling the bowel through the 12 mm port site. Once the resected bowel segment was mobilized, the mesentery was closed intracorporeally with biting clips and the ureteral anastomoses were accomplished extracorporeally by suturing techniques after mobilizing the ureters. Securing the conduit to the retroperitoneum was again accomplished by biting clips applied intracorporeally. Two subsequent patients have had ileal loop diversion with entirely intracorporeal bowel resections and reanastomosis using these staplers.[15] In all 3 patients, the ureteroileal anastomoses were sutured extracorporeally. This same technique has been repeated by others.[246] Other applications for these techniques would be urologic reconstructions utilizing other gastrointestinal segments. Augmentation cystoplasty can be performed with harvested gastric, small bowel, or large bowel segments. Ureteral interposition or replacement could theoretically be performed. Finally, supravesical diversions with ileal conduits represent only one of many methods of noncontinent and continent heterotopic or orthotopic bladder replacement techniques. Automatic, linear cutting staplers have the potential to make such urologic reconstructions possible. The lithogenic properties of metallic staples used for urinary tract reconstruction are well known. Stone formation attributed to exposed steel staples occurs in 3.2 to 4.2% of patients with ileal conduits and 4.9 to 10% of patients with Kock pouches.[247–250] The lithogenic potential of tita-

nium staples exposed to human urine is not known. Kerbl and colleagues have used a linear titanium stapling device to excise a bladder cuff during nephroureterectomy in 6 adult humans.[28] Three patients have been followed more than a year without complication and/or endoscopic evidence of staple exposure. Endoscopic verification of lack of exposed staples and oversewing the staple line are recommended by some authors. Prototypic automated staplers using dissolvable staples are currently under study. Julian and Ravitch compared stone formation on exposed stainless steel and Polysorb (U.S. Surgical, Norwalk, CT) absorbable staples used to close the bladder in dogs. Although staple exposure was much higher in bladders closed with absorbable staples (56% vs 2%), crystal formation more commonly occurred on exposed stainless steel staples (25% vs 7%).[251]

Laparoscopic augmentation cystoplasty has also been investigated. Early efforts attempted to use novel biomaterials such as intestinal submucosa.[252] Others have utilized tissue expansion techniques to expand the native ureter and augment the bladder with this laparoscopically.[253] The small bowel has been utilized during a transverse hemicystectomy with ileocystoplasty in porcine model.[254] Finally, Siqueria and colleagues described the synchronous correction of small bladder capacity by laparoscopically augmenting the bladder with ileum, but also performing a continent ileovesicostomy in the porcine model.[255] The next step of course was clinical application. The first reported case of laparoscopic ileocystoplasty was Sanchez de Badajoz and colleagues' case report of a patient with urinary tuberculosis. An isolated segment of ileum was taken using EndoGIA staplers. The enterocystoplasty was performed with two firing of the EndoGIA stapler plus the addition of holding sutures.[256] Three patients were described by Gill and colleagues using different bowel segments in each of these cases. The functionally reduced bladder capacities were augmented using the ileum, the sigmoid, and the cecum and proximal ascending colon in these patients.[257] In reporting the application of laparoscopic ileal cystoplasty, Elliott and colleagues noted some important technical considerations. Important to this operation included (a) preoperative evaluation of compliance and videourodynamics; (b) cystoscopic placement of externalized ureteral catheters; (c) transperitoneal placement of trocars; (d) identification of the cecum; (e) proximal mobilization of the ileum sufficient for pelvic placement; (f) measurement of ileal length with segment of precut vessel loop; (g) vertical cystostomy after incision of the peritoneum and entering the space of Retzius; (h) ileal division and side-to-side anastomosis using EndoGIA stapler; (i) detubularization and freehand intracorporeal suturing into a U-shaped configuration; (j) fixing ileal patch at the 6- and 11-o'clock positions; (k) completion of ileal-bladder anastomosis in quadrants with running sutures; (l) irrigation of bladder and placement of a closed suction drain into the pelvis; and (m) cystogram at 4 weeks postoperatively.[258] Because of the hazards associated with enterocystoplasty, the search for an ideal substitute continues even in the minimally invasive era. One recent investigation used a variety of different biodegradable grafts in an animal model. Thirty-one minipigs underwent transperitoneal laparoscopic partial cystectomy and augmentation cystoplasty using nothing (6 controls), porcine bowel acellular tissue matrix (ATM) (6), bovine pericardium (BPC) (6), human placental membranes (HPM) (6), or porcine small intestinal submucosa (SIS) (6). All 3 grafts had only mucosal regeneration at 12 weeks postoperatively and all had contracted to between 60 and 75% of their original sizes.[259]

The bladder has not only been the target of intense endourologic research interest, but also it has finally been reconstructed in a variety of methods. This bring the discussion full circle, as is fitting, Wolf and Taheri have recently reported a laparoscopic undiversion. This was in a 25-year-old man who had undergone an open ileal conduit diversion and colostomy with mucous fistula for a gunshot wound 11 months prior to presentation. The colostomy and mucous fistula were taken down first and an extracorporeal bowel anastomosis was performed. Next, laparoscopic trocars were positioned and the bladder dome and abdominal portion of the ileal conduit were mobilized. A single-layered ileovesical anastomosis was performed using a 4-0 absorbable suture.[260]

VESICOURETHRAL ANASTOMOSIS Laparoscopic reconstructive surgery has been applied to one of the most difficult repairs urologists perform, vesicourethral reanastomosis following radical prostatectomy. First attempted clinically in 1992, research work in animal models continues.[261] In combined canine series of 20 animals, the radical retropubic prostatectomy and reconstruction was accomplished with a mean operative time of 294.5 minutes.[262,263] In the study by Moran and colleagues, the laparoscopic reconstruction was performed with the laparoscope closely approximated to the tissues for a microscopic repair. Six to 8 fluorescently colored polyglactin intracorporeal sutures were placed utilizing microsurgical suspension techniques to convert square knots to slip configurations and back (see Figure 50-35).[132] No Foley catheters were positioned so as to evaluate the completeness of the microlaparoscopic repair (Figure 50-57, cystogram). One anastomotic leak occurred in 6 animals available for long-term follow-up. Minimal scarification was noted grossly or on trichrome stained sections in animals at necropsy.

Clinical application of laparoscopic repair of the vesicourethral anastomosis has been widely performed. There appears to be two basic approaches by review of the literature. There are those who favor an interrupted anastomosis and those who prefer a running anastomosis. There are no prospective randomized data to support either philosophy at present. Claims for almost any belief suggesting an advantage or disadvan-

tage for each technique can be found. For instance, there are those who suggest that the running anastomosis simplifies and facilitates the repair. But there is a large series that argues the opposite.[264] There are investigators who believe that the anastomosis capable laparoscopically is potentially better than its open counterpart. Large series are just beginning to be able to investigate this possibility. The complications from the vesicourethral anastomosis should be fewer. Urinary extravasation should be minimal. In one current series, Menon's group has now begun to leave no postoperative drains when they use a running anastomosis.[265] Bladder neck contracture should likewise be lowered, but the exact incidence even in open series is not known.[266] One such investigation noted contracture in 11% of radical prostatectomy patients.[267] This data is not yet fully available, but there are groups suggesting that symptomatic bladder neck contractures are fewer following the laparoscopic repair. Is this due to the anastomotic technique or rather secondary to the method of prostatobladder neck division or to the method of mobilization of the bladder for performing a laparoscopic radical prostatectomy? Innovative investigations that might answer this question are beginning to emerge, but follow-up remains short.[268] A new semiautomatic suturing device has recently been reported from Yamada and colleagues, called Maniceps. Using this device in 15 patients, the urethrovesical anastomosis was completed in 8.1 minutes (range 5–12). They report 1 bladder neck contracture at short follow-up.[269] Another recent investigational method used 2-octyl cyanoacrylate adhesive for an in vivo canine study to glue the anastomosis in 12 dogs. Four anastomoses were performed with 8 interrupted sutures compared with 8 using the adhesive. Only 1 of the adhesive animals anastomoses had leak pressures 70 mm Hg or greater, whereas all 4 control suture animals achieved this expected outcome.[270] Laser welding has also been attempted in the canine model to facilitate this anastomosis. This was an open radical prostatectomy model, but 4 animals had a conventional 8 interrupted suture technique, while the experimental group had 4 support sutures followed by a diode laser welded anastomosis using a chromophore doped albumin solder. They noted superphysiologic leak pressures in all of these animals with no other differences in healing.[271]

ROBOTIC RECONSTRUCTION

INTRODUCTION The next generation of surgical robotics required the downsizing of mechanized instruments to reproduce the complex ability of the surgeon's arms and hands.[272] Next, the surgical tools themselves needed to be added or subtracted from the devices so that surgical multitasking was possible. To control and coordinate the functions of the robot requires a computer. The computer is responsible for interpreting the surgeon's actions and transforming them into the movements of the robotic arms and hands. This requires incredible fidelity and incorporates a

wide range of motion. The computer is translating the surgeon's movements into precise codes to smoothly and rapidly manipulate the robot (Figure 50-50A). Here the robot is in direct contact with the patient and the surgeon is removed to the controlling station. As with the laparoscopic surgery removing the surgeon from actually seeing the surgical field, the robotic hands are removing the laparoscopic instruments from actually touching and performing the surgery (see Figure 50-50B). The actual robotic tools, or end effectors, are located at the distal end of long instruments, which are inserted into the patient through laparoscopic trocars (see Figure 50-50C). The movement of the instruments is controlled manually at the work station. To allow the end effector to be maximally effective, at least 6 degrees of freedom are necessary (see Figure 50-50D).

A great deal of research effort has been applied to solve the problem of the actual surgical interface.[273–275] That is what type of device is best for the surgeon to manipulate that will provide the computer with the information necessary to perform the surgery. Possibilities include scissor-like hand pieces that provide the computer with the data necessary to manipulate the end effector. Glove-like input devices have been proposed, and view-directed controls utilizing the endoscopic image itself to be the frame of reference are being investigated. Some input devices are position controlled and others are direction controlled. In the former, the movement of the end effector is coupled to the movement of the input device by the surgeon. A continuous movement of the input device is needed to achieve continuous movement of the end effector. In the direction-controlled interface, the input device controls the velocity of the end effector. Therefore, no continuous movement is necessary to achieve continuous movement of the end effector. One study evaluating various input devices included a spacemouse, free-flying joystick, immersion probe, and head-tracking systems. Wapler suggested that for guiding the endoscope a head-tracking system would allow a more intuitive method of control.[276] For manipulating the end effector, the following requirement should be met: The manipulator must be compact enough to allow at least three systems to work independently without danger of collision, the patient should be manually accessible at all times, the insertion point must be kept invariant when moving the end effector, allowance must be made for patient movements, all endoscopes and instruments must be manually controllable in case of manipulator failure, and the movement of the end effector must not be self-locking. In addition, there are three options for supporting such a robotic system in the operating room, these include a stand-alone system, a ceiling-mounted system, or a system that attaches to the operating room table. Both the stand-alone and ceiling-mounted systems would require more room and have special precautions to ensure that no relative movement occur between the operating room table and the manipulator's base. At the beginning

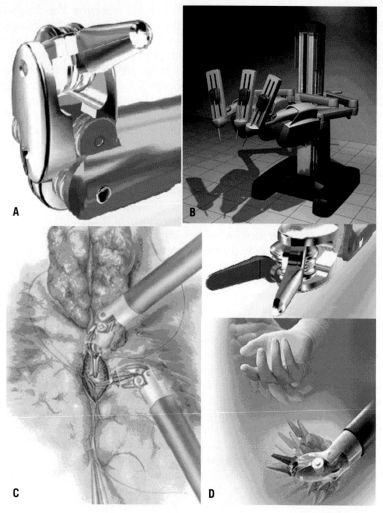

Figure 50-50 The da Vinci robotic surgical assist system. A, The needle driver en fasse. B, The patient-side surgical system. C, The system shown diagrammatically during sutured reconstruction. D, The patented EndoWrist system mimicking a human hand and then some for increased degrees of freedom. (Intuitive Surgical, Mountain View, CA)

complex, necessitating the 8 mm trocar portals. The da Vinci surgeon console does not approximate anything like standard laparoscopic instruments. The surgeon's hands, wrists, and fingers manipulate a patented articulated EndoWrist. This type of system is necessary to take advantage of the laparoscopic instrument's dexterity. The other major difference of the two surgical robotic systems lies in the da Vinci ergonomic viewing console (see Figure 50-50). The surgeon sits at the console, which is designed to support the surgeon's head while viewing the 3-D image and has a separate adjustable surface on which the surgeon can rest his/her arms. The vision system is fully three-dimensional and integrated in the performance of the two robotic arms. The da Vinci system is a stand-alone device that moves in toward and over the patient, whereas the Zeus system is a component and attaches to the sides of the operating room table, as does the separate and independent Aesop arm. In both robotic systems, the fidelity of movement is superb, and the time delay from surgeon's movement to the robotic instrument movement is imperceptible. The cost of each system is above $900,000 (US) currently.

GENERAL APPLICATIONS Numerous cardiothoracic, general surgical, gynecologic, and urologic procedures have been attempted either in animate laboratories or clinically.[277–288] Most of these studies have been case reports with series only available for evaluation of outcomes in cardiac surgery. A case report of computer-assisted robotic Heller's myotomy in a 76-year-old female with progressive dysphagia was performed in Columbus, OH.[278] The da Vinci system was utilized using 4 operative cannulas (5 mm liver retractor, two 10 mm working ports in the patient's midline and left midclavicular line, and one 5 mm port in the left anterior axillary line). An assistant surgeon stayed at the patient's bedside and controlled retraction and changed instruments on the robotic arm. The total operative time was 160 minutes and she was discharged the following day. Another case report again utilized the da Vinci system to perform a Nissen fundoplication on a 56-year-old female with long-standing gastroesophageal reflux.[279] This was performed using 5 trocar ports; 12 mm supraumbilical 30 degree camera (used a robotic camera system), 10 mm right anterior axillary port for liver retraction (used a mobile table-mounted mechanical self-retaining device), and two 10 trocars for the right and left hands of the da Vinci robot. The patient's position was in low lithotomy position with the table in steep reverse Trendelenburg's setting. The surgeon was approximately 10 feet away from the patient, and the assistant was stationed between the patient's legs. The assistant performed the instrument changes and utilized a harmonic scalpel. There was no operative time listed, but the patient was discharged from the hospital in under 24 hours. The largest general surgical series has recently been reported from the group in Strasbourg, France, on laparoscopic robotic cholecystectomy.[280] These authors reported the

of surgery, the abdomen is prepped and draped in the same fashion for laparoscopic surgery. When the trocars have been positioned, the manipulators are attached to the operating room table. Each manipulator is manually brought into position such that the invariant point is exactly at the trocar. When all the manipulators are in place, the actual surgical procedure is begun. Currently the surgeon has only visual feedback from the videomonitor. There are ongoing efforts to include force-feedback (ie, haptic input) into the robotic manipulators so the surgeon can perceive subtle nuances of the laparoscopic environment.

There currently are two available laparoscopic robotic units in use, the Zeus system and the da Vinci systems; however, others are in the works. The Zeus system has recently been acquired by Intuitive Surgical and the systems may possibly merge, but the da Vinci system was approved in July 2000 in the United States. The Zeus Robotic Surgical System has an ergonomic workstation with rather conventional-appearing handles. The surgeon's movements are scalable to the surgeon's specifications. A ratio of 5:1 means that for every inch the surgeon moves the handles

on the console, the robotic surgical instruments would move one-fifth of an inch. Tremors can be filtered out as well. The Zeus computer translates the surgeon's movements to the end effectors placed via trocars inside of the patient. The instruments themselves act similarly to conventional laparoscopic devices except that the surgeon does not actually touch them. The monitor on the Zeus system is a standard video image, the surgeon does have the option of wearing specialized binoculars to view the image in 3-D. The da Vinci company has the capability to add 3-D imaging full time without the need for the special glasses, but current research has not demonstrated a significant advantage for these image systems. The other robotic system is da Vinci. This robotic surgical system has an articulated wrist that allows 6 degrees of freedom during the performance of laparoscopic surgery (Figure 50-59B). This wrist addition allows for the 2 additional degrees of freedom, and there is some basic evidence that that additional motion translates into more adaptive ability by skilled and nonskilled surgeons. The downside to the da Vinci instrument tips would be that they are more laparoscopic, robotic cholecystectomy in 25 patients (16 women and 9 men) with a median age of 59 (range 28–81). They used the Zeus surgical robotic system with 4 laparoscopic trocar sites (one 10 mm umbilical camera port and three 5 mm ports for retraction and robotic surgery). The Zeus instruments were 3 mm in diameter and the surgeon was remote (4 meters) from the patient, and Aesop was used to voice control the camera. The assistant stayed at the operating room table to aid in retraction, clip application, and exchange instruments. Completely robotic cholecystectomy was accomplished in 24 of 25 patients, and 1 patient was completed with standard laparoscopic methods. The median time for the dissection was 25 minutes (range 14–109). The median time to set up and take down the robotic system was 18 minutes (range 13–27). An engineer was present in 22 of the cases, making 3 minor technical adjustments (2 nonfunctional graspers and 1 malfunctioning robotic arm sensor). Laparoscopic splenectomy, an extirpative surgical procedure, has recently been accomplished with the da Vinci robot.[281] A 69-year-old female was seen with idiopathic thrombocytopenia purpura (ITP). The patient was placed in steep reverse Trendelenberg's position after placing one 11 mm camera port, two 8 mm robotic arm ports, and one 11 mm assistant port. The surgeon was 10 feet from the operating room table and used a hook dissector and Cadiere grasping forceps. Short gastric vessels were taken via the 10 mm trocar with an ultrasonic dissector. The spleen was 1,000 g and was extracted via morcellation from the 10 mm site after entrapment. The procedure time was 65 minutes, operating room time was 90 minutes, and actual splenic dissection time was 31 minutes. Robotic setup and draping took just 9 minutes. One final surgical case has also been reported, robotic pancreatic surgery.[282] A 46-year-old female presented with a symptomatic 2.5 cm complex solid/cystic mass at the tail of her pancreas. The robotic surgery was performed in the modified lithotomy position using 4 laparoscopic ports. The total operating room time was 275 minutes with actual surgery time of 185 minutes. The pathology was a benign neuroendocrine tumor and the patient left the hospital on postoperative day 2. Robotic bowel and vascular surgery is being investigated.[283]

Gynecologic surgeons have also performed robotically assisted laparoscopic hysterectomies, adnexal surgeries, and microsurgical tubal and uterine horn anastomosis. This gynecologic work has been performed at the Cleveland Clinic utilizing Zeus and Aesop in a series of porcine experiments.[284–286] Both uterine and adnexal surgeries have been described, including microscopic reanastomis of the fallopian tubes.[287] At the University of Texas Medical Branch, Galveston, 11 patients were enrolled into a laparoscopic, computer-enhanced robotic hysterectomy trial.[288] Six patients had CIN or well-differentiated endometrial carcinoma, 4 had medically nonresponsive postmenopausal bleeding, and 1 had unstaged ovarian cancer. The mean age was 55 (range 27–77). Four trocars were ustilized and operative times were 4.5 to 10 hours. Blood loss averaged 300 cc (range 50–1,500). Hospital stay was 2 days (range 1–3). There was 1 open conversion, the fifth patient in this series.

Just to push the envelope a little further, robotic surgery is beginning to be applied to pediatric surgery as well. Recent reports of robotic Nissen fundoplications have been published.[289] Eleven children with a mean age of 12 years (range 7–16) presented with gastroesophageal reflux. The mean operating time for the robotic fundoplication was 136 minutes (range 105–180). Four ports were utilized, including one 12 mm optical trocar, two 8 mm robotic trocars, and one 5 mm assistant port. There have been 2 children who have had robotic cholecystectomies with an averate time of 137 minutes. Finally, 1 child has had a robotic bilateral salpingo-oopherectomy for gonadoblastoma taking 95 minutes.

UROLOGIC APPLICATIONS Urologic applications have also begun.[290–301] In work by Louis Kavoussi's group at Johns Hopkins University, Aesop has been utilized for telementoring and teleproctoring advanced laparoscopic procedures.[290] In 1998, Bowersox and Cornum first used a robotic surgical telemanipulator to perform an open urological surgery in swine.[291] Sung and colleagues, in 1999, performed robotic-assisted laparoscopic pyeloplasties in a porcine model utilizing the Zeus system.[293] Guillonneau's group in Paris began a program in utilizing the Zeus system in the animate laboratory and started to accrue patients into clinical applications performing laparoscopic pelvic lymphadenectomies in 20 consecutive patients with stage T3M0 disease.[294] They noted no need for open conversions, and the average operative time was 2.1 hours, 1 full hour longer than their usual laparoscopic times. They noted that the time for robotic setup was 30 minutes. Abbou and colleagues from Creteil, France, have also been exploring urologic applications.[295] They recently reported the use of the da Vinci robotic system to perform a laparoscopic radical prostatectomy in a 63-year-old man with Gleason's sum score of 6 prostatic adenocarcinoma, clinically staged T1c and a PSA of 7 ng/mL. They utilized 5 trocars (one 12 mm umbilical camera port, two 8 mm trocars located at the lateral rectus sheath, and 2 lateral 5 mm trocars at the iliac position for the assistant). Robotic instruments used were the Cadiere and DeBakey forceps, 2 needle drivers, long and round tip forceps, scalpel, electrocautery, and a prototype bipolar forceps. The operating time was 420 minutes, well in excess of their standard operative time of 240 minutes. Assembly of the robot took 30 minutes and disengaging the unit took 15 minutes. The vesicourethral running 3-0 polyglactin suture anastomosis took 30 minutes. These authors mention that the 3-D imaging system and the full 6 degrees of freedom of the da Vinci robotic system made in vitro training on animals streamlined to the point that they could proceed to clinical applications quickly. Drawbacks of the system were pointed out to include, lack of tactile feedback, the high cost of the robotic equipment, the cost of disposables ($1,800 [US]) for this radical prostatectomy case, and the time lost to replace the surgical instruments. Guillonneau and the Montsouris group have recently published the first case of robot-assisted laparoscopic nephrectomy.[296] They utilized their Zeus robotic system in a 77-year-old female with a nonfunctioning, hydronephrotic right kidney secondary to a UPJ obstruction. They performed a transabdominal nephrectomy utilizing 3 robotic arms (Zeus and Aesop). A 10 mm trocar was placed at the right pararectal line for the camera port and Aesop. Two 5 mm trocars in the right flank in a triangular fashion for the robotic instruments (mainly a forceps in the left and monopolar scissors in the right). A 5 mm trocar was placed at the umbilicus, and a 12 mm trocar was placed in the right subcostal region for suction/irrigation, retraction, and application of clips and/or endovascular gastrointestinal stapler. The operative time was 200 minutes, anesthesia time was 245 minutes, blood loss was less than 100 mL, and the patient's postoperative course was uneventful.[296]

The probable proliferation of computer-enhanced robotic surgery is beginning to materialize in urologic practice. From robotic-assisted adrenalectomies and retroperitoneal lymphadenectomies to robotic sacrocolpoplasty, all urologic applications are beginning to be reported.[297–299] As with surgical applications, these are mostly anecdotal case reports. One group's pioneering efforts deserves special attention, from Creteil, France. Hoznek and colleagues have been attempting to use the da Vinci robot to perform kidney transplant surgery.[300] A 26-year-old male received a cadaver donor transplant, which was performed with a hybrid open/robotic technique. The operative time was 178 minutes with a robotic vascular anastomosis time of 57 minutes. The authors present several interesting features of eliminating the surgeon from contact with the patient, including reduction in the risk of infectious transmission to the surgeons.

There are two urologic surgeries that are begging the attention of the computer-enhanced robotic application: pyeloplasty and radical prostatectomy with urethrovesical reanastomosis. Guilloneau and colleagues first published on robotic techniques for pyeloplasty in 2000.[301] Currently, series are beginning to be reported. Gettman and colleagues have presented preliminary work on 9 patients using the da Vinci robotic system to perform 4 Anderson-Hynes and 2 Fengerplasty ureteropelvic junction repairs.[302] The estimated blood loss was < 50 cc, the mean overall operating room time was 140 minutes, and the mean suture time was 70 minutes. There were no open conversions. They have subsequently updated their Anderson-Hynes dismembered pyeloplasty series to 9, with a mean operating room time of 138.8 minutes (range 80–215). The mean suturing time was 62.4 minutes (range 40–115).[303] Other groups with the available technology can be expected to rapidly follow with series.[304] Radical prostatectomy with urethrovesical anastomosis is the next frontier. Abbou and colleagues first reported a case in 2001 as noted previously.[295] They have expanded their series and have been performing the entire robotic surgery extraperitoneally.[305] This prefaces the astounding data beginning to flow from the Vattikuti Urology Institute at Henry Ford Hospital in Detroit.[306] The number of reported robotic radical prostatectomies is over 400 cases currently, with rigid follow-up strategies for solving operative problems that are constantly associated with this surgery, incontinence, and impotence.[307] The remarkable aspect of this experience is that innovations are already being reported that might enhance the operative technique even more, such as the single knot, 2-color running suture.[308] Ahlering and colleagues at U.C. Irvine have shown that open surgical skills might be rapidly transferred into the laparoscopic environment with the use of the da Vinci robot.[309] They report on 12 robotic radical prostatectomies all completed successfully with no open conversions and no blood transfusions. They have been able to equate this skill transfer to approximately the equivalent of a laparoscopic surgeon performing > 100 laparoscopic radical prostatectomies. The questions remaining are how well can this operation be performed, what is the learning curve, and can the complications of radical prostatectomy be minimized. All of these are approaching the event horizon. Shrivastava's group has estimated that the operative time for a robotic radical prostatectomy is below 150 minutes.[310] As their series expands and follow-up times accrue, data regarding impotence, incontinence, and bladder neck contractions will all be reported. Others should be able to confirm these findings rapidly, and the much anticipated results of brightly illuminated, magnified controlled environment will materialize.[311]

REMOTE TELEROBOTIC SURGERY It would appear from the previous discussion that most of the framework for operating on people with minimally invasive techniques could be accomplished from remote locations. The ethical, financial, and educational potential for this type of surgery is staggering. But as complex a scenario as this sounds, much basic groundwork is already being done for both research and clinical applications. The term telemedicine has become quite fashionable secondary to the world's rapid acceptance of computerized media and internet connectivity.[312–319] Recall the significance of the year 1999, when computers outsold televisions in the United States. In fact, the U.S. government has been a strong supporter of pioneering efforts in the telemedicine field with research grants. The great potential for telecommunications is being realized in digital radiology practices, where the radiologist can view and comment on clinical radiographs of patients at the hospital from his/her home. Robotic surgery, as we have just seen, is a technology based on computer integration of a transducer station and the robotic

instrument is the end effector. The ability to combine these essentially digital computerized modalities is both obvious and possible.[320–322] The first problem for interfacing telecommunications and robotic surgery is linking for real-time interaction. Several methods are possible, including regular telephone lines, fiberoptic cables, microwave transmission, satellite linkages, and broadband communication (integrated services digital network [ISDN], local area networks [LANs], and dedicated T-1 lines). Recently the surgical group at Virginia Commonwealth University used regular internet connections to interact with surgeons in Ecuador and the Dominican Republic to perform 6 laparoscopic cholecystectomies.[323] These surgeons used 33.6 K bps to 64 K bps lines to transmit voice and video.

Telementoring has already been performed for multiple surgeries as well as urologic laparoscopic cases. Dr. Kavoussi's group at Johns Hopkins has gained significant recognition for these pioneering efforts. In their initial studies, the surgeon mentor was located in a control room > 1,000 feet from the operating room; 14 advanced and 9 basic laparoscopic procedures were performed.[290] Telementoring was accomplished using real-time computer video images, 2-way audio communication links, and a robotic arm to control the videoendoscope. Success was achieved in 22 of 23 cases without increased operative times or complications. They then extended their investigations and distances between the Johns Hopkins Bayview Medical Center and the Johns Hopkins Hospital (distance = 3.5 miles) for 27 more telementoring laparoscopic procedures utilizing public phone lines. Finally, they have extended their novel surgical instruction capabilities to the international arena with cases in Austria, Italy, and Thailand. Others have reported on the technology necessary for successful telementoring. The U.S. Navy recently studied the feasibility of laparoscopic hernia repairs aboard the *USS Abraham Lincoln* while cruising the Pacific Ocean.[324] Telementoring was possible from remote locations in Maryland and California. In a recent research investigation, Broderick and colleagues at the Virginia Commonwealth University reported that decreasing transmission bandwidth does not significantly affect laparoscopic image clarity or color fidelity as long as the laparoscopes are positioned and maintained at their optimal working distance.[324]

It was only a matter of time before the da Vinci or the Zeus systems were linked to a remote surgical effector in another place, and the actual surgery was performed with the aid of an assistant. The first laparoscopic cholecystectomy done remotely was down the hall in Montreal, Canada. Kavoussi was the first to perform a surgery remotely from another hospital in the same town. Finally, a surgeon in New York City successfully removed the gallbladder of a patient in Strasbourg, France, with a 155 millisecond time lag. The operation took 1 hour and 16 minutes. The robotic machines can with little doubt accomplish complex surgical interventions and function with-

out fatigue. Since the surgeon already has given up all visual information to the technology of laparoscopic surgery, the next great step is passing the surgical dissection to the machines.

INCISIONLESS (OR NATURAL ORIFICE) SURGERY The limits of minimally invasive surgery are being stretched by the ever-inquisitive surgical pioneer. Threre is no reason to believe that the preliminary results of endoluminal and/or transluminal surgeries will stop with the easiest types of procedures to more sophisticated endeavors.[325] Now add a dextrous multidegrees of freedom robotic interface and the future should rapidly evolve into sophisticated surgical reconstructive arena. Lest the reader think this is the stuff of scinence fiction, and not scientific reality, a brief overview is necessary. Serpentine robots are devices that were originally designed off the kinesiology of another complex biologic joint, the spine. The purpose of the serpentine robots is to make a device that has more degrees of freedom than does the normal human arm. As computer-control algorithms advance and the means to control the complex maneuvers of greater than 10 to 20 or 30 degrees of freedom become available, these systems have become increasingly complex. The first such systems were called serpentine because of the needed ability for robotic arms to "snake" through passages and pipes to inspect nuclear reactors, fuel tank baffles, and wing spars. To overcome the multiple joint control issues and prevent restrictive backlash, Miyake in 1986 described innovative solutions in control.[326] The U.S. Navy funded a spine-like arm for ocean exploration in 1968, which has been called the Scripps Tensor Arm. Another such ultrahigh dexterity robotic arm was developed by Ralph Mosher in 1969, called the Articulating Mechanism. It was a modular and low-cost alternative to the Scripps design, but was not as precise as the former. Many of the space arms for use on the United States Space Shuttle were serpentine. The Frederick Wells arm, designed in 1970 at the Marshall Space Flight Center in Huntsville, Alabama, was such a device. This arm has continued to evolve with improvements by Iwatsuka, in 1986, and by Wuenecher. Wuenecher called his device the Remote Control Manipulator intended to aid astronauts. The Spine Robot is a Swedish-made serpentine robotic arm invented by Ove Larson and Charles Davidson in 1983. It consists of stacked ovoidal discs controlled by opposable cables. There are now many versions of this design using bellows, U-joints, and pressurized capillary systems (Sheinman). In 1984, Motohiko Kuura designed the Expandable and Contractible Arms for serpentine applications. The final addition in this series is the 1991 Modular Robotic Joint (MJR) robotic arm invented by Mark Rosheim.[327] The advantages of this system are that it allows for more degrees of freedom than the human arm, increases modularity, and is fault tolerant—if one joint fails another is capable of providing the needed mobility to accomplish its task. Why would surgeons be at all interested in more degrees of freedom you might wonder. Another coming technologic tour de force is woundless surgery (Figure 50-51, left). This type of complex surgery is also called peroral, transgastric endoscopic surgery, and cholecystectomies, appendectomies, and tubal bandings have already been performed[328,329] In order to achieve more complex tasks, such as nephrectomy or radical prostatectomy, an ultrahigh dexterity robotic arm will be necessary (see Figure 50-51, right).

CONCLUSIONS

Minimally invasive urologic reconstructive surgery is rapidly expanding at numerous centers around the world. The ability to reconstruct every urologic organ by laparoscopic methods has been reported, and replacement via robotic-enhanced methods is well underway. The technology to accomplish these dextrous maneuvers is changing substantially since the first edition of this textbook. Suturing technology and techniques are the leading methods that are fostering these reconstructions, but the skills and talents of innovators in this field cannot be denied. Mechanical-assist technologies certainly offer the capacity to potentiate or facilitate the complex laparoscopic reconstructions necessary for laparoscopic urologic surgery. In one recent report, Antiphon and colleagues describe the use of Aesop and another mechanical arm (Lina arm, Lina Medical, Denmark) to perform complete solo laparoscopic radical prostatectomy.[330] Robotic surgery offers the potential to rapidly integrate these skills to a much broader range of urologists, perhaps even bringing these now sophisticated techniques into the hands of all urologists. In one recent investigation, skill performance between standard instruments and two surgical robotic systems was compared. It was noted that general task performance utilizing standard laparoscopic instruments is faster but with similar precision to either the da Vinci or the Zeus robots. In performing the more sophisticated reconstructive task of suturing, neither robotic system improved the efficiency (as measured by time to complete the task) as compared with a trained laparoscopic surgeon. However, precision was improved by the addition of the robotic interface. In addition, with knot tying, which involves even more intricate intracavitary manipulations, an improvement was noted in both efficiency and precision with only the da Vinci robotic system. These authors conclude that current robotic systems are not *cost* justifiable currently when compared with skilled, highly trained endoscopic surgeons.[331] But one must always filter claims based on current knowledge and current costs, especially when Luddite tendencies or fear of advanced technologies in replacing fundamental human methods is perceived. It therefore seems obvious that laparoscopic suturing skills, no matter how difficult to master, have some merit, and there is little doubt that transfer of skills from the laparoscopic realm to the robotic environment is possible. Almost everything in the operating

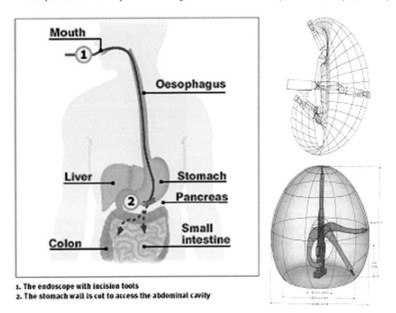

Figure 50-51 Serpentine robot with a view for use during per oral, transgastric intra-abdominal surgery.

environment at present for the urologic laparoscopist can be considered a barrier to the rapid acquisition of the skills necessary to master suturing. Yet the brightly illuminated, magnified view beckons for microsurgical reconstruction that may be better than our open counterparts can achieve without the routine use of loupes.[132] Recently the group from Cleveland has used the da Vinci to perform a sural nerve graft during a laparoscopic radical prostatectomy with a mean operative time of 6.5 hours in 3 patients.[332] Again, robots should be able to augment our ability here as well.

Unique opportunities exist for further continued improvement in reconstructive technologies. Several intriguing technologies will be reviewed for their potential application in the future. Starting with suture technology, it now appears possible that an absorbable suture can be manufactured that does not require knots at all, and may obviate all potential disadvantages of running suturing. Medical textiles research has become increasingly aware of the limitations imposed by minimally invasive surgery. In 1967, McKenzie published a little-known technique of a multiple-barbed nylon suture to repair tendons with greater strength and less inflammatory reaction.[333] Ruff from Duke University began work in 1992 of an absorbable barbed suture for cosmetic repairs.[334] A barbed suture, in theory, removes tension from the apposing suture line, decreasing the foreign-body reaction. Further evolution of this suture is reported by Dattilo and colleagues with a barbed bidirectional absorbable monofila-

ment suture.[335] In this investigation, the authors used a unique suture of monofilament polydioxanone containing 78 barbs in a spiral pattern around the circumference of the suture (Quill Medical, Research Triangle Park, NC). The bidirectional barbed nature of this suture does not require knots for adequate tissue strength (Figure 50-52). The barbed configuration anchors the suture into the tissue and provides adequate apposition while the wound heals with minimal tension and pressure. Preliminary work suggests that the knotless suture material may result in less scar tissue formation.

It would be a major advance in reconstructive surgery if the advantages of the robotic arm-wrist-hand mechanism could be incorporated into a simpler mechanical device. Such a prototype is being investigated by Olympus Medical (Figure 50-53). But it is the control systems themselves that set the current generation of surgical robotic systems apart from a mere multidegree of free-

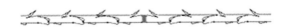

Figure 50-52 Quill Medical Inc.'s bidirectional barbed suture material. (Quill Medical Inc., Research Triangle Park, NC)

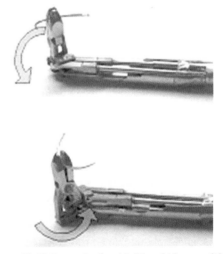

Figure 50-53 Innovative hand-held multidegree of freedom suturing device prototype from Olympus.

dom instrument. As mentioned previously, it is the inherent ability to think, formulate strategy, come up with innovative solutions, and instinctively know what to do and when that separates the surgeon from the machine. Yet, as soon as each caveat is stated, there are fundamental research activities in artificial intelligence that are looking to replicate and even go beyond human capacity. The hallmark feature of the Intelligence Age, of which we find ourselves at the inception, is that change is going to occur with exponential frequency.[336] Surgery and medicine should be natural applications of advanced intelligence systems; because the cost of health care is rising so dramatically and the nuances of requiring fault tolerance, indefatigable effectors are in our machines, not us. We cannot achieve the micron degree of accuracy that our robots will.

ADDENDUM: SHORT HOME SUTURING COURSE

Intracorporeal suturing represents a difficult task in experienced hands. A robotic interface certainly helps overcome many of the barriers to skill, but there is no evidence that the robot can replace skill to overcome a flawless anastomosis. How then can the average urologist hope to obtain these skills and apply them whenever the situation calls for intracorporeal placement of sutures? There are two alternatives. You can either practice utilization of laparoscopic suturing skills or utilize any of the included shortcuts discussed in this chapter. If your goal is to obtain skills that can be used time and time again for increasingly complex laparoscopic intracorporeal reconstructions, your time is better spent learning how to suture without opting for shortcuts. This can be accomplished by spending time and money at courses, or you can utilize simple equipment and practice inanimately at home, the office, or in the operating room. It sounds ridiculous to memorize the 12 steps that we presented in Figure 50-22. This represents only a starting place for you to master the choreographed utilization of both your hands. After over a decade and a half of teaching others advanced reconstructive skills, I've yet to find a simpler method than these readily mastered microsurgical steps that provide a practioner the skills to universally master suturing in every environment (even using the da Vinci Surgical System). To do this you will require a camcorder and tripod. A tennis ball will serve as the targeted "organ" for reconstruction. You may utilize any suturing instruments or a disposable grasper that is available, or contact your local manufacturer's representative to borrow one. Cut sutures to a prescribed length and you can procede. Slow down first and try to get a feel for the instrument's tip motions. Once you get proficient at handling the needle, make things progressively more difficult by covering your camera and tennis ball with a blanket. Finally, add a pelvic trainer (again, obtainable from a manufacturer's representative), trocars, and a plastic human pelvis (scale models are obtainable from many biological supply houses for under $35 [US]). Your best bet is to keep both

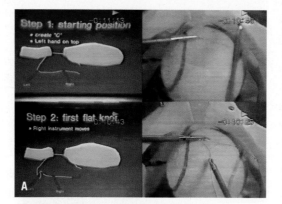
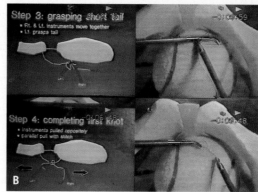
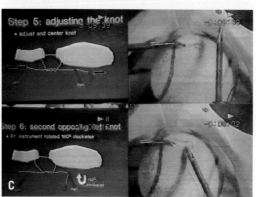
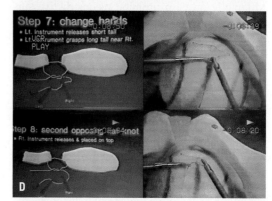
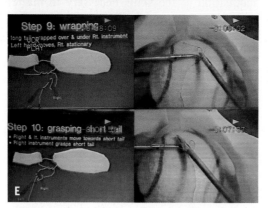
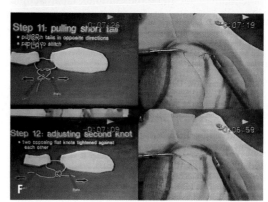

Figure 50-54 A-F, Still photographs of a home-study course in suturing.

hands on either side of the camera, but as skills advance you should move to the side as is required for most animate applications. I have taken still photographs from a video recorder during just such a home-study course to demonstrate each step again (Figure 50-54). Every time you get frustrated take a rest. Each time you start, things should get easier. The hand-eye coordination to function in the videolaparoscopic environment will develop.

Ran Katz and colleagues recently described a simple method of training for performing the vesicourethral anastomosis using chicken skin. A model urethra and bladder neck are prepared by folding and tabularizing a 5 × 4 cm piece of skin over a 14F catheter. Training again is performed in a pelvic trainer. The single knot method of Van Velthouven can be easily adapted to this training technique. As described by the authors, the initial attempts require the longest times for neophytes (residents and urologists with minimal laparoscopic experience). Needle passage was easier, followed by knotting and suturing, in terms of

skill acquisition. They noted in 10 neophytes who followed their 5-step regimen that all were able to advance and perform complete, accurate urethrovesical anastomoses.[337] Yet chicken skin is not human tissue, it smells (not intended to be species biased) and takes some time to prepare. In addition, a good model should seek to be robust for applications in research necessary to advance suture-based research. We have recently presented a microfiber model using a cheap, flexible, moldable, water resistant, and odorless material (Miracle Towel, Turtle Wax, Chicago, IL, but located at most stores).[338] You can also mark on it to improve your accuracy.

Good luck!

REFERENCES

1. Das S. Urologic laparoscopy: the future is now. Urol Clin North Am 2001;NA 28:1–3.
2. Carroll PR. Laparoscopic urologic surgery: differentiating what should be done from what can be done [editorial]. J Urol 1994;151:1603–4.

3. Harrell AG, Heniford BT. Minimally invasive abdominal surgery: lux et veritus past, present, and future. Am J Surg 2005;190:239–43.
4. Clarke HC. Laparoscopy. New instruments for suturing and ligation. Fertil Steril 1972;23:274–7.
5. Ko ST, Airan MC. Therapeutic laparoscopic suturing techniques. Surg Endosc 1992;6:41–6.
6. Mettler L, Semm K. Pelviscopic uterine surgery. Surg Endosc 1992;6:23–31.
7. Marrero MA, Corfman RS. Laparoscopic use of sutures. Clin Obstet Gynecol 1991;34:387–94.
8. Petrovsky B, Perelman M, Kuznichev A. Resection and plastic surgery of bronchi [translation]. Russia: Mir Publications; 1968. p. 202–21.
9. Steichen FM, Ravitch MM. Contemporary stapling instruments and basic mechanical suturing techniques. Surg Clin North Am 1984;64:425–40.
10. Fowler DL, White RA. Laparoscopic-assisted sigmoid resection. Surg Laprosc Endosc 1991;1:183–8.
11. Jacobs M, Verdeja JC, Goldstein HS. Minimally invasive colon resection (laparoscopic colectomy). Surg Laparosc Endosc 1991;1:144–50.
12. Chiu AW, Chen M-T, Huang WJS, et al. Case report: laparoscopic nephroureterectomy and endoscopic excision of bladder cuff. Min Invas Ther Allied Tech 1992;1:299–303.
13. Clayman RV, Kavoussi LR, Figenshau RS, et al. Laparoscopic nephroureterectomy: initial case report. J Laparoendosc Surg 1991;1:343–9.
14. Kerbl K, Chandhoke PS, McDougall E, et al. Laparoscopic stapled bladder closure: laboratory and clinical experience. J Urol 1993;149:1437–9.
15. Kozminski M, Partamian KO. Case report of laparoscopic ileal loop conduit. J Endourol 1992;6:147–50.
16. Grainger DA, Meyer WR, DeCherney AH, Diamond MP. Laparoscopic clips: evaluation of absorbable and titanium with regard to hemostasis and tissue reactivity. J Reprod Med 1991;36:493–5.
17. Klein RD, Jessup G, Ahart F, et al. Comparison of laparoscopic titanium and absorbable polymeric ligating clips. Surg Endosc 1993;7:124A.
18. Ravo B, Rosales C, Serino F, Castagneto M. The use of absorbable staples for construction of a bladder tube. Surgery 1991;173:29–32.
19. Corman ML, Prager ED, Hardy TG Jr, Bubrick MP. Comparison of the Valtrac biofragmentable anastomosis ring with conventional suture and stapled anastomosis in colon surgery. Results of a prospective, randomized clinical trial. Dis Colon Rectum 1989;32:183–7.
20. Smith AD, Bubrick MP, Mestitz ST, et al. Evaluation of the biofragmentable anastomotic ring following preoperative irradiation to the rectosigmoid in dogs. Dis Colon Rectum 1988;31:5–9.
21. Moran ME, Bowyer DW, Szabo Z. Laparoscopic suturing in urology: a model for vesicourethral anastomosis. Min Invas Ther Allied Tech 1993;2:165–70.
22. Frede T, Stock C, Rassweiler JJ, Alken P. Retroperitoneoscopic and laparoscopic suturing: tips and strategies to improve efficiency. J Endourol 2000;14:905–13.
23. Moran ME. Laparoscopic suturing and skills acquisition: methods to improve efficiency. J Endourol 2000;14:913–4.
24. Gomella LG. Laparoscopy and urologic oncology—I now pronounce you man and wife [editorial]. J Urol 2003;169: 2057–8.
25. Moran ME. Robotic surgery: urologic implications. J Endourol 2006. [In press]
26. Costi R, Denet C, Sarli L, et al. Laparoscopy in the last decade of the millennium. Have we really improved? Surg Endosc 2003;17:791–7.
27. Meilahn JE. The need for improving laparoscopic suturing and knot tying. J Laparoendosc Surg 1992;2:267.
28. Bisson J, Vinson RK, Leadbetter GW Jr. Urolithiasis from stapler anastomosis. Amer J Surg 1979;137:280–2.
29. Ravo B, Rosales C, Serino F, Castagneto M. The use of absorbable staples for construction of a bladder tube. Surg Gynecol Obstet 1991;173:29–32.
30. Low RK, Moran ME. Argon beam coagulation: implications for reconstructive urology. Min Invas Ther Allied Tech 1993;2:75–8.
31. Kirker-Head CA, Steckel RR, Schwartz A, Williams R. Evaluation of surgical staples for ligation of the renal pedicle during nephrectomy. Urol Res 1988;16:63–6.
32. Sugarbaker DJ, Mentzer SJ. Improved technique for hilar vascular stapling. Ann Thorac Surg 1992;53:165–6.
33. Kerbl K, Chandhoke PS, McDougall E, et al. Laparoscopic clips and staples: vascular application. J Endourol 1992; 6:S142.
34. Moran ME. Theory of vascular pedicle hemostasis during laparoscopic nephrectomy. Min Invas Ther Allied Tech 1991;1:A69.
35. Nathanson LK, Easter DW, Cuschieri A. Ligation of the structures of the cystic pedicle during laparoscopic cholecystectomy. Am J Surg 1991;161:350–4.
36. Nathanson LK, Nathanson PDK, Cuschieri A. Safety of vessel ligation in laparoscopic surgery. Endoscopy 1991;23: 206–9.
37. Nelson MT, Nakashima M, Mulvihill SJ. How safe are laparoscopically placed clips? An invitro and in vivo study. Arch Surg 1992;127:718–20.
38. Beltran KA, Foresman PA, Rodeheaver GT. Quantitation of force to dislodge endoscopic ligation clips: EndoClip II vs. LigaClip ERCA. J Laparoendosc Surg 1994;4:253–6.
39. Feldman SL, Presman D, Kandel GL. Renal arteriovenous fistula following nephrectomy. Br J Urol 1985;57:592.
40. Goldstein AG, Delaurentis DA, Schwarz AJ. Post-nephrectomy arteriovenous fistula. J Urol 1967;98:44–7.
41. Lacombe M. Renal arteriovenous fistula following nephrectomy. Urology 1985;25:13–6.
42. Baniel J, Schein M. Partial nephrectomy using a linear stapling device. Br J Urol 1992;69:218.
43. Avant LO, Starr GA. Vesicourethral reanastomosis by mechanical stapling and transurethral deep dorsal venous ligation: a new technique for radical retropubic prostatectomy. J Endourol. [Submitted]
44. Dziki AJ, Duncan MD, Harmon JW, et al. Advantages of handsewn over stapled bowel anastomosis. Dis Colon Rectum 1991;34:442–8.
45. Jansson OK, Zilling TL, Walther BS. Healing of colonic anastomoses: comparative experimental study of glued, manually sutured, and stapled anastomoses. Dis Colon Rectum 1991;34:557–62.
46. Moritz E, Achleitner D, Holbling N, et al. Single vs. double stapling technique in colorectal surgery. A prospective randomized trial. Dis Colon Rectum 1991;34:495–7.
47. West of Scotland and Highland Anastomosis Study Group. Suturing or stapling in gastrointestinal surgery: a prospective randomized study. Br J Surg 1991;78:337–41.
48. Griffith DP, Gleeson MJ. The prosthetic bladder—perhaps the technology has arrived. Scand J Urol Nephrol Suppl 1992;142:109–22.
49. Clayman RC, McDougall E, Chandhoke PS, et al. Laparoscopic ureteral reimplantation: laboratory studies. J Endourol 1992;6:S144.
50. Das S. Laparoscopic removal of bladder diverticulum. J Urol 1992;148:1837–9.
51. Parra RO, Jones JP, Andrus CH, Hagood PG. Laparoscopic diverticulectomy: preliminary report of a new approach for the treatment of bladder diverticulum. J Urol 1992; 148:869–71.
52. Parra RO, Andrus CH, Jones JP, Boullier JA. Laparoscopic cystectomy: initial case report on a new treatment for the retained bladder. J Urol 1992;148:1140–4.
53. Schuessler WW, Vancaillie TG, Preminger GM. Laparoscopic dismembered pyeloplasty [abstract B-30]. Min Invas Ther Allied Tech 1992;1 Suppl:A68.
54. Gluckman OR, Stoller M, Irby P. Laparoscopic pyelocaliceal diverticula ablation. J Endourol 1993;7:315–7.
55. Levinson AK, Greskovich FJ, Swanson DA, et al. Fibrin glue for partial nephrectomy. Urolology 1991;38:314–6.
56. Winfield HN, Donovan JF, Godet AS, Clayman RV. Human laparoscopic partial nephrectomy: initial case report for benign disease. J Endourol 1993;7:521–6.
57. Satava RM. Surgery 2001: a technologic framework for the future. Surg Endosc 1993;7:111–3.
58. Halsted W. The training of the surgeon. Bull Johns Hop Hosp 1904;15:267–76.
59. Rothschild JG. What alternatives has minimally invasive surgery provided the surgeon? Arch Surg 1998;133:1156–9.
60. Derossis AM, Fried GM, Abrahamowicz M, et al. Development of a model for training and evaluation of laparoscopic skills. Am J Surg 1998;175:482–7.
61. Hanna GB, Drew T, Clinch P, et al. Psychomotor skills for endoscopic manipulations: differing abilities between right and left-handed individuals. Ann Surg 1997;225:333–8.
62. Hanna GB, Cuschieri A. Influence of the optical axis-to-target angle on endoscopic task performance. Surg Endosc 1999;13:371–5.
63. Holden JG, Flach JM, Donchin Y. Perceptual-motor coordination in an endoscopic surgery simulation. Surg Endosc 1999;13:127–32.
64. Hanna GB, Shimi S, Cuschieri A. Influence of direction of view, target-to-endoscope distance and manipulation angle on endoscopic knot tying. Br J Surg 1997;84: 1460–4.
65. Breedveld P, Stassen HG, Meijer DW, Stassen LPS. Theoretical background and conceptual solution for depth perception and eye-hand coordination problems in laparoscopic surgery. Min Invas Ther Allied Tech 1999;8:227–34.
66. Kum CK, Goh P, Alexander DJ, Moochala S. Three-dimensional versus two-dimensional imaging for laparoscopic suturing. Br J Surg 1997;84:35.
67. Barnes RW. Surgical handicraft: teaching and learning surgical skills. Am J Surg 1987;153:422–7.
68. Reznick RK. Teaching and testing technical skills. Am J Surg 1993;165:358–61.
69. Dent TL. Training and privileging for new procedures. Surg Clin North Am 1996;76:615–21.
70. Macmillan AIM, Cuschieri A. Assessment of innate ability and skills for endoscopic manipulations by the advanced Dundee endoscopic psychomotor tester: predictive and concurrent validity. Am J Surg 1999;177:274–7.
71. Lang NP, Rowland-Morin PA, Coe NP. Identification of communication apprehension in medical students starting surgery rotation. Am J Surg 1998;176:41–5.
72. Smith DM, Kolb DA. A user's guide for the learning-style inventory. A manual for teachers and trainers. Boston: McBer and Co; 1986.
73. Lynch TG, Woelfl NN, Steele DJ, Hanssen CS. Learning style influences student examination performance. Am J Surg 1998;176:62–6.
74. Kaufman HH, Wiegand RL, Tunick RH. Teaching surgeons to operate-principles of psychomotor skills training. Acta Neurochir 1987;87:1–7.
75. Jones MB, Kennedy RS. Isoperformance curves in applied psychology. Hum Factors 1996;38:167–82.
76. Melvin WS, Johnson JA, Ellison EC. Laparoscopic skills enhancement. Am J Surg 1996;172:377–9.
77. Sammarco MJ, Youngblood JP. A resident teaching program in operative endoscopy. Obstet Gynecol 1993;81:463–6.
78. Schirmer BD, Edge SB, Dix J, Miller AD. Incorporation of laparoscopy into a surgical endoscopy training program. Am J Surg 1992;163:46–52.
79. Wolfe BM, Szabo Z, Moran ME, et al. Training for minimally invasive surgery: need for surgical skills. Surg Endosc 1993;7:112–4.
80. Heniford BT, Backus CL, Matthews BD, et al. Optimal teaching environment for laparoscopic splenectomy. Am J Surg 2001;181:226–30.
81. Anastakis DJ, Regehr G, Reznick RK, et al. Assessment of technical skills transfer from the bench training model to the human model. Am J Surg 1999;177:167–70.
82. Ko CY, Whang EE, Karamanoukian R, et al. What is the best method of surgical training? A report of America's leading senior surgeons. Arch Surg 1998;133:900–5.
83. Martin JA, Regehr G, Reznick R, et al. Objective structured assessment of technical skill (OSATS) for surgical residents. Br J Surg 1997;84:273–8.
84. Rosser JC, Rosser LE, Savalgi RS. Skill acquisition and assessment for laparoscopic surgery. Arch Surg 1997;132:200–4.
85. Steele RJC, Walder C, Herbert M. Psychomotor testing and the ability to perform an anastomosis in junior surgical trainees. Br J Surg 1992;79:1065–7.
86. Medina M. Formidable challenges to teaching advanced laparoscopic skills. JSLS 2001;5:153–8.
87. Macmillan AIM, Cuschieri A. Assessment of innate ability and skills for endoscopic manipulations by the advanced Dundee endoscopic psychomotor tester: predictive and concurrent validity. Am J Surg 1999;177:274–7.
88. Francis NK, Hanna GB, Cuschieri A. Reliability of the Dundee endoscopic psychomotor tester (DEPT) for dominant hand performance. Surg Endosc 2001;15:673–6.
89. Fried GM, Derossis AM, Bothwell J, Sigmann HH. Comparison of laparoscopic performance in vivo with performance measured in a laparoscopic simulator. Surg Endosc 1999;13:1077–81.
90. Rosser JC, Rosser LE, Savalgi RS. Objective evaluation of a laparoscopic surgical skill program for residents and senior surgeons. Arch Surg 1998;133:657–61.
91. Derossis AM, Antoniuk M, Fried GM. Evaluation of laparoscopic skills: a 2-year follow-up during residency training. Can J Surg 1999;42:293–6.
92. Olinger A, Pistorius G, Lindemann W, et al. Effectiveness of a hands-on training course for laparoscopic spine surgery in a porcine model. Surg Endosc 1999;13:118–22.
93. Meier AH, Rawn CL, Krummel TM. Virtual reality: surgical application—challenge for the new millennium. J Am Coll Surg 2001;192:372–84.
94. Ramshaw BJ, Young D, Garcha I, et al. The role of multimedia interactive programs in training for laparoscopic procedures. Surg Endosc 2001;15:21–7.
95. Rosser JC, Herman B, Risucci DA, et al. Effectiveness of a CD-ROM multimedia tutorial in transferring cognitive

knowledge essential for laparoscopic skill training. Am J Surg 2000;179:320–4.

96. Rogers DA, Regehr G, Howdieshell TR, et al. The impact of external feedback on computer-assisted learning for surgical technical skill training. Am J Surg 2000;179:341–3.

97. Mann CC. The end of Moore's Law? Tech Rev 2000;1:42–8.

98. Haluck RS, Krummel TM. Computers and virtual reality for surgical education in the 21st Century. Arch Surg 2000; 135:787–92.

99. Krummel TM. Surgical simulation and virtual reality: the coming revolution Ann Surg 1998;228:635–7.

100. Marescaux J, Clement JM, Tassetti V, et al. Virtual reality applied to hepatic surgery simulation: the next revolution. Ann Surg 1998;228:627–34.

101. Trunkey DD, Botney R. Assessing competency: a tale of two professions. J Am Coll Surg 2001;192:385–95.

102. Rosser JC, Murayama M, Gabriel NH. Minimally invasive surgical training solutions for the twenty-first century. Surg Clin North Am 2000;80:1607–24.

103. Satava RM, Jones SB. Preparing surgeons for the 21st century. Surg Clin North Am 2000;80:1353–65.

104. Moore RG, Adams JB, Partin AW, et al. Telementoring of laparoscopic procedures: initial clinical experience. Surg Endosc 1996;10:107–10.

105. Lee BR, Bishoff JT, Janetschek G, et al. A novel method of surgical instruction: international telementoring. World J Urol 1998;16:367–70.

106. Cubano M, Poulose BK, Talamini MA, et al. Long distance telementoring. A novel tool for laparoscopy aboard the USS Abraham Lincoln. Surg Endosc 1999;13:673–8.

107. Broderick TJ, Harnett BM, Merriam NR, et al. Impact of varying transmission bandwidth on image quality. Telemed J E Health 2001;7:47–53.

108. Gandsas A, Draper K, Chekan E, et al. Laparoscopy and the internet. A surgeon survey. Surg Endosc 2001;15:1044–8.

109. Durst L. The center for minimal access surgery—teaching for tomorrow. J Telemed Telecare 2000;6 Suppl 2:S14–5.

110. Green LS, Loughlin KR, Kavoussi LR. Management of epigastric vessel injury during laparoscopy. J Endourol 1992;2:99–101.

111. Nathanson LK, Cuschieri A. The falciform lift: a simple method for retraction of falciform ligament during laparoscopic cholecystectomy. Surg Endosc 1990;4:186.

112. Mettler L, Semm K. Pelviscopic uterine surgery. Surg Endosc 1992;6:23–31.

113. Reich H, Clarke C, Sekel L. A simple method for ligating with a straight and curved needles in operative laparoscopy. Obstet Gynecol 1992;79:143–7.

114. Nathanson LK, Nathanson PDK, Cuschieri A. Safety of vessel ligation in laparoscopic surgery. Endoscopy 1991; 23:206–9.

115. Cuschieri A, Shimi S, Nathanson LK. Laparoscopic reduction, crural repair, and fundoplication of large hiatal hernia. Amer J Surg 1992;163:425–30.

116. McComb PF. A new suturing instrument that allows the use of microsuture at laparoscopy. Fertil Steril 1992;57: 936–8.

117. Oko M, Rosin RD. Extracorporeal knotting with a new instrument. Min Invas Ther Allied Tech 1993;2:1–3.

118. Puttick MI, Nduka BA, Darzi A. Extracorporeal knot tying using an atraumatic Babcock clamp. J Laparoendosc Surg 1994;4:339–41.

119. Kennedy JS. A technique for extracorporeal suturing. J Laparoendosc Surg 1992;2:269–72.

120. Andrews S, Lewis JL. Minimal access suturing: an assessment of knot substitutes. Min Inv Ther 1992;1:309.

121. Moran ME. Stationary and automated laparoscopically assisted technologies. J Laparoendosc Surg 1993;3:221–7.

122. Tonietto G, Pintaldi S. Finger-assisted laparoscopic surgery. J Laparoendosc Surg 1994;4:205–7.

123. Tan HL, Hutson JM. Case report: laparoscopically-assisted cysto-prostatectomy. Min Invas Ther Allied Tech 1994;3: 207–10.

124. Daum IW. "EndoHand," an manipulator for M.I.S. [abstract O-86]. Min Invas Ther Allied Tech 1994;3 Suppl 1:7.

125. Schurr T, Melzer A, Dautzenberg P, et al. Development of steerable instruments for minimal invasive surgery in modular conception. Acta Chir Belg 1993;63:73–7.

126. Durrani AF, Preminger GM. Advanced endoscopic imaging: 3-D laparoscopic endoscopy. In: Szabo Z, Kerstein MD, Lewis JE, editors. Surgical Technology International II. San Francisco: Universal Medical Press; 1994. p. 141–7.

127. Cartmill J, Patkin M, Graber JG, et al. Ergonomics and needle holding ability of laparoscopic needle holders [abstract 132]. Surg Endosc 1993;128.

128. Agarwal DK, Gaur DD, Agarwal M. A new concept of laparoscopic suturing. Min Invas Ther Allied Tech 1994; 227–9.

129. Cuschieri A, Szabo Z. Tissue approximation in endoscopic surgery. Oxford: Isis Medical Media; 1995. p. 90–4.

130. Waninger J, Kauffmann GW, Shah IA, Farthmann EH. Influence of the distance between interrupted sutures and the tension of sutures on healing of experimental colonic anastomoses. Am J Surg 1992;163:319–23.

131. Szabo Z, Rose EH, Ellis MS, Burch BH. Slip-knot suspension technique: a fail-safe microanastomosis for small-caliber vessels. Microsurgery 1992;13:100–2.

132. Bowyer DW, Moran ME, Szabo Z. Laparoscopic suturing in urology: a model for the lower urinary tract. J Endourol 1992;6:S142.

133. Szabo Z, Bowyer DW. Laparoscopic suturing: principles and techniques. In: Das S, Crawford ED, editors. Urologic laparoscopy. Philadelphia: W.B. Saunders; 1994. p. 225–44.

134. Pietrafitta JJ. A technique of laparoscopic knot tying. J Laparoendosc Surg 1992;2:273–5.

135. Kozminski M, Richards,WH 3rd. Fly-casting method of intracorporeal knot tying. Urology 1994;44:577–8.

136. Cuschieri A. Tissue approximation. Probl Gen Surg 1991;8:366–77.

137. Soper NJ, Hunter JG. Suturing and knot tying in laparoscopy. Surg Clin North Am 1992;72:1139–52.

138. Bowyer DW, Moran ME, Szabo Z. Laparoscopic suture materials. Western Section AUA, 1st Prize Round Table, Kuaui, HI, October, 1992.

139. Abrahams HM, Kim DH, Moran ME. Intracorporeal interrupted suturing: the ideal length of suture material. JSLS 2001;5:383–4.

140. Moran ME, Abrahams HM, Kim DH. Suture length is a key variable in suturing efficiency. J Endourol 2001;15: A22,A1–P5.

141. Meizer A, Lirici MM, Reuthebuch O, et al. New knotting, ligature, and purse string techniques. Min Invas Ther Allied Tech 1992;1:74.

142. Gomes da Silva E. Suturoscope: a new device that allows endoscopic sutures to be performed with traditional threads. Surg Endosc 1990;4:220–3.

143. Saclarides TJ, Smith L, Ko S-T, et al. Transanal endoscopic microsurgery. Dis Colon Rectum 1992;35:1183–91.

144. Hoznek A, Solomon L, Rabi R, et al. Vesicourethral anastomosis during laparoscopic radical prostatectomy: the running suture method. J Endourol 2000;14:749–53.

145. Van Velthoven RF, Ahlering TE, Peltier A, et al. Technique for laparoscopic running urethrovesical anastomosis: the single knot method. Urology 2003;61:699–702.

146. Menon M, Tewari A, Peabody JO. Vattikuti Institute prostatectomy: technique. J Urol 2003;169:2289–92.

147. Desai PJ, Moran ME, Parekh AR, Calvano CJ. Running suturing: the ideal suture length facilitates this task. J Endourol 2000;14:191–4.

148. Moran ME, Marsh C, Perrotti M. Theory of veiscourethral anastomoses. J Endourol 2006. [In press]

149. Bariol SV, Stewart GD, Tolley DA. Laparoscopic suturing: effect of instrument handling on suture strength. J Endourol 2005;19:1127–33.

150. Moran ME, Marsh C, Perrotti M. Achilles' heel of Van Velthoven anastomosis. J Endourol 2006. [In press]

151. Moran ME, Marsh C, Perrotti M. Running vesicourethral anastomosis: number of bites. J Endourol 2006. [In press]

152. Moran ME, Marsh C, Perrotti M. Running circular anastomosis after radical prostatectomy: solving potential disadvantages using bidirectional barbed knotless suture. J Endourol 2006. [In press]

153. Riskin DJ, Schwaitzberg SD. A comparison of holding strength of various surgical clips. Surg Endosc 2003;17:654–6.

154. Kumar U, Albala DM. Newer techniques in intracorporeal tissue approximation: suturing, tissue adhesives, and microclips. Urol Clin North Am 2001;28:15–21.

155. Tarnoff M, Rosen M, Brody F. Planned totally extraperitoneal laparoscopic Spigelian hernia repair. Surg Endosc 2002;16:359.

156. Hill AC, Maroney TP, Virmani R. Facilitated coronary anastomosis using a nitinol U-Clip device: bovine model. J Thorac Cardiovasc Surg 2001;121:859–70.

157. Von Maszewski M, Sucher JF, Macfadyen BV Jr. Laparoscopic instrumentation: linear cutters, clip appliers, and staplers. Semin Laparosc Surg 2001;8:69–76.

158. Murr MM, Gallagher SF. Technical considerations for transabdominal loading of the circular stapler in laparoscopic Roux-en-Y gastric bypass. Am J Surg 2003;185:585–8.

159. Waage A, Gagner M, Feng JJ. Early experience with computer-mediated flexible circular stapling technique for upper gastrointestinal anastomosis. Obes Surg 2003;13:88–94.

160. Chan D, Bishoff JT, Ratner L, et al. Endovascular gastrointestinal stapler device malfunction during laparoscopic nephrectomy: early recognition and management. J Urol 2000;164:319–21.

161. Hsu TH, Su LM, Ratner LE, Kavoussi LR. Renovascular complications of laparoscopic donor nephrectomy. Urology 2002;60:811–5.

162. Meng MV, Freise CE, Kang SM, et al. Techniques to optimize vascular control during laparoscopic donor nephrectomy. Urology 2003;61:93–7.

163. Murayama KM, Grune MT, Matamoro A Jr, et al. Staple occlusion of the infrarenal aorta: a videoscopic retroperitoneal approach. J Vasc Surg 1997;25:786–90.

164. Lund GO, Winfield HN, Donovan JF, Narepalem N. Laparoscopically-assisted penile revascularization for vasculogenic impotence [abstract V5124]. J Endourol 1994;8:S64.

165. Jordan GH. Pediatric genitourinary laparoscopic surgery. AUA Today 1994;7:14–5.

166. Denes FT, Mendonca BB, Arap S. Laparoscopic management of intersexual states. Urol Clin North Am 2001; 28:31–42.

167. Markovich R, Jacobson A, Aldana JP, et al. Practice trends in contemporary management of adult ureteropelvic junction obstruction. Urology 2003;62:22–5.

168. Baldwin DD, Dunbar JA, Wells N, McDougall EM. Single-center comparison of laparoscopic pyeloplasty, acucise endopyelotomy, and open pyeloplasty. J Endourol 2003; 17:155–60.

169. Schuessler WW. Laparoscopic pyeloplasty. AUA Today 1994;7:15.

170. Jarrett TW, Chan DY, Charambura TC, et al. Laparoscopic pyeloplasty: the first 100 cases. J Urol 2002;167:1253–6.

171. Gaur DD, Agarwal DK, Purohit KC, Darshane AS. Retroperitoneal laparoscopic pyelolithotomy. J Urol 1994;151:927–9.

172. Ramakumar S, Lancini V, Chan DY, et al. Laparoscopic pyeloplasty with concomitant pyelolithotomy. J Urol 2002;167:1378–80.

173. Sundaram CP,Grubb RL 3rd, Rehman J, et al. Laparoscopic pyeloplasty for secondary ureteropelvic junction obstruction. J Urol 2003;169:2037–40.

174. Kaouk JG, Kuang W, Gill IS. Laparoscopic dismembered tabularized flap pyeloplasty: a novel technique. J Urol 2002;167:229–31.

175. Gill IS, Savage JJ, Senagore AJ, Sung GT. Laparoscopic ileal ureter. J Urol 2000;163:1199–202.

176. Gettman MT, Lotan Y, Roerhborn CG, et al. Cost-effective treatment for ureteropelvic junction obstruction: a decision tree analysis. J Urol 2003;169:228–32.

177. Gill IS, Matin SF, Desai MM, et al. Comparative analysis of laparoscopic versus open partial nephrectomy for renal tumors in 200 patients. J Urol 2003;170:64–8.

178. Klopukh BV, Shama S, Picken M, Turk TM. Comparison of laparoscopically assisted partial nephrectomy using digital compression versus purely laparoscopic nephrectomy using vacular pedicle clamp in a porcine model. J Endourol 2003;17:313–5.

179. Simon SD, Ferrigni RG, Novicki DE, et al. Mayo Clinic Scottsdale experience with laparoscopic nephron sparing surgery for renal tumors. J Urol 2003;169:2059–62.

180. Phelan MW, Perry KT, Gore J, Schulam PG. Laparoscopic partial nephrectomy and minimally invasive nephron-sparing surgery. Curr Urol Rep 2003;4:13–20.

181. Cherullo EE, Gill IS, Ponsky LE, et al. Laparoscopic ureterocalicostomy: a feasibility study. J Urol 2003;169:2360–4.

182. Grubb Rl 3rd, Sundaram CP, Yan Y, et al. Use of titanium staples during upper tract laparoscopic reconstructive surgery: initial experience. J Urol 2002;168(4 Pt 1):1366–9.

183. Vanlangendouch R, Clayman RV, et al. Laparoscopic ureterocalicostomy: development of a technique simplified by application of nitinol clips and a wet monopolar electrosurgery device. J Endourol 2006. [In press]

184. Kane CJ, Bolton DM, Stoller ML. Current indications for open stone surgery in an endourology center. Urology 1995;45:218–21.

185. Kaouk JH, Gill IS, Desai MM, et al. Laparoscopic anatrophic nephrolithotomy: feasibility study in a chronic porcine model. J Urol 2003;169:691–6.

186. Kuhlmann U, Gruntzug A,Vetter W, et al. Percutaneous transluminal dilation : a new treatment of renovascular hypertension? Klinische Wochenschrift 1978;56:703–7.

187. Hsu THS, Gill IS, Sung GT. Laparoscopic aortorenal bypass: a feasibility study. J Laparoendosc Adv Surg Tech 2000; 10:55–8.

188. Gill IS, Murphy DP, Hsu THS, et al. Laparoscopic repair of renal artery aneurysm. J Urol 2001;166:202–5.

189. Sung TS, Abreu JC, Gill IS, et al. Laparoscopic splenorenal bypass: survival study [abstract]. J Urol 2003;169:500.

190. Ng CS, Abreu SC, Steinberg AP, et al. Laparoscopic management of intra-parenchymal renal artery aneurysm [abstract]. J Urol 2003;169:500.

191. Hoznek A, Gettman M, Antiphon P, et al. Robot assisted kidney transplantation [abstract]. J Urol 2003;169:499.

192. Gluckman GR, Stoller M, Irby P. Laparoscopic pyelocaliceal diverticula ablation. J Endourol 1993;7:315–7.
193. Ruckle HC, Segura JW. Laparoscopic treatment of a stone-filled, caliceal diverticulum: adefinitive, minimally invasive option. J Urol 1994;151:122–4.
194. Miller SD, Ng CS, Streem SB, Gill IS. Laparoscopic management of caliceal diverticular calculi. J Urol 2002;167:1248–52.
195. White R, Rosenberg DJ, Moran ME. Type II pyelocaliceal diverticula: endourologic implications of this rare type of caliceal eventration. J Endourol 2006. [In press]
196. Moss SW. Floting kidneys: a century of nephroptosis and nephropexy. J Urol 1997;158:699–702.
197. Urban DA, Clayman RV, Kerbl K, et al. Laparoscopic nephropexy for symptomatic nephroptosis: initial case report. J Endourol 1993;6:147–50.
198. Elashry OM, Nakada SY, McDougall EM, Clayman RV. Laparoscopic nephropexy: Washington University experience. J Urol 1995;154:1655–9.
199. Plas E, Daja K, Riedl CR, et al. Long-term followup after laparoscopic nephropexy for symptomatic nephroptosis. J Urol 2001;166:449–52.
200. Szekely JG. Letter to the editor. J Urol 1997;157:266.
201. Kaynan AM, Rehman J, Hoenig DM. Laparoscopic ureteral surgery. Sem Laparosc Surg 2000;7:166–75.
202. Nezhat C, Nezhat F, Green B. Laparoscopic treatment of obstructed ureter due to endometriosis by resection and ureteroureterostomy: a case report. J Urol 1992;148:865–8.
203. Wickham JEA. The surgical treatment of renal lithiasis. In: Wickham JEA. Urinary calculous disease. New York: Churchill Livingstone; 1979. p.145–98.
204. Wuernschimmel E, Lipsky H. Laparoscopic treatment of an upper ureteral stone. J Laparoendosc Surg 1993;3:301–7.
205. Baba S, Oya M, Miyahara M, et al. Laparoscopic surgical correction of circumcaval ureter. Urology 1994;44:122–6.
206. Ramalingam M, Selvarajan K. Laparoscopic transperitoneal repair of retrocaval ureter: report of two cases. J Endourol 2003;17:85–7.
207. Kavoussi LR, Clayman RV, Brunt LM, Soper NJ. Laparoscopic ureterolysis. J Urol 1992;147:426–9.
208. Atala A, Goldstein DS, Kavoussi LR, et al. Laparoscopic correction of vesicoureteral reflux. J Urol 1993;149:453A.
209. Puppo P, Carmignani G, Gallucci M, et al. Bilateral laparoscopic ureterolysis. Eur Urol 1994;25:82–4.
210. Nezhat CH, Nezhat F, Seidman D, Nezhat C. Laparoscopic ureteroureterostomy: a prospective follow-up of 9 patients. Prim Care Update Ob Gyns 1998;5:200.
211. Reich H, McGlynn F. Laparoscopic repair of bladder injury. Obstet Gyn 1990;76:909–10.
212. Low RK, Moran ME. Laparoscopic use of the ureteral illuminator. Urology 1993;42:455–7.
213. Parra RO. Laparoscopic repair of intracorporeal bladder perforation. J Urol 1994;151:1003–5.
214. Ehrlich RM, Gershman A, Fuchs G. Laparoscopic vesicoureteroplasty in children: initial case reports. Urology 1994;43:255–61.
215. Ehrlich RM, Gershman A. Laparoscopic seromyotomy (autoaugmentation) for non-neurogenic neurogenic bladder in a child: initial case report. Urology 1993;42:175–8.
216. McDougall EM, Clayman RV, Figenshau RS, Pearle MS. Laparoscopic retropubic auto-augmentation of the bladder. J Urol 1995;153:123–6.
217. Bowyer DW, Moran ME, Szabo Z. Laparoscopic augmentation cystoplasty using two graft materials [abstract 957]. J Urol 1993;149:452A.
218. Jordan GH, Winslow BH. Laparoscopically assisted continent catheterizable cutaneous appendicovesicostomy. J Endourol 1993;7:517–20.
219. Anderson KR, Fadden PT, Kerbl K, et al. Laparoscopic continent urinary diversion in a porcine model [abstract PXXII-11]. J Endourol 1993;7:S197.
220. Nezhat CH, Nezhat FR, Freiha F, Nezhat CR. Laparoscopic vesicopsoas hitch for infiltrative ureteral endometriosis. Fertil Steril 1999;71:376–9.
221. Fugita OD, Dinlenc C, Kavoussi L. The laparoscopic Boari flap. J Urol 2001;166:51–3.
222. Harewood LM. Laparoscopic needle colposuspension for genuine stress incontinence. J Endourol 1993;7:319–22.
223. Vancaillie TG, Schuessler WW. Laparoscopic bladder neck suspension. J Laparoendosc Surg 1991;1:169–173.
224. Harden M, Vancaillie TG. Laparoscopic bladder neck suspension. Infect In Urol 1994;147–50.
225. Burton GA. A randomized comparison of laparoscopic and open colposuspension. Neurourol Urodyn 1994;13:487–98.
226. McDougall EM, Portis A. The laparoscopic bladder neck suspension fails the test of time [abstract]. J Urol 1999;161:105.
227. Seman EI, Cook JR, O'Shea RT. Two-year experience with laparoscopic pelvic floor repair. J Am Assoc Gynecol Laparosc 2003;10:38–45.
228. Deval B, Haab F. What's new in prolapse surgery? Curr Opin Urol 2003;13:315–23.
229. Yano H, Iwazawa T, Monden T. Excision of a urachal sinus with use of a voice-controlled laparoscope. J Laparoendosc Adv Surg Tech A 2003;13:45–9.
230. Khurana S, Borzi PA. Laparoscopic management of complicated urachal disease in children. J Urol 2002;168(4 Pt 1): 1526–8.
231. Cadeddu JA, Boyle KE, Fabrizio MD, et al. Laparoscopic management of urachal cysts in adulthood. J Urol 2000; 164:1526–8.
232. Gerridzen GR, Futter NG. Ten-year review of vesicle diverticula. Urology 1982;20:33–5.
233. Kelalis PP, Mclean P. The treatment of diverticulum of the bladder. J Urol 1967;98:349–52.
234. Kutzmann AA. Diverticulum of the urinary bladder: an analysis of 100 cases. Surg Gynec Obstet 1933;56:898.
235. Peterson LJ, Paulson DF, Glenn JF. The histopathology of vesical diverticula. J Urol 1973;110:62–4.
236. Anderson KR, Clayman RV. Laparoscopic lower urinary tract reconstruction. World J Urol 2000;18:349–54.
237. Kaouk JH, Gill IS, Desai MM, et al. Laparoscopic orthotopic ileal neobladder. J Endourol 2001;15:131–42.
238. Baldwin DD, Herrell SD, Dunbar JA, et al. Simplified laparoscopic radical cystectomy with orthotopic ileal neobladder creation in a porcine model. J Endourol 2003; 17:307–12.
239. Simonato A, Gregori A, Lissiani A, et al. Laparoscopic radical cystoprostatectomy: a technique illustrated step by step. Eur Urol 2003;44:132–8.
240. Abdel-Hakim AM, Bassiouny F, Abdel Azim MS, et al. Laparoscopic radical cystectomy with orthotopic neobladder. J Endourol 2002;16:377–81.
241. Matin SF, Gill IS. Laparoscopic radical cystectomy with urinary diversion: completely intracorporeal technique. J Endourol 2002;16:335–41.
242. Gill IS, Kaouk JH, Meraney AM, et al. Laparoscopic radical cystectomy and continent orthotopic ileal neobladder performed completely intracorporeally: the initital experience. J Urol 2002;168:13–8.
243. Guputa NP, Gill IS, Fergany A, Nabi G. Laparoscopic radical cystectomy with intracorporeal ileal conduit diversion: five cases with a 2-year follow-up. BJU Int 2002;90: 391–6.
244. Turk I, Davis JW, Deger S, Winkelmann B, et al. Laparoscopic radical cystectomy with intracorporeal creation of a continent urinary diversion. Future or present? Urologe A 2002;41:107–12.
245. Bohm B, Milsom JW, Stolfi VM, Kitigo K. Laparoscopic intraperitoneal anastomosis. Surg Endosc 1993;7:194–6.
246. Thorbeck CV, Sanchez de Badajoz S, Toscano R. Laparoscopic ileal conduit. Surg Endosc 1993;2:257A.
247. Brenner M, Johnson DE. Ileal conduit calculi from stapler anastomosis: a long-term complication? Urology 1985; 26:537–40.
248. Ginsberg D, Huffman JL, Lieskowsky G, et al. Urinary tract stones: a complication of the Kock pouch continent urinary diversion. J Urol 1991;145:956–9.
249. Lieskovsky G, Boyd SD, Skinner DG. Cutaneous Kock-pouch urinary diversion. Probl Urol 1991;5:268.
250. Myers RP, Rife CC, Barrett DM. Experience with the bowel stapler for ileal conduit urinary diversion. Br J Urol 1982; 54:491–3.
251. Julian TB, Ravitch MM. Closure of the urinary bladder with stainless steel and absorbable staples. Ann Surg 1986; 204:186–92.
252. Calvano CJ, Moran ME, Parekh AR, et al. Laparoscopic augmentation cystoplasty using novel biomaterial Surgisis: small-intestinal submucosa. J Endourol 2000;14:213–7.
253. Desai MM, Gill IS, Goel M, et al. Ureteral tissue balloon expansion for laparoscopic bladder augmentation: survival study. J Endourol 2003;17:283–93.
254. Lifshitz DA, Beck SDW, Barret E. Laparoscopic transverse hemicystectomy with ileocystoplasty in a porcine model. J Endourol 2001;15:199–203.
255. Siqueria TM Jr, Paterson RF, Kuo RL, et al. Laparoscopic ileocystoplasty and continent ileovesicostomy in a porcine model. J Endourol 2003;17:301–5.
256. Sanchez de Badajoz E, Mate Hurtado A, Jimenez Garrido A, Gutierrez de la Cruz JM. Laparoscopic cystoplasty. Arch Esp Urol 1993;46:615–9.
257. Gill IS, Rackley RR, Meraney AM, et al. Laparoscopic enterocystoplasty. Urology 2000;55:178–81.
258. Elliott SP, Meng MV, Anwar HP, Stoller ML. Complete laparoscopoic ileal cystoplasty. Urology 2002;59:939–43.
259. Portis AJ, Elbahnasy AM, Shalhav AL, et al. Laparoscopic augmentation cystoplasty with different biodegradable grafts in an animal model. J Urol 2000;164:1405–11.
260. Wolf JS Jr, Taheri PA. Laparoscopic urinary undiversion. J Urol 1998;159:198–9.
261. Schuessler WW, Kavoussi LR, Clayman RV, Vancaillie TG. Laparoscopic radical prostatectomy: initial case report [abstract 130]. J Urol 2002;147:246A.
262. Moran ME, Bowyer DW, Szabo Z, Higgins RJ. Laparoscopic microsurgical reconstruction following radical prostatectomy [abstract 791]. J. Urol 1993;149:410A.
263. Price DT, Chari RS, Neighbors JD, et al. Laparoscopic radicalprostatectomy in the canine model [abstract 03-34]. J. Endourol 1994;8:S53.
264. Rassweiler J, Seemann O, Hatzinger M, et al. Technical evolution of laparoscopic radical prostatectomy after 450 cases. J Endourol 2003;17:143–54.
264. Menon M, Tewari A, Peabody J. Vattikuti Institute prostatectomy: technique. J Urol 2003;169:2289–92.
266. Borboroglu PG, Sands JP, Roberts JL, Amling CL. Risk factors for vesicourethral anastomotic stricture after radical prostatectomy. Urology 2000;56:96–100.
267. Kochakarn W, Ratana-Olarn K, Viseshsindh V. Vesicourethral stictures after radical prostatectomy: review of treatment and outcome. J Med Assoc Thai 2002;85:63–6.
268. Bhayani SB, Pavlovich CP, Hsu TS, et al. Prospective comparison of short-term convalescence: laparoscopic radical prostatectomy versus open radical retropubic prostatectomy. Urology 2003;61:612–6.
269. Yamada Y, Honda N, Nakamura K, et al. Vesicourethral anastomotic suture placement during radical prostatectomy using Maniceps. Urol Int 2003;70:181–5.
270. Grummet JP, Costello AJ, Swanson DA, et al. Vesicourethral anastomosis with 2-octyl cyanoacrylate adhesive in an in vivo canine model. Urology 2002;60:935–8.
271. Grummet JP, Costello AJ, Swanson DA, et al. Laser welded vesicourethral anastomosis in an in vivo canine model: a pilot study. J Urol 168:281-284,2002.
272. Partin AW, Adams JB, Moore RG, Kavoussi LR. Complete robot-assisted laparoscopic urologic surgery: a preliminary report. J Am Coll Surg 1995;181:552–7.
273. Rovetta A, Sala R, Wen X, Togno A. Remote control in telerobotic surgery. IEEE Trans Syst Man Cyber 1996;26: 438–44.
274. Lazeroms M, Jongkind W, Honderd G. Telemanipulator design for minimally invasive surgery. Proc Am Control Conf 1997;June:2982–6.
275. Dowler NJ, Holland SRJ. The evolutionary design of an endoscopic telemanipulator. IEEE Robotics Automat 1996;Dec:38–45.
276. Wapler M. Medical manipulators—a realistic concept? Min Invas Ther Allied Tech 1995;4:261–6.
277. Prasad SM, Ducko CT, Stephenson ER, er al. Prospective clinical trial of robotically assisted endoscopic coronary grafting with 1-year follow-up. Ann Surg 2001;233:725–32.
278. Melvin WS, Needleman BJ, Krause KR, et al. Computer-assisted robotic Heller myotomy: initial case report. J Laparoendosc Adv Surg Tech 2001;11:251–3.
279. Chapman WHH 3rd, Young JA, Albrecht RJ, et al. Robotic Nissen fundoplication: alternative surgical technique for treatment of gastroesophageal reflux disease. J Laparoendosc Surg Adv Surg Tech 2001;11:27–30.
280. Marescaux J, Smith MK, Folscher D, et al. Telerobotic laparoscopic cholecystectomy: initial clinical experience with 25 patients. Ann Surg2001;234:1–9.
281. Chapman WHH 3rd, Albrecht RJ, Kim VB, et al. Computer-assisted laparoscopic splenectomy with the da Vinci surgical robot. J Laparoendoscop Adv Surg Tech 2002;12:155–9.
282. Melvin WS, Needleman BJ, Krause KR, Ellison EC. Robotic resection of pancreatic neuroendocrine tumor. J Laparoendosc Adv Surg Tech 2003;13:33–6.
283. Hollands CM, Dixey LN, Torma MJ. Technical assessment of porcine enteroenterostomy performed with ZEUS robotic technology. J Pediatr Surg 2001;36:1231–3.
284. Margossian H, Falcone T. Robotically assisted laparoscopic hysterectomy and adnexal surgery. J Laparoendosc Adv Surg Tech A 2001;11:161–5.
285. Margossian H, Garcia-Ruiz A, Falcone T, et al. Robotically assisted laparoscopic microsurgical uterine horn anastomosis. Fertil Steril 1998;70:530–4.
286. Margossian H, Falcone T. Robotically assisted laparoscopic hysterectomy and adnexal surgery. J Laparoendosc Surg Adv Surg Tech 2001;11:161–5.
287. Krapohl BD, Reichert B, Machens HG, et al. Computer-guided microsurgery: surgical evaluation of a telerobotic arm. Microsurgery 2001;21:22–9.
288. Diaz-Arrastia C, Jurnalov C, Gomez G, Townsend C Jr. Laparoscopic hysterectomy using a computer-enhanced surgical robot. Surg Endosc 2002;16:1271–3.

289. Gutt CN, Markus B, Kim ZG, et al. Early experiences of robotic surgery in children. Surg Endosc 2002;16:1083–6.

290. Kavoussi LR, Moore RG, Partin AW, et al. Telerobotic assisted laparoscopic surgery: initial laboratory and clinical experience. Urology 1994;44:15–9.

291. Bowersox JC, Cornum RL. Remote operative urology using a surgical telemanipulator system. Urology 1998;52:17–22.

292. Kavoussi LR, Moore RG, Adams JB, Partin AW. Comparison of robotic versus human laparoscopic camera control. J Urol 1995;154:2134–6.

293. Sung GT, Gill IS, Hsu TH. Robotic-assisted laparoscopic pyeloplasty: a pilot study. Urology 1999;53:1099–103.

294. Guillonneau B, Cappele O, Martinez JB, et al. Robotically assisted, laparoscopic pelvic lymph node dissection in humans. J Urol 2001;165:1078–81.

295. Abbou CC, Hoznek A, Salomon L, et al. Laparoscopic radical prostatectomy with a remote controlled robot. J Urol 2001;165:1964–6.

296. Guillonneau B, Jayet C, Tewari A, Vallancien G. Robot assisted laparoscopic nephrectomy. J Urol 2001;166:200–1.

297. Pautler SE, McWilliams GW, Harrington FS, Walther MM. An articulating retractor holder to facilitate laparoscopic adrenalectomy and nephrectomy. J Urol 2001;166:198–9.

298. Di Marco DS, Chow GK, Gettman MT, Elliott DS. Robotic sacrocolpopexy [abstract V707]. J Urol 169:183.

299. Yohannes P, Gu Y. Combined robotic-assisted and manual laparoscopic left retroperitoneal lymph node dissection for nonseminomatous testicular cancer [abstract V1873]. J Urol 169:500.

300. Hoznek A, Zaki SK, Samadi DB, et al. Robotic assisted kidney transplantation: an initial experience. J Urol 2002; 167:1604–6.

301. Guillonneau B, Cappele O, Bosco J. Pyeloplastie laparoscopique avec assistance robotisee: premier cas. Prog Urol 2000;10:61A.

302. Gettman MT, Peschel R, Neururer R, Bartsch G. A comparison of laparoscopic pyeloplasty performed with a daVinci robotic system versus standard laparoscopic techniques: initial clinical results. Eur Urol 2002;42:453–8.

303. Gettman MT, Neururer R, Bartsch G, Peschel R. Anderson-Hynes dismembered pyeloplasty performed using daVinci robotic system. Urology 2002;60:509–13.

304. Yohannes P, Burjonrappa SC. Laparoscopic Anderson-Hynes dismembered pyeloplasty using the daVinci robot technical considerations. J Endourol 2003;17:79–83.

305. Antiphon P, Hoznek A, Gettman M, et al. Extraperitoneal laparoscopic robot assisted radical prostatectomy [abstract V965]. J Urol 2003;169:249.

306. Tewari A, Peabody J, Sarle R, et al. Technique of daVinci robot-assisted anatomic radical prostatectomy. Urology 2002;60:569–72.

307. Tewari A, Peabody JO, Fischer M, et al. An operative and anatomic study to help in nerve sparing during laparoscopic and robotic radical prostatectomy. Eur Urol 2003;43:444–54.

308. Van Velthoven RF, Ahlering TE, Peltier A, et al. Technique for laparoscopic running urethrovesical anastomosis: the single knot method. Urology 2003;61:699–702.

309. Ahlering TE, Skarecky DW, Lee D, Clayman RV. Successful transfer of open surgical skills to a laparoscopic environment using a robotic interface: initial experience with laparoscopic radical prostatectomy [abstract]. J Urol 2003;169:441,1649.

310. Shrivastava A, Peabody JO, Menon M. Vattikuti institute prostatectomy: can we predict time taken for performing new procedures? [abstract DP24]. J Urol 2003;169:344–5.

311. Moran ME, Bowyer DW, Szabo Z. Laparoscopic suturing in urology: a model for vesicourethral anastomosis. Min Invas Ther Allied Tech 1993;2:165–70.

312. Healy JC. The global impact of telematics for health-care professionals. Min Invas Ther Allied Tech 1998;7:105–9.

313. Huang HK. Telemedicine and teleradiology technologies and applications. Min Invas Ther Allied Tech 1997;5/6:387–92.

314. Wilson D. Teleradiology at the 121st general hospital in Yongsan, Korea. Min Invas Ther Allied Tech 1997;5/6:404–7.

315. Dayhoff R, Siegel E. Digital imaging among medical facilities. Min Invas Ther Allied Tech 1997;5/6:408–15.

316. Lyche D. Telemedicine: technology versus the business case. Min Invas Ther Allied Tech 1997;5/6:416–20.

317. Ecken BK, Harbick RF, Pease A. Uses and benefits of telemedicine. Min Invas Ther Allied Tech 1997;5/6:444–7.

318. Crowe B. Establishing the costs of telemedicine services. Min Invas Ther Allied Tech 1997;5/6:432–5.

319. Wooton R. Telemedicine: the current state of the art. Min Invas Ther Allied Tech 1997;5/6:393–403.

320. Lemaster H, Meylor J, Meylor F. Internet technologies and requirements for telemedicine. Min Invas Ther Allied Tech 1997;5/6:436–43.

321. Etter M, Feussner H, Siewert JR. Guidelines for teleconsultation in surgery. Surg Endosc 1999;13:1254–5.

322. Lirici MM, Papaspyropoulos V, Angelini L. Telerobotics in medicine and surgery. Min Invas Ther Allied Tech 1997;5/6:364–78.

323. Marescaux J, Mutter D. Inventing the future of surgery. Min Invas Ther Allied Tech 1998;7:69–70.

324. Broderick TJ, Harnett BM, Doam CR, et al. Real-time internet connections: implications for surgical decision making in laparoscopy. Ann Surg 2000;234:165–71.

325. Richards WO, Rattner DW. Endoluminal and transluminal surgery: no longer if, but when. Surg Endosc 2005;19:461–3.

326. Miyake N. 1986. U.S. Patent 4,568,311. "Flexible Wrist Mechanism." Filed 11 January 1983 and issued 4 February 1986.

327. Rosheim ME. Robot evolution. The development of anthrobotics. New York: John Wiley & Sons; 1994.

328. Awan AN, Swain CP. Endoscopic vertical band gastroplasty with an endoscopic sewing machine. Gastrointest Endosc 2002;55:254–6.

329. Kalloo AN, Singh VK, Jagannath SB, et al. Flexible transgastric peritoneoscopy: a novel approach to diagnostic and therapeutic interventions in the peritoneal cavity. Gastrointest Endosc 2004;60:114–7.

330. Antiphon P, Hoznek A, Benyoussef A, et al. Complete solo laparoscopic radical prostatectomy: initial experience. Urology 2003;61:724–9.

331. Dakins GF, Gagner M. Comparison of laparoscopic skills performance between standard instruments and two surgical robotic systems. Surg Endosc 2003;17:574–9.

332. Kaouk JH, Desai MM, Abreu SC, et al. Robotic assisted laparoscopic sural nerve grafting during radical prostatectomy: initial experience. J Urol 2003;170:909–12.

333. McKenzie AR. An experimental multiple barbed suture for long flexor tendons of the palm and fingers. Preliminary report. J Bone Joint Surg Br 1967;49:440–7.

334. US patents 5,342,376 and 6,241,747 B1.

335. Dattilo PP Jr, King MW, Cassill NL, Leung JC. Medical textiles: application of an absorbable barbed bi-directional surgical suture. J Text Appar Tech Manag 2002;2:1–5.

336. Moran M. The law of accelerating returns. J Endourol 2006. [In press]

337. Katz R, Nadu A, Olsson LE, et al. A simplified 5-step model for training laparoscopic urethrovesical anastomosis. J Urol 2003;169:2041–4.

338. Firoozi F, Moran ME, Kolios E, et al. Modeled system for evaluating robotic running vesicourethral anastomosis. 23rd World Congress on Endourology. J Endourol 2005;19:A132.

51

Exiting the Abdomen: The Importance of a Methodical and Meticulous Approach

Sejal S. Quayle, MD

Jaime Landman, MD

A systematic approach to exiting the abdomen is an essential component of all laparoscopic procedures, which helps to minimize postoperative complications. Careful inspection of the operative field for adequate hemostasis and appropriate closure of abdominal wall defects are critical. Trocar and hand-assist device defects continue to be a major source of postoperative morbidity following laparoscopic surgery. In contrast to open surgery, laparoscopy offers a distinct advantage in closure of abdominal wall defects, as direct endoscopic viewing of the peritoneal surface of the abdominal wall affords the surgeon the opportunity to evaluate from the "inside out" deficiencies in the closure and closure-related complications, such as incorporation of visceral structures.

A systematic and methodical approach to minimizing bleeding and closure-related abdominal wall complications is provided in this chapter. Devices designed to facilitate trocar-site closure have been developed and will also be reviewed.

SYSTEMATIC EXIT OF THE ABDOMEN AFTER LAPAROSCOPIC PROCEDURES

STEP 1: INSPECTION After completion of the surgical objectives, inspection of the entire surgical field is performed. The goals of inspection include identification of hemostasis and unrecognized damage to visceral structures.

The reduced haptic feedback associated with current conventional laparoscopic technology makes it critical to check for unsuspected visceral injury. The entire surgical field should be meticulously inspected. Unsuspected injuries are frequently located just outside the working operative field where retractors have been positioned during the procedure. In the course of renal laparoscopic procedures, the liver and spleen commonly require prolonged cephalad retraction for exposure. During retraction, the liver or spleen may be inadvertently lacerated or otherwise traumatized. Similarly, during laparoscopic pelvic procedures, it is common for a retractor to be applied to the sigmoid colon and small bowel to achieve adequate surgical exposure. These structures are usually outside the active visual operative field for prolonged periods of time and can be lacerated or rendered ischemic as a result of zealous retraction. Careful inspection of the surgical field and all areas of retraction outside

the immediate surgical field allow for early recognition and management of injuries.

After inspection for organ injury, inspection for adequate hemostasis should be systematically performed throughout the entire operative field. Although arterial bleeding is usually readily apparent during all stages of laparoscopy, the typical pneumoperitoneum of 12 to 15 mm Hg applied to insufflate body cavities and develop a surgical working space provides a very effective form of venous tamponade. Indeed, transient elevations in pneumoperitoneum are frequently purposely applied for temporary control of venous bleeding during laparoscopic surgery. As venous bleeding can be obscured by the standard pressures of the pneumoperitoneum, inspection for hemostasis must be performed under conditions of low insufflation pressure. The insufflation pressure should be reduced to ≤ 5 mm Hg pressure prior to inspection. The entire operative field—including retraction sites—should be carefully examined under these conditions.

Occasionally, due to the limitations of currently available aspiration devices, it can be difficult to completely aspirate all fluids from the operative field to discern if there is active venous bleeding. Under these conditions, the surgical field can be filled with saline and reinspected. Active arterial or venous bleeds appear as small rivulets of swirling blood in the pool of irrigant. Identification of these rivulets should prompt an aggressive search for the source of bleeding.

After inspection of the active operative field and retraction sites, body wall access sites should similarly be inspected for hemostasis. Trocar sites should be inspected by removing the trocar and inspecting the abdominal wall site for bleeding under low insufflation pressure. Particular care should be taken during inspection of the primary access site, as this is the only trocar that is not placed under direct vision. Trocar site bleeding can usually be easily controlled without conversion to an open procedure. Placement of full-thickness, hemostatic sutures under endoscopic control is usually adequate for abdominal wall hemostasis. Application of a Carter-Thomason device (Inlet Medical, Inc., Eden Prarie, MN) is very useful in this regard. The technique for suture passage is described later in this chapter and is the same as the technique for fascial closure. Occasionally, a figure-of-eight suture is

required to stop abdominal wall bleeding. On rare occasions, if the bleeding cannot be adequately controlled by endoscopic techniques, trocar sites should be extended to allow for direct, visual hemostatic control.

STEP 2: TROCAR EXTRACTION In the adult, trocar site closure is dependent on the size of the fascial defect created by the trocar. Traditional "cutting" trocars use a sharp blade to penetrate the body wall. These trocars create a defect in the fascia equal to the diameter of the trocar. More recently, trocars that use a blunt surface to spread body wall tissues radially or axially ("dilating trocars") have been introduced. These trocars create a fascial defect half the size of the diameter of the trocar.

To prevent incisional hernia formation, all trocar sites with fascial defects > 6 mm are closed. Trocar sites with fascial defects ≤ 6 mm do not require fascial closure in the adult with normal tissues. In pediatric cases, and in patients with poor quality fascia (eg, history of abdominal wall herniation, poor nutritional status, history of exogenous steroid usage), all trocar sites should be closed. Thus, in the majority of patients, application of dilating trocars obviates the need for fascial closure, even when 12-mm trocars are applied; only skin closure is required.

Several clinical studies have demonstrated that it is safe and effective to simply remove dilating trocars without closing the fascia. Shalhav and colleagues compared fascial non-closure after the use of dilating trocars to fascial closure after the use of traditional cutting trocars in one study and demonstrated no evidence of hernia formation in either group with a mean follow-up of 4.8 months.[1] In another study, Liu and McFadden reported results of 180 non-midline laparoscopic trocar sites created by dilating trocars that were not closed. With a median follow-up of 11 months, no hernias were identified.[2] Recently, Venkatesh and colleagues prospectively compared dilating trocars to cutting trocars among 56 patients and demonstrated both significantly faster abdominal closure times for dilating trocars and no evidence of hernia formation in any trocar sites at a mean follow-up of 5 months.[3]

A number of techniques are currently available for closure of fascial defects > 6 mm in diameter. Elashry and colleagues performed a prospective, randomized study in which they evaluated laparoscopic trocar closure techniques. The Carter-Thomason device was found to be the fastest and the least commonly associated with trocar closure related complications.[4] In this study, 95 trocars were randomized to one of eight trocar-site closure techniques, and the Carter-Thomason device described below was significantly faster (mean closure time of 2.5 minutes) than closure with any other device with the exception of the standard hand closure, which took an average of 1.9 minutes. This device also had no associated complications, and this made it more effective than any of the other devices with the exception of the angiocatheter technique described below.

Standard Technique of Hand-Sutured Closure This closure involves first the removal of the trocar followed by the use of a Sinn or other small retractor for visualization of the fascial edges. Kocher clamps are then placed on the fascial edges, and a figure-of-eight stitch is placed using 0-absorbable suture on a CT-1 needle with tooth forceps. As trocar sites are small, this technique can be quite challenging, and frequently, incorporation of the fascia in the closure is not accomplished. For very thin patients, this technique is expeditious and useful, but for patients with significant abdominal girth, alternative closure techniques should be employed.

Carter-Thomason Needle-Point Suture Passer (CTNSP) The Carter-Thomason device consists of a cone shaped metal guide and a small needle grasper that is used to pass the suture (Figure 51-1). Insertion of the cone-shaped metal guide tube follows removal of the trocar. This cone shape of the device has a tamponade effect on the abdominal wall defect and thus prevents loss of the pneumoperitoneum. The CTNSP, carrying 24 inch, 0-absorbable suture, is then passed through a predrilled hole in the cone-shaped guide, and thus, the suture traverses the muscle, fascia, and peritoneum. The CTNSP is observed entering the abdominal cavity under endoscopic vision to minimize the chances of visceral injury. The suture is then released, and the CTNSP is moved to the other hole in the guide. The suture is re-grasped and brought out 180° away from the other end. After the guide is removed, the suture can be tied. Needle passage and grasping must be performed under direct endoscopic vision to prevent visceral injury. (Figure 51-2A to Figure 51-2D)

Maciol Suture Needle Set The trocar is kept in place during the use of this non-disposable device (ConMed, Utica, NY), which includes three needlepoint suture carriers: one curved suture introducer, one straight-tip suture introducer, and one open-grooved suture retriever (Figure 51-3A to Figure 51-3C). A 24-inch, 0-absorbable suture is passed through the hole in the introducer, and the introducer is then passed into the peritoneal cavity between the trocar and the skin incision. Again, entrance into the abdominal cavity is performed under direct endoscopic vision to minimize the chances of visceral injury. The retrieval needle, placed into the peritoneal cavity 180° from the initial suture passage, grasps the suture and removes one end from the peritoneal cavity. All instruments, including the trocars, are then removed from the site, and the suture can be secured. (Figure 51-4)

Puncture Closure Device The disposable PCD (ConMed, Utica, NY) inserts through a 10-mm trocar (Figure 51-5). Turning the knob leads to exposure of a J-shaped needle; the configuration of this needle precludes damage to internal organs. The J-shaped needle is then brought through one fascial edge, and a suture is loaded onto the needle. The device is then advanced, and the needle is rotated such that it can penetrate the opposite fascial edge. The device is then withdrawn, and the suture is left in place. This suture can then be tied. (Figures 51-6A and 51-6B).

Tahoe Surgical Instruments Ligature Device The TSIL (Tahoe Surgical Instruments, San Juan, PR) is a disposable device constituted by a handle with a locking button and two sharp hollow metal needles 2 cm apart (Figure 51-7). The trocar is removed, and a 24-inch, 0-absorbable suture is placed into the TSIL's delivery needle.

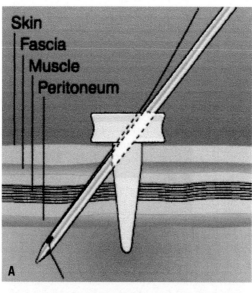

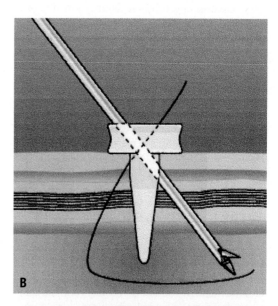

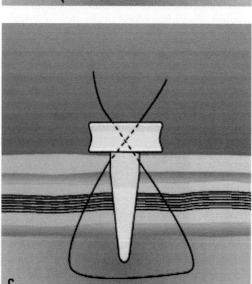

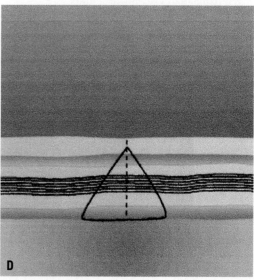

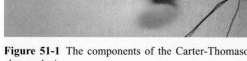

Figure 51-1 The components of the Carter-Thomason closure device.

Figure 51-2 The grasper and suture are passed through one side of the cone-shaped device (A). The suture is released, the grasper is inserted on the opposite side. The grasper is used to hold the suture (B). The suture is pulled through the fascia (C). The suture is tied (D).

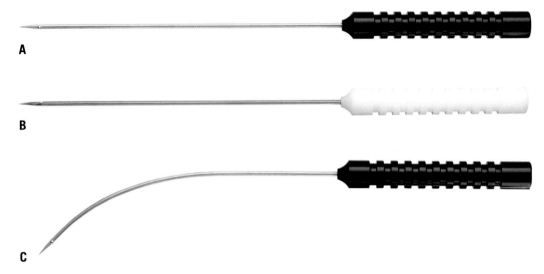

Figures 51-3 The curved suture introducer (A), the straight-tip suture introducer (B) and the open-grooved suture retriever (C) of the Maciol Suture Needle Set.

Both needles then pierce the fascia on either side of the port site. Depression of the handle causes a metal retrieval loop to be extended from the other hollow needle, and this encompasses the tip of the delivery needle. The suture is extended and is thus fed through the metal loop. The retrieval loop is then closed, and the entire device is removed. In this way, the suture is brought through the abdominal wall and can be tied. (Figure 51-8)

Angiocatheter Closure Device   Use of an angiocatheter can facilitate trocar site closure. A 5-inch, 14-gauge intravenous catheter and needle are introduced into the abdomen on one side of the 10 mm port. Once the catheter is visualized, the needle obturator is removed and a 24-inch 0-absorbable suture is passed into the abdomen. The angiocatheter is then removed and reinserted through the other fascial edge. After the catheter is visualized, the obturator is removed, and a 36-inch, 0-polyprolene suture is looped in half and inserted into the catheter. The 24-inch suture is passed through the loop, and the angiocatheter is removed. The suture can then be tied to itself.

Trocars that create fascial defects ≤ 6 mm do not typically require fascial closure, as described above, but endoscopic inspection for hemostasis of each trocar site should still be performed. For the final trocar that is removed, the endoscope and sheath are removed as one unit, with the endoscope protruding just beyond the trocar. In this way, the surgeon can inspect the fasciotomy and subcutaneous tissues for bleeding. If bleeding is noted, trocars can be replaced through the prior trocar sites and hemostasis can be obtained as described previously. Prior to complete closure of all trocar sites, efforts should be made to extract as much of the carbon dioxide insufflant as possible because the gas can result in irritation of the peritoneum or diaphragm and may increase postoperative pain.

STEP 3: CLOSURE OF HAND-ASSIST DEVICE OR ORGAN EXTRACTION SITES   A hand-assist device incision or an incision made for intact organ extraction after a laparoscopic procedure is typically closed prior to trocar removal. These larger incisions are treated like any standard surgical incision and should be closed in a standard meticulous fashion. After closure of the larger incision, the body cavity can be re-insufflated and again inspected for hemostasis. Each trocar site can then be closed as previously described.

STEP 4: SKIN CLOSURE   Subcuticular 4-0 absorbable sutures can be used to approximate the skin edges of 12 mm trocar sites. Five millimeter trocar sites may be approximated by an adhesive strip without a subcuticular closure. Tissue adhesives may also be employed for rapid skin closure. The tissue adhesive 2-octylcyanoacrylate (Dermabond, Ethicon Inc., Somerville, NJ) has been compared to standard subcuticular closure with a running 4-0 poliglecaprone 25 (Monocryl, Ethicon Inc., Somerville, NJ) in a prospective randomized trial.[5] Although closure with Dermabond (Ethicon, Inc.) was significantly faster than standard closure, 155 seconds versus 286 seconds, respectively, several wound separations were noted in the Dermabond group and no wound complications were noted in the standard closure group. Bernard and colleagues noted no difference in wound complication rate in another prospective randomized study comparing Dermabond to conventional sutures for excisional wound closure. However, the suture group did score significantly higher on the visual analog scale than the Dermabond group.[6] Tissue adhesives are available, but further studies comparing these adhesives to standard closure in a surgical setting are still needed.

If Dermabond trocar site closure is elected, use of several techniques can help facilitate the closure. Trocar sites should be irrigated with sterile saline and excellent hemostasis should be ensured, for even a small amount of blood intermingled with the Dermabond "glue" may result in a cosmetically unappealing closure. The patient should be repositioned so skin edges can be

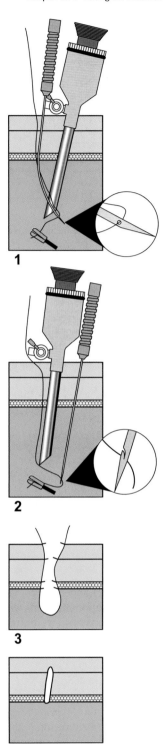

Figure 51-4 Use of the Maciol Suture Needle Set for trocar site closure.

brought together in a tension free manner. Although digital approximation of the skin edges usually allows for good skin edge approximation and closure, occasionally forceps are required to evert the skin edges. The authors have incorporated Dermabond glue skin closure into their technique because it allows for an expeditious skin closure that is watertight. This allows patients to bathe on the first postoperative day if desired.

While Dermabond glue closure has been very effective for the majority of trocar sites that run

Figure 51-5 The Puncture Closure Device.

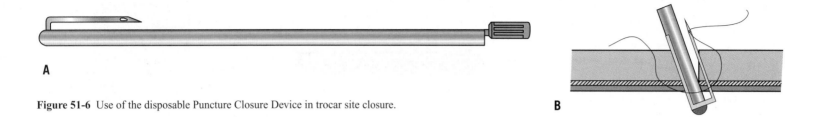

Figure 51-6 Use of the disposable Puncture Closure Device in trocar site closure.

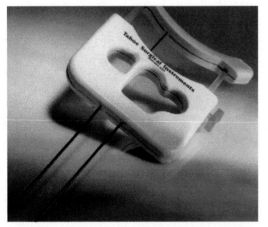

Figure 51-7 Tahoe Surgical Instruments Ligature device.

transverse along Langer's lines, we have experienced skin separation problems with cephalocaudal midline incisions (ie, extraction site for laparoscopic radical prostatectomy). We thus close these incisions with subcuticular sutures.

CONCLUSIONS

A systematic and thorough approach to exiting the abdomen constitutes an integral component of successful laparoscopy and is critical in order to avoid a number of complications. Thorough inspection of the operative field and recognition of any intraoperative organ injury, as well as identification of bleeding, will help prevent immediate postoperative morbidity. Appropriate closure of all trocar sites and hand-assist device sites, with or without the use of port-site closure devices, will prevent complications such as wound dehiscence and evisceration in the short-term, and hernia formation in the long-term.

REFERENCES

1. Shalhav AL, Barret E, Lifshitz DA, Lingeman JE, et al. Transperitoneal laparoscopic renal surgery using blunt 12 mm trocar without fascial closure. J Endourol 2002;16:43.

2. Liu CD, McFadden DW. Laparoscopic port sites do not require closure when non-bladed trocars are used. Am Surg 2000;66:853–4.

3. Venkatesh R, Landman J, Rehman J, et al. Prospective randomized comparison of traditional cutting and dilating disposable trocars for laparoscopic access. J Urol 2003. [Submitted]

4. Elashry OE, Nakada SY, Wolf JS, et al. Comparative clinical study of port-closure techniques following laparoscopic surgery. J Am Coll Surg 1996;183:335–44.

5. Switzer EF, Dinsmore RC, North JH. Subcuticular closure versus Dermabond: a prospective randomized trial. Am Surg 2003;69:434–6.

6. Bernard L, Doyle J, Friedlander SF, et al. A prospective comparison of octyl cyanoacrylate tissue adhesive (Dermabond) and suture for the closure of excisional wounds in children and adolescents. Arch Dermatol 2001;137:1177–80.

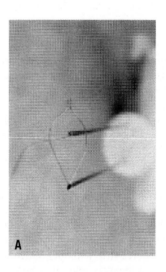
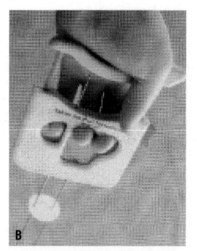
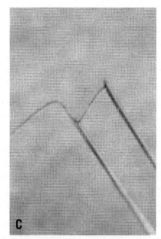
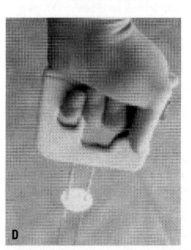

Figure 51-8 Use of the Tahoe Surgical Instruments Ligature Device in trocar site closure.

52

Postoperative Care

Marlene Corujo, MD
Kevin R. Anderson, MD

The goal of laparoscopic surgery is to decrease the morbidity and recuperative time associated with the equivalent open procedure. Thus, patients who have undergone laparoscopic surgery should be released from the hospital sooner and resume regular activity without the prolonged postoperative pain that is often associated with a large incision. To take full advantage of this new technology, postoperative management must also be modified to achieve two important goals: (1) to ensure that no complications related to laparoscopy have occurred in the perioperative and postoperative periods and (2) to discharge the patient home as soon as is medically indicated. This chapter will briefly list specific complications that can occur during laparoscopic surgery as they relate to the postoperative recognition, management, and prevention of these complications.

Laparoscopy can be divided into four phases: placement of the Veress needle and trocars, insufflation of the peritoneum with carbon dioxide (CO_2), dissection, and closure of the trocar sites. Complications may occur intraoperatively or postoperatively relative to any of these four phases. Careful perioperative and postoperative management is necessary not only to prevent complications from occurring, but also to recognize early signs and symptoms of complications that might have resulted at any stage of laparoscopic surgery.[1]

Incorrect placement of the Veress needle or trocar could cause injury to bowel, bladder, or vessels. When persistent abdominal pain, fever, or peritoneal signs occur postoperatively, consider perforation of a viscus. If the bowel injury is small and recognized immediately, and the bowel was prepared preoperatively, intracorporeal techniques can be used to repair the injury laparoscopically. Otherwise, conversion to an open procedure is necessary. The occurrence of intraoperative or postoperative hematuria and/or pneumoturia (gas expansion of the urinary drainage bag) indicates a possible bladder injury. Again, this can sometimes be repaired laparoscopically before converting to an open procedure.

Puncture of the aorta and inferior vena cava, although rare, is life threatening and requires immediate laparotomy and repair. Injury to an abdominal wall vessel (ie, inferior epigastric artery or vein) may not be apparent during the laparoscopic procedure because of the tamponade effect of the port. Once the port is removed, delayed bleeding may become clinically detectable based on the finding of abdominal distention and/or a decrease in the postoperative hematocrit. Anterior abdominal wall hematoma and ecchymosis can also form subsequent to disruption of anterior abdominal wall vessels and should be suspected if there is continued abdominal pain with swelling around the trocar sites. Injury to abdominal wall vessels, when diagnosed intraoperatively, can be repaired directly under laparoscopy using intracorporeal suturing techniques or by transabdominal wall passage of a needle that carries a ligature to occlude the bleeding vessel. This can be done percutaneously with a nonabsorbable suture passed via Stamey needle and tied over a dental roll bolster. Alternatively, an Endo Close device (United States Surgical, Norwalk, CT) can be used to pass and retrieve an absorbable suture around the injured vessel through the port site incision so that the knot remains in the subcutaneous tissue layers. If a nonabsorbable suture is used over a bolster, the suture is removed on postoperative day 10 to prevent a foreign body reaction.[2]

Insufflation of the peritoneum with CO_2 can lead to acute pneumothorax or pneumomediastinum, and in the postoperative period, can dissect along the subcutaneous tissue planes and result in ecchymosis and pain. At the end of the operation, all CO_2 is allowed to escape from the abdomen to prevent irritation of the peritoneum and diaphragm, which can lead to abdominal and referred shoulder pain.

Postoperative complications that relate to dissection misadventures vary depending on the laparoscopic surgery performed. The unique management strategies relative to the type of procedure will be discussed below.

Adequate closure of the fascial defects of the trocar sites ≥ 10 mm (≥ 5 mm in children) will prevent incisional hernias. But if the patient is unable to tolerate oral intake and develops nausea and vomiting, a small bowel obstruction through one of the trocar sites may have occurred. Such a bowel obstruction can be corrected by either open surgery or laparoscopic technique. Newer trocars avoid blind cutting altogether and use radial dilation instead. The advantage is that the resulting port site does not require fascial closure.

UPPER URINARY TRACT SURGERY

NEPHRECTOMY FOR BENIGN AND MALIGNANT DISEASE   In the immediate postoperative period, the nasogastric tube is removed in the operating room. The Foley catheter may be left in place overnight since post-laparoscopy diuresis often occurs after a prolonged pneumoperitoneum. Patients may begin oral intake (starting with clear liquids) within 24 to 48 hours (Table 52-1). Pneumatic compression stockings are used intraoperatively, and patients should begin ambulation the day after surgery to prevent thromboembolic com-

Table 52-1 Postoperative Management after Major Laparoscopic Procedures			
	Day 0	Day 1	Day 2
Patient Care			
Foley catheter	Remove in OR or in evening*	Remove in AM after diuresis†	
Nasogastric tube	Remove in OR		
Antibiotics	One dose before OR	Continue for 24 hours	
Parenteral narcotics	Morphine	Change to oral pain medication	Minimal oral pain medication needed
Diet	Clear liquids	Advance to regular	Regular diet
Ambulation	Remove pneumatic stockings	Increase ambulation	Ready for discharge
Physical examination			
Abdominal distention	None	Slightly increased	Resolved
Abdominal pain	Present	Minimal	Minimal
Ecchymosis	Present	Slightly increased	No change
Crepitus	Present	Non	Non
Laboratory findings			
Hematocrit	No change in the evening	No change	None needed

*Pneumoperitoneum ≤ 2 hr.
†Pneumoperitoneum ≥ 2 hr.

plications. Clayman and colleagues[3] and Winfield and Schuessler[4] reviewed their initial 10 cases and reported one case of pulmonary embolus. Intravenous antibiotics are given as a prophylactic dose preoperatively and then continued for 24 hours. Parenteral narcotic requirements may be diminished if the trocar sites are infiltrated with 0.5% bupivacaine. By the second postoperative day, many patients require only oral pain medications, and others need no further pain management.

The patient is placed in the modified flank position for a prolonged period of time (3 to 5 hours) and injuries relating to patient positioning may become apparent postoperatively. These can include brachial plexus injury, vastus lateralis compartment syndrome, atelectasis, hip pain, and asymmetric facial and periorbital edema. Many of these conditions require only supportive and pain management, but incentive spirometry and prompt mobilization should be encouraged to resolve the atelectasis.

The dissection required to perform a laparoscopic nephrectomy can potentially injure vessels such as the adrenal artery and vein, renal artery and vein, gonadal vessels, and venae cavae. Small and large bowel injury may occur as a result of puncture injury caused by dissecting instruments or from diathermy burns caused by direct contact with an instrument conducting electrocautery current or by capacitive coupling. Recent advances in instrumentation avoid monopolar electrocautery. These include bipolar dissection and vibrational energy (harmonic scalpel).

In the Clayman and colleagues series, the average blood loss was 250 mL. A decrease in hematocrit postoperatively is a sign of an intraoperative vascular injury. Postoperative hematocrit levels should be monitored for the first 24 hours. Careful abdominal examinations should include assessment for rebound or other peritoneal signs that might indicate a viscous injury. The average length of hospital stay varies from 2 to 5 days with a convalescence period of 1 to 3 weeks.[3]

Ureterectomy In most cases, ureterectomy is performed in combination with a nephrectomy for both benign and malignant disease. The nasogastric tube is removed immediately after the operation. Oral intake begins 1 to 3 days after the operation on average. In the case of nephroureterectomy for malignant disease, a cuff of bladder is taken with the ureter. The Foley catheter remains in place until cystography is performed (prior to the patient's discharge from the hospital). On postoperative day 1, the pneumatic compression stockings are removed and the patient is encouraged to ambulate. Intravenous antibiotics are continued for 24 hours after the operation. Parenteral narcotics may be necessary during the first 24-hour period, but only oral pain medication was necessary for many patients after the first day.[4]

In an initial report by Chandhoke and colleagues in three patients who underwent complete nephroureterectomy for malignant disease, the average operative time was 8 hours.[6] Patients are placed in the Trendelenburg position and rotated so the contralateral side is down and cushioned on a beanbag. Given the length of the procedure, however, care must be taken to avoid brachial plexus neuropathy. The average blood loss was reported to be 200 mL. Again, should the hematocrit decrease postoperatively, the possibility of a vascular injury should be considered. The mean hospital stay was 6 days. A cystogram was performed on postoperative day 2 or 3. If extravasation did not occur, the Foley catheter was removed. However, if extravasation did occur, the Foley catheter remained in place for 1 week.

Adrenalectomy The incidence of laparoscopic adrenalectomy has rapidly increased and is now being performed by both urologists and general surgeons. Both the retroperitoneal and transperitoneal approaches have been used. The technique for insufflation and patient positioning is similar to that for laparoscopic nephrectomy; however, there is marked variation in port placement reported in the literature. Suzuki and colleagues described the cases of 12 patients undergoing laparoscopic adrenalectomy.[7] The operative time was similar to that for laparoscopic nephrectomy (average of 278 minutes [range 182 to 470 minutes]) and the average blood loss was higher (370 ml); therefore the same considerations regarding positioning and potential hemorrhage should be observed. Hematocrit levels should be monitored for the first 24 hours. A complete abdominal as well as neurologic examination is essential in these patients. During laparoscopic dissection for adrenalectomy potential areas of injury are the renal capsule vessels and adrenal vessels. Serum amylase is included in the laboratory evaluations considering the proximity of the adrenal glands to the tail of the pancreas on the left and the head of the pancreas on the right. The nasogastric tube can be removed postoperatively by the anesthesiologist prior to transfer to the recovery room and the Foley catheter can be removed that evening or the following morning. Most patients can ambulate the following morning and often are discharged on postoperative day 2. Specific considerations are the same as for open adrenal surgery; in patients in whom pheochromocytomas are removed blood pressure should be monitored closely postoperatively.

Laparoscopic Pyeloplasty Laparoscopic pyeloplasty has been done since 1993 with results that are equal to that of the "gold standard", open pyeloplasty. The reported success rate is 94 to 96% with a two year follow-up. Techniques used include the Anderson-Hynes dismembered pyeloplasty, Y-V plasty, Heineke-Mirhulicz and Davis intubated ureterotomy, with the former being the most common approach. Concominant pyelolithotomy can also be performed. The closure is done over a double pigtail catheter. A drain (Jackson Pratt or Penrose) is placed through a lateral port site and left near the repair.[8,9]

Postoperatively, diet is usually resumed within the first 24 hours. The drain is removed on the second day, and most patients are discharged by the third day. Bleeding, requiring transfusion, is rare, as are urine leaks. The stent is removed at 4 weeks and should be followed by a functional study (intravenous urogram vs renal scan) to evaluate drainage.

LOWER URINARY TRACT SURGERY

Pelvic Lymph Node Dissection Laparoscopic pelvic lymph node dissection is often performed to stage adenocarcinoma of the prostate. In the immediate postoperative period, the nasogastric tube can be removed in the operating room. Oral intake begins on the day of surgery. The Foley catheter is removed on the first postoperative day. Pneumatic compression stockings are also removed about 4 to 6 hours after the operation, at which time the patient is encouraged to ambulate. Patients are given an intravenous dose of antibiotics just before surgery and continue on oral antibiotics for 5 days after the operation. The use of scrotal supports and ice packs postoperatively may prevent hydrocele formation.[10] Pain is usually controlled well with oral analgesics, although in one study, patients required an average of 1.5 mg of intravenous morphine in the postoperative period.[11] The majority of patients did not need analgesics after discharge.

The exposure for a pelvic lymph node dissection can potentially injure the bladder, ureter, external iliac artery or vein, obturator nerve, large and small bowel, and a variety of smaller vessels such as the circumflex vein or an accessory obturator vein. Small vessel injuries are repaired immediately with occlusive clips; a large vascular injury, however, requires open exploration and repair. The average operative time was 150 minutes.[12] Prior to removal of the laparoscope, the urine in the urinary drainage bag tubing should be visually inspected for hematuria. If present, the diagnosis of a bladder injury can be confirmed by filling the bladder with a saline/indigo carmine solution. Iatrogenic bladder injuries can be repaired laparoscopically. If hematuria is observed postoperatively, an intravenous pyelogram and cystogram are necessary to rule out a bladder or ureteral injury. A small bladder injury may be managed with prolonged urethral catheter drainage. The best way to avoid bladder injury is to keep the dissection medial to the obliterated median umbilical ligament. Obturator nerve palsy can result from sharp dissection, electrocautery, or stretch injury damage to the obturator nerve that lies inferior to the nodal tissue during dissection.

Persistent postoperative fever, abdominal pain, or prolonged ileus may signal an unrecognized viscous injury that may have occurred during trocar placement or tissue dissection either from mechanical injury (blunt retraction or sharp dissection) or electrothermal injury with delayed necrosis of the bowel wall. Ileus may also be caused by herniation of the bowel through one of the port sites, resulting in obstruction. Fever may indicate a pelvic abscess. A complete radiologic evaluation should be done. Abdominal radiography (flat plate, upright, and decubitus films) is necessary to assess for obstruction or free air. An abdominal and pelvic computed tomography scan may show a pelvic abscess or abdominal wall hernia. A complete blood count is done; a decrease in hematocrit indicates ongoing hemorrhage, whereas an elevated white blood cell count can be associated with abscess formation or ischemic bowel injury.

The average hospital stay after a laparoscopic node dissection is 2 days. Patients generally resume their normal activities between 5 and 7 days and are fully recovered in about 11 days.[12]

VARICOCELE LIGATION Laparoscopic ligation is indicated for varicoceles (unilateral or bilateral) in patients with subfertility problems, pain, or adolescent testicular growth retardation. This operation is generally performed in the ambulatory center, and patients are discharged on the same day. Both the nasogastric tube and the Foley catheter are removed either in the operating room or in the recovery room. Clear liquids are given to the patient as soon as he is awake. Patients are encouraged to ambulate within 4 to 6 hours after the operation. An average of 8 or 9 Tylenol tablets with codeine are used within the first postoperative week. One group showed that 5 of 14 patients did not require any analgesics after the third postoperative day.[13]

The average length of the operation was 101 to 105 minutes for a unilateral varix and 153 to 167 minutes for bilateral varices.[13–16] The increased time was attributed to the identification and preservation of the testicular artery. If scrotal swelling persists in the postoperative period, a hydrocele or a recurrent varix should be suspected.

LAPAROSCOPIC RADICAL PROSTATECTOMY Recent experience has seen the rapid increase in the use of laparoscopic techniques for the treatment of prostate cancer. This approach, in the hands of a skilled laparoscopist, can provide improved visualization and decreased intraoperative blood loss. The urethrovesical anastomosis can be done with either an interrupted or running suture technique. Purportedly, the urethral catheter can be removed within the first week after surgery.[17–18]

Patients usually resume a full diet within 2 to 3 days of surgery. Pain control is facilitated by patient-controlled analgesia devices for narcotics but generally is rapidly converted to oral pain medication within the first 24 hours. A single Jackson-Pratt drain is left postoperatively and removed when the output becomes minimal (generally less than 30 cc in an 8-hour period).

Long term results assessing continence and potency, as yet appear to be equivalent to the open approach for radical prostatectomy.

PEDIATRIC PROCEDURES

NEPHRECTOMY AND NEPHROURETERECTOMY FOR BENIGN DISEASE Performing a nephrectomy or nephroureterectomy for benign disease in the pediatric population has the distinct advantage of improved access to the kidney because there is less perirenal fat. Many nonfunctional kidneys in children are associated with both a small renal artery and a small renal vein. These dysgenic kidneys may also have an abnormal number and location of renal vessels. If a nephroureterectomy is being performed for reflux nephropathy, the ureter is dissected down to the level of the bladder, at which point it can be occluded with a vascular clip. Removal of a bladder cuff is unnecessary. If a nephroureterectomy is being performed for obstruction at the ureterovesical junction in a single system, the transected end of the ureter near the bladder is left open. In neither case is a postoperative cystogram necessary prior to removal of the Foley catheter. In the immediate postoperative period the oral gastric or nasogastric tube is removed immediately. The Foley catheter is removed on the first postoperative morning. The patient may have a limited amount of clear liquids on the night of surgery; most children, however, will experience some abdominal distention on the first postoperative day. In most cases, this distention resolves by the second postoperative day (if the child is encouraged to ambulate), and a regular diet is begun, after which the child can be discharged. Parenteral narcotics are generally not necessary after the first 24 hours and may be unnecessary if the trocar sites are infiltrated with 0.5% bupivacaine. Pneumatic compression stockings are not necessary in the pediatric population.

DIAGNOSIS OF CRYPTORCHIDISM OR INTERSEX STATES The earliest use of laparoscopy in urology was for the diagnosis of cryptorchidism.[19] The laparoscope allows the surgeon to verify the presence or absence of a testicle through a 2 mm port at the umbilicus. The procedure takes approximately 15 minutes and has very few reported complications. In young boys (less than 2 years of age) a Foley catheter is not necessary. The bladder can be emptied completely using Crede's method. An oral gastric tube is placed by the anesthesiologist preoperatively and removed at the end of the procedure. The 2 mm fascial defect at the umbilicus does not require fascial closure. The majority of these patients can be discharged on the same day of the procedure. Complete evacuation of any remaining CO_2 will prevent postoperative peritoneal irritation.

A similar technique is used for the diagnosis of intersex conditions with careful evaluation of any rudimentary müllerian duct structures such as the vagina, cervix, uterus, and/or fallopian tube. The postoperative management for diagnostic laparoscopy of intersex states is the same as that for cryptorchidism.

LAPAROSCOPIC ORCHIDOPEXY After laparoscopic diagnosis of an intra-abdominal testis, the gonad is then brought into the scrotum using laparoscopic techniques. The testis is completely dissected such that it is attached only to the testicular vessels and vas deferens. A Dartos pouch in the scrotum is developed and a long Jakes clamp is passed through this incision, over the ipsilateral pubic ramus and into the peritoneal cavity lateral to the medial umbilical ligament and medial to the inferior epigastric vessels. The testis is then grasped and brought into the dartos pouch. Optionally, the testis may be secured in place with a 3-0 silk tie brought through the inferior scrotum and affixed over a bolster. The patient is discharged home from the recovery room and may resume a regular diet immediately. The bolster is removed in 10 to 14 days. Oral pain medications are sufficient and generally required for only the first two days postoperatively.

ORCHIECTOMY If an intra-abdominal testis or gonad is to be removed, this is usually accomplished by placement of at least two more ports (one 2 mm and one 5 mm). In general, minimal dissection is required to remove an intra-abdominal testis (similar to that of laparoscopic varicocele ligation). These patients can be discharged the same day of surgery after ensuring that good hemostasis on the gonadal vessels is secured by use of vascular clips. The oral gastric or nasogastric tube is immediately removed after surgery, as is the Foley catheter. A regular diet is begun immediately and the patient is encouraged to return to normal activities.

The best treatment of postoperative complications is prevention. Adherence to proper principles of postoperative management will allow patients undergoing laparoscopic procedures to benefit from shorter hospital stays while avoiding preventable complications through early detection and treatment.

REFERENCES

1. Kavoussi LR, Sosa RE, Capelouto C. Complications of laparoscopic surgery. J Endourol 1992;6:95–8.
2. Green LS, Loughli KR, Kavoussi LR. Management of epigastric vessel injury during laparoscopy. J Endourol 1992; 61:99–101.
3. Clayman RV, Kavoussi LR, Soper NJ, et al. Laparoscopic nephrectomy: Review of the initial 10 cases. J Endourol 1992;6:127–31.
4. Winfield HN, Schuessler WW. Laparoscopic renal surgery. In: Clayman RV, McDougall EM, editors. Laparoscopic urology. St. Louis: Quality Medical Publishing; 1993. p. 272–308.
5. Winfield HN, Schuessler WW. Laparoscopic ureteral surgery. In: Clayman RV, McDougall EM, editors. Laparoscopic urology. St. Louis: Quality Medical Publishing; 1993. p. 322–70.
6. Chandhoke PS, Clayman RV, Kerbl K, et al. Laparoscopic ureterectomy: initial clinical experience. J Urol 1993;149: 992–7.
7. Suzuki K, Kageyama S, Ueda D, et al. Laparoscopic adrenalectomy: clinical experience with 12 cases. J Urol 1993; 150:1099–102.
8. Siqueira TM Jr, Nadu A, Kuo RL, et al. Laparoscopic treatment for ureteropelvic junction obstruction. Urology 2002;60:973–8.
9. Jarrett TW, Chan DY, Charambura TC, et al. Laparoscopic pyeloplasty: the first 100 cases. J Urol 2002;167:1253–6.
10. Winfield HN, Schuessler WW. Pelvic lymphadenectomy: limited and extended. In: Clayman RV, McDougall EM, editors. Laparoscopic urology. St. Louis: Quality Medical Publishing; 1993. p. 225–59.
11. Kerbl K, Clayman RV, Petros JA, et al. Staging pelvic lymphadenectomy for prostate cancer: a comparison of laparoscopic and open techniques. J Urol 1993;150:396–9.
12. Ruckle H, Hadley R, Lui P, Stewart S. Laparoscopic pelvic lymph node dissection: assessment of intraoperative and early postoperative complications. J Endourol 1992;6: 117–9.

13. Donovan JF, Winfield HN. Laparoscopic varix ligation. J Urol 1992;147:77–81.

14. Donovan JF, Winfield HN. Laparoscopic varix ligation with Nd:Yag laser. J Endourol 1992;6:165–71.

15. Winfield HN, Schuessler WW. Laparoscopic varix ligation. In: Clayman RV, McDougall EM, editors. Laparoscopic urology. St. Louis: Quality Medical Publishing; 1993. p. 260–71.

16. Winfield HN, Schuessler WW. Laparoscopic varix ligation. In: Clayman RV, McDougall EM, editors. Laparoscopic urology. St. Louis: Quality Medical Publishing; 1993. p. 371–82.

17. Bhayani SB, Pavlovich CP, Hsu TS, et al. Prospective comparison of short-term convalescence: laparoscopic radical prostatectomy versus open radical retropubic prostatectomy. Urology 2003;61:612–6.

18. Guillonneau B, Cathelineau X, Doublet JD, et al. Laparoscopic radical prostatectomy: assessment after 550 procedures. Crit Rev Oncol Hematol 2002;43:123–33.

19. Cortesi N, Ferrari P, Zumbarda E, et al. Diagnosis of bilateral abdominal cryptorchidism by laparoscopy. Endoscopy 1976;8:33–5.

53

Prevention and Management of Laparoscopic Complications

Benjamin R. Lee, MD
Thomas W. Jarrett, MD

Complications are a potential occurrence with any surgical procedure. Even with experience, surgeons may face individual factors such as a patient's anatomy, disease status, and comorbidities. The potential for laparoscopic complications is the same as for open surgical procedures, in addition to specific complications related to laparoscopic techniques. Over the past decade, there has been an exponential rise in the application and advances in urologic laparoscopy, with the ability to perform virtually every open abdominal urologic surgery laparoscopically. Inevitably, complications will occur with any surgical practice, and the goal of this chapter is to review the prevention, identification and management of laparoscopic complications.

Data from large multi-institutional series have reported major complication rates ranging from 2 to 6.9% overall (Table 53-1).[1–4] With stratification of the difficulty level of these procedures into categories of easy (diagnosis of and treatment of cryptorchidism and varicocelectomy), difficult (renal cyst decortication, lymphocele marsupialization, pelvic lymph node dissection, nephropexy), and very difficult (nephrectomy, adrenalectomy, retroperitoneal lymph node dissection, pyeloplasty, and radical prostatectomy), the complication rates differ to 1.3%, 6.8% and 13.6%, respectively.[4]

As would be expected, mortality rates for laparoscopic procedures have declined dramatically over the past three decades. A review of over 20,000 cases from multiple series from 1951 through 1968 showed a previous mortality rate of about 1 in 1,000 cases, or 0.1%. Several more recent reviews, however, showed a decrease of up to 12-fold, with mortality rates now ranging from 0.02% to 0.08% of cases.[5,6]

PREVENTION

The key for preventing complications is preoperative planning and patient selection. With careful evaluation and imaging studies when indicated, complications can be minimized. Absolute contraindications to laparoscopy include (1) intestinal obstruction and/or substantial distention, (2) massive hemoperitoneum, (3) history of, or active, peritonitis, (4) abdominal wall infection, (5) uncorrected coagulopathy, and (6) large abdominal hernias that may prevent effective pneumoperitoneum.[8,9]

Special considerations may be necessary for the following conditions:

1. **Previous abdominal surgery.** The nature of the procedure, the location of the old incision, and the location of the planned laparoscopic procedure should be considered. Prior operative reports are helpful to delineate the precise extent of surgery. The entry point for the Veress needle or the initial trocar should be at least 6 to 8 cm away from prior surgical sites. Use of open access techniques may allow primary trocar insertion under direct vision, or alternatively, the retroperitoneal approach can be employed. The effect of previous abdominal surgery on urological laparoscopy was reviewed in a series of 700 patients at a single institution. In this series, 366 (52%) had never undergone surgery, 105 (15%) had a history of abdominal surgery at the same anatomical region, and 229 (33%) had a history of abdominal surgery at a different region. There were no significant differences in operative blood loss, rate of conversion to open procedure, or rate of operative complications.[10] Therefore, previous abdominal surgery is not an absolute contraindication to a laparoscopic procedure depending on location of the previous incision and current operative location.

2. **Diaphragmatic hernia.** This may allow the pneumoperitoneum to extend into the thoracic cavity with resultant pneumomediastinum. The large hiatal hernia may allow herniation of intra-abdominal contents into the chest with cardiorespiratory impairment.[11] Larger symptomatic hiatal hernias that may need surgical repair should have evaluation prior to an elective procedure.[12]

3. **Obesity.** Morbid obesity was once considered a relative contraindication to laparoscopy. In obese patients, the increased thickness of the abdominal wall may hinder initial placement of the Veress needle and insertion of working trocars. In addition, it may be necessary to increase the intra-abdominal pressure to 20 mm Hg to have an adequate working space. For renal procedures, shifting the trocar positions laterally may facilitate application. Furthermore, once the pneumoperitoneum is established and trocar insertion is achieved, a large amount of intraperitoneal fat may make the procedure more difficult. Several studies have shown, however, that laparoscopy can be safely performed in the obese patient with some technical modifications.[13,14]

4. **Irreducible external hernia.** This may result in vascular compromise of the incarcerated viscus.

5. **Ascites.** In ascites, the gas-filled intestinal loops float on the surface of the fluid in the peritoneal cavity, increasing the likelihood of injury. Furthermore, patients with ascites may represent metastatic disease[15] and should be fully evaluated prior to therapy. Ascitic fluid suspicious for malignancy should be sent for cytologic evaluation.

6. **Organomegaly.** In patients with organomegaly, the surgeon should remain 6 to 8 cm away from the edge of any palpable organ.

Further cornerstones for prevention of complications include experience in laparoscopic techniques and adequate preoperative planning. If the surgeon has minimal laparoscopic experience, he should be mentored by a more experienced surgeon. Practice before entering the operating room on the pelvic trainer, taking courses on laparoscopy, and practice in the animal lab all contribute to decreasing the learning curve. By thoroughly and systematically learning the technique of laparoscopy, with the gradual expansion

Table 53-1 Multi-institutional Series of Laparoscopic Complications

Author	N	Overall Incidence	Vascular	Bowel	Conversion to Open
Fahlenkamp et al[4]	2,407	4.4%	1.7%	1.1%	0.8%
Soulie et al[3]	1,085	6.9%	0.4%	0.6%	2.1%
Meraney et al[2]	404	2%	1.7%	0.25%	0.7%
Vallancien et al[1]	1,311	0.7%	0.5%	1.2%	1.2%
Total / Average	**5,207**	**3.5 ± 2.7%**	**1.08 ± 0.7%**	**0.79 ± .44%**	**1.2 ± .064%**

of difficulty of cases, complications can be kept to a minimum. A current stepwise training program has been defined by the German Urologic Association,[4] which includes modules on theoretical knowledge and handling of instruments, practice on the pelvic trainer, supervised laparoscopic surgeries on laboratory animals, assisting in laparoscopic surgeries, and independently performing surgeries under the supervision of experienced surgeons.

The surgeon and the entire operating team should be prepared to convert the laparoscopic procedure to laparotomy in case of intraoperative difficulties. The patient should be fully informed of this possibility, and this risk should be included in the patient consent. All operating room personnel should be experienced with laparoscopic equipment and procedures. The equipment should be tested thoroughly before initiating the procedure, gas canisters for CO_2 should be checked for adequate volume, and backup equipment should be readily available.

PATIENT PREPARATION Patient preparation is a vital factor in avoidance of complications. Informed consent should involve a thorough discussion of the alternative treatments and the risks, benefits, and potential complications of the procedure. The patient should be clearly informed about the possibility of converting the procedure to open surgery in case of difficulties, complications or inability to complete the procedure laparoscopically. Routine bowel preparation such as the use of magnesium citrate and a clear liquid diet the day before surgery will help decompress the lower intestine and may be helpful for complex laparoscopic surgical procedures such as nephrectomy and retroperitoneal lymph node dissection, in which there is potential of bowel injury. Orogastric and urinary catheters are standard for laparoscopic urologic procedures to decompress the stomach and bladder respectively, and facilitate laparoscopic visualization. Perioperative antibiotics are administered on call to the operating room. The patient should be secured to the table, all pressure points appropriately padded, and the rotation of the table tested. The anterior abdominal wall should be prepped so as to allow immediate open surgical intervention if needed. Intermittent pneumatic compression stockings will help prevent deep venous thrombosis.

Even with optimal patient selection and preparation, complications may occur. We will discuss complications encountered in laparoscopic surgery and present strategies for both prevention and management.

COMPLICATIONS OF VERESS NEEDLE PLACEMENT

Placement of the Veress needle and establishment of an adequate pneumoperitoneum is a critical step in laparoscopy. Penetration complications are reported at 0.18%[16,17] and include those induced by either the Veress needle or trocar. The insufflation needle is most commonly introduced at the

umbilicus. The following initial needle insertion points are the most hazardous: right upper quadrant (liver and vessels), right iliac fossa (appendicular adhesions), rectus muscle (epigastric vessels), and anywhere in the vicinity of scars.[11] A common initial difficulty in laparoscopy is the proper placement of the Veress needle. Several maneuvers to confirm proper positioning of the needle prior to starting the insufflation are the following, although none are truly foolproof:

1. Aspiration of colored (red, yellow, green, and brown) or malodorous fluid suggests improper placement.
2. Drop test: apply a drop of saline solution inside the hub of the needle and attempt to aspirate. Inability to aspirate the fluid suggests the fluid has dispersed into the abdomen and the needle is in the correct position.
3. Palmer test: inject 10 mL of saline solution into the needle and attempt to aspirate. Inability to aspirate the fluid suggests the fluid has dispersed into the abdomen and the needle is in the correct position.
4. An initial pressure reading < 8 mm Hg suggests intraperitoneal positioning.
5. A decrease in pressure with elevation of the abdominal wall indicates proper positioning within the peritoneal cavity.
6. Use of the "stirring technique" (rotation of the needle after insertion to see if it moves freely) must be discouraged since a small puncture wound can become a more serious laceration.
7. Advancement test: if the Veress needle is in the correct intraperitoneal location, it can be advanced 1 cm deeper without resistance.

PREPERITONEAL PLACEMENT The most common incorrect needle placement site is the preperitoneal space. Although rarely injurious to the patient, this increases the distance between the skin and the intraperitoneal cavity, resulting in difficult trocar placement, CO_2 absorption, and a decrease in working space. If the angle of placement of the Veress needle is too oblique, the needle may slide over the peritoneum without penetrating it, and the tip of the needle will be placed between the fascia and the peritoneum (Figure 53-1). The preperitoneal potential space can expand enough to accommodate as much as 3 to 4 L of gas. If it expands symmetrically, the abdomen will appear distended as after corrected intraperitoneal insufflation. It will also have convincing tympani upon percussion of the abdomen. Unfortunately, this complication is usually identified after the initial trocar is placed, when endoscopic inspection reveals preperitoneal fat. The peritoneum can easily be observed intact over the viscera. Attempts to evacuate the preperitoneal space with needle and syringe and reinsertion of the needle at the same or another location may be successful. Repositioning the Veress needle to the superior umbilical region may allow successful insufflation (Figure 53-2). If discovered at the time of the trocar insertion,

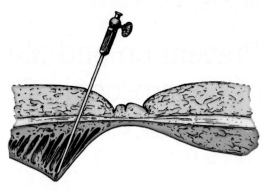

Figure 53-1 Example of tenting of the peritoneum during Veress needle placement. Reproduced with permission from Hulka JF.[47]

preperitoneal insufflation can also be managed by carefully opening the peritoneum with laparoscopic scissors and riding the tip of the trocar beneath it. Alternatively, the open Hasson technique can be performed. Once the proper pneumoperitoneum is achieved, preperitoneal gas will usually be compressed and will not interfere with the completion of the procedure.

VISCERAL INJURY Perforation of the stomach, bowel, or bladder is indicated by the aspiration of intestinal gas or unclear or malodorous fluid through the needle with a syringe. If perforation occurs, the Veress needle should be immediately removed and discarded. The surgeon may choose either to use a new needle and reinsert at another location or to perform open laparoscopy using the Hasson technique. One should keep in mind that this perforation might be the result of adhesions of the viscus to the anterior wall, not just the result of random puncture.[18] After insufflation, the injury should be examined with the laparoscope and a decision made as to the appropriate management. Because of the small size of the Veress needle, the majority of injuries do not

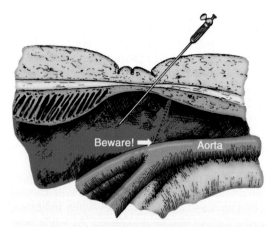

Figure 53-2 Placing the Veress needle in the supraumbilical position may allow successful placement into the peritoneal cavity despite the properitoneal insufflation. This diagram also demonstrates that the bifurcation is at the approximate level of the umbilicus, and Veress needles and trocars should be directed into the hollow of the pelvis to help prevent injury to the great vessels. Reproduced with permission from Hulka JF.[47]

require operative intervention.[8] At the end of the procedure, the site of injury should be reexamined. If there is any question regarding the injury, a laparotomy should be performed and the perforation examined directly.

VASCULAR INJURY The Veress needle may injure the omental or mesenteric blood vessels or major abdominal or pelvic vessels. Thin individuals, adolescents, and infants are more prone to vascular injury. The bifurcation of the great vessels is approximately at the level of the umbilicus; therefore, Veress needles and trocars should be directed into the hollow of the pelvis (see Figure 53-2). After the placement of the Veress needle, if blood appears at its hub or if blood is withdrawn into a syringe, the needle should be withdrawn slightly. The new position should be retested before the pneumoperitoneum is established to prevent intravascular gas administration.[19]

Management of major vessel injury caused by insertion of the Veress needle is controversial. Because of the narrow diameter of this needle, some surgeons believe it should be treated as a perforation of intestinal loop by removal and then reinsertion at another location.[8] On the other hand, some recommend immediate laparotomy when major vessel injury is suggested.[20] Still others take an intermediate approach. Their management depends on the amount of bleeding, and ranges from observation to cauterization to exploration with suturing or to the use of laparoscopically placed clips to control the bleeding.[11,21] The authors believe that clean needle penetration of even a major vessel will not usually cause significant bleeding unless the situation is made worse by lateral motion of the needle. This confirms the importance of not moving the needle after insertion until proper position has been confirmed.

COMPLICATIONS OF INSUFFLATION AND PNEUMOPERITONEUM

SUBCUTANEOUS EMPHYSEMA, PNEUMOMEDIASTINUM, AND PNEUMOTHORAX The establishment of an adequate pneumoperitoneum is critical to successful laparoscopic surgery. Failure to establish pneumoperitoneum is the most common cause of failed laparoscopy for the novice surgeon. Most surgeons use the Veress needle to access the peritoneal cavity and create pneumoperitoneum. Strict attention to technique will avoid more complications of insufflation. Insufflation injuries account for a minority of cases[22] and are usually the result of either incorrect Veress needle position or prolonged high-pressure pneumoperitoneum. The needle may be incorrectly placed in the subcutaneous tissue, preperitoneal space, or viscus. Subcutaneous emphysema is most often secondary to Veress needle placement anterior to the abdominal fascia or CO_2 leakage around the trocar port. It is not a serious problem and is easily diagnosed by asymmetric distention, crepitus, and a sharp increase in pressure when the abdominal wall is grasped. It is easily and safely evacuated through the needle or trocar sheath by pressing the skin against the abdominal fascia.[11] Extensive subcutaneous emphysema, however, may be due to pneumothorax or pneumomediastinum.[23,24]

If crepitus extends off the chest wall to the neck, termination of the laparoscopic procedure should be strongly considered. A continuum of fascial planes exists between the cervical soft tissue and the mediastinum, meaning that gas in the subcutaneous tissues can track upward into the neck and then course down into the mediastinum.[25] Subcutaneous emphysema of the neck space and chest wall may also be a sign of pneumothorax or pneumomediastinum. Just as gas may track into the mediastinum from the subcutaneous tissues, the reverse may occur as well. Pneumomediastinum may occur if the needle is inserted in the retroperitoneal space or the base of the mesentery. Insufflated air may escape the abdominal cavity, connecting it with the mediastinum. Undetected pneumothorax or pneumomediastinum can be life-threatening. If they are suspected, a chest x-ray film should be obtained immediately. If tension pneumothorax develops, the abdominal gas should be evacuated and immediate decompression of the pleural space is warranted via either a 16-gauge needle placed into the second intercostal space in the midclavicular line or by a tube thoracostomy. Pneumomediastinum usually can be managed conservatively by close observation.[24]

Pneumoscrotum is frequently encountered with pelvic laparoscopy. It is advisable to manually compress the scrotum at the end of the procedure at the time of evacuation of the pneumoperitoneum. Alternatively, wrapping the scrotum with an elastic bandage will reduce gas passage into the scrotum. Most cases of subcutaneous emphysema, scrotal emphysema, and pneumomediastinum will usually resolve spontaneously within 24 to 36 hours with no significant morbidity. Patients should be informed of these possibilities to decrease anxiety in the postoperative period should they occur.

BOWEL INSUFFLATION If the bowel is penetrated by the needle and insufflated, asymmetric abdominal distention, belching, or passage of flatus during the induction of pneumoperitoneum strongly suggests entry into the gastrointestinal tract. Insufflation should be stopped, the gas line disconnected, and the gas allowed to escape. When proper pneumoperitoneum is established, reinspect the suspected penetration site thoroughly. Particular attention should be paid to through-and-through injuries to the bowel, since the exit site of the needle often sustains more damage than the entry site.[19]

PROLONGED HIGH INTRA-ABDOMINAL PRESSURE High pneumoperitoneal gas pressure can cause decreased venous return due to caval compression and can result in decreased cardiac output leading to hypotension. Additionally, the increased pressure on the diaphragm requires increased ventilation pressure that may lead to pneumothorax. This increased pressure can rupture bullae or thin-walled alveoli, especially in patients with underlying pulmonary disease. Moreover, the increased intra-abdominal pressure may result in the passage of gas through the weak points or defects in the diaphragm or retroperitoneally along the great vessels into the mediastinum and subsequent pneumothorax or pneumomediastinum.[24,26] The abdominal contents may also be forced into the chest through a hiatal hernia. High initial pressure suggests improper positioning of the Veress needle, either preperitoneal placement, within an organ or a clogged needle tip. Pressure sensors on the insufflator should detect this problem. If high pressure develops during the procedure, it may be caused by a faulty insufflator, improper pressure setting of the insufflator, or overpressuring from the use of a CO_2 cooled laser or argon beam coagulator. The latter problem is caused by the air-cooled device generating pressure too rapidly for the insufflator to compensate. Intermittent venting through a trocar valve will correct the high pressure. Faulty insufflator problems can be corrected by always having backup equipment available.

GAS EMBOLISM Gas embolism is an infrequent, but potentially devastating, complication of laparoscopy. Although intravasation of gas resulting from elevated intra-abdominal pressure has been suggested as a cause of gas embolism, the most likely cause is incorrect Veress needle placement.[27] Many of the early reported fatalities due to gas embolism occurred when air was used as the insufflating medium. CO_2 has much greater solubility than air and can be cleared more rapidly by hyperventilation. Nevertheless, CO_2 embolism can occur. The diagnosis of a gas embolism may be difficult, and there is often no warning prior to acute cardiovascular collapse.

The presenting features of gas embolism include sudden profound hypotension, cyanosis, tachycardia, and other dysrhythmias. Less frequently, the first indication of gas embolism is pulmonary edema or even delayed sudden death. Sudden development of a mill wheel murmur over the pericardium can occur.[28] This murmur may occur in the absence of clinical signs and even before changes in the heart sounds. Intraoperative end-tidal CO_2 monitoring has improved the potential for early embolism detection. In the case of CO_2 embolism, it would show an abrupt increase in end-tidal CO_2. The most sensitive monitor and fastest detector of intracardiac gas is the precordial Doppler stethoscope. Capnography is a useful monitoring technique that accurately reflects the arterial CO_2 tension. Other indicators of gas embolism are the presence of blood on aspiration from the Veress needle, pulsations of the flowmeter with the patient's pulse during insufflation, and absence of signs of distention of the abdomen, despite an adequate volume of insufflated gas. Aspiration of gas or foaming blood from the central venous line will establish the diagnosis. The verification of Veress needle placement prior to insufflation to avoid intravascular injection of gas is of the utmost importance. Finally, the Veress needle must never be inserted with the gas tubing connected to it.[29]

If gas embolism is suspected, emergency measures include:

1. Immediate discontinuation and deflation of the pneumoperitoneum to prevent progression of the hemodynamic decompensation.
2. Placement of the patient in the left lateral decubitus position (Durant's position) to minimize right ventricular outflow problems.
3. Hyperventilation with 100% oxygen.
4. Introduction of a central venous catheter for aspiration of the gas.
5. Hyperbaric oxygen and cardiopulmonary bypass.[30,31]

TROCAR INJURIES

Trocar injuries are most likely to occur during the blind insertion of the first trocar.[32] Injuries can be minimized with use of a visual obturator trocar[33] which consists of an optical obturator with a clear, blunt window at its distal tip, and either a recessed knife blade (Visiport, U.S. Surgical Corp., Norwalk, CT) or two sharpened ridges on the tip of the trocar (Optiview, Ethicon Endo-Surgery, Cincinnati, OH) to divide the fascia and enter the peritoneum. Secondary trocars can be placed practically anywhere in the abdomen under laparoscopic guidance. Injury of the gastrointestinal tract, abdominal wall vessels, major intra-abdominal blood vessels, and urinary tract have all been described.[34] The likelihood of such injuries increases in the presence of underlying adhesions from prior abdominal surgery. In these cases, the surgeon may choose to perform open Hasson laparoscopy.

Several steps should be taken to help avoid trocar injuries:

1. Verify an adequate skin incision that will accommodate the trocar so that undue force is not needed to penetrate the skin and underlying fascial planes.
2. Spread the subcutaneous tissue with a hemostat to allow the blade of the trocar to abut directly into the fascia.
3. Check that there is full pneumoperitoneum before trocar insertion. A transient increase in the intra-abdominal pressure to 20 mm Hg in adults may ensure an adequate pneumoperitoneum.
4. Verify proper equipment function and trocar safety shield function.
5. Use a trocar with a sharp point to minimize the force necessary to enter the peritoneal cavity. Disposable trocars ensure sharp points and the added benefit of a safety shield often not found on reusable trocars.
6. Direct the trocar into the pelvis in the midline.
7. Hold the elbow of the thrusting arm close to the rib cage to better stabilize the wrist and hand. The index finger should be extended on the sheath to act as a break on the abdominal wall to prevent the thrust from pushing the trocar too deeply.
8. Use a gentle twisting motion of the trocar to allow it to pass more smoothly through the rectus fascia.
9. Always insert secondary trocars under direct vision. Transillumination of the abdominal wall with the laparoscope can help identify superficial abdominal wall vessels.
10. Avoid trocar placement in the mid-rectus area where the epigastric vessels and major branches may be inadvertently injured.

In contrast to Veress needle injuries, significant perforation of a major blood vessel or gastrointestinal tract with the trocar usually requires open laparotomy. The trocar and sheath should be left in place while performing laparotomy to minimize further contamination or blood loss and locate the injury site. Trocar injuries should be managed like any other penetrating injury to the abdomen. Intestinal injuries should be repaired with purse-string or double-layer silk sutures if the laceration is less than one half the diameter of the lumen. With expanding laparoscopic techniques, the recent introduction of laparoscopic stapling devices, non-crushing bowel clamps, and larger laparoscopic cannulas, laparoscopic management of hollow viscous injury is becoming more common for experienced laparoscopists.[35,36] For other laparoscopists, however, particularly the novice, immediate laparotomy may be wiser in such circumstances.

ABDOMINAL WALL INJURY

The inferior epigastric vessels are particularly at risk. Such injury may result in bleeding around the sheath into the abdominal cavity or formation of abdominal wall hematoma. To reduce the likelihood of this potential complication, the room should be darkened and the abdominal wall transilluminated with the laparoscope to identify the vessels and select the proper trocar site. Additionally, placement of trocars lateral to the rectus muscle can minimize the potential for injury to these vessels. If an abdominal wall vessel injury occurs, the trocar sheath should be left in place to tamponade the vessel and allow it to seal. The bleeding may be controlled by a clamp applied tightly near the trocar. If a metal trocar is used, careful cauterization applied to the sheath may control the bleeding. If bleeding persists, a through-and-through abdominal wall polypropylene suture may control the bleeding.[37] This can be accomplished with a Keith needle passed adjacent to the trocar and back up through the skin.

COMPLICATIONS OF OPEN ACCESS (HASSON TECHNIQUE)

Although the Hasson technique is extremely useful in reducing laparoscopic complications, it does not obviate risks. The wider incision leads to an increased incidence of abdominal wall injuries (bleeding, hematoma, gas leakage) and wound infection. The small bowel may be injured while opening the peritoneum sharply, since this technique is used mainly in patients with a history of previous abdominal surgery and/or infection in whom intestinal adhesions are more common. Incomplete or improper sealing around the laparoscopic sheath leads to escape of insufflation gas and an inadequate pneumoperitoneum.[38] Simply allowing the high-flow insufflator to keep up with the gas loss is probably the best management option because attempts at sealing the leak may result in subcutaneous emphysema. Another solution is to use a Hasson-style cannula with an internal balloon that seals at the peritoneal surface as opposed to the skin surface.

OPERATIVE INJURIES

This class of complications occurs after initial trocar placement and during the course of the procedure. It should be noted that the two-dimensional image produced by current laparoscopic video systems results in a loss of depth perception for the surgeon. The laparoscopic instruments are extremely long and thin and therefore can easily penetrate most abdominal organs if they are manipulated within the peritoneal cavity without direct visual guidance. To minimize injury, the laparoscopist and assistants should closely coordinate movement of the camera and instruments. Complete visualization of the tips of the instruments at all times, as well as careful attention while passing instruments through the trocars, must be maintained.

THERMAL INJURY Even though fiberoptic light sources are used, the high-intensity light source can sometimes make the end of the laparoscope extremely hot. If the tip is allowed to remain in contact with the viscera for a long time, a thermal injury may occur. This is most likely to occur with any rapid loss of pneumoperitoneum, such as accidental removal of the laparoscopic sheath, which may bring the abdominal viscera into direct contact with the tip of the laparoscope.[39]

ELECTROCAUTERY INJURY Electrical injury represents one of the most serious complications of laparoscopy surgery. Failure to recognize a bowel burn injury can result in significant morbidity and mortality. Early recognition of the injury and surgical exploration when warranted is crucial in avoiding disasters.[40] The vast majority of electrocautery injuries result from error in technique rather than uncontrolled events. The injuries occur by one of the following two mechanisms: a spark may jump from the grasping forceps during coagulation or the laparoscopic forceps may brush directly against the bowel, either with the tip or the heel of the scissors, causing a burn.[41] Thermal spread from prolonged monopolar electrocautery can spread several centimeters. Even bipolar electrocautery may spread up to 6 mm.[42]

Avoidance of bowel burn injuries is dependent on careful cautery technique. The insulation of each instrument should be checked to make sure that it is intact. Moreover, when applying electrocautery, the entire tip of the instrument should be in the visual field to be certain that the conducting metal is not lying on the bowel.

Finally, when using cautery, be sure the area to be cauterized is completely dissected free and isolated from the surrounding tissues to prevent thermal injury. Minor thermal injuries identified intraoperatively may be managed conservatively with observation, hyperalimentation, and intravenous antibiotics. Wheeless reported on 33 patients known to have sustained electrocautery bowel injuries at laparoscopy.[43] In the first six cases in which the bowel was visibly burned, immediate laparotomy revealed that in only two was an actual perforation identified. In the next 27 patients, conservative treatment alone was used, and none of these required laparotomy. Thus, only 2 of 33 patients (6%) required laparotomy for thermal bowel injuries. Such an injury, if identified at operation, may appear as a whitish area on the serosa. This does not usually require laparotomy. If the serosa is separated and the muscularis or the mucosa or even the lumen of the intestine is seen, laparotomy is indicated.

Unfortunately, bowel burn injuries are often unrecognized at the time of laparoscopy. The majority of patients with unrecognized injuries present 2 to7 days postoperatively with vague abdominal discomfort, trocar site pain, nausea, low-grade fever, and moderate leukocytosis and bandemia (release of immature neutrophils in the circulation).[44] A plain x-ray film of the abdomen may reveal an ileus. Free air is not always a helpful early sign since it is often seen up to 2 weeks after laparoscopy (Figure 53-3). Early recognition or suspicion can be aided with a manual differential white blood cell count and an abdominal computed tomography (CT) scan with intravenous (IV) and oral contrast. If a postoperative patient does not respond quickly to antibiotics and signs of peritonitis develop, laparotomy is mandated. The area of injury may undergo necrosis in the range of 18 hours to 14 days, and perforation may result. The immune response following laparoscopy may be altered compared to open surgery.[45] Aldana and colleagues reported that white blood cell apoptosis following laparoscopic bowel injury is elevated compared to controls, but only at half the level of open bowel injury at one day and one week. Furthermore, these levels equilibrated to similar levels after 2 weeks.[45] Since animals who have undergone laparoscopic bowel injury often develop neutropenia, a decrease in white blood cell count may be the outcome of a net loss of circulating neutrophils. The associated increased bandemia further supports this concept. Theoretically, a net decrease in peripheral neutrophil count is likely to occur as a result of either sequestration of a large amount of neutrophils in a particular organ, such as the lung, or enhanced margination of neutrophils to the vascular endothelial bed. Since sympathetic stimulation and/or stress often causes demargination of neutrophils from the vascular bed and is associated with leukocytosis, laparoscopic surgery-induced neutropenia may not be the outcome of either.

At exploration, intestinal burn injuries may be more extensive than visual inspection shows, and thus, simple oversewing of the injury should not be attempted. The crater itself is a small part of devitalized tissue caused by electrocoagulation spreading through the bowel wall. Since tissue damage can be detected as far as 5 cm away from the injury site by monopolar cautery, resection of a 6 cm margin on either side of the injury and end-to-end anastomosis is recommended.[46] Bipolar injury, in contrast to unipolar cautery injury, is usually localized to the visualized burn area. Conservative management is usually sufficient for small burned areas. If the burn is severe, excision of the burn and suturing of the defect (if it is small) or simple end-to-end anastomosis (if the lesion involves over half of the bowel lumen) will suffice.[47]

Although small and large bowel injuries are the most frequently reported visceral injuries, laceration to the liver, spleen, stomach, and colonic mesentery may occur. These injuries may be encountered during Veress needle placement, trocar insertion, or surgical dissection. Previous abdominal surgery is a risk factor for intestinal injuries. Bowel or omentum may adhere under areas of abdominal scars. In these high-risk patients, open trocar placement (Hasson technique) should be considered.

A mechanical bowel preparation is advised in patients scheduled for laparoscopy who have had prior abdominal surgery. Gastric injury usually results from trocar insertion in a distended stomach due to esophageal intubation or during mask induction with an inhalation anesthetic. To avoid gastric injury, patients should withhold oral intake for 8 to 12 hours prior to surgery and a nasogastric or oral gastric tube should be inserted before Veress needle placement.

VASCULAR INJURY Vascular injuries are the most common complication reported in the urologic laparoscopic literature. In several large reviews, the overall incidence of vascular injuries was 0.4 to1.8%.[1,3,4,48] During initial Veress needle placement, the aorta and common iliac vessels are more liable to injury. The inferior vena cava is somewhat less likely to be injured because

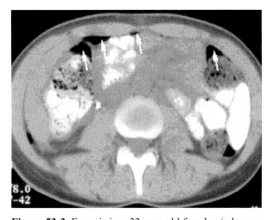

Figure 53-3 Free air in a 32-year-old female s/p laparoscopic pyeloplasty and pyelolithotomy. CT scan on postoperative day 4 to exclude residual stones shows persistent, non-pathologic, free intraperitoneal gas following surgery. The CO_2 is usually absorbed by the third postoperative day but can persist longer in the absence of pathologic findings. s/p = status post

of its retrolateral relationship to the aorta. Avoidance of major vessel injury depends on the strict adherence to the basic rules of Veress needle and trocar insertion. Additionally, proper patient selection will identify those at increased risk. The laparoscopist should be especially careful in very thin patients and children since the aorta may lie only 2 to 3 cm from the skin.[20,49] Diagnosis of major vascular injury is easily confirmed by the return of frank blood from the Veress needle or trocar sheath. Bleeding may be concealed if the injury is confined to the retroperitoneum.[50,51] Immediate laparotomy is indicated if major vascular injury is diagnosed or strongly suspected or the patient is hemodynamically unstable. The Veress needle or trocar sheath should be left in place and the stopcock closed, since this will tamponade bleeding and help localize the site of injury. Movement of the Veress needle or trocar should be avoided, because this may convert a puncture injury into a large tear. In cases of severe hemorrhage, the aorta should be compressed immediately on entering the peritoneal cavity followed by prompt proximal and distal control of the bleeding vessels. A suture repair will suffice for a minor arterial injury. In larger arterial injuries, débridement and a graft repair may be needed. It is important to fully mobilize and inspect the back wall of a major vessel to rule out a through-and-through injury.

Renal vascular injuries are possible during laparoscopic renal surgery. The management of renal vascular injury depends on the severity. Most vascular injuries related to the upper urinary tract involve branches of the renal vein or vena cava, although arterial branches are possible. A minor hole may be occluded with atraumatic grasping forceps before applying laparoscopic clips or ligatures.[52] If bleeding cannot be tamponaded for adequate visualization, immediate open exploration is indicated.[53] Undue traction on the renal hilum during dissection of the adjacent tissue may result in an avulsion injury with subsequent retraction of the end of the vessel. Significant torque on an instrument may be transmitted to the end of the instrument and result in an increased force of dissection. With venous bleeding, increasing the pneumoperitoneum temporarily to between 20 and 25 mm Hg may help tamponade vessels and improve visualization. Intermittent application of the irrigator/aspirator can clear the blood and identify the vessel. Insertion of a gauze sponge through the 12 mm trocar to temporarily tamponade the area may also help improve visualization. When use of a gastrointestinal stapling device on the renal vein or artery is performed, one must ensure that there are no inadvertent surrounding clips that might cause a misfire.[54] Use of a Ligasure vessel sealing system will provide ligation and division of arteries up to 6 mm and veins up to 12 mm in diameter.[42] Alternatively, the Harmonic scalpel (Ethicon Endo-Surgery) will seal vessels up to 3 mm and induce comparatively less collateral thermal heat damage at 6 mm.[55] Use of either of these modalities can ligate surrounding perihilar lymphatic tissue or lumbar vessels and decrease the need for placement of titanium clips, which potentially could cause a GIA misfire.

Mesenteric hematoma has been reported as a complication of laparoscopic surgery.[56] If such a hematoma is identified during laparoscopy, it must be closely monitored during the procedure. Evidence of expansion of the hematoma or compromised bowel circulation requires immediate laparotomy. Injuries to the superficial and deep epigastric vessels are becoming increasingly more common with the use of multiple trocar sites and usually occur during lateral trocar placement. The diagnosis and management of such injuries were discussed earlier in this chapter (see "Abdominal Wall Injury").

Occasionally injury to the abdominal wall or pelvic vessels may not be recognized until the postoperative period. Decreased hematocrit levels following laparoscopic surgery should alert the surgeon to the possibility of ongoing hemorrhage. An inordinate amount of pain around the trocar site, ecchymosis, or a palpable paramedian mass are signs of a rectus sheath hematoma. Conservative management with close monitoring of the patient's hematocrit and correction of any underlying coagulopathy is usually sufficient. On the other hand, if the hematoma is expanding or the hematocrit continues to drop, exploration of the wound and ligation of the bleeding vessel are mandated.

URINARY TRACT INJURIES

BLADDER The bladder may be perforated or lacerated during Veress needle placement, trocar placement, or laparoscopic dissection. Previous abdominal surgery with displacement of the bladder dome or any congenital anomalies of the lower urinary tract may increase the risk of bladder injury. The placement of a Foley catheter for gravity drainage prior to the procedure should all but obviate the risk of bladder perforation. Verifying that the pelvic lymphadenectomy is carried out lateral to the median umbilical ligament should also help prevent this problem. Aspiration of urine from the Veress needle is an obvious sign of bladder perforation. Should bladder injury occur, a decision must be made between nonoperative management with catheter drainage versus formal repair. Veress needle injuries usually require no specific intervention other than catheter drainage and antibiotics, unless a large laceration is present. Trocar placement may result in significant bladder injury. Intraoperative pneumaturia, distention of the Foley bag or hematuria should alert the laparoscopist to potential bladder injury. If a bladder injury is suspected, instillation of indigo carmine or methylene blue dye into the bladder may help identify the site of injury. Laparoscopic repair of the perforation may be performed using 2-0 polyglactin on a UR-6 needle. However, if the adequacy of the closure is unsatisfactory, open repair should be performed.[57]

URETER Ureteral injury is reported sporadically in non-urologic laparoscopy and is mainly attributable to electrocautery injury and rarely to direct trocar injury. A thorough knowledge of normal ureteral anatomy is mandatory, as is an awareness that variations in the normal anatomy can occur in patients with previous abdominal surgery or congenital anomalies such as ureteral duplication or horseshoe kidney. The ureter is at risk during pelvic lymph node dissection, particularly proximally near the beginning of the external iliac vein where the ureter crosses the bifurcation of the iliac artery. In addition to early identification of the ureter during lymphadenectomy, keeping the dissection lateral to the medial umbilical ligament may decrease the risk of bladder and ureteral injuries.

Electrocautery should be avoided in the vicinity of the ureter. Hemorrhage in this area should be controlled with surgical clips or ligators when possible. Unfortunately, the diagnosis of ureteral injury is usually not made at the time of surgery. Ureteral injuries usually become evident 1 to 5 days postoperatively. Intravenous urography and/or retrograde pyelography may help confirm the diagnosis and locate the site of injury. The management of ureteral injuries depends on many factors, such as the nature of the injury, the site of injury, and the timing of diagnosis. Treatment should be individualized for each patient. If injury is recognized intraoperatively, it is wiser to open and repair it. Small burns or lacerations, however, may be managed by ureteral stenting. A major thermal burn injury to the ureter requires wide débridement and repair. The choice of repair depends on the length and level of injury. If the diagnosis of the ureteral injury is made postoperatively, adequate drainage should be obtained. Since retrograde stent placement is often difficult,[58] percutaneous nephrostomy drainage with or without antegrade placement of a ureteral stent can be attempted initially. If a large urinoma is identified, percutaneous drainage could be performed. Gomel and James reported complete laparoscopic intervention for repair of a ureteral injury discovered intraoperatively.[59] The ureter was stented, and the edges of the laceration were approximated with a single laparoscopic suture to facilitate healing. The ureter healed within 2 weeks.

RECTAL INJURIES Rectal injury is a potential complication of radical prostatectomy with an incidence of 1.3%.[60] Inadvertent opening of the rectum during radical prostatectomy converts the case from clean to contaminated surgery, and therefore, increases the risk of septic complications, including wound infection, pelvic abscess, peritonitis, recto-urinary fistula, and even death.[61] Intraoperative recognition of rectal injury is a crucial step in management. Following copious irrigation with saline and povidone-iodine, the prostatectomy is completed. The margins of the rectal defect are clearly identified with an intrarectal metal bougie. The rectal wall is closed in two layers; the inner mucosal and outer seromuscular layers are closed with continuous or interrupted sutures with a 3-0 polyglactin 910, 17 mm half circle needle, tied extraluminally. The integrity of the repair can then be checked by filling the rectum with air through a rectal catheter to distend the lumen and look for air bubbles in the fluid-filled pelvic cavity. Two suction tube drains are placed, one anteriorly in Retzius' space, and another posteriorly through the pouch of Douglas at the location of the rectal injury. Antibiotics are broadened to include a third-generation cephalosporin and anaerobic coverage. All patients undergoing laparoscopic radical prostatectomy should undergo preoperative bowel prep and clear liquid diet. If there is any question regarding the integrity of the repair or contamination of the site, open conversion with either primary repair or diverting colostomy should be considered.

LIVER/GALLBLADDER AND SPLENIC INJURIES Liver/gallbladder and spleen injuries have been reported during right and left laparoscopic renal procedures, respectively.[34] Minor capsular tears of the liver and spleen can usually be addressed via coagulation with the argon beam coagulator or electrocautery. Oxidized cellulose can be applied for additional hemostasis. Deeper injuries may require more attention. For the spleen, open control may be necessary, or even splenectomy for cases of persistent bleeding. For the liver, compression sutures may be necessary. In cases refractory to simple maneuvers, general surgical consultation is recommended. Tears of the gallbladder usually occur secondary to retraction and require concomitant cholecystectomy.

PANCREATIC INJURY Pancreatic injuries have been described with left-sided dissections where the pancreatic tail crosses the upper pole of the kidney and adrenal.[4] Intended distal pancreatectomy may be necessary for upper pole pathology and may be safely performed with a stapling device. General surgical consultation is recommended prior to such procedures. If an injury is recognized or even suspected, the defect should be closed if possible and ample drainage of the area with closed suction drainage established.

DIAPHRAGMATIC INJURIES Injuries to the diaphragm have been described with both right- and left-sided procedures and can be lethal if unrecognized.[62] With a transperitoneal approach, the injury is usually due to electrocautery injury of the adjacent diaphragm during upper pole/adrenal dissection. With a retroperitoneal approach, the injury may be a result of supracostal trocar placement. The injury may be identified if an obvious pleurotomy with concomitant floppy diaphragm sign from CO_2 passage into the pleural cavity is seen. In other cases, the injury may be more subtle, with increased ventilatory pressures or hypercarbia. In severe cases, cardiopulmonary arrest may occur due to a tension pneumothorax. When suspected, the anesthesiologist should be informed in order to closely monitor the patient's cardiopulmonary status. If the patient's condition is stable, pneumoperitoneum should be decreased to 10 mm Hg, and the procedure should be completed before addressing the pleurotomy. The pleurotomy should be closed under direct vision, ensuring that air is evacuated from the pleural cavity. A low threshold for tube thoracostomy should be maintained if the patient's condition becomes unstable after diaphragmatic injury is sustained.

During trocar removal and closure of the fascia, a segment of bowel can become caught in the end of the trocar and become entrapped in the fascial defect, or the fascial closure needle may pass through the bowel. Bowel entrapment can be easily avoided by direct observation of trocar removal, as well as closing the fascia under laparoscopic visualization.

Orthopedic and/or neurologic injury may occur if the patient is not properly positioned and padded. Of all the nerve groups, the brachial plexus is the most susceptible to nerve damage from malposition during anesthesia. The use of shoulder braces with the patient in the Trendelenburg position pushes the clavicle into the retroclavicular space, which in turn, exerts pressure on the brachial plexus.[63] Careless positioning of the patient's arm, particularly abduction of more than 90°, may also cause a brachial plexus injury. Extreme outward rotation of the head of the humerus will exert excessive pressure on the brachial plexus; therefore, the patient's arm should be pronated (facing the side) when the arms are placed next to the trunk. Femoral neuropathy after laparoscopy has been attributed to abduction and extreme lateral rotation of the hip joint in the dorsal lithotomy position.[64] To avoid such complications, careful attention to patient positioning and proper padding of bony prominences is mandatory.

We prefer to avoid the use of shoulder braces, and instead, place a rolled towel behind the shoulder and hip for upper tract laparoscopy, subsequently securing the patient to the table at the level of the ankles, hips, and shoulders using 3-inch silk tape. Since the patient's arms are draped across the chest on a folded blanket or pillow, the elbows should be carefully padded so as to protect the ulnar nerve. Prior to initiation of the procedure, the table is rotated to test the tape and final position of the table. Each time the surgical table is moved, it is important to ensure that the patient clears all surrounding structures, such as the nurses' Mayo stand and monitors, and be certain that the patient is still properly padded.

Injury of the obturator nerve can result from pelvic lymphadenectomy for staging of prostate cancer. Complete transection should be managed by standard open repair using 6-0 polypropylene suture. Electrocautery should be used with caution—if at all—in the vicinity of the obturator nerve.

POSTOPERATIVE COMPLICATIONS

ABDOMINAL PAIN The occurrence of significant abdominal pain during the postoperative period should raise the suspicion of an underlying injury.

Rectus sheath hematoma may be suspected in any patient complaining of severe abdominal pain and who has a subcutaneous bulge. The tenderness and the guarding associated with hematoma may be confused with localized peritonitis. CT can confirm the diagnosis of abdominal wall hematoma (Figure 53-4). Since spontaneous resolution of hematoma is typical, an initial period of conservative treatment is appropriate. If there is any evidence of infected hematoma or fascial necrosis, immediate surgical exploration is recommended. Abdominal pain may also be the result of bleeding at the site of abdominal wall puncture. If incisional bleeding is identified, removal of the sutures and repeat suturing under local anesthesia may be necessary. It may be difficult to distinguish deep bleeding from bowel injury. A drop in hematocrit or an abdominal CT scan that reveals blood or a large fluid collection can help in the diagnosis (Figure 53-5).

Intestinal injury caused by electrocautery usually reveals itself within 48 hours postoperatively but may be delayed. Prompt diagnosis and management is critical to avoid major long-term sequelae. Patients may develop the classic signs of abdominal pain, fever, and signs of peritonitis that usually fail to respond to antibiotics. Many patients, however, present only with diarrhea and non-specific abdominal findings, such as specific trocar site tenderness.[44] Thus, any reasonable clinical suspicion of enteric injury needs to be investigated expediently, because morbidity and mortality increase significantly with a delay in diagnosis. Suspicion of intestinal injury necessitates continuous postoperative monitoring of vital signs, repeated abdominal exams, serial serum blood work, including complete blood counts and manual differentials, and a CT scan with oral Gastrograffin to determine if there is any evidence of bowel injury. Exploratory laparoscopy and/or laparotomy should be performed, regardless, if there is still strong clinical suspicion or unexplained findings.[65]

Interpretation of the CT scan is crucial and requires special attention to abnormal fluid col-

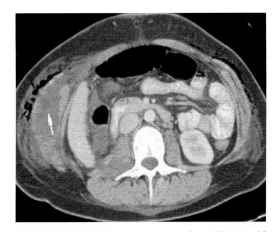

Figure 53-4 Flank wall hematoma in a 54-year-old woman s/p right laparoscopic nephrectomy with tachycardia and decreasing hemoglobin. Computed tomography on postoperative day 2 showed a hematoma (*arrow*) at the lateral trocar site. s/p = status post

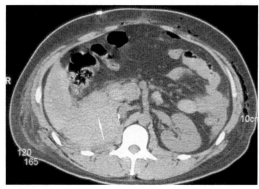

Figure 53-5 Retroperitoneal hematoma in a 43-year-old patient s/p left nephrectomy with tachycardia and decreasing hematocrit. Computed tomography shows hematoma (*arrow*) in renal fossa bed. s/p = status post

lections (urine, stool, blood) extraluminal oral contrast and/or the presence of intraperitoneal air. Oral Gastrograffin alone is usually sufficient, unless urinoma is strongly suspected. Intravenous contrast may be helpful in such situations. Free air in the abdomen is not always pathologic. Draper and colleagues studied 57 patients postlaparoscopy and found that air resolved in 46 patients by day 3 but persisted up to 7 days in 9 patients and beyond that in 2 patients.[66] Thus, the presence of free air alone does not warrant surgical exploration.

URINARY EXTRAVASATION WITH URINOMA Urinary extravasation and subsequent urinoma may occur after any perforation of the urinary drainage system. This is usually a consequence of inadequate drainage after procedures such as pyeloplasty, partial nephrectomy or radical prostatectomy. Less commonly, the cause may be an unrecognized ureteral or bladder injury. Patients frequently present with abdominal pain, ileus, leukocytosis, and fever, and less frequently, with flank tenderness and hematuria. Diagnosis can be made by intravenous urography, or abdominal/ pelvic CT scan. Once properly diagnosed, most problems can be addressed without surgical exploration. Antegrade or retrograde stenting of the ureter and bladder drainage can be used to address the acute injury. Any persistent or infected collections outside the urinary tract may require additional percutaneous drainage (Figure 53-6). Persistence of symptoms and or clinical deterioration may necessitate surgical exploration, drainage and repair.

SHOULDER PAIN Some degree of postoperative shoulder pain may be expected as a result of peritoneal diaphragmatic irritation from CO_2 due to conversion to carbonic acid. The pain is usually described as an arthralgic-like discomfort in one or both shoulders. It may occur in as many as one-third of patients but is severe in less than 5%. This pain can usually be managed with oral analgesics before resolving in 24 to 48 hours. To minimize the frequency and severity of shoulder pain postoperatively, CO_2 should be completely evacuated from the peritoneal cavity at the conclusion of the pro-

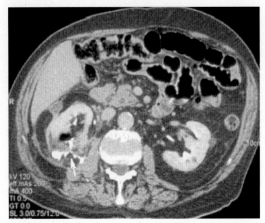

Figure 53-6 Urinoma in a 73-year-old male with ileus and flank pain following laparoscopic partial nephrectomy. Computed tomography scan with intravenous contrast shows extravasation of contrast consistent with urine leakage and urinoma at the tumor removal site. A percutaneous drain was placed, and the fistula resolved by postoperative day 21 with drainage of the urinoma.

cedure. Directing the laparoscope to the pocket of intra-abdominal gas, as well as having the anesthesiologist give some large tidal volumes, will help to evacuate the pneumoperitoneum.

INCISIONAL HERNIA   The risk of herniation in adults has primarily been associated with larger trocars, 10 to 12 mm (Figure 53-7). The 5-mm trocar seldom causes incisional hernia in adults, but can be a problem in children. Patients with chronic cough and umbilical hernia are at increased risk. To decrease the likelihood of postoperative incisional hernia, the use of a smaller diameter trocar has been suggested. Piercing the skin and fascia at different angles to create a Z tract will avoid the direct communication between the skin and fascial tracts and diminishes the chance of herniation. Proper closure of 10-mm and larger trocar sites, and taking adequate precautions to prevent infection at the trocar sites, will also help avoid incisional hernia.

We advocate use of the Carter-Thomason needlepoint fascial closure device (Inlet Medical, Eden Prairie, MN) to close incision greater than 5 mm in adults.[67] This device has a single-action jaw at the end of a sharp, needle-pointed grasper. This construction allows 3 "degrees of freedom"—translational movement in and out of the abdomen, rotational movement, and an end-effector jaw that allows it to grasp the suture. The jaw is open in the activated state to allow a double-stranded No. 1 polyglactin suture to be secured within the jaws of the device. By retracting the spring-loaded, handheld grip, one can open the jaw and grasp the suture.

The first pass of the Carter-Thomason device should start on the side of the incision away from the camera to optimize visualization and location of the suture during the second pass. Under direct visualization, the needle tip is pierced lateral to the incision (under direct vision) into the abdomen and is advanced away from the camera. The suture is dropped free, and the instrument withdrawn,

leaving one loop of the suture passed through the fascial edge. The device is then inserted on the contralateral side of the incision, the loop of suture grasped and pulled up through the incision. The suture edges are drawn up, the incision is probed with a finger to determine if a persistent fascial defect greater than 5 mm is encountered, and then the peritoneal view of the fascia is examined for bleeding and trapped viscera.

INTERNAL HERNIA   For patients with signs of a bowel obstruction where no clear fascial defect is identified, the possibility of an internal, especially mesenteric, hernia should be considered. Small bowel obstruction due to incarcerated small bowel through the large bowel mesentery is a possibility (Figure 53-8). CT scan is helpful in making the diagnosis. Knoepp and colleagues reported the possibility of this problem, as well as the need to close all mesenteric defects (even large bowel) during procedures.[68]

DEEP VENOUS THROMBOSIS   Deep venous thrombosis is a potential complication of any surgical procedure but does not appear to have a higher incidence in laparoscopic surgery. To minimize the risk of these complications, we use a sequential compression hose at 40 mm Hg. Early ambulation is also effective in preventing deep venous thrombosis.

ANESTHETIC COMPLICATIONS

Although anesthetic complications related to laparoscopic surgery are beyond the scope of this chapter, we will present a brief overview of such potential complications.

CHANGES IN CARDIOVASCULAR AND PULMONARY FUNCTION   Most of the anesthetic complications seen in laparoscopic surgery are related to CO_2 pneumoperitoneum and positioning. CO_2 insufflation of the peritoneal cavity will lead to an increase in the total peripheral resistance due to compression of the abdominal aorta, an increase

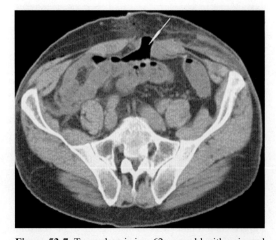

Figure 53-7 Trocar hernia in a 62-year-old with pain and fluid drainage from the umbilical trocar site. Computed tomography scan shows loop of small bowel which has herniated through midline trocar site.

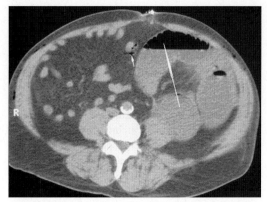

Figure 53-8 Mesenteric hernia in a 46-year-old patient returns 2 weeks postoperatively with nausea and vomiting. Abdominal computed tomography with oral contrast shows herniated loops of small bowel (*large arrow*) through small iatrogenic defect in descending colon during left laparoscopic nephrectomy. The diagnosis was made because these loops of small bowel are clearly lateral to the descending colon (*small arrow*).

in the sympathetic activity, and increased venous resistance. Compression of the inferior vena cava will lead to a decrease of venous return, decreased cardiac output, and eventually to hypotension.[69]

The effect of patient positioning and pneumoperitoneum on venous return and blood pressure is largely dependent on the state of the patient's intravascular volume prior to insufflation of CO_2. Factors such as preoperative bowel prep and decreased insensible loss of fluids compared to open surgery may play a role in assessing volume status.

Again, the insufflation pressure used for laparoscopy can result in significant changes in respiratory function. Hypercarbia is common during laparoscopic surgery due to absorption of CO_2 from the peritoneal cavity.[70] The degree of hypercarbia during laparoscopic surgery is related to the length of the procedure, as well as the development of significant subcutaneous emphysema.[71] Controlled ventilation can effectively maintain a normal $PaCO_2$ by maintaining adequate alveolar ventilation through increasing minute ventilation and respiratory rate.[70] Hypoxia may result from the elevated intra-abdominal pressure associated with the Trendelenburg position. Close monitoring of oxygen saturation with pulse oximetry (and correction by increasing the inspired oxygen concentration and with hyperventilation) can often correct this problem.

CARDIOVASCULAR COMPLICATIONS Cardiac Arrhythmia   Cardiac arrhythmias are common during laparoscopic surgery. In one study, 47% of patients developed arrhythmia, which was associated with bradycardia in 30% of patients.[72] The most common causes for arrhythmia during laparoscopic surgery include hypercarbia and hypoxia from hypoventilation during anesthesia with a decreased cardiac output and consequently lower coronary artery perfusion secondary to elevated intra-abdominal pressure and also to a profound vagal reflex response to the peritoneal distention.[73] Other rare causes of cardiac arrhythmias include gas embolism and endobronchial intubation. The management of arrhythmia includes (1) medication such as lidocaine, (2) reducing the anesthetic agent, especially if it is halothane, (3) administration of 100% oxygen in inspired air, (4) release of intra-abdominal pressure, and (5) verifying endotracheal tube placement.

Hypotension The most common causes of hypotension during laparoscopic surgery are hemorrhage, gas embolism, hypoxia, pneumothorax, or pneumomediastinum.

Hypertension Hypertension may result from hypercarbia, insufficient general anesthesia, or occasionally from high intra-abdominal pressure.

GASTRIC ASPIRATION It is possible that the combination of pneumoperitoneum and Trendelenburg's position predisposes to passive regurgitation, particularly in the relatively obese. The incidence, however, appears to be as low as 0.2%.[74] Preoperative administration of 10 mg metoclopramide hydrochloride orally or intravenously may decrease the incidence of regurgitation and aspiration. If the patient has a history of esophageal reflux, ranitidine or omeprazole will reduce the gastric acidity, and hence, minimize the potential consequences of pulmonary aspiration of gastric contents. In addition, a rapid-sequence induction of anesthesia can be used to reduce the risk of such aspiration.

HYPOTHERMIA The range and duration of operative laparoscopic techniques are expanding. This expansion exposes the patient to longer operative times, large volumes of CO_2 to maintain a pneumoperitoneum, and higher gas flow rates. CO_2 is obtained from cylinders or operating room lines and is routinely delivered unwarmed and dry. This may cause a reduction in the patient's body core temperature, which has been evaluated and found to be 0.3° to 3°C for each 50 L of CO_2 delivered.[75] Warming the CO_2 to a temperature of approximately 30°C prior to abdominal delivery has therefore been suggested and shown to be of value.[76]

OLIGURIA Transient intraoperative oliguria is a constant phenomenon during laparoscopic procedures due to compression of the pneumoperitoneum on the renal vein.[77] The effects of pneumoperitoneum at different pressures on the urinary output, creatinine clearance, and renal tubular cells were assessed in different experimental animal studies.[78,79] These studies demonstrated a significant decrease of urine output and creatinine clearance at an intra-abdominal pressure ≥ 10 mm Hg. These changes largely normalize 2 hours following desufflation.[80] Lee and colleagues demonstrated that there were no long-term effects or signs of chronic ischemic histologic changes detected for a period of 3 months after up to 5 hours of pneumoperitoneum.[81] As well, there was no change in the serum creatinine concentration after prolonged

pneumoperitoneum periods. Clinical trials are needed to determine the feasibility of operating at an intra-abdominal pressure of 10 mm Hg, rather than the standard 15 mm Hg.

RETROPERITONEAL APPROACH COMPLICATIONS

Since the majority of urologic procedures are performed in the retroperitoneal space, laparoscopic intervention in this area has expanded since the description of the balloon dilation technique of Gaur.[82] In the setting of previous abdominal surgery, or as a primary approach, the retroperitoneal approach is an alternative for therapeutic intervention. The retroperitoneal approach differs from the transperitoneal approach in terms of limited working space, orientation, and anatomic landmarks.[83] The open (Hasson) technique is used routinely for the retroperitoneal approach, thus eliminating the complications related to insertion of the Veress needle or initial blind trocar placement (such as perforation of a solid or hollow viscus, blood vessel injury, and gas embolism).

In a series of 404 retroperitoneal procedures (Meraney et al), vascular injuries were identified in 1.7% and bowel injuries in 0.25% of patients. Treatment of vascular incidents must incorporate several crucial factors regarding the etiology and extent of the injury, as well as the surgeon's level of laparoscopic experience. Conversion to an open procedure is always an option. Temporary packing of the area with gauze sponges placed through the 12-mm trocar can improve visualization. Furthermore, increasing the pneumoperitoneum to 20 mm Hg can also tamponade venous bleeding. Introduction of an additional port may facilitate tissue retraction, providing better exposure. Meraney and colleagues describe placement of a locking Allis clamp to grasp surrounding tissue in the area of bleeding, and twist 90 degrees, in order to aid hemostatic control. The risk of a serious electrocautery injury to a visceral organ is decreased, but one must still be conscious of their presence behind a thin veil of peritoneum.

ANALYSIS OF COMPLICATIONS

Laparoscopy is now firmly established in urology and is a standard of care for procedures for the kidney and adrenal gland. As with other surgical procedures, there is clearly an effect from the learning curve in developing one's laparoscopic skills, techniques, and familiarity with the instrumentation. The more difficult the procedure, the higher the complication rate. As one progresses from a simple case to the most difficult procedure, the complications increase ninefold. As experience grows, however, the incidence of complications decreases markedly. Fahlenkamp and colleagues reported a complication rate of 13.3% for the first 100 procedures, and subsequently, this rate decreased to 3.6%.[4]

Studies have compared one versus two proficient laparoscopic surgeons in order to determine if overall outcomes and complications were dif-

ferent. There was a decrease in total operative time (143 vs. 218 minutes) and estimated blood loss, (92 vs. 158 cc) favoring a surgical team with two proficient laparoscopic surgeons.[84] Early in the learning curve for complex procedures, such factors may help decrease it.

CONCLUSION

Recent data suggest that completion of a single post-residency instructional course, typically attended by practitioners interested in laparoscopy, may not be sufficient for optimal performance of a new skill, as measured by complication rates. See and colleagues suggest that ongoing educational experience through affiliation with others performing similar procedures can decrease long-term complication rates.[85] This may indicate that training and granting of privileges should be accompanied by a long-term commitment to study and work with those in urology with similar laparoscopic interests. With increasing laparoscopic experience, improvement in instrumentation, and further development of specialty-specific techniques, the complication rates should continue to decline. Laparoscopy will continue to evolve and become an increasingly important technique for the management of urologic disease.

REFERENCES

1. Vallancien G, Cathelineau X, Baumert H, et al. Complications of transperitoneal laparoscopic surgery in urology: review of 1,311 procedures at a single center. J Urol 2002;168:23–6.
2. Meraney AM, Samee AA, Gill IS. Vascular and bowel complications during retroperitoneal laparoscopic surgery. J Urol 2002 Nov;168:1941–4.
3. Soulie M, Salomon L, Seguin P, et al. Multi-institutional study of complications in 1,085 laparoscopic urologic procedures. Urology 2001;58:899–903.
4. Fahlenkamp K, Rassweiler J, Fornara P, et al. Complications of laparoscopic procedures in urology: experience with 2,407 procedures at 4 German centers. J Urol 1999;162:765–71.
5. Mintz M. Risks and prophylaxis in laparoscopy: a survey of 100,000 cases. J Reprod Med 1977;18:269–72.
6. Hulka JF, Peterson HB, Phillips JM. American Association of Gynecologic Laparoscopists' 1988 membership survey on laparoscopic sterilization. J Reprod Med 1990;35:584–6.
7. Vilardell F, Seves I, Marti-Vicente A. Complications of peritoneoscopy. A survey of 1,455 examinations. Gastrointest Endosc 1968;14:178–80.
8. Bailey RW. Complications of laparoscopic general surgery. In: Zucker KA, editor. Surgical laparoscopy. St. Louis: Quality Medical Publishing; 1991. p. 311–42.
9. Winfield HN, Donovan JF, See WA, et al. Urological laparoscopic surgery. J Urol 1991;146:941–8.
10. Parsons JK, Jarrett TJ, Chow GK, Kavoussi LR. The effect of previous abdominal surgery on urological laparoscopy. J Urol 2002;168:2387–90.
11. Pentecoast MP, Curtis EM. Laparoscopy. In: Ridley JH, editor. Gynecologic survey: errors, safeguards, salvage. Baltimore: Williams & Wilkins; 1981. p. 135–57.
12. Loffer F, Pent D. Indications, contraindications and complications of laparoscopy. Obstet Gynecol Surg 1975;30:4037–47.
13. Fujta O, Chan DY, Kavoussi LR, Jarrett TW. Laparoscopic nephrectomy in the markedly obese living renal donor. Urology 2000;56:926–9.
14. Yap RL, Chan DY, Fradin J, Jarrett TW. Intraoperative ultrasound guided retroperitoneal laparoscopic renal biopsy in the morbidly obese patient. J Urol 2000;163:1197–8.
15. Castilho LN, Fugita OE, Mitre AI, Arap S. Port site tumor recurrences of renal cell carcinoma after videolaparoscopic radical nephrectomy. J Urol 2001;165:519.

16. Schafer M, Lauper M, Krahenbuhl L. Trocar and Veress needle injuries during laparoscopy. Surg Endosc 2001;15:275.

17. Catarci M, Carlini M, Gentileschi P, Santoro E. Major and minor injuries during the creation of pneumoperitoneum. A multi-center study on 12,919 cases. Surg Endosc 2001;15:566–9.

18. De Cherney AH. Laparoscopy with unexpected viscus penetration. In: Nichols DH, editor. Clinical problems, injuries and complications of gynecologic surgery. 2nd ed. Baltimore: Williams & Wilkins; 1988. p. 62–3.

19. Gomel V, Taylor P, Yuzpe A, et al. Indications, contraindications and complications. In: Gomel V, editor. Laparoscopy and hysterectomy in gynecologic practice. Chicago: Year Book; 1986. p. 59–74.

20. Malinak LR, Wheeler JM, Simolke G. Vascular injuries at laparoscopy. In: Nichols DH, editor. Clinical problems, injuries and complications of gynecologic surgery. 2nd ed. Baltimore: Williams & Wilkins; 1988. p. 58–61.

21. McDonald PT, Rich NM, Collins GJ Jr, et al. Vascular trauma secondary to diagnostic and therapeutic procedures: laparoscopy. Am J Surg 1978;135:651–5.

22. Chamberlain GVP, Carron-Brown J. Gynecological laparoscopy. London: Royal College of Obstetricians and Gynecologists; 1978.

23. Kent RB. Subcutaneous emphysema and hypercarbia following laparoscopic cholecystectomy. Arch Surg 1991;126:1154–6.

24. Kalhan SB, Reaney JA, Collins RI. Pneumomediastinum and subcutaneous emphysema during laparoscopy. Cleve Clin J Med 1990;57:639–42.

25. Maunder RJ, Pierson DJ, Hudson LD. Subcutaneous and mediastinal emphysema, pathophysiology, diagnosis, and management. Arch Intern Med 1984;144:1447–1453.

26. Doctor NH, Hussain Z. Bilateral pneumothorax associated with laparoscopy: a case report of a rare hazard and review of the literature. Anaesthesia 1973;28:75–81.

27. McKenzie R. Laparoscopy. N Z Med J 1971;74:87–91.

28. Keith L, Silver A, Becker M. Anesthesia for laparoscopy. J Reprod Med 1974;12:227–33.

29. Fishburne JI Jr, Keith L. Anesthesia. In: Phillips JM, editor. Laparoscopy. Baltimore: Williams & Wilkins; 1977. p. 69–86.

30. McGrath RB, Zimmerman JF, Williams JF, et al. Carbon dioxide embolism treated with hyperbaric oxygen. Can J Anaesth 1989;36:586–9.

31. Diakun TA. Carbon dioxide embolism: successful resuscitation with cardiopulmonary bypass. Anesthesiology 1991;74:1151–3.

32. Phillips J, Hulka D, Hulka BJ, et al. Laparoscopic procedures: a national survey for 1975. J Reprod Med 1977;181:219–25.

33. Thomas MA, Rha KH, Ong AM, et al. Optical access trocar injuries in urological laparoscopic surgery. 2003;170:61–3.

34. Schafer M, Lauper M, Krahenbuhl L. Trocar and Veress needle injuries during laparoscopy. Surg Endosc 2001;15:275–80.

35. Kavoussi LR, Sosa RE, Capelouto C. Complications of laparoscopic surgery. J Endourol 1992;6:95–8.

36. Cooperman AM, Zucker KA. Laparoscopic guided intestinal surgery. In: Zucker KA, editor. Surgical laparoscopy. St. Louis: Quality Medical Publishing; 1991. p. 295–310.

37. Green LS, Loughlin KR, Kavoussi LR. Management of epigastric vessel injury during laparoscopy. J Endourol 1992;9:117–9.

38. Hasson HM. Open laparoscopy: a report of 150 cases. J Reprod Med 1974;12:234–8.

39. Ruckle H, Hadley R, Lui P, et al. Laparoscopic pelvic lymph node dissection: assessment of intraoperative and early postoperative complications. J Endourol 1992;6:117–9.

40. Hu JF, Soderstrom RM, Corson SL, et al. Complications committee of the American Association of Gynecologic Laparoscopists, first annual report. J Reprod Med 1973;10:301–6.

41. Lackritz RM. Bowel burn with laparoscopy. In: Nichols DH, editor. Clinical problems, injuries and complications of gynecologic surgery. 2nd ed. Baltimore: Williams & Wilkins; 1988. p. 64–5.

42. Landman J, Kerbl K, Rehman J, et al. Evaluation of a vessel sealing system, bipolar electrosurgery, harmonic scalpel, titanium clips, endoscopic gastrointestinal anastomosis vascular staples and sutures for arterial and venous ligation in a porcine model. J Urol 2003;169:697–700.

43. Wheeless CR. Thermal gastrointestinal injuries. In: Phillips JM, editor. Laparoscopy. Baltimore: Williams & Wilkins; 1977. p. 231–235.

44. Bishoff JT, Allaf M, Kirkels W, et al. Laparoscopic bowel injury: incidence and clinical presentation. J Urol 1999;161:887–90.

45. Aldana JP, Marcovich R, Singhal P, et al. Immune response to laparoscopic bowel injury. J Endourol 2003;17:317–22.

46. Wheeless CR Jr, et al. Gastrointestinal injuries associated with laparoscopy. In: Phillips JM, editor. Endoscopy in gynecology. American Association of Gynecologic Laparoscopists; 1978. p. 317–24.

47. Hulka JF. Complications. In: Hulka JF, editor. Textbook of laparoscopy. New York: Grune & Stratton; 1985. p. 119–30.

48. Theil R, Adams J, Schulum P, et al. Venous dissection injuries during laparoscopic urologic surgery. J Urol 1996;155:1874–6.

49. Montero M, Tellado MG, Rios J, et al. Aortic injury during diagnostic pediatric laparoscopy. Surg Endosc 2001;15:519.

50. Peterson HB, Greenspan JR, Ory HW. Death following puncture of the aorta during laparoscopic sterilization. Obstet Gynecol 1982;59:133–4.

51. McDonald PT, Rich NM, Collins GJ, et al. Vascular trauma secondary to diagnostic and therapeutic procedure: laparoscopy. Am J Surg 1978;135:652–5.

52. McGinnis DE, Strup SE, Gomella LG. Management of hemorrhage during laparoscopy. J Endourol 2000;14:915–21.

53. Capeluto CC, Kavoussi LR. Complications of laparoscopic surgery. Urology 1993;42:2–12.

54. Chan D, Bishoff JT, Ratner L, et al. Endovascular gastrointestinal stapler device malfunction during laparoscopic nephrectomy: early recognition and management. J Urol 2000;164:319–21.

55. Tulikangas PK, Beesley S, Boparai N, Falcone T. Assessment of laparoscopic injuries by three methods. Fertil Steril 2001;76:817–9.

56. Esposito JM. Hematoma of the sigmoid colon as a complication of laparoscopy. Am J Obstet Gynecol 1973;117:581–2.

57. Reich H, McGlynn F. Laparoscopic repair of bladder injury. Obstet Gynecol 1990;76:909–10.

58. Dowling RA, Corriere JN, Sandler CM. Iatrogenic ureteral injury. J Urol 1986;135:912–5.

59. Gomel V, James C. Intraoperative management of ureteral injury during operative laparoscopy. Fertil Steril 1991;55:416–9.

60. Guillonneau B, Gupta R, El Fettouh H, et al. Laparoscopic management of rectal injury during laparoscopic radical prostatectomy. J Urol 2003;169:11694–6.

61. Sabiston DC Jr. Antisepsis, technique, sutures and drains. In: Principles of operative surgery. 11th ed. Philadelphia: WB Saunders Co.; 1977. p. 323–9.

62. Del Pizzo JJ, Jacobs SC, Bishoff JT, et al. Pleural injury during laparoscopic renal surgery: early recognition and management. J Urol 2003;169:41–4.

63. Prentice JA, Martin JT. The Trendelenburg position—Anesthesiologic considerations. In: Positioning in anesthesia and surgery. Philadelphia: WB Saunders; 1987. p. 127–45.

64. Hershlag A, Loy RA, Lavy G, et al. Femoral neuropathy after laparoscopy. J Reprod Med 1990;35:575–76.

65. Yayciogly O. Early repeated exploration after laparoscopic urologic surgery: comparison of clinical, radiologic, and surgical findings. Urology 2002;;59:190–4.

66. Draper K, Jefson R, Jongeward R Jr, McLeod M. Duration of postlaparoscopic pneumoperitoneum. Surg Endosc 1997;11:809–11.

67. Lee BR. Closure techniques and exiting the abdomen. In: Bishoff JT, Kavoussi LR, editors. Atlas of laparoscopic retroperitoneal surgery. WB Saunders; 2000.

68. Knoepp L, Smith M, Huey J, et al. Complication after laparoscopic donor nephrectomy: a case report and review. Transplantation 1999;68:449–51.

69. Johannsen G, Anderson M, Juhl B. The effect of general anesthesia on the hemodynamic events during laparoscopy with CO2 insufflation. Acta Anaesthesiol Scand 1989;33:132–6.

70. Curlik M. Anesthetic considerations in urologic laparoscopy. In: Gomella LH, Kozminski M, Winfield H, eds. Laparoscopic urologic surgery. New York: Raven Press, 1994.

71. Sosa E, Weingram J, Stein B, et al. Hypercarbia in laparoscopic pelvic lymph node dissection. J Urol 1992;147:246A.

72. Myles PS. Bradyarrhythmias and laparoscopy: a prospective study of heart rate changes with laparoscopy. Aust N Z J Obstet Gynaecol 1991;31:171–3.

73. Harris NME. Cardiac arrythmias during anaesthesia for laparoscopy. Br J Anaesth 1984;56:1213–6.

74. Duffy BL. Regurgitation during pelvic laparoscopy. Br J Anaesth 1979;51:1089–90.

75. Ott DE. Laparoscopic hypothermia. J Laparoendosc Surg 1991;1:127–31.

76. Ott DE. Correction of laparoscopic insufflation hypothermia. J Laparoendosc Surg 1991;1:183–6.

77. Harman PK, Kron IL, McLachlan HD. Elevated intra-abdominal pressure and renal function. Ann Surg 1982;196:594–9.

78. Kirsch AJ, Hensle TW, Chang DT, et al. Increased intra-abdominal pressure causes oliguria and apoptosis secondary to vascular compromise in the rat pneumoperitoneum model. J Urol 1994;151:343A.

79. Vukasin A, Lopez M, Shicman S, et al. Oliguria in laparoscopic surgery. J Urol 1994;151:343A.

80. McDougall MM, Monk TG, Hicks M, et al. Effect of pneumoperitoneum on renal function in an animal model. J Urol 1994;151:462A.

81. Lee BR, Cadeddu JA, Molnar-Nadasdy G, et al. Effect of pneumoperitoneum on renal histology. J Endourol 1999;13:279–82.

82. Gaur DD. Laparoscopic operative retroperitoneoscopy: Use of a new device. J Urol 1992;148:1137–9.

83. Gill IS, Clayman RV, Albala DM, et al. Retroperitoneal and pelvic extraperitoneal laparoscopy: an international perspective. Urology 1998;52:566–71.

84. Siqueira TM, Gardner TA, Kuo RL, et al. One versus two proficient laparoscopic surgeons for laparoscopic live donor nephrectomy. Urology 2002;60:406–9.

85. See WA, Cooper CS, Fisher RJ. Predictors of laparoscopic complications after formal training in laparoscopic surgery. JAMA 1993;270:2689–92.

54

Encrusted Urinary Drains: Evaluation and Endourologic Management

Brian A. VanderBrink, MD

Encrustation is a clinical problem occurring with indwelling urinary drainage devices both external and internal. The chemical constituents of the urine combine with the tubing to form a matrix upon which further calcification occurs, with the end result being encrustation (Figure 54-1). A variety of factors contribute to the rate at which this process occurs, including the material of the stent or catheter, urine composition, and duration of contact of the drain with urine. This phenomenon can be observed with suprapubic and nephrostomy tubes as well as ureteral stents.

Ureteral stents have been used extensively in urology since their first description in 1967.[1] Their main application is towards preventing or treating obstruction within the urinary tract secondary to a variety of causes (eg, calculus disease, malignancy, edema following reconstructive surgeries). Attendant to their use are their associated morbidities, such as pain, infection, and encrustation.[2] The encrusted stent has many names throughout the literature: the retained stent, forgotten stent, and the overlooked stent.[3,4] The "forgotten" stent may be asymptomatic and "remembered" only when its presence is incidentally revealed with abdominal imaging. Conversely, a patient with ureteral obstruction from an encrusted stent can present with urosepsis that can prove lethal in some cases.[5]

This chapter is intended to review the literature on the subject of the encrusted stents and drainage catheters, discuss the risk factors for

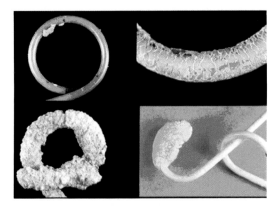

Figure 54-1 Encrustation of varying composition and severity on ureteral stents. Reproduced with permission from Roupret M, Daudon M, Hupertan V, et al. Can ureteral stent encrustation analysis predict urinary stone composition? Urology 2005;66:246–51.

encrustation, and describe the endourologic evaluation and management of these encrusted and retained urinary drainage devices.

RISK FACTORS FOR ENCRUSTATION

While no formal consensus exists as to the maximum indwelling time for internal ureteral stents, prior studies have shown increasing rates of encrustation with increasing indwelling time. El-Faqih and colleagues, in a series of 290 stone patients with 141 stents retrieved and examined, discovered that encrustation occurred in 9.2% of the stents retrieved prior to six weeks, in 47.5% when indwelling for 6 to 12 weeks, and which rose to 76.3% at longer than 12 weeks.[6] Clinical obstruction, however, as evidenced by urography or isotope studies, was recorded in only 5% of the patient population and was absent with indwelling periods of less than 6 weeks. Most case reports and patent series of encrusted stents consistently show that the stent had been in place for more than three months.

There are conflicting reports about whether the composition of the stent is a factor in degree of encrustation. *In vitro* studies have shown that hydrophilic-coated polyurethane stents encrust faster and to a larger extent than silicone or non–hydrophilic-coated polyurethane stents.[7] The hydrophilic coating is used to reduce the coefficient of friction of the stent during endourologic placement, but this hydrogel coating is permeable to inorganic salts and may account for the enhanced risk of encrustation. In a separate study, Wollin and colleagues demonstrated that stent type and duration of insertion did not correlate significantly with the amount of encrustation observed from stents retrieved from humans after 11 to 17 days.[8]

A history of urolithiasis also predisposes one to develop encrustations. In a clinical study of 40 patients, Robert and colleagues found that patients with a history of urolithiasis had a nearly threefold increased risk of encrustation of ureteral stents compared to non-stone formers.[9] Formation of encrustations is also dependent on both the urinary constituents and bacterial colonization.[10] When in contact with urine, the stents are rapidly covered by a bacterial biofilm and, with continued growth, can lead to obstruction of the urine flow and possibly urinary tract sepsis (Figure 54-2).[8] In the presence of urease-

producing organisms—especially a species of Proteus—hydrolysis of urea occurs, and the corresponding elevation of pH induces the deposition of calcium and magnesium phosphate crystals along this biofilm. In non-infected urine, the encrustations often result from accumulation of calcium oxalate on the surface.[11]

Investigators have recently developed a novel method to specifically target this chemical reaction to reduce calcium deposition. Watterson and colleagues coated circular silicone disks with oxalate-degrading enzymes and implanted these disks in a rabbit model for 30 days.[12] There was a 21% and 40% reduction in dry weight of encrustation and calcium within the encrustation, respectively, in the experimental group compared to the control group. Other attempts to eliminate or reduce encrustation of urinary drainage devices have been pursued using a variety of techniques. Hyaluronic acid, heparin and pentosan polysulfate sodium are types of glycosaminoglycans, which are compounds that are extremely potent inhibitors of nucleation, crystal growth, and aggregation.[13–15] Glycosaminoglycan-coated stents and catheters have demonstrated increased resistance to encrustations in

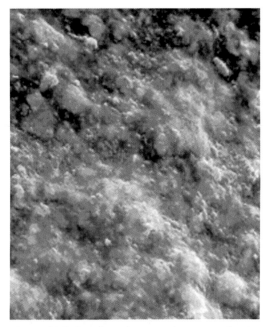

Figure 54-2 Scanning electron microscopy of polyurethane ureteral stent following use demonstrating biofilm and surface irregularities from encrustations.

experimental studies.[16,17] Other methods demonstrated in vitro to reduce encrustations in urinary catheters include electrified catheters,[18] inflation of balloon retention devices with the antibacterial solution triclosan,[19] intermittent, rather than continuous, drainage through the catheter,[20] and irrigations with Suby G solution.[21]

EVALUATION OF ENCRUSTED STENT AND SELECTION OF EXTRACTION TECHNIQUE

Imaging plays a pivotal role in determining the appropriate surgical management of the encrusted and retained stent. The principal chemical composition of the encrustation surrounding the stent is typically calcium-based, and a plain film such as a kidney, ureter, and bladder (KUB) should suffice enough to assess the degree of encrustation along with any associated stone burdens on the proximal or distal coils (Figure 54-3). Quantifying the stone burden associated with encrustation by multiplying the width of encrustation around the stent by the length expressed in millimeters squared (mm^2) or direct measurement can have some prognostic significance. Some authors have suggested that a severe stone burden (> 400 mm^2) or calcifications > 3 mm over one-third of the stent are more likely to require a multimodal or percutaneous therapeutic approach to render the patient stone-free.[22–24] Computerized tomography or ultrasonography can also help assess stone burden, especially in the uric acid stone former, where the stones are radiolucent and the extent possibly underestimated by radiograph (Figure 54-4). If the stone burden is large, assessment of differential renal function with radionucleotide studies is prudent. This test serves a twofold purpose; to determine pre-procedural

function in what may be potentially a litigious situation, and to evaluate the function of the affected renal unit. A poorly functioning kidney with significant stone burden may be better suited with a nephrectomy rather than multiple procedures to eliminate all stones. However, case series have reported significant recovery of renal function following endourologic management of severely encrusted ureteral stents.[25]

If there is no encrustation visible on radiograph, an attempt to remove the stent in a retrograde fashion may be attempted. Ideally, fluoroscopy should be available to see if there is uncoiling of the proximal curl during removal, as this may be a site of resistance. If there is any resistance, or if the patient complains of significant pain during attempts at cystoscopic removal, one should stop immediately since the risk of stent fracture or ureteral injury cannot be ignored. At times, it may be possible to remove the stent outside the urethral meatus prior to meeting resistance. If this occurs a guidewire can be passed retrograde through the lumen of the stent in an attempt to determine its patency or to straighten the proximal curl. If these measures prove unsuccessful, then a procedure to address likely encrustation of the proximal curls will be required. In cases where encrustation is minimal, extracorporeal shock wave lithotripsy (ESWL) has been used with high success rate.[26–29] After adequate treatment, repeat cystoscopy can be performed and retrieval of stent attempted in the same setting.

Significant stone encrustation of the vesical portion of the stent can be addressed by performing

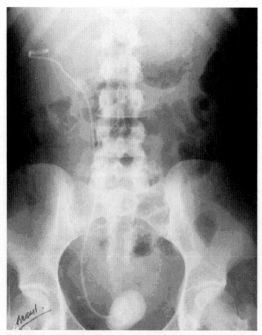

Figure 54-3 Plain film of a patient with a retained ureteral stent and bladder stones. Reproduced with permission from Lam JS, Gupta M.[34]

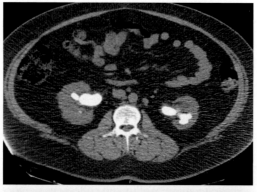

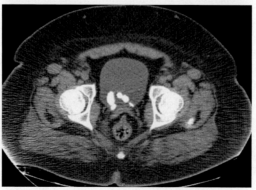

Figure 54-4 Computerized tomography images of the proximal and distal ends of a completely encrusted stent from a patient whose severity of encrustation was significantly underestimated by plain films. Stone composition on stents was uric acid.

transurethral cystolitholapaxy using either laser, electrohydraulic, or pneumatic lithotripsy. Calcifications along the ureteral component of the stent can be treated with retrograde ureteroscopy and laser lithotripsy (see the video clip on the accompanying CD-ROM).[30,31] In certain cases, it can be difficult for the ureter to accommodate both the ureteroscope and stent. When this occurs, placing a new ureteral stent alongside the encrusted stent and waiting for the ureter to passively dilate, and performing interval ureteroscopy may be beneficial.[32] Some authors have reported high success rates in treating calcified stents using endourologic techniques in a single anesthetic setting,[31,33,34] but it is not unusual to need multiple sessions to successfully render the patient stent- and stone-free, depending upon which modalities are used.[22,24,25]

Antegrade nephroscopy and ureteroscopy can also serve as alternative means to access the proximal collecting system to perform lithotripsy on a calcified ureteral stent.[35] The percutaneous route, as with uncomplicated nephrolithiasis, is the preferred primary approach when stone size is greater than 2 cm and/or if there is associated significant encrustation on the proximal ureteral end of the stent.[22,23,35] In the case of simultaneous large proximal and distal encrustations, the issue of which encrusted end to address first (proximal or distal) is a matter of both preference and severity of stone burden. Treating the lower coil first transurethrally, placing a ureteral catheter retrograde, and repositioning the patient to the prone position to obtain percutaneous access to treat the upper coil is an efficient and logical approach.

An alternative non-surgical option to treating the encrustation is the instillation of chemolytic agents via nephrostomy tube. Case reports using hemiacidrin and Suby's G solution to dissolve associated stones and encrustation followed by successful cystoscopic retrieval of the stent have been described.[36,37] These agents should be reserved for extreme cases, given their irritating effects on the lower urinary tract and the need for close monitoring secondary to potential electrolyte imbalances from systemic absorption.

EVALUATION AND MANAGEMENT OF ENCRUSTED AND RETAINED NEPHROSTOMY TUBE

Percutaneous nephrostomy and suprapubic tubes are also subject to the same complication of encrustation as ureteral stents with prolonged indwelling times precluding their removal (Figure 54-5). Several reports are in the literature detailing the inability to remove the nephrostomy tubes and their respective management.[38–44] The type of drainage catheter can affect the etiology behind the entrapment. A common finding with a retained Malecot nephrostomy tube is that the flange of the Malecot catheter can become anchored to the urothelium by tissue bridges or adhesions. This can be due to either prolonged use or from an unusual complication, perforation of the renal pelvis from the Malecot nephrostomy tube, and resulting inflammatory response to the

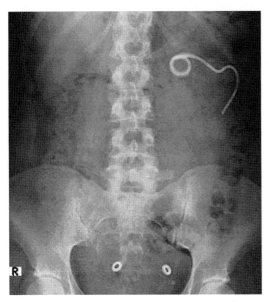

Figure 54-5 Calcified nephrostomy from a female patient who had it placed for symptomatic nephrolithiasis during pregnancy.

injury to the renal pelvis entrapping the flange within the renal sinus (Figure 54-6).

Tasca and Cacciola describe a case report of entrapped nephrostomy tube in a 61-year-old woman where a nephrostomy tract was created alongside the Malecot catheter, and the overgrown tissue bridging the wings of the tube was incised with a urethrotome.[38] In a similar fashion, Koolpe and Lord described the dilation of an eccentric

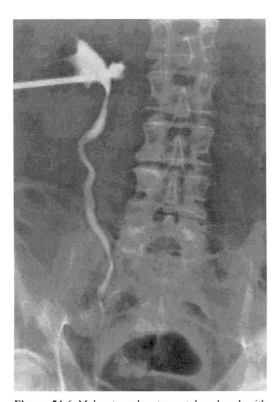

Figure 54-6 Malecot nephrostomy tube placed with unrecognized renal pelvis perforation. Attempts to remove it were met with resistance, and the incorrect positioning was revealed with nephrostogram. The tube was removed percutaneously after removing the adhesions from the tube and the renal sinus.

nephrostomy tract alongside the existing nephrostomy tube with lysis of calcifications and tissue bridges using nephroscopy.[39] Less invasive methods have been described utilizing the tube as the conduit for passing instruments. Bellman and colleagues described a novel method of treating a retained nephrostomy tube that had been in place for a nine-week period for bacilli Calmette-Guérin instillation.[40] The authors passed a stone-grasping forceps through the Malecot nephrostomy tube under fluoroscopic guidance to straighten the flanges and applied electrocautery to incise tissue, enabling easy removal. (Figure 54-7) Sardina and colleagues described a similar minimally invasive approach by placing a 9 French pediatric cystoscope though the lumen and utilized a Bugbee electrode to incise a tissue bridge in 3 patients.[41]

Once again, during the evaluation, imaging helps to determine the extent of calcification and the operative approach. Large stone burdens on the proximal end of the nephrostomy tube may necessitate ESWL, ureteroscopic lithotripsy, percutaneous nephrolithotomy, or a combined approach. Percutaneous access through an adjacent calix may be necessary to perform lithotripsy on the calcified portion of the nephrostomy tube to allow for removal. Intraluminal pneumatic lithotripsy within the encrusted nephrostomy tube under fluoroscopic guidance in concert with ureteroscopic lithotripsy has been described to straighten and remove a nephrostomy tube.[42]

CONCLUSIONS

The combination of potential significant morbidity associated with neglected internal stents and the increased mobility of our society and patients, has provided the impetus for the pursuit of novel methods to limit such complications. A computerized tracking system for patients with indwelling ureteral stents has been advocated to reduce the number of forgotten stents.[45,46] Ather and colleagues noted the incidence of long-term indwelling stents decreased to 1.2% from 12.5% with the use of a software program that alerted the urologist that the stent needed to be addressed.[45] Altering the manner in which ureteral drainage is achieved is another way to reduce the number of patients lost to follow-up. Mydlo and Streater employed straight ureteral stents exteriorized through the urethral meatus and connected to a urethral catheter following ureteroscopy in presumably non-compliant patients.[47] In this study, all patients with straight ureteral stents returned for follow-up, whereas only 45% of those with internal stents did. Of course, this increased compliance comes at the expense of added morbidity from exteriorized stent and catheter.

Absorbable and biodegradable ureteral stents have been proposed as the ideal way to accomplish temporary drainage without the need for removal or follow-up.[48] Unfortunately, these stents have not been without problems. In a phase II multi-institutional clinical trial of temporary biodegradable ureteral drainage stents, 4.5% of patients had

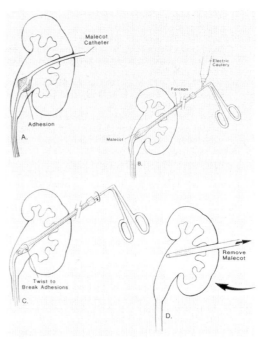

Figure 54-7 Diagram of nephrostomy tube removal. *A*, Malecot tip of nephrostomy tube entrapped in the renal pelvis by adhesions. *B*, Stone-grasping forceps straightening Malecot flanges and positioned for incision of tissue with electrocautery. *C*, Forceps are rotated in both directions to free the nephrostomy tube. Reproduced with permission from Bellman GC, et al.[40]

a severe adverse event related to the stent resulting from stent migration or problems with stent fragment passage.[49] Fortunately, all patients were treated endoscopically with no adverse sequelae. Nonuniform and incomplete dissolution are technical hurdles still needing to be overcome prior to widespread applicability of this technology.

Finally, it is of paramount importance that the treating urologist communicates clearly to the patient the presence of any internal urologic stents, the temporary intent of their use, risks with prolonged indwelling times and need for appropriate follow-up. While external draining catheters, such as nephrostomy or suprapubic tubes, are not hidden, these patients must also be educated about the need for regular maintenance and follow-up if they are to be kept in situ for prolonged periods of time. Unfortunately, with all of these precautions exercised, stenting and draining of the urinary tract will continue to be an essential part of the practice of urology, and until an improved way to accomplish this task evolves, there will be patients who will inevitably encounter complications from their use.

REFERENCES

1. Zimskind PD, Fetter TR, Wilkerson JL. Clinical use of long-term indwelling silicone ureteral splints inserted cystoscopically. J Urol 1967;97:840–4.
2. Saltzman B. Ureteral stents. Indications, variations, and complications. Urol Clin North Am 1988;15:481–91.
3. Monga M, Klein E, Castañeda-Zúñiga WR, Thomas R. The forgotten indwelling ureteral stent: a urological dilemma. J Urol 1995;153:1817–9.
4. Persky L, Lockhart JJ, Karp R, et al. The overlooked, retained double-J stent. Urology 1990;36:519–521.
5. Singh V, Srinivastava A, Kapoor R, Kumar A. Can the com-

plicated forgotten indwelling uretric stents be lethal? Int Urol Nephrol 2005;37:541–6.

6. El-Faqih SR, Shamsuddin AB, Chakrabarti A, et al. Polyurethane internal ureteral stents in treatment of stone patients: morbidity related to indwelling times. J Urol 1991;146:1487–91.

7. Tunney MM, Keane PF, Jones DS, Gorman SP. Comparative assessment of ureteral stent biomaterial encrustation. Biomaterials 1996;17:1541–6.

8. Wollin TA, Tieszer C, Riddell JV, et al. Bacterial biofilm formation, encrustation and antibiotic adsorption to ureteral stents indwelling in humans. J Endourol 1998;12:101–11.

9. Robert M, Boularan AM, El Sandid M, Gasset D. Double-J ureteral stent encrustations: clinical study on crystal formation on polyurethane stents. Urol Int 1997;58:100–4.

10. Ramsay JWA, Crocker RP, Ball AJ. Urothelial reaction to ureteric intubation. Br J Urol 1987;66:66.

11. Reid G, Davidson R, Denstedt JD. XPS, SEM and EDX analysis of conditioning film deposition on ureteral stents. Surf Interface Anal 1994;21:581–6.

12. Watterson JD, Cadieux PA, Beiko DT, et al. Oxalate-degrading enzymes from oxalobacter formingenes: a novel device coating to reduce urinary tract biomaterial-related encrustation. J Endourol 2003;17:269–74.

13. Kitamura T, Zerwekh J, Pak C. Partial biochemical and physiochemical characterization of organic macromolecules in urine from patients with renal stones and control subjects. Kidney Int 1982;21:379–86.

14. Leal J, Finlayson B. Absorption of naturally occurring polymers on to calcium oxalate surfaces. Invest Urol 1977;14:278–83.

15. Robertson WG, Peacock M, Nordin B. Inhibitors of the growth and aggregation of calcium oxalate crystals in vitro. Clin Chem Acta 1973;43:31.

16. TenkeP, Riedl CR, Jones GL, et al. Bacterial biofilm formation on urologic devices and heparin coating as preventive strategy. Int J Antimicrob Agents 2004;23:67–74.

17. Zupkas P, Parsons CL, Percival C, Monga M. Pentosanpolysulfate coating of silicone reduces encrustation. J Endourol 2000;14:483–8.

18. Chakravarti A, Gangodawila S, Long MJ, et al. An electrified catheter to resist encrustation by Proteus mirabilis biofilm. J Urol 2005;174:1129–32.

19. Sticker DJ, Jones GL, Russell AD. Control of encrustation and blockage of Foley catheters. Lancet 2003;361:1435–7.

20. Sabbuba NA, Sticker DJ, Long MJ, et al. Does the valve regulated release of urine from the bladder decrease encrustation and blockage of indwelling catheters by crystalline proteus mirabilis biofilms? J Urol 2005;173:262–6.

21. Getliffe KA. The use of bladder wash-outs to reduce urinary catheter encrustation. Br J Urol 1994;73:696–700.

22. Singh I, Gupta NP, Hemal AK, et al. Severely encrusted polyurethane ureteral stents: management and analysis of potential risk factors. Urology 2001;58:526–31.

23. Somers WJ. Management of forgotten or retained indwelling ureteral stents. Urology 1996;47:431–5.

24. Borboroglu PG, Kane CJ. Current management of severely encrusted ureteral stents with a large associated stone burden. J Urol 2000;164:648–50.

25. Mohan-Pillai K, Keeley FX, Moussa SA, et al. Endourological management of severely encrusted ureteral stents. J Endourol 1999;13:377–9.

26. Smet G, Vandeursen H, Baert L. Extracorporeal shock wave lithotripsy for calcified ureteral catheter. Urol Int 1991;46:211.

27. Cass AS, Kavaney PB, Smith CL. Multiple cystine stone formations on an indwelling ureteral stent treated by extracorporeal shock wave lithotripsy. J Urol 1992;147:1076.

28. Lupu AN, Fuch GJ, Chaussy CG. Calcification of ureteral stent treated by extracorporeal shock wave lithotripsy. J Urol 1986;136:1297–8.

29. Flam TA, Debre B, Brochard M, et al. Extracorporeal shock wave lithotripsy to remove calcified stents. Urology 1990;36:164–5.

30. Killeen KP, Bihrle W. Ureteroscopic removal of retained ureteral double-J stents. Urology 1990;35:354–9.

31. Bukkapatnam R, Seigne J, Helal M. 1-step removal of encrusted retained ureteral stents. J Urol 2003;170:1111–4.

32. Hubert KC, Palmer JS. Passive dilation by ureteral stenting before ureteroscopy: eliminating the need for active dilation. J Urol 2005;174:1079–80.

33. Teichman JM, Lackner JE, Leveillee J, Hulbert JC. Total endoscopic management of encrusted ureteral stent under a single anesthesia. Can J Urol 1997;4:456–9.

34. Lam JS, Gupta M. Tips and tricks for the management of retained ureteral stents. J Endourol 2002;16:733–41.

35. LeRoy AJ, Williams HJ Jr, Segura JW, et al. Indwelling ureteral stents: percutaneous management of complications. Radiology 1986;158:219–22.

36. Abber JC, Kahn RI. Pyelonephritis from severe incrustations on silicone ureteral stents: management. J Urol 1983;130:763–4.

37. Schulze KA, Wettlaufer JN, Oldani G. Encrustation and stone formation. Complication of stents. Urology 1985;25:616–8.

38. Tasca A, Cacciola A. Mini-invasive management of a rare complication of percutaneous stone treatment: entrapped nephrostomy tube. Urol Int 2004;72:165–7.

39. Koolpe HA, Lord B. Eccentric nephroscopy for the incarcerated nephrostomy. Urol Radiol 1990;12:96–8.

40. Bellman GC, Pardalidas N, Smith AD. Endourologic management of retained surgical drains and nephrostomy tubes. J Endourol 1994;8:115–7.

41. Sardina JI, Bolton DM, Stoller ML. Entrapped Malecot nephrostomy tube: etiology and management. J Urol 1995;153:1882–3.

42. Canby-Hagino ED, Caballero RD, Harmon WJ. Intraluminal pneumatic lithotripsy for the removal of encrusted urinary catheters. J Urol 1999;162:2058–60.

43. Rudy DC, Seigel RS, Woodside JR. Removal of incarcerated nephrostomy tube with Gruntzig catheter. Urology 1983;21:188–9.

44. Stewart LH, Kernohan RM, Loughridge WG. Nephrostomy tubes resistant to removal. Br J Urol 1992;70:213–4.

45. Ather MH, Talati J, Biyabani R. Physician responsibility for removal of implants: the case for a computerized program for tracking overdue double-J stents. Tech Urol 2000;6:189–92.

46. McChay PJ, Ramsden PD. A computerized ureteric stent retrieval system. Br J Urol 1996;77:147–8.

47. Mydlo JH, Streater S. The applicability of using straight ureteral stents for the treatment of ureteral stones in presumably non-compliant patients. Urol Int 2001;66:107–12.

48. Auge BK, Ferraro RF, Madenjian AR, Preminger GM. Evaluation of a dissolvable ureteral drainage stent in a swine model. J Urol 2002 168:808.

49. Lingeman JE, Preminger GM, Berger Y, et al. Use of a temporary ureteral drainage stent after uncomplicated ureteroscopy: results from a phase II clinical trial. J Urol 2003;169:1682–8.

Pelvic Lymphadenectomy

Chandru P. Sundaram, MD, FRCS

In 1991, Schuessler and associates first reported laparoscopic pelvic lymph node dissection (LPLND) for staging of prostate cancer.[1] In the early '90s, LPLND was the most frequently performed urologic laparoscopic surgery. With the stage migration in prostate cancer because of widespread screening of patients, LPLND is not frequently performed. The operation provides useful information in a patient with prostate cancer where pathologic involvement of the pelvic lymph nodes will alter definitive management of the prostate cancer. Today, although LPLND is most commonly performed for the surgical staging of prostate cancer (CaP), extended versions of this staging modality are performed in a few selected patients with malignancy of the bladder, urethra and penis, where confirmation of nodal metastases could significantly alter management. LPLND is increasingly performed as part of laparoscopic radical prostatectomy with or without robotic assistance. For patients with urologic pelvic malignancy, the status of the pelvic lymph nodes will have a major impact on prognosis as well as the determination of appropriate therapeutic intervention. It is generally agreed that extensive lymphatic dissemination of malignancy in a patient with neoplastic disease involving the prostate, bladder, urethra, or penis is a sign that the cancer is likely incurable in most patients. To empirically forge ahead with an aggressive course of treatment when the lymph node status is unknown could subject the patient to unwarranted morbidity since the outcome of the disease will not be significantly altered if lymphatic dissemination has occurred. This eventuality underscores the importance of obtaining accurate histopathologic staging information prior to developing a treatment plan.

In the past, attempts at detecting pelvic lymphatic metastases using noninvasive diagnostic modalities such as computed tomography (CT), magnetic resonance imaging, and pelvic lymphangiography have been unsatisfactory as a result of unacceptably low sensitivity and specificity.[2–5] Ultrasound and CT-guided transcutaneous fine-needle aspiration biopsy can be effective when evaluating enlarged pelvic lymph nodes. Unfortunately, these interventions are highly operator-dependent, and in the absence of gross lymphadenopathy are incapable of determining the presence of micrometastasis following early dissemination of malignancy. Therefore pelvic lymph node dissection remains the gold standard for accurate staging of patients with urologic pelvic malignancy. Procedures performed with the intention of sampling pelvic lymphatic tissue are only indicated for those patients in whom knowledge of the lymph node status is needed to direct further therapeutic decisions. Specifically, in patients of advanced age or who have severe comorbidity to such an extent that radical surgery or the administration of radiation therapy with curative intent would be intolerable, the benefit of evaluating the lymph node status is negligible.

INDICATIONS

ADENOCARCINOMA OF THE PROSTATE In a 1959 landmark study that evaluated the common lymphatic pathways by which metastatic adenocarcinoma of the prostate spreads, Flocks and colleagues clearly demonstrated a direct correlation between the clinical stage of disease and an increased likelihood of lymphatic metastasis.[6] This was especially true in patients in whom periprostatic extension involved the seminal vesicles; pelvic lymph node metastasis was noted in 50 to 80% of patients under these circumstances. Similarly, elevation of serum tumor markers, including enzymatic prostatic acid phosphatase and prostate-specific antigen (PSA), may suggest an increased likelihood of lymph node involvement. Stamey and Kabalin demonstrated a strong correlation between advanced clinical stage and increasing serum PSA to advancing pathologic stage.[7] Similarly, others reported studies that focused on the correlation between serum PSA and pathologic stage.[8,9] Partin and colleagues confirmed that the prevalence of pelvic lymph node involvement correlated with serum PSA, clinical stage and histologic grade.[10]

Although these important studies have greatly increased the urologist's ability to predict the extent of disease in patients with CaP, the associations are by no means absolute. Unfortunately, the relationship between serum tumor markers and actual pathologic stage is not clear cut. A markedly elevated PSA level is strongly indicative of advanced disease, whereas a PSA of less than 10 ng/mL suggests early local disease. To rely on these values alone, however, may lead to an under- or overstaging of CaP, resulting in erroneous therapeutic intervention and unwarranted morbidity with no clinical improvement in the patient's outcome.[10] For this reason, histopathologic evaluation of the pelvic lymph node specimen remains the gold standard for making therapeutic decisions.[11] Before 1980, the surgical staging of CaP included a lymph node dissection of all fibrofatty lymph–node-bearing tissue within the space bounded by the genitofemoral nerve laterally, the common iliac vessels proximally, and Cloquet's node distally. This extensive lymphadenectomy effectively removed the common and external iliac, hypogastric, and obturator lymph node groups. Unfortunately, the extent of this dissection led to an early complication rate of 12 to 24%, with patients experiencing lymphocele formation, lymphedema, and thromboembolic phenomena.[12] Over the last 20 years, a less extensive lymphadenectomy has been advocated. This modification in the margins of dissection was based on the knowledge that 85 to 95% of lymph node positivity in patients with lymph node metastases was found within the obturator-hypogastric node packets. Furthermore, the incidence of so-called metastatic skip lesions, which bypass the primary obturator-hypogastric landing zones to involve the more proximal iliac or aortic chains, was reported to be only 6 to 14%.[13,14] These findings have led to the standardization of obturator-hypogastric lymphadenectomy as an acceptable procedure for the pathologic staging of patients with CaP.

Clark and colleagues from Vanderbilt University, randomized 123 patients undergoing radical prostatectomy to an extended node dissection on the right versus the left side of the pelvis with the other side being a limited dissection.[15] The limited dissection only included nodes along the external iliac vein and the obturator nerve. Pelvic nodal metastases were found in eight patients (6.5%). Positive nodes were found in four patients on the side of the extended dissection and in three patients on the side of the limited dissection, and on both sides in one patient. They concluded that extended node dissection in patients undergoing radical prostatectomy identifies few patients with nodal involvement that are not detected by a limited dissection. Complications, which included lymphocele in four patients, lower extremity edema in five, deep venous thrombosis in two, and ureteral injury and pelvic abscess in one each, occurred three times more often on the side of the extended dissection. This was, however, a group of patients with a low probability for nodal metastases.[15] A 2002 report, however, advocates a more medial boundary that includes the lymphatic tissue along the hypogastric vessels. In the study of 365 patients who underwent meticulous lymph node dissection along the external iliac vein, the obturator nerve, and the hypogastric vessels during an open radical retropubic prostatectomy, positive lymph nodes were found in the nodes along the hypogastric artery in 58% of patients, and exclusively at that site in 19%.[16]

LPLND is most useful in a patient in whom metastatic prostate cancer is detected and the morbidity of treatment for presumed localized prostate cancer is avoided. Conversely, patients who undergo LPLND and do not have nodal metastases have had an unnecessary procedure. Wolf used cost and patient preference end points and a decision analysis model, and determined that LPLND before intended open radical retropubic prostatectomy was beneficial only in patients with at least a 39% risk of lymph node metastases.[17] The risk of pelvic nodal metastases had to be only 20% to justify LPLND in patients prior to a radical perineal prostatectomy. At Indiana University, in patients undergoing laparoscopic radical prostatectomy, a PSA of greater than 10, a Gleason score ≥ 7, or Clinical Stage T2b, are indications for LPLND during the same procedure.

Similar analyses have not been performed for patients considering radiotherapy. Obvious nodal involvement portends poor prognosis following radiotherapy, but the benefit of LPLND before radiotherapy is not clear. Gerber and associates compared the outcome of 31 men who had localized prostate cancer and negative LPLND with 42 men who had localized prostate cancer and who underwent radiotherapy without lymph node dissection. There was no significant difference in follow-up PSA or development of skeletal metastases between the two groups after controlling for PSA levels, Gleason scores and clinical stage.[18]

Nomograms by Partin and associates, which are based on over 4,000 patients treated for prostate cancer, can be used to determine the risk of nodal metastases in a patient based on PSA, clinical stage, and Gleason score. The risk of nodal involvement obtained from these tables may be used to determine the indication for an LPLND in an individual patient.[19] As was previously suggested, the likelihood of encountering lymphatic metastasis in patients with low-stage/low-grade disease (T1a, T1c, T2a, and/or well-differentiated) is less than 25%. In this cohort, if surgical intervention is elected, it is generally considered appropriate to proceed directly to radical retropubic prostatectomy with concomitant open pelvic lymph node dissection. Alternatively, if radical perineal prostatectomy is considered, the minimally invasive nature of LPLND makes it the ideal procedure if pathologic staging is warranted based on preoperative physical examination and laboratory evaluation.

Patients who may be considered for LPLND before definitive treatment of prostate cancer include those with:

1. Clinical stage T2b or higher,
2. Gleason scores of > 7,
3. Serum PSA of ≥ 20 ng/mL (Hybritech assay),
4. Positive seminal vesicle biopsy (T3c),
5. Enlarged lymph nodes on pelvic imaging, when percutaneous biopsy was not possible.

As will be discussed elsewhere in this chapter, a more extensive pelvic lymphadenectomy is appropriate for staging cancers involving primary sites with a more proximal lymphatic drainage (see "Cancer of the Penis"). Although extended lymphadenectomy is usually advocated for the pathologic staging of neoplasia arising in the urinary bladder, urethra, or penis, there are certain clinical situations in which extensive lymph node dissection is also advisable in men with CaP. Patients with a profoundly elevated serum PSA (> 40), a Gleason score of 8 or higher, and advanced clinical stage (T3) are at a high risk of demonstrating advanced disease. In these patient cohorts, a negative intraoperative histopathologic evaluation of obturator lymph node frozen sections should alert the urologist to the possibility that "skip lesions" involving more proximal lymph node chains may be present. In such instances where clinical and laboratory evidence strongly suggest advanced CaP, but frozen section pathologic studies show the obturator lymph nodes are free of metastatic disease, extended LPLND may be considered.

CARCINOMA OF THE URINARY BLADDER It has been demonstrated that the perioperative morbidity and mortality following radical cystectomy with concomitant pelvic lymphadenectomy does not significantly differ from that of cystectomy alone. Furthermore, this radical approach may improve the accuracy of staging and potentially increase the survival of patients demonstrating micrometastatic nodal disease.[20–23] If, during radical cystectomy, intraoperative frozen section evaluation reveals extensive lymphatic metastasis from primary transitional cell carcinoma (TCC) of the bladder, it is advocated that the procedure be terminated and chemotherapy initiated unless the cystectomy can be advised to prevent symptoms from progression of bladder cancer. The vast majority of these patients with advanced nodal metastases can be identified with preoperative imaging. Similarly, in a patient with lymphatic dissemination of adenocarcinoma or squamous cell carcinoma of the urinary bladder, extirpative surgery is unlikely to have any curative potential. For these reasons, the lymph node status of patients with primary cancer of the urinary bladder can be a major determinant in selecting the optimal therapeutic approach for each individual.[20–24]

There have, however, been reports demonstrating that a proportion of patients with grossly node-positive bladder cancer can be cured with radical cystectomy and an extended pelvic lymph node dissection.[25] In a study of 84 patients with grossly node-positive bladder cancer (N2–3), who underwent cystectomy and extended PLND, 24% survived with a follow-up of up to 10 years.[26] Extended LPLND in patients with transitional cell carcinoma of the bladder is therefore likely to be indicated in an occasional patient. LPLND as part of laparoscopic radical cystectomy with urinary diversion has been performed successfully in a few centers.[27,28]

In the coming years, cystectomy with urinary diversion performed with intracorporeal suturing will likely be performed at several institutions, because of the advances in laparoscopic instrumentation and robotic assistance. During such an operation, a meticulous extended LPLND is essential for staging, as well as for therapeutic reasons. In a study of 83 patients with node-positive TCC of the bladder who underwent cystectomy and PLND, the median five-year survival rate was 29%. All patients in this study were preoperatively staged as N0M0.[23]

The urinary bladder has a more proximal primary lymphatic drainage route than the prostate. Extended pelvic lymph node dissection appropriate for the pathologic staging of bladder cancer will be described later in this chapter.

CANCER OF THE URETHRA Although exceedingly rare, isolated carcinoma of the urethra is the only urologic cancer more commonly seen in the female population.[29] Tumors involving the distal urethra generally metastasize to the superficial and deep inguinal nodes. More proximal urethral lesions metastasize first to the external and internal iliac, as well as the obturator, lymph node chains, although some overlapping of the respective drainage fields is not unusual. In several series, lymphatic involvement at initial presentation can be as high as 35 to 50%, foreshadowing a bleak prognosis for patients with this disease.[30] In 80 to 96% of cases in which palpable inguinal lymphadenopathy is found at the initial assessment, the disease has already metastasized.

As with other genitourinary malignancies, radical exenterative surgery is contraindicated in patients with evidence of metastatic urethral carcinoma because the disease course will not be improved and the prognosis at this stage is grim. Extended LPLND may be considered in a selected group of:

1. patients who present with radiologic evidence of pelvic lymphadenopathy that is not accessible to percutaneous needle biopsy;
2. patients being considered for radiotherapy as a primary modality for urethral cancer.

CANCER OF THE PENIS   The superficial and deep inguinal lymph node chains provide the lymphatic drainage for the skin (including the prepuce and frenulum) and subcutaneous tissues of the penis. The corpus cavernosum penis and corpus spongiosum penis, urethra, and glans penis drain primarily into the external iliac nodes via the deep inguinal lymphatic chain. In 25% of cases, palpable inguinal lymphadenopathy harboring metastatic disease is present at the time of initial presentation. Pathologic evaluation of bilateral inguinal lymph node dissection specimens from patients presenting with non-palpable nodes reveals an additional 12 to 20% of patients with metastatic disease at the time of presentation.[31,32] The five-year survival rate of patients with inguinal lymph node metastases who are left untreated is roughly 19%. The prognosis is improved to an approximately 45% five-year survival rate if an early bilateral ilioinguinal lymphadenectomy is performed.[33] This signifies the possibility of surgical cure even in the face of early disseminated disease. Unfortunately, this procedure is not without significant risk. The 10 to 40% morbidity and 3% mortality associated with ilioinguinal lymphadenectomy needs to be weighed against the possibility of failing to obtain a surgical cure through the excision of occult metastatic disease.[32–34] Since tumor metastases found within the iliac or more proximal lymph nodes are associated with an exceedingly dismal prognosis, Mukamel and deKernion recommend that bilateral pelvic lymphadenectomy should be the initial pathologic staging procedure for patients with penile cancer.[35] They describe an extended dissection encompassing the removal of all lymphatic tissue from the femoral canal to the bifurcation of the iliac vessels. The boundaries of lymphadenectomy are similar to the dissection with bladder cancer. More distal lymphatic dissection, however, should include the perivascular lymphatics overlying the pubic bone and underneath the inguinal ligament.[36]

Pelvic lymph node positivity revealed during this procedure would obviate the need for subjecting the patient to the attendant morbidity and mortality of the groin dissection as the probability of obtaining a surgical cure at this point is essentially zero. The therapeutic benefit of complete pelvic lymphadenectomy has not been established. It can, however, provide useful staging information that can identify patients for adjuvant therapy. In the event that the pelvic lymphadenectomy reveals no metastasis in the excised tissue, ilioinguinal node dissection is recommended.

Extended LPLND is an option for patients with a high risk of pelvic nodal metastases. Risk factors include extensive inguinal nodal involvement, CT evidence of pelvic lymphadenopathy that is inaccessible to needle biopsy/aspiration cytology, and high-grade invasive primary neoplasm. It can be performed with the inguinal lymphadenectomy or it can be staged, depending on the likelihood and extent of pelvic and inguinal lymph node involvement. Furthermore, it is suggested that the dissection is first made on the side ipsilateral to the penile lesion so that an intraoperative frozen section pathologic evaluation of all lymphatic tissue specimens can be performed. Dissection of the contralateral side would be deemed unnecessary in the event of ipsilateral lymph node positivity.

SURGICAL ANATOMY

The parietal peritoneum covers the structures of the pelvis and forms ligaments and folds that are recognized during laparoscopy (Figures 55-1A and 55-1B).[37] The median umbilical ligament is in the midline and extends from the dome of the bladder to the umbilicus. It contains the obliterated remnant of the urachus. Occasionally, this may be patent or form cysts. The medial umbilical ligaments are formed by the obliterated umbilical arteries that originate from the internal iliac arteries (hypogastric artery). The lateral umbilical ligaments overlie the inferior epigastric vessels. The gonadal vessels from the lateral aspect and the vas deferens or the round ligament (in females) from the medial aspect converge to the internal inguinal ring (Figure 55-2). The femoral canal may be visible medial to the external iliac vein. The iliac vessels are exposed on incision of the peritoneum. The common iliac arteries bifurcate into the external and internal iliac arteries about the level of the sacroiliac joint (Figure 55-3). The external iliac artery exits through the femoral canal to form the femoral artery. The internal iliac artery supplies the pelvic viscera through the following branches: superior vesical artery, inferior vesical artery, middle rectal, uterine and vaginal arteries (in the female), and the obturator arteries. The external iliac vein runs medial to the external iliac artery. The ureter crosses the iliac vessels in the region of the bifurcation of the iliac artery. The ureter proceeds medially to the trigone of the bladder posterior to the vas deferens. In the female, the ureter forms the posterior boundary of a shallow depression named the ovarian fossa, in which the ovary is situated. The vas deferens runs medially from the internal inguinal ring, crossing the external iliac vessels. In the female, the round ligament is a homologous structure that runs from the internal ring to the uterus. The obturator nerve emerges from the medial border of psoas muscle at the brim of the pelvis, runs along the lateral wall of the pelvis, above the obturator vessels, to the upper part of the obturator foramen, where it enters the thigh. It runs posterior to the iliac vessels close to the bifurcation. The obturator nerve distributes muscular branches to the adductor muscles. The genitofemoral nerve runs on the psoas major muscle in the retroperitoneum medial to the gonadal vessels. It divides into the genital and femoral branches. The genital branch descends on the external iliac artery and passes through the internal ring along the back of the spermatic cord to supply the cremasteric muscle in the male. The femoral branch passes along the inner margin of the psoas muscle beneath the inguinal ligament and is distributed to the upper and anterior aspect of the thigh.

The pelvic lymph nodes and lymphatics parallel the vessels after which they are named (Figure 55-4). The obturator nodes lie along the pelvic sidewall adjacent to the obturator nerve. The external and internal iliac lymph nodes drain into the common iliac lymph nodes, which communicate with the pre-sacral nodes and drain into the para-aortic nodes. There is also some secondary convergence of the pelvic nodes to the deep inguinal nodes and the femoral nodes.

The anatomic basis for the LPLND follows the lymphatic drainage of the prostate, as follows:[38,39]

1. Lymphatic drainage of the prostate.
2. Primary echelon: obturator, hypogastric, external iliac.
3. Secondary echelon: pre-sciatic, pre-sacral, distal common iliac.
4. Tertiary echelon: proximal common iliac, aortic.

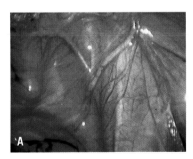

Figure 55-1 Laparoscopic view of the right hemipelvis (A) and a diagram of the pelvic peritoneum with the underlying structures.

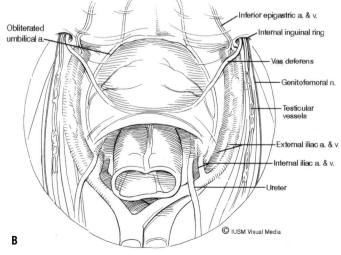

B

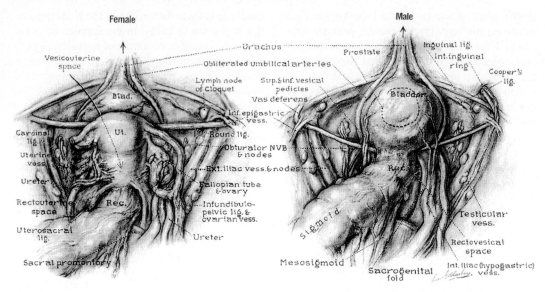

Figure 55-2 The peritoneal surfaces of the male and female pelves. In the female, the ureter is medial to the ovarian vessels, and deep to the uterine artery. (Reproduced with permission from Brooks JD. Anatomy of the lower urinary tract and male genitalia. In: Campbell's urology, 7th ed. W.B. Saunders Company; 1997. p. 98.)

INFORMED CONSENT

Potential major complications to be discussed include vascular injury causing severe hemorrhage necessitating emergency transfusion or open exploration, plus visceral injury including bowel, bladder, and ureteral injury, all of which may require open repair. The potential dangers of CO_2 insufflation should also be discussed. The risks include hypercarbia resulting in cardiopulmonary embarrassment, painful subcutaneous emphysema, pneumothorax, and intravascular CO_2 insufflation. Unsatisfactory dissection may result in poor lymphatic tissue yield. This may be more common during a surgeon's early experience with the surgery. The inability to obtain adequate exposure of the obturator-iliac regions secondary to anatomic confounders such as obesity, large-scale adhesions, or anomalous vascular architecture would also oblige the surgeon to convert the procedure to open surgery.

Potential postoperative complications, including lymphedema and lymphocele formation that may require percutaneous drainage and that can result in deep venous thrombosis and pulmonary embolism, should be understood by the patient. The possibility of hematoma formation which, if infected, may require open evacuation and drainage. As with all surgical operations requiring general anesthesia, the attendant risks of pneumonia, myocardial infarction, stroke, and death are discussed. Other less common complications encountered following LPLND include wound infection or dehiscence, lower extremity deep venous thrombosis, and obturator nerve palsy. In addition, alternative treatment plans that would negate the need for a lymph node dissection (eg, watchful waiting for prostate cancer) should be discussed.

PREOPERATIVE PREPARATION

Prior to LPLND, the standard presurgical evaluations are appropriate. This includes a general screen of the blood chemistry as well as a hemogram, coagulation studies, a recent chest radiograph and electrocardiogram. A blood typing and antibody screen are mandatory, since LPLND is not without significant risk of vascular injury and hemorrhage requiring emergency transfusion. If further radical surgery is planned pending a lymph node biopsy that is negative for metastatic disease, many surgeons advise the patient to bank autologous blood in the event that transfusion becomes necessary during the procedure.

The LPLND candidate is given specific instructions regarding the appropriate preoperative routine. The healthy patient scheduled to undergo LPLND alone who has no previous abdominopelvic pathology, surgery, or radiotherapy is instructed to self-administer either an oral laxative such as magnesium citrate or an enema on the evening before surgery. Decompressing the bowel in this manner decreases the risk of enterotomy. In addition, the patient should be instructed to cease oral intake past midnight and to report for admission to the hospital on the morning of surgery. In certain clinical situations, a more intensive mechanical and antibiotic bowel preparation should be administered the evening before surgery, if more extensive surgery such as radical cystectomy with urinary diversion is planned if the nodes are negative on frozen section examination.

All patients are administered one dose of a broad-spectrum parenteral antibiotic (eg, 1 gm cefazolin intravenously) 1 hour preoperatively. On arrival in the operating room, anti-embolic, pneumatically cycled compression boots are placed on the patient. For improved positioning, muscle relaxation, exposure, and analgesia, general anesthesia is considered most appropriate for LPLND.

The patient is placed in a supine position on the operating table (Figure 55-5). After adequate

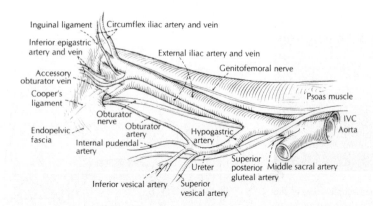

Figure 55-3 The right iliac vessels, with the branches of the hypogastric artery. A knowledge of the location of the obturator nerve, the ureter, and the accessory obturator vein is important during laparoscopic pelvic lymph node dissection. (Reproduced with permission from deVere White RW, Huang A. Pelvic lymphadenectomy. In: Graham SD Jr, editor. Glenn's urologic surgery, 5th ed. Lippincott Williams and Wilkins; 1998. p. 271.)

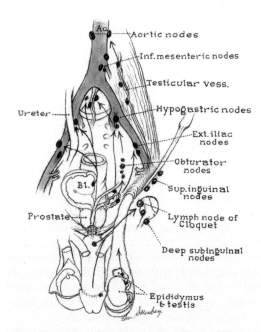

Figure 55-4 The male pelvis with lymphatic drainage of the pelvic organs, with the relationship to the vessels. (Reproduced with permission from Campbell's urology, 7th ed. W.B. Saunders Company; 1997. p. 103.)

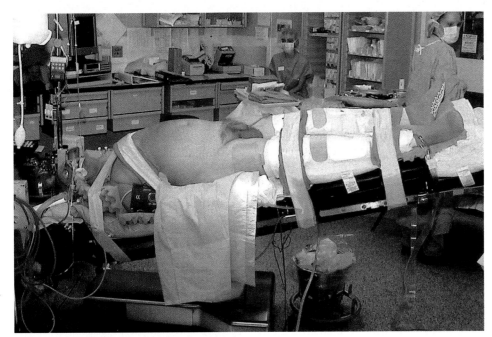

Figure 55-5 The patient is securely taped and well padded. A Trendelenburg's position with a rotation to the right facilitates dissection of the left pelvic nodes.

general anesthesia is obtained, a Foley urethral catheter and an oro/nasogastric tube are inserted. Both patient arms are carefully padded and secured at the sides. Wide adhesive tape placed across the chest and thigh secures the patient to the operating table. The entire abdomen, including the groin and genitals, is then antiseptically prepared and draped in a manner suitable for standard laparotomy. Access to the genitalia during surgery may be helpful in an occasional patient, especially those who are obese, since tugging on the testis can help identify the internal inguinal ring.

INSTRUMENTATION

The 10 mm 0° laparoscope is used. The video monitoring equipment should be placed to allow a comfortable and unobstructed view by all members of the surgical team. Ideally, dual monitors should be used on each side of the patient off the foot end of the operating table. For LPLND, the standard diamond configuration of four laparoscopic ports requires two 10/12-mm and two 5-mm trocar-sheath units (Figure 55-6). For the obese patient, an additional 5-mm trocar-sheath unit is required for the suggested inverted U or fan configuration of five laparoscopic ports (Figure 55-7). The fan configuration is required when a laparoscopic radical prostatectomy is planned if the LPLND is negative for malignancy. These port configurations will be discussed later in this chapter (see "Transperitoneal Pelvic Lymph Node Dissection"). If the extraperitoneal approach to LPLND is elected or the closed Veress needle technique for obtaining CO_2 pneumoperitoneum is unsuccessful, a Hasson-type, open-placement cannula is required.

Instruments that we use extensively include the Harmonic Scalpel with the curved shears

(Ethicon Endo-Surgery, Cincinnati, OH), laparoscopic dissectors, and a suction irrigator. The bipolar forceps are invaluable to assist with hemostasis. A 5-mm three-prong or fan-shaped retractor aids in holding loops of bowel cephalad. Five- or 10-mm laparoscopic vein retractors or "minicurved" retractors are helpful in retracting the iliac vessels laterally to facilitate improved access to the pelvic sidewall and obturator fossa. Additionally, 10-mm spoon-shaped laparoscopic forceps have proven ideal for the delivery of the resected lymph node packet after dissection is complete (Karl

Storz Endoscopy, Tuttlingen, Germany). The 10-mm specimen bag (Endopouch, Ethicon Endo-Surgery) is used when the specimen is large, the lymph nodes capsule violated, and with extended LPLND. Finally, a laparoscopic suction/irrigation device is essential for maintaining a clear field of dissection, for blunt dissection during the operation, and for assessing hemostasis at the conclusion of the procedure. We also use an absorbable "cigarette" sponge constructed from a piece of Gelfoam gelatin sponge that is wrapped in Surgicel oxidized regenerated cellulose (Ethicon Inc., Somerville, NJ) and tied with two 2/0 polyglactin sutures at each end. This is helpful for applying direct pressure on minor bleeding, and can be introduced through a 10-mm trocar.

As a precaution, particularly during the surgeon's early experience, the surgical nursing staff should have a standard laparotomy tray set up in the operating room should the need for emergency laparotomy arise. As experience with laparoscopic surgical technique is gained, the need to convert to an open procedure will decrease, but the open set should always be in the room ready to be used if required.

TECHNIQUE

TRANSPERITONEAL PELVIC LYMPH NODE DISSECTION After adequate pneumoperitoneum has been obtained and the placement of a 10/12-mm subumbilical port has been accomplished, a 0° (or 30°) telescope is then introduced into the abdominal cavity and a thorough and systematic survey of the abdominal contents is performed to rule out injury or gross metastatic disease. Any extensive adhesions or fatty tissue deposits in the vicinity of the umbilical ligaments

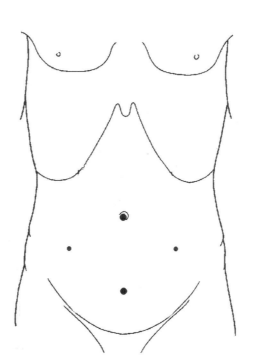

Figure 55-6 A diamond configuration of the trocar position. The larger solid circles and the smaller circles depict the position of the 10/12-mm and 5-mm trocars, respectively.

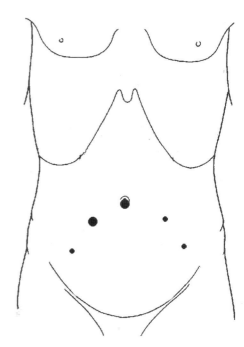

Figure 55-7 This trocar configuration is used for a laparoscopic radical prostatectomy and can be used for extended laparoscopic pelvic lymph node dissection (LPLND) or LPLND in obese patients.

are noted, since these findings may indicate the need for a modification of the standard diamond configuration of working port placement. Adhesions near the sites selected for working port positions may require lysis before port placement can be completed.

For most patients, the diamond configuration of four laparoscopic ports is well suited to transperitoneal LPLND (see Figure 55-6). This arrangement features two lateral 5-mm working ports placed midway between the umbilicus and anterior superior iliac spines along the lateral edge of the rectus muscle and a 10/12 mm suprapubic midline port placed 3 to 5 cm above the symphysis pubis. We routinely use the Ethicon Endopath trocars (Ethicon Inc.) with a non-bladed visual obturator. The primary trocar is inserted under direct vision with the laparoscope within the visual obturator during the trocar insertion. All working ports are placed under direct laparoscopic visualization, and transillumination of the abdominal wall during the selection of puncture sites should reduce the risk of transecting abdominal wall vessels during port placement. An alternative arrangement for port placement in obese patients with an abundance of urachal fatty tissue is the inverted U or fan configuration (see Figure 55-7). The disadvantage of this alternative placement is that an additional 5-mm laparoscopic port is needed. The patient is placed in a 30° Trendelenburg's position and a 15° to 30° lateral rotation to elevate the side of dissection (see Figure 55-5), thus gravitating loops of bowel away from the operative field. At this point, adhesions interfering with proper exposure of the obturator fossa may require lysis. This is particularly true of dissection on the left side, since sigmoid colonic diverticular inflammation may create adhesions of the sigmoid colon to the pelvic sidewall. Incising along the white line of Toldt should easily mobilize the sigmoid colon to allow a clear view of the iliac-obturator region.

It is necessary to accurately identify several important landmarks before beginning dissection of the pelvic lymph nodes (see Figures 55-1A and 55-1B). The testicular vessels and vas deferens should be identified as they enter the pelvis via the deep inguinal ring. The testicular vessels continue cephalad while the vas deferens runs posteromedially over the iliac vessels and the obliterated umbilical artery (ligament) en route to its position alongside the seminal vesicles deep within the pelvis. The umbilical ligament should be seen extending from the anterior abdominal wall on its way to join the internal iliac artery near the bifurcation of the common iliac artery. It should be noted that the "obliterated" umbilical artery is often widely patent near its junction with the internal iliac artery and has been the source of significant hemorrhage following accidental transection. In non-obese patients, pulsation of the external iliac artery may indicate its position beneath the peritoneum.

LIMITED PELVIC LYMPH NODE DISSECTION

Limited lymphadenectomy including the obturator and hypogastric nodes is the appropriate procedure for the pathologic staging of patients with prostate cancer (Figure 55-8). Dissection should begin on the side that is more likely to harbor nodal metastases. This includes the side of the positive prostate biopsies or prostate nodule. If there is no preference for the side based on preoperative data, the right side is performed first since adhesions requiring colonic mobilization are more common on the left side. The initial incision through the posterior peritoneal membrane begins at a point approximately midway between the obliterated umbilical artery and the internal inguinal ring high over the pubic bone. It is then extended cephalad, medial to the external iliac artery, toward a point near the bifurcation of the common iliac artery (Figures 55-9A and 55-9B). The anatomic relationship of the ureter to the bifurcation of the common iliac artery must be well conceptualized by the surgeon to avoid transection requiring stenting or possibly open repair. The vas deferens with its deferential artery is then identified, dissected free, and transected using electrocautery.

The external iliac vein is then exposed by careful dissection of all fibrofatty, lymph–node-bearing tissue medial to the external iliac artery. With the use of blunt and sharp dissection techniques, the lateral border of dissection is formed by clearing all fibro-lymphatic tissue from the anterior and medial surfaces of the external iliac vein (Figures 55-10A and 55-10B).

Gentle medial traction placed on the obliterated umbilical artery forms a plane delineating the medial boundary of the obturator node packet. Blunt dissection lateral to the obliterated umbilical artery is continued inferiorly to develop this plane to the level of the pubic bone and Cooper's

ligament. This completes the inferior apex of the dissection. In this area, venous variations are frequently encountered. Not uncommonly an accessory obturator vein may be identified as it joins the external iliac vein just after the iliac vessels enter the pelvis through the femoral canal. With careful manipulation, the inferior apex of the obturator lymph node packet may be maneuvered beneath this tributary, but as is often the case, 5- or 10-mm Hem-o-Lok clips (Weck Closure System, Research Triangle Park, NC) should be placed on the accessory vein proximally and dis-

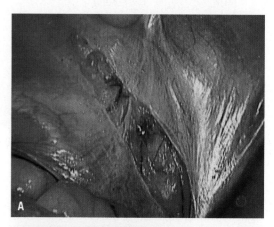

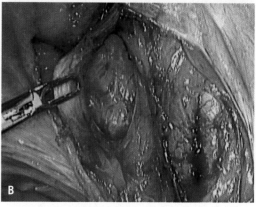

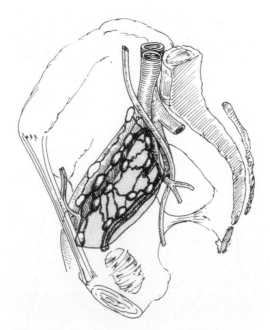

Figure 55-8 The shaded area depicts the iliac and obturator nodes that are excised for a limited pelvic node dissection. (Reproduced with permission from deVere White RW, Huang A. Pelvic lymphadenectomy. In: Graham SD Jr. Ed. Glenn's urologic surgery, 5th ed. Lippincott Williams and Wilkins; 1998. p. 271.)

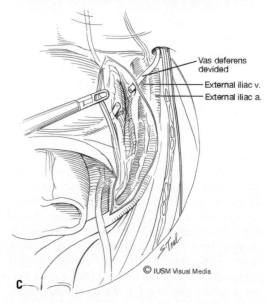

Vas deferens divided
External iliac v.
External iliac a.

© IUSM Visual Media

Figure 55-9 *A*, Incision is made between the medial umbilical ligament and the internal inguinal ring. *B*, The vas deferens is divided and the iliac vessels and obturator fossa exposed.

tally, followed by division, before the distal lymph node packet can be freed. These locking hemoclips are recommended since they are less prone to dislodge during further dissection in the region.

The distal extent of the lymph node packet is freed with judicious use of electrocautery or the ultrasonic shears. A clip is used at the distal end to occlude lymphatics and minimize the risk of a postoperative lymphocele. The free distal apex of the node packet is then grasped and elevated using proximal traction. With blunt dissection at the base of the node packet, the underlying obturator nerve and vessels should come into view as gentle traction draws the packet superiorly (see Figures 55-10A and 55-10B). The hypogastric nodes deep to the obturator nerve and overlying the hypogastric artery are carefully included in the nodal specimen. During dissection of the lymph node packet toward the bifurcation of the common iliac artery, any small blood or lymphatic vessels encountered should be sealed with electrocautery or the ultrasonic shears. Normally, the obturator vessels are preserved as their course is medial and slightly posterior to the obturator nerve. These vessels may be controlled and divided if required. Again, it must be remembered that, as the dissection nears the bifurcation of the common iliac artery, the proximity of the ureter puts it at risk of unintentional injury.

When the level of the common iliac bifurcation is reached, the proximal lymphatic vessels are cauterized and/or clamped with a hemoclip, and divided, resulting in a free lymph node packet. With 10-mm, spoon-shaped laparoscopic forceps, the free lymph node packet is delivered through a 10/12 mm port using a gentle twisting motion. The flap valve at the entrance to the port must be manually opened during extraction of the lymph node packet to avoid shearing and loss of lymphatic tissue within the barrel of the sheath. Laparoscopic visualization of the intracorporeal open end of the sheath during extraction of the lymph node packet will further ensure that no lymphatic tissue was dislodged from the packet during removal and facilitate immediate location and recovery of any lymphatic tissue accidentally sheared from the packet during extraction. If the lymphatic tissue is large or there is concern of violation of the lymph node capsule, a 10-mm Endopouch entrapment sack may be used for specimen retrieval.

If immediate radical surgery is planned pending a negative histopathologic evaluation of the lymphatic tissue specimen, the lymph node packet is sent for immediate frozen section analysis and attention is then turned to the opposite side. If radical surgery is not planned, we rarely order frozen section histopathologic evaluation of the lymph node specimens. If immediate radical surgery is not planned, we send the nodes from the first side for frozen section analysis because a positive node on the first side could obviate dissection on the contralateral side. False negative rate of frozen section evaluation of lymph node sampling can be as high as 19%.[40] The table is rotated in the opposite direction, and a similar dissection proceeds on the contralateral side.

At the conclusion of the laparoscopic procedure, a thorough evaluation of the abdomen is necessary. Particular attention is directed to the operative sites to ensure that meticulous hemostasis has been achieved. Intra-abdominal pressure is lowered to approximately 5 mm Hg to permit identification of any venous bleeding formerly tamponaded during the higher intra-abdominal pressures maintained throughout the procedure. Since the physical presence of the ports may tamponade any potential bleeding from a lacerated abdominal wall vessel, the secondary ports are all removed under direct laparoscopic visualization. The primary port is removed over the laparoscope, the laparoscope being the last instrument to exit the intra-abdominal space. This guards against herniation of abdominal contents and allows for a final inspection for hemorrhage formerly tamponaded by the camera port. In addition, digital exploration of all 10 or 12 mm port incisions may be performed to rule out herniation before closure. Any residual CO_2 is expressed out of the abdominal cavity, and all fascial defects 10 mm or larger are closed separately with a single 0 polydioxanone suture on the fascia using a Carter Thomasson device (Inlet Medical, Eden Prairie, MN). Closure of the fascia may be avoided if dilating trocars were used and the fascial defects at the end of the surgery are less than 10 mm. We now routinely close all trocar site skin incisions with 2-octyl cyanoacrylate topical skin adhesive (Dermabond, Ethicon Inc.). Three to four thin layers of the adhesive are applied to the incision after approximating the wound edges with a forceps or the fingers. Ten to 15 seconds are required after each layer is applied. The wound edges are held together until the adhesive has set. The oro/nasogastric tube is removed before the patient emerges from the anesthesia. The patient is then transferred to the post-anesthesia care unit for routine postoperative monitoring.

EXTENDED PELVIC LYMPH NODE DISSECTION

As previously mentioned, certain clinical indications merit a more extensive lymph node dissection. The extended LPLND includes the excision of all lymphatic tissues found within any boundaries as noted in Table 55-1. Obviously, to gain access to this broader region of dissection, a more extensive mobilization of the sigmoid colon and ceco-appendiceal regions are required. Alternatively, an inverted V peritoneotomy has been described that may provide greater exposure of the iliac-obturator region.[41]

This includes a second peritoneal incision that originates at the same point over the pubic bone as the initial incision and continues posteromedially and equidistant to the initial incision. This forms a triangular peritoneal free flap based along the medial umbilical ligament and the spermatic cord, which, when elevated, allows a more thorough exposure of the underlying obturator-iliac region. Full access to the lymphatic tissue deep to these vessels is facilitated by gentle medial retraction of the external iliac artery and vein.

EXTRAPERITONEAL PELVIC LYMPH NODE DISSECTION

It is evident that by maintaining the integrity of the peritoneal membrane the risks of visceral injury, intraperitoneal spillage of potentially tumor-laden lymphatic tissue, and postoperative development of intra-abdominal adhesions associated with direct instrumentation and manipulation of the intraperitoneal contents may be decreased or avoided. Additionally, tedious and time-consuming adhesiotomy, followed by mobilization of sigmoid colonic and ceco-appendiceal regions that often must precede exposure of the

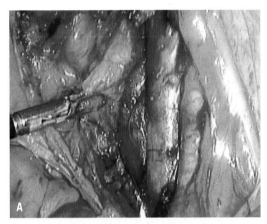

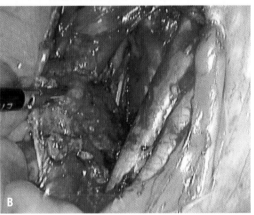

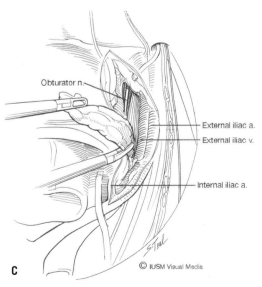

Obturator n.

External iliac a.

External iliac v.

Internal iliac a.

© IUSM Visual Media

Figure 55-10 *A*, The external iliac vein and *B*, the obturator nerve are exposed after the nodal tissue is distally detached.

TABLE 55-1 Boundaries of Pelvic Lymphadenectomy

Boundaries	Limited	Extended
Lateral	External iliac vein	Genitofemoral nerve
Medial	Medial umbilical ligament	Ureter, Bladder
Inferior	Pubis	Pubis
Superior	Bifurcation of common iliac artery	Distal Common Iliac Artery
Posterior	Obturator nerve and hypogastric artery	Obturator nerve and pre-sciatic tissue

obturator-iliac regions, is avoided with the extraperitoneal approach. Furthermore, the intact peritoneum may help ameliorate the difficulty of obtaining adequate exposure commonly encountered in the obese patient. By retaining the fat-laden loops of bowel and omentum (that tend to fall into the operative field) within the peritoneal cavity, the intact peritoneum passively facilitates exposure of the iliac-obturator region. This, in turn, may lessen the need for the extreme Trendelenburg's position typically used to gravitate these barriers away from the operative site.

On the other hand, several disadvantages of this alternative approach have been noted. The working space available for extraperitoneal LPLND is limited by the ability to successfully develop and insufflate the properitoneal space. Even with excellent expansion and CO_2 insufflation, the properitoneal working area is much more confined than in the intraperitoneal space. The balloon dissection required to develop the properitoneal space also produces a shearing effect between the parietal surface of the peritoneal membrane and the overlying fascial layer. This results in a tattered appearance of the properitoneal space. This effect, combined with the cephalad displacement of the vas deferens, may present a confusing picture to the laparoscopic surgeon.

In a patient with a history of lower abdominal or pelvic intra- or extraperitoneal surgery, the resultant postoperative sequelae of fibrosis and scarring within the tissue planes of the abdominal wall may severely limit expansion of the properitoneal space. Similarly, the fibrosis and scarring following extraperitoneal LPLND may complicate future regional procedures such as radical retropubic prostatectomy. In addition, the potentially higher likelihood of lymphocele formation and extensive subcutaneous CO_2 emphysema may complicate the extraperitoneal LPLND candidate's postoperative course.

The patient is placed supine under general anesthesia with endotracheal intubation. About 2 cm below the umbilicus, a 3-cm vertical midline incision is carried inferiorly and deepened to the level of the rectus abdominis fascia. The properitoneal space is then entered by splitting the musculus rectus abdominis and fascia transversalis. The latter fascial layer is deep to the musculus rectus abdominis below the umbilicus and arcuate line. A properitoneal space is developed using blunt finger dissection to the extent that a balloon dilation device can be introduced.

A modification of the device described by Gaur and colleagues for creation of the retroperitoneal working space while attempting the first extraperitoneal laparoscopic nephrectomy proved successful in expanding the properitoneal space.[42] This device features the finger cot of a transurethral resection drape secured to a 20 French red rubber (Robinson) catheter by silk free ties. The thicker polyethylene natural rubber material has demonstrated the ability to withstand pressure exerted by injection of the 800 to 1,000 mL of saline solution required to adequately expand the properitoneal space. This is important, since balloon rupture during expansion will mandate a thorough search of the properitoneal space for fragments. Fortunately, if the polyethylene balloon ruptures, the fragments tend to be large and easily recoverable. Latex fractures into smaller pieces, which may lead to a serious inflammatory or allergic response if retained. A commercially available preperitoneal balloon (U.S. Surgical Corp, Norwalk, CT) may be used to create the extraperitoneal working space.

With successful dilation of Retzius' space, the pubic bone and external iliac vessels become visible. We use a self-retaining, 10 or 12-mm Blunttip trocar, which has a inflatable balloon and a foam sponge/collar assembly. (U.S. Surgical). Twelve to 15 mm Hg of CO_2 is insufflated through the cannula. In the standard diamond configuration, the working ports are then placed carefully into the properitoneal space so as to avoid traversing the peritoneal membrane. The working ports are placed under direct laparoscopic guidance. Should the peritoneal membrane be violated, properitoneal space will likely be obliterated. This situation will necessitate conversion of the port placement from the extra- to an intraperitoneal position.

Afferent lymphatics are controlled with clips to minimize the possibility of a postoperative lymphocele. With the exception of creating a peritoneotomy, extraperitoneal LPLND proceeds in the same sequence as described for the intraperitoneal approach to obturator lymph node dissection once the ports are in place.

POSTOPERATIVE CARE

All patients are admitted to the hospital following laparoscopic surgery. They receive two additional postoperative doses of a parenteral broad-spectrum antibiotic at an 8-hour interval and their diet is advanced as tolerated. The Foley catheter should be removed as soon as the patient is alert and oriented. Ambulation should be tolerated on the evening of surgery, and any postoperative pain should be manageable with oral analgesics; parenteral narcotics are rarely indicated. Most patients are discharged from the hospital within 24 hours of surgery and should be able to resume normal activity within 1 week.

RESULTS

The results of several series of patients who underwent LPLND are summarized in Table 55-2. The transperitoneal approach is most widely used. Compared to the extraperitoneal approach, there is more operating space and the anatomic landmarks are easier to identify with the transperitoneal approach. In experienced hands, LPLND retrieves a number of nodes that is similar to the open approach. Compared to open surgery, there is a shorter convalescence and hospital stay.[43,44]

There are few reported series of patients who underwent the extraperitoneal approach. In a series of 36 patients from Das in 1996, the operating time was between 50 and 110 minutes, with a blood loss of 30 to 65 cc. In three patients, the procedure was not possible via the laparoscopic approach. The mean number of nodes harvested was 12.2, and in 16.6% of patients, metastatic prostate cancer was detected on frozen section analysis. Postoperative complications included a parietal hematoma in one patient and a lymphocele in another.[45]

The theoretical benefits include less risk of bowel injury, a decreased incidence of postoperative ileus, and a shorter operative time. Twenty-two patients were randomized to transperitoneal or extraperitoneal approaches. The duration of surgery was less with the extraperitoneal group (87 vs. 117 minutes). Four patients in the extraperitoneal group were converted to the open approach due to epigastric artery bleeding and problems with gas leakage. Lymphoceles developed in two patients in the extraperitoneal group.[46]

In a comparative study between similar groups of 12 and 6 patients who underwent transperitoneal LPLND and extraperitoneal LPLND, respectively, it was determined that the absorption of carbon dioxide was significantly greater and more rapid during extraperitoneal LPLND. In all but one patient, hypercarbia and acidemia were prevented by an increased ventilatory rate. The extraperitoneal approach may not be the preferred option in patients with cardiopulmonary disease.[47] The operating time should be minimized, and subcutaneous emphysema avoided to decrease the incidence of hypercarbia.

The effectiveness of LPLND has been documented with similar nodal yields when compared to open PLND.[13,44] Rukstalis and associates performed open surgery immediately following LPLND to determine the completeness of the laparoscopic approach.[48] They found that 87 to 95% of the nodes could be removed laparoscopically. The effect of inadequate nodal excision during the learning curve was demonstrated by Guazzoni and colleagues in 1994.[49] Open surgical revision of the lymphatic tissue during RRP in 30 patients who underwent LPLND, revealed a mean of over six residual lymph nodes in each patient. The number of residual nodes progressively decreased, especially after the first 20 patients.

TABLE 55-2 Results of Transperitoneal LPLND in English Literature

Authors	No. of Patients	No. of Nodes	Mean Operating Time	Mean Hosp. Stay	No. Complications (%)	No. of Conversions (%)
Winfield et al 1992[13]	66	9.6	150	1.5	17 (26)	11 (16)
Bowsher et al, 1992[63]	20	10	100	1	–	3 (15)
Schuessler et al, 1993[51]	147	45.8	158	2	46 (31)	4 (3)
Kerbl et al, 1993[43]	30	–	199	1.7	6 (20)	0
Rukstalis et al, 1994[48]	103	8.9	156	1.6	14 (14)	10 (10)
Guazzoni et al, 1994[49]	30	14.8	–	–	7 (23)	0
Doublet et al, 1994[64]	29	8.4	90	2[†]	6 (21)	3 (10)
Lang et al, 1994[53]	100	9.3	138	1.1	9 (9)	0
Klän et al, 1995[65]	70	13.6	136	–	11 (16)	2 (3)
Maffezzini et al, 1995[66]	158	11	–	–	–	7 (4.5)
Perroti et al, 1996[60]	20	9	190	1.2	4 (20)	1 (5)
Brant et al, 1996[67]	60	10	120	1	2 (3)	2 (3)
Lezin et al, 1997[68]	22	–	175	1.6	7 (32)	1 (5)
Kava et al, 1998[69]	24	10.8	174	1.2	3 (13)	0
Stone and Stock, 1999[70]	189	9	75	1[†]	17 (9)	0
Shackley et al, 1999[71]	27	6.5	55	1[†]	–	0
Parkin J et al, 2002*[72]	50	–	110	1.8	9 (22)	1 (2)

LPLND = laparoscopic pelvic lymph node dissection.

*Both transperitoneal and extraperitoneal approaches were used.

[†]Median.

COMPLICATIONS

Complication rates reported for LPLND range from 3.7 to 33%, with most complications being minor.[48,50–52] The complication rate decreased markedly with the surgeon's experience with the operation. In a study by Lang and associates, the complication rate was 14% in the first 15 cases and only 4% in the next 50 cases.[53] In recent years, increasing numbers of residents are being trained in advanced urologic laparoscopy during their residencies. Furthermore, many more advanced laparoscopic procedures like nephrectomies and prostatectomies are being performed. The learning curve for this operation is likely to be much less.

In an Italian study in 1994, the number of residual lymph nodes following LPLND decreased considerably after the first 20 cases.[49] The effectiveness of LPLND when compared by many investigators to the open approach, was satisfactory.[13,44,48] It is, however important to follow the principles of open surgery and follow the anatomic boundaries to ensure completeness of the dissection.

Most complications reported following LPLND are listed in Table 55-3. Lymphoceles are infrequently reported following LPLND. Subclinical lymphoceles, however, have been detected in 30.4% of patients (7) who underwent pelvic CTs following LPLND prior to undergoing radiotherapy. Only 3.5% of patients (2) developed symptomatic lymphoceles, one of whom required percutaneous drainage with sclerotherapy, whereas the lymphocele resolved spontaneously in the other patient.[54] Symptomatic lymphoceles are more frequently seen following extraperitoneal LPLND, since the peritoneal drainage of the lymphatic fluid is not available. Subcutaneous mini-dose heparin, which has been identified as a predisposing factor, is not recommended. Prophylaxis against deep venous thrombosis requires the use of an intermittent pneumatic compression device during and after surgery. The incidence of scrotal and penile edema, and leg edema was 28% and 10%, respectively, in patients undergoing extended pelvic lymphadenectomy.[55]

Vascular injuries specific to the PLND can occur during dissection of the nodal tissue in the vicinity of the external iliac vein and aberrant obturator vessels. The external iliac vein may be compressed by the intra-abdominal pressure, and therefore, may not be readily apparent. The intra-abdominal pressure can be reduced to 10 or 5 mm Hg for better visualization of the vein. The pulsation of the external iliac artery is a landmark that can help with localization of the vein that lies medial to the artery. Should vascular injury occur, increasing the intra-abdominal pressure to 20 mm Hg and direct compression on the bleeding surface should be the initial maneuver. If bleeding continues, other measures, including conversion to open surgery, can be required.

Injury to the bladder may occur during extended LPLND where the medial boundary can extend to the bladder. The bladder can be repaired in two layers with intracorporeal suturing using 2/0 polyglactin suture. Ureteral injury should be avoided at the bifurcation of the external iliac artery by identification of the ureter. During more caudal dissection, the ureter should not be encountered if the dissection remains lateral to the medial umbilical ligament. Ureteral injury can be repaired laparoscopically if the injury is immediately identified and if the distal segment is healthy and viable. If there is any doubt of the viability of the distal ureter, open conversion and ureteral reimplantation is recommended.

PORT SITE METASTASES Port site metastases have been reported (to my knowledge) in three cases of LPLND for urologic malignancies: one for prostate cancer, and two for bladder cancer.[56–58] An entrapment sack was not used in all these cases. Both the bladder transitional carcinomas were T3 lesions. It is therefore advisable that, when LPLND is being performed for TCC or advanced high-grade prostate cancer, an entrapment sack be used to minimize contamination of the port site during specimen retrieval. The risk of port-site metastases is, however, exceedingly small. When the risk for recurrence is high, other precautions that have been recommended include avoidance of nodal capsular rupture, trocar fixation to prevent dislodgment, avoiding gas leakage along and around the trocar, placing drainage when needed before desufflation, povidone-iodine irrigation of instruments, trocars and port site wounds, and suturing 10-mm and larger trocar wounds.[59]

MINILAPAROTOMY Surgeons without laparoscopic skills can perform the PLND via a small midline 6 cm incision. Bilateral inguinal incisions with aggressive retraction have also been successful. Perrotti and associates compared the minilaparotomy with LPLND and standard open surgery and found that nodal yield with minilaparotomy was similar to standard surgery and morbidity, and hospital stay was similar to LPLND. The operating time was 90 minutes with the minilaparotomy,

Table: 55-3 Complications of Transperitoneal Laparoscopic Pelvic Lymph Node Dissection

Total number of patients (multiple centers): 442
Total number of complications: 59 (13%)

Intraoperative complications (N = 19)

Anesthetic complications: 1
  Unable to access peritoneum: 1
  Organ Injuries
    Vascular: 9
    Bladder: 3
    Ureter: 2
    Obturator nerve: 2
    Bowel: 1

Postoperative complications (N = 40)

Urinary retention: 7
Lymphocele/lymphedema: 5
Prolonged ileus: 5
DVT: 5
Prolonged scrotal edema: 3
Bleeding requiring transfusion: 3
Significant echymosis: 2
Wound infection: 2
Delayed diagnosis of bowel injury: 2
Small bowel obstruction: 2
Anesthetic complications: 1
Fascial dehiscence: 1
Pelvic hematoma: 1
Retroperitoneal abscess: 1
Secondary open surgical intervention: 13
Complete lymphadenectomy could not be done: 17

Adapted from Gill IS, Clayman RV. Laparoscopic pelvic lymphadenectomy. Surg Oncol Clin North Am 1994;3:323.
DVT =

compared to 190 minutes for LPLND.[60] Herrell and colleagues in a similar study noted no difference in number of nodes obtained by either of these approaches.[61] Multiple complications occurred in the standard open group with no complications in the other two groups.

RECENT ADVANCES During the last two years, almost every urologic laparoscopic surgery has been performed with robotic assistance. Guillonneau and associates compared robotically assisted LPLND (RLPLND) with conventional LPLND in 10 patients for each procedure and confirmed the feasibility of the approach.[62] Though robotics for this surgery has not been shown to be superior to conventional laparoscopy, it may be the future of laparoscopy with further advancement in robotic instrumentation. Robotically assisted laparoscopic radical prostatectomy and radical cystoprostatectomy has been performed, and lymph node dissection as part of these surgeries will also be performed with robotic assistance. Robotics may also makes telesurgery a reality in routine surgical care.

CONCLUSION

Laparoscopic pelvic lymph node dissection as a procedure for staging of prostate cancer is being performed in few patients since most patients with prostate cancer in developed countries have early localized malignancy. Lymph node dissection as part of laparoscopic radical prostatectomy, with or without robotic assistance, is being performed in increasing numbers as definitive treatment of localized prostate cancer. Extended pelvic node dissection is indicated in patients with malignancy of the bladder, urethra and penis. A meticulous dissection that duplicates open surgery is required when this operation is performed.

ACKNOWLEDGEMENT

This chapter was written by J. Mathew Glascock and Howard N. Winfield in the first edition of *Smith's Textbook of Endourology*.

REFERENCES

1. Schuessler WW, Vancaillie TG, Reich H, et al. Transperitoneal endosurgical lymphadenectomy in patients with localized prostate cancer. J Urol 1991;145:988–91.
2. Mukamel E, Hannah J, Barbaric Z, et al. The value of computerized tomography scan and magnetic resonance imaging in staging prostatic carcinoma: comparison with the clinical and histologic staging. J Urol 1986;136:1231–3.
3. Benson KH, Watson RA, Spring DB, et al. The value of computerized tomography in evaluation of pelvic lymph nodes. J Urol 1981;126:63–4.
4. Loening SA, Schmidt JD, Brown RC, et al. A comparison between lymphangiography and pelvic node dissection in the staging of prostate cancer. J Urol 1977;117:752–6.
5. Paulson DF, Piserchia PV, Gardner W. Predictors of lymphatic spread in prostatic adenocarcinoma: uro-oncology research group study. J Urol 1980;123:697–9.
6. Flocks RH, Culp D, Porto R. Lymphatic spread from prostatic cancer. J Urol 1959;81:194–6.
7. Stamey TA, Kabalin JN. Prostate specific antigen in the diagnosis and treatment of adenocarcinoma of the prostate. I. Untreated patients. J Urol 1989;141:1070–5.

8. Lange PH, Ercole CJ, Lightner DJ, et al. The value of serum prostate specific antigen determinations before and after radical prostatectomy. J Urol 1989;141:873–9.
9. Hudson MA, Bahnson RR, Catalona WJ. Clinical use of prostate specific antigen in patients with prostate cancer. J Urol 1989;142:1011–7.
10. Partin AW, Yoo J, Carter HB, et al. The use of prostate specific antigen, clinical stage, and Gleason score to predict pathologic stage in men with localized prostate cancer. J Urol 1993;150:110–4.
11. Paulson DF. The prognostic role of lymphadenectomy in adenocarcinoma of the prostate. Urol Clin North Am 1980; 7:615–22.
12. Lieskovsky G, Skinner DG, Weisenberg T. Pelvic lymphadenectomy in the management of carcinoma of the prostate. J Urol 1980;124:635–8.
13. Winfield HN, Donovan JF, See WA, et al. Laparoscopic pelvic lymph node dissection for genitourinary malignancies: indications, techniques, and results. J Endourol 1992;6:103–11.
14. McLaughlin AP, Saltzstein SL, McCollough DL, et al. Prostatic carcinoma: incidence and location of unsuspected lymphatic metastases. J Urol 1976;115:89–94.
15. Clark T, Parekh DJ, Cookson MS, et al. Randomized prospective evaluation of extended versus limited lymph node dissection in patients with clinically localized prostate cancer. J Urol 2003;169:145–7.
16. Bader P, Burkhard FC, Markwalder R, Studer UE. Is a limited lymph node dissection an adequate staging procedure for prostate cancer? J Urol 2002;168:514–8.
17. Wolf JS Jr. Indications, technique, and results of laparoscopic pelvic lymphadenectomy. J Endourol 2001;15:427–35.
18. Gerber GS., Bales GT, Gornik HL, et al. Treatment of prostate cancer using external beam radiotherapy after laparoscopic pelvic lymph node dissection. Br J Urol 1996;77:870–5.
19. Partin AW, Kattan MW, Subong EN, et al. Combination of prostate-specific antigen, clinical stage, and Gleason score to predict pathological stage of localized prostate cancer. A multi-institutional update. Erratum in JAMA 278(9). JAMA 1997;278:118.
20. Whitmore WF Jr, Marshall VF. Radical total cystectomy for cancer of the bladder: 230 consecutive cases five years later. J Urol 1962;87:853–68.
21. Dretler SP, Ragsdale BD, Leadbetter WF. The value of pelvic lymphadenectomy in the surgical treatment of bladder cancer. J Urol 1973;109:414–6.
22. Skinner DG. Management of invasive bladder cancer: a meticulous pelvic node dissection can make a difference. J Urol 1982;128:34–6.
23. Mills RD, Turner WH, Fleischmann A, et al. Pelvic lymph node metastases from bladder cancer: outcome in 83 patients after radical cystectomy and pelvic lymphadenectomy. J Urol 2001;166:19–23.
24. Lieskovsky G, Skinner DG. Role of lymphadenectomy in the treatment of bladder cancer. Urol Clin North Am 1984; 11:709–16.
25. Konety BR, Joslyn SA, O'Donnell MA. Extent of pelvic lymphadenectomy and its impact on outcome in patients diagnosed with bladder cancer: analysis of data from the Surveillance, Epidemiology and End Results Program database. J Urol 2003;169:946–50.
26. Herr HW, Donat SM. Outcome of patients with grossly node positive bladder cancer after pelvic lymph node dissection and radical cystectomy. J Urol 2001;165:62–4.
27. Gill IS, Kaouk JH, Meraney AM, et al. Laparoscopic radical cystectomy and continent orthotopic ileal neobladder performed completely intracorporeally: the initial experience. J Urol 2002;168:13–8.
28. Turk I, Deger S, Winkelmann B, et al. Laparoscopic radical cystectomy with continent urinary diversion (rectal sigmoid pouch) performed completely intracorporeally: the initial 5 cases. J Urol 2001;165(6 Pt 1):1863–6.
29. Levine RL. Urethral cancer. Cancer 1980;45:1965–72.
30. Grabstald H, Hilaris B, Henschke U, et al. Cancer of the female urethra. JAMA 1966;197:835–42.
31. Skinner DG, Leadbetter WF, Kelly SB. The surgical management of squamous-cell carcinoma of the penis. J Urol 1972;107:273–7.
32. Kossow JH, Hotchkiss RS, Morales PA. Carcinoma of penis treated surgically: analysis of 100 cases: Urology 1973; 2:169.
33. Beggs JH, Spratt JS. Epidermoid carcinoma of the penis. J Urol 1964;91:166–72.
34. deKernion JB, Tynberg P, Persky L, et al. Carcinoma of the penis. Cancer 1973;32:1256–62.
35. Mukamel E, deKernion JB. Early versus delayed lymph node dissection versus no lymph node dissection for carcinoma of the penis. AUA Update Series 9:No. 2, 1990.

36. Culkin DJ, Beer TM. Advanced penile carcinoma. J Urol 2003;170:359–65.
37. Scott-Conner CE, Hedican S. Laparoscopic anatomy of the pelvis. Sem Lap Surg 1999;6:43–50.
38. Catalona WJ. Prostate cancer. New York: Grune and Stratton Inc; 1984.
39. Lieber MM. Pelvic lymphadenopathy. In: Crawford ED, Borden TA, editors. Genitourinary cancer surgery. Philadelphia: Lea & Febiger; 1982.
40. Catalona WJ, Stein AJ. Accuracy of frozen section detection of lymph node metastases in prostatic carcinoma. J Urol 1982;127:460–1.
41. See WA, Cohen MB, Winfield HN. Inverted V peritoneotomy significantly improves nodal yield in laparoscopic pelvic lymphadenectomy. J Urol 1993;149:772–5.
42. Gaur DD, Agarwal DK, Purohit KC. Retroperitoneal laparoscopic nephrectomy: initial case report. J Urol 1993;149: 103–5.
43. Kerbl K, Clayman RV, Petros JA, et al. Staging pelvic lymphadenectomy for prostate cancer: a comparison of laparoscopic and open techniques. J Urol 1993;150(2 Pt 1):396–9.
44. Parra RO, Andrus C, Boullier J. Staging laparoscopic pelvic lymph node dissection: comparison of results with open pelvic lymphadenectomy. J Urol 1992;147(3 Pt 2):875–8.
45. Das S. Laparoscopic staging pelvic lymphadenectomy: extraperitoneal approach. Semin Surg Oncol 1996;12: 134–8.
46. Persson BE, Haggman M. Minimally invasive techniques for prostate cancer pelvic lymph node dissection. A randomized trial of trans and extraperitoneal methods. J Urol 1996;155:1388A.
47. Glascock JM, Winfield HN, Lund GO, et al. Carbon dioxide homeostasis during transperitoneal or extraperitoneal laparoscopic pelvic lymphadenectomy: a real-time intraoperative comparison. J Endourol 1996;10:319–23.
48. Rukstalis DB, Gerber GS, Vogelzang NJ, et al. Laparoscopic pelvic lymph node dissection: a review of 103 consecutive cases. J Urol 1994;151:670–4.
49. Guazzoni G, Montorsi F, Bergamaschi F, et al. Open surgical revision of laparoscopic pelvic lymphadenectomy for staging of prostate cancer: the impact of laparoscopic learning curve. J Urol 1994;151:930–3.
50. Fahlenkamp D, Rassweiler J, Fornara P, et al. Complications of laparoscopic procedures in urology: experience with 2,407 procedures at 4 German centers. J Urol 1999;162(3 Pt 1): 765–71.
51. Schuessler WW, Pharand D, Vancaillie TG. Laparoscopic standard pelvic node dissection for carcinoma of the prostate: is it accurate? J Urol 1993;150:898–901.
52. Kavoussi LR, Sosa E, Chandhoke P, et al. Complications of laparoscopic pelvic lymph node dissection. J Urol 1993;149:322–5.
53. Lang GS, Ruckle HC, Hadley HR, et al. One hundred consecutive laparoscopic pelvic lymph node dissections: comparing complications of the first 50 cases to the second 50 cases. Urology 1994;44:221–5.
54. Freid RM, Siegel D, Smith AD, Weiss GH. Lymphoceles after laparoscopic pelvic node dissection. Urology 1998; 51(Suppl 5A):131–4.
55. Stone NN, Stock RG, Unger P. Laparoscopic pelvic lymph node dissection for prostate cancer: comparison of the extended and modified techniques. J Urol 1997;158:1891–4.
56. Stolla V, Rossi D, Bladou F, et al. Subcutaneous metastases after coelioscopic lymphadenectomy for vesical urothelial carcinoma. Eur Urol 1994;26:342.
57. Bangma Chr H, Kirkels WJ, Chadha S, Schröder FH. Cutaneous metastasis following laparoscopic pelvic lymphadenectomy for prostatic carcinoma. J Urol 1995;153:1635.
58. Altieri V, D'Armiento M, DeSio M, et al. Can laparoscopic lymphadenectomy disseminate bladder cancer? Acta Urol Ital 1998;12:231.
59. Tsivian A, Sidi AA. Port site metastases in urological laparoscopic surgery. J Urol 2003;169(4):1213–8.
60. Perrotti M Gentle DL Barada JH et al. Mini-laparotomy pelvic lymph node dissection minimizes morbidity, hospitalization and cost of pelvic lymph node dissection. J Urol 1996;155:986–8.
61. Herrell SD, Trachtenberg J, Theodorescu D. Staging pelvic lymphadenectomy for localized carcinoma of the prostate: a comparison of 3 surgical techniques. J Urol 1997;157:1337–9.
62. Guillonneau B, Cappele O, Martinez JB, et al. Robotic assisted, laparoscopic pelvic lymph node dissection in humans. J Urol 2001;165(4):1078–81.
63. Bowsher WG, Clarke A, Clarke DG, Costello AJ. Laparoscopic pelvic lymph node dissection for carcinoma of

the prostate and bladder. Aust N Z J Surg 1992;62: 634–7.

64. Doublet JD, Gattegno B, Thibault P. Laparoscopic pelvic lymph node dissection for staging of prostatic cancer. Eur Urol 1994;25:194–8.

65. Klan R, Meier T, Knispel HH, et al. Laparoscopic pelvic lymphadenectomy in prostatic cancer: an analysis of seventy consecutive cases. Urol Int 1995;55:78–83.

66. Maffezzini M, Carmignani G, Perachino M, et al. Benefits and complications of laparoscopic pelvic lymphadenectomy for detection of stage D1 prostate cancer: a multicenter experience. Eur Urol 1995;27:135–7.

67. Brant LA, Brant WO, Brown MH, et al. A new minimally invasive open pelvic lymphadenectomy surgical technique for the staging of prostate cancer. Urology 1996;47: 416–21.

68. Lezin MS, Cherrie R, Cattolica EV. Comparison of laparoscopic and minilaparotomy pelvic lymphadenectomy for prostate cancer staging in a community practice. Urology 1997;49:60–4.

69. Kava BR, Dalbagni G, Conlon KC, Russo P. Results of laparoscopic pelvic lymphadenectomy in patients at high risk for nodal metastases from prostate cancer. Ann Surg Oncol 1998;5:173–80.

70. Stone NN, Stock RG. Laparoscopic pelvic lymph node dissection in the staging of prostate cancer. Mt Sinai J Med 1999;66:26–30.

71. Shackley DC, Irving SO, Brough WA, O'Reilly PH. Staging laparoscopic pelvic lymphadenectomy in prostate cancer. BJU Int 1999;83:260–4.

72. Parkin J, Keeley FX Jr, Timoney AG. Laparoscopic lymph node sampling in locally advanced prostate cancer. BJU Int 2002;89:14–7.

56

Laparoscopic Varix Ligation

Timothy Mulholland, MD

INTRODUCTION

A varicocele is a dilation of the pampiniform plexus, the primary venous drainage of the testicles. Regarded as a progressive lesion, the deleterious effects in spermatogenesis caused by a varicocele increases over time.[1] Some investigators indicate that a varix can affect the contralateral testis as well.[2]

PREVALENCE, POSSIBLE CAUSES, AND IMPLICATIONS OF VARICOCELE

The assumed mechanisms of varicocele formation include increased venous pressure in the left renal vein, collateral venous anastomoses, and incompetent valves of the internal spermatic vein. Varicoceles occur predominantly on the left side, probably because of the difference in anatomy in the internal spermatic veins on the left and right sides. Unlike the right testicular vein that enters the vena cava obliquely, the left spermatic vein enters the left renal vein at a right angle. The venous insertion on the left is also 8 to 10 centimeters more cephalad than the insertion on the right. Presumably this increases the hydrostatic pressure within the left spermatic vein when compared with the right.[3]

A varix is usually asymptomatic, but occasionally causes orchalgia. Becoming evident initially in adolescence, a varicocele is present in 15% of all men.[3] The World Health Organization (WHO) reports varicocele present in 25.4% of men with abnormal semen and in 11.7% of men with normal semen.[4] Varicoceles are a contributing factor in up to 40% of primary cases and up to 80% of secondary cases of male factor subfertility.[3] It is unknown why some men with varicocele suffer impaired spermatogenesis and steroidogenesis while other men are unaffected.[3]

The exact mechanism of impaired fertility owing to the varix is unknown and probably multifactorial. Investigators propose that one of the principal mechanisms of testis dysfunction in the presence of a varicocele is increased testicular temperature resulting from the reverse venous blood flow in the spermatic veins, which disrupts counter-current testicular temperature modulation. Zorgniotti has demonstrated increased testicular temperature is associated with varices,[5] and Wright reports a decrease in testis temperature following varicocelectomy.[6]

DIAGNOSIS OF VARICOCELE The diagnosis of a varicocele is based primarily on a careful physical examination of the patient in both a supine and a standing position. Our patients stand for 10 to 15 minutes in a warm room. To limit the effect of cremasteric retraction, the testes are gently supported; inspection and palpation of the scrotum starts at a point just superior to the testes. Veins are easily distinguished from lipoma of the spermatic cord: while veins compress, a lipoma will tend to slip from grasp when gently pinched. Traditionally, varices are graded with respect to size and/or appearance. A large or grade III varicocele is visible on inspection. A medium or grade II varicocele is palpable without a Valsalva maneuver. A small or grade I varicocele is palpable only during a Valsalva maneuver. Small varicoceles can be difficult to detect on physical exam, but nevertheless may be responsible for reductions in male reproductive function. A thorough physical exam will establish the diagnoses in the majority of cases. However, in the appropriate patient with an equivocal exam, color Doppler sonography may be helpful. A subclinical varicocele is one found only on scrotal sonography and not on physical exam. Results following ligation of a subclinical varicocele are unpredictable. We do not attempt to identify subclinical varices routinely and use sonography only in equivocal cases or to examine the contralateral spermatic cord (Figure 56-1).

TREATMENT OPTIONS Treatment of a varix includes several options. Transvenous sclerosis or embolization of varices by an interventional radiologist is a nonsurgical treatment option. Embolization is accomplished using either balloons or coils to obstruct venous flow or by instilling a sclerosing agent, such as boiling hot contrast media or absolute ethanol, to induce thrombosis of the varix. Both embolization and sclerosis are performed under local anesthesia with supplementary intravenous sedation. Rates of success for transvenous embolization and sclerosis vary, but generally do not approach those reported for operative varix ligation, especially when patients in whom sclerotherapy cannot be performed are included. Some European investigators, however, promote sclerotherapy as better than or equal to surgical therapy.

Surgical treatment options for a varix include the inguinal approach of Ivanissevich,[10] the subinguinal approach of Marmar,[11] or the retroperitoneal approach of Palomo.[12] With the inguinal and subinguinal procedures, the spermatic vessels are identified as they course through the inguinal canal and below the external ring, respectively. Spermatic and cremasteric veins encountered at these sites are carefully exposed and ligated with attention toward preservation of the testicular artery and lymphatics.

The Palomo approach can be done by open or laparoscopic techniques. One disadvantage of this technique is the lack of access to the cremasteric vein, which, according to Enquist and Stein, will contribute to a higher recurrence rate when compared with the subinguinal microscopic technique described by Goldstein. However, the retroperitoneal approach does permit ligation of spermatic veins without the attendant risk of injuring arterial collaterals, specifically the cremasteric and deferential arteries. In comparison with the open approach, the laparoscopic varix ligation offers several advantages: (1) improved visualization of the vessels via a transperitoneal approach, especially in the obese patient; (2) fewer veins present to ligate (and fewer arteries to spare in the cephalad spermatic vascular bundle if one so chooses); (3) magnification of vascular structures, which facilitates identification and preservation of the spermatic artery and lymphatics; (4) a panoramic view of the retroperitoneal structures, which permits identification and ablation of aberrant collateral veins that arise from the kidney, iliac vein, or sigmoid colon to traverse the internal inguinal

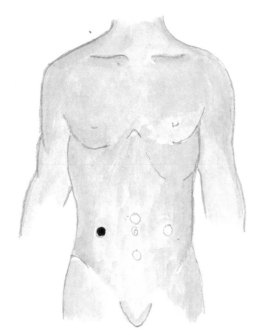

Figure 56-1 Port position. A 5 mm trocar is placed in the supraumbilical midline and serves as the camera port in all cases. Unilateral left varix ligation is performed with left lateral and suprapubic midline 5 mm ports. Bilateral varix ligation is performed with right and left lateral 5 mm ports.

ring; and (5) access to right or left varicocele with the same number of access ports.

Additionally, the risk of testicular ischemia is presumably reduced because collateral arterial flow to the testis joins the spermatic cord well below the level of ligation, compared with the subinguinal approach, where the risk of ligation of arterial collaterals is increased. As a technical point, it is important to make sure any ligation occurs below the L4 level because the spermatic vein can often branch above this level. Proponents of the retroperitoneal approach are divided regarding the utility of sparing the spermatic artery. Several reports have found no difference in testis volume after laparoscopic clipping of the entire retroperitoneal spermatic vascular bundles without arterial sparing. Both Kattan and Ng reported increased rates of varix recurrence and hydrocele when the spermatic artery is spared. Conversely, many surgeons have excellent success with the arterial sparing technique.

The laparoscopic Palomo approach has been compared with the open Palomo approach by several investigators. In comparing these two retroperitoneal procedures, most have found the laparoscopic approach equal or superior in efficacy and patient tolerance. Cost analysis has shown the laparoscopic approach to be more expensive than the open approach, but costs associated with laparoscopy have subsequently decreased because of reduction in both operating time and cost of laparoscopic equipment. We routinely use the transperitoneal approach to laparoscopic varix ligation, though a retroperitoneal approach has been reported. Demirci has shown the transperitoneal approach to be equivalent to the extraperitoneal approach. This discussion focuses on the transperitoneal laparoscopic approach to varix ligation.

INDICATIONS AND CONTRAINDICATIONS

Treatment of a varix by any approach is indicated when a patient demonstrates a varicocele and one of the following conditions: male factor subfertility verified on semen analysis, adolescent testis growth disparity or retardation, or intractable pain not attributable to other causes. A varix ligation is reportedly the most cost-effective treatment when diagnosed in a man suffering subfertility.[30]

Practical contraindications to laparoscopic varix ligation are limited to patients who have undergone a prior retroperitoneal varix ablation. The site of laparoscopic transperitoneal and open retroperitoneal Palomo varix ligation is the same. Repeat exposure of the spermatic veins cephalad to the internal ring negates the benefit of ligation in the case of persistent or recurrent varicocele. Patients with persistent varix following retroperitoneal ligation should be treated by alternate methods: either spermatic vein sclerosis by transvenous access or by spermatic vein ligation via the inguinal (Ivanissovitch) or subinguinal (Marmar-Goldstein) approach. We have, however, successfully performed salvage varicocelectomy in patients who have undergone failed transvenous

or inguinal varix ablation. Other investigators have found that previous groin surgery, such as a hernia or orchidopexy, was not a contraindication to laparoscopic varicocelectomy. Obesity, previous abdominal surgery, or umbilical hernia are considered relative contraindications that can be disregarded with appropriate experience and precautions at the time of peritoneal access.

PATIENT PREPARATION

In addition to completing the standard patient-specific preoperative work-up, preoperative discussion includes review of alternate treatment options (including no treatment), and their associated risks (complications, recurrence, cost) and benefits (success, response in seminal fluid analysis, pregnancy). Potential risks specific to laparoscopic varix ligation are clearly delineated. Since an exhaustive review of all possible complications is impractical, we particularly emphasize the remote possibility of injury to the intestine and/or blood vessels, which would mandate open repair. Additionally, we inform each patient of the potential need to convert the laparoscopic procedure to an open approach because of unanticipated operative findings, such as bleeding, adhesions, or inflammation. In our series to date, all varix ligations have been completed laparoscopically. Each patient should be aware that, despite successful varix ligation, improvement in seminal fluid parameters and/or reduction in pain is not assured. In fact, there is a nominal risk of testicular atrophy because of compromised testicular arterial blood flow. The anticipated success of varicocelectomy should be addressed. Varicocelectomy will result in improved seminal fluid characteristics in the majority of (but not all) patients. In patients presenting with pain, varix ligation will improve or eliminate orchalgia in approximately 50%. The treatment of orchalgia by varix ligation demands careful patient selection and each patient must be informed of the possibility of persistent pain.

PREOPERATIVE PREPARATION

Although this procedure has been done under both epidural and local anesthesia, we feel that laparoscopy with pneumoperitoneum is best tolerated under general anesthesia. Chiu has shown that epidural anesthesia is inferior when compared with general anesthesia for laparoscopic varicocele ligation. After induction of anesthesia, we place an oral gastric tube to evacuate the stomach. The patient's abdomen and genitalia are prepped and draped. The bladder is drained by a catheter after the patient is draped. Access to the external genetilia allows gentle intermittent manual traction on the testis/spermatic cord during the procedure, which aids in identification of spermatic vessels and collateral veins that traverse the internal ring.

INSTRUMENTATION

We have used both the Veress needle and the open Hasson technique to gain initial pneumoperitoneum. Currently we use the Ver-

ess needle and feel this is safe when appropriate precautions are taken. The principal instruments that we use during laparoscopic varix ligation are a curved dissector, a curved scissors, and a right-angle dissector. A 5 mm, 45° laparoscopic lens is used. We no longer routinely use a 5 mm laparoscopic Doppler probe to assist in identification and isolation of the spermatic artery, since several investigators have shown no benefit from sparing the internal spermatic artery. We use 5 mm ports because they have been shown to decrease morbidity when compared with 10 mm ports The veins are ligated with 2-0 silk ligature using intracorporeal tying techniques (Figure 56-2).

TECHNIQUE

We place the patient in the supine position with arms adducted. Skin preparation includes the abdomen and genitals. After infiltrating 0.25% marcaine, a 5 mm skin incision is made just above the umbilicus. The Veress needle is passed through this incision and into the peritoneal cavity. Proper position of the Veress needle is confirmed using appropriate tests and insufflation proceeds to reach an intraperitoneal pressure of 20 mm Hg. Once proper pneumoperitoneum is achieved, a 5 mm trocar is advanced into the peritoneal cavity and a 45° camera inserted. Inspection of the peritoneal contents is completed, giving special attention to the peritoneal contents deep to the site of Veress needle insertion and first trocar. If the internal ring is obscured by the sigmoid colon on the left or the cecum and appendix on the right, these structures must be mobilized carefully. Once the internal ring is exposed, the spermatic vessels

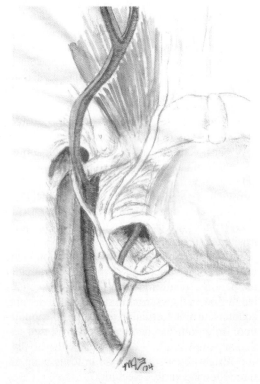

Figure 56-2 The anatomy as seen from the laparoscope during varix ligation.

are identified deep to the peritoneal membrane passing cephalad over the psoas muscle. The vas deferens is seen curving medially and caudad over the external iliac artery and vein. Next we place two 5 mm ports. In the case of a left side varix, we insert one port lateral to the rectus muscle just below the level of the umbilicus and the other in the midline midway between the pubis and the umbilicus. For bilateral varices, both ports are placed lateral to the right and left rectus muscle just below the level of the umbilicus. Once the ports are placed, the patient is put in Trendelenburg's position. We mobilize the colon as necessary to expose underlying spermatic vessels just above the internal ring. We incise the peritoneal membrane lateral and parallel to the spermatic vascular bundle. This incision is 3 to 5 cm in length and positioned 3 to 5 cm above the internal ring to avoid the confluence of spermatic vessels and vas as they join to traverse the inguinal canal. The iliac artery will be just medial to the spermatic vessels at this level. The medial flap of the peritoneum is grasped, and the underlying spermatic vessels are bluntly swept from the underside of the peritoneal membrane. From the midpoint of this incision, a second "T" incision is made perpendicular and medial to the first, dividing the peritoneal membrane overlying the spermatic vessels and extending to the lateral edge of the iliac artery, thus providing excellent exposure of the spermatic vascular bundle. External traction on the testis/cord at this point will aid in identifying all veins that contribute to the varicocele. The entire spermatic vascular bundle is then freed from the underlying psoas muscle using both sharp and blunt dissection. With 2 to 3 cm freely mobile, the spermatic vascular bundle is then separated into medial and lateral components. The artery is not specifically identified, though typically will lie posterior and medial. Using an intracorporeal knotting technique, we ligate and divide each vascular segment. Following completion of the of the varix ligation, the pneumoperitoneum is reduced (< 8 mm Hg) and the operative field assessed for hemostasis. We remove each trocar while examining insertion sites from within as desufflation proceeds. Once all trocars and scope are removed, the subcutaneous tissues are reapproximated and the skin closed with a subcuticular 3-0 Vicryl Rapide (Figure 56-3).

RESULTS Successful treatment has been shown to improve semen parameters in 60 to 80% of men.[7,35–37] Pregnancy rates are variable: authors report a 20 to 60% pregnancy rate when varicocele ligation is performed for infertility. Pain resolved in 50 to 86% of patients who were treated for pain.[35,39–41] Complications include hydrocele (0–5.6%) and recurrent varicocele (0–10%). The majority of investigators report recurrent varix in less that 5% of patients. Other complications are rare and include the following: (1) bleeding either from inferior epigastric vessel

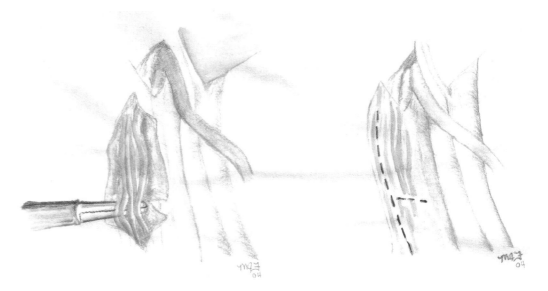

Figure 56-3 The peritoneal incision and gonadal vein dissection; the spermatic vessels are visible deep to the peritoneal membrane – it's the visible spermatic vessels that determine the location of the incision.

secondary to trocar placement or delayed bleeding from the spermatic vessel because of incomplete ligation or thermal injury, and (2) visceral injury because of trocar or instrument mishap. Very few surgeons report conversion to an open approach. Conversion is usually due to colonic adhesions. To date, we have not converted any laparscopic varix ligation to an open approach.

REFERENCES

1. Fretz P, Sandlow JI. Varicocele: current concepts in pathophysiology, diagnosis, and treatment. Urol Clin North Am 2002;29:921–37.
2. Kass EJ, Stork BR, Steinert BW. Varicocele in adolescence induces left and right testicular volume loss. BJU Int 2001;87:499–501.
3. Goldstein M. Surgical management of male infertility and other scrotal disorders. In Walsh PC, Retik AB, Vaughan ED, Wein AJ, editors. Campbell's Urology. 8th ed. Philadelphia: WB Saunders; 2002. p. 1532–87.
4. World Health Organization. The influence of varicocele on parameters of fertility in a large group of men presenting to infertility clinics. Fertil Steril 1992;57:1289–93.
5. Zorgniotti AW. Testis temperature, infertility, and the varicocele paradox. Urology 1980;16:7–10.
6. Wright EJ, Young GP, Goldstein M. Reduction in testicular temperature after varicocelectomy in infertile men. Urology 1997;50:257–9.
7. Abdulmaaboud MR, Shokeir AA, Farage Y, et al. Treatment of varicocele: a comparative study of conventional open surgery, percutaneous retrograde sclerotherapy, and laparoscopy. Urology 1998;52:294–300.
8. Sautter T, Sulser T, Suter S, et al. Treatment of varicocele: a prospective randomized comparison of laparoscopy versus antegrade sclerotherapy. Eur Urol 2002;41:398–400.
9. Tauber R, Johnsen N. Antegrade scrotal sclerotherapy for the treatment of varicocele: technique and late results. J Urol 1994;151:386–90.
10. Ivanissevich O. Left varicocele due to reflux; experience with 4,470 operative cases in forty-two years. J Int Coll Surg 1960;34:742–55.
11. Marmar JL, DeBenedictus TJ, Praiss D. The management of varicoceles by microdissection of the spermatic cord at the inguinal ring. Fertil Steril 1985;43:583–8.
12. Palomo A. Radical cure of varicocele by a new technique: preliminary report. J Urol 1949;61:604.
13. Enquist E, Stein BS, Sigman M. Laparoscopic versus subinguinal varicocelectomy: a comparative study. Fertil Steril 1994;61:1092–6.
14. Goldstein M, Gilbert BR, Dicker AP, et al. Microsurgical inguinal varicocelectomy with delivery of the testis: an artery and lymphatic sparing technique. J Urol 1992;148:1808–11.
15. Donovan JF Jr. Laparoscopic varix ligation. Urology 1994;44:467–9.
16. Wishahi MM. Detailed anatomy of the internal spermatic vein and the ovarian vein. Human cadaver study and operative spermatic venography: clinical aspects. J Urol 1991;145:780–4.
17. Belloli G, Musi L, D'Agostino S. Laparoscopic surgery for adolescent varicocele: preliminary report on 80 patients. J Pediatr Surg 1996;31:1488–90.
18. Student V, Zatura F, Scheinar J, et al. Testicle hemodynamics in patients after laparoscopic varicocelectomy evaluated using color Doppler sonography. Eur Urol 1998;33:91–3.
19. Sun N, Cheung TT, Khong PL, et al. Varicocele: laparoscopic clipping and color Doppler follow-up. J Pediatr Surg 2001;36:1704–7.
20. Ng WT. Testicular artery sparing laparoscopic varicoceletomy (LV) in adolescents. J Pediatr Surg 2002;37:142–3.
21. Kattan S. The impact of internal spermatic artery ligation during laparoscopic varicocelectomy on recurrence rate and short post operative outcome. Scand J Urol Nephrol 2001;35:218–21.
22. Lynch WJ, Badenoch DF, McAnena OJ. Comparison of laparoscopic and open ligation of the testicular vein. Br J Urol 1993;72(5 Pt 2):796–8.
23. Cohen RC. Laparoscopic varicocelectomy with preservation of the testicular artery in adolescents. J Pediatr Surg 2001;36:394–6.
24. Esposito C, Monguzzi G, Gonzalez-Sabin MA, et al. Results and complications of laparoscopic surgery for pediatric varicocele. J Pediatr Surg 2001;36:767–9.
25. Podkamenev VV, Stalmakhovich VN, Urkov PS, et al. Laparoscopic surgery for pediatric varicoceles: randomized controlled trial. J Pediatr Surg 2002;37:727–9.
26. Rashid TM, Winfield HN, Lund GO, et al. Comparative financial analysis of laparoscopic versus open varix ligation for men with clinically significant varicoceles. J Urol 1994;151:310A.
27. Gaur DD, Agarwal DK, Purohit KC. Retroperitoneal laparoscopic varicocelectomy. J Urol 1994;151:895–7.
28. Gurpinar T, Sariyuce O, Balbay MD, et al. Retroperitoneoscopic bilateral spermatic vein ligation. J Urol 1995;153:127–8.
29. Demirci D, Gulmez I, Hakan NA, et al. Comparison of extraperitoneoscopic and transperitoneoscopic techniques for the treatment of bilateral varicocele. J Endourol 2003;17:89–92.
30. Schlegel PN. Is assisted reproduction the optimal treatment for varicocele-associated infertility? A cost-effective analysis. Urology 1997;49:83–90.
31. Barqawi A, Furness P 3rd, Koyle M. Laparoscopic Palomo varicocelectomy in the adolescent is safe after previous ipsilateral inguinal surgery. BJU Int 2002;89:269–72.
32. Chiu AW, Huang WJ, Chen KK, Chang LS. Laparoscopic ligation of bilateral spermatic varices under epidural anesthesia. Urol Int 1996;57:80–4.

33. Matsuda T, Horri Y, Takeuchi H, Yoshida O. Laparoscopic Varicocelectomy. J Urol 1991;145:325A.

34. Matsuda T, Ogura K, Uchida J, et al. Smaller ports result in shorter convalescence after laparoscopic varicocelectomy. J Urol 1995;153:1175–7.

35. Donovan JF. Laparoscopic varix ligation. Urol Clin North Am 1993;1:15–32.

36. Jarow JP, Assimos DG, Pittaway DE. Effectiveness of laparoscopic varicocelectomy. Urology 1993;42:544–7.

37. Ulker V, Garibyan H, Kurth KH. Comparison of inguinal and laparoscopic approaches in the treatment of varicocele. Int Urol Nephrol 1997;29:71–7.

38. Schlesinger MH, Wilets IF, Nagler HM. Treatment outcome after a varicocelectomy. A critical analysis. Urol Clin North Am 1994;21:517–29.

39. Peterson AC, Lance RS, Ruiz HE. Outcomes of varicocele ligation done for pain. J Urol 1998;159:1565–7.

40. Maghraby HA. Laparoscopic varicocelectomy for painful varicoceles: merits and outcomes. J Endourol 2002;16:107–10.

41. Itoh K, Suzuki Y, Yazawa H, et al. Results and complications of laparoscopic palomo varicocelecctomy. Arch Androl 2003;49:107–10.

42. Esposito C, Monguzzi GL, Gonzalez-Sabin MA, et al. Laparoscopic treatment of pediatric varicocele: a multicenter study of the Italian society of video surgery in infancy. J Urol 2000;163:1944–6.

43. Nyirady P,Kiss A, Pirot L, et al. Evaluation of 100 laparoscopic varicocele operations with preservation of testicular artery and ligation of collateral vein in children and adolescents. Eur Urol 2002;42:594–7.

44. Riccabona M, Oswald J, Koen M, et al. Optimizing the operative treatment of boys with varicocele: sequential comparison of 4 techniques. J Urol 2003;169:666–8.

57

Renal Surgery: Benign Disease, Cyst Ablation, and Calicealectomy

Sean P. Hedican, MD

Stephen Y. Nakada, MD

Benign renal disease processes represent an ideal application for the laparoscopic approach owing to the significant morbidity associated with large flank or subcostal incisions required for their corresponding open procedures. Improvements in the understanding of laparoscopic anatomy, instrumentation, and laparoscopic training have made many of these operations commonplace at both community and university centers. We outline the major procedures now being performed for benign renal diseases and provide a stepwise guide for approaching these operations that we hope will prove useful for both experienced and inexperienced laparoscopic surgeons.

GENERAL

INDICATIONS **Simple Nephrectomy** Laparoscopic simple nephrectomy is often far from "simple" even for the most experienced laparoscopic surgeon because the conditions for which it is performed often result in significant perinephric scarring. The end result of these conditions is typically a kidney with marginal function and associated pain, hematuria, recurrent infections, or renovascular hypertension. Initiating conditions include chronic obstruction from an undiagnosed or inadequately treated ureteropelvic junction (UPJ) narrowing, stone disease, extrinsic compression, or iatrogenic strictures of the ureter.[1,2] Patients with persistent infections in poorly functioning kidneys from vesicoureteral reflux (VUR) or associated stone disease may require a nephrectomy to halt recurrence of the infectious process or pain associated with the condition. Similar symptoms may occur in patients with acquired renal cystic disease, autosomal dominant polycystic kidney disease (ADPKD), or multicystic dysplastic kidneys, ultimately necessitating removal. Atherosclerosis, fibromuscular abnormalities, or prior trauma to the renovascular system can result in a poorly functioning renal unit associated with renin-mediated hypertension not alleviated by medical management. This condition requires surgical removal of the affected side in order to control blood pressure. A large angiomyolipoma not amenable to a partial nephrectomy would be another condition for which laparoscopic simple nephrectomy could be considered. Xanthogranulomatous pyelonephritis (Figure 57-1) and renal

tuberculosis are two infectious conditions of the kidney that are relative contraindications to laparoscopic removal, as will be discussed later in this chapter.

Heminephrectomy Laparoscopic removal of an upper- or lower-pole moiety is performed for certain benign disease processes in kidneys with a complete duplication of the collecting system. Upper-pole obstruction and a differential decline in function most commonly occur in association with an ectopic ureter, with or without associated reflux, or an obstructing ureterocele.[3,4] Isolated loss of lower-pole function in the setting of a complete duplication of the collecting system most often is the result of a chronic UPJ obstruction or reflux nephropathy.[4,5] Presenting symptoms include flank pain, recurrent infections, incontinence, or more subtle signs of chronic infection.[4] In such cases, the amount of residual function in the remaining moiety of the affected side justifies whether preservation or removal of that portion of the renal unit should be performed. In cases of reflux or ectopia with obstruction, the associated ureteral segment is also removed as low down as possible to prevent it from serving as a potential reservoir for infection.

Benign Cyst Disease The primary indications for decortication of a renal cyst or cysts include pain, hematuria, collecting system obstruction, or associated bowel or respiratory complaints.[6–8] There are four categories of cysts that have been treated with regularity laparoscopically: simple, complex, peripelvic, or cysts associated with ADPKD.

Simple Cysts A possible cause and effect relationship between a large simple renal cyst and one of the above noted presenting symptoms is usually established by first performing a percutaneous puncture under ultrasound or computed tomographic (CT) guidance with aspiration of the cyst. If the symptoms improve following the aspiration, then a causal relationship is implied. Unfortunately, puncture and aspiration alone are often inadequate to prevent reaccumulation of the cyst fluid with recurrence of symptoms (Figure 57-2A and B). Instillation of sclerosing agents such as alcohol, providone-iodine, tetracycline, and minocycline increases the overall success rate of percutaneous management to 75 to 97%.[9–13] Despite the high reported success rate of this minimally invasive procedure, laparo-

scopic decortication of such cysts is often required as a salvage procedure if symptomatic reaccumulation occurs following percutaneous drainage and sclerosis.[7]

Complex Renal Cysts Bosniak[14] provided diagnostic groupings of cysts based on radiographic findings on enhanced and unenhanced CT scan imaging that could be used to predict the risk of cystic renal malignancy (Table 57-1). The incidence of malignancy in Bosniak I lesions is negligible, and the high risk of cystic renal cancer in Bosniak IV lesions (90%) requires approaching them as if they were a malignancy. The use of laparoscopy for treating these types of lesions, therefore, is not controversial. The controversy exists on whether or not laparoscopy should be utilized for the diagnostic evaluation and treatment of symptomatic Bosniak II and III lesions, given their risk of malignancy. Obvious concerns exist regarding the possibility of tumor spillage should a lesion prove to be a cystic renal cancer, especially when a transperitoneal approach is utilized. Catastrophic cases of diffuse tumor seeding following transperitoneal laparoscopic decortication have been described.[15] Attempts to define the presence of malignancy via predecortication cyst aspiration cytology have a reported false-negative predictive value of 20%.[6] Tradi-

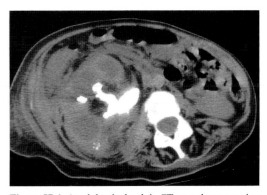

Figure 57-1 An abdominal-pelvic CT scan demonstrating the classic "bear paw" appearance of a patient with xanthogranulomatous pyelonephritis (XGP) of the right kidney. Note the presence of renal calcifications along with replacement of the collecting system with a fatty soft tissue mass representing lipid-ladened macrophages. Although perinephric stranding is visible, the intensity of the adhesion formation is not readily apparent, as open removal of this kidney required resection of a portion of the liver and mass clamping and oversewing of the hilar structures.

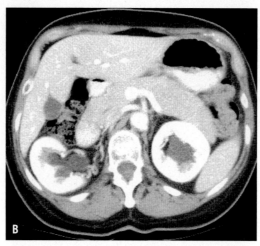

Figure 57-2 An abdominal-pelvic CT scan revealing reaccumulation of a large symptomatic simple cyst of the right kidney that failed two prior percutaneous aspiration attempts, the last involving sclerosis with alcohol (A). Note the intimate association and extension of the cyst beneath the inferior edge of the liver (B). This patient eventually underwent successful laparoscopic cyst decortication.

tionally, the safest approach to these lesions has been an open excision, treating the lesions as if they were a malignancy; however, several recent series have suggested the potential utility of the laparoscopic approach.[7,16]

Peripelvic Cysts Approximately 6% of all simple renal parenchymal cysts can be found immediately adjacent to or abutting the renal pelvis.[17] Although it is not clear what percentage will become symptomatic, cysts located in these areas can result in obstruction of the collecting system with resultant caliceal distention, pain, hematuria, recurrent infections, and stone formation.[18–20] Percutaneous aspiration and marsupialization as well as retrograde ureteroscopic treatment of these cysts have been employed with variable success.[7,21,22] The use of sclerosing agents in this scenario is risky owing to the close proximity of the collecting system and the potential for injury.[23,24] Because of their location, laparoscopic decortication of these lesions is associated with an increased risk of collecting system injury relative to simple cyst excision[7,19] and often requires additional operative maneuvers to prevent such occurrences.

Cysts Associated with Autosomal Dominant Polycystic Kidney Disease Unilateral and bilateral decortications of multiple cysts associated with ADPKD have been shown to improve flank and abdominal pain and, in some cases, associated gastrointestinal and diaphragmatic complaints in these patients.[8] As many as 60% of patients with ADPKD will suffer from chronic flank pain, which is largely thought to be a result of capsular distention providing noxious stimulus of visceral afferent nerves to the kidney.[25] Other potential causes of painful stimulus include episodes of cyst infection, as well as acute hemorrhage.[26] Compression of normal surrounding areas of renal parenchyma has also been hypothesized to create ischemia within the affected kidneys, leading to activation of the renin-angiotensin system with resultant hypertension and progressive decline of renal function over time.[27,28]

Percutaneous aspiration of these cysts often leads to rapid reaccumulation and recurrence of pain. Aggressive open decortications have resulted in more durable pain relief in 80 to 90% of patients at 1 year; however, progressive recurrence over time has been reported as new cysts form and others enlarge.[29,30] Ye and colleagues[30] reported initial pain relief in 92% of their patients at 1 year, but this declined to 81% by 5 years. Unfortunately, open decortications were also associated with significant morbidity and even mortalities, with several published series in the late 1950s reporting mortality rates of 11%.[31,32] A more contemporary series by Fleming and Barry[33] described their series of 28 patients who underwent open decortications resulting in 1 patient death, while 13% suffered prolonged ileus, and 10% cardiac dysrhythmias. In 1995, Teichman and Hulbert[34] reported the successful use of laparoscopy to perform cyst decortications in 6 patients with ADPKD. Lee and colleagues[8] recently reported durable pain relief in ADPKD patients 3 years following laparoscopic decortication with additional improvements in blood pressure, quality of life, and stabilization of renal function during the study period.

Calicealectomy Caliceal diverticula are transitional cell-lined, dilated chambers that connect with the collecting system via a narrow opening. Their etiology is unclear, but the leading theories include a failure of fusion of one of the branchings of the ampulla of the ureteric bud[35,36]

versus rupture into the collecting system of an adjacent abscess.[37] Approximately 40% have associated calculi.[35,36] Patients with this condition often present with pain, infections, or hematuria.[37] Occasionally, diverticula are asymptomatic and discovered incidentally on imaging procedures performed for other reasons. These may not require surgery, depending on their size, patient age, comorbidities, and preference. Stone clearance success rates for percutaneous approaches to a stone-bearing diverticulum have been reported to be as high as 70 to 95%, but 20 to 33% may have persistence of the diverticulum.[38–42] This technique can be extremely challenging in patients with anteriorly located lesions owing to the difficulty of accessing the diverticulum without passing tangentially through a significant portion of the renal parenchyma.

Alternative treatment approaches include shock wave lithotripsy (SWL) and a retrograde ureteroscopic approach. SWL has a low stone clearance rate of 6 to 58%,[38,39,43–46] but a surprisingly high percentage of symptomatic patients (75%) have reported resolution of their symptoms with this technique.[44] If it can be accessed from below, an alternative approach is to incise or balloon dilate the neck of the diverticulum, and to then attempt to ablate the diverticulum with laser energy or electrocautery. This technique can be cumbersome for large stone burdens, and often the neck of the diverticulum cannot be readily identified. In addition, adequate collapse and ablation of the diverticulum often does not occur. Pang and colleagues[47] described a successful stone clearance rate of 66% using this approach.

The laparoscopic approach to caliceal diverticula was first described in 1993[37] and has proven to be ideally suited for anterior or lateral-based diverticula with associated large stone burden and minimal overlying parenchyma (Figure 57-3). This approach can also be applied to posterior-based lesions, but is arguably more invasive than the percutaneous approach.

Nephropexy The condition of nephroptosis (pathologic hypermobility of the kidney) typically presents as intermittent pain in the flank or lower quadrant with standing activities that improves when supine. This condition can also be associated with hematuria, upper or lower tract urinary infections, urinary calculi, or hypertension.[48–52] Classically, it occurs in the right kidney of thin women or patients who have recently experienced a significant amount of weight

Table 57-1 Bosniak Criterion*[6,14,150]					
Type	I. II. Wall	III. IV. Septa	V. VI. Calcification	VII. VIII. Enhancement	Malignant Potential
I	Thin	Absent	Absent	Absent	< 0.7%
II	Thin	Few	Few	Absent	24%
III	Slightly Thickened	Multiple	Multiple	Absent	41%
IV	Thickened	Multiple with Nodularity	Extensive with Nodularity	Present	90%

*Determined by computed tomographic imaging with and without contrast.

loss,[53] with some series reporting as high as a 10:1 female predominance.[54]

Laparoscopic fixation of the kidney to the retroperitoneal fascia (nephropexy) is performed to prevent rotation and/or descent of the kidney to alleviate episodes of pain-inducing obstruction or ischemia. Downward displacement is thought to cause stretching and partial luminal narrowing of the main renal artery, which has been supported by nuclear renal scan and angiographic findings.[50,55,56] Previously, nephroptosis was felt to warrant surgery if radiographic descent of the kidney by > 2 vertebral spaces (5 cm) on standing relative to supine images was demonstrated.[53,57,58] The historic lack of clinical improvement in patients operated on using this diagnostic criterion has lead to a more functional stratification of surgical candidates.[53] Patients with the greatest likelihood of benefiting from a nephropexy have now been defined as symptomatic individuals with documented obstruction (prolonged one-half excretion times [$t_{1/2}$]), decreased relative function, and/or renal ischemia (poor 1- to 2-minute perfusion times) on a diuretic renal scan on the affected side that improve on the supine relative to the upright study (Figure 57-4A, B, and C).[53,58] Fornara and colleagues defined the minimum requirements prior to performing a nephropexy as a symptomatic patient with a documented functional difference of at least 10% between the supine and sitting nuclear renal scans.[53]

PATIENT PREPARATION Patient preparation should include a complete history and physical examination with specific attention to prior transperitoneal or retroperitoneal surgical procedures, episodes of associated peritonitis, locations of abdominal scarring, and other conditions, which could add complexity to a laparoscopic approach.[59] Conditions resulting in hepato- or splenomegaly such as fatty liver infiltration or portal vein hypertension, respectively, can also complicate laparoscopic operations on retroperitoneal structures. Prior lumbar fixations, kyphoscoliosis, or a depressed flattened diaphragm associated with severe cases of chronic obstructive pulmonary disease can also impact the positioning and exposure required for laparoscopic operations. Laparoscopic surgery in the morbidly obese patient, although previously thought to be a relative contraindication,[60] has subsequently been shown to be efficacious and to yield results superior to open surgery.[61] This condition does, however, require minor modifications in port placement owing to the thickness and mobility of the large abdominal pannus.

Appropriate imaging studies to assist in surgical planing and patient selection should be performed. Our preferred study for patients undergoing laparoscopic simple nephrectomy is a CT scan with and without contrast, which is extremely helpful in outlining the anatomy of the kidney and its surrounding organs. In patients with atherosclerotic disease, careful attention should be given to the artery of the affected renal unit to make sure there is not calcified plaque, which can result in clip or staple fracturing and uncontrolled hemor-

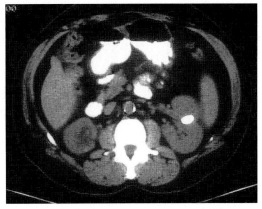

Figure 57-3 A stone-containing, anterolateral-based caliceal diverticulum demonstrated on CT scan imaging. Note the marked thinning of the overlying parenchyma and resultant indentation of the renal surface.

rhage during laparoscopic attempts at securing the vessel.[62] In patients with renal cystic disease, delayed contrast sequences delineating separation between the collecting system and the cyst wall are particularly helpful, especially in cases of ADPKD in whom multiple cysts are decorticated. These delayed images define the relationship of renal pathology to the collecting system and help determine whether or not preoperative ureteral catheter placement is indicated. A plain film prior to and at the end of acquiring the delayed images can also be used to provide coronal imaging of the collecting system when evaluating such nuances as whether or not a stone is located within a diverticulum. Alternative modalities to image patients with a contrast allergy or poor overall renal function include a noncontrast CT scan or magnetic resonance imaging (MRI) with and without gadolinium administration.

Nuclear renal scan imaging to document poor function in the affected side or moiety prior to nephrectomy or heminephrectomy, respectively, is often performed in addition to the above noted studies. This is a critical study for patients with a duplicated system in whom a potential heminephrectomy is planed. Patients with suspected renin-mediated hypertension can be evaluated using provocative captopril nuclear renal scan imaging or renal vein renin samplings with ultimate gold standard confirmation provided by angiography.[63] In patients with radiographically confirmed nephroptosis, the critical study is the nuclear renal scan performed in both a supine and sitting position. The initial study performed is often an intravenous pyelogram, as the symptoms are difficult to differentiate from an ureteropelvic junction obstruction or an intermittently obstructing calculus. The two nuclear renal scans need to be performed on two different dates and comparisons made between the 1- and 2-minute perfusion times, relative renal function, and the $t_{1/2}$ excretion times. A reduction in the perfusion or prolongation of the drainage times in the sitting position, in addition to symptomatic changes and demonstrated descent of greater than 2 vertebral bodies (5 cm) on intravenous pyelogram are diagnostic (see Figure 57-4A, B, and C).[53,58]

Laboratory and additional patient performance assessments are identical to those used for open operations. These should include routine hematologic, chemistry, and coagulation studies, as well as a dipstick and microscopic urine assessment. Patients with atherosclerotic renovascular disease should undergo careful cardiovascular assessment, as concomitant carotid and coronary artery disease is often present and may need correction prior to nephrectomy.

We typically perform a type and screen for blood products. Rarely, when more significant bleeding is anticipated, a type and cross or autologous blood donation should be considered. This latter approach may also be applied to all patients early in an individual surgeon's laparoscopic experience. Patients are instructed to avoid the use of aspirin for 1 week and nonsteroidal anti-inflammatory medications for 72 hours prior to surgery. If the patient is on oral anticoagulant therapy, this should be discontinued at least 5 days prior to surgery, if feasible, or the patient admitted and converted to heparin in cases where the duration of blood-thinning agents must be minimized.

A mechanical bowel preparation consisting of a clear liquid diet the day prior to surgery and administration of a bottle of magnesium citrate is utilized for all laparoscopic procedures. Cleansing of the bowel is important because it decompresses the large bowel, aiding in visualization and facilitating dissection. In addition, it also limits fecal soiling should a bowel injury occur and anecdotally appears to speed recovery of bowel function.

INFORMED CONSENT Every procedure, which is scheduled to be performed laparoscopically, should include the phrase "laparoscopic, possible open _" on the surgical posting and consent form. It should also be thoroughly explained to the patient that if it becomes unsafe or deemed impossible to progress laparoscopically, then the procedure will be converted to an open operation. Although a complication such as a bowel injury or uncontrolled hemorrhage can lead to an open conversion of a laparoscopic case, conversion in and of itself should not be viewed by the patient as a complication, but rather a safe alternative for completion of the proposed procedure. Similar to open operations, informed consents for laparoscopic surgical procedures should include a specific discussion of all potential major and minor complications. It should also include an accurate revelation of the individual surgeon's experience with laparoscopy and the particular surgical procedure being performed. If the surgeon will have a proctor or more experienced laparoscopic surgeon assisting him or her, this should also be clearly discussed, including that individual's qualifications. Utilization of specialized equipment that is new to the operating surgeon, such as robotics, which could significantly alter the flow or outcome of the operation, should also be revealed. The elements in Table 57-2 should be included within the informed consent for all laparoscopic renal procedures, including several additions specific for heminephrectomy, renal cyst ablation, calicealectomy, and nephropexy.

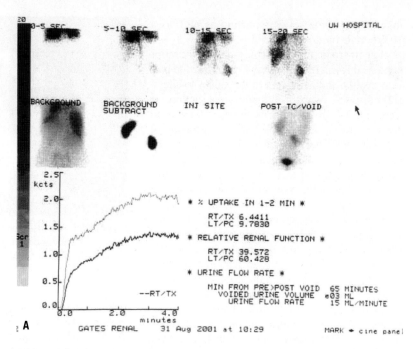

Figure 57-4 Diagnostic nuclear renal Lasix scans of a patient with clinical nephroptosis. *A,* A preoperative supine study reveals reasonable perfusion (1- to 2-minute uptake: right, 6.4%; left, 9.8%) and relative function (right, 39.6%; left, 60.4%). *B,* Preoperative sitting study demonstrates classic declines of perfusion (1- to 2-minute uptake: right, 2.0%; left, 8.6%) and relative function of the ptotic right kidney (right, 19%; left, 81%). Note the low-lying position of the right kidney on the sitting relative to the supine images. *C,* Postlaparoscopic nephropexy, sitting study demonstrates corrected position of the right kidney and marked improvements in perfusion (1- to 2-minute uptake: right, 11.0%; left, 8.8%) and relative function (right, 55%; left, 45%).

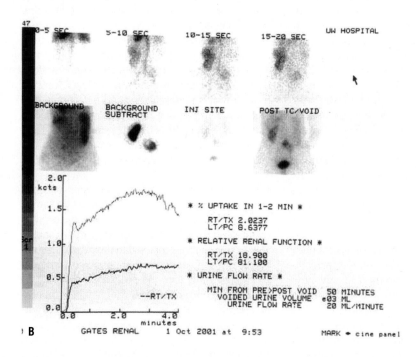

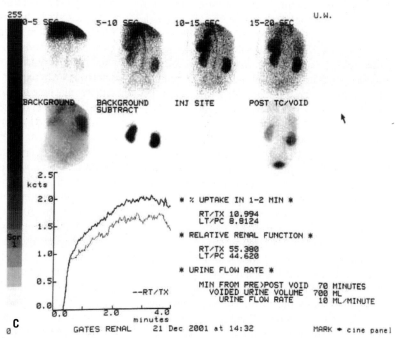

PREOPERATIVE PREPARATION On call to the operating room, a broad-spectrum parenteral antibiotic (second-generation cephalosporin) is usually administered. The pneumoperitoneum has been shown to reduce venous velocity and blood return from the lower extremities.[64] To improve the mechanical return of blood from the lower extremities and to stimulate the release of plasminogen activators,[65] TED Hose and sequential compression devices are applied to the lower extremities in all patients undergoing prolonged laparoscopic procedures.

The operative table should be equipped with a kidney rest and push button electric controls, allowing for flexion, airplaning, and Trendelenburg's positioning. We utilize 3-inch foam padding and a second layer of eggcrate on the entire surface of the operative table to limit pressure points during the operation. Obese patients with a large abdominal pannus may also require the use of a beanbag to assist in low pressure, contoured securing of all aspects of their excess girth. In cases where the beanbag is utilized, the large gel pad can be placed over its surface and supplemented using additional foam.

Patient Positioning: Transperitoneal Procedures After the endotracheal tube has been secured, the patient is placed with their down kidney directly over the kidney rest in the flank position with slight (15-degree) posterior tilt from the vertical. This degree of angulation improves access to the surface of the abdomen for port placement and lessens medial rotation of the kidney as dissection progresses. Some surgeons prefer vertical flank positioning and then adjust the position by actively airplaning the table at the beginning of the case to assist in port placement, or during the case when medial rotation of the kidney occurs. A posterior gel-pad roll covered by a towel can be positioned lengthwise across the patient's lower back and secured to the table using a double-jointed support arm to provide reliable stabilization of the patient even during full airplaning away from the operating surgeon. The patient's lower leg is flexed and the upper leg is kept straight as ample pillows are placed between the legs to keep them at a comfortable neutral separation without abduction. Pillows should be placed perpendicular to the lower extremities to limit the possibility of the lower legs rolling off the operative table as it is airplaned. Care must be taken to minimize the amount of pillow end protruding from between the upper thighs, as these can inhibit the downward excursion of instru-

Table 57-2

Risk Elements of the Informed Consent for all Laparoscopic Renal Procedures
Bleeding requiring transfusion
Infection (retroperitoneal of superficial)
Injury to adjacent structures (eg, bowel, adrenal, spleen, liver, pancreas, etc.)
Renal insufficiency
Thromboembolism
Cardiovascular event
Postoperative bowel obstruction or prolonged ileus
Neuromuscular injury
Hernia formation
Persistent pain
Additional Risk Elements
Heminephrectomy
Persistent urinary leakage
Need for additional drainage procedure (eg, stent or percutaneous drainage)
Renal Cyst Ablation
Injury of the collecting system
Persistent urinary leakage
Need for additional drainage procedure (eg, stent or percutaneous drainage)
Cyst recurrence
Calcicealectomy
Injury to the collecting system
Persistent urinary leakage
Need for additional drainage procedure (eg, stent or percutaneous drainage)
Stone extrusion
Caliceal or stone recurrence
Persistent pain
Nephropexy
Continued hypermobility

ments inserted through lower quadrant ports. Foam should be utilized to pad the tubing of the sequential compression devices to prevent contact between the body and these firm structures.

We utilize two arm boards placed adjacent to one another on the opposite side of the table from the patient's pathology to support their arms. An axillary roll made from eggcrate foam or gel-pad material is inserted 2 finger-breadths beneath the axilla to prevent excessive stretch of the brachial plexus while minimizing contact pressure. The kidney rest is elevated slightly and the table is flexed minimally to increase the working space between the lower ribcage and the iliac crest, thus facilitating separation of trocars on the abdomen or flank. Excessive kidney rest elevation and flexion of the table is discouraged as it can actually reduce the working space within the abdomen and may lead to neuromuscular injury to the flank in contact with the operative table.[66] A sufficient number of pillows should be placed between the arms to allow comfortable shoulder-width separation. These pillows are oriented in line with the arms and are inserted deep into the axilla of the upper arm; otherwise, they will take up too much space along the abdomen and limit upward movements of the laparoscopic instruments.

A strap is placed across the lower legs of the patient in the area of the midcalf, and the electrocautery pad is adhered to the upper thigh. Two towels are folded lengthwise and one is placed at the hip just above the cautery pad extending downward to cover the genitalia while the other passes from the elbow to across the shoulder of the upper arm. Two to three passes of 3-inch cloth tape are brought from table edge to table edge across the towels, with care taken not to place too much compressive force at the point of body contact. After the tape passes over the shoulder of the upper arm and approaches the elbow, it is split from the far end and wrapped on either side of the tower of pillows on the arm boards (Figure 57-5). This secures the arms, the pillows on which they rest, and the upper torso to the operative table. A foam or gel-pad ring may be required to keep the patient's head in a neutral location after they have been positioned. Airplaning and Trendelenburg's movements of the table should be tested prior to prepping the abdomen and flank to ensure that all areas of the patient are adequately secured.

When a beanbag is utilized, it is pushed up around the patient's abdomen and back in a cradling fashion with care taken not to elevate the edges so high that they may inhibit downward movements of the laparoscopic instruments. Care must also be exercised to keep the supporting edges broad as suction is being applied to solidify the beanbag, otherwise narrow edges of contact can produce excessive pressure and result in myonecrosis. Two-inch foam strips can be inserted along contact points to provide necessary extra padding.

Bilateral simple nephrectomy is occasionally indicated, with the most common clinical scenario being persistent hypertension, pyelonephritis, vesicoureteral reflux, protein-wasting nephropathy, hematuria, or painful cystic disease associated with the native kidneys in kidney transplant recipients.[67,68] In these cases, the operative table is prepared in similar fashion to unilateral cases with the exception that the arm boards are opened on either side at almost 90 degrees to the table. Large foam wedges are placed on each arm board on which the patient's arms rest and are secured at the forearms. The patient is positioned with their umbilicus at the level of the break in the operative table, the kidney rest is elevated to a neutral position, and the table is flexed slightly. This allows the patient to be fully airplaned to the right or left to elevate the side on which the kidney is being removed and prevents the need for patient repositioning between nephrectomies.[67,68]

Patient Positioning: Retroperitoneal Procedures Patient positioning for retroperitoneal procedures is similar to that for transperitoneal operations with several noteworthy exceptions. Since the retroperitoneal space presents a smaller overall working environment and a more limited region of port entry, several maneuvers are critical to optimize both. The patient is placed in a flank position without angulation. This position displaces the lateral peritoneal reflection along with the colon in an anterior direction,[69] doubling the undisturbed anterior-to-posterior length of the retroperitoneal space.[70] Chiu and colleagues demonstrated that merely placing a patient in the flank position increased the distance between the quadratus lumborum and the colon 8.7 to 27.3 mm on the left and 4.6 to 18.1 mm on the right side.[71] The kidney rest is elevated until it is in contact with the flank and more table flexion is utilized than with the transperitoneal approach to enlarge the space between the lower ribs and the iliac wing. This is an important step to enlarge the much more limited surface area for retroperitoneal port insertion. The remainder of the patient padding and positioning is identical to that performed for transperitoneal surgery, with the exception that beanbags and posterior gel-pad rolls are not utilized, as they can limit the excursion of instruments during retroperitoneal laparoscopic procedures.

Anesthesiology Preparations The anesthesiologists should be encouraged to calculate and replace fluid deficits prior to insufflation of the abdomen to minimize the hemodynamic effects of the pneumoperitoneum that are more pronounced with hypovolemia.[72–74] Nitrous oxide inhalants should be avoided as they can lead to bowel distention, making visualization difficult and increasing the potential for bowel injury.[75,76] The use of nitrous oxide inhalant during laparoscopy has also been shown to create a gaseous environment in the peritoneum supportive of combustion, which can be potentially catastrophic if electrocautery is being utilized.[77] A urinary drainage (Foley) catheter and oro- or nasogastric tube are inserted prior to patient positioning to decompress the bladder and stomach, respectively. The Foley catheter should be secured with tape to the lower leg for patients in

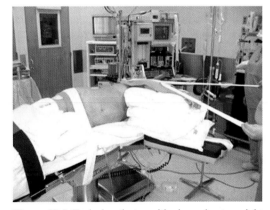

Figure 57-5 Typical patient positioning prior to a right transperitoneal laparoscopic renal procedure. The extremities are comfortably separated utilizing stacks of pillows, and there is only minimal flexion applied to the operative table without significant kidney rest elevation. Several strips of wide cloth tape secure the patient to the operative table at the hip and across the shoulder and upper arm. The skin is protected with towels, and the tape passing over the shoulder is split to the elbow and secured on either side of the stack of pillows. A leg strap is passed across the lower legs.

the flank position. Oliguria during prolonged laparoscopy is common, and the anesthesiologist must be well versed on this issue and avoid "chasing the urine output," as this can lead to fluid overload.[78–81] The upper arm should be the site for placement of the blood pressure cuff and parenteral lines for which rapid access may be necessary. A pneumatic patient warming device can be adhesed to the upper extremities and torso or on the lower extremities up to the level of the hips to assist in maintaining patient temperature throughout the case. Even though the peritoneal surface and bowel is not exposed through a large incision during laparoscopy, heat exchange can still be significant because of the convection flow of the insufflant. Warming of the patient utilizing these devices or insufflant warmers is important to maintain body temperature throughout the case, especially in older patients.

Operative Site Preparation and Draping The ipsilateral abdomen and flank are shaved from the area of the xiphoid to pubis. A solution of providone-iodine (Betadine) or a similar surface preparation is used to paint the surgical area. The preparation should be wide enough to include the possibility of an open conversion via a flank, subcostal, or midline incision. Special laparoscopic drapes with widened apertures, Velcro straps for cords and tubing, and instrument pockets are commercially available, although a standard paper flank drape can be utilized and the aperture enlarged with scissors to give adequate exposure. Channels can also be created for the light and camera cords, as well as the insufflation tubing, by pulling up redundant drape and clamping it to itself while the cords are brought out through the ends.

Operating Room Setup The operative site and the laparoscopic approach determine the variables of the operating room setup for the procedure. The patient is positioned on the operating room table in the flank or semiflank orientation with their affected side up as outlined above. The surgeon and the first assistant stand on the contralateral side of the table to the patient's pathology for transperitoneal procedures and the ipsilateral side for retroperitoneal procedures. The scrub nurse or technician stands on the opposite side of the table from the primary surgeon, which facilitates passage of equipment directly across the operative table. This arrangement eliminates the need for the operative surgeon to take their eyes away from the primary monitor to reach behind or to their side to receive instruments.

The primary tower containing the insufflator, light source, and camera box is positioned across from the operating surgeon so he or she can visually inspect the settings as well as the pressure readings throughout the case. The secondary tower is placed on the same side as the primary surgeon for use by the scrub nurse or second assistant. Monitor towers are positioned toward the head of the table and angled back toward the operating surgeon. The height of the monitor must be appropriate for the operating surgeon so

upward tilting of the head and subsequent neck fatigue can be avoided. Irrigation fluids are hung on one of the intravenous poles near the head of the patient and the suction canisters are also situated near the anesthetic machine. The scrub nurse places their working table directly over the patient's lower legs. This consists of a Mayo stand on which all frequently used equipment is placed. The back equipment tables are placed end to end just lateral to the patient's feet, forming an L-configuration with the table on the same side as the scrub nurse. The most lateral table contains the open instrumentation (Figure 57-6).

PROCEDURES

SIMPLE NEPHRECTOMY The major advantages of the transperitoneal approach to laparoscopic simple nephrectomy over the retroperitoneal approach are a larger working space and anatomy that is familiar to most surgeons. Disadvantages of this approach include the need to dissect and retract the colon, spleen, and pancreas on the left and the liver and duodenum on the right. There is also an increased risk of visceral complications as a result.[62,82] Limited dissection of the bowel, avoidance of areas of intraperitoneal adhesion, and rapid posterior access to the main renal artery

when performing nephrectomy are the main advantages of the retroperitoneal approach.

Instrumentation (University of Wisconsin, Madison)

Four non-bladed trocars: two 5 mm and two 10/12 mm (with reducers)

Two 10 mm laparoscopes: one 0-degree and one 30-degree

Two 5 mm laparoscopes: one 0-degree and one 30-degree (available in the room)

One 14-gauge Veress needle (transperitoneal)

One trocar-mounted balloon dilation device (Origin Medsystems, Menlo Park, CA) (retroperitoneal)

One 10/12 mm blunt tip cannula (available in the room)

One 10/12 mm visual introducing cannula

One 5 mm curved electrocautery scissors

One 5 mm curved Maryland dissector

One 5 mm curved Harmonic scalpel and generator

One 10 mm locking Babcock

One 5 mm dolphin-nosed grasper

One 10 mm right-angle dissector

One 5 mm toothed locking grasper

One 5 mm electrocautery hook

Two 5 mm laparoscopic needle drivers (available in the room)

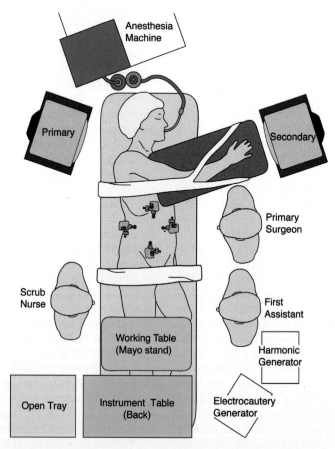

Figure 57-6 Standard operating room set-up for a laparoscopic right-sided transperitoneal renal procedure. The scrub nurse or assistant is positioned across the table, providing easy transfer of instruments to the operating surgeon. During retroperitoneal procedures the setup is essentially a mirror image of the transperitoneal arrangement with the exception of the patient position, which remains unchanged. Placement of generators toward the foot of the bed minimizes cord interference with surgeon movements around the operative table.

One 5 mm diamond flex triangle retractor (Genzyme, Tucker, GA) (available in the room)

One 10 mm PEER retractor (Jarit, Hawthorne, NY)

One Martin arm (available in the room)

One GIA vascular stapler and two reloads

One 11 mm multiload clip applier

One 5 mm irrigator/aspirator

One LapSac (Cook Urological, Spencer, IN) (5 × 8 and 8 × 10 inches) (optional for morcellation of specimens)

One Endocatch II bag (U.S. Surgical, Norwalk, CT) (optional for intact specimen removal)

One grasping needle port closure device

One smoke evacuator valve (Plume-Away: Stryker Endoscopy, San José, CA) (optional)

One No. 15 blade scalpel and handle

Two fine-toothed pickups

One Tonsil clamp

Two S-retractors

Three 0-Vicryl ties

Four 4-0 absorbable sutures on a cutting needle

One-quarter-inch Steri-Strips

Benzoin

Open nephrectomy surgical pan

STEPS OF THE PROCEDURE: TRANSPERITONEAL

Step 1: Creation of the Pneumoperitoneum and Initial Entry Access The patient is positioned on the table in a modified flank position, as described above, with the side of the operative pathology placed up. A 1 cm incision is made through the skin in the lower quadrant just lateral to the rectus muscle midway between the umbilicus and the anterior-superior iliac crest in nonobese patients. This location may need to be shifted cephalad and lateral in obese patients owing to the large abdominal pannus. A small clamp is utilized to spread the underlying subcutaneous tissues down to the level of the fascia. A Veress needle is then inserted perpendicular to the fascial surface. The initial audible "pop" is the puncturing of the fascia, whereas the second represents entry into the peritoneal cavity. This secondary sound is generated by the snap of the internal obturator of the needle and often can be felt in the introducing hand as well as heard. The tip of the Veress needle should move freely side to side with no perceived resistance, and gentle irrigation and aspiration of saline via a 10 cc syringe should confirm correct positioning of the needle in the peritoneal space. Saline injected into the hub of the Veress needle should flow freely, and on removal of the syringe the column of saline should drain readily into the abdomen via gravity alone ("drop test"). Aspiration of air or enteric contents heralds entry into the bowel with the Veress needle. The abdomen is insufflated to 15 mm Hg pressure, elevating the flow rate of CO_2 once it is clear that the initial peritoneal pressures are appropriately low. Initial insufflation pressures should be less than 10 mm Hg, and higher pressures often indicate entrapment of the needle in omentum, mesentery, or the preperitoneal space.

Vascular and enteric injuries on initial trocar entry of the abdomen have been reported to occur in 0.3% of laparoscopic cases.[83] A review of

3 series in which 617 access entry injuries occurred demonstrated a 3% death rate following this occurrence, with 59% owing to vascular and 41% resulting from bowel injuries, respectively.[83] For this reason, we utilize a visual obturator such as the OptiView (Ethicon Endo-Surgery, Cincinnati, OH) or Visiport (U.S. Surgical, Norwalk, CT) to establish initial access. Both allow insertion of the laparoscope into a pistol-shaped introducer placed through the top of a 10/12 mm standard laparoscopic port. The OptiView introducer also comes in a 5 mm size and is shaped like a standard obturator rather than the pistol configuration. Both devices allow visualization of each layer of the abdominal wall as it is traversed. Entry through the peritoneum is heralded by a widening black hole in the center of the visual field through which the device is advanced. During trocar insertion, it is important to angle ports toward the area of interest to prevent limitations on excursion and to ensure that the peritoneal and fascial entry points do not line up, therefore limiting the potential for herniation following their removal.

Another option for entry access is utilization of a Hasson cannula via an open technique. This approach usually requires a slightly larger incision to allow adequate exposure of the underlying fascia using the S-retractors. The fascia is incised and a 0 absorbable suture mounted on a semicircular needle, such as a UR-6, is utilized to place a tacking suture through each corner of the fascial incision. The underlying muscular fibers are split using a tapered clamp and the posterior fascial layer is incised exposing the preperitoneal fat. The thickness of this layer can vary markedly depending on the habitus of the patient. The preperitoneal fat is spread to expose the underlying peritoneum, which is grasped and incised to reveal the peritoneal contents. At this point, we usually replace the tacking sutures to include all of the transected layers. A blunt-tipped open cannula (eg, Hasson) is then inserted through the peritoneal opening. Variations of this type of trocar are available; however, they usually pass through a cuff that is shaped like an inverted cone that is snugged down into the fascial opening and locked in place on the shaft of the trocar. The fascial corner sutures are then wrapped around circular guides on the conical cuff to secure the port in position. Universal or flip-top reducers are placed to allow utilization of 5 mm instruments via the 10/12 mm ports.

Step 2: Secondary Port Placement After initial access to the peritoneum, a thorough inspection of the abdomen is performed to assess for the presence of adhesions, organomegaly, or altered location of the kidney, which could impact positioning of secondary ports. A skin incision is made for each port that corresponds to the width of the port itself, which can be determined by pressing the mouth of the port into the skin and indenting the epidermis. If the skin incision is too small, it can result in difficult trocar insertion. The increased force generated to insert the trocar can ultimately cause rapid uncontrolled entry into the abdomen through a partially collapsed

body wall with resultant injury of the underlying viscera or vasculature. If the skin incision is too large, it can result in leakage of the pneumoperitoneum or inadvertent port dislodgment from the peritoneum. In patients with a nonobese body habitus, a 10/12 mm port is inserted in the periumbilical region. An additional 5 mm trocar is inserted approximately 2 cm below the subcostal margin in the midclavicular region. As mentioned above, all ports are shifted lateral and slightly cephalad in markedly obese patients to avoid the abdominal pannus. Placement of ports too close to the ribs or attached cartilage can inhibit movement of the instruments as they encounter the ribcage. The location of secondary port placement is identical for right- and left-handed surgeons.

Three ports are often adequate for performing left-sided nephrectomies; however, an optional 5 mm port can be placed between the twelfth rib and the iliac crest in the posterior axillary line to allow for kidney and ureteral retraction by an assistant if so desired. For right-sided nephrectomies, a similarly located fourth port is often necessary for liver retraction (Figure 57-7). Some surgeons prefer lowering the upper midclavicular port on the right and moving it more medial while placing an additional 5 mm port above to use for liver retraction. This is accomplished by passing a locking instrument through this port, under-

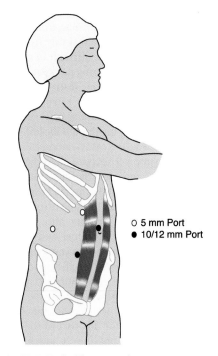

Figure 57-7 Typical laparoscopic port arrangement for a right-sided transperitoneal renal procedure. Trocars are usually inserted near the umbilicus, midway between the iliac crest and umbilicus, just below the costal margin in the midclavicular line, and at the anterior axillary line midway between the twelfth rib and the iliac crest. Procedure-based determinations of port size are discussed in each individual operative section within the chapter. In general, 10/12 mm ports are used at the umbilicus and lower quadrant, whereas 5 mm ports are used at the costal and lateral margins. Modification of port location for obesity involves shifting ports cephalad and lateral to avoid the abdominal pannus.

○ 5 mm Port
● 10/12 mm Port

neath the liver, and grasping the cut edge of the peritoneum on the lateral body wall.

In cases where a bilateral simple nephrectomy is being performed, a total of 5 trocars are utilized in an "X"-configuration.[67,68] A 10/12 mm port is inserted at the umbilicus, or several centimeters above, with 2 ports inserted in the right and left midclavicular line several centimeters below the costal margin and at the level of the anterior superior iliac spine.[67,68] These can either be all 10/12 mm ports or, for a right-handed surgeon, the left subcostal and right anterior superior iliac midclavicular ports can be replaced by 5 mm trocars. Conversely, for left-hand-dominant surgeons, the left anterior superior iliac spine and right subcostal midclavicular ports can be replaced with 5 mm ports. Minor upward adjustments to the location of the ipsilateral lower quadrant port may be required when a transplant kidney is present.

The trocars are appropriately positioned within the abdomen by pulling them back until the insufflation port is just within the peritoneal cavity. Ports can be secured to the abdominal wall by placing a 2-0 absorbable or nonabsorbable suture through the skin, tying an air-knot, then wrapping the suture once around the stopcock and tying it securely. If securing sutures are utilized, the port is rotated so the stopcock is furthest away from the area of dissection prior to placing the suture. This prevents the stitch from limiting upward movements of the instruments during dissection. Fascial splitting trocars with a grooved shaft are usually held firmly by the split edges of the fascia and are difficult to dislodge, obviating the need for securing sutures.

Step 3: Exposure of the Retroperitoneum
Adequate exposure of the retroperitoneum requires mobilization of several key structures. On the left side, upper quadrant adhesions of the omentum or bowel are often encountered and require mobilization to expose the edge of the splenic flexure and descending colon. The laparoscopic lens is usually inserted through the lower quadrant port and the operating surgeon utilizes the Maryland grasper and dissecting instrument via the periumbilical and subcostal port, depending on their dominant hand. The camera can also be inserted via the periumbilical port site and the lower-quadrant port used for working instruments, depending on the area of the dissection and what port access gives the best visualization. Usually for this part of the dissection the 0-degree lens provides a better view of the area of interest, especially as the avascular line of Toldt is incised and mobilization of the colon is carried inferiorly across the pelvic inlet. We typically utilize the Harmonic scalpel for most of the dissection, although the electrocautery shears can also be utilized. The Harmonic scalpel coagulates and divides structures utilizing heat generated from vibrations of the jaws of the instrument at a frequency of 55,500 Hertz.[84,85] This results in intracellular water vaporization, protein denaturation, and release of water vapor instead of smoke. The advantage of this device

over electrocautery is its reduced amount of collateral damage, lack of arcing to adjacent structures, reduced impairment of visualization, and its ability to seal and divide vessels as large as 4 mm in diameter.[86–88]

In older patients, additional adhesions may be encountered adjacent to the sigmoid colon owing to previous bouts of diverticulitis, and care must be exercised not to inadvertently transect enlarged diverticula in this region. The dissection should be carried cephalad to release all lateral attachments of the spleen while gently lifting it up using the shaft of an instrument inserted through the upper port. Splenic mobilization should continue until the greater curvature of the stomach is visualized (Figure 57-8). This is a critical step on the left side because the spleen will act as a dead weight to draw the pancreas and colon medial, thus giving better exposure of the kidney and preventing these structures from being injured. The plane between Gerota's fat and the posterior aspect of the colonic mesentery is often easily discernable and usually can be teased apart by a combination of blunt and cautery dissection. The vessels within the mesenteric fat and the smoother surface of the thin layer of Gerota's fascia overlying the retroperitoneal fat often provide additional clues to differentiating between these two layers. Separation along this plane should continue down across the pelvic inlet and the colon folded back on its mesentery until the pulsation of the aorta is visualized.

On the right side, the line of Toldt is similarly incised down around the cecum extending into the pelvis. The upper midclavicular and periumbilical ports are usually utilized for the dissection. The liver is mobilized by transecting the triangular ligament laterally and the coronary ligament below its lower edge. A 5 mm Diamond

Flex Triangle retractor (Genzyme, Tucker, GA) can be utilized for broad-based secure elevation of the liver via the lateral port between the twelfth rib and iliac crest. Once positioned beneath the liver, the retractor is secured to the operating table using a robotic (eg, Martin) arm. The right colon and its mesentery are separated from Gerota's fascia as described for the left-sided dissection. As the colon is rolled medially, the duodenum can be visualized in the upper portion of the retroperitoneum and is kocherized to reveal the underlying inferior vena cava (IVC). It is important to realize that, with rare exception, the duodenum overlies the vena cava and requires medial mobilization to adequately expose the right renal vein and upper IVC.

Step 4: Securing the Ureter The remaining steps of the operation are typically performed using a 30-degree laparoscopic lens inserted via the lower-quadrant port. The surgeon operates through the subcostal and periumbilical ports with the dominant hand usually controlling the dissecting instruments. The ureter is identified as one of two tubular structures running in a craniocaudal direction in the retroperitoneum. It usually lies deep and lateral to the similar-appearing blue-tinged gonadal vein. After adequate mobilization of the sigmoid colon, the ureter can almost always be visualized after it crosses the iliac vessels and heads into the pelvis. If it cannot be directly visualized, sometimes it provides enough tactile sensation as a firm "band-like" structure in the retroperitoneum to allow localization when a laparoscopic instrument is drawn across it from lateral to medial. Gentle squeezing of a nonpulsatile tubular structure that produces a peristaltic wave confirms that the observed structure is the ureter.

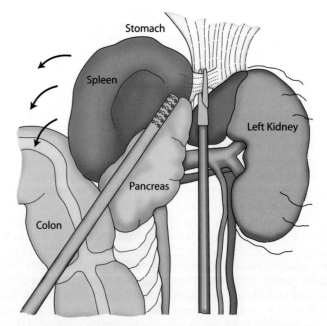

Figure 57-8 Complete exposure of the left retroperitoneum involves complete release of all lateral splenic attachments until the edge of the greater curvature of the stomach is visible. Once released, the weight of the spleen pulls the attached pancreas and bowel medially, protecting these structures while giving complete access to the renal hilum.

The upward-directed tips of the Maryland dissector are used to elevate the ureter either together or separate from the gonadal vein. On the right side it is preferable to release the gonadal vein medially, so it is not placed on any significant traction during the dissection, as this can result in aneurysmal dilation or rupture of its very weak entry point into the IVC. The peri-ureteral tissues can be separated using gentle downward blunt dissection together with Harmonic coagulation and division whenever more substantial tissue bands are encountered, as these often contain ureteral feeding vessels. Complete creation of a window beneath the ureter is facilitated by first opening Gerota's fascia lateral over the psoas musculature. The dissection is carried up along the top of the psoas to the region of the lower pole of the kidney. At this point, we typically secure and divide the ureter by placing a total of three 11 mm clips and cutting between the first and second clips. If easy separation of the gonadal vein and ureter cannot be performed, we will divide the ureter, gonadal vein, and peri-ureteral tissues together utilizing the Endo-GIA staple with a vascular (2.5 mm) load.

Step 5: Dissection and Securing of the Hilum Differences in the vascular anatomy between the right and left kidney require slight alterations in hilar dissection techniques between the two sides. On the left side, the gonadal vein drains into the left renal vein; it therefore can be utilized as a convenient method for identifying the surface of this structure. The tissue overlying the anterior surface of the gonadal vein is divided starting at the most proximal part of the vein that is visible. The Harmonic scalpel is ideal for performing this part of the operation, as there can be small branches that enter the gonadal vein medially and can cause troublesome bleeding if the tissues are merely transected. The gonadal vein is traced cephalad until the surface of the main renal vein is exposed on the left.

On the right side, the gonadal vein drains into the vena cava and can be used in similar fashion to identify the caval surface, although extreme care should be utilized in dissecting around this structure because of the fragility of its entry point into the IVC and risk of avulsion. It is important to separate the gonadal vein from the ureter so it can be swept medially, or to clip and divide it several centimeters distal to the IVC to prevent traction at its entry point. Often the surface of the IVC is readily visible after medial mobilization of the duodenum, and tracing the gonadal vein is unnecessary. The medial surface of the vena cava should then be exposed and followed cephalad to the entry point of the right renal vein, which often lies higher than one would anticipate relative to the predicted midregion of the kidney. Once the renal vein is identified, the correct dissection plane directly on the surface of the vein is established by incising the overlying adventitial tissue. The surrounding fibro-fatty and lymphatic tissue is grasped and the vein is rolled away and peeled out of the confines of this tissue on both its superior and inferior surfaces using blunt dissection.

On the left side, the adrenal vein branch is identified entering the cephalad surface of the main renal vein and is usually slightly medial to the entry site of the gonadal vein below, although the two sites can emerge from the same location. During this portion of the dissection, the assistant can elevate the kidney by grasping the ureter from the lateral-most port if one has been placed. Alternatively, a 2-0 nylon mounted on a Keith needle can be passed through the abdominal wall, followed by the wall of the ureter or periureteral tissues, and back out through the abdominal wall. The suture is then secured with a clamp (Figure 57-9). This can be elevated and lowered as desired to place the hilum on stretch and prevents the need for a lateral trocar on the left and on the right, which enables continuous maintenance of liver retraction through the lateral trocar during this portion of the dissection.

Completion of the hilar dissection can be performed utilizing either an anterior-inferior or a posterior approach to the renal artery.

Anterior-Inferior Approach This approach usually requires clipping and dividing of the gonadal, adrenal, and underlying ascending lumbar vein branches on the left side. The ascending lumbar vein branch invariably crosses over the renal artery and tethers the renal vein down making anterior exposure to the artery difficult. A total of 4 clips are placed on large branch veins, and endoshears are used to divide between the third and fourth clips. The Harmonic shears can be utilized to divide vein branches up to 4 mm in size by placing the Harmonic generator at a variable setting of 2. It is then used to create a coagulative seal at two widely spaced spots on the vessel, followed by coagulation and transection between the sealed areas. Care should be utilized not to inadvertently contact the main renal vein with any portion of the Harmonic shears, as this can lead to a thermal puncture.

The adrenal vein branch is similarly isolated and the overlying lymphatic and fibro-fatty tissues dissected until a right angle can be passed behind it. If the degree of fibrosis around the kidney allows it, we will release the edge of the adrenal gland from the medial aspect of the kidney prior to clipping and dividing the adrenal vein branch. The Harmonic shears are the ideal instrument for performing this portion of the procedure, as they efficiently seal the large number of small arteries that feed the adrenal gland. The jaws of the Harmonic are opened and the lower noninsulated jaw is pushed several millimeters into the tissues with the backside of the instrument flush on the adrenal gland to prevent injury to an early arterial branch or late upper-pole vein confluence of the renal vasculature. The jaws are then closed and activated. If bleeding occurs from a partially transected vessel, then advancement of the jaws across the area of bleeding is performed to complete the coagulation and transection. The adrenal gland does not swell and ooze as much utilizing this approach, as it does if the main adrenal vein branch is transected prior to dividing the medial arterial twigs. If the medial adrenal plane is difficult to establish, the adrenal vein branch is

clipped and transected and dissection of the main renal vasculature is continued. The adrenal vein branch can also be spared in cases where there is adequate vein length between the gonadal and adrenal vein branch entry points to allow either straight or angled application of the Endo-GIA stapler across the main renal vein (Figure 57-10).

As the assistant lifts the ureter and lower pole lateral to place the hilar vessels on stretch, the packet of lymphatic tissue between the artery and vein can be grasped and the artery and vein peeled away. The tissue between the vessels can then be divided by sequential transection using the Harmonic dissector until a right-angle clamp can be readily passed behind the artery and vein. Spreading of the right-angle dissector should confirm the presence of approximately 2 to 2.5 cm of space to allow easy passage of the Endo-GIA stapler. The hilum is placed on stretch by inserting the irrigator-aspirator through the upper port and placing it between the artery and vein and then lifting (Figure 57-11).

We prefer use of the 2.5 mm vascular Endo-GIA stapler to secure and divide the artery and vein; however, the interlocking Weck clips (Weck Closure Systems, Research Triangle Park, NC) also provide a safe means of controlling the arterial and, in some cases, the venous stump. Three Weck clips are placed on the artery and endos-

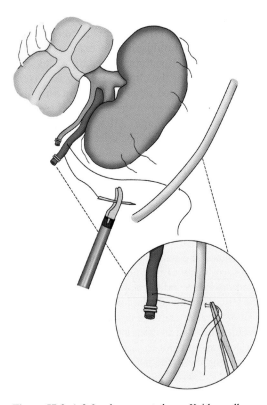

Figure 57-9 A 2-0 nylon mounted on a Keith needle can be utilized to provide variable amounts of kidney elevation without the need of an assistant's instrument. For the left side, this can alleviate the need for a lateral-most trocar. The needle is passed through the abdominal wall, then through the upper ureter or pelvis, and back out the abdominal wall. The needle is removed and tension on the suture can be altered to provide varying amounts of internal retraction as needed. (Insert) A clamp is placed on the suture ends at skin level to maintain the desired position.

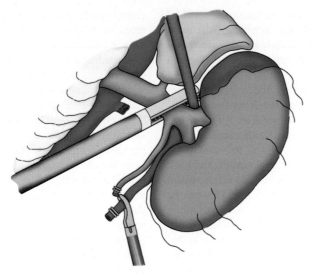

Figure 57-10 Once the renal artery has been secured and transected via a posterior approach, it is often easiest to approach the renal vein anteriorly. The kidney is flipped back into its lateral position and is slightly elevated by the assistant's grasper or a transabdominal nylon suture. The adrenal vein branch can usually be left intact with this approach. To gain extra venous length lateral to the adrenal vein branch to allow application of the Endovascular stapler, a blunt instrument such as the irrigator-aspirator can be inserted posterior to the kidney along its medial edge for elevation and lateral retraction, maximizing the space between the edge of the adrenal gland and the upper pole of the kidney.

hear division is performed leaving two clips on the stay side. Five clips are placed on the vein dividing between clips, so remain on the stay side. Caution should also be exercised when applying Weck clips to make certain the toe and recipient latch of the clip are entirely across the vessel being secured, otherwise the clip can puncture through the wall of the vessel and result in significant hemorrhage. All surrounding lymphatic tissue should also be released to prevent it from being entrapped in the locking mechanism of the clip, resulting in incomplete closure and possible delayed opening.

The device used to secure the hilar vessels can be introduced via the periumbilical or lower-quadrant port, depending on which provides the best angle of approach to the hilum. This is especially important if the stapler is not an articulating type. The narrow jaw of the stapler is slid between the artery and vein and the stapler advanced until the black marking line on the lower jaw passes the far wall of the artery and the device is clamped. Visualization of what is contained within the jaws of the instrument prior to firing the staple line and transecting the tissue is facilitated by rotating the device clockwise and then counterclockwise.[89] This careful inspection is necessary as 50% of the 1.7% of vascular Endo-GIA misfirings are due to application on previously placed clips.[89]

Once the artery is transected, the vein should appear collapsed and the specimen loses some of its turgor. If these changes are not observed, then a careful inspection for accessory arteries should be performed. Once the surgeon is confident that the kidney no longer has arterial flow, the vascular Endo-GIA stapler is passed across the vein in

an area free of clips, as well as the distal arterial staple line, and the vein is secured and divided.

The anterior-inferior approach to the right kidney is identical to what is performed on the left with the exception that no branches usually enter the main renal vein, and if they do, they are usually small secondary vessels that can be divided using the Harmonic scalpel. Although it is short, the right renal vein will usually accom-

modate the stapler. Another advantage on the right side is that many times the right renal artery lies slightly below the main renal vein, thus facilitating its identification and isolation.

Posterior Approach The posterior approach, or posterior renal artery control,[90] is usually employed anytime the artery cannot be readily controlled from the anterior-inferior exposure. The advantage of this maneuver on the left side is that it gives excellent access to the entire length of the artery, many times obviating the need to transect the lumbar vein as the artery can be secured and transected distally. If the renal vein segment is lengthy between the gonadal vein branch and the entry point into the hilum, it may be possible to leave all branches of the left renal vein intact with this approach.

During this maneuver, Gerota's fascia and fat are divided over the lateral aspect of the kidney using the Harmonic shears as outlined in Step 6 below. The fat is released laterally as the kidney is rolled medially. A blunt instrument such as the suction-irrigator should be utilized to roll the kidney, preventing parenchymal injury. If this plane cannot be established because of fibrosis, then a dissection and release lateral to Gerota's, as done during a radical nephrectomy, can be performed. Division of the more cephalad attachments is also required to allow the kidney to be completely flipped medially. Careful inspection of the hilar area usually reveals pulsations of the artery. The fibro-fatty tissues overlying the artery are grasped and divided until the smooth surface of the arterial wall is visible. The artery is then shelled out of the surrounding lymphatic tissue until a right angle can be completely passed behind it and spread to allow placement of the vascular Endo-GIA stapler or Weck clips. The assistant can utilize the lateral port, if present, to push the kidney medial and

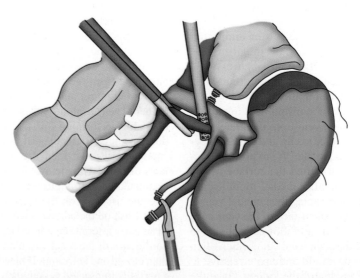

Figure 57-11 The anterior-inferior approach to the renal artery usually requires division of the adrenal vein branch to provide enough mobilization of the vein to enable cephalad retraction. Simultaneous elevation of the kidney and separation of the artery and vein can be achieved by insertion of the tip of the irrigator-aspirator between these two structures. The narrow jaw of the Endovascular stapler can then be passed between the artery and vein while the wider jaw passes inferior to the artery. Once the jaws of the stapler are closed, the instrument can be roticulated to confirm correct positioning.

keep the hilum on stretch during dissection and securing of the artery.

Once the artery is divided, the kidney is flipped lateral and the assistant elevates the ureter and lower pole of the kidney via the lateral port, or the primary surgeon elevates it via the upper port, to visualize the vein. The upper edge and posterior surface of the main renal vein are dissected free of all surrounding tissue lateral to the gonadal vein branch until a right angle can be easily passed and spread behind it. This enables clear placement of the Endo-GIA around the vein, which is then transected. The posterior approach to the hi\lar dissection on the right side is identical to that described on the left.

In cases of severe perivascular fibrosis, several groups have described early en bloc ligation and division of the renal artery and vein.[91,92] The hilum must be skeletonized as much as possible to allow application of the stapler. Shekarriz and colleagues[91] described use of the wider (3.5 mm) clips to accommodate the increased bulk of the dual vasculature and associated hilar tissue. In their series, 5 patients were managed in this fashion without a significant bleeding event or delayed fistula formation after 2 years of follow-up. Hrebinko and Phelan[92] described similar en bloc division of the hilar vasculature using a laparoscopic Endo-GIA stapler application during hand-assisted renal procedures for cancer in 12 patients, none of whom suffered a fistula or catastrophic bleeding event on short follow-up of 3 to 33 months. We do not generally advocate this approach as other authors have demonstrated the possibility of acute bleeding or delayed arteriovenous fistula formation in a pig model.[93]

Step 6: Release of the Lateral and Cephalad Renal Attachments   Once the hilum has been secured, the lateral attachments are released if they have not already been freed using the Harmonic scalpel. If the amount of scarring around the kidney does not allow easy dissection between Gerota's fat pad and the renal capsule, the dissection should proceed outside Gerota's similar to a radical nephrectomy. An alternative is to perform a subcapsular dissection for cases of severe perinephric fibrosis.[94] In this technique, the parenchyma and collecting system is "shelled out" of the capsule, leaving the posterolateral capsule and all of the surrounding tissue behind. The lateral attachments are released by incising Gerota's fascia parallel to the lateral border of the kidney. The lower pole is then elevated by the surgeon grasping the ureter, or bluntly retracting it, while teasing and transecting tissue from superficial to deep layers. The kidney is rolled medially and the dissection is carried cephalad. Often complete release of the cephalad attachments requires flipping the kidney to approach it from the anterior and then posterior. If poor planes exist, an alternative to separation of the cephalad attachments is to create windows in the tissue, separating it into smaller bundles that can be secured using the Endo-GIA stapler. Once it is completely released, the kidney is placed adjacent to the spleen on the left or on the surface of the liver on the right to facilitate entrapment of the specimen.

Step 7: Entrapment with Morcellation or Intact Removal of the Specimen   *Entrapment with Morcellation*   It is our preference to morcellate noninfected specimens for which we typically use an Endocatch II (15 mm) bag (U.S. Surgical Inc., Norwalk, CT); however, the smaller Endocatch I (10 mm) (U.S. Surgical Inc., Norwalk, CT) bag can also be utilized. It is easier to operate and is safe for benign specimens. Both bags are mounted on a metal ring, which is delivered by advancing an inner core handle to spring the bag open. An encircling drawstring is then pulled to close the bag on the specimen, tearing it away from the metal ring. The inner core handle is then pulled back, withdrawing the metal ring, and the device is removed, leaving the bagged specimen and drawstring in the peritoneum or retroperitoneum.

Alternatively, a LapSac (Cook Urological, Spencer, IN) can be utilized. The LapSac is made of nylon with a polyurethane inner coating and has been shown to be impermeable to substances such as indigo carmine and albumin, which are smaller than uropathogenic bacteria, providing the option for morcellating specimens that have a strong likelihood of containing infectious organisms.[95] The LapSac should also be utilized if a high-speed tissue morcellator is utilized, as it has the highest resistance to mechanical perforation.[96] The 8 × 10-inch LapSac will hold most specimens with the exception of very large > 1,000 g kidneys. Noninfected specimens can be morcellated in either a nonpermeable LapSac or Endocatch II bag, although the latter is less resistant to perforation.[96]

The Endocatch II bag is inserted through the lower-quadrant port site after removing the port, as it is too large to fit through the lumen of a 10/12 mm trocar. The assistant opens the Endocatch II bag with the mouth of the ring just below the kidney as the surgeon grasps the ureter with the dominant hand and slides the lower pole of the kidney off the spleen or liver into the bag. The upper pole is guided into the bag using a dissector inserted through the subcostal port. Once the kidney and attached tissues are completely within the bag, the drawstring is then pulled, closing the device, which is then withdrawn as described above. Care must be utilized when morcellating specimens in the Endocatch bag as its resistance to perforation is minimal compared with the LapSac.[96] An empty sponge stick is an excellent instrument for fracturing and removing the kidney while the bag is kept under careful inspection from the peritoneal side. The entrapment sac is elevated through the trocar site and its edges rolled back to feed it out as the specimen dissipates. Eventually the entire bag will be released and the port site is then irrigated and the trocar reinserted using the appropriate obturator.

The LapSac is also too large to pass through a standard 10/12 mm trocar so the periumbilical port is removed, and the sac is rolled and stuffed manually or with the aid of an introducer deeply into the abdomen. The port is reintroduced and the sac is unwound within the peritoneal cavity. A standard .035-inch glidewire can be passed twice through the drawstring holes of the LapSac skipping every other hole on the first pass and traversing the skipped holes on the second pass. The mouth of the sack is positioned below the spleen or liver, depending on the side of the nephrectomy. The bottom of the bag is pulled down onto the psoas, and the inferior lip of the sac is slightly elevated as the laparoscopic lens is inserted into the bag and moved in circular motions to open the sac. The posterior tab of the sac is held up with a grasper inserted through the upper port, and the anterior tab of the sac is held open via the lower-quadrant port with the laparoscopic lens inserted via the periumbilical port. The lower pole of the kidney is then slid into the sac with the aid of a grasper inserted via the lateral-most port. Once the kidney is pushed deeply into the sac, the drawstring is brought out via the lower-quadrant port site and the bag elevated through the skin. If a potentially infected specimen is morcellated, antibiotic soaked towels are placed around the port site as the morcellation process proceeds, and gloves and gowns should be changed following the morcellation and the port sight irrigated with antibiotic solution. Dirty instruments used in the morcellation process should be removed from the surgical field. Large ADPKD kidneys require fluid decompression prior to extraction by either morcellation or intact specimen removal.

Entrapment with Intact Removal   In some cases, such as an infected kidney bearing a large staghorn calculus, it may be desirable to remove the specimen intact. Elashry and colleagues[97] demonstrated that removal of the specimen via a lower-quadrant incision connecting the port sites resulted in an increased incidence of hernia formation. We prefer to use a periumbilical or Pfannenstiel incision for intact extractions. In this technique, a standard incision is made in one of these two locations down to, but not through, the peritoneum. A purse-string 2-0 Vicryl suture is placed in the exposed center of the peritoneum or around the periumbilical port site if utilized. The peritoneum is then incised with the cautery, or the port removed, and a large Endocatch II bag is inserted through the peritoneal opening. The purse-string suture is tied allowing reestablishment of the pneumoperitoneum. The kidney is then captured in the Endocatch as previously described, and the peritoneal incision is widened and the specimen removed. Alternatively, the surgeon's arm can be inserted into the incision until the forearm prevents loss of the pneumoperitoneum and the kidney can be grasped with the introduced hand and removed.[98] In this method, the peritoneal incision should be just large enough to allow introduction of the forearm. After removal of the specimen, the peritoneum is closed using a running 2-0 Vicryl and a moistened laparotomy pad is placed in the incision.

Step 8: Exiting the Abdomen and Port Closure   Final inspection of all areas of dissection is performed under low insufflation pressures of 5 mm Hg pressure to look for venous hemorrhage that might otherwise be compressed by the pneumoperitoneum. Careful inspection of the hilar vessel stumps is also performed. The Harmonic shears can be utilized for obtaining hemostasis of localized areas of bleeding away from the main hilar vascular stumps. We place a half-sheet of oxidized regenerated cellulose (Surgicel, Johnson and Johnson, Arlington, TX) at the area of the transected vessels, along the margin of the adrenal gland, and any other areas where persistent venous oozing is noted. After hemostasis is deemed adequate, the pressure of the pneumoperitoneum is increased to 15 mm Hg. It is not necessary to reperitonealize the colon, as this occurs rapidly with or without suture placement.

We place a 0-Vicryl closure suture at each of the 10/12 mm port sites with the aid of a fascial closure device such as the Carter-Thomason (Inlet Medical, Eden Prairie, MN),[99] which has been shown to be one of the more efficient means of closing the fascia in animal and clinical studies.[100,101] The other advantage of this type of device is that it allows full-thickness closure of the port site, including both fascia and peritoneum, which is important because subfascial herniations have been reported following laparoscopy.[102,103] The Carter-Thomason can be utilized in one of several ways, the easiest is to grasp the Vicryl closure stitch 1 to 2 cm back from its end and to pass a full-thickness simple suture through the center of the cut fascial edges on either side of the port, leaving the port in place. A grasper is utilized by the assistant via one of the other ports to hold the end of the suture, and the device is then removed. The Carter-Thomason grasping needle is reinserted through the other side of the fascia, the suture is transferred to the jaws of the device within the abdomen, and it is withdrawn and tagged with a clamp. A conical guide with holes for passage of the closure needle through the fascia is also available to facilitate use of this device, but it can be utilized only after removal of the port, which then needs to be reinserted after placement of the stitch. The final alternative is to remove the port and use the index finger of the nondominant hand inserted into the fascial defect to guide insertion of the needle, which is pinched between the thumb and the inserted index finger while maintaining the pneumoperitoneum. An advantage to utilizing the finger is the ability to feel the edges of the fascial split, which are not always parallel to the skin incision when fascial splitting or nonlinear cutting trocars are utilized. The instrument companies and some surgeons advocate that it is not necessary to close the fascia for fascial-splitting trocars[104]; however, we recently described a case of port site herniation via such a port site following a laparoscopic donor nephrectomy.[105] As a result, we now place a closure suture at nearly all 10/12 mm fascial defects. The 5 mm port is removed first under vision, so a suture can be placed using the other ports if bleeding is observed.

The last port closed is the lower-quadrant port, through which the pneumoperitoneum is evacuated to prevent CO_2 irritation of the diaphragm. The patient is placed in slight Trendelenburg's

positioning and is given several extended large-volume respirations to evacuate as much of the retained insufflant as possible. Once complete evacuation of the CO_2 has been performed, the closure suture is elevated and the port is pulled out of the abdomen while the laparoscope is left within the peritoneum. The laparoscope is then slowly withdrawn in a perpendicular axis to the patient, making sure bowel and omentum drop away as the laparoscope passes out through the fascial opening. The final fascial suture is then tied and the incisions are irrigated with antibiotic solution. If a Pfannenstiel incision was created, the fascia is closed using a No. 1 polydioxanone suture, and the subcutaneous tissues reapproximated with several interrupted 3-0 absorbable sutures. Each incision site is injected with 0.25% Marcaine, and a subcuticular closure is performed using 4-0 absorbable suture. Steri-Strips are placed with the aid of benzoin followed by a Band-Aid at each of the port sites.

STEPS OF THE PROCEDURE: RETROPERITONEAL
Step 1: Initial Entry Access and Creation of the Pneumoretroperitoneum McDougall and colleagues[106] describe the use of a Veress needle inserted into the retroperitoneum at Petit's triangle (inferior lumbar triangle) just above the iliac crest in the posterior axillary line. A CO_2 pneumoretroperitoneum is created to 15 mm Hg pressure and the initial 10/12 mm port is inserted at this site. More commonly, an open retroperitoneal access is utilized by first making a 1.5 to 2 cm incision just below the tip of the twelfth rib, then spreading the underlying fat down to the lumbodorsal fascia using two S-retractors. The lumbodorsal fascia is then punctured using a Tonsil clamp and the underlying muscle fibers split until the fat of the retroperitoneal space can be visualized. A 0-Vicryl suture mounted on a semicircular (UR-6) needle can be inserted through each fascial edge to assist in securing the Hasson-type cannula. The surgeon inserts an

index finger into the retroperitoneum, sweeping away the underlying fat until the smooth surfaces of the psoas and quadratus lumborum musculature are palpated and the edge of the peritoneal envelope is swept as far medially as the length of the inserted finger will allow. At this point many authors favor use of a trocar-mounted balloon dissection device (eg, Origin Medsystems, Menlo Park, CA) to facilitate creation of the retroperitoneal space.[107] This device consists of a trocar with an attached lucent balloon that is positioned between the posterior surface of Gerota's fascia and the psoas muscle and is then inflated with air while performing direct vision monitoring via a laparoscope inserted through its lumen (Figure 57-12). The amount of instilled air depends on the size of the patient, with 400 to 600 cc instilled in pediatric and 800 to 1,000 cc in adult patients.[69] Positioning of the balloon outside of Gerota's fascia has been shown to give rapid and reliable access to the posterior aspect of the renal hilum.

Alternative methods for creating the retroperitoneal space include insertion of a red rubber catheter on which the cut index finger of a No. 7 surgical glove has been tied.[71] The fashioned finger balloon is sequentially filled with saline to the desired volume ≤ 500 cc to facilitate dissection. Pressure-volume laboratory studies demonstrated similar intraballoon pressures between the index finger of a No. 7 and the middle finger of a No. 8 surgical glove after inflating with 500 cc saline.[71] No ruptures were noted in vitro. During clinical cases, a total of 38 patient procedures were performed using this method; however, finger balloon rupture occurred in 3; all had undergone prior retroperitoneal surgery.[71] In 1 patient, all of the fragments could not be retrieved; however, no complications resulted during 6 months of follow-up.

McDougall and colleagues[106] advocate use of the middle finger of a No. 8 Triflex surgical glove (Baxter Healthcare Corporation, Valencia, CA) in

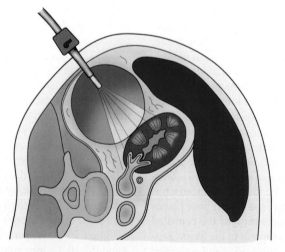

Figure 57-12 Several trocar-mounted retroperitoneal balloon dilators through which the laparoscope can be inserted are commercially available. These dilators allow confirmation of correct balloon positioning and direct inspection of the retroperitoneal contents as the dilation is being performed.

which laboratory tests demonstrated that balloon pressures never exceeded 20 mm Hg during filling to 2,000 cc, and the burst point was approximately 4,000 cc. They reported the use of their finger balloon in 12 retroperitoneal renal procedures during which they inflated it with 1,000 cc of saline and experienced no balloon ruptures.

The initial port can also be inserted at the retroperitoneal entry site and the CO_2 insufflation begun at 15 mm of Hg pressure, while the laparoscope is used to push into and sweep down the attachments between the posterior surface of Gerota's fascia and the psoas muscle.[108] These latter two methods do not, however, provide the same degree of anteromedial displacement of the kidney within Gerota's fascia that is so critical for rapid identification and access to the hilar structures.

A blunt-tip Hasson cannula may be utilized as the primary port at the initial entry site for insertion of the laparoscope. The fascial tacking sutures are wrapped around the guides on the inverted conical sleeve of the Hasson cannula, which is then seated down into the incision prior to locking it on the port sleeve to help prevent leakage of the pneumoretroperitoneum. Other authors favor use of the Origin 10/12 mm blunt-tip cannula (Origin Medsystems, Menlo Park, CA) at the initial entry site, as the internal retention balloon snugs tight against the inner aspect of the abdominal wall by sliding down the adjustable external cuff, creating an excellent seal resistant to leakage of CO_2.[108] The retroperitoneum is insufflated to 15 mm Hg pressure and the 10 mm 30-degree laparoscope is inserted.

Step 2: Identification of Anatomic Landmarks and Secondary Port Placement In a review of visualized anatomic landmarks following initial retroperitoneal access in 18 patients at the Cleveland Clinic, Sung and colleagues[109] reported visualizing the psoas muscle (100%), lateral peritoneal reflection (83%), ureter (61%), renal artery pulsations (56%), aortic pulsations (90% on the left), and inferior vena cava (25% on the right).[108] Because of the proximity of the port site placement during retroperitoneal procedures (6–8 cm),[69] it is often difficult to adequately visualize the site of port entry when introducing additional trocars, even with the 30-degree lens.

A reliable method of bimanual controlled introduction has been described.[107] In this method, the primary port is removed and the index finger of the nondominant hand is inserted and used to ensure that the peritoneal envelope is swept away, as two ports are introduced at the midaxillary line, one approximately 2 fingerbreadths above the iliac crest and one just off the tip of the eleventh rib (Figure 57-13). Placement of the lower midaxillary port too close to the edge of the iliac wing will result in frustrating limitations of instrument excursion by the bone. The inserted finger can be protected using an S-retractor as described by Gill,[69] which is especially important if bladed trocars are used. The use of fascial splitting trocars reduces the risk when performing this maneuver. A third trocar is then inserted just lateral to the palpated edge of

the psoas muscle. The size of the inserted ports is dependent on the dominant hand of the primary surgeon and the side on which the operation is being performed (see Figure 57-13).

Step 3: Incision of Gerota's Fascia and Identification of Hilar Vessels The laparoscope is inserted through the trocar located just off of the tip of the twelfth rib and the surgeon works through the lower midaxillary and posterior ports. The assistant retracts the kidney anterolaterally through the upper midaxillary port to place the hilum on stretch (see Figure 57-13). A longitudinal incision is made through Gerota's fascia and the psoas muscle is traced cephalad until the vigorous pulsations of the renal artery are visible beneath their fibro-fatty, lymphatic covering. Early posterior identification of the artery is one of the primary advantages of the retroperitoneal approach. Once the artery is identified, the Harmonic scalpel is utilized to gently tease and divide the overlying fibro-fatty tissue until the wall of the artery is encountered. The artery is then dissected circumferentially at the surface of its muscular coat until a right-angle or Maryland dissector can be readily passed behind it and spread to provide adequate space to secure and divide the vessel.

Step 4: Securing of Hilar Vessels As described previously for the transperitoneal approach, options for securing the main renal artery include the 2.5 mm Endovascular-GIA stapler or self-locking Weck clips. As always, care must be exercised to be certain the tips of the stapler are visualized, as inadvertent clamping of cephalad and medial tissue on the right can result in partial transection of the inferior

vena cava, and on the left the superior mesenteric artery can be injured.

Once the artery has been divided, the kidney should become noticeably less tense, and the more anteriorly located main renal vein can be visualized. On the left side, it may be necessary to circumferentially dissect, clip, and divide the adrenal, gonadal, and/or the lumbar vein branches to allow adequate dissection and mobilization of the main renal vein for application of the Endovascular-GIA stapler. The vein should appear collapsed and the kidney decompressed, if it does not, a thorough inspection caudal and cephalad to the main renal artery should be performed to ensure that no accessory arteries are present. If accessory arteries are identified, these must be secured and transected prior to stapling the main renal vein to prevent engorgement and vigorous bleeding from the kidney and vein stump. Once the collapsed main renal vein has been adequately mobilized, the 2.5 mm Endovascular-GIA stapler is utilized to secure and divide it. Again, it is critical to observe the entire length of the stapling device to prevent accidental injury of anteromedial structures.

Step 5: Transection of Ureter and Release of Inferior Attachments The fibro-fatty tissues above and below the transected hilar vessels are teased away with the Harmonic scalpel. The ureter and gonadal vein, if its entry point remains with the specimen, are identified medially on the psoas, dissected circumferentially, clipped, and divided. At this point the ureter can be grasped and retracted laterally, while the entire lower pole is freed of all its attachments using the Harmonic scalpel.

○ 10/12 mm Blunt-tip Trocar
● 10/12 mm or 5 mm Trocar
⊗ 5 mm Trocar

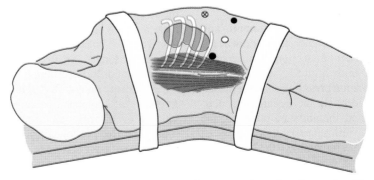

Figure 57-13 Typical trocar arrangement for a retroperitoneal renal procedure. The initial port is a blunt-tip Hasson-type inserted several fingerbreadths below the tip of the twelfth rib. Once the retroperitoneal space has been created and the peritoneal envelope swept medially, an additional port is inserted several fingerbreadths below the twelfth rib just lateral to the paraspinal muscles and slightly below the blunt-tip port in the posterior axillary line. For right-sided procedures, this is a 5 mm port for a right-handed surgeon and a 10/12 mm port for a left-handed surgeon. For left-sided procedures, this is a 10/12 mm port for a right-handed surgeon and a 5-mm port for a left-handed surgeon. A 5 mm port is inserted just off the tip of the eleventh rib in the midaxillary line. A fourth port is inserted two fingerbreadths (~ 3 cm) above the iliac wing in the midaxillary line. For right-sided procedures, this is a 10/12 mm port for a right-handed surgeon and a 5 mm port for a left-handed surgeon. For left-sided procedures, this is a 5 mm port for a right-handed surgeon and a 10/12 mm port for a left-handed surgeon.

Step 6: Release of Cephalad Attachments and Adrenal Gland   Downward traction on the ureter helps to expose the upper pole of the kidney, which is then separated from the adrenal gland by inserting the jaws of the Harmonic scalpel along the juncture of the two, allowing time for adequate hemostasis. The ureter is alternately held lateral and medial while applying downward retraction as indicated to provide adequate exposure of the dissection plane. Once the adrenal gland is released, no significant attachments to the kidney should remain, and it can be moved freely in the retroperitoneum.

Step 7: Entrapment with Morcellation or Intact Removal of the Specimen   Once the specimen is free within the retroperitoneum, it can be placed in an entrapment sac and either delivered intact by enlarging the primary or lower midaxillary port,[69] or it can be morcellated as described for transperitoneal procedures. Use of the LapSac is cumbersome given the confines of the retroperitoneal space, but it can be introduced via the 10/12 mm port site and positioned with the closed end directed deep into the pelvic extent of the extraperitoneal space, while the kidney is kept high in the retroperitoneum. The ureter and lower pole are gently swept into the bag in a longitudinal orientation as the surgeon holds two of the tabs on the mouth of the bag to keep it open as the kidney is delivered inside. As discussed for the transperitoneal approach, the advantage to use of this bag for removal of benign specimens include its resistance to mechanical perforation and lack of permeability to uropathogens when morcellating infected specimens.[95,96] Gill[69] describes the use of one of the ring-mounted entrapment sacs (eg, Endocatch I or II), which can be inserted at one of the 10/12 mm port sites, the specimen entrapped, and the port site enlarged to allow intact removal. If the port site is enlarged to deliver the specimen intact, the fascial incision is then closed using a running No. 1 polydioxanone suture.

Step 8: Exiting the Retroperitoneum and Port Closure   The pneumoretroperitoneum is lowered and the areas of dissection are once again inspected under both high (15 mm) and low (5 mm Hg) insufflation pressures. Once hemostasis is felt to be adequate the pneumoretroperitoneum is evacuated, the ports are removed, and the S-retractors are utilized to put a simple fascial closure stitch at the remaining 10/12 mm port site. Since the peritoneum is not violated, full-thickness closure utilizing a device such as the Carter-Thomason is not required and is often difficult to use owing to the proximity of the ports. The remainder of the skin closure and dressings are identical to what was described for transperitoneal nephrectomy.

POSTOPERATIVE CARE   The patient is usually encouraged to begin ambulation or to at least sit up in a chair the night of their surgery. That night, or the following day, clear liquids are initiated if bowel sounds are present and the patient is ambulated at least per shift. Pain is controlled with the use of parenteral agents or a patient-controlled analgesia device. We maintain compression devices and TED Hose while the patient is at rest in the bed or chair. The orogastric tube is removed immediately following the operation and the Foley catheter is typically removed once the patient is ambulating on postoperative day 1. If the patient has a history of voiding abnormalities, we often wait to remove the Foley catheter until the second postoperative day. Broad-spectrum antibiotic coverage is continued for 24 hours following surgery and is converted to a week-long course of an oral agent appropriate for the patient's situation should a suspected infection exist. We typically use a sulfa-based agent or a fluoroquinolone. If clear liquids are tolerated without bloating and active bowel sounds are present, the patient's diet is advanced to general on postoperative day 2 and they are switched to oral pain medication. Once the patient is tolerating a regular diet, their pain is well-controlled on oral agents, and they are passing flatus they are discharged from the hospital. Typically, discharge occurs on postoperative day 2 or 3, and is most commonly delayed by slow return of bowel function. If active flatus is not occurring by day 2, we help stimulate its return by administering a bisacodyl suppository.

RESULTS   Laparoscopy for benign disease is being offered at many academic centers, as well as community-based hospitals. The results of contemporary series of laparoscopic simple transperitoneal and retroperitoneal nephrectomy are summarized in Tables 57-3 and 57-4. Recent series reveal average operative times of 2.5 hours,[110] although reported average times of 7 hours demonstrate the potential complexity of these dissections.[111] A fivefold reduction in the amount of narcotic analgesia relative to open nephrectomy as demonstrated by McDougall and Clayman,[112] with convalescence times of 2 to 4 weeks, reflects the benefits of laparoscopy. Mean length of stay in most reported series still averages slightly more than 3 days[111] whereas European and Asian series are slightly longer, which in large part may be a reflection of differing criterion for discharge.[113]

A recent review by Landman and colleagues[114] of 3 comparative series (one European) totaling 67 laparoscopic simple (50 transperitoneal; 17 retroperitoneal) versus 55 retroperitoneal open nephrectomies for benign disease demonstrated mean operative times of 241 and 146 minutes, respectively. Length of stay and time to full recovery averaged 5.1 and 30.8 days for the laparoscopic group and 8.5 and 145 days for the open group, respectively. Open conversion was required in 5 (7.5%) of the 67 patients, which is similar to the 8% open conversion rate in 106 transperitoneal laparoscopic simple nephrectomies reported by Eraky and colleagues.[2] As stated earlier in the chapter, many simple nephrectomies are far from simple owing to the scarring associated with the pathologic process. Indeed, the underlying renal pathology has been shown to have a direct correlation to the incidence of conversion with renal tuberculosis, post-traumatic renal atrophy, infarcted kidneys, and xanthogranulomatous pyelonephritis having an open conversion rate of 89% in one large multi-institutional German study.[115]

Eraky and colleagues[2] reported one of the largest single-institution experiences with transperitoneal laparoscopic simple nephrectomy (see Table 57-3). These authors performed a total of 106 laparoscopic transperitoneal nephrectomies for primary indications consisting of chronic pain, recurrent infection, or associated hypertension. The open conversion rate in their series was 8% with 5 owing to failure to progress secondary to adhesions, 3 for bleeding, and 1 owing to inability to entrap the specimen. All specimens were entrapped and manually morcellated in a LapSac. Mean operative time was 186 minutes overall, but averaged 217 minutes for the initial half of the series and 154 minutes for the latter half. There were 4 major complications, including a pulmonary embolism, colonic perforation requiring colostomy, and an infected hematoma requiring percutaneous drainage. The mean hospital stay was 2.9 days.

Hemal and colleagues[1] reported one of the largest single-institution experiences with retroperitoneal laparoscopic simple nephrectomy (see Table 57-4). These authors performed a total of 185 laparoscopic retroperitoneal nephrectomies or nephroureterectomies for benign conditions, including 154 nephrectomies for such indications as ureteropelvic junction obstruction (77), stone disease (53), ureteral stricture (9), tuberculosis (7), dysplasia (4), ectopic ureterocele (2), and renovascular hypertension (2).[1] A total of 18 patients required conversion to open surgery (9.72%), with 14 of these conversions occurring during the first 100 cases. Four conversions were urgent (3 bleeding; 1 colon injury), and 14 were elective owing to failure to progress as a result of adhesions (12), or loss of the pneumoretroperitoneum secondary to a peritoneal rent (2). The average operative time for completed laparoscopic procedures was 100 minutes, and the mean blood loss was 133 cc. Four patients required a blood transfusion. Seven major complications (3.78%) were reported, including the 4 that led to an open conversion and a retroperitoneal collection requiring exploration and drainage. Thirty-two minor complications (16.2%) occurred, including the 2 peritoneal violations that led to open conversion.[1]

Fornara and colleagues[67] reported their series of 11 kidney transplant patients who underwent bilateral laparoscopic transperitoneal native nephrectomies. Mean operative time was 195 minutes and blood loss was 345 cc. One patient required open conversion owing to bleeding from the renal artery. Complications included a retroperitoneal hematoma requiring a 2-unit blood transfusion, fever of unclear etiology, and a urinary tract infection. Postoperative renal function was stable in all patients, and the mean analgesia requirement was 14 mg morphine equivalent and hospital stay of 4.2 days. This

Table 57-3   Results of Laparoscopic Simple Nephrectomy: Transperitoneal

Series	Number	OR Time (Mean: min)	EBL (Mean: cc)	Open Conversions	Extraction Method(s)	Analgesia (Morphine Equiv: mg)	Complications (minor)	Complications (major)	LOS (Mean: days)	Convalescence (Mean: days)
Eraky et al[2]	106	186	–	9 (8%)	Morcellated	–	24 (33%)	4 (3.8%)	2.9	–
Keeley et al[110]	79	146	–	4 (5%)	Intact	–	13 (16.5%)	1 (1.3%)	4.7	–
Ono et al[167]	27	265	455	3 (11.1%)	Morcellated	12.9 mg* pentazoline IM	–	6 (22%)	10*	17
Kerbl et al[111]	20	355	200	1 (5%)	Morcellated	54	2 (10%)	5 (25%)	3.6	28
Rassweiler et al[113]	18	206.5	–	2 (11.1%)	Intact	1 vial over 2d	3 (16.7%)	4 (22.2%)	6.6	24
Parra et al[168]	12	145	140.7	1 (8.0%)	Morcellated	14	1 (8.3%)	1 (8.3%)	3.5	16
Totals	262	187.9†	–	20 (7.6%)	–	–	43 (16.4%)	21 (8%)	4.3†	–

*Twenty-one patients not requiring a laparotomy.
†Weighted averages.
EBL = estimated blood loss; LOS = length of stay.

compared favorably with 10 patients at the same institution who had bilateral open nephrectomies. The open surgery group required 3 times the amount of postoperative analgesia and had a mean hospital stay of 10.7 days.[67]

As mentioned previously, two infectious conditions of the kidney for which the laparoscopic approach has demonstrated questionable results include xanthogranulomatous pyelonephritis (XGP) and renal tuberculosis. XGP is an intense infectious/inflammatory condition of the kidney associated with chronic infection, obstruction, and the presence of renal calculi. CT scan imaging usually demonstrates enlargement of the kidney with a "bear-paw" appearance resulting from fat-laden macrophage replacement of the collecting system (see Figure 57-1). The disease results in an intense fibrotic response around the kidney with adhesion to adjacent structures, including bowel, adrenal gland, liver, IVC, aorta, spleen, pancreas, and psoas muscle. Fistula formation to the colon or skin of the flank has been reported.[116,117] A recent review by Bercowsky and colleagues[118] demonstrated a 60% complication rate in 5 patients undergoing laparoscopic removal, with a mean operative time of 6 hours, bringing to question the utility of laparoscopy in this setting.

Reported open conversion rates for attempted laparoscopic nephrectomy for renal tuberculosis are as high as 80% in the most experienced of hands,[115] with spillage of caseating material reported by several groups.[119,120] The need for extended multidrug therapy following this type of occurrence and the difficulty of these operations makes this another questionable disease for which laparoscopic nephrectomy should be utilized.

ADPKD represents a challenging case because of the size of the kidneys, with many extending across the midline or deep into the pelvis.[26,121] The significant size of these specimens requires initial cyst decompression utilizing the Harmonic shears with irrigation and aspiration performed of the released fluid to allow adequate exposure of the hilum for dissection.[122] A recent comparison of 10 ADPKD kidneys removed laparoscopically compared with 10 removed open demonstrated no complications in the laparoscopic group with a significant reduction in hospital stay (2.6 vs 6.6 days, respectively).[123] Mean laparoscopic times were, however, significantly longer than in the open group (247 vs 205 minutes), with one case converted to an open procedure.

COMPLICATIONS   The reported complications with establishment of transperitoneal and retroperitoneal access for any laparoscopic approach can also occur during laparoscopic simple nephrectomy. In a review of 2,407 laparoscopic cases in urology, Fahlenkamp and colleagues[124] demonstrated a 0.2% incidence of adjacent organ perforation. This is similar to the 0.3% access-related injuries reported during gynecologic surgery.[125,126] The use of an open blunt-tip trocar access as described by Hasson[127] is not a guarantee against injury. Penfield reported a .06% bowel injury rate using an open access technique during 10,840 laparoscopic cases.[128] Two aortic injuries have also been reported using the Hasson technique.[129]

Several reviews have specifically assessed the complications inherent to nephrectomy and stratified them relative to the type of nephrectomy performed.[62,115,130] Siquiera and colleagues[62] described their experience with 213 laparoscopic nephrectomies, which included 84 live donor nephrectomies, 61 radical nephrectomies, 55 simple nephrectomies, and 13 nephroureterectomies. The majority (196) were performed via a transperitoneal approach with the exception of 17 retroperitoneal simple nephrectomies. A total of 16 major (7.5%) complications occurred, which included 3 (1.4%) that were access related, 9 (4.2%) intraoperative, and 4 (1.9%) postoperative complications. Only 1 complication occurred in the group undergoing a laparoscopic simple nephrectomy, which was a liver laceration on initial trocar insertion, but this group had the highest rate of elective conversion (12.7%) owing to lack of progression (7 of the 8 elective conversions).

Table 57-4   Results of Laparoscopic Simple Nephrectomy: Retroperitoneal

Series	Number	OR Time (Mean: min)	EBL (Mean: cc)	Open Conversions	Extraction Method(s)	Analgesia (Morphine Equiv: mg)	Complications (minor)	Complications (major)	LOS (Mean: days)	Convalescence (Mean: days)
Hemal et al[1]	185	100	133	18 (9.7%)	Intact	–	30 (16.2%)	7 (3.8%)	3.0	–
Gaur[169]	38	131.8	83.5	6 (16%)	–	Mean 2.4 d	16 (42.1%)	1 (2.6%)	2.7	13.3
Doublet et al[170]	36	95	–	0	Intact	–	0	1 (2.7%)	3.7	–
Ono et al[171]	20	198	135	0	Morcellated	None–4, 33 mg pentazocine-16	0	1 (5%)	8.0	18.9
Rassweiler et al[113]	17	211.2	–	1 (5.9%)	–	.5 vials over 1 d	2 (11.8%)	3 (17.6%)	6.3	21
McDougall et al[106]	9	348	235	0	Morcellated	39	1 (11.1%)	1 (11.1%)	3.5	7
Gasman et al[172]	8	120	65	0	Intact	22.5 mg	0	0	2.6	–
Total	308	125.2*	–	25 (6.6%)	–	–	49 (15.9%)	14 (4.5%)	3.6*	–

*Weighted averages.
EBL = estimated blood loss; LOS = length of stay.

Gill and colleagues[130] performed a multi-institutional review of 185 patients who underwent a laparoscopic nephrectomy, 153 of which were for benign disease. Complications were 3-fold higher among patients undergoing radical nephrectomy (34%) versus the simple (12%), respectively. Access-related complications occurred in 2%, including 1 abdominal wall lesion, 1 trocar injury to a hydronephrotic kidney, and 1 hernia at a port site. Intraoperative complications included an ipsilateral pneumothorax attributed to transpleural insertion of a secondary port requiring a chest tube. Another patient suffered a splenic laceration that appeared to resolve with direct pressure, but ultimately led to a postoperative bleed and need for an open splenectomy. Other authors have successfully utilized a fibrin sealant to achieve adequate hemostasis laparoscopically when splenic laceration occurs.[131] Three patients (2%) developed a postoperative ileus, 2 (1.3%) cardiovascular complications, 2 (1.3%) urinary retention, and 2 (1.3%) neurologic complications. The incidence of elective conversion during laparoscopic simple nephrectomy was 3.3%, with no emergent conversions.

Dissection and securing of the hilar vessels is the step related to the greatest number of "crash" conversions owing to uncontrollable hemorrhage. In the series by Siqueira and colleagues,[62] all 5 emergency conversions, 3 during live donor and 2 during radical laparoscopic nephrectomy, occurred while dissecting and/or securing the hilar vessels or their branches. Two of these episodes resulted from a misfired or misplaced Endovascular-GIA stapler. Similarly, Gill and colleague's series reported emergency conversions for 3 vascular injuries all within the laparoscopic radical nephrectomy group and none in the simple nephrectomy group.[130] One of these vascular injuries occurred as a result of a malfunction of the Endovascular-GIA stapler. Malfunctions during securing the hilar vessels with the Endovascular-GIA stapler have been reported with an incidence of 1.7%, with 50% resulting from misplacement over previously placed clips.[89] As a result of such occurrences, several authors advocate use of devices such as the LigaSure (Valley Labs, Boulder, CO),[89] bipolar coagulation,[132] or the Harmonic scalpel to secure the branches of the main renal vein to prevent incorporation of clips within the Endovascular-GIA stapler.

In a review of 2,407 laparoscopic cases in urology, Fahlenkamp and colleagues[124] demonstrated a 0.8% incidence of adjacent organ perforation. They also noted a 3:1 ratio for the incidence of visceral injury during the transperitoneal versus the retroperitoneal approach, respectively.[124] In Siqueria's series of 213 laparoscopic nephrectomies, visceral injuries included 2 (0.9%) liver and 1 (0.5%) splenic injury.[62] Bowel injury occurred in 2 patients (0.9%), which is similar to the 0.8% incidence of bowel complications reported by Bishoff and colleagues[133] in a group of 915 patients who underwent assorted laparoscopic urologic procedures. Unfortunately, 70% of laparoscopic bowel injuries are not recognized intraoperatively and present with an unusual constellation of signs and symptoms unique to laparoscopic-associated perforations. These include disproportionate single trocar site pain, abdominal distention, diarrhea, and leukopenia followed rapidly by cardiopulmonary collapse.[133]

HEMINEPHRECTOMY Complete duplication of the collecting system is found in 1 of 125 individuals.[3] The primary indications for surgical intervention include an ectopic ureter associated with a poorly functioning dysplastic upper-pole moiety or an upper-pole moiety with chronic obstruction and resultant poor function. Destruction and hydronephrosis of the lower-pole system can also result from reflux nephropathy or an obstructing ureteropelvic junction.[5] Recurrent infections, flank or abdominal pain, and incontinence may also be present.[4] Surgical intervention includes removal of the diseased moiety as well as all or a portion of the associated ureter. The laparoscopic approach to upper-pole heminephrectomy was first described by Jordan and Winslow in 1993.[134] This has since become an increasingly popular technique for the treatment of patients with this condition. Both the transperitoneal and retroperitoneal approach have been described,[5,134–137] although most authors seem to favor the transperitoneal exposure because of the more familiar orientation of the hilum and improved working space in children.[135]

INSTRUMENTATION (University of Wisconsin, Madison)

Standard cystoscopic pan (optional)
.035-inch floppy-tip wire (optional)
Six French (F) open-ended catheter (optional)
Ampule of methylene blue (optional)
Four nonbladed trocars:
    Two 5 mm and two 10/12 mm (with reducers)
Two 10 mm laparoscopes: one 0-degree and one 30-degree
Two 5 mm laparoscopes: one 0-degree and one 30-degree (available in the room)
One 14-gauge Veress needle
One 10/12 mm blunt-tip cannula (available in the room)
One trocar-mounted balloon dilation device (Origin Medsystems, Menlo Park, CA) (retroperitoneal)
One 10/12 mm visual introducing cannula
One 5 mm curved electrocautery scissors
One 5 mm curved Maryland dissector
One 5 mm curved Harmonic scalpel and generator
One 10 mm locking Babcock
One 5 mm dolphin-nosed grasper
One 10 mm right-angle dissector
One 5 mm toothed locking grasper
One 5 mm electrocautery hook
Two 5 mm laparoscopic needle drivers (available in the room)
One 5 mm laparoscopic handpiece for the argon beam coagulator and generator (available in the room)
One 5 mm Diamond Flex Triangle retractor (Genzyme, Tucker, GA) (available in the room)
One 10 mm PEER retractor (Jarit, Hawthorne, NY)
One Martin arm (available in the room)
One 11 mm multiload clip applier (available in the room)
One 5 mm irrigator/aspirator
One grasping needle port closure device
One smoke evacuator valve (Plume-Away: Stryker Endoscopy, San José, CA) (optional)
15F round Davol drain
One No. 15 blade scalpel and handle
Two fine-toothed pickups
One Tonsil clamp
Two S-retractors
Three 0-Vicryl ties
Four 4-0 absorbable suture on a cutting needle
One-quarter-inch Steri-Strips
Benzoin
Open nephrectomy surgical pan

STEPS OF THE PROCEDURE **Step 1: Placement of a Ureteral Catheter** Some authors favor initial cystoscopic insertion of a ureteral catheter into the ureter draining the nondiseased moiety prior to performing the laparoscopic portion of the procedure.[134,136] Others do not believe this is a necessary step of the operation, as the two ureters are often easy to differentiate at the time of laparoscopy.[5] The catheter does, however, aid in the identification of the normal ureter, while dissecting out the dilated ureter draining the diseased moiety. It also allows injection of indigo carmine after excising the parenchyma of the upper or lower pole to help in the intraoperative identification of any inadvertent injuries to the normal collecting system of the remaining moiety. Recognition of this occurrence is important as it can usually be repaired laparoscopically, and further complications can be avoided by placement of a drain with or without a stent.

For insertion of an external ureteral catheter, the patient is placed in the dorsal lithotomy position and a rigid or flexible cystoscope is utilized to introduce a .035-inch floppy-tip wire under fluoroscopic control up the ureter of interest. A 6F open-ended catheter is then passed over the wire into the intrarenal collecting system. The wire is removed and a contrast injection performed to confirm accurate positioning. The Foley catheter is inserted and the open-ended catheter is then secured to the Foley catheter using one-hal-inch Steri-Strips and benzoin or several silk ties. A piece of intravenous line extension tubing is connected to the open-ended catheter and attached to a 3-way stopcock on which a 60 cc syringe filled with methylene blue-colored saline is mounted. This allows easy access for injection during the laparoscopic procedure. The methylene blue-colored saline is created by adding an ampule of methylene blue to 250 cc of sterile saline. A ureteral drainage bag is attached to the remaining port on the stopcock. The patient is then positioned for laparoscopic renal surgery as outlined for simple nephrectomy.

Step 2: Creation of the Pneumoperitoneum and Initial Entry Access This step is identical to that outlined for laparoscopic nephrectomy, utilizing either the transperitoneal or retroperitoneal approach.

Step 3: Placement of Secondary Port Sites This step is identical to what was outlined for the laparoscopic nephrectomy, utilizing either a transperitoneal or retroperitoneal approach.

Step 4: Exposure of the Retroperitoneum This step is identical to that outlined for laparoscopic nephrectomy, utilizing either the transperitoneal or retroperitoneal approach. Mobilization allowing unobstructed access to the hilar structures is critical, as dissection and securing of the upper-pole blood supply is necessary, as is the ability to pass the transected ureter behind the renal artery and vein as described below for an upper-pole heminephrectomy. Deep hilar visualization and identification of these structures are also important when resecting the lower-pole system, although passage of the resected collecting system behind the vessels is not necessary.[5]

Step 5: Identification and Dissection of the Upper- or Lower-Pole Ureter The dilated upper- or lower-pole ureter is usually readily identifiable as a medial torturous tubular structure, which may be intimately attached to the ureter draining the normal moiety. This latter structure can usually be differentiated by gently drawing an instrument across the surface of the suspected location of the ureter and feeling the resistive catch as it passes over the underlying stent. The two ureters can be intimately attached and the proximal aspect of the dilated system is dissected out with care taken not to injure the wall or vasculature supplying the normal system. Dissection and exposure of the hilar vessels is identical to what was described for nephrectomy. In this procedure it is not necessary to transect the main renal vessels, but to mobilize them as they cross anterior to the upper-pole collecting system and to identify and dissect out the branches supplying the upper- or lower-pole moiety.

Complete mobilization is facilitated by performing the dissection prior to transection of the ureter, as distention of the diseased moiety often helps to define the correct plane. This dissection should continue until a right-angle clamp can be passed freely behind the vessels for an upper-pole heminephrectomy. Gerota's fat is usually attenuated overlying the hydronephrotic moiety. The fascia is incised and Gerota's fat is split over the extent of the diseased segment. The Harmonic scalpel is utilized to separate the adrenal gland from the upper-pole system when performing an upper-pole heminephrectomy. Complete mobilization of the affected moiety to the edge of the normal pole parenchyma should be performed to facilitate eventual removal of the diseased portion of the kidney.

Step 6: Division of the Ureter and Vasculature of the Involved Moiety The ureter is then transected at the point where it can be easily separated from the normal ureter to prevent inadvertent injury to this structure. If the diseased ureter is associated with an obstructing ureterocele or an intermittently obstructing ectopic ureter that passes through the region of the bladder neck, the proximal end can be left open and all contained urine aspirated.[135] This allows for collapse of the remaining ureteral segment and prevents the establishment of a closed chamber of stagnant urine, which can lead to infection of the distal ureteral remnant. If reflux is present, most advocate removal of the involved ureter as distal as possible, leaving a strip of ureter attached to the normal ureter if necessary to prevent injury. The distal stump is then ligated or clipped adjacent to the bladder.[5,134] Janetschek and colleagues[5] advocate performing the distal ureteral dissection first, prior to any renal manipulation. Their rationale is that the likelihood of conversion is greatest during the renal portion of the surgery, and if an open flank incision is required after laparoscopic securing of the distal ureter, this approach saves the patient a possible second incision for the ureterectomy.[5]

Once the ureter is transected, if the upper-pole moiety is involved, the lowest portion of the exposed pelvis and lower ureter is grasped from above and is pulled up from behind the vessels. Additional connections between the hilar vessels and a portion of the pelvis may remain and are divided. If the lower pole is being removed the hilar-based medial margin of the hydronephrotic moiety is identified and may lie close to the main renal vasculature.

Two 11 mm titanium clips or Weck interlocking clips are placed both proximally and distally on the arterial branches arising from the main renal artery or separately from the aorta to supply the involved moiety, which were dissected out as outlined above. The branches are then transected. Venous branches less than 4 mm in diameter can usually be secured using the Harmonic scalpel alone or with clips placed on the stay side to ensure adequate hemostasis. An Endovascular-GIA stapler can also be utilized to secure and divide more substantial polar vessels.

Step 7: Excision of the Hydronephrotic Remnant The diseased remnant can usually be identified visually by its darkened poorly perfused appearance following transection of the polar vessels. It can also be delineated by palpation with the laparoscopic instruments, which reveals a more ballotable yielding character relative to the firmer quality of the normal renal parenchyma. The ureter and attached pelvis can be elevated and the moiety entered at the lateral juncture of the two poles away from the hilar structures. The Harmonic shears are ideal for removing the tissue of the diseased pole and providing adequate hemostasis. The edge of the resection is elevated and gently extended circumferentially palpating opposite the planed line of incision to make certain normal parenchyma is appreciated at this level. Other devices such as the paddle cautery and argon beam coagulator can also be utilized to assist with hemostasis. On occasion, bleeding from the cut margin may be vigorous and unresponsive to the above-noted measures. An absorbable suture on an SH needle may be introduced to place a figure-of-eight or short running suture to secure areas of bleeding.

Knots are tied intracorporeally or, alternatively, the ends of the suture can be secured using Lapra-Tys (Ethicon EndoSurgery, Cincinnati, OH), which are small absorbable Vicryl securing clips placed using a specially designed applier. Another alternative for removing the tissue and obtaining simultaneous hemostasis is to use the LigaSure (Valley Lab, Boulder, CO) bipolar vessel sealer for performing the resection of the hydronephrotic parenchyma in what has been reported to be a "bloodless resection."[138] Others have described the use of the Endovascular-GIA stapler, which can be fired sequentially around the line of demarcation between the two poles or used to secure and divide the upper pole in a single firing of the GIA stapler.[139] The obvious potential complication with this latter approach is the creation of a small isolated chamber of urine with the potential for infection, although this apparently did not occur in the 2 renal units in which this method was employed.[139]

Step 8: Inspection for Injury to the Normal Collecting System and Drain Placement Once the specimen has been completely excised, it is placed above the spleen on the left or the liver on the right, while further inspection and hemostasis is obtained. A member of the circulating personnel is then asked to use the previously assembled methylene blue irrigation system to inject blue-tinged saline into the collecting system.[136] Careful inspection of the bed of the resection site is performed laparoscopically to evaluate for any areas of normal collecting system injury. Any areas of leakage are closed using intracorporeal suturing and knot tying or placement of Lapra-Tys to secure the suture ends as outlined above. Small violations of the collecting system in regions where the surrounding tissue is insubstantial can be managed effectively by use of gelfoam soaked in fibrin glue products.[140,141] This requires that low pressures are maintained within the collecting system, which can be facilitated by converting the open-ended catheter to an indwelling double-pigtail stent at the end of the procedure.

Step 9: Entrapment and Removal of the Specimen and Drain Placement Once final inspection has been performed under both high and low insufflation pressures and hemostasis is deemed adequate, the Carter-Thomason closure device is utilized to place a fascial closure stitch at all of the 10/12 mm port sites. If the amount of resected tissue is small, it may be possible to deliver it through one of the 10/12 mm port sites. For larger specimens, a ring-attached entrapment bag (eg, Endocatch I) can be utilized. The entrapment device is inserted through the lower-quadrant 10/12 mm port site. An instrument is then passed via the epigastric/subcostal port and utilized to grasp the specimen to deliver it into the bag. The entrapment sac is then closed and drawn out through the port and the ring is detached. The port is removed and the bag, with contained specimen, is removed. If the bagged specimen is too large to fit through the established port incision, it is drawn up tight against the abdominal wall and judicious enlargement of the skin and fascial incisions is performed to allow delivery of the specimen. S-retractors are inserted to provide adequate exposure of the fascia once the skin incision is enlarged. A right-angle clamp can be inserted carefully at the corner of the incision with the backside of the right angle used to protect the bag. The electrocautery or Metzenbaum scissors are utilized to enlarge the incision with great care taken not to incise or rupture the entrapment bag. The sac can be gently rocked back and forth to deliver it from the incision while maintaining visual monitoring of the bag to ensure that it does not rupture, and that advancement of the neck of the bag correlates with progression within and not simply stretching.

Some authors[133,136] advocate placement of a postoperative drain while others[5,135] do not. The perforated end of a 15F round Davol drain, with the spike removed and a clamp placed on the opposite end, can be advanced through the lateral-most 5 mm port and positioned in the retroperitoneum. The 5 mm port is removed and the drain is secured to the skin using a 3-0 nylon suture.

Step 10: Exiting the Abdomen, Port Closure, and Ureteral Catheter Management Once the specimen is delivered, the insufflation is turned off, the S-retractors are reinserted, and the previously placed full-thickness fascial closure stitch is placed on traction to facilitate placement of several additional closure stitches. A 0-Vicryl suture mounted on a UR-6 needle works well for this purpose. The pneumoperitoneum is then reestablished and the organ extraction site reinspected. Provided the closure is adequate and no intraperitoneal structures are incorporated, the remainder of the port closure and exiting the abdomen process is identical to what was previously described for laparoscopic nephrectomy.

If no collecting system injury to the normal moiety is demonstrated, the ureteral catheter may be removed at the end of the procedure[134] or left in place until the following day if dissection around the normal ureter was extensive or the orifice noted to be tight on cannulation. Male patients can be repositioned supine and female patients frog-legged to allow fluoroscopic exchange of the stent using a metal-tipped pusher when a collecting system injury is identified and repaired. The Benson 0.035-inch wire is inserted into the external ureteral catheter after its securing Steri-Strips or sutures are removed. The access catheter is removed and an appropriate-sized stent is inserted followed by a metal-tipped pusher, which is then advanced until the radiopaque band is positioned at the level of the inferior pubic symphysis under fluoroscopic guidance. The wire is removed and pigtail formation in the renal pelvis and bladder confirmed.

POSTOPERATIVE CARE The postoperative care following laparoscopic heminephrectomy is identical to that for nephrectomy, with the only noteworthy exception being management of the external stent. If an external stent was placed at the beginning of the operative procedure and no obvious collecting system injury to the normal moiety was demonstrated, it may be removed at the end of the operation or the next day. If a collecting system injury was demonstrated and repaired intraoperatively, the catheter can be exchanged for a double-pigtail stent using a metal-tip pusher under fluoroscopy at the end of the laparoscopic portion of the operation. If a stent is inserted, it is usually left in place for 1 to 2 weeks to allow adequate closure and healing of the collecting system repair.

If a drain was placed, output is monitored until it is less than 30 cc on 2 consecutive shifts following removal of the Foley catheter on postoperative day 1. If the drain output remains elevated, a drain fluid creatinine level should be checked. The patient can be sent out with the drain in place until outputs decline if fluid creatinine is markedly elevated above the serum level. Large outputs that persist beyond 1 week are usually a result of a substantial injury to the normal collecting system that was unrecognized or inadequately repaired, or it may be due to persistent production of urine from a retained portion of the resected moiety.[142] A retrograde pyelogram into the normal ipsilateral ureter will differentiate between these two clinical scenarios by demonstrating a leak in the case of an injury and no leakage if urine is being produced by retained parenchyma. Confirmation and management of this scenario can be made by selective angiography to demonstrate residual perfused parenchyma of the resected pole, which can then be embolized.[142] An alternative management option would be a repeat laparoscopic or an open exploration and repair.

RESULTS The first case of laparoscopic heminephrectomy for ureteral ectopia was reported by Jordan and Winslow[134] in 1993. Janetschek and colleagues[5] performed 14 laparoscopic heminephrectomies in 14 patients with a mean age of 5.4 years, all via a transperitoneal approach. An upper-pole heminephrectomy was performed in 5 children with an associated refluxing ectopic megaureter and 2 with an obstructive ectopic megaureter. Five patients had nonfunctioning hydronephrotic lower poles secondary to reflux nephropathy and 2 a nonfunctioning upper pole owing to an obstructing ureterocele. The average operative time was 222 minutes in 12 cases undergoing heminephrectomy alone, and 427 minutes in 2 cases combined with a Pfannenstiel incision through which an ureterocelectomy and reimplantation of the lower-pole ureter was performed.[5] In this series, blood loss was minimal (10–30 cc) and the mean length of hospital stay was 4.4 days in the 12 patients undergoing laparoscopy alone, and 7 to 8 days in the 2 patients who also underwent a reimplantation. This surprisingly long stay was thought to be a reflection of differing European standards for discharge. There were no significant intraoperative or postoperative complications reported.

More recently, Horowitz and colleagues[135] reported their series of 14 laparoscopic upper-pole heminephrectomies in 13 patients with a mean age of 3.8 years. Twelve were associated with an ectopic ureter (2 refluxing) and 2 with ureteroceles. All procedures were performed via a transperitoneal approach. Their mean operative time was 100 minutes for the unilateral procedures and 125 minutes for the bilateral. The mean estimated blood loss was < 30 cc with a length of hospital stay of 2.6 days. No major intraoperative or postoperative complications were reported. Wang and colleagues[142] recently reported their series of 4 patients undergoing laparoscopic upper-pole heminephrectomy for a poorly functioning upper-pole segment associated with an ectopic ureter. One patient developed a urinary fistula owing to persistence of a small amount of functioning upper-pole parenchyma, which was identified on super-selective angiography and treated successfully with embolization.

COMPLICATIONS All of the complications reported above for laparoscopic nephrectomy are possible following laparoscopic heminephrectomy. Although hilar dissection is required, as well as securing of the upper-pole vasculature, major intraoperative or postoperative hemorrhage did not occur in any of the series mentioned above.[5,134,135,142] Urinary leakage owing to a lower-pole collecting system injury was not reported in these series, although Wang and colleagues[142] presented a case of persistent urine drainage from a retained portion of upper-pole parenchyma that was confirmed on super-selective angiography and successfully embolized.

CYST ABLATION The goal of laparoscopic cyst ablation for patients with ADPKD or large solitary or peripelvic cysts is relief of symptoms generated by the compressive effects of the cyst. These cysts often take up significant amounts of the retroperitoneal space or are located medially within the hilum, making a transperitoneal exposure ideal for their management. A retroperitoneal approach to posterior-based cysts has also been described.[143]

INSTRUMENTATION (University of Wisconsin, Madison)

Standard rigid or flexible cystoscopic pan (optional: peripelvic cyst)

.035-inch floppy-tip wire (optional: peripelvic cyst)

6F open-ended catheter (optional: peripelvic cyst)

Ampule of indigo carmine (optional: peripelvic cyst)

Ampule of methylene blue (optional: peripelvic cyst)

Four nonbladed trocars:

Three 5 mm and one 10/12 mm (with reducer) (no ultrasound anticipated)

Two 5 mm and two 10/12 mm (with reducers) (ultrasound anticipated)

Two 10 mm laparoscopes: one 0-degree and one 30-degree

Two 5 mm laparoscopes: one 0-degree and one 30-degree (available in the room)

One 14-gauge Veress needle

One 10/12 mm blunt-tip cannula (available in the room)

One trocar-mounted balloon dilation device (Origin Medsystems, Menlo Park, CA) (retroperitoneal)

One 10/12 mm visual introducing cannula

One 5 mm curved electrocautery scissors

One 5 mm curved Maryland dissector

One 5 mm curved Harmonic scalpel and generator

One 10 mm locking Babcock

One 5 mm dolphin-nosed grasper

One 10 mm right-angle dissector

One 5 mm toothed locking grasper

One 5 mm electrocautery hook

Two 5 mm laparoscopic needle drivers (available in the room)

One 5 mm laparoscopic handpiece for the argon beam coagulator and generator (available in the room)

One 5 mm Diamond Flex Triangle retractor (Genzyme, Tucker, GA) (available in the room)

One 10 mm PEER retractor (Jarit, Hawthorne, NY)

One Martin arm (available in the room)

One 11 mm multiload clip applier (available in the room)

One 5 mm irrigator/aspirator

One 10 mm laparoscopic biopsy forceps (Snowden-Pencer Inc., Tucker, GA)

One 5 mm laparoscopic injecting needle

One 10 mm deflectable laparoscopic ultrasound probe (Tetrad, Tetrad Corp., Englewood, CO)

One grasping needle port closure device

One smoke evacuator valve (Plume-Away: Stryker Endoscopy, San Jose, CA) (optional)

15F round Davol drain

One No. 15 blade scalpel and handle

Two fine-toothed pickups

One Tonsil clamp

Two S-retractors

Three 0-Vicryl ties

Four 4-0 absorbable suture on a cutting needle

One-quarter-inch Steri-Strips

Benzoin

Open nephrectomy surgical pan

STEPS OF THE PROCEDURE   Step 1: Placement of a Ureteral Catheter or Administration of Indigo Carmine   Decortication of renal cysts that arise in, or extend deep into, a peripelvic location run the risk of entry into the collecting system. Recognition of this occurrence is important as it can usually be repaired laparoscopically and further complications avoided by placement of a drain with or without a stent. Two methods can be utilized to identify entry into the collecting system, one requires cystoscopic placement of a ureteral catheter at the beginning of the operation and repositioning, the other involves simple administration of indigo carmine prior to insufflation. If an external ureteral catheter technique is desired, a cystoscopic insertion and methylene blue irrigation system is performed identical to what was described for laparoscopic heminephrectomy. The patient is then positioned for laparoscopic renal surgery as outlined for simple nephrectomy.

An alternative to the above-noted technique is the administration of indigo carmine prior to creation of the pneumoperitoneum. Because of the relative oliguria that occurs during laparoscopic procedures, the indigo carmine will remain present within the collecting system for the duration of the procedure. Aspiration of the cyst with examination of the aspirated fluid for the presence of blue discoloration can be utilized to determine if the aspirated structure is a portion of the collecting system prior to decortication.[144] Compression of the renal pelvis with release of blue-tinged fluid after decortication confirms an injury to the collecting system and also helps to define its location. We prefer this method for peripelvic cyst decortication because of the thin layer of separation between the collecting system and the base of the cyst that can be perforated during wire manipulations and catheter insertion (Figure 57-14). In addition, this latter technique obviates the need for repositioning of the patient, thus reducing overall operative times.

Step 2: Creation of the Pneumoperitoneum and Initial Entry Access   This step is identical to that outlined for laparoscopic nephrectomy, utilizing either the transperitoneal or retroperitoneal approach.

Step 3: Secondary Port Placement   There are no significant alterations to the secondary port placements as described for laparoscopic nephrectomy. Although an Endo-GIA stapler is not necessary for this operation, we maintain the left lower-quadrant 10/12 mm port to use for the 10 mm lens and for removal of cyst-wall specimens. Liver elevation is almost always necessary for right-sided procedures owing to the cephalad extent or multiplicity of lesions requiring the lateral port as described for right-sided nephrectomies.

Secondary ports for the retroperitoneal approach are identical to those described for nephrectomy. If intraoperative ultrasound is anticipated, the 10/12 mm working port used to introduce the Endovascular-GIA stapler during nephrectomy can be utilized to insert the deflectable laparoscopic ultrasound probe.

Step 4: Exposure of the Retroperitoneum   This step is identical to that outlined for laparoscopic nephrectomy, utilizing either the transperitoneal or retroperitoneal approach, as the majority of cysts requiring decortication are large or multiple and require access to all areas of the renal surface.

Step 5: Identification and Exposure of Cyst Surface   Complete mobilization of the surface of the cyst wall from surrounding structures is easier to perform prior to decompression of the cyst unless exposure is limited owing to its expanse. This is especially true for a large upper-pole cyst on the right side secondary to overlap of the liver edge (see Figure 57-2A). Identification of a peripelvic, or primarily intraparenchymal, cyst can be difficult, especially in male patients with a thickened and adherent Gerota's fat layer. In such patients, use of a deflectable ultrasound probe can help to facilitate locating the margins of the cyst and guide the unroofing process. This

may also prove helpful in identifying deeper parenchymal cysts during extensive decortications performed for ADPKD, or assessing wall nodularity within indeterminate cysts. Intraoperative ultrasound requires insertion via the 10/12 mm port in the left lower quadrant and moving the laparoscope to the periumbilical port site, which may require switching to a 5 mm lens if a 5 mm port was placed at this location.

Once the cyst has been exposed, confirmation that there is no connection with the collecting system should be established for a peripelvic or any cyst that extends deep along portions of the collecting system. This can be determined by puncture and aspiration using a laparoscopic needle inserted via the 5 mm port when indigo carmine was administered prior to insufflation or following a retrograde injection of methylene blue if a preoperative ureteral catheter was placed. The aspirated fluid can be placed on a clean surgical gauze to facilitate identification of a ring of blue staining when visual inspection of the syringe is equivocal secondary to pigment contained within the cysts. If concern exists regarding the possibility of malignancy, the aspirated cyst fluid can be sent for cytopathologic assessment.

It is important to make every effort to aspirate as much of the released material as possible from pigmented cysts associated with ADPKD, since peritoneal contact with this material has been shown to result in a chemical peritonitis (Figure 57-15A and B).[145] If spillage occurs, contact areas are repetitively irrigated using the irrigator-aspirator. The postoperative clinical course of these patients can be difficult to differentiate from patients suffering an unrecognized bowel injury and can also result in a profound ileus.

Step 6: Cyst Unroofing, Biopsy, and Specimen Extraction   The Harmonic scalpel is the ideal device for unroofing large simple cysts, as well as multiple cysts associated with ADPKD, because it limits bleeding from the cut edge of the cysts, yet minimizes collateral damage to struc-

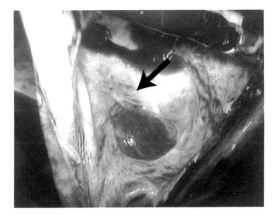

Figure 57-14 Collecting system identification during laparoscopic cyst decortication for a multichambered cyst with deep hilar extension. An ample of indigo carmine was administered intravenously by the anesthesiologist prior to creation of the pneumoperitoneum. Note the blue-tinged urine that can be seen through the thin wall of the base of the cyst (arrow), yet no urine leakage is identified.

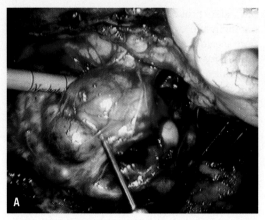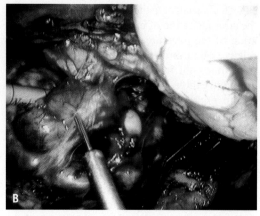

Figure 57-15 Laparoscopic cyst decortication in a patient with ADPKD and numerous pigmented cysts. *A,* To prevent postdecortication peritonitis syndrome induced by release of pigmented fluids into the peritoneal cavity, needle puncture of each pigmented cyst and *B,* aspiration of its contents should be performed prior to unroofing with the Harmonic shears and thorough irrigation.

tures such as the collecting system.[122] It is safest to begin opening the cyst at its thinnest point, which typically is found far from the edges. This is appreciated as a translucent-appearing area that is often darker than surrounding regions of the kidney because of the underlying cavity. A laparoscopic aspirating needle can be inserted in this area as described above. Incision of the cyst wall is continued down to its border with normal parenchyma or collecting system and the entire margin is circumferentially excised. This can be removed in sequential strips if a question exists regarding what is parenchyma and what is cyst wall. More vigorous edge bleeding often implies entry into normal parenchyma and can usually be controlled using the Harmonic device, bipolar electrocautery, pressure with a sheet of Surgicel, or the argon beam coagulator. On rare occasion, a figure-of-eight suture or a short interlocking running stitch along the edge may be required for hemostasis.

If a concern exists regarding the possibility of malignancy, as occurs with decortication of complex cystic lesions, the cyst fluid should be completely aspirated and sent for cytology. The excised cyst walls should be sent for pathologic inspection along with a biopsy of the base of the cyst. The cyst base biopsies are taken from regions that are not immediately adjacent to the collecting system. If a region of obvious thickening or nodularity is noted, specimens should be taken from these regions. Careful scrutiny of preoperative imaging studies can help locate concerning areas within the base of the cyst and guide sites for biopsy.

Smaller cyst-wall and biopsy specimens can be removed directly via 10/12 mm ports. Larger cyst-wall specimens for which there is not a concern for malignancy can be cut into strips and removed through the 10/12 mm port. Alternatively, an Endocatch I or II bag can be utilized to bag and remove the specimen. The Endocatch I bag can be inserted via a 10/12 mm port, but requires ultimate removal of the port for specimen extraction. An Endocatch II bag can be utilized when the specimen(s) is especially large, but requires initial removal of the port and inser-

tion via the port incision. We prefer to perform specimen extraction via the lower-quadrant port site as it is the most elevated in the flank position, preventing contact with bowel or deep intraperitoneal displacement of the specimen should a perforation of the bag occur. Morcellation can be performed as outlined for simple nephrectomy.

Decortication of all visible superficial and deeper cysts as well as final ultrasound inspection with a 10 mHz deflectable Tetrad ultrasound unit (Tetrad Corp., Englewood, CO) to help identify any other previously unrecognized cysts within several millimeters of accessible surfaces has been advocated by several authors.[8] These additional cysts are also marsupialized, and the average number of cysts decorticated using this approach was 220 cysts per procedure in one review.[8] Because of the degree of mobilization and the resultant volume reduction following the procedure, some authors performed a postdecortication nephropexy in 77% of their patients using a 0 polyglactin suture passed through the posterior abdominal wall fascia and capsule of the kidney and secured at each end with a Lapra-Ty.[8,146] This helps prevent hypermobility and torsion of the decompressed kidney on its hilar structures.

Step 7: Final Inspection, Exiting the Abdomen, and Port Closure Final inspection for hemostasis following cyst decortication is identical to what was previously described for laparoscopic nephrectomy. In addition, the areas of decortication and base biopsies should also be carefully inspected for evidence of urine leakage. If an externalized ureteral catheter was utilized, the circulating nursing staff or assistant can inject dilute methylene blue to help identify any leaks. If injected indigo carmine was utilized, gentle compression of the renal pelvis will identify any injury. An attempt at suture closure should be performed for all substantial collecting system lacerations utilizing a 4-0 Vicryl or polydioxanone suture. Smaller injuries involving the calices will often seal with stent drainage alone. Closure sutures are placed at each of the 10/12 mm port sites using the Carter-Thomason device. If a collecting system injury occurs, a 15F round Davol drain with the

spike removed can be inserted via the 5 mm lateral port site. A clamp is secured to its end to prevent leakage of the CO_2 as it is fed into the abdomen and positioned in the retroperitoneum. The 5 mm port is then removed and the drain is secured to the skin using a 3-0 nylon suture. The abdomen is desufflated, fascial entry sites are secured, and the peritoneal cavity is exited as previously described for laparoscopic nephrectomy.

If a collecting system repair was required, a ureteral catheter can be inserted at the end of the procedure. A simple stent exchange can be performed under fluoroscopy if an open-ended catheter was utilized without repositioning by utilizing a .035-inch floppy-tip wire, a metal-tip pusher, and an appropriate-sized stent. In this approach the stent is inserted, followed by the metal-tip pusher, which is advanced to the inferior edge of the pubic symphysis and the wire is removed under fluoroscopy, confirming proper position of the proximal and distal pigtails. If an external catheter was not utilized, the patient can be repositioned in the dorsal lithotomy, reprepped and draped, and a wire and subsequent stent introduced via the cystoscope in standard fashion. A Foley catheter is then inserted at the end of the procedure to minimize reflux along the stent.

POSTOPERATIVE CARE The immediate postoperative care of patients having undergone renal cyst decortication is identical to that after laparoscopic simple nephrectomy with the following noteworthy exceptions. If a collecting system injury occurred and a drain and stent were inserted, the Foley catheter is left in place for 24 hours provided the drain output is minimal (ie, < 30 cc per 8 hours). The Foley catheter is removed on postoperative day 2 and the drain output is monitored. If the drain output increases markedly, the source of the fluid can be evaluated by sending it for a creatinine level. If it is significantly above the measured serum creatinine level, then a portion of the fluid is urine and the Foley catheter should be left in place or replaced if it was removed. Once the Foley catheter has been discontinued and there is no significant increase in the drain output over the next 8-hour shift, the drain can be removed. Patients are usually sent home on postoperative day 2 or 3. The stent is left in place for approximately 1 week, and a retrograde pyelogram can be performed at the time of removal if concern exists regarding continued leakage.

The other exception to the standard postoperative care of patients following renal cyst decortication are those patients with ADPKD and a large number of hemorrhagic cysts. These patients can have a very protracted course secondary to a chemical peritonitis from the contents of the cysts and, as a result, can require up to 50% more parenteral analgesics than patients undergoing laparoscopic removal of their entire kidney.[145] The clinical postoperative presentation of these patients can include distention, diffuse abdominal pain, fevers, elevated white blood cell count, and a profound ileus. In these patients, supportive care with intravenous fluids, pain medication, and tincture of time lead to ultimate resolution, although this can significantly prolong the hospital stay.

RESULTS *Simple Symptomatic Parenchymal Cysts* In a review of 5 series totaling 74 patients with large symptomatic cysts, the radiographic success rate of laparoscopic decortication was noted to be 90% over a mean follow-up of 7 months.[6] Lifson and colleagues[147] reported their series of 5 patients undergoing cyst decortication for a symptomatic large cyst with all 5 remaining pain free on a mean follow-up of 33 months. Roberts and colleagues[7] reviewed their series of laparoscopic decortication of large symptomatic parenchymal cysts in 21 patients. Thirteen patients in their series had a transperitoneal and 8 a retroperitoneal approach with a mean operative time of 164 minutes, operative blood loss of 98 cc, and a hospital stay of 1.9 days. They noted a 5% recurrence rate over a mean follow-up period of 15.8 months, although only 58% of the patients in their entire series underwent follow-up imaging.[7]

Peripelvic Cysts Most reported series do not clearly delineate between peripelvic and parenchymal cysts; however, Roberts and colleagues compared their series of 21 parenchymal with 11 peripelvic cysts for which a laparoscopic decortication was performed.[7] A similar distribution of approaches (7 transperitoneal and 4 retroperitoneal) was noted for the peripelvic operations relative to what was mentioned above for the parenchymal lesions. There was a statistically significant longer mean operative time (233 minutes) and (blood loss 182 cc) noted for the peripelvic cyst decortications, which was felt to reflect the more technically challenging nature of this operation. Mean follow-up of 22.4 months did not demonstrate any evidence of recurrence. Not surprisingly, the percentage of patients with inadvertent entry into the collecting system was higher for the patients with peripelvic (18%) relative to simple parenchymal cysts (14.3%).[7] Rubenstein and colleagues[148] described 1 patient in their series of 10 laparoscopic cyst decortications with a large peripelvic cyst extending between the renal artery and vein that was decorticated and a wick of 6 × 1 cm polytetrafluoroethylene was placed to help prevent reformation of the cyst. This patient developed a small recurrent cyst, but remained asymptomatic at 10 months.

Hoenig and colleagues[19] reviewed their experience of laparoscopic ablation of symptomatic peripelvic cysts in 4 patients. Cyst size ranged from 4 to 6 cm and 2 patients had concomitant stone disease. Three of the 4 underwent a transperitoneal approach and 1 a retroperitoneal approach with a mean operative time of 338 minutes, estimated blood loss of 90 cc, and length of stay of 2.75 days. One patient suffered a laceration of the renal pelvis, which was recognized and repaired intraoperatively. All patients had initial resolution of their preoperative pain, but 1 patient developed a symptomatic recurrence at 2 months, requiring an open decortication.

Another patient developed an asymptomatic recurrence of a 2 cm peripelvic cyst at 9 months.

Recently, Doumas and colleagues[149] reported their series of 5 patients with peripelvic cysts ranging from 4.5 to 6.5 cm in size. All underwent transperitoneal laparoscopic decortication with a mean operative time of 155 minutes and estimated blood loss < 150 cc. No intraoperative complications and only 1 minor postoperative complication (subcutaneous hematoma) occurred. All patients remained free of symptoms and radiographic evidence of obstruction at a mean follow-up of 23 months.

Indeterminate Complex Cystic Lesions Most surgeons advocate treating Bosniak IV (see Table 57-1) lesions identical to cystic renal cancer owing to the 90% risk of reported malignancy.[6,14,150] Controversy exists in the use of laparoscopy to evaluate and manage asymptomatic or symptomatic Bosniak II and III lesions with their associated 24% and 41% risk, respectively, of malignancy. Even though completion nephrectomy can be performed when cancer is identified in resected wall segments or aspirated fluids, a recent case report by Meng and colleagues[15] illustrates the possibility that laparoscopic decortication may alter the progression pattern of disease if it goes undiagnosed. In their case, a patient with a symptomatic 20 cm Bosniak I lesion underwent a laparoscopic cyst decortication and analysis of the cyst wall demonstrated benign tissue. Seven months later, the patient presented with a large renal mass involving the spleen and colon, liver, subcutaneous port site, lymph node, and peritoneal metastases, and pathology revealed Fuhrman grade 4 chromophil and sarcomatoid renal carcinoma.[15] The diffuse spread of disease over a relatively short period of time suggests that tumor spillage and possibly convection-related dissemination from the pneumoperitoneum likely contributed.

In contrast to this case, Santiago and colleagues[16] reported their series of 35 patients who underwent laparoscopic assessment and management of Bosniak II and III lesions. A total of 5 (14.3%) were discovered to harbor malignancy, and 4 underwent immediate partial or radical nephrectomy, and 1 a delayed partial nephrectomy. No recurrences were identified after a mean follow-up of 20.2 months. Roberts and colleagues[7] described their series of laparoscopic management of renal cystic disease, which included 8 patients with Bosniak II and III lesions. One patient (12.5%) was identified on final pathology to have a small < 1 cm focus of papillary renal cancer and underwent eventual open radical nephrectomy with excision of the trocar site used for specimen extraction. In a similar case, Lifson and colleagues[147] discovered a small focus of papillary carcinoma in the cyst wall of a Bosniak I lesion and the patient underwent immediate open radical nephrectomy. A prior negative cyst fluid aspiration cytology had been obtained on the patient and he remains free of disease recurrence at 58 months of CT scan follow-up.[147]

The results of these last 3 series indicate that, in select patients with indeterminate cysts,

laparoscopy may provide a reasonable diagnostic and therapeutic approach provided a careful inspection of the cyst base with biopsy, cytologic evaluation of aspirated fluid, and meticulous pathologic review of the resected cyst wall is performed. The finding of positive aspiration cytologies in only 14% of proven cystic malignancies,[151] and the case report by Meng and colleagues[15] illustrates that accurate diagnosis at the time of laparoscopy may not be feasible and misdiagnosis may have a disastrous effect on the ultimate course of disease.

Autosomal Dominant Polycystic Kidney Disease Symptomatic recurrence requiring repeat surgical therapy occurs more frequently following decortications performed for ADPKD owing to the multifocal, progressive nature of the disease. Subsequent treatment, including repeat laparoscopic decortication, cyst puncture and aspiration, and nephrectomy, is required in 10.3 to 37.5% of patients.[8,122,147,152] Overall improvement in pain, bowel, or pulmonary complaints has been defined and reported in variable fashion (Table 57-5). Lee and colleagues[8] utilized analog pain scores to calculate the relative pain relief (RPR) value for each patient, which equaled (preoperative pain score) – (postoperative pain score)/(preoperative pain score). The RPR was calculated as 58%, 47%, and 63% at 12, 24, and 36 months, respectively. Greater than 50% reduction in pain was noted in 73%, 52%, and 81% of patients at 12, 24, and 36 months, respectively. These authors also showed significant improvements in 6 of 8 Quality of Life domains 1 year following laparoscopic decortication.[8]

Intrarenal ischemia from cyst growth, renal handling of sodium, inappropriate activity of the renin-angiotensin-aldosterone system, volume expansion, and increased atrial natriuretic peptide and plasma endothelin levels have been postulated to contribute to the hypertension noted in 50 to 70% of ADPKD patients before renal function is impaired.[27] Lee and colleagues[8] evaluated the impact of laparoscopic decortication on hypertension in their patients using the antihypertensive therapeutic index (ATI) defined as (dose of blood pressure medication 1/maximum dose 1) + (dose medication 2/maximum dose 2) + etc. A total of 5 (23.8%) of the initial 21 patients with hypertension became normotensive following their procedure. Nine additional patients had a mean 49% improvement in their ATI; however, 6 patients had a mean worsening of 53%. The impact on creatinine clearance was also assessed by these authors using pre- and postoperative Cockcroft and Gault calculations of renal function, which demonstrated changes of +4%, +7%, and –2% at 1, 2, and 3 years, respectively.[8]

COMPLICATIONS The potential complications that can occur with cyst decortications include all of those mentioned previously for laparoscopic nephrectomy with the exception of Endovascular-GIA malfunction. Complications that occur with greater frequency following decortication procedures include collecting system injury with

Table 57-5 Results of Laparoscopic Cyst Decortication in ADPKD Patients

Series	Pts. (Proc.)	TP/RP	OR Time (Mean: min)	Analgesia (Morphine Equiv: mg)	LOS (days)	EBL	Transfusion	Symptomatic Success	F/U (Mean: months)	Repeat Treatment	Complications
Lee et al[8]	29 (35)	33/2	294	61.1	3.2	124	0	> 50% pain reduction 73% (12 m) 52% (24 m) 81% (36 m)	32.3	10.3%	3 (8.6%): Major 7 (20%): Minor
McNally et al[122]	7 (8)	8/0	–	–	3.9	< 200	25%	51% pain reduction (14 m)	14	14.3%	3 (37.5%): Major
Lifson et al[147]	8 (11)	10/1	~ 137	–	~ 2.2	~ 116	9%	Pain free 87.5% (6 m) 71.4% (12 m) 66.7% (24 m) 25% (36 m)	24	37.5%	1 (9%)
Brown et al[152]	8	8/0	164	–	< 2	< 150	–	50% (12–28 m)	12–28 m	37.5%	0

EBL = estimated blood loss; F/U = follow-up; LOS = length of stay; RP = retroperitoneal; TP = transperitoneal.

resultant urinoma in as high as 8.5% of patients with ADPKD,[8] 14.3% of simple parenchymal, and 18% of peripelvic cysts.[7] Hemorrhage requiring transfusion occurred more commonly in patients undergoing decortication procedures in association with ADPKD (see Table 57-5). Several of these cases were associated with the administration of heparin following concomitant insertion of a dialysis catheter.[122] The discovery of malignancy in < 0.7% of simple cysts[150] and 12.5 to 14.3% of patients undergoing laparoscopic decortication for Bosniak II and III lesions[7,16] could potentially lead to the catastrophic spread of disease as described by Meng and colleagues.[15]

CALICEALECTOMY The laparoscopic approach to stone-bearing caliceal diverticula is best suited to anterior-based lesions as mentioned above under indications.[153] For this reason, we prefer a transperitoneal approach for this operation, although retroperitoneal exposure of the kidney with access and trocar distribution as described above have been described.[154] The purported advantages of the retroperitoneal approach are the lack of manipulation of the bowels as well as the reduced potential for intraperitoneal extrusion of stone or infectious material.

INSTRUMENTATION (University of Wisconsin, Madison)

Standard rigid or flexible cystoscopic pan
.035-inch floppy-tip wire
6F open-ended catheter
Ampule of indigo carmine
Ampule of methylene blue
Three nonbladed trocars (left); 4 nonbladed trocars (right)
Two 5 mm and one 10/12 mm (with reducer) (left)
Three 5 mm and one 10/12 mm (with reducer) (right)
Two 10 mm laparoscopes: one 0-degree and one 30-degree
Two 5 mm laparoscopes: one 0-degree and one 30-degree (available in the room)

One 14-gauge Veress needle
One 10/12 mm blunt-tip cannula (available in the room)
One trocar-mounted balloon dilation device (Origin Medsystems, Menlo Park, CA) (retroperitoneal)
One 10/12 mm visual introducing cannula
One 5 mm curved electrocautery scissors
One 5 mm curved Maryland dissector
One 5 mm curved Harmonic scalpel and generator
One 10 mm locking Babcock
One 5 mm dolphin-nosed grasper
One 10 mm right-angle dissector
One 5 mm toothed locking grasper
One 5 mm electrocautery hook
Two 5 mm laparoscopic needle drivers (available in the room)
One 5 mm triradiate grasping forceps
One 5 mm laparoscopic injecting needle
One 5 mm laparoscopic argon beam coagulation probe
One 10 mm PEER retractor (Jarit, Hawthorne, NY)
One 11 mm multiload clip applier (available in the room)
One 5 mm irrigator/aspirator
One Endocatch I bag (stone specimen removal)
One grasping needle port closure device
One smoke evacuator valve (Plume-Away: Stryker Endoscopy, San Jose, CA) (optional)
One 5 mm Diamond Flex Triangle retractor (Genzyme, Tucker, GA) (available in the room) (right)
One Martin arm (available in the room) (right)
One No. 15 blade scalpel and handle
Two fine-toothed pickups
One Tonsil clamp
Two S-retractors
Three 0-Vicryl ties
Four 4-0 absorbable sutures on a cutting needle
One-quarter-inch Steri-Strips
Benzoin
Open nephrectomy surgical pan

STEPS OF THE PROCEDURE Step 1: Placement of a Ureteral Catheter or Administration of Indigo Carmine This step is identical to that

outlined above for renal cyst decortications when cysts closely approximate the collecting system.

Step 2: Creation of the Pneumoperitoneum and Initial Entry Access This step is identical to that outlined for laparoscopic nephrectomy, utilizing either the transperitoneal or retroperitoneal approach.

Step 3: Secondary Port Placement The only alteration to the secondary port placements as described for laparoscopic nephrectomy is the replacement of the periumbilical 10/12 mm port with a 5 mm port, as GIA stapler insertion is not necessary. Ultimately, this will require the use of a 5 mm laparoscopic lens during placement of the stone(s) into the Endocatch I bag and for fascial closure of the 10/12 mm port site. Depending on the location of the diverticulum on the right, liver elevation may not be necessary provided the lesion is located in the midregion of the kidney or the kidney sits lower in the retroperitoneum. This eliminates the need for the lower lateral port for right-sided procedures, which is used almost exclusively for liver elevation.

Secondary port placement for the retroperitoneal approach is identical to that described for nephrectomy with the exception of replacing the 10/12 mm trocars with 5 mm ports. Again, this will require the use of a 5 mm laparoscope for bagging of the stone specimen.

Step 4: Exposure of the Retroperitoneum This step is identical to that outlined for laparoscopic nephrectomy, utilizing either the transperitoneal or retroperitoneal approach, with the following exceptions. Complete splenic mobilization may not be necessary for diverticulum in the midregion of the left kidney as complete upper-pole exposure is often unwarranted. Alternatively, on the left, the line of Toldt can be incised around the splenic flexure, leaving the pancreas and spleen in situ. This usually provides adequate exposure and requires less dissection. On the right, the duodenum does not have to be kocherized unless it closely approximates the area of involved parenchyma, as access to the great vessels is not necessary for this procedure.

Step 5: Renal Dissection and Identification of the Diverticulum A 30-degree 10 mm laparoscope is inserted through the 10/12 mm port in the lower quadrant for the transperitoneal approach. In the retroperitoneal approach, a 30-degree lens is also utilized via the 10/12 mm port off the tip of the twelfth rib. The surgeon operates via the 5 mm ports utilizing the Maryland dissector held in the nondominant hand and the Harmonic shears in the dominant hand. If the location of the diverticulum on the right requires liver elevation for adequate exposure during the transperitoneal approach, the Diamond Flex retractor is inserted through the lateral 5 mm port between the tip of the twelfth rib and iliac crest. The retractor handle is twisted until the appropriate triangle configuration is obtained, and it is then placed beneath the liver edge, elevated into position, and secured to the operative table utilizing the Martin robotic arm or an endo holder. Care should be exercised to prevent unnecessary pressure on the gallbladder or porta hepatis.

The kidney contained within Gerota's fascia and fat is usually easily identified by palpation of a firm structure in the retroperitoneum. The Harmonic shears are utilized to divide Gerota's fascia and fat overlying the lateral margin of the kidney beginning at the lower pole and progressing cephalad. Frequent infections and inflammatory events may make exposure of the smooth capsular surface of the kidney difficult. The Harmonic device is ideal for performing this separation as it limits the amount of capsular oozing. The relative location of the calculus within the kidney is known as a result of the preoperative CT scan imaging confirming its regional position (see Figure 57-3). The exact location is identified laparoscopically as a parenchymal indentation on the surface of the kidney[154] (Figure 57-16A), although this area can also appear raised relative to the surrounding parenchyma.[153] If inflammatory events have occurred within the diverticulum, the overlying fat may adhere to and fill the parenchymal depression. This can be probed with a laparoscopic aspirating needle to confirm the presence of the underlying stone as a hard area of contact feedback. Theories regarding thinning of the parenchyma in this region include a lack of induction of the metanephric blastema in this region for those who believe in congenital origins versus resultant scarring and atrophy from inflammation.[35–37]

Step 6: Incision of the Diverticulum and Stone Extraction Regardless of the origin, the parenchyma in this region is usually thin and devoid of significant blood supply, allowing incision with the electrocautery or Harmonic shears (Figure 57-16B) without marked hemorrhage.[154] Once the overlying parenchyma has been incised, the diverticulum is irrigated gently to reveal the contained stone. The 10 mm laparoscope is exchanged for the 30-degree 5 mm lens, which is inserted in the subcostal region for the transperitoneal approach and in the posterior axillary line 5 mm port for the retroperitoneal approach. The Endocatch I bag is introduced via the 10/12 mm port and the other 5 mm port is utilized to extract the stone(s) using the percutaneous three-prong graspers and to place all stone material into the entrapment sac (Figure 57-17A and B). The drawstring is then pulled tight on the sac, the port is removed, and the drawstring clamped near the skin level. The stones within the entrapment sac are left in situ within the peritoneum or retroperitoneum and the port is then reintroduced.

Step 7: Diverticulum Ablation and Closure of Collecting System The diverticulum is inspected to find its communication with the collecting system. Identification is facilitated by injection of methylene blue via the externalized ureteral catheter or by gentle compression of the renal pelvis if preinsufflation indigo carmine was utilized instead. Both techniques result in a stream of blue-tinged urine emitting from the area of the connection. If the opening is not identified using these techniques, then it is likely extremely small, and fulguration of the area alone or application of fibrin glue products (see Figure 57-16C) will usually suffice to prevent leakage of urine. The 5 mm laparoscopic argon beam coagulator is ideal for complete ablation of the urothelial lining of the diverticulum, although the back of the electrocautery or Harmonic shears can also be utilized. Once the entire surface has been ablated, a 3-0 Vicryl on an RB-1 needle is inserted via the 10/12 mm port and a figure-of-eight closure suture is placed across the mouth of the diverticulum. A total of 3 throws are placed in the suture, with the first being a surgeon's knot. Repeat injection of methylene blue via the externalized stent (or compression of the pelvis if intravenous indigo carmine is utilized) confirms a water-tight closure.

One option when a large, gaping cavity is created that is unlikely to collapse following fulguration is to insert a tongue of Gerota's fat into the base of the diverticulum. It is then secured with one or more sutures of 3-0 Vicryl to the wall of the diverticulum utilizing intracorporeal suturing techniques.

Step 8: Exiting the Abdomen, Drain Placement, and Port Closure The area of the dissection is inspected for hemostasis once again at low insufflation pressures, and all bleeding points are cauterized. The perforated end of a 15F round Davol drain with the spike removed is inserted via the lower-quadrant port in the transperitoneal approach and the lateral-most port in the retroperitoneal approach. Placing a clamp on the back end of the drain prevents release of the pneumoperitoneum during this maneuver. A grasper is inserted via the port used to bag the specimen and is utilized to position the drain lateral and behind the kidney to monitor for any leakage of urine. The specimen is removed under vision of the 5 mm laparoscope inserted via the remaining 5 mm port with the fascial incision enlarged if necessary. If enlargement of the fascial site is not anticipated, then the fascial closure needle can be utilized to place a closure stitch at the port site prior to insertion of the drain. The final port is removed as previously described after evacuation of the pneumoperitoneum. As with other retroperitoneal procedures, the blunt-tip trocar site is usually closed under vision, while the fascial incisions of the 5 mm ports are not sutured. The skin incisions are closed as previously described.

POSTOPERATIVE CARE The postoperative care following laparoscopic calicealectomy is identical to that for cyst decortication. If an external stent was placed at the beginning of the operative procedure, it is removed at the end of the operation or exchanged for a double-pigtail stent using

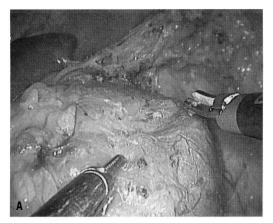
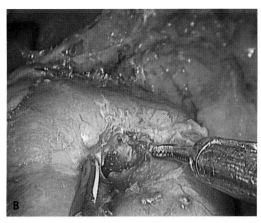
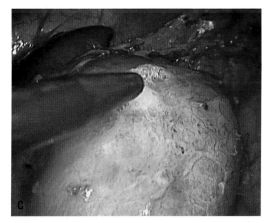

Figure 57-16 Laparoscopic calicealectomy *A*, An indentation on the surface of the renal parenchyma marks the location of the diverticulum. *B*, Harmonic shears are utilized to unroof the overlying parenchyma. *C*, The small ostium of the diverticulum is occluded utilizing fibrin glue products.

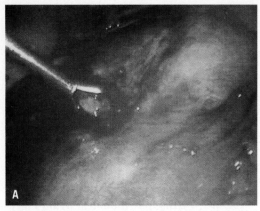
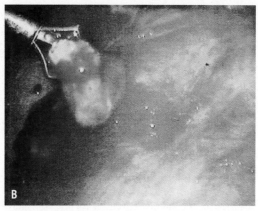

Figure 57-17 Laparoscopic calicealectomy and stone extraction. *A,* The thinned area of parenchyma has been incised and the stone can be visualized as it is being engaged utilizing the three-prong percutaneous stone graspers. *B,* The stone is extracted from the diverticulum and deposited into an entrapment sac.

a metal-tip pusher under fluoroscopy when closure of the ostium of the diverticulum is in question. The drain output is monitored until it is less than 30 cc on two consecutive shifts following removal of the Foley catheter on postoperative day 1. If the drain output remains elevated, a drain fluid creatinine level should be checked, and if it is markedly elevated above serum levels, the patient can either be sent out with the drain until outputs decline or a double-pigtail stent inserted if large volume urine-laden drainage continues. If a stent is inserted, it is usually left in place for 1 week to allow adequate coaptation and closure of the mouth of the diverticulum.

RESULTS   There have been limited published series on laparoscopic caliceal diverticulectomy amounting to a total of 5 patients.[35,153,154] Approaches were split between the transperitoneal (2) and retroperitoneal approach (3), with all 5 reported cases noted to be stone free and asymptomatic on limited mean reported follow-up of 3.5 months (2–5 months). One of these 5 patients suffered a recurrence of their diverticulum; however, it was 90% reduced from its original size.[154] Mean operative time of approximately 127 minutes was reported.[154]

COMPLICATIONS   Any of the intraoperative or postoperative complications related to access entry, retraction, dissection, or port closure as described for simple nephrectomy are possible with laparoscopic diverticulectomy. The one exception would be the absent risk of a major vascular event secondary to Endovascular-GIA stapler misadventure, because no major vascular structures should require transection during this procedure. A total of 3 complications among 5 patients who underwent laparoscopic caliceal diverticulectomy have been reported in the literature. One patient had a significant hemorrhage requiring a 3-unit blood transfusion.[154] This presumably occurred at the site of incision of the diverticulum. Another had a persistent discharge from their port site for 2 months.[154] The source of this prolonged drainage was not detailed further and was said to resolve spontaneously without any

described intervention. Another patient was noted to have prolonged crepitance that was thought to be a result of using the argon beam coagulator, since it persisted for 1 week, which exceeds what would be expected from rapidly absorbed CO_2.[37]

Another potential complication, not observed among these 5 patients, that has occurred following laparoscopic diverticulectomy is a persistent urine leak or urinoma development in the flank (T. J. Moon personal communication, 2003). This results from either inadequate suture closure of the neck of the caliceal diverticulum or inadvertent dissection into the collecting chamber at a site other than the connection. Drainage usually abates rapidly following insertion of a ureteral stent (T. J. Moon personal communication, 2003). If stent placement is unsuccessful in resolving a urinary fistula, more invasive methods extrapolated from similar scenarios following partial nephrectomy, such as percutaneous drainage, tissue adhesive injection, or open exploration, could be required.[155,156]

Nephropexy   In 1993, Urban and colleagues[157] reported the first case of laparoscopic nephropexy for the treatment of clinically significant nephroptosis. It has since been shown to be equally efficacious with superior postoperative pain, morbidity, and convalescence in comparison with the open approach.[53] Laparoscopic fixation of the kidney to the quadratus lumborum fascia can be accomplished via a transperitoneal or retroperitoneal exposure. We, along with other groups, advocate upper-pole fixation to the cut margin of the coronary ligament of the liver, which is best accomplished via a transperitoneal exposure.[158] A retroperitoneal exposure with fixation to the quadratus fascia has been described only with the port distribution as outlined for retroperitoneal nephrectomy.[159] As previously mentioned, the majority of nephropexy procedures are performed on the right, with only 10% of cases isolated to the left kidney.[48,58]

INSTRUMENTATION   (University of Wisconsin, Madison)

Four nonbladed trocars
Three 5 mm and one 10/12 mm (with reducer)

Two 10 mm laparoscopes: one 0-degree and one 30-degree
Two 5 mm laparoscopes: one 0-degree and one 30-degree (available in the room)
One 14-gauge Veress needle
One 10/12 mm blunt-tip cannula (available in the room)
One trocar-mounted balloon dilation device (Origin Medsystems, Menlo Park, CA) (retroperitoneal)
One 10/12 mm visual introducing cannula
One 5 mm curved electrocautery scissors
One 5 mm curved Maryland dissector
One 5 mm curved Harmonic scalpel and generator
One 10 mm locking Babcock
One 5 mm dolphin-nosed grasper
One 10 mm right-angle dissector
One 5 mm toothed locking grasper
One 5 mm electrocautery hook
Two 5 mm laparoscopic needle drivers
One 5 mm laparoscopic argon beam coagulation probe
One 10 mm PEER retractor
One 11 mm multiload clip applier (available in the room)
One 5 mm irrigator/aspirator
One grasping needle port closure device
One smoke evacuator valve (Plume-Away: Stryker Endoscopy, San Jose, CA) (optional)
One 5 mm Diamond Flex Triangle retractor (Genzyme, Tucker, GA)
One Martin arm (available in the room)
One No. 15 blade scalpel and handle
Two fine-toothed pickups
One Tonsil clamp
Two S-retractors
Three 0-Vicryl ties
Four 4-0 absorbable suture on a cutting needle
one-quarter-inch Steri-Strips
Benzoin
Open nephrectomy surgical pan

STEPS OF THE PROCEDURE   **Step 1: Creation of the Pneumoperitoneum and Initial Entry Access**   This step is identical to that outlined for laparoscopic nephrectomy, utilizing either the transperitoneal or retroperitoneal approach. Care must be exercised in these cases on initial entry with the Veress needle in the lower quadrant, as the kidney can be displaced into this area in some cases of extreme mobility. Usually airplaning the table slightly away from the operating surgeon will cause the kidney to roll into a more normal location.

Step 2: Secondary Port Placement   This step is identical to that outlined for laparoscopic nephrectomy, utilizing either the transperitoneal or retroperitoneal approach, with the exception that only the periumbilical port needs to be a 10/12 mm to enable insertion of the needle-mounted sutures, whereas all others can be substituted with 5 mm ports. This requires the use of a 5 mm laparoscopic lens. Alternatively, the same port sizes and configuration for laparoscopic nephrectomy can be utilized for this procedure, allowing use of the 10 mm laparoscope if desired.

Step 3: Exposure of the Retroperitoneum

This step is identical to that outlined for laparoscopic nephrectomy, utilizing either the transperitoneal or retroperitoneal approach. In the transperitoneal approach it is not necessary to kocherize the duodenum, as access to the hilar vessels is unnecessary and this structure is widely separated from the lateral margin of the kidney. The Genzyme liver retractor is inserted via the lateralmost port and is utilized by the assistant surgeon to elevate the liver edge to expose the coronary ligament. Care should be exercised when transecting the infrahepatic peritoneal attachments to the liver to leave enough of a shelf-like edge beneath which the upper pole of the kidney can be inserted and two securing sutures to the renal capsule placed as described by Elashry and colleagues.[158]

Step 4: Exposure of the Renal Capsule and Quadratus Fascia and Patient Positioning

Once the kidney is exposed within Gerota's, it should be elevated back into its standard position, as it may be found flipped into a medial or inferior location. Appropriate positioning of the kidney in the retroperitoneum is facilitated by placing the patient into deep Trendelenburg's position and airplaning the table away from the operating surgeon. The lateral and superior border of the kidney are identified and Gerota's fascia is incised over this area and the anterior fat peeled back from the surface of the kidney, while several centimeters of the posterior layer of fat is excised to expose the capsule of the kidney. The contact region between the edge of the kidney and the retroperitoneal fat is noted, and the Harmonic shears are utilized to remove all of the fat overlying this region so the broad fascial surface of the Quadratus musculature is available for suturing. The lack of intervening fat allows for better visualization during suture placement through the Quadratus fascia and renal capsule and creates better contact between the surfaces of these structures. The use of an intervening strip of Gerota's fat as a bolster over which the securing sutures are tied can result in necrosis of the fat and resultant mobility. Differing thickness of fat bolsters can also result in poor contact points, stress at the remaining sutures, tear outs, and subsequent failure of the procedure.

Step 5: Bolster Preparation and Suturing

Two-inch Surgicel bolsters are created by rolling cut segments and securing each end with a 3-0 Vicryl tie. Nephropexy sutures are spaced approximately 1.5 inches apart so a total of 2 sutures are tied down over each bolster. Longer bolsters can be utilized, but are more cumbersome. We prefer the use of 2-0 silk suture mounted on an SH needle for our nephropexy stitches because of its permanence, induced tissue response, and ease of tying. The SH needle is ideal for this procedure owing to its tapered point and relatively flat curvature, allowing gentle, yet lengthy passage beneath the renal capsule. Each suture is cut into a 7-inch length, which is optimal for throwing a single intracorporeal suture.

The upper pole of the kidney is secured to the cut edge of the infrahepatic peritoneal edge by placing 2 sutures first through the peritoneum then through the adjacent region of renal capsule. This step is the reason why it is important to cut the peritoneum low enough to leave an adequate shelf beneath which the upper pole can be inserted and sutured. Care should be exercised to place these renal capsular sutures just where the convexity becomes the anterior surface of the upper pole, as more posterior placement will force the kidney into slight anterior rotation. While these sutures are being placed, the patient remains in deep Trendelenburg's position with full lateral rotation to help keep the kidney in its anatomic position. The assistant utilizes the Genzyme liver retractor to elevate the liver edge to expose this region for suture placement. The needle is passed initially from outside to inside through the infrahepatic peritoneal edge and is pulled through to the appropriate length prior to passage through the capsule of the kidney to prevent sawing through this delicate structure. The needle is scythed just below the capsule for as long a length as the arc of the needle will allow. Care must be exercised to avoid entry into the substance of the renal parenchyma, which can result in vigorous and persistent bleeding, making visualization during the operation difficult. A second suture is then placed in identical fashion approximately 1.5 inches medial to the first. Prior to tying either suture, a 2-inch Surgicel bolster is placed between the capsule of the kidney and the cut infrahepatic peritoneal edge. This not only aids in hemostasis, but also stimulates tissue reaction and clotting between the two structures with eventual fibrous fixation. These sutures are then carefully tied down over the bolsters to a degree of visual tension that brings both into firm contact with the bolster, but is not enough to lacerate the capsule.

Once these sutures are placed, the operative assistant removes the Genzyme retractor and replaces it with a blunt instrument such as the irrigator-aspirator. This instrument is then utilized to provide temporary liver elevation, when necessary, but more importantly, to provide lateral kidney retraction while the sutures are being planed and tied down. This is especially important when tying down the sutures on the convexity of the lower pole. The kidney is first held into position by the assistant and, beginning along the lateral border of the upper pole, the site for fascial and renal capsular suture placement is then mentally visualized and the assistant relaxes retraction of the kidney enough to allow better exposure of these surfaces. The sutures are then placed first through the Quadratus fascia and then through the capsule of the kidney. A second suture is then placed approximately 1.5 inches lower on the convexity of the kidney, and a Surgicel bolster is then positioned between the quadratus fascia in this area and the capsule of the kidney. The assistant then retracts the kidney into its appropriate position and the sutures are sequentially tied down over the bolster as described above. The process is then repeated until the kidney is firmly fixed to the Quadratus fascia. This usually requires approximately 4 or 5 laterally based sutures in addition to the 2 that were placed through the infrahepatic peritoneal edge (Figure 57-18).

Fornara and colleagues[53] described a similar technique but placed only a single nonabsorbable polyester suture through the upper pole and a second through the convexity of the kidney, fixing each to the Quadratus fascia. McDougall and colleagues[57] utilize a braided polyester suture with a preformed loop on the end. The suture-mounted needle is passed initially through the capsule of the kidney then through the Quadratus fascia, and the needle is brought through the loop to allow cinching into place. Once all of the securing

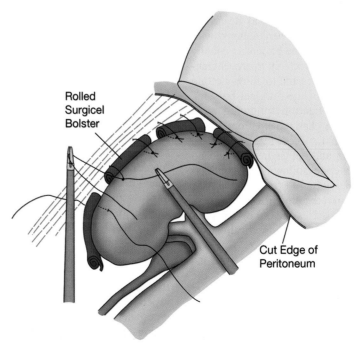

Figure 57-18 Right laparoscopic nephropexy. Two sutures are placed at a time through the quadratus fascia and renal capsule and are tied over rolled Surgicel bolsters.

Series	Technique	TP/RP	OR Time (Mean: min)	Analgesia (Morphine Equiv: mg)	LOS (Mean: days)	Radiographic Success	Symptomatic Success	Follow-up	Complications
Plas et al[58]	Mesh Graft	30/0	154	16	6	9/10 (90%)	11/3 (85%) Cured	5.9 years (median)	1 symptomatic recurrence
McDougall et al[57]	Suturing	12/2	246	37	2.6	13/14 (92.8%)	21% Cured 71% Improved	3.3 years (mean)	1 vomiting & dehydration
Fornara et al[53]	Suturing (2 sutures)	23/0	49	15 & 550 mg Ibuprofen	–	–	91% Improved 2 Not assessed	13 m (mean)	3 (13%): 1 UTI, 2 retroperitoneal hematoma

Table 57-6 Results of Laparoscopic Nephropexy

LOS = length of stay; RP = retroperitoneal; TP = transperitoneal.

sutures have been placed utilizing this technique, they are then tightened and secured using a Lapra-Ty suture clip. The cephalad-to-caudal approach for suture placement and securing of the kidney allows fixation to occur first in the areas of least tension and proceeds toward the area of maximum tension in the lower pole.

Instead of tacking sutures, Plas and colleagues[58] utilized a polypropylene mesh shaped like an ellipse to cover the kidney in its sagittal extension, and then secured the mesh to the abdominal wall with staples. Previously, an absorbable polyglactin mesh had been utilized for their initial 6 patients; however, this was ultimately abandoned after a patient developed symptomatic recurrent mobility 3 months following surgery.[58]

Step 6: Exiting the Abdomen and Port Closure After tying the final suture, the operative table is returned to its neutral position and the kidney is visually monitored to ensure that it maintains its fixed position in the retroperitoneum. Final inspection of the areas of dissection for hemostasis, exiting the abdomen, and port site closure are then performed in identical fashion to what was described for laparoscopic nephrectomy.

POSTOPERATIVE CARE The immediate postoperative care for patients having undergone nephropexy is identical to what was described following laparoscopic simple nephrectomy with the following exceptions. The patient is usually kept in a supine position overnight to prevent tension at the securing sutures and to allow clotting to begin in the region of the Surgicel bolsters. Postoperative immobilization following open nephropexy procedures has ranged from 1.5 to 10 days, with resultant success rates of 36.3 to 83%.[160–163] Fornara and colleagues[53] noted no difference in success rates following immobilization for 3 days in their initial 11 patients, and their next 12 patients who were immobilized anywhere from 1 to 3 days. This series and our own experience indicate that protracted immobilization following the procedure is not necessary. Ambulation is initiated the following day, and once the patient has demonstrated stable mobility the Foley catheter is removed. If bowel sounds are present, the diet can usually be advanced rapidly because of the limited mobilization of the bowel.

The patient is typically discharged home on postoperative day 1 or 2 and is instructed to refrain from all "vertical jarring" activities, such as jogging or horseback riding, for 4 to 6 weeks to allow

stable fixation of the kidney. A follow-up nuclear renal scan is then performed in the sitting position and is compared with the patient's preoperative sitting images. This should demonstrate a postoperative position of the kidney in the sitting position nearly identical to the supine images and resolution of any previously demonstrated reduction in 1- to 2-minute perfusion, relative renal function, or tracer excretion (see Figure 57-4A, B, and C).

RESULTS The long-term results of 3 of the larger published series of laparoscopic nephropexy (Table 57-6) reveal that symptomatic improvement or cure is noted in 92 to 100%, with radiographic improvement in 90 to 100% of those with sufficient follow-up using suturing and mesh graft fixation techniques.[53,57,58] In Plas and colleagues' series, 1 patient out of 30 developed a symptomatic recurrence when she felt a "tearing" sensation in her flank during vigorous exercise 3 months following her surgery and once again developed symptomatic nephroptosis.[58] This was one of the patients who had an absorbable mesh graft fixation performed. A comparison of 23 laparoscopic with 12 prior open nephropexy procedures performed at a single institution demonstrated only slightly longer mean operative time of 61 versus 49 minutes, but reductions of postoperative pain medication (15 vs 38 mg morphine equivalent), mean hospital stay (3.7 vs 16 days), and complications (13 vs 33%) for the laparoscopic relative to the open approach.[53]

COMPLICATIONS As with the other renal laparoscopic procedures, any of the intraoperative or postoperative complications related to access entry, dissection, or port closure as described for simple nephrectomy are possible with laparoscopic nephropexy, with the exception of Endovascular-GIA stapler misadventure. Summarizing the laparoscopic series outlined in (see Table 57-6), complications include minor retroperitoneal hematoma (2.9%), urinary tract infection (1.5%), nausea/vomiting (1.5%), and symptomatic recurrence following exercise (1.5%).[53,57,58] Other complications reported for open nephropexy, though not occurring in these series, remain theoretic possibilities and include genitofemoral entrapment or neuralgia, costal osteomyelitis, hydronephrosis, and obstruction or stenosis of the ureteropelvic junction.[53,54,164] Another potential risk when utilizing a permanent mesh would be the risk of infection or rejection of the mesh, which

was reported to be 1% in a review of 500 cases during which it was used for hernia repair.[58,165]

CONCLUSIONS Fifteen years after Clayman and colleagues[166] ushered in the new era of laparoscopic surgery in urology with their report of the first case of laparoscopic nephrectomy, the procedure is now commonplace at many university and community hospitals. Increased experience with this operation has resulted in a more refined understanding of the anatomy and ergonomics of laparoscopic renal surgery, leading to further application to other forms of benign disease. Partial extirpative and reconstructive renal procedures such as heminephrectomy, renal cyst ablation, calicealectomy, and nephropexy are now being performed laparoscopically with regularity and have led to improvements in postoperative morbidity and convalescence similar to laparoscopic nephrectomy. In the process, urologists have had to familiarize themselves with physiologic responses, anatomic exposures, and complications that are unique to the laparoscopic approach.

The expansion of patient educational materials available via the Internet, health maintenance organizations seeking shorter hospital stays, and the desire for employers to minimize periods of convalescence have further fueled the growth of laparoscopic renal surgery. Technological advances in instrumentation, robotics, tissue welding, hemostatic agents, and ablative devices have already begun to impact how we are currently performing these operations. These advances combined with the limitless vision of the urologist's mind will ultimately determine how the term "minimally invasive renal surgery" is defined in the next 15 years.

REFERENCES

1. Hemal AK, Gupta NP, Wadhwa SN, et al. Retroperitoneoscopic nephrectomy and nephroureterectomy for benign nonfunctioning kidneys: a single-center experience. Urology 2001;57:644–9.
2. Eraky I, el-Kappany HA, Ghoneim MA. Laparoscopic nephrectomy: Mansoura experience with 106 cases. Br J Urol 1995;75:271–5.
3. Malek RS, Kelalis PP, Stickler GB, Burke EC. Observations on ureteral ectopy in children. J Urol 1972;107:308–13.
4. Schlussel RN, Retik AB. Ectopic ureter, ureterocele, and other anomalies of the ureter. In: Walsh PC, Retik AB, Vaughn ED Jr, Wein AJ, editors. Campbell's urology, 8th ed. Philadelphia: W. B. Saunders; 2002. p. 2007–52.
5. Janetschek G, Seibold J, Radmayr C, Bartsch G. Laparoscopic heminephroureterectomy in pediatric patients. J Urol 1997;158:1928–30.

6. Wolf JS Jr. Evaluation and management of solid and cystic renal masses. J Urol 1998;159:1120–33.
7. Roberts WW, Bluebond-Langner R, Boyle KE, et al. Laparoscopic ablation of symptomatic parenchymal and peripelvic renal cysts. Urology 2001;58:165–9.
8. Lee DI, Andreoni CR, Rehman J, et al. Laparoscopic cyst decortication in autosomal dominant polycystic kidney disease: impact on pain, hypertension, and renal function. J Endourol 2003;17:345–53.
9. Ohkawa M, Tokunaga S, Orito M, et al. Percutaneous injection sclerotherapy with minocycline hydrochloride for simple renal cysts. Int Urol Nephrol 1993;25:37–43.
10. Fontana D, Porpiglia F, Morra I, Destefanis P. Treatment of simple renal cysts by percutaneous drainage with three repeated alcohol injection. Urology 1999;53:904–7.
11. Hanna RM, Dahniya MH. Aspiration and scerotherapy of symptomatic simple renal cysts: value of two injections of a sclerosing agent. AJR Am J Roentgenol 1996;167: 781–3.
12. Ohta S, Fujishiro Y, Fuse H. Polidocanol sclerotherapy for simple renal cysts. Urol Int 1997;58:145–7.
13. Reiner I, Donnell S, Jones M, et al. Percutaneous sclerotherapy for simple renal cysts in children. Br J Radiol 1992; 65:281–2.
14. Bosniak MA. The current radiological approach to renal cysts. Radiology 1986;158:1–10.
15. Meng MV, Grossfeld GD, Stoller ML. Renal carcinoma after laparoscopic cyst decortication. J Urol 2002;167:1396.
16. Santiago L, Yamaguchi R, Kaswick J, Bellman GC. Laparoscopic management of indeterminate renal cysts. Urology 1998;52:379–83.
17. Amis ES Jr, Cronan JJ, Pfister RC. The spectrum of peripelvic cysts. Br J Urol 1983;55:150–3.
18. Hinman F Jr. Obstructive renal cysts. J Urol 1978;119:681–3.
19. Hoenig DM, McDougall EM, Shalhav AL, et al. Laparoscopic ablation of peripelvic renal cysts. J Urol 1997;158:1345–8.
20. Barloon TJ, Vince SW. Caliceal obstruction owing to a large parapelvic cyst: excretory urography, ultrasound and computerized tomography findings. J Urol 1987;137:270–1.
21. Hulbert JC, Hunter D, Young AT, Castaneda-Zuniga W. Percutaneous intrarenal marsupialization of a perirenal cystic collection—endocystolysis. J Urol 1988;139:1039–41.
22. Kavoussi LR, Clayman RV, Mikkelsen DJ, Meretyk S. Ureteronephroscopic marsupialization of obstructing peripelvic renal cysts. J Urol 1991;146:411–4.
23. Lang EK. Renal cyst puncture and aspiration: a survey of complications. AJR Am J Roentgenol 1977;128:723–7.
24. Camacho MF, Bondhus MJ, Carrion HM, et al. Ureteropelvic junction obstruction resulting from percutaneous cyst puncture and intracystic isophendylate injection: an unusual complication. J Urol 1980;124:713–24.
25. Gabow PA. Autosomal dominant polycystic kidney disease. N Engl J Med 1993;329:332–42.
26. Elashry OM, Nakada SY, Wolf JS Jr, et al. Laparoscopy for adult polycystic kidney disease: a promising alternative. Am J Kidney Dis 1996;27:224–33.
27. Wang D, Strandgaard S. The pathogenesis of hypertension in autosomal dominant polycystic kidney disease. J Hypertens 1997;15:925–33.
28. Chapman AB, Johnson A, Gabow PA, Schrier RW. The renin-angiotensin-aldosterone system and autosomal dominant polycystic kidney disease. N Engl J Med 1990;323:1091–6.
29. Elzinga LW, Barry JM, Torres VE, et al. Cyst decompression surgery for autosomal dominant polycystic kidney disease. J Am Soc Nephrol 1992;2:1219–26.
30. Ye M, Chen JH, Zhang L, et al. Long-term results of cyst decapitating decompression (CDD) operation for autosomal dominant polycystic kidney disease (ADPKD) [abstract 1114]. J Urol 1997;157:286.
31. Dalgaard O. Bilateral polycystic disease of the kidneys: a follow-up of 284 patients and their families. Acta Med Scand 1957;158:1–255.
32. Yates-Bell JG. Rovsing's operation for polycystic kidney. Lancet 1957;1:126–8.
33. Fleming TW, Barry JM. Bilateral open transperitoneal cyst reduction surgery for autosomal dominant polycystic kidney disease. J Urol 1998;159:44–7.
34. Teichman JM, Hulbert JC. Laparoscopic marsupialization of the painful polycystic kidney. J Urol 1995;153:1105–7.
35. Wulfsohn MA. Pyelocaliceal diverticula. J Urol 1980;123:1–8.
36. Middleton AW Jr, Pfister RC. Stone-containing pyelocaliceal diverticulum: embryogenic, anatomic, radiologic and clinical characteristics. J Urol 1974;111:2–6.
37. Gluckman GR, Stoller M, Irby P. Laparoscopic pyelocaliceal diverticula ablation. J Endourol 1993;7:315–7.
38. Hendrikx AJ, Bierkens AF, Bos R, et al. Treatment of stones in caliceal diverticula: extracorporeal shock wave lithotripsy versus percutaneous nephrolitholapaxy. Br J Urol 1992;70:478–82.
39. Jones JA, Lingeman JE, Steidle CP. The roles of extracorporeal shock wave lithotripsy and percutaneous nephrostolithotomy in the management of pyelocaliceal diverticula. J Urol 1991;146:724–7.
40. Bellman GC, Silverstein JI, Blickensderfer S, Smith AD. Technique and follow-up of percutaneous management of caliceal diverticula. Urology 1993;42:21–5.
41. Hedelin H, Geterud K, Grenabo L, et al. Percutaneous surgery for stones in pyelocaliceal diverticula. Br J Urol 1988; 62:206–8.
42. Hulbert JC, Reddy PK, Hunter DW, et al. Percutaneous techniques for the management of caliceal diverticula containing calculi. J Urol 1986;135:225–7.
43. Streem SB, Yost A. Treatment of caliceal diverticular calculi with extracorporeal shock wave lithotripsy: patient selection and extended followup. J Urol 1992;148(3 Pt 2): 1043–6.
44. Ritchie AWS, Parr NJ, Moussa SA, Tolley DA. Lithotripsy for calculi in caliceal diverticula? Br J Urol 1990;66:6–8.
45. Psihramis KE, Dretler SP. Extracorporeal shock wave lithotripsy of caliceal diverticula calculi. J Urol 1987;138:707–11.
46. Wilbert DM, Jenny E, Stoeckle M, et al. Calyceal diverticular stones: is ESWL worthwhile? [abstract 316]. J Urol 1986; 42:183A.
47. Pang K, David RD, Fuchs GJ. Treatment of stones in caliceal diverticuli using retrograde endoscopic approach: critical assessment after 2 years. J Endourol 1992;6 Suppl 1:S80.
48. Hubner WA, Schramek P, Pfluger H. Laparoscopic nephropexy. J Urol 1994;152:1184–7.
49. Hoenig DM, Hemal AK, Shalhav AL, Clayman RV. Nephroptosis: a "disparaged" condition revisited. Urology 1999; 54:590–6.
50. O'Reilly PH, Pollard AJ. Nephroptosis: a cause of renal pain and a potential cause of inaccurate split renal function determination. Br J Urol 1988;61:284–8.
51. Thomson WN, Innes JA, Munro JF, et al. Renal mobility in women attending a pyelonephritis clinic and in controls. Br J Urol 1978;50:73–5.
52. Clorius JH, Huber W, Kjelle-Schweigler M, et al. Evidence of possible association of nephrolithiasis and nephroptosis. Nephron 1978;22:382–5.
53. Fornara P, Doehn C, Jocham D. Laparoscopic nephropexy: 3-year experience. J Urol 1997;158:1679–83.
54. Moss SW. Floating kidneys: a century of nephroptosis and nephropexy. J Urol 1997;158(3 Pt 1):699–702.
55. de Zeeuw D, Donker AJ, van Herk G, Kremer E. Nephroptosis and kidney function. Nephron 1978;22:366–73.
56. Donaldson IM, Doig A, Knight IC. Nephroptosis with nocturnal polyuria. Am J Med 1967;43:289–93.
57. McDougall EM, Afane JS, Dunn MD, et al. Laparoscopic nephropexy: long-term follow-up—Washington University experience. J Endourol 2000;14:247–50.
58. Plas E, Daha K, Riedl CR, et al. Long-term followup after laparoscopic nephropexy for symptomatic nephroptosis. J Urol 2001;166:449–52.
59. Seifman BD, Dunn RL, Wolf JS Jr. Transperitoneal laparoscopy into the previously operated abdomen: effect on operative time, length of stay and complications. J Urol 2003;169:36–40.
60. Mendoza D, Newman RC, Albala D, et al. Laparoscopic complications in markedly obese urologic patients (a multi-institutional review). Urology 1996;48:562–7.
61. Fazeli-Matin S, Gill IS, Hsu TH, et al. Laparoscopic renal and adrenal surgery in obese patients: comparison to open surgery. J Urol 1999;162(3 Pt 1):665–9.
62. Siqueira TM Jr, Kuo RL, Gardner TA, et al. Major complications in 213 laparoscopic nephrectomy cases: the Indianapolis experience. J Urol 2002;168(4 Pt 1):1361–5.
63. Novick AC, Fergany A. Renovascular hypertension and ischemic nephropathy. In: Walsh PC, Retik AB, Vaughn ED Jr, Wein AJ, editors. Campbell's urology. 8th ed. Philadelphia: W. B. Saunders; 2002. p. 229–71.
64. Jorgensen JO, Hanel K, Lalak NJ, et al. Thromboembolic complications of laparoscopic cholecystectomy. BMJ 1993;306:518–9.
65. Inada K, Koike S, Shirai N, et al. Effects of intermittent pneumatic leg compression for prevention of postoperative deep venous thrombosis with special reference to fibrinolytic activity. Am J Surg 1988;155:602–5.
66. Wolf JS Jr, Marcovich R, Gill IS, et al. Survey of neuromuscular injuries to the patient and surgeon during urologic laparoscopic surgery. Urology 2000;55:831–6.
67. Fornara P, Doehn C, Fricke L, et al. Laparoscopic bilateral nephrectomy: results in 11 renal transplant patients. J Urol 1997;157:445–9.
68. Fuchs GJ, Beck HW, Chong TW. Simultaneous bilateral simple nephrectomy. J Endourol 2000;14:805–10.
69. Gill IS. Retroperitoneal laparoscopic nephrectomy. Urol Clin N Am 1998;25:343–60.
70. Capelouto CC, Moore RG, Silverman SG, Kavoussi LR. Retroperitoneoscopy: anatomical rationale for direct retroperitoneal access. J Urol 1994;152:2008–10.
71. Chiu AW, Chen KK, Wang JH, et al. Direct needle insufflation for pneumoperitoneum: anatomic confirmation and clinical experience. Urology 1995;46:432–7.
72. Kashtan J, Green JF, Parsons EQ, Holcroft JW. Hemodynamic effects of increased abdominal pressure. J Surg Res 1981; 30:249–55.
73. Ho HS, Saunders CJ, Corso FA, Wolfe BM. The effects of CO_2 pneumoperitoneum on hemodynamics in hemorrhaged animals. Surgery 1993;114:381–7.
74. Cullen DJ, Coyle JP, Teplick R, Long MC. Cardiovascular, pulmonary, and renal effects of massively increased intra-abdominal pressure in critically ill patients. Crit Car Med 1989;17:118–21.
75. Eger EI 2nd, Saidman LJ. Hazards of nitrous oxide anesthesia in bowel obstruction and pneumothorax. Anesthesiology 1965;26:61–6.
76. Scheinin B, Lindgren L, Scheinin TM. Peroperative nitrous oxide delays bowel function after colonic surgery. Brit J Anaesth 1990;64:154–8.
77. Neuman GG, Sidebotham G, Negoiana E, et al. Laparoscopy explosion hazards with nitrous oxide. Anesthesiology 1993;78:875–9.
78. Cisek LJ, Gobet RM, Peters CA. Pneumoperitoneum produces reversible renal dysfunction in animals with normal and chronically reduced renal function. J Endourol 1998;12:95–100.
79. Harman PK, Kron IL, McLachlan HD, et al. Elevated intra-abdominal pressure and renal function. Ann Surg 1992; 196:594–7.
80. Dunn MD, McDougall EM. Renal physiology. Laparoscopic considerations. Urol Clin N Am 2000;27:609–14.
81. Wolf JS Jr. Pathophysiologic effects of prolonged laparoscopic operation. Sem Surg Oncol 1996;12:86–95.
82. Meraney AM, Samee AA, Gill IS. Vascular and bowel complications during retroperitoneal laparoscopic surgery. J Urol 2002;168:1941–4.
83. Chandler JG, Corson SL, Way LW. Three spectra of laparoscopic entry access injuries. J Am Coll Surg 2001; 192:478–91.
84. Jackman SV, Cadeddu JA, Chen RN, et al. Utility of the Harmonic scalpel for laparoscopic partial nephrectomy. J Endourol 1998;12:441–4.
85. Loughlin KR, Maranchie J, Steele G, et al. Application of the Harmonic scalpel to perform partial nephrectomies in a porcine model [abstract 1635]. J Urol 1997;157:419.
86. Helal M, Albertini J, Lockhart J, Albrink M. Laparoscopic nephrectomy using the harmonic scalpel. J Endourol 1997;11:267–8.
87. Voyles CR, Tucker RD. Education and engineering solutions for potential problems with laparoscopic monopolar electrosurgery. Am J Surg 1992;164:57–62.
88. Landman J, Kerbl K, Rehman J, et al. Evaluation of a vessel sealing system, bipolar electrosurgery, Harmonic scalpel, titanium clips, endoscopic gastrointestinal anastomosis vascular staples and sutures for arterial and venous ligation in a porcine model. J Urol 2003;169:697–700.
89. Chan D, Bishoff JT, Ratner L, et al. Endovascular gastrointestinal stapler device malfunction during laparoscopic nephrectomy: early recognition and management. J Urol 2000;164:319–21.
90. Nakada SY. Techniques in endourology: hand-assisted laparoscopic nephrectomy. J Endourol 1999;13:9–15.
91. Shekarriz B, Meng MV, Lu HF, et al. Laparoscopic nephrectomy for inflammatory renal conditions. J Urol 2001; 166:2091–4.
92. Hrebinko R, Phelan M. En masse stapling of renal hilar vessels during laparoscopic nephrectomy does not result in arteriovenous fistula [abstract P10-16]. J Endourol 2002;16:A43.
93. Kerbl K, Chandhoke PS, Clayman RV, et al. Ligation of the renal pedicle during laparoscopic nephrectomy: a comparison of staples, clips, and sutures. J Laparoendosc Surg 1993;3:9–12.
94. Moore RG, Chen RN, Hedican SP. Laparoscopic subcapsular nephrectomy. J Endourol 1998;12:263–4.
95. Urban DA, Kerbl K, McDougall EM, et al. Organ entrapment and renal morcellation: permeability studies. J Urol 1993; 150:1792–4.
96. Rassweiler J, Stock C, Frede T, et al. Organ retrieval systems for endoscopic nephrectomy: a comparative study. J Endourol 1998;12:325–333.

97. Elashry OM, Giusti G, Nadler RB, et al. Incisional hernia after nephrectomy with intact specimen removal: caveat emptor. J Urol 1997;158:363–9.

98. Shalhav AL, Siqueira TM Jr, Gardner TA, et al. Manual specimen retrieval without a pneumoperitoneum preserving device for laparoscopic live donor nephrectomy. J Urol 2002;168:941–4.

99. Carter JE. A new technique of fascial closure for laparoscopic incisions. J Laparoendosc Surg 1994;4:143–8.

100. Nakada SY, McDougall EM, Gardner SM, et al. Comparison of newer laparoscopic port closure techniques in the porcine model. J Endourol 1995;9:397–401.

101. Elashry OM, Nakada SY, Wolf JS Jr., et al. Comparative clinical study of port-closure techniques following laparoscopic surgery. J Am Coll Surg 1996;183:335–44.

102. Montz FJ, Holschneider CH, Munro MG. Incisional hernia following laparoscopy: a survey of the American Association of Gynecologic Laparoscopists. Obstet Gynecol 1994;84:881–4.

103. Kadar N, Reich H, Liu CY, et al. Incisional hernia after major laparoscopic gynecologic procedures. Am J Obstet Gynecol 1993;168:1493–5.

104. Shalhav AL, Barret E, Lifshitz DA, et al. Transperitoneal laparoscopic renal surgery using blunt 12-mm trocar without fascial closure. J Endourol 2002;16:43–6.

105. Lowry PS, Moon TD, D'Alessandro A, Nakada SY. Symptomatic port site hernia associated with a non-bladed trocar following laparoscopic live donor nephrectomy. J Endourol 2003;17:493–4.

106. McDougall EM, Clayman RV, Fadden PT. Retroperitoneoscopy: the Washington University Medical School experience. Urology 1994;43:446–52.

107. Gill IS, Grune MT, Munch LC. Access technique for retroperitoneoscopy. J Urol 1996;156:1120–4.

108. Gill IS, Rassweiler JJ. Retroperitoneoscopic renal surgery: our approach. Urology 1999;54:734–8.

109. Sung GT, Gill IS, Soble JJ, Schweizer D. Anatomical landmarks and time management during retroperitoneoscopic radical nephrectomy [abstract P7-10]. J Endourol 1998;12 Suppl 1:S151.

110. Keeley FX, Tolley DA. A review of our first 100 cases of laparoscopic nephrectomy: defining risk factors for complications. Br J Urol 1998;82:615–8.

111. Kerbl K, Clayman RV, McDougall EM, et al. Transperitoneal nephrectomy for benign disease of the kidney: a comparison of laparoscopic and open surgical techniques. Urology 1994;43:607–13.

112. McDougall EM, Clayman RV. Advances in laparoscopic urology. Part 1. History and development of procedures. Urology 1994;43:607–13.

113. Rassweiler J, Frede T, Henkel TO, et al. Nephrectomy: a comparative study between the transperitoneal and retroperitoneal laparoscopic versus the open approach. Eur Urol 1998;33:489–96.

114. Landman J, McDougall EM, Gill IS, Clayman RV. Adult laparoscopic urology. In: Gillenwater JY, Grayhack JT, Howards SS, Mitchell ME, editors. Adult and pediatric urology. 4th ed. Philadelphia: Lippincott Williams & Wilkins; 2002. p. 660–753.

115. Rassweiler J, Fornara P, Weber M, et al. Laparoscopic nephrectomy: the experience of the laparoscopy working group of the German Urologic Association. J Urol 1998; 160:18–21.

116. Chuang CK, Lai MK, Chang PL, et al. Xanthogranulomatous pyelonephritis: experience in 36 cases. J Urol 1992; 147:333–6.

117. Eastham J, Ahlering T, Skinner E. Xanthogranulomatous pyelonephritis: clinical findings and surgical considerations. Urology 1994;43:295–9.

118. Bercowsky E, Shalhav AL, Portis A, et al. Is the laparoscopic approach justified in patients with xanthogranulomatous pyelonephritis? Urology 1999;54:437–3.

119. Gupta NP, Agrawal AK, Sood S. Tubercular pyelonephritic nonfunctioning kidney—another relative contraindication for laparoscopic nephrectomy: a case report. J Laparoendosc Adv Surg Tech A 1997;7:131–4.

120. Kim HH, Lee KS, Park K, Ahn H. Laparoscopic nephrectomy for nonfunctioning tuberculous kidney. J Endourol 2000;14:433–7.

121. Dunn MD, Portis AJ, Elbahnasy AM, et al. Laparoscopic nephrectomy in patients with end-stage renal disease and autosomal dominant polycystic kidney disease. Am J Kidney Dis 2000;35:720–5.

122. McNally ML, Erturk E, Oleyourryk G, Schoeniger L. Laparoscopic cyst decortication using the harmonic scalpel for symptomatic autosomal dominant polycystic kidney disease. J Endourol 2001;15:597–9.

123. Seshadri PA, Poulin EC, Pace D, et al. Transperitoneal laparoscopic nephrectomy for giant polycystic kidneys: a case control study. Urology 2001;58:23–7.

124. Fahlenkamp D, Rassweiler J, Fornara P, et al. Complications of laparoscopic procedures in urology: experience with 2,407 procedures at 4 German centers. J Urol 1999; 162(3 Pt 1):765–71.

125. Leonard F, Lecuru F, Rizk E, et al. Perioperative morbidity of gynecological laparoscopy. A prospective monocenter observational study. Acta Obstet Gynecol Scand 2000; 79:129–34.

126. Jansen FW, Kapiteyn K, Trimbos-Kemper T, et al. Complications of laparoscopy: a prospective multicentre observational study. Br J Obstet Gynaecol 1997;104:595–600.

127. Hasson HM. A modified instrument and method for laparoscopy. Am J Obstet Gynecol 1971;110:886–7.

128. Penfield AJ. How to prevent complications of open laparoscopy. J Reprod Med 1985;30:660–3.

129. Hanney RM, Carmalt HL, Merrett N, Tait N. Use of the Hasson cannula producing major vascular injury at laparoscopy. Surg Endosc 1999;13:1238–40.

130. Gill IS, Kavoussi LR, Clayman RV, et al. Complications of laparoscopic nephrectomy in 185 patients: a multi-institutional review. J Urol 1995;154(2 Pt 1):479–83.

131. Canby-Hagino ED, Morey AF, Jatoi I, et al. Fibrin sealant treatment of splenic injury in open and laparoscopic left radical nephrectomy. J Urol 2000;164:2004–5.

132. Schuster TG, Wolf JS Jr. Use of bipolar electrocautery during laparoscopic donor nephrectomy. J Urol 2001;165 (6 Pt 1):1968–70.

133. Bishoff JT, Allaf ME, Kirkels W, et al. Laparoscopic bowel injury: incidence and clinical presentation. J Urol 1999; 161:887–90.

134. Jordan GH, Winslow BH. Laparoendoscopic upper pole partial nephrectomy with ureterectomy. J Urol 1993;150:940–3.

135. Horowitz M, Shah SM, Ferzli G, et al. Laparoscopic partial upper pole nephrectomy in infants and children. BJU Int 2001;87:514–6.

136. Wang DS, Bird VG, Cooper CS, et al. Laparoscopic upper-pole heminephrectomy for ectopic ureter: surgical technique. J Endourol 2003;17:469–73.

137. El-Ghoneimi A, Valla JS, Steyaert H, Aigrain Y. Laparoscopic renal surgery via a retroperitoneal approach in children. J Urol 1998;160(3 Pt 2):1138–41.

138. Lifshitz DA, Powsner E, Lask D, Livne PM. Laparoscopic nephroureterectomy of a non-functioning upper pole moiety. Utilizing the LigaSure device. J Endourol 2003;17 Suppl 1:A282.

139. Cybulski P, Honey RJ, Pace K. Laparoscopic staged bilateral upper pole partial nephrectomies for bilateral complete duplication anomaly with ectopic ureters. J Endourol 2003;17 Suppl 1:A283.

140. Patel R, Caruso RP, Taneja S, Stifelman M. Use of fibrin glue and gelfoam to repair collecting system injuries in a porcine model: implications for the technique of laparoscopic partial nephrectomy. J Endourol 2003;17:799–804.

141. Pruthi RS, Chun J, Richman M. The use of a fibrin tissue sealant during laparoscopic partial nephrectomy. BJU Int 2004;93:813–7.

142. Wang DS, Bird VG, Cooper CS, et al. Laparoscopic upper-pole heminephrectomy for ectopic ureter. J Endourol 2003;17 Suppl 1:A283.

143. Ou YC, Yang CR, Chang YY, et al. The clinical experience of gaseous retroperitoneoscopic and gasless retroperitoneoscopy-assisted unroofing of renal cyst. Zhonghua Yi Xue Za Zhi (Taipei) 1997;59:232–9.

144. Hedican SP. Laparoscopy in urology. Surg Clin N Am 2000; 80:1465–85.

145. Landman J, Lee D, Rehman J, et al. Peritonitis following laparoscopic cyst decortication in patients with autosomal dominant polycystic kidney disease (ADPKD):

evaluation of the inflammatory properties of renal cyst fluid [abstract 87]. J Urol 2002;167:21.

146. Dunn MD, Portis AJ, Naughton C, et al. Laparoscopic cyst marsupialization in patients with autosomal dominant polycystic kidney disease. J Urol 2001;165(6 Pt 1):1888–92.

147. Lifson BJ, Teichman JM, Hulbert JC. Role and long-term results of laparoscopic decortication in solitary cystic and autosomal dominant polycystic kidney disease. J Urol 1998;159:702–6.

148. Rubenstein SC, Hulbert JC, Pharand D, et al. Laparoscopic ablation of symptomatic renal cysts. J Urol 1993;150: 1103–6.

149. Doumas K, Skrepetis K, Lykourinas M. Laparoscopic ablation of symptomatic peripelvic renal cysts. J Endourol 2004;18:45–8.

150. Chapple CR, Newman J, O'Brien JM, Considine J. Adenocarcinoma in the free wall of a simple renal cyst. J R Coll Surg Edinb 1987;32:320–1.

151. Hayakawa M, Hatano T, Tsuji A, et al. Patients with renal cysts associated with renal cell carcinoma and the clinical implications of cyst puncture: a study of 223 cases. Urology 1996;47:643–6.

152. Brown JA, Torres VE, King BF, Segura JW. Laparoscopic marsupialization of symptomatic polycystic kidney disease. J Urol 1996;156:22–7.

153. Ruckle HC, Segura JW. Laparoscopic treatment of a stone-filled, caliceal diverticulum: a definitive minimally invasive therapeutic option. J Urol 1994;151:122–4.

154. Harewood LM, Agarwal D, Lindsay S, et al. Extraperitoneal laparoscopic caliceal diverticulectomy. J Endourol 1996;10:425–30.

155. Tekin MI, Peskircioglu L, Boyvat F, Ozkardes H. Practical approach to terminate urinary extravasation: percutaneous fistula tract embolization with N-butyl cyanoacrylate in a case with partial nephrectomy. Tech Urol 2001;7:67–9.

156. Stephenson AJ, Haikimi AA, Snyder ME, Russo P. Complications of radical and partial nephrectomy in a large contemporary cohort. J Urol 2004;171:130–4.

157. Urban DA, Clayman RV, Kerbl K, et al. Laparoscopic nephropexy for symptomatic nephroptosis: initial case report. J Endourol 1993;7:27–30.

158. Elashry OM, Nakada SY, McDougall EM, Clayman RV. Laparoscopic nephropexy: Washington University experience. J Urol 1995;154:1655–9.

159. Rehman J, Hoenig DM. Laparoscopic nephropexy. J Endourol 2000;14:881–8.

160. Walther V, Wieland WF, Hein I. [Ren mobilis. Pathogenesis, symptoms and therapy.] Fortschr Med 1981;99:2002–5.

161. Hagmaier V, Heberer M, Leibundgut B, et al. [Long-term observations on different methods of nephropexy.] Helv Chir Acta 1979;46:351–5.

162. Schmitz W, Boeminghaus F. [Nephroptosis and nephropexy.] Zentalbl Chir 1970;95:705–8.

163. Mayor G, Zingg EJ. Nephropexy. In: Mayor G, Zingg EJ, editors. Urologische Operationen. New York: Thieme; 1990. p. 34–8.

164. Bernt O, Griepentrog U, Pohl M. [Surgical treatment of nephroptosis.] Z Urol Nephrol 1974;67:667–71.

165. Hofbauer C, Anderson PV, Juul P, Qvist N. Late mesh rejection as a complication to transabdominal preperitoneal laparoscopic hernia repair. Surg Endosc 1998;12:1164–5.

166. Clayman RV, Kavoussi LR, Soper NJ, et al. Laparoscopic nephrectomy: initial case report. J Urol 1991;146:278–82.

167. Ono Y, Katoh N, Kinukawa T, et al. Laparoscopic nephrectomy, radical nephrectomy and adrenalectomy: Nagoya experience. J Urol 1994;152(6 Pt 1):1962–6.

168. Parra RO, Perez MG, Boullier JA, Cummings JM. Comparison between standard flank versus laparoscopic nephrectomy for benign renal disease. J Urol 1995;153:1171–4.

169. Gaur DD. Simple nephrectomy: retroperitoneal approach. J Endourol 2000;14:787–91.

170. Doublet JD, Peraldi MN, Monsaint H, et al. Retroperitoneal laparoscopic nephrectomy of native kidneys in renal transplant recipients. Transplantation 1997;64:89–91.

171. Ono Y, Katoh N, Kinukawa T, et al. Laparoscopic nephrectomy via the retroperitoneal approach. J Urol 1996;156:1101–4.

172. Gasman D, Saint F, Barthelemy Y, et al. Retroperitoneoscopy: a laparoscopic approach for adrenal and renal surgery. Urology 1996;47:801–6.

58

Laparoscopic Live Donor Nephrectomy

Peter A. Pinto, MD

Gary W. Chien, MD

Arieh L. Shalhav, MD

Following the pioneering work of Clayman and associates performing the first laparoscopic nephrectomy in 1990,[1] the role of minimally invasive surgery was introduced into renal transplantation with the first laparoscopic live donor nephrectomy (LLDN) in 1995.[2] Multiple reports have demonstrated the benefit and long-term success of this procedure.[3–6] The Annual Report of the U.S. Organ Procurement and Transplantation Network and the Scientific Registry of Transplant Recipients has collected data over the 10-year period from 1992 to 2001 and reports that cadaveric donors rose from 7,202 in 1992 to 8,202 in 2001, an increase of 14%, while the number of transplants from living donors more than doubled, from 2,535 in 1992 to 5,969 in 2001 (a 135% increase).[7] This trend can possibly be attributed to the application of new technologies, such as laparoscopic techniques, along with the less stringent criteria for potential donors.[8,9] Regardless of the reason, the number of living donors has increased considerably over the last 10 years, and LDN has played a role. It has become an alternative to open nephrectomy and arguably the standard of care for living renal procurement.

INDICATIONS AND PREOPERATIVE EVALUATION

The patient selection and preoperative work-up for LDN are similar to the open donor nephrectomy. However, the patient selection should be matched to the surgeon's experience. During the learning curve, the surgeon should select only "ideal" cases: left kidney, single renal artery with normal left renal vein, and patients with normal body habitus. Following the first 20 to 50 cases, the surgeon may expand his/her patient selection to include kidneys with multiple arteries, venous anomalies, obese patients, and right-sided kidneys. Traditional imaging studies performed to evaluate the renovascular anatomy included conventional renal angiography and excretory urography. Recently these studies have been replaced by computed tomographic (CT) angiography with three dimensional reconstructions[10–12] (Figure 58-1). Three dimensional CT angiography can demonstrate arterial as well as venous vascular anomalies, which do not preclude a laparoscopic approach, but aid in preplanning (Figures 58-2 and 58-3).

SURGICAL TECHNIQUE

The patient is placed flat on the operating table, and a Pfannenstiel incision is marked after the patient undergoes general anesthesia. The patient is then placed left side up in a right lateral decubitus position and the table flexed at the level of the flank (Figure 58-4). The patient's abdomen and left flank are then prepped and draped. The suprapubic area is included in the surgical field so the Pfannenstiel incision can be made later. Pneumoperitoneum is established with a Veress needle initially after a skin incision is made at the anterior axillary line 8 to 12 cm caudal to the rib cage (Figure 58-4B). An initial trocar is then placed 5 to 8 cm caudal to the rib cage at the lateral border of the rectus muscle (Figure 58-4A) using a 12 mm optical viewing non-bladed access trocar as described by Marcovich and colleagues;[13] this is the camera port. The second trocar is placed through the Veress needle site (see Figure 58-4B). This is the surgeon's right-hand working port. Three additional 5 mm trocars are placed, one about 2–3 cm caudal to the rib cage at the lateral border of the rectus muscle (Figure 58-4C). This is the surgeon's left-hand working port. Another 5 mm trocar is placed on the midline at the level of the planned Pfannenstiel incision. (Figure 58-4D). This port is used for the retraction of bowel by the first assistant and is included in the Pfannenstiel incision for organ procurement. The last port is placed on the mid-axillary line about 4 to 8 cm caudal to the rib cage (Figure 58-4E) after the colon has been reflected medially. This port is used for lateral retraction to allow easier dissection of the renal hilum and upper pole. The variability in the port placement relates to the size of the patient. In smaller patients, the distance from the rib cage increases, and in larger patients, it decreases.

Dissection begins with incising the line of Toldt and reflecting the colon medially together with medial reflection of the spleen dividing the splenorenal, splenodiaphragmatic, and splenocolic ligaments. The dissection continues at the level of Gerota's fascia and is extended down to the true pelvis, where the psoas muscle, ureter, and gonadal vessels are identified. At this point, the dissection is focused around the ureter, preserving the ureteral sheath with the ureteral intrinsic vessels intact. Some surgeons prefer taking the gonadal vein with the ureter to reduce ureteral compromise (Figure 58-5). The ureter is dissected down to the crossing point of the iliac artery. We prefer an ultrasonic rather than a monopolar dissector because it has been shown that the lateral thermal damage is significantly reduced with the ultrasonic dissection.[14] The gonadal vessels are

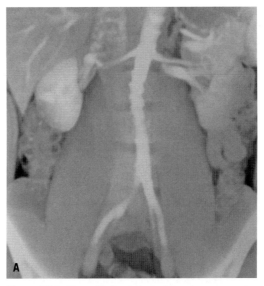 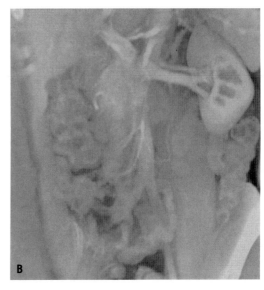

Figure 58-1 Normal left renal arterial and venous anatomy.

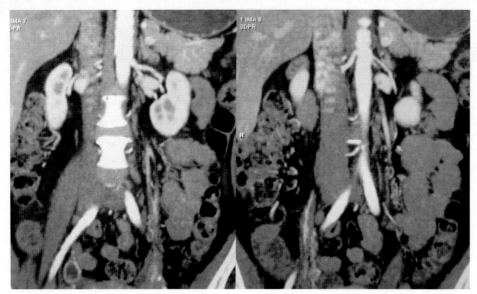

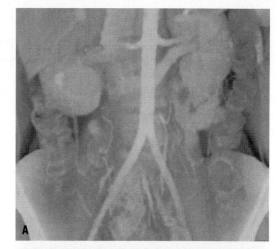

Figure 58-2 Early branching of the main left renal artery is seen (A) with an additional renal artery arising from the aorta (B).

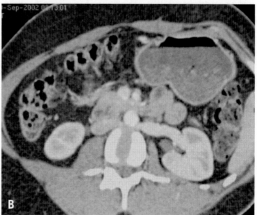

Figure 58-3 CT revealed a left retroartic renal vein.

reflected medially off the ureter. If there are difficulties with identifying or dissecting the ureter, this portion of the dissection is postponed, and dissection is focused around the renal hilum. In thin patients, the renal vein is seen through Gerota's fascia as the landmark. In patients with a large amount of perinephric fat, the gonadal vein can be dissected and followed cranially in order to identify the renal vein. Alternatively, meticulous blunt and sharp dissection through Gerota's fascia and perihilar fat after identifying the lower and upper poles of the kidney can reveal the renal vein through its presumed location. For hilar dissection, the first assistant holds the camera with the left hand. With the right hand, he/she holds a kittner, blunt grasper, or a suction, allowing for medial retraction and/or suction to optimize hilar exposure. A second assistant can use a kittner through the lateral 5 mm port to gently retract the kidney laterally to better expose the renal hilum. The surgeon holds the 5 mm ultrasonic scalpel in his/her dominant hand and either a grasper or a suction tip in the left hand. Gerota's fascia is incised over the renal vein and dissection is continued until the correct plane on the renal vein is reached. Dissection then continues along the renal vein medially, exposing the gonadal, lumbar, and adrenal veins. Dissection of the adrenal vein is performed while gentle traction is applied on the upper pole of the kidney laterally. The adrenal vein is dissected from its origin on the renal vein into the adrenal gland until there is sufficient length to apply at least one clip on each side and leaving a 3 mm adrenal vein stump off the renal vein. The adrenal vein is then divided (Figure 58-6). The gonadal and lumbar veins are circumferentially dissected, clipped, and divided using the same principle. The reason for the stump left on the renal vein is to allow reclipping or suturing of the stump in case the clip slips off during manipulation. The Hem-o-lok clip (Weck Closure Systems, Research Triangle Park, NC) may have an advantage over the metal clip in that

it has a self-locking mechanism that is designed to ligate and stay on the vessel securely. An alternative technique for dividing the renal vein branch is preferred by the senior author. The bipolar electrocautery is used to cauterize the branches of the renal vein before they are divided using the ultrasound scalpel.[15] The absence of laparoscopic clips on these renal vein stumps allows for easier and safer placement of the endostapler device on the renal vein. It also avoids the risk of including a surgical clip within the stapler line and allows a longer renal vein to be harvested. In the senior author's series of 160 laparoscopic live donor nephrectomy cases, no complications resulted from the use of this technique.

The renal vein is then circumferentially dissected free, and then gently retracted superiorly, exposing the neurolymphatic tissue covering the renal artery. Dissection continues through the neurolymphatic tissue until the renal artery is exposed. Once the renal artery is identified, dissection is performed to reveal the origin of the

renal artery off the aorta, and about 2 cm of renal artery is circumferentially dissected. The medial border of the ureter is then exposed, while the lower pole of the kidney and the proximal ureter is retracted laterally with a kittner through the lateral port. The posterior wall muscles are exposed, which connect in a plane at the level of the medial aspect of the ureter and the inferior aspect of the renal artery. Next, dissection between the adrenal and the upper pole of the kidney is carried out, again using a kittner from the lateral port to retract

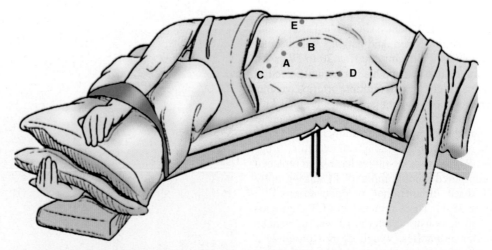

Figure 58-4 Patient position for left laparoscopic donor nephrectomy. Trocar sites: *A,* initial trocar site (12 mm) for camera. *B,* 2nd trocar (12 mm) for right hand of surgeon. *C,* 3rd trocar (5 mm) for left hand of surgeon. *D,* 4th trocar (5 mm) for 1st assistant retraction. *E,* 5th trocar (5 mm) for 2nd assistant retraction.

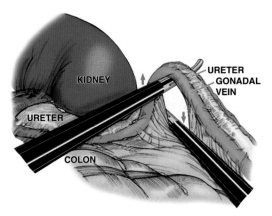

Figure 58-5 Diagram illustrating dissection of the intact ureteral-gonadal packet.

the upper pole of the kidney inferior laterally. This is performed until a plane connects the posterior abdominal muscles with the superior aspect of the renal vessels at the level of the upper pole of the kidney. The medial aspect of the upper pole is freed from all attachments using a combination of blunt and sharp dissection with the ultrasound dissector. At this point, dissection continues by peeling the perinephric fat off the kidney at the level of the renal capsule starting at the lower pole of the kidney, then laterally, and finally posteriorly. The perinephric fat is kept intact around the renal hilum and between the lower pole and the ureter. This is done to avoid any injury to small vessels that may feed the ureter or cause bleeding. The first assistant retracts the perinephric fat as the surgeon dissects it. The kidney is reflected medially to complete dissection of the posterior aspect of the kidney. Dissection continues around the renal hilum to ensure that the renal vessels are circumferentially free, and in one plane with the rest of the kidney. The upper pole dissection is continued until it is entirely free and off the posterior abdominal muscles. About 2 cm of the renal vein is freed medial to the adrenal vein stump to allow the GIA stapler to be placed medial to the adrenal

vein stump without having the renal vein clips within the staple line. The ureter is then clipped at the level of the iliac artery and sharply divided 2 mm above the clip while the assistant retracts the bowel medially. No clip is placed on the proximal side of the ureter when incised. If bleeding is noted from the incised ureteral vessels, clips or bipolar electrocautery can be used for hemostasis. The surgeon holds the kidney in place with the left-hand instrument and uses the ultrasonic dissector with the right hand while the first assistant aspirates the fluid accumulating around the renal hilum to allow a clear surgical field.

Once the kidney is attached to the body only by the renal artery and vein, and there is sufficient space to place the GIA stapler on the vessels, a modified Pfannenstiel incision[16] is made (Figure 58-7). This 7.5 cm skin incision is made at the pubic hairline and taken down to the fascia, and then the subcutaneous fat is dissected off the fascia along the midline. The fascia is incised vertically between the rectus muscle for approximately 7 cm, and the first assistant's right hand is introduced into the abdominal cavity after bluntly opening the peritoneum with his/her fingers. The pneumoperitoneum is preserved since the skin and fascial incisions are crossed and seal when the arm is snugly inserted. The hand is used for retraction of the bowel medially while the 5 mm lateral port is used to retract the kidney laterally. Alternatively, the hand can be used to hold the kidney laterally, exposing the entire length of the vessels (Figure 58-8). Both of these maneuvers will allow for safe placement of the GIA stapler under vision on the artery and vein sequentially.

At this point, the surgeon's left hand is holding the 5 mm suction, which is needed because of the urine output from the incised ureter. In addition, the suction probe can be gently placed between the artery and the vein, retracting the kidney laterally to maximize the length of the vessels and to ensure excellent visibility once the GIA stapler is engaged around the origin of the renal artery off the aorta. The same principle is used to get maxi-

mal length around the renal vein. The GIA stapler is inserted through the lateral 12 mm port using the articulation of the device so the jaws of the stapler are parallel to the axis of the aorta. Alternatively, the renal artery can be doubly clipped, preferably with Hem-o-lok clips, using no clips on the specimen side. The renal artery is divided using cold scissors. Once the renal artery is divided, the GIA stapler is removed and another GIA stapler is positioned on the renal vein (Figure 58-9). Again, with the help of the hand, the GIA stapler is placed so that there are no clips crossing the staple line, and the GIA stapler is as medial as possible to get maximal length. Once the vein is divided, the assistant gently grasps the kidney and removes it through the modified Pfannenstiel incision. The kidney is placed on ice and given to the transplant surgery team.

The incision is then packed with a lap pad, and pneumoperitoneum is re-established. Hemostasis of the renal hilar stump, renal, and ureteral bed is verified under vision with the pneumoperitoneum pressure reduced to 4 mm Hg. The fascia of the rectus muscles is then closed using a running No. 1 PDS suture. Pneumoperitoneum is re-established and accumulation of blood in the abdominal cavity is ruled out. The trocars are removed under vision and the skin of the modified Pfannenstiel and the 12 mm incision is closed using 3-0 monocryl sutures, while that of the 5 mm trocar incisions is closed with SteriStrips.

To minimize delayed graft function related to early acute tubular necrosis of the graft, the senior author's team uses the following methods:

1. Dissection at 10 mm Hg of pneumoperitoneum for as long as possible
2. Avoid pneumoperitoneum pressures > 20 mm Hg
3. Clipless division of left renal vein branches for safer organ procurement and longer renal vein
4. Use of ultrasound dissection to minimize lateral thermal damage
5. Manual retrieval rather than endo-bag retrieval

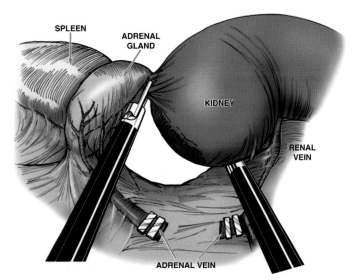

Figure 58-6 Diagram illustrating division of the adrenal vein, allowing mobilization of the renal upper pole.

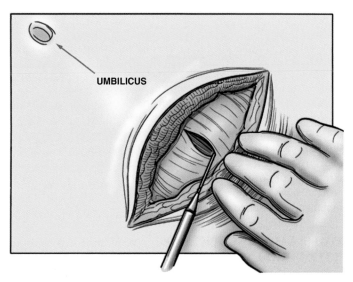

Figure 58-7 Diagram showing a modified Pfannnenstiel incision after a laparoscopic living donor nephrectomy.

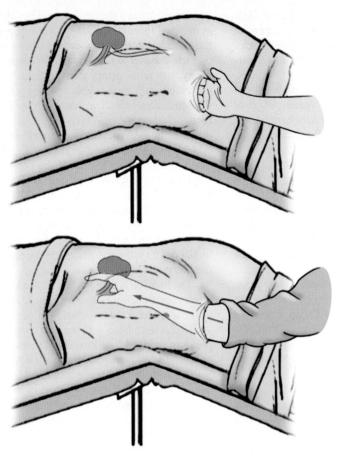

Figure 58-8 Diagram demonstrating insertion of a hand through the Pfannenstiel incision to retract the kidney.

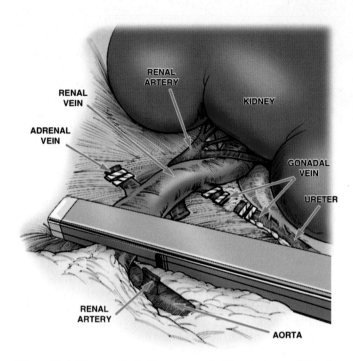

Figure 58-9 Diagram illustrating placement of the stapler parallel to the aorta and vena cava.

6. Collaboration of two proficient laparoscopic surgeons with an active assistant to decrease operating time and warm ischemia time, at least during the initial learning curve
7. Use of 2 doses of 12.5 g of Mannitol: first at the beginning of arterial dissection, second before reflecting the kidney medially
8. Furosemide 10 mg IV is given prior to ligation of the renal artery
9. Reduce pneumoperitoneum to 0 mm Hg for 5 to 10 minutes before dividing the artery

POSTOPERATIVE MANAGEMENT

Before extubation, the orogastric tube is removed. After routine observation in a post-anesthesia care unit, the patients are transferred to a nonmonitored floor bed. In the morning of the first postoperative day, the urinary catheter is removed, routine blood work is performed, ambulation is encouraged, and oral liquids are started. The diet is then advanced as tolerated throughout the day. Routine discharge is in the morning of postoperative day 2 if blood work and vital signs are stable, and the patient is able to ambulate and tolerate oral diet.

OUTCOMES: LAPAROSCOPIC AND OPEN LIVE DONOR NEPHRECTOMY

Since the first case by Kavoussi and Ratner in 1995, laparoscopic live donor nephrectomy is quickly establishing itself as the standard of care for living renal procurement. Compared with open surgery, laparoscopy provides the donor less postoperative pain, shorter hospital stays, better cosmesis, and more rapid return to normal activities. This is not surprising, as the results of laparoscopic nephrectomy for benign and malignant conditions compared with open nephrectomy have demonstrated this.[17–21]

Donor morbidity has recently been examined on a national level. Matas and colleagues recently surveyed 234 United Network for Organ Sharing (UNOS) listed kidney transplant programs to determine current living donor morbidity and mortality for open nephrectomy, hand-assisted LLDN, and standard LLDN.[22] The number of responding programs was 171, and morbidity was comparable between the different techniques. Complications requiring reoperation occurred in 0.4% of open cases, 1.0% of hand-assisted LLDN, and 0.9% of standard LLDN cases. Complications that did not necessitate reoperation occurred in 0.3% of open cases, 1.0% of hand-assisted LLDN, and 0.8% of standard LLDN cases. There were two reported mortalities following standard LLDN.

Regarding graft function, kidneys procured laparoscopically have been shown to function well in the short and long term. The largest initial series from the University of Maryland and Johns Hopkins have demonstrated excellent long-term graft function in the recipient.[23,24] No differences were observed in patient or allograft survival rates or long-term creatinine clearance rates when compared with open cases.

FINANCIAL CONSIDERATIONS

When analyzing the entire finances regarding LLDN, one has to look past the initial operative and hospital costs. Studies have demonstrated the laparoscopic approach does not provide cost savings to the hospital, and in some reports may be more costly than open surgery.[25–27] Yet, when factoring into the financial equation the shorter recuperative period, allowing the donor to return to work sooner, LLDN overall has been shown to be more cost effective.[28]

CONCLUSION

As in other fields of surgery, laparoscopy has had a profound impact on renal transplantation. No longer in its infancy, LLDN has become the procedure of choice for the majority of transplant centers nationally and abroad. Although less than 10 years old, the benefit to the donor, overall financial considerations, and recipient outcomes have made LLDN the standard of care.

REFERENCES

1. Clayman RV, Kavoussi LR, Soper NJ, et al. Laparoscopic nephrectomy. N Engl J Med 1991;324:1370–1.
2. Ratner LE, Ciseck LJ, Moore RG, et al. Laparoscopic live donor nephrectomy. Transplantation 1995;60:1047–9.

3. Ratner LE, Montgomery RA, Kavoussi LR. Laparoscopic live donor nephrectomy: the four year Johns Hopkins University experience. Nephrol Dial Transplant 1999;14:2090–3.

4. Flowers JL, Jacobs S, Cho E, et al. Comparison of open and laparoscopic live donor nephrectomy. Ann Surg 1997; 226:482–9.

5. Ratner LE, Montgomery RA, Kavoussi LR. Laparoscopic live donor nephrectomy. A review of the first 5 years. Urol Clin North Am 2001;28:709–19.

6. Siqueira TM, Shalhav AL, Stevens LH, et al. Laparoscopic live donor nephrectomy: comparing the results with the standard open donor nephrectomy. [In press]

7. University Renal Research and Education Association; United Network for Organ Sharing. 2002 Annual Report of the U.S. Organ Procurement and Transplantation Network and the Scientific Registry of Transplant Recipients: Transplant Data 1992–2001. Rockville (MD): Department of Health and Human Services, Health Resources and Services Administration, Office of Special Programs, Division of Transplantation; 2003.

8. Schweitzer EJ, Wilson J, Jacobs S, et al. Increased rates of donation with laparoscopic donor nephrectomy. Ann Surg 2000;232:392–400.

9. Kasiske BL, Cangro CB, Hariharan S, et al. The evaluation of renal transplant candidates: clinical practice guidelines. Am J Transplant 2001;1 Suppl 2:3–95.

10. Cochran ST, Krasny RM, Danovitch GM, et al. Helical CT angiography for examination of living renal donors. AJR Am J Roentgenol 1997;168:1569–73.

11. Smith PA, Ratner LE, Lynch FC, et al. Role of CT angiography in the preoperative evaluation for laparoscopic nephrectomy. Radiographics 1998;18:589–601.

12. Kawamoto S, Montgomery RA, Lawler LP, et al. Multidetector CT angiography for preoperative evaluation of living laparoscopic kidney donors. AJR Am J Roentgenol 2003;180:1633–8.

13. Marcovich R, Del Terzo MA, Wolf JS Jr. Comparison of transperitoneal laparoscopic access techniques: optiview visualizing trocar and Veress needle. J Endourol 2000;14:175–9.

14. Lamm P, Juchem G, Weyrich P, et al. The harmonic scalpel: optimizing the quality of mammary artery bypass grafts. Ann Thorac Surg 2000;69:1833–5.

15. Orvieto M, Chien GW, Harland R, et al. Bipolar electrocoagulation for clipless division of left renal vein branches during laparoscopic live donor nephrectomy. Transplant Proc 2004;36:2625–7.

16. Shalhav AL, Siqueira TM Jr, Gardner TA, et al. Manual specimen retrieval without a pneumoperitoneum preserving device for laparoscopic live donor nephrectomy. J Urol 2002;168:941–4.

17. Siqueira TM Jr, Kuo RL, Gardner TA, et al. Major complications in 213 laparoscopic nephrectomy cases: the Indianapolis experience. J Urol 2002;168(4 Pt 1):1361–5.

18. Gill IS, Meraney AM, Schweizer DK, et al. Laparoscopic radical nephrectomy in 100 patients: a single center experience from the United States. Cancer 2001;92: 1843–55.

19. Chan DY, Cadeddu JA, Jarrett TW, et al. Laparoscopic radical nephrectomy: cancer control for renal cell carcinoma. J Urol 2001;166:2095–9.

20. Ono Y, Kinukawa T, Hattori R, et al. Long-term outcome of laparoscopic radical nephrectomy [abstract 81]. J Urol 2000;163:19.

21. Dunn MD, Portis AJ, Shalhav AL, et al. Laparoscopic versus open radical nephrectomy: a 9-year experience. J Urol 2000;164:1153–9.

22. Matas AJ, Bartlett ST, Leichtman AB, Delmonico FL. Morbidity and mortality after living kidney donation, 1999–2001: survey of United States Transplant Centers. Am J Transplant 2003;3:830–4.

23. Nogueira JM, Cangro CB, Fink JC, et al. A comparison of recipient renal outcomes with laparoscopic versus open live donor nephrectomy. Transplantation 1999;67:722–8.

24. Ratner LE, Montgomery RA, Maley WR, et al. Laparoscopic live donor nephrectomy: the recipient. Transplantation 2000;69:2319–23.

25. Sosa JA, Albini TA, Powe NR, et al. Laparoscopic vs. open live donor nephrectomy: a multivariate patient outcome analysis [abstract]. Transplantation 1998;65:S85.

26. Odland MD, Ney AL, Jacobs DM, et al. Initial experience with laparoscopic live donor nephrectomy. Surgery 1999;126:603–6.

27. Wolf JS, Tchetgen MB, Merion RM. Hand-assisted laparoscopic live donor nephrectomy. Urology 1998;52:885–7.

28. Pace KT, Dyer SJ, Phan V, et al. Laparoscopic versus open donor nephrectomy. A cost utility analysis. Surg Endosc 2003;17:134–42.

59

Renal Surgery: Malignant Disease

David I. Lee, MD

Elspeth M. McDougall, MD

Ralph V. Clayman, MD

The initial report of a transperitoneal laparoscopic nephrectomy occurred in 1991.[1] The obvious benefits of decreased morbidity from laparoscopy teamed with demonstrated equivalent cancer control have validated laparoscopic radical nephrectomy as a standard of care.[2] Retroperitoneal approaches have also been well established as approaches to malignant renal tumors. Technological advances have allowed the performance of hand-assisted laparoscopic nephrectomy as well as laparoscopic partial nephrectomy and wedge excision of small exophytic renal masses and nephroureterectomy. This chapter will review the current applications of laparoscopic approaches to renal malignancies.

INDICATIONS

The indications for radical versus partial nephrectomy parallel those of open surgery. Indications for retroperitoneal nephrectomy over transperitoneal radical nephrectomy include previous abdominal surgery that has likely resulted in significant intraabdominal adhesions. Contraindications for laparoscopic radical nephrectomy include the extension of tumor thrombus above the level of the renal vein. Reports of control of the renal vein with tumor thrombus limited to this structure, or barely entering the inferior vena cava (IVC), have been published.[3] Tumors up to 15 cm in size have also been removed laparoscopically, as have tumors affecting the perirenal fat or adrenal.

PATIENT PREPARATION

The patient is advised to take a clear liquid diet the day before the procedure. A formal bowel preparation is not performed in anticipation of any the laparoscopic renal ablative procedures, although a Dulcolax suppository is advised the day before the procedure.

PREOPERATIVE PREPARATION

After the patient arrives in the hospital, the patient receives antibiotic prophylaxis usually in the form of cefazolin intravenously. In the patient with an increased risk of deep vein thrombosis, 5,000 units of heparin are administered subcutaneously; this is continued every 12 hours until the patient is ambulatory. After the induction of general anesthesia, an orogastric tube and Foley catheter are placed. The patient is then gently turned into a nearly full flank position (70°) with the affected side up. With the operating table flexed and kidney rest raised, the patient's pressure points are carefully padded and the patient is secured to the table with padded table straps. The use of orthopedic table braces has become standard in our operating room; the patient is gently rolled against these at the shoulder and the hip. We do not use the bean bag because the firmness this device obtains once deflated has, in our hands, been associated with transient nerve paresis and, in one patient, a compartment syndrome.

INSTRUMENTATION

For a transperitoneal nephrectomy, the list of our usual instrumentation is displayed in Table 59-1. For retroperitoneal nephrectomy, the disposable Hasson-type inflatable trocar (Bluntport, U.S. Surgical, Norwalk, CT) is used as the primary port after the retroperitoneal space is created. The

Table 59-1 Laparoscopic Instrumentation for Standard Transperitoneal Radical Nephrectomy (University of California, Irvine)

Disposable Equipment
12-mm Endopath ETS45 articulating laparoscopic stapler (Ethicon Endosurgery, Cincinnati, OH)
10-mm Ligasure Atlas device (Valleylab, Boulder, CO)
12-mm Stability Sleeve Trocars with axially dilating obturator (3) (Ethicon)
5 by 8- and 8 by 10-inch LapSacs (Cook Urological, Spencer, IN)
Veress needle (150 mm) (Ethicon)
CO_2 Insufflation Tubing
10 Sponges (Raytex)
5-mm Harmonic Shears (curved) (Ethicon)
5-mm Argon Beam Coagulator probe (Valleylab)

Non-disposable equipment
5-mm Endotip Trocars (2) (Storz, Culver City, CA)
Endoholder (Codman (division of Johnson & Johnson)
Extra long (46 cm) suction irrigator probe, 5 mm (Davol)
Laparoscope: 10-mm 0° and a 10-mm 30° lens and a 5-mm 0° and a 5-mm 30° lens (Storz)
5-mm bowel grasper (Storz)
Atraumatic, non-locking 5-mm smooth tip (duckbill) grasping forceps (3) (Storz)
Traumatic (toothed), locking, 5-mm grasping forceps (4) (Storz)
LapSac introducer (Cook)
Electroshield device to attach to electrocautery for active electrode monitoring (Encision, Boulder, CO)
5-mm Diamond L hook electrode and cord (Encision, Boulder, CO)
5-mm and 10-mm PEER retractors (Jarit Surgical Instruments, Hawthorne, NY)
5-mm laparoscopic needle drivers (Storz)
10-mm soft curved angled forceps (Maryland dissector) (Storz)
10-mm right angle dissector (Storz)
Carter Thomason needle suture grasper and closure cones (Inlet Medical, Eden Prairie, MN)
5-mm Diamond Flex Angulating Triangle retractor (Snowden-Pencer)

Available But Not Opened Equipment
10-mm Clip Appliers with 9-mm and 12-mm clips (Ethicon)
5-mm disposable reticulating Endoshears (U.S. Surgical, Norwalk, CT)
Endostitch and suture (0, 2-0, 4-0, Polysorb, Polydac, and Prolene) (U.S. Surgical)
Disposable Hasson Trocar 12-mm Blunt Tip (U.S. Surgical)
3-0 cardiovascular silk (RB-1 needle) and 0-Vicryl suture for fascial closure
Lapra-Ty clips and 10-mm Lapra-Ty clip applier (Ethicon)
Gauze rolls (5) (Carefree Surgical Specialties)
10-mm Satinsky clamp with flexible port (Aesculap, Center Valley, PA)
One set of laparoscopic bulldog clamps (Kline, San Antonio, TX)

remaining trocars that are used are all dilating trocars; bladed trocars are no longer used in our operating room. Thus the fascia is only closed for those ports placed in the midline. Only one port site hernia using these dilating trocars has been reported to our knowledge.[4] Otherwise, the laparoscopic instrumentation for the retroperitoneal approach is the same. The laparoscopic partial nephrectomy, however, has a somewhat higher demand for instrumentation (Table 59-2).

STEP-BY-STEP DESCRIPTION OF OPERATIVE PROCEDURE

LAPAROSCOPIC TRANSPERITONEAL RADICAL NEPHRECTOMY ACCESS For access on either kidney, our preference is to make the initial skin incision approximately 2 fingerbreadths cranial, and medial to the anterior superior iliac spine. The subcutaneous tissue is spread with a Kelly clamp, and the underlying fascia is grasped with two Allis clamps. These clamps are then used to stabilize, not lift, the abdominal wall, while the Veress needle is introduced. A pneumoperitoneum of 25 mm Hg is obtained to provide a tense abdominal wall for subsequent trocar placement. A 12-mm endoscopic dilating non-bladed trocar is placed via the initial 12-mm incision; a zero-degree lens is used to observe the safe passage of the trocar across the abdominal wall. Then a 10-mm 30° laparoscope is introduced and used to examine the intra-abdominal contents for signs of inadvertent injury and planning of subsequent trocar placement. The surgeon then reduces the pneumoperitoneum to 15 mm Hg. Next a non-bladed 12-mm trocar is placed 2 cm below the costal margin in the midclavicular line. Another non-bladed 12-mm trocar is placed lateral to the margin of the rectus muscle approximately three to five fingerbreadths above the umbilicus. Further along in the procedure, a non-bladed 5-mm trocar is typically placed below the costal margin in the posterior axillary line once the colon has been mobilized. (Figures 59-1 and 59-2)

RIGHT SIDE **Step 1: Peritoneal Incisions and Pararenal Dissection** The dissection of the right kidney can be thought of as a wedge (Figure 59-3). The thin edge of the wedge is aligned along the lateral border of the dissection, the line of Toldt. This edge is incised using the Harmonic shears from the pelvic brim to the lower pole of the kidney. Upon careful inspection of the abdomen, the kidney outline is commonly visualized from underneath the ascending colon. The kidney is not freed at this point from the sidewall; rather, the incision is continued from the upper pole of the kidney, cephalad to the level of the

Table 59-2 Additional Instrumentation for Laparoscopic Partial Nephrectomy
Tissuelink (Tissuelink, Dover, NH) (available, unopened)
Tisseal and Floseal with laparoscopic applicators (Baxter, Irvine, CA)
Surgicel (prepare Floseal at outset of case – 2 vials)

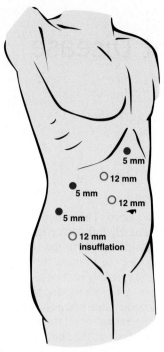

Figure 59-1 Diagram demonstrating port sites used for right transperitoneal nephrectomy. White circles represent 12-mm port sites. Black circles represent 5-mm port sites. The optional upper midline 5-mm port may be used for liver retraction, while the lower lateral optional 5-mm port is only used if there is difficulty with specimen entrapment in a LapSac.

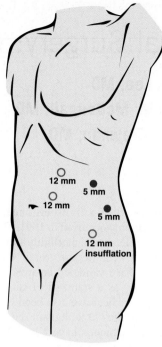

Figure 59-2 Diagram demonstrating port sites used for left transperitoneal nephrectomy. The 12-mm insufflation port is marked. White circles represent 12-mm port sites. Black circles represent 5-mm port sites. The lower 5-mm port site is optional; it is only placed if there is difficulty with specimen entrapment in a LapSac

diaphragm; the triangular ligament of the liver is also divided at this time. Meanwhile, the colonic reflection overlying the anterior surface of the kidney is identified by gently lifting the colon. This plane is entered and the ascending colon is thus freed from the underlying Gerota's fascia. In general, this plane lies well lateral to the lateral half of the anterior surface of the kidney.

This mobilization of the colon represents the first of three layers of dissection required to complete the broad side of the wedge configuration. The second layer of the wedge is comprised of a Kocher maneuver to move the duodenum medially off of the middle to lower anterior medial surface of the kidney, and extreme caution must be exercised at this portion of the dissection. The duodenum is uniformly present, but it often appears flattened and sometimes seems imbued with a bluish tint reminiscent of the vena cava. In all cases, however, the duodenum must be mobilized in this area of the lower half of the kidney before the surgeon is able to visualize the inferior vena cava. After the surgeon mobilizes the duodenum medially, the inferior vena cava should then begin to come into view. The dissection over the inferior vena cava represents the third layer of the wedge. This part of the dissection can be carried cephalad beneath the lower edge of the liver.

Next, the posterior coronary hepatic ligament can be incised from the line of Toldt laterally to the lateral border of the inferior vena cava. In some cases, it is easier to do this prior to the Kocher maneuver on the duodenum. This incision is usually carried just 1 to 2 cm caudal to the liver edge. This incision will meet the inferior

vena cava well above the level of the right adrenal vein, thus ensuring the en bloc removal of the adrenal and kidney within Gerota's fascia if a radical, rather than total, nephrectomy is deemed necessary by the surgeon.

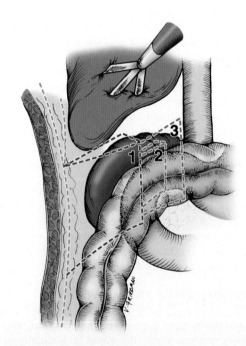

Figure 59-3 Diagram of the right-sided nephrectomy demonstrating the wedge-shaped configuration. The numbers refer to the 3 distinct levels of dissection along the medial aspect of the kidney: colon, duodenum, and inferior vena cava. Note that, on the right side, the line of Toldt paralleling the kidney is left intact; this is done to preclude the kidney from falling medial and obscuring the renal hilum.

Step 2: Securing the Gonadal Vein The gonadal vein can usually be identified at its origin on the IVC, caudal and anterior to the renal vein. The gonadal vein is circumferentially dissected and ligated with the 10 mm bipolar Ligasure Atlas device (Valleylab, Boulder, CO) or alternatively by dividing it between two pairs of vascular clips. It is often helpful to realize that if caval bleeding is encountered during dissection along the anteromedial surface of the IVC, it is most often actually from the gonadal vein. Increasing the pneumoperitoneum temporarily to 25 mm Hg will effectively slow down—or even stop—significant venous injuries, aiding in identification and control of troublesome bleeding. The argon beam coagulator can also greatly aid in the control of small (ie, < 3 mm) venous and 1- to 2-mm arterial injuries. The argon gas expelled from the tip of the instrument helps to clear the field of blood but can quickly increase the intra-abdominal pressure. This argon gas must be frequently vented during the use of this instrument.

Step 3: Securing the Ureter The ureter usually lies just posterior and lateral to the gonadal vein. Once dissected from retroperitoneal tissues, it is usually divided with a load of the vascular stapler. The use of the Ligasure on the adrenal and gonadal veins and the stapler on the ureter, renal artery, and renal vein, precludes the use of the clip applier in most of the laparoscopic nephrectomies performed at our institution. Alternatively, three Hem-o-lok clips (Weck Closure Systems, Research Triangle Park, NC) can be placed on the renal artery; a less expensive option than a stapler load or clip applier.

Step 4: Securing the Adrenal Vein The adrenal vein can be identified by marching the dissection up along the IVC cranially. If a clip applier is employed, the surgeon must be sure to leave two clips on the IVC side, however we now secure and divide the adrenal vein with the 10 mm Ligasure device. If the adrenal gland is to be spared, then the upper medial border of the kidney should be dissected free at this time. Gerota's fascia must be entered in this area, and the Ligasure or vascular stapler can be insinuated along the renal border to "push away" the adrenal gland medially.

Step 5: The Renal Hilum In preparation for dissecting the renal hilum, we have found it to be helpful to utilize the PEER retractor (Jarit Surgical Instruments, Hawthorne, NY) attached to the Endoholder to provide lateral retraction of the kidney along the renal hilum. By placing the kidney on stretch thusly, the hilar dissection is greatly facilitated. The retractor is placed such that the legs straddle the renal hilum (ie, one leg cranial and one leg caudal to the hilum) (Figure 59-4). Once attached to the Endoholder, the retraction is firm and reliable (Figure 59-5).

The right angle hook electrode is a favorite instrument for this part of the dissection. The hook can be used to engage tissue and then retract it away from underlying vascular structures before the electrocautery is engaged. The active electrode monitoring system (Encision Inc, Boulder, CO) is utilized to avoid the possibility of arc-

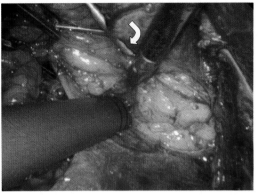

Figure 59-4 The right renal vein is stapled and cut with a laparoscopic vascular stapler. Note the PEER retractor (white arrow) straddling the hilum providing lateral traction on the kidney.

ing from the shaft of the instrument to adjacent bowel or other structures. The vein is usually first identified in this dissection with the artery usually lying just posterior and often slightly superior to the vein. Once the artery is identified, it is skeletonized sufficiently to allow the placement of the vascular stapler for ligation. Alternatively, five clips can be used to ligate this vessel; three clips are placed on the stay side and the artery is divided with two clips on the kidney side. Recently, the locking clips have been used; in which case only three clips are applied: two on the stay side and one on the renal specimen side. The renal vein is taken with another load of the vascular stapler. Chan and colleagues described an alternative technique to expedite the hilum dissection.[5] The superior and inferior border of the renal artery is dissected cleanly so that the retroperitoneal musculature can be identified. The jaws of the vascular stapler can then be placed in these dissected areas and the artery can then be divided, thus avoiding the posterior dissection of the renal artery.

If the dissection of the artery cannot be completed in this orientation, the kidney itself can be freed of its posterior attachments and thus "flipped" forward. The artery can then be approached from the posterior direction. The artery in this case may be dissected further medi-

ally to where it crosses beneath the posterior surface of the IVC; the potential for injury to the IVC must remain in the surgeon's mind during this part of the procedure.

Another possibility is to divide the ureter first; this structure can then be retracted upward, and the hilum can be more easily accessed along the broad expanse of its inferior surface. This approach provides simultaneous access to the underside of the renal artery and vein. This access to the renal hilum, albeit somewhat awkward, at times may be very helpful in certain situations, such as extensive perihilar adhesions.

Step 6: Freeing the Specimen and Securing the Ureter Once all vascular attachments have been divided, the specimen is freed from the retroperitoneum by incising the remainder of the lateral and posterior attachments. The ureter is secured by either a load of the vascular stapler or the Ligasure device. A sufficient length of ureter should be left in order to grasp it using a locking grasper passed via the 5-mm subcostal port. The specimen, once completely freed, should be placed on top of the liver using the ureter as the handle. Once satisfactorily positioned, the locking grasper can be placed into the Endoholder to maintain the kidney's position on the anterior surface of the liver.

Step 7: Entrapment for Morcellation The laparoscope is now moved to the upper midclavicular port. If morcellation is to be performed, the impermeable 8 by 10-inch LapSac (Cook Urological, Spencer, IN) is used. Just prior to introduction, a nitinol guidewire (eg, Terumo) is threaded twice around the sack via every other hole in the top of the sack (Figure 59-6).[6] Now when the LapSac is introduced via the paramedian port, the neck of the sack will spring open, enabling the surgeon to complete the entrapment process with only two, rather than three, graspers. The sack is unfurled in the abdomen with two atraumatic grasping forceps and opened just below the lower edge of the liver. Specimens up to 1,700 grams have been successfully entrapped in the LapSac.

If the specimen is to be removed whole, then one of the available, rapidly opening plastic entrapment sacks can be used. The 15-mm entrap-

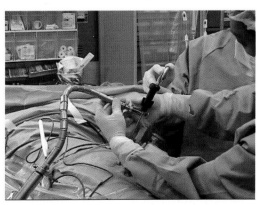

Figure 59-5 The Endoholder is being fastened onto a PEER retractor to provide lateral traction on the renal hilum.

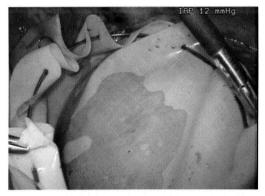

Figure 59-6 LapSac for renal entrapment. Note a guidewire has been inserted through the same holes through which the nylon drawstring passes; the guidewire facilitates opening the sack.

ment sack cannot be passed through a trocar but may be placed after one 12-mm trocar is removed.

Step 8: Morcellation Versus Intact Removal Upon successful entrapment of the kidney, the mouth of the sac is delivered through the upper midclavicular line port. A specialized draping system is used to help prevent any tumor spillage during the morcellation process. The surgical field around the port site is covered with a "10,10" drape, a fenestrated absorbent towel, and a nephrostomy drape, sequentially. A hole is placed in the center of all three of these layers, and the neck of the sack is pulled through this hole.

The 12-mm port site through which the sack is exiting is enlarged to 2 cm to enable a larger piece of kidney to be removed under direct vision. Mechanical morcellation is then performed with a ring forceps. The camera operator must remain vigilant during this step to quickly identify any loss of pneumoperitoneum or puncture of the LapSac. If any puncture is noted, the port site is immediately enlarged to deliver the remaining specimen intact. After the sack is withdrawn, the team members involved in the morcellation re-gown themselves. The triple drape is removed from the table.

These plastic sacks can be easily punctured during intra-abdominal morcellation; indeed, in a decade, the authors have had only two acute bowel injuries during laparoscopic renal surgery, both occurred when attempting morcellation with the kidney in a plastic sack. Work by Eichel and colleagues has shown that puncture of a plastic sack, even with a ring forceps, can occur with only 19 lbs of pressure versus 43 lbs of pressure when using a LapSac.[7] Landman and colleagues reported a compromise situation in which the specimen was entrapped in a plastic sack and then via a 3-cm incision, only the portion of the specimen above the abdominal wall (ie, extra-abdominal morcellation) was morcellated under direct vision. With this approach, entrapment and morcellation time could be reduced to 13 minutes, and fragment size was increased from 1.5 to 4.5 g.[8]

For intact removals, we prefer to proceed with entrapment in a plastic sack and then to create a lower midline abdominal incision or Pfannenstiel incision. Larger incisions higher up on the abdomen tend to be more painful, and incisions created by connecting port sites may lead to poorer healing and delayed postoperative hernias.

Step 9: Exiting the Abdomen Once the procedure is complete, the pneumoperitoneum should be reduced to 5 mm Hg, and the abdomen carefully inspected for bleeding. Copious irrigation is useful in decreasing the amount of residual small clots and for detecting any rivulets of red streaming through clear irrigant. The rivulet is a sure sign of continued bleeding, and the sources should be controlled. Once no further bleeding is detected, a 5-mm laparoscopic injection needle is used to instill 30 cc of 1/4% Marcaine to the bed of the kidney and the diaphragm for possible pain control. All ports are removed under direct vision. The non-bladed, non-midline trocar sites do not require closure. The morcellation site and

any midline port greater than 10 mm is closed using a fascial closure device such as the Carter-Thomason needle grasper (Inlet Medical, Grand Prairie, MN). Skin sites are closed with a subcuticular suture of 4-0 absorbable suture, Steristrips, and a Band-aid or, more simply, with a tissue glue (eg, Dermabond).

LEFT SIDE Step 1: Peritoneal Incisions and Pararenal Dissection The template for anatomic dissection of the left kidney most resembles an inverted cone or a water scooper (Figure 59-7). The lateral side of the cone is formed by the line of Toldt that is incised from the pelvic brim, cephalad to the level of the diaphragm. Unlike the right side, the colon covers more of the anterior kidney on the left side. Thus, the incision in the line of Toldt is made uninterrupted for the length of the retroperitoneum at the outset. There is a remarkably constant attachment from the descending colon at the splenic flexure to the anterior abdominal wall; this attachment must be incised to gain access to the upper portion of the line of Toldt. The most cephalad portion of this incision must be carried along the underside of the diaphragm above the spleen. This allows the spleen to fall medially away from the side wall aiding in the upper pole renal dissection.

The medial portion of the cone is then created by developing the plane between Gerota's fascia and the colonic mesentery. The descending colon is bluntly retracted medially. The plane is often appreciated most easily at the lower pole of the kidney. The upper anterior broad base of the cone is defined by the splenocolic ligament, which is incised to allow further medial retraction of the colon. The upper posterior base of the cone is defined by the splenorenal ligament, which is also incised, thereby releasing the spleen to move medially. The extensive freeing of the spleen protects it from damage during the remainder of the procedure. Indeed, incidental splenectomy is rare with a laparoscopic versus an open approach.[9]

Step 2. The Gonadal Vein The left gonadal vein is the key to the renal hilum because it reliably drains into the left renal vein. Early identification and subsequent cephalad dissection give the surgeon confidence as the hilum is approached. Tributaries to the gonadal vein are quite rare, and thus, the vein provides a safe plane of dissection all the way to the hilum. If there is difficulty in identifying this vein, it can be picked up caudal, either at the level of the internal ring in the male or the ovary in the female, and then traced cephalad.

Step 3. Securing the Ureter This is handled in a manner similar to a right nephrectomy.

Step 4. Securing the Renal Hilum Once the renal vein is identified, the gonadal vein is circumferentially dissected and divided using the Ligasure device (Figure 59-8). Alternatively, it may be taken with four clips. Next, the ascending lumbar vein entering the posterior aspect is likewise individually dissected and secured. Then the superior border of the renal vein is dissected, and the adrenal vein is located, circumferentially dissected, and secured. If clips are indeed used, they must be

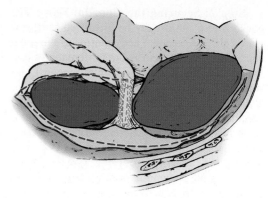

Figure 59-7 Diagram demonstrating the inverted cone template for en bloc dissection during left radical nephrectomy. Unlike on the right side, the reflection of the colon comes to the lateral sidewall, and thus, an incision in the line of Toldt parallel to the kidney needs to be made; this incision is not carried deeply in an effort to hold the kidney lateral, which helps somewhat with the hilar dissection.

placed at least 1 cm away from the body of the renal vein. This allows easy placement of the vascular stapler on the renal vein. If the stapler is fired across a clip, the stapler may freeze-up and may not be able to be properly released.[10] Remedies to this situation include more medial dissection of the renal vein to allow placement of second stapler medial to the first; if this is not possible then conversion to open surgery is often necessary.

The renal artery is usually exposed by retracting the renal vein caudally. The artery is taken with a load of the vascular stapler or with five vascular clips, leaving three on the stay side, or with locking clips (eg, Hem-o-lok) leaving two on the stay side. The vein is taken with a second load of the stapler.

The remaining dissection, entrapment, morcellation, and intact removal are identical to the right side. Obviously, the specimen is placed over the spleen rather than the liver for entrapment.

SURGICAL TECHNIQUE: RETROPERITONEAL NEPHRECTOMY

An alternative approach for radical nephrectomy is the retroperitoneal approach. Although this is the preferred approach for open surgery, the

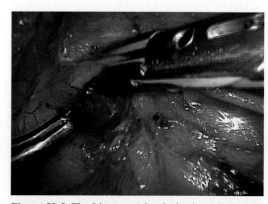

Figure 59-8 The Ligasure Atlas device is applied to the left gonadal vein. This device is used on the renal vein tributaries to avoid inadvertent placement of clips that would make stapler placement difficult.

abundance of adipose tissue in the retroperitoneum makes identification of anatomic landmarks more difficult. In patients with extensive prior abdominal surgeries, however, the retroperitoneal approach may yield a much easier dissection. Indeed, avoidance of violation of the peritoneal cavity may reduce intraoperative and postoperative morbidity. This approach has become the preferred approach for most simple nephrectomies for small kidneys and, in some centers, is the primary approach for all renal laparoscopic surgery regardless of the size of the kidney or the nature of the disease process (ie, benign vs. malignant).

ACCESS The initial skin incision is created just below and posterior to the tip of the twelfth rib (ie, in the midaxillary line). The incision should be 2 cm to admit the surgeon's index finger for blunt dissection. Under direct vision, the flank muscles are bluntly divided, and the thoracolumbar fascia is incised. "Army-Navy" or "S" retractors are helpful to gain entry to and visualization of the retroperitoneal space. The surgeon should be able to feel 180° around the space created as well as palpate the psoas muscle. Adequate dissection is performed to admit a balloon dilator (eg, Bluntport) that is inflated to 800 cc with room air. During inflation, a 0° or 30° lens can be introduced to view the anatomy as the fat in the retroperitoneum is bluntly dissected by the expanding transparent balloon. If needed, the balloon can be deflated and then replaced higher in the retroperitoneum and reinflated. The balloon is removed and replaced with a Hasson-type trocar or a 12-mm cannula with a balloon and soft collar sealing mechanism (Bluntport). The latter appears to limit the development of subcutaneous emphysema and CO_2 absorption. A pneumoperitoneum of 15 mm Hg is established and a 10-mm, 30° laparoscope is inserted. The psoas muscle at this point should be relatively easy to visualize. Gerota's fascia and the ureter may also be visible.

Accessory non-bladed ports are placed with endoscopic guidance. A 12-mm port is placed at the lower midaxillary line 2 cm cephalad to the iliac crest; a 12-mm port is placed at the tip of the 12th rib in the posterior axillary line and a 5-mm port is placed at the 11th rib on the anterior axillary line. This creates a "T" configuration (Figure 59-9). Alternatively, ports can be placed in a subcostal array only ("I" configuration) or a 5th port can be added anterior creating a "W".[11] Alternatively, these ports can be placed under digital control. The surgeon can place his/her index finger through the initial incision and guide the blunt ports into one of the previously described arrays.

OPERATIVE TECHNIQUE Initially the psoas muscle is cleared of remaining adipose tissue to help orient the surgeon. The clearing of the psoas muscle should proceed in a cephalocaudal manner and then medially to clearly delineate the medial border of the psoas. This is an essential maneuver, as failure to perform this part of the dissection may result in "missing" the kidney

entirely. Indeed, when the psoas muscle is not dissected to its identifiable medial border, retraction of the retroperitoneal tissues anteriorly at this point misses the kidney and it remains posterior. Only after dissection of the medial border of the psoas muscle can the kidney be reliably retracted anterior and the hilum put on stretch.

After dissecting along the medial border of the psoas muscle, a retractor passed via the most medial port can be used to sweep all tissue bordering the medial aspect of the psoas muscle anteriorly; this will put traction on the kidney and place the renal hilum on stretch. Then, as the dissection is continued medially and cephalad along the psoas muscle, the pulsations of the renal hilum should be appreciated. After the hilum's location has been determined, the posterior leaflet of Gerota's fascia is entered 1 to 2 cm from the psoas. The artery is dissected circumferentially and then taken first, either with clips or the vascular stapler. The renal vein is then dissected circumferentially and taken with a vascular stapler.

One caveat: on the left side, caution must be exercised as the ascending lumbar vein may be encountered early, prior to identification of the renal artery. This vein is dissected and secured with two pairs of clips and divided. Also on the left side, the adrenal and gonadal veins will need to be taken; this can be done with four clips or with the Ligasure device. The ureter is transected in a similar fashion.

The specimen is entrapped in a rapidly deployable plastic bag (Endocatch II, U.S. Surgical). Very large specimens or specimens for morcellation may require that a purposeful opening into the peritoneal cavity be made in order for entrapment to occur.

Intact removal of the specimen is performed by one of a few variations. The initial port site can be extended transversely to 8 cm or larger, and the specimen delivered. Alternatively in males, a Pfannenstiel incision is made and access is gained to Retzius' space. Blunt finger dissection allows joining of this space to the retroperitoneum, and the specimen can then be delivered via this lowlying incision as described by Gill. Alternatively in females, a generous peritoneotomy can be created; the patient is then placed into a steep Trendelenburg's position. The vagina is prepared and a sponge stick is placed in the vagina. A 3 cm colpotomy is created laparoscopically and the drawstring of the entrapment sack is passed into the vagina. The specimen is thus delivered transvaginally and the colpotomy is closed.

Contrary to initial concerns, inadvertent entry into the peritoneal cavity does not mandate conversion to a transperitoneal technique. Indeed, these openings into the peritoneal cavity are usually small, and the resulting pneumoperitoneum seldom compromises the retroperitoneal space.

Systematic inspection and removal of ports is important in retroperitoneal surgery. The CO_2 pressure is decreased to 5 mm, and the abdomen and port sites are examined for hemostasis. No fascial sutures need be placed except to help close the initial 2-cm incision.

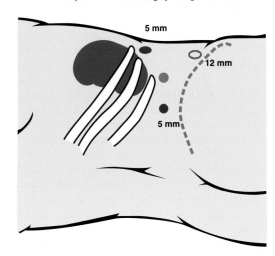

Figure 59-9 Diagram demonstrating the 'T' configuration for port placement for a right retroperitoneal nephrectomy. The central gray circle is the access site. The kidney is represented as the grey shadow underneath the costal margin.

SURGICAL TECHNIQUE: LAPAROSCOPIC PARTIAL NEPHRECTOMY

The approach to the laparoscopic partial nephrectomy is guided by the location and depth of the tumor. Generally, tumors located on the anterior portion of the kidney are approached transperitoneally, while those located posterior are approached retroperitoneally.

In addition to the location of the tumor, the depth of tumor penetration into the kidney is of importance. In general, exophytic tumors (ie, > 60% of the tumor lying above the surface of the kidney and well away from the collecting system), can usually be managed without the need for vascular clamping. In contrast, tumors that are endophytic (ie, > 60% of the tumor lying below the surface of the kidney and likely requiring entry into the collecting system for removal) usually require vascular clamping. For those tumors that are neither truly exophytic or endophytic (ie, mesophytic), in general, vessel clamping is recommended; even here, however, if the lesion is small and well away from the collecting system, a nonischemic approach can be used. Laparoscopic methods for vascular clamping include laparoscopic and standard bulldog clamps and laparoscopic and standard Satinsky clamps. For a hand-assist approach, the standard bulldog clamps can be used. For a standard laparoscopic approach, the laparoscopic bulldogs can be applied. A Satinsky clamp can be used either with a 12-mm flexible port or by the method of Turk. The latter method comprises placing and removing a 5-mm port; through the resulting incision and peritoneotomy, the Satinsky clamp can be passed under endoscopic guidance. The small amount of clearance between the clamp and the peritoneotomy does not significantly compromise the pneumoperitoneum. With this approach, risks of warm ischemia and renal vascular intimal damage must remain on the surgeon's mind. Should overall anticipated ischemic time exceed 30 minutes, then renal cooling should be employed. This can be done laparoscopically using an ice slush around the kidney or by a ureteral access sheath for intrarenal cooling.[12,13]

OPERATIVE TECHNIQUE The patient positioning, port positioning, and access are similar to the transperitoneal or retroperitoneal nephrectomy given appropriate circumstances. A ureteral stent is not placed unless extensive entry into the collecting system is anticipated. In most cases, if there is concern of entry into the collecting system, then indigo carmine and mannitol or Lasix is administered intravenously just prior to excising the tumor. In all cases, the laparoscopic ultrasonography unit is essential to guide the surgeon during excision of the base of the tumor in order to obtain a margin-free specimen. The exposure of the kidney is similar to that of the radical nephrectomy. Once the area of the tumor is localized, Gerota's fascia is entered 1 to 2 cm away from the tumor, and the renal capsule is cleared of perinephric fat. The fat is dissected circumferentially around the border of the tumor, pushing the fat up onto the tumor itself. Any of the peritumor fat that is detached during this part of the procedure is sent for separate pathologic analysis. The borders of the tumor should be cleared of fat until the renal capsule is clearly visualized. The patient is given mannitol, indigo carmine, and copious fluids intravenously to maximize renal perfusion and to help identify any entry into the collecting system during the subsequent excision of the tumor.

If renal vascular control needs to be obtained, it should be done so at this point. The renal hilum should be neatly dissected. The artery and vein are separated. If a Satinsky clamp is to be placed, then a lower midline pararectus position provides an appropriate acute angle of approach to the hilum. Either the artery alone or the artery and vein together are secured. The former is preferred (Figure 59-10).

The renal capsule is then scored with either the open active blade of the harmonic shears, the harmonic scalpel or with the hook electrocautery (Figure 59-11). Any bleeding is immediately controlled with the argon beam coagulator. After a circumferential incision in the peritumor renal capsule has been made, the renal parenchyma is incised with the harmonic scalpel in its most dependent portion; this insures that any bleeding will have less of a tendency to obscure the surgeon's path of dissection. A negative margin is assured by careful visualization to avoid entry into the capsule of the tumor. Active suctioning with the non-dominant hand is usually necessary to maintain good visualization. The suction unit can also be used to gently retract the tumor, thereby exposing the deeper parenchymal line of resection. The tumor can essentially be "rolled out" of the renal parenchyma in this manner. Once excised, the tumor is captured in a 5-mm rapidly deployable entrapment sack, delivered from the abdomen intact, and sent for pathologic analysis of the margins.

Attention is then turned to gaining hemostasis. This can be done with one of several modali-

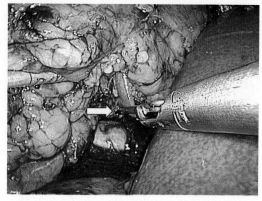

Figure 59-10 Laparoscopic view of laparoscopic bulldog clamp (white arrow) being applied to renal hilum.

ties. If the vessels have been clamped, then the Tissuelink "floating ball" radiofrequency device (Tissuelink, Dover, NH) can be used to seal the incised parenchyma.[14] The tip of the instrument contains a "floating ball" around which saline drips at 1 cc/s (Figure 59-12). The saline provides tissue cooling so the radiofrequency delivered can cauterize without charring. The energy then penetrates deeper into the tissue and can control even small arterial bleeding. Small circular motions around the center of the bleed are most effective in delivering the energy.

When the vessels have not been clamped, there are several means available for achieving hemostasis. While the "floating ball" can be used, it is tedious. The argon beam coagulator works rapidly. It is used to lightly "paint" the raw parenchymal surface. It provides electrocoagulation to a depth of 2 to 3 mm. Next, a layer of fibrin glue is delivered to the resection bed, followed by a layer of regenerated oxidized cellulose (Surgicel) followed by another layer of fibrin glue. This "hemostatic sandwich", as described by Wolf and colleagues, provides a solid bed of hemostatic sealant that appears to seal even small urine leaks.

If a large rent in the collecting system is noted due to blue urine escaping from the kidney, the edges can be sewn together with an Endostitch device or more commonly with free-hand suturing using a curved needle (eg, CT1). Application of a Lapra-Ty clip to the end of the suture and again after closing the collecting system provides excellent closing tension on the suture without the need for intracorporeal or extracorporeal knotting. The clip, also acts as a bolster, preventing the suture from pulling through the parenchyma. If warm ischemia is being used, then after securing hemostasis and closure of the collecting system; the vascular clamps that have been placed should then be removed and the kidney reinspected for hemostasis.

Other variations exist for the resection of renal masses. Many authors routinely clamp the renal vessels and excise the renal mass using standard laparoscopic shears.[15,16] Variations also abound for hemostasis. Although standard electrocautery has not been effective, the argon beam coagulator and the Tissuelink have been used.[14,17] Hemostatic agents or methods such as fibrinogen-soaked

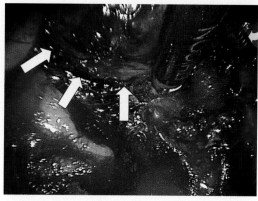

Figure 59-11 The Harmonic Shears are used to excise a renal tumor. The tumor at the top of the frame (white arrows at the margin) is being retracted upward by a suction device (yellow arrow).

Gelfoam[18], microwave[19], holmium laser[20], RF ablation[21], FloSeal[22] have been used with varying degrees of success. Some authors advocate the use of bolster sutures placed through the edges of the capsule.[23,24] Transparenchymal sutures are then tied down over Gelfoam pieces or bolsters, thereby duplicating the open technique that many surgeons use. The necessity of this standard open surgical maneuver is debatable, given the advent and successful use of the aforementioned hemostatic alternatives.

As with all laparoscopic procedures, at the end of the case, the pneumoperitoneum is reduced to 5 mm Hg. Careful inspection of the hilum, kidney and other dissection areas is performed to ensure hemostasis. A 10-mm round drain is placed in the retroperitoneum. The abdomen is then exited.

POSTOPERATIVE CARE Patients receive 15 mg of ketorolac (Toradol) intravenously every 6 hours as requested, for 36 hours, as well as an oral narcotic as necessary. Diet is resumed immediately with clear fluids and advanced as tolerated. The patient is ambulated on the first post-operative day. If there is scant drainage, the drain is removed on postoperative day 1. Discharge is routinely planned for the evening of postoperative day 1 or the morning of postoperative day 2, provided the patient is passing flatus. Parenteral antibiotics are

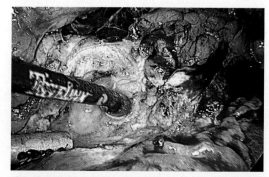

Figure 59-12 The renal tumor has been excised and the Tissuelink is being used to help achieve hemostasis. Note the white discoloration of the renal tissue as it is being coagulated.

stopped on postoperative day 1. The patient is discharged on oral analgesics. Of note, it is not uncommon for these patients to develop some constipation postoperatively; as such, use of a Dulcolax suppository as needed, and sending the patient home on a stool softener (eg, Colace one tablet twice a day) is recommended.

TRANSPERITONEAL RADICAL NEPHROURETERECTOMY

INDICATIONS Transitional cell carcinoma (TCC) of the upper ureter and/or the renal pelvis commonly necessitates nephroureterectomy. Although many surgeons have had success with ureteroscopic or percutaneous resection of upper tract TCC, these tumors are typically either less than 1 to 2 cm in size or of low grade, often in patients with other extenuating circumstances (eg, renal insufficiency, high risk, solitary kidney). For high-grade bulky disease, nephroureterectomy is the gold standard treatment. Laparoscopic nephroureterectomy was first reported by Clayman and colleagues in 1991.[25]

PATIENT PREPARATION AND POSITIONING The patient preparation is identical to that for laparoscopic radical nephrectomy. Because the final pathologic stage plays an important role in the postoperative care, the patient is informed that an incision will definitely be made in order to retrieve the specimen intact. As such, many surgeons perform this case with the hand-assisted approach. The hand allows rapid manual dissection to be performed especially with regard to dissection of the distal ureter. Prior to nephroureterectomy, cystoscopy should be performed to evaluate the lower urinary tract for TCC, and an upper tract study should have been obtained to clear the contralateral kidney and ureter.

SURGICAL TECHNIQUE **Insufflation and Port Placement** Insufflation is performed as described previously for the radical nephrectomy in the anterior axillary line three to four fingerbreadths above the iliac crest. A template for trocar positioning is presented in Figure 59-13. With hand-assisted nephrectomy, however, a myriad of different possibilities exist. Many surgeons will prefer a right nephrectomy to place the handport in the right lower quadrant and allow the camera to be more centrally located. Later on during the case, another 12-mm port may be placed either in the midline between the umbilicus and the symphysis pubis or in the midclavicular line 2 to 3 cm below the level of the umbilicus. Other urologists may prefer to place the handport in the midline from the umbilicus caudally.

Renal Dissection The laparoscopic dissection of the kidney mirrors that of the laparoscopic radical nephrectomy. The adrenal gland is spared in all cases, except when the tumor involves and invades an upper-pole calix. The only difference is that the ureter is not divided near the kidney but instead is left intact and mobilized toward the pelvis.

Ureteral Dissection The patient is placed in Trendelenberg's position, and the ureter is gently grasped. The dissection of the ureter is taken more distally over the course of the iliac vessels; the superior vesical vessels that are seen crossing over the ureter are divided. The vas or round ligament is encountered next and divided, along with the ipsilateral medial umbilical ligament. This should bring the surgeon down to the ureterovesical junction.

There are several techniques for distal ureteral management at this point. The authors recommend fine dissection of the distal ureter to the level of the intramural ureter or ureteral tunnel. The harmonic shears are used to make a vertical incision through the intramural tunnel at 12, 3, 6, and 9 o'clock, thereby allowing the surgeon to dissect the ureter down to, but not through, the ureteral tunnel (method of Y. Ono, Nagoya, Japan). A laparoscopic stapler with articulating head (tissue load) is then applied to the distal ureter/bladder cuff to complete the dissection (Figure 59-14). Alternatively, a more generous cuff of bladder can be taken using laparoscopic scissors. The cystotomy is then sutured closed with free-hand suturing or an Endostitch device. Again, Lapra-Ty clips may be very helpful here to expedite the closure.

Cystoscopic Management of the Distal Ureter/Bladder Cuff After completion of the laparoscopic portion, the patient is repositioned into a dorsal lithotomy position. If staples are visualized by flexible cystoscopy and no ureteral orifice is seen, the procedure can be terminated.

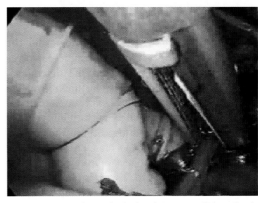

Figure 59-14 The articulating laparoscopic stapler is used to ligate the ureter with a cuff of bladder during this hand-assisted laparoscopic nephroureterectomy.

More commonly, the ureteral orifice is visualized and a ureteral catheter is gently placed into the remaining short intramural ureteral segment. A Collings knife is then used to unroof the intramural ureter over the ureteral catheter until staples are seen (Figure 59-15). After staple identification, a resectoscope equipped with a roller-ball electrode is used to fulgurate for a radius of 1 cm around the site of unroofing. Finally, a Foley catheter is left to gravity drainage for 48 hours. Alternatively, as described independently by Leveillee and Nadler, flexible cystoscopy can be performed either during or after the ureteral dissection. The former is very helpful in guiding the surgeon to make sure the entire ureter has been taken, thereby precluding the need for use of the Collings knife or roller electrode.

ALTERNATIVE APPROACH: RETROPERITONEAL LAPAROSCOPIC NEPHROURETERECTOMY Ono and Gill independently described a retroperitoneal approach during which a total retroperitoneoscopic nephrectomy is performed. In the Gill method, the ureter, having been released from the bladder at the outset of the procedure, is then plucked cephalad, and the specimen delivered via the same method used for total nephrectomy with intact removal.[26] In the Ono method, the kidney is mobilized downward, and a Gibson incision is

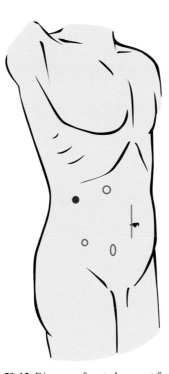

Figure 59-13 Diagram of port placement for right hand-assisted nephroureterectomy. The white circles are 12-mm ports while the black circles are 5-mm ports. The insufflation would begin in the right lower quadrant. The arrangement for the left would be essentially a mirror image. An optional right lower quadrant 12-mm trocar (red circle) is placed if the ureterovesical junction cannot be easily reached with the stapler.

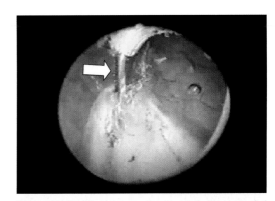

Figure 59-15 The intramural ureter is being unroofed transurethrally with a Collings knife (white arrow) via a standard resectoscope. Note the placement of a green ureteral catheter into the ureteral stump to help guide the knife.

utilized both to deliver the renal specimen and to excise a cuff of bladder.[27]

Alternative Management Strategies for the Distal Ureter The "pluck technique" involves transurethral ureteral resection of the ureteral orifice, tunnel, and ureterovesical junction to the perivesical fat prior to the laparoscopic component of the procedure; it is performed with the patient in a dorsal lithotomy position. The ureter is thereby released from the bladder, and a Foley catheter is placed. As soon as is feasible during the laparoscopic portion, the ureter is clipped to prevent further leakage of urine into the retroperitoneum. Once the kidney is freed, the surgeon can "pluck" the ureter cephalad, thereby precluding any pelvic dissection of the ureter. The major drawback of this approach is leakage of malignant cell-laden urine into the retroperitoneum. Reports of seeding after an open "pluck" procedure have been published by several urologists.[28–30]

Next, the application of a needlescopic technique for management of the distal ureter was described by Gill and colleagues in 1999.[31] The patient first undergoes cystoscopy to rule out a concomitant bladder tumor and to ensure adequate bladder capacity. Diminished bladder capacity (less than 200 mL) increases the technical difficulty due to limited working space. Under direct cystoscopic vision, two needlescopic trocars (2 mm) are inserted suprapubically into the bladder. A 2-mm Endoloop is inserted through the needlescopic trocar. A 6 French ureteral catheter is passed through the loop and into the affected ureter with the assistance of a guidewire. A 24F continuous-flow resectoscope is then passed into the bladder alongside the ureteral catheter. A Collings knife is used to electrosurgically score circumferentially the urothelium around the intramural ureter such that a 2- to 3-cm cuff is outlined. Then using a 2-mm grasper, the ureteral orifice and hemitrigone are retracted anteriorly and a full-thickness incision is made with the Collings knife, thereby freeing approximately 3 to 4 cm of ureter. The Endoloop is then positioned over the ureter and closed tightly, occluding the lumen as the ureteral catheter is withdrawn. The tail of the Endoloop is then cut with 2-mm laparoscopic scissors. The bladder edges about the excised ureter are then coagulated. Instruments are removed from the bladder and a Foley catheter is left indwelling. The laparoscopic retroperitoneal nephrectomy component of the procedure is then performed, and the ureter is pulled up and delivered intact with the kidney.

A similar theoretical concern also exists with this approach as the ureteral dissection is performed at the outset rather than the end of the procedure, thereby allowing leakage of potentially tumor–cell-laden urine. In addition, leakage can occur along the two intravesical port sites.

Many other methods for dealing with the distal ureteral cuff have been described. Nadler described using an electrosurgical probe via flexible cystoscopy to transurethrally free the ureter from the bladder at the end of the procedure. In this case, much of the leakage of tumor–cell-laden

urine should be largely precluded. Alternatively, Breda adopted the method of ureteral intussusception to the laparoscopic approach, thereby avoiding a formal dissection of the distal ureter.[32]

Other authors, after completing the nephrectomy portion of the procedure and clipping the ureter, make a small Pfannenstiel-type incision. Via cystotomy, a formal excision of the ureter and cuff of bladder is accomplished. Through the same incision, the specimen is extracted.

POSTOPERATIVE CARE The postoperative care is identical to the care rendered following a laparoscopic nephrectomy. The only difference is that, if a pluck or a formal transvesical resection of a cuff of bladder was completed, then the Foley catheter should be left in place for 5 to 7 days; a cystogram can be done during catheter removal. If intussusception was used, then the catheter can be removed on day 3. In contrast, if the cuff was taken with a stapler and no further treatment of the ureteral orifice or tunnel is required, then the Foley catheter can be removed on postoperative day 2; if further transurethral treatment of the ureteral tunnel is needed, then the catheter can be left in place for 5 days.

In these patients, a regimen of routine surveillance cystoscopy (every 3 to 4 months for 2 years, every 6 months for 2 years, and then annually, if there has not been a recurrence) is indicated owing to the 40% chance of developing a bladder tumor. The role of follow-up intravenous urograms is more controversial because the 1 to 2% of patients who develop contralateral upper tract TCC usually present with signs of their disease, and it is quite rare for the intravenous pyelogram to serendipitously reveal an otherwise "silent" occult upper tract lesion.[33] Urine cytology can be obtained at each surveillance visit.

RESULTS

LAPAROSCOPIC RADICAL NEPHRECTOMY The advantages related to minimally invasive procedures have been borne out for the laparoscopic radical nephrectomy. Four areas are of particular importance: efficacy, efficiency, equanimity, and economy. The efficacy of laparoscopic radical nephrectomy has now been documented by a long-term, multi-institutional study showing equivalent cancer-free and recurrence-free survival at greater than 4 years in a cohort of 60 patients.[34] Earlier studies by Kavoussi (3-year follow-up) and Ono (2-year follow-up) also documented equivalent results between open and laparoscopic groups.[35,36]

As the experience with this approach has grown, laparoscopic nephrectomy has become more efficient. Indeed, at some institutions (eg, Cleveland Clinic) the laparoscopic nephrectomy is quicker than the open, while at many other major medical centers, it has come down in time until it is within an hour of the time needed to do a standard open nephrectomy. In another regard, the laparoscopic approach has proven far superior to the open approach in recovery and mor-

bidity for the patient. McDougall and colleagues showed that laparoscopic radical nephrectomy was associated with a more rapid return of oral intake, a significantly decreased postoperative analgesic requirement, and a shorter hospital stay. Additionally, the laparoscopic population had a speedier return to normal activity and to full recovery. Additional subsequent articles have further corroborated these findings (Table 59-3).

Lastly, with regard to economy, Lotan and colleagues showed that laparoscopic nephrectomy is cost-effective if the procedure is completed in less than 4.7 hours, if operating room costs are kept under $5,500, and the patient leaves the hospital in less than 5 days. If these conditions are met, the overall savings are over $1,000 for the laparoscopic approach.[37] These conditions are routinely met or exceeded at many medical centers today; indeed, the average operative time is routinely less than 4.5 hours, with a hospital stay of only 1 to 2 days. In sum, given the results that have been corroborated at multiple centers, the laparoscopic radical nephrectomy has truly superseded its open counterpart as the current standard of care for non nephron-sparing therapy for renal cell cancer.

LAPAROSCOPIC PARTIAL NEPHRECTOMY When examining laparoscopic partial nephrectomy, Gill and colleagues reported the most comprehensive series in this regard. A retrospective comparison of 100 laparoscopic versus 100 open partial nephrectomies at the Cleveland Clinic was completed.[16] The groups were not equal, with the mean size of the mass being larger in the open group, and more solitary kidneys in the open group. As far as efficacy in this group, there were three positive margins in the laparoscopic group compared to none in the open group. Whether this will translate into survival differences or not, only time will tell. The efficiency was comparable, with the operative times being longer in the open group, but warm ischemia times longer in the laparoscopic group. Serum creatinines, both preoperative and postoperative, were not different between groups. The superior equanimity of the laparoscopic approach was well shown, with analgesia requirements, hospital stay, and time to full convalescence all being less for the laparoscopic group. The emergence of laparoscopic partial nephrectomy as a viable treatment option for nephron-sparing renal cancer surgery continues (Table 59-4). Nuances in techniques with regard to hemostatic and ablative energy modalities will continue to push the curve towards less invasive surgery. At present, however, this approach, while an alternative to open, has yet to become widely accepted as standard of care.

LAPAROSCOPIC NEPHROURETERECTOMY In regard to nephroureterectomy, the results are less extensive than with nephrectomy owing to the relative paucity of upper tract transitional cell cancer. Table 59-5 reviews results of three comparative trials contrasting open nephroureterectomy and laparoscopic or hand-assisted nephroureterectomy. Overall, 66 laparoscopic or hand-assisted

Table 59-3 Laparoscopic Radical Nephrectomy: Worldwide Experience

Report	n	OR Time (hrs)	EBL (cc)	Specific Weight (g)	Stage	Hospital Stay (d)	Recovery (wk)	Follow-up (mo)	Comp (major/minor)	Seeding
Peschel/Janetschek[47]	31	2.4	NA	NA	T1/T2	2.9	NA	18	0% / 0%	None
Ono/Kinukawa[36]	91	4.9	300	289	T1/T2	NA	3.0	22	11%	None
Barrett/Fentie[39]	72	2.9	NA	402	T1/T2	4.4	NA	21	1 death 3%/ 8%	One
Clayman/McDougall[40]	61	5.5	172	452	T1/T2 /T3b(r.v.)	3.4	3.6	25	3%/ 34%	None
Gill[2]	100	2.8	212	403	T1/T2/T3	1.6	4.2	16	3%/ 11%	None
Kavoussi/Chan[35]	67	4.3	289	NA	T1/T2/T3	3.8	NA	36	15% overall	None
Total	422	3.8	243	387	T1/T2 T3a/T3b	3.2	3.6	23	Mort. 0.3%	0.3%

laparoscopic procedures were compared to 54 open nephroureterectomies. With regard to efficacy, Shalhav's report, which has follow-up out to 24 months, demonstrates that overall cancer survival appears to be similar, as well as the bladder recurrence rate. In that study, however, there was longer follow-up in the open than in the laparoscopic group. This particular area needs further attention over the coming years given the small numbers of patients treated. The efficiency of the procedure still favors the open approach by upwards of 2 hours. But the equanimity again favors the laparoscopic approach: hospital stay and postoperative analgesic requirements were significantly decreased in the cohort undergoing laparoscopy. Most striking, however, full convalescence was expedited by more than 6 weeks. Lastly, with regard to economy, Meraney and Gill showed that, in their first 14 laparoscopic nephroureterectomy cases, there was a 28% greater cost to laparoscopy. As operative times dropped, however, their last 14 cases were 6% less

expensive than for open nephroureterectomy.[38] However, in none of the communications in which the procedure was performed transperitoneally has the laparoscopic approach been shown to be cost-effective. As such, unlike laparoscopic radical/total nephrectomy, the laparoscopic nephroureterectomy is still in need of further evaluation in order to determine its position vis-à-vis open nephroureterectomy. The most important of these aspects remain: efficacy and cost.

COMPLICATIONS

In published series of laparoscopic transperitoneal standard nephrectomy the complications have included transfusion, ileus, bowel obstruction, wound infection, medical complications, and other organ injuries. Barrett and colleagues reported two patients requiring transfusions and two bowel obstructions in their series. Another patient had a wound infection and another had unstable angina.[39] In the Ono and colleagues

report, two patients out of 60 required blood transfusions. There were intraoperative injuries to the left renal artery, duodenum, spleen, adrenal gland, and a periureteral artery. The duodenal and left renal artery injuries required open conversion. Postoperative complications included two patients with ileus and another with a pulmonary embolus.[36] The group from Washington University also critically examined their series of 61 laparoscopic nephrectomies and found 2 major complications (ligation of the superior mesenteric artery and bleeding requiring conversion). There were 21 minor complications, including several nerve palsies due to positioning, congestive heart failure, ileus, incisional hernia, atelectasis, a torn LapSac in two cases, and pleural effusion.[40] Overall, the complication rate for laparoscopic radical nephrectomy runs 8 to 15%. This compares favorably with the open experience in general, but the incidence of blood transfusions and wound complications is understandably less with the laparoscopic approach.

Table 59-4 Laparoscopic Partial Nephrectomy: Worldwide Experience

Report	n	Approach (TP/RP/HA)	OR Time (hr)	EBL (cc)	Mean Tumor Size (cm)	Hosp. Stay (d)	Recovery (wk)	Follow-up (mo)	Comp	% Benign
Kim et al.[48]	48	TP/RP	3.5	NA	2.1	3	NA	12	14.5%	21%
McDougall et al[49]	9	TP	6.5	217	NA	5.3	4.2	NA	33%	20%
Winfield et al[50]	6	TP	6.1	525	NA	8	NA	NA	16%	NA
Gill et al[51]	100	RP	3	125	2.8	2	4	7.2	5%	30%
Hoznek et al[52]	13	RP	1.9	72	NA	5.3	4.2	22	15%	NA
Wolf et al[53]	10	HA	3.3	460	2.4	2	1.2	3	30%	28%
Stifelman et al[18]	11	HA	4.55	319	1.9	3.3	< 4	NA	18%	55%
Totals	197	–	3.4	179	2.5	2.9	3.8	9.4	35%	29%

HA = hand-assisted; NA = data not available; OR = operating room; TP = transperitoneal; RP = retroperitoneal.

Table 59-5 Comparative Nephroureterectomy Trials (Laparoscopic and Hand-Assisted Laparoscopic versus Open Trials)

Series	n	Operative Approach	OR Time (hr)	EBL (cc)	Analgesic (mg MSO4)	Hosp. Stay (d)	Recovery (wk)	Follow-up (yr)	Major Complications (%)
Shalhav et al[45]	25	Laparoscopic	7.7	199	37	3.6	2.8	2.0	8
	17	Open	3.9	441	144	9.6	10	3.6	29
Seifman et al[54]	16	Hand-assist	5.3	557	48	3.9	2.5	1.5	19
	11	Open	3.3	345	81	5.2	7.5	1.2	27
Keeley and Tolley[55]	22	Laparoscopic	2.4	NA	NA	5.5	NA	NA	NA
	26	Open	2.3	NA	NA	10.8	NA	NA	NA
Total	66	Laparoscopic	5.1	339	41.3	4.4	2.7		10
Total	54	Open	3.0	403	119	9.3	9.0		28

*Alteration in distal ureteral management secondary to recurrences.
NA = data not available.

In regard to retroperitoneal nephrectomies, Abbou and his group summarized an experience of 50 such cases. Two patients had minor complications of atelectasis and local inflammation. Two major complications were encountered: one colon injury requiring temporary diversion and one conversion due to bleeding.[41] Gill reported on his series of 53 retroperitoneal nephrectomies and had 2 major complications, including splenectomy and renal arterial injury requiring conversion. Eight minor complications occurred, including infection, hematoma, ileus, atelectasis, skin rash, and cutaneous hyperesthesia.[42] On average, the complication rate with the retroperitoneal route is very similar to that of the transperitoneal route: 7 to 14%.[43]

In Gill's review of 200 open and laparoscopic partial nephrectomies, a higher major intraoperative complication rate was noted mainly consisting of renal hemorrhage. Postoperatively, no difference was seen in the rate of complications between the two groups.[16] Kim and colleagues from John Hopkins reviewed their series of 73 laparoscopic partial nephrectomies versus a group of 35 laparoscopic nephrectomies.[44] They found that there was no difference in the hospital stay, blood transfusion rate, or surgical complications. There was, however, a significant increase in postoperative serum creatinine levels in the radical nephrectomy, which was not seen in the partial nephrectomy group. These authors felt that, based on this data, partial nephrectomy should be performed whenever possible. Overall, the complication rate with wedge excisions is similar to that of nephrectomy: 8 to 16%.[43]

Shalhav and colleagues' review of 25 nephroureterectomy cases revealed 2 major complications and 10 minor complications. This compared favorably with an open cohort that had 5 major and 5 minor complications.[45] Gill and colleagues reported 42 retroperitoneal cases.[46] Two major complications were noted, consisting of bleeding requiring conversion and extravasation of excessive retroperitoneal bladder irrigant after cystoscopic disarticulation of the ureter. Overall complication rates are higher for nephroureterectomy than for nephrectomy, ranging from 12 to 48%.[43]

CONCLUSIONS

Laparoscopic renal surgery, with its unquestioned benefits on patient pain and recovery, has been established for renal cell carcinoma as being equally efficacious as its open counterpart. In many centers, it is the unquestioned standard of care. For partial nephrectomy and nephroureterectomy, the tide is also turning and will continue to do so as data accumulates. Wave upon wave of progress in minimally invasive surgery continues to fall upon the urological shores; the tide continues to rise.

REFERENCES

1. Clayman RV, Kavoussi LR, Soper NJ, et al. Laparoscopic nephrectomy. N Engl J Med 1991;324:1370.

2. Gill IS, Meraney AM, Schweizer DK, et al. Laparoscopic radical nephrectomy in 100 patients: a single center experience from the United States. Cancer 2001;92:1843.

3. Sundaram CP, Rehman J, Landman J, Oh J. Hand assisted laparoscopic radical nephrectomy for renal cell carcinoma with inferior vena caval thrombus. J Urol 2002; 168:176.

4. Lowry PS, Moon TD, D'Alessandro A, Nakada SY. Symptomatic port-site hernia associated with a non-bladed trocar after laparoscopic live-donor nephrectomy. J Endourol 2003;17:493.

5. Chan DY, Su LM, Kavoussi LR. Rapid ligation of renal hilum during transperitoneal laparoscopic nephrectomy. Urology 2001;57:360.

6. Sundaram CP, Ono Y, Landman J, et al. Hydrophilic guide wire technique to facilitate organ entrapment using a laparoscopic sack during laparoscopy. J Urol 2002;167:1376.

7. Eichel L, Abdelshehid C, Lee DI, et al. In vitro comparison of burst tension and puncture pressure in commonly used organ retrieval bags. 2003. [Submitted]

8. Landman J, Venkatesh R, Kibel A, Vanlangendonck R. Modified renal morcellation for renal cell carcinoma: laboratory experience and early clinical application. Urology 2003;62:632.

9. Cooper CS, Cohen MB, Donovan JF Jr. Splenectomy complicating left nephrectomy. J Urol 1996;155:30.

10. Chan D, Bishoff JT, Ratner L, et al. Endovascular gastrointestinal stapler device malfunction during laparoscopic nephrectomy: early recognition and management. J Urol 2000;164:319.

11. Cicco A, Salomon L, Saint F, et al. [Retroperitoneal laparoscopic surgery and carcinogenic risk]. Prog Urol 2001;11:8.

12. Gill IS, Abreu SC, Desai MM, et al. Laparoscopic ice slush renal hypothermia for partial nephrectomy: the initial experience. J Urol 2003;170:52.

13. Landman J, Venkatesh R, Lee D, et al. Renal hypothermia achieved by retrograde endoscopic cold saline perfusion: technique and initial clinical application. Urology 2003; 61:1023.

14. Sundaram CP, Rehman J, Venkatesh R, et al. Hemostatic laparoscopic partial nephrectomy assisted by a water-cooled, high-density, monopolar device without renal vascular control. Urology 2003;61:906.

15. Guillonneau B, Bermudez H, Gholami S, et al. Laparoscopic partial nephrectomy for renal tumor: single center experience comparing clamping and no clamping techniques of the renal vasculature. J Urol 2003;169:483.

16. Gill IS, Matin SF, Desai MM, et al. Comparative analysis of laparoscopic versus open partial nephrectomy for renal tumors in 200 patients. J Urol 2003;170:64.

17. Simon SD, Ferrigni RG, Novicki DE, et al. Mayo Clinic Scottsdale experience with laparoscopic nephron sparing surgery for renal tumors. J Urol 2003;169:2059.

18. Stifelman MD, Sosa RE, Nakada SY, Shichman SJ. Hand-assisted laparoscopic partial nephrectomy. J Endourol 2001;15:161.

19. Yoshimura K, Okubo K, Ichioka K, et al. Laparoscopic partial nephrectomy with a microwave tissue coagulator for small renal tumor. J Urol 2001;165:1893.

20. Lotan Y, Gettman MT, Ogan K, et al. Clinical use of the holmium:YAG laser in laparoscopic partial nephrectomy. J Endourol 2002;16:289.

21. Corwin TS, Cadeddu JA. Radio frequency coagulation to facilitate laparoscopic partial nephrectomy. J Urol 2001; 165:175.

22. User HM, Nadler RB. Applications of FloSeal in nephron-sparing surgery. Urology 2003;62:342.

23. Gill IS, Desai MM, Kaouk JH, et al. Laparoscopic partial nephrectomy for renal tumor: duplicating open surgical techniques. J Urol 2002;167:469.

24. Wilhelm DM, Ogan K, Saboorian MH, et al. Feasibility of laparoscopic partial nephrectomy using pledgeted compression sutures for hemostasis. J Endourol 2003;17:223.

25. Clayman RV, Kavoussi LR, Figenshau RS, et al. Laparoscopic nephroureterectomy: initial clinical case report. J Laparoendosc Surg 1991;1:343.

26. Kaouk JH, Savage SJ, Gill IS. Retroperitoneal laparoscopic nephroureterectomy and management options for the distal ureter. J Endourol 2001;15:385.

27. Kamihira O, Aichi K, Ono Y, et al. Retroperitoneoscopic nephroureterectomy for transitional cell carcinoma of the renal pelvis and ureter: Nayoga experience. J Urol 164 Suppl. 20, 2002.

28. Jones D, Moisey C. A cautionary tale of the modified "pluck" nephroureterectomy. British J Urol 1993;71:486.

29. Hetherington J, Ewing R, Philip N. Modified nephroureterectomy: a risk of tumor implantation. Br J Urol 1986;58:368.

30. Arango O, Bielsa O, Carles J, Smith S. Massive tumor implantation in the endoscopic resected area in modified nephroureterectomy. J Urol 1893;157:157.

31. Gill IS, Soble J, Miller SD, Smith S. A novel technique for management of the en bloc bladder cuff and distal ureter during laparoscopic nephroureterectomy. J Urol 1999;161:430.

32. Dell'Adami G, Breda G. Transurethral or endoscopic ureterectomy. Eur Urol 1976;2:156.

33. Holmang S, Hedelin H, Anderstrom C, et al. Long-term followup of a bladder carcinoma cohort: routine followup urography is not necessary. J Urol 1998;160:45.

34. Portis AJ, Yan Y, Landman J, et al. Long-term followup after laparoscopic radical nephrectomy. J Urol 2002;167:1257.

35. Chan DY, Cadeddu JA, Jarrett TW, et al. Laparoscopic radical nephrectomy: cancer control for renal cell carcinoma. J Urol 2001;166:2095.

36. Ono Y, Kinukawa T, Hattori R, et al. Laparoscopic radical nephrectomy for renal cell carcinoma: a five-year experience. Urology 1999;53:280.

37. Lotan Y, Gettman MT, Roehrborn CG, et al. Cost comparison for laparoscopic nephrectomy and open nephrectomy: analysis of individual parameters. Urology 2002;59:821.

38. Meraney AM, Gill IS. Financial analysis of open versus laparoscopic radical nephrectomy and nephroureterectomy. J Urol 2002;167:1757.

39. Barrett PH, Fentie DD, Tarager LA. Laparoscopic radical nephrectomy with morcellation for renal cell carcinoma: the Saskatoon experience. Urology 1998;52:23.

40. Dunn MD, Portis AJ, Shalhav AL, et al. Laparoscopic versus open radical nephrectomy: a 9-year experience. J Urol 2000;164:1153.

41. Cicco A, Salomon L, Hoznek A, et al. Results of retroperitoneal laparoscopic radical nephrectomy. J Endourol 2001;15:355.

42. Gill IS. Laparoscopic radical nephrectomy for cancer. Urol Clin North Am 2000;27:707.

43. Eichel L, Clayman RV. Laparoscopic renal surgery: coming of age. 2003. [Submitted]

44. Kim FJ, Rha KH, Hernandez F, et al. Laparoscopic radical versus partial nephrectomy: assessment of complications. J Urol 2003;170:408.

45. Shalhav AL, Dunn MD, Portis AJ, et al. Laparoscopic nephroureterectomy for upper tract transitional cell cancer: the Washington University experience. J Urol 2000; 163:1100.

46. Gill IS, Sung GT, Hobart MG, et al. Laparoscopic radical nephroureterectomy for upper tract transitional cell carcinoma: the Cleveland Clinic experience. J Urol 2000; 164:1513.

47. Janetschek G, Jeschke K, Peschel R, et al. Laparoscopic surgery for stage T1 renal cell carcinoma: radical nephrectomy and wedge resection. Eur Urol 2000;38:131.

48. Kim FJ, Hsu TH, Su LM, et al. Laparoscopic partial nephrectomy. J Urol 2002;167(4 Suppl):3.

49. McDougall EM, Elbahnasy AM, Clayman RV. Laparoscopic wedge resection and partial nephrectomy—the Washington University experience and review of the literature. J Soc Laparoendosc Surg 1998;2:15.

50. Winfield HN, Donovan JF, Lund GO, et al. Laparoscopic partial nephrectomy: initial experience and comparison to the open surgical approach. J Urol 1995;153:1409.

51. Gill IS, Desai MM, Kaouk JH, et al. Laparoscopic partial nephrectomy for renal tumor: duplicating open surgical techniques. J Urol 2002;167:469.

52. Hoznek A, Salomon L, Antiphon P, et al. Partial nephrectomy with retroperitoneal laparoscopy. J Urol 1999;162:1922.

53. Wolf JS Jr, Seifman, BD, Montie JE. Nephron sparing surgery for suspected malignancy: open surgery compared to laparoscopy with selective use of hand assistance. J Urol 2000;163:1659.

54. Seifman BD, Montie JE, Wolf JS Jr. Prospective comparison between hand-assisted laparoscopic and open surgical nephroureterectomy for urothelial cell carcinoma. Urology 2001;57:133.

55. Keeley FX, Tolley DA. Laparoscopic nephroureterectomy: making management of upper-tract transitional-cell carcinoma entirely minimally invasive. J Endourol 1998; 12:139.

60

Laparoscopic Adrenalectomy

Yeh Hong Tan, MD, FRCS
David M. Albala, MD

Since it was described in 1992,[1] laparoscopic adrenalectomy (LA) has become the standard of care for a variety of adrenal lesions in many centers around the world. Multiple studies have reported significant advantages with the laparoscopic approach when compared with the traditional open approach. This minimally invasive approach offers patients less postoperative pain, a shorter hospital stay, a faster return to normal activities, and a better cosmetic result.

Depending on the surgeon's expertise, different approaches have been employed. These include either removing the gland with a transperitoneal (lateral and anterior) or a retroperitoneal (lateral and posterior) laparoscopic technique. In addition to being efficacious, these procedures have also been proven to be safe. The learning curve with these techniques is reasonable, although previous laparoscopic experience greatly facilitates a safe and timely operation and avoids unnecessary conversions to open surgery. The current techniques and results of laparoscopic adrenalectomy will be reviewed.

INDICATIONS

Laparoscopic adrenalectomy is a safe and effective method for removal of most adrenal lesions. Current indications for laparoscopic adrenalectomy include functioning adrenal lesions such as aldosteronoma, pheochromocytoma, and androgen/estrogen, glucocorticoid-producing adenomas. Occasionally, symptomatic adrenal cysts and myelolipomas may be removed laparoscopically. Bilateral LA may also be performed in patients with bilateral adrenal hyperplasia (Cushing syndrome or disease). Nonfunctioning adrenal lesions larger than 4 to 5 cm or tumors that have shown growth in size on serial imaging may also be excised laparoscopically.

The use of laparoscopy in the management of larger malignant masses is somewhat controversial. The lack of a true capsule around the adrenal gland greatly increases the risk of local invasion of these highly aggressive tumors. This makes complete excision and adherence to basic oncologic principles a difficult task, even during open surgical approaches. It is not surprising that long-term survival rates for any surgical approach have been poor, especially when coupled with the lack of effective chemotherapeutic agents.

In light of these difficulties, many surgeons advocate an open approach to known adrenal malignancies or for large lesions (> 8–10 cm). In spite of these fears, there have been multiple reports of effective and complete laparoscopic surgical excision of malignant masses.[2] Prospective, randomized trials are lacking, however, and may be slow in coming because of the relative rarity of these tumors (0.3% of all cancers). Laparoscopic adrenalectomy for adrenal metastasis has also been reported.

CONTRAINDICATIONS

General contraindications for a laparoscopic approach include those patients with an uncorrected coagulopathy, peritonitis, intestinal obstruction, and severe cardiopulmonary disease. However, there are two absolute contraindications for a laparoscopic adrenalectomy. These include patients with an uncontrolled or malignant pheochromocytoma and patients with an adrenal cortical carcinoma with local invasion. Locally advanced tumors with obvious extension to surrounding structures or those with venous involvement are not candidates for laparoscopic excision and should be approached through an open approach.

As noted earlier, adrenal carcinoma remains a relative contraindication for LA because of the concern of tumor clearance and intraoperative spillage. Although the risk of malignancy increases with size, the maximum size of an adrenal lesion suitable for LA is still debatable. Most surgeons agree that tumors greater that 8 cm should be removed with an open approach. Other relative contraindications for LA include morbid obesity and previous abdominal surgery.

Obesity has been suggested to be a relative contraindication of a laparoscopic approach to the adrenal gland. Indeed, early series have shown a higher rate of complications (especially minor) in patients with an elevated body mass index (BMI). While more recent investigators have noted that obesity is associated with longer operating room times and slight increases in complication rates, most authors feel that obese patients are easily managed as the surgeon gains operative experience and advances along the learning curve.[3]

Finally, significant previous abdominal surgery can be a relative contraindication to transperitoneal laparoscopy if adhesions are so dense as to create an unacceptably high risk of inadvertent enterotomy. In this instance, the surgeon can opt for a retroperitoneal approach, either through a standard flank incision or through retroperitoneal laparoscopy.[2]

PREOPERATIVE STUDIES

A complete, step-by-step discussion of the evaluation of a patient with an adrenal lesion is beyond the scope of this textbook. Clearly, each patient requires an assessment of any lesion from a radiologic perspective as well as a full metabolic evaluation.

A complete endocrinologic assessment will entail measurement of serum electrolytes, serum hormone levels, serum catecholamines, urine studies for catecholamines and their metabolites, and urine levels of steroid hormones and their metabolites.

The exact tests ordered will of course depend on observed clinical signs and symptoms and the patient history and physical exam. In addition, stimulation studies such the low- and high-dose dexamethasone suppression tests and plasma renin activity can also be applied as necessary and appropriate. Provided that the surgical lesion has been evaluated completely, patients will require a recent serum chemistry panel prior to surgery to search for significant electrolyte disturbances. Many surgeons advocate checking a complete blood count as well. In the absence of a history of a significant bleeding or coagulopathy disorder, most patients do not require routine coagulation studies (eg, bleeding time, PT, PTT). Any patient who is suspected of harboring a malignant mass should be evaluated for occult metastatic lesions using a chest radiograph and measurement of liver enzymes and alkaline phosphatase.

The development of computed tomography (CT) and magnetic resonance imaging (MRI) has led to improvements in the ability to detect and characterize adrenal lesions with accuracy (Figure 60-1). These imaging studies can provide valuable information on the size of the lesion and extension of the tumor into surrounding structures. Adrenal lesions are commonly found serendipitously on imaging studies performed for other complaints, especially on CT scans. CT imaging using thin cuts, both before and after intravenous contrast, can greatly aid in the assessment of these lesions. Small lesions without enhancement after contrast and Hounsfield measurements of 15 units or less are rarely malignant and do not require further evaluation in the absence of clinical symptoms. MRI scanning can also give useful information on certain lesions such as pheochromocytoma, which has a typical bright light-bulb appearance on T2-weighted images. In certain instances, ^{131}I-metaiodoben-

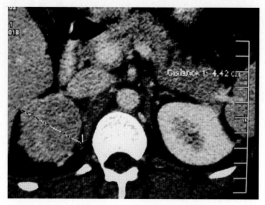

Figure 60-1 CT Scan of a right adrenal tumor.

zylguanidine scintigraphy (MIBG) may be helpful, especially in localizing small or recurrent pheochromocytoma.

PREOPERATIVE PREPARATION

Informed consent is obtained before the surgery. The risks and complications of the procedure, including the possibility of conversion to open surgery, are explained to the patients. A mechanical and antibiotic bowel preparation is given to all patients. This helps decompress the intestines to facilitate exposure during dissection and allows for conservative repair of any inadvertent bowel injury. Broad spectrum antibiotic should be given perioperatively. The patients should be typed and cross-matched for 2 units of blood.

Patients with a functioning tumor require endocrinologic assessment and metabolic correction. In patients with primary hyperaldosteronism, spironolactone may be given preoperatively. The serum potassium levels and blood pressure should be carefully monitored. In patients with Cushing's syndrome, a serum glucose level needs careful monitoring and glucocorticoid replacement may be necessary. In patients with pheochromocytoma, control of blood pressure and cardiac arrhythymias are essential. This usually entails the use of alpha-adrenergic blockade with the subsequent addition of beta-blockade in the presence of arrhythmias. This sequence of blockade is very important as primary beta-blockade can lead to severe hypertension from unopposed alpha agonist activity. Some endocrinologists advocate the use of the tyrosine hydroxylase inhibitor metyrosine as preoperative medical blockade, but this regimen can be difficult to tolerate owing to side effects. As always, close intraoperative monitoring of vitals signs through the use of invasive lines is crucial. This includes arterial lines, central lines, and large-bore catheters for rapid fluid infusion. Anesthesiologists should also be prepared for rapid and drastic shifts in blood pressure (intraoperative hypertension and hypotension after removal of the lesion) and should have vasoactive medications drawn and ready for immediate infusion in the event that the preoperative blockade is incomplete.

OPERATIVE PREPARATION

When performing a laparoscopic adrenalectomy, general anesthesia with endotracheal intubation is used with controlled ventilation to ensure adequate oxygenation and to avoid hypercarbia. Nitrous oxide can lead to bowel distention and should be avoided during this procedure. Intraoperative monitoring of vital signs is important. Central venous lines and arterial lines are placed when necessary. In addition, a nasogastric tube and urinary catheter are inserted to decompress the stomach and bladder prior to creation of the pneumoperitoneum.

INSTRUMENTATION

Operating room requirements for this procedure are relatively straightforward and do not require instrumentation and equipment that should not already be available at most hospitals. A room large enough to accommodate all of the equipment is essential, as the video tower and any additional devices can quickly fill a small room.

Standard laparoscopic equipment is used in all approaches to the adrenal gland. This equipment includes: a 0° or 30° laparoscope, Veress needle, electrocautery, endoscopic retractors, graspers, dissectors and scissors, suction irrigation device, and clip appliers (5 mm or 10 mm). Typically, three to four 10 mm trocars are placed for the dissection of the adrenal gland. A laparoscopic video tower with a video monitor, camera system (single or three chip), and gas insufflator is used. Digital imaging or video recording devices may also be useful. Two video monitors should be used to provide an unobstructed view for the surgeon and the rest of surgical team. We frequently employ a curved dissecting scissors that are connected to electrocautery as the main dissecting instrument. Some advocate the use of hook cautery instead of curved scissors, but this is clearly a matter of personal choice and experience.

Some surgeons advocate the use of high-frequency (harmonic) instruments to divide the adrenal vessels (except the main adrenal vein) and the surrounding fatty tissue. Although we have not routinely used these devices, they clearly can offer an advantage in those patients with excessive retroperitoneal fat. Small bleeders within this redundant fat can be bothersome and difficult to control during a search for the adrenal gland and its vasculature.

Intraoperative ultrasound is occasionally helpful when searching for a small lesion to enucleate. Current devices can be passed intra-abdominally, but require a larger trocar. These instruments can be difficult to use and clearly benefit from operator experience.

A retractor is also necessary to move the spleen or the liver off the adrenal to allow for the complete dissection. A fan device works well and should be safe on the surrounding organs if used appropriately. Malleable, shepherd's crook retractors are also available and are particularly

helpful at raising the liver off Gerota's fascia and the hepatic flexure of the colon. We frequently employ a large, blunt grasper, which can be used to sweep tissues aside as well as to grasp an edge of exposed peritoneum and thereby lift and retract the offending object or tissues.

At the end of the procedure, a specimen entrapment bag is used to retrieve the adrenal tissue. The Endocatch device (US Surgical Corp., Norwalk, CT) is easy to open and has a nice, fixed open mouth into which the specimen is delivered. The LapSac (Cook Urological, Spencer, IN), however, has been proven to be impervious and is the bag of choice for any lesion that is possibly malignant. This device can be cumbersome and requires skill to keep the mouth of the bag open while passing the specimen into its interior. In all cases, open surgical instruments should be available in the operating room in the event a conversion to an open procedure is necessary.

SURGICAL TECHNIQUES

The respective merits of a transperitoneal versus a retroperitoneal laparoscopic approach to the adrenal gland have been greatly discussed in the literature. Most surgeons recognize the inherent difficulties of the reduced operating space with a retroperitoneal route, but espouse the advantages that come with avoidance of the peritoneal cavity and its risk of adhesions and trocar-site hernias. Importantly, retroperitoneal access allows for the rapid mobilization and early ligation of the adrenal vein (especially on the left side). This is particularly important for pheochromocytomas and malignant masses.

Published series have reported the need for increased surgeon experience with retroperitoneoscopy, but have not necessarily noted differences in overall complication rates.[3-6] It is important to note, however, that the retroperitoneal portions of some of these series were performed after the transperitoneal cases, making it difficult to differentiate between the importance of surgeon experience versus the importance of operative approach.

Nevertheless, there are currently no series that specifically address the benefits of one approach over the other when applied to laparoscopy of the adrenal gland. It does seem intuitive to recommend that each case should be planned on an individual basis, accounting for the size of the lesion, the side of the pathology, the patient's past surgical history, and the experience of the surgeon.

POSITIONING The patient is placed in the lateral decubitus (45°–60°) position, with the side of lesion up, and supported with an inflatable beanbag and a protective axillary roll. The operative table is not routinely flexed. The beanbag allows for stabilization of the patient and is further aided by the use of wide silk tape secured to the rails of the bed. The bottom leg is flexed at the hip and knee while the upper leg remains straight. It is important to fully pad all pressure points, including both the top and bottom legs as well as the axilla. The upper arm can be supported on pillows or on a specifically designed holder secured to the bed rail. This position should be very familiar to most urologic surgeons, as it is the same as for a flank approach for extirpative and reconstructive renal surgery.

Pneumatic compression stockings are placed over both legs to reduce venous stasis. The patient's abdomen is then prepped and draped in a conventional fashion.

The surgeon stands facing the patient's abdomen, and the first assistant stands facing the back of the patient. Both the camera operator and scrub nurse stand alongside with the surgeon. The surgeon typically holds an atraumatic grasper in his/her nondominant hand while the dominant hand controls the working instrument.

INSUFFLATION AND TROCAR PLACEMENT For the creation of the pneumoperitoneum, a Veress needle or open Hasson technique may be used, depending on the surgeon's experience. When the Veress needle is placed in the subcostal region along the anterior axillary line, caution should be exercised to prevent a liver or spleen injury. The abdomen is initially distended to 20 mm Hg pressure before insertion of trocars.

The sites of trocar placement vary with the surgeon's preference, taking into account the size and side of the lesion and the body habitus of the patient. In general, four trocars are used for this procedure. Trocars are placed under the ipsilateral costal margin. Two 10/12 mm trocars can be used for the center trocars allowing the surgeon to exchange the laparoscope and a large clip-applier in either position, depending on the best angle of attack. Five mm trocars are generally used at either end of the line to allow for a retractor or a grasper. The center trocars are positioned at the anterior axillary line and the midclavicular line, while the outer trocars are placed in the midline and the posterior axillary line. Except for the initial trocar, all should be placed under direct laparoscopic vision. The pneumoperitoneum is then reduced and maintained at 15 mm Hg pressure throughout the procedure (Figures 60-2 and 60-3).

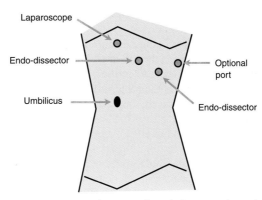

Figure 60-3 Port placement for a left transperitoneal laparoscopic adrenalectomy.

RIGHT TRANSPERITONEAL ADRENALECTOMY After adequate insufflation using a Veress needle, the entire abdomen should be tympanitic after the pneumoperitoneum surrounds the liver. Care must be taken during lateral insufflation to avoid placement of the Veress needle into the liver parenchyma. The abdominal cavity is initially inspected and any overlying adhesions are lysed. The exposure of the right adrenal gland depends on the adequate mobilization of the liver (Figure 60-4). The triangular ligaments of the liver are incised, and the liver is gently retracted in the cephalad direction. The posterior peritoneum is incised close to the liver edge from the line of Toldt laterally to the inferior vena cava medially. The ascending colon and hepatic flexure are routinely mobilized. Gerota's fascia is then incised.

The upper pole of the kidney is identified, and the perinephric fat is dissected superiorly close to the inferior vena cava to expose the adrenal gland. The superior and anterior aspects of the adrenal gland are mobilized. Small blood vessels are controlled with electrocautery and laparoscopic clips. Dissection along the lateral border of the vena cava allows for identification of the right adrenal vein. Meticulous dissection is required to avoid tearing of the adrenal vein (Figure 60-5). When the adrenal vein is isolated, laparoscopic clips are applied, with at least 2 clips on the vena cava side and 1 or 2 clips on the adrenal side. The adrenal vein is then sharply divided between the clips. The

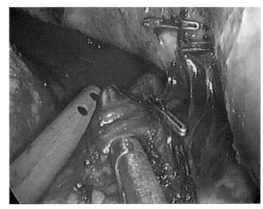

Figure 60-5 Dissection of the right adrenal vein.

inferior and lateral aspects of the adrenal gland are mobilized. The harmonic scalpel is a useful adjunct to facilitate dissection of the adrenal gland. The adrenal gland is dissected free from the surrounding structures. The specimen is placed into an organ entrapment bag before removal through one of the trocar sites (Figure 60-6). The abdominal pressure is then lowered to 5 mm Hg and the operative site is carefully inspected for bleeding before closure of the abdominal trocar sites. The 10/12 mm trocar sites require fascial closure with a 2-0 absorbable suture. A fascial closure device, such as the Puncture Closure Device (ConMed Corp., Utica, NY) can be very helpful and avoids difficult and often blind suturing of the abdominal fascia. The skin is re-approximated with a subcuticular 4-0 absorbable suture. The surgical specimen is then sent to pathology for further examination (Figure 60-7).

LEFT TRANSPERITONEAL ADRENALECTOMY For a left adrenalectomy, the patient is placed in a right lateral decubitus position. After the trocars have been placed as described, the abdominal cavity is similarly inspected with a 30° laparoscope. Using endoscopic scissors or a harmonic scalpel, the splenic flexure of the colon is incised along the line of Toldt. The dissection is continued superiorly to mobilize the spleen to the level of the gastric fundus. The upper pole of the kidney is exposed by freeing the posterolateral attachment

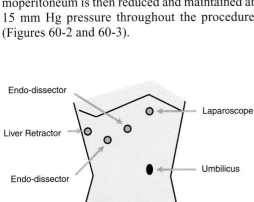

Figure 60-2 Port placement for a right transperitoneal laparoscopic adrenalectomy.

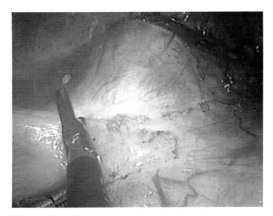

Figure 60-4 Mobilization of a right adrenal tumor.

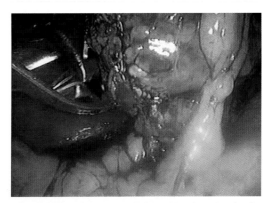

Figure 60-6 Placement of the adrenal tumor in the entrapment sack.

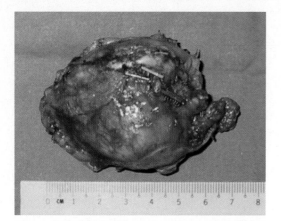

Figure 60-7 The adrenal tumor after removal. Note the clips on the adrenal vein.

of the lienorenal ligament in the direction of the diaphragm. The plane between Gerota's fascia and the pancreatic tail should be developed. The spleen is retracted superiorly and medially to expose the adrenal gland in the retroperitoneal space. This maneuver exposes the adrenal gland and will allow the dissection to begin in the correct plane.

The superior aspect of the adrenal gland is dissected and this dissection is continued medially. The dissection of the inferior portion of the gland should be performed last, as starting here will lead to superior gland retraction and unnecessary bleeding. Small inferior phrenic vessels are ligated with clips after mobilization of the superior pole of the adrenal gland. Medially, the adrenal vein can be identified as it joins the left renal vein. The left adrenal vein is dissected, isolated, and occluded with laparoscopic clips, with at least 2 clips on the patient's side. The vein is then sharply divided between clips. The dissection is then continued along the inferior aspect of the gland. Small vessels should be controlled and divided. The gland is freed after the lateral and posterior attachments have been released. The adrenal gland is placed in a specimen retrieval bag before removal. The bag is removed through the most inferior trocar site with minimal spreading of the oblique muscles using a Kelly clamp. The operative field is inspected at 5 mm Hg pressure to check for hemostasis. The trocar sites are closed in the similar fashion as described previously.

RETROPERITONEAL ADRENALECTOMY Retroperitoneoscopic adrenalectomy can be performed either by lateral flank approach[3,4] or posterior lumbar approach.[5] The retroperitoneal laparoscopic adrenalectomy avoids entering the peritoneal cavity and possible injury to the abdominal organs. The lateral flank approach allows a more spacious working cavity, but a large tumor may obscure the surgical plane to the adrenal vessels. The posterior lumbar approach allows direct access to the main adrenal vascular supply before the gland is manipulated.[6] Depending on the surgeon's experience, a retroperitoneal approach may be used for obese patients and patients with previous abdominal surgery. However, the working space is smaller than the trans-

peritoneal route, and this approach requires a longer learning curve.

In the more common lateral approach, the patient is placed in the full lateral decubitus position (90°) and secured in the standard fashion. The surgeon faces the back of the patient and the assistant stands on the opposite side. Initially, a small incision (2 cm) is made at the midaxillary line above the iliac crest. The incision is deepened until the retroperitoneal space is entered. The posterior pararenal space is developed using digital dissection. An adequate working space can be further developed using a commercially available balloon dilator. The pararenal space is expanded just outside the Gerota's fascia. A 10/12 mm trocar is inserted and the posterior pararenal space is expanded with carbon dioxide gas insufflation at the pressure of 15 mm Hg. The laparoscope is inserted and the other trocars are inserted under direct vision. A trocar (5 mm or 10/12 mm) is placed just below the costal margin in the posterior axillary line.

Using blunt dissection, the peritoneal membrane is reflected medially. A 10/12 mm trocar is inserted at the anterior axillary line below the costal margin. If necessary, an additional 5 mm trocar may be placed above the iliac crest along the anterior axillary line to facilitate intraoperative retraction (Figure 60-8).

After insertion of all trocars, the insufflation pressure is then lowered and maintained at 10 to 12 mm Hg. Gerota's fascia is incised widely in the cephalo-caudad direction. Caution should be taken to avoid inadvertent opening of the peritoneal membrane. Early entry into the perirenal fat to identify the adrenal gland should be avoided, as it can produce hemorrhage, which may obscure the operative field. The perirenal fat is dissected free from the surrounding structures, which include the diaphragm (superiorly), psoas muscle (posteriorly), and medially, the pancreas (left) or liver (right). In some cases, a laparoscopic ultrasound probe may be useful in identifying the adrenal gland.

The perirenal fat is dissected to expose the plane between adrenal gland and the upper pole of the kidney. The adrenal gland is gently lifted superiorly, and the kidney is retracted inferiorly. Small vessels are secured using electrocautery or

clips. The adrenal vein and inferior vena cava are exposed. The adrenal vein is isolated and secured with clips before it is divided. Great care must be taken during lateral retraction of the adrenal gland to avoid tearing the adrenal vein and vena cava on the right side. The rest of the adrenal gland is then freed from the surrounding structures. The specimen is removed using an entrapment bag through the largest trocar site. The insufflation pressure is lowered to 5 mm Hg, and the operative field is then inspected for hemostasis before removal of the trocars. The trocar sites are closed with absorbable suture.

POSTOPERATIVE CARE

In the recovery room, the nasogastric tube and urinary catheter may be removed. All fluids are begun on the day of surgery, if tolerated. Postoperative pain is usually minimal and oral analgesics are prescribed as necessary. Any excessive pain should raise the suspicion of an intra-abdominal complication. Sequential compression devices and stockings are kept in use until the patient is ambulatory. Patients should be encouraged for early ambulation. Patients can be discharged within 1 to 2 days after surgery. Patients may resume their normal activities as tolerated.

In selected patients, a postoperative endocrinologic consultation may be required.

RESULTS

Since 1992, many studies have reported the safety and efficacy of LA. The results of contemporary series are presented[7–13] (Table 60-1). Published results from peer-reviewed journals have consistently shown that LA is both safe and efficacious. Furthermore, operative times have begun to rival those of open procedures as surgeons become more experienced with this technique and with laparoscopy in general. Prospective randomized controlled trials comparing LA with conventional open surgery are unlikely to be undertaken under the present situation, where both surgeons and patients are inclined to adopt a minimally invasive surgical approach.

However, several studies have compared these two approaches retrospectively[14–22] (Table 60-2). These studies have reported a reduced blood loss and lower morbidity. These patients had less pain and fewer analgesic requirements and also reported a faster oral intake and earlier ambulation, shorter hospital stay, and a quicker return to normal activity.

In general, LA takes longer to perform than open surgery. A review of the recent literature demonstrates mean operative times that range from 94 to 188 minutes for the transperitoneal approach and 114 to 178 minutes for retroperitoneal laparoscopy. However, the mean operative times of LA can improve with experience.[14,17] Complication rates in these series have ranged from a low of 2.6% up to 16%, while mortality rates have been reported from 0.0 to 1.3%. Con-

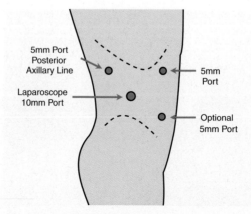

Figure 60-8 Port placement for a retroperitoneal laparoscopic adrenalectomy.

Table 60-1 Contemporary Results of Laparoscopic Adrenalectomy

Authors	No.	Approach	Mean Operative Time (min)	Complications (%)	Hospital Stay (days)	Conversion to Open Surgery (%)
Meria et al[7]	212	Trans	102	10	3.6	14
Castilho et al[8]	94	Trans	117	21.3	6.1	5.1
Pillinger et al[9]	59	Trans	175	6.8	3.8	5.1
Porpiglia et al[11]	72	Trans	130–140	16.7	4.3	4
Kebebew et al[12]	176	Trans/Retro	168	5.1	1.7	0
Salomon et al[10]	115	Retro	118	15.5	4	0.8
Bonjer et al[13]	111	Retro	114	11	2	4.5

version rates for both approaches have been low: 0.9 to 7% for transperitoneal laparoscopy and 0.8 to 5.1% for the retroperitoneal route.

Most striking are the patient comfort parameters. Mean analgesic use, length of hospital stay, and time of convalescence are all markedly lower in the laparoscopic groups. Further improvements in these parameters have been noted in several series of needlescopic patients, although the authors admit that this is more likely related to improving surgeon skill and experience than true superiority of the instrumentation.

For functional adrenal lesions, numerous studies have reported favorable outcomes. In primary hyperaldosteronism, patients who underwent LA experienced fewer complications and a shorter hospital stay. They were equally likely to improve their blood pressure and hypokalemia.[23,24] In patients with Cushing syndrome, the cure rate and operative and long-term morbidity were similar for the laparoscopic and open adrenalectomy approaches.[25] Patients with pheochromocytoma have been successfully treated with LA.[26] Intraoperative hemodynamic values during laparoscopic adrenalectomy for pheochromocytoma were comparable to those of traditional open surgery. Patients who underwent a laparoscopic procedure had a faster post-operative recovery.[27]

Morbid obesity has been associated with increased operative times and with increased blood loss. However, Fazeli-Martin and colleagues reported that laparoscopic adrenal surgery is technically feasible in the markedly and morbidly obese patient. Compared with open surgery, it results in a quicker return of bowel function, less analgesic requirements, shorter convalescence, and a reduced hospital stay.[2]

COMPLICATIONS

As with any laparoscopic surgical procedure, patient selection and the surgeon's experience are extremely important. Judicious patient selection is probably the most important factor that can decrease the morbidity of a laparoscopic adrenalectomy. Patients with relative or absolute contraindications to laparoscopic surgery should be considered for an open surgical procedure.

The size of the lesion and the endocrinologic disorder being treated have had a significant impact on outcomes. In general, tumors larger than 6 cm have an increased risk of malignancy. Larger lesions are also technically challenging. Patients with Conn syndrome are likely to develop electrolyte abnormalities and require monitoring of blood pressure. Patients with Cushing syndrome may require postoperative steroid supplement. In patients with pheochromocytoma, close perioperative monitoring of blood pressure is essential. Cardiovascular complications, including stroke, may develop if appropriate measures are not taken.

To avoid complications, care should be taken during creation of the pneumoperitoneum. The Veress needle should be placed in proper position to avoid injury to the liver, spleen, and intestines. Alternatively, a Hasson technique for initial trocar placement can be used. During dissection, caution should be exercised to avoid injury to the surrounding structures such as the bowel and pancreas. These injuries should be recognized and repaired accordingly. When indicated, either a laparoscopic repair or open laparotomy should be performed.

Vascular complications are the most serious and may involve injury to the adrenal vessels, renal arteries and veins, and the inferior vena cava. Laparoscopic control of a vascular injury may be attempted with electrocautery or clips. In some cases, intracorporeal suturing may be used. When the patient is hemodynamically unstable or control is difficult, it is mandatory to proceed with open exploration to control the bleeding.

In the postoperative period, early ambulation is encouraged to reduce the risk of a deep vein thrombosis. In selected patients, chest physiotherapy is required to prevent lung atelectasis. Postoperative shoulder pain is a common, though usually a self-limited complication.

CONCLUSION

Laparoscopic adrenalectomy is a safe, proven, and effective option for treating patients with small-sized benign adrenal tumors. This is an advanced laparoscopic procedure and should be undertaken only by those with extensive laparoscopic experience. Small solitary adrenal metastasis may also be excised laparoscopically. The greatest controversy surrounding laparoscopic adrenalectomy is its application for adrenal cancer. The literature is replete with case reports and small series, but lacks direct comparisons with open, oncologic surgery. The final decision over the relevance of laparoscopy for adrenal cancer will be determined by time and increasing experience, but it appears highly likely that it will grow to replace open surgery at many centers.

Table 60-2 Comparative Studies of Open and Laparoscopic Adrenalectomy

Authors	Approach	No.	Operative Time (min)	Complications (%)	Blood Loss (mL)	Hospital Stay (days)
Tan et al[14]	Open	48	87	27	—	7.2
	Lap	58	128	5.2	—	3.2
Dudley et al[15]	Open	23	85	52	426	8.5
	Lap	36	158	5.6	194	3.5
Gill et al[16]	Open	100	219	27	563	7.6
	Lap	110	189	10	125	1.9
Vargas et al[17]	Open	20	178	25	283	7.2
	Lap	20	193	10	245	3.1
Winfield et al[18]	Open	17	140	5.8	266	6.2
	Lap	21	219	14	183	2.7
Thompson et al[19]	Open	50	126	18	—	5.7
	Lap	50	168	6	—	3.1
Hazzan et al[20]	Open	28	139	39	—	7.5
	Lap	28	188	16	—	4.0
Hallfeldt et al[21]	Open	30	106	27	380	10
	Lap	40	135	13	260	7
Imai et al[22]	Open	40	127	50	162	18
	Lap	41	180	0.5	40	12

REFERENCES

1. Gagner M, Lacroix A, Bolte E. Laparoscopic adrenalectomy in Cushing's syndrome and pheochromocytoma. N Engl J Med 1992;327:1033.
2. Fazeli-Martin S, Gill IS, Hsu TH, et al. Laparoscopic renal and adrenal surgery in obese patients: comparison to open surgery. J Urol 1999;162:665–9.
3. Suzuki K. Laparoscopic adrenalectomy: retroperitoneal approach. Urol Clin North Am 2001;28:85–95.
4. Sung GT, Hsu TH, Gill IS. Retroperitoneoscopic adrenalectomy: lateral approach. J Endourol 2001;15:505–11.
5. Baba S, Miyajima A, Uchida A, et al. A posterior lumbar approach for retroperitoneoscopic adrenalectomy: assessment of surgical efficacy. Urology 1997;50:19–24.
6. Baba S, Iwamura M. Retroperitoneal laparoscopic adrenalectomy. Biomed Pharmacother 2002;56 Suppl 1:113s–9s.
7. Meria P, Kempf BF, Hermieu JF, et al. Laparoscopic management of primary hyperaldosteronism: clinical experience with 212 cases. J Urol 2003;169:32–5.
8. Castilho LN, Mitre AI, Arap S. Laparoscopic adrenal surgery in a Brazilian center. J Endourol 2003;17:11–8.
9. Pillinger SH, Bambach CP, Sidhu S. Laparoscopic adrenalectomy: a 6-year experience of 59 cases. ANZ J Surg 2002;72:467–70.

10. Salomon L, Soulie M, Mouly P, et al. Experience with retroperitoneal laparoscopic adrenalectomy in 115 procedures. J Urol 2001;166:38–41.
11. Porpiglia F, Garrone C, Giraudo G, et al. Transperitoneal laparoscopic adrenalectomy: experience in 72 procedures. J Endourol 2001;15:275–9.
12. Kebebew E, Siperstein AE, Duh QY. Laparoscopic adrenalectomy: the optimal surgical approach. J Laparoendosc Adv Surg Tech A 2001;11:409–13.
13. Bonjer HJ, Sorm V, Berends FJ, et al. Endoscopic retroperitoneal adrenalectomy: lessons learned from 111 consecutive cases. Ann Surg 2000;232:796–803.
14. Tan YH, Yip SK, Chee C, Cheng CW. Comparison of laparoscopic and open adrenalectomy—a Singapore experience. Asian J Surg 2002;25:330–4.
15. Dudley NE, Harrison BJ. Comparison of open posterior versus transperitoneal laparoscopic adrenalectomy. Br J Surg 1999;86:656–60.

16. Gill IS. The case for laparoscopic adrenalectomy. J Urol 2001;166:429–36.
17. Vargas HI, Kavoussi LR, Bartlett DL, et al. Laparoscopic adrenalectomy: a new standard of care. Urology 1997;49:673–8.
18. Winfield HN, Hamilton BD, Bravo EL, Novick AC. Laparoscopic adrenalectomy: the preferred choice? A comparison to open adrenalectomy. J Urol 1998;160:325–9.
19. Thompson GB, Grant CS, van Heerden JA, et al. Laparoscopic versus open posterior adrenalectomy: a case-control study of 100 patients. Surgery 1997;122:1132–6.
20. Hazzan D, Shiloni E, Golijanin D, et al. Laparoscopic vs open adrenalectomy for benign adrenal neoplasm. Surg Endosc 2001;15:1356–8.
21. Hallfeldt KK, Mussack T, Trupka A, et al. Laparoscopic lateral adrenalectomy versus open posterior adrenalectomy for the treatment of benign adrenal tumors. Surg Endosc 2003;17:264–7.

22. Imai T, Kikumori T, Ohiwa M, et al. A case-controlled study of laparoscopic compared with open lateral adrenalectomy. Am J Surg 1999;178:50–3.
23. Duncan JL 3rd, Fuhrman GM, Bolton JS, et al. Laparoscopic adrenalectomy is superior to an open approach to treat primary hyperaldosteronism. Am Surg 2000;66:932–5.
24. Shen WT, Lim RC, Siperstein AE, et al. Laparoscopic vs open adrenalectomy for the treatment of primary hyperaldosteronism. Arch Surg 1999;134:628–31.
25. Acosta E, Pantoja JP, Gamino R, et al. Laparoscopic versus open adrenalectomy in Cushing's syndrome and disease. Surgery 1999;126:1111–6.
26. Janetschek G, Finkenstedt G, Gasser R, et al. Laparoscopic surgery for pheochromocytoma: adrenalectomy, partial resection, excision of paragangliomas. J Urol 1998;160:330–4.
27. Sprung J, O'Hara JF Jr., Gill IS, et al. Anesthetic aspects of laparoscopic and open adrenalectomy for pheochromocytoma. Urology 2000;55:339–43.

61

Laparoscopic Ureteral Reconstructive Surgery

John M Varkarakis, MD

Louis R. Kavoussi, MD

Laparoscopic cholecystectomy heralded a new era of surgical practice. This procedure demonstrated that extirpative abdominal surgery could be successfully accomplished through small incisions while significantly decreasing postoperative analgesic requirements, length of hospital stay, and duration of convalescence.[1] This seminal application led to the widespread adoption of laparoscopy in other surgical specialties, including urology, where it was first used for diagnostic pelvic lymph node dissection in patients with prostate cancer.[2] Evolution in instrumentation design and operative techniques shifted focus from an extirpative to a reconstructive focus. One of the most challenging areas of urologic surgery involves ureteral surgery. The small caliber and delicate nature of this organ, makes reconstruction particularly challenging, but modern methods now provide for successful laparoscopic management of a variety of ureteral pathologies, including ureteral malignancies, ureteropelvic junction obstruction (UPJ), impacted ureteral calculi, strictures, and retroperitoneal fibrosis. Worldwide experience has demonstrated that a laparoscopic approach to urologic disease of the ureter is an effective and equivalent minimally invasive alternative to traditional open surgical repair.

ANATOMIC CONSIDERATIONS

A comprehensive knowledge of ureteral anatomy is essential when performing a laparoscopic procedure. For surgical purposes, the ureter is divided into the abdominal, or upper portion, and the pelvic, or lower portion. The abdominal ureter extends from the kidney to the iliac vessels. It originates at the UPJ and courses along the psoas muscle before crossing the genitofemoral nerve at the level of the fourth lumbar vertebra. The gonadal vessels pass anteriorly over the mid upper ureter. The ureter extends toward the pelvic brim to cross the external iliac vessels on the right and the common iliac vessels on the left. Once the ureter has entered the pelvis, it courses posterior and medial to the medial umbilical ligament and enters the detrusor muscle just posterior to the superior vesicle artery. Important structures adjacent to the distal ureter include the vas deferens in the male and the round ligament, uterine artery, and broad ligament in the female. These structures lie anteriorly and may need to be divided to gain access to the distal ureter.

The upper ureter derives its blood supply from the renal artery, the mid-ureter is fed by branches from the aorta and gonadal artery, while the lower portion of the ureter is served by branches of the common iliac, internal iliac and vesical arteries. Once these vessels reach the ureter, they course longitudinally within the periureteral adventitia, forming an extensive plexus. As such, ligation of much of the blood supply will not impact on viability in a healthy ureter.

It is important to recognize the normal relationship between the renal pelvis and hilar vessels. The renal artery and vein are anterior to the renal pelvis, with the vein located most anterior. The renal artery divides into several branches, with the posterior being the most consistent and the first to branch. The anterior branch divides into four segmental arteries (apical, upper, middle, and lower). Anomalous blood vessels can supply segments of the kidney. Lower-pole vessels causing ureteropelvic junction (UPJ) obstruction usually course anterior to the ureter.

Gerota's fascia is connected to the lateral parietal peritoneum by the lateroconal fascia. The space between this fascia and the posterior peritoneum is the anterior pararenal space, whereas the space dorsolateral to this fascia is the posterior pararenal space. This is the space entered during retroperitoneoscopy.

Of importance is the way the posterior peritoneum and the lateral peritoneal reflection behave when the patient changes position. Moving the patient from a supine to a flank position displaces the peritoneal reflection from the posterior axillary line, anteriorly because of the downward movement of the colon. This increases the retroperitoneal space and decreases the potential of entering the peritoneal cavity when placing the trocars for retroperitoneoscopy.

The pelvic extraperitoneal space where the lower ureter will be found is the preperitoneal space caudal to the pelvic brim and between the parietal peritoneum and the fascia transversalis. Retzius' space is also considered a part of this space.

PATIENT SELECTION

Patients with uncorrectable bleeding abnormalities, abdominal wall infection, generalized peritonitis; malignant ascites, and massive hemoperitoneum are at higher risk during laparoscopic surgery. Large aortic and iliac aneurisms, a history of previous renal trauma, and a history of prior retroperitoneal or transperitoneal surgery, can increase the difficulty of the procedure but do not preclude laparoscopy from being performed

by a surgeon with laparoscopic expertise. Informed consent should always be obtained, not only for the laparoscopic procedure but for an open procedure as well, in case conversion becomes necessary. The patient should know the procedure-dependent complications as well as the complications involved with laparoscopy itself.

PREOPERATIVE EVALUATION AND PREPARATION

Laboratory testing should be individualized, but urine should be collected for microscopic analysis and/or culture. A blood type and screen should be performed on all patients. No aspirin or aspirin-like compounds should have been taken within 5 days of surgery.

Radiographic and other specialized preoperative studies will be discussed for each surgical technique. X-ray films should be available and placed on the view box in the operating suite before beginning the procedure.

Pyelography should be a starting point in the evaluation of a patient with ureteral pathology. The intravenous or computed tomography (CT) pyelograms define the anatomy of the collecting system on the affected side. A diuretic nuclear renal scan is helpful in quantifying the degree of obstruction, if present, and documents the relative percentage of kidney function. The function in kidneys with high-grade obstruction is best assessed after the kidney is drained. A retrograde pyelogram before laparoscopic intervention is helpful in evaluating the ureter and delineating the length of obstruction if not seen on other imaging.

OPERATIVE PREPARATION

Many of the preoperative steps are common to all laparoscopic ureteral surgery procedures. Attention to these details will facilitate successful visualization of the ureter and minimize complications. A combination of ampicillin and gentamicin or a single dose of a third-generation cephalosporin is administered intravenously on arrival at the operating room. Pneumatic compression stockings are placed before induction of general anesthesia. A nasogastric or orogastric tube should be placed and the stomach emptied. The bladder should also be emptied using a Foley catheter.

For upper ureteral laparoscopic procedures, the patient is placed in a 60° lateral decubitus position. A roll is placed behind the back to support the patient, and the contralateral arm is padded and tucked alongside the patient (Figure 61-1). The ipsilateral arm is draped across the chest over egg crate padding with the elbow gently bent cephalad. The ipsilateral shoulder is also rotated cephalad to move the arm away from the operative field, allowing maximal mobility of the laparoscope and operating instruments. The hips and legs are kept supine, with a pillow placed behind the knees and padding the heels. Wide cloth tape is placed across the shoulder and hip to secure the patient to the table. The lower legs should be secured with tape or straps below the knees. The table should be test-rolled prior to placing drapes to be certain that the patient is secured to the operating table.

The abdomen and exposed flank are shaved and prepared from the xiphoid to mid-thigh, including the genitals. Monitors are positioned at the upper one-third of the table across from the surgeon and assistant (Figure 61-2).

For lower ureteral laparoscopic procedures, the patient is placed in the supine position. Each arm is positioned alongside the patient. Additional padding is placed along the arms, under the knees, and underneath the heels. The monitors are positioned at the foot of the table (Figure 61-3).

TRANSPERITONEAL ACCESS

Port placement is individualized for each procedure. The trocar size chosen varies with each case and according to surgeon preference. The upper ureter can most easily be accessed with the patient in the flank position (see Figure 61-2). To establish a pneumoperitoneum, a Veress needle is introduced in the umbilicus. The peritoneal cavity is insufflated to a pressure of 15 to 20 mm Hg. Three midline trocars are used for upper ureteral surgery: a 10-mm umbilical trocar, a 5-mm trocar 1/3 inferior to the xiphoid, and a 12-mm trocar half way between the umbilicus and pubis (Figure 61-4).

Trocar placement to approach the lower pelvic ureter is accomplished with the patient in the supine position. A Veress needle is placed through the umbilicus, and pneumoperitoneum is established to a pressure of 15 to 20 mm Hg. Initial trocar placement is performed through a semicircular 1-cm incision at the umbilicus. One or two ports are positioned in each lower quadrant 2 cm medial to the corresponding anterior superior iliac spine. This configuration provides optimal access to the pelvic ureter from the iliac vessels to the ureterovesical junction (Figure 61-5). When approaching the entire ureter, a combination port placement is required (Figure 61-6). All ports are secured in position with 2-0 Vicryl sutures. In case of scars due to prior surgery, either the Hasson cannula or the Veress needle is initially placed in a scar-free area of the abdomen, preferably the upper left or right quadrant.

RETROPERITONEAL ACCESS

With the patient in a flank position, the table is flexed, opening the costoiliac space. A 2-cm skin

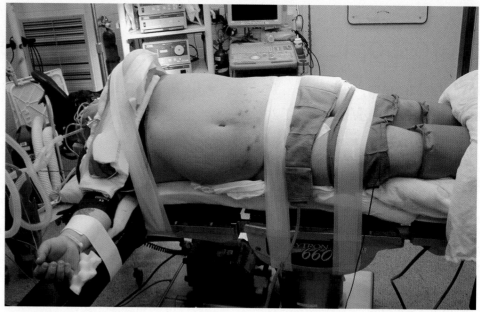

Figure 61-1 60° flank position.

incision is made below the tip of the 12th rib. The flank muscle fibers are bluntly separated using the S-retractors. After the anterior thoracolumbar fascia is opened and access to the retroperitoneum is gained, finger dissection between the psoas muscle and the posterior Gerota's fascia is performed in order to create the initial space where the balloon dilator will be placed. Mobilization can be carried anteromedially in order to bluntly detach the lateral peritoneal deflection from the undersurface of the anterolateral abdominal wall to allow more space for the trocar placement. A trocar-mounted silicone balloon distention device[3] (Origin Medsystems, Menlo Park, CA) is placed in the space made in the retroperitoneum. Installation of 800 mL of air in the balloon will create adequate space. In the pediatric population 400 mL is sufficient. For ureteral surgery, secondary balloon dilation cau-

dal to the initial site of dilatation is done in order to create access to the middle and lower ureter.

Following balloon deflation and removal of the device, a 10-mm Bluntport trocar (Origin Medsystems) is placed in the 2-cm incision. This trocar has an internal fascial retention balloon and an external foam cuff, which provides an airtight seal. Pneumoperitoneum is then achieved and the remaining ports are placed with a combination of direct camera guidance and manual control.

The limited retroperitoneal space forces trocars to be placed closer one to another. This can lead to limited visualization of the entry tip of the secondary trocars. Although individualized, the camera is placed through the 10-mm primary port while a set of secondary ports are placed, one at the anterior axillary line, two to three fingerbreadths above the anterosuperior iliac spine, and the other at the lateral border of the paraspinal muscles along the inferior border of the 12th rib.

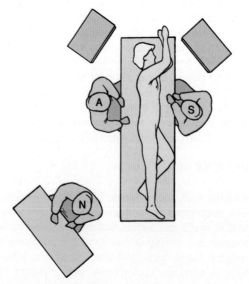

Figure 61-2 Positioning of operating room equipment and personnel for laparoscopic approach to right abdominal ureter.

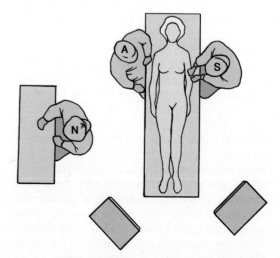

Figure 61-3 Positioning of operating room equipment and personnel for laparoscopic approach to right pelvic ureter.

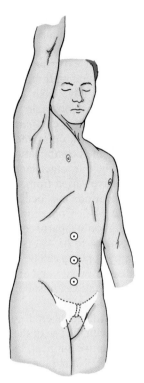

Figure 61-4 Port placement for approach to abdominal ureter. The optional 5-mm port is used for retraction.

LAPAROSCOPIC DISMEMBERED PYELOPLASTY

Ureteropelvic junction obstruction can be caused by a congenital intrinsic narrowing of the lumen or by external compression, usually by a crossing vessel. Preoperative evaluation includes a diuretic renogram, and an intravenous pyelogram (IVP). Confirmation can be obtained at the time of surgery with a retrograde pyelography. Other diagnostic methods such as CT angiography,[4] endoluminal ultrasonography,[5] and contrast-enhanced color Doppler ultrasonography[6] can be used in

case an obstructing vessel is suspected. When laparoscopic repair is scheduled, the abovementioned tests are not mandatory. Direct intraoperative observation obtained with laparoscopy will make the diagnosis of the crossing vessel.

Open pyeloplasty for the repair of UPJ obstruction was the standard treatment for several decades, with success rates of > 90% having been reported in several large series.[7,8] The morbidity associated with a flank incision, however, has led to the development of minimally invasive retrograde and antegrade approaches to UPJ repair. These endoscopic techniques have success rates of 70 to 88%.[9–11] A fluoroscopically placed ureteral cutting balloon (Acucise, Applied Medical Resources, Laguna Hills, CA) provided an even less invasive alternative, although early success rates of only 70% had been reported.[12]

In 1993, laparoscopic pyeloplasty was introduced to reconstruct the UPJ under direct vision.[13,14] The rationale was to develop a procedure that had the advantages of minimal morbidity achieved with endourologic approaches while maintaining the high success rate of open pyeloplasty. This approach has been successful in a variety of pathologies, including patients with UPJ obstruction secondary to a crossing vessel, a high ureteral insertion, a large redundant renal pelvis, or those who failed a prior endoscopic repair.

TECHNIQUE Transperitoneal Approach The patient is positioned in a lateral position for access to the upper ureter. A retrograde pyelogram is obtained and a 7 French double pigtail ureteral stent is placed. It is important to select a stent that can extend from the bladder to the upper pole collecting system to prevent the curl of the stent from lying at the anastomosis because

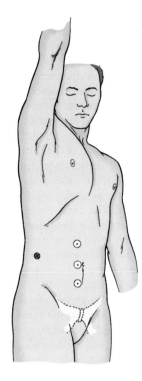

Figure 61-7 Port placement for dismembered pyeloplasty. The optional 5-mm port is used for retraction.

this will make reconstruction more challenging. Port placement for access to the UPJ may be augmented by an additional 5-mm trocar placed in the anterior axillary line midway between the costal margin and the iliac crest (Figure 61-7).

The kidney and renal pelvis are identified lateral to the colon just beneath the peritoneum. The peritoneum overlying the kidney is incised from upper pole to 4 cm below the lower pole, and the colon retracted medially (Figure 61-8). Positioning the patient laterally allows the colon to fall medially. The ureter can usually be identified by following the psoas muscle medially from the lower pole of the kidney. A sweeping motion with graspers perpendicular to the course of the ureter is used to bluntly dissect loose areolar tissue and identify the ureter. Dissection around the ureter distal to the UPJ should be minimized to preserve blood supply. Palpation of the indwelling ureteral stent aids in following the course of the ureter to the UPJ. Care should be taken not to confuse the gonadal vessels and the ureter. If these vessels are impeding ade-

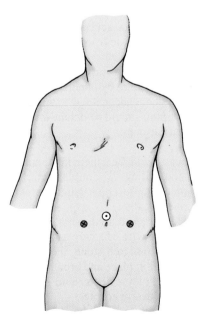

Figure 61-5 Port placement for approach to pelvic ureter.

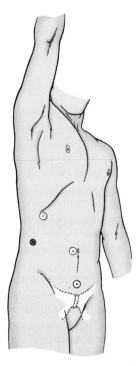

Figure 61-6 Combination port placement for access to entire ureter.

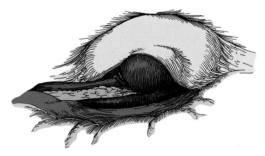

Figure 61-8 Incision of peritoneal reflection and medial mobilization of colon to expose the right ureteropelvic junction.

quate visualization, they can usually be swept medially, but on occasion, they need to be ligated and transected. Once the renal pelvis is identified, it should be dissected free to obtain adequate length to perform a tension-free repair. If a lower pole crossing artery is encountered, we recommend preservation to maximize future renal function.

Scissors are used to transect the renal pelvis above the UPJ and care should be taken not to spiral the incision or cut the ureteral stent. The proximal end of the stent is pulled from the pelvis after the anterior incision in the renal pelvis is completed. The posterior wall of the pelvis is then transected. The ureter is spatulated using the 5-mm scissors, and the diseased portion is incised and removed. Care must be taken not to pull the stent out of the ureter during this maneuver. A reduction pyeloplasty can be performed at this time if necessary.

If an anterior lower pole vessel is encountered, it is transposed behind the renal pelvis. A 4-0 Vicryl suture is placed between the apex of the spatulated ureter and the dependent portion of the renal pelvis. The posterior row of sutures are then placed using interrupted or running 4-0 Vicryl sutures. The proximal end of the ureteral stent is then repositioned in the renal pelvis, and the anterior row of interrupted or running sutures are placed (Figure 61-9). The excess pyelotomy incision above the repair is closed using a running 4-0 Vicryl suture.

A 5-mm suction drain is passed through the lateral 5-mm port site. This drain is positioned near the posterior aspect of the reconstructed UPJ and secured externally to the skin with a 3-0 silk suture. The colon is replaced in its original position over the repair, and the procedure is concluded in a standard fashion.

The nasogastric tube is removed in the operating room, and the Foley catheter is taken out on the second postoperative day. The flank drain is removed when the drainage becomes negligible, usually on the second postoperative day. If drain output increases, the Foley catheter is placed again for 48 hours. A clear liquid diet is begun on the night of surgery and advanced as tolerated. Parenteral antibiotics are continued for 24 hours. The ureteral stent is removed 3 weeks postoperatively. The repair is evaluated on an IVP 6 weeks after stent removal, and a nuclear renal scan is obtained 3 months postoperatively.

Retroperitoneal Approach The patient is placed in a flank extended position. After developing the retroperitoneal space off the tip of the 12th rib, two secondary ports are placed at the anterior and posterior axillary line and at the same axial plane. Additional trocars can be placed making the port configuration a T or W shape.

The retroperitoneal approach although offering less space than the transperitoneal, has the theoretical advantage of identification of the ureter immediately after entering the retroperitoneal space. If the ureter is not readily seen, attention is paid to the hilar fat in order to identify the pulsating renal artery, and this will lead to the renal pelvis. Further ureteral dissection and

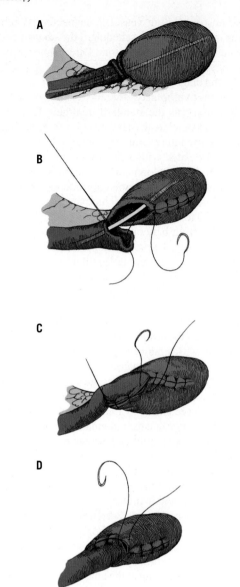

Figure 61-9 Reconstruction of a ureteropelvic junction obstructed by a lower-pole vessel. *A*, Proposed incision. *B*, Apex of spatulated ureter is anastomosed to dependent portion of renal pelvis after lower-pole vessel posterior transposition. *C*, Rotation of ureter to provide access for posterior rows of interrupted sutures. *D*, Completion of anterior row of sutures to complete anastomosis.

pyeloplasty technique are performed as described previously for the transabdominal approach.

RESULTS Several large series of laparoscopic pyeloplasties demonstrate success rates equivalent to open surgery (Table 61-1). Jarrett and colleagues addressed the question of durability of this procedure in a review of 99 patients who underwent laparoscopic pyeloplasty and had up to a 6-year follow (mean 2.2 years).[15] Their success rate was 96%, and all cases that failed did so in the first year. There were no late recurrences.

Compared to other minimally invasive techniques, improved results are seen due to the fact that both open surgery and laparoscopy can definitively address a crossing vessel.

In a comparative study, Brooks and colleagues demonstrated lower analgesic requirements, shorter hospital stays, and faster recover-

ies for laparoscopic surgery compared with other minimally invasive techniques.[16] Operation time was the highest for the laparoscopic approach, but with increasing experience and improved instrumentation, operating times decreased.

Complications have also decreased with experience and are comparable with rates seen with open surgery. In a comparative study by Bauer and colleagues, open and laparoscopic pyeloplasty presented complications at 11% and 12%, respectively.[17] In other large series, complication rates have varied from 4% to 30%. All type of complications can occur and are presented in Table 61-2. Conversion rates depend upon each surgeon's laparoscopic experience and range from 1.4 to 45.4% (see Table 61-1). Laparoscopic pyeloplasty can be performed both by the transperitoneal and retroperitoneal approach. Complications, hospital stay, and success rates are comparable.

Laparoscopic dismembered pyeloplasty has been performed with the use of the da Vinci Surgical System (Intuitive Surgical, Inc., Sunnyvale, CA) in 9 patients.[18] No intraoperative complications occurred, and open conversion was not necessary. The only postoperative complication was an open exploration required to repair a defect in the renal pelvis. Mean operating time was 138.8 minutes (range, 80 to 215 minutes), and hospital stay was 4.7 days (range, 4 to 11 days). Operating times decreased due to diminished suturing times (mean 62.4 minutes). Long-term efficacy data were not available due to short follow-up (mean 4.1 months).

URETEROLITHOTHOMY

The development of extracorporeal shock wave lithotripsy and improvements in endoscopic, ultrasonic, laser, pneumatic, and electrohydraulic-lithotripsy devices have greatly reduced the need for open ureteral stone extractions. A small number of patients still fail these techniques and may require open removal. Raboy and colleagues first described a laparoscopic method for ureterolithotomy that is an acceptable alternative to open surgery when less invasive endourologic approaches fail.[19]

Ureteral anatomy must be clearly defined prior to the procedure by obtaining an IVP. If the distal ureter is not adequately visualized, a retrograde pyelogram should be obtained to rule out a concomitant stricture.

TECHNIQUE With the patient in the supine position, an indwelling 7F double-pigtail stent is placed under fluoroscopic guidance. An open-ended ureteral catheter can be advanced to the level of the stone and used to assist in bypassing the stone with a wire. If a wire cannot be maneuvered past an impacted stone, then the external stent can be left in place and brought out through a council tip Foley catheter and secured via a Tuohy-Borst sidearm adapter.

The patient is positioned on the table according to the position of the stone. A stone located in

Table 61-1 Laparoscopic Pyeloplasty

Study	Number of Patients	Operative Times	Approach (minutes)	Conversion Rate (%)	Complications (%) Intraop	Complications (%) Postop	Postop Hospital Stay (days)	Success Rate (%)
Schuessler et al[13]	5	Transperitoneal	330, 210–240	—	—	20	3	80
Kavousssi & Peters[14]	1	Transperitoneal	480	—	—	—	3	100
Recker et al[58]	5	Transperitoneal	305, 190–390	20	—	—	8, 7–10	100
Nakada et al[59]	4	Transperitoneal	530, 465–645	—	—	—	4, 3–11	100
Janetschek et al[60]	11	Transperitoneal & retroperitoneal	215, 120–360	9	—	18.1	5.1, 3–11	100
Chen et al[61]	13	Transperitoneal	340, 240–360	—	15	15	3.2, 2–4	100
Moore et al[62]	30*	Transperitoneal	270, 135–480	—	3.3	6.6	3.4, 2–6	96.6
Puppo et al[63]	11	Retroperitoneal	190, 150–240	45.4	—	—	3.3, 4–7	63.4
Chen et al[61]	57*	Transperitoneal	258, 138–480	—	3.5	8.8	3.3, 2–6	—
Bauer et al[17]	42*	Transperitoneal	—	—	2.4	9.5	—	98
Ben Slama et al[64]	15*	Retroperitoneal	178, 100–250	6.6	—	20	4.8, 1–14	100
Janetchek et al[65]	67*	Transperitoneal & retroperitoneal	119, 189–210	1.4	—	—	4.1	98.5
Soulie et al[66]	55*	Retroperitoneal	185, 100–260	5.4	—	12.7	4.5, 1–14	88.9
Eden et al[67]	50	Retroperitoneal	164, 120–240	4	—	4	2.6, 2–7	98
Jarrett et al[15]	100*	Transperitoneal	252, 120–480	—	2	11	3.5, 2–8	96

Intra = intraoperatively; Postop = postoperatively.

*Patients with non-dismembered pyeloplasty included.

the upper ureter is approached with the patient in the lateral position, and port placement is similar to that for laparoscopic pyeloplasty (see Figure 61-4). For lower ureteral stones, the patient can be maintained in the supine position with the trocars placed as shown in Figure 61-10.

The line of Toldt is incised as previously described in the region near the position of the stone. The retroperitoneal course of the ureter is exposed once the colon or sigmoid is reflected medially. Tilting the table away from the side of the stone allows the bowel to fall away from the operative field. Gentle grasping or transverse sweeping movements can be used to identify the position of the ureteral calculus, since the stone is usually palpable. Moreover, the ureter is usually visually dilated above the point of obstruction. Radiographic localization of the stone using fluoroscopy may be helpful if the stone is not readily apparent.

Once the stone is located, a longitudinal incision is made in the ureter using 5-mm scissors. The incision is made just large enough to allow the stone to be removed intact. By gently milking the ureter, the stone can be delivered through the incision (Figure 61-11). Every attempt should be made to remove the stone intact. An organ entrapment sack may be used for large stones.

An internal stent should be positioned in patients in whom a preoperative stent could not be passed beyond the stone. This is accomplished by passing a wire through the external stent and guiding it under direct vision up the proximal ureter. The external stent is removed and an indwelling double-pigtail stent can be passed over the wire. Position should be verified both cystoscopically and radiographically.

The ureterotomy can be loosely reapproximated over the ureteral catheter using interrupted 4-0 Vicryl sutures (see Figure 61-11). Alternatively, if the incision is less than 1 cm, it may be left open to heal over a stent. A urethral

catheter is placed. A retroperitoneal suction drain may be placed in a fashion similar to that described for laparoscopic pyeloplasty.

For the retroperitoneal technique, the patient is in the flank position. A small incision is made at the tip of the 12th rib, through which the retroperitoneal space is balloon-dissected. If the stone is located lower, the balloon dissector is repositioned so dissection continues more distally. The first port is placed in this incision. Two more ports are placed with a combination of direct vision and manual guidance. One 10-mm port is placed at the superior edge of the iliac crest, the other 5-mm trocar posterior and lateral to the lumbar muscles at the one end of a line that passes over a standard subcostal incision. After balloon dissection, the stone location is usually evident and few further dissection is needed to reach the bulging ureter. The following steps are similar to those followed in the transabdominal approach.

Once drainage has become minimal, the drain should be removed. The stent is removed 4 to 6 weeks postoperatively. Follow-up studies include an IVP at 3 and 6 months after stent removal.

RESULTS A small number of patients have undergone laparoscopic ureterolithotomy to date. Harewood and colleagues successfully removed ureteral calculi laparoscopically in five patients.[20] These patients required minimal pain medication and stayed only 2 days in the hospital.

A similar result was reported in six patients with large impacted ureteral stones that were successfully removed laparoscopically.[21] Rabou and colleagues performed a laparoscopic ureterolithotomy in a patient with distal cystine stones and reported no evidence of obstruction or leakage on 4-week postoperative IVP.[19]

The only comparative study of laparoscopic versus open ureterolithotomy by Skrepetis and colleagues confirmed the advantages of less analgesic requirements, shorter hospital stay and faster recovery, of laparoscopy over open surgery.[22] In the largest series of 24 patients by Feyaerts and colleagues only one case failed due to accidental push-back of the stone to the kidney.[23] All other studies (Table 61-3) had success rates of 100%.

Complications were minor and mainly constituted short-term postoperative fever, ileus, deep venous thrombosis, incisional hernias, subcutaneous emphysema, and subcutaneous hematomas. Urinary leak was seen. Harewood and colleagues reported a urinary leak in 55.5%,[20] but this was only of 3 days duration. Keeley and colleagues[24] and Skrepetis and colleagues[22] reported patients with leakage of 12 and 10 days, respectively, which were treated conservatively. Of note, both of these cases were performed without stents. A urinoma requiring drainage was reported by Micali and colleagues, but in this case no drain was left postoperatively.[21]

There are no long-term results concerning the incidence of ureteral stricture postoperatively. In

Table 61-2 Laparoscopic Pyeloplasty: Complications

Complications during Laparoscopic Pyeloplasty

Serosal tear	Transient ureteral edema	Myocardial infarction
Abdominal wall hematoma	Stent migration	Congestive heart failure
Clipped colonic diverticulum	Transient ileus	Pneumonia
Urinoma formation	Pyelonephritris	Thrombophlebitis
Retroperitoneal bleeding	Stone recurrence	—

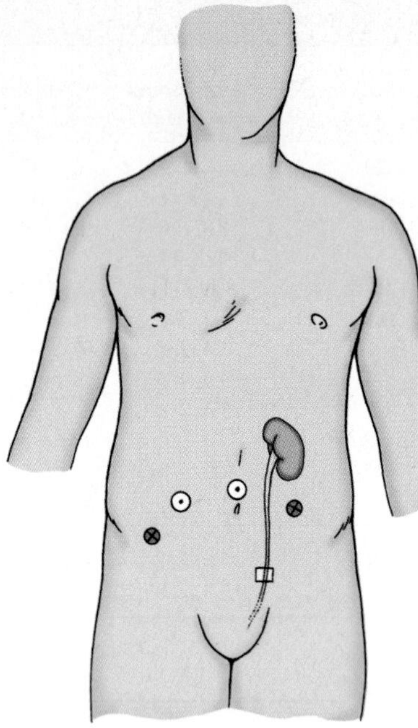

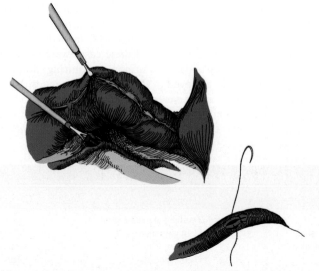

Figure 61-10 Port placement for laparoscopic ureterolithotomy of left lower ureteral stone. The 10-mm port should be placed contralateral to the side to be approached.

most cases, the ureterotomy was made with a cold knife, but some authors used the diathermy hook[20] or a neodymium:yttrium-aluminum-garnet (Nd:YAG) laser.[25]

URETEROLYSIS

Retroperitoneal fibrosis is an inflammatory condition of the retroperitoneum that occurs as either a primary (idiopathic) form or secondary to conditions such as inflammatory bowel disease, endometriosis, radiation therapy, neoplasm, vascular aneurysms, or drug therapy (ie, methysergide).[26,27] The goals of ureterolysis include relief of ureteral entrapment, preservation of renal function, prevention of recurrent obstruction, and diagnosis of underlying pathologic causes.

To evaluate the extent of retroperitoneal disease and to rule out the possibility of occult malignancy, a CT scan of the abdomen and pelvis with oral and intravenous contrast must be obtained. A search for malignant conditions in adult men should include a digital rectal examination, stool guaiac test, prostate-specific antigen assay, and a chest x-ray film. Adult women should have a pelvic examination, stool guaiac test, breast examination, mammogram, and chest x-ray film. The addition of an erythrocyte sedimentation rate may provide a tool for following the activity of the inflammatory process. An IVP should be obtained to define the degree of medial ureteral displacement. Renography should be performed to assess the residual function and degree of obstruction on the affected side. A retrograde pyelogram just prior to the laparoscopic procedure may also be helpful to delineate the entire course of the ureter and rule out possible distal ureteral strictures.

TECHNIQUE After placement of an indwelling ureteral stent, the patient is positioned in a fashion similar to that described for laparoscopic pyeloplasty. A supine position may be used if both ureters are involved. The table can be rotated to allow the bowel to fall out of the operative field. An ex-dwelling ureteral stent or lighted stent helps in identifying the course of the involved ureter. In experienced hands, an indwelling ureteral catheter is usually sufficient. It should be of sufficient length to allow lateral displacement of the ureter.

A pneumoperitoneum is established and trocars placed as illustrated in Figure 61-7 to allow access to the upper ureter. An additional 5-mm port may be placed in the anterior axillary line midway between the costal margin and iliac crest. This port aids in retraction during dissection of the ureter.

With the use of grasping forceps and dissecting scissors, the colon is retracted medially and the peritoneal reflection incised across the iliac vessels ending distal and medial to the medial

Figure 61-11 Stone delivered through a ureteral incision and ureterotomy closed with interrupted sutures.

umbilical ligament. The incision is then extended proximally to the hepatic flexure on the right or the splenic flexure on the left. A sweeping motion brings the colon medially and exposes the psoas muscle (Figure 61-12A). It is important to remember that the fibrotic process may retract the ureter over the great vessels. The ureter should be first identified in the portion uninvolved by the fibrotic process. This is usually in the area medial to the medial umbilical ligament near the bladder or proximally in the region of the UPJ.

The assistant retracts the periureteral tissues laterally while the surgeon develops a window around the ureter. A right-angle forceps is used to pass a 4-inch piece of umbilical tape around the freed segment of the ureter (Figure 61-12B). The ends of the umbilical tape are fastened together using a single 9-mm clip. This maneuver facilitates retraction of the ureter to aid in dissection. Care must be taken not to pull too vigorously to avoid avulsing the ureter.

Every attempt should be made to rule out malignancy as a cause of obstruction. Biopsies of the periureteral tissues must be taken using laparoscopic biopsy forceps and specimens should be sent for frozen and permanent sections.

A combination of blunt and sharp dissection is used to shell the ureter out of the fibrotic process. To prevent compromise of the ureteral blood supply, cauterization should be used with great caution. The gonadal vessels can be involved in the inflammatory process and should be dissected off the ureter. If necessary, they may be clipped and transected. The dissection is continued until the ureter is freed from the renal pelvis to below the fibrotic process.

Once the ureter is free, it is necessary to isolate it from the fibrotic process. The medial and lateral cut edges of the peritoneum are re-approximated after the ureter is transposed into the peritoneal cavity. A hernia stapler or suture placement can be used to re-approximate the incised peritoneal edges (Figure 61-12C). Using a GIA stapler inserted through the umbilical port to split the omentum, an omental wrap can be created. The tissue is used to create a sleeve that can be positioned around the ureter and secured to itself using 9-mm clips or 3-0 Vicryl sutures. Drains are not necessary. An IVP is performed 2 weeks following surgery, at which time the ureteral stent is removed. Follow-up radiographic studies (IVP and diuretic renal scan) are then obtained at 3, 6, and 12 months, postoperatively. Regular activities are resumed after removal of the stent.

RESULTS Kavoussi and colleagues first reported a laparoscopic technique to dissect and intraperitonealize the ureter of a patient with idiopathic retroperitoneal fibrosis.[28] Since then, a limited number of laparoscopic ureterolysis procedures have been performed.[29,30] In one of the largest series (reported by Fugita and colleagues), 13 patients underwent laparoscopic ureterolysis.[31] It was necessary to convert in 15% of the cases; complications occurred in 30% of the patients, but they were all minor and managed conserva-

Table 61-3 Laparoscopic Ureterolithotomy

Study	Number of Patients	Approach	Stone Size (mm)	Suture Placement	Stent Placement	Mean Operative Times (min)	Conversion Rate (%)	Postop Hospital Stay (days)	Success Rate (%)
Rabou et al[19]	1	Transabdominal		No	+	—	—	1	100
Bellman et al[68]	2	Transabdominal	11–10	No	+	—	—	—	100
Gaur et al[69]	8	Retroperitoneal	20–12	No	±	40	37.5	1	62.5
Harewood et al[20]	9	Transabdominal & retroperitoneal	28–5	Yes	±	158	—	5.2	100
Fahlenkamp et al[25]	2	Transabdominal	18–11	Yes	+	—	—	2	100
Micali et al[21]	6	Transabdominal	18–10	Yes	+	222	20	3.3	83.3
Keeley et al[24]	14	Transabdominal	40–18	Yes/No	±	105	—	5.6	100
Skrepetis et al[22]	18	Transabdominal	31–12	Yes	±	130	—	3.2	100
Feayaerts et al[23]	24	Transabdominal & retroperitoneal	33–7	Yes/No	±	111	—	3.8	100

Postop = postoperative.

tively. Transfusion was necessary in 8%; analgesic requirements were minimal, and mean hospital stay was 4 days. After a mean follow-up of 30 months, 92% of the patients showed relief of their obstruction.

URETEROVESICAL REIMPLANTATION

Open ureteral reimplantation is performed in children mainly for vesicoureteral reflux disease. In adults a refluxing anastomosis is usually performed for the treatment of distal ureteral strictures or endometriosis where endoscopic therapy is inappropriate or has failed.

TECHNIQUE With the patient in a supine position, flexible cystoscopy is performed, and a ureteral stent is placed in the ureter. It is important also to see the location of the ureteral orifices and the length of the posterior wall available to create the extravesical detrusor tunnel.

The pneumoperitoneum is obtained in the standard fashion, and four ports are usually used. One 10-mm port for the camera (5-mm for children) is placed just below the umbilicus, while two working ports (10-mm or 3-mm) are positioned in the lower quadrant in the midclavicular line and 1 inch below the umbilicus. The last trocar (3- to 5-mm) is placed suprapubically or in the contralateral lower quadrant. Alternatively, the three working ports can be placed along an imaginary shallow Pfannenstiel incision; two lateral at the midclavicular line and one in the midline. The advantage of this configuration is that it allows for inconspicuous conversion. With the surgeon on the contralateral side, the colon is reflected, and the ureter is identified above the bifurcation of the iliac vessels and dissected caudally.

In case of a ureteral stricture, the dome of the bladder is transilluminated with the help of the cystoscope, and a guidewire is passed transvesically through the location of the new orifice in a controlled fashion. A ureteral catheter is placed over the wire, into the abdominal cavity and through the open-ended ureter. The cystotomy is widened with laparoscopic scissors, and the previously transected ureter is anastomosed with the bladder.

When the length of the ureter is insufficient for primary anastomosis, mobilization of the bladder may be needed. This includes ligation of the contralateral pedicle. A Boari flap procedure can then be performed using an anterior bladder flap created as in open surgery. This flap is anastomosed with the ureter.

If the ureter is going to be reimplanted in an antireflux way, the most commonly described technique has been the laparoscopic Lich-Gregoir reimplantation. When the mobilization has reached the bladder wall, scissors score the bladder serosa for 3 cm in a straight line. The bladder musculature is dissected to the mucosal layer, and the flaps of the trough are developed. The dissection proceeds around the ureter onto the lateral and medial aspects of the ureterovesical junction, resulting in an inverted Y configuration. At this point, the bladder mucosa can be seen bulging outward.

The ureter is tucked in the tunnel, and the muscle sutured over it with interrupted 3-0 polyglactin 910 at 0.5 cm intervals. The first suture should not be placed at the very end of the inverted Y in order to avoid kinking of the ureteral orifice. The ratio of tunnel length to ureteral diameter should be 5:1.[32] Assessment of the ureteral position is made with the bladder variably distended. Greatly distending the bladder will further flatten the posterior bladder wall, producing a straight ureteral course along the retroperitoneum.

For adults with a cystotomy, a cystogram is performed prior to catheter removal usually at 72 hours. The stent is usually removed 15 to 30 days, postoperatively. A drain placed near the anastomosis is removed when output is minimal. For children with a Lich-Gregoir reimplantation, the stent can be left in place and removed with the catheter on postoperative day one.

RESULTS Laparoscopic ureteral reimplantation is feasible and was first performed in 1993 by Ehrlich and colleagues in children with high-grade ureterovesical reflux.[33] Operative time was reasonable (170 to 195 minutes), and the advantages of short hospital stay, fast recovery, and minimal postoperative pain were confirmed. Short follow-up at 2 months showed resolution of the reflux. Unfortunately, even in the largest series presented, long-term results are lacking.[34]

The first case of ureteral reimplantation in adults was presented by Reddy and Evans.[35] The primary difference between children and adults is that, during dissection, in children the ureter is readily identified due to the paucity of retroperitoneal fat.

As laparoscopic urologists gain more and more experience, more technically challenging approaches to reimplant the ureter are being reported. Examples include the laparoscopic Boari flap procedure presented by Fugita and colleagues,[36] or a transvesical cross-trigonal Cohen antireflux ureteroneocystostomy performed by Gill and colleagues.[37]

URETEROURETEROSTOMY FOR RETROCAVAL URETER

Eight case reports have been presented of this rare entity. The diagnosis is made by IVP and the

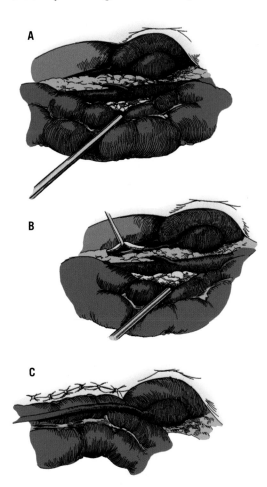

Figure 61-12 *A*, Incision of the peritoneum and medial retraction of colon to expose retroperitoneal fibrosis with encased right ureter. *B*, Umbilical tape aids in retraction for dissection of the ureter. *C*, The ureter is intraperitonealized and the cut edges of the peritoneum re-approximated.

characteristic S shaped course of the ureter. Both transabdominal[38–40] and retroperitoneal[41–43] approaches have been reported.

TECHNIQUE After a stent is passed, the patient is placed in a modified right lateral flank position, and after abdominal insufflation with the Veress needle, three ports are placed, one in the umbilicus, one midway between the xiphoid and the umbilical port, and one at the low midline. The line of Toldt is incised, the colon reflected medially, and the ureter identified and separated from the posterior surface of the vena cava. The proximal ureter is often dilated.

The ureter is divided at the most distal segment of the dilated ureter. The distal ureteral stump is dissected anterior to the vena cava and spatulated. The two ends are sutured either freehand or with the help of an automated suturing device. A drain is placed, and the operation is concluded in the standard fashion.

Postoperatively, the drain is removed when output is minimal; oral intake starts on postoperative day one, and the patient's activities are advanced as tolerated. Follow-up includes an IVP 3 months after the procedure.

RESULTS This procedure is feasible and presents with all the advantages of laparoscopy, such as less postoperative pain, shorter hospital stay, and faster recovery, without compromising surgical outcome. With advances in experience and suturing, operating times have decreased significantly. Initial reports needed 9 hours,[44] while more recent ones have decreased the time to 3 hours and 45 minutes.[45] No major complications have been reported.

URETERORURETEROSTOMY/ LAPAROSCOPIC REPAIR OF URETERAL INJURY

Closed injury of the ureter is usually iatrogenic, most often occurring during endoscopic manipulation[46] or laparoscopic gynecological procedures.[47,48] Small perforations can heal spontaneously with stenting; larger injuries, however, require definitive repair. Laparoscopy allows minimal invasive correction of the injury, either by suturing the ureteral tear or by performing an end-to-end ureteroureteral anastomosis.

Although short-term follow-up shows good results, limited postoperative data are available to define stricture recurrence and other complications.[49,50]

LAPAROSCOPIC CUTANEOUS URETEROSTOMY

Cutaneous ureterostomies are performed for palliation from advanced malignant disease. Open surgery is quite morbid in these patients.[51] Placement of nephrostomy tubes has considerably decreased the complication rate. Nevertheless, the quality of life is often poor, with tube changes

required and problems arising due to obstruction and dislodgement.

Laparoscopic cutaneous ureterostomy has been reported with good results.[52] The technique is more complex than placing a nephrostomy tube, and Puppo and colleagues suggest that this procedure be offered only when life expectancy is more than 6 months.[53]

The technique involves standard laparoscopic dissection of the ureter, which is cut as low as possible. The ureter free in the abdominal cavity is grasped with an endo-Babcock and withdrawn through one of the lateral ports after the abdomen is deflated. The cutaneous ureterostomy nipple is then performed in the usual manner.

ANASTOMOSIS BETWEEN THE BOWEL AND THE URETER

Isolated case reports of laparoscopic formation of an ileal ureter[54] and formation of an ureteroileal anastomosis[55–57] completely intra-abdominally have been published. Although, at this writing, these techniques are performed at highly specialized centers, they hold promise in dealing with complex integration of the bowel into the urinary tract.

COMPLICATIONS

General complications of laparoscopic surgery have been well documented and should always be kept in mind.[16,17] Complications specific to laparoscopic ureteral reconstruction occur as a result of injury to the ureter and can be minimized by adhering to basic laparoscopic dissection techniques and experience. Excess traction during dissection can cause ureteral avulsion. Moreover, prolonged tension in one area can lead to ischemic injury with resultant necrosis, extravasation, and stricture formation. If an anastomosis has been performed, excess manipulation of the ureter can result in disruption of the suture line. At the conclusion of any procedure, the ureter should be carefully inspected to rule out ureteral extravasation.

Vigorous retraction of the ureter can cause proximal or distal migration of an indwelling ureteral stent resulting in ineffective postoperative drainage. Possible complications from inadequate drainage include ureteral fistulas, urinoma formation, and severe postoperative abdominal pain. These may be prevented by using a stent of adequate length such that traction will allow both ends to remain in proper position. An abdominal radiograph and cystoscopy should be performed after each procedure to document stent position. Closed drainage can be effective, postoperatively, if leakage occurs. This usually takes place within 48 hours of surgery. Management consists of converting the leak into a controlled fistula by maintaining drainage for at least 1 week. Prior to removing the drain it should be taken off suction to be sure output decreases over 24 to 48 hours.

As in open ureteral surgery, care should be taken to perform a tension-free repair to avoid

increasing the risk of ureteral stricture. A follow-up IVP or renal scan after stent removal is recommended to evaluate if there is stricture formation.

As laparoscopic ureteral reconstruction procedures become more common, accurate assessment of complication rates will be possible.

REFERENCES

1. Soper MJ, Barteau JA, Clayman RV, et al. Comparison of early postoperative results for laparoscopic versus standard open cholecystectomy. Surg Gynecol Obstet 1992;174:114.
2. Griffith DO, Schuessler WW, Vancaille TH, Reich H. Transperitoneal endosurgical lymphadenectomy in patients with localized prostate cancer. J Urol 1991;145:988.
3. Gill IS. Retroperitoneal laparoscopic nephrectomy. Urol Clin North Am 1998;25:343.
4. Quillin SP, Brink JA, Heiken JP, et al. Helical (spiral) CT angiography for identification of crossing vessels at the ureteropelvic junction. Am J Roengenol 1996;166:1125.
5. Bagley DH, Liu JB, Goldberg B. Endoluminal sonographic imaging of the ureteropelvic junction. J Endourol 1996; 10:105.
6. Frauscher F, Janetschek G, Klauser A, et al. Laparoscopic pyeloplasty for UPJ obstruction with crossing vessels: contrast-enhanced color Doppler findings and long term results. Urology 2002;59:500.
7. Notely RG, Beaugie JM. The long-term follow-up of Anderson-Hynes pyeloplasty for hydronephrosis. Br J Urol 1973;45:464.
8. Persky L, Krause JR, Boltuch RL. Initial complications and late results in dismembered pyeloplasty. J Urol 1977;118:162.
9. Motola JA, Badlani GH, Smith AD. Results of 221 consecutive endopyelotomies: an eight-year follow up. J Urol 1993;149:453.
10. Nakada SY, Johnson M. Ureteropelvic junction obstruction: retrograde endopyelotomy. Urol Clin North Am 2000; 27:677.
11. McClinton S, Steyn JH, Hussey JK. Retrograde balloon dilatation for pelviureteric junction obstruction. Br J Urol 1993;71:152.
12. Lechevallier E, Eghazarian C, Ortega JC, et al. Retrograde Acucise endopyelotomy: long term results. J Endourol 1999;13:575.
13. Schuessler WW, Grune MT, Tecuanhuey LV, Preminger GM. Laparoscopic dismembered pyeloplasty. J Urol 1993;150: 1795.
14. Kavoussi LR, Peters CA. Laparoscopic pyeloplasty. J Urol 1993;150:1891.
15. Jarrett TW, Chan DY, Charambura TC, et al. Laparoscopic pyeloplasty. J Urol 2002;167:1253.
16. Brooks JD, Kavoussi LR, Preminger GM, et al. Comparison of open and endourological approaches to the obstructed ureteropelvic junction. Urology 1995;46:791.
17. Bauer JJ, Bishoff JT, Moore RG, et al. Laparoscopic versus open pyeloplasty: assessment of objective and subjective outcome. J Urol 1999;162:692.
18. Gettman M, Neururer R, Bartsch G, Peschel R. Anderson-Hynes dismembered pyeloplasty performed using the da Vinci robotic system. Urology 2002;60:509.
19. Rabou A, Ferzli GS, Ioffreda R, Albert P. Laparoscopic ureterolithotomy. Urology 1992;39:223.
20. Harewood LM, Webb DR, Pope AJ. Laparoscopic ureterolithotomy: the results of an initial series, and an evaluation of its role in the management of ureteric calculi. BJU Int 1994;74:170–6.
21. Micali S, Moore RG, Averch TD, et al. The role of laparoscopy in the treatment of renal and ureteral calculi. J Urol 1997;157:463.
22. Skrepetis K, Doumas K, Siafakas I, Lykourinas M. Laparoscopic versus open ureterolithotomy. A comparative study. Eur Urol 2001;40:32.
23. Feayaerts A, Rietbergen J, Navarra S, et al. Laparoscopic ureterolithotomy for ureteral calculi. Eur Urol 2001;40:609.
24. Keeley FX, Gialas I, Pillai M, et al. Laparoscopic ureterolithotomy: the Edinburgh experience. BJU Int 1999;84:765.
25. Fahlenkamp D, Schonberger B, Liebetruth L, et al. Laparoscopic laser ureterolithotomy. J Urol 1994;152:1549.
26. Lepro H, Walsh PC. Idiopathic retroperitoneal fibrosis. J Urol 1979;122:1.
27. Sosa RE, Vaughan ED, Gibbons RP. Retroperitoneal fibrosis. AUA Update Series 1987; Vol 6: Lesson 21.
28. Kavoussi LR, Clayman RV, Brunt M, Soper NJ. Laparoscopic ureterolysis. J Urol 1992;147:426.

29. Monev S. Idiopathic retroperitoneal fibrosis: prompt diagnosis preserves organ function. Cleve Clin J Med 2002;69:160.

30. Matsuda T, Arai Y, Muguruma K, et al. Laparoscopic ureterolysis for idiopathic retroperitoneal fibrosis. Eur Urol 1994;26:286.

31. Fugita OE, Jarrett TW, Kavoussi P, Kavoussi LR. Laparoscopic treatment of retroperitoneal fibrosis. J Endourol 2002;16:571.

32. Duckett JW. Update on vesicoureteral reflux. AUA Update Series 1993; Vol 12: Lesson 5.

33. Ehrlich RM, Gershman A, Fuchs G. Laparoscopic vesicoureteroplasty in children: initial case reports. Urology 1994;43:255.

34. Lakshmanan Y, Fung LCT. Laparoscopic extravesical ureteral reimplantation for vesicoureteral reflux: recent technical advances. J Endourol 2000;14:589.

35. Reddy PK, Evans RM. Laparoscopic ureteroneocystostomy. J Urol 1994;152:2057.

36. Fugita OE, Dinlenc C, Kavoussi L. The laparoscopic Boari flap. J Urol 2001;166:51.

37. Gill IS, Ponsky LE, Desai M, et al. Laparoscopic crosstrigonal Cohen ureterocystostomy: novel technique. J Urol 2001;166:1811.

38. Ameda K, Kakizaki H, Harabayashi T, et al. Laparoscopic ureteroureterostomy for retrocaval ureter. Int J Urol 2001;8:71.

39. Ishitoya S, Okubo K, Arai Y. Laparoscopic ureterolysis for retrocaval ureter. Br J Urol 1996;77:162.

40. Matsuda T, Yasumoto R, Tsuijno T. Laparoscopic treatment of a retrocaval ureter. Eur Urol 1996;29:115.

41. Miyazato M, Kimura T, Ohyama C, et al. Retroperitoneoscopic ureterostomy for retrocaval ureter. Hinyokika Kiyo 2002;48:25.

42. Salomon L, Hoznek A, Balian C, et al. Retroperitoneal laparoscopy of a retrocaval ureter. BJU Int 1999;84:181.

43. Mugigya S, Suzuki K, Ohhira T, et al. Retroperitoneoscopic treatment of retrocaval ureter. Int J Urol 1999;6:419.

44. Baba S, Oya M, Miyahara M, et al. Laparoscopic surgical correction of circumcaval ureter. Urology 1994;44:122.

45. Polashik TJ, Chen RN. Laparoscopic ureteroureterostomy for retrocaval ureter. J Urol 1998;160:121.

46. Holman E. Laparoscopic management of ureteral perforation during ureterolithotripsy. J Endourol 1998;12:259.

47. Tulikangas PK, Gill IS, Falcone T. Laparoscopic repair of ureteral injuries. J Am Assoc Gynecol Laparosc 2001; 8:259.

48. Liu CY, Kim JH, Bryant JF. Laparoscopic ureteroureteral anastomosis of the distal ureter. J Am Assoc Gynecol Laparosc 2001;8:412.

49. Tulikangas PK, Goldberg JM, Gill IS. Laparoscopic repair of ureteral transection . J Am Assoc Gynecol Laparosc 2000; 7:415.

50. Liu CH, Wang PH, Lin NM, Yaan CC. Ureteral injury after laparoscopic surgery. J Am Assoc Gynecol Laparosc 1997;4:503.

51. Brin EN, Shiff M, Weiss RM. Palliative urinary diversion for pelvic malignancy. J Urol 1975;113:619.

52. Liosides P, Grasso M, Lui P. Laparoscopic cutaneous ureterostomy: technique for palliative upper urinary tract drainage. J Endourol 1995;9:315.

53. Puppo P, Ricciotti G, Bozzo W, et al. Videoscopic cutaneous ureterostomy for palliative urinary diversion in advanced pelvic cancer. Eur Urol 1995;28:328.

54. Gill IS, Savage SJ, Senagore AJ, Sung GT. Laparoscopic ileal ureter. J Urol 2000;163:1199.

55. Gupta NP, Gill IS, Fergany A, Nabi G. Laparoscopic radical cystectomy with intracorporeal ileal conduit diversion: five cases with a 2-year follow up. BJU Int 2002;90:391.

56. Matin SF, Gill IS. Laparoscopic radical cystectomy with urinary diversion: completely intracorporeal technique. J Endourol 2002;16:335.

57. Gill IS, Fregany A, Klein EA, et al. Laparoscopic radical cystoprostatectomy with ileal conduit performed completely intracorporeally: the initial 2 cases. Urology 2000;56:26.

58. Recker F, Subotic B, Goepel M, Tscholl R. Laparoscopic dismembered pyeloplasty: preliminary report. J Urol 1995; 153:1605.

59. Nakada SY, McDougall EM, Clayman RV. Laparoscopic pyeloplasty for secondary ureteropelvic junction obstruction: preliminary experience. Urology 1995;46:257.

60. Janetschek G, Peschel R, Altarc S, Bartsch G. Laparoscopic and retroperitoneoscopic repair of ureteropelvic junction obstruction. Urology 1996;47:311.

61. Chen RN, Moore RG, Kavoussi LR. Laparoscopic pyeloplasty. Indications, technique, long term outcome. Urol Clin North Am 1998;25:323.

62. Moore RG, Averch TD, Schulam PG, et al. Laparoscopic pyeloplasty: experience with the initial 30 cases. J Urol 1997;157:459.

63. Puppo P, Perachino M, Ricciotti G, et al. Retroperitoneoscopic treatment of ureteropelvic obstruction. Eur Urol 1997;31:204.

64. Ben Slama MR, Salomon L, Hoznel A, et al. Extraperitoneal laparoscopic repair of ureteropelvic junction obstruction: initial experience in 15 cases. Urololgy 2000; 56:45.

65. Janetschek G, Peschel R, Franscher F. Laparoscopic pyeloplasty. Urol Clin North Am 2000;27:695.

66. Soulie M, Salomon L, Patard JJ, et al. Extraperitoneal laparoscopic pyeloplasty: a multicenter study of 55 procedures. J Urol 2001;166:48.

67. Eden CG, Cahill D, Allen JD. Laparoscopic dismembered pyeloplasty: 50 consecutive cases. BJU Int 2001;88:526.

68. Bellman GC, Smith AD. Special considerations in the technique of laparoscopic ureterolithotomy. J Urol 1993; 151:146.

69. Gaur DD. Retroperitoneal laparoscopic ureterolithotomy. World J Urol 1993;11:175.

62

Laparoscopic Techniques for the Correction of Pelvic Organ Prolapse

Li-Ming Su, MD

E. James Wright, MD

Pelvic organ prolapse encompasses various conditions resulting from weakening of the endopelvic fascia and muscles of the pelvic diaphragm (the major pelvic fascial support system) when organs within the pelvis protrude into the vaginal canal. This can include prolapse of the bladder, uterus and cervix, small bowel, rectum, or various combinations of these organs. Many factors can lead to damage, separation, and attenuation of the pelvic fascial support system resulting in pelvic organ prolapse. Such risk factors include childbirth, pelvic surgery, obesity, respiratory disorders, hypoestrogenemia, occupational and recreational stress, connective tissue disorders, and pelvic neuropathy.

For simplification, pelvic organ prolapse can be divided into defects in the support of (1) the anterior vaginal wall, (2) vaginal apex, (3) posterior vaginal wall, (4) perineal body, or (5) various combinations of the four. Pelvic organ prolapse can present along a continuum, from slight loss of support to complete eversion of the vagina. As the pelvic floor subtends bladder, bowel, and sexual function, a wide range of signs and symptoms can develop. In order to plan successful treatment, symptoms and subjective complaints must be correlated as accurately as possible with the anatomic defects observed.

The previous edition of this text focused primarily on laparoscopic procedures for treating stress incontinence. Since then, the isolated indication for laparoscopic continence surgery has found limited utility. This is partly owing to the great variability in success of such procedures.[1–3] Likely the greater influence has come from the increasing ease and feasibility of various pubovaginal sling techniques. With a more uniform success profile and minimally invasive technique, these procedures have, in our opinion, made laparoscopic colposuspension (bladder neck suspension) a less attractive option for effectively treating stress incontinence.

While enthusiasm wanes for laparoscopic continence surgery, techniques for laparoscopic repair of pelvic organ prolapse continue to expand. As many urologists now include within their scope of practice repair of complex pelvic organ prolapse, pelvic laparoscopy offers a new horizon. As it is generally believed that abdominal repair of many prolapse conditions offers greater durability and a lower recurrence rate,

laparoscopic techniques may find a role in bridging the gap between vaginal and abdominal approaches. In this context, the value of laparoscopic prolapse repair in terms of durability, recurrence, complication, recovery, quality of life, cosmesis, and other parameters continues to be investigated. We find the techniques described in this chapter to be successful in many of these respects. They are in no way exhaustive, as many in the areas of female urology and urogynecology continue to explore new laparoscopic solutions to age-old problems.

PATIENT EVALUATION

An algorithm for history-taking, physical examination and specialized testing is useful for efficiently diagnosing prolapse and related pelvic floor disorders. With adequate diagnostic assessment, treatment strategies and expectations for functional and anatomic outcome can be more accurately determined. The history should focus on identifying risk factors previously mentioned, along with assessment of urinary, bowel and sexual function.

With increasing degrees of pelvic organ prolapse, women often report the sensation of pressure in the introitus (or a vaginal "bulge"). Many will describe the need to manually reduce a protruding vaginal segment in order to void or defecate (splinting). If sexually active, some women will relate difficulties with intercourse due to obstruction of the vagina or a change in positional comfort. Voiding dysfunction is often coincidental with loss of pelvic support. This may include stress or urge incontinence, urgency and frequency syndromes, and even varying degrees of obstruction and urinary retention. A frequency and volume voiding diary maintained for 24-72 hours may be useful in objectifying the voiding history and guiding treatment. A number of self-administered, validated questionnaires, such as the Urogenital Distress Inventory (UDI and UDI-6), the Incontinence Impact Questionnaire (IIQ and IIQ-7), the Pelvic Floor Distress Inventory (PFDI), and the Pelvic Floor Impact Questionnaire (PFIQ) have been developed to help standardize incontinence and pelvic floor complaints, their severity, and impact on quality of life.[4,5] With regard to bowel function, the history should include inquiries about anal incontinence, fecal urgency, constipation, tenesmus, and any need for splinting. Such signs and

symptoms may indicate varying degrees of anal sphincteric injury, pelvic neuropathy and posterior compartment prolapse.

Because the signs and symptoms of pelvic prolapse are often not organ or compartment specific,[6] the physical examination is critical for identifying and staging anatomic defects. The physical examination specific to assessment of pelvic organ prolapse begins with visual inspection of the external genitalia while the patient is in lithotomy position. Estrogen status, dermatologic lesions and loss of resting pelvic tone can be assessed. Sensory neural evaluation can be done with a cotton swab in the S2-S4 dermatomes to determine loss or lateralizing signs. With forceful straining, any vaginal protrusion, perineal descent, rectal prolapse or urine leak can be observed.

Further assessment of pelvic organ prolapse makes use of either a Sims speculum or the posterior blade of a separated Graves speculum. These instruments allow sequential reduction of the posterior and then anterior vaginal walls to isolate specific compartments. One of the most useful and descriptive classifications for pelvic organ prolapse is the Pelvic Organ Prolapse Quantification (POP-Q) scale.[7] This grading system allows for a systematic and reproducible accounting of anatomic defects and provides for a mental picture of prolapse severity. The system uses six reference points along the anterior and posterior vaginal walls to describe compartment descent in relation to the hymenal ring. An additional three measurements include length of the perineal body, genital hiatus, and vagina. These measurements are made during maximal strain and, taken in total, define an anatomic, patient-specific assessment of prolapse severity for diagnosis and surgical planning. The system requires some practice to use comfortably, but its accuracy warrants familiarity. It is sometimes helpful or confirmatory to evaluate the patient in the upright position if valsalva or strain maneuvers do not reproduce the reported prolapse signs.

Following prolapse assessment, a bimanual exam is done to evaluate the uterus and adnexa, if present, as well as to palpate a full or tender bladder. Assessment of levator function and strength is also made during the pelvic examination. This can be done transvaginally along the posterior and lateral vaginal walls, taking into account the force of contraction and its duration.[8]

The need for additional testing to evaluate pelvic organ prolapse is variable. Multichannel urodynamic assessment is often included in the workup if urinary incontinence or other voiding complaint is present. With increasing stages of pelvic organ prolapse, urodynamic testing can be done with maneuvers designed to simulate anatomic correction. Such "reduction" maneuvers include supporting a prolapsing vaginal segment with a Sims speculum, tampon, or sponge stick during valsalva and cough events. While the sensitivity of reduction maneuvers is unclear, they may be helpful when valsalva leakage is observed. The role of cystoscopy in this setting is also unclear unless there is concomitant microhematuria or new onset of irritative voiding complaints.

NONSURGICAL TREATMENT OPTIONS

As with many disease processes, management of pelvic organ prolapse depends largely on the severity of presenting symptoms. Other factors, including patient age, general health, lifestyle, motivation, and outcome expectations help guide management. Many nonsurgical therapies are available for treating the various symptoms attributed to pelvic organ prolapse. These include pelvic floor exercises and lifestyle modification, pharmacotherapy, and pessaries.

The concept of pelvic floor exercises to strengthen the muscles of pelvic support originates from Kegel's description in 1948 of exercises for postpartum pelvic rehabilitation.[9] Kegel's exercises remain in the treatment algorithm for patients with low-stage pelvic organ prolapse and varying degrees of dysfunction, including stress and urge urinary incontinence. Complementary measures to reinforce proper contraction of the pelvic musculature include biofeedback, weighted vaginal cones, and direct intravaginal electrical stimulation of the levator musculature. Incorporating the patient's awareness of the pelvic floor musculature and the reliability of performing effective pelvic floor contractions into activities of daily living can be helpful in modulating severity or progression of symptoms. This may be especially important in patients with physically active lifestyles, including laborers and athletes. Appropriate instruction in performing pelvic floor contractions during different body positions and activities (eg, standing from a sitting position, jumping, lifting, coughing) can enhance effectiveness.[10]

Patients must also understand the risk factors that contribute to voiding dysfunction and urinary incontinence, and what measures they can take to limit them. This includes avoiding excessive fluid intake, alcohol, and caffeine, as well as instituting timed voiding. Although pelvic floor exercises and lifestyle modification can be useful in treating patients with mild symptoms of urinary incontinence, compliance remains a significant limiting factor, and more severe degrees and symptoms of pelvic floor prolapse are often resistant to such therapy.

The use of pharmacotherapy in the treatment of pelvic floor prolapse is limited to alleviating associated symptoms, such as urinary incontinence and constipation, without directly addressing the anatomic defect leading to prolapse. Pharmacotherapy may be used primarily, or as an adjunct following surgical correction of pelvic organ prolapse. Anticholinergic medications are the mainstay of medical therapy for patients suffering from urinary frequency syndromes and urge incontinence.

Treatment of bowel dysfunction associated with pelvic organ prolapse can be divided into therapies for fecal incontinence and constipation. Regular intake of a high-fiber diet or stool-bulking supplements may produce more formed stools that are less problematic than liquid stools in patients with fecal incontinence. Antidiarrheal agents such as loperamide hydrochloride and simethicone (Imodium) and diphenoxylate and atropine (Lomotil) decrease gastrointestinal motility and are helpful in patients with fecal incontinence and diarrhea. Treatment of constipation relies on preparations that increase the bulk of the stool but soften its consistency, examples being concentrated wheat germ or bran. Laxatives such as magnesium hydroxide increase bowel frequency and the water content in stool.

Pessaries have long been used for the nonsurgical treatment of women suffering from pelvic organ prolapse. Many types are available in two broad categories: support pessaries and space-filling pessaries. An example of a support pessary is the ring, which uses a spring mechanism to elevate the posterior fornix with its opposite end, firmly supported by the posterior aspect of the pubic symphysis. Alternatively, space-filling pessaries act by either creating a suction effect between the pessary and the vaginal wall or by occupying the vaginal fornix with a structure of larger diameter than the genital hiatus. Pessaries are effective in many women with varying degrees of pelvic organ prolapse and can be used in patients awaiting definitive surgery, or in those who are unfit or decline surgical management. Complications that can arise with the use of pessaries include vaginal wall ulceration, fistula formation, and bowel herniation, all of which can be minimized by proper sizing, routine cleansing, and regular surveillance. Although pessaries can be effective in addressing the anatomic defect(s) of prolapse, there are no studies specifically addressing their effectiveness in alleviating the associated symptoms. Neither are there studies comparing the effectiveness of pessaries versus surgical correction of prolapse.

SURGICAL TREATMENT OPTIONS

Restoring the fascial support system is the basis for surgical correction of pelvic organ prolapse. Although categorization of prolapse based on anterior, apical, posterior, or perineal body defects exists, correction of more than one or all of these defects is often necessary. Surgery can be undertaken vaginally or abdominally. The choice of

approach can be influenced by many factors, but should be dictated primarily by detailed pelvic examination, documenting the degree or stage of prolapse (see "Patient Evaluation"). The patient's desires and expectations regarding preservation of sexual function, postoperative recovery, risk of recurrence, and cosmesis may also influence the surgical approach. Women who desire to maintain sexual function require repair that avoids compromising the vaginal axis, length, and capacity, while in the frail or elderly woman, colpocliesis may be effective. The patient's lifestyle (sedentary vs. active) and coexisting medical conditions (eg, chronic obstructive pulmonary disease, steroid use, diabetes, connective tissue disorders) may direct the surgical approach. Patients with severe degrees of prolapse associated with extreme attenuation of local tissues may benefit from additional support measures afforded by inclusion of exogenous material. Such "fascial replacement" can be accomplished abdominally or transvaginally. Taken together, a single surgical route or procedure may be inadequate to address all support defects, and a combination "above and below" strategy may be useful.

With improvements in endoscopic instrumentation and video technology, laparoscopic techniques continue to evolve as an alternative to abdominal repair of pelvic organ prolapse. Procedures such as uterosacral suspension, culdoplasty, and abdominal sacral colpopexy are feasible laparoscopically. As less invasive surgical techniques, these laparoscopic repairs have low morbidity, with excellent anatomic restoration.[11-15] The following sections will focus on these procedures, outlining informed consent, patient preparation, instrumentation, surgical technique, postoperative care, results, and potential complications. Although laparoscopic Burch colposuspension (the Burch procedure) and paravaginal repair (for correction of an anterior defect) and laparoscopic levator myorraphy (for correction of posterior vaginal defect) have been described,[16] the specific focus of this chapter will be on correction of apical (ie, vaginal vault) and perineal body support defects. We believe that correction of isolated anterior and posterior compartment defects is more easily addressed by the vaginal approach, and higher failure rates have been reported for laparoscopic Burch colposuspension compared to traditional open surgery.[1-3] Recommended instrumentation and equipment for laparoscopic pelvic surgery is listed in Table 62-1.

INDICATIONS FOR LAPAROSCOPIC REPAIR OF PELVIC ORGAN PROLAPSE

Laparoscopic pelvic organ prolapse repair is indicated in individuals with symptomatic pelvic organ prolapse who desire to maintain sexual function. Patients should be free of medical comorbidities that preclude abdominal laparoscopy (ie, severe pulmonary or cardiovascular disease, bleeding diatheses). In addition, patients must be able to tolerate a general anesthesia, as laparoscopic repair of pelvic organ prolapse can-

Table 62-1 Instrumentation and Equipment for Laparoscopic Pelvic Surgery

Laparoscopic Equipment	General Equipment
Endoscopic camera	Hand-held electrocautery device and unit
High-powered endoscopic light source	2-0, 3-0, 4-0 and 0-polyglactin suture
Fiberoptic light cable	2-0 polyethylene terephthalate suture (TI-CRON, U.S.
Color video monitor (2)	Surgical Corp.) or other non-absorbable suture material
Carbon dioxide gas insufflator	Pelvicol porcine dermal xenograft (Bard, Covington GA)
Veress needle	or other suitable graft material
10-mm 0° and 30° laparoscope	Sterile measuring tape
12-mm Visiport device (United States Surgical Corp.)	No. 15 scalpel blade
12-mm trocar (1)	16 French Foley catheter
5-mm trocar (3)	Ampule of methylene blue or indigo carmine
5-mm atraumatic grasping forceps	**Equipment for Vaginal Surgery:**
5-mm curved monopolar electrocautery scissors	
5-mm electrocautery hook	Weighted vaginal speculum
5-mm bipolar electrocautery forceps	End-to-end anastomosis (EEA) sizer or sponge-stick for
Laparoscopic Kitner dissectors	vaginal manipulation
5-mm needle drivers (2)	
5-mm irrigator/aspirator device	**Optional Equipment:**
5- and 10-mm vascular clip appliers	
Carter-Thomason fascial closure device	AESOP Robotic Arm (Computer Motion, Inc., Goleta, CA)
Anti-fog lens solution and/or sterile hot water thermos	5-mm ultrasonic shears
	10-mm endoscopic linear stapling device (for vaginal
	hysterectomy)

not be performed under a regional anesthetic. Prior abdominal or pelvic surgery (eg, abdominal hysterectomy, appendectomy) is not an absolute contraindication to laparoscopic pelvic floor reconstruction, but patients with a "frozen pelvis" or who have received prior radiotherapy should be approached with caution.

INFORMED CONSENT

For any laparoscopic procedure, the patient should be aware of the possibility of conversion to an open technique. Patients should be informed about the possibility of bleeding and the need for transfusion, cardiovascular event, infection, adhesions, and adjacent vascular and organ injury (including the colon, rectum, small bowel, ureters, or bladder). For patients undergoing sacral colpopexy with graft interposition, additional risks of erosion, infection, bowel fistulization, reoperation and explantation should be discussed. With concurrent vaginal surgery, such as colporrhaphy or pubovaginal sling, the possibility of postoperative urinary retention should be discussed. Instructions on clean intermittent catheterization should be given to these patients preoperatively. Lastly, the possibility of recurrent prolapse should always be discussed with the patient prior to surgery.

PREOPERATIVE PREPARATION

In preparation for laparoscopic pelvic surgery, patients are instructed to maintain a clear liquid diet one day prior to surgery. Bowel preparation includes one bottle of citrate of magnesium taken the day prior to surgery and a cleansing enema the morning of surgery. Patients are instructed to discontinue blood thinners (including aspirin, warfarin, vitamin E) and all nonsteroidal anti-inflammatory medications at least 7 days prior to

surgery. One dose of intravenous antibiotics to cover skin and bowel flora as well as vaginal anaerobes (eg, cefoxitin and clindamycin) is administered prior to surgery.

SURGICAL TECHNIQUES

PATIENT POSITIONING AND OBTAINING ACCESS
To allow vaginal and abdominal access during surgery, the patient is placed in lithotomy position in Allen stirrups with the hands and arms padded and tucked at the sides of the abdomen. Sequential compression devices are placed on the patient's padded lower extremities. After establishment of general anesthesia, the patient is secured to the operating table with shoulder sleds and tape at the level of the chest. Steep Trendelenburg's position is induced to encourage cephalad migration of the bowel contents out of the pelvic cavity. An orogastric tube and Foley catheter are placed to decompress the stomach and bladder. If available, the AESOP robotic arm (Intuitive Surgical Inc., Sunnyvale, CA) is attached to the operating table at the level of the patient's right shoulder; otherwise, the laparoscope is held and controlled by the assistant surgeon.

Insufflation of the peritoneal cavity is achieved using a Veress needle. Alternatively, the Hassan technique may be used, especially if the patient has had prior pelvic surgery making Veress access more risky. Trocars are placed as shown in Figure 62-1. Initially, a 12-mm trocar is inserted at the level of the umbilicus with the use of a Visiport device (U.S. Surgical Corp., Norwalk, CT). The remaining trocars are inserted under laparoscopic view. Most laparoscopic pelvic reconstruction can be done with a transperitoneal four-trocar technique. Although much of the operation requires only the 5-mm trocars, a 12-mm trocar is required at the right pararectus site to allow for insertion of an endoscopic linear

stapling device (if needed for laparoscopic-assisted hysterectomy), 10-mm vascular clips, and for introduction of sutures and other necessary instrumentation into the operative field. A fifth 5-mm trocar may be placed just medial to the left anterior superior iliac spine if needed for retraction of the sigmoid colon. An insufflation pressure of 15 mm Hg with carbon dioxide gas is used during the duration of the operation. A 10-mm 0° laparoscope is placed through the umbilical trocar and its movement controlled by the AESOP robotic arm. The operating surgeon stands on the left side of the patient, operating through the two pararectus trocars with the table rotated slightly towards the left. The assistant surgeon stands on the right side of the patient providing retraction, suction, and irrigation via the right–lower-quadrant 5-mm trocar.

CORRECTION OF APICAL (VAGINAL VAULT) SUPPORT DEFECT
Vaginal vault prolapse is estimated to occur in 0.1 to 45% of patients following hysterectomy[17,18] and is associated with attenuation of the uterosacral and cardinal ligament complex when the uterus is present. For women with symptomatic uterovaginal prolapse, laparoscopic-assisted vaginal hysterectomy can be performed in conjunction with a gynecology team prior to pelvic reconstruction. The indications and technique of laparoscopic-assisted vaginal hysterectomy are beyond the scope of this chapter and can be found in gynecologic surgical texts elsewhere.[19] Two laparoscopic techniques for the correction of apical support defects include transperitoneal laparoscopic sacral colpopexy and uterosacral ligament suspension.

Laparoscopic Sacral Colpopexy Laparoscopic sacral colpopexy is performed transperitoneally, modeling the conventional abdominal sacral colpopexy. While we prefer acellular porcine dermis (Pelvicol) for grafting between the prolapsed vagina and anterior sacrum, other

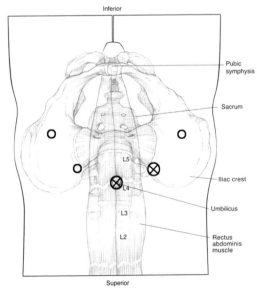

Figure 62-1 Trocar configuration for laparoscopic pelvic surgery, with 12-mm trocars (*larger circle with X*) and 5-mm trocars (*smaller circle*).

options are available. The procedure is described in a step-wise fashion.

Step 1 – Exposure of the pelvic cavity As many patients will have had prior pelvic surgery (ie, hysterectomy, tubal ligation, prolapse repair) extensive adhesiotomy may be required. The pelvic cavity should be cleared of any small bowel. With the patient in a steep (30° to 40°) Trendelenburg's position, blunt retraction of the small bowel out of the pelvic cavity is usually sufficient for exposure to the true pelvis. Adhesions that commonly occur between the sigmoid colon and lateral pelvic sidewall should be carefully lysed with laparoscopic scissors to allow for retraction of the sigmoid colon to the left side of the pelvis and exposure of the sacral promontory. For patients with a redundant sigmoid colon, this segment may be pexed to the left anterior abdominal wall for enhanced exposure. A 3-0 silk suture on a Keith needle is first passed through the left abdominal wall lateral to the left pararectus trocar, through an epiploic appendage of the sigmoid and passed back out of the left abdominal wall near the insertion site. As the suture is tied externally, the sigmoid is retracted anteriorly and superiorly out of the pelvis. Alternatively, a 5th trocar (5-mm) placed two finger breadths medial to the left anterior superior iliac spine, can accommodate instruments for retracting the sigmoid colon.

Step 2 – Delineation of the vaginal apex An EEA sizer or sponge-stick is inserted into the vagina to delineate the vaginal apex and its relationship to the bladder, rectum, and sacrum (Figure 62-2) and to manipulate the vagina during laparoscopic dissection and suturing.

Step 3 - Exposure of the vaginal cuff A transverse incision is made in the peritoneum overlying the vaginal apex. The peritoneum is dissected circumferentially, exposing the serosal surface of the vaginal apex. Care should be taken in mobilizing the bladder from the anterior surface and the rectum from the posterior surface of the vagina so as to minimize the risk of iatrogenic injury to these structures with subsequent fistula. As a blunt device, a laparoscopic Kitner dissector can be useful for this maneuver. If the plane between the bladder and anterior vagina is difficult to define, the bladder can be partially filled to delineate the margin between the two structures. The anterior and posterior portion of the vaginal apex should be adequately exposed (ie, approximately 3 to 4 cm) to allow the V-shaped graft to be adequately secured (see Step 5).

Step 4 – Exposure of the sacrum After mobilizing and retracting the sigmoid colon to the left, a vertical peritoneal incision is made overlying the midline of the sacrum starting from the sacral promontory and extending to the vaginal cuff. Dissection along the midline minimizes possible injury to the sacral nerves. Superficial peritoneal flaps are raised to allow for proper coverage of the graft once in place. Laparoscopic forceps can be used to "palpate" the underlying bony sacrum. In certain cases, the use of a 10-mm 30° laparoscopic lens may provide a better perspective for visualizing the sacrum. Careful blunt dissec-

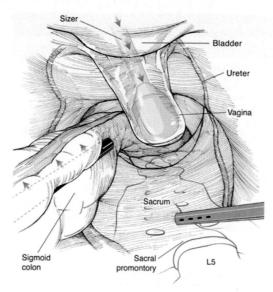

Figure 62-2 Laparoscopic assessment of anatomic relationship of vaginal apex to rectum, bladder, and sacrum.

tion of the fatty tissue over the sacrum reveals the longitudinal glistening white fibers of the anterior sacrococcygeal ligament. The middle sacral vessels coursing along the midline of the sacrum can be a source of troublesome bleeding and should be avoided. Only a small 2-cm window exposing the sacrococcygeal ligament overlying the first and second sacral segments is necessary.

Step 5 – Insertion and fixation of graft support With an EEA sizer or sponge-stick placed into the vagina to simulate the normal vaginal axis, a sterile measuring tape can be inserted into the operative field to define the length between the vaginal apex and mid-sacrum. A suitable length graft (approximately double the length measured between the vaginal apex and sacrum) is introduced into the operative field through a 12-mm trocar. To support the vaginal apex, we use a single piece of graft folded into a V-shaped strut (Figure 62-3). The authors prefer acellular porcine dermis (xenograft) for this purpose, although use of synthetic and allograft tissue has been described.[20] First, two to three interrupted permanent sutures are placed between the graft and the vaginal fibromuscular serosa (excluding

the vaginal epithelium) of the posterior vagina using laparoscopic intracorporeal suturing techniques. Once this is completed, the graft is fixed approximately at its midpoint to the anterior sacrococcygeal ligament overlying the first or second sacral body with two to three sutures. Tension should be applied to each suture to determine if adequate bites of the anterior sacrococcygeal ligament anchor the graft strut. Alternatively, titanium staples or spiral tacks can be used to secure the graft.[12,15] Finally, the remaining length of graft is folded forward on itself and secured to the anterior vagina (Figure 62-4). Any redundancy of graft material can be trimmed. Using an EEA sizer or sponge-stick, the assistant can elevate the vaginal apex towards the sacrum to simulate the normal vaginal axis and reduce tension on the graft during fixation. Excessive tension on the graft strut should be avoided because failure of the repair may occur due to disruption of the vaginal or sacral sutures postoperatively. Patients may also experience pelvic pain or defecation dysfunction if the graft is under tension.

Step 6 – Retroperitonealization of the graft and culdoplasty The graft strut is retroperitonealized by using a continuous 3-0 polyglactin suture to re-approximate the peritoneal flaps (Figure 62-5) and a modified Moschcowitz and Halban culdoplasty is performed to close the rectovaginal and paravaginal spaces using (3-0 polyglactin) purse-string sutures to minimize the risk of postoperative enterocele formation.[21,22]

Step 7 – Cystoscopic evaluation Cystoscopy is routinely performed following the above laparoscopic repair to assess patency of the ureters. Methylene blue or indigo carmine may be administered intravenously for this purpose. If any concern exists regarding the integrity of either ureter, the ureters must be evaluated by either fluoroscopic (ie, retrograde pyelography) and/or laparoscopic means.

Step 8 - Exiting the abdomen The insufflation pressure is dropped to 8 to 10 mm Hg, and the pelvis is inspected closely for bleeding. After

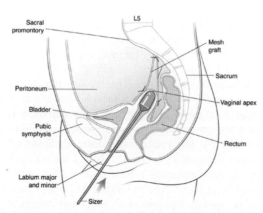

Figure 62-3 Sagittal view of inverted V-shaped graft bridging the vaginal apex and sacrum.

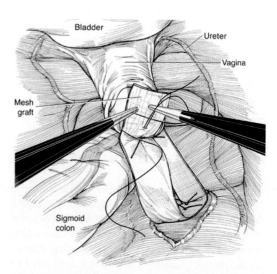

Figure 62-4 Laparoscopic intracorporeal suturing of graft to the posterior vagina, followed by the sacrum, and lastly, the anterior vagina.

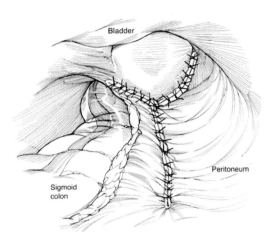

Figure 62-5 Retroperitonealization of graft.

obtaining hemostasis and only after confirming bilateral ureteral efflux, the 12-mm trocar sites are closed using the Carter-Thomason fascial closure device (Inlet Medical, Eden Prairie, MN), and the trocars are removed under laparoscopic view. All trocar sites are closed with 4-0 polyglactin subcuticular stitches and sterile dressings applied.

Laparoscopic Uterosacral Ligament Suspension Uterosacral ligament suspension is an alternative method for correction of vaginal vault prolapse. This repair is best performed in the setting where uterosacral ligaments are well defined with little attenuation. Unilateral suspension of the vaginal apex to the right uterosacral ligament is often sufficient, but bilateral uterosacral ligament suspension can be performed. The first two steps of laparoscopic uterosacral ligament suspension follow that of laparoscopic sacral colpopexy described above. Since the vaginal apex is sutured directly to the uterosacral ligament(s), the steps for exposure of the vagina, sacrum and use of interposing graft material are not necessary. The following steps continue from Steps 1 & 2 described above:

Step 3 – Defining the uterosacral ligaments The fold of the right uterosacral ligaments can be easily defined by pushing the vaginal apex to the left side of the pelvis using an EEA sizer or sponge-stick placed within the vagina. Alternatively, a tenaculum or an Allis clamp placed on the vaginal apex can be used to evert the vagina, thus placing tension on the uterosacral ligaments. As the uterosacral ligaments normally coalesce and insert at the level of the cervix, they will appear as two folds coursing laterally between the vagina, along the pelvic sidewall, and toward the sacrum. These folds *should not* be mistaken for the ureteral fold lying just anterior and lateral. As the uterosacral ligament lies in close proximity to the ureter (at times within 1 to 2 cm), care should be taken to avoid entrapping the ureter or distorting its course during placement and fixation of the sutures between the uterosacral ligament and vagina.

Step 5 – Fixation of the vaginal apex to the uterosacral ligament Two to three permanent interrupted sutures are placed between deep bites of the serosal layer of the lateral aspect of the vaginal apex and the ipsilateral uterosacral ligament (Figure 62-6). A similar fixation is performed between the vagina and uterosacral ligament on the contralateral side. An EEA sizer or sponge-stick is placed into the vagina to elevate the vaginal apex toward the uterosacral ligaments, reducing tension during fixation.

Step 6 – Culdoplasty and exiting the abdomen As in laparoscopic sacral colpopexy, a modified Moschcowitz and Halban culdoplasty is performed to close the rectovaginal space with 3-0 polyglactin purse-string sutures.[21,22] Following laparoscopic repair and prior to exiting the abdomen, a cystoscopy is performed to ensure patency of the ureters. Only after efflux from the ureters is confirmed are the trocar sites closed and abdomen exited.

CORRECTION OF PERINEAL DESCENT Perineal body descent was originally described by Parks and colleagues in 1966.[23] Since their observation, the condition has been linked to a variety of anorectal and gastrointestinal disorders, including constipation, fecal incontinence, rectocele, and enterocele. The association of these various bowel conditions to perineal body descent is thought to result from stretching of the pudendal nerve, with subsequent neuropraxia. Surgical repairs that do not reestablish perineal body support in those patients with excessive perineal body laxity may result in worsening pudendal neuropraxia and denervation of the pelvic floor musculature. As a consequence, persistent or recurrent prolapse may occur. In women with symptomatic perineal descent associated with vaginal vault prolapse, sacral colpoperineopexy reconstitutes support of the perineum, posterior compartment and vagina.

Laparoscopic Sacral Colpoperineopexy As in laparoscopic sacral colpopexy described above, the vaginal apex and sacrum are defined and exposed by the transperitoneal laparoscopic route. In order to restore perineal body support, a longer segment of graft is required to span the length from perineum to sacrum. Again a V-

shaped configuration is used, with a longer arm extending down and attaching to the perineal body. Pressure on the perineum is applied with a sponge-stick to provide laparoscopic visualization of the perineal body. Two interrupted permanent sutures are placed between secure bites of the perineal body and the anchoring graft. The long arm of the graft strut is then secured to the posterior vagina followed by the anterior sacrococcygeal ligament overlying the sacrum. Once support of the perineal body and posterior vagina are established, the graft is then folded forward on itself and secured to the anterior vagina. As previously described, the graft is retroperitonealized, and a culdoplasty is performed.

POSTOPERATIVE CARE

Following laparoscopic repair of pelvic organ prolapse, a 16 French Foley catheter is left in place and removed on the first postoperative day. If a simultaneous cystocele, rectocele, or pubovaginal sling procedure has been performed, an estrogen or clindamycin-impregnated vaginal packing is left in place for 24 hours and then removed. Intravenous ketorolac is administered for postoperative pain control, and patients are begun on clear liquids on the first postoperative day. Patients are discharged once tolerating a diet and ambulating without assistance. If patients are unable to void, a Foley catheter is reinserted and a voiding trial performed in 3 to 5 days on an outpatient basis. Alternatively, patients can be taught clean intermittent catheterization until normal voiding returns.

Patients are instructed to avoid heavy lifting for 6 to 8 weeks postoperatively. Intercourse should be avoided for the first 6 weeks after surgery. Stool softeners may be given to prevent constipation.

RESULTS

The technique of laparoscopic sacral colpopexy was first described by Nezhat and colleagues in 1994.[12] In their series, the laparoscopic approach to correction of vaginal vault prolapse was applied to 12 women with symptomatic post-hysterectomy vaginal prolapse and 3 women with genital prolapse who required hysterectomy. Using modifications of conventional abdominal sacral colpopexy, vaginal vault suspension to the sacrum was performed laparoscopically using either Gore-Tex (W.L. Gore and Associates, Inc., Phoenix, AZ) or mersilene mesh interposition. Mean operative time was 170 minutes, estimated blood loss was 226 mL, and length of stay was 2.3 days. Within a follow-up period ranging from 3 to 40 months, all patients described relief of their symptoms and had excellent vaginal support without coital difficulties or prolapse recurrence. One bleeding complication requiring open conversion occurred during application of staples for sacral graft fixation. Since the report by Nezhat and colleagues, several other series have been published addressing laparoscopic management of pelvic organ prolapse. These are summarized in Table 62-2. As many of the series included women who required

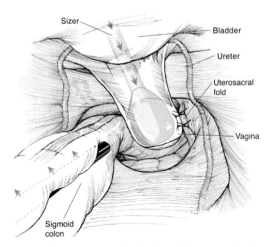

Figure 62-6 Laparoscopic fixation of the vagina to the right uterosacral ligament.

Table 62-2 Clinical Results of Laparoscopic Series Addressing Vaginal Vault Prolapse

Clinical Series	Prolapse Procedure(s)[a]	No. Patients	Mean Follow-up (mos.)	Mean Operating Time (min)	Mean EBL (mL)	Mean Hospital Stay (days)	Objective Success (%)[b]	Subjective Success (%)[b]
Nezhat et al.[12]	Lap sacral colpopexy	15	range 3–40	170	226	2.3	N/A	100
Ross[11]	Lap sacral colpopexy[c]	19	12	N/A	N/A	<1	100	N/A
Montironi et al.[15]	Lap sacral colpopexy[c]	35	14.6	112	N/A	4.3	N/A	100
Cosson et al.[13]	Lap sacral colpopexy[c]	77 (65 patients)	11.4	276	N/A[d]	3.5	N/A	94
Seman et al.[14]	Lap uterosacral suspension[e]	73	8	155.8	129	5.4	90	90.4

[a] Listed surgical procedure addresses technique used to correct vaginal vault prolapse.
[b] Success defined as no recurrence of vaginal vault prolapse.
[c] Various procedures including laparoscopic Burch, paravaginal repair, enterocele repair, posterior vaginal repair also performed.
[d] Only one patient with perioperative hemorrhage over 500 mL.
[e] 73 patients underwent combined procedures of which 47 patients underwent laparoscopic uterosacral ligament suspension to address vaginal vault prolapse.

EBL = estimated blood loss; N/A = not available

concurrent procedures such as laparoscopic Burch colposuspension, laparoscopic paravaginal repair, transvaginal anterior vaginal repair, and hysterectomy, objective comparison of clinical outcomes is difficult. In addition, duration of follow-up is relatively short in these series, and the criteria for defining success of prolapse surgery are subjective. In an effort to use objective criteria, Seman and colleagues reviewed their two-year experience with laparoscopic pelvic floor repair using POP-Q stage quantification preoperatively and at 6 weeks and every 6 months postoperatively to evaluate the outcome of prolapse repair.[14] Patients were treated with site-specific repairs, many requiring multiple concurrent procedures. Overall objective success rates were 90%. For those patients presenting with defects only in the apical compartment (ie, vaginal vault) the objective success rate was 100%.

Comparing the available published series on laparoscopic pelvic prolapse repairs, mean operative times ranged from 112 to 276 minutes, estimated blood loss 129 to 226 mL, and length of hospital stay at < 1 to 5.4 days.[11–15] To date, no prospective randomized comparison exists between laparoscopic and open approaches to vaginal vault prolapse repair, but results from the currently available laparoscopic series approach those of open techniques. Cumulative results of abdominal and vaginal approaches to vaginal vault prolapse reveal a mean operative time ranging from 107 to 247 minutes, estimated blood loss of 168 to 374 mL, and length of hospital stay of 1.5 to 3.7 days.[24–28] The objective and subjective success rates for correction of vault prolapse with laparoscopic techniques range from 80 to 100% and 90 to 100%, respectively. Lefranc and colleagues reported on 85 patients who underwent open abdominal sacral colpopexy for the treatment of post-hysterectomy vaginal vault prolapse performed over a 20-year period.[29] With a median follow-up of 10.5 years, the success rate

for correction of vaginal vault prolapse was 97.7%, with only 2 patients experiencing recurrence of vault prolapse. Others have reported similar success rates for curing vaginal vault prolapse with abdominal sacral colpopexy ranging from 90 to 100%.[24,27,30,31] Similar results (82–100% success rates) with uterosacral suspension via a vaginal approach have also been reported.[18,25,26,28,33] Longer follow-up in the laparoscopic series is certainly needed to determine the durability of their results compared to conventional open surgical techniques.

COMPLICATIONS

While intraoperative complications are rare during laparoscopic pelvic organ prolapse repair, a wide array of events has been reported. These include cystitis; prosthetic mesh erosion; infective lumbar diskitis; trocar injury to colon, rectum, and epigastric artery; ureteral injury; bladder injury; bleeding from paravaginal varices and presacral vessels; blood transfusion; and open conversion.[12–16,34,35] Most of these complications are limited to case reports, making valid comparison with open series impossible. Four complications and their management, however, are worthy of further discussion: (1) prosthetic mesh erosion, (2) ureteral injury, (3) bladder injury, and (4) bleeding from presacral vessels.

Prosthetic mesh erosion following laparoscopic sacropexy was first reported by Cosson and colleagues, when mersilene mesh was interposed between the vagina and sacrum.[35] Staples were used to fixate the mesh to the vagina and cervix. Although full-thickness penetration of the vagina was not noted at the time of surgery by digital assessment, the patient experienced two separate episodes of vaginal pain and bleeding with staples visible by vaginal inspection. The staples were removed vaginally with no sequelae. The

authors concluded that staples should not be used to secure the mesh to the vagina and have since used nonabsorbable sutures. Montironi and colleagues also reported one case of vaginal erosion by polypropylene mesh.[15] Mesh erosion is not unique to the laparoscopic approach, since one series reported a 12% rate of erosion (7 patients in 57) following abdominal sacral colpopexy.[36] Of the 7 patients, 2 patients had asymptomatic erosion of nonabsorbable suture through the posterior vagina, and were treated conservatively with estrogen cream with no sequelae. The remaining 5 patients experienced erosion of prosthetic mesh at the vaginal apex and presented with symptoms of vaginal bleeding or malodorous discharge. The average time to erosion was 14 months (range 4 to 24 months). Although mobilization of the eroded mesh and vaginal advancement was initially tried on 2 patients, all 5 eventually required partial mesh excision and vaginal advancement. No patient experienced recurrence of vault prolapse. From their experience, Kohli and colleagues modified their technique to use cadaveric fascia lata instead of synthetic mesh and avoid placement of permanent sutures at the vaginal apex, which is often attenuated and poorly vascularized. Of note, the overall incidence of synthetic mesh erosion following abdominal sacral colpopexy is 9%.[20]

Ureteral injury and/or obstruction can also occur during prolapse repair. Seman and colleagues reported one case of bilateral ureteral occlusion by suture that occurred during laparoscopic uterosacral suspension that required open conversion.[14] Ureteral injury is more common during uterosacral suspension due to the proximity of the ureters to the uterosacral ligament. The incidence of ureteral injury during vaginal uterosacral suspension has been reported between 2.4 and 11%.[18,28] Buller and colleagues reported that, near the cervix, the ureter courses within 0.9 cm of the anterior portion of the uterosacral ligament.[37] The precise course of the ureters with respect to the uterosacral ligaments is difficult to appreciate vaginally. Laparoscopy may provide better visualization of the course of the ureter and reduces the incidence of ureteral injury. Barber and colleagues concluded that suspension sutures should be placed in the inferomedial portion of the uterosacral ligament at a level just cephalad to the ischial spine in order to avoid ureteral kinking or injury and emphasized that all patients should undergo intraoperative cystoscopy to assess ureteral patency. When ureteral kinking is suspected, ipsilateral sutures should be removed, cystoscopy repeated to confirm ureteral efflux, and sutures placed more medial along the uterosacral ligament. If ureteral injury has occurred, ureteral stenting or reimplantation may be required, depending on the extent of injury.

Bladder injury is rare but most often occurs during dissection of the vesicovaginal plane or in dissection into Retzius' space in patients undergoing concurrent laparoscopic Burch colposuspension or paravaginal repairs. As many patients have had prior pelvic surgery or previous attempts at prolapse repair, scarring may result in obliteration of the natural tissue planes. During dissection between the anterior vagina and bladder, the authors recommend placement of a Foley catheter and either an EEA sizer or sponge-stick to define the limits of the two structures. After initial reflection of the parietal peritoneum off of the vaginal apex, blunt dissection with a laparoscopic Kitner dissector can be used to define the vesicovaginal plane by hugging the anterior vagina and rolling the bladder off of the vagina. Dissection should be carried out medial to lateral, but dissection too lateral may risk injury to the ureters. Small cystotomies can be closed laparoscopically with absorbable sutures with no sequelae.[11]

The presacral vessels can be a source of troublesome bleeding and this has been reported as a cause for open conversion.[12,16] During dissection of the anterior sacrococcygeal ligament, abundant presacral fat may obscure the ligament. Small venous bleeding may be controlled with bipolar electrocautery. If the larger middle sacral vessels are exposed, they should be avoided, and dissection carried out to the right of midline. Sharp dissection should be minimized. Gentle blunt dissection with a suction-irrigator device may be useful in defining the anterior sacrococcygeal ligament. If bleeding is encountered, direct pressure should be applied to the source, and insufflation pressure increased temporarily. Additional trocars may be placed for exposure and control of the bleeding points. Electrocautery and sutures may be used when feasible, but proper judgment is essential for conversion to open surgery if these measures fail.

CONCLUSIONS

Laparoscopic techniques for the correction of vaginal vault prolapse and perineal descent are well defined and adhere to the surgical principles of conventional abdominal sacral colpopexy, uterosacral suspension, and abdominal sacral colpoperineopexy.

The laparoscopic approach provides excellent visualization of the pelvic anatomy, allowing for site-specific repair of pelvic organ prolapse.

Longer-term follow-up is required to critically evaluate the durability, recurrence rate, and morbidity of laparoscopic prolapse repair as compared to conventional open surgical techniques.

REFERENCES

1. el-Toukhy TA, Davies AE. The efficacy of laparoscopic mesh colposuspension: results of a prospective controlled study. BJU Int 2001;88:361–6.
2. Su T-H, Wang H-G, Hsu C-Y, et al. Prospective comparison of laparoscopic and traditional colposuspensions in the treatment of genuine stress urinary incontinence. Obstet Gyenecol 1998;91:55–9.
3. McDougall EM, Heidorn CA, Portis AJ, Klutke CG. Laparoscopic bladder neck suspension fails the test of time. J Urol 1999;162:2078–81.
4. Uebersax JS, Wyman JF, Shumaker SA, et al. Short forms to assess life quality and symptom distress for urinary incontinence in women: the Incontinence Impact Questionnaire and the Urogenital Distress Inventory. Continence Program for Women Research Group. Neurourol Urodyn 1995;14:131–9.
5. Barber MD, Kuchibhatla MN, Pieper CF, Bump RC. Psychometric evaluation of 2 comprehensive condition-specific quality of life instruments for women with pelvic floor disorders. Am J Obstet Gynecol 2001;185:1388–95.
6. Ellerkmann RM, Cundiff GW, Melick CF, et al. Correlation of symptoms with location and severity of pelvic organ prolapse. Am J Obstet Gynecol 2001;185:1332–8.
7. Bump RC, Mattiasson A, De Brubaker LP, et al. The standardization of terminology of female pelvic organ prolapse and pelvic floor dysfunction. Am J Obstet Gynecol 1996;175:10–7.
8. Romanzi LJ, Polaneczky M, Glaxer HI. Simple test of pelvic muscle contraction during pelvic examination: correlation to surface electromyography. Neurourol Urodyn 1999;18:603–12.
9. Kegel AH. Progressive resistance exercise in the functional restoration of the perineal muscles. Am J Obstet Gynecol 1948;56:238–44.
10. Wyman JF, Fantl JA. Bladder training in ambulatory care management of urinary incontinence. Urol Nurse 1991;11:7–11.
11. Ross JW. Techniques of laparoscopic repair of total vault eversion after hysterectomy. J Am Assoc Gynecol Laparosc 1997;4:173–83.
12. Nezhat CH, Nezhat F, Nezhat C. Laparoscopic sacral colpopexy for vaginal vault prolapse. Obstet Gynecol 1994;84:885–8.
13. Cosson M, Rajabally R, Bogaert E, et al. Laparoscopic sacrocolpopexy, hysterectomy, and Burch colposuspension: feasibility and short-term complications of 77 procedures. JSLS 2002;6:115–9.
14. Seman EI, Cook JR, O'Shea RT. Two-year experience with laparoscopic pelvic floor repair. J Am Assoc Gynecol Laparosc 2003;10:38–45.
15. Montironi PL, Petruzzelli P, Di Noto C, et al. Combined vaginal and laparoscopic surgical treatment of genito-urinary prolapse. Minerva Ginecol 2000;52(7–8):283–288.
16. Wattiez A, Canis M, Mage G, et al. Promontofixation for the treatment of prolapse. Urol Clin North Am 2001;28:151–7.
17. Cruikshank SH. Sacrospinous fixation – should this be performed at the time of hysterectomy? Am J Obstet Gynecol 1991;180:859–65.
18. Karram M, Goldwasser S, Kleeman S, et al. High uterosacral vaginal vault suspension with fascial reconstruction for vaginal repair of enterocele and vaginal vault prolapse. Am J Obstet Gynecol 2001;185:1339–43.
19. Nezhat C, Siegler A, Nezhat F, et al. Operative gynecologic laparoscopy, 2nd ed. New York: McGraw-Hill; 2000. p. 272–94.
20. Iglesia C, Fenner D, Brubaker L. The use of mesh in gynecologic surgery. Int Urogynecol J 1997;8:105–15.
21. Moschcowitz AV. The pathogenesis, anatomy and cure of prolapse of the rectum. Surg Gynecol Obstet 1912;15:7–14.
22. Halban J. Gynakologische operationslehre. Berlin: Urban and Schwarzenberg, 1932.
23. Parks AG, Porter NH, Hardcastle J. The syndrome of the descending perineum. Proc R Soc Med 1966;59:477–82.
24. Scarpero HM, Cespedes RD, Winters JC. Transabdominal approach to repair of vaginal vault prolapse. Tech Urol 2001;7:139–45.
25. Amundsen CL, Flynn BJ, Webster GD. Anatomical correction of vaginal vault prolapse by uterosacral ligament fixation in women who also require a pubovaginal sling. J Urol 2003;169:1770–4.
26. Jenkins VR 2nd. Uterosacral ligament fixation for vaginal vault suspension in uterine and vaginal vault prolapse. Am J Obstet Gynecol 1997;177:1337–44.
27. Winters JC, Cespedes RD, Vanlangendonck R. Abdominal sacral colpopexy and abdominal enterocele repair in the management of vaginal vault prolapse. Urol 2000; 56(Supp 6A):55–63.
28. Barber MD, Visco AG, Weidner AC, et al. Bilateral uterosacral ligament vaginal vault suspension with site specific endopelvic fascia defect repair for treatment of pelvic organ prolapse. Am J Obstet Gynecol 2000;183:1402–11.
29. Lefranc J-P, Atallah D, Camatte S, Blondon J. Longterm followup of posthysterectomy vaginal vault prolapse abdominal repair: a report of 85 cases. J Am Coll Surg 2002;195: 352–8.
30. Addison WA, Livengood CH, Sutton GP, Parker RC. Abdominal sacral colpopexy with mersilene mesh in the retroperitoneal position in the management of posthysterectomy vaginal vault prolapse and enterocele. Am J Obstet Gynecol 1985;153:140–6.
31. Timmons MC, Addison WA, Addison SB, Cavnar MG. Abdominal sacral colpopexy in 163 women with posthysterectomy vaginal vault prolapse and enterocele. Evolution of operative techniques. J Reprod Med 1992;37:323–7.
32. Cundiff GW, Harris RL, Coates K, et al. Abdominal sacral colpoperineopexy: a new approach for correction of posterior compartment defects and perineal descent associated with vaginal vault prolapse. Am J Obstet Gynecol 1997;177:1345–55.
33. Shull, BL, Bachofen C, Coates KW, Kuel TJ. A transvaginal approach to repair of apical and other associated sites of pelvic organ prolapse with uterosacral ligaments. Am J Obstet Gynecol 2000;183:1365–74.
34. Kapoor B, Toms A, Hooper P, et al. Infective lumbar discitis following laparoscopic sacrocolpopexy. J R Coll Surg Eding 2002;47:709–10.
35. Cosson M, Vinatier D, Rajabally R, et al. Rejection of stapled prosthetic mesh after laparoscopic sacropexy. Int Urogynecol J 1999;10:349–50.
36. Kohli N, Walsh PM, Roat TW, Karram MM. Mesh erosion after abdominal sacrocolpopexy. Obstet Gynecol 1998; 92:999–1004.
37. Buller JL, Thompson JT, Cundiff GW, et al. The uterosacral ligament: an anatomic description including adjacent structures [abstract]. Int Urogynecol J 1999;10 (Suppl 2):9.

63

Laparoscopic Radical Cystectomy and Urinary Diversion

Andrea Sorcini, MD

Ingolf Tuerk, MD, PhD

Radical extirpative surgery of the bladder remains the treatment of choice for muscle-invasive carcinoma.[1] Bladder cancer is the second most common genitourinary malignancy, with transitional-cell carcinoma (TCC) comprising nearly 90% of all primary bladder tumors. It was estimated that 54,200 new patients would be diagnosed with bladder cancer in 1999 and that there would be 12,100 projected deaths from the disease.[2] The majority of patients present with superficial bladder tumors, 20 to 40% either present with or develop invasive disease. Most TCCs that are or become invasive are high-grade tumors. These tumors originate in the bladder mucosa, progressively invade the lamina propria, and move sequentially into the muscularis propria, perivesical fat, and contiguous pelvic structures, with increasing incidence of lymph node involvement with progression.[3,4] During the past 30 years, radical cystectomy has emerged as one of the standard forms of therapy for patients with high-grade, invasive bladder cancer. However, early results of radical cystectomy indicated that only about 50% of patients treated for high-grade invasive disease were cured and that most patients subsequently died of metastatic disease within 3 years of diagnosis. Lack of universal acceptance of this procedure was due to its morbidity, in particular the need for urinary diversion.[5] This is certainly true of the laparoscopic approach to this procedure.

Laparoscopy, as it applies to urologic surgery, is here to stay. It is quickly becoming a more accepted and popular form of treatment for urologic disease. From the community urologist to the academic specialist, it is an essential tool in the armamentarium of our specialty. Training programs realize the importance and need to incorporate these techniques in educating residents if they are to be competitive in the work force. Urologists' gained confidence in their laparoscopic skills has allowed them to attempt more complex and challenging procedures. Recent technical developments, improved tools for training and learning, as well as patient demand have rendered this field an exciting aspect of urologic medicine. The present day urologist cannot ignore laparoscopy as an important integral surgical tool.

From the time of the first reported laparoscopic radical cystectomy (LRC) by Parra in 1992 to the present, this approach to bladder surgery has gained momentum.[6] Throughout the 1990s, there has been widespread interest in treating invasive bladder carcinoma using minimally invasive approaches. Advances in laparoscopic urologic surgery are most adequately represented by the advent and establishment of laparoscopic prostatectomy (LRP). The overall decrease in patient morbidity and hospital stay is well documented.[7,8] However, the long-term oncologic results, continence, and potency data remain to be determined. With the advent of urologic laparoscopy as it applies to other organs, such as the kidney, the adrenal gland, and, most recently, the prostate, it is a logical progression to apply these techniques to the last frontier: the bladder.

SURGICAL TECHNIQUE

PATIENT'S PREPARATION Bowel preparation is initiated at home by self-administration of 4 liters of polyethylene glycol with electrolytes the day before the surgical procedure. The day of surgery, the patient receives antibiotic prophylaxis with a second generation cephalosporin. The antibiotic is administered at the induction of anesthesia and for 24 post-operative hours. Lower extremity compressive devices are applied before induction of anesthesia.

The patient is placed in a supine position, a nasogastric tube is inserted, and a 16 French (F) Foley catheter is placed to drain the bladder.

MALE RADICAL CYSTOPROSATECTOMY Laparoscopic Access Pneumoperitoneum is first introduced with a Veress needle. A primary 10 mm laparoscopic trocar is then placed at the level of the umbilicus. After inspection of the abdominal cavity, four trocars are placed in a "fan-shape" fashion. Two 10 mm trocars are then placed under laparoscopic control on the lateral pararectal lines about 10 cm above the symphysis pubis. Finally, two 5 mm trocars are positioned 2 to 3 cm medial to the anterior-superior iliac spine bilaterally (Figure 63-1). The patient is then placed in Trendelenburg's position.

Incision of Denonvilliers' Fascia The peritoneum is incised at the level of the Douglas pouch. The tips of the seminal vesicles are dissected to expose the Denonvilliers' fascia. The fascia is incised in the midline to expose the perirectal fat. The fibers of the rectum are bluntly pushed posteriorly away from the prostate. This dissection is carried down as far as the apex of the prostate. Complete mobilization of the rectum is fundamental to better define the prostatic and vesical pedicles and to prevent rectal injuries.

Exposure of Endopelvic Fascia Incision of the peritoneum is carried out along the external iliac artery and extended distally to the abdominal wall lateral to the umbilical ligaments, and proximally to the common iliac artery. At the level of the pubic bone, the bladder and perivesical fat are dissected off the pelvic wall with exposure of the endopelvic fascia. The fascia is incised bilaterally and the fibers of the levator muscle carefully dissected. This maneuver facilitates greatly the identification of the lateral aspect of the vesicoprostatic pedicles.

Dissection of the Ureters The ureters are found at the crossing over of the common iliac artery. The ureters are dissected down to the bladder wall with care to preserve their vascular supply. The ureters are clipped distally, divided, and the distal ureteral margins sent for frozen section. Two 4-0 Vicryl holding sutures of different colors are placed at the distal end of the ureters. The dissected distal ureters are positioned above the level of iliac vessels.

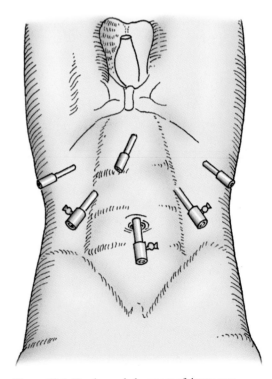

Figure 63-1 Number and placement of the trocars.

Transection of Vesical and Prostatic Pedicles After the previously described complete mobilization of rectum and lateral dissection of the bladder off the pelvic wall, the vascular pedicles of the bladder and prostate are well defined. It is important to note that the bladder is purposely left attached to the anterior abdominal wall in the midline to facilitate the exposure of the vascular pedicles. The vascular pedicles of the bladder and prostate are divided using endo-GIA laparoscopic vascular staplers. Three or four reloads are necessary to completely divide the pedicle in each side (Figure 63-2).

Incision of the Endopelvic Fascia and Control of the Prostatic Dorsal Venous Complex The umbilical ligaments and urachus are incised to enter the Retzius' space. The bladder is dissected from the abdominal wall to expose the anterior aspect of the prostate and the endopelvic fascia. The incision of the endopelvic fascia is completed toward the puboprostatic ligaments. The ligaments are sharply divided to expose the apex and the dorsal venous complex of the prostate. Once the membranous urethra and the dorsal venous complex are exposed, the complex is suture ligated with 0-Vicryl on a CT-1 needle and divided. The urethra and the apex of the prostate are fully dissected. The transection of the urethra depends on the planed urinary diversion and full urethra preservation (orthotopic neobladder) to complete urethra resection at the level of the pelvic floor muscle (supravesical urinary diversion). After transection of the urethra, it is important to close it at the prostatic apex to avoid urine spillage in the peritoneal cavity. The closure is performed with a figure-of-eight 2-0 Vicryl suture. The rectourethralis muscle is divided and radical cystoprostatectomy completed.

The specimen is immediately placed in an endo bag and positioned in the upper abdomen.

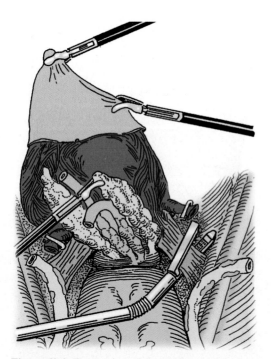

Figure 63-2 Transection of the bladder pedicles with endo-GIA.

FEMALE ANTERIOR EXENTERATION Because of the different anatomy of the female pelvis and reproductive organs, the technique for laparoscopic radical cystectomy has to be adjusted. In preparation for the lithotomy, the female patient must be in a position that allows access to the vagina, which is filled with a vaginal patch.

After establishing peritoneal access, as in male patients, it is easier to handle the bladder, uterus, and ovaries when these organs are fixed together en bloc.

Suture of Fundus Uteri and Bladder After careful inspection of the abdominal cavity, the ovaries are identified. The infundibulopelvic ligaments are exposed and the overlaying peritoneum incised and divided between Weck clips. The broad ligaments are incised bilaterally, parallel to the tubes. The tubo-ovaric complex is completely free. In order to facilitate the excision en bloc of the anterior pelvic organs, the bladder, fundus of the uterus, and ovaries are sutured together. This maneuver allows easy retraction of the uterus anteriorly otherwise performed by the assistant.

Mobilization of the rectum of the posterior vaginal wall, lateral bladder mobilization, and transection of the bladder pedicles is similar to the male technique.

Dissection of Bladder Neck and Proximal Urethra After bilateral incision of the endopelvic fascia, the pubovesical ligaments and the bladder neck are exposed. The ligaments are sharply divided to expose the dorsal venous complex. Once the membranous urethra and the dorsal venous complex are exposed, the complex is suture ligated with 0-Vicryl on a CT-1 needle and divided. Now the urethra is transected at the level of the pelvic floor and immediately closed to avoid urine spillage in the peritoneal cavity. The closure is performed with a figure-of-eight 2-0 Vicryl suture. With the help of the suture, the bladder is retracted toward the peritoneal cavity and dissected off the anterior vaginal wall as far as possible. A vaginal patch in the vagina facilitates the identification of the vagina. At the level of the cervix, the anterior vaginal wall is divided and the vaginal patch is removed. At this point, the vagina is open and the first assistant has to press a sterile sponge against the introitus to avoid gas loss. After transection of the postior vaginal wall, the specimen is completely mobilized and can be removed. Therefore, the first assistant moves between the legs in order to introduce an endocatch bag over the open vagina into the pelvis. The specimen is located into the bag and after closing removed through the vagina. After this maneuver, the vagina is closed with a 0-Vicryl suture on a CT-1 needle using the intracorporeal suturing technique.

Bilateral Pelvic Lymph Node Dissection It is much easier to perform an extended pelvic lymph node dissection after the bladder is removed from the pelvis and the ureter is mobilized and moved away from the iliac vessels. An extended bilateral pelvic lymph node dissection is then performed. The limits of the dissection are the pubic bone caudally, the aortic bifurcation cranially, the genitofemoral nerve anteriorly, and the

internal iliac artery posteriorly. The removal of the lymph nodes is performed using a small endo bag.

SPECIMEN RETRIEVAL Specimen removal in female patients has been previously described. In male patients, bladder retrieval depends on the planed urinary diversion. With the use of a rectosigmoid pouch (Mainz pouch II), the opened rectum offers a unique way to remove the specimen in an endo bag via the anal canal. If an ileal conduit is the proposed urinary diversion, a 4 to 5 cm incision is then performed at the level of the previously selected stoma site (usually at the right pararectal region) to retrieve the bladder. In patients who are selected for an orthotopic neobladder, a 4 to 5 cm incision infraumbilical in the midline is most appropriate for the removal of the specimen.

URINARY DIVERSION Once laparoscopic radical prostatectomy has been mastered, radical cystectomy only involves the additional simple step of taking down the lateral pedicles with the endo-GIA stapler. The challenge is the urinary diversion.

The ileal loop urinary diversion has been the standard type of urinary diversion since it was described by Bricker in 1950.[9] The first laparoscopic ileal loop urinary conduit was reported by Kozminski and Partamian.[10] Their procedure did not include a cystectomy. A total of five port sites were used, one of which served as the stoma site. Laparoscopically, both ureters were mobilized and transected. The bowel anastomosis was performed extracorporeally by gently elevating a small loop of ileum through a port site. The initial operation took 6 hours and 20 minutes. De Badajoz and colleagues and Puppo and colleagues provided their patients with an ileal conduit after laparoscopic cystectomy as described before.[11,12]

To date, most authors perform a laparotomy after lap cystectomy to remove the specimen and construct the urinary diversion (ileal conduit). However, Gill and colleagues have reported successful ileal conduit urinary diversion by laparoscopy alone, performed in two men.[13] The surgical time of the complete procedure (laparoscopic cystectomy and ileal conduit) was 11.5 and 10 hours, blood loss was 1,200 and 1,000 mL, respectively.

Most patients who are motivated and healthy enough to undergo a 10-hour laparoscopic procedure will also be the type of patients who desire the long-term quality-of-life benefits of a continent urinary diversion as well as the short-term recovery benefits of a laparoscopic approach.

The first experimental laparoscopic ureterosigmoidostomy for urinary diversion using pigs was reported by Trinchieri and colleagues.[14] Anderson and colleagues published their experience constructing a laparoscopically assisted sigma rectum pouch as a continent urinary diversion in an animal model (pig).[15] The laparoscopically mobilized sigma was extracorporally positioned via a laparotomy. The pouch was formed by side-to-side anastomosis of the bowel segment opened with a stapler, and the ureterocolonic anastomoses were done extracorporeally. Postoperative function of the pouch was good. However, in 44% of the cases, the formation of stones was diagnosed in the area of titan clips, and in 33%, stenosis of the ureterocolic anastomosis occurred. Denewer and colleagues used the same technique in 1999 for continent urinary diversion after laparoscopic cystectomy in their 10 patients.[16] An 8 cm long incision in the lower abdomen was required to construct the sigma-rectum pouch extracorporally using a stapling technique, and the ureters were implanted in an antireflux fashion. No postoperative follow-up information was provided regarding stone formation.

The most noticeable benefit of the sigma-rectum pouch diversion is the easy construction and the nearly 100% day- and nighttime continence of properly selected patients. The sigma-rectum pouch is a modification of the ureterosigmoidostomy and was first described by Fisch and colleagues as an alternative continent urinary diversion.[17] Several authors reported excellent functional results of this continent urine reservoir after open radical cystectomy.[18–20]

To our knowledge, we performed in April 2000 the first continent urinary diversion completely laparoscopically using the Mainz pouch II technique.[21] Another issue of the laparoscopic procedure is how to remove the cystectomy specimen. Usually laparoscopists make a minilaparotomy incision for specimen removal. The opening of the sigmoid and rectum or the vagina also allows for removal of the specimen without enlarging any of the abdominal port sites.

Despite the simplicity of the Mainz pouch II and the good quality of life provided by this kind of continent urinary diversion, the orthotopic neobladder remains the gold standard of urinary diversion in patients undergoing radical cystectomy owing to muscle invasive bladder cancer. Until 2 years ago, technical obstacles were too great for creating a neobladder laparoscopically. Gill and colleagues first described the technique and the successful outcome of laparoscopic-performed orthotopic neobladder. They used a completely intracorporeal technique and needed 8.5 to 10 hours of operating time.[22] More recently, the majority of laparoscopic surgeons use a laparoscopic-assisted technique for building an orthotopic neobladder.[23–25] This means using the necessary incision for specimen removal to create most of the neobladder extraperitoneally and going back to the laparoscopic approach for the anastomisis between urethra and neobladder. This seems to be the most logical procedure, providing patients with the most desirable urinary diversion, while maintaining the advantages of minimally invasive surgery and significantly reducing operating time.

SURGICAL TECHNIQUE

LAPAROSCOPIC ILEAL CONDUIT: EXTRACORPO-REAL Before performing the minilaparotomy for specimen removal, it is helpful to mark the ureters with different stained holding sutures (white/blue, 4-0 Vicryl), for two reasons: (1)

crossing of the left ureter underneath the sigmoid colon, and (2) identifying the ureters in the minilaparotomy (adipose patients).

The distal 5 to 6 cm of the left ureter is dissected with care to preserve the periureteral tissue and its vascular supply. A space is bluntly created just anterior to the sacrum and posterior to the mesentery of the sigmoid colon to allow the passage of the left ureter to the right using the previously placed holding suture. Just before specimen removal, both holding sutures are placed extracorporeally and secured with a clamp.

Using the minilaparotomy (3–4 cm extension of the right side 10 mm pararectal port) for specimen removal, the distal ileum is identified and brought in front of the abdominal wall. A small bowel segment of 12 to 15 cm is isolated with a GIA 55 stapler. The continuity of the bowel is reestablished by performing a functional end-to-end anastomosis using GIA 55 mm and TA 55 mm intestinal staplers. The mesentery is reapproximated using absorbable sutures and the distal ileum relocated in the abdomen. The distal ureters are brought in the operative field and properly aligned using the color-coded holding sutures. The spatulated ureters are stented and anastomosed in a Bricker fashion to the ileal conduit utilizing 4-0 Monocryl sutures. The proximal end of the conduit is replaced in the abdomen. The fascia of the rectus muscle is partially closed leaving just the space to allow the passage of the conduit. The loop is secured to the muscle fascia and the stoma is matured.

Pneumoperitoneum is reestablished and the proper placement of the ileal conduit is confirmed. The conduit is sutured to the anterolateral abdominal wall to prevent potential internal hernias. A Jackson-Pratt (JP) drain is left in the small pelvis. The fascia of the 10 mm port site is closed under direct vision with 0-Vicryl. The pneumoperitoneum is drained and the procedure completed.

Postoperative Care The Jackson-Pratt drain is removed sequentially as drainage decreases and no urine leakage is confirmed by determination of creatinine in the drain fluid. The patient starts on fluids on postoperative day 2 and oral intake of food starts on postoperative day 4, according the clinical situation. The patient is discharged between days 6 and 8 with both double J-stents in place. In 2 to 3 weeks, the ureteral stents are removed as an outpatient procedure.

LAPAROSCOPIC MAINZ II POUCH (SIGMA-RECTUM POUCH): INTRACORPOREAL Before surgery, patients undergo outpatient sigmoidoscopy to exclude diverticulosis.

Further selection criteria include a competent anal sphincter, assessed by the ability to hold a 200 to 300 mL water enema for 2 hours, and adequate renal function (serum creatinine < 1.5).

An antimesenteric enterotomy is made with an electric hook at the rectosigmoid junction and extended 10 cm proximally and 10 cm distally (Figure 63-3). In men, this allows for transanal removal of the specimen (Figure 63-4). The posterior walls of the rectum and sigmoid are then

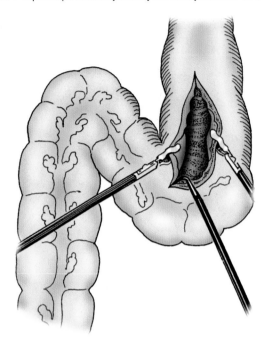

Figure 63-3 Opening of the sigmoid intestine (antimesenterically) with electric hook.

anastomosed side-to-side with a running 3-0 Maxon to form the posterior wall of the pouch (Figure 63-5). Nonrefluxing ureteral anastomoses are formed by preparing a 3 to 4 cm submucosal bed in the posterior plate of the pouch, and then drawing the mobilized ureters through the pouch plate and securing with 3-4 sutures (4-0 Vicryl) in this previously formed bed. After insertion of 8 F monopigtail ureteral catheters (via the opened rectum), the submucosal tunnels are completed by suturing the mucosa over the ureters (4-0 Vicryl) (Figure 63-6). The ureteral stents are brought out of the anus and the pouch is drained with a transanal 26 F Nélaton catheter. The anterior wall of the pouch is closed with a

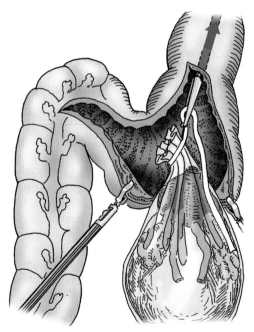

Figure 63-4 Removal of the specimen in the endo bag via the opened rectum.

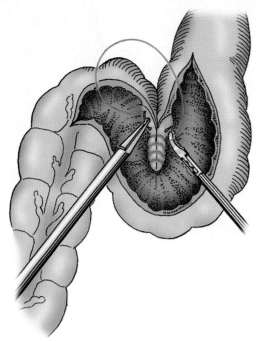

Figure 63-5 Side-to-side anastomoses of rectum and sigmoid to form the posterior wall of the pouch.

running 3-0 Maxon (Figure 63-7). The pelvis is drained with a single JP through one of the lateral 5 mm trocar incisions. The fascia of the 10 mm port sites is closed under direct vision with 0-Vicryl. The pneumoperitoneum is drained and the procedure completed. The Foley catheters as well as both single J-stents are fixed with sutures to the skin close to the anus.

Postoperative Care The JP drain is removed sequentially as drainage decreases and no urine leakage is confirmed by determination of creatinine in the drain fluid. The patient starts on fluids on postoperative day 2 and oral intake of food starts on postoperative day 4, according to the clinical situation. The ureteral stents are removed on day 7 and the pouch catheter on day 8 with discharge of the patient.

ILEAL NEOBLADDER (STUDER): EXTRA-/INTRA-CORPOREAL Similar to the creation of an ileal conduit before carrying out the minilaparotomy for specimen removal, the left ureter needs to be crossed underneath the sigmoid colon toward the right side.

The incision for the removal of the bladder should be located in the midline subumbilical (4 cm extension of the subumbilical 10 mm trocar). Through the same incision, the distal ileum is exteriorized and 60 cm of bowel is isolated 15 cm proximal to the ileocecal junction. Vascularization of the bowel segment needs to be preserved using the standard transillumination technique. Isolation of the loop as well as side-to-side anastomosis of the distal ileum is carried out using GIA 55 and TIA 55 intestinal staplers. The window in the mesenterium needs to be closed to avoid an internal hernia with 4 to 5 interrupted stitches (3-0 Monocryl). The re-anastomosed distal ileum is dropped back into the intraperitoneal cavity while the isolated ileum segment remains

extracorporeal. The distal 50 cm of the isolated ileum segment is detubularized along the antimesenteric line using the Bowie knife. The proximal 10 cm length of the isolated loop remains intact for the Studer limb. The detubularized part of the ileum is folded in a U-shape, and the posterior plate of the neobladder is created with a running suture on the corresponding edges of the detubularized ileum using 3-0 Monocryl. Starting from the chimney, the anterior wall of the pouch is closed with a running suture (3-0 Monocryl), except for the remaining opening at the most distal part, which will be used for the anastomosis with the urethra. The almost completely fashioned neobladder is then carefully reinserted into the abdomen and the minilaparotomy is closed except for the opening of the subumbilical camera port.

After reestablishing the pneumoperitoneum the remaining distal opening of the neobladder is identified and selected for the urethroileal anastomosis. Care must be taken to ensure that the mesenterium of the ileal neobladder is not under tension and the mesenteric pedicle is not twisted. The anastomosis is performed with two running sutures using 2-0 Monocryl on a UR-6 needle (similar to an LRP). Fixing the neobladder to the urethra facilitates the subsequent ureterointestinal anastomosis.

The ureteroileal anastomosis is than carried out completely intracoporeally using free-hand laparoscopic suturing techniques exclusively. After identifying the Studer chimney, the left ureter is brought into the operative field and properly aligned to the length and spatulated. After performing an ileotomy on the left side of the chimney, the left ureter (corner of spatulation) is fixed with one stitch (4-0 Vicryl, RB-1 needle) to the ileotomy. A double J-stent (26/7) is delivered into the intraperitoneal cavity over the right lateral

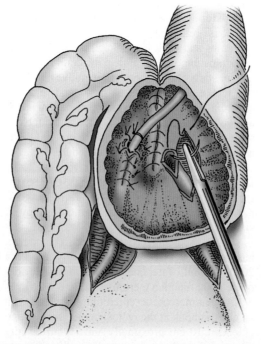

Figure 63-6 Suturing of the mucosa of the sigmoid over the already implanted ureter to create the submucosal tunnel (non-refluxing anastomoses).

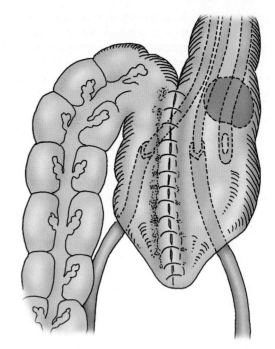

Figure 63-7 The anterior wall of the pouch is closed with running suture (3-0 Maxon) and both ureters were stented with 8 F ureteral catheters and the pouch was drained with 26 F Nélaton catheter.

5 mm port. The proximal loop of the stent is inserted into the ureter and advanced into the renal pelvis, using a guide wire. The distal loop is inserted into the Studer chimney. The ureteroileal anastomosis is completed with two running sutures (4-0 Monocryl, RB-1 needle). The right ureteroileal anastomosis is completed on the right side of the chimney in a similar manner. The constructed orthotopic ileal neobladder is irrigated through the Foley catheter to check for any leakage. After hemostasis is confirmed and the small pelvis irrigated and cleaned, a JP drain is inserted through the left lateral 5 mm port and placed in the pelvis. All trocars are than removed and the port site incisions are closed as usual.

Postoperative Care The urethral Foley catheter is irrigated every 4 to 6 hours for the first 3 days and 3 to 4 times the day after. The JP drain is removed sequentially as drainage decreases and no urine leakage is confirmed by determination of creatinine in the drain fluid. The patient starts on fluids on postoperative day 2 and oral intake of food starts on postoperative day 4, according to the clinical situation. The patient will be discharged between days 6 and 8 with the Foley catheter and both double J-stents in place. Three weeks after the surgery, a cystoscopy will be performed as an outpatient procedure to remove the ureteral stents.

SUMMARY

Clearly, the last decade has seen promising advances in laparoscopic urologic surgery. What once was thought technically impossible is now becoming a reality. Earlier, laparoscopy was used mostly for ablation of diseased tissue, and now it has become a tool for reconstruction as well. Although reconstructive laparoscopy still remains challenging, advances in clip and suture technology have been of great benefit. These advances made it possible for radical cystectomy and construction of a continent urinary diversion to be performed by the laparoscopic approach alone, while maintaining established oncologic and reconstructive principles. But laparoscopic cystectomy and urinary diversion are still in their infancy. A number of problems need to be addressed before such complicated procedures become commonplace. The future will surely see further improvements in instruments for reconstruction plus the application of novel energy sources to achieve more rapid, yet accurate, approximation of tissue.

REFERENCES

1. Messing EM, Young TB, Hunt VB, et al. Comparison of bladder cancer outcome in men undergoing hematuria home screening versus those with standard clinical presentations. Urology 1995;45:387–96.
2. Landis SH, Murray T, Bolden S, et al. Cancer statistics. Cancer J Clin 1999;49:8–31.
3. Lerner SP, Skinner DG, Lieskovsky G, et al. The rationale for en bloc pelvic lymph node dissection for bladder cancer patients with nodal metastases: long-term results. J Urol 1993;149:758–65.
4. Ghoneim MA, el-Mekresh MM, el-Baz MA, et al. Radical cystectomy for carcinoma of the bladder: critical evaluation of the results in 1,026 cases. J Urol 1997;158:393–9.
5. Malavaud B, Vaessen C, Mouzin M, et al. Complications for radical cystectomy. Impact of the American Society of Anesthesiologists score. Eur Urol 2001;39:79–84.
6. Parra RO, Andrus CH, Jones JP, Boullier JA. Laparoscopic cystectomy: initial report on a new treatment for the retained bladder. J Urol 1992;148:1140–4.
7. Guillonneau B, Vallancien G. Laparoscopic radical prostatectomy: the Montsouris experience. J Urol 2000;163:418–22.
8. Jacob F, Salomon L, Hoznek A, et al. Laparoscopic radical prostatectomy: preliminary results. Eur Urol 2000;37:615–20.
9. Bricker EM. Bladder substitution after pelvic evisceration. Surg Clin North Am 1950;30:1511–21.
10. Kozminski M, Partamian KO. Case report of laparoscopic ileal loop conduit. J Endourol 1992;6:147–50.
11. Sanchez de Badajoz E, Gallego Perales JL, Recho Rosado A, et al. Laparoscopic cystectomy and ileal conduit: case report. J Endourol 1995;9:59–62.
12. Puppo P, Perachino M, Ricciotti G, et al. Laparoscopically assisted transvaginal radical cystectomy. Eur Urol 1995;27:80–4.
13. Gill IS, Fergany AMR, Klein EA, et al. Laparoscopic radical cystectomy with ileal conduit performed completely intracorporally: the initial 2 cases. Urology 2000;56:26–9.
14. Trinchieri A, Zannetti G, Montanari E, et al. Experimental and clinical urinary diversion. Ann Urol (Paris) 1995;29:113–6.
15. Anderson KR, Fadden PT, Kerbl K, et al. Laparoscopic assisted continent urinary diversion in the pig. J Urol 1995;154:1934–8.
16. Denewer A, Kotb S, Hussein O, el-Maadawy M. Laparoscopic assisted cystectomy and lymphadenectomy for bladder cancer: initial experience. World J Surg 1999;23:608–11.
17. Fisch M, Wammack R, Steinbach F, et al. Sigma-rectum pouch (Mainz pouch II). Urol Clin North Am 1993;20:561–9.
18. Fisch M, Wammack R, Hohenfellner R. The sigma rectum pouch (Mainz pouch II). World J Urol 1996;14:68–72.
19. Gerharz EW, Kohl UN, Weingartner K, et al. Experience with the Mainz modification of ureterosigmoidostomy. Br J Surg 1998;85:1512–6.
20. Gilja I, Kovacic M, Radej M, et al. The sigmoidorectal pouch (Mainz pouch II). Eur Urol 1996;29:210–5.
21. Turk I, Deger S, Winkelmann B, et al. Laparoscopic radical cystectomy with continent urinary diversion (rectal sigmoid pouch) performed completely intracorporeally: the initial 5 cases. J Urol 2001;165:1863–6.
22. Gill IS, Kaouk JH, Meraney AM, et al. Laparoscopic radical cystectomy and continent orthotopic ileal neobladder performed completely intracorporeally: the initial experience. J Urol 2002;168:13–8.
23. Gaboardi F, Simonato A, Galli S, et al. Minimally invasive laparoscopic neobladder. J Urol 2002;168:1080–3.
24. Menon M, Hemal AK, Tewari A, et al. Nerve-sparing robot-assisted radical cystoprostatectomy and urinary diversion. BJU Int 2003;92:232–6.
25. Basillote J, Abdeshehid C, Ahlering TA, Shanberg A. Laparoscopic assisted radical cystectomy and ileal neobladder: a comparison with the open approach. J Urol 2004;172:489–93.

Laparoscopic Abdominal Wall Hernias: Incisional, Parastomal, and Inguinal Hernia Repairs

Thai T. Nguyen, MD
Howard N. Winfield, MD

ABDOMINAL WALL INCISIONAL AND PARASTOMAL HERNIAS

Abdominal wall hernia following major genitourinary or abdominal surgery is a significant surgical problem. It has been reported that up to 26% of patients who undergo major abdominal surgery can develop an abdominal wall hernia.[1–3] Factors that may predispose a patient to the formation of such hernias include multiple abdominal surgeries, infection, obesity, poor nutritional status, and chronic medical problems, especially pulmonary, all of which interfere with the normal healing process.

Traditionally, the repair of abdominal wall hernias has been approached via an open technique. A wide variety of techniques have been developed, such as those described by Stoppa and Wantz.[4,5] However, the recurrence rate after open suture incisional hernia repair has been reported to be as high as 54%.[6,7] While the introduction of prosthetic material in incisional hernia repair has decreased the recurrence rates, the risk of wound infections and local wound complications may be increased.[8–13] Owing to the high recurrence rates, and subsequent reattempts at repair followed by increasingly higher recurrence rates, an alternative to open surgery is attractive.

With the advent of laparoscopic surgery, a new form of hernia repair is now available to surgeons. The goal of the laparoscopic approach to abdominal hernia repair should be to decrease recurrence rates and wound complications, while offering the patient the advantages of a minimally invasive procedure. The first laparoscopic incisional hernia repair was reported in 1993.[14] Since that time, studies comparing open and laparoscopic abdominal wall hernia repair have suggested that patients who undergo laparoscopic hernia repair experience the predicted advantages of less pain and shorter hospitalization, while the recurrence rate and complication rates are lower.[15,16]

Parastomal hernia following formation of an ileostomy or colostomy is not uncommon. This condition is associated with 1.8 to 28.3% of end ileostomies and 4 to 30.8% of end colostomies.[17] These rates are somewhat lower following loop ileostomies and colostomies. The site of stoma formation (through or lateral to the rectus abdominis), trephine size, fascial fixation, and closure of lateral space are not proven to affect the incidence of hernia. If repair is required, a prosthetic mesh technique should be considered, especially if the hernia is recurrent[17,18] (Figure 64-1).

INDICATIONS The laparoscopic approach may be considered for repair of any form of incisional abdominal, flank, or parastomal hernia that might occur following genitourinary surgery. However, general recommendations would be that if the hernia size is greater than 15 cm in transverse dimension that a laparoscopic approach may not be optimal and may be severely limited in working space requirements. In this case, an open approach such as myofascial rectus abdominis flaps (the separation of parts technique) may be preferable for incisional hernias.[19] For very large parastomal hernias, an open approach with mesh and/or relocation of the stoma may be preferred. Mesh should be generally avoided in the presence of suspected infection or a history of radiation. Comorbidities such as obesity, peripheral vascular disease, or heart disease may favor the laparoscopic approach, because the speed of the procedure, lack of significant third spacing of fluids, avoidance of significant ileus, and decreased pain all help the more ill patient with a symptomatic hernia.[19]

PATIENT PREPARATION All patients undergo preoperative imaging by computed tomography (CT) scan, with a concurrent loopogram performed in the case of parastomal hernias, to determine the contents of the hernia and define the extent of the fascial defect (Figure 64-2). All patients receive oral antibiotics, a full mechanical bowel preparation with Golytely, and are typed and screened for blood products. Patients are routinely given 1 dose of broad-spectrum antibiotics on call to the operating room.

SURGICAL TECHNIQUE Prior to performing the laparoscopic repair, an orogastric tube is placed for gastric decompression and a 16 French (F) Foley catheter is placed in the bladder or stoma of the urinary diversion in the case of a parastomal hernia repair.

Under general anesthesia, the Hasson cannula technique is used to obtain an initial pneumoperitoneum. The location of the initial entry port is in a site farthest away from the hernia defect and surgical incision so as to minimize the risk of entry into an area of adhesions or bowel. In other words, if the hernia were in the right mid-/lower abdomen, the Hasson cannula entry would be the left upper quadrant. The working port size, number, and placement are dependent on the location, type, and size of the hernia. Generally 3 to 4 ports (5–11 mm) are required. The basic objective is to space out the ports in a triangular fan shape configuration with the apex of the triangle directed to the hernia. Adhesiolysis is achieved with both blunt and sharp dissection. The hernia contents are emptied and the fascial edges are freed circumferentially of overlying tis-

Figure 64-1 Parastomal hernia following ileal conduit formation.

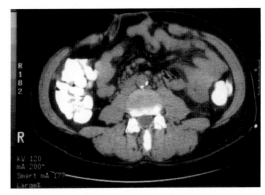

Figure 64-2 Incisional hernia following radical cystectomy.

sue beyond 3 cm (Figure 64-3). The mesentery supplying the ileal or colonic conduit is carefully identified and preserved, with separation from surrounding herniated bowel in the case of parastomal hernia repairs (Figure 64-4).

The circumferential dimensions of the hernia defect are measured by percutaneously placing an 18-gauge spinal needle under laparoscopic guidance through the edge of the fascial defect. Once the size of the defect is determined, a piece of polytetrafluoroethylene Gore-Tex DualMesh product (W.L. Gore & Associates, Flagstaff, AZ) is cut 2 to 4 cm larger. Four quadrant stitches of 2-0 Gore-Tex are placed on the mesh that is then rolled up and inserted into the abdominal cavity through a 10/11 mm port site. The DualMesh has a smooth side with a pore size of < 3 μm, which diminishes adhesion formation to bowel, and a rough side with a pore size of 22 μm, which creates more ingrowth of fibroblast and collagen. The smooth side is oriented toward the bowel contents and the rough side toward the abdominal wall. The mesh is positioned and the quadrant stitches brought out percutaneously using the Carter Tomlinson (Inlet Medical, Eden Prairie, MN) device. The helicoidal staples (ProTack, Autosuture Inc., Norwalk, CT) secures the Gore-Tex mesh to the fascia edge beyond the defect. Tacks are placed every 1.5 cm around the outer edge of the defect. In the case of a parastomal hernia, a radial incision is made in the Gore-Tex mesh such that the wings can be wrapped behind the stomal loop of bowel and secured in place (Figure 64-5). We have found it easiest to fashion the radial incision within the abdominal cavity after the mesh has been partially secured rather than trying to anticipate the location ex vivo. Final hemostasis is obtained and the port sites are closed in the usual fashion.

POSTOPERATIVE CARE An abdominal wall compressive dressing is placed at the termination of the procedure so as to reduce the development of postoperative seromas, and the patient is encouraged to wear an abdominal wall binder as much as possible over the ensuing 6 weeks. Discharge from hospital is variable, but usually occurs within 1 to 3 days, depending on the size

of the hernia repair, postoperative pain, and resolution of any adynamic ileus. Strenuous or lifting activities are discouraged for 6 weeks.

RESULTS Laparoscopic incisional hernia repair has gained increasing popularity as a result of the low recurrence and complication rate of the procedure as well as improved patient postoperative course. Table 64-1 lists some recent studies of laparoscopic incisional hernia repair. Most surgeons are using expanded polytetrafluoroethylene (PTFE) in their repairs. The recurrence rates appear to be 2 to 4%, but have been reported as high as 9%, depending on the study and the surgeon's experience. Mean follow-up is reasonable at 22.5 months. The most frequent complications with laparoscopic incisional hernia repair consist of unresolving seromas (1–36%), wound infections (0–6%), ileus (1–10%), bowel injury (0–6%), and prolonged pain (0–2%).[20]

Finally, four recent studies comparing laparoscopic mesh and open mesh incisional hernia repair suggest that the recurrence, complication, and hospitalization rates are lower with the laparoscopic approach (Table 64-2). However, only one of these clinical studies is randomized.[21]

Sizeable studies of laparoscopic parastomal hernia are currently unavailable in the literature. Most studies consist of case reports or small series. Our own study consists of 4 patients who have all done well with the use of DualMesh at greater than 12 months follow-up.[22] There have been no complications or recurrences noted in this small series.

The most dangerous and time consuming portion of the procedure is the lysis of bowel and omental adhesions from the abdominal wall, and the reduction of the hernia contents. Adhesiolysis should be performed with judicious use of electrocautery or the Harmonic Shears (Ethicon Endosurgery, Cincinnati, OH), especially in close proximity to the bowel. Careful inspection of the abdominal cavity after placement of the mesh for bleeding or bowel injury is mandatory. In the event of an iatrogenic enterotomy, the original standard of care would be repair of the injury by laparoscopic means or laparotomy and removal

of the mesh. Placement of the mesh (ie, foreign body) in this situation would be discouraged. Some authors, however, have recently reported placing the mesh laparoscopically in the face of only an isolated bowel injury in patients who have undergone a very thorough bowel preparation, and who have no other risk factors such as steroids, the injury not being recognized immediately, and spillage not having occurred.[23]

In the presence of potentially contaminated abdominal wall defects, the use of Surgisis (Cook Surgical, Bloomington, IN), a new four-ply bioactive, prosthetic mesh derived from porcine smallintestine submucosa might be considered.[24]

Of the currently available prosthetic materials, GoreTex mesh has been shown to have a lower foreign body reaction, lower rate of adhesion formation, and decreased infection rate compared with other commonly used materials.[25,26] An alternate popular material is the Composix E/X mesh (Davol Inc., Cranston, RI).

LAPAROSCOPIC INGUINAL HERNIORRHAPHY

As pointed out by Schlegel and Walsh, inguinal hernias may be present in 5 to 12% of men with clinical prostate cancer.[27] In the urologic community these authors popularized the transabdominal preperitoneal repair of inguinal and femoral hernias at the time of pelvic surgery. Subsequent reports have confirmed the usefulness of preperitoneal herniorrhaphy concurrent with urologic procedures in both children and adults.[28–30] The logical extension, then, is to perform laparoscopic herniorrhaphy concurrently with urologic laparoscopic procedures. With the growing interest in minimally invasive techniques in urology, especially in the area of laparoscopic and robotically assisted radical prostatectomy, and given that 1 in 10 men undergoing laparoscopic pelvic lymphadenectomy or prostatectomy might have an inguinal hernia, proficiency in laparoscopic herniorrhaphy would obviate the need for reoperation under a second anesthetic, and the need to minimize morbidity for the patient and reduce overall costs to the health care system.

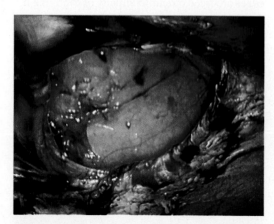

Figure 64-3 Intraperitoneal borders of incisional hernia defined.

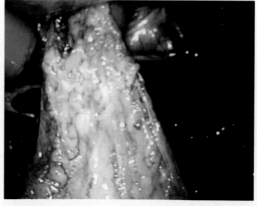

Figure 64-4 Borders of parastomal hernia defined with preservation of mesentery of ileal conduit.

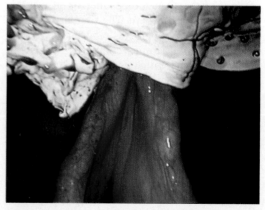

Figure 64-5 Gore-Tex DualMesh wrapped around ileal conduit and tacked to close off parastomal hernia.

Table 64-1 Studies of Laparoscopic Incisional Hernia Repair

Study	Type of Mesh	No. of Patients	Recurrence (%)	Follow-Up (months)
Franklin et al[77]	Polypropylene	176	1	30
Toy et al[78]	PTFE	144	4	7
Carbajo et al[79]	PTFE	100	2	30
Chowbey et al[80]	Polypropylene	202	1	35
Heniford and Ramshaw[81]	PTFE	100	3	22
Heniford et al[82]	PTFE	407	3	23
LeBlanc et al[83]	PTFE	96	9	51

As improvements in technology and refinements in techniques improve the outcomes of laparoscopic inguinal hernia repair, the procedure will be performed more often. In the future, urologists will encounter more and more patients who have undergone such repairs. Indeed, there have been recent reports of laparoscopic inguinal herniorrhaphy complicating subsequent radical retropubic prostatectomy, even forcing the procedure to be aborted in some cases.[31–33] It would therefore benefit any urologist to be familiar with laparoscopic inguinal herniorrhaphy.

INDICATIONS Laparoscopic inguinal herniorrhaphy may be performed for direct or indirect defects, including primary, recurrent, and bilateral inguinal hernias, as well as for femoral hernias.

PATIENT PREPARATION **Preoperative Studies** For the patient in whom laparoscopic urologic surgery is planned, careful examination of the inguinal region with the patient in the upright position during a Valsalva maneuver may reveal the presence of an otherwise asymptomatic hernia. As for all laparoscopic surgery, routine blood work and radiologic imaging is obtained based on the patient's age and medical history. Even if the urinalysis is not suggestive of infection, a urine culture is necessary to exclude this avoidable source of prosthetic infection, especially if the hernia repair is to be done concurrently with a urologic procedure that allows urine into the surgical field (ie, radical prostatectomy).

Medications All nonsteroidal anti-inflammatory agents and aspirin-containing products are discontinued for 7 days preoperatively. Bowel preparation is administered at the discretion of the surgeon, but some mechanical regimen to decrease the volume of luminal contents (eg, magnesium citrate) is recommended. Intravenous broad-spectrum antibiotics, although not strictly required in a "clean" surgical case, are prudent when prosthetic material is to be implanted.

Informed Consent Assuming that the patient is to undergo laparoscopic herniorrhaphy concurrently with another laparoscopic procedure, a discussion of the risks and benefits of laparoscopy in general should have already taken place. Potential complications specific to laparoscopic inguinal hernia repair are discussed later. The patient is advised that the primary urologic procedure takes precedence; if laparoscopic herniorrhaphy at the conclusion of the procedure does not appear likely to proceed uneventfully

because of a difficult previous dissection in the pelvis, bleeding, anesthetic considerations, or other reasons, then it may be postponed. The patient is preoperatively given the option of an open hernia repair under the same anesthetic if the urologist decides against the laparoscopic approach intraoperatively.

Positioning of Equipment and Personnel The main video monitor, insufflator, video unit, light source, and electrosurgical generator are located on a movable cart placed at the foot of the operating table, thereby allowing the surgeon an unobstructed view of the monitor and instrument indicators.

Patient Positioning The patient is placed supine in a moderate head-down tilt with the ipsilateral side rotated upward. Arms should be tucked by the side so that they do not impede movement of the primary surgeon. A Foley catheter should be placed to drain the bladder and an orogastric tube placed to decompress the stomach.

INGUINAL-PELVIC ANATOMY The key to successful and safe laparoscopic herniorrhaphy is a thorough understanding of the inguinal-pelvic anatomy. Urologists familiar with laparoscopic pelvic lymphadenectomy are experienced in identifying these structures from a laparoscopic perspective. A brief review will nonetheless facilitate subsequent explanation of the procedural steps.

The first landmarks evident from the intraperitoneal perspective are the three umbilical ligaments, all formed by peritoneal folds overlying preperitoneal tubular structures. The median umbilical ligament, over the obliterated urachus, is directly in the midline extending from the dome of the bladder to the umbilicus. The medial umbilical ligaments, representing the obliterated umbilical arteries, are usually the most prominent structures, but may be obscured by preperitoneal fat in some patients. They are oriented in an inverted V shape,

running from the deep pelvic space medial to the external iliac vessels and lateral to the bladder up along the anterior abdominal wall toward the midline. All dissection for unilateral laparoscopic herniorrhaphy is performed lateral to the medial umbilical ligaments. Between the medial and inferior epigastric vessels lies the medial fossa, where direct inguinal hernias occur. The lateral fossa is just lateral to the inferior epigastric vessels, wherein lies the internal inguinal ring, the site of indirect inguinal hernias.

Within the preperitoneal space, the plane external to the peritoneal membrane, lie the structures responsible for creating the umbilical ligaments: the urachus, umbilical arteries, and inferior epigastric vessels. Other pelvic structures in this space are the vas deferens, external iliac vessels, the deep circumflex iliac vessels, and pubic or accessory branches of the inferior epigastric vessels. The courses of these arteries and veins are best understood in terms of their relationship to the transversalis fascia analogs (the iliopubic tract, Cooper's ligament, and iliopectineal arch), which are the thickenings and condensations of the transversalis fascia that define the layer external to the preperitoneal space. Whereas the inguinal ligament is the landmark often used by inguinal surgeons, the best landmark for the laparoscopist performing herniorrhaphy is the iliopubic tract. This strong fascia runs from the iliac crest and anterior superior iliac spine inferiorly and medially to curve around the femoral sheath and attach to Cooper's ligament and the pubic tubercle. It forms the medial border of the internal inguinal ring and the lateral border of the femoral ring (Figures 64-6 and 64-7). Cooper's ligament is seen by the laparoscopist as the white ligament coursing back from the pubic ramus under the distal portion of the external iliac vessels to lie at the inferomedial border of the femoral ring. The iliopectineal arch and the underlying aponeurotic arch of the transversus abdominis run lateral to the iliopubic tract, forming the lateral border of the internal inguinal ring, and then insert along with the iliopubic tract on the pubis and Cooper's ligament. The triangular space created by the iliopubic tract and aponeurotic arch inferior (distal) to the inferior epigastric vessels and internal inguinal ring is the weak point in the medial fossa through which direct herniation occurs. An indirect hernia is seen laparoscopically as an orifice lateral and superior to the inferior epigastric vessels (see Figure 64-7).

Table 64-2 Studies Comparing Laparoscopic Mesh and Open Mesh Incisional Hernia Repair

Study	Type of Repair	No. of Patients	Recurrence (%)	Follow-Up (months)
Carbajo et al[79]	Open	30	7	27
	Laparoscopic	30	0	27
Ramshaw et al[15]	Open	174	21	21
	Laparoscopic	79	3	21
Chari et al[84]	Open	14	0	6–27
	Laparoscopic	14	0	6–27
Zanghi et al[85]	Open	15	0	40
	Laparoscopic	11	0	18

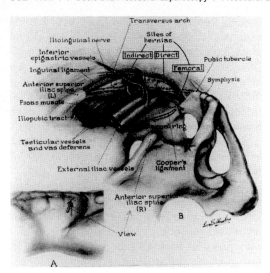

Figure 64-6 Anatomy of preperitoneal structures in the left inguinal space. (From Schlegel PN and Walsh PC.[27])

The testicular vessels laterally and the vas deferens medially form the "triangle of doom" for the novice surgeon performing laparoscopic herniorrhaphy (see Figure 64-7). This triangle containing the proximal portion of the external iliac vessels is the area where the urologist performs laparoscopic pelvic lymphadenectomy. Deep dissection in this area during laparoscopic herniorrhaphy is unnecessary and risks vascular injury. To avoid neurovascular injury during laparoscopic herniorrhaphy, however, the "triangle of doom" is an inadequate warning zone. The area just lateral to the testicular vessels or medial to the iliopubic tract contains nerves (femoral nerve, lateral femoral cutaneous nerve, and femoral branch of the genitofemoral nerve) and vessels (deep circumflex) that lie just external to the transversalis fascia.[34] When fixing the prosthesis in place, it is unnecessary and unsafe to place staples medial to the iliopubic tract in the area superior and lateral to the inguinal ring. The inferior epigastric vessels, distal portion of the external iliac vessels, and their pubic or accessory obturator branches all lie within areas that must be approached when properly stapling the prosthesis to the anterior abdominal wall and Cooper's ligament. Close inspection of all sites before stapling is essential.

SURGICAL OPTIONS Five major types of laparoscopic herniorrhaphy have been described: closure of the internal ring without prosthesis, plug repairs, intraperitoneal onlay mesh (IPOM), transabdominal preperitoneal repair (TAPP), and totally extraperitoneal repair (TEP). The first laparoscopic hernia repair, performed by closing the internal inguinal ring with clips to treat an indirect hernia, was reported by Ger[35] in 1982 with a later report published in 1990.[36] Simple suture closure of an indirect hernia defect and reapproximation of the peritoneum over the repair with clips was subsequently reported by others.[37,38] These repairs were applicable only to indirect hernias and subsequently abandoned owing to unacceptably high early recurrence rates.

The next step in laparoscopic inguinal herniorrhaphy was reported in 1989 by Bogojavlensky,[39] who placed a roll of polypropylene mesh into indirect and femoral hernia defects and closed the peritoneum over the defect. Excision of the hernia sac prior to plugging of the defect with mesh was reported by Schultz and colleagues in 1990.[40] Several other modifications of plug repairs have been described, including the application of a patch over the proximal end of the plug over which the neck of the inverted hernia sac was stapled,[41] formation of the plug into a fan[42] or mushroom shape,[43] attachment of the patch to the plug prior to implantation,[44] and suturing of the aponeurotic arch to the iliopubic tract over the plugged defect.[45] Although the patch is sewn or stapled to transversalis fascia analogs in several of these repairs to improve fixation,[45–47] methods incorporating a prosthetic plug have been abandoned because of high recurrence rates and migration of the plug into the inguinal canal, mimicking recurrence.[34]

The remaining three techniques of laparoscopic hernia repair are based on the open preperitoneal prosthetic repair of Stoppa. The first of these techniques, the IPOM repair, was reported in 1990 when Popp described the laparoscopic suturing of the margins of a direct inguinal hernia followed by the intraperitoneal placement of a patch of dehydrated dura mater.[48] Subsequent techniques have involved the intraperitoneal fixation of a nonabsorbable prosthesis over the hernia defect.[49–54] Despite the minimal dissection required and associated decreased operative time, interest in this technique has been limited by concerns of possible adhesion formation or erosion of mesh into the abdominal viscera.[34] IPOM is still considered investigational, and materials that are less prone to adhesion formation and tissue reactivity are being evaluated.

Currently, the most popular approach to laparoscopic herniorrhaphy is TAPP. Through an intraperitoneal approach, the peritoneum is widely incised and reflected to expose the transversalis fascia analogs supporting the inguinal

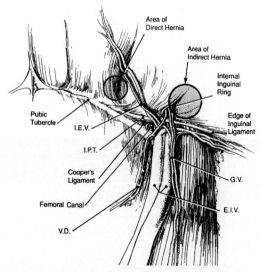

Figure 64-7 Anatomy of preperitoneal structures in the right inguinal space. (From Geis WP et al.[95])

area. A large patch of prosthetic material is then placed overlying the medial and lateral fossae with generous overlap. The mesh is usually stapled in place taking care to avoid nerve entrapment, after which the peritoneum is closed (Figure 64-8). The first large series describing this standard technique was reported by Arregui and colleagues[55] in 1992, and numerous publications since then attest to its popularity. The advantage of TAPP over IPOM is that the peritoneum is interposed between the abdominal contents and the prosthesis, presumably diminishing the risk of adhesion formation and viscera erosion.

TEP is based on the same anatomic principles as TAPP, but attempts to avoid the potential complications of transperitoneal laparoscopy. Although Popp[56] in 1991 proposed the use of percutaneous aquadissection to help develop the preperitoneal space prior to insertion of a prosthesis transabdominally, McKernan and Laws[57] and Ferzli and colleagues[58] in 1992 first described a totally extraperitoneal approach in the literature. Some have reported visualizing the inguinal site from the intraperitoneal perspective; while inserting and then fixing the prosthesis extraperitoneally,[59,60] others perform the entire procedure in the extraperitoneal space.[57,58,61–63] The extraperitoneal space can be developed with a balloon dissector,[61,63] fluid,[60] or gas,[57–60,62] with or without the use of a blunt probe[57–59,62] to aid in the dissection. The proponents of TEP argue that the risk of intraperitoneal complications is reduced compared with the transperitoneal approach. Difficulties with TEP include a limited working space and indistinct anatomic structures. The learning curve for the strictly extraperitoneal approach may be longer than for other techniques. Urologists who perform extraperitoneal laparoscopic radical prostatectomy, however, will be experienced with this approach.

Transabdominal Preperitoneal Herniorrhaphy A skin incision is made at the inferior crease of the umbilicus, and pneumoperitoneum is created with a Veress needle, following which a 10 to 12 mm port is inserted. Alternatively, access can be obtained via the Hasson technique in the same location. After inspecting the abdominal cavity with a 10 mm 30° laparoscope, two secondary ports are inserted, one on each side of the patient a few centimeters below the level of the umbilicus in the anterior axillary line. The contralateral port is 10 to 12 mm in size, while the ipsilateral port can be 5 mm in size. For bilateral repairs, both should be 10 to 12 mm. Alternate port configurations include replacing the contralateral port with one in the midline half the distance between the umbilicus and pubis, or placing the lateral secondary ports lower in the abdomen.

The peritoneum is incised transversely across the anterior margin of the hernia defect(s) from the medial umbilical ligament to the anterior superior iliac spine. Care is taken to keep the incision horizontal and not allow it to drift anteriorly. This incision will place the hernia approximately in the middle of the operative field and will allow subsequent exposure of the transversalis fascia analogs (see Figure 64-8). The only significant structures crossed by the incision are the inferior epigastric vessels and the iliopubic tract. Injury to the former usually can be avoided with careful dissection. Although not necessary in most instances, these vessels can be clipped and transected if troublesome. The iliopubic tract serves as an important landmark for staple placement later in the procedure.

The peritoneal flaps are developed by retracting the peritoneal edges and bluntly dissecting them free from the body wall and underlying structures. If adherent areas are encountered, the surgeon can either use retraction and countertraction by grasping the adherent band of tissue with a second instrument and separating the structures, or the band—if it is judged not to be vascular—may be transected. The vas deferens must be identified and preserved during these maneuvers if it has not already been divided during laparoscopic pelvic lymphadenectomy or radical prostatectomy. The posterior peritoneal flap is developed first. The posterior limit of the dissection is Cooper's ligament inferomedially. Superolaterally, the flap should be reflected only as far as the iliopectineal arch and testicular vessels. Next, the anterior half of the peritoneal flap is reflected. The only structures at risk of injury here are the inferior epigastric vessels, which should be left on the anterior abdominal wall. The flap should be reflected only 3 to 4 cm above the peritoneal incision.

A direct hernia sac, unless recurrent after a failed inguinal repair or particularly large, usually is reducible. An indirect sac is more frequently narrow and deep. If not reducible, the sac should be incised in a circumferential fashion just at or inside the neck of the sac. A wide incision might compromise later closure of the peritoneum. Dissection and attempted removal of the amputated sac are unnecessary and pose a risk of neurovascular injury. The retained sac may fill with fluid postoperatively (groin seroma or scrotal hydrocele), but the collection usually resolves within a few weeks without sequelae. The preperitoneal area that has been exposed is next cleared of fatty tissue, with special attention paid to Cooper's ligament and the iliopubic tract, which will serve as the main anchoring points of the prosthesis. Small vessels, branches of the inferior epigastric or external iliac vessels, will often be seen crossing near Cooper's ligament. These should be avoided if possible, since they may retract under the tension of the pneumoperitoneum and result in hemorrhage during attempted ligation.

The prosthetic material (usually polypropylene) is now introduced into the abdomen through one of the larger ports. A 7 × 12 cm section usually is adequate to generously cover indirect, direct, and femoral hernia sites, but the surgeon should not hesitate to use a larger piece or even two separate pieces if additional coverage is required. The mesh is inserted by rolling or folding it so that it can be passed down the port with a fine-tipped curved dissector. Once in the peri-

toneal cavity, the mesh is unfurled and manipulated into the preperitoneal space. A third instrument port can sometimes be useful since it can be frustratingly awkward at times to get the prosthesis into the proper position. Some surgeons incise the mesh on one side so that it can slip around the spermatic cord. Others believe that this is unnecessary and place the prosthesis over the cord.

The nonocclusive 12 mm clip applier (hernia stapler) is inserted through the midline or contralateral port and used to staple the anterior edge of the prosthesis first, avoiding the epigastric vessels. A bimanual technique using the nonoperating hand to palpate the head of the stapler through the abdominal wall facilitates exact placement. Applied pressure must not be too firm

or staples will penetrate too deeply, risking nerve entrapment. Another trick is to partially deploy the staple and use one end to "hook" the mesh and then guide it into place. The superolateral staples are placed next, extending from the upper corner of the prosthesis only as far down as the iliopubic tract. The last staple(s), placed in the iliopubic tract itself, must not be placed too deeply lest nerves become entrapped. Staples should not be placed medial to the iliopubic tract in this location for the same reason. When applying staples lateral to the internal ring, the surgeon must be able to palpate the stapler head through the abdominal wall to ensure that staples are not placed posterior to the inguinal ligament. Inferomedially, staples are placed from the corner of the

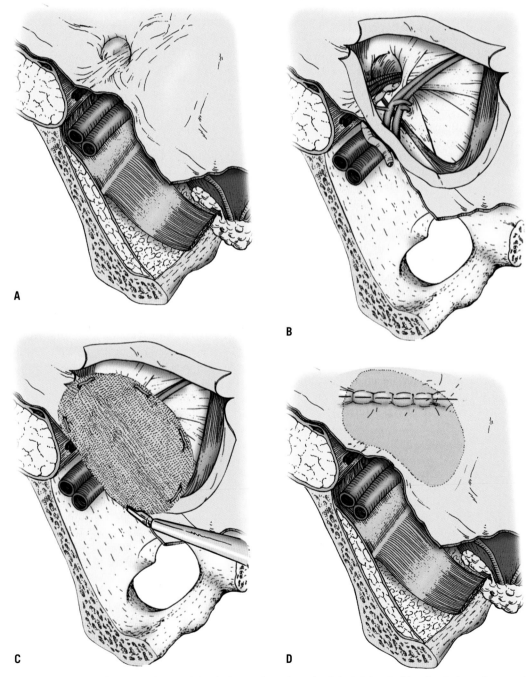

Figure 64-8 Steps in laparoscopic transabdominal preperitoneal repair of the left inguinal hernia: *A,* the peritoneum is incised transversely over the hernia defect (*dotted line*), *B,* peritoneal flaps are reflected to expose the inguinal floor, *C,* the prosthetic mesh is stapled into place, *D,* the peritoneum is closed over the mesh. (From Soper NJ et al.[96])

prosthesis down to the pubic tubercle and Cooper's ligament. Exact visualization of each staple deployment also is imperative to avoid injury to vessels coursing above, below, and over Cooper's ligament and the iliopubic tract. Finally, staples are placed in the iliopubic tract running between the inferior edge of the prosthesis and the internal inguinal ring. Again, inexact or excessively deep staple placement risks neurovascular injury. Figure 64-9 demonstrates appropriate staple fixation of the prosthesis.

Although fixation of the mesh is usually included as an integral step in descriptions of laparoscopic inguinal herniorrhaphy, the necessity of this step is controversial. Many surgeons feel that fixation is crucial to reducing hernia recurrence by preventing the mesh from rolling up and uncovering the hernia defect. Mesh fixation, on the other hand, has been linked to an increased incidence of nerve injury, incurs the increased cost of the stapling device (or increased costs associated with longer operative times if fixation is accomplished by suturing), and necessitates at least one 10 to 12 mm working port if using a stapler. Recent retrospective studies as well as prospective, randomized trials have reported no significant differences in operative time, nerve entrapment, complications, or recurrences between fixed and unfixed mesh repairs.[64–66]

The intra-abdominal pressure is decreased to inspect for hemorrhage and reduce tension on the peritoneum. The peritoneal incision and any defects created during reflection of the peritoneum or incision of the hernia sac are closed over the prosthesis either with the stapler or by suturing. The staples or sutures must be placed sufficiently close together to prohibit internal herniation through the peritoneotomy.

The port sites are inspected for bleeding from the inner aspect of the abdominal wall. Ports are removed one by one under vision at 5 mm Hg intra-abdominal pressure, and the gas is then evacuated from the abdomen. The 5 mm skin incisions are closed with subcuticular absorbable sutures and/or sterile skin tape. The larger incisions are closed with fascial sutures followed by skin closure.

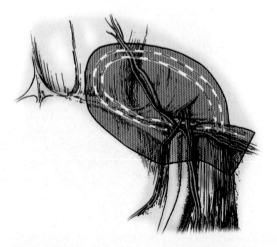

Figure 64-9 Stapled mesh over the right inguinal floor. (From Geis WP et al.[95])

Totally Extraperitoneal Herniorrhaphy

TEP starts with a small subumbilical incision that is carried down through the anterior rectus sheath to expose the rectus muscles. The muscles are split in the midline, and gentle finger dissection creates a tunnel down toward the pubis. Inferior to the arcuate line, this tunnel becomes the preperitoneal space. Choices at this stage are to insert a Hasson-type cannula and start insufflating with gas to open up the preperitoneal space, to dissect with a blunt probe placed through an operating laparoscope, or to use a dilating balloon to gradually lift the peritoneum off the body wall and expand the preperitoneal space. This mechanical expansion breaks strands of connective tissue that often persist when gas alone is used. These strands otherwise prevent full expansion of the preperitoneal space, requiring tedious dissection to transect them and allow complete visualization of the preperitoneal space. The simplest and least expensive dilating balloon is made on the operating table by tying the middle finger of a large sterile surgical glove over the end of a 16F red rubber catheter or other available sterile tubing. Slow inflation of the balloon with approximately 1 L of saline or gas from the insufflator will safely expand the space to adequate dimensions. Alternatively, a commercially prepared dilating balloon can be purchased from one of several manufacturers. One advantage of some of the commonly available devices, the ability to look through and direct the balloon as it dilates, can be duplicated as well by the surgeon at the operating table by tying the finger of the glove over a long 10 mm laparoscopic cannula instead of a catheter. The balloon-cannula is inserted into the tunnel beneath the rectus muscles and the insufflator is connected. When the laparoscope is inserted into the balloon-cannula and the gas insufflated, the pelvic structures can be visualized through the balloon (albeit not too clearly). A final option for creation of the preperitoneal space is to insert a Veress needle, Hasson-type cannula, or dilating balloon directly into the preperitoneal space either at the hernia site or, preferably, just above the symphysis pubis. If the bladder is drained by a catheter, as it should be prior to all extraperitoneal herniorrhaphies, the suprapubic site is fairly safe for gaining access.

Secondary ports are inserted under vision from a 10 mm laparoscope placed through the primary port as in transperitoneal procedures. The secondary ports should be placed lower down on the abdominal wall compared with placement during transperitoneal procedures to avoid violation of the peritoneum. Some authors have recommended placing all three ports in the midline: one at the umbilicus, one just above the symphysis pubis, and the third halfway between the other two. If inadvertent entry into the peritoneal cavity occurs, the gas can be allowed to escape continuously by inserting a Veress needle percutaneously into the peritoneal cavity. This will allow successful completion of the procedure in an extraperitoneal fashion if the peritoneotomy is small.

The anatomic structures are often difficult to identify from the preperitoneal perspective

because the fatty and connective tissues are not uniformly compressed by a membrane (ie, the peritoneum) and therefore obscure the distinctions that can be appreciated from the intraperitoneal perspective. Nonetheless, with continued insufflation and gentle manipulation of the peritoneum off the pelvic sidewall, the appropriate landmarks can be ascertained. The shiny white Cooper's ligament and bluish external iliac vein are often the best structures to identify first. Once oriented, the surgeon cleans off the transversalis fascia analogs and addresses the hernia sac as described earlier. Again, a deep indirect hernia sac should be amputated if it cannot be dissected easily off the spermatic cord. A significant cord lipoma should be resected to allow a better fit of the mesh around the spermatic cord.

The mesh is inserted and positioned as previously described. The same admonitions as for stapling the prosthesis during the transperitoneal procedure apply here. Always proceed with caution on the iliopubic tract and Cooper's ligament. Again, the necessity of mesh fixation is controversial.

The pneumoproperitoneum is released after removal of the ports under direct vision at a pressure of 5 mm Hg, and sites are closed as described earlier.

POSTOPERATIVE CARE If only a laparoscopic herniorrhaphy has been performed, patients are discharged home from the recovery room unless unusual circumstances suggest the need for inpatient observation (eg, abdominal discomfort, need for parenteral analgesics, or medically unfit for rapid discharge). A small number of oral pain relievers are prescribed routinely, although they often are used for only a few days, if at all. The patient is encouraged to resume normal activity the next day, except for heavy lifting, which is restricted for the first week. There may be some abdominal bloating after transperitoneal procedures, and an over-the-counter laxative may be helpful.

RESULTS A few large series on laparoscopic herniorrhaphy have been recently published (Table 64-3). Operative times,[67–69] morbidity, reoperation rates, and recurrence rates[70] have been shown to decrease as surgeon experience increases. The mean operative time may be as low as 30 minutes in experienced hands, but may be over twice that time for those still learning the procedure. Overall minor and major complication rates were 4.2% and 1.6% for this series of studies. Nearly 95% of the patients underwent laparoscopic herniorrhaphy on an outpatient basis. The overall recurrence rate was less than 1%, though only two of the studies report their follow-up time. Prolonged follow-up is necessary to determine the true rate of recurrence following laparoscopic repair.

Several randomized, prospective trials[71–75] have attempted to compare the various techniques of laparoscopic inguinal herniorrhaphy with their open counterparts (Tables 64-4 and 64-5). Operative times were consistently and significantly longer for laparoscopic herniorrhaphy

Table 64-3 Results of Laparoscopic Inguinal Herniorrhaphy

	Schwab et al[67]	Schultz et al[68]	McCloud and Evans[69]	Bittner et al[70]	Total
Period of surgery	5/91–4/01	12/92–11/99	6/94–4/00	4/93–12/01	–
No. patients	1,388	1,952	769	6,479	10,588
No. hernias	1,903	2,500	984	8,050	13,437
Technique	1,561 TEP				–
	324 TAPP	TAPP	TAPP	TAPP	
	18 IPOM				
Mean surgical time (min)	75.4*	32	25 unilateral	47 uninlateral	–
	33.6†		38 bilateral	70 bilateral	
EBL (mL)	22‡	–	–	–	
Converted	17	5	3	10	35 (0.3%)
No. complications	101	89	164	255	609 (5.8%)
Minor	83	70	157	131	441 (4.2%)
Major	18	18	7	124	167 (1.6%)
Mortality	0	1	0	1	2 (0.2%)
Admitted	79	–	39	–	118/2,157 (5.5%)
Hospital stay (days)	0.07	2.1	–	–	
No. recurrences	11	26	8	60	105/13,437 (0.8%)
Follow-up	–	39 mos. (mean)	–	22 mos. (median)	–

*Resident as primary surgeon with attending assisting.
†Attending surgeon only.
‡$n = 433$.

Table 64-4 Randomized Controlled Trials of Laparoscopic versus Open Inguinal Herniorrhaphy

	Taniphat et al[71]			Picchio et al[72]			Tschudi et al[73]		
Enrollment period	8/92–1/96			11/96–12/97			2/93–11/94		
Technique	TAPP	Mod. Bassini	P Value	TAPP	Lichtenstein	P Value	TAPP	Shouldice	P Value
No. patients	60	60	–	53	52	–	51	49	–
No. hernias	60	60	–	53	52	–	66	61	–
Mean surgical time (min.)	95 ± 28	67 ± 27	< .001	49.6 ± 5.4	33.9 ± 6.2	< .001	87.2 ± 27.3†	58.2 ± 14.6†	< .0001
							124 ± 45.3‡	79 ± 16.6	
Mean hospital stay (days)	2.6 ± 1.2	3.0 ± 1.5	.10	2.3 ± 0.1	2.2 ± 0.1	.38	4.8 ± 1.6	6.2 ± 2.5	.0064
Analgesia	27*	18*					2.5 ± 4.5 g	4.6 ± 4 g	.048
	22	21		40.4**	50.0**		paracetamol	paracetamol	
	6	17	.016	40.4	30.8	.69			
	3	4		15.4	17.3		6.5 ± 11.2 mg	19.0 ± 23.7 mg	.0005
	2	0		3.8	1.9		morphine	morphine	
Return to work (days)	14	15	.14	6.1 ± 0.1	6.5 ± 0.2	< .03	–	–	–
Return to full activity (days)	28	35	.25	45.5	42.7	.04	24.3 ± 14.5	41.7 ± 28.7	.0003
% Recurrence	1.7	0	1.0	–	–	–	3.0	8.2	
Follow-up	32 months (mean)	–		–	–	–	4.9 years (median)	–	–

*No. of patients requiring 0, 1, 2, 3, and > 3 pethidine injections, respectively.
**Percentage of patients receiving 0, 1, 2, and > 2 doses of intramuscular diclofenac over 2 days postoperatively.
†Unilateral repair.
‡Simultaneous bilateral repair.

Table 64-5 Randomized Controlled Trials of Laparoscopic versus Open Inguinal Herniorrhaphy (continued)

	Berndsen et al[74]			Lal et al[75]		
Enrollment period	2/93–3/96			5/00–12/01		
Technique	TAPP	Shouldice	P Value	TEP	Lichtenstein	P Value
No. patients	518	524	–	25	25	–
No. hernias	518	524	–	25	25	–
Mean surgical time (min.)	65	55	< .001	75.7 ± 31.6	54 ± 15	< .0001
Mean hospital stay (days)	–	–	–	1.48	1.4	> .05
Analgesia	4 tablets	12 tablets	< .001	2.6 tablets	5.76 tablets	< .001
	Distalgesic	Distalgesic		Voveran	Voveran	
	1st postop	1st postop		(50 mg)	(50 mg)	
	week	week				
Return to work (days)	10	14	< .001	12.8 ± 7.1	19.3 ± 4.3	< .001
Return to full activity (days)	–	–	–	–	–	–
% Recurrence	1.2	0.6	.339	0	0	–
Follow-up	3 months		–	13 months		–

as compared with open repair. Analgesic requirement may be lower for the laparoscopic repair as compared with open herniorrhaphy; however, there appear to be no significant differences in hospital stay, or recurrence rates. Three of five studies found decreased convalescence in the laparoscopy group, one study was equivocal, and one study found no significant difference. No significant differences in major or minor complications were demonstrated except for the study by Tanphiphat and colleagues, which found an increased rate of postoperative parasthesia in the open repair group as compared with the laparoscopic herniorrhaphy group (33% vs 12%, $P = .008$).[71] In addition, Lal and colleagues found that all 25 patients in the laparoscopic group reported being "very satisfied" with the cosmetic results of their surgery, while only 7 patients (28%) in the open group reported being "very satisfied" ($P < .001$).[75]

Most of the randomized, controlled trials comparing open repair with laparoscopic herniorrhaphy contain relatively small numbers of patients, thereby lacking the power to provide statistically reliable results. To enhance the value of individual studies, a meta-analysis of the individual trials was performed by the EU Hernia Trialists Collaboration, which involved 70 investigators in 20 countries.[76] Forty-one trials were identified involving 7,161 patients. Individual patient data were available for 25 trials (4,165 participants). Operative times were longer for laparoscopic repairs by an overall weighted mean difference of 14.81 minutes (95% CI 13.98–15.64, $P < .0001$). Of 3,130 laparoscopic repairs, 85 (2.7%) were converted to open, while 5 (0.1%) among 3,541 open procedures were converted to a laparoscopic repair.

Postoperative complications were uncommon. There appeared to be fewer hematomas (8.7% vs 10.5%, $P < .01$) and more seromas (5.8% vs 3.8%, $P = .001$) in the laparoscopy group. Wound or superficial infection also appeared less frequently in the laparoscopic groups (Peto's odds ratio 0.45, $P < .0001$). There were only 3 cases of deep infection: 1 case of mesh infection in each group as well as a deep infection in an open, non-mesh group. Potentially serious visceral injury or vascular injury was more common in the laparoscopy group compared with the open group (15 vs 5). Six of 7 visceral injuries occurred in the laparoscopic groups, consisting of 4 bladder injuries, 1 small bowel injury, and 1 punctured stomach. A single small bowel injury occurred in the open group. Two postoperative bowel obstructions were both in the laparoscopic arms. Only 6 port site hernias were reported.

In all trials with data, time to return to normal activity was shorter in the laparoscopic groups with a difference of about 7 days ($P < .0001$). There were also fewer cases of persisting pain 1 year following hernia repair in the laparoscopic groups (13.8% vs 19.1%, $P < .0001$). There were also fewer cases of persisting numbness in the laparoscopic groups (7.2% vs 13.4%, $P < .0001$).

In the laparoscopy groups, 86 (2.7%) recurrences were reported among 3,138 repairs compared with 109 (3.1%) recurrence among 3,504 open procedures ($P = .16$). The nature of the open repair influenced the comparative performance of both TAPP and TEP laparoscopic herniorrhaphy. Hernia recurrence was less common after laparoscopic procedures than after open non-mesh repair, but no difference was noted in comparison with open mesh repairs.

COMPLICATIONS General laparoscopic complications are reviewed in Chapter 53 and will not be covered here. A number of complications relatively specific to laparoscopic abdominal wall herniorrhaphy are examined in detail in Tables 64-6 to 64-12.

ACKNOWLEDGMENTS

We would like to acknowledge the efforts of J. Stuart Wolf, Jr., MD, and Nathaniel J. Soper, MD, whose "Herniorrhaphy" chapter in the first edition of *Smith's Textbook of Endourology* provided a foundation upon which this chapter was expanded and updated.

Tables 64-6 to 64-12 Complications of Laparoscopic Abdominal Wall Herniorrhaphy

Hematoma, Seroma and Hydrocele

- **Diagnosis** Postoperative swelling in the groin, scrotum, or abdominal wall may represent hematoma, seroma, hydrocele, or early hernia recurrence. Subcutaneous fluid collections may be noted within a few days postoperatively, but collections deep to the abdominal fascia may not become apparent for a week or more. Hematomas may be painful and tender or may become firmer with time. Erythema, tenderness, and fluctuation should prompt the consideration of infection.
- **Etiology** Undetected or inadequately addressed laceration of abdominal wall vessels (inferior epigastric, circumflex iliac), inguinal-pelvic vessels (deferential, gonadal, external spermatic, cremasteric, obturator, external iliac), or their branches may produce hematomas. Interrupted lymphatics combined with postsurgical inflammatory processes or a retained hernia sac predispose to seromas and hydroceles. Gentle tissue handling minimizes these complications.
- **Prevention** Larger vessels are avoided with careful dissection. Risk of undetected vessel trauma, which may lead to postoperative hematoma formation, is minimized by limiting dissection of the hernia defects and cord structures. Mobilization of deep or large hernia sacs offers no therapeutic advantage.
- **Treatment** Conservative management is usually sufficient, as uninfected fluid collections will likely resolve. In the event of disabling symptoms or suspected infection, operative drainage may be required. If the fluid contains bacteria and is isolated from the mesh, antibiotic therapy and percutaneous drainage are indicated. If the fluid is infected and in contact with the mesh, open exploration and removal of the mesh is indicated.

Infection of the Prosthesis

- **Diagnosis** Erythema, tenderness, swelling, warmth, and fluctuance are the usual external signs of localized infection. Pain, fever, malaise, gastrointestinal disturbances, and leukocytosis may be the presenting signs if a deep abscess forms. Aspiration with microscopic and bacteriologic examination is indicated if infection is suspected.
- **Etiology** A prosthesis may become infected during manipulation or subsequently from direct or hematogenous spread.
- **Prevention** Although there are no specific data regarding mesh herniorrhaphy, the Infectious Diseases Society of America lists procedures that include the implantation of permanent prosthetic materials under the category "moderate evidence to support a recommendation for use" of surgical antimicrobial prophylaxis.[86] Broad-spectrum intraoperative antibiotic coverage of both skin and enteric organisms, such as a second-generation cephalosporin is recommended. The usefulness of continuing antibiotic administration postoperatively is doubtful. There is disagreement as to the need for antimicrobial prophylaxis to prevent hematogenous seeding during later invasive procedures (dental procedures, endoscopy, etc.) in a patient with implanted prosthetic mesh.
- **Treatment** Incision and drainage with removal of the prosthesis are required.

Bowel Adhesion to the Prosthesis and Bowel Obstruction

- **Diagnosis** Abdominal pain, abdominal distension, and gastrointestinal disturbances are the signs associated with bowel adherence to the mesh, with subsequent bowel obstruction.
- **Etiology** Most experimental evidence in animal models suggests that bowel adhesion to the prosthesis is most likely to occur after intraperitoneal herniorrhaphy and least likely to occur following TEP.[87,88] Although PTFE is generally thought to incite less tissue reaction than polypropylene, one group found no difference between the two materials when placed intraperitoneally in a pig model.[89] However, adhesions in experimental animals after transperitoneal prosthesis placement, when they do occur, appear flimsy and do not involve the bowel.[87,88,90] Clinical experience suggests that this complication is unusual in humans.
- **Prevention** Based on the experimental findings noted above, careful closure of the peritoneum over the hernia defect is advised, if possible.
- **Treatment** Repeat laparoscopy with visualization of the repair site is appropriate for the patient who does not respond to a course of conservative management with intravenous hydration, bowel rest, and nasogastric suction. This will allow diagnosis of the cause of the bowel obstruction. Laparoscopic adhesiolysis may be considered, but open laparotomy is advised if there is any question of the ability to safely identify and manage the problem laparoscopically.

continued

Chapter 64 / Laparoscopic Abdominal Wall Hernias: Incisional, Parastomal, and Inguinal Hernia Repairs **587**

Tables 64-6 to 64-12 continued

Nerve Entrapment

- **Diagnosis** Pain due to nerve entrapment may be constant or intermittent, dull or sharp, burning or tingling. Hip flexion often diminishes the pain. There may be pain over the actual site of injury, and a light tapping at this site may cause an "electric" sensation down the course of the nerve.[91] Pain may be noted immediately after surgery or may become apparent over the next few weeks.
- **Etiology** A number of nerves are at risk of entrapment injury during laparoscopic herniorrhaphy, including almost any branch of the lumbar plexus. Entrapment most commonly involves the lateral femoral cutaneous nerve (causing meralgia paresthetica) or femoral branch of the genitofemoral nerve.[91,92] These injuries occur when staples are placed medial to the iliopubic tract in the area lateral to the testicular vessels. Staples around the internal inguinal ring can entrap the ilioinguinal nerve, iliohypogastric nerve, and genital branch of the genitofemoral nerve if staples are placed too deeply (through the transversalis fascia analogs into the internal oblique musculature).[91]
- **Prevention** Careful staple placement, not using excessive pressure when firing staples into the abdominal wall, and avoiding the area medial to the iliopubic tract and lateral to the testicular vessels will prevent nerve entrapment. As discussed above, some surgeons have abandoned mesh fixation altogether.
- **Treatment** With analgesics and avoidance of activities that exacerbate the symptoms, most problems will resolve within 6 weeks. Local injections of anesthetics and corticosteroids may be helpful. If the symptoms persist beyond this period, laparoscopic removal of the offending staples may provide relief. If the duration since herniorrhaphy is prolonged (> 3 months), neurolysis or neurectomy may be required since perineural fibrosis complicates the condition and may preclude resolution by staple removal alone.[91]

Testicular Pain or Atrophy

- **Diagnosis** The complaint of a painful scrotum should prompt an evaluation with a careful physical examination and urinalysis. Suspected epididymitis should be treated appropriately. Testicular torsion is unlikely in this setting but must be considered, especially if the onset of pain is acute.
- **Etiology** Neurovascular injury during manipulation of the spermatic cord or indirect hernia is presumably the cause of postoperative testicular complications.
- **Prevention** Avoiding unnecessary manipulation of the cord structures and indirect hernia sac will reduce the incidence of testicular injury.
- **Treatment** If infection and testicular torsion appear unlikely, then scrotal support and oral anti-inflammatory medication can be offered to provide symptomatic relief since the testicular pain will likely spontaneously resolve over the course of 1 to 2 weeks. Testicular atrophy is a potential complication of any hernia procedure and the patient should be counseled accordingly during the preoperative visit.

Internal Herniation

- **Diagnosis** The patient will present with signs and symptoms of bowel obstruction.
- **Etiology** Failure to adequately close the peritoneum over the prosthesis during transperitoneal herniorrhaphy may allow bowel to slip through the peritoneotomy and produce obstruction.[93,94] Herniation of bowel through the larger trocar sites is more common.
- **Prevention** Careful closure of the peritoneal defect and ensuring that each staple has a generous bite of tissue should prevent internal herniation. Similarly, fascial closure of larger port sites must be secure.
- **Treatment** Laparoscopy or laparotomy, as described earlier, will allow surgical correction of the problem. The repair can be left intact underneath the repaired peritoneal defect. Likewise, for a port site hernia, the bowel contents are laparoscopically reduced and the hernia site closed by intracorporeal or extracorporeal suturing techniques.

Inguinal Hernia Recurrence

- **Diagnosis** A groin mass should be considered to be an inguinal hernia recurrence if there are no signs of infection and the mass is pulsatile with a Valsalva maneuver.
- **Etiology** Most recurrences of inguinal hernias following laparoscopic repair have been attributed to the use of prosthetic mesh of inadequate size early in the surgeon's experience.
- **Prevention** A sufficiently large piece of mesh should be used to cover all potential sites of herniation with generous overlap. A 7 × 12 cm piece of mesh is recommended as the minimum size for laparoscopic herniorrhaphy.
- **Treatment** Several authors have reported successful repeat laparoscopic herniorrhaphy following a recurrence. The urologist performing laparoscopic herniorrhaphy should refer a patient with a suspected recurrence to a general surgeon.

REFERENCES

1. Mudge M, Hughes LE. Incisional hernia: a 10-year prospective study of incidence and attitudes. Br J Surg 1985;72:70–1.
2. George CD, Ellis H. The results of incisional hernia repair: a twelve-year review. Ann R Coll Surg Engl 1986;68:185–7.
3. Israelsson LA. The surgeon as a risk factor for complications of midline incisions. Eur J Surg 1998;164:353–9.
4. Stoppa RE. The treatment of complicated groin and incisional hernias. World J Surg 1989;13:545–54.
5. Wantz G. Incisional hernioplasty with Mersilene. Surg Gyn Obst 1991;172:129–37.
6. Paul A, Korenkov M, Peters S, et al. Unacceptable results of the Mayo procedure for repair of abdominal incisional hernias. Eur J Surg 1998;164:361–7.
7. Luijendijk RW, Lemmen MH, Hop WC, Wereldsma JC. Incisional hernia recurrence following "vest over pants" or vertical Mayo repair of primary hernias of the midline. World J Surg 1997;21:62–5.
8. McLanahan D, King LT, Weems C, et al. Retrorectus prosthetic mesh repair of midline abdominal hernia. Am J Surg 1997;173:445–9.
9. Temudom T, Siadati M, Sarr M. Repair of complex giant recurrent ventral hernias by using tension free intraperitoneal prosthetic mesh (Stoppa technique): lessons learned from our initial experience (fifty patients). Surgery 1996;120:738–43.
10. Koller R, Miholic J, Jakl RJ. Repair of incisional hernias with expanded polytetrafluoroethylene. Eur J Surg 1997;163:261–6.
11. Amid PK, Shulman AG, Lichtenstein IL. A simple stapling technique for prosthetic repair of massive incisional hernias. Am Surg 1994;60:934–7.
12. Leber GE, Garb JL, Alexander AL, Reed WP. Long-term complications associated with prosthetic repair of incisional hernias. Arch Surg 1998;133:378–82.
13. White TJ, Santos MC, Thompson JS. Factors affecting wound complications in repair of ventral hernias. Am Surg 1998;64:276–80.
14. LeBlanc KA, Booth WV. Laparoscopic repair of incisional abdominal hernias using expanded polytetrafluoroethylene: preliminary findings. Surg Laparosc Endosc 1993;3:39–41.
15. Ramshaw BJ, Esartia P, Schwab J, et al. Comparison of laparoscopic and open ventral herniorrhaphy. Am Surg 1999;65:827–31.
16. Park A, Birch DW, Lovrics P. Laparoscopic and open incisional hernia repair: a comparison study. Surgery 1998;124:816–21.
17. Carne PW, Robertson GM, Frizelle FA. Parastomal hernia. Br J Surg 2003;90:784–93.
18. Rubin MS, Schoetz DJ Jr, Matthews JB. Parastomal hernia. Is stoma relocation superior to fascial repair? Arch Surg 1994;129:413–8.
19. Dumanian GA, Denham W. Comparison of repair techniques for major incisional hernias. Am J Surg 2003;185:61–5.
20. Cassar K, Munro A. Surgical treatment of incisional hernia. Br J Surg 2002;89:534–45.
21. Carbajo MA, Martin del Olmo JC, Blanco JI, et al. Laparoscopic treatment vs open surgery in the solution of major incisional and abdominal wall hernias with mesh. Surg Endosc 1999;13:250–2.
22. Kozlowski PM, Wang PC, Winfield HN. Laparoscopic repair of incisional and parastomal hernias after major genitourinary or abdominal surgery. J Endourol 2001;15:175–9.
23. Koehler RH, Voeller G. Recurrences in laparoscopic incisional hernias repairs: a personal series and review of the literature. JSLS 1999;3:293–304.
24. Franklin ME, Gonzalez Jr JJ, Michaelson RP, et al. Preliminary experience with new bioactive prosthetic material for repair of hernias in infected fields. Hernia 2002;6:171–4.
25. Bauer JJ, Salky BA, Gelernt IM, Kreel I. Repair of large abdominal wall defects with expanded polytetrafluoroethylene (PTFE). Ann Surg 1987;206:765–9.
26. Law NW. A comparison of polypropylene mesh, expanded polytetrafluoroehtylene patch and polyglycolic acid mesh for the repair of experimental abdominal wall defects. Acta Chir Scand 1990;156:759–62.
27. Schlegel PN, Walsh PC. Simultaneous preperitoneal hernia repair during radical pelvic surgery. J Urol 1987;137:1180–3.
28. Abarbanel J, Kimche D. Combined retropubic prostatectomy and preperitoneal inguinal herniorrhaphy. J Urol 1988;140:1442–3.
29. Fernandes E, Gonzalez R. Preperitoneal approach for hernia repair: clinical application in pediatric urology. J Urol 1991;146:1099–100.
30. Choi BB, Steckel J, Denoto G, et al. Preperitoneal prosthetic mesh hernioplasty during radical retropubic prostatectomy. J Urol 1999;161:840–3.
31. Katz EE, Patel RV, Sokoloff MH, et al. Bilateral laparoscopic inguinal hernia repair can complicate subsequent radical retropubic prostatectomy. J Urol 2002;167:637–8.
32. Liedberg F. Re: Bilateral laparoscopic inguinal hernia repair can complicate subsequent radical retropubic prostatectomy [letter]. J Urol 2002;168:661.
33. Foley CL, Kirby RS. Re: Bilateral laparoscopic inguinal hernia repair can complicate subsequent radical retropubic prostatectomy [letter]. J Urol 2003;169:1475.
34. Annibali RG, Fitzgibbons RJ Jr, Filipi CJ, et al Laparoscopic inguinal hernia repair. In: Greene FL, Ponsky JL, editors. Endoscopic surgery. Philadelphia: WB Saunders; 1994.
35. Ger R. The management of certain abdominal hernia by intra-abdominal closure of the neck of the sac. Ann R Coll Surg Engl 1982;64:342–4.
36. Ger R, Monroe K, Duvivier R, Mishrick A. Management of indirect inguinal hernias by laparoscopic closure of the neck of the sac. Am J Surg 1990;159:370–3.
37. Dion Y-M, Morin J. Laparoscopic inguinal herniorrhaphy. Can J Surg 1992;35:209–12.

38. Dion Y-M. Laparoscopic inguinal herniorrhaphy: an individualized approach. Surg Laparosc Endosc 1993;3:451–5.

39. Bogojavlensky S. Laparoscopic treatment of inguinal and femoral hernias [video]. Presented at the Eighteenth Annual Meeting of the American Association of Gynecological Laparoscopists, Washington, DC, 1989.

40. Schultz L, Graber J, Pietrafitta J, Hicock D. Laser laparoscopic herniorrhaphy: a clinical trial preliminary results. J Laparoendosc Surg 1990;1:41–5.

41. Corbitt JD Jr. Laparoscopic herniorrhaphy. Surg Laparosc Endosc 1991;1:23–5.

42. Nolen M, Melichar R, Jennings WC, McGee JMC. Use of a Marlex fan in the repair of direct and indirect hernias by laparoscopy. J Laparoendosc Surg 1992;2:61–4.

43. Hawasli A. Laparoscopic inguinal herniorrhaphy: the mushroom plug repair. Surg Laparosc Endosc 1992;2:111–6.

44. Seid AS, Deutsch H, Jacobson A. Laparoscopic herniorrhaphy. Surg Laparosc Endosc 1992;2:59–60.

45. Gazayerli MM. Anatomical laparoscopic hernia repair of direct or indirect inguinal hernias using the transversalis fascia and iliopubic tract. Surg Laparosc Endosc 1992;2:49–52.

46. Sailors DM, Layman TS, Burns RP, et al. Laparoscopic hernia repair: a preliminary report. Am Surg 1993;59:85–9.

47. Hawasli A. Laparoscopic inguinal herniorrhaphy: classification and 1 year experience. J Laparoendosc Surg 1992;2:137–43.

48. Popp LW. Endoscopic patch repair of inguinal hernia in a female patient. Surg Endosc 1990;5:10–2.

49. Toy FK, Smoot RT Jr. Toy-Smoot laparoscopic hernioplasty. Surg Laparosc Endosc 1991;1:151–5.

50. Spaw AT, Ennis BW, Spaw LP. Laparoscopic hernia repair: the anatomic basis. J Laparoendosc Surg 1991;1:269–77.

51. Toy FK, Smoot RT Jr. Laparoscopic hernioplasty update. J Laparoendosc Surg 1992;2:197–205.

52. Campos L, Sipes E. Laparoscopic hernia repair: use of a fenestrated PTFE graft with endo-clips. Surg Laparosc Endosc 1993;3:35–8.

53. Rosenthal D, Franklin ME. Use of percutaneous stitches in laparoscopic hernioplasty. Surg Gynecol Obstet 1993;176:491–2.

54. LeBlanc KA, Booth WV. Avoiding complications with laparoscopic herniorrhaphy. Surg Laparosc Endosc 1993;3:420–4.

55. Arregui ME, Davis CJ, Yucel O, Nagan RF. Laparoscopic mesh repair of inguinal hernia using a preperitoneal approach: a preliminary report. Surg Laparosc Endosc 1992;2:53–8.

56. Popp LW. Improvement in endoscopic hernioplasty: transcutaneous aquadissection of the musculofascial defect and preperitoneal endoscopic patch repair. J Laparoendosc Surg 1991;1:83–90.

57. McKernan JB, Laws HL. Laparoscopic preperitoneal prosthetic repair of inguinal hernias. Surg Rounds 1992;7:597–610.

58. Ferzli GS, Massad A, Albert P. Extraperitoneal endoscopic inguinal hernia repair. J Laparoendosc Surg 1992;2:281–6.

59. Phillips EH, Carroll BJ, Fallas MJ. Laparoscopic preperitoneal inguinal hernia repair without peritoneal incision. Surg Endosc 1993;7:159–62.

60. Popp LW. Hernioscopic stuffing of direct inguinal hernia in female patients using absorbable mesh. Surg Endosc 1993;7:22–5.

61. Eubanks S, Newman L 3rd. Gasless laparoscopic herniorrhaphy. In: Smith RS, Organ CH Jr, editors. Gasless laparoscopy with conventional instruments. San Francisco: Norman Publishing; 1993. p. 53–71.

62. McKernan JB, Laws HL. Laparoscopic repair of inguinal hernias using a totally extraperitoneal prosthetic approach. Surg Endosc 1993;7:26–8.

63. Cable RL, Gilling PJ. Laparoscopic extraperitoneal inguinal hernia repair using a balloon dissection technique. Aust N Z J Surg 1994;64:431–3.

64. Smith AI, Royston CMS, Sedman PC. Stapled and nonstapled laparoscopic transabdominal preperitoneal (TAPP) inguinal hernia repair. Surg Endosc 1999;13:804–6.

65. Ferzli GS, Frezza EE, Pecoraro AM Jr, Ahern KD. Prospective randomized study of stapled versus unstapled mesh in a laparoscopic preperitoneal inguinal hernia repair. J Am Coll Surg 1999;188:461–5.

66. Khajanchee YS, Urbach DR, Swanstrom LL, Hansen PD. Outcomes of laparoscopic herniorrhaphy without fixation of mesh to the abdominal wall. Surg Endosc 2001;15:1102–7.

67. Schwab JR, Beaird DA, Ramshaw BJ, et al. After 10 years and 1903 inguinal hernias, what is the outcome for the laparoscopic repair? Surg Endosc 2002;16:1201–6.

68. Schultz C, Baca I, Götzen V. Larparoscopic inguinal hernia repair: a review of 2500 cases. Surg Endosc 2001;15:582–4.

69. McCloud JM, Evans DS. Day-case laparoscopic hernia repair in a single unit. Surg Endosc 2003;17:491–3.

70. Bittner R, Schmedt CG, Scharz J, et al. Laparoscopic transperitoneal procedure for routine repair of groin hernia. Br J Surg 2002;89:1062–6.

71. Tanphiphat C, Tanprayoon T, Sangsubhan C, Chatamra K. Laparoscopic vs open inguinal hernia repair: a randomized, controlled trial. Surg Endosc 1998;12:846–51.

72. Picchio M, Lombardi A, Zolovkins A, et al. Tension-free laparoscopic and open hernia repair: randomized controlled trial of early results. World J Surg 1999;23:1004–9.

73. Tschudi JF, Wagner M, Klaiber C, et al. Randomized controlled trial of laparoscopic transabdominal preperitoneal hernioplasty vs Shouldice repair. Surg Endosc 2001;15:1263–6.

74. Berndsen F, Arvidsson D, Enander LK, et al. Postoperative convalescence after inguinal hernia surgery: prospective randomized multicenter study of laparoscopic versus Shouldice inguinal hernia repair in 1042 patients. Hernia 2002;6:56–61.

75. Lal P, Kajla RK, Chander J, et al. Randomized controlled study of laparoscopic total extraperitoneal vs open Lichtenstein inguinal hernia repair. Surg Endosc 2003;17:850–6.

76. EU Hernia Trialists Collaboration. Laparoscopic versus open groin hernia repair: meta-analysis of randomized trials based on individual patient data. Hernia 2002;6:2–10.

77. Franklin ME, Dorman JP, Glass JL, et al. Laparoscopic ventral and incisional hernia repair. Surg Laparosc Endosc 1998;8:294–9.

78. Toy FK, Bailey RW, Carey S, et al. Prospective, multicenter study of laparoscopic ventral hernioplasty. Preliminary results. Surg Endosc 1998;12:955–99.

79. Carbajo MA, del Olmo JC, Blanco JI, et al. Laparoscopic treatment of ventral abdominal wall hernias: preliminary results in 100 patients. JSLS 2000;4:141–5.

80. Chowbey PK, Sharma A, Khullar R, et al. Laparoscopic ventral hernia repair. J Laparoendosc Adv Surg Tech A 2000;10:79–84.

81. Heniford BT, Ramshaw BJ. Laparoscopic ventral hernia repair: a report of 100 consecutive cases. Surg Endosc 2000;14:419–23.

82. Heniford BT, Park A, Ramshaw BJ, Voeller G. Laparoscopic ventral and incisional hernia repair in 407 patients. J Am Coll surg 2000;190:645–50.

83. LeBlanc KA, Booth WV, Whitaker JM, Bellanger DE. Laparoscopic incisional and ventral herniorrhaphy: our initial 100 patients. Hernia 2001;5:41–5.

84. Chari R, Chari V, Eisenstat M, Chung R. A case controlled study of laparoscopic incisional hernia repair. Surg Endosc 2000;14:117–9.

85. Zanghi A, Di Vita M, Lomenzo E, et al. Laparoscopic repair vs. open surgery for incisional hernias: a comparison study. Ann Ital Chir 2000;71:663–7.

86. Dellinger EP, Gross PA, Barrett TL, et al. Quality standard for antimicrobial prophylaxis in surgical procedures. Clin Infect Dis 1994;18:422–7.

87. Schlechter B, Marks J, Shillingstad RB, Ponsky JL. Intraabdominal mesh prosthesis in a canine model. Surg Endosc 1994;8:127–9.

88. Attwood SE, Caldwell MT, Marks P, et al. Adhesions after laparoscopic inguinal hernia repair. A comparison of extra versus intra peritoneal placement of a polypropylene mesh in an animal model. Surg Endosc 1994;8:777–80.

89. Layman TS, Burns RP, Chandler KE, et al. Laparoscopic inguinal herniorrhaphy in a swine model. Am Surg 1993;59:13–9.

90. Eller R, Twaddell C, Poulos E, et al. Abdominal adhesions in laparoscopic hernia repair. An experimental study. Surg Endosc 1994;8:181–4.

91. Seid AS, Amos E. Entrapment injury in laparoscopic herniorrhaphy. Surg Endosc 1994;8:1050–3.

92. Eubanks S, Newman L 3rd, Goehring L, et al. Meralgia paresthetica: a complication of laparoscopic herniorrhaphy. Surg Laparosc Endosc 1993;3:381–5.

93. Felix EL, Michas CA, McKnight RL. Laparoscopic herniorrhaphy. Transabdominal preperitoneal floor repair. Surg Endosc 1994;8:100–4.

94. Hendrickse CW, Evans DS. Intestinal obstruction following laparoscopic hernia repair. Br J Surg 1993;80:1432.

95. Geis WP, Crafton WB, Novak MJ, Malagro M. Laparoscopic herniorrhaphy: results and technical aspects in 450 consecutive procedures. Surgery 1993;114:765–74.

96. Soper NJ, Brunt LM, Kerbl K. Laparoscopic general surgery. N Engl J Med 1994;330:409–19.

65

Laparoscopic Retroperitoneal Lymph Node Dissection

Brian Fong, MD

David Chan, MD

James Porter, MD

The feasibility of laparoscopic retroperitoneal lymph node dissection (LRPLND) in men with cancer of the testis has been demonstrated by several investigators.[1–3] At present the primary indication for LRPLND is to evaluate the retroperitoneal lymph nodes in men with clinical stage 1 nonseminomatous germ cell tumors (NSGCT). However, stage IIa-IIc patients (2–5 cm nodes) after chemotherapy have undergone LRPLND with acceptable results.[4,5]

For patients with stage I NSGCT, controversy surrounds their management, and strong arguments are presented for open RPLND,[6] chemotherapy, and for surveillance protocols.[7] Open RPLND offers the advantage of providing accurate staging information since approximately 25 to 30% of men with stage I NSGCT harbor micrometastases.[6] In addition, many patients with small volume retroperitoneal nodal disease can be cured by surgery alone and will not require adjuvant chemotherapy.[6] The primary argument against open RPLND has been the potential for ejaculatory dysfunction; however, this has been largely addressed since surgical modifications permit the preservation of antegrade ejaculation in up to 98% of patients.[6]

Proponents of surveillance in men with localized cancer of the testis argue that 70 to 75% of such patients are already cured and are thus unnecessarily exposed to the risks and morbidity of surgery. Complications have been reported in 6 to 19% of patients undergoing open RPLND.[8,9] The strongest argument for surveillance, however, is that the overall survival in men with stage I NSGCT who are participants in surveillance studies is 98%, although as many as 7 to 10% of patients who develop recurrent disease may not be successfully salvaged with chemotherapy.[10–12] The limitations of surveillance protocols include the potential for patient anxiety about having cancer and not being treated and the "need to know" that some patients may experience. In addition, in order for surveillance protocols to be successful, these young men must be highly motivated and committed to frequent and extended follow-up. This can sometimes be a challenge in this patient population.

Chemotherapy has been used routinely in patients with advanced NSGCT and in patients with recurrences after RPLND. Chemotherapy has also been applied as primary therapy to patients with stage 1 NSGCT. In most cases, two cycles of chemotherapy are given as primary therapy and three cycles for advanced disease or for recurrence after RPLND. Disease recurrence after primary chemotherapy for stage I NSGCT is extremely rare, with success rates of 95 to 98%. The disadvantages of chemotherapy are that it is ineffective for teratoma, and 50 to 70% of patients with stage 1 disease will receive it needlessly. In addition, chemotherapy has been shown to decrease fertility in patients with testis cancer. Concerns have also been raised about the long-term consequences of chemotherapy and the potential for the development of secondary malignancies.[13]

INDICATIONS

The goal of treating patients with stage 1 NSGCT should be the timely recognition and treatment of those men with metastatic disease. To avoid overtreatment, this goal is best accomplished by the availability of accurate staging information. Of the three treatment options presented—surveillance, chemotherapy, and open RPLND—the latter meets these criteria better than the other two options. Open RPLND provides accurate staging information and is curative in 75 to 80% of patients with stage II disease. However, the morbidity of open RPLND can be significant with prolonged bowel dysfunction, pain and convalescence, and complications in 6 to 19% of patients.[8,9] LRPLND has the potential to provide the same benefits of open RPLND, but with a marked reduction in morbidity. Thus, LRPLND could provide the diagnostic and therapeutic advantages of open RPLND, but with morbidity less than that of chemotherapy and slightly more than that of surveillance.

The role of LRPLND in the treatment of patients with stage 1 NSGCT has evolved. Early in the experience, LRPLND was performed mainly as a diagnostic procedure and was viewed as an extension of clinical staging with the primary goal of reducing the incidence of relapse in patients who might otherwise be considered for surveillance protocols.[14] All patients who were found at LRPLND to have pathologic stage II disease received chemotherapy. However, this approach made it impossible to determine the therapeutic role of LRPLND, and many were critical of the need for dual therapy in patients receiving LRPLND. Despite these critics, it was clear that LRPLND as a diagnostic procedure was allowing patients with pathologic stage I disease to avoid needlessly receiving chemotherapy and the morbidity of open surgery. Once it was determined that open RPLND could be reliably reproduced laparoscopically, investigators began following patients with micrometastatic disease (stage IIa), and in limited numbers of patients, there have been no recurrences in the retroperitoneum to date.

Based on the above considerations, our current indications for LRPLND include patients with clinical stage 1 NSGCT and who would otherwise be considered candidates for open RPLND. These criteria include pathologic stage T1-3 tumors, no evidence of metastatic disease on radiographic staging of the chest and abdomen, and normal tumor markers. LRPLND can also be applied in patients with postchemotherapy residual pathologic stage II disease with negative markers (Table 65-1).

PATIENT PREPARATION

Patients being considered for LRPLND should have a complete staging evaluation of the testicular malignancy which consists of chest radiography, abdominal computed tomography (CT), and measurement of serum markers. Those patients with suspicion of disease on chest radiography are further evaluated with chest CT. In most cases, LRPLND should be limited to those men without evidence of metastases. Other preoperative studies may be indicated based on the individual patient history or findings on physical examination.

Table 65-1 Indications for Laparoscopic Retroperitoneal Lymph Node Dissection

Clinical stage I nonseminomatous testis tumor
Negative testis tumor markers
Candidate otherwise considered for surveillance
No absolute contraindications to laparoscopic surgery
Residual isolated abdominal or pelvic mass after chemotherapy in the presence of negative test tumor markers. These cases must be individualized and approached very cautiously.

From Campbell's Urology, 8th Edition, 2002

The presence of significant obesity, a history of multiple abdominal surgeries, or previous episodes of peritonitis are relative contraindications to LRPLND. In such cases, open surgical approaches should be considered. As is true for all laparoscopic procedures, patients should be counseled that a larger incision might be necessary to complete the procedure or to repair vascular or intestinal injuries. In addition, patients should be counseled about alternative management options. The option of open RPLND should be discussed. Preoperative sperm banking should be recommended.

Patients should undergo a complete mechanical bowel preparation, including oral antibiotics to minimize the risk of complications in the event of a bowel injury and to decompress the small intestine. Autologous blood donation should also be considered since the risk of significant hemorrhage appears to be higher with LRPLND than with an open retroperitoneal lymphadenectomy.[15–20]

PREOPERATIVE PREPARATION

ANESTHESIA AND PATIENT POSITIONING LRPLND is performed using general endotracheal anesthesia. A Foley catheter and orogastric tube are placed to decompress the bladder and stomach, respectively, to decrease the risk of injury to these structures. Antiembolic pneumatic boots should be placed on the lower extremities. The patient is placed in a torque position similar to that used for a thoracoabdominal approach to the kidney and retroperitoneum. The ipsilateral side is rotated approximately 35 degrees off the operating table and the pelvis remains flat. The ipsilateral arm is draped across the chest and is suspended on a portable stand or fixed support (Figure 65-1). The patient should be carefully secured to the operating table since the table will be rotated severely during the procedure.

POSITIONING OF OPERATING ROOM PERSONNEL AND EQUIPMENT Standard laparoscopic equipment is used to perform LRPLND. The majority of the dissection is performed bluntly using grasping forceps or hook cautery. Endoscopic scissors, blunt grasping instruments (endoscopic Babcock clamp), and a clip applier are also used as needed. In some cases, a broad retractor (fan retractor) is helpful to elevate the liver to facilitate the superior

portion of the dissection. Tissue is easily removed through a 10 to 12 mm trocar, making an endoscopic bag or sack unnecessary. In addition, laparoscopic needle drivers should be available and facility with laparoscopic suturing to repair vascular injury is necessary. It is also helpful to have tissue sealants available in the event of minor bleeding and to assist with sealing lymphatic channels. As with any laparoscopic procedure, a laparotomy tray should be immediately available in the event of an emergency.

Since LRPLND is performed in the mid- to upper abdomen, it is best to have a television monitor positioned on each side of the patient. The surgeon and first assistant stand on the contralateral side of the operating table (left side for right-sided LRPLND); the second assistant maintains the endoscope from the ipsilateral side of the table. The scrub nurse stands next to the second assistant. If there are only two surgeons, they are positioned on opposite sides of the table, with the primary surgeon in the contralateral position.

TECHNIQUE

PORT PLACEMENT AND ASSIGNMENT LRPLND is an advanced laparoscopic procedure, and considerable experience with other laparoscopic procedures is recommended before attempting this operation. Because most of the procedure involves dissection around the great vessels, the risk of vascular injury is high, and as mentioned previously, facility with laparoscopic suturing is essential to safely repair injuries that may occur.

Four or five laparoscopic ports are generally used to perform LRPLND. It is best to use at least 10 mm trocars at all sites since this allows maximal flexibility in moving instruments to facilitate the dissection. In addition, a single 12 mm trocar is also useful since there may be occasions when a trocar of this size is necessary for the placement of large grasping forceps or endoscopic staplers.

The initial port is placed in the infraumbilical position. For purposes of discussion, the ports will be referred to by the numbers that appear in Figure 65-2. The patient is positioned for a right-sided LRPLND. A 12 mm trocar is placed at site 5 with 10 mm trocars at the remaining sites. The port in the left lower quadrant (port 4) is optional for a right-sided dissection. A 10 mm endoscope with a 0- or 30-degree lens is moved to site 2 after all the laparoscopic ports have been inserted. If three persons are performing the procedure, the surgeon uses instruments placed through ports 1 and 5 while standing in the cephalad position on the contralateral side of the table. The first assistant uses instruments placed through ports 3 and 4 and stands next to the surgeon. The second assistant stands on the contralateral side and maintains the endoscope, which is repositioned through port 2 following trocar placement.

RIGHT-SIDED PROCEDURE Following patient positioning, the pneumoperitoneum may be established using a closed (Veress needle) or open (Hasson trocar) technique. Intra-abdominal pressure is

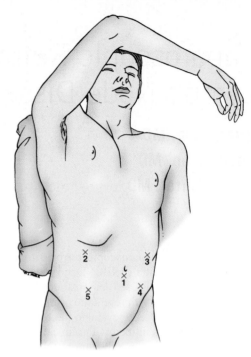

Figure 65-2 Patient position for right-sided LRPLND. Numbers refer to trocar sites.

maintained at 15 to 20 mm Hg throughout the procedure. After the placement of all operative ports, the operating table is rotated approximately 35° toward the surgeon so that the right side of the patient is elevated. The first assistant then uses an endoscopic Babcock clamp or other large, blunt grasping instrument through port 3 to pull the cecum toward the left side of the abdomen. The surgeon uses endoscopic scissors placed through port 1 and a grasping forceps placed through port 5. If five ports are used, the first assistant also uses forceps placed through port 4. This countertraction allows for an incision to be made along the white line of Toldt lateral to the right colon (Figure 65-3).

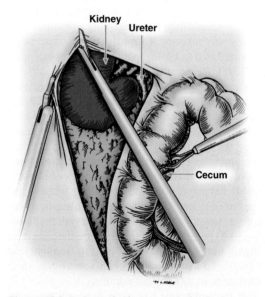

Figure 65-3 Endoscopic shears are used to incise along the white line of Toldt lateral to the cecum for a right-sided LRPLND. The bowel is retracted medially to help expose the right kidney and ureter.

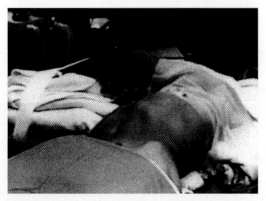

Figure 65-1 Patient position for left-sided LRPLND.

The bowel is continually retracted medially as the incision is taken to the level of the hepatic flexure. The undersurface of the colonic mesentery, the ureter, and iliac and gonadal vessels will come into view. Care must be taken to avoid injury to these structures. The limits of the dissection are the ureter laterally, the renal hilum superiorly, the medial aspect of the vena cava or aorta medially (left-sided and right-sided RPLND, respectively), and the level of the origin of the inferior mesenteric artery inferiorly (Figure 65-4). Nodal tissue is removed to the bifurcation of the common iliac vessels on the ipsilateral side and the stump of the spermatic cord is excised.

After the right colon has been completely mobilized, it may be unnecessary for the first assistant to continue to maintain retraction on the bowel using the endoscopic Babcock clamp. If this is the case, then the assistant can use a blunt grasping forceps to facilitate the dissection. The surgeon exchanges the scissors for a grasping forceps and continues to work through ports 1 and 5. The dissection is generally begun inferiorly by identifying the ureter, gonadal vessels, and lateral surface of the inferior vena cava (IVC). The gonadal vessels may be clipped and divided, leaving the distal aspect to be dissected later as the stump of the spermatic cord is excised. Since the ureter and gonadal vessels may be easily confused, it is essential that the gonadal vein be dissected carefully toward its junction with the IVC before it is divided. Alternatively, a ureteral catheter may be placed at the outset of the procedure to facilitate identification of this structure. The lymphatic and fatty tissue between the IVC and ureter is dissected bluntly in a cephalad direction until the right renal vein is identified (Figure 65-5). It is best to maintain the dissection directly on the surface of the IVC so that small vessels can be identified and controlled using electrocautery or the endoscopic clip applier. Occasionally an accessory or aberrant lower pole renal artery will be encountered during this portion of the dissection. Alternatively, the dissection may be begun superiorly by identifying the renal vein and its junction with the IVC. Tissue is then removed in a caudad direction on the anterior surface of the

IVC and between this structure and the ureter. Inferiorly, the dissection is continued along the ipsilateral common iliac vein to its bifurcation.

Tissue is then dissected in the interaortocaval region beginning at the level of the renal hilum (Figure 65-6). Gentle lateral retraction on the aorta and IVC facilitates this dissection as grasping forceps are used to bluntly remove the tissue until the anterior spinous ligament is clearly visualized. Some nodal tissue posterior to the great vessels can be carefully resected as the lumbar veins are clipped to prevent tearing, which can lead to troublesome hemorrhage (Figure 65-7). A complete dissection posterior to the great vessels is not performed. The interaortocaval dissection is taken inferiorly to the level of the inferior mesenteric artery. The contralateral renal vessels are generally easily visualized. Care must be taken to clip as many of the main lymphatic channels as possible to decrease the risk of postoperative lymphatic leakage. Using the "split and roll" technique, the retrocaval (for the right LRPLND) and retroaortic (for the left LRPLND) tissue should be removed to ensure a complete clean out.

The final step in the procedure is the excision of the ipsilateral stump of the spermatic cord. The gonadal vessels have generally been clipped and divided earlier, and the proximal cut end of these vessels is gently grasped by the first assistant. The surgeon continues to operate through ports 1 and 5. Sharp and blunt dissection is used in and around the internal inguinal ring to expose and remove the stump of the cord (Figure 65-8). A long silk suture on the distal aspect of the cord that remains from the inguinal orchiectomy is generally evident. The nodal tissue and excised spermatic cord are then easily removed from the abdomen using grasping forceps (endoscopic entrapment bag).

The lymph nodes are sent for frozen section analysis to determine whether metastatic disease is present. If evaluation of the lymph nodes shows multifocal cancer or any involved lymph node greater than 2 cm, then the procedure is concluded and chemotherapy is recommended. If the lymph nodes show evidence of micrometastatic disease, then the trocar sights are closed and the patient is repositioned for contralateral

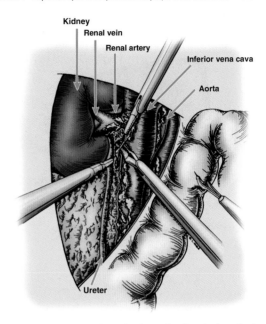

Figure 65-5 Blunt dissection is used to free the lymphatic and fatty tissue between the L and ureter (right-sided inferior vena cava RPLND).

LRPLND. When performing a bilateral dissection, it is important to identify and preserve the post-ganglionic sympathetic fibers in order to avoid ejaculatory dysfunction.

The area of dissection is carefully inspected to ensure that adequate hemostasis has been achieved. The intraperitoneal pressure is lowered to 5 mm Hg to help visualize any small venous bleeding. The small and large bowels are also inspected for any signs of injury. Laparoscopic clips are liberally applied to all areas where lymphatic channels were divided in an effort to decrease lymphatic leakage. The pneumoperitoneum is then evacuated and the trocars are removed under direct vision. The fascia at each port site is closed using 2-0 absorbable suture and the skin is reapproximated using 4-0 suture.

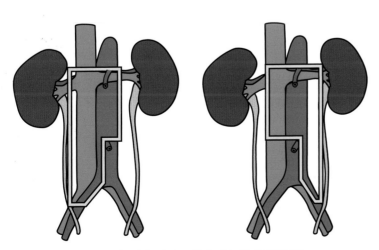

Figure 65-4 Templates for right- (A) and left- (B) sided LRPLNP.

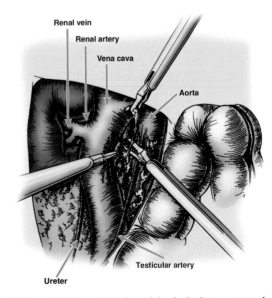

Figure 65-6 Lymphatic tissue lying in the interaortocaval region is dissected bluntly.

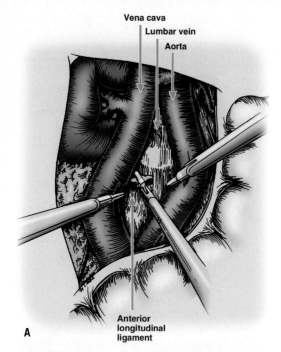

Vena cava
Lumbar vein
Aorta

Anterior
longitudinal
ligament

A

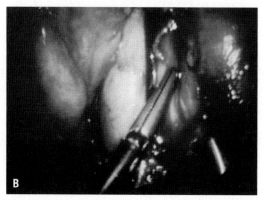

B

Figure 65-7 *A,* The anterior spinous (longitudinal) ligament is exposed as the interaortocaval dissection is completed. Clips have been placed on the lumbar vein. *B,* Grasping forceps are in contact with the anterior spinous ligament as the interaortocaval dissection is completed. The inferior vena cava is to the left and the aorta to the right as one views the intraoperative photograph.

MODIFICATIONS TO THE TECHNIQUE As experience with LRPLND has improved, several modifications to the technique have been made.[21] Identification of the ureter can be augmented by placement of a 6-F ureteral catheter over a 0.038-inch Amplatz super-stiff guide wire into the ipsilateral ureter and secured to the Foley catheter. Manipulation of the catheter can help locate the ureter. An infrared light emitting stent for the same purpose has also been described.[22] Open conversion is often required for significant vascular injuries, but successful control of bleeding has been accomplished using clips and fibrin glue.[23] With regard to the limits of dissection, retroaortic and retrocaval tissue are not routinely removed. It is technically feasible but it adds at least 1 hour to the dissection.[24] Moreover, studies have noted that when nodal packets are taken separately, all positive nodes are found ventral to the lumbar vessels.[25,26] No reports have documented metastatic disease only in the retroaortic and retrocaval regions. In terms of approaches to

LRPLND, the anterior extraperitoneal approach has been described to have satisfactory clinical outcomes,[27] and a nerve-sparing approach has also been noted.[29] However, further studies are necessary to evaluate its potential as an alternative to the transperitoneal and retroperitoneoscopic approaches.

POSTOPERATIVE CARE

The orogastric tube is removed at the completion of the procedure. The Foley catheter is generally left indwelling for at least 24 hours to help monitor urine output and hemodynamic status. The hematocrit is obtained during the first 24 hours postoperatively. A liquid diet can generally be initiated on the first postoperative day with rapid advancement as tolerated to solid food. Patients are generally hospitalized for 2 to 3 days with return to normal activity levels within 2 to 4 weeks. The most frequently encountered serious complications of LRPLND are hemorrhage, chylous ascites, and undetected bowel injury. Significant abdominal tenderness, unexplained fever, or gastrointestinal symptoms may indicate an intestinal injury and early exploration and repair are necessary. Radiographic evaluation may be considered prior to exploration but may be difficult to interpret in the immediate postoperative period. Patients are followed postoperatively with chest radiography, abdominal CT scans, and tumor markers at regular intervals to assess for signs of tumor recurrence.

RESULTS

After the feasibility of LRPLND was demostrated in case reports,[2,3,29] the safety, reproducibility, and long-term results were investigated in the initial case series. The first series was reported by Janetschek and colleagues[15] based on a single institutional experience of 15 patients in Austria. Their technique involved a combined anterior and lateral transperitoneal approach. Operative time was slightly less than 6 hours for left-sided tumors and 9 hours for right-sided tumors. Two required open conversion; several had bleeding controlled laparoscopically; none required transfusions. Mean hospitalization was 5.5 days and patients returned to normal activities in 12 to 22 days. All patients preserved antegrade ejaculation. The three patients found to have positive nodes were treated with adjuvant chemotherapy, while the remaining patients had no relapse at 1 to 19 months follow-up. The second series was a multi-institutional experience from four centers in the United States.[20] The technique involved a limited removal of nodal tissue posterior to the aorta and IVC. Successful procedures were performed in 18 of 20 patients with a mean duration of 6 hours with a median blood loss of 250 mL. The average number of lymph nodes removed was 14.5 nodes. Antegrade ejaculation was preserved in all men and they were discharged from hospital in 3 days or less with return to full activity in 2 to 3 weeks. Significant complications occurred in 20% of patients with the most common complica-

tion being bleeding. Two patients required laparotomy because of bleeding from the gonadal vessels. Three node-positive patients were given adjuvant chemotherapy with no recurrence at 5 to 14 months. However, one patient with negative abdominal lymph nodes developed a new pulmonary nodule at 4 months, and was salvaged by chemotherapy. No recurrent abdominal disease was noted at median follow-up of 10 months.

Since these initial series, several institutions have published and updated their experience with LRPLND.[24,28,30–34] A summary of the results is presented in Table 65-2. There have been over 260 LRPLND procedures performed worldwide and the number of patients with extended follow-up continues to increase. Amongst patients with clinical stage I disease, LRPLND has been performed safely without the need for open conversion in 88 to 100% of patients. Mean operative times ranged from 3.5 to 5.5 hours and mean estimated blood loss varied from less than 50 cc to 398 cc. Hospitalization in uncomplicated cases was usually under 4 days and return to normal activities can be achieved within 2 weeks. Preservation of antegrade ejaculation was maintained in 97 to 100% of patients and parallels that of the open nerve-sparing technique. The technique of the laparoscopic nerve-sparing RPLND should allow antegrade ejaculation to be maintained in those patients requiring a bilateral dissection.[28,35] The efficacy of LRPLND as a staging modality is supported by the low retroperitoneal recurrence rate, and the single local recurrence reported by Janetschek was due to a tumor in the primary landing site that had been removed at surgery but was missed on histological examination. This patient was cured with two cycles of chemotherapy and additional contralateral LRPLND.[23] If the dissection performed during LRPLND was inadequate, as posed by some critics, then a higher rate of retroperitoneal recurrence would be expected. The vast majority of recurrences

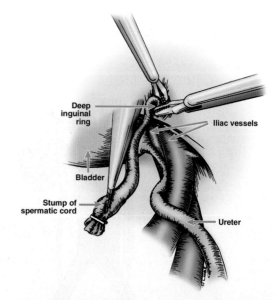

Deep
inguinal
ring

Iliac vessels

Bladder

Stump of
spermatic cord

Ureter

Figure 65-8 Blunt dissection is used to free the lymphatic and fatty tissues between the inferior vena cava anhd ureter (right-sided LRPLND).

reported in these series were noted in the lungs. The therapeutic efficacy of LRPLND remains to be determined, as most patients in these series with pathologic stage IIa disease undergo chemotherapy. About 50 to 65% of patients with low volume retroperitoneal disease treated by open RPLND are cured of disease.[36] In order to determine if LRPLND offers similar therapeutic benefit, a group of such patients must be followed closely under a surveillance protocol instead of receiving immediate chemotherapy. However, in series of one of the author's (JRP) 4 patients with stage IIa disease did not receive chemotherapy after LRPLND and at a mean follow-up of 20 months, there have been no recurrences.

The complications associated with LRPLND are reported to occur in 6 to 17% of patients, and the majority of the complications are minor. The most common major complication was bleeding owing to vascular injury. However, chylous ascites occurred in 13% of patients in one of the author's series (JRP). One hypothesis for the high rate of chylous leak may be because LRPLND patients eat the day after surgery, and therefore the lymphatic channels may not have time to seal and are more prone to leaking. Patients are now routinely placed on a low-fat diet for 1 week preoperatively and 2 weeks postoperatively with no further cases of chylous ascites. There clearly is an extended learning curve with LRPLND, with both complications and operative time decreasing with experience. Janetschek reported a mean operative time of 476 min (range 240–630 min) in the first 15 cases, which was reduced to a mean of 219 min in later series.[23] Cost analysis was performed by Ogan and colleagues, revealing that open RPLND was less costly ($7,162 USD vs 7,804 USD) owing to operating room time and equipment. However, LRPLND showed cost advantage when performed in less than 5 hours or when the patient was discharged within 2 post-operative days.[37]

Postchemotherapy LRPLND in stage IIb-IIc disease has been demonstrated by several institutions, but the complication rate and operative times are considerably higher than for stage I disease.[4,23,38] Complications usually involved vascular injuries requiring open conversion; however, bowel injuries are also more likely due to the scarring induced by the chemotherapy.[4,39] With the higher rate of complications, the continued role of LRPLND in postchemotherapy patients is being questioned. Janetschek has evaluated the role of LRPLND in stage IIb disease in decreasing the dosing regimen of chemotherapy to two cycles preoperatively, but the long-term result of this protocol remains to be determined.[23]

CONCLUSION

LRPLND is an advanced laparoscopic procedure and, as such, there is a learning curve with longer operative times and more complications early in the experience. Bleeding from vascular injury appears to be the most frequent complication and laparoscopic suturing skills are helpful in dealing with this problem. Operative times are longer than

Table 65-2 Summary of Worldwide Clinical Series for Laparoscopic RPLND[4,20,24,28,30-34]

Author	No. Patients	Side R	Side L	Success Rate (%)	Complications Minor	Complications Major	Mean Operative Time Min (range)	Mean Blood Loss mL (range)	Mean Hospital Stay Days (range)	Convalescence Days (range)	Antegrade Ejaculation (%)	Recurrences Local (%)	Recurrences Distant (%)	Median Follow-Up Months (range)
Klotz[34]	4	0	4	75	0	0	285	–	1–2	10	–	–	–	–
Gerber et al[20]	20	12	8	90	20	0	360 (240–600)	250 (30–3000)	3 (1–5)	14 (5–24)	100	0	10	10 (2–25)
Guisti et al[33]	6	3	3	100	17	0	325 (275–420)	minimal	18 + 4.8 (4–6)	16.2 (12–27)	–	0	0	27 (12–42)
Zhuo et al[31]	13	8	5	92	0	0	292 (210–400)	250	6.4	–	100 (3 no f/u)	–	–	–
Nelson et al[24]	29	18	1	93	6.9	0	258 (157–380)	389 (75–3000)	2.6 (1–5)	17	96.6	0	6.9	16 (1–65)
Rassweiler et al[32] – Transperitoneal + Extraperitoneal	34	–	1	88	8.8	5.9	248	–	–	5.3	97	0	5.9	40
Leblanc et al[28] – Extraperitoneal	25	12	1	100	0	0	230 (180–300)	> 50	1.2 (1–3)	15	100	0	0	15 (3–35)
Janetschek[23]	Stage I: 20	3		98	10	0	219		3.3	–	–	1.3	0	46
	Stage IIA: 5		–				226		3.5	–	–	0	0	35
Palese et al[4]	125 Stage I: 75 Stage II: 49 Stage IIA+: 7	3	4	71	14	43	396 (188–700)	1053 (75–2800)	13 (1–68)	–	–	0	0	24 (12–60)

for open RPLND but patients experience a faster recovery of bowel function, shorter hospital stay, and earlier return to normal activities. The rate of retroperitoneal recurrence after LRPLND is low, with most recurrences occurring in the chest.

The role of LRPLND in the treatment of patients with stage I NSGCT is evolving. Studies have demonstrated that it is a safe and reproducible technique with clear advantages over open RPLND with regard to patient morbidity. The low rate of retroperitoneal recurrence with LRPLND suggests that it has the ability to accurately stage patients with NSGCT, and thus, identify those patients who can avoid chemotherapy as well as those who will benefit from this treatment. What has not been answered is the therapeutic efficacy of LRPLND and, therefore, what the role of laparoscopy is in the overall treatment of patients with stage I NSGCT. In order to determine the ability of LRPLND to cure patients with stage IIa disease, these patients must be followed closely and not receive chemotherapy. If the therapeutic role of LRPLND can be proven, then this procedure has the potential to offer our patients the advantages of open RPLND with much less morbidity and, at the same time, avoid unnecessary exposure to chemotherapy. This would truly be an advance for our patients and maintain the role of urologists in the treatment of this disease.

REFERENCES

1. Janetschek G, Reissigl A, Peschel R, et al. [Laparoscopic retroperitoneal lymph node excision in clinical stage I non-seminomatous testicular cancer]. Urologe A 1994;33:24–30.
2. Rukstalis DB, Chodak GW. Laparoscopic retroperitoneal lymph node dissection in a patient with stage 1 testicular carcinoma. J Urol 1992;148:1907-10.
3. Stone NN, Schlussel RN, Waterhouse RL, Unger P. Laparoscopic retroperitoneal lymph node dissection in stage A nonseminomatous testis cancer. Urology 1993;42:610–4.
4. Palese MA, Su LM, Kavoussi LR. Laparoscopic retroperitoneal lymph node dissection after chemotherapy. Urology 2002;60:130–4.
5. Janetschek G, Hobisch A, Hittmair A, et al. Laparoscopic retroperitoneal lymphadenectomy after chemotherapy for stage IIB nonseminomatous testicular carcinoma. J Urol 1999;161:477–81.
6. Donohue JP, Thornhill JA, Foster RS, et al. Retroperitoneal lymphadenectomy for clinical stage A testis cancer (1965 to 1989): modifications of technique and impact on ejaculation. J Urol 1993;149:237–43.
7. Oliver RT, Hope-Stone HF, Blandy JP. Justification of the use of surveillance in the management of stage I germ cell tumours of the testis. Br J Urol 1983;55:760–3.
8. Sago AL, Ball TP, Novicki DE. Complications of retroperitoneal lymphadenectomy. Urology 1979;13:241–3.
9. Donohue JP, Rowland RG. Complications of retroperitoneal lymph node dissection. J Urol 1981;125:338–40.
10. Sogani PC, Fair WR. Surveillance alone in the treatment of clinical stage I nonseminomatous germ cell tumor of the testis (NSGCT). Semin Urol 1988;6:53–6.
11. Thompson PI, Nixon J, Harvey VJ. Disease relapse in patients with stage I nonseminomatous germ cell tumor of the testis on active surveillance. J Clin Oncol 1988;6:1597–603.
12. Raghavan D, Colls B, Levi J, et al. Surveillance for stage I non-seminomatous germ cell tumours of the testis: the optimal protocol has not yet been defined. Br J Urol 1988;61:522–6.
13. Grossfeld GD, Small EJ. Long-term side effects of treatment for testis cancer. Urol Clin North Am 1998;25:503–15.
14. Richie JP. Editorial comment. Urology 1994;44:391.
15. Janetschek G, Reissigl A, Peschel R, et al. Laparoscopic retroperitoneal lymph node dissection for clinical stage I nonseminomatous testicular tumor. Urology 1994;44:382–91.
16. Dunphy CH, Ayala AG, Swanson DA, et al. Clinical stage I nonseminomatous and mixed germ cell tumors of the testis. A clinicopathologic study of 93 patients on a surveillance protocol after orchiectomy alone. Cancer 1988;62:1202–6.
17. Freedman LS, Parkinson MC, Jones WG, et al. Histopathology in the prediction of relapse of patients with stage I testicular teratoma treated by orchidectomy alone. Lancet 1987;2:294–8.
18. Costello AJ, Mortensen PH, Stillwell RG. Prognostic indicators for failure of surveillance management of stage I non-seminomatous germ cell tumours. Aust N Z J Surg 1989;59:119–22.
19. Read G, Stenning SP, Cullen MH, et al. Medical Research Council prospective study of surveillance for stage I testicular teratoma. Medical Research Council Testicular Tumors Working Party. J Clin Oncol 1992;10:1762–8.
20. Gerber GS, Bissada NK, Hulbert JC, et al. Laparoscopic retroperitoneal lymphadenectomy: multi-institutional analysis. J Urol 1994;152:1188–92.
21. Janetschek G. Laposcopic retroperitoneal lymph node dissection: evolution of a new technique. World J Urol 2000;18:267–71.
22. Kim K, Schwaitzberg S, Onel E. An infrared ureteral stent to aid in laparoscopic retroperitoneal lymph node dissection. J Urol 2001;166:1815–6.
23. Janetschek G. Laparoscopic retroperitoneal lymph node dissection. Urol Clin North Am 2001;28:107–14.
24. Nelson JB, Chen RN, Bishoff JT, et al. Laparoscopic retroperitoneal lymph node dissection for clinical stage I nonseminomatous germ cell testicular tumors. Urology 1999;54:1064–7.
25. Holtl L, Peschel R, Knapp R, et al. Primary lymphatic metastatic spread in testicular cancer occurs ventral to the lumbar vessels. Urology 2002;59:114–8.
26. Janetschek G, Hobisch A, Holtl L, Bartsch G. Retroperitoneal lymphadenectomy for clinical stage I nonseminomatous testicular tumor: laparoscopy versus open surgery and impact of learning curve. J Urol 1996;156:89–94.
27. Hsu TH, Su LM, Ong A. Anterior extraperitoneal approach to laparoscopic retroperitoneal lymph node dissection: a novel technique. J Urol 2003;169:258–60.
28. LeBlanc E, Caty A, Dargent D, et al. Extraperitoneal laparoscopic para-aortic lymph node dissection for early stage nonseminomatous germ cell tumors of the testis with introduction of a nerve sparing technique: description and results. J Urol 2001;165:89–92.
29. Janetschek G, Reissigl A, Peschel R, Bartsch G. Laparoscopic retroperitoneal lymphadenectomy in the pig: initial report. J Endourol 1993;7:243–7.
30. Janetschek G, Peschel R, Hobisch A, Bartsch G. Laparoscopic retroperitoneal lymph node dissection. J Endourol 2001;15:449–55.
31. Zhuo Y, Klaen R, Sauter TW, Miller K. Laparoscopic retroperitoneal lymph node dissection in clinical stage I nonseminomatous germ cell tumor: a minimal invasive alternative. Chin Med J (Engl) 1998;111:537–41.
32. Rassweiler JJ, Frede T, Lenz E, et al. Long-term experience with laparoscopic retroperitoneal lymph node dissection in the management of low-stage testis cancer. Eur Urol 2000;37:251–60.
33. Giusti G, Beltrami P, Tallarigo C, et al. Unilateral laparoscopic retroperitoneal lymphadenectomy for clinical stage I nonseminomatous testicular cancer. J Endourol 1998;12:561–6.
34. Klotz L. Laparoscopic retroperitoneal lymphadenectomy for high-risk stage 1 nonseminomatous germ cell tumor: report of four cases. Urology 1994;43:752–6.
35. Peschel R, Gettman MT, Neururer R, et al. Laparoscopic retroperitoneal lymph node dissection: description of the nerve-sparing technique. Urology 2002;60:339–43.
36. Donohue JP, Thornhill JA, Foster RS, et al. The role of retroperitoneal lymphadenectomy in clinical stage B testis cancer: the Indiana University experience (1965 to 1989). J Urol 1995;153:85–9.
37. Ogan K, Lotan Y, Koeneman K, et al. Laparoscopic versus open retroperitoneal lymph node dissection: a cost analysis. J Urol 2002;168:1945–9.
38. Rassweiler JJ, Seemann O, Henkel TO, et al. Laparoscopic retroperitoneal lymph node dissection for nonseminomatous germ cell tumors: indications and limitations. J Urol 1996;156:1108–13.
39. Winfield HN. Laparoscopic retroperitoneal lymphadenectomy for cancer of the testis. Urol Clin North Am 1998;25:469–78.

66

Laparoscopic Radical Prostatectomy

Osamu Ukimura

Andrew P. Steinberg

Sidney C. Abreu

Inderbir S. Gill

In 1999-2000, Guillonneau and Vallancien established a sophisticated reproducible transperitoneal antegrade technique of laparoscopic radical prostatectomy (LRP).[1,2] At this writing, several worldwide teams have proven that LRP is becoming an acceptable treatment option for organ-confined prostate cancer.[3–7] The techniques of LRP appear in line with the established principles of open radical prostatectomy. Reports regarding early oncologic outcomes and measurements of quality of life after LRP are encouraging.

PATIENT SELECTION

Proper patient selection is important in assuring good surgical and oncologic outcomes. Patients need to fulfill criteria for undergoing prostatectomy and criteria for undergoing laparoscopy. Open or laparoscopic radical prostatectomy, in many centers, is reserved for patients with clinically localized prostate cancer (T1, T2). The surgical treatment of locally advanced or metastatic prostate cancer remains controversial. Patients with a life expectancy of less than 10 years are generally not considered candidates because of the slow growth rate of prostate cancer. Since there is an obvious learning curve, prior hormonal treatment, huge prostate size, and patient obesity may be considered as relative contraindications by the novice laparoscopist. Even for the expert laparoscopic surgeon, relative contraindications include prior open retropubic surgery, or radiation therapy, and uncorrected coagulopathy.

OPERATIVE TECHNIQUE

Both transperitoneal and extraperitoneal approaches to LRP are used, each with its inherent advantages and disadvantages. The transperitoneal technique as popularized by Guillonneau and Vallencien begins retrovesically, with a transverse peritoneotomy in the retrovesical cul-de-sac and subsequent mobilization of the vas deferens and seminal vesicles.[1,2] Subsequently, an anterior peritoneotomy is performed and dissection of the prostate is undertaken. This technique continues to be used with success in many centers worldwide. In an attempt to avoid potential bowel complications and potential risk of anastomotic urine leak in the transperitoneal approach, some centers are using an extraperitoneal approach.[7–10]

OPERATIVE PREPARATION On the day prior to surgery, the patient is started on a diet of clear fluids, and bowel preparation is performed with two bottles of magnesium citrate. The patient is given parenteral antibiotic (first-generation cephalosporin), and bilateral sequential compression devices are placed. Following general anesthesia, the patient is placed in a supine, modified lithotomy position with thighs abducted to allow simultaneous intraoperative perineal access. The arms are adducted by the side of the patient. All bony prominences are meticulously padded, and the patient is secured to the table with safety straps. A 22 French Foley catheter is inserted to decompress the bladder, and the patient is placed in a 30° Trendelenburg's (head down) position.

OPERATING ROOM SETUP The surgeon stands to the left of the patient (Figure 66-1). The first assistant is across from the surgeon (on the right side of the patient) and the second assistant on the surgeon's left side. If an AESOP robotic arm is used to hold the laparoscope, the second assistant is not necessary. One monitor is placed on either side of the patient's pelvis.

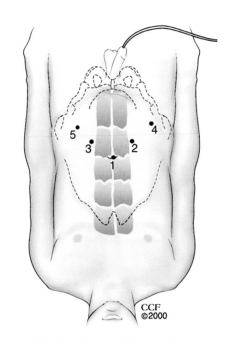

Figure 66-1 The five-port "fan array" transperitoneal approach is shown.

LAPAROSCOPIC ACCESS A 1-cm incision is made under the umbilicus. Veress needle CO_2 pneumoperitoneum is obtained to 15 mm Hg. In total, five laparoscopic ports (three 5-mm ports and two 12-mm ports) are placed in an inverted "V" shape configuration (see Figure 66-1). In our experience, trocar-related injury to the inferior epigastric artery has occurred more frequently on the right side. In order to minimize this complication, we recommend laparoscopic transillumination for careful identification of inferior epigastric arterial pulsations, and use of the step-port, a non-bladed port (Ethicon, Cincinnati, OH). In event of significant bleeding, prompt and meticulous suture ligature of the vessel, proximally and distally, using a Carter-Thomason suture passer should be performed.

The bladder is distended with 200 mL saline via the Foley catheter, and an inverted U-shaped peritoneotomy is performed extending across both medial umbilical ligaments to enter Retzius' space. Dissection is performed immediately along the undersurface of the rectal fascia to expose the pubic arch, and finally the endopelvic fascia and periprostatic fat. Upon completion of this step, the bladder is decompressed.

PELVIC (OBTURATOR) LYMPH NODE DISSECTION A pelvic lymph node dissection is undertaken when indicated (PSA ≥ 10, Gleason score ≥ 7, large-volume tumors, or palpable Prostatic nodule). The standard anatomic boundaries of limited obturator lymphadenectomy are used. Larger lymphatics are clipped, but most can be easily controlled with electrocautery. Lymph nodes are routinely sent for frozen section analysis. If lymphatic metastases are confirmed, prostatectomy is not performed

LIGATION OF DORSAL VENOUS COMPLEX The superficial dorsal vein is coagulated with bipolar forceps and divided. The endopelvic fascia is incised bilaterally, maintaining the puboprostatic ligaments intact. (Figure 66-2) A laparoscopic Kittner, or "peanut," can be used to tease the levator muscle fibers off the prostatic apex. Dissection distal to the apex is minimized in order to prevent injury to this nerve-rich, sphincter-active area. If a wide complex remains, the puboprostatic ligaments can be shaved down using electrocautery with the heel of the "J" hook. The Foley catheter is replaced with a metallic urethral dilator (22F). With

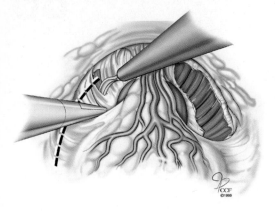

Figure 66-2 Incision of endopelvic fascia is performed bilaterally until the puboprostatic ligaments are visualized.

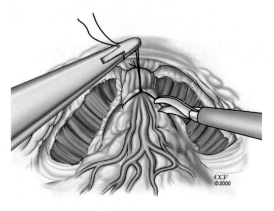

Figure 66-4 The back-bleeding stitch is placed and the bladder neck is transected. The dotted line demonstrates the plane of dissection between the base of the prostate and the anterior bladder neck.

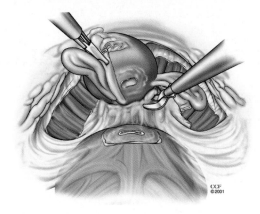

Figure 66-6 Incision of Denonvilliers' fascia is performed with "cold" Endoshears, and extreme care is taken to avoid injury to the rectum.

an assistant placing posterior traction on the dilator (thereby separating somewhat the deep dorsal vein complex from the urethra), two stitches (CT-1 needle, 2-0 Vicryl) are placed across the dorsal venous complex (Figure 66-3). Contact between the needle and dilator alerts the surgeon that the stitch is entering the urethral lumen. In an attempt to improve postoperative continence, retropubic urethropexy is performed by suspending the sutures from the pubic periosteum anteriorly.

BLADDER NECK TRANSECTION A back-bleeding stitch (CT-1 needle, 2-0 Vicryl) across the anterior surface of the prostate is placed (Figure 66-4). In a nerve-sparing procedure, the lateral pelvic fascia covering the prostate is incised superficially with "cold" Endoshears (US Surgical) in order to release the tethering of the neurovascular bundles. This fascial incision must remain superficial, thus not compromising either the prostate capsule or the prostate gland itself.

Several "tricks" have been developed in order to assist the surgeon in locating the bladder neck. An assistant retracts the back-bleeding stitch anteriorly towards the symphysis pubis, tenting the prostate anteriorly while the bladder is retracted cephalad and posteriorly. By performing this maneuver, one can identify where the prevesical fat ends, signifying the prostatovesical junction. Repeated in-and-out movements of the urethral dilator can also aid in visualization of the bladder neck.

The anterior and posterior bladder neck is sequentially incised with J-hook electrocautery. The posterior bladder neck is transected precisely at its junction with the prostate. The ureteral orifices must be visualized prior to transection in order to avoid injury. In the case of a large median lobe, the posterior incision should be high up on the convex surface of the lobe. The posterior bladder neck can then be dissected off the lobe until the correct posterior plane is reached.

VAS DEFERENS AND SEMINAL VESICLES DISSECTION The plane between the posterior base of the prostate and the bladder neck is dissected until the vasa deferentia are seen (Figure 66-5). The vasa are individually grasped and transected. With continuous cephalad traction on each vas, the seminal vesicles are dissected using the Harmonic Scalpel (Ethicon Inc.). The vesicular artery, located at the tip of the seminal vesicles, is secured with Hem-o-lok clips (Weck Closure Systems, Research Triangle Park, NC) and transected. Denonvilliers' fascia is incised below the junction of the seminal vesicles and the prostate (Figure 66-6). Care must be taken as to the exact position of this incision. A high incision close to

the prostate may result in positive margins at this location, while a low incision may cause rectal injury.

TRANSECTION OF LATERAL PEDICLES In a non–nerve-sparing procedure, the lateral pedicles are widely transected with an Endo-GIA stapler (US Surgical) (Figure 66-7). Care must be exercised during the non–nerve-sparing portion of the surgery to remain anterior to the rectum, since this is a primary situation for a rectal injury.[11] We currently perform nerve-sparing by an energy-free, completely athermal technique. Our technique involves transient control of the lateral prostate pedicles with an atraumatic vascular bulldog clamp (Figure 66-8A).[12] Pedicles are divided by precise cold cutting, and neurovascular bundles are teased away with gentle blunt and sharp dissection (Figure 66-8B). Throughout the transection of lateral pedicles and release of neurovascular bundles, our bulldog technique completely eliminates any form of electrocautery, thermal energy, clips, or bioadhesives. After bulldog unclamping, hemostasis is secured with meticulous, superficial suturing of transected blood vessels with 4-0 Vicryl (Figure 66-8C).

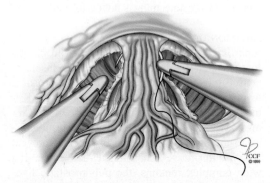

Figure 66-3 Two dorsal vein stitches are placed. Retropubic urethropexy is then performed by suspending these sutures to the puboprostatic ligaments above.

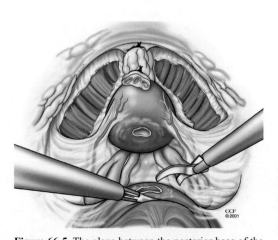

Figure 66-5 The plane between the posterior base of the prostate and the bladder neck is dissected until the vasa deferens are seen.

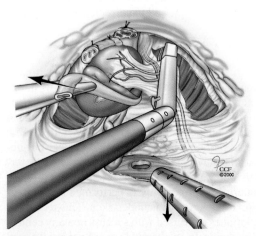

Figure 66-7 In a non–nerve-sparing transection of lateral pedicles, the articulating Endo-GIA stapler is used to widely transect the lateral pedicle and neurovascular bundle from the prostate.

TRANSECTION OF DORSAL VENOUS COMPLEX, URETHRA AND APICAL DISSECTION While maintaining constant cephalad retraction of the prostate, the dorsal venous complex is transected with the Harmonic Scalpel. If bleeding ensues, a figure-of-eight stitch (2-0 Vicryl, CT-1 needle) is placed. Anterior and posterior urethral transection is performed carefully using cold-cutting scissors (Figure 66-9). In an asymmetric apical contour, care must be taken in tailor dissection to the anterior and posterior contours of the individual prostate apex, maintaining the maximum urethral stump without compromising apical surgical margin. Once dissection of the prostate is completed, the speci-

men is placed in a 10-mm Endocatch bag (US Surgical) for subsequent extraction.

REAL-TIME TRANSRECTAL ULTRASOUND GUIDANCE Tactile feedback is somewhat attenuated during laparoscopy as compared to open surgery. Real-time intraoperative transrectal ultrasonography (TRUS) guidance during laparoscopic radical prostatectomy can help offset this perceived technical disadvantage. (see Figure 66-8B) Intraoperative TRUS navigation is helpful in the following specific technical aspects: (1) visualization of hypoechoic prostate cancer nodule, (2) precision during lateral pedicle transection and release of neurovascular bundles, (3) calibrated wider dissection at the site of suspected extracapsular extension of cancer nodule in order to achieve negative margins, (4) tailored apical dissection according to the individual prostate apex, and (5) facilitating posterior bladder neck transection.

URETHROVESICAL ANASTOMOSIS The bladder neck is carefully inspected and if necessary, reconstructed in a "tennis racket" fashion. If compromise of the ureteral orifices is suspected, the patient is given intravenous indigo carmine and furosemide. Both orifices are then observed until blue-colored urine is visualized, confirming patency. The urethrovesical anastomosis can be performed by interrupted or running techniques. We initially used a two-stitch running technique (2-0 Vicryl, UR-6 needles). The urethral dilator has an end-on hollowed tip and is used to guide the needle into the urethral stump. The first suture is placed at 5 o'clock and runs in a clockwise direction towards the 12 o'clock position (Figure 66-10). At this point, the dilator is replaced by a 22F Foley catheter. The second stitch is placed at 5 o'clock and runs in a counter-clockwise direction. The two stitch ends are tied at 12 o'clock, allowing immediate watertight approximation (Figure 66-11). We are using a single-stitch, double-needle technique, as described by Van Velthoven.[13] The stitch is pre-prepared on the back table by tying two 10-inch lengths of 2-0 monofilamentous sutures with a UR-6 needle (dyed 2-0 Monocryl and un-dyed 2-0 Caprosyn). Both ends of the stitch are passed outside-in at the posterior bladder neck

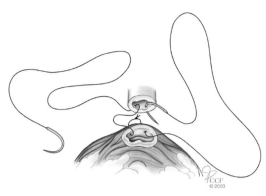

Figure 66-10 First stitch. The first anastomotic stitch starts at 5 o'clock and runs in a clockwise direction until the 11 o'clock position

(6 o'clock). Each end is run for three to four passes in opposite directions. Both stitches are then pulled tight, bringing the posterior bladder neck anastomotic plate tightly and uniformly in contact with the urethra. The metal sound is removed and Foley catheter reinserted. The suture ends are then run until they meet anteriorly and tied together. This method has enhanced the intraoperative watertightness of the anastomosis, allowing early catheter removal on day 3. The Foley balloon is filled with 30 mL and the bladder is filled to 120 mL to test the integrity of the anastomosis.

LAPAROSCOPIC EXIT AND POSTOPERATIVE CARE The specimen is extracted through a circumumbilical extension of the primary port site. The fascia in this incision is closed with interrupted figure-of-eight sutures (0 Vicryl). A Jackson-Pratt drain is placed through a lower 5-mm port site. The fascia of the right-sided 12-mm port is closed under direct visualization with a Carter-Thomason needle and an 0 Vicryl suture. Skin incisions are closed with subcuticular stitches. All skin incision sites are infiltrated with bupivacaine hydrochloride 0.25% to aid in postoperative pain management. Additionally, patients with normal renal function are given 30 mg of intravenous ketorolac, followed by 15 mg every 6 hours postoperatively. On the evening of surgery, patients are instructed to ambulate, and oral intake is gradually introduced. Typically, the hospital stay is between 1 and 2 days. The patient returns on the 3rd postoperative day for cystogram. The Foley catheter is removed if no leakage is detected. If contrast extravasation is noted,

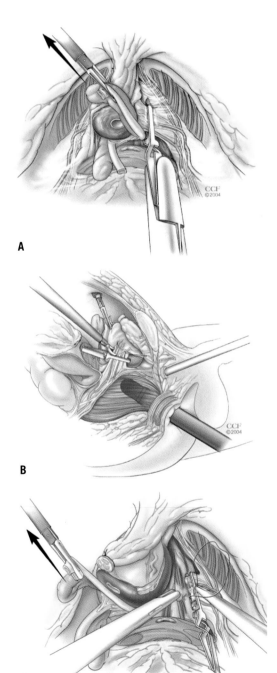

Figure 66-8 *A*, Transient bulldog clamp on right lateral pedicle. *B*, Energy-free nerve sparing using cold cutting under TRUS monitoring. *C*, Superficial hemostatic 4-0 suturing of transected lateral pedicle.

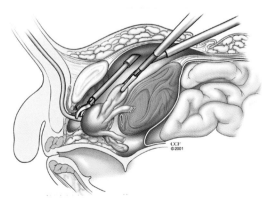

Figure 66-9 Urethral transection and prostatic apical dissection is carefully performed using cold-cutting Endoshears.

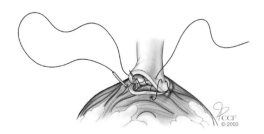

Figure 66-11 The second anastamotic stitch runs counterclockwise, and the two stitch ends are tied at 12 o'clock, allowing immediate watertight approximation.

the Foley catheter is maintained, and repeat cystogram performed in 1 week.

PERIOPERATIVE DATA

INTRAOPERATIVE DATA The difficulty, in the initial attempts to perform LRP, was due in part, to the long operative times. The initial series of Schuessler and colleagues had an average operative time of 9.4 hours.[14] As both cumulative and individual experiences have grown, the operative times for LRP have approached those of open surgery. At the Cleveland Clinic, our first 50 cases averaged 5.4 hours, while the next 100 cases averaged 3.7 hours. Our current operative times range from 2 to 3.5 hours. Guillonneau and colleagues reported decreasing operative times of 4.6 hours in their first 50 cases, 4.0 hours in their next 50, and 3.4 hours in the last 140 cases (Table 66-1).[15]

High operative blood loss and transfusion rates have been common problems in open retropubic radical prostatectomy. Laparoscopy affords excellent vision of the dorsal venous complex and a tamponade effect of the pneumoperitoneum, which minimizes blood loss. In our experience, average estimated blood loss was 355 mL for our initial group of 50 patients, and close to 300 mL for the next 100 patients. The blood transfusion rate remains below 3%. Other experienced laparoscopic urologists have similarly reported blood losses of less than 400 mL, with a transfusion rate below 5%.[8,10,16–18]

PERIOPERATIVE COMPLICATIONS Reported major and minor complication rates of 2 to 4% and 9 to 23%, respectively,[8,10,16–18] compare favorably to open surgical complication rates. Yao and Lu-Yao performed a pooled analysis of 101,604 conventional open prostatectomies and reported overall complication rates between 26.3 and 31.3% depending on hospital surgical volumes.[19] The rate of open conversion in LRP remains less than 5% in most larger series.[8,10,16–18] Comparing transperitoneal versus extraperitoneal approaches, no significant difference was found in perioperative data analysis,[10,20] although potential bowel complications and potential risk of anastomotic urine leak in the transperitoneal approach may remain controversial.[8,21]

POSTOPERATIVE RECOVERY Compared to open prostatectomy, LRP has the potential to decrease treatment-related morbidity and accelerate recovery. Hospital stay after LRP at the Cleveland Clinic decreased to an average of 1.6 days. In a comparative study at a single institution of 219 open radical prostatectomies versus early series of 219 LRP versus late series of 219 LRP, Rassweiler and colleagues reported that the amount of postoperative analgesia (51 vs. 34 vs. 30 mg, respectively) and number of days back to normal activity (52 vs. 31 vs. 27 days, respectively) were significantly greater after open surgery, even though the mean operative time was significantly

shorter after open surgery than early LRP series, but not more significant than late LRP series (196 vs. 288 vs. 218 minutes, respectively). [22]

ONCOLOGIC OUTCOME

SURGICAL PATHOLOGY Guillonneau and colleagues examined 1,000 consecutive patients who underwent LRP and reported positive surgical margins in 6.9%, 18.6%, 30%, and 34% for pathological stages pT2a, pT2b, pT3a, and pT3b, respectively, without an increase in positive margin rate when a nerve-sparing procedure was performed.[23] A German laparoscopic working group demonstrated multi-institutional data of 5,824 patients undergoing LRP by 50 urologists in 18 institutions. [24] Rate of positive margins averaged 10.6% (range, 3.2 to 18%) for pT2, 32.7% (range, 20 to 38.5%) for pT3a, and 56.2% (range, 40 to 75%) for pT3b. [24] Recent reported positive surgical margin of LRP ranged 8 to 31% in overall (Table 66-2).[17,18,21,23,24,30–32] Removal of an intact prostate with negative margins is important for long-term cure. Pathologically revealed extracapsular extension in clinically localized prostate cancer is associated with adverse prognosis.

Since most prostate cancers arise in the peripheral zone close to the prostatic capsule, attempts to achieve wide surgical margins may risk damage to the neurovascular bundle or the urethral sphincteric mechanism. Concern has recently been raised that the muted tactile feedback during LRP may potentially compromise such individualized intraoperative assessment of a prostatic cancerous nodule suggestive of extracapsular extension, which may be achieved subjectively by digital palpation during open radical prostatectomy. [25] We have described the use of intraoperative real-time TRUS guidance during LRP. [26,27] Intraoperative TRUS is capable of imaging a substantial percentage of non-palpable prostate cancers, but also periprostatic anatomy such as the course, dimensions, and vascularity of the neurovascular bundles. The use of real-time TRUS guidance during laparoscopic radical prostatectomy resulted in a significant overall improvement of our positive margin rates of 8%.[28,29]

LONG TERM Because of the slow-growing nature of most prostate cancers, declaring "cure" requires long follow-up. Currently available data for long-term oncologic outcomes after LRP are

Table 66-1 Perioperative Data

	Guillonneau[15]	Erdogru[10]	Ruiz[8]	Stolzenburg[17]		Rozet[18]	
Approach	Trans	Trans	Extra	Trans	Extra	Extra	Extra
No. of Patients	567	53	53	165	165	700	600
OR time (hr)	3.5	4.25	3.5	4.1	3.7	2.5	3.0
Blood loss (mL)	380	185	322	678	803	220	380
Transfusion rate	4.9%	2%	1.3%	1.2%	5.4%	0.9%	1.2%
Complication	Major 3.7%/ Minor 14.6%	3.7%	7.5%	9.1%	6.1%	Major 2.4%/ Minor 9.7%	Major 2.3% / Minor 9.2%
Illeus	1%	1.8%	—	2.4%	0.6%	—	0.3%

Table 66-2 Oncologic Outcome after LRP

	Rassweiler[24]	Hoznek[21]	Rozet[18]	Guillonneau[23]	Stolzenburg[17]	Gill[28,29]	Curto[38]
No. of Patients	500	134	600	1000	700	157	413
Pathological Stage							
pT2	59%	75%	72%	78%	55%	71%	59%
pT3	34%	24%	28%	22%	44%	29%	41%
Positive Surgical Margin Rate							
Overall	19%	25%	18%	19%	20%	8%	31%
pT2	7%	17%	15%	15%	11%	4%	22%
pT3	32%	49%	26%	31%	31%	18%	43%
Biochemical Progression-Free Survival Rate							
At 3 yrs	83%	—	—	91%	—	—	—
At 5 yrs	73%	—	—	—	—	—	—
Clinical Progression Rate							
At 3 yrs	4.1%	—	—	—	—	—	—
At 5 yrs	9.8%	—	—	—	—	—	—

still intermediate term of biochemical (PSA) free survival. Guillonneau and colleagues followed 1,000 patients after LRP and reported an overall biochemical progression-free survival rate of 90.5% at 3 years.[23] Rassweiler and colleagues reported initial 500 LRP experiences with a minimal follow-up of 23 months, revealing PSA recurrence in 55 patients (11%). PSA progression-free rates were 83.0% at 3 years and 73.1% at 5 years, and the clinical progression rate was to 4.1% at 3 years and 9.8% at 5 years.[30] A report from three German centers (Heilbronn, Basel, and Zurich) demonstrated PSA recurrence rates of 8.6% for pT2 and 17.5% for pT3a at 5 years.[24]

FUNCTIONAL OUTCOMES

URINARY CONTINENCE Urinary continence remains a cause of serious morbidity in a small number of patients following prostatectomy. Recent large series from German multi-center studies demonstrated a continence (no pad) rate of 84.9% (range, 72 to 94%) at 12 months after LRP.[24] Reported continence at 12 months after LRP ranged from 85 to 97% (Table 66-3).[17,23,24,31-33]

POTENCY Potency is a primary concern for preoperatively potent men contemplating treatment options for localized prostate cancer. Laparoscopy, with its magnified vision, allows for precise identification and handling of the neurovascular bundles. But use of thermal energy (ultrasonic or electrical) during neurovascular

bundle release can potentially cause collateral thermal damage to the delicate cavernous nerves.[34] Erectile function recovery after radical prostatectomy is variable, with reported potency outcomes ranging from 9 to 86% after open radical prostatectomy,[31,35,36] and from 48 to 66% after laparoscopic surgery (Table 66-4).[18,29,32,37-41] Multiple factors are pertinent in this regard, including the employed definition of potency, patient age and preoperative potency status, type of nerve-sparing performed, surgeon experience, use of oral medical aids, postoperative interval, and method of data collection. The emerging data with nerve-sparing LRP are encouraging. With further modifications and advances, it is likely to improve further, closely aligned with sophisticated open nerve-sparing techniques. Authors are proposing our energy-free nerve-sparing technique, completely eliminating any form of electrocautery, thermal energy, clips, or bioadhesives.

SURAL NERVE GRAFTING We have employed robotic-assistance to perform the microsurgical task of sural nerve grafting during LRP.[42] Employing the da Vinci System, the surgeon's hand movements are sensed, filtered, scaled, and transferred to the lateral arms, where they are translated into precise and smooth surgical moves at the tips of the robotic instruments. There are no natural hand tremors or unintended movements due to fatigue. In addition to this capability, the ×10 magnified, threedimensional view helps to precisely place four to six interrupted perineural

stitches of 7-0 nylon sutures to bridge the gap of the neurovascular bundle.

Kaouk and colleagues reported the procedure successfully in 3 potent men 48, 49, and 59 years old.[42] In the first case, the entire procedure was performed robotically, and in the subsequent cases, the robot was used only for the sural nerve grafting and urethrovesical anastomosis, while radical prostatectomy was accomplished by conventional laparoscopy. During radical prostatectomy, deliberate wide resection of both neurovascular bundles was performed in the first and third cases, and only the left neurovascular bundle was resected in the second case. Total operative time was 6.5 hrs, 7 hrs, and 6 hrs, respectively, and hospital stay was 2 days, 3 days, and 2 days, respectively. Surgical margins were focally positive at the apex in the first and third cases. The first patient was having semi-rigid erections with sildenafil citrate, although still not adequate for penetration (7 months postoperatively); the second patient was potent without any medication (5 months postoperatively); the third did not have any degree of erection as of 1 month postoperatively. Long-term potency data are essential to validate the technical success of this approach.

CONCLUSION

As increasingly mature experiences are published from institutions worldwide, laparoscopic radical prostatectomy is gaining acceptance as an alternative to treatment for clinically localized prostate cancer, with its advantages of shorter convalescence and less operative blood loss, as well as comparable early oncologic outcomes to open radical prostatectomy. Careful prospective evaluations of long-term oncologic outcomes, as well as further improvement for quicker and/or better functional recovery, are awaited.

Table 66-3 Urinary Continence Recovery Rate after LRP

	Salomon[32]	Rassweiler[33]	Guillonneau[23]	Eden[43]	Stolzenburg[17]	German Group[24]
Continence at 6 months	75%	74%	73%	85%	84%	—
Continence at 1 year	90%	97%	86%	90%	92%	85% (range, 72 to 94%)

Table 66-4 Potency Recovery Rate after LRP

	Guillonneau[38]	Menon[39]	Salomon[32]	Roumeguere[40]	Rozet[18]	Su[41]	Gill[29]	Curto[37]
Overall Patient Undergoing Nerve-Sparing LRP								
6-mo intercourse rate	—	32%	43%	—	—	40%	43%	43%
1-yr intercourse rate	66%	59%	57%	65%	—	48%	65%	59%
Preoperatively Excellent Potent Patient Undergoing Nerve-Sparing LRP								
6-mo intercourse rate	—	—	57% (< 60 yrs)	—	43% (IIEF > 20)	54% (IIEF>21)	64% (IIEF>21)	—
1-yr intercourse rate	—	—	65% (< 60 yrs)	—	—	64% (IIEF > 21)	82% (IIEF > 21)	—

REFERENCES

1. Guillonneau B, Vallancien G. Laparoscopic radical prostatectomy: initial experience and preliminary assessment after 65 operations. Prostate 1999;39:71–5.
2. Guillonneau B, Vallancien G. Laparoscopic radical prostatectomy: the Montsouris experience. J Urol 2000;163:418–22.
3. Abbou CC, Salomon L, Hoznek A, et al. Laparoscopic radical prostatectomy: preliminary results. Urology 2000;55:630–4.
4. Rassweiler J, Sentker L, Seemann O, et al. Laparoscopic radical prostatectomy with the Heilbronn technique: an analysis of the first 180 cases. J Urol 2001;166:2101.
5. Gill IS, Zippe CD. Laparoscopic radical prostatectomy: technique. Urol Clin North Am 2001;28:423–36.
6. Hara I, Kawabata G, Miyake H, et al. Comparison of quality of life following laparoscopic and open prostatectomy for prostate cancer. J Urol 2003;169:2045–8.
7. Stolzenburg JU, Do M, Pfeiffer H, et al. Endoscopic extraperitoneal radical prostatectomy: initial experience after 70 procedures. J Urol 2003;169:1694.
8. Ruiz L, Salomom L, Hoznek A, et al. Comparison of early oncologic results of laparoscopic radical prostatectomy by extraperitoneal versus transperitoneal approach. Eur Urol 2004;46:50–4.
9. Cathelineau X, Cahill D, Widmer H, et al. Transperitoneal or extraperitoneal approach for laparoscopic radical prostatectomy: a false debate over a real challenge. J Urol 2004;171:714–6.
10. Erdogru T, Teber D, Frede T, et al. Comparison of transperitoneal and extraperitoneal laparoscopic radical prostatectomy using match-pair analysis. Eur Urol 2004;46:312–9.
11. Guillonneau B, Gupta R, El Fettouh H, et al. Laproscopic management of rectal injury during laproscopic radical prostatectomy. J Urol 2003;169:1694.
12. Gill IS, Ukimura O, Rubinstein M, et al. Lateral pedicle control during laparoscopic radical prostatectomy: refined technique. Urology 2005;65:23–7.
13. Van Velthoven RF, Ahlering TE, Peltier A, et al. Technique for laparoscopic running urethrovesical anastomosis: the single knot method. Urology 2003;61:699.
14. Schuessler WW, Schulam PG, Clayman RV, et al. Laparoscopic radical prostatectomy: initial short-term experience. Urology 1997;50:854.
15. Guillonneau B, Rozet F, Barret E, et al. Laparoscopic radical prostatectomy: assessment after 240 procedures. Urol Clin North Am 2001;28:189.
16. Guillonneau B, Rozet F, Cathelineau X, et al. Perioperative complications of laparoscopic radical prostatectomy: the Montsouris 3-year experience. J Urol 2002;167:51–6.
17. Stolzenburg JU, Rabenalt R, Do M, et al: Endoscopic extraperitoneal radical prostatectomy: oncological and functional results after 700 procedures. J Urol 2005;174:1271–5.
18. Rozet F, Galiano M, Cathelineau X, et al. Extraperitoneal laparoscopic radical prostatectomy: a prospective evaluation of 600 cases. J Urol 2005;174:908–11.
19. Yao S-L, Lu-Yao G. Population-based study of relationships between hospital volume of prostatectomies, patient outcomes, and length of hospital stay. J Natl Cancer Inst 1999;91:1950.
20. Brown JA, Rodin D, Lee B, Dahl DM. Transperitoneal versus extraperitoneal approach to laparoscopic radical prostatectomy: an assessment of 156 cases. Urology 2005;65:320–4.
21. Hoznek A, Menard Y, Salomon L, Abbou CC. Update on laparoscopic and robotic radical prostatectomy. Curr Opin Urol 2005;15:173–80.
22. Rassweiler JM, Seemann O, Schulze M, et al. Laparoscopic versus open radical prostatectomy: a comparative study at a single institution. J Urol 2003;169:1689–93.
23. Guillonneau B, el-Fettouh H, Baumert H, et al. Laparoscopic radical prostatectomy: oncological evaluation after 1,000 cases a Montsouris Institute. J Urol 2003;169:1261–6.
24. Rassweiler J, Stolzenburg J, Susler T, et al. Laparoscopic radical prostatectomy—the experience of the German Laparoscopic Working Group. Eur Urol 2006;49:113–9.
25. Hernandez DJ, Epstein JI, Trock BJ, et al. Radical retropubic prostatectomy. How often do experienced surgeons have positive surgical margins when there is extraprostatic extension in the region of the neurovascular bundle? J Urol 2005;173:446–9.
26. Ukimura O, Gill IS, Desai MM, et al. Real-time transrectal ultrasonography during laparoscopic radical prostatectomy. J Urol 2004;172:112–8.
27. Ukimura O, Gill IS. Pictorial essay: real-time transrectal ultrasound guidance during nerve-sparing laparoscopic radical prostatectomy. J Urol 2006. [In press]
28. Ukimura O, Magi-Galluzzi C, Gill IS. Real-time transrectal ultrasound guidance during nerve-sparing laparoscopic radical prostatectomy: Impact on surgical margins. J Urol 2006. [In press]
29. Gill IS, Ukimura O. Thermal energy-free laparoscopic radical prostatectomy: 1 year potency outcomes. [Submitted]
30. Rassweiler J, Schulze M, Teber D, et al. Laparoscopic radical prostatectomy with the Heilbronn technique: oncological results in the first 500 patients. J Urol 2005;173:761–4.
31. Penson DF, McLerran D, Feng Z, et al: 5-year urinary and sexual outcomes after radical prostatectomy: results from the prostate cancer outcomes study. J Urol 173 2005;1701–5.
32. Salomon L, Anastasiadis AG, Katz R, et al. Urinary continence and erectile function: a prospective evaluation of functional results after radical prostatectomy. Eur Urol 2002;42:338–43.
33. Rassweiler J, Sentker L, Seemann O et al. Laparoscopic radical prostatectomy with the Heilbronn technique: an analysis of the first 180 cases. J Urol 2001;166:2101–8.
34. Ong AM, Su LM, Varkarakis I, et al. Nerve sparing radical prostatectomy: effects of hemostatic energy sources on the recovery of cavernous nerve function in a canine model. J Urol 2004;172:1318–22.
35. Walsh PC, Marschke P, Ricker D, Burnett AL. Patient-reported urinary continence and sexual function after anatomic radical prostatectomy. Urology 2000;55:58–61.
36. Kundu SD, Roehl KA, Eggener SE, et al. Potency, continence and complications in 3477 consecutive radical retropubic prostatectomies. J Urol 2004;172:2227–31.
37. Curto F, Benijts J, Pansadoro A, et al. Nerve sparing laparoscopic radical prostatectomy: our technique. Eur Urol 2006;49:344–52.
38. Guillonneau B, Cathelineau X, Doublet JD, et al. Laparoscopic radical prostatectomy: assessment after 550 procedures. Crit Rev Oncol Hematol 2002;43:123–33.
39. Menon M, Shrivastava A, Sarle R, et al. Vattikuti Institute prostatectomy: a single-team experience of 100 cases. J Endourol 2003;17:785–90.
40. Roumeguere T, Bollens R, Vanden Bossche M, et al. Radical prostatectomy: a prospective comparison of oncological and functional results between open and laparoscopic approaches. World J Urol 2003;20:360–6.
41. Su LM, Link RE, Bhayani SB, et al Nerve-sparing laparoscopic radical prostatectomy: replicating the open surgical technique. Urology 2004;64:123–7.
42. Kaouk JH, Desai MM, Abreu SC, et al. Robotic assisted laparoscopic sural nerve grafting during radical prostatectomy: initial experience.J Urol 2003;170:909–12.
43. Eden CG, Cahill D, Vass JA, et al. Laparoscopic radical prostatectomy: the initial UK series. BJU Int 2002;90:876.

Part VI

Lower Urinary Tract Procedures

67

Ultrasound Anatomy of the Prostate and Seminal Vesicles

Keith W. Kaye, MD

Following meticulous studies by McNeal,[1] Myers and colleagues,[2] Oelrich,[3] and others[4–7] and catalyzed by interest in transrectal ultrasound (TRUS), our understanding of prostate anatomy and especially ultrasound anatomy has increased dramatically. This chapter discusses the current understanding of normal prostate anatomy, the simplified ultrasound physics underlying the TRUS technique, the ultrasound anatomy of normal prostate and seminal vesicles, the anatomy and ultrasound anatomy of benign prostatic hyperplasia (BPH), and the use of TRUS in the alternative treatments of BPH.

NORMAL ANATOMY PROSTATE AND STRIATED EXTERNAL SPHINCTER

McNeal[1] has shown that in the normal 20- to 30-year-old man, the prostate consists of four glandular zones and four fibromuscular structures. These lie around the prostatic urethra. The prostatic urethra is divided into a proximal urethral segment above the verumontanum and is angled about 30 degrees anterior to the line of the distal urethral segment, which contains the verumontanum. The glandular areas are the peripheral, central, and transition zones as well as the periurethral glands. The fibromuscular structures are the anterior fibromuscular stroma, preprostatic sphincter, external sphincter, and longitudinal smooth muscle of the urethra.

The peripheral zone (PZ) in the normal prostate is the largest, forming about 70% of the glandular volume and occupying the most posterior or rectal surface of the gland (Figure 67-1). The central zone (CZ), which surrounds the ejaculatory ducts, is cone shaped with its base at the base of the prostate and apex extending up to the verumontanum where its ducts drain into the urethra. Forming only about 5% of the normal glandular volume, the paired transition zones (TZ) lie on either side of the proximal prostatic urethra,

above the verumontanum, and immediately outside the preprostatic sphincter. The periurethral glands form about 1% of glandular volume and lie interspersed with the smooth muscle fibers of the proximal urethral segment.

The anterior fibromuscular stroma (AFS) covers the anterior and lateral aspects of the glandular tissue, much like a shield, and is made up of the downward continuation of the smooth muscle fibers of the detrusor as well as, to varying degrees, an upward continuation of the striated external sphincter. The preprostatic sphincter (PPS), once believed to be a continuation of the superficial trigone but now considered a downward extension of the detrusor into the prostate, surrounds the posterior and lateral aspects of the proximal urethral segments and prevents retrograde ejaculation.

Until recently, the concept of the striated external urethral sphincter (SEUS) was that this is a flat plate of muscle sandwiched between a superior and inferior layer of fascia forming a "urogenital diaphragm," and that the prostate rests on this much like an apple on a table. Studies by Oelrich,[3] Myers and colleagues,[2] and Kaye and colleagues[6] have shown this to be incorrect. There is *no such structure as a urogenital diaphragm* and *this term should no longer be used.*

The inferior fascial layer *does* exist. This is the perineal membrane, which is well documented and can clearly be seen during perineal operations, such as total penectomy, that expose the bulb of the penis. The concept of a superior layer of a "urogenital diaphragm" arose from erroneous dissection artifacts and descriptions by Henle (1873)[8] and Holl (1897),[9] which have been perpetuated in the literature ever since. Oelrich,[3] Myers and colleagues,[2] and Kaye and colleagues[6] have clearly demonstrated there is no such superior membrane.

The striated external urethral sphincter is now known to be a circumferential cylinder of striated muscle surrounding the smooth muscle of the

membranous urethra. It extends inferiorly from the perineal membrane above the bulb of the penis up to the apex of the prostate and then continues up on the anterior aspect of the prostate as part of the anterior fibromuscular stroma (Figure 67-2 and Figure 67-3). This anatomy can best be understood from a good appreciation of the embryological development of the prostate and membranous urethra. As Oelrich has pointed out, the primordium of the striated external sphincter is laid down around the urethra prior to development of the prostate. This primordium extends anteriorly from the perineal membrane (immediately above the corpus spongiosum and bulbospongiosus muscle) to the bladder and posteriorly from the perineal membrane to the mesonephric ducts (which

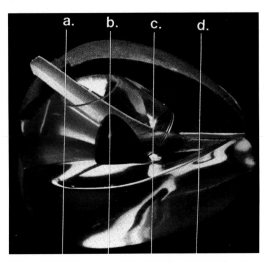

Figure 67-1 Prostate model of McNeal. Note the clear cylinder of preprostatic sphincter surrounding the proximal urethral segment, anterior fibromuscular stroma (brown), paired transition zones (blue), peripheral zone (yellow), and cone-shaped central zones (red) surrounding ejaculatory ducts. Levels a and b correspond to those in Figures 67-3 and 67-4. (Reproduced with permission from McNeal JE.[1])

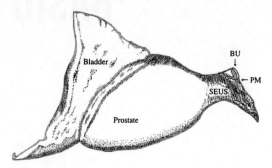

Figure 67-2 Lateral view of a young adult prostate showing a striated external urethral sphincter (SEUS) extending from the perineal membrane (PM) at the base of the bulbar urethra (BU), as a circumferential cylinder of muscle, to the apex of the prostate and then continuing on the anterior aspect of the prostate to the bladder. (Adapted from Oelrich TM.[3])

become the ejaculatory ducts). Subsequently, the prostate, which develops as a posterolateral diverticulum from the urethra, grows into the developing sphincter and causes it to become attenuated in all areas where the prostate develops.

At term, because the prostate has not yet surrounded the anterior part of the urethra, the sphincter still extends on its anterior aspect from the perineal membrane to the bladder. Laterally the fibers cover the prostate to its posterolateral border, and below the prostate the fibres are truly sphincteric and completely surround the urethra, being thickest anteriorly. The sphincter reaches the peak of development before puberty, when pubertal growth of the prostate results in further attenuation of much of the muscle.

With puberty, the prostate develops laterally and also begins to fuse anteriorly to cover the urethra to varying degrees. Myers has demonstrated that at times the prostatic tissue may only fuse anteriorly over the urethra for a fairly short distance, resulting in a prostate with a short anterior

commissure and a prominent anterior notch (Figure 67-4A), whereas in other individuals the prostate fuses along the length of the urethra anteriorly as far as the prostate extends posteriorly, and there is a long anterior commissure with no anterior notch (Figure 67-4B).

Within the striated external urethral sphincter is the longitudinal smooth muscle, which is part of the urethra itself. Immediately outside the submucosa and above the verumontanum, it contains fibers of the downward extension of the superficial trigone.

SIMPLIFIED ULTRASOUND PHYSICS

Ultrasound images depend on the degree of reflection of sound waves back from various tissues to the transducer emitting the sound. The three degrees of ultrasound image, or echogenicity, of the prostate are as follows:

1. Isoechoic: Glandular tissue tends to reflect a medium number of the sound waves back to the transducer and the images appear as low-level grays.
2. Hypoechoic: Fibrous and muscular tissues, such as the true capsule or sphincters, tend to reflect few sound waves back and they appear darker gray or blackish.
3. Hyperechoic: Fat surrounding the prostate or calculi within the gland tends to reflect most of the sound waves back to the transducer and appear as light gray or white.

NORMAL ULTRASOUND ANATOMY

When performing transrectal ultrasound of the prostate (TRUSP), the prostate is visualized in two planes. Initially, starting high up above the base of the gland, scanning is performed in the transverse plane. The transducer is then gradually withdrawn

to visualize in succession the bladder, ampullae of the vas and seminal vesicles, base of the prostate, midgland, and then the apex and external sphincter. Next, the longitudinal plane is scanned to look at the midline structures. By rotating or angling the transducer, the more lateral aspects of the right and left sides can be visualized.

TRANSVERSE SCANNING With the transducer high in the rectum, the bladder lumen containing urine is seen as an anterior black structure with a dark gray representing the surrounding bladder wall. Between the rectum and bladder the round-to oval-shaped ampullae of the vas are situated medially and somewhat anteriorly, with the hypoechoic seminal vesicles represented as either short bow tie–like structures or sometimes longer structures drooping around the rectum (Figure 67-5).

Slightly lower down, immediately below the bladder neck, the normal prostate has a triangular shape and is surrounded by white hyperechoic fat. Two broad areas are seen: an inner area that is somewhat darker, or hypoechoic, with a central isoechoic center, and an outer area closer to the rectal surface that is more isoechoic or lighter. These are called the inner gland and the outer gland, respectively[4,10] (Table 67-1, Figure 67-6). It should be noted and stressed that the term "zone" is used only when specifically referring to one of the glandular zones of McNeal. The inner gland at this level is seen as a dark hypoechoic ring, which posterolaterally is the smooth muscle preprostatic sphincter joining with the anterior fibromuscular stroma more anteriorly. Within this dark ring, the central isoechoic area consists of urethral mucosa, periurethral glands, and the longitudinal smooth muscle of the urethra. The outer gland is mainly central zone with a small amount of peripheral zone more laterally. Within the central zone, toward the rectal surface of the

Figure 67-3 Prostate apex, membranous urethra, and striated external sphincter. Longitudinal (sagittal) section, immediately lateral to the midline from prostate apex (P) to corpus spongiosum (CS). Note significant vascular and fibrous infiltration of the striated sphincter (SEUS) of this 85-year-old man. C = Cowpers gland; FD = fascia of Denonvilliers; SM = smooth muscle of membranous urethra.

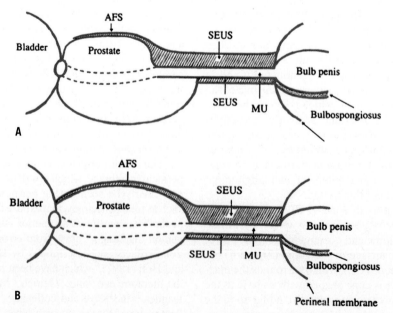

Figure 67-4 Striated external urethral sphincter. *A,* Prostate with short anterior commissure and prominent apical notch. Lateral view. Note SEUS extending to the bladder as part of the anterior fibromuscular stroma (AFS). MU = membranous urethra. *B,* Prostate with long anterior commissure and no apical notch.

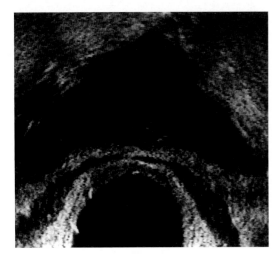

Figure 67-5 Transverse scan above the base of the prostate with symmetric seminal vesicles drooping around the rectum.

prostate base, the ejaculatory duct complex can sometimes be seen as a hypoechoic (containing muscle) round or oval area.

As the transducer is withdrawn farther to the level between bladder and verumontanum, the prostate anatomy becomes more complex (Figure 67-7). Immediately outside the hypoechoic ring of the preprostatic sphincter is the isoechoic transition zone. There is less central zone at this level as one moves toward the apex of the cone and more peripheral zone. Thus, the outer gland at this level is made up of the three main glandular areas (ie, transition, central, and peripheral zones), whereas the inner gland consists of the preprostatic sphincter, periurethral glands, and longitudinal smooth muscles. Moving down toward the apex, the prostate becomes smaller and rounder. The outer gland is formed entirely by the peripheral zone, whereas the inner gland is made up of the anterior fibromuscular stroma.

LONGITUDINAL SCANNING Imaging usually commences in and around the midline where it is easy to identify the anechoic bladder neck. For this reason, it is advisable for the patient to have some urine in the bladder during the examination. Extending from bladder neck to verumontanum,

Table 67-1 Prostate Constituents

Normal	BPH
Inner Gland	
Transition zone	Normal constituents
Anterior fibromuscular stroma	+ Transition zone
Preprostatic sphincter	
Periurethral glands	
Longitudinal smooth muscle	
Striated external sphincter	
Outer Gland	
Transition zone	Central zone
Central zone	Peripheral zone
Peripheral zone	

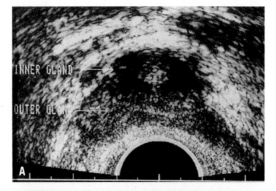

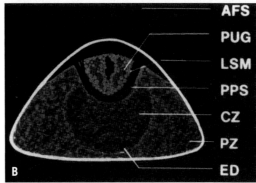

Figure 67-6 Transverse scan of the normal prostate below the bladder neck (level a, Figure 67-1). Note prominent inner and outer glands. AFS = Anterior fibromuscular stroma; PUG = periurethral glands; LSM = longitudinal smooth muscle; PPS = preprostatic sphincter; CZ = central zone; PZ = peripheral zone; ED = ejaculatory duct complex.

the preprostatic sphincter appears as a diffuse hypoechoic area. The prostatic urethra itself is not usually visible. More distally, the hypoechoic external sphincter can be seen extending from the base of the bulbar urethra to the apex of the prostate and may be seen extending over the anterior surface of the prostate for varying distances (Figure 67-8, and see Figures 67-2, 67-3, and 67-4). These landmarks can often be better delineated by having the patient contract the external sphincter. As mentioned above, the degree of development of the striated external sphincter varies from patient to patient, and thus, so will its visualization on ultrasound. Moving the transducer slightly more laterally above the base of the prostate, the ampulla of the vas is visualized along with the seminal vesicle more posteriorly toward the rectum. Fat surrounding the seminal vesicle can penetrate the prostate base to varying degrees and may be seen as hyperechoic white lines. This is called the invaginated extraprostatic space (IES).[11] Careful study may reveal the hypoechoic ejaculatory duct extending toward the verumontanum.

Moving the transducer more laterally, some transition zone may be seen. Finally, at the most lateral part of the gland the prostate image becomes more oval and is made up entirely of the isoechoic peripheral zone surrounded by hyperechoic fat.

BENIGN PROSTATIC HYPERPLASIA

ANATOMY The transition zone, which is situated just outside the preprostatic sphincter, begins to hypertrophy with age, constituting the bulk of the

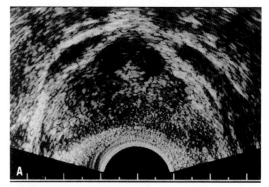

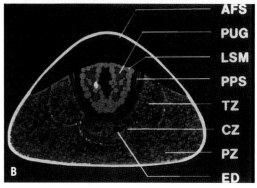

Figure 67-7 Transverse scan of the normal prostate above the verumontanum (level b, Figure 67-1). Note the central zone becoming smaller and transition zones appearing on either side of preprostatic sphincter. AFS = Anterior fibromuscular stroma; PUG = periurethral glands; LSM = longitudinal smooth muscle; PPS = preprostatic sphincter; TZ = transition zone; CZ = central zone; PZ = peripheral zone; ED = ejaculatory duct complex.

area affected by BPH. As it hypertrophies, it expands laterally, medially, and anteriorly as well as proximally and distally and eventually forms the two "lateral lobes" seen at surgery. As BPH progresses, the hypertrophied transition zone glands and the smooth muscle of the preprostatic sphincter intermingle to such a degree that most of the nodules become embedded within the sphincter. Thus the major inner area of BPH consists of hypertrophied glandular transition zone tissue together with varying amounts of fibromuscular tissue.

The periurethral glands, which are within the preprostatic sphincter, may also contribute to BPH

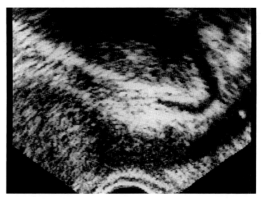

Figure 67-8 Longitudinal scan of the apex of a normal prostate. The well-developed hypoechoic external sphincter extends from the anechoic bulbar urethra at right to the apex of the prostate and then on to the anterior aspect of the prostate as part of the anterior fibromuscular stroma.

tissue. When they begin to hypertrophy, they do so in a different fashion from the transition zone and do so by projecting inside the bladder to form the middle lobe. The central and peripheral zones play no part in BPH, but become compressed by the enlarging benign tissue and form the false capsule.

ULTRASOUND ANATOMY On transverse scanning, the major change seen is that the prostate becomes more oval and eventually round in shape. Although it increases in transverse diameter, the greatest increase occurs in anteroposterior diameter.[5] Interestingly, the TRUS image of the prostate with BPH reveals an inner and outer gland just as in the normal prostate (see Table 67-1). The exact constituents, however, are different. In the older man with BPH, the major portion of the hypoechoic inner gland reflects hypertrophy of the transition zone. This usually remains hypoechoic because of the significant amount of fibromuscular tissue incorporated with the glandular tissue (Figure 67-9). On both transverse and longitudinal scanning, a middle lobe may often be seen projecting into the bladder to varying degrees (Figure 67-10). Transurethral resection of the prostate (TURP) removes both the lateral and middle lobes. It has been shown on TRUS

that some months after TURP the prostate largely regains the shape of a normal gland, except that instead of a well-developed inner gland there is a TURP defect that is anechoic and contains urine.[5]

USE OF TRUS FOR ALTERNATIVE THERAPIES Prostate volume must be determined before treatment of BPH to serve as a baseline. Digital rectal examination is notoriously inaccurate for this, whereas TRUS has been shown to be an excellent way of fairly accurately determining the volume. Several methods may be used. The planimetric method, which involves taking transverse images at 0.5 cm intervals from base to apex, is the most accurate but also the most cumbersome and time consuming. The most common is the biplanar method. Maximum transverse (T), anteroposterior (A), and longitudinal (L) planes are measured and the volume calculated using the following formula:

$$\text{Volume} = T \times A \times L \times 0.52^{12,13}$$

This same formula may be used for measuring the volume of the BPH tissue alone, that is, the hypertrophied transition zone or inner gland, and may be particularly important for the medical treatment of BPH.

In any of the newer modalities for treating BPH, especially when no tissue samples are obtained (eg, medical treatments, stent placement, some laser prostatectomies), it is important to use TRUS in conjunction with prostate-specific antigen to help rule out carcinoma.

Another use of TRUS is for laser prostatectomy, either during planning or treatment. When lasing, especially posteriorly toward the rectum, it is advisable to know the thickness of the outer gland, and TRUS is the best way to ascertain this. Some authors have used TRUS as an integral part of laser prostatectomy procedures.[14]

It can thus be seen that TRUS provides a better understanding of the normal and pathologic gland and has now become an indispensable adjunct in both the evaluation and treatment of prostatic disease.

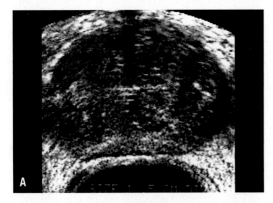

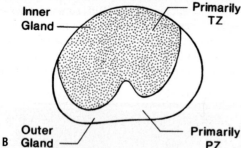

Figure 67-9 Transverse scan of BPH tissue. Note globular shape. Inner gland is somewhat hypoechoic since it consists primarily of hypertrophied transitional zone and a compressed outer gland. (Reproduced with permission from Kaye KW.[5])

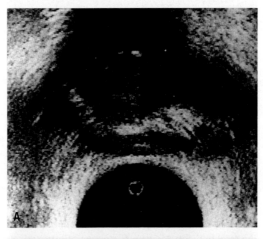

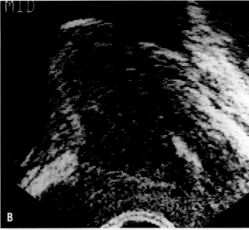

Figure 67-10 *Left:* Transverse scan at bladder neck with prominent middle lobe projecting into bladder. *Right:* Longitudinal scan of same patient.

REFERENCES

1. McNeal JE. The prostate gland: morphology and pathobiology. Monogr Urol 1983;4:3–33.
2. Myers RP, Goellner JR, Cahill DR. Prostate shape, external striated urethral sphincter and radical prostatectomy: the apical dissection. J Urol 1987;138:543–50.
3. Oelrich TM. The urethral sphincter muscle in the male. Am J Anat 1980;158:229–46.
4. Kaye KW, Richter L. Ultrasonographic anatomy of normal prostate gland: reconstruction by computer graphics. Urology 1990;35:12–7.
5. Kaye KW. Changing concepts of sonographic prostate anatomy with benign hyperplasia. J Endourol 1989;3:103–7.
6. Kaye KW, Milne N, Creed K, van der Werf B. The 'urogenital diaphragm', external urethral sphincter and radical prostatectomy. Aust NZ J Surg 1997;67:40–4.
7. Villers A, Terris MK, McNeal JE, Stamey TA. Ultrasound anatomy of the prostate: the normal gland and anatomical variations. J Urol 1990;143:732–8.
8. Henle J. Handbuch der systematischen Anatomie des Menschen. Braunschweig: F. Vieweg and Sons; 1873.
9. Holl M. Die muskeln und fascine des Beckenausganges. In: Handbuch der Anatomie des Menschen. Jena: G. Fischer; 1897.
10. Lee F, Siders DB. Prostate cancer: staging by transrectal ultrasonography. In: Resnick MI, editor. Prostate ultrasonography. Philadelphia: BC Decker; 1990. p. 85–95.
11. Lee F, Torp-Pedersen ST, Siders DB. Use of transrectal ultrasound in diagnosis, guided biopsy, staging, and screening for prostate cancer. Urology 1989;33(6 Suppl):7–12.
12. Greene DR, Egawa S, Hellerstein DK, Scardino PT. Sonographic measurements of transition zone of prostate in men with and without benign prostatic hyperplasia. Urology 1990;36:293–9.
13. Stone NN, Ray PS, Smith JA. Ultrasound determination of prostate volume: a comparison of transrectal (ellipsoid versus planimetry) and suprapubic methods. J Endourol 1990;4:5–11.
14. Childs SJ. Techniques of laser assisted TURP. Laser-assisted transurethral resection of the prostate. Baltimore: Williams & Wilkins; 1993. p. 56–66.

68

Clinical Application of Transrectal Ultrasound in Diagnosis and Treatment

Mahesh Desai, MD

Ultrasonography has gained popularity in the diagnosis and treatment of various urological diseases. Increasingly, it is used by many urologists as an extension of routine physical examination. Ultrasonography is a dynamic investigation that is operator-dependent, and hence, may be optimally utilized if performed by the urologists themselves. Development in instrumentation and imaging has increased diagnostic ability of transrectal ultrasonography (TRUS). Technological advancement in ultrasound equipment, gray scale imaging, high frequency transducer (7.5 KHz) and color Doppler have resulted in significant improvements in the visualization in prostate. TRUS of the prostate may have an important part to play in the management of virtually all prostatic diseases (Figure 68-1).

TECHNOLOGY

TRUS is performed with a hand-held endorectal probe. Most transducers have high frequency, which provides a spatial resolution of up to 0.2 mm. Biplanar scanning in sagittal and transverse axial planes is performed for complete scanning of the prostate. Recent technical refinements include color and power Doppler enhancement and, more recently, three-dimensional scanning along with the use of contrast agents such as micro bubbles, which enables the operator to assess the blood flow within various regions of the prostate.

TRUS ANATOMY OF THE NORMAL PROSTATE

The image of the prostate produced by modern ultrasonographic equipment is simply a picture of the low-power microscopic anatomy of the gland. McNeal's zonal anatomy is well reproduced by TRUS.[1] The normal pubertal prostate is a triangularly shaped gland. The urethra and ejaculatory ducts are structures around which the glandular components of the prostate gland form. Fibromuscular stomas cover the gland anteriorly. The prostatic urethra is divided into anterior and posterior segments by the verumontanum. The transitional zone (TZ) is in relation to the anterior prostatic urethra, while the peripheral zone (PZ) is in relation to the posterior urethra (Figure 68-2). The central zone (CZ) surrounds the ejaculatory duct. periprostatic sphincter is a sleeve around the anterior urethra, seen as a thin linear

hypoechoic area. The TZ lies just outside the periprostatic sphincter. It only comprises 5% of glandular tissue in the adult prostate before the age of 40. Ultrasonographically, the TZ appears inhomogenous and is surrounded by the PZ. TZ is the site of origin of benign prostatic hypertrophy (BPH). An increase in the TZ due to BPH changes the shape of the gland only. About 20% of prostate cancer originates from the TZ. PZ occupies the posterior and lateral region of the prostate, extending from the base to the prostate's apex and is in relation to the posterior portion of the prostatic urethra. It is separated from the TZ by the surgical capsule and comprises 70% of the glandular prostate. Epithelial cells are uniformly small and round with smooth walls, giving the PZ a homogenous echotexture on trans imaging. The PZ is the most common site of origin of prostate cancer and infection. The trapezoid area, distal to the apex, bordered cephalad by the PZ, anteriorly by memberanous urethra, caudally by the rectourethralis and posteriorly by the rectum, is a well-demarcated area on TRUS. It is seen as a bright echogenic area because it only contains fat and few blood vessels. The capsule here is deficient, and therefore, cancer can escape early from this area. The landmark CZ is triangular in shape and surrounds the ejaculatory duct along its entire course, extending from the base of the gland to the verumontanum. Ultrasonographically, the CZ is seen as the tissue surrounding the hypoechoic muscle of the ejaculatory duct. Seminal vesicle and ejaculatory ducts the prostate.

They are surrounded by a thin layer of fat. This gives the appearance of the beak of a bird and is therefore called the beak sign. Again, there is deficiency in the prostate capsule, and cancer can escape early from this region. Therefore obliteration of beak signs has surgical importance. Usually the CZ is not associated with any pathology and only 5 to 10% of cancer arises from this area.

TRUS TECHNIQUE

TRUS is normally performed with the patient in a lateral decubitus position. The rectum should be empty to avoid artifacts produced by rectal content. A digital examination per rectum should be performed prior to inserting the TRUS probe to rule out any painful, anal or sphincter condition. The sphincter should be lubricated generously. Systematic digital examination of the prostate should be performed and normal and abnormal findings noted. Usually a biplanar, multifrequency transducer is used. A disposable latex condom is placed over the entire portion of transducer to be placed in the rectum and is generously lubricated. Most transducers have a water pathway to distend a balloon at the tip of the probe. This increases the distance between the prostate and the transducer thereby giving a window in which to examine the PZ at a variable distance, keeping the area of interest in the sharpest zone of focus. The examination of the prostate begins using a 7.5 MHz frequency in transverse section. This is usually done by pie-shaped, sector-type

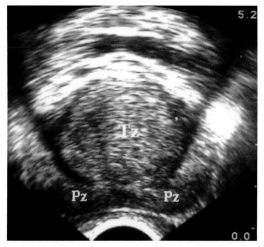

Figure 68-1 Normal prostate scan shows large (80%) peripheral zone and small (5 to 10%) transitional zone.

Figure 68-2 Longitudinal scan showing large circular transitional zone (Tz) with compressed peripheral zone (Pz).

scanner. Sagittal or longitudinal scanning nowa-days is done by a linear array scanner. Newer probes have multiple-frequency and multiple-plane scanning capabilities, so that the complete prostate can be effectively imaged.

PROSTATE AND SEMINAL VESICLE SIZE DETERMI-NATION An accurate estimation of the size and weight of the prostate is necessary for a number of reasons (eg, planning therapy, assessing the importance of prostate-specific antigen (PSA) levels, monitoring success of treatment). The weight of the prostate (in grams) is essentially equivalent to the volume of the prostate (in cubic centimeters) because the specific gravity of the prostate is between 1.0 and 1.05. The simplest method of assessing the prostate size is by assum-ing the gland to be spheroidal in shape. The three largest dimensions, namely, the transverse (r^1), cephalocaudal (r^2) anterioposterior (r^3) dimen-sions are measured.

The prostate volume is calculated by the formula:

$$\text{Volume} = r^1 \times r^2 \times r^3 \ (cc^3)/2$$

PLANIMETRIC VOLUME CALCULATION The prostate is examined from apex to base at 0.5 cm. Using a computer, electronic planimetric calcula-tions of the area of each scanned sections are obtained, and all sections are summed to obtain the total volume.[2] If a "stepper" type device (which automatically moves the transducer in and out of the prostate at a set interval) is used, the accuracy of the planimetric technique is improved.

TRUS IN BPH

BPH is one of the many causes of lower urinary tract symptoms (LUTS) in elderly men. Obstruc-tive BPH is the result of an age-related growth of the transitional zone of the prostate. It is essen-tial to identify an obstructive prostate as BPH develops in the TZ. The TZ is non- existent in the pubertal prostate and starts developing slowly after age 40. Therefore, it is logical that morpho-logical parameters that assess TZ growth in terms of pattern and volume should correlate with obstructive BPH. Transrectal ultrasonogra-phy is an excellent imaging modality for prostate anatomy that could potentially measure such TZ volume or pattern-related parameters. We stud-ied two such TRUS-based parameters, presumed circle area ratio (PCAR) and transitional zone area ratio (TZAR), in evaluation of LUTS.[3] Ohe proposed that it was the shape rather than the size of the prostate that determined obstruction. It was proposed that the normal non-obstructed prostate gland is semilunar, with the transverse diameter being greater than the anterioposterior (AP) diameter. With enlargement of the gland, there is an increase in both the AP and transverse diameters. With development of obstruction, however, the AP diameter increases more than the transverse diameter, giving the prostate gland a more circular shape .The PCAR measures how

closely the shape of a given prostate resembles a sphere. Watanabe has shown that a PCAR of > 70 correlates well with the diagnosis of obstruction, and that a PCAR of > 0.8 correlates with a 97% favorable response to transurethral prostatic resection (TURP) as determined by improvement in the AUA symptoms score. Our study had also demonstrated that PCAR corre-lates well with the physiological parameters of obstruction, and a PCAR of 0.78 was a good predictor of prostate obstruction with sensitivity of 75% and specificity of 92%.

Kaplan and colleagues proposed that the TZ volume rather than total prostate volume corre-lates well with obstruction, and that the TZ index (TZI), which is a ratio of TZ volume to the total gland volume, correlates best with obstruction. They showed that a TZI of 0.5 is an accurate cut of point for diagnosing prostatic obstruction. How-ever, we noticed that the length of TZ as measured by sagittal scanning was prone to significant interobserver variation. Moreover, we saw that TZ dimension on transverse scanning was associated with the least variation. We, therefore, put forward the concept of transitional zone area ratio (TZAR), which is based solely on transverse scan measurement of the prostate gland. The concept of TZAR is similar to that of TZI where, in obstructive BPH, there is greater proportion of TZ in relation to the total prostate gland. A PCAR (> 0.76) and TZAR of (> 0.50) were shown to cor-relate with prostatic obstruction.

MEASUREMENT OF PCAR AND TZAR The PCAR is calculated by measuring the area and circumference of the prostate gland at the level of its transverse diameter (Figure 68-3).

The TZAR is calculated using the formula:

$$\text{TZAR} = - \text{ Maximum area of transitional zone on transverse scan/Maximum area of total prostate on transverse scan}$$

Predicting response to therapy is an important aspect of any evaluation modality for BPH. Patients with no evidence of obstruction on pressure flow studies show a 36 to 70% failure rate after TURP. Watanabe and colleagues have shown a 97% suc-cess rate of TURP in patients with PCAR > 0.80. In

our experience, patients with high pressure and low flow on urodynamic evaluation, most patients with a PCAR > 0.75, and all patients with a TZAR > 0.50 showed a good to average improvement after TURP. The most important predictive value of PCAR and TZAR in the underactive (low-pressure, low-flow) detrusor group. Pressure flow studies in this group do not distinguish between a primary underactive detrusor or underactive detrusor sec-ondary to decompensation following chronic obstruction, the latter having favorable response to TURP. Our study showed that both PCAR and TZAR were useful in predicting which patient in this subset would respond to TURP. Based on our data, we recommend the use of TRUS in routine evaluation of BPH and reserve more invasive uro-dynamic studies for patients showing a discrepancy between TRUS and clinical findings.

ACUTE BACTERIAL PROSTATITIS In acute pro-statitis, TRUS should be performed carefully as it may be painful. Ultrasonographic features of acute prostatitis include an enlarged, round and usually symmetric capsule with decreased echogenicityechogenicity. The entire gland is edematous, and therefore, internal differentiation is lost giving the entire gland a uniform hypoe-chogenicity. The normal, bright hyperechoic appearance of the periprostatic fat is lost due to inflammation and is diagnostic. After treatment, improvement can be monitored by reappearance of normal configuration.

PROSTATIC ABSCESS Prostatic abscess should be suspected clinically and on digital rectal examina-tion. TRUS can be painful and should be done gently. TRUS can show areas of irregularity and abnormal echogenicity of different sizes in the prostate. An abscess focus is usually hypoechoic, with thin or thick septate sometimes, suggesting areas of liquification. Fluid-filled collection sur-rounded with a thick rim suggests inflammation or infection. TRUS-guided prostatic abscess drainage is both diagnostic and therapeutic and is the treatment of choice (Figure 68-4).

Steps for TRUS-Guided Prostatic Abscess Drainage Prepare the rectum with low enema and treat with a broad spectrum antibiotic at least 30 minutes prior to aspiration. The patient is

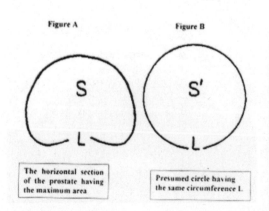
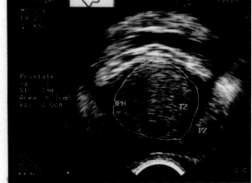

Figure 68-3 PCAR concept and formula for its calculation.

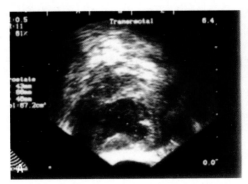 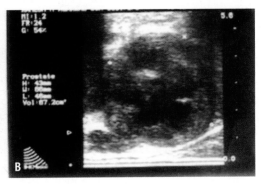

Figure 68-4 Prostatic abscess and hypoechoic area, *A*, in transverse and *B*, longitudinal scan.

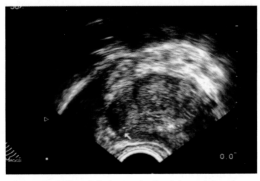

Figure 68-5 Hypoechoic area in the right peripheral zone proved malignant on biopsy.

placed in left lateral position. Using TRUS guidance, an No. 18 needle is introduced in the abscess cavity. The contents are aspirated and sent for culture. An antibiotic solution is instilled in the abscess cavity.

TRUS is repeated in 48 hours and repeat aspiration may be required.

CHRONIC PROSTATITIS Chronic prostatitis cannot be diagnosed with certainty by TRUS, although many abnormalities may be present in patients with documented chronic inflammation. Circumvent the hypoechoic area between TZ and PZ; ejaculatory duct calcification and periurethral zone irregularity or thickening are some of the features that are present. Normal ultrasonography, however, does not exclude diagnosis of prostatitis, and TRUS helps to select patients who require further investigations involving prostatic fluid analysis leading to appropriate treatment.

PROSTATE CANCER The majority (80%) of prostate cancer originates in the peripheral zone. The PZ can be evaluated accurately by TRUS. Although not a primary means to diagnosing prostate cancer, TRUS may help clarify the diagnosis further and help obtain a precise biopsy of the prostate.

The hypoechoic appearance of prostate cancer on ultrasonography results from the pathologic features of prostate cancer (Figure 68-5). Most cancers consist of a dense mass of cells differing in structure from the normal prostate gland.[4] Cancer destroys the normal glandular structure, replacing it with a packed mass of cells, either in the form of small glands or as a sheet without discernible structure. The malignant tissue contains few sonographically detectable interfaces and therefore appears hypoechoic in relation to the adjacent normal tissue. Prostate cancer on TRUS is usually hypoechoic (60 to 70%) but can also be isoechoic (40%) or hyperechoic (rare) depending upon the grade of the tumor. Hypoechoic tumors are more likely to be moderately or poorly differentiated, whereas isoechoic tumors tend to be well or poorly differentiated. Overall, the tumor was seen by USG in only 10% of prostates with tumors with a Gleason score of 2, 3 and 4 (well differentiated), in 74% of tumors with a Gleason score of 5, 6 and 7 (moderately differentiated),

and in all cases with poorly differentiated tumors (a score of 8 to 10).[5] The most common hypoechoic lesion is close to the capsule. These lesions are well delineated because they are adjacent to the more echogenic areas outside the prostate (fat, muscle).

Isoechoic lesions are the most difficult to distinguish. Several features may contribute to cancer being undetectable by ultrasonography, such as tumor size, grade, location, stage and pattern of growth. Higher frequency transducers produce finer resolution, and consequently, improve the identification of such small tumors (Figure 68-6).

It is important to detect extracapsular spread to improve negative surgical margins in radical prostatectomy specimens. There are some TRUS findings that are suggestive of the presence of extracapsular extension (ECE). These include protrudance and irregular borders at the capsule, and obliterance of fat plane just outside of the prostatic capsule. Involvement of the seminal vesicle is suspected when there is asymmetry, loss of beak sign or interruption of the linea alba. However, ECE by a small microscopic cluster of tumor cells may be impossible to see on TRUS.

Identification of very small tumor (< 4 mm) is beyond the capability of any ultrasound study. Some smaller tumors do not completely replace the normal prostate structure, but infiltrate among normal acini, producing a relatively normal echo pattern.[6] A tumor occupying most of the prostate may not be visible on ultrasonography. This reflects the superscan phenomenon, where a tumor virtually replaces the prostate so that there is little normal tissue left for comparison. As a result, the gland has a uniform echopattern, and the cancer is not appreciated. Absence of normal margin between the peripheral and transitional zones in a rounded prostate may indicate the possibility of such large volume cancer. Stage A tumors are transitional zone tumors and are isoechoic, and therefore, less likely to be distinguished from the surrounding echo image of normal TZ. It may also be difficult easy to detect a peripheral zone cancer in patients with a large TZ adenoma because the peripheral zone is markedly compressed. Many patients with Stage A cancer in the peripheral zone, that may not be seen in preoperative TRUS scanning, will become visible on repeat ultrasonography after the transurethral resection of the prostatic adenoma.[7] Presumably,

the compressed peripheral zone tissue and contained cancer expand, and the contrast between benign and malignant tissue becomes apparent. Similar compression of the peripheral zone can be seen when the transrectal probe is pressed firmly against the back of the prostate, making a small hypoechoic area virtually disappear.[8]

TRUS has a doubtful role in screening of the prostate but it is useful in staging of prostate cancer,[9] monitoring the response to therapy,[10] and guidance to prostatic biopsy or interstitial radiation seed implementation.

ULTRASOUND-GUIDED BIOPSY Possibly, the greatest clinical application of TRUS is to obtain systematic tissue biopsy samples in a patient with elevated PSA and/or abnormal DRE. TRUS is capable of providing accurate biopsy needle placement within a specific area of the prostate. Ultrasound-guided prostate biopsy can be performed via transperineal or transrectal approach using a trucut biopty gun. Usually biopsy is performed in the lateral decubitus position. The marker on the viewing screen corresponds to the path of the needle and proper alignment leads to accurate biopsies. Patients experience less discomfort with the transrectal biopsy, especially when spring-loaded devices are used.[11] The risk of infection and sepsis appears to be reduced by the use of bowel preparation and prophylactic antibiotics.

THREE-DIMENSIONAL ULTRASOUND IMAGING OF THE PROSTATE A limitation of conventional TRUS images are their two-dimensional charac-

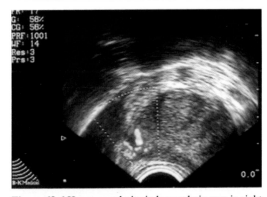

Figure 68-6 Hypervascularity in hypoechoic area in right peripheral zone on color Doppler.

ter. The prostate is imaged in transverse and sagittal views. It is difficult to locate the same image plane in subsequent examinations, but 3D ultrasound imaging of the prostate may overcome these limitations, providing an estimation of prostate and tumor volume with great accuracy and consistency.[12] With a 3D ultrasound imaging system, the patient's prostate can be scanned in only a few seconds and viewed interactively on a computer, after the patient has departed, and prostate and tumor volume can be measured with better accuracy.

Color Doppler transrectal ultrasonography depicts blood flow within the prostate and has been used during evaluation of various pathologic conditions.[13,14] Cancer in general grows more rapidly than normal prostate tissue or benign adenoma. Tissues that grow at a faster rate require increased blood supply to the rapidly dividing cells. Color Doppler has shown that cancer in general has the following characteristics:

1. An increased number of visualized vessels.
2. An increase in the size of the vessels.
3. An increase in the irregularity and contour of the vessels.
4. Increased flow rates.

Color Doppler evaluation may potentially help to differentiate cancer from benign tissue and identify malignant tumors of the prostate in both abnormal and normal areas. This may also allow more direct biopsies, easier tissue diagnosis, and fewer false positive and false negative biopsies.

Power Doppler may be more sensitive in low–blood-flow areas of prostate cancer, thus being more informative than color Doppler alone. Contrast-enhanced Doppler ultrasound studies may help to delineate tumors by discovering increased angiogenesis, and hence, increased aggressiveness of tumor.

REFERENCES

1. McNeal J. The zonal anatomy of the prostate. Prostate 1981: 2:35–9.
2. Hastak SM, Gammelgaard J, Holm HH. Transrectal ultrasonic volume determination of the prostate—a preoperative and postoperative study. J Urol 1981;127:1115–8.
3. Desai MM. Transrectal ultrasound parameters: presumed circle area ratio and transitional zone area in the evaluation of patients with lower urinary tract symptoms. J Endourol 1999;13:317.
4. Wheeler TM, Scardino PT; Cantini M. Whole organ mapping of radical prostatectomy specimens. J Urol 1987;137:224A.
5. Shinohara K, Scardino PT, Carter SSt C, Wheeler TM. Pathologic basis of the sonographic appearance of the normal and malignant prostate. UCNA 1989;16:675.
6. Shinohara K, Scardino PT, Wheeler TM. The appearance of the prostate cancer on transrectal ultrasonography: correlation of imaging and pathological examination. J Urol 1989;142:76.
7. McNeal JE, Price HM, Redwine EA, et al. Stage A vs. stage B adenocarcinoma of the prostate: morphological comparison and biological significance. J Urol 1998;139:61.
8. Bartsch G, Egender G, Hubscher H, Rohr H. Sonometrics of the prostate: J Urol 1982;127:1119–21.
9. Resnick MI, Willard JW, Boyce WH. Transrectal ultrasonography in the evaluation of patients with prostatic carcinoma. J Urol 1980;124:4482.
10. Parra RO, Wolf RM, Huben RP. Echogenic patterns of local pelvic recurrences following radical pelvic surgery as evaluated by transrectal ultrasonography [Abstract]. America Urological Association Report, May 17-21, 1987. Anaheim (CA): AUA.
11. Ragde H, Aldape HC, Blasko JC. Biopsy: an automatic needle biopsy device. Covington (GA): CR Bard; 1987.
12. Newman JS, Bree RL, Rubin JM. Prostate cancer; diagnosis with color Doppler sonography with histologic correlation of each biopsy site. Radiology 1995;195:86–90.
13. Rifkin M , Sudakoff G, Alexander A. Color Doppler imaging of the prostate; techniques, results and potential applications. Radiology 1993;186:509–13.

69

Physiology and Assessment of Outflow Obstruction: A Urodynamic and Fluroscopic Perspective

Jerry G. Blaivas, MD

Benign prostatic hypertrophy (BPH) describes a pathoanatomical condition, whereas prostatism denotes the constellation of voiding symptoms commonly associated with this condition. Prostatism is a clinical syndrome consisting of irritative and obstructive bladder symptoms. Filling symptoms include urinary frequency, urgency, urge incontinence, nocturia, and dysuria. Voiding symptoms include hesitancy, straining, decreased stream, and postvoid dribbling. In most instances, the patient has more than one complaint. It has generally been assumed that obstructive symptoms are caused by prostatic obstruction and that irritative symptoms are caused by inflammation or detrusor overactivity. Despite the logic implied, most clinical studies that document the relationship between symptoms and underlying pathophysiology can establish no such correlation. It is not even known, for example, whether urethral obstruction is the primary mechanism by which BPH causes symptoms. Nor is it known whether relief of obstruction is a prerequisite to successful treatment of symptoms. Likewise, the relationship between symptoms and commonly used indices of prostatism, such as uroflow and postvoid residual urine, is unknown.

Recent evidence suggests that the etiology of prostatic symptoms is multifactorial involving (1) prostatic urethral obstruction, (2) impaired detrusor contractility, (3) detrusor overactivity, and (4) sensory urgency.[1–8] For decades it has been assumed that the cause of symptoms in patients with prostatism was prostatic obstruction and that relief of obstruction was accompanied by relief of symptoms. Nevertheless, this simple hypothesis has never been subjected to any rigorous clinical trial. A number of investigators have stated that, in the absence of prostatic obstruction, neither detrusor overactivity nor impaired detrusor contractility is improved after prostatectomy, but only a few clinical studies addressing this issue can be found in the literature. We need larger and more complete studies to determine:

1. Is prostatic obstruction the sine qua non of prostatism?
2. Is relief of obstruction necessary for a successful treatment outcome?
3. Is prostatectomy indicated only in patients with documented outlet obstruction or does a nonspecific effect of prostatectomy amelio-

rate symptoms, regardless of the underlying condition?
4. Is there a relationship between individual symptoms of prostatism and the urodynamic findings?
5. Should treatment be selected on the basis of symptoms or the underlying pathophysiology?
6. Can specific therapies be directed at one particular condition, such as detrusor instability or impaired detrusor contractility?

With the advent of reliable instruments to document symptoms (questionnaires and diaries) and the ability to define and quantitate the underlying pathophysiology (multichannel video-urodynamic studies), we now have the technical ability to answer these questions. We believe that specific treatments should be tailored to the underlying pathophysiology, but well-done clinical trials are necessary to determine if we are correct.

DEFINING AND QUANTIFYING SYMPTOMS

To evaluate outcomes in any meaningful way, it is necessary to tabulate relevant data before and after treatment. This should include:

1. A structured micturition history and/or questionnaire including:
   - The day and nighttime inter-voiding interval.
   - The number of micturitions day and night.
   - The reported strength of the urinary stream.
   - The need to push or strain.
   - Hesitancy.
   - Urgency of urination.
   - Urge incontinence.
   - Postvoid dribbling.
2. A "bother index" for each symptom.
3. A global assessment score, such as the American Urologic Association (AUA) or International Continence Society (ICS) symptom scores. The AUA BPH symptom index is a seven-item, five-point questionnaire with a maximum score of 35. It has been validated with respect to test-retest validity and as an outcome measure before and after treatment.[9]
4. A quality-of-life score
5. A physical examination including:
   - A general examination.
   - A brief screening neurologic examination

(to discriminate normal, paraplegic, quadriplegic, hemiplegic, dementia, etc., status).
   - A focused neurourologic examination (perianal sensation, anal sphincter tone and control, and bulbocavernosus reflex).
   - A prostate examination (size and consistency of the prostate).
6. A micturition diary (self-reported by patient) including:
   - The time of micturition
   - A description of symptoms
   - The voided volume

Urodynamic parameters: currently, no single measure of either prostatic obstruction or detrusor contractility is available to compare patients in clinical trials. The parameters discussed below do permit patients to be classified as having prostatic obstruction or impaired detrusor contractility, or both, but since they are not represented as a single number, it is difficult to present data comparing one series of patients with another. We believe that the following urodynamic parameters are the most useful for comparison purposes:

1. Maximum uroflow
2. Detrusor pressure at maximum flow
3. Voided volume
4. Presence of detrusor instability

INTERPRETATION OF URODYNAMIC STUDIES

The main purpose of urodynamic evaluation is to document the underlying cause of the patient's complaints and to correlate symptoms to urodynamic findings. To do so, it is essential to understand the nature of the patient's complaints and to use the urodynamic evaluation as a provocative test to mimic the symptoms. The history, physical examination, and micturition diary should clearly document the patient's symptoms prior to beginning the urodynamic evaluation.

The urodynamic study is an interactive process between the examiner and the patient. The examiner should know at the time of the study whether the patient's symptoms have been reproduced, and if so, before completion of the study, the underlying cause should be clearly understood. The possible causes for each kind of complaint will be listed below.

Before starting the urodynamic study, the following information should be known:

1. What symptoms are you trying to reproduce?
2. What is the functional bladder capacity (the usual voided volume, based on the voiding diary)?
3. Does the patient usually empty the bladder (based on examinations and measurement of postvoid residual urine)?
4. Is the uroflow normal; that is, is there a likelihood of either urethral obstruction or impaired detrusor contractility?
5. Could a neurologic lesion be causing detrusor-sphincter dyssynergia, neurogenic detrusor overactivity, or detrusor areflexia?

Voiding symptoms generally have one or more of three basic underlying etiologies: bladder outlet obstruction, impaired detrusor contractility, and detrusor overactivity.

Filling symptoms may be caused by detrusor overactivity, sensory urgency, low bladder compliance, or polyuria.

A careful evaluation should be performed to exclude underlying causes of filling symptoms, including urinary tract infection, bladder and prostate cancer, urolithiasis, and neurologic conditions. Polyuria can be caused by excessive fluid intake, diabetes mellitus, diabetes insipidus, and other less common conditions. Nocturia may be the result of abnormal drinking patterns, a reversal of the normal diurnal antidiuretic hormone cycle, congestive heart failure, or venous insufficiency.

Bladder outlet obstruction is characterized by a detrusor contraction of adequate magnitude (pressure) and duration and a diminished uroflow. Impaired detrusor contractility is characterized by a weak or poorly sustained detrusor contraction and a low flow. Uroflow, without synchronous measurement of detrusor pressure, cannot distinguish between urethral obstruction, impaired detrusor contractility, and normal function.[10,11] Nevertheless, there are no strict criteria for defining these terms. The final diagnosis is based on clinical judgment, taking the following factors into account:

1. Numeric data from the pressure flow tracings:[12] bladder outlet obstruction is defined as a sustained detrusor contraction of over 40 cm H_2O associated with a uroflow of < 12 mL/sec. Impaired detrusor contractility is a detrusor contraction of < 30 cm H_2O associated with a uroflow of < 12 mL/sec. Indeterminate detrusor contraction is a pressure between 30 and 40 cm H_2O associated with a uroflow of < 12 mL/sec.

2. Visual inspection of the pressure flow curves (Figure 69-1).

3. Radiographic appearance of the urethra during voiding: once obstruction has been defined by pressure-flow studies, the narrowest segment of the urethra during voiding at maximum uroflow is usually the site of obstruction (Figure 69-2).

4. Abrams-Griffiths nomogram[13] (Figure 69-3).

5. Micturitional urethral pressures[12,14,15]: in patients in whom the diagnosis or site of obstruction is uncertain, the micturitional urethral pressure profile is usually definitive. The procedure is performed with a triple-lumen catheter under fluoroscopic guidance. One lumen is used for bladder filling, one for measuring detrusor pressure, and one for measuring urethral pressure. During voiding, the catheter is gradually pulled along the urethra and the urethral pressure measured from the vesical neck to the proximal bulb. Normally the bladder and prostatic urethra are isobaric during voiding. The point of obstruction is defined by a sudden drop in pressure (Figure 69-4). When combined with voiding cystourethrography, this technique may be the only method for distinguishing vesical neck from prostatic obstruction.[16–18]

6. Computerized indices of detrusor contractility and urethral obstruction.

DETRUSOR CONTRACTILITY Most methods of evaluating detrusor contractility are based on the Hill equation, which expresses the relation between the force generated by an actively contracting muscle and its velocity of shortening. The Hill equation always has the same form, but the numeric values differ from muscle to muscle depending on two unique properties of each muscle: its maximal velocity of shortening and maximum force. For the bladder, maximum velocity of shortening is expressed as maximum uroflow and maximum force by maximum detrusor pressure. Using these values, Griffiths described the bladder output relation, which is analogous to the Hill equation.[19] For the bladder, maximum uroflow occurs when urethral resistance is zero, and maximum detrusor pressure occurs when there is no flow. Thus, for any given bladder and urethra, there is an inverse relation between detrusor pressure and uroflow: the higher the pressure, the lower the flow, and vice versa. Two other variables must be taken into account, bladder volume and the level of muscle activation. Each bladder has an optimal volume (muscle length) at which it achieves maximum flow. At higher or lower volumes, it generates a lower flow. Detrusor pressure is also dependent on bladder volume. Maximum isometric detrusor pressure occurs at low bladder volumes. Finally, detrusor contractility is dependent on the degree of muscle activation. For any given bladder volume and urethral resistance, isometric detrusor pressure depends on the degree of muscle activation; the greater the activation, the greater the pressure generated by the detrusor.

A number of different methods for assessing detrusor contractility have emerged over the last decade (the stop test, bladder output relation, bladder working function, force velocity plots, pressure/velocity plots, the parameter U/L, and the Watt factor), but none has widespread clinical utility.[8,12,20–29] This is partly due to the complicated interrelationships between detrusor pressure, uroflow, bladder volume, urethral resistance, and detrusor contractility. To be clinically useful, any detrusor contractility factor must take urethral resistance into account. Low detrusor contractility may be sufficient for a patient with low urethral resistance, but it may result in urinary retention when resistance is high.

The Watt factor (WF) is probably the most widely used measure of detrusor contractility.[30] It is determined by calculating detrusor pressure (force) in relation to bladder volume (muscle length) and urinary flow rate (contraction velocity), all measured at the same instant. The maximum WF is a measure of detrusor contraction strength at a single instant in time, but it is necessary to obtain a WF curve throughout micturition to assess overall detrusor contractility. Normally WF increases sharply at the initiation of micturi-

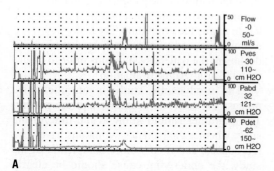

A

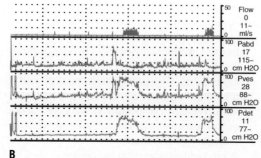

B

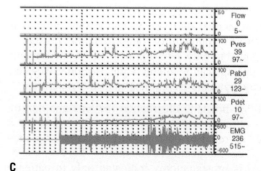

C

Figure 69-1 Detrusor pressure/uroflow study. *A*, Normal. *B*, Prostatic obstruction. *C*, Impaired detrusor contractility. *Pves* = Vesical pressure; *Pabd* = abdominal pressure; *Pdet* = detrusor pressure.

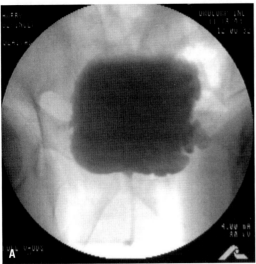

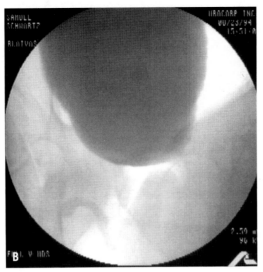

Figure 69-2 Voiding cystourethrograms of the same patients as in Figure 69-1, *B* and *C*. *A*, Prostatic obstruction. *B*, Impaired detrusor contractility.

tion and rises gently, reaching a peak when the bladder is nearly empty (Figure 69-5).

URETHRAL OBSTRUCTION Urethral Resistance Factors The first attempts to quantify urethral resistance involved mathematical definitions of bladder outlet obstruction obtained by calculating "resistance coefficients." All published urethral resistance factors are based on a hydrodynamic understanding of voiding, in which the bladder outlet is considered to be a rigid pipe.[31,32] Various hydrodynamic parameters (including Reynold's number) with respect to laminar or turbulent flow, boundary shear, or wall shear resistance owing to fluid viscosity and urethral wall roughness, along with eddy formation (resulting from geometric and directional changes in fluid) were derived and used in complex formulas. However, in a strict mathematical and physical sense, urethral flow is neither laminar nor turbulent, and many of the assumptions are not relevant to urethral flow. Thus, the clinical and scientific value of these formulations was limited.[25] Moreover, all resistance factors are calculated for a single point of the voiding cycle, and thus, do not reflect time-dependent changes.

Passive Urethral Resistance Relation (PURR) The urethral resistance relation (URR) was introduced by Griffiths to denote a plot of pressure versus flow rate for each moment of time during the voiding cycle.[21] Mathematical analysis of the resulting curves results in the formulation of a urethral resistance relationship to define outlet resistance. These numerical relationships are based on his theory of flow in collapsible tubes (ie, flow is controlled by the elastic properties of the urethra and this control is exerted by local elastic constrictions or compressions at the flow controlling zone).

The PURR was developed by Schafer and constitutes a simplified model of the URR.[25] The PURR has a mathematical form that is described by a reduced form of the Bernoulli equation:

$$Pressure = Puo + Q2(1/C)$$

where Puo is the urethral opening pressure (which characterizes the elasticity/distensibility of the urethra), Q is the flow, and C is a constant (determined by a computer program) reflecting the effective outlet size. According to the underlying model, the PURR exactly defines the impact of the passive bladder outlet during voiding when the outlet is maximally open. Based on this model, Schafer found that the PURR allows differentiation between constrictive and compressive obstructions, independent of bladder function.[25] He further divided the PURR graph

into seven zones that indicate increasing urethral obstruction. Schafer developed a simplified version of the PURR that can be read directly from detrusor/pressure uroflow studies without computer analysis.[27] The works of both Griffiths and Schafer have been modified by others.[8,22,33]

It is important to view the pressure-flow urodynamic studies in proper clinical perspective. The presence of a urethral catheter during voiding has a variable effect on uroflow. Some patients have a normal uroflow without a catheter and a markedly impaired flow with a urethral catheter in place. It may be necessary to perform a number of uroflow studies and then use clinical judgment as to whether the pressure-flow urodynamics are representative of the patient's normal micturition. In general, if a patient has pressure-flow criteria for obstruction, but the uroflow without a catheter in the urethra is normal, one would recognize that the urethra has low compliance (which may be an early manifestation of urethral obstruction) but not make a diagnosis of obstruction.

DETRUSOR OVERACTIVITY Involuntary detrusor contractions are seen in over 50% of patients with BPH, but their presence does not correlate with urethral obstruction.[1,2,34] In other words, a patient with clinical BPH may have detrusor instability in the presence of prostatic obstruction. Even in the absence of prostatic obstruction, detrusor overactivity may cause obstructive symptoms. In this scenario, at a relatively low bladder volume, the patient develops an involuntary bladder contraction that is perceived as an urge to void. He rushes to the bathroom, but when he gets there, the involuntary bladder contraction has subsided and he no longer has the urge to void. He attempts to void by straining and pushing, but is unable to do so because of the small bladder volume.

Once it has been determined that there are overactive detrusor contractions, it is important to determine the following.

1. Does the patient empty the bladder?
   - Whether or not the patient has a significant postvoid residual on a daily basis should have been determined prior to the urodynamics study based on a voiding diary and physical examination and postvoid residual measurement (ultrasound or catheter).

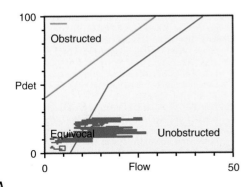

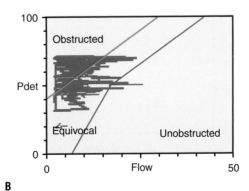

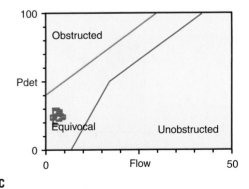

Figure 69-3 Abrams-Griffiths nomograms of the same patients as in Figure 69-1. *A*, Normal. *B*, Prostatic obstruction. *C*, Impaired detrusor contractility.

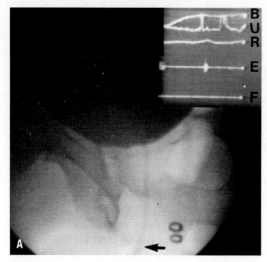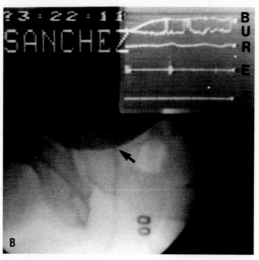

Figure 69-4 Micturitional urethral pressure profile. *A*, The patient is in the midst of a detrusor contraction. The detrusor and urethral channels are zeroed to the same baseline, and at this instant in time, urethral pressure is measured just distal to the membranous urethra (arrow). Urethral pressure measures 30 cm H_2O and detrusor pressure is 100 cm H_2O. This means that the site of obstruction is somewhere between the vesical neck and membranous urethra. *B*, The urethral measure port was moved up and down the urethra, and the site of obstruction was identified as 1 cm distal to the vesical neck. The detrusor and urethral pressure are isobaric with the bladder at this point (arrow).

sphincter and interrupt the stream, but as soon as the sphincter fatigues, incontinence ensues because the detrusor contraction itself remains unabated.

URINARY INCONTINENCE

Urinary incontinence occurs in about 5 to 10% of men with clinical BPH. Sphincteric incontinence is only seen in patients who have had prior prostatic surgery or abdominoperineal resection of the rectum or have a neurologic condition. Usually a clear differentiation can be made between sphincteric incontinence and detrusor overactivity on a clinical basis.

There is great variability in the amount of postvoid residual urine; accordingly, repeated measurements are necessary. If it is clear from these data that incomplete bladder emptying is not a clinical problem, the presence of postvoid residual during the urodynamic examination is clinically insignificant. If there is clinically significant residual urine, the cause must be determined. There are only two possibilities: impaired detrusor contractility and urethral obstruction. The conditions are distinguished by analyzing the pressure-flow characteristics. One can argue that detrusor contractility is impaired any time there is incomplete emptying, but clinically the diagnosis is made based on the strength and duration of the detrusor contraction. If the patient has involuntary detrusor contractions and impaired detrusor contractility, the diagnosis is detrusor overactivity with impaired contractility.

2. What is the degree of the patient's awareness, concern, and control?
   - Once it has been determined that involuntary detrusor contractions are the cause of the patient's symptoms, more information is needed about these factors. At the time of the first involuntary detrusor contraction it should have been determined whether the patient is aware of the contraction, whether he is concerned, and whether he perceived it as an urge, pain, etc. The bladder should be refilled and the patient instructed to try to abort the involuntary detrusor contraction should it occur again during filling. His ability to interrupt the stream and abort the contraction should be noted. Some patients perceive the involuntary detrusor contraction as an urge to void and once aware of it can contract the sphincter, interrupt the stream, and prevent incontinence by aborting the detrusor contraction. Other patients can contract the

REFERENCES

1. Abrams P. In support of pressure-flow studies for evaluating men with lower urinary tract symptoms. Urology 1994; 44:153.
2. Blaivas JG. Pathophysiology and differential diagnosis of benign prostatic hypertrophy. Urology 1988;32:5.
3. George N, Slade N. Hesitance and poor stream in men without bladder outflow obstruction—the anxious bladder. Br J Urol 1979;51:506.
4. Jensen KME, Bruskewitz R, Iversen P, Madsen PO. Predictive value of voiding pressure in benign prostatic hyperplasia. Neurourol Urodynam 1983;2:117.
5. Kuo HC, Tsai TC. Assessment of prostatic obstruction and bladder function by urodynamic pressure flow study. J Formosan Med Assoc 1987;86:1084.
6. Kuo HC, Tsai TC. The predictive value of urine flow rate and voiding pressure in the operative outcome of benign prostatic hypertrophy. J Formosan Med Assoc 1988;87:323.
7. Neal DE, Ramsden PD, Sharples L, et al. Elective prostatectomy. Br Med J 1989;99:62.
8. Rollema HJ, van Mastrigt R. Improved indication and follow-up in transurethral resection of the prostate using the computer program CLIM: a prospective study. J Urol 1992; 148:111.
9. Barry MJ, Fowler FJ Jr, O'Leary MP, et al. AUA Measurement Committee: correlation of the American Urologic Association Symptom Index with self-administered versions of the Madsen-Iverson, Boyarsky, and Maine Medical Assessment Program Symptom Indexes. J Urol 1992; 148:1558.
10. Chancellor MB, Blaivas JG, Kaplan SA, Axelrod S. Bladder outlet obstruction versus impaired detrusor contractility: role of uroflow. J Urol 1991;145:810.
11. Gerstenberg TC, Andersen JT, Klarskov P, et al. High-flow infravesical obstruction. J Urol 1982;127:943.
12. Blaivas JG. Multichannel urodynamic studies in men with benign prostatic hyperplasia: indications and interpretation. Urol Clin North Am 1990;13:543.
13. Abrams PH, Griffiths DJ. The assessment of prostatic obstruction from urodynamic measurements and from residual urine. Br J Urol 1979;51:129.
14. Yalla SV, Sharma GVRK, Barsamian EM. Micturitional urethral pressure profile during voiding and the implications. J Urol 1980;124:649.
15. Yalla SV, Blute R, Waters W, et al. Urodynamic evaluation of prostatic enlargements with micturitional vesicourethral static pressure profiles. J Urol 1981;125:685.
16. Blaivas JG. Urodynamic diagnosis of primary bladder neck obstruction. World J Urol 1984;2:191.
17. Norlen L, Blaivas JG. Unsuspected proximal urethral obstruction in young and middle-aged men. J Urol 1986;135:972.
18. Yalla SV, Waters WB, Snyder H, et al. Urodynamic localization of isolated bladder neck obstruction in men: studies with micturitional vesicourethral static pressure profiles. J Urol 1981;125:677.
19. Griffiths DJ. Assessment of detrusor contraction strength or contractility. Neurourol Urodynam 1991;10:1.
20. Coolsaet BRLA, Blok C. Detrusor properties related to prostatism. Neurourol Urodynam 1986;5:435.
21. Griffiths DJ. Urodynamics: the mechanics and hydrodynamics of the lower urinary tract. In: Medical Physics Handbooks. Vol 4. Bristol: Adam Hilger; 1980.
22. Rollema HJ, van Mastrigt R. Detrusor contractility before and after prostatectomy. Neurourol Urodynam 1987;6:220.

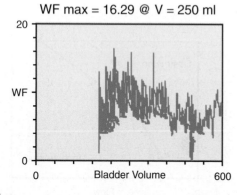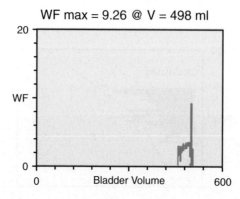

Figure 69-5 Detrusor contractility measured by Watt's factor. *A*, Normal. *B*, Impaired detrusor contractility.

23. Sarky MS, Blaivas JG. Low-pressure low-flow syndromes: a computer-based classification on functional basis. Neurourol Urodynam 1988;7:223.

24. Schafer W. The contribution of the bladder outlet to the relationship between pressure and flow during micturition. In: Hinman F Jr, editor. Benign prostatic hypertrophy. New York: Springer-Verlag; 1983.

25. Schafer W. Urethral resistance? Urodynamic concepts of physiological and pathological bladder outlet function during voiding. Neurourol Urodynam 1985;4:161.

26. Schafer W, Waterbar F, Langen PH, Deutz FJ. A simplified graphical procedure for detailed analysis of detrusor and outlet function during voiding. Neurourol Urodynam 1989;8:405.

27. Schafer W. Analysis of active detrusor function during voiding with the bladder working function. Neurourol Urodynam 1991;10:19.

28. van Mastrigt R, Griffiths DJ. The contractility of the urinary bladder. Urol Int 1979;34:410.

29. van Mastrigt R. Urodynamic analysis using an on-line computer. Neurourol Urodynam 1987;6:206.

30. Griffiths D, van Mastrigt R, Bosch R. Quantification of urethral resistance and bladder function during voiding, with special reference to the effects of prostate size reduction on urethral obstruction due to benign prostatic hyperplasia. Neurourol Urodynam 1989;8:17.

31. Bruskewitz R, Jensen KME, Iversen P, Madsen PO. Relevance of minimum urethral resistance in prostatism. J Urol 1983;129:769.

32. Gleason DM, Lattimer JK. The pressure-flow study: a method for measuring bladder neck resistance. J Urol 1962; 87:844.

33. Spangberg A, Terio H, Engberg A, Ask P. Quantification of urethral function based on Griffiths' model of flow through elastic tubes. Neurourol Urodynam 1989;8:29.

34. Andersen JT. Prostatism: Clinical, radiologic, and urodynamic aspects. Neurourol Urodynam 1982;1:241.

Laser Prostatectomy

Richard Lee, MD

Jaspreet Sandhu, MD

Ricardo R. Gonzalez, MD

Alexis E. Te, MD

Since their introduction into the field of urology approximately two decades ago, lasers have undergone an evolution from theory to practical application. One of the more recent applications lies in the treatment of benign prostatic hyperplasia, or BPH, via laser prostatectomy.

Currently, the gold standard for treatment of BPH is represented by electrocautery-based transurethral resection of the prostate (TURP). TURP, however, is associated with complications and side effects, including fluid absorption, electrolyte imbalance, intraoperative and postoperative bleeding, and inadequate resection. This led to the development of safer, and more effective, alternatives for treatment. Laser therapy promised several advantages over standard TURP, including technical simplicity and the absence or minimization of complications such as intraoperative fluid absorption, bleeding, retrograde ejaculation, impotence, and incontinence. Laser therapy also required a shorter hospital stay and faster recovery. The lack of bleeding and irrigant absorption also theoretically allows laser prostatectomy to treat larger glands with less physiologic stress, suggesting a role for laser therapy in patients with a high burden of coexisting medical disease. Recent estimates suggest an increasing number of practicing urologists are in fact already performing laser prostatectomies on patients with symptomatic BPH, and this number is certain to continue increasing.

It is interesting to note, then, that despite great fanfare, laser prostatectomy failed to maintain its initial appeal owing to an inability to meet high expectations as well as the emergence of some unexpected side effects. To fully appreciate the influences driving the effectiveness as well as morbidities of laser therapies for BPH, one must first examine how the physics of laser energy impacts clinical performance.

LASER THEORY

LASER PHYSICS The word "laser" actually represents an acronym standing for Light Amplification by Simulated Emission of Radiation. An external energy source is used to excite electrons in a medium with an inherently large population of unstable electrons, causing the electrons to reach a higher energy state, called a metastable level. As the electrons return to ground state, they release an amount of energy equal to that initially absorbed, resulting in spontaneous emission of photons.[1–2] Minimal escape of these photons is then achieved by use of a tilted mirror mechanism. Unlike normal white light, which is composed of the entire visible electromagnetic spectrum, laser energy is monochromatic, that is, all of its photons originate from the same energy level transition with both spatial and temporal coherence.[1–3] Additionally, laser rays are parallel to each other and hence do not converge or diverge unless reflected or focused by a lens or mirror. However, once transmitted through flexible fibers by internal reflection, the laser beam will become divergent as it exits the fiber.

Laser energy may be defined by a core set of characteristics, including wavelength (λ) and frequency (ι). Energy (E), in units of joules (J), is defined as the product of Planck's constant (h) and frequency, that is, $E = h\iota$, or alternatively a product of Planck's constant (h), the speed of light (c), and 1/wavelength, that is, $E = hc/\lambda$. Power (P), in units of watts (W), is defined as energy (E) per unit time (t).

Laser energy affects tissue by inducing coagulation, vaporization, or even a mechanical tearing of tissue.[3] Power directly influences the temperature level created, and thereby speed, by which a surgical effect is achieved. Generally, a temperature of greater than 50°C is required to produce a coagulative effect, whereas a temperature of greater than 100°C is required to produce a vaporization effect. Medical laser sources usually possess a maximum power output of 20 to 100 W, although some newer sources can reach a power of 280 W.

Power density, defined as power per unit area (P/A), represents the most important parameter that expresses the strength of the laser at a fixed location. The importance of this concept is emphasized with the two types of side-firing fibers that are available: (1) fibers with 15- to 20-degree divergent beams and (2) fibers with 70- to 90-degree divergent beams.[1–3,5,6] Fibers with narrowly divergent beams will have a much higher power density than fibers with widely divergent beams owing to the difference in the size of target areas. As a corollary, this also implies that maximum power density arises when the tip of a laser fiber is almost in contact with tissue, that is, at the distance where divergence is minimized.[1–3,4,5]

LASER-TISSUE INTERACTION Four major interactions occur when laser energy is applied to human tissue.

Reflection Up to 50% of the incident energy of a laser beam is reflected away. After the initial reflection, the remaining energy is then transmitted through the tissue for a specific distance, depending on the type of laser used as well as the particular type of tissue being treated, for example, 8 to 10 mm in the prostate for the Nd:YAG laser. After absorption, the laser energy is then converted to thermal energy, or heat.

Scattering As laser energy strikes the irregularities of a tissue surface, diffuse reflection, also known as scattering, occurs. Scattering may occur in either forward or backward directions. The amount of scatter that occurs depends on tissue characteristics such as water content, cell constituents, and pigments. Scattering also depends on the resonant absorption and re-emission of radiation by the atoms of the receiving tissue as well as the diffraction or radiation of laser energy in directions away from the line of propagation of the advancing wave. As a result of scattering, a laser beam does not merely continue to penetrate in a straight line, but also dissipates its energy within the surrounding area, beginning when it hits the first tissue interface and continuing to create a zone of heat along the path of the beam. For example, forward scatter in front of an Nd:YAG beam created from the sidewalls of the lased crater increases the power density over the first 1 to 3 mm beneath the surface, causing the point of maximum power density to be ahead of beam contact. This results in rapid vaporization of cells just under the surface, causing the "popcorn effect," or a mini explosion of escaping vapors.

Penetration Laser energy may alternatively penetrate tissue. The depth of penetration by laser energy depends on the wavelength and composition of the receiving tissue. Penetration is often described by "extinction length," the depth of penetration of an incident beam beyond which only 10% of the initial beam energy is left, that is, 90% absorption. Therefore, after one extinction length, 10% of the beam will penetrate further, whereas after two extinction lengths, 1% of the beam will penetrate further, and so on.

Absorption Laser energy may finally be absorbed by tissue. Absorption of laser energy is often described by "absorption length," the depth of tissue through which 63% of the incident beam energy is absorbed. It is important to note that the different components of living tissue absorb different types of laser energy wavelengths in variable fashion. Water, constituting 75 to 85% of soft tissue, absorbs both Nd:YAG and KTP laser energy very poorly, resulting in deep penetration of laser beam into tissue. In contrast, holmium:YAG energy is very well absorbed by water, resulting in less penetration and increased surface vaporization. Pigments, such as hemoglobin, bilirubin, and melanin absorb Nd:YAG energy poorly, but KTP energy very efficiently. Tissue proteins absorb Nd:YAG energy moderately well. Finally, carbon, an abundant constituent of all living tissue, is a final breakdown product of pyrolysis and represents a strong absorber of all wavelengths of laser energy.

LASER-INDUCED TISSUE EFFECTS The predominant mechanism of laser-induced tissue effect is the thermal conversion of laser energy, or photothermolysis, which results in the elevation of target tissue temperature. Laser tissue effects may be subsequently categorized as either (1) coagulation, or photopyrolysis, followed by delayed tissue sloughing or (2) vaporization, that is, photovaporolysis, with resulting immediate tissue ablation.

Coagulation represents the process of raising the temperatures of organic compounds to the point of molecular breakdown, usually greater than 50°C. Once tissue has been coagulated and further laser energy applied, absorption does not appear to be affected, but scattering may be doubled. The backscatter and reflection cause greater diversion of energy, and therefore a wider and longer zone of coagulation. This may be useful if a limited depth of penetration with a wider width of laser effect is desired. For BPH therapy, however, the use of coagulation alone makes the procedure imprecise and can be especially hazardous when working close to the external urethral sphincter.

Vaporization refers to the change from solid to gaseous state of a material. Human tissue requires approximately 2,500 J/g to change its temperature from 37° to 100°C. With laser prostatectomy, gaseous vapors and tissue proteins that are converted to smoke are washed away with irrigation. The kinetic energy of escaping vapor causes mini-explosions within tissue, further adding to mechanical rupture of membranes.

The overall rate of tissue ablation is determined by the rate of laser energy deposition into tissue, which in turn is driven by the laser light wavelength (λ). In laser prostatectomy, one attempts to quickly deliver a sufficient amount of energy per unit volume of tissue to bring cells to vaporization temperature. If the cells are brought only to coagulation temperature, they then become half as penetrable to laser energy, thus increasing backscatter and surrounding coagulation and thereby halting the forward progress of ablation. This directly implies that applying laser light energy at lower power densities for increasing periods of time will only result in a greater depth of coagulation and possible periprostatic injury rather than creation of a channel defect.

LASER DELIVERY SYSTEMS A standard Nd:YAG, holmium, or KTP laser source is used to provide energy for laser prostatectomy. It should be capable of at least 40 watts of power output and continuous laser emission without interruption. Some older machines may also require an external water source attachment for cooling; newer machines with internal cooling mechanisms, which do not require an external water source attachment, are generally much more convenient and versatile. The connector on the laser source for the attachment of surgical delivery fibers must match the delivery fiber chosen for use. The majority of marketed surgical lasers accept any delivery fiber with an industry standard "SMA905" connector.

Generally, standard 21 to 22 French (F) rigid cystoscopes have been used to perform laser prostatectomy. In cases where continuous-flow irrigation is required because of a small bladder capacity, one may place a suprapubic catheter intraoperatively to permit fluid outflow. Some surgeons have also reported using a pressurized irrigation system, though others have found this counterproductive because the pressurized flow may fill the bladder too quickly and limit continuous laser application time before bladder emptying is required. Recently, several purpose-designed "laser cystoscopes" have been introduced, including designs by Circon ACMI, Olympus America, Karl Storz, and Richard Wolf Medical Instruments. These new endoscopes all incorporate continuous-flow irrigation designs in a relatively small sheath, generally a 23 to 23.5F size. Some possess a distinctive beak designed to hold the opposite prostate lobe away from the laser element.

Fiberoptics Fiberoptics are used as the mainstay of laser energy delivery in prostatectomy. Once laser energy has been produced, it travels via total internal reflection through the length of a flexible fiber that is passed through a rigid cystoscope. The most commonly used fiber for laser transmission has an inner core of silicon dioxide (quartz) and an outer coat (cladding) of Teflon FEP (tetrafluoroethylene-hexafluoropropylene), which has a higher index of refraction (1.35) than quartz. The surrounding medium (water or air) in which the fiber is placed has the highest refractive index as compared with quartz, cladding, or medium. This arrangement of sequential reduction of the refractive index from the outside is essential for the total internal reflection required in laser beam transmission. If this arrangement is reversed, or if rays entering the fiber strike at an angle that is greater than the critical angle (angle of acceptance), the laser beam will not have total internal reflection and, rather, will escape through the wall of the fiber, which is dangerous. As a practical matter, for example, laser energy will escape from the sides of the quartz fiber if it is bent too acutely.

Although total internal reflection is essential for transmission of laser energy through a fiber, it ultimately does impact negatively on beam quality at the tip of the fiber, that is, the distal beam no longer remains collimated. Ultimately, there is a loss of spatial coherency, leading to a slightly divergent beam and decline in power density profile. At present, even among the best fibers, only 20 to 25% of the energy reaches the tip, while the rest is lost in transmission. Attempts are in progress to find a core material that can transmit laser energies of longer wavelengths while still retaining flexibility, a suitable refractive index, and nontoxicity toward living tissue.

Side-Firing Delivery Systems For effective use in the prostate, fiber tips that reflect, refract, or deflect the beam perpendicular to its long axis are optimal. These fibers are termed side-firing fibers. There are several manufacturers that make a variety of side-firing laser fibers. These vary in terms of the mechanisms that cause side-firing, power density, durability, size of the tip, angle of beam emergence, arc of beam divergence, capacity to be used in contact mode, and cost. Side-firing tips have two components: (1) reflecting or deflecting mechanisms and (2) encasing and cooling mechanisms.

Fiber tips may be made of quartz, pure gold, or gold-plated alloy. These materials vary in their ability to withstand heat and melting. For right-angle delivery of the beam, the metal tip fiber uses either (1) a mirror of glass or polished gold or (2) total internal reflection from a prismatic tip. The angle of deflection may vary from 45° to 105°, and the arc of beam divergence from 7° to 38°. A major drawback of metallic tips is that after they are used in contact with tissue, carbonization results, facilitating the absorption of very high levels of laser energy. This often leads to an elevation of temperature to greater than the melting point of the metal (melting point of gold = 1,064°C), leading to tip melting or fracture. This in fact occurs more rapidly if irrigant flow is low or if a gas pocket forms around the tip. It is therefore recommended that metal-tipped fibers be used 2 to 3 mm away from tissue, thereby substantially lowering the power density.

The nonmetallic quartz tip achieves right-angle delivery by prismatic internal reflection from a highly polished cut at 45°. The angle of deflection is approximately 78° to 90°. These deflecting tips are encased in heat-protective glass cladding. One manufacturer has created an area of vacuum in the tip, thereby enhancing the difference in optical densities between the internal fiber and the cladding, which makes internal reflection more efficient. Quartz tips can be used in contact with tissue to achieve high power density and vaporization. They can also withstand high temperatures, as the melting point of quartz is 1,610°C. In these fibers, the inner reflective core is additionally shielded by an outer cladding of heat-resistant material; the outer cladding additionally prevents excessive tissue adherence, and thereby heating of the tip. When brought into contact with tissue, these tips deliver a minimally diverted beam and high power density suitable for vaporization. When drawn away from tissue, these fibers produce a divergent beam with low power density suitable for coagulation. They can therefore be used for both vaporization and coagulation as required. After prolonged use, the glass cladding of these fibers develops microfractures that make energy delivery inefficient.

End-Firing Delivery Systems The ends on noncontact-tip, end-firing laser fibers are of limited use for prostatic ablation because the laser beam cannot be adequately directed. Additionally, when in contact with tissue, thermal tissue breakdown results in carbonaceous deposits on the tip, thus causing tip melting, changing the shape from a tapered (sculptured) stylus to a misshapen blob. The ends on fibers have been used as "contact tips" for prostatic treatment by attaching a highly heat-resistant material such as sapphire to the tip of the fiber.[6,7] These can be designed in various shapes, such as slender or obtuse cones,

bullet-nosed, hemispheric, or blunt-ended, depending on the intended use. Laser energy is used to heat the tips, which are then used as cutting, coagulating, or evaporating instruments. Pointed tips tend to have the highest power density, blunt ends the lowest. Minor modifications such as frosting of the distalmost tip by end etching can allow leakage of laser energy ahead of the distal end, and thus can produce better first-pass hemostasis as a result of coagulation. Similarly, incorporation of reflective geometry at the tip may increase the power density at the treatment surface and improve vaporization. Currently available contact probes, however, are inefficient. At the high power densities that are required for vaporization of the prostate, the sapphire stylus itself heats up significantly as a result of significant absorption of laser energy. Some manufacturers have coated the distal sapphire tip with a ceramic coating and/or have used a liquid coolant system to cool the tip. Many think that the time required for tissue vaporization using contact instrumentation, however, is too long, and often supplementary procedures, such as punching out of prostate tissue or mini-TURP, are necessary. End-firing fibers can be used effectively to incise the prostate, however, and are an important part of enucleation-type operations.

EVOLUTION OF LASER THERAPY

A variety of lasers have been developed to treat BPH. Each capitalized on unique optical characteristics that resulted in significantly different clinical outcomes.

Nd:YAG Laser During the early 1990s, the 1,064 nm wavelength neodymium:yttrium-aluminum-garnet (Nd:YAG) laser was first utilized in a laser technique known as visual laser ablation of the prostate (VLAP). Close to the infrared portion of the electromagnetic spectrum, the Nd:YAG wavelength is poorly absorbed by both water and hemoglobin and is transmitted as a free beam through the liquid endoscopic environment with little or no diminution of energy. Because it is poorly absorbed by tissue water, it has a very long absorption length in tissue, penetrating more deeply into tissues than other surgical laser wavelengths and is accompanied by relatively slow absorption by tissue proteins over a depth of several millimeters. The predominant laser-tissue interaction in most soft tissue surgical applications consists of laser light energy absorption and conversion to heat or thermal energy. The relatively slow and nonselective absorption of Nd:YAG laser energy by melanin, pigmented tissues, and proteins translates into a relatively gradual transfer of thermal energy to tissues, producing slow tissue cooking or coagulation as the predominant effect. The Nd:YAG laser thus became an inherently excellent tissue coagulator.

Taking full advantage of the tissue-coagulating ability of the Nd:YAG laser wavelength, several studies have shown the ability to heat large volumes of the prostatic transition zone to tempera-

tures resulting in cell death (≥ 608°C), tissue necrosis, and subsequent substantial mechanical tissue loss through slough and resorption.[8,9] This was facilitated by the application of extended laser application times at low to moderate power settings by divergent, relatively low energy density Nd:YAG beams resulting in large amounts of total laser energy delivered to tissues. Subsequent iterations of the VLAP technique began using higher wattage lasers in contact mode for resection in larger glands.[3]

VLAP became popular amongst urologists because it represented a low morbidity procedure compared with electrocautery-based TURP. Early data in fact demonstrated good short-term subjective and objective outcomes. Despite low morbidities, however, the VLAP procedure developed a reputation for long-term dysuria and urinary retention requiring extended postoperative catheterization. It became clear that VLAP was limited in its ability to effectively treat BPH with effective durability: Although the Nd:YAG laser was capable of reaching power outputs as high as 120 watts in continuous wave mode, its predominant coagulative effect on tissue leading to slough and resorption resulted in prolonged postoperative catheterization and dysuria. Early during the VLAP era, it became evident that this coagulative laser could not unseat the gold standard of care, the electrocautery TURP.

The demise of the coagulative VLAP technique heralded a new trend toward developing laser delivery systems with higher energies and power densities; these would possess "vaporizing" capabilities with the ability to create immediate tissue defects within the prostatic fossa.[10] Initial attempts involved using the Nd:YAG wavelength at higher powers to vaporize tissue in a side-firing approach. Despite being able to vaporize tissue away with the higher power, however, the issue of coagulation necrosis and charring persisted because of the nonselective tissue absorption characteristics of the Nd:YAG wavelength. Additionally, the char created at the surface limited vaporization efficiency past this layer and increased the depth of coagulation necrosis. Thus, despite achieving a TURP-like defect within the prostatic fossa, the problem of postoperative dysuria persisted, making this procedure still patient unfriendly.

Holmium:YAG Laser The next evolution in laser therapy, the 2,140 nm wavelength holmium:YAG solid state laser, appeared poised to better achieve an electrocautery TURP-like result.[11,12] Available in several power configurations, the Ho:YAG laser is capable of tissue vaporization at the highest power setting. Compared with Nd:YAG laser's coagulative effect, the holmium laser wavelength penetrates less than 500 μm into tissue, is highly absorbed in water, and can be used for tissue cutting and vaporization. Because of the high absorption in water, a vapor bubble is formed in front of the optical fiber during each laser pulse, consuming part of the laser energy. The bubble produces an initial photomechanical effect, tearing the tissue apart, followed by a tissue vaporization effect occurring in the vapor environment of the bubble that is associated with superficial coagulation of the target tissue. The high absorption of the Ho:YAG laser beam in the aqueous irrigant implies close contact between the optical fiber and the tissue must be constantly maintained for efficient tissue vaporization effect.

Gilling and colleagues first described the use of the Ho:YAG laser in a side firing mode.[13] The first studies of holmium laser ablation of the prostate (HoLAP) described successful early removal of catheters and good clinical outcomes with this "vaporizing" wavelength, either alone or combined with the Nd:YAG laser. While the laser was able to achieve vaporization, however, removal of large tissue volumes was tedious and time consuming, since true vaporization occurred in thin layers with a relatively thin underlying coagulation zone.

Holmium-Nd:YAG combination laser prostatectomy was quickly supplanted by a pure Ho:YAG vaporization of the prostate, as the latter demonstrated superior clinical outcomes.[14] Holmium laser technique was further refined by directly incising and mobilizing the prostatic lobes in a manner familiar to resectionists with clinical results in fact rivaling those of electrocautery TURP.[15] This holmium laser enucleation of the prostate (HoLEP) approach takes advantage of the cutting capabilities of the Ho:YAG laser. The Ho:YAG laser makes precise incisions in prostate tissue to extract a lobe from the prostatic capsule and then push it into the bladder. The tissue is then extracted by an evacuator or by pulling pieces out manually. To reduce the time, special morcellators cut and aspirate pieces of prostate tissue. Average operative times typically range from 60 to 80 minutes in the hands of well-experienced surgeons and are comparable to TURP. Hemostasis is well controlled. The major disadvantage of the HoLEP technique, however, lies with the associated high learning curve; a surgeon must perform an estimated 20 to 25 procedures in a short period of time to gain proficiency. Prostatic perforations may occur during the first few cases or even over an extended period of time if infrequently performed. There is also a small but finite risk of bladder perforation requiring open cystotomy closure owing to the need for a morcellator. As a result, the HoLEP procedure has had lower acceptance in the urology community than other systems. Recently, a 100 W side-firing holmium laser system has been released and promoted as an ablative treatment for small glands. However, it is a new technology that will still require scrutiny and long-term assessment.

KTP LASER The latest advance in laser technology for prostatectomy involves the potassium-titanyl-phosphate (KTP) laser. Doubling the frequency of pulsed Nd:YAG laser energy with a KTP crystal led to creation of a 532 nm wavelength laser with substantially different tissue interaction properties compared with its parent.[16]

Unlike the Nd:YAG wavelength, the KTP wavelength is selectively absorbed by hemoglobin, which acts as an intracellular chromophore. KTP laser energy is transparently delivered through a fluid medium, such as water, into the cell where it is absorbed by hemoglobin, then rapidly heated, leading to rapid vaporization of tissue. This in addition to the wavelength's short optical penetration into tissue confines high power laser energy to a superficial layer of prostatic tissue that is vaporized rapidly and hemostatically with only a 1 to 2 mm rim of coagulation. The thin coagulation zone arises as a result of the quasi-continuous emission characteristics of the KTP laser: Typically, continual irradiation of a single point causes heat to diffuse into deeper tissue layers, creating coagulation wherever there is enough convection thermal energy for protein denaturation, but insufficient energy for vaporization. This usually occurs at low laser powers since the heat created is insufficient to vaporize tissue, and heat diffusion into deeper tissue layers competes noticeably with persistent superficial energy deposition. However, given the efficient energy transfer characteristics of the KTP laser wavelength in addition to the continual bladder irrigation used to cool the tissue between the pulses of laser energy, these effects are minimized to create only a thin layer of coagulated tissue. These selective characteristics led to the use of the KTP laser in prostatectomy being coined as "photoselective vaporization of the prostate" (PVP).

The initial trials involved the comparison of the KTP laser against the Nd:YAG laser in 41 canines.[30] Both techniques were hemostatic in nature, with no irrigant absorption detected. KTP laser vaporization produced a prostatic defect with a mean diameter of 3.0 and 2.4 cm at 2 days and 8 weeks postoperatively, respectively. Statistically smaller defects were produced by Nd:YAG laser vaporization (2.0 and 1.4 cm, respectively) and coagulation (0.5 and 0.9 cm, respectively). No dog treated with KTP laser vaporization was incontinent or developed urinary retention postoperatively. The use of the KTP laser thus appeared safe and effective in small-scale animal series.

Nd:YAG/KTP Laser Hybrid Low power KTP lasers were initially used in conjunction with older Nd:YAG lasers. The former provided ancillary cutting, sculpting, or incising capabilities, while the latter induced tissue loss through coagulative necrosis.

Kollmorgen and colleagues reported on the use of a 40 W Nd:YAG laser in 32 men with BPH, 15 of whom also received adjunct treatment with a 34 W KTP laser with a 2.5-year follow-up period.[17] All but one patient were treated on an outpatient basis. Durable improvements in peak urinary flow rate, that is, Qmax, (10 to 21 mL/s), postvoid residual, that is, PVR, (167 to 64 mL), and AUA symptom score (24 to 9) were seen up to 2.5 years after treatment. Twelve (70.5%) of these patients required recatheterization, but once adjunct treatment with the KTP laser was initiated in the series, the incidence of recatheter-

ization fell to 33% (5 of 15 patients). Multiple side effects common to Nd:YAG treatment were noted: 4 patients went into postoperative retention, 4 experienced prolonged dysuria, 2 experienced bladder neck contractures, and 5 experienced retrograde ejaculation.

Shingleton and colleagues measured the performance of 60 W Nd:YAG/40 W KTP hybrid laser prostatectomy against that of electrocautery TURP in a randomized, prospective fashion for 100 patients with BPH in 1999.[18] They noted durable improvements in AUA symptom score (22 to 7) and Qmax (7.6 to 15.4 mL/s) for Nd:YAG/KTP hybrid laser prostatectomy out to 1-year follow-up, comparable with that of electrocautery TURP (21 to 3 and 6.5 to 16.7 mL/s, respectively). Of note, the study revealed that patients who underwent laser treatment required a longer period to achieve maximum improvement compared with traditional TURP, a reflection of the lack of tissue debulking at the time of surgery for the former. The authors also note that the low power of the KTP laser made it of only limited utility in the study.

Carter and colleagues performed a comparable study measuring 60 W Nd:YAG/30 W KTP hybrid laser prostatectomy against that of electrocautery TURP in 204 patients residing in the UK.[19] As with the Shingleton study, the authors noted comparable operative times, 37.4 minutes for laser resection versus 35.7 minutes for electrocautery TURP. They also noted comparable, durable results between laser and electrocautery TURP at 1-year follow-up, in terms of Qmax, PVR, and International Prostate Symptom Score (IPSS). The laser group had no patients requiring postoperative transfusions, whereas the electrocautery TURP group had 5 patients requiring postoperative transfusions. KTP laser treatment was thought to decrease the obstructive effect of the early prostatic swelling associated with the Nd:YAG coagulation effect. Nevertheless, 26 (28%) patients from the laser prostatectomy group still required prolonged postoperative catheterization versus 5 (5%) from the electrocautery TURP group.

60 W KTP Laser Experiments with a higher power 60 W KTP laser began with both in vivo canine studies as well as cadaveric canine and human trials.[20] The KTP laser had proven its ability to vaporize tissue while minimizing accompanying coagulation effects. Kuntzman and colleagues performed anterograde laser prostatectomy in 10 dogs using a 60 W KTP laser; the same study also measured the effects of the 60 W KTP laser in dog and human cadavers. The higher powered KTP laser produced the largest tissue cavity in the shortest period of time, (average diameter of 3 cm in 26 minutes), compared with the 80 W Nd:YAG (2 cm diameter in 30 minutes) as well as the Ho:YAG (1.9 cm diameter in 90 minutes) lasers. The 60 W KTP laser also produced a minimum zone of necrosis (0.2 cm) as well as a lower rate of postoperative urinary retention compared with Nd:YAG laser vaporization. The 60 W KTP laser also demonstrated faster mean resection times (29 minutes) compared with 38 W KTP laser treatment

(36 minutes). Cadaveric data from the same study implied that the KTP laser could be as effective in living human prostatic tissue as in canine tissue in vivo. These were the first signs that the 60 W KTP laser could be used as a safe and effective tool in laser prostatectomy.

The first human trials with the 60 W KTP laser came in a series of 10 patients described by Malek and colleagues in 1998.[21] No patients suffered postoperative TURP syndrome or urinary retention; in fact, all patients were catheter-free in less than 24 hours after the procedure. Patients experienced a significant improvement in Qmax (142%) by 24 hours postoperatively. Although the follow-up described was preliminary in nature, initial results have suggested enduring results in terms of Qmax, mean AUA symptom score, and mean PVR at the 3-month follow-up period. Mean operative time was recorded at 29 minutes.

A slightly larger series of 22 patients treated with prostatectomy using the 60 W KTP laser presenting the UK experience was published in 1999 by Carter and colleagues.[22] The KTP laser demonstrated superior efficacy compared with the Nd:YAG laser as measured by both urinary flow rate and symptom scores; there was also a decreased period of postoperative catheterization and urinary tract infections. Mean operative time was recorded at 39 minutes.

The first human trials with the 60 W KTP laser were followed by a larger series of 55 patients in 2000.[23] The 2-year experience with the higher powered KTP laser again corroborated initial findings. Patients experienced statistically significant, enduring improvements in postoperative AUA symptom score (mean = 14, 82% improvement), Qmax (mean = 29.1mL/s, 278% improvement), and PVR (27 mL, 75% improvement) at 2-year follow-up, comparing favorably with published results for conventional TURP. Mean operative time was 44 minutes. All patients in the series were catheter-free 24 hours after the procedure; none required recatheterization. None experienced TURP syndrome. Hematuria was negligible despite the use of antiplatelet agents by many patients. A 9% incidence of retrograde ejaculation at 2-year follow-up was noted, an expected side effect given the authors' deliberate attempt to widely resect the bladder neck. These results demonstrated that prostatectomy with the 60 W KTP laser was as effective as conventional TURP and in fact demonstrated postoperative complications comparable to TURP and even to other laser therapies, such as Ho:YAG.

80 W KTP Laser Despite the effectiveness of the 60 W KTP laser in prostatectomy, its less-than-ideal speed of vaporization inherently limited the size of prostate that could be resected given time constraints. The next logical improvement, therefore, lay in increasing laser power to speed tissue ablation. It is interesting to note that to preserve a thin coagulation zone while still maintaining a high vaporization efficiency, a unique laser pulsing technology was incorporated into the 80 W high power KTP laser system. A high frequency

modulation of laser light generates a continuous stream of short micropulses with a duration of 4.5 ms and a peak power of 280 W, that is, 3.5 times the average laser power of regular 80 W laser. The short duration of the micropulses does not allow time for heat to diffuse from the superficial layer, thus confining energy to a small volume of tissue, in a situation referred to as thermal confinement. As each micropulse generates a very fast temperature increase inside tissue, the tissue water is not only rapidly vaporized, but the surrounding tissue matrix is torn apart as well, allowing for efficient removal of prostatic tissue. Continuous bladder irrigation is thus required to cool the tissue as well as to provide a clear aqueous medium for laser light to transmit to target tissue sans loss of energy.

The first experiments with a higher powered 80 W KTP laser began with ex vivo animal models.[24] Twenty perfused porcine kidneys were used as a model for human prostatic tissue. High power KTP laser resection was compared with high frequency current, that is, TURP-like, resection. The 80 W KTP laser technique showed a statistically significant decrease in hemorrhage compared with traditional TURP-like resection, demonstrating that essentially bloodless ablation of tissue could occur. The slower ablation performance of the KTP laser compared with electrocautery (100 vs 20 seconds per 16 cm^3) seen in the series could be attributed to the particular drag speeds, sweeping modes, and repetition of applications chosen for the KTP laser in the experiment.

PHOTOSELECTIVE LASER VAPORIZATION PROSTATECTOMY

Currently, photoselective laser vaporization prostatectomy (PVP) is performed with the 80 W KTP laser. Hai and Malek presented the first human experience with 80 W KTP laser prostatectomy.[25] Ten patients were followed for 1 year after their prostatectomy in a pilot study. Patients experienced statistically significant improvements in AUA symptom score (23.2 to 2.6), quality of life (QOL) scores (4.3 to 0.5), Qmax (10.3 to 30.7 mL/s), and PVR (137.6 to 3 mL). No patient experienced postoperative urinary retention, infection, incontinence, or erectile dysfunction; none subsequently developed bladder neck contractures or urethral stricture. Two patients in fact did not require postoperative catheterization at all. Only one patient, on active anticoagulation, experienced mild transient postoperative hematuria requiring recatheterization for 24 hours. The mean operative time was 19.8 minutes.

In a US multicenter study published in 2004, Te and colleagues expanded the experience with the 80 W KTP in laser prostatectomy with a series of 145 patients treated by PVP with 1-year follow-up.[26] Significant and durable improvements in AUA Symptom Index (AUA SI) scores, QOL scores, Qmax, and PVR were

demonstrated up to 12 months postoperatively. Mean AUA symptom scores declined from 24 to 1.8 at 12 months; mean QOL scores improved from 4.3 to 0.4, Qmax from 7.7 to 22.8 mL/s, and PVR from 114.2 to 7.2 mL. Mean prostate volume, as determined by ultrasound, decreased from 54.6 to 34.4 mL. Mean operative time was 36 minutes, and no patient required a blood transfusion. More than 30% of patients were sent home without a catheter; those with postoperative catheters had them removed in a mean of 14 hours. Reported morbidities were generally minor. Eight percent of patients experienced mild-to-moderate dysuria lasting more than 10 days. Eight percent had transient hematuria, and 3% had postoperative retention. Among the 56 men who were potent prior to the procedure, 27% experienced retrograde ejaculation, but none experienced impotence.

Te and colleagues then expanded the experience with 80 W KTP laser prostatectomy to 200 patients, the largest and most recent data series to study PVP.[27] All but 5 patients were discharged within 23 hours of laser prostatectomy sans significant complications or postoperative electrolytes changes. Follow-up was available for 156, 104, 87, and 42 men at 1, 3, 6, and 12 months, respectively. Mean Qmax increased from 8.5 mL/s preoperatively to 19.4, 19.3, 20.9, and 16.6 mL/s postoperatively, while mean IPSS decreased from 18.4 preoperatively to 10.7, 8.9, 7.4, and 7.9 in the same timeframe. Mean PVR decreased from 178 mL preoperatively to 77, 69, 75, and 91 mL postoperatively. Complications included retrograde ejaculation in 14 patients, short-term dysuria in 9 patients, urinary tract infections in 7 patients, clot retention in 3 patients, and bladder neck contracture in 2 patients with urodynamically proven bladder dysfunction. Reoperation was required for symptoms in only 3 patients.

Predictors of Success with PVP An effort was made by Monoski and colleagues in 2005 to define those patients who would benefit most from laser prostatectomy by using preoperative urodynamic parameters.[28] Forty-four patients with acute urinary retention secondary to BPH were stratified into groups based on the presence or absence of detrusor overactivity (DO) and impaired detrusor contractility (IDC). Although all patients benefited from laser prostatectomy, with expected improvements in IPSS, flow rate, and PVR, men with preoperative DO, however, had a significantly higher IPSS than those without preoperative DO (11.6 vs 7.3, $p = .049$). These patients were also twice as likely to require the use of postoperative anticholinergics. Additionally, the flow rate in men with preoperative IDC was significantly lower at 1 month postoperatively than in those sans preoperative IDC (7.8 vs 17.6, $p = .026$). Patients with preoperative IDC also had a significantly higher PVR at 1 month compared with baseline (309.6 mL vs 99.9 mL, $p = .001$). Three men required reoperation for bladder neck contractures within the first year, and all 3 had preoperative IDC; although preoperative IDC is not a contraindication for PVP, patients should be counseled that there is an increased risk of bladder neck contractures and reoperation (3/8 patients; 37.5%) when IDC is identified.

Te and colleagues similarly studied the ability of preoperative prostate volume and PSA to predict the effect of laser prostatectomy upon patients.[29] A total of 139 patients with obstructive lower urinary tract symptoms induced by BPH were stratified into multiple groups based on preoperative PSA levels. A significant difference in AUA symptom score and Qmax was observed in patients with PSA > 6.0 ng/mL at 12 and 24 months compared with those with PSA < 6.0 ng/mL. In addition, mean prostate volumes for patients with PSA > 6.0 ng/mL, that is, 83.1 ± 30.6 cc (n = 52), were significantly larger than those for PSA < 6.0 ng/mL, that is, 48.3 ± 16.7 cc (n = 87). Mean AUA SI improvement was 69%, 74%, and 76% versus 86%, 92%, and 85% in these groups at 1-, 2-, and 3-year follow-up, respectively. Similarly, improvement in Qmax was 124%, 145%, and 139% versus 194%, 185%, and 179% at 1-, 2-, and 3-year follow-up, respectively.

Special Populations: Patients with Large Glands and on Anticoagulants One of the advantages with the faster resection time of the 80 W KTP laser lies in the ability to perform laser prostatectomy on larger glands in reasonable times. Sandhu and colleagues detailed large prostate volume resection with the 80 W KTP laser in 2004.[30] Sixty-four men with BPH prostates of at least 60 mL in volume by ultrasound who had failed medical therapy were taken for resection with the 80 W KTP laser. The mean preoperative prostate volume was 101 mL with a mean operative time of 123 minutes. IPSS decreased from 18.4 to 6.7 at 12 months; Qmax increased from 7.9 mL/s to 18.9 mL/s, whereas PVR decreased from 189 to 109 mL. No transfusions were required nor was there evidence of postoperative hyponatremia. All 62 patients were discharged within 23 hours. This was the first evidence that the 80 W KTP laser could be used as a safe and effective means for with durable results for large volume prostatectomy.

Sandhu and Te then described a modification of large volume laser prostatectomy, dubbed the vaporization incision technique (VIT) in 2005.[31] The standard laser prostatectomy technique was modified to include a midline incision in the median lobe carried down to trigone, two incisions made immediately lateral to the medial lobe, as well as two high lateral lobe incisions. The two halves of the median lobe are first vaporized, then the lateral lobes, and finally the apex. The VIT was evaluated in 20 patients with high volume prostates and compared with 64 prior patients with similar volume prostates who had been treated with standard laser prostatectomy. VIT was found to better delineate prostate anatomy, improve intraoperative visualization, and decrease operative time per volume of prostate from 1.24 min/mL tissue to 1.10 min/mL tissue. IPSS and flow rates at 1 and 3 months postoperatively showed no significant differences between the two techniques. No perioperative complications were noted, nor were any blood transfusions required.

The final safety aspect of the 80 W KTP laser to be studied in detail was its use in anticoagulated patients at high risk of clinically significant bleeding. A series of 24 anticoagulated patients with BPH treated with laser prostatectomy using the 80 W KTP laser was studied.[32] Of these, 8 were on warfarin, 2 on clopidogrel, and 14 on aspirin. Eight (33%) of these patients had a previous myocardial infarction, 7 (29%) cereberovascular disease, and 7 (29%) peripheral vascular disease. No patients developed clinically significant hematuria postoperatively, and none developed clot retention. No transfusions were required, nor were there any thromboembolic events. One patient had transient postoperative urinary retention requiring discharge with a catheter. Two patients developed retrograde ejaculation, and 2 patients had urinary tract infections postoperatively. Mean operative time was 101 minutes. Follow-up revealed a decrease in IPSS from 18.7 to 9.5, as well as an increase in Qmax from 9.0 to 20.1 mL/s at 12 months. PVR decreased from 134 to 69 mL at 1 month, but changes were not statistically significant beyond that timepoint. In this study, all patients underwent PVP safely without any adverse thromboembolic or bleeding events. Significantly, more energy and time was used for lasing per gland size in these patients. Additionally, the major difference between anticoagulated and non-anticoagulated patients lay in the safe and effective use of the perineal prostate block instead of regional anesthesia otherwise contraindicated by anticoagulation status.

The efficacy and safety of the laser prostatectomy in high-risk anticoagulated patients was then expanded to 83 patients by Malloy and colleagues in 2005.[33] Eighty-one of such high-risk patients had some type of measurable hematologic deficiency at the time of surgery. Immediate postoperative lab values, however, showed no significant changes from baseline, in terms of both hemoglobin or electrolyte abnormalities. No transfusions were required, nor were there any thromboembolic events. Four patients experienced postoperative clot retention whereas 5 patients experienced urinary retention. Four patients required a second operation: 2 for clot evacuation, 1 for excessive bleeding, and 1 for bladder neck contracture. Overall, studies of 80 W KTP laser prostatectomy reveal it to be safe and of benefit in patients with coagulopathies, platelet disorders, or in those considered to be high cardiopulmonary surgical risks.

Clinically, the PVP KTP laser prostatectomy appears to possess many advantages. Its efficacy appears to be equivalent or nearly equivalent to that of standard transurethral resection of the prostate, because an instant tissue defect can be created with excellent hemostasis, sans absorption of hypotonic fluid. Utilizing normal saline irrigation also removes the risk of dilutional hyponatremia. The procedure can be performed with a wide range of anesthesia from a prostate block with IV sedation to regional anesthetic to general anesthesia. It can be used in high-risk patients such as those anticoagulated with heparin, warfarin, nonsteroidal anti-inflammatory drugs, and aspirin. Often, no postoperative irrigation is required, and catheter time is relatively short. Many patients do not even require postoperative catheters.

PATIENT PREPARATION Very little special patient preparation is needed prior to laser prostatectomy. Many patients today are routinely taking aspirin, nonsteroidal anti-inflammatory drugs (NSAIDs), and other medications that may affect platelet function. Others may be actively receiving chronic anticoagulation with agents such as warfarin. Although these patients might have raised concerns in the era of electrocautery TURP, the hemostasis associated with laser prostatectomy allows select patients to be treated without stopping or changing their medical regimen.[46,34,35] The risks of treatment on anticoagulation therapy should be clearly stated to the patient, particularly when using relatively less hemostatic approaches such as the holmium laser.

Age-appropriate patients should be screened with both digital rectal examination (DRE) and serum prostate-specific antigen (PSA) levels. Abnormalities may be evaluated with transrectal prostatic ultrasound and biopsy as indicated, depending on the age and health. Such screening is important in laser prostatectomy since pathology is not adequately sampled for histologic examination.[36]

A minority of patients with bladder outlet obstruction because of BPH will present with active urinary tract infection or with significant pyuria. This should be treated preoperatively prior to laser prostatectomy, especially with VLAP where a significant volume of coagulated, nonperfused, necrotic tissue left in situ for several weeks postoperatively may become seeded with bacteria in the presence of active infection. This can produce a recalcitrant prostatitis that can be difficult to treat and may result in urosepsis. For the typical patient who presents with sterile urine, routine antibiotic prophylaxis is recommended prior to laser resection of the prostate.

The consent for laser prostatectomy is very similar to that obtained for other transurethral operations. Patients are informed that they will require an anesthetic, and thus will be subject to the standard risks associated with anesthesia. They are informed of potential complications associated with any invasive urologic procedure such as bleeding, urinary tract perforation, infection, urinary incontinence, erectile dysfunction, retrograde ejaculation, and urethral stricture or bladder neck contracture. Finally, the patient should be informed that remaining tissue can grow back, causing recurrent voiding symptoms and additional prostate surgery may be required.

Patients are also informed that the results of laser treatment of the prostate have been documented to be durable only for at least 2 to 3 years, and that its durability over a longer period of time await 5- or 10-year follow-up data.

PREOPERATIVE PREPARATION Special preparation for laser prostatectomy is not required. Standard patient positioning in the dorsal lithotomy position with sterile draping and cleansing preparation as for routine cystoscopy or any other transurethral operation are used. Video display is routinely utilized. A properly functioning laser source and compatible laser delivery fiber are required. The surgeon should understand the tissue effects of the particular laser wavelength chosen as well as the desired treatment parameters and operative technique for the delivery fiber to be used.

Laser safety should be of paramount importance in the operating room. Laser energy can cause significant thermal injury to human tissues, including irreversible retinal damage if the eye is struck. All operating room personnel and the patient must wear proper eye protection. Operating room windows should be covered to prevent the inadvertent passage of stray laser light; doors should be appropriately marked to warn outside personnel that laser energy is in use. Special filters are available to cap the cystoscope lens, serving to protect videoendoscopy equipment from retrograde transmission of laser light. One must note that many laser accidents are related to disruption of the fiberoptic delivery systems outside the patient and often away from the operative field entirely, resulting in the transmission of stray laser light. Similarly, when the laser is not being actively used, and in particular when the delivery fiber is removed from the cystoscope and the working end lies free on the operative field, the surgeon should remove his foot from over the laser pedal, and nursing personnel should close the shutter on the laser machine to prevent accidental firing. Paper drapes can be easily ignited and patients burned by the laser beam.

TECHNIQUE Laser prostatectomy requires either local, regional, or systemic anesthesia because of pain associated with acute laser burns to the prostatic urethra. Leach and colleagues have in addition described a transperineal injection technique using lidocaine and bupivacaine to achieve local prostatic and pudendal nerve blockade, which when combined with intravenous sedation may also provide adequate anesthesia to perform laser prostatectomy.[37]

Cystourethroscopy is performed with a standard 21 to 26F cystoscope. Specialized continuous-flow cystoscopes purposely designed for laser prostatectomy have also been developed. If continuous-flow irrigation is inadequate to provide a clear field of vision, a suprapubic catheter can be placed to provide continuous intraoperative irrigation flow as well as for postoperative urinary drainage. Since clinically negligible fluid absorption occurs during laser prostatectomy, special irrigation solutions are not required; normal saline provides crisp visualization, is relatively inexpensive, and thus represents the fluid of choice compared with osmolar solutions. Room temperature, as opposed to warmed, irrigation provides cooling for the laser delivery fiber, limiting thermal damage as well as prolonging the usable lifespan of fibers. The irrigant is hung at a normal height, generally 30 cm above the bladder, and allowed to flow under gravity. Suction irrigation to the outflow port should be avoided, is unnecessary, and may increase the risk of inadvertent bladder perforation. The laser fiber is fixed in a convenient location on the drapes, generally on the left patient legging for a right-handed surgeon, and the proximal connector passed off the operative field to be attached to the laser source. Care should be taken not to clamp or crimp the fiberoptic cable when fixing it to the drape to avoid damage. The prostatic anatomy is carefully assessed and the prostatic urethral length from the bladder neck to the proximal aspect of the verumontanum is inspected. The laser fiber is then passed through the working port of the cystoscope and visualized in the prostatic urethra in preparation to begin laser application.

Laser tissue interaction operative principles apply for laser prostatectomy. Laser energy is directed at the locations along the prostatic urethra that are obstructive such as medial, lateral, and anterior lobe tissue. To optimize energy transfer to prostatic tissue, these applications should be continuous and uninterrupted. A systematic and aggressive approach to laser prostatectomy will ensure complete laser treatment of all obstructive tissue elements. Laser resection may begin with either the medial lobe or lateral lobes, but should always be started proximally and continued distally, working away from the bladder neck and toward the verumontanum. After the proximal prostate near the bladder neck is opened by superficial tissue vaporization, there will be improved irrigation flow for the more distal laser treatment.

For the VLAP laser technique utilizing an Nd:Yag laser with a side-firing metal mirror, laser application must be performed for at least a minimum of 60 to 90 seconds at a point location for adequate tissue coagulation. This VLAP technique involves the application of laser energy at 1 to 2 cm intervals, such that the tissue coagulation effects will overlap. For the lateral lobes, laser energy may be applied in a 4-quadrant approach at 4, 8, 2, and 10 o'clock positions at 1 to 2 cm intervals until the verumontanum is approached. The addition of 3 and 9 o'clock laser applications may be needed in larger glands where the anteroposterior dimension of the prostatic urethra may also be increased. Medial lobe resection usually involves 6 o'clock, or alternatively 5 and 7 o'clock, applications of VLAP laser energy, again at 1 to 2 cm intervals. As a rough guideline, every gram of prostate tissue to be resected requires approximately 1,000 J of VLAP energy. This technique has generally fallen out of current urologic practice and is not recommended since it generally results in a greater degree of unwanted coagulation necrosis.

HoLAP, HoLEP, or PVP laser energy may be applied in a continuous fashion over an area, barring excessive tissue resection (eg, perforation). HoLAP consists of "painting" systematically over the surface of the prostate until a TURP-like cavity is formed. The high powered holmium laser is used with a maximum average power of 60 W at an energy setting of 2.4 J at 25 Hz. The prostate is ablated circumferentially to achieve a satisfactory channel.

HoLEP, on the other hand, consists of enucleating the prostate. This is performed by using an end-firing fiber to dissect the adenoma from the surgical capsule. The intact median and lateral lobes, or alternatively, subtotal fragments of the lobes are pushed into the bladder and further morcellated using a mechanical morcellator or an electrosurgical loop. If an electrosurgical loop is used to further fragment the devascularized lobes, irrigation should be changed to glycine. HoLEP is performed at a maximum average power setting of 80 W (2.0 J at 40 Hz) or 100 W (2.0 J at 50 Hz). After morcellation or fragmentation, the tissue is evacuated or aspirated by the easiest means—transuretherally or suprapubically.

PVP is similar to HoLAP in technique, but the KTP wavelength and power is more efficient at vaporization. The KTP laser source is used at a setting of 80 W to vaporize the median lobe first to the level of the trigone. Once a channel has been created that allows adequate irrigation, the lateral lobes are next vaporized. This is followed by apical vaporization. At the end of the PVP procedure, a cavity should be present where adenoma once was. If bleeding is encountered during the PVP, the laser setting is lowered to 40 W to allow coagulation instead of vaporization, and the target area coagulated.

Prolonged contact of laser fibers with tissue during active laser application should be avoided whenever possible. Optimally, the fiber tip should be held just off the mucosal surface such that a clear plane of water stands between the tip and tissue; by moving the beak of the cystoscope close to the fiber tip, the scope can be used to hold tissue away from the tip in many instances. In addition, resecting proximal before distal prostate tissue aids in freeing up tissue away from the fiber, especially in longer and larger, more occlusive prostates. Finally, when all else fails and occlusive prostate tissue must remain in contact with the metal mirror during treatment, a very slight vibratory motion of the fiber tip, that is, no more than 1 to 2 mm longitudinal oscillation, such that the laser application is still held stable over a single constant tissue focus, combined with good water flow can keep tissue from adhering to the metal fiber tip. For all fibers with a mirror reflecting mechanism, routine cleaning of the fiber is recommended. The buildup of spattered particulate on the fiber surface during treatment can cause superheating with fiber degradation, loss of efficiency of laser transmission, and eventually degradation of the fiber requiring replacement. Prophylactic cleaning between each laser application and ensuring adequate room temperature water flow throughout the duration of each individual laser application are the most important and simplest means of preserving the integrity of these devices.

Additionally, fibers relying on an internal quartz reflector require special handling. The quartz tips of these devices are relatively brittle and susceptible to mechanical trauma, even with the capillary tube covering that most employ. Therefore, greater care should be taken during passage of these fibers through the cystoscope to prevent breakage. Similarly, aggressive cleaning of these devices during use is not recommended as this may also damage the tip; only very excessive tissue buildup should be gently wiped away with a gauze sponge. In general, laser fibers are resistant to thermal damage and will therefore tolerate tissue contact. However, the resistance to thermal damage is not unlimited, and if buried in tissue at high power settings or subject to poor irrigation flow, the fiber will eventually be degraded to the point of requiring replacement. In addition, some of the quartz reflecting fibers still incorporate a metal cap or cover, which can easily melt if buried in tissue during laser application even while the underlying quartz fiber is relatively unaffected.

POSTOPERATIVE CARE   At the conclusion of laser prostatectomy, a urinary catheter is left in place to provide drainage. A suprapubic catheter may be left in place to facilitate early or repeated voiding trials if desired. Catheter drainage is required for most patients treated with the Nd:YAG laser since its effects essentially represent a burn injury to the prostatic parenchyma and are therefore associated with an acute phase of tissue edema that tends to cause urinary retention.

Many routinely discharge patients following complete recovery from anesthesia, making laser prostatectomy essentially an outpatient procedure. Catheter drainage to a urinary leg bag if necessary can be maintained and easily mastered by most patients. Patients should note that if they possess a history of preoperative urinary retention or a history of detrusor hypocontractility with a large preoperative residual urine volume, as is commonly seen in diabetes mellitus, they may require longer catheterization times. Postoperative management with suprapubic catheter drainage in these individuals may be ideal to allow easy or repeated voiding trials if needed.

When the urinary catheter is removed, patients should receive a 5- to 7-day course of a broadspectrum oral antibiotic, usually trimethoprimsulfamethoxazole or a fluoroquinolone, to clear the urine of any bacterial colonization that may have occurred during catheterization. Following catheter removal, immediate improvement in voiding may not immediately occur, especially with the VLAP or HoLAP techniques or in any laser procedure where vaporization is not efficient, resulting in a greater degree of coagulation necrosis. In fact, patients might have little or no change in voiding during the first 1 to 2 weeks postoperatively, and they may experience slightly worse symptoms while the treated prostatic transition zone sloughs. During this time, patients may notice a cloudy, white appearance in the urine, caused by proteinaceous material from the dissolving prostate; others may note the passage of minute particulate matter in the urine. This phase of active tissue dissolution can be associated with symptoms of mild dysuria, which are usually relieved by nonsteroidal anti-inflammatory drugs as needed. Phenazopyridine (Pyridium) seems to be much less effective for this syndrome, but may also be used as needed. Patients with intractable dysuria may have pyuria, requiring appropriate antibiotic therapy. By 4 to 6 weeks following such a laser prostatectomy, most patients begin to notice a significant improvement in their voiding pattern. Improvement will continue in most men for an additional 6 to 12 weeks and longer, until maximum voiding outcome is achieved. By 3 months, voiding outcomes are similar to those expected after electrocautery TURP. With efficient vaporization and limited coagulation necrosis that routinely occur with high power KTP applications, improvement may occur as short as a few days to a week with minimal dysuria.

Because of the superior surgical hemostasis associated with laser prostatectomy, no restrictions on physical activity are needed, even in the immediate postoperative period. After catheter removal, sexual intercourse is allowed immediately if desired, but recommended at about 1 month postoperatively. Patients should be warned of the possibility that the ejaculate may be temporarily dark or bloody.

Serum levels of PSA rise approximately tenfold following laser prostatectomy, generally peaking on the first postoperative day.[38,39] This seemingly corresponds with the height of capillary leakage and tissue edema after the laser burn injury. By 3 months, serum PSA levels have been observed to be at or below baseline in more than half of our patients. Approximately 90% have returned to or are below baseline values by 6 months. Those with significant and persistent elevations of PSA levels beyond this time probably should be evaluated for subclinical prostatic infection or occult carcinoma.

COMPLICATIONS   All reported studies have noted markedly less morbidity associated with laser prostatectomy compared with traditional surgical approaches.

Bleeding is the main complication of traditional electrocautery TURP, often necessitating transfusion and causing associated problems such as clot retention, premature termination of the procedure, and inadequate relief of obstruction.[40] Bleeding can also result in continuous catheter irrigation and complications such as stricture secondary to traction on the Foley catheter. Rarely, uncontrolled bleeding can even require open packing of the prostatic fossa. Poor visibility because of bleeding is also thought to be a cause of sphincteric damage and incontinence resulting from TURP. The incidence of hemorrhage requiring blood transfusion is 3.9% and increases twofold if the amount of resected tissue exceeds 45 mL or if the resection time is longer than 90 minutes. In contrast to transurethral electroresection, which cuts across the prostatic parenchyma and opens prostatic venous sinuses, laser prostatectomy seals blood vessels as it coagulates the transition zone and prevents both absorption of irrigating fluid and hemorrhage; the hemostasis associated with laser prostatectomy is thus superior, with multiple studies of anticoagulated patients undergoing resection demonstrating lack of bleeding complications.[46,41,42]

Irrigant fluid absorption during electrocautery TURP results in a 2% incidence of TURP syndrome because of dilutional hyponatremia, glycine-induced ammonia intoxication, or the direct toxic effect of glycine.[54] As with bleeding, fluid absorption increases with larger glands and longer resection times. Laser prostatectomy minimizes this complication, again through its sealing zone of coagulative effect on tissue, which prevents fluid absorption.

The incidence of urethral stricture after electrocautery TURP is 3.1%; if bladder neck contractures are included, this figure approaches 5%.[54] Stricture formation is thought to be secondary to trauma induced by the large size of the resectoscope as well as the use of low-intensity, coagulating current, which penetrates deeper into tissue than cutting currents. Since laser procedures do not use electrical current, the cystoscopes utilized are smaller in size, and the overall operative time is usually shorter, the incidence of stricture is lower following laser procedures.[43,44] The incidence of reoperation for residual obstructive tissue is difficult to determine since most published series of laser prostatectomy have documented initial experiences with this technology, which involves not only a learning curve factor, but also a relatively short postoperative follow-up, that is, generally a year or less.

Postoperative infections may also occur after TURP. The median incidence of urinary tract infection following TURP is 15.5%, whereas epididymitis occurs in 1.2%.[54] Urinary tract infections have been reported in 1 to 20% of patients following laser prostatectomy and epididymitis in 5 to 7% of patients.[45,46] The treatment of such infections may be more problematic in VLAP-type prostatectomies secondary to the residual necrotic prostate tissue that remains in situ for several weeks after laser coagulation. Although postoperative urinary tract infection may occur as an uncomplicated cystitis, the coagulated and necrotic prostate may also become infected. When this occurs, the most common manifestation is subacute prostatitis, characterized by significant and persistent irritative voiding symptoms, with mild prostatic and/or epididymal tenderness on examination, persistent pyuria, and positive urine cultures. Two cases of frank urosepsis have in fact been reported following laser prostatectomy, both requiring TURP to remove infected necrotic prostate tissue.[47] Aggressive antibiotic therapy is therefore warranted in these patients.

Residual necrotic prostate tissue is also responsible for the 20 to 32% incidence of postoperative urinary retention, which may last from a few days to several weeks postoperatively after VLAP treatment. This incidence far exceeds that of the 6.5% incidence of urinary retention following electrocautery TURP.[54] To overcome this problem, some investigators have resorted to the use of stents in the postoperative phase following VLAP.[48] Postoperative urinary retention, however, does not appear to be as great a problem with more recent KTP-driven PVP, where the incidence of postoperative retention was noted to be as low as 3%.[40]

Another complication unique to VLAP is the high incidence of irritative voiding symptoms during the initial few weeks following surgery, again owing to coagulated necrotic tissue that has not yet sloughed, as well as raw and unepithelialized mucosa.

The HoLEP technique is uniquely susceptible to bladder or prostatic perforations secondary to the use of tissue morcellators that cut and aspirate pieces of prostate tissue, as well as from the cutting laser technique. A bladder perforation will likely require an open cystotomy closure, often requiring moving the patient from a cystoscopy suite to an operating room.

Finally, retrograde ejaculation represents another potential side effect of electrocautery TURP, occurring in up to 90% of patients. The most recent high power (80 W) KTP laser data show that retrograde ejaculation also represents a potential problem in laser prostatectomy, with a 27% incidence of retrograde ejaculation.[40] Similarly, the incidence of impotence following electrocautery TURP ranges from 4 to 13%.[54] Such impotence is thought to be due to either (1) the diffusion of electrical current into the cavernosal nerves, which travel close to the prostatic apex or (2) interference with penile arterial flow, which occasionally depends in part on prostatic vascularity. The overall incidence of impotence following all forms of laser prostatectomy is rare. Norris and colleagues reported that of 108 patients who underwent VLAP, 56 were sexually active prior to the procedure (intercourse more than once a month) and 37 patients were sexually active postoperatively at 3 to 6 months; outcomes in the remaining 19 patients was not specified.[49] Other VLAP studies cite a 4.3 to 9.5% rate of impotence.[4,50,51] The most recent 80 W KTP in contrast data shows no loss of potency in patients treated with laser prostatectomy.[40]

CONTRAINDICATIONS   There are scenarios when laser coagulation of the prostate is not indicated, where electrocautery resection may still be advantageous. These include certain cases of bladder cancer, in which acute electrocautery resection of the bladder neck or enlarged prostate may be necessary to access tumors behind the bladder neck, especially anteriorly. Rarely, this maneuver may also be needed for ureteroscopic access. In cases in which histologic assessment of the prostate for invasion by transitional cell carcinoma is required for staging of malignancy, electrocautery resection is indicated. Finally, in the uncommon case of chronic, recurring prostatitis where electroresection of the prostate may be used to remove infected tissue and/or prostatic

calculi, laser prostatectomy cannot substitute for an aggressively performed TURP. In the rare case of a prostatic abscess that must be unroofed transurethrally, electrocautery resection is similarly indicated.

CONCLUSIONS

Laser prostatectomy has proved to be a safe and efficacious surgical intervention to relieve symptomatic bladder outlet obstruction. Overall morbidity contrasts favorably with standard surgical approaches. Moreover, laser technology is generally accessible to the practicing urologist, and the transurethral endoscopic approach and operative techniques are not complex. Collectively, these attributes have positioned laser prostatectomy as an accepted and often preferred surgical alternative for the treatment of BPH.

One should note that concerns have been raised regarding the cost effectiveness of laser prostatectomy because of the expense of the delivery systems ($50,000 to $80,000 [US] for a laser system vs $8400 [US] for electrocautery) as well as the recurring cost of laser fibers ($225 to $850 [US]).[52] Although the delivery system is expensive, it is a one-time expenditure, and the source can be used for other urologic and/or specialty applications. A recent survey found that more than 42% of urologists in the United States reported already having a laser delivery system within their medical center. With the ongoing competition among manufacturers of laser fibers, these fibers are expected to become more durable, efficient, and inexpensive. From a financial standpoint, the main advantage of laser prostatectomy lies in its ability to offer an outpatient procedure without TURP syndrome or bleeding problems. The lower incidence of other complications such as urinary retention, impotence, and incontinence will result in overall reduced costs because of lower morbidity. The ability to resect larger glands, even in patients who are anticoagulated or who possess a high burden of comorbid disease, also lends additional versatility to the procedure.

REFERENCES

1. Milam DF. Physical principles of laser energy. In: Smith JJ, Stein B, Benson RJ, editors. Physical principles of laser energy. St. Louis: Mosby; 1994. p. 1–9.
2. Childs SJ. Laser-assisted transurethral resection of the prostate (TURP). Philadelphia: Lippincott, Williams & Wilkins; 1993. p. 1–81.
3. Dixon CM, Lepor H. Laser ablation of the prostate. Semin Urol 1992;10:273–7.
4. Narayan P, Fournier G, Indudhara R, et al. Transurethral evaporation of prostate (TUEP) with Nd:YAG laser using a contact free beam technique: results in 61 patients with benign prostatic hyperplasia. Urology 1994;43:813–20.
5. Fournier G Jr, Narayan P. Factors affecting size and configuration of neodymium:YAG (Nd:YAG) laser lesions in the prostate. Lasers Surg Med 1994;14:314–22.
6. Anvari B, Rastegar S, Motamedi M. Modeling of intraluminal heating of biological tissue: implications for treatment of benign prostatic hyperplasia. IEEE Trans Biomed Eng 1994;41:854–64.
7. Watson G, Anson K, Janetschek G, et al. An in depth evaluation of contact laser vaporization of the prostate. J Urol 1994;151:231A.
8. Assimos DG, McCullough DL, Woodruff RD, et al. Canine transurethral laser-induced prostatectomy. J Endourol 1991;5:145–9.
9. Kabalin JN, Gong M, Issa MM, Sellers R. Insight into mechanism of neodymium:Yttrium-aluminum-garnet laser prostatectomy utilizing the high power contact free beam technique. Urology 1995;45:421–6.
10. Shanberg A, Lee I, Tansey L, Sawyer D. Extensive neodymium-YAG photoirradiation of the prostate in men with obstructive prostatism. Urology 1994;43:467–71.
11. Johnson DE, Cromeens DM, Price RE. Use of the holmium:YAG laser in urology. Lasers Surg Med 1992;12:353–63.
12. Kabalin JA. Holmium:YAG laser vaporization prostatectomy. J Urol 1995;153:229A.
13. Gilling P, Cass C, Malcolm A, Fraundorfer M. Combination holmium and Nd:YAG laser ablation of the prostate: initial clinical experience. J Endourol 1995;9:151–3.
14. Gilling P, Cass C, Cresswell M, et al. The use of the holmium laser in the treatment of benign prostatic hyperplasia. J Endourol 1996;10:459–61.
15. Mackey M, Chilton C, Gilling P, et al. The results of holmium laser resection of the prostate. Br J Urol 1998;81:518–9.
16. Kuntzman RS, Malek R, Barret DM, Bstowick DG. Potassium-titanyl-phosphate laser vaporization of the prostate: a comparative functional and pathologic study in canines. Urology 1996;48:575–83.
17. Kollmorgen TA, Malek RS, Barrett DM. Laser prostatectomy: two and a half years' experience with aggressive multifocal therapy. Urology 1996;48:217–22.
18. Shingleton WB, Terrell F, Renfroe DL, et al. A randomized prospective study of laser ablation of the prostate versus transurethral resection of the prostate in men with benign prostatic hyperplasia. Urology 1999;54:1017–21.
19. Carter A, Sells H, Speakman M, et al. A prospective randomized controlled trial of hybrid laser treatment or transurethral resection of the prostate, with a 1-year follow-up. BJU Int 1999;83:254–9.
20. Kuntazman RS, Malek RS, Barrett DM, Bostwick DG. High-power (60-watt) potassium-titanyl-phosphate laser vaporization prostatectomy in living canines and in human and canine cadavers. Urology 1997;49:703–8.
21. Malek RS, Barrett DM, Kuntzman RS. High power potassium-titanyl-phosphate (KTP/532) laser vaporization prostatectomy: 24 hours later. Urology 1998;51:254–6.
22. Carter A, Sells H, Speakman M, et al. A prospective randomized controlled trial of hybrid laser treatment or transurethral resection of the prostate, with a 1-year follow-up. BJU Int 1999;83:254–9.
23. Malek RS, Kuntzman RS, Barrett DM. High power potassium-titanyl-phosphate laser vaporization prostatectomy. J Urol 2000;163:1730–3.
24. Reich O, Bachmann A, Schneede P, et al. Experimental comparison of high power (80W) potassium titanyl phosphate laser vaporization and transurethral resection of the prostate. J Urol 2004;171:2502–4.
25. Hai MA, Malek RS. Photoselective vaporization of the prostate: initial experience with a new 80W KTP laser of the treatment of benign prostatic hyperplasia. J Endourol 2003;17:93–6.
26. Te A, Malloy TR, Stein BS, et al. Photoselective vaporization of the prostate for the treatment of benign prostatic hyperplasia: 12-month results from the first United States multicenter prospective trial. J Urol 2004;172:1404–8.
27. Te AE, Sandhu JS, Reddy B, et al. The first 200 patients treated with high-power KTP photoselective laser vaporization prostatectomy: the New York Presbyterian experience [abstract 1561]. AUA Annual Meeting 2005.
28. Monoski MA, Sandhu JS, Gonzalez RR, Te AE. Urodynamic predictors of success with photoselective laser vaporization prostatectomy in patients with benign prostatic hyperplasia and pre-operative retention [abstract 1305]. AUA Annual Meeting 2005.
29. Te AE, Malloy TR, Stein BS, et al. Impact of prostate-specific antigen and prostate volume as predictors of efficacy outcomes in photoselective vaporization prostatectomy (PVP): analysis and results of ongoing prospective multicenter study at 3 years [abstract 1554]. AUA Annual Meeting 2005.
30. Sandhu JS, Ng C, VanderBrink BA, et al. High power potassium-titanyl-phosphate (KTP) photoselective laser vaporization of the prostate (PVP) for the treatment of benign prostatic hyperplasia (BPH) in men with large prostates. Urology 2004;64:1155–9.
31. Sandhu JS, Te AE. Photoselective vaporization of the prostate—the vaporization incision technique for large volume prostates [abstract V1346]. AUA Annual Meeting 2005.

32. Sandhu JS, Ng CK, Gonzalez RR, et al. Photoselective laser vaporization prostatectomy in anticoagulated men. J Endourology. [Submitted]

33. Malloy TR, Sandhu JS, Smith AL, et al. Photoselective vaporization of the prostate (PVP) in anticoagulated patients: a multicenter retrospective evaluation of feasibility [abstract 1562]. AUA Annual Meeting Abstract 2005.

34. Kabalin JN, Gill HS. Urolase laser prostatectomy in patients on warfarin anticoagulation: a safe treatment alternative for bladder outlet obstruction. Urology 1993;42:738–40.

35. Bolton DM, Costello AJ. Management of benign prostatic hyperplasia by transurethral laser ablation in patients treated with warfarin anticoagulation. J Urol 1994;151: 79–81.

36. Kabalin JN. Stage A prostate cancer today. J Urol 1993;150: 1749–50.

37. Leach GE, Sirls L, Ganabathi K, et al. Outpatient visual-assisted prostatectomy under local anesthesia. Urology 1994;43:149–53.

38. Kabalin JN. Laser prostatectomy performed with a right angle firing neodymium:YAG laser fiber at 40 watts power setting. J Urol 1993;150:95–9.

39. Kabalin JN, Gill HS, Bite G. Laser prostatectomy performed with a right angle firing neodymium:YAG laser fiber at 60 watts power setting. J Urol 1995;153:1502–5.

40. Mebust WK, Holtgrewe HL, Cockett ATK, et al. Transurethral prostatectomy: immediate and postoperative complications. A cooperative study of 13 participating institutions evaluating 3,885 patients. J Urol 1989;141:243–7.

41. Kabalin JN, Gill HS. Urolase laser prostatectomy in patients on warfarin anticoagulation: a safe treatment alternative for bladder outlet obstruction. Urology 1993;42: 738–40.

42. Bolton DM, Costello AJ. Management of benign prostatic hyperplasia by transurethral laser ablation in patients treated with warfarin anticoagulation. J Urol 1994;151: 79–81.

43. Cowles RS, Kabalin JN, Childs S, et al. A prospective randomized study comparison of transurethral resection to visual laser ablation of the prostate for the treatment of benign prostatic hyperplasia. Urology 1995;46:155–60.

44. Kabalin JN, Bite G. Three-year experience with Nd:YAG laser coagulation prostatectomy in 225 patients. J Urol 1995;153:229A.

45. McCullough DL, Roth RA, Babayan RK, et al. Transurethral ultrasound-guided laser-induced prostatectomy: National Human Cooperative Study results. J Urol 1993;150: 1607–11.

46. Narayan P, Tewari A, Fournier G, Toke A. Impact of prostate size on the outcome of transurethral laser evaporation of the prostate for benign prostatic hyperplasia. Urology 1995;45:776–82.

47. Haupt G, Herde T, Senge T. Visual laser ablation for benign prostatic hyperplasia. J Endourol 1993;7:S127.

48. Petas A, Talja M, Tammela T, et al. Bioresorbable PGA-urospiral preventing urinary retention in VLAP. J Urol 1995;153:534A.

49. Norris JP, Norris DM, Lee RD, Rubenstein MA. Visual laser ablation of the prostate: clinical experience in 108 patients. J Urol 1993;150:1612–4.

50. Dixon C, Machi G, Theune C, et al. A prospective double-blind, randomized study comparing the safety, efficacy and cost of laser ablation of the prostate and transurethral prostatectomy for the treatment of BPH. J Urol 1994;151:229A.

51. Dixon CM. Right-angle free beam lasers for the treatment of benign prostatic hyperplasia. Semin Urol 1994;12:165–9.

52. Perlmutter AP, Muschter R. The optimization of laser prostatectomy. Part I: Free beam side fire coagulation. Urology 1994;44:847–55.

Interstitial Laser Therapy

Rolf Muschter, MD, PhD

Interstitial laser therapy of the prostate—also named interstitial laser coagulation (ILC) or laser-induced interstitial thermotherapy (LITT)—was originally developed to generate coagulation necrosis of a large volume *inside* the adenomatous tissue of the prostate without damaging the urethra and the internal sphincter to achieve a physiologic volume reduction of the obstructive prostate tissue by secondary atrophy rather than by tissue sloughing. After some years of clinical experience and growing knowledge on ILC and related techniques, such as transurethral needle ablation (TUNA), it became obvious that laser energy, which is administered to tissues by placing a laser radiation applicator inside ("interstitial" laser application), can achieve different quantitative and qualitative effects, and in the case of treating benign prostatic hyperplasia (BPH), different clinical effects might occur.[89] These depend not only on the type of laser source, laser applicator, and irradiation parameters, but also, and in particular, on the "treatment scheme" (eg, number of applicator placements) the surgeon is following. ILC is surgeon-dependent. Therefore, interstitial laser therapy can be performed as a procedure in which a large tissue volume is coagulated with or without preserving the urethra, resulting in a significant volume reduction of the prostate. It can also be performed, however, by use of the same laser, applicator, and irradiation parameters, with the result of a low-volume coagulation. If the first type of interstitial laser therapy, "high-volume" interstitial laser coagulation (HV-ILC), is performed, the surgeon might achieve a clinical effect comparable to transurethral resection of the prostate (TURP); in the latter case, "low-volume" interstitial laser coagulation (LV-ILC), or LITT, clinical effects that might occur are probably not related to a relevant volume reduction or tissue ablation, respectively. Unfortunately, the literature published to date does not discriminate between HV-ILC and LV-ILC, nor does it mention that ILC is a procedure for which clinical outcome depends highly on the surgeon. The terminology used in the past does not even reflect these differences.

If laser energy is administered by irradiating an outer or inner surface, for example, in transurethral free-beam laser application such as visual laser ablation of the prostate (VLAP), the amount of tissue that can be necrotized is limited by two factors: the relatively shallow penetration depth of laser radiation, and the limited size of the organ surface that is accessible.[1-3] By contrast, in interstitial laser irradiation the applicator can be inserted as deep and as often as necessary to the desired region to coagulate any amount of tissue.

INDICATIONS

Patients selected for interstitial laser therapy have moderate to severe lower urinary tract symptoms (LUTS) and mild to moderate, or in HV-ILC, even severe bladder outlet obstruction (BOO) related to BPH, with moderate to pronounced benign prostatic enlargement (BPE), and would otherwise be candidates for surgical intervention, either transurethral or open, or other minimally invasive procedures. In principle, there is no limit to the prostate volume that can be treated by this approach; even large middle lobes can be treated (Table 70B-1).[91]

Concomitant diseases, such as strictures of the urethra or bladder calculi, can be treated in the same session.

Patients with chronic urinary retention or with poor detrusor function will need to have a catheter in place for a longer period after the procedure because of the time required for the prostate to shrink sufficiently to clear the obstruction. Of course, longer catheterization is necessary in any type of treatment in which there is no immediate tissue removal.

Virtually no intraoperative morbidity is associated with interstitial laser therapy, and in principle it can be performed with the patient under local anesthesia (as far as it seems acceptable to perform a cystoscopy with minor transurethral manipulation under local anesthesia). Thus, even high-risk patients who would not be candidates for transurethral resection need not be excluded from this treatment modality. Recurrent or residual BPH after previous prostate surgery, laser treatment, or microwave treatment can also be treated by interstitial laser coagulation.

Although interstitial laser coagulation alone is a sufficient treatment, in smaller prostates with median bar obstruction, an additional incision of the bladder neck may be useful.[4] This can be done in the 5- and 7-o'clock or in the 6-o'clock positions using either a Collings knife or a bare laser fiber. Other combination treatments such as interstitial laser coagulation of the side lobes plus subtotal transurethral resection (eg, of the median lobe) may be beneficial for selected patients to shorten postprocedure catheter time. An interesting concept might also be the combination of ILC and TURP in such manner that ILC is performed just before standard TURP in order to improve hemostasis. In recent times, some authors have used ILC as a separate procedure sometime before TURP for the same reason. The combination of simultaneous interstitial laser therapy and visual laser ablation of the prostate might increase the efficacy of each procedure,[5] but so far no major series have been published on the subject. Combination of ILC with temporary stents was often discussed, but so far only limited experiences were reported.

Antegrade ejaculation was preserved in approximately 80% of the patients who underwent the laser procedure.[8-12] This represents a significant improvement over TURP, but the risk of retrograde ejaculation occurring after interstitial laser therapy cannot be eliminated completely.

Interstitial laser therapy should therefore be the choice for high-risk patients who need surgical intervention and for patients who require surgical treatment but in whom it is essential to minimize surgical risks. Patients desiring rapid symptom relief after treatment should be excluded from laser coagulation therapy and preferably treated with TURP.

Patients whose primary concern is normal ejaculation should be treated medically. If surgery for them is unavoidable, interstitial laser therapy is the treatment of choice, and there is a very fair chance of preserving ejaculation. The surgeon can increase this chance by not treating the bladder neck; however, the consequence is the risk of a suboptimal result in correction of voiding symptoms. In any case, the patient should be advised that the loss of prograde ejaculation is a possible side effect of interstitial laser therapy.

Patients with obstructive symptoms from carcinoma of the prostate are also candidates for interstitial laser therapy.[13,14] Indications are the

Table 70B-1 Indications and Contraindications for Interstitial Laser Therapy
Indications
BPH of any degree that would require surgical intervention Any gland size and configuration Normal and high-risk patients
Contraindications
Curable prostate cancer Bladder cancer at the bladder outlet or infiltrating the prostate Active uriniary tract infection, acute epididymitis, prostatitis, or prostate abscess
BPH = bengn prostatic lyperplasia.

same as those for a palliative transurethral resection to treat bladder outlet obstruction, such as locally advanced disease. Interstitial laser therapy is definitely not an alternative to radical prostatectomy or curative radiotherapy or any other treatment with curative intent.

Patients with symptomatic BPH who are suspected of having prostate cancer because of their elevated serum prostate-specific antigen (PSA) level, but who are not candidates for curative treatment, can be treated with interstitial laser coagulation, but should have a biopsy of the prostate immediately after treatment during the same session. If curative therapy is possible, a screening biopsy should be performed and evaluated before laser treatment. If biopsy results are positive, the patient should not receive interstitial laser therapy.

Patients who have bladder cancer close to or at the bladder neck or in whom invasion of the prostate is uncertain should not receive interstitial laser therapy. The procedure is also contraindicated in cases of acute prostatitis or epididymitis and when there is an abscess of the prostate. Chronic prostatitis, however, which is frequently present in BPH patients, is not a contraindication to interstitial laser therapy.

PATIENT PREPARATION

As in most minimally invasive modalities for the treatment of BPH, in interstitial laser therapy no tissue is sampled for pathologic examination. Therefore, a digital rectal examination and serum PSA level evaluation are essential. If either of these is suspicious of cancer, a transrectal ultrasound examination and a screening biopsy should be performed before or after interstitial laser therapy, depending on the patient's age and physiologic status and the potential treatment consequences.

A patient with an active urinary tract infection must be treated with appropriate antibiotics before interstitial laser therapy. Patients with acute epididymitis or acute prostatitis should not undergo interstitial laser therapy until they have completely recovered from these conditions. If there is significant residual urine volume or if the patient has chronic or acute retention, a suprapubic or Foley catheter should be inserted and left in place after treatment until voiding is sufficient. Routine perioperative antibiotic prophylaxis is recommended[9] to produce sterile urine preoperatively, particularly if a prostate biopsy is to be performed transrectally at the time of laser therapy.

As in any other BPH treatment, the success of interstitial laser treatment should be monitored during follow-up. Therefore, the patient's AUA symptom score, urinary flow rate, residual urine volume, and prostate volume should be measured before treatment. Additional urodynamic measures (pressure-flow studies) are helpful for assessing the decrease in obstruction after laser therapy.

The common diagnostic procedures usually required for TURP are sufficient for interstitial laser therapy. Special radiologic or endoscopic examinations are not necessary. In general, it is recommended to follow the specific guidelines for the diagnosis of BPH or BPS (benign prostatic hyperplasia syndrome), respectively.

As for other procedures, informed consent should include information about the different treatment options, including transurethral resection, and the specific advantages, disadvantages, risks, and potential complications of each method. Patients should be informed that surgical risks such as significant bleeding or TURP syndrome are rare or nonexistent. The chance of the patient's retaining normal sexual function is approximately 80%. The patient should be aware that the failure rate for this procedure is about 10 to 15% within 1 year (for an unselected group of patients), and that postprocedure catheterization will be necessary for some time. The patient should know that only few studies on long-term results are published, showing approximately 70% durable success for up to 9 years.

Published reports of the complications associated with interstitial laser therapy and their incidence include complicated urinary tract infection with fever or epididymitis or prostatitis (0.5%), transient stress incontinence (0.1%), urgency, and strictures of the urethra or bladder neck (2–5%), including recurrences of preexisting, simultaneously treated strictures.[6–11] More frequent are uncomplicated urinary tract infections in about 10 to 35% of patients and transient irritative symptoms in 9 to 15%; tissue sloughing also has been noted. Permanent incontinence has never been reported, but should not be excluded from the list of potential risks.

Some risks can only be theorized, such as coagulation of the rectum with consequent fistulas, damage to the neurovascular bundle, and fiber breakage during irradiation that produces fiber fragments that must be removed by electroresection. With correct application techniques and equipment, these risks can be avoided. The incidence of these risks, however, was never reported.

PREOPERATIVE PREPARATION

Interstitial laser therapy can be performed with a local, regional, or systemic anesthetic.[134] If local anesthesia is chosen, such as by transperineal injection of lidocaine to achieve a blockade of the prostate and pudendal nerves, overfilling of the bladder, which could cause discomfort, should be avoided. Although no permanent irrigation is necessary during this procedure, a suprapubic catheter can be useful.

After adequate anesthesia is induced, the patient is put in the dorsal lithotomy position. Routine disinfection and an inflammable drape, as generally required for any laser surgery, should be used. If not previously done, a routine urethrocystoscopy is performed. A video camera and monitor are useful but not required. All general laser safety measures (eg, warning signs and signals and wavelength-specific eye protection) must be observed before, during, and after interstitial laser therapy.

Interstitial laser applicators can be placed using several different approaches.[11,15] In practice, endoscopically controlled transurethral placement has proved most useful. The percutaneous placement from the perineum guided by transrectal ultrasound was not used in the recent series.

INSTRUMENTATION

Several laser wavelengths have been studied for use in interstitial laser therapy[6,16–18]; published reports have demonstrated that 800 to 1,100 nm wavelengths offer relatively deep penetration depths in water and efficient volumetric heating, which permits delivering necrotic temperatures deep into tissues (Table 70B-2). These wavelengths can be delivered by flexible optical fibers; consequently, Nd:YAG lasers (1,064 nm) were first used for interstitial laser therapy.[19–24] Recent experiments have shown that diode lasers emitting at approximately 805, 830, 940, 980, and 1000 nm, and even the Ho:YAG laser (2,100 nm), are also suitable for generating large interstitial coagulation volumes.[6,16–18,96,102,131,135] Clinical trials using these diode lasers and the Ho:YAG laser are still ongoing.[6,16]

Bare fibers—as used by Littrup and colleagues[25,26] and McNicholas and colleagues[27] in animal experiments to evaluate interstitial laser therapy for prostate cancer and later by McNicholas and colleagues[15,28–31] for BPH treatment—emit all laser energy from a very small area (0.3 mm² with a 600 μm fiber). Even with low laser power, high-power densities are achieved (330 watts/cm² with 1 watt), leading to immediate carbonization and vaporization. Experiments have demonstrated that interstitial irradiation with a bare fiber at up to a 20-watt power setting produces only a small spherical lesion of 5 to 10 mm total diameter, consisting of a central cavity filled with debris and adjacent char and a small coagulated rim.[15,20,22–24,32–37] For LV-ILC this might be sufficient. To achieve HV-ILC, a very high number of applications is required.

To avoid charring and to achieve large-volume coagulation, the power density of an interstitial applicator must be much lower (5–10 watts/cm²).[24,38] Since Bown[39] first discussed interstitial laser therapy for cancer treatment in 1983, several types of applicators with larger irradiating surfaces have been used in lab-

Table 70B-2 Instruments for Interstitial Laser Therapy

Transurethral Approach
Any cystoscope; integrated cystoscope described by Miller[57] is recommended
No auxiliary instruments required
No continuous irrigation required

Perineal Approach
Transrectal ultrasound scanner with aiming grid
Trocar cannula
Cystoscope not required

oratory or clinical experiments,[35,40–47] but these have produced similarly unimpressive results.

Interstitial laser therapy for BPH was a completely new concept first described by Hofstetter and Muschter and colleagues.[19–21,23] New types of applicators were specially designed (Figure 70B-1). Two technical principles have been elucidated to extend the emitting surface.[38,48] One solution is a diffusor tip that emits the radiation circumferentially and randomly in all directions in a more or less even pattern along the entire length of the applicator.[48] Another solution is a system emitting the laser radiation circumferentially in a forward direction (with a ring- or cone-shaped beam profile at an angle of approximately 45 degrees in water, Figure 70B-2). This is achieved by eliminating the transversal modes of the laser beam.[38] In tissue, by light reflection and predominantly scattering, the latter type of applicator almost acts like a diffusor tip, too. Both types of applicators create rather homogeneous coagulation zones around the emitting tip. These increase in size by conduction of heat to the periphery. Their final shape is ovoid, ellipsoid, or spherical[2,16,17,20,24] (Figure 70B-3). Lesion length depends on the emitting length of the applicator; the radius of the lesion can be up to 1 cm (ie, up to diameter 2 cm), depending on laser wavelength, laser power, and radiation time (in vivo maximal single lesion volume approximately 4–10 cm[3]).[2,20,24,49–54]

Interstitial applicators consist of an emitter (eg, transparent quartz glass cylinder or teflon coating) affixed to the distal end of a flexible 600 µm quartz glass fiber, in some types with specific cut of the tip. Different dimensions have been tested; for routine use in the prostate, an emitter length of 2 cm and a diameter of approximately 2 mm were found to be the best compromise based on the technical requirements (large radiating surface) and the surgical requirements (small size for simple handling). For ease in placement, the tip of the applicator is exaggerated.[20] The actual design of the interstitial applicators may vary among manufacturers.[55,56]

The goal of interstitial laser therapy is to achieve a relevant coagulation volume in the shortest time. Although this can be achieved with multiple (successive or simultaneous) applicator placements, each single treatment volume should be large. Therefore, radiation parameters must be chosen to fulfill this requirement.[115] Optimal parameters vary for different laser wavelength and applicator combinations.[2,6,16–18]

Using constant laser power in the range from 5 to 7 watts, the maximum coagulation volume can be expected within approximately 10 minutes of irradiation time without the risk of carbonization.[20,21,23,24] Some laser/applicator combinations may be operated with a constant power of up to 10 watts for 10 minutes.

More rapid heating by using higher laser power would reduce irradiation time but increase the risk of carbonization or even make carbonization a certainty by using a power density above the carbonization threshold. For short irradiation times, however, high powers are tolerable. Therefore various power formatting programs were designed and tested to achieve the maximum coagulation volume within the minimum total irradiation time[2,16–18] (Table 70B-3). In this type of laser energy application, irradiation starts with a relatively high power that is reduced by repeated steps or continuously to maintain the temperature in the center of the lesion at the highest level just below the carbonization threshold. This allows further energy influx to increase the size of the lesion, and this power is maintained until a temperature balance is reached in the periphery[2] (Figure 70B-4).

A feedback system further optimizes energy application; in such a system the actual emitted laser power depends on the temperature generated and measured at the applicator (Indigo 830e, Johnson & Johnson). Different optical feedback devices are also available for detecting carbonization that occurs at the applicator, thereby preventing thermal damage of fibers by automatically terminating laser irradiation.

The Ho:YAG laser can also be used in combination with an applicator specifically designed for interstitial laser therapy (Auriga, Wavelight, Starnberg, Germany). Experiments demonstrated that lesion volumes eqivalent to those achieved by the Nd:YAG or diode lasers could be generated by use of high pulse energies and relatively long pulse durations. Sufficiently large lesions were achieved in relatively short application times (10 seconds to 1 minute). Depending on the pulse frequency, the average laser power can be calculated. Interstitial lesions generated with the Ho:YAG laser consist of a central cavity and adjacent zone of coagulation.

To achieve large lesions inside the prostate lobes, the laser applicator needs to be placed deep inside. The ideal angle would be perpendicular, however, in transurethral placement the applicator comes in at a rather tangential angle. Because the laser fiber is flexible with a rigid or fragile tip, if not properly guided, the fiber might slide along the surface, bend, and even break. Transurethral interstitial laser therapy requires a rigid scope with a working channel large enough to accommodate the fiber, usually between 5 and 7F. The viewing angle of the scope can range from 0 to 30 degrees. An ideal instrument has a small separate working channel that ends at the level of the telescope for optimal stabilization of the fiber during puncture, such as the atraumatic urethrocystoscope described by Miller and colleagues[57] or the Gilling laser resectoscope. If a standard cystoscope with the usual "half-pipe" sheath tip is used, rotation might improve fiber placement.[113]

Continuous irrigation is not required throughout the procedure. While placing the applicator, irrigation will optimize visualization of the prostate and laser fiber. Any sterile irrigation fluid can be used, such as saline solution or water. Auxiliary instruments for placing the fibers are not necessary. Any type of urinary catheter can be used for bladder drainage.

For percutaneous (perineal) interstitial laser therapy, a transrectal ultrasound scanner is helpful, preferably one with an aiming device (eg, template) as is used for the perineal placement of

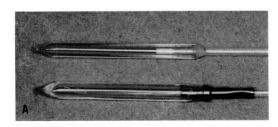
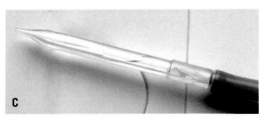
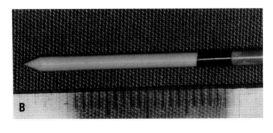
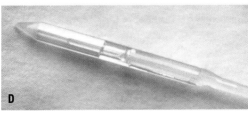

Figure 70B-1 *A,* Interstitial applicator for Nd:YAG laser. Top: Applicator with cone-shaped beam pattern (ITT light guide). Bottom: Applicator with diffuse beam pattern. *B,* Interstitial applicator for 830 nm diode laser with diffuse beam pattern (diffuser tip). *C,* Interstitial applicator for 940 nm diode laser (ITT light guide) with cone-shaped beam pattern. *D,* Interstitial applicator for Auriga Ho:YAG laser with wide-angled cone-shaped beam pattern mounted to a low-OH quartz-glass fiber.

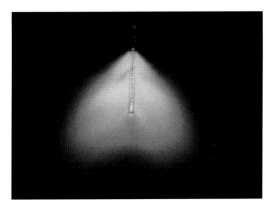

Figure 70B-2 Beam pattern of ITT light guide in water.

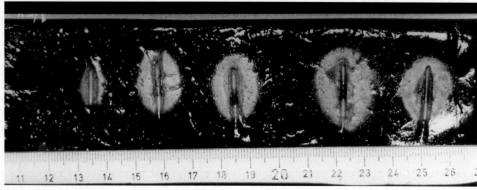

Figure 70B-3 Lesions induced by interstitial laser coagulation in vitro (in porcine liver with an Nd:YAG laser and ITT light guide) showing the results of different irradiation parameters.

seeds for local radiation therapy of prostate cancer.[138] For penetrating the skin and guiding the fiber into position into the prostate, a special cannula large enough to accommodate the applicator is used. With an outer diameter of approximately 2.1 mm and a sharpened tip, this cannula can be inserted without dilation.[8,9,11,24]

OPERATIVE STEPS

TRANSURETHRAL APPROACH

1. Administer local anesthetic or initiate spinal or general anesthesia.
2. Prepare the operative field and instruments.
3. Instill lubricant gel into the urethra, connect the cystoscope to a light source and an irrigation container, and attach a video camera to the scope if appropriate. Insert and advance the cystoscope under direct vision into the bladder.
4. Fill the bladder and place a suprapubic catheter if appropriate.
5. Empty the bladder.
6. Attach the laser fiber connector to the laser aperture.
7. Activate the laser unit and set in the standby mode.
8. Insert the applicator into the cystoscope's working channel and advance until it is visible.
9. Retract the cystoscope and fiber together back into the prostatic urethra (wide-angle view).
10. Choose a treatment point and advance the fiber to just contact, but not penetrate the urethra. Hold the cystoscope's tip close to the treatment point and advance the cystoscope if necessary (almost to or to tissue contact).
11. Tilt the cystoscope laterally in the desired angle from the center axis of the urethra. In the sagittal plane, keep the cystoscope aligned in the direction of the urethra or, in voluminous lobes, angle it ventrally or moderately dorsally (Figure 70B-5A).
12. Advance the fiber to puncture the urethra (Figure 70B-5B). Observing the applicator's proximal end or fiber depth marker, insert the applicator completely or further to the desired depth (Figures 70B-6a, b, and c).
13. Activate the laser beam for the prescribed treatment duration.
14. Put the laser in the standby mode. Retract the applicator into the cystoscope.
15. Repeat steps 10 through 14 at additional sites within the same and other prostate lobes until the desired volume of tissue has been treated (see Figures 70B-6a, b, and c). The order of punctures should follow a scheme.
16. Inactivate the laser unit and remove all instruments.
17. Place a transurethral catheter if appropriate.

PERINEAL APPROACH

1. Administer local anesthetic or initiate spinal or general anesthesia.
2. Prepare the operative field and instruments.
3. If necessary, perform a urethrocystoscopy. Place a suprapubic or transurethral catheter.
4. Insert the transrectal ultrasound scanner and scan the prostate. Attach the aiming device (template).
5. Attach the laser fiber connector to the laser aperture.
6. Activate the laser unit and set in the standby mode.
7. Choose a treatment point, insert the trocar cannula, and advance it to the desired depth and location under ultrasound guidance (Figure 70B-7).
8. Remove the trocar, insert the applicator into the cannula, and retract the cannula.
9. Activate the laser beam for the prescribed treatment duration.

10. Put the laser in the standby mode; remove the applicator.
11. Repeat steps 7 through 10 at additional sites within the same and other prostate lobes until the desired volume of tissue has been treated.
12. Inactivate the laser unit and remove all instruments.

TECHNIQUE

The goal of HV-ILC is to necrotize a large volume in each lateral lobe and the median lobe (if needed) to produce therapeutic results while preserving healthy tissues (Figure 70B-8).[90,130] The total number of fiber placements is dictated by the total prostate volume and configuration and finally dependent on the discretion of the surgeon. Any number of placements can be used. Generally it is better to treat one extra site than one too few, because some overlapping of the lesions needs to be taken into account. A general guideline would be one to three applicator placements for each estimated 5 to 10 cm^3 of BPH tissue. Individual placements (in the tissue, not points of puncture) of the laser fiber should be spaced by about 0.5 to 1 cm and at different angles (Figure 70B-9) to minimize substantial overlap of treatment volumes (which is not harmful but wastes time), but close enough so there are no gaps of untreated tissue. The points where the fibers are inserted can be close to each other.

Although the final result of a successful HV-ILC regarding prostate volume reduction and decrease of BOO could be compared with TURP, LV-ILC is comparable with transurethral needle ablation (TUNA) or transurethral microwave thermotherapy (TUMT). The treatment effect of LV-ILC is predominantly symptomatic improvement and probably not related to volume reduction, but to potential destruction of afferent nerves, although this is not based on experimental data. The goal of LV-ILC is to generate symptomatic improvement in mildly obstructed patients with no or little unwanted side effects, such as the requirement of other than local anesthesia and the need for prolonged catheterization. The application technique is identical to HV-ILC with fewer numbers of fiber placements and/or different laser parameters (eg, lower laser power, shorter irradiation time).

Table 70B-3 Power Formatting Programs

Laser/Applicator	Power (W)	Time (sec)	Total Irradiation Time (min)	Total Energy (J)
Nd:YAG with ITT light guide	20	30	3	1,980
	15	30	–	–
	10	30	–	–
	7	90	–	–
Nd:YAG with ITT fiber (2 cm diffuser)	10	60	5	1,920
	7	60	–	–
	5	180	–	–
Diode 830 nm with diffuser tip	10	30	4	1,460
	7.4	30	–	–
	7.4–5	30	–	–
	5	150	–	–
Diode 940 nm with ITT light guide	50–9	–	1.5	–

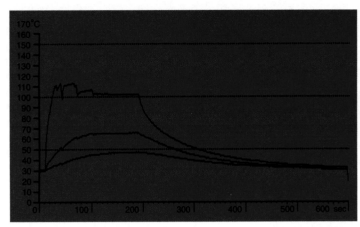

Figure 70B-4 Temperature profile for in vivo laser-treated canine prostate (Nd:YAG laser, ITT light guide, formatted laser power of 20/15/10/7 watts, 3-minute irradiation time). Top: Temperature at 4 nm distance from the applicator; middle: temperature at 8 nm; bottom: temperature at 12 nm.

Fiber placement is basically limited by proximity of the produced treatment volume to the (1) prostatic urethra, (2) prostatic capsule, and (3) points along the prostatic urethra distal to the bladder neck and proximal to the external sphincter. With the ultrasound-guided perineal approach, this can easily be achieved by measuring and keeping the distance between the applicator and the urethra or the capsule on all sides at approximately 1 cm (the expected radius of coagulation). Likewise, staying within the limits with the transurethral approach is not difficult.

In general, the sites for fiber placement should be chosen where the mass or bulk of hyperplastic tissue is found. In the sagittal plane,

fiber penetration should be in the direction of the urethra. With the patient in the lithotomy position, the direction of the prostatic urethra in most cases is approximately parallel to the operating table at the apex, turning anteriorly near the bladder. Therefore, in the apical zone it is best to puncture the lateral lobes at the 3- and 9-o'clock positions and penetrate parallel to the operating

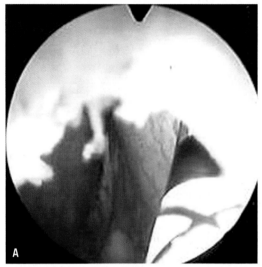

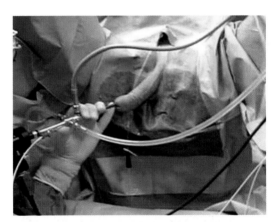

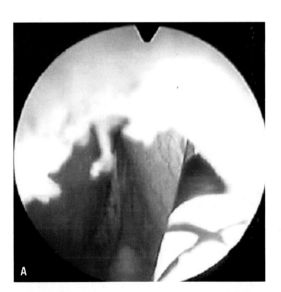

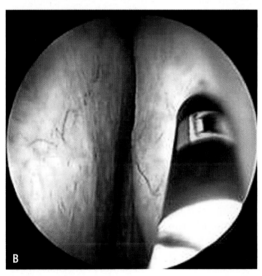

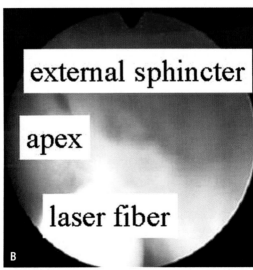

Figure 70B-5 *A*, Cystoscope angled for puncture of the anterior part of apex of left lobe. *B*, Corresponding endoscopic view (laser fiber is in tissue contact).

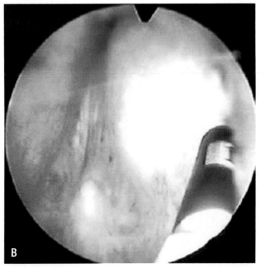

Figure 70B-6a Endoscopic view, *A*, anterior and *B*, posterior placement of laser fiber, apex left lobe.

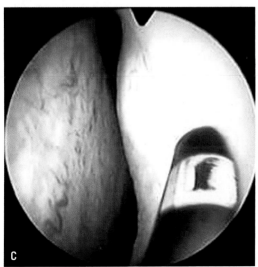

Figure 70B-6b Endoscopic view, anterior placements of laser fiber: left lobe, *A*, apex; *B*, center-part; *C*, base.

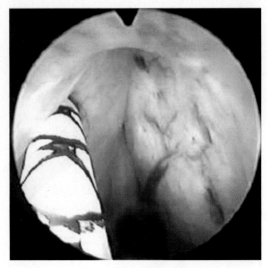

Figure 70B-6c Endoscopic view, anterior placement of laser fiber apex right lobe, after treatment of left lobe (points of puncture circled, apex and base anterior and posterior).

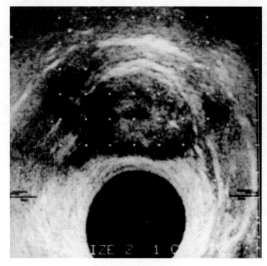

Figure 70B-7 Transrectal ultrasound image of the prostate with the laser fiber placed in the left lateral lobe.

table. When closer to the bladder neck, it is suitable to penetrate more anteriorly at the 10- and 2-o'clock positions. In larger prostates, multiple punctures at different fan-shaped angles are required (Figure 70B-10). If present, anterior tissue can also be treated.

It could be important to preserve the urethra to minimize symptoms following the procedure. If the urethra is accidentally necrotized, however, ordinary tissue sloughing may occur and is not harmful (the treatment effect is then much like that of deep transurethral free-beam coagulation).[8–11] Avoiding damage to the urethra requires both a minimum depth and angle of fiber penetration. The applicator should be inserted to a depth of at least 0.5 cm beyond the irradiating part. In most types of applicators this corresponds to their proximal end (see Figure 70B-1A, C, and D) and in others to a fiber depth marker (see Figure 70B-1B). The fiber penetration angle in relation to the longitudinal axis of the urethra should be the maximum achievable; in the apical zone this is approximately 45 degrees. Closer to the bladder neck it is often less (20 degrees in big prostates) because of the convex shape of the lobe (see Figure 70B-8C). For effective treatment of this part of the lobe it is also possible to insert the fiber at a point closer to the apex at a lower angle and then carefully penetrate deeper toward the

bladder neck (Figure 70B-11).

Coagulating the prostate capsule is unnecessary and should be avoided. In practice, fiber penetration to the lateral or anterior parts of the capsule is almost impossible because of the limited penetration angle and depth achievable, but is probably not harmful or of clinical significance if it should occur. In addition, the highly vascular nature of the prostate capsule acts as a heat sink and contributes to preventing potential coagulation of the capsule itself and adjacent structures. However, for maximum safety one should always avoid advancing the applicator dorsally (see Figure 70B-10) because there is little or no BPH tissue to treat, and yet there is a potential risk of affecting structures adjacent to the prostate (eg, neurovascular bundles and rectum) or inducing subtrigonal lesions with subsequent (relative) bladder neck strictures.

All puncture points must be within the length of the prostatic urethra between the external sphincter and the bladder neck. The puncture point closest to the bladder neck should be no closer than 1.5 cm from the bladder neck so that it will not penetrate the bladder. Accidental penetration of the applicator through the prostate into the bladder can be detected by feeling resistance to fiber penetration. If the laser is activated and the bladder is full, there is no effect because of light diffusion and low laser power. If the bladder is

empty and the fiber is in contact with the bladder wall, there is a chance of coagulating the bladder wall, which can be, but is not necessarily, a problem. If fiber penetration occurs, the fiber can simply be pulled back into the prostate and that site can be treated. The most apical puncture point should be in the prostatic urethra just in front of the proximal end of the external sphincter (see Figure 70B-6) so that no apical tissue goes untreated. As discussed earlier, care must be taken to insert the applicators to the required depth.

When the median lobe is being treated, the fiber should be advanced in the direction of the bladder (Figures 70B-12 and 70B-13) to prevent subtrigonal penetration. A large median lobe should be treated with more than one puncture. Depending on its size and shape, punctures can be made at different levels and angles. When puncturing the median lobe, pressure from the fiber can push the lobe before the fiber penetrates, resulting in tangential placement of the fiber. This can be avoided by directing the fiber somewhat dorsally. For the effective treatment of a median lobe, several fiber placements are necessary because of the great surface area with consequent cooling by the fluid in the bladder.

Adopting an order scheme for punctures can be helpful. There can be any starting point: bladder neck, apex, median lobe, or lateral lobe. If the first lesion is produced in the apex, the prostate becomes a little harder in that area because of coagulation. This firmness facilitates subsequent penetrations toward the bladder neck, which is a bit more difficult to reach because of the limited space in the prostatic urethra.

While laser energy is being delivered into the prostate tissue through the applicator, it is better to stabilize the fiber and cystoscope by holding them manually rather than mechanically anchoring them (eg, with a tripod). If a mechanical anchor is used, patient motion could pull the fiber out of the prostate.

Bleeding at a treatment site is usually slight or nil. Irrigation keeps the field clear. Deep punctures might bleed after the fiber is withdrawn because not all of the puncture channel is coagulated. Typically, all bleeding stops in a short time, and cautery is usually not required.

If a laser feedback system is used and detects carbonization during treatment, it will terminate irradiation at that treatment site. The applicator

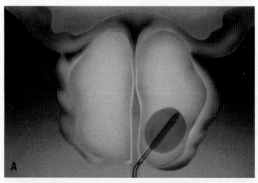

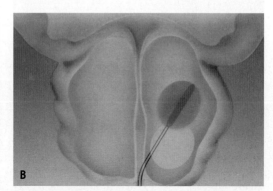

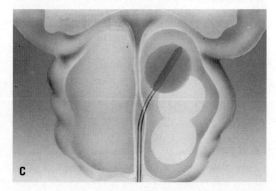

Figure 70B-8 Scheme of repeated applicator placements at the apex (A), center (B), and base (C) of the left lateral lobe.

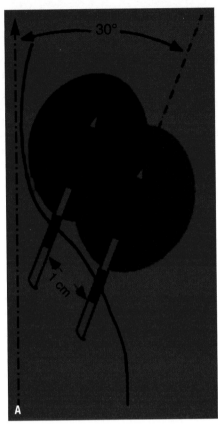
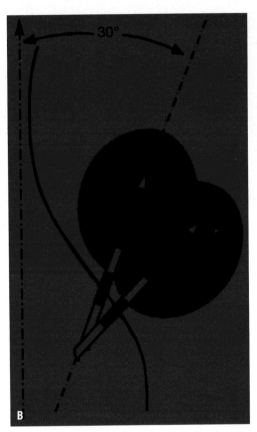

Figure 70B-9 Scheme of applicator placements at 1 cm spacing with the same angle (A), and at the same puncture point with different angles (B).

should be withdrawn and inspected. Usually it can be cleaned and used for subsequent treatment sites. Burned fibers should not be used anymore because fiber damage increases rapidly with subsequent use. Resumption of treatment with either the same or a new fiber should always proceed at a new puncture spot.

Other approaches than that described are the transrectal[11,15,58] and the laparoscopic/pelvioscopic[11] approach. The transrectal approach has no advantages over the perineal approach but entails such risks as infection or bowel injury,[15] so the latter approach might be suitable for the treatment of cancer but seems to be too aggressive for BPH.

Online treatment control is possible with the use of MRI,[59] as shown by several authors treating malignancies with interstitial laser therapy[53,54,60–63] and BPH.[121–123,127] In the treatment of cancer, it is critical to leave malignant tissue untreated, and therefore online treatment control is required; in BPH treatment, however, this would be too costly and is not necessary. Transrectal ultrasound is not suitable for online control because changes are detectable only when tissue is carbonized or vaporized.[21,23,25,58,64,65] Multichannel rectal temperature monitoring can be performed for additional safety; direct temperature measurements in several patients in the tissue, prostate capsule, and rectum[8–11,24] proved that (1)

the desired temperatures with temporal and spatial distributions, as expected based on animal experiments,[2,3,20] were achieved in the treatment volume, and (2) that no critical increases in temperatures were detectable in the capsule or surrounding organs, in particular the rectum.[24] Computerized calculations or simulations of the temporal and spatial temperature profiles[66,67] provide no additional information and are not required for monitoring interstitial laser therapy of BPH.

Animal experiments demonstrated that the combination of a systemically administered photosensitive drug and laser therapy using a specific laser wavelength and a nonthermal energy range (photodynamic therapy [PDT]) could be useful for treating BPH.[68] Early trials with interstitial PDT using different photosensitive agents were undertaken some years ago to treat prostate cancer.[69,70] Although no major breakthrough was achieved, the concept seems promising, but requires further investigation.

POSTOPERATIVE CARE

Following interstitial laser therapy, a catheter (either a 10–14F suprapubic catheter or a 14–20F urethral catheter) is left in place to provide urinary drainage. Since bleeding seldom occurs, bladder irrigation is usually not required, but can be useful in individual cases for a few hours to prevent clot retention.

Heuck and Mueller-Lisse and colleagues[51,52,121–124] report that postprocedure

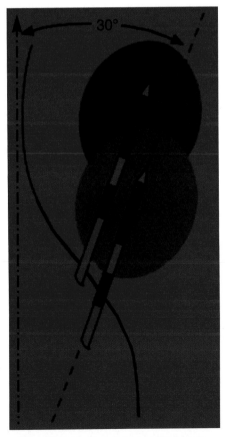

Figure 70B-11 Alternative applicator placement for treating the central or basal parts of a lateral lobe (compare with Figure 70B-9A).

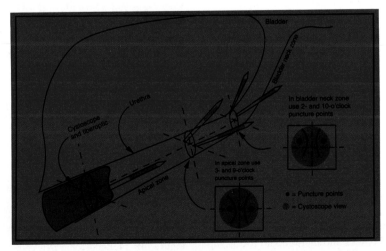

Figure 70B-10 Applicator penetration orientations along the prostate urethra.

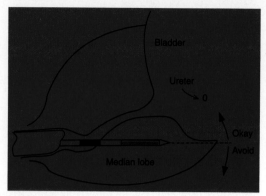

Figure 70B-12 Sagittal view of the applicator penetration orientation.

MRI demonstrates a marked increase in prostate volume, returning to the preprocedure value within about 5 to 7 days. In addition, because of the coagulation, the consistency of the prostate tissue becomes firmer, thus usually resulting in a temporary increase in the degree of obstruction. Consequently, voiding function and obstructive symptoms usually become temporarily worse, somewhat correlating with the coagulation volume. Therefore, the majority of patients require urinary drainage for a few days. Patients with moderate to good detrusor function are able to compensate the acutely increased obstruction. In this group the catheter can be removed early. Patients with chronic retention or with poor or decompensated detrusor function, however, will require the catheter for a longer time. In principle this is not specific to interstitial laser therapy, but applies to all procedures without substantial immediate tissue removal. The need for and duration of catheterization is different in HV- and LV-ILC.

If a transurethral catheter is used, it should be taken out after 1 to 7 days. Patients who fail to void should be catheterized for another few days. If a suprapubic catheter is used, it is usually clamped on the first day. Continuous voiding training can be done during the day with regular control of the residual urine volume, while at night sufficient drainage can be achieved. If voiding function becomes satisfactory, the suprapubic catheter should be removed. This can be expected within 1 week for most patients.

During the weeks following high-volume interstitial laser therapy a continuous volume reduction of the prostate is observed with shrinking of the coagulated lesions.[8-11,20,24] Only small residues are detectable after 6 weeks and vanish completely within another 4 to 6 weeks.[51,52] In this period, symptoms and voiding function continue to improve in most patients. A few patients show a more stepwise, often dramatic improvement that can occur at any time during follow-up, even after 3 months.

Subjective satisfaction is usually achieved within 2 to 6 weeks, and a substantial objective improvement in urinary flow rate and prostate volume in HV-ILC can usually be measured after 4 to 8 weeks. The final outcome can be judged after approximately 3 months (Figure 70B-14).

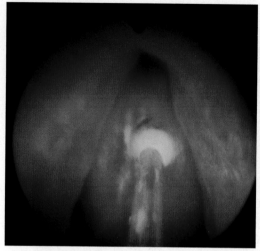

Figure 70B-13 Interstitial applicator inserted in the middle lobe.

RESULTS

Several studies indicated the effectiveness of interstitial laser coagulation of BPH regarding all of the three characteristics of the disease: symptoms, obstruction, and enlargement[5,7-11,71-77,99] (Tables 70B-4, 70B-5, and 70B-6). This was summarized in several review articles.[80,90,124,130,136,139,140]

In the initial study, 239 patients[8-11] were treated at Grosshadern Hospital of Munich University from July 1991 through October 1993. During this time, many technical and procedural improvements were made and the difficulties that arose from the learning curve had been overcome. However, the results were encouraging and compared nicely with published reports of TURP.[9,12,76] The multivariate analysis showed no factors predicting final success or failure, such as initial symptoms, flow rates, residual volumes or prostate volumes, and endoscopic or perineal access, except the number of cases previously performed (reflecting the learning curve). Interstitial laser therapy was safe, with a low potential for severe side effects. Re-treatment for persistent voiding problems was necessary within 1 year in 9.6% of patients. For the early treatment group, follow-up was up to 30 months at the time of evaluation, with only a few more patients requiring retreatment.

Urodynamic measurements could be done in a limited number of patients before and after treatment. Pressure-flow studies demonstrated a sufficient decrease of the urethral opening pressure and the urethral resistance.[76,78,101,107,114]

In a later series (October 1993 through December 1993), 48 patients were treated interstitially with standard instrumentation (Nd:YAG laser and ITT light guide), application technique (transurethral application with the integrated cystoscope), and laser parameters (power reduced stepwise from 20 to 7 watts; 3 minutes' total irradiation time per single fiber placement), and compared prospectively with 49 TURP patients (who preoperatively had no statistically significant group differences and included no follow-up losses).[4,6,7] On average, within 12 months AUA

scores improved for these patients from 31.0 to 2.3 points (TURP group, 31.1–3.5 points), life quality index from 4.7 to 0.6 points (TURP group, 4.7–1.3 points), peak flow rates from 9.4 to 19.7 mL/s (TURP group, 8.9–25.6 mL/s), residual urine volume from 128 to 17 mL (TURP group, 167–7 mL), and prostate volumes from an average of 47.1 to 27.5 mL (TURP group, 40.2–21.2 mL) (Figure 70B-15). Four laser-treated patients were not completely satisfied with results and were re-treated by transurethral resection. The resected weight in these patients was minimal (8.6 g average) compared with the original volume of the prostate before laser treatment. The persistence of obstruction was usually caused by small tissue residues in unfavorable locations such as the apex or the bladder neck.

Another consecutive study (January 1994 through June 1994) compared interstitial laser coagulation alone, interstitial laser coagulation plus bladder neck incision, and transurethral resection.[4,6,7] Symptoms were evaluated at 2-week intervals. From about the sixth week after treatment, average results in the three groups were not significantly different statistically. Symptom relief was achieved earlier in the TURP patients than in the interstitial laser therapy patients, but not in the combination treatment group.

During the initial phase, several other authors have used interstitial laser therapy for the treatment of BPH.[5,71-77] Orovan and Whelan,[71] Arai and colleagues,[72] Neuhaus and colleagues,[5] and Bloch[73] have used the ITT light guide and transurethral application technique. Henkel and colleagues,[74] Janetschek and colleagues,[75] and Horninger and colleagues[76] employed ITT light guides as well, but inserted them exclusively from the perineum under transrectal ultrasound guidance. The latter group used a three-dimensional imaging system.[75,76] Handke and colleagues,[77] who also performed interstitial laser therapy transperineally, were using another application system[55] specifically designed for interstitial treatment. McNicholas and colleagues[15] employed bare fibers, which they inserted under

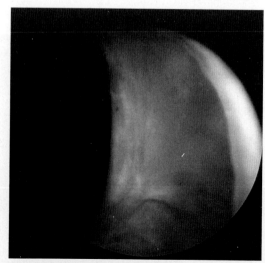

Figure 70B-14 Endoscopic view of the prostate urethra 3 months after interstitial laser therapy.

Table 70B-4 Symptom and Urinary Flow Rate Chages after ILC

Author/Year of Publication	n	Follow-Up (months)	AUA Score Preop	AUA Score Postop	Peak Flow Preop (mL/s)	Peak Flow Postof (mL/s)
Arai et al, 1998[72,92–95]	76	12	19.7	7.4	7.1	11.1
Conn et al, 1996[98]	12	3	22.6	6.0	7.1	14.1
Conn et al, 1999[97]	165	12	22.4	8.3	8.6	14.2
Daehlin and Hedlund, 1999[100,101]	49	12	22	11	8.6	9.9
de la Rosette et al, 1997[103,104]	25	3	20.6	6.9	9.1	20.3
Floratos et al, 2000[108]	53	12	20	7	8.8	13.5
		24		7		10.7
		36		10		12.0
Greenberger and Steiner, 1998[109]	25	6	20.2	8.8	8.3	14.1
Henkel et al, 1995[74,110]	35	12	21	8	5.3	10.3
Horninger et al, 1995[76,113]	12	12	29	6	8.3	16.9
Knoll et al, 2003[87]	72	84	18.8	8.8	n/a	n/a
Lynch and Williams, 2000[117]	39	6	23.5	6.1	8.4	18.4
Martov and Kilchunov, 1996[117]	25	6	19.9	13.5	8.7	13.5
Martov et al, 1998[118]	42	24	23.7	9.2	6.5	13.9
Matsuta et al, 2003[85]	45	24	18.0	5.7	7.6	11.6
McNicholas and Alsudani, 1996[120]	36	12	22	7	9.4	14.6
Muschter and Hofstetter et al, 1995[8,9,10,11,129]	239	12	25.4	6.1	7.7	17.8
Muschter et al, 1995[7]	48	12	31.0	2.3	9.4	19.7
Muschter, 1996[125,126]	112	6	20.9	7.9	8.0	14.2
Muschter et al, 1996[128]	42	3	22.1	4.2	8.2	24.9
Muschter and Whitfield, 1999[80]	394	12	24.2	6.3	7.9	17.2
		24		6.8		15.7
		36		7.9		15.2
Nishizawa et al, 2003[83,84]	28	3	23.1	8.0	AUR	11.2
Orovan and Whelan, 1994[71]	16	3	16.3	5.8	8.8	11.9
Roggan et al, 1994[134]	27	2	14	5	8.0	13.0
Schettini et al, 1996[135]	20	3	22.6	9.2	7.9	15.0
Whelan, 1997[143]	112	6	18.2	8.2	10.4	17.0
Whitfield, 1996[144,145]	40	6	19.0	8.1	8.4	14.3
Williams 1998[147]	25	12	23.2	7.2	8.4	16.8
Williams 1996[146]	165	18	22.1	8.8	8.6	14.6
Zhenghua and Ciling 1996[148]	78	3	22.5	8.5	9.8	16.5

AUR = acute urinary retention; n/a = not applicable.

transrectal ultrasound guidance, either transrectally into the side lobes or transurethrally for isolated median bar obstruction.

All authors reported good clinical results (Table 70B-7). Horninger and colleagues[76] treated a selected group of 12 patients with large prostate glands (average volume 57 mL). After 12 months they noted an AUA score decrease from 29 to 6 points, a urinary peak flow increase from 8.3 to 16.9 mL/s, and a decrease in average residual volume from 119 to 30 mL. Urodynamic measurements showed a decrease of the intravesical pressure from 59 to 48 cm H_2O. Henkel and colleagues[74] treated 38 high-risk patients and recorded an AUA score improvement of 26 to 9 points after 6 months. Transrectal ultrasound volumetry of the prostate showed a decrease in prostate volume of 5 to 48%. The peak flow rate improved to over 15 mL/s in 50% of patients, and detrusor pressure became normal in 45% of patients. Bloch[73] treated 28 outpatients, 14 of whom had chronic retention. Urinary peak flow rates improved from 5.0 to 14.3 mL/s (9.0–41.0), and the residual urine volume from 152 to 54 mL on average. Arai and colleagues[72] treated 50 patients. Although they performed only 2 to 6 fiber placements, they found that 80% of their patients were completely satisfied and had an AUA score improvement from 20.1 to 10.0 points,

a peak flow increase from 7.0 to 9.5 mL/s, and a decrease of the residual urine volume from 90 to 45 mL within 3 months. The prostate volume decreased from 33.5 to 27.5 mL. The retrospective analysis of these results leads to the interpretation that this was the first report on LV-ILC.

Handke and colleagues[77] re-treated 2 of 13 patients within the first 2 months of follow-up,

Henkel and colleagues[74] re-treated 3 of 22 patients within 6 months, and Bloch[73] re-treated 1 of 28 patients. In other series, the authors did not report that any re-treatment was necessary during follow-up.[71,72,75,76]

A prospective international multicenter study (interstitial laser therapy vs transurethral resection of the prostate) using a diode laser emitting at 830 nm combined with the diffusor tip started in early 1995.[6] Results at 3 months in 47 patients showed an average AUA score improvement of 20.0 to 6.8 points, urinary peak flow rate from 8.1 to 15.0 mL/s, residual urine volume from 121 to 60 mL, and prostate volume from 39.5 to 29.9 mL. In 4% of patients, re-treatment was necessary. By now, this laser system is well established worldwide.[82,85,89,97–99,103–106,109,113,116,125,126,133,142–145]

Results of the more recent studies are summarized in Tables 70B-4, 70B-5, and 70B-6. Other studies were performed using ILC focused on specific topics, such as management of urinary retention,[83] postprocedural catheterization,[84] and cost-effectiveness.[79]

COMPLICATIONS

Specific complications of interstitial laser therapy are extremely rare. McNicholas and colleagues[31] observed the only serious complication reported in the literature, which was a small bowel injury that occurred in 1 patient treated with a bare fiber that was inserted transrectally. In theory, it is possible when using interstitial applicators and transurethral or perineal access that coagulation of the prostate capsule and adjacent organs might occur, but even if they do, this would probably not be of clinical significance in most cases. Coagulation of the neurovascular bundle and the rectum (the latter resulting in a fistula) could occur, but by avoiding extremely deep fiber placement, especially in a dorsal direction, it is highly unlikely these complications would occur. No reports on such events can be found in the literature.

In interstitial laser therapy, the light applicators are placed into the tissue. Theoretically, they can

Table 70B-5 Volume Reduction after Interstitial Laser Coagulation (ILC)

Author/Year of Publication	Before ILC (mL)	After ILC (mL)	%
Arai et al, 1996[93]	42.6	35.6	16.4
Henkel et al, 1995[74,111,112]	67	43	35.8
Horninger et al, 1997[113]	57.0	52.3	8.25
Krautschick et al, 1999[115]	40/62/104*	n/a	18
Kursh et al, 2003[82]	41.5	35.1	15.4
Martov und Kilchunov, 1996[118]	53.8	42.1	21.75
Muschter and Hofstetter, 1994[8]	47.4	29.1	38.6
Muschter et al, 1995[7]	47.1	27.5	41.6
Nishizawa et al, 2003[83]	54.6	44.0	19.4
Norby et al, 2002[81]	44	26	41.0
Roggan et al, 1994[134]	49	36	26.5
Schettini et al, 1996[135]	66.6	49.0	26.4
Tsui et al, 2003[79]	46.6	34.1	26.8
Whelan, 1997[143]	n/a	n/a	26.1
Zhenghua and Ciling, 1996[148]	40	28	30

*pretreatment volumes were stratified in 3 groups: < 50 mL, 50-80 mL, > 80 mL; listed are the mean values of each group.
n/a = not applicable.

Table 70B-6 Symptom and Urinary Flow Rate Changes after ILC Compared with Controls in Nonrandomized and Randomized Studies

Author/Year of Publication	Procedure/n	Follow-Up (months)	AUA Score Preop	AUA Score Postop	Peak Flow Preop (mL/s)	Peak Flow Postop (mL/s)
Muschter et al, 1995[124]	TURP 49	12	31.1	3.5	8.9	25.6
	ILC 48	12	31.0	2.3	9.4	19.7
de la Rosette et al/Whitfield, 1996[105,144,145]	TURP 56	6	22.4	6.5	8.3	20.3
	ILC 110	6	21.5	9.7	8.3	14.0
Fay et al, 1997[106]	TURP 24	6	22.5	8.6	8.8	18.9
	ILC 20	6	23.0	10.8	7.5	11.6
AFU multicenter, 1998[136]	TURP 16	12	?	9.3	?	18.7
	ILC 27	12	?	6.9	?	15.4
Norby et al, 2002[81]	TURP/TUIP 24	6	21.3	6.8	9.6	20.6
	TUMT 46	6	20.5	9.5	9.1	13.2
	ILC 48	6	21.4	9.5	10.2	16.2
Kursh et al, 2003[82]	TURP 37	24	23.0	7.0	9.1	16.5
	ILC 35	24	24.0	9.0	9.2	13.9
Liedberg et al, 2003[86]	TURP 11	12	n/a	n/a	n/a	n/a
	ILC 20	12	n/a	n/a	n/a	n/a

ILC = interstitial laser coagulation; TUIP = transurethral incision of the prostate; TUMT = transurethral microwave thermotherapy; n/a = not applicable; TURP = transurethral resection of the prostate.

break for either of two reasons: mechanical stress or overheating. A high degree of straining of the fiber can result in mechanical damage. In some types of applicators damage can occur inside only and no parts can break off. If the tip were to break off, the stress point would always be outside the tissue at its surface. Therefore, the broken-off part of the applicator could easily be removed with a forceps. Overheating because of the formation of char at the applicator tip could lead to a fiber breaking off inside the tissue. Most laser systems for interstitial therapy, therefore, have feedback systems that detect charring and switch the system off before the applicator can break. In the unlikely event of broken fiber fragments remaining in the tissue, they can be removed by electroresection, but in the experience of several authors this has never happened.[21,23,24,74,76]

Other possible complications and side effects are not specific to interstitial laser therapy. Bleeding, if it occurs, is most often caused by mechanical trauma (eg, of varicose veins on the urethral surface resulting from motion of the cystoscope). Minor bleeding from puncture sites is also possible. Bleeding usually stops within a short time without further treatment. To prevent clot retention, postoperative irrigation can be done for several hours. Significant bleeding from interstitial laser therapy is extremely rare; in all reported

cases it has been caused by the suprapubic catheter.[9] Unintentional infusion of irrigation fluid or a significant TURP syndrome has not occurred in interstitial laser therapy.[9,10] A mechanical perforation of the bladder or the prostate capsule is extremely unlikely to occur and has never been reported.

Frequently in the early postoperative period, a transient increase in obstruction and a concomitant increase in obstructive symptoms occurs. Transient irritative symptoms such as urgency can also occur. This is usually caused by edema, but can also be associated with either secondary uncomplicated urinary tract infection or urethral necrosis. In the latter case, parts of the urethra were most likely coagulated as a result of placement of the applicator close to the urethra. This is often accompanied by tissue sloughing.[9,10] No specific treatment of these conditions is required. Permanent incontinence has never been reported. The rate of urinary tract infection, which can occur because of postprocedure catheterization, can be kept low by simple antibiotic prophylaxis.[9] Significant urinary tract infection with fever, epididymitis, or prostatitis can occur after interstitial laser therapy with probably the same frequency as after any other transurethral procedure.

Urethral strictures or bladder neck strictures, which occurred in approximately 5% of

patients in the first series, resulted from instruments and application technique that required further refinement and development.[9,10] In the more recent series, the urethral strictures observed were recurrences of previously treated strictures.[6,7]

Patients' sexual function regarding libido and erection has not been affected by interstitial laser therapy in the initial or later studies.[9,10] A loss of prograde ejaculation is possible. In the first series of patients,[9–12] 93.3% of the sexually active patients responding to a questionnaire indicated that they had retained normal ejaculation patterns. Most authors either did not report on retrograde ejaculation or inability to ejaculate or did not encounter this complication.[71,73,74,76,77] Arai and colleagues[72] found retrograde ejaculation in 2 of 50 patients. In an international multicenter study this complication was observed in 6% of patients.[6] If an additional bladder neck incision is performed, however, loss of prograde ejaculation can be higher.[4,7]

The serum concentration of PSA increases dramatically after interstitial laser therapy; within a short time, however, it returns to the pretreatment level.[10] A late recurrence of increased PSA level during follow-up must be looked at carefully. In conjunction with digital rectal examination, PSA can still be used for cancer screening.

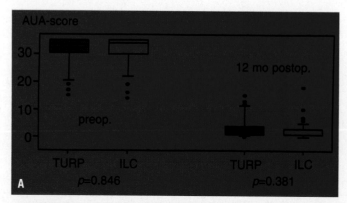

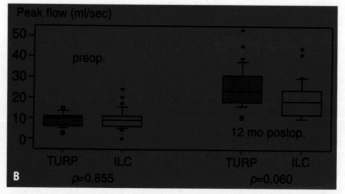

Figure 70B-15 *A*, Treatment results of TUPR vs interstitial laser therapy in 49 and 48 patients with BPH. AUA symptom score is given before and 12 months after treatment. *B*, Urinary peak flow rate before and 12 months after treatment.

Table 70B-7 Retherapy after Interstitial Laser Coagulation (as reported in studies with at least 12 months' follow-up)

Author/Year of Publication	Follow-Up (months)	Retherapy (%)
Conn et al, 1999[97]	12	6
Floratos et al, 2000[108]	36	24.3
Henkel et al, 1995[74]	12	13.6
Horninger et al, 1995[112]	12	0
Knoll et al, 2003[87]	84	15.8 TURP 15.8 medication
Krautschick et al, 1999[115]	24	11.9
Kursh et al, 2003[82]	24	16
McNicholas and Alsudani, 1996[120]	12	0
Muschter and Hofstetter, 1994[8]	12	9.6
Muschter et al, 1995[7]	12	8.3
Terada et al, 2004[88]	48.4	22.0 TURP 13.0 medication

REFERENCES

1. Perlmutter AP, Muschter R. The optimization of laser prostatectomy. Part I: Free beam side fire coagulation. Urology 1994;44:847–55.
2. Muschter R, Perlmutter AP. The optimization of laser prostatectomy. Part II: Other lasing techniques. Urology 1994; 44:856–61.
3. Muschter R, Perlmutter AP. Vergleichende Untersuchungen zur Laserkoagulation und vaporisation der Prostata. Akt Urol 1995;26 Sonderheft 1:113–6.
4. Muschter R, Ehsan A, Baumhackl D, Stepp HG. Interstitielle Laserkoagulation versus transurethrale Resektion—Ergebnisse eines prospektiven Vergleichs. Urologe A 1995;34:574.
5. Neuhaus L, Lietz L, Borkowski M. Erfahrungsbericht über die kombinierte Behandlung der Prostata mit interstitieller und endourethraler Laserkoagulation. Lasermedizin [in press].
6. Muschter R, Hofstetter A, Anson K, et al. Nd:YAG and diode lasers for interstitial laser coagulation of benign prostatic hyperplasia: experimental and clinical evaluation. J Urol 1995;153:229A.
7. Muschter R, Ehsan A, Stepp HG, Hofstetter A. Clinical results of LITT in the treatment of benign prostatic hyperplasia. In: Müller G, Roggan A, editors. Laser-induced interstitial thermotherapy, vol PM25. Bellingham, WA: SPIE Press; 1995. p. 434–42.
8. Muschter R, Hofstetter A. Erfahrungen mit der interstitiellen Laserkoagulation in der Therapie der benignen Prostatahyperplasie. Lasermedizin 1994;10:133–9.
9. Muschter R, Hofstetter A. Interstitial laser therapy outcomes in benign prostatic hyperplasia. J Endourol 1995;9:129–35.
10. Muschter R, Hofstetter A. Technique and results of interstitial laser coagulation. World J Urol 1995;13:109–14.
11. Muschter R, Zellner M, Hessel S, Hofstetter A. Die interstitielle laserinduzierte Koagulation (ILK) der Prostata zur Therapie der benignen Hyperplasie (BPH). Urologe A 1995;34:90–7.
12. Muschter R, Zellner M, Hofstetter A. Lasers and benign prostatic hyperplasia—experimental and clinical results to compare different application systems. J Urol 1994;151:230A.
13. Muschter R. Laser-induced interstitial thermotherapy of benign prostatic hyperplasia and prostate cancer. SPIE Proc 1994;2327:287–92.
14. Muschter R, Hofstetter A. Interstitial laser coagulation for local palliation of prostate cancer. J Urol 1995;153:240A.
15. McNicholas TA, Aslam M, Lynch MJ, O'Donoghue N. Interstitial laser coagulation for the treatment of urinary outflow obstruction. J Urol 1993;149:465A.
16. Muschter R, Perlmutter AP, Anson K, et al. Diode lasers for interstitial laser coagulation of the prostate. SPIE Proc 1995;2395:77–82.
17. Muschter R, Hessel S, Jahnen P, et al. Evaluation of different laser wavelengths and application systems for LITT, vol PM25. Bellingham, WA: SPIE Press; 1995. p. 212–23.
18. Muschter R, Perlmutter AP, Anson K, et al. Experimentelle Untersuchungen zur Eignung von Halbleiterlasern für die interstitielle Laserkoagulation der Prostata—Erste Ergebnisse. Lasermedizin 1995;11:150–6.
19. Hofstetter A. Interstitielle Thermokoagulation (ITK) von Prostatatumoren. Lasermedizin 1991;7:179.
20. Muschter R, Hofstetter A, Hessel S, et al. Hi-tech of the prostate: Interstitial laser coagulation of benign prostatic hypertrophy. SPIE Proc 1992;1643:25–34.
21. Muschter R, Hofstetter A, Hessel S, et al. Interstitial laser coagulation of the prostate. Lasers Surg Med 1992;4:25.
22. Muschter R, Hofstetter A. “Thermische” Therapie der benignen Prostatahyperplasie. Munch Med Wochenschr 1992;134:630–4.
23. Muschter R, Hofstetter A, Hessel S, et al. Interstitial laser prostatectomy—experimental and first clinical results. J Urol 1992;147:346A.
24. Muschter R, Hessel S, Hofstetter A, et al. Die interstitielle Laserkoagulation der benignen Prostatahyperplasie. Urologe A 1993;32:273–81.
25. Littrup PJ, Lee F, Borlaza GS, et al. Percutaneous ablation of canine prostate using transrectal ultrasound guidance. Invest Radiol 1988;23:734–9.
26. Littrup PJ, Sacknoff EJ, Lee F, et al. Comparison of Nd:YAG laser and absolute ethanol in the percutaneous ablation of canine prostate. Laser Med Surg News Adv 1988;4:21–5.
27. McNicholas TA, Charig C, Steger AC, Bown SG. Interstitial laser coagulation of the prostate: an experimental study. Lasers Med Sci 1988;3:446A.
28. McNicholas TA, Lynch MJ, Parkinson MC, O'Donoghue NE. Interstitial laser coagulation (ILC) of the prostate. J Endourol 1992;6:137.
29. McNicholas TA, Pope AJ, Timoney A, et al. Interstitial laser coagulation of the prostate: experimental and clinical studies. J Urol 1992;147:210A.
30. McNicholas TA, Pope AJ, Timoney A, et al. Hyperthermia of the prostate by interstitial laser coagulation. J Urol 1992; 147:345A.
31. McNicholas TA, Steger AC, Bown SG. Interstitial laser coagulation of the prostate. An experimental study. Br J Urol 1993;71:439–44.
32. Matthewson K, Coleridge-Smith P, Northfield TC, Bown SG. Comparison of continuous-wave and pulsed excitation for interstitial neodymium-YAG laser-induced hyperthermia. Lasers Med Sci 1986;1:197–201.
33. Matthewson K, Barton T, Lewin MR, O'Sullivan JP, Northfield TC, Bown SG. Low power interstitial Nd:YAG laser photocoagulation in normal and neoplastic rat colon. Gut 1988;29:27–34.
34. Masters A, Bown SG. Interstitial laser hyperthermia. Semin Surg Oncol 1992;8:242–9.
35. Godlewski G, Bourgeois JM, Sambuc P, et al. Ultrasonic and histopathological correlations of deep focal hepatic lesions induced by stereotaxic Nd:YAG laser applications. Ultrasound Med Biol 1988;14:287–91.
36. Steger AC, McNicholas TA. Interstitial hyperthermia of the prostate. In: McNicholas TA, editor. Lasers in urology: principles and practice. New York: Springer; 1990. p. 141–9.
37. Bown SG. New approaches to local destruction of tumours—interstitial laser hyperthermia and photodynamic therapy. SPIE Proc 1991;1525:325–30.
38. Hessel ST, Frank F. Technical prerequisites for the interstitial thermo-therapy using the Nd:YAG laser. SPIE Proc 1990;1201:233–8.
39. Bown SG. Phototherapy of tumors. World J Surg 1983;7: 700–9.
40. Arnfield M, Gonzalez S, Lea P, et al. Cylindrical irradiator fiber tip for photodynamic therapy. Lasers Surg Med 1986;6:150–4.
41. Daikuzono N, Joffe SN, Tajiri H, et al. Laserthermia: a computer-controlled contact Nd:YAG system for interstitial local hyperthermia. Med Instrum 1987;21:275–7.
42. Van Eeden PJ, Steger AC, Bown SG. Fibre tip considerations for low power laser interstitial hyperthermia. Lasers Med Sci 1988;3:A336.
43. Godlewski G, Rouy S, Pignodel C, et al. Deep localized neodymium (Nd)-YAG laser photocoagulation in liver using a new water cooled and echoguided handpiece. Lasers Surg Med 1988;8:501–9.
44. Panjehpour M, Overholt BF, Milligan AJ, et al. Nd:YAG laser-induced interstitial hyperthermia using a long frosted contact probe. Lasers Surg Med 1990;10:16–24.
45. Matsumoto R, Selig AM, Colucci VM, Jolesz FA. Interstitial Nd:YAG laser ablation in normal rabbit liver: trial to maximize the size of laser-induced lesions. Lasers Surg Med 1992;12:650–8.
46. Nolsoe CP, Torp-Pedersen S, Olldag PES, Holm HH. Bare fibre low power Nd-YAG laser interstitial hyperthermia. Comparison between diffuser tip and non-modified tip. An in vitro study. Lasers Med Sci 1992;7:1–7.
47. Shi X, Dachmann AH. In vitro diode laser photocoagulation: comparison of fiber tips. Lasers Surg Med Suppl 1995; 7:70.
48. Slatkine M, Mead D, Konwitz E, Johnson ED. A neodymium: YAG fiber delivery system for interstitial photothermal therapy. SPIE Proc 1994;2129:56–66.
49. Johnson DE, Cromeens DM, Price RE. Interstitial laser prostatectomy. SPIE Proc 1994;2129:67–71.
50. Johnson DE, Cromeens DM, Price RE. Interstitial laser prostatectomy. Lasers Surg Med 1994;14:299–305.
51. Heuck A, Müller-Lisse U, Muschter R, et al. Einsatz der Magnetresonanz-Tomographie für die Darstellung der interstitiellen Laserkoagulation bei der benignen Prostatahyperplasie: Erste Erfahrungen. Lasermedizin 1995;11:27–33.
52. Heuck A, Müller-Lisse U, Schneede P, et al. Value of MR imaging for the monitoring of laser-induced interstitial thermotherapy in benign prostatic hyperplasia. Eur Radiol 1995;5:S293.
53. Ascher PW. Interstitial thermotherapy of brain tumors with Nd:YAG laser under real time MRI control. SPIE Proc 1990;1200:242–5.
54. Ascher PW, Justich E, Schröttner O. Interstitial thermotherapy of central brain tumors with the Nd:YAG laser under real-time monitoring by MRI. J Clin Laser Med Surg 1991;9:79–83.
55. Beuthan J, Müller G, Schaldach B, Zur CH. Fiber design for interstitial laser treatment. SPIE Proc 1991;1420:234–41.
56. Gomella L, Lotfi A, Tulleners E, et al. Interstitial contact laser photocoagulation of the canine prostate: preliminary studies. Lasers Surg Med Suppl 1994;6:60.
57. Miller RA, Coptcoat MJ, Parry J, et al. The integrated cystoscope: an alternative to conventional and fibreoptic cystoscopy. Br J Urol 1987;60:128–31.
58. Hoopes JP, Williams JC, Harris RD, et al. Interstitial laser coagulation (ILC) of the canine prostate with transrectal ultrasound (TRUS) and thermal monitoring. J Urol 1994; 151:334A.
59. Heuck A, Müller-Lisse U, Schneede P, et al. Dynamic assessment of laser-induced temperature effects in bovine prostatic tissue with MRI: an experimental approach. Eur Radiol 1995;5:S362.
60. Jako GJ, Jolesz FA. The control of neodymium:YAG laser fiber optics hyperthermia with magnetic resonance imaging. SPIE Proc 1986;712:72–7.
61. Castro DJ, Saxton RE, Layfield LJ, et al. Interstitial laser phototherapy assisted by magnetic resonance imaging: a new technique for monitoring laser-tissue interaction. Laryngoscope 1990;100:541–7.
62. Anzai Y, Lufkin RB, Saxton RE, et al. Nd:YAG interstitial laser phototherapy guided by magnetic resonance imaging in an ex vivo model: dosimetry of laser-MR-tissue interaction. Laryngoscope 1991;101:755–60.
63. Amin Z, Lees WR, Bown SG. Technical note: interstitial laser photocoagulation for the treatment of prostatic cancer. Br J Urol 1993;66:1044–7.
64. Hashimoto D, Takami M, Idezuki Y. In-depth radiation therapy by YAG laser for malignant tumors in the liver under ultrasonic imaging. Gastroenterology 1985;88:1663A.
65. Steger AC, Shorvon P, Walmsley K, et al. Ultrasound features of low power interstitial laser hyperthermia. Clin Radiol 1992;46:88–93.
66. Wilson BC, Adam G. A Monte Carlo model for the absorption and flux distributions of light in tissue. Med Phys 1983; 10:824–30.
67. Whiting P, Dowden J, Kapadia P. A mathematical analysis of the results of experiments on rats' livers by local laser hyperthermia. Lasers Med Sci 1989;4:55–64.
68. Johnson S, Motamedi M, Egger N, et al. Photosensitizing the canine prostate with 5-aminolevulinic acid: a new laser prostatectomy? J Urol 1995;153:298A.
69. McPhee MS, Thorndyke CW, Thomas G, et al. Interstitial applications of laser irradiation in hematoporphyrin derivative-photosensitized Dunning R3327 prostate cancers. Lasers Surg Med 1984;4:93–8.
70. Camps JL Jr, Powers SK, Beckman WC Jr, et al. Photodynamic therapy of prostate cancer: an in vitro study. J Urol 1985;134:1222–6.
71. Orovan WL, Whelan JP. Neodymium:YAG laser treatment of BPH using interstitial thermotherapy: a transurethral approach. J Urol 1994;151:230A.
72. Arai Y, Ishitoya S, Okubo K, Suzuki Y. Interstitial laser coagulation for benign prostatic hyperplasia: treatment outcome and quality of life (QOL). J Urol 1995;153:415A.
73. Bloch M. Ambulante Laserbehandlung bei benigner

Prostatathyperplasie. Erste Erfahrungen [abstract]. Tagung Vereinigung Norddeutscher Urol (Neumünster) 1994;17:6.
74. Henkel TO, Greschner M, Luppold T, et al. Perineal interstitial laser of the prostate (PILP). SPIE Proc 1995;2327:1–3.
75. Janetschek G, Strasser H, Horninger W, Bartsch G. 3-D ultraschallgesteuerte Plazierung der Sonden für die interstitielle Lasertherapie der Prostatahyperplasie. Urologe A 1994;33:S81.
76. Horninger W, Janetschek G, Pointner J, et al. Are TULIP, interstitial laser and contact laser superior to TURP? J Urol 1995;153:413A.
77. Handke A, Roggan A, Andreesen R, Miller K. Laserinduzierte interstitielle Thermotherapie (LITT) bei BPH. Urologe A 1994;33:S81.
78. Zellner M, Muschter R. Initiale urodynamische Ergebnisse nach interstitieller Laserkoagulation der Prostata bei benigner Hyperplasie. Lasermedizin 1994;10:141–4.
79. Tsui KH, Chang PL, Chang SS, Cheng HL. Interstitial laser photocoagulation for treatment of benign prostatic hypertrophy: outcomes and cost effectiveness. Chang Gung Med J 2003;26:799–806.
80. Muschter R, Whitfield H. Interstitial laser therapy of benign prostatic hyperplasia. Eur Urol 1999;35:147–54.
81. Norby B, Nielsen HV, Frimodt-Moller PC. Transurethral interstitial laser coagulation of the prostate and transurethral microwave thermotherapy vs transurethral resection or incision of the prostate: results of a randomized, controlled study in patients with symptomatic benign prostatic hyperplasia. BJU Int 2002;90:853–62.
82. Kursh ED, Concepcion R, Chan S, et al. Interstitial laser coagulation versus transurethral prostate resection for treating benign prostatic obstruction: a randomized trial with 2-year follow-up. Urology 2003;61:573–8.
83. Nishizawa K, Kobayashi T, Watanabe J, Ogura K. Interstitial laser coagulation of the prostate for management of acute urinary retention. J Urol 2003;170:879–82.
84. Nishizawa K, Kobayashi T, Mitsumori K, et al. Intermittent catheterization time required after interstitial laser coagulation of the prostate. Urology 2004;64:79–83.
85. Matsuta Y, Ichioka K, Terada N, et al. Interstitial laser coagulation for benign prostatic hyperplasia: clinical results of the Indige diode laser system. Hinyokika Kiyo 2003;49: 195–200.
86. Liedberg F, Adell L, Hagberg G, Palmqvist IB. Interstitial laser coagulation versus transurethral prostate resection of the prostate for benign prostatic enlargement—a prospective randomized study. Scand J Urol Nephrol 2003;37:494–7.
87. Knoll T, Michel MS, Trojan L, et al. Langzeitergebnisse der interstitiellen Laserkoagulation zur Behandlung der benignen Prostatahyperplasie. Akt Urol 2003;34:48–51.
88. Terada N, Arai Y, Okubo K, et al. Interstitial laser coagulation for management of benign prostatic pyperplasia: long-term follow-up. Int J Urol 2004;11:978–82.
89. Muschter R, Hofstetter A. Die interstitielle Laserkoagulation mit dem Diodenlaser der Wellenlänge 830 nm zur Therapie der benignen Prostatahyperplasie—High- versus Low-Volume-Koagulation. Lasermedizin 2000;15:72–80.
90. Muschter R. Current status of laser treatment of BPH. Med Laser Appl 2001;16:5–14.
91. Muschter R, Gilling P. Lasers for median lobe hyperplasia. Curr Urol Rep 2002;2:306–10.
92. Arai Y, Ishitoya S, Okubo K, Suzuki Y. Interstitial laser coagulation for benign prostatic hyperplasia: 1-year follow-up and analysis of patient profile linked to clinical response. J Urol 1996;155:319A.
93. Arai Y, Ishitoya S, Okubo K, Suzuki Y. Transurethral interstitial laser coagulation for benign prostatic hyperplasia: treatment outcome and quality of life. Br J Urol 1996;77:93–8.
94. Arai Y, Kanba T, Ishitoya S, et al. Interstitial laser coagulation for benign prostatic hyperplasia: preliminary clinical results. Int J Urol 1995;2:104–9.
95. Arai Y, Okubo K, Okada T, et al. Interstitial laser coagulation for management of benign prostatic hyperplasia: a Japanese experience. J Urol 1998;159:1961–5.
96. Bhatta KM, Perlmutter A, Cho G, et al. A new technique of subsurface and interstitial laser therapy using a diode laser (wavelength = 1000 nm) and a catheter delivery device. J Urol 1996;155:310A.
97. Conn RL, Kursh ED, Williams JC, et al. One year outcomes of interstitial laser coagulation of the prostate in 100 men: a multicenter experience. J Urol 1999;161:390.
98. Conn RL, Muschter R, Adams CS, Esch VC. International registry results for an interstitial laser BPH treatment device. SPIE Proc 1996;2671:316–20.
99. Costello AJ, Agarwal DK, Crowe HR, Lynch WJ. Evaluation of interstitial diode laser therapy for treatment of benign prostatic hyperplasia. Tech Urol 1999;5:202–6.
100. Daehlin L. Interstitial laser coagulation and transurethral needle ablation in the management of lower urinary tract symptoms due to benign prostatic obstruction. Scand J Urol Nephrol 1999;203:21–4.
101. Daehlin L, Hedlund H. Interstitial laser coagulation in patients with lower urinary tract symptoms from benign prostatic obstruction: treatment under sedoanalgesia with pressure flow evaluation. BJU Int 1999;84:628–36.
102. Daidoh Y. [A basic study of the interstitial laser prostatectomy using pulsed holmium:yttrium-aluminum-garnet (Ho:YAG) laser]. Nippon Hinyokika Gakkai Zasshi 1996;87:650–9.
103. de la Rosette JJMCH, Muschter R, Lopez MA. Interstitial laser coagulation in the treatment of BPH using a tissue adaptive laser system. J Endourol 1996;10 Suppl 1:S93.
104. de la Rosette JJMCH, Muschter R, Lopez MA, Gillatt D. Interstitial laser coagulation in the treatment of benign prostatic hyperplasia using a diode-laser system with temperature feedback. Br J Urol 1997;80:433–8.
105. de la Rosette JJMCH, Muschter R, Whitfield HN, et al. Report of a prospective multicenter randomized study evaluating interstitial laser coagulation for BPH. J Endourol 1996;10 Suppl 1:S125.
106. Fay R, Chan SL, Kahn R, et al. Initial results of a randomized trial comparing interstitial laser coagulation therapy to transurethral resection of the prostate. J Urol 1997;157:41.
107. Floratos DL, de la Rosette JJMCH. The value of urodynamics in laser prostatectomy. Eur Urol 2000;37:509–16.
108. Floratos DL, Sonke GS, Francisca EA, et al Long-term follow-up of laser treatment for lower urinary tract symptoms suggestive of bladder outlet obstruction. Urology 2000;56:604–9.
109. Greenberger M, Steiner MS: The University of Tennessee experience with the Indigo 830e laser device for the minimally invasive treatment of benign prostatic hyperplasia: interim analysis. World J Urol 1998;16:386–91.
110. Henkel TO, Greschner M, Luppold T, et al. Perineal interstitial laser of the prostate (PILP). In: Bown SG, Escourrou J, Frank F, et al, editors. Medical applications of lasers II. SPIE Proc 1994;2327:293–5.
111. Henkel TO, Niedergethmann M, Alken P. Laserinduced interstitial thermotherapy (LITT): in vitro and in vivo studies. J Endourol 1995;9 Suppl 1:S56.
112. Henkel TO, Niedergethmann M, Alken P. Perfusion rate and perfusion medium: how important is their influence during interstitial laser coagulation (ILC)? J Endourol 1995;9 Suppl 1:S151.
113. Horninger W, Janetschek G, Watson G, et al. Are contact laser, interstitial laser, and transurethral ultrasound-guided laser-induced prostatectomy superior to transurethral prostatectomy? Prostate 1997;31:255–63.
114. Issa MM, Townsend M, Jiminez VK, et al. A new technique of intraprostatic fiber placement to minimize thermal injury to prostatic urothelium during indigo interstitial laser thermal therapy. Urology 1998;51:105–10.
115. Krautschick AW, Köhrmann KU, Henkel TO, et al. Interstitial laser coagulation in benign prostatic hyperplasia: a critical evaluation after 2 years of follow-up. Urol Int 1999;62:76–80.
116. Lopez M, Vargas JC, Muschter R, Perlmutter AP. The size of prostatic interstitial laser lesions can be controlled by temperature. J Urol 1997;157:41.
117. Lynch WJ, Williams JC. Physician's dialogue: interstitial laser coagulation technique clinical research updates. World J Urol 2000;18 suppl 1:S14–5.
118. Martov AG, Kilchukov ZI. Interstitial laser-induced coagulation of BPH: 6 months follow-up. J Endourol 1996;10 Suppl 1:S191.
119. Martov AG, Kilchukov ZI, Gushchin BL. Long-term follow-up in interstitial laser coagulation in BPH treatment. J Endourol 1998;12 Suppl 1:S195.
120. McNicholas T, Alsudani M. Interstitial laser coagulation therapy for benign prostatic hyperplasia. SPIE Proc 1996;2671:300–8.
121. Mueller-Lisse UG, Heuck AF, Schneede P, et al. Postoperative MRI in patients undergoing interstitial laser coagulation thermotherapy of benign prostatic hyperplasia. J Comput Assist Tomogr 1996;20:273–8.
122. Mueller-Lisse U, Heuck A, Stehling MK, et al. MRT-Monitoring vor, während und nach der laserinduzierten Thermotherapie der benignen Prostatahyperplasie. Erste klinische Erfahrungen. Radiologe 1996;36:722–31.
123. Mueller-Lisse UG, Heuck AF, Thoma M, et al. Predictability of the size of laser-induced lesions in T1-weighted MR images obtained during interstitial laser-induced thermotherapy of benign prostatic hyperplasia. J Magn Res Imag 1998;8:31–9.
124. Mueller-Lisse UG, Thoma M, Faber S, et al. Coagulative interstitial laser-induced thermotherapy of benign prostatic hyperplasia: online imaging with a T2-weighted fast spin-echo MR sequence—experience in six patients. Radiology 1999;210:373–9.
125. Muschter R. Current status of laser treatment of BPH. Med Laser Appl 2001;16:5–14.
126. Muschter R. Interstitial laser therapy. Curr Opinion Urol 1996;6:33–8.
127. Muschter R, de la Rosette JJMCH, Whitfield H, et al. International multi-center study results of interstitial laser coagulation (ILC) using an 830 nm diode laser. J Urol 1996;155:318A.
128. Muschter R, de la Rosette JJMCH, Whitfield H, et al. Initial human clinical experience with diode laser interstitial treatment of benign prostatic hyperplasia. Urology 1996;48:223–8.
129. Muschter R, Schneede P, Müller-Lisse UG, Heuck A. Magnetresonanztomographie zur Therapiesteuerung bei thermisch-ablativer Prostatatherapie mittels interstitieller Laserkoagulation. Urologe [B] 1999;39:227–30.
130. Muschter R, Sroka R, Perlmutter AP, et al. High power interstitial laser coagulation of benign prostatic hyperplasia. J Endourol 1996;10 Suppl 1:S197.
131. Muschter R, Zellner M, Hessel S, Hofstetter A. Interstitial laser coagulation of the prostate: experiences in the treatment of benign prostatic hyperplasia. Prog Clin Biol Res 1994;386:521–7.
132. Perlmutter AP, Muschter R. Interstitial laser prostatectomy. Mayo Clin Proc 1998;73:903–7.
133. Perlmutter AP, Muschter R, Anson K, et al. Semiconductor diode lasers in the canine prostate: laser-tissue-interaction. In: Anderson RR, editor. Lasers in surgery: advanced characterization, therapeutics, and systems V. SPIE Proc 1995;2395:42–6.
134. Roggan A, Handke A, Miller K, Müller G. Laser-induced interstitial thermotherapy of benign prostatic hyperplasia: basic investigations and first clinical results. Minimal Invasive Medizin 1994;5:55–63.
135. Schettini M, Diana M, Fortunato P, et al. Results of interstitial laser coagulation of the prostate. J Endourol 1996;10 Suppl 1:S191.
136. Schulman C, Simon J, Zlotta AR. Interstitial laser coagulation for treatment of benign prostatic hyperplasia using local anesthesia only. J Endourol 1998;12 Suppl 1:S196.
137. Sroka R, Perlmutter AP, Martin T, Muschter R. LITT on canine prostates: an in-vivo study to compare the effects of different wavelengths. SPIE Proc 1996;2671:335–8.
138. Stein BS, Altwein JE, Muschter R, et al. Laser prostatectomy. In: Denis L, Griffiths K, Khoury S, et al, editors. Fourth International Consultation on Benign Prostatic Hyperplasia (BPH): proceedings 4, Plymouth: Plymbridge Distributors Ltd; 1998. p. 529–40.
139. Steiner MS. Physician's dialogue: interstitial laser coagulation technique: executive summary. World J Urol 2000;18 Suppl 1:S4–5.
140. Strasser H, Janetschek G, Horninger W, Bartsch G. Three-dimensional sonographic guidance for interstitial laser therapy in benign prostatic hyperplasia. J Endourol 1995;9:497–501.
141. Volpe MA, Fromer D, Kaplan SA. Holmium and interstitial lasers for the treatment of benign prostatic hyperplasia: a laser revival. Curr Opin Urol 2001;11:43–8.
142. Wheelahan J, Scott NA, Cartmill R, et al. Minimally invasive laser techniques for prostatectomy: a systematic review. The ASERNIP-S review group. Australian Safety and Efficacy Register of New Interventional Procedures—Surgical. BJU Int 2000;86:805–15.
143. Whelan JP. Interstitial laser coagulation of the prostate: transrectal ultrasound findings 3 months after treatment. J Urol 1997;157:435.
144. Whitfield HN. A randomized prospective multicenter study evaluating the efficacy of interstitial laser coagulation. J Urol 1996;155:318A.
145. Whitfield HN. The use of an interstitial diode laser (Indigo) in laser prostatectomy: a randomized, controlled, prospective study. J Endourol 1995;9 Suppl 1:S149.
146. Williams JC. Interstitial laser coagulation of the prostate. Tech Urol 1996;2:130–5.
147. Williams JC. Interstitial laser coagulation of the prostate: introduction of a volume-based treatment formula with 12-month follow-up. World J Urol 1998;16:392–5.
148. Zhenghua G, Ciling C. ITT combined with vaporized incision for treatment of BPH. J Endourol 1996;10 Suppl 1:S192.

Holmium Laser Prostatectomy

Andrew Tan, FRACS(Urol)

Peter Gilling, FRACS(Urol)

TURP (transurethral resection of the prostate) and open prostatectomy have dominated the surgical treatment of bladder outlet obstruction secondary to benign prostatic hyperplasia (BPH) for many decades. Although many "less invasive modalities" have been promoted in recent times, most have been proven to lack the equivalent clinical efficacy.

Holmium laser prostatectomy has stood out as the one alternative to TURP and open prostatectomy that matches both procedures in clinical outcomes, but is associated with less morbidity. The development of the technique that is currently in use—holmium laser enucleation of the prostate (HoLEP), has been aided by the development of a transurethral tissue morcellator. As a result, very large prostates can be dealt with endoscopically with low perioperative morbidity.

PROPERTIES OF THE HOLMIUM WAVELENGTH

The holmium:yttrium-aluminium-garnet (Ho: YAG) laser possesses several properties that make it an ideal incisional tool for soft tissue. It is a pulsed laser in the near infrared range of the wavelength spectrum (2,140 nm), allowing it to be transmitted down fine flexible optical fibers. Each pulse of energy is in the kilowatt range, and as it is highly absorbed by water, the depth of penetration is relatively short at 0.4 mm. These properties create a high-intensity thermal effect in tissue vaporization at the tip of the fiber, with very little in the way of forward scatter of energy into deeper tissue. As a result, when removing tissue with the holmium laser, "what you see is what you get," in contrast to the Nd:YAG laser where coagulation at deeper tissue planes leads to delayed tissue sloughing and characteristic irritative voiding symptoms postoperatively. The holmium laser also possesses good hemostatic properties, thereby decreasing the need for postoperative irrigation, and is able to be used with saline irrigation, which diminishes the risk of dilutional hyponatremia (Table 70C-1).

HOLMIUM LASER IN THE TREATMENT OF BPH

The holmium laser was originally introduced into urology to treat urinary stones.[1] Its precise cutting properties soon led to its use in the treatment of strictures and bladder tumors.[2,3] Animal studies confirmed the ability of the holmium laser to cre-ate an immediate ablative defect in dog prostates without causing deep-tissue coagulation.[4]

The initial experience of using the holmium laser for prostatectomy was in combination with the Nd:YAG laser. This was known as the CELAP procedure (combined endoscopic laser ablation of the prostate).[5] The holmium laser was used to create a channel in the prostate following a coagulation prostatectomy with the Nd:YAG laser. This procedure was developed in an attempt to decrease catheter times associated with the VLAP procedure (visual laser ablation of the prostate), which solely relied on the Nd:YAG laser. Patients in this series were compared with a similar group of patients undergoing VLAP, and mean catheter times were shortened from 11.6 days with VLAP to 4.1 days with CELAP.[5]

Holmium-only prostatectomy was developed when it became apparent that the holmium wavelength itself possessed excellent hemostatic properties. The first holmium-only prostatectomy was an ablative, or vaporization, procedure termed the HoLAP (holmium laser ablation of the prostate). The initial series of 79 patients undergoing this procedure at our institution experienced an improvement at 3 months in peak urinary flow from an average of 9.2 mL/s to 14.5 mL/s and a decrease in AUA symptom score from an average of 18.8 to 8.3.[6] Catheterization times were decreased compared with CELAP to an average of 2.6 days. Mottet and colleagues carried out a randomized trial comparing HoLAP with TURP.[7] They showed that postoperative improvements in peak urinary flow rates and symptom relief were equivalent between the two groups. HoLAP took longer to perform than TURP, but was associated with less perioperative bleeding and decreased catheterization times.

A follow-up study of the original cohort of patients who underwent HoLAP at our institution was recently carried out with an average follow-up period of over 7 years.[8] Although a large number of patients were lost to follow-up because of death or lack of availability, analysis of the patients who were available revealed that HoLAP produces durable results in symptom relief and improvement in maximal urinary flow rate. The reoperation rate was 15% over the period of follow-up. This compares well with studies that have involved the use of other contact vaporization modalities to perform a prostatectomy. Although the HoLAP procedure had a short learning curve, it was tedious, with a slow rate of tissue ablation, and remains suitable only in small prostates (< 40 g).

To overcome some of the inefficiencies of holmium laser ablation, the technique of holmium laser resection of the prostate naturally evolved (HoLRP).[9] This procedure involves partially enucleating each lobe of the prostate and then dividing the lobe into small pieces while it is still attached to the capsule. One of the benefits of this procedure is that tissue is retrieved for histological analysis, although the quality tends to be less than that of a TURP specimen owing to thermal artifact.[10] Typically a third of the resected volume of the prostate is lost to vaporization.

A randomized trial was carried out in which 44 patients were randomized to either HoLRP or VLAP using the Nd:YAG laser.[11] Patients were well matched in urodynamic parameters and symptoms. Clinical outcomes, apart from reoperations, between the two groups were essentially equivalent at 12 months of follow-up, although there were significant differences in flow rates at 1, 3, and 6 months of follow-up, which favored HoLRP. The amount of dysuria and postoperative discomfort was significantly less in the HoLRP group, even when the length of time the catheter was left in the VLAP patients (5 days) was taken into account. Relief of urodynamic obstruction when measured by peak detrusor pressure at maximal flow (PdetQmax) and Schafer grade was greater in the HoLRP group when measured at 3 months. There were fewer reoperations and all other perioperative parameters apart from operative time favored the HoLRP group.

A randomized trial comparing HoLRP with TURP has been carried out at our institution with 2-year and 4-year follow-up.[12,13] The clinical outcomes were similar in urodynamic improvement, symptom assessment, continence, and potency. All the perioperative factors such as nursing contact time, catheter time, length of hospital stay, and transfusion rate were less in the holmium group. Operative time was again longer

---

Table 70C-1 Properties of the Holmium:YAG Laser

Wavelength of 2,140 nm: absorbing chromophone water.

Short penetration depth – 0.4 mm: minimal energy absorption beyond the tip of the fiber.

High power density at the tip of the fiber: leads to tissue vaporization.

Excellent hemostatic properties: decreased need for postoperative bladder irrigation.

Able to be used with saline irrigation: decreases risk of dilutional hyponatremia.

in the holmium group. Despite the increase in operative time, HoLRP was found to be more cost effective than TURP when a cost-benefit analysis of the two procedures was carried out using data from this trial.[14] Other investigators evaluating the HoLRP technique have had similar results to ours.[15–19]

The main reason the operative time is longer for HoLRP than TURP is because of the time taken to incise the lateral lobe fragments into pieces small enough to be safely extracted through the urethra. To overcome this, a transurethral tissue morcellator was developed and a true enucleation procedure then became possible.[20,21]

HOLMIUM LASER ENUCLEATION OF THE PROSTATE

The current technique of holmium laser prostatectomy involves the enucleation of whole anatomical lobes of the prostate. The holmium laser fiber thus becomes analogous to the surgeon's index finger during an open prostatectomy, shelling the adenoma from the surgical capsule. The lobes are then chopped up into small fragments by a transurethral soft tissue morcellator that simultaneously removes the tissue.

The operative times have been shortened considerably, and tissue retrieved significantly increased when compared with HoLRP.[20–22]

HOLEP: SURGICAL TECHNIQUE

PROCEDURE INDICATIONS Patients are selected on the basis of symptoms and voiding uroflowmetry with the addition of pressure flow urodynamics where indicated. Although HoLEP is relatively bloodless, it is advisable (but not mandatory) for patients to discontinue warfarin prior to surgery. Our practice is to routinely assess the prostate volume by ultrasound prior to surgery. This gives an indication of the duration of the procedure and helps to identify other pathology such as bladder stones that can be dealt with by the holmium laser in the same setting. Although there is no upper limit of prostate size that can undergo holmium laser enucleation, size correlates well with the difficulty and length of the procedure.[23]

PATIENT PREPARATION Patients with an active urinary tract infection should be deferred until they have completed a course of antibiotics and have sterile urine. Those patients with a raised PSA or an abnormal rectal examination should undergo a prostate biopsy prior to surgery to rule out the presence of prostate cancer. It is not necessary to crossmatch blood for this procedure as the transfusion rate in our institution is less than 0.2%. All patients undergo a spinal or general anesthetic with 160 mg of gentamicin given intravenously at the time of anesthesia induction.

INFORMED CONSENT All patients are informed of the risks and benefits of HoLEP. The benefits include improvement in urinary flow and

decrease in symptom scores as well as urodynamic relief of bladder outlet obstruction. As with any type of surgery aimed at removing obstructing tissue, patients should routinely be advised that although voiding symptoms such as flow and hesitancy may improve noticeably as soon as the catheter is removed, storage symptoms such as frequency, urgency, and nocturia may take weeks to months to improve and may require adjuvant treatment with anticholinergic medication. Patients with suspected poor detrusor contractility should be told that they might require a period of intermittent self-catheterization postoperatively to aid with bladder emptying. The risks and potential complications of HoLEP include the risks of anesthesia, infection, bladder perforation during morcellation, bleeding, late development of urethral stricture and bladder neck stenosis, stress incontinence, and decreased potency.

PREOPERATIVE PREPARATION Patients are placed in the lithotomy position under general or spinal anesthetic with standard cardio-respiratory monitoring and protection of pressure points. Intravenous gentamicin is given at the induction of anesthesia, and the genitalia are swabbed with aqueous povidone iodine or chlorhexidine.

INSTRUMENTATION The holmium laser currently in use at our institution is the 100 W Versapulse Holmium Laser (Lumenis, Tel Aviv, Israel) with a 550 μm end-firing fiber. The power is set at 2.0 J at 50 Hz (100 W). A trained laser safety officer operates the holmium laser. The fiber is placed through a 6 French (F) ureteric catheter (Cook, Spencer, IN) to protect the telescope and stabilize the fiber.

We perform HoLEP with a 27F continuous-flow resectoscope that has been designed specifically for this procedure. The inner sheath is modified to incorporate a laser fiber channel at the tip to guide the fiber, and a bridge at the other end through which the laser fiber and ureteric catheter are stabilized with a Luer-Lok port (Baxter, Deerfield, IL). Through this resectoscope we place a 30-degree telescope. The irrigating solution is normal saline. The 26F nephroscope (Storz, Germany) is used. An adaptor is used to connect this to the outer sheath. The Versacut morcellator (Lumenis) is composed of a handpiece with hollow reciprocating blades, high suction roller-pump/control box, and a variable-speed foot pedal. So far this is the only commercially available transurethral morcellator (Table 70C-2).

HoLEP: A STEP-BY-STEP APPROACH

STEP 1: BLADDER NECK INCISIONS The first step of the HoLEP procedure is to create bladder neck incisions (BNIs) at 5 and 7 o'clock down to the surgical capsule (Figure 70C-1). In small prostates (< 40 mL), this may be all that is needed. A review of the initial 69 patients treated at our institution with this technique alone has been published.[12] The average prostate size was

24.4 mL. There were no adverse events, and all patients were able to void the next day following removal of the catheter. Average flow rate improved from 7.9 mL/s preoperatively to 19.0 mL/s at 3 months of follow-up. Mean International Prostate Symptom Scores (IPSS) decreased from 22.3 preoperatively to 8.1 after 3 months. Cornford and colleagues performed single-incision holmium bladder neck incisions as a day case in 100 men less than 30 g in size, and found good long-term improvements in symptom scores and flow rates at up to 2 years of follow-up.[25] Only 3 patients failed to void spontaneously after catheter removal.

The bladder neck incisions are performed down to the depth of the surgical capsule, which is identified by circular fibers running transversely. It is important to define the capsule accurately at this stage, as this will serve as the landmark for the correct depth for the rest of the procedure. The incisions are continued down and medially to a point on each side of the verumontanum. The laser fiber is kept close to the end of the resectoscope so that the ceramic beak can be used to separate tissue during the dissection. The incisions are widened laterally by undermining the lateral lobes. This helps to define the plane for the dissection of these lobes later on and improves the flow of irrigant, thereby enhancing visibility. If the median lobe is particularly large and there is a long distance between the verumontanum and the bladder neck, the correct plane may be found initially just proximal to the

Table 70C-2 Equipment Required for Holmium Laser Enucleation of the Prostate
80–100 W holmium laser
550 micrometer laser fiber through 6F ureteric catheter
27F continuous-flow resectoscope modified with laser fiber guide
26F telescope/nephroscope with 5 mm straight working channel
Transurethral morcellator

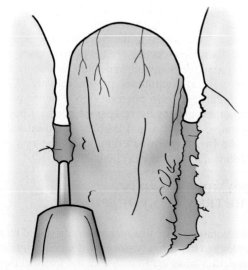

Figure 70C-1 Bladder neck incisions are made at 5 and 7 o'clock down to the surgical capsule of the prostate.

verumontanum, and then this incision can be connected up with one made at the bladder neck.

Bleeding vessels are often encountered just each side of the verumontanum, and these can be coagulated effectively by pulling back and defocusing the beam slightly.

STEP 2: ENUCLEATION OF THE MEDIAN LOBE
The median lobe is dissected off the surgical capsule in a retrograde fashion by joining the two bladder neck incisions just proximal to the verumontanum with a transverse incision (Figure 70C-2). The beak of the resectoscope comes into play here to push the adenoma up toward the bladder as dissection takes place. Care must be taken not to undermine the bladder neck. The median lobe is detached at the bladder neck and allowed to float into the bladder.

STEP 3: ENUCLEATION OF THE LATERAL LOBES
Extending the initial bladder neck incisions laterally at the verumontanum commences the undermining of the lateral lobes. The dissection continues in a circumferential manner toward the 11- and 1-o'clock positions on each side. If the correct plane is found, the lobes can be peeled off the capsule with the laser in an analogous manner to the index finger of a surgeon during an open prostatectomy. A third bladder neck incision is next made at 12 o'clock, and the upper part of the lateral lobes is detached from the surgical capsule using a lateral sweeping motion. These are continued downward and distally until the incisions can be joined at the apex (Figure 70C-3). The step that most novices find challenging is judging where the upper and lower incisions will meet up. Coming back too far with the top incision may damage the sphincter,

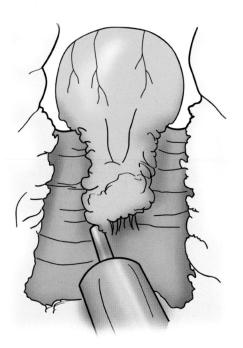

Figure 70C-2 The median lobe is dissected off the surgical capsule in a retrograde manner with a side-to-side movement of the laser fiber.

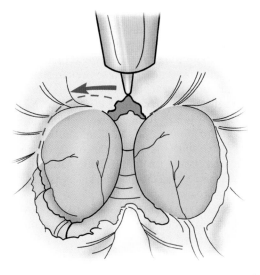

Figure 70C-3 After the lateral lobe has been undermined, an incision is made at 11 o'clock and is swept down to meet with the lower incision.

whereas failure to extend the top incision enough before sweeping down will create a false dissection plane and lead to an inefficient and more troublesome enucleation.

Once the two incisions are joined, the dissection carries on along this broad front in a retrograde fashion toward the bladder neck where the lobe is detached and left to float into the bladder.

Throughout the enucleation, the holmium laser coagulates small veins and arteries as they are encountered. Once all the adenoma has been enucleated, pulling the laser fiber back slightly and defocusing the beam coagulate any ongoing bleeders. Excellent hemostasis is vital prior to morcellation.

STEP 4: MORCELLATION OF ENUCLEATED FRAGMENTS
Morcellation of the enucleated fragments takes place through a nephroscope with a 5 mm working channel. The morcellator produces suction through the hollow blades, which engages the lobes with the blades. The high-speed blades then reciprocate back and forth to slice off fragments with a guillotine action. The fragments are suctioned through the blades and on through tubing attached to the back of the handpiece to the roller pump and then into a sieve.

Morcellation is best performed with a full bladder to avoid the bladder wall being trapped in the morcellator blades. If injury to the bladder wall does occur, it is generally minor and does not interfere with the procedure. More major injuries are very rare, but may lead to troublesome bleeding or extravasation of saline irrigant. Occasionally morcellation is difficult because of the fibrous nature of the prostatic tissue, because visibility is not optimal or because extravasation of fluid has led to inability to adequately distend the bladder. In these cases, two options are available:

1. A catheter may be left in for a week and the patient brought back to theater for morcellation of tissue fragments. In our experience the prostate tissue softens remarkably over a few

days and is very easily morcellated at this later setting.
2. A small suprapubic cystotomy can be made and the tissue fragments removed through this incision. This small incision does not tend to add significantly to morbidity or to the recovery period.[26]

Morcellation can remove tissue at a rate of up to 10 g/min, although 4 g/min is the average, and any small remaining fragments are evacuated with a Toomey syringe. The size of the prostate gland does not seem to have an impact on the efficiency of morcellation.[27]

POSTOPERATIVE CARE At the conclusion of the case we insert a 2-way 20F Foley catheter with the balloon inflated to 20 mL with sterile water. The patient is usually given a 20 to 40 mg dose of intravenous frusemide in order to promote a diuresis. The vast majority of patients require no bladder irrigation. Catheters are removed the following day if hematuria is satisfactorily light, and the patients are discharged from hospital after they have had 2 or 3 successful voids.

RESULTS HoLEP has been compared with TURP for prostates in the 40 to 200 g range in a randomized trial with 12 months' follow-up.[28] Although the mean operative times for the HoLEP cases were longer than in the TURP cases, HoLEP patients on average had their catheters out earlier, spent less time in hospital, and suffered less adverse events than those in the TURP group. More prostate tissue was removed in the HoLEP group compared with the TURP group. The clinical outcomes at the 12-month follow-up mark were equivalent in both groups with respect to improvements in symptom scores and peak flow rates. Relief of urodynamic obstruction when measured by the reduction in detrusor pressure at maximal flow rate (PdetQmax) and passive urethral resistance relationship (Schafer grade) was significantly better in the HoLEP group, which is probably a reflection of the greater amount of tissue removed. The average morcellation rate in this study was 3.4 g/min.

Two other randomized trials have been performed comparing HoLEP with TURP.[29,30] Both trials confirm that morbidity is significantly less with HoLEP than TURP, and that efficacy in smaller glands is at least equivalent up to 12 months.

Prostate glands that are greater than 100 g in size can be safely enucleated without the risks of bleeding or glycine irrigant absorption that are present when TURP is performed on a prostate of this size. The initial series of 43 patients undergoing HoLEP with prostates greater than 100 g were studied at our institution.[23] The mean follow-up interval was 6 months. Twelve of the patients had urinary retention at the time of surgery. The mean laser time was 66.4 minutes (range 24–146 minutes). The mean morcellation time was 16.1 minutes (range 4–65 minutes). The average resected weight was 61.8 g of tissue (range 20–152 g).

Catheter time was an average of 19.7 hours (range 10–44 hours), and the average hospital stay was 28.4 hours (range 17–48 hours). Four of the patients required irrigation for hematuria and only 1 patient required recatheterization.

In a more recent review of 86 patients from the Indiana University unit undergoing HoLEP with a mean prostatic volume of 170 mL (range 125–309 mL) and an average preoperative AUA score of 19.6, Matlaga and colleagues reported a mean operative time of 128 minutes to resect an average of 140 g of tissue per case.[31] At a follow-up interval of 12 months, the average AUA score had decreased to 5.1.

Moody and Lingeman compared the outcomes of 10 patients who underwent open prostatectomy with 10 patients who underwent HoLEP.[32] All patients had a prostate gland size of greater than 100 g. There was no significant difference in operative times, but on average a greater weight of resected tissue was actually removed in the HoLEP group (151 vs 106 g, $p = .07$)! Patients in the HoLEP group on average spent less time in hospital (2.1 vs 6.1 days). All of the HoLEP patients left hospital without a catheter, whereas all of the open prostatectomy patients had a catheter in when they left hospital.

Kuntz and Lehrich have performed the first randomized trial of HoLEP versus open prostatectomy.[33] Although operative times were longer in the HoLEP group (138.4 vs 90 minutes), catheterization times and hospital stay were both significantly less in the HoLEP group (24 vs 144 hours and 48 vs 240 hours, respectively). At the 12-month follow-up, the clinical outcomes in both groups was equivalent. HoLEP is therefore as effective as open prostatectomy in matched patients, but is associated with much less perioperative morbidity.

A comparison of perioperative data and clinical outcomes in several HoLEP series is outlined in Table 70C-3.

Kuo and colleagues have reported on the morbidity associated with HoLEP in a series of 206 patients.[34] In this series the resected weight of prostatic tissue ranged from 3 to 376 grams (mean 68.2 g). The blood transfusion rate was 1%, compared with a rate of 3.9% for TURP. The transfusion rate doubles if the resected volume is larger than 45 mL or the resection time exceeds 90 minutes.[35] A comparison of various complications from several series is shown in Table 70C-4.

Smaller prostates have also been treated with HoLEP. In a recent randomized trial, Aho and colleagues compared HoLEP with HoNNI for prostates < 40 g.[36] Although HoLEP took longer to perform (7.0 vs 29.7 minutes), morbidity was no greater and urodynamic outcomes were significantly better in the HoLEP patients. All patients were treated on a day-stay basis.

FINANCIAL IMPLICATIONS AND THE LEARNING CURVE Although HoLEP offers serious competition to TURP and open prostatectomy for the surgical treatment of lower urinary tract symptoms secondary to benign prostatic hyperplasia, there are probably three perceived reasons, apart from marketing issues, that are preventing it becoming used more widely.

The first of these is the perception that acquiring the high-powered holmium laser requires considerable capital expenditure. Any cost-effectiveness analysis must take into account the cost savings of performing a procedure that incurs less time in hospital and less adverse events. As mentioned above, HoLRP has been found to be more cost effective than TURP in our institution if at least 93 cases are performed per year.[14] A cost-effectiveness analysis of HoLEP versus TURP is currently being undertaken at our institution and we expect that HoLEP will prove slightly more expensive than TURP on a per case basis (because of morcellator costs), but that cost savings may occur over the longer term because of what is likely to be a lower reoperation rate compared with TURP, given the larger proportion of the adenoma removed.

The holmium laser can also be used to perform lithotripsy, bladder tumor resection, and incision of ureteric and urethral strictures. These procedures account for around 25% of the use of the holmium laser at our institution and this helps to decrease the utilization cost of the holmium laser for BPH therapy.

Larner and colleagues have also investigated the feasibility of HoLEP as a day case procedure.[37] They reported a series of 38 patients where the mean stay after the procedure was 302 minutes. In each case a community nurse removed the catheter at the patient's home 48 hours after the procedure. Three men had to be admitted to hospital for complications.

The second major reason that surgeons are reluctant to take up HoLEP is because it is perceived to be more difficult than TURP. There is certainly a learning curve associated with HoLEP. This is because it requires a different technique to that of loop resection. El-Hakim and Elhilali found that after performing 20 procedures under supervision, a urology resident could reasonably be expected to achieve outcomes similar to that of a more experienced surgeon.[38] Our experience would tend to agree with this finding, and we have found that it is best to start with prostate gland sizes in the 40 to 50 g range. Anecdotally, the residents rotating through our unit who are relatively inexperienced in both TURP and HoLEP tend to find HoLEP easier to learn because of the improved visibility and the intuitive nature of dissecting along a surgical plane.

Hochreiter and colleagues have published the technique whereby the adenoma is enucleated until the lobe is attached by a narrow stalk to the capsule; they called this the "mushroom technique."[39] The electrocautery unit is then introduced, the irrigating solution changed to glycine, and the lobe is resected in a piecemeal fashion as in a TURP. This is essentially the HoLRP technique performed with the aid of electrocautery. It may have a place in units where a morcellator is not available, but it is unlikely that it affords any benefit over standard HoLEP and morcellation.

The third reason relates to procedural reimbursement, which varies country by country. HoLEP is rarely reimbursed to a level that reflects the time and skill required, and this becomes a further deterrent for many urologists.

CONCLUSIONS

Holmium laser prostatectomy has evolved into an enucleation technique, which is combined with transurethral morcellation of whole prostatic lobes. It is associated with less intraoperative

Table 70C-3 Perioperative Data and Clinical Outcomes from Some Recent HoLEP Series

Author	n	Average Prostate Size (mL)	Average Operating Time (min)	Average Resected Tissue Weight (g)	Mean Qmax (mL/s)	Mean AUA Score	Mean Postvoid Residual Volume (mL)
Kuntz and Lehrich[33]	60	114.6	135.9	83.9	Baseline: 3.8 6 months: 29.9	Baseline: 22.1 6 months: 2.4	Baseline: 280 6 months: 4.4
Hurle et al[27]	155	54 ± 33 (8–186)	87 ± 44 (19–260)	37 ± 26 (4–130)	Baseline: 9.3 ± 3.0 18 months: 21.9 ± 7	Baseline: 26.5 ± 5.3 18 months: 1.2 ± 1.0	–
Hochreiter et al[39]	156	38 (20–70)	62 (20–120)	–	Baseline: 8 24 months: 20	Baseline: 20 24 months: 3	Baseline: 190 24 months: 30
Moody and Lingeman[32]	10	> 100 (estimate)	197 ± 16	151 ± 14		Baseline: 19.6 6 months: 6	–
Kuo et al[26]	108	–	166.8 (75–376)	120.6 (75–376)		Baseline: 20.3 + 6.4 (6–35) 10 months (mean): 4.7 + 3.8 (0–16)	–
Elzayat et al[40]	552	83.7 (20–351)	86 (15–255)	52.1 (5–340)	200% improvement from baseline to 12 months	75% improvement from baseline to 12 months	–

Table 70C-4 Comparison of Perioperative and Postoperative Complications of Holmium Laser Enucleation of the Prostate

Series	No. of Patients	Clot Retention	Lower Urinary Tract Infection	Bladder Mucosal Injury	Bladder Perforation	Urethral Stricture	Bladder Neck Stenosis	Reoperation	Recatheterization	Blood Transfusion
Kuntz and Lehrich[33]	60	–	–	–	–	1 (1.7%)	–	6 (10%)	3 (5%)	0 (0%)
Hochreiter et al[39]	125	2 (2%)	10 (8%)	–	–	2 (2%)	–	–	–	–
Hurle et al[27]	155	0 (0%)	6 (3.8%)	13 (8.3%)	1 (0.6%)	5 (3.2%)	1 (0.6%)	3 (1.9%)	–	–
Kuo et al[34]	206	5 (2.4%)	–	4 (1.9%)	1 (0.5%)	5 (2.4%)	8 (3.9%)	–	16 (7.8%)	2 (1%)
Tan et al[28]	31	2 (6.5%)	–	–	–	1 (3.2%)	0 (0%)	0 (0%)	5 (16%)	0 (0%)

bleeding, shorter hospital stay, and shorter catheterization times compared with TURP. Although the operative times are generally longer than those seen in TURP, this is because, on average, more tissue is removed with the HoLEP procedure. Efficiency is actually superior! Clinical outcomes in terms of symptom relief and improvement in peak urinary flow rate are equivalent to TURP, but HoLEP has been shown to be more effective at relieving urodynamic obstruction. HoLEP is also able to deal with larger glands than TURP and is the endourologic equivalent of an open prostatectomy. HoLEP is cost effective and is teachable, with an average of 20 supervised cases being required to conquer the learning curve. HoLEP is emerging as a genuine and durable alternative to TURP and open prostatectomy for the surgical treatment of bladder outlet obstruction secondary to benign prostatic hyperplasia.

REFERENCES

1. Sayer J, Johnson DE, Price RE, Cromeens DM. Ureteral lithotripsy with the holmium:YAG laser. J Clin Laser Med Surg 1993;11:61–5.
2. Webb DR, Kockelburgh R, Johnson WF. The Versapulse holmium surgical laser in clinical urology: a pilot study. Minim Invasive Ther 1993;2:23–6.
3. Razvi HA, Chun SS, Denstedt JD, Sales JL. Soft-tissue applications of the holmium:YAG laser in urology. J Endourol 1995;9:387–90.
4. Kabalin JN. Holmium:YAG laser prostatectomy canine feasibility study. Lasers Surg Med 1996;18:221–4.
5. Gilling PJ, Cass CB, Malcolm A, Fraundorfer MR. Combination holmium and Nd:YAG laser ablation of the prostate: initial clinical experience. J Endourol 1995;9:151–3.
6. Gilling PJ, Cass CB, Cresswell MD, et al. The use of the holmium laser in the treatment of benign prostatic hyperplasia. J Endourol 1996;10:459–61.
7. Mottet N, Anidjar M, Bourdon O, et al. Randomized comparison of transurethral electroresection and holmium:YAG laser vaporization for symptomatic benign prostatic hyperplasia. J Endourol 1999;13:127–30.
8. Tan AHH, Gilling PJ, Kennett KM, et al. Long-term results of high-power holmium laser vaporization (ablation) of the prostate. BJU Int 2003;92:707–9.
9. Gilling PJ, Cass CB, Cresswell MD, Fraundorfer MR. Holmium laser resection of the prostate: preliminary results of a new method for the treatment of benign prostatic hyperplasia. Urology 1996;47:48–51.
10. Das A, Kennett KM, Sutton T, et al. Histologic effects of holmium:YAG laser resection versus transurethral resection of the prostate. J Endourol 2000;14:459–62.
11. Gilling PJ, Cass CB, Malcolm A, et al. Holmium laser resection of the prostate versus neodymium:yttrium-aluminium-garnet visual laser ablation of the prostate: a randomised prospective comparison of two techniques for laser prostatectomy. Urology 1998;51:573–7.
12. Gilling PJ, Kennett KM, Fraundorfer MR. Holmium laser resection v transurethral resection of the prostate: results of a randomised trial with 2 years of follow up. J Endourol 2000;14:757–60.
13. Westenberg A, Gilling P, Kennett K, et al. Holmium laser resection of the prostate versus transurethral resection of the prostate: results of a randomized trial with 4-year minimum long-term followup. J Urol 2004;172:616–9.
14. Fraundorfer MR, Gilling PJ, Kennett KM, Dunton NG. Holmium laser resection of the prostate is more cost effective than transurethral resection of the prostate: results of a randomized prospective study. Urology 2001;57:454–8.
15. Kabalin JN. Holmium:YAG laser prostatectomy: results of a U.S. pilot study. J Endourol 1996;10:453–7.
16. Matsuoka K, Iida S, Tomiyasu K, et al. Holmium laser resection of the prostate. J Endourol 1998;12:279–82.
17. Bukala B, Denstedt JD. Holmium:YAG laser resection of the prostate. J Endourol 1999;13:215–8.
18. Mackey MJ, Chilton CP, Gilling PJ, et al. The results of holmium laser resection of the prostate. Br J Urol 1998; 81:518–9.
19. Kitagawa M, Furuse H, Fukuta K, Aso Y. Holmium:YAG laser resection of the prostate versus visual laser ablation of the prostate and transurethral ultrasound-guided laser induced prostatectomy: a retrospective comparative study. Int J Urol 1998;5:152–6.
20. Gilling PJ, Kennett KM, Das AK, et al. Holmium laser enucleation of the prostate (HoLEP) combined with transurethral tissue morcellation: an update on the early clinical experience. J Endoruol 1998;12:457–79.
21. Fraundorfer MR, Gilling PJ. Holmium:YAG laser enucleation of the prostate combined with mechanical morcellation: preliminary results. Eur Urol 1998;33:69–72.
22. Moody JA, Lingeman JE. Holmium laser enucleation of the prostate with tissue morcellation: initial United States experience. J Endourol 2000;14:219–23.
23. Gilling PJ, Kennett KM, Fraundorfer MR. Holmium laser enucleation of the prostate for gland larger than 100g: an endourologic alternative to open prostatectomy. J Endourol 2000;14:529–31.
24. Gilling PJ, Cass CB, Cresswell MD, et al. The use of the holmium laser in the treatment of benign prostatic hyperplasia. J Endourol 1996;10:459–61.
25. Cornford PA, Biyani CS, Powell CS. Transurethral incision of the prostate using the holmium:YAG laser: a catheterless procedure. J Urol 1998;159:1229–31.
26. Kuo RL, Kim SC, Lingeman JE, et al. Holmium laser enucleation of prostate (HoLEP): the Methodist Hospital experience with greater than 75 gram enucleations. J Urol 2003;170:149–52.
27. Hurle R, Vavassori I, Piccinelli A, et al. Holmium laser enucleation of the prostate combined with mechanical morcellation in 155 patients with benign prostatic hyperplasia. Urology 2002;60:449–53.
28. Tan AH, Gilling PJ, Kennett KM, et al. A randomized trial comparing holmium laser enucleation of the prostate for the treatment of bladder outlet obstruction secondary to benign prostatic hyperplasia in large glands (40 to 200 grams). J Urol 2003;170(4 Pt 1):1270–4.
29. Montorsi F, Naspro R, Salonia A, et al. Holmium laser enucleation versus transurethral resection of the prostate: results from a 2-center, prospective, randomized trial in patients with obstructive benign prostatic hyperplasia. J Urol 2004;172(5 Pt 1):1926–9.
30. Kuntz RM, Ahyai S, Lehrich K, Fayad A. Transurethral holmium laser enucleation of the prostate versus transurethral electrocautery resection of the prostate: a randomized prospective trial in 200 patients. J Urol 2004; 172:1012–6.
31. Matlaga BR, Kim SC, Kuo RL, et al. Holmium laser enucleation of the prostate of > 125 mL. BJU Int 2006;97:81–4.
32. Moody JA, Lingeman JE. Holmium laser enucleation for prostate adenoma greater than 100gm: comparison to open prostatectomy. J Urol 2001;165:459–62.
33. Kuntz RM, Lehrich K. Transurethral holmium laser enucleation versus transvesical open enucleation for prostate adenoma greater than 100 gm: a randomized prospective trial of 120 patients. J Urol 2002;168(4 Pt 1):1465–9.
34. Kuo RL, Paterson RF, Siqueira TM Jr, et al. Holmium laser enucleation of the prostate: morbidity in a series of 206 patients. Urology 2003;62:59–63.
35. Mebust WK, Holtgrewe HL, Cockett ATK, Peters PC. Transurethral prostatectomy: immediate and postoperative complications. A cooperative study of 13 participating institutions evaluating 3,885 patients. J Urol 1989;141:243–7.
36. Aho TF, Gilling PJ, Kennett KM, et al. Holmium laser bladder neck incision versus holmium enucleation of the prostate as outpatient procedures for prostates less than 40 grams: a randomized trial. J Urol 2005;174:210–4.
37. Larner TRG, Agarwal D, Costello AJ. Day-case holmium laser enucleation of the prostate for gland volumes of < 60 mL: early experience. BJU Int 2003;91:61–4.
38. El-Hakim A, Elhilali MM. Laser enucleation of the prostate can be taught: the first learning experience. BJU Int 2002;90:863–9.
39. Hochreiter WW, Thalmann GN, Burkhard FC, Studer UE. Holmium laser enucleation of the prostate combined with electrocautery resection: the mushroom technique. J Urol 2002;168(4 Pt 1):1470–4.
40. Elzayat EA, Habib EI, Elhilali MM. Holmium laser enucleation of the prostate: a size-independent new "gold standard." Urology 2005;66:108–13.

Electrosurgery of the Prostate: Improvements in TURP—Treatments and Outcomes

Jonathan D. Schiff, MD

Alexis E. Te, MD

INTRODUCTION

Transurethral resection of the prostate (TURP) has been the gold standard to relieve the obstructive symptoms associated with benign prostatic hyperplasia (BPH). The TURP is a commonly performed urological procedure. However, its frequency is declining with the advent of medical and minimally invasive therapies. In 1993, 227,120 TURPs were performed in US hospitals according to data from the Agency for Health Care Research and Quality. By 2000, the number had fallen to 118,224.[1] Clearly, the alternatives to surgery are impacting patient and physician therapeutic decisions.

In spite of the array of microwave, laser, thermal and medical therapies for the management of the enlarged prostate, TURP continues to be the preferred procedure to remove prostate obstruction to urine flow. Additionally, technological and medical advances have improved the outcomes expected after TURP over its half decade history of use. This chapter will review some of the major improvements in instrumentation and patient care that have made the TURP a safer and still very effective procedure.

EQUIPMENT IMPROVEMENTS

Developments in lighting and cystoscopy, the combination electrical power and a high resistance loop, all culminated in the 1932 apparatus put together by McCarthy with an oblique lens system cystoscope with a tungsten loop for resection.[2] In the 1970s, significant advances were made with the development of the Hopkins rod-lens system and of fiberoptic lighting systems, both of which vastly improved visualization.[3] The use of video as an adjunct and teaching tool greatly facilitated the surgical education of urologists in the 1980s, and new developments in video cameras have helped with visualization. Improved electrical generators allowed for more precise and efficient application of cutting and coagulation power during the resection. Higher power generators allow for improved vaporization and appropriate coagulation and desiccation of tissue during the procedure. Finally, the development of the thick loop electrode allowed for increased coagulation while removing tissue (Figure 71A-1). These improvements have been enthusiastically adopted. The most recent signif-

icant improvements in TURP outcomes also come from improved pre-, intra-, and postoperative patient care.

ELECTROSURGICAL PRINCIPLES

Electrosurgery utilizes a radio frequency electric current to cut and fulgurate tissue.[4] The chosen frequency is very important in achieving the desired effect without complications. Current electrosurgical tools operate between 400,000 and 1 million Hz. The characteristics of the electric current, including waveform, peak voltage, and power, determine whether cutting or coagulation results from the application of the electrosurgical tool. A continuously alternating radio frequency sine wave delivers a high current and high power (Figure 71A-2). The continuous application of such a current generates enough heat to cut tissue, but the heat is dissipated so quickly that surrounding tissue is not coagulated and hemostasis is poor. Fulguration results from short bursts of high-voltage radio frequency sine waves with a pause between each burst. This pause allows for dispersal of energy, resulting in coagulation of surrounding tissue. While both waveforms deliver the same peak voltage, the discontinuous nature of the coagulation current results in less average power delivery.[4]

The generator chosen is very important in governing the current delivered during a procedure. The power generated is dependent on the current delivered by the generator and the tissue resistance. Modern generators have the ability to adjust the current supplied based on the tissue's resistance in order to keep power constant. Older generators did not have this capability. Generators also differed in their ability to deliver constant power. For example, the ValleyLabs Force 40 generator generates more power over a broader range of tissue resistance and is efficient in vaporization, while the older Force 2 was originally designed with limits on power delivery to prevent deep coagulation owing to persistent detected by increasing levels of tissue resistance in specific surgical applications. The FX generators now use microprocessors to monitor resistance changes and adjust power over a broader range of encountered resistance.[5,6]

Desiccation occurs by the slow process of driving water particles out of a cell. Steam and

bubbles, and the change in tissue color to a light brown are the visual effects of desiccation. Importantly, changes in tissue characteristics during an electrosurgical procedure affect the performance of the instruments. Tissue charring has an insulating effect, lowering the efficiency of vaporization. Persistent application of power to one area results in large-scale desiccation and then coagulation necrosis. Again, as charring occurs with persistent application, resistance increases and further desiccation requires increased power levels. Fulguration is a superficial charring of tissue. A coagulation waveform is sparked to the tissue surface and the heat is widely dispersed by long sparks and intermittent current application, thus the energy does not penetrate deeply and a superficial effect is obtained. The cells dry out quickly, but do not vaporize, thus a char effect is achieved, yielding a hemostatic effect. Cutting or vaporization results when the tissues are rapidly heated causing cells to explode into steam, thus leaving a void where the

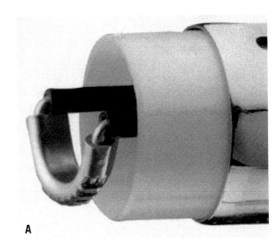

A

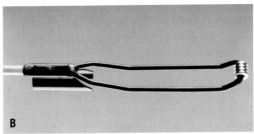

B

Figure 71A-1 Advances in TURP equipment. *A*, Thick loop electrode. *B*, Grooved roller ball electrode.

Figure 71A-2 Electrosurgical waveforms (radiofrequency sine waves) and demonstration of physiologic application of tissue vaporization. *A*, Cutting waveform. *B*, Coagulation waveform. *C*, Blend waveform. *D*, Demonstration of tissue vaporization, resistance, and dessication. *A* to *C* from Te AE and Kaplan SA.[35]

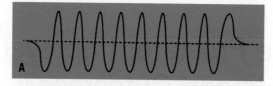

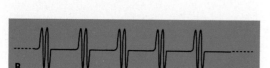

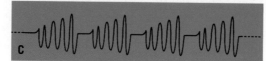

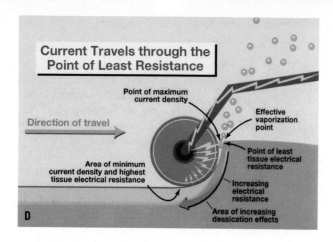

cells were previously present. A high current is delivered to the cutting loop. Surface area is extremely important such that a high current density must be delivered to affect a concentrated focus of power, which is instantly translated into heat at the surface. With the instantaneous delivery of high energy, the majority of energy is dissipated into steam and is carried away by an aqueous irrigant. This heat energy should not be conducted into deeper tissue, or it would desiccate these tissues.

INDICATIONS

Historically, the strict indications for TURP were (and continue to be) refractory urinary retention, azotemia secondary to bladder outlet obstruction, gross hematuria from the prostate, and bladder stone formation. While these symptoms underlie the possible severity of prostatic enlargement, the current armamentarium of medical and minimally invasive therapies forestalls the development of severe symptoms. Today, the most common indication for TURP today is relief of symptoms secondary to outlet obstruction. A large, single-center review found that 81% of patients who underwent TURP from 1991 through 1998 had lower urinary tract symptoms only. Urinary retention was the indication in 15% and recurrent prostatitis for 10%. Gross hematuria (4%) and bladder stones (6%) completed the five most common indications.[7]

This contrasts importantly with the transurethral prostatectomy outcomes study reported by Mebust and colleagues in 1989. This review included men from 13 operating centers from 1978 to 1987. They found that lower urinary symptoms alone were found in 30% of men at TURP, while 27% had recurrent retention and 12% suffered from recurrent prostatitis. A full 12% underwent TURP for hematuria and 3% for bladder stones.[8] In less than 10 years, the indications for TURP shifted dramatically, from predominantly correcting physiological derangements to improving symptoms and quality of life.

Shifting the indications more to quality of life concerns from medial necessity means that subjective decisions about quality of life must be made by patient and physician. The Agency for Health Care Policy and Research (AHCPR) created clinical guidelines for urologists and patients to help in the decision process.[9] Patients with minimal symptoms, including an AUA symptom score less than 7 or a urinary flow rate greater than 15 mL/s should be counseled to undergo watchful waiting. Men with higher symptom scores (greater than 7) or impaired urinary flow (flow rate less than 15 mL/s) with symptoms were considered for intervention, after discussing possible therapeutic benefits and risks. Importantly, and not surprisingly, those with the most severe preoperative voiding symptoms report the greatest postoperative improvements after TURP.[10]

PATIENT PREPARATION

The performance of a TURP can entail the potential loss of at least 1 unit of blood. Therefore, many patients undergo extensive preoperative medical evaluations. A complete blood count, chemistry profile, chest radiograph, and electrocardiogram are mandatory to evaluate general health and concomitant disease. Coagulation parameters should be checked prior to surgery and aspirin should be discontinued for 7 to 10 days preoperation.

Mebust and associates found an elevated risk of postoperative complications if serum creatinine level was greater than 1.5 mg/dL.[8] Any history of renal dysfunction or cardiac or pulmonary disease must be aggressively investigated prior to surgery, and physiologic function optimized as appropriate. Death from sepsis was the most common cause of mortality in AUA cooperative study, thus evaluation for possible urinary tract infection with a careful history and a urinalysis and culture is warranted prior to TURP.[8] Treatment with at least 7 days of a culture-specific antibiotic prior to TURP for any positive midstream culture is warranted. Patient with indwelling urinary catheters should be treated with preoperative antibiotics, even in the absence of symptoms of urinary infection, as many are chronically colonized.

Cystoscopy prior to TURP allows for the evaluation of prostate size, length, and configuration. Bladder stones or tumors may also be visualized, and better operative planning can be performed. Small bladder tumors can safely be resected at the time of TURP, but larger or more aggressive-appearing lesions should be removed at another time.

Prostates larger than 100 g based on cystoscopic and transrectal ultrasound measurements are generally managed in an alternate fashion with open procedures such as an open prostatectomy. Standard loop TURP should be reserved for glands up to 80 to 100 g, the upper limit of safe resection based on an operative time of 90 minutes.[11] Glands smaller than 30 g in younger men may be better managed with transurethral incision.

Prostate-specific antigen (PSA) levels should also be measured prior to TURP, and any result greater than normal should prompt a biopsy. Routine prostate cancer screening with PSA and biopsy preoperatively has decreased the number of men with cancer diagnosed on TURP specimen from 22% in the 1980s to 6.3% by the 1990s.[7,8] Men diagnosed with cancer and obstructive voiding symptoms often elect to undergo radical prostatectomy or radiotherapy with hormonal therapy, both of which can ameliorate symptoms.

Recent evidence suggests patients before TURP would benefit from pretreatment with finasteride. It has been reported that finasteride, a 5α-reductase inhibitor, can control and treat hematuria associated with prostatic enlargement.[12] Since this reported observation, trials have been undertaken to determine if finasteride taken prior to TURP helped to decrease blood loss. A recent randomized, placebo controlled trial compared blood loss for patients who received finasteride for 2 weeks pre-TURP with a placebo-treated group.[13] They found that mean blood loss and blood loss per gram of tissue resected was significantly less in the group treated with finasteride. While transfusion requirements were not reported, this study and other reports suggest that finasteride 2 weeks prior to TURP should be strongly considered for all patients.

INFORMED CONSENT

It is important to inform patients of the risks of TURP prior to undergoing the procedure. This aspect is important since the majority of men are operated electively primarily for symptomatic indications to improve their quality of life. Since medical necessity is not a priority in many, we as physicians are obligated to inform patients of the worst potential complications up front.

Death either during or immediately after the procedure is the most severe possible complication. Fortunately, mortality rates associated with TURP are low. The average in-hospital mortality for TURP has been approximately 0.4% over the past decade, without much change.[1] A recent single institution review of 520 TURPs found no mortalities either intra- or postoperatively.[7] The slightly older AUA cooperative study reported a 0.1% mortality rate in 3,385 patients.[8] Therefore, mortality should be mentioned, but is a rare occurrence.

Blood transfusions are not infrequently required during or immediately following TURP. Older studies reported transfusion rates of 6%, and more recent series found only a 0.4% transfusion rate.[7,8] However, the average gland size in patients requiring transfusion was larger, and those patients with glands larger than 45 g should specifically be counseled that their transfusion risk approaches 10%.[8]

Cardiac complications should also be discussed. Myocardial dysrhythmia occurs more commonly in 1 to 2% of patients, but acute myocardial infarction occurs in only 0.1 to 0.2% of patients. Postoperative risks are predominantly infection related with a frequency of 2 to 3% reported. Failure to void after catheter removal occurs in 2 to 7% of patients, and can be predicted based on preoperative history and urodynamic studies. Patients at risk should be counseled appropriately.

Finally, the risk of dilutional hyponatremia or "TUR syndrome" associated with the TURP procedure must be considered. This complication is due to absorption of the hypotonic nonionic glycine irrigation fluid required for the procedure. Clinically significant absorption is associated with larger prostates and longer resection times as reported in the AUA cooperative study.[8] This syndrome, associated with absorption of hypotonic irrigation fluid, occurs in 0.8 to 2% of patients. Often, the syndrome can be limited/prevented by intraoperative use of diuretics, if capsular perforation is noted, by using saline as the intravenous fluid and limiting resection time.

PREOPERATIVE PREPARATION

The patient is brought into the operating room and positioned in the dorsal lithotomy position in preparation for TURP. Anesthesia is made in consultation with the anesthesiologist and based on patient preference and medical history. Two studies evaluated the difference in outcomes between TURP performed under epidural or spinal anesthesia compared with general anesthesia. Although these studies found no difference in blood loss, postoperative morbidity, or mortality,[14,15] a theoretical advantage exists to monitoring patients for mental status changes under a spinal anesthetic for an early sign of TUR syndrome. Therefore, in the absence of any spinal or neuromuscular problems with the patient, the selection of general or spinal/epidural anesthesia is a risk/benefit discussion involving the patient, surgeon, and anesthesiologist.

Preoperative antibiotic use has become the standard of care prior to TURP. Patients without a history of positive urinary culture or symptoms preoperatively can be given a single parenteral dose of a first-generation cephalosporin. Several studies have evaluated the use of antibiotics preoperatively, and the majority support the use of a single parenteral dose.[14,16–18] Those with symptoms and a positive culture should be treated with culture-specific antibiotics prior to undergoing TURP. Penicillin-allergic patients can receive either gentamicin alone or a DNA gyrase inhibitor class antibiotic such as ciprofloxacin. If the patient has any prosthetic devices or mitral valve prolapse, the use of ampicillin and gentamicin should be considered. All patients should be given a single parenteral dose of antibiotics prior to TURP. Many authors recommend continuing at least oral antibiotic therapy until after the Foley catheter is removed.[3]

Once the appropriate anesthesia is induced, the patient should be positioned in the dorsal lithotomy position with the knees bent to approximately 70 degrees. The buttocks should be slightly off the operating table. Adequate padding must be placed underneath the patient's backside, where most of the pressure is exerted, and at the point where the lateral calf may contact the leg supports. Compression stockings should be placed. Prior to the onset of surgery, the operating physician and assistant should perform a rectal examination on all patients. The penis and perineum are then scrubbed with a germicidal soap solution and betadine for 5 minutes. Next, an O'Connor rectal drape is placed to facilitate sterile access to the rectum for prostatic manipulation during the procedure as needed. The patient is then draped in a sterile fashion.

INSTRUMENTATION

Historically, water was used as the irrigant fluid during a TURP. However, since water is hypotonic, any absorption causes rapid hemolysis in addition to other electrolyte imbalances. While water is still less expensive than other irrigants, the majority of urologists use a solution with a higher osmolality, such as 1.5% glycine or mannitol, as the irrigant. Although these fluids still can cause electrolyte disturbances if absorbed into the blood stream, they do not cause hemolysis with an osmolality of approximately 200 mOsm/L.[3]

We prefer to begin with a 26 French (F) resectoscope. This instrument can be passed either blindly or with a visual obturator. Our preference is to pass the scope under visual guidance, or to begin with the Timberlake obturator in order to gently dilate the fossa navicularis and then switch to the visual obturator once the scope is into the bulbar urethra. If the meatus or distal urethra is too narrow, male urethral sounds are often adequate to calibrate the urethra up to 30F. Calibrating to 30F will usually allow for accommodation of a 26F resectoscope sheath. Occasionally, the distal urethra cannot be calibrated adequately and an internal urethrotomy is required, or a 24F resectoscope is used. An internal urethrotomy can be performed using either an Otis urethrotome or a curved No. 12 scalpel blade to make a dorsal urethrotomy.[3] If the calibration is still inadequate or the patient has a penile prosthesis, a perineal urethrostomy can be temporarily created to perform the TURP (Figure 71A-3).[11]

An important choice for resectoscope sheaths is whether to use continuous flow or a standard sheath. The advantage of continuous flow is increased speed, as one does not have to intermittently stop to empty the bladder. Another advantage is that the pressure in the bladder and prostate is constant at filling, and the bladder should not become overdistended during the procedure. However, several important considerations exist with the use of continuous flow. The prostatic fossa is continuously dilated during the procedure, which can lead to a false sense of progress to the less experienced. The dynamic widening and then falling back with emptying that is seen using the standard resectoscope is absent with continuous flow. To overcome this problem and to gauge progress, one can intermittently stop inflow with the continuous flow sheath and allow the prostate gland to "fall back" in and determine the adequacy of resection. Another problem can occur when bleeding is encountered. Since the continuous flow sheath has in and out flow ports, the outflow may not be as brisk since it may be blocked by a clot and debris. When managing brisk bleeding, limiting outflow will increase invesical pressure and decrease bleeding. However, the risk of fluid absorption increases and one must be cognizant of this risk during the procedure. With the continuous flow scope, suction is utilized by some to increase outflow. Caution is required when utilizing this technique, since outflow with limited inflow may result in a bladder collapse with risk of bladder perforation during resection. Use of gravity drainage decreases this risk of perforation. With the proper foreknowledge of these drawbacks, they can easily be overcome. Our current preference is to use the continuous flow sheath under gravity drainage.

Another important choice is the use of the thick versus the thin loop electrode. The thin loop allows for efficient vaporization and better control of cutting during the procedure. The electrical cutting current is not dissipated over as large a surface area, so the cutting current is applied over a thinner front to the tissue. This high current density allows efficient vaporization and improved ease of cutting. The thick loop has a larger surface area and disperses the energy over a broad area. This causes current density to be less and results in coagulation and desiccation to occur in the trailing edge after the initial leading edge cut is made. This improved hemostasis. If resistance is significant while cutting, a higher power level is required to increase leading edge vaporization efficiency for cutting with a thick loop. Clearly, choice of loop is a surgeon's preference, and is dictated by one's experience with the technique and comfort with the technology.

OPERATIVE PROCEDURE

After the instruments are chosen and the patient is positioned and anesthetized, the case begins. A standard cystoscopy is performed with a 30-degree lens. The relevant anatomy is identified, including the ureteral orifices, the bladder neck, the location of the verumontanum, and external urethral sphincter. We also evaluate the height of the bladder neck and the angle at which the scope is placed to navigate this landmark. The bladder is also visually inspected in its entirety. Next, the resectoscope sheath is passed with either the Timberlake or visual obturator, or some combination. After the resectoscope sheath is in place, the resectosope is passed and the dimensions of the prostate are again inspected. We take approximate measurements of the dimensions of the prostate in relation to the ureteral orifices and verumontanum and external sphincter with the loop out to roughly gauge the extent of resection (see Figure 71A-3). The presence of a large median lobe or a high bladder neck can impair the pace of resection and the visualization of landmarks. If this situation is encountered, we begin by carefully resecting the bladder neck from 5 o'clock to 7 o'clock.

The most important principle in performing a TURP is to formulate a plan and then proceed in an orderly, stepwise fashion. Most urologists prefer to resect ventral adenomatous tissue first, which allows the dorsal adenoma tissue to drop down. Again, the presence of a high bladder neck or median lobe may necessitate partial resection of the floor first to improve irrigant flow by creating a channel for fluid and adenoma chips to flow through. The initial procedure described by Nesbit and then reviewed and revised by Holtgrewe is the method most commonly applied.[19,20] The resectoscope is positioned in the midprostatic fossa, and the loop is extended out to ensure adequate clearance of the bladder neck.

Resection begins at approximately 1 o'clock and is continued in a clockwise fashion to 6 o'clock (see Figure 71A-3). The depth of resection should be approximately far down enough to expose the fibers of the prostatic capsule around the bladder neck. Once this area is adequately resected, attention is turned to the 11-o'clock position, and a similar resection is carried out counterclockwise to the 6-o'clock position. Hemostasis should be achieved at each area prior to advancing to the next point area of resection. The posterior aspect of the vesical neck is the most frequent area at which the trigone is undermined. This results in extravasation of irrigant, and may lead to TUR syndrome development. If a narrow bladder neck results at the end of the procedure, the 6-o'clock position can be incised to decrease the risk of bladder neck contracture.[21]

After the bladder neck has been resected, the prostate adenoma tissue is debulked in quadrants.

The verumontanum is visualized, and the resectoscope is placed just proximal to this important landmark. Resection begins at the 12-o'clock position, and is carried around to the 3-o'clock position. We prefer to take long, deep swipes, often angling the scope contralaterally to get adequate depth of the resection. The fibrous capsule

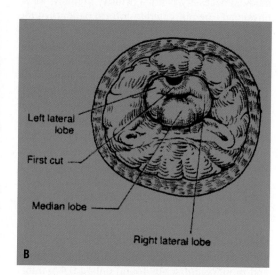

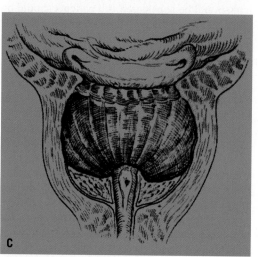

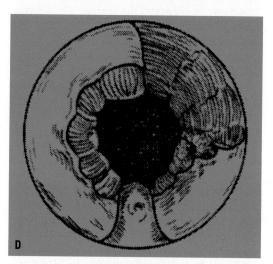

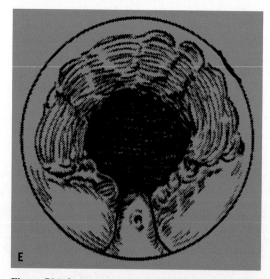

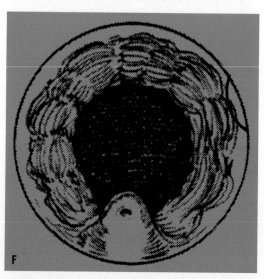

Figure 71A-3 Anatomic overview of the prostate and general TURP strategy. *A*, Lateral view of prostate prior to resection. *B*, Coronal view of prostate prior to resection. *C*, Schematic of prostate after TURP completion. *D*, Resection begins at left lateral lobe superiorly (12 o'clock to 6 o'clock clockwise). *E*, Resection continued at right lateral lobe (12 o'clock to 6 o'clock counterclockwise). *F*, Resection completed at base and apex. From Santarosa et al[36] (Figures 37-1 and 37-2).

can be visualized after resection to assess completeness. Prostatic stones, which usually form between the capsule and the hypertrophied tissue, usually signal that the appropriate depth has been reached. Pulsatile arterial bleeding often is encountered near the capsule and at the bladder neck, as the prostate blood supply arises peripherally. These bleeders are very distinct from the venous oozing that is encountered first. Arteries should be cauterized immediately as the blood loss obscures the view and prevents precise resection. Venous bleeding may be dealt with later, but should be controlled if significant. The length of resection should be premeasured, with the resection swipes falling just short of the verumontanum. After the 12-o'clock to 3-o'clock quadrant is completely resected, the remainder to 6 o'clock is resected in a similar fashion, thus completing resection of the left lobe of the prostate. Hemostasis is then achieved, and then the right lobe is resected in a similar fashion from 12 o'clock counterclockwise to 6 o'clock.

Apical tissue that is just proximal to the external sphincter may remain and may extend distal to the veru.[22] Resection in this area carries an increased risk of incontinence, and discretion is utilized. The verumontanum must not be cut or coagulated, as this can result in painful ejaculation secondary to ejaculatory duct obstruction. Care must be taken not to injure the sphincter during resection because this may cause postoperative urinary incontinence. The tissue is carefully resected with short sweeps. At the completion of resection, the bladder should easily be visible with the resectoscope in at the level of the verumontanum.

Once resection is completed, an Ellick evacuator is used to remove all adenoma chips from the bladder. All chips must be removed, as any left in the bladder may later occlude the urinary catheter, causing obstruction, bladder spasms, and increased postoperative hemorrhage. After several evacuations with the Ellick, the resectoscope is then replaced and the bladder visually inspected. Any remaining chips can be snared with the loop and removed, with care taken to inspect all bladder diverticula if present. Final hemostasis is achieved with careful coagulation of any bleeding points. The resectoscope is then removed with a final visual inspection of the bladder, prostatic fossa, and urethra. The bladder should be left full, and overly aggressive irrigation is not needed, as this can disrupt clots that formed and increase bleeding.

We typically leave a 24F 3-way Foley catheter with 30 to 60 cc in the balloon at a slow rate of continuous bladder irrigation for 12 to 24 hours. More fluid can be placed in the balloon if a larger resection has been performed, but more volume often leads to increased number and severity of bladder spasms. If persistent bleeding results that does not readily clear with slow irrigation, gentle traction is placed on the catheter until the irrigant is clear. Traction can be placed with as gentle a maneuver as placing the hub of the Foley in one of a variety of catheter-securing devices on the leg or with the more traditional use of cloth tape on the calf. We

believe that the minimum amount of traction to clear the irrigant of gross bleeding is the best used. Traction may also cause involuntary contractions that may contribute to bleeding. Short-acting antimuscurinic agents may be considered.

If vigorous bleeding continues despite irrigation and gentle traction, arterial bleeding may be the cause. Prior to leaving the operating room, the resectoscope should be reintroduced, and the prostatic fossa and bladder neck should be inspected for arterial bleeding.

POSTOPERATIVE CARE

Immediately post-TURP, the patient is brought to the recovery room where an electrolyte panel and complete blood counts are sent. The patients are monitored until the lab results return and the spinal/epidural anesthesia has begun to wear off. Unless capsular perforation occurred, a large venous sinus entered or the bladder neck was undermined, electrolyte abnormalities are uncommon.

Any electrolyte imbalances are corrected. If hyponatremia results, but the patient is clinically stable, intravenous normal saline and fluid restriction often slowly corrects any problem. If the patient evidences any change in mental status or has other signs of clinical deterioriation, a loop diuretic such as furosemide can be given as well. We reserve the use of hypertonic saline for serious hyponatremia with a serum sodium less than 120 or if the patient becomes obtunded and has seizure activity. The patient should be monitored in a critical care setting until symptoms resolve and the sodium level begins to correct in this case. Care should be taken not to correct the electrolyte abnormality too rapidly as this can result in cerebral damage and central pontine myelinolysis. Usually, we aim to replace half the deficit in the first 8 to 16 hours, with the remainder corrected over the ensuing 24 hours. Contemporary series report a 0.8 to 2% incidence of TUR syndrome.[7,8]

Blood counts are also checked immediately postoperatively, and transfusions are very judiciously given. We use a hematocrit cutoff of 28 to 30% in a healthy, asymptomatic patient before considering a transfusion. Patients with a history of coronary or cerebral vascular disease or with any ischemic symptoms should be transfused promptly and considered for intensive monitoring. Most contemporary series have low rates of blood transfusion after TURP, with rates from 0.4 to 6.4% in the two most recent, large scale series.[7,8]

More routine postoperative care consists of monitoring the patient for bladder spasms, which frequently occur, especially with aggressive cauterization or resection at the bladder neck. We often prescribe antimuscarinic agents post-TURP to prevent these spasms. Vigilance is also required as the Foley balloon, in spite of being overinflated, can slip into the prostatic fossa. This should be suspected if the drainage ceases, the patient becomes acutely distended, and manual irrigation is difficult. At this point, the balloon should be taken down, and the catheter should be advanced into the bladder. Overfilling the balloon can also

cause ureteral orifice obstruction, especially if traction is maintained, and this would manifest as flank discomfort similar to acute renal colic.

Patients are given an oral antibiotic, usually trimethoprim-sulfamethoxazole or flouroquinolone until the Foley catheter is removed. We ambulate patients as soon as possible after traction has been removed. A regular diet is given as soon as the patient has fully recovered from anesthesia, and stool softeners are used immediately as well. Since resection is very close to the rectum, we do not allow any rectal suppositories or examinations in the immediate postoperative period.

Traction is usually released by 12 to 24 hours postoperation, and continuous bladder irrigation is slowly weaned off over the next 12 to 24 hours. If the effluent is clear after irrigation is off for 3 to 5 hours, the catheter can be discontinued. Our patients are usually given a trial of voiding on postoperative day 2, and if they void, they are discharged home with stool softeners and antimuscarinics as needed. The average length of stay in US hospitals after TURP is reported as 3.2 days.[1]

RESULTS

Nearly all of the published studies evaluating TURP find this to be a highly effective procedure in improving urinary flow rates and decreasing symptom scores. The AHCPR panel guideline meta-analysis found that patients had an 88% chance of symptomatic improvement after TURP.[9] A recent large review of 520 TURPs performed at the Naval Medical Center in San Diego found an average improvement in International Prostate Symptom Score from 23.8 preoperatively to 6.4 postoperatively.[7] Other recent studies, often comparing TURP with another minimally invasive modality, found average improvements in IPSS scores ranging from 13.6 to 19 at 6 to 24 months postoperation.[23–26] These studies also document large average improvements in flow rate (Q_{max} mL/s) of 5.7 mL/s at 12 months[23] and 9.1 mL/s to 10.7 mL/s at 24 months.[25,26]

An interesting finding in most contemporary series is that the mean weight of resection specimens has declined compared with older series. The landmark AUA study reported an average specimen weight of 22 g, while a more recent series by Borboroglu and colleagues reported a mean specimen weight of 18.8 g.[7,8] Another recently reported series found an average resection weight of 15 g of tissue.[27] Although this trend is not completely linear, especially outside the United States, the suggestion is that TURPs done in more recent series are removing less tissue.[28,29] In these studies, the majority of patients are treated for symptomatic relief rather than absolute medical indications, and this may temper the aggressiveness of resection.

Quality of life is now a major factor in the consideration of outcomes after any surgery, especially in TURP, where recent reports find the overwhelming majority of men choosing this operation for symptomatic relief and not for absolute medical indications. Our own experience finds that greater than 90% of men are satisfied with the outcomes of TURP. Others have found substantial and significant improvements in quality of life scores after TURP. Quality of life improved by an average of 3.42 at 12 months,[23,27] and an average of 2.91 units at 24 months.[5,26] Therefore, by either IPSS, quality of life, or Qmax data, TURP is an extremely effective procedure in reducing symptoms and improving quality of life. TURP is still considered, and rightly so, the gold standard in minimally invasive treatment of BPH.

COMPLICATIONS

Intraoperative complications occur infrequently. Two recent large series of TURP, one reviewing a large experience in the 1980s and the other covering the 1990s, found intraoperative complication rates of 6.0% and 2.5%, respectively.[7,8] The most common intraoperative complications reported include transfusion requirement in 0.2 to 2%, which decreased significantly in the more modern series; irrigant extravasation leading to TUR syndrome in 0.8 to 2% of cases; and myocardial arrhythmia in 1.1 to 1.3% of patients. Importantly, no intraoperative deaths were reported in either series.

Intraoperative arterial bleeding may also occur, usually manifesting as jets of blood with pulsatile flow. This should be controlled with coagulation, as loss of visualization can quickly occur with arterial bleeding. Transfusion requirement was found to be related to prostate size and operative time in the AUA cooperative study.[8] Glands over 45 g and resections lasting more than 90 minutes were both associated with higher rates of transfusion. These two risk factors were also found to be associated with an increased likelihood of suffering from TUR syndrome. Both complications require symptomatic treatment as described in the preceding section on postoperative care, and vigilance as to their potential occurrence, especially in the presence of large glands and extended operative times.

Irrigant extravasation occurs with perforation of the prostatic capsule. The symptoms associated with this problem include restlessness, nausea, vomiting, and abdominal or lower back pain. If extravasation is suspected, hemostasis should be achieved and the procedure terminated promptly. Catheter drainage and observation are usually sufficient, especially when recognized early. Bladder perforation may also occur with overdistension of the bladder with irrigant (especially if a concomitant small transurethral resection of the bladder [TURB] was performed) or from injury with the resecting loop. Signs include lower abdominal rigidity, and if an intraperitoneal perforation occurred, shoulder pain from intraperitoneal and diaphragmatic irritation, with abdominal pain, nausea, and possible vomiting. Again, prompt termination, catheter drainage (without bladder irrigation) and close observation usually suffice. A cystogram can be performed on the cystoscopy table with fluoroscopy to determine whether any perforation is intra- or extraperitoneal. Large

intraperitoneal perforations may require open cystotomy repair, especially if they fail to improve with serial observation.

Mortality both intra- and postoperative are not common after TURP. The AUA cooperative study found a 0.2% mortality in 3,885 patients, with no intraoperative deaths.[8] A more contemporary series of 520 TURPs performed at a single institution had no deaths intraoperatively or at 30 days.[7] Importantly, mortality has declined with time, having been 2.5% in a large series from the 1950s and 1.3% reported in a large series from the 1960s to 1970s.[30,31] Other contemporary series report mortality rates comparable with the more recent series between 0 and 1.3%, with the Healthcare Cost and Utilization Project (HCUP) database reporting a 0.4% mortality reported for all TURPs in the year 2000.[1] Regarding mortality, TURP appears to be a very safe procedure.

A variety of other postoperative complications may occur. The risk of failing a trial of void and requiring a catheter on discharge was 6.5% and 2.4% in the AUA cooperative study.[8] A more recent series found 7.1% of patients were discharged home with catheters.[7] This difference is most likely due to changes in hospitalization patterns, where patients who failed a trial of void in the contemporary series were immediately discharged home with a catheter for repeat voiding trials in an outpatient setting. In the earlier series with longer mean length of stay, patients who failed trials of voiding were often kept in the hospital for repeat voiding trials prior to discharge. Failing a trial of void is often due to bladder hypotonicity, which can be documented with cystometrogram usually done preoperatively. Extended catheter drainage for up to 7 to 10 days often improves this condition. Some urologists have tried bethanecol chloride to hasten the return of bladder contractility, but we prefer more catheter drainage and patience. Residual adenoma may also be the culprit, especially if the procedure was prematurely terminated from a complication. The only cure for this problem is to re-resect the tissue.

Postoperative bleeding can occur, requiring clot evacuation and continued irrigation. Bleeding is often precipitated by straining to defecate or coughing, both of which can be avoided with the use of stool softeners or cough suppressants (non-narcotic). If bleeding does occur with clots, clot evacuation and possible cystoscopy with evacuation may be required to stop bleeding. In our experience, a discrete bleeding site is rarely found.

Urinary tract infections have been reported in 2.1 to 2.3% of patients in the early postoperative period.[7,8] For this reason, we leave patients on oral antibiotics until the catheter is removed and the patient has a successful trial of void. If the patient is recatheterized after failing the voiding trial, a prescription for antibiotics is given for the patient to begin 24 hours prior to and for 48 hours after the next trial of void is planned.

Other more severe late post-TURP complications include bladder neck contractures, ure-

theral strictures, and late postoperative bleeding. Bladder neck contractures were reported in 1.9 to 2.1% of patients in two large studies.[7,8] The usual presentation is of a patient who initially had a strong stream followed by progressive reduction with increasing urinary frequency and nocturia. Treatment consists of bladder neck incision with a Collings knife, cold urethrotome, or resectoscope incision of the bladder neck, which can be done at 12 o'clock. Urethral strictures were found in 1% and 3.7% of patients, respectively, and are usually due to resectoscope trauma.[7,8] Treatment consists of uretheral dilation or visual urethrotomy. Late postoperative bleeding occurs in less than 2% of patients, and is usually managed conservatively with irrigation, and recent reports suggest that finasteride may play an important role.[12]

Other serious complications associated with TURP include urinary incontinence and impotence. Incontinence results from damage to the external sphincter, but can also occur from detrusor contractions and instability, or if residual adenoma tissue blocks the external sphincter. Early incontinence associated with detrusor irritability and spasms resolves with time, and is treated with antimuscurinic medications. Kegel exercises can help strengthen the external sphincter, but results vary with severity of damage. Collagen injections may be needed in patients with severe sphincter damage. A comparison of patients with BPH who were treated with either watchful waiting or TURP found no difference in urinary incontinence or impotence between the groups.[32]

Impotence was also thought to occur as a result of TURP, being reported in up to 4% of patients post-TURP.[8] The close relationship of the cavernous nerves to the floor of the prostate highlights the potential for injury. However, more recent literature does not support a causal link between TURP and impotence, and some studies even suggest that TURP, by improving quality of life in patients with severe symptoms from BPH, may improve erectile function.[33,34] Therefore, in the absence of severe complications and perforation, TURP does not worsen and may improve sexual function.

CONCLUSION

TURP is the gold standard for the treatment of lower urinary tract symptoms from BPH. Advances in instrumentation and patient care have made the performance of TURP safer over the past two decades, without lessening the therapeutic benefit. This is especially important because the indications for TURP shifted from being predominantly medical necessity to quality of life issues over the past two decades. Recent use of finasteride prior to TURP will likely further reduce morbidity of this procedure. Still, the potential for complications and even death postoperatively exists, so all patients must be carefully counseled about the risks of the procedure as well as the benefits. Care must be taken, especially in patients with larger glands undergoing TURP, to minimize potential problems. In experienced hands, TURP remains an excellent choice for the alleviation of moderate to severe symptoms of BPH, and for patients who have failed medical therapy. Further innovations in instrumentation and medical care will undoubtedly make this procedure safer and possibly even more effective.

REFERENCES

1. Agency for Healthcare Research and Quality. Healthcare Cost and Utilization Project, 2003. HCUPnet, available at: http://hcup.ahrq.gov/HCUPnet.asp (accessed April 13, 2006).
2. Nesbit RM. A history of transurethral prostatectomy. Rev Mex Urol 1975;35:349–62.
3. Fitzpatrick JM, Mebust WK. Minimally invasive and endoscopic management of benign prostatic hyperplasia. In: Walsh PC, Retik AB, Vaughan ED, et al, editors. Campbell's urology. Vol. 2. 8th ed. Philadelphia: Saunders; 2003. p. 1379–422.
4. Kramolowsky EV, Tucker RD. The urological application of electrosurgery. J Urol 1991;146:669–74.
5. ValleyLab, editor. ValleyLab Force 40 instruction manual. Colorado: ValleyLab Inc.; 1993.
6. ValleyLab, editor. ValleyLab Force 2 instruction manual. Colorado: ValleyLab Inc.; 1985. Vol. 7.1–7.11.
7. Borboroglu PG, Kane CJ, Ward JF, et al. Immediate and postoperative complications of transurethral prostatectomy in the 1990s. J Urol 1999;162:1307–10.
8. Mebust WK, Holtgrewe HL, Cockett AT, Peters PC. Transurethral prostatectomy: immediate and postoperative complication. A cooperative study of 13 participating institutions evaluating 3,885 patients. J Urol 1989;141:243–7.
9. McConell J, Barry M, Bruskewitz R, et al. Benign prostatic hyperplasia: diagnosis and treatment. Clinical practice guidelines no. 8. AHCPR Publication 94-0582. AFH Services, editor. Rockville, MD: US Department of Health and Human Services; 1994.
10. Greene LF, Holcumb GR. Transurethral resection in special situations. In: Greene LF, Segura JW, editors. Transurethral surgery. Philadelphia: WB Saunders; 1979. p. 216.
11. Santarosa RP, Te AE, Kaplan SA. Transurethral resection, incision, and ablation of the prostate. In: Graham SDJ, editor. Glenn's urologic surgery. 5th ed. Philadelphia: Lippincott-Raven; 1998. p. 921–31.
12. Puchner PJ, Miller MI. The effects of finasteride on hematuria associated with benign prostatic hyperplasia: a preliminary report. J Urol 1995;154:1779–82.
13. Donohue JF, Sharma H, Abraham R, et al. Transurethral prostate resection and bleeding: a randomized, placebo controlled trial of the role of finasteride for decreasing operative blood loss. J Urol 2002;168:2024–6.
14. Nielsen OS, Maigaard S, Frimodt-Moller N, Madsen PO. Prophylactic antibiotics in transurethral prostatectomy. J Urol 1981;126:60–2.
15. McGowan SW, Smith GF. Anesthesia for transurethral prostatectomy. A comparison of spinal intradural anesthesia with two methods of general anesthesia. Anaesthesia 1980;35:847–53.
16. Gibbons RP, Stark RA, Correa RJ Jr, et al. The prophylactic use—or misuse—of antibiotics in transurethral prostatectomy. J Urol 1978;119:381–3.
17. Leroy A, Humbert G, Fillastre JP, Grise P. Penetration of lomefloxacin into prostatic tissue. Am J Med 1992;92:12S–14S.
18. Viitanen J, Talja M, Jussila M, et al. Transurethral resection of the prostate and related topics: randomized controlled study of chemoprophylaxis in transurethral prostatectomy. J Urol 1993;150:1715–7.
19. Nesbit RM. Transurethral prostatectomy. Springfield, IL: Charles C. Thomas; 1943.
20. Holtgrewe L. Transurethral prostatectomy. Urol Clin North Am 1995;22:357–68.
21. Kulb TP, Kainer M, Lingeman JE, Foster RS. Prevention of post-prostatectomy vesical neck contracture by prophylactic vesical neck incision. J Urol 1987;137:230–1.
22. Shah PJ, Abrams PH, Feneley RC, Green NA. The influence of prostatic anatomy on the differing results of prostatectomy according to the surgical approach. Br J Urol 1979;51:549–51.
23. Wagrell L, Schelin S, Nordling J, et al. Feedback microwave thermotherapy versus TURP for clinical BPH—a randomized, controlled multicenter study. Urology 2002; 60:292–9.
24. Norby B, Nielsen HV, Frimodt-Moller PC. Cost-effectiveness of new treatments for benign prostatic hyperplasia: results of a randomized trial comparing the short-term cost-effectiveness of transurethral interstitial laser coagulation of the prostate, transurethral microwave thermotherapy and standard transurethral resection or incision of the prostate. Scand J Urol Nephrol 2002;36:286–95.
25. Tkocz M, Prajsner A. Comparison of long-term results of transurethral incison of the prostate with transurethral resection of the prostate, in patients with benign prostatic hypertrophy. Neurourol Urodyn 2002;21:112–6.
26. Hindley RG, Mostafid AH, Brierly RD, et al. The 2-year symptomatic and urodynamic results of a prospective randomized trial of interstitial radiofrequency therapy vs transurethral resection of the prostate. BJU Int 2001;88: 217–20.
27. Ekengren J, Haendler L, Hahn RG. Clinical outcome 1 year after transurethral vaporization and resection of the prostate. Urology 2000;55:231–5.
28. Estey EP, Mador DR, McPhee MS. A review of 1486 transurethral resections of the prostate in a teaching hospital. Can J Surg 1993;36:37–40.
29. Horninger W, Unterlechner HJ, Strasser H, Bartsch G. Transurethral prostatectomy: mortality and morbidity. Prostate 1996;28:195–200.
30. Holtgrewe HL, Valk WL. Factors influencing mortality and morbidity of transurethral prostatectomy: a study of 2,015 cases. J Urol 1962;87:450–9.
31. Melchior J, Valk WL, Foret JD, Mebust WK. Transurethral prostatectomy: computerized analysis of 2,223 consecutive cases. J Urol 1974;112:634–42.
32. Wasson JH, Reda DJ, Bruskewitz RC, et al. A comparison of transurethral surgery with watchful waiting for moderate symptoms of benign prostatic hyperplasia. N Engl J Med 1995;32:75–9.
33. Soderdahl DW, Knight RW, Hansberry KL. Erectile dysfunction following transurethral resection of the prostate. J Urol 1996;156:1354–6.
34. Brookes ST, Donovan JL, Peters RJ, et al. Sexual dysfunction in men after treatment for lower urinary tract symptoms: evidence from a randomised controlled trial. BMJ 2002;324:1059–61.
35. Te AE, Kaplan SA. Electrovaporization of the prostate. Curr Opin Urol 1996;6:2–9, specifically p. 3.
36. Santarosa RP, Te AE, Kaplan SA. Transurethral resection of the prostate. In: Krane R, Siroky M, Fitzpatrick J, editors. Operative urology. New York: Churchill Livingstone; 2000. p. 248–9.

Electrosurgery of the Prostate: Improvements in ESU, TUEVP and Bipolar Resection

Anup Patel MS, FRCS (Urol)

The safe application of electrical energy to living organisms has underpinned many important surgical advances in the past two centuries. Once scientists had discovered the main requisites for storing electrical and magnetic energy (an electrical resistor, a capacitor, and an inductor), the next step was to induce an alternating current and apply this to human tissues in order to cut tissue without neuromuscular stimulation. The earliest pioneer of prostate electrotherapy was perversely, a gynecologist, Tripier (1861), who applied pulses of electrical energy to the prostate through a rectal electrode to treat gonococcal prostatitis. The first transurethral application of electricity to the human prostate was credited to the Italian, Enrico Bottini in 1874, who used staged treatments to incise and ablate morbidly enlarged prostates. The next major advance was to apply electrosurgical energy to the prostate under direct visual control, initially through a perineal urethrostomy (Wishard), and later through an air-dilating cystoscope. By 1897, the introduction of an irrigating cystoscope by Freudenberg allowed thermo-galvanic prostatic destruction under visual endoscopic control for the first time. The next challenge was to develop an energy source that emits a high-frequency current that works reliably in a fluid environment. The Poulsenlampe was the first such source. It was originally developed for radiotelegraphy, and was subsequently used by deForest who accidentally produced the first high-frequency cutting effect. Later on, deForest patented the triode tube but he never used it for this application. After Edwin Beer's pioneering work on cystoscopic ablation of bladder tumors with insulated copper wire electrodes coupled to a Wappler Excell generator (1910), endoscopic transurethral prostatic ablation of small and medium-sized prostates began in earnest on both sides of the Atlantic with Stevens, and Luys with his technique of "forage de la prostate."

Hugh Hampton Young used a cautery punch device in 1911 for removing prostate tissue and incorporated the principle of a continuous flow of water between inner and outer sheaths to keep the instrument cool. Over the next 15 years, various tube and spark-gap electrosurgical generators were developed by Wappler with Wyeth. Max Stern then introduced the first resectoscope fitted with a tungsten thin-wire loop and coupled to such generators. His instrument was 27 French in size, bipolar, and although it permitted a clean cut through the tissue, bleeding from large arterioles was frequent since the cutting current only produced a shallow depth of coagulation. Theodore Davis, a general surgeon with urological interest from South Carolina introduced several innovations. The first was a thicker, larger, stronger loop, which was moved slowly through the tissue from within the sheath towards the bladder. The second was a more powerful cutting current, and the third was the simultaneous use of two generators, one for cutting and the other for coagulating tissue, using an electromagnetic footswitch to interchange from one to the other. This led to the next and most important change in electrosurgical generator design, that of combining two separate currents (a powerful cutting current and a highly damped spark-gap coagulating current) into a single device, with footswitch control of each different mode. Although he died a relative pauper, William T. Bovie's pioneering design of an electrosurgical unit (ESU) developed in conjunction with the Liebel-Flarsheim Company of Cincinatti, endures as the basis for all modern generators used in transurethral electrosurgery of the prostate to this day. McCarthy modified Stern's resectoscope to cut from the bladder towards the operator, and incorporated this working element, which had to be manipulated with both hands, into a non-conductive bakelite sheath (first introduced in England). Thereafter, there was a veritable explosion of interest in transurethral resection of the prostate (TURP) in the early 1930s, but the morbidity of the procedure remained high. Later in the same decade, Reed Nesbit introduced the concept of a single-handed resectoscope, but his instrument never gained popularity due to sticking of the working element mechanics. Eventually, this led to the acknowledgement by most, that there was a definite learning curve, even in the hands of eminent urologists of the time, and that training in resection techniques was essential. In 1948, Iglesias de la Torre of Havana (a student of McCarthy) designed a spring mechanism that allowed full control over the forward excursion of the electrode with one hand, while the return excursion was passively controlled by the spring.[1] Earlier, during World War II, Captain George Baumrucker of the US Army Medical Corps had taught resection techniques in Europe whilst on active duty, and designed a spring mechanism for the working element with an action that was the reverse of the Iglesias mechanism. Hence, the Baumrucker working element became more popular in Europe and is virtually unknown in America today. Further improvements in telescope optics incorporating glass fiber bundles (and later, the Hopkins rod lens system) and high-intensity external light sources, together with improved antibiotic drugs, anesthetic techniques, and the wider availability of blood transfusion, helped to establish the place of the modern day TURP.

The foundation for transurethral electrovaporization of the prostate began with the discovery by Kirwin in 1934 that, by varying the dimensions of the active electrode surface, different tissue effects such as cutting and coagulation could be obtained simultaneously with pure cutting current.[2] Using the Comprex Oscillator developed by the Wappler company (which emitted only a pure cutting current) and a continuous flow resectoscope to dissipate the surface heat, he was able to "shrink open" the obstructing prostate. This was the first electrodesiccation prostate treatment, but only resurfaced 30 years later, when Irving Bush and, later, Winston Mebust, both succeeded in "shrinking open" the prostate in debilitated patients. Within the decade of the late 1980s and early 1990s, disappointing results with neodymium:yttrium-aluminum-garnet (Nd:YAG) laser ablation of the prostate set the scene for transurethral electrovaporization of the prostate (TUEVP) to make a resurgence through modification of monopolar electrode surface configuration. The credit for this goes to Irving Bush in 1993.[3]

TUEVP has mounted a firm challenge to the domain of loop resection, with the prospect of reducing both morbidity and inpatient stay costs, but it has not yet managed to gain ascendancy except in the hands of a few enthusiasts. Its early development, however, has many parallels to that of its venerable predecessor, and brings to mind the words of Day, who stated, "Transurethral resection will be abandoned by hosts of urologists after giving it a short trial," something that many believe to be true today of transurethral electrovaporization of the prostate. Only time will tell if the days of TURP as the "gold standard" are numbered, for history teaches us that many new technologies progress through phases of amazement, skepticism, and scorn before they gain widespread acceptance.

IMPACT OF ESU AND ELECTRODE CONFIGURATIONS

In clinical practice, electrosurgical frequencies greater than 100,000 Hertz (in the radiofrequency range) are used because lower frequencies are unsafe and can produce undesirable neuromuscular contractions. Tissue is heated through the phenomenon of ohmic resistance. When cutting current is applied to a tissue bed by an active electrode with a small surface contact area, as the high-frequency alternating current travels through the tissue to the large surface area of the return electrode and then to ground, there are rapidly reversing cyclical changes in molecular polarity (Figure 71B-1). This leads to rapid heating of intracellular water closest to the active electrode to a temperature above the boiling point, resulting in instantaneous steam production. As the steam escapes, the cells explode to leave a powdery residue, and a tissue defect ensues. This is the mechanism of monopolar electrosurgical tissue cutting. In a fluid environment, the irrigant must be non-conductive in order to localize the current effect to the site of application. Conductive thermal transfer means that the flow of irrigant serves to dissipate surface heat, while the circulation of the tissue provides a variable heat sink that dissipates heat generated deeper within the tissue. The final thermal tissue effects are governed by the maximum temperature achieved, the total time that this temperature is sustained, and most importantly, the temperature rise time (rate of increase to the maximum temperature). If the temperature rise is slow and/or the total thermal dose is low, tissue cellular proteins are denatured, the cell is desiccated, but the cell wall is left intact in a shrunken denatured state, leading to coagulated necrosis of tissue according to the thermal sensitivity of its component cell types. In contrast, a rapid increase in temperature to a value greater than 100°C causes a loss of intracellular water, which is rapidly boiled and turns to steam. Under these conditions of tissue heating, it is the power density with which the energy is applied, that governs whether the cells are desiccated, carbonized, or vaporized. Low-power density results in cell death by desiccation and carbonization with delayed sloughing, while high-power density vaporizes cells directly, producing an instant tissue defect.

Different tissue effects, such as cutting and coagulation, can be produced by modifying the way that the electrical energy is delivered, either by the source electrosurgical unit, the active electrode shape, or by the surgical technique. For a tissue-cutting or vaporization effect, the current voltage must be high enough to produce an electrical arc from the active electrode to the tissue surface (ie, at least 200 peak volts). It is important to remember that the formation of this arc is hampered if the active electrode is in direct contact with the tissue at this point (ie, when activating the foot-pedal). This aspect of surgical technique, where the cut pedal is activated just before contact with the tissue to get the most efficient

arcing sufficient to form a plasma vapor to conduct subsequent current more efficiently, is of paramount importance when an active electrode of large surface area is used for a cutting effect, as in TUEVP.

In contrast, the coagulation current waveform is very different from the cutting current by virtue of being damped and pulsed to increase its peak voltage for deeper penetration into the tissues. This damped higher voltage waveform produces a slower heat rise time and results in hemostasis through desiccation and coagulation below the tissue surface. Nevertheless, tissue cutting can still be achieved with this damped coagulation waveform if the power is increased, but this is self-limiting as there is rapid electrode and tissue surface carbonization, which insulates deeper tissue from further efficient vaporization. A better way to achieve simultaneous tissue vaporization and coagulation during transurethral surgery is to utilize the principles of cutting current density by altering active electrode size and surface configuration, first discovered through serendipity by Kirwin in 1934.[2] For a pure sine wave current (such as cutting current), the contact area of the active electrode is the principal determinant of the current density delivered to the target tissue. Hence, for the same current in the cutting mode, a point electrode (or a thin-wire loop in endourology) provides excellent cutting, while a flat electrode with a larger surface area (or a barrel roller electrode) provides good surface coagulation. The unique combination of small, high-current density contact prominences (ridges or spikes) with low-current density areas (from larger contact points of the electrode surface) in a single electrode allowed simultaneous tissue cutting and surface coagulation using only a pure cutting-current waveform for the first time. TUEVP and transurethral electro-vapor-resection of the prostate (TUEVRP) are both "new" treatments that evolved through a modification of conventional electrosurgical tissue desiccation by virtue of an innovative and unique electrode design. The credit for this development must go to Robert H. Quint of ACMI, who worked closely with many urological innovators in the past half century and ignited the spark that lit the fire of my own interest in the basic science and history of electrosurgery. He has offered us affordable surgical technology with the prospect of reduced bleeding and lower morbidity from fluid absorption for

prostate tissue removal in patients with bothersome lower urinary tract symptoms (LUTS) associated with benign prostatic hyperplasia (BPH). Similar endoscopic benefits have also widened the application of this unique technology to several other specialities, such as gynecology, where troublesome luminal endometrial fibroids can be vaporized without the need for a hysterectomy, and colorectal surgery, where symptomatic large unresectable tumors can be palliated with low patient morbidity and short hospitalization.

OVERCOMING THE CHALLENGES OF HIGH TISSUE IMPEDANCE DURING TUEVP

No new technology is "born" perfect, and thus it was for prostate electrovaporization. During the early clinical phase of TUEVP, there was recognition that repeated applications of a smooth 3-mm diameter roller electrode desiccated the tissue and quickly limited tissue removal and the size of the cavity that could be created. In fact, the larger the electrode (eg, 5-mm roller electrodes), the greater the desiccation effect predominated over the vaporization effect. However, it was this very same desiccation effect that conferred some of the clinical advantages of electrovaporization over loop resection, such as reduced bleeding from surface coagulation with cutting current. The main consequences of such limited tissue removal in the early days of TUEVP, were frustrated urologists, poor clinical outcomes, and unhappy patients with morbidity from irritative symptoms as a consequence of having excessively coagulated tissue left to separate through a process of unpredictable sloughing (just as was seen previously with the Nd:YAG lasers or, for that matter, any other energy source that produced tissue coagulation as a predominant effect). Although the incorporation of surface grooves and ridges, as in the first generation of VaporTrode electrodes (3-mm Grooved Bar—Figure 71B-2) improved the efficiency of tissue removal compared to a smooth surfaced electrode, some tissue desiccation still occurred with repeated passes, eventually limiting the amount of tissue that could be removed. At the time, there was no clear understanding amongst the profession of the impact on tissue impedance, of electrode size and surface configuration, of endoscopic technique or of the impact of different generator designs. As a result, a variety of smooth and grooved roller electrodes of different size-and-surface configurations (Figure 71B-3) coupled to routinely available electro-

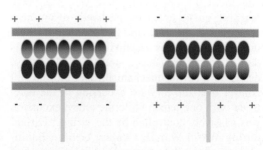

Figure 71B-1 Molecular hysteresis from rapidly alternating high frequency monopolar current causing ohmic heating.

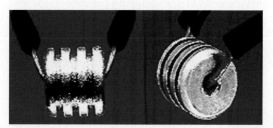

Figure 71B-2 3-mm VaporTrode Grooved Bar.

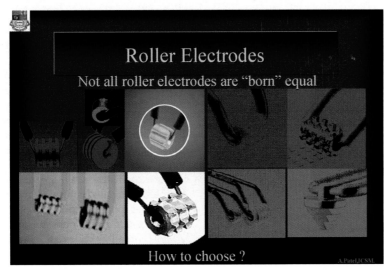

Figure 71B-3 Variety of vaporization electrode configurations available after introduction of the VaporTrode electrode.

surgical units, and the old loop technique of resection, was in use for TUEVP. Clinicians entering the learning curve of transurethral prostate electrovaporization TUEVP, therefore, responded (instinctively and according to the limited published literature of the time) by increasing dial power settings on their traditional generators (Figure 71B-4), sometimes to a value double that which was traditionally used for thin-wire loop resection (up to 300 watts cut power setting and 80 W coagulation power setting). Although not well understood at the time, the result of the initial reaction to use higher power was to compound the problem, for the increase in the dial power settings led to faster desiccation of the tissue bed, driving up the tissue impedance, and finally, leading to surface charring and carbonization. Furthermore, early advice from certain "expert" clinicians on points of TUEVP technique, where use of coagulation current whilst simultaneously rolling the electrode over the tissue bed was recommended in order to clean the grooved roller electrodes of adherent surface debris, also worsened the increase in tissue impedance and further limited subsequent tissue removal through any vaporization effect, for the coagulating current desiccated the cells, reducing their water content and making it difficult to subsequently vaporize them.

Although it almost became a basic tenet of this treatment modality, high dial power settings also raised new and purely hypothetical fears about effects on potency and continence. Furthermore, when electrodes were reused (as with loops) at these higher dial power settings, loss of insulation material from the suspensory wires, also led to damage by arcing of current from this bare metal to various components of the resectoscope, either the insulated tip (Figure 71B-5), or the sides of the tip of the rod lens. Expensive repair bills ensued.

At this point, with suboptimal results from what seemed to be a very promising new technique, with an energy source everyone was "familiar with and thought they understood well,"

many abandoned the technique, while others reverted to the use of sandwich and combination techniques alternating between a vaporization electrode and a loop.[4-6] Indeed, some of the early exponents of TUEVP even switched to thicker loops (of a fashion which had been tried as long ago as the early 1930s by Theodore Davis of North Carolina, who was an early proponent of TURP).[7] This left a few lingering enthusiasts who began a phase of basic research in order to try to understand the reasons for some of the clinical problems. The prime thrust of this work was to study some of the variables that might have impacted on tissue removal during TUEVP, for without doubt, the interplay of these variables was far more critical during electrovaporization due to the larger electrode size, than with loop resection.

VARIABLES AFFECTING TISSUE REMOVAL DURING ELECTROVAPORIZATION

Several studies investigated the effects of the many variables that could affect the electrovaporization process.[8-13] Two of these were in vivo studies (canine prostate and rabbit bladder), and the rest were ex vivo in human cadaver prostate, surgical prostatectomy specimens, or bovine tissue. Certain trends to optimize tissue removal by vaporization were highlighted by each study. An

electrode configuration with surface ridges was undoubtedly superior to a smooth electrode of equivalent size with respect to tissue removal even under multiple pass conditions. At the same time, these roller electrodes produced more coagulation than a regular loop.[8,9] A slower electrode drag speed compared to that of a normal loop, improved tissue vaporization, but repeated electrode passes desiccated the tissue and reduced subsequent vaporization.[8,9,13] Reuse of vaporization electrodes also diminished the vaporization effect by 50%,[8] presumably as the electrode surface became coated with caramelized tissue debris, which reduced current transfer. Excessive pressure by digging the electrode into the tissue produced less tissue removal through electrovaporization than a medium contact pressure, presumably by interfering with plasma arc formation. Limits of generator power setting were established for the change in effect from controlled vaporization, to either desiccation at one extreme or uncontrolled resection at the other. The two in vivo studies confirmed that, as electrosurgical tissue heating occurred instantaneously, the presence of blood flow did not significantly change the findings of the ex-vivo laboratory studies.[11,12] Furthermore, the importance of knowledge of the power curves of different generators was emphasized for the first time.[9] This was later reaffirmed by van Swol and associates,[10] who reminded us of the fact that most generators perform optimally according to the dial setting in the pure cut mode at a resistance of only 400 ohms, which matches the impedance of fresh tissues. They and others demonstrated the differences in power output between conventional generators and the newer generation of microprocessor-controlled, impedance-independent units.[14] In Figure 71B-6, the results of our own bench tests show the impact of rising impedance on the real power output of an electrosurgical unit of conventional design as an example of type (Force 2, Valleylab), compared to the dial power setting. Clearly, there was a large disparity between the panel setting and the true output of the machine as impedance increased. The results of this kind of testing were confirmed by limited testing in actual patients during a transurethral electrovaporization procedure with a VaporTrode 3-mm grooved bar electrode.

Hypothetical concerns that electrovaporization was associated with a greater risk of deep tissue heating than TURP were dispelled by the

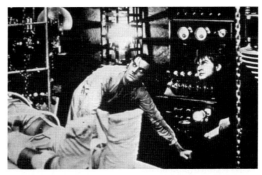

Figure 71B-4 Increased power on generator panel setting.

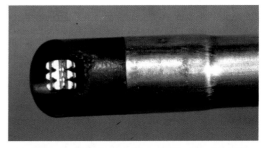

Figure 71B-5 Damage to insulated resectoscope tip from reuse of electrode. This may lead to further arcing of current onto rod-lens at high panel power settings of the ESU.

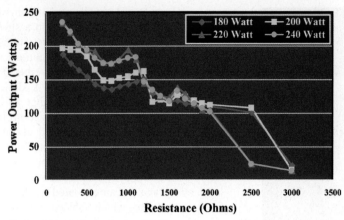

Figure 71B-6 Bench test results of actual power output of Force 2 ESU in pure cut mode over wide range of impedance compared to panel setting.

finding that neither treatment produced histologic thermal damage deeper than 1 mm when a pure cutting current was used.[9] Two clinical studies of interstitial thermometry during both loop resection and electrovaporization with a variety of different electrodes and electrosurgical units also confirmed the findings that there was no excessive heating of the neurovascular bundles, while reaffirming the surface heat sink effect of continuous flow irrigation (Figure 71B-7).[15,16] Importantly, both sets of authors cautioned against prolonged applications of coagulating current, either at the level of the prostatic capsule or at the apex, for the coagulating waveform had higher peak voltage than cutting current. This higher voltage peak facilitates deeper penetration into the thin tissue barrier beyond the lumen of the resection cavity and risks indirect unseen damage to the neurovascular bundles at the prostatic apex or in the region of posterior capsular perforations, particularly in small glands. In summary, these studies both highlighted and reaffirmed the fact that urologists must pay greater attention to many variables, such as electrode size and configuration (the balance struck between the size, shape, and number of high current density prominences on the electrode surface), the slower speed of electrode, and the different contact pressure on the tissue. Furthermore, they must seek to have a full understanding of basic electrosurgical principles and the power curve limitations of their own operating room electrosurgical units, if they were to get the most efficient tissue removal and the best clinical results with transurethral electrovaporization of the prostate. The outcomes of six prospective randomized studies evaluating TUEVP are summarized in Table 71B-1.

IMPROVEMENTS IN ESU TECHNOLOGY

Within the past decade or so, manufacturers of traditional solid state electrosurgical units have incorporated various changes in the design of these units, driven by the surgical observations on inconsistency of tissue effect during different kinds of electrosurgical applications, and the need to limit or control the extent of collateral tissue damage, both with respect to increased application times and applications in different media (as in gaseous or fluid phases). One of the earliest examples of these changes was the adoption of integrated computer-controlled technology. The purpose of this technology was to monitor both current and voltage in "real time" and auto-regulate feedback in order to make it possible to rapidly vary either one or the other according to the impedance (resistance) of the tissue. This meant that, in accordance with Ohm's law, the newer generation of electrosurgical units were capable of maintaining either constant voltage by automatically varying current and power (eg, Erbe ICC 350), or constant power by automatically varying current and voltage output (eg, Valleylab Force Fx) in order to retain the consistency of the effect at the tissue interface, regardless of variations of the active electrode configuration, within certain tolerances. The main difference between these two types of machines with respect to prostate electrovaporization, was that the one that maintained constant voltage usually still required a higher dial power setting of a range similar to older design units.

The role of the generator as an important variable affecting the efficiency of tissue removal during the electrovaporization process was first studied in detail by Lim and colleagues.[9] In a laboratory ex vivo study, they demonstrated that, when all other variables were standardized, use of a computer-controlled constant power output generator allowed equivalent tissue removal during electrovaporization with a grooved roller electrode, but at a pure cut power setting a third lower than that used on a conventional device (ie, 150 W for Force FX vs 220 W for Force 40). Since that time, we and a few others have reported clinical experience of prostate electrovaporization at pure cut settings below 200 W using these new computer-controlled electrosurgical units.[10] In our study, it was routinely possible to create excellently sized cavities in the prostatic lumen with a panel setting equivalent to that used for regular loop resection (130 to 170 W), using a computer-controlled constant power output generator (Force Fx, Valleylab—Figure 71B-8), provided, of course, that the right electrode and surgical technique were also employed.[17] Experience of necessary panel settings in the pure cut mode with several other ESUs tested in our center have shown that a wide range of panel settings was necessary for adequate electrovaporization, as shown in Table 71B-2. Better affordability should come hand-in-hand for purchasers, with a wide choice of commercially available machines. During some of our clinical studies, where real-time measurements were taken during activations of the electrode at different time points during TUEVP procedures, measurements of current, voltage, and impedance, reemphasized the large discrepancies between panel settings in the cut mode and the actual generator output in older style generators (Figure 71B-9).

In a subsequent study, we evaluated two different electrosurgical generators to determine the lowest panel power setting at which prostate electrovaporization could be sustained in vivo, and then studied their power output curves at bench tests. With the experience gained from our previously reported prospectively randomized double-blind clinical study we picked and standardized the electrode configuration and used an operative technique that had been shown to give tissue removal equivalent to loop resection.[17] One of these, the Excalibur Plus (Conmed USA), permitted prostate electrovaporization at panel settings below 100 W for the first time, without compromising satisfactory early clinical outcomes. It was clinically effective for TUEVP with

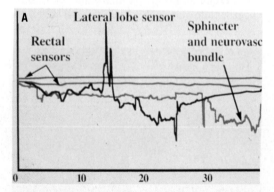

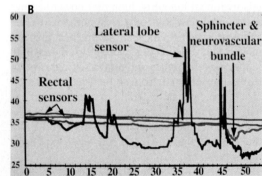

Figure 71B-7 *A,* Interstitial optical thermometry demonstrating temperature changes during TURP, and *B,* during TUEVP confirming no unseen deep heating of vital structures, and protective cooling effect of continuous flow irrigation at apex as cavity is created.

Table 71B-1   TUEVP Morbidity Outcome Data: Meta-analysis of 6 Prospectively Randomized Studies of Standard Loop Resection Versus Prostate Electrovaporization

	Loop Resection		Electrovaporization		Number of Studies
Number of patients	300		292		6
	Mean	Range	Mean	Range	
Baseline symptom score	22.4	18–27	23.2	19–27	5
Baseline peak flow (mL/s)	8.9	6.9–11.4	8.4	7.3–10.3	5
Operation time (min)	40.7	21.6–53	46	25.9–60	4
Catheter time (hr)	74.25	46.6–65	40.3	20.9–48	6
Hospital stay (d)	4	2.5–4.8	2.6	1.1–4.9	6
Transfusion	6.4%	2–11.6	0%	0	3
Clots or macroscopic hematuria	13.6%	8.8–20	4.2%	3–5.7	3
Postoperative urinary retention (transient)	7.9%	3.8–12	15%	6–23	3
Urinary tract infection	5.2%	0–11.6	8%	0–18	3
Epididymitis	2.5%	0–5	0.7%	0–1.4	2
Retrograde ejaculation	85%	81–89	74%	72–76	2
Impotence	9%	7–11	14%	11–17	2
Postoperative irritative symptoms	22.5%	10–35	20%	15–25	2
Urinary incontinence	1.3%	0–3.8	7.2%	3–18.6	4
Reoperation within 1 year	5.5%	4–7	5.5%	4–7	3
Bladder neck sclerosis	4%	3–5	1.4%	0–4.2	4
Urethral stricture	2%	0–4	2%	0–4	3

Two studies were performed with grooved-roller electrodes (Hammadeh et al,[45] Gallucci et al,[46] Kupeli S et al[47]), two with spiked-roller electrodes (Shokeir et al,[48] Patel et al[49]), and one with a fluted-roller electrode (McAllister et al [50]). Another study by Hammadeh et al[51] maintains the advantages seen with electrovaporization over 5 years of follow-up, while both groups had a 4% incidence of urethral strictures, the rate of bladder neck stenosis was 4% for TURP and only 2% for TUEVP, while the reoperation rates were 13% for both cohorts, with respective impotence and retrograde ejaculation rates of 11% and 89% for TURP, compared to 17% and 72% for TUEVP (not significant).
Operating time was longer for vaporization in the three studies performed with regular generators with panel power set above 200 watts. It was equivalent in the two where a constant power output generator with panel power set below 200 watts was used (Patel et al,[49] McAllister et al[50]). The influence of a learning curve for a new procedure on the morbidity outcomes is not clear for the vaporization data (except in study 4, which was started after a learning curve experience of 1 year). Operative techniques were not standardized. Prostate volume was not limited to small or medium-sized glands in study 4, but was limited in the other studies.
Trends are highlighted in red text (favoring electrovaporization) or blue text (favoring TURP) provided data from at least three studies was available. The highest incontinence and impotence rates were seen where a standard TURP technique and generator were used for electrovaporization.

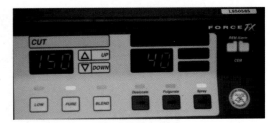

Figure 71B-8 Panel settings on Force Fx ESU used for effective TUEVP (results comparable to TURP), when coupled to a VaporTrode Spiked Bar.

future modifications in monopolar electrode design coupled with use of a generator that could either maintain constant power output or slowly increase actual power output as impedance increased. In this way, the routine use of low panel settings for transurethral electrovaporization could be assured on a routine basis, and patients would have the potential benefit of fewer postoperative irritative symptoms as the amount of coagulated desiccated tissue left for delayed sloughing would be minimized.

RECENT IMPROVEMENTS IN ELECTRODE DESIGN FOR TUEVP

A poor electrode design may be ineffective at removing sufficient tissue, may cause prolonged irritative symptoms leading to excessive patient morbidity and a higher re-treatment rate, and may damage the resectoscope. Indeed, even in some randomized studies where relatively inefficient VaporTrode fluted electrodes were used, there was no advantage accrued to patients treated with TUEVP, compared to those treated with TURP, and the two treatments were found to be equivalent.[19] Several solutions have been tried to overcome these problems, including sandwich techniques where vaporization is followed by loop resection with an option of following on with more vaporization,[20] and the use of different generator special effects.[21] Many urologists have also been frustrated by the lack of tissue for histologic analysis after TUEVP with plain and grooved roller electrodes and, being more comfortable with the technique of loop resection, have reverted back either to regular loop resection or to modified loop resection (eg, thicker, wider, flatter loops with mini-rollers).[22,23] Furthermore, it "seemed" that prostate electrovaporization involved a longer procedure time than for TURP, although this was

a VaporTrode Spiked Bar at panel settings between 60 to 80 W in the pure cut mode.[18] In subsequent bench tests, we used a Metron QA-ES electrosurgical analyzer (Metron, Travbaneveien, Trondheim, Norway) to measure actual power output, comparing the power output curves in the clinically effective panel power setting range for each ESU. The most obvious difference between the two generators was the shape of these curves. The Force 2 (Valleylab) generator overestimated actual power output as impedance increased from 200 to 3,000 Ω, while the Excalibur Plus unit underestimated it compared to the panel setting. The actual power output started 33% below the panel setting at the lowest impedance (200 Ω), peaked at 60% above an incident panel setting of 80 W, and then fell away gradually once more between an impedance of 1,300 to 3,000 Ω (Figure 71B-10). This shape of power output curve was a new variation on power curve design and was the opposite of that seen with most commonly used ESUs. This difference in power curve design seemed to offer an explanation as to why tissue could be vaporized at such low panel settings, even without the use of computer-controlled technology, for in reality, the output was slightly higher as we described above.

Furthermore, also during our study, we observed that, in a small number of cases and

regardless of prostate size, the 3-mm spiked-bar VaporTrode - Force 2 combination, permitted effective electrovaporization at a lower dial power setting (180 W) than had been previously described when this ESU had been coupled by others with the 3-mm grooved-bar VaporTrode. Our observation showed for the first time that a more efficient electrode could even compensate for the shortcomings of a generator of suboptimal power curve design, and allow the use of lower panel settings on these older type machines, for those who could not afford the extra expense of replacing an older model in their operating room.

Taken together, these findings indicated a real potential for improving the safety and efficiency of tissue clearance during prostate electrovaporization by limiting excessive desiccation through

Table 71B-2   Clinical Experience of Lowest ESU Panel Settings in the Pure Cut Mode Required to Perform Transurethral Prostate Electrovaporization in our Unit for a Range of Commonly Available Electrosurgical Generators

Generator	Pure Cut Panel Power Setting (Watts)
Bard 5000	250–300
Valleylab Force 2 or 40	220–280
ERBE ICC 350 (Microprocessor-controlled constant voltage)	180–240 Effects 1–2 (No high cut)
Valleylab Force FX (Microprocessor-controlled constant power output)	130–170
Maxim Bovie X 30 and 40	150–170 (TURP Micro-fixed panel setting)
Conmed Excalibur Plus	60–120

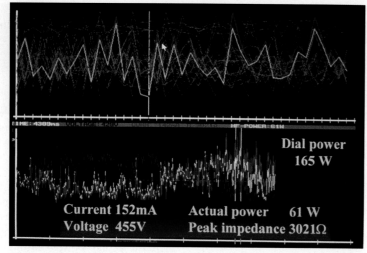

Figure 71B-9 Real time monitoring data during TUEVP with Force 2 ESU showing difference between dial power (165 W) and actual power output (61 W) at higher tissue impedance.

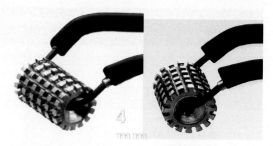

Figure 71B-11 ResecTrode Electrode with 96 surface prominences and 384 vaporizing surface edges.

ity and shorter hospitalization after TUEVP over either regular or modified loop resection, are retained with this newer electrode without compromising clinical outcomes and has allowed the safe, expeditious treatment of glands in excess of 100 cc in volume.

FURTHER INNOVATIONS IN ESU DESIGN FOR REGULAR LOOP PROSTATE ELECTROSURGERY

not necessarily the case in a prospective randomized study if the right equipment and technique were used.[16] Many electrodes had been tried by several different manufacturers in the interim in the search of a configuration that struck the right balance between design, number of surface prominences, and electrode size. None of these had lived up to the required expectations in clinical evaluation. Hence, cognizant of the fact that the majority were not able to emulate our outcomes, a new roller electrode design was developed and evaluated in our center in association with the inventor of the original VaporTrode electrodes (Robert H. Quint). This electrode, known as the ResecTrode was a wider version of the 3-mm Spiked VaporTrode we had previously preferred in clinical studies. In order to allow for more tissue removal per pass, it was a third larger in width, at 4 mm, without increasing thickness diameter compared to the 3-mm VaporTrodes that preceded it. The disadvantage others had found who had previously tried larger electrodes up to 5 mm in diameter (width), was that this translated to more tissue desiccation due to a drop in current density with the larger electrode surface area which, of course, limited tissue

removal. Hence in the new ResecTrode design, 96 mini square-edged surface prominences were incorporated as a result of computer-generated surface design according to electrical field theory (Figure 71B-11) giving 384 mini cutting edges for tissue resection. This electrode, through its larger width, not only allowed the vaporization of 33% more tissue per pass that its 3-mm predecessors, but clinical tests showed that it also allowed unhindered resection of tissue chips for the first time with a barrel electrode (albeit with more tissue drag than with a loop), whilst retaining the clinical benefits of TUEVP, in comparison to modified loop resection. This, of course, meant that, not only was tissue available for histologic analysis (Figure 71B-12), but the TUEVP procedure was now capable of being performed even more expeditiously than before, so that the possibility to tackle larger glands was open to more urologists. Furthermore, the ResecTrode could also compensate for the deficiencies of an average electrosurgical generator with less than ideal power curves during TUEVP. Our experience to date in a two-center experience[24] with over 50 cases treated in our own center, has shown that the benefits of lower morbid-

Some electrosurgical units have incorporated special voltage-driven effects to improve tissue coagulation with loop and point electrodes. The ICC350 unit from Erbe is one such device, and has several incremental "High-Cut" modes which provide peak voltages between 400 and 700 V for deeper tissue penetration and coagulation. Combination of such units with loops that are thicker, may produce marginally better hemostasis although, so far in the published literature, this has not been significantly better than that obtained by an electrovaporization electrode coupled to an efficient generator and correct operative technique.

In an extension of the use of blended currents to reduce the bleeding associated with standard monopolar resection, in the mid 1990s, "coagulating cutting" was developed by Karl Storz (Tuttlingen, Germany), whereby phases with predominant cutting was alternated with shorter defined phases of coagulation. In clinical trials, however, the technique was disadvantaged by longer operating times related to a slower cutting speed due to a tissue drag effect during the phases of coagulation. To counteract this drawback, high voltage pulses

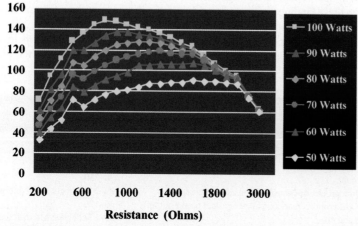

Figure 71B-10 Power curves of Excalibur Plus ESU.

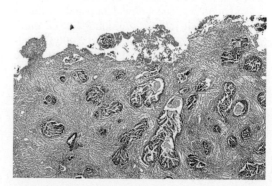

Figure 71B-12 Histology of chip cut with ResecTrode, showing benign prostatic hyperplasia.

were introduced for the phases of coagulation, and coagulating intermittent cutting (CIC) came into existence. The output signal of the generator was a pulse-modulated sinusoidal wave of variable high amplitude voltage "tuned" for optimized cutting, but this time, due to sparking from the high voltage pulses in a minority of cases, gas bubble formation increased and impeded the operator's vision. The last modification of the CIC generator deployed a controlled but variable (rather than fixed) pause between the cutting and coagulating pulses, each of which were of fairly constant voltage. In so doing, if power output decreased, the lag between the two pulses increased so that less power was delivered to the patient (Figure 71B-13), but once again, the energy load applied to the patient was higher, as with TUEVP, and as before, no disadvantage was accrued.[25]

A different strategy has been used by Aesculap with the Focus 640 ESU, to try to reduce excessive tissue charring during monopolar electrosurgical cutting with thin wire electrodes. Their laboratory tests had apparently shown that the

intensity of the monopolar electrode sparking, though well-defined at the moment of contact and at release of tissue contact, was variable through the duration of the cut itself (Figure 71B-14). Consequently, they developed Microcut modes, which reduced the internal dosage voltage in a way that a predetermined spark limit would not be exceeded if extensive sparking was detected. Thus, the Microcut modes limited the spark intensity and minimized the effective power at the electrode to a value sufficient for an excellent cutting effect, but which avoided unintended collateral tissue damage. This control principle (set peak dosage 150 V) is shown and explained in Figure 71B-15. The only difference between the two Microcut modes was, that there were different predefined values for the spark limit (higher spark intensity—hence more tissue carbonization with Microcut 2 mode than for Microcut 1). This can also be interpreted as an element in a general "dial-down" philosophy, which was also defined in the international standard IEC601–2-2. Unfortunately, this advantage with Microcut, as with CIC, is not applicable to vaporization electrodes.

BIPOLAR PROSTATE ELECTROSURGERY

This newly introduced technology updated and revitalized something that was tried in the early decades of the last century. What then was the attraction of such technology over standard monopolar loop resection? It permitted electrosurgical tissue cutting in a conductive saline medium, and this immediately offered urologists tackling larger glands the possibility of using more endoscopic resection time without risking

morbidity from the effects of water absorption and TUR syndrome. How was this achieved in electrosurgical terms? As with monopolar cutting, the generator must initially produce a momentary high-energy spike to initiate a plasma vapor layer ionized in the form of a non-equilibrium plasma, where plasma ions and electrons are responsible for current flow. But unlike monopolar surgery, the current does not arc to the tissue and then pass to a large surfaced return electrode applied to the skin heating the intervening tissue by ohmic resistance. Instead, the active electrode and return are in close proximity to each other separated by an insulator. The electron emission from the smaller active electrode vaporizes the adjacent liquid to form a thin gas layer (plasma pocket) that grows to form a larger bubble containing energetic species that can dissociate both water and organic molecules.[26] It is likely that the thermal effect probably occurs at much lower temperatures ($< 70°C$) compared to monopolar surgery (300 to 400°C). All bipolar technologies use radio frequency (RF) energy output from specialized electrosurgical generators (320 to 450 kHz for Gyrus Plasma Kinetic [Figure 71B-16], 100 kHz square wave for the Vista Coblation system [ACMI Corp. Southborough, MA, Figure 71B-17]—the latter being 5 times lower than for monopolar systems), and 350 kHz for the Olympus Surgmaster generator. At the time of writing, the frequency of the newest system from Storz is not published. The energy passes down the active electrode, through the plasma pocket and thence through the conductive solution to the tissue bed before returning to the thicker return, before finally returning to ground through the active cord. Hence, there is no need for a return plate, and the risk of inadvertent burns at this site

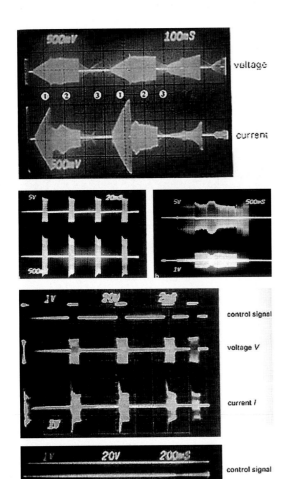

Figure 71B-13 Coagulation intermittent cutting waveform evolution.

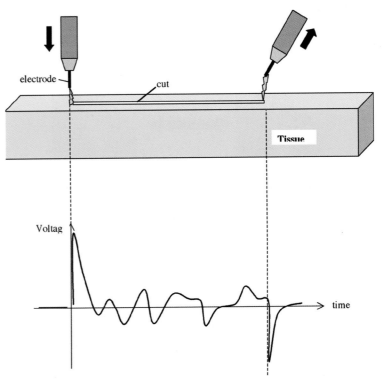

Figure 71B-14 Analysis of spark intensity voltage showing variability during cut but relatively constant voltage peaks at start and end of cut.

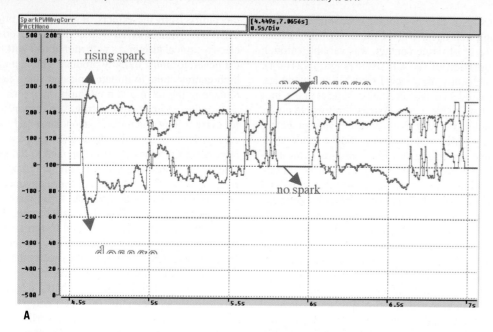

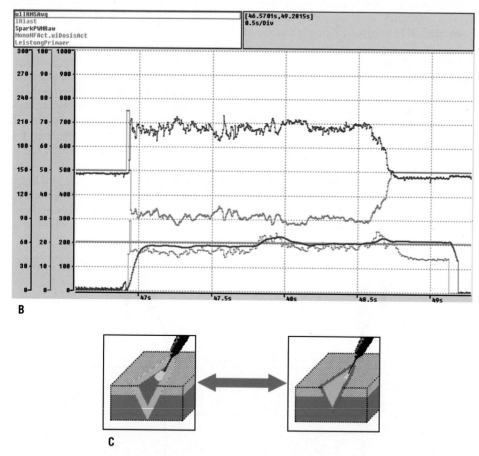

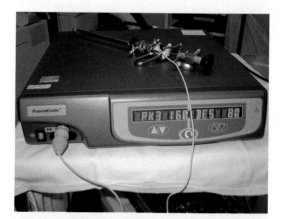

Figure 71B-16 Plasma Kinetic Bipolar Electrosurgical Generators 1st Generation and SuperPulse (Gyrus).

Figure 71B-15 Real time monitoring data during prostatic resection sequence with Aesculap Focus 640 ESU showing constancy of sparking in Micro Cut 2 mode when voltage is preset, and impact on tissue effect with regard to precision of cut.

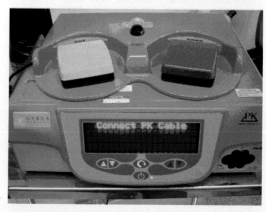

Figure 71B-17 Coblation (Vista) Bipolar Electrosurgical System (ACMI Corp.).

available systems, though there are certain basic similarities (eg, active electrode slightly thinner and separated from thicker return electrode component by an insulator), but resectoscope sizes, design of the electrode housings, plus coupling to the active and return cords differ.

At the moment of fire-up by foot-pedal activation, if the activated component of the bipolar electrode is not in contact with the tissue, if the gap is too wide, or if there is insufficient power, current flow is simply dissipated by the large volume of electrolyte solution in a full bladder, and there is no effect. On the other hand, if the power/voltage spike is not high enough to both form and maintain the plasma vapor pocket, stuttered cutting will result depending on the quality of tissue contact. As a result of these challenges, the initial plasma kinetic (PK) Gyrus system, which was the first to encounter some of these difficulties, has been modified in recent years culminating in the availability of the latest Gyrus SuperPulse Generator. This newer device is preconfigured for maximal allowable current under low impedance conditions. However, the surgeon is able to choose between two sets of cut voltages, which are preset (represented by SP1 and SP2 mnemonics). The SuperPulse Generator is designed to recognize the active electrode and offers default settings that are optimal for a range of conditions at the tip (eg, SP2 160, corresponding to a maximum voltage of 307 Volts Root

from inadequate contact is eliminated. Furthermore, the combination of low operating frequency and low voltage in bipolar prostate electrosurgery should also eliminate the possibility of interference with all types of cardiac pacemakers.

The common challenges faced by each of the four systems commercially available regardless of manufacturer, are to reliably establish a cutting plasma corona preferentially at the distal active

electrode, to achieve a plasma condition with acceptably short delays from the time of footswitch activation by the surgeon (ie, instantaneous fire-up), to maintain this under all cutting conditions, and to provide adequate hemostasis from both cut and coagulation sources of footswitch operation.

The configuration and size of the active electrode for prostate resection and incision (Figure 71B-18) is unique for each of the commercially

Mean Square (Vrms) sinusoidal [434V peak] and 160 W maximum average power). The Super-Pulse Generator contains an energy reservoir facility in the form of a bank of internal capacitors. In this way, there is provision of sufficient voltage for both instant fire-up at the start of each cut and for power ride-through under challenging conditions of impedance. In this way, this manufacturer has resolved the problems of stuttered cutting that occurred with the previous generation of the device. The reservoir bank is quickly pre-charged before foot pedal RF voltage initiation by the surgeon. Tests have shown that under high flow and cold saline conditions, more power than normal is required to initiate and maintain plasma conditions at the active electrode tip. The capacitor reservoir can provide up to 4,000 W of power for short periods (≈10 ms), but only if the tip impedance is low enough.

At baseline, before RF voltage application, the impedance differential between bipolar active and return electrodes is between 23 to 60 Ω depending on the saline temperature and the proximity of the active electrode to the tissue bed. At high power (4,000 W) and low impedance (23 Ω), a voltage of close to 300 Vrms can be sustained by the SuperPulse Generator long enough to allow saline immediately surrounding the active loop to be actively heated to reach boiling point in a few milliseconds. This phenomenon is due to current crowding at the reduced surface area of this part of the active electrode and creates a non-equilibrium vapor pocket containing charged sodium ions as shown in Figure 71B-19. A plasma can then be established inside the enveloping vapor pocket. This plasma of activated sodium ions is visible to the naked eye as an orange glow in saline solution (Figure 71B-20), as confirmed by optical emission spectroscopic analysis (whereas a blue glow is visible in a potassium chloride solution). There is a time delay of 1 to 2 μs from the initial negative current spike until light is emitted. Once formed, the impedance of this plasma is higher and ranges from 500 to 3,000 Ω, depending on how much of the loop is in the vapor pocket, as opposed to being in local contact with saline, and depending on the length of the vapor pocket (higher impedances with longer plasma vapor pocket lengths). Power delivery now becomes focused around the active loop rather than being dissipated in the saline and tissue between active and return components of the active electrode. Thereafter, sustaining the plasma requires much less power, the energy reservoir is no longer required and is automatically replenished, while output voltage falls by being repetitively formed during each half cycle of the high-frequency exciting voltage waveform. Plasma volume is smaller and impedance is lower at the lower preset voltage setting of SP1. This is detected visually by a less intense orange glow around the active electrode. The SP2 setting gives the surgeon the option of larger plasma volume and slightly higher preset voltage if cutting becomes difficult under the conditions encountered. Fire-up should usually take no more

than 20 ms after activation by the surgeon as a result of the capabilities of the capacitor reservoir bank. In vivo saline-tissue-based models have shown that, in practice, once an activated loop is in contact with tissue, no more than 100 W are usually required to sustain the user defined maxi-

mum voltages. It is likely that, in future, newer waveform algorithms could also be developed for different clinical scenarios requiring better hemostasis, such as novice system users or in cases where there is a particular interest in minimizing bleeding, as in large vascular prostates. Hence, the

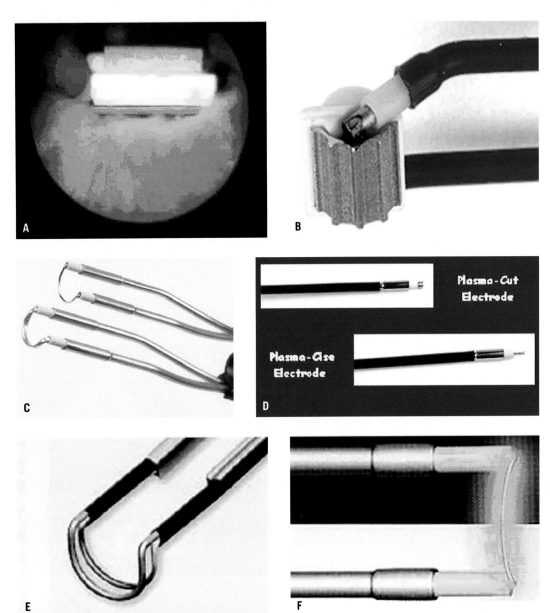

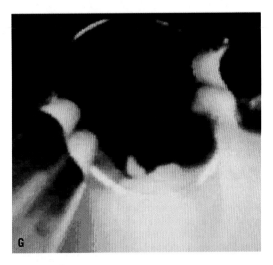

Figure 71B-18 Bipolar electrode configurations of *A* and *B*, Plasma V vaporization electrode (Gyrus Medical, Maple Grove, MN), *C*, PlasmaSect thick and thin resecting loops (Gyrus Medical), *D*, PlasmaCise thick and thin incision electrodes (Gyrus Medical), *E*, Vista Coblation resecting double loop (ACMI Corp., Southborough, MA), *F*, Surgmaster single resecting loop (Olympus), and *G*, Storz double resecting loop (Karl Storz, Tuttlingen, Germany).

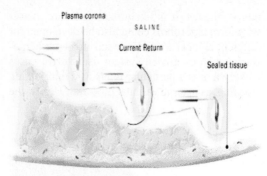

Figure 71B-19 Formation of plasma pocket around active electrode and return pathway of current.

natural evolution of this technology will be in the direction of greater versatility of application.

With all available systems, an ionized plasma vapor layer is formed at high energy around the active component of the electrode. Once formed the vapor pocket can be maintained at low voltages (100 to 350 Vrms) just as the electrode is close to making contact with the tissue. Molecular disassociation takes place as carbon-carbon and carbon-nitrogen bonds are broken down. The end result is production of elementary molecules and low molecular weight gases of oxygen, nitrogen, hydrogen, and carbon dioxide. Clinically, there is a precision tissue effect with minimal collateral damage, as the charged ions have only a short estimated range of 50 to 100µm of penetration. The extent of the collateral tissue damage depends on resistive heating caused by any current flowing through the tissue, and by limited thermal transfer from the electrode sources. The end result is excellent localized cutting, with little in the way of the burnt smell traditionally associated with monopolar cutting (especially for the Coblation system). The depth of the surface coagulation is determined principally by the electrode configuration and by the system design, as well as by the technique used by the operator (time and pressure of contact). Coagulation has to take place with this technology at low peak voltage (in direct contrast to monopolar coagulation: 80 to 100 V for the plasma kinetic system and 65 to 115 V for the Vista system—Figure 71B-21), as

higher peak voltages convert the liquid into a gaseous phase of higher impedance. This, in turn, changes impedance from a resistive to a capacitive mode, which reduces energy flow, reduces dissipated heat and limits the final coagulation effect.

Despite its presence in the marketplace for several years, there is a paucity of peer-reviewed published data with regard to bipolar technology in prostate treatment beyond a learning curve experience, and one or two small single-center randomized trials. Published clinical data is only available for the Gyrus and Vista systems and this review will be confined to these systems only.

The Plasma Kinetic (PK Gyrus, Bucks, UK) system has been in clinical use for bipolar transurethral vaporization for at least half a decade now. In a recent publication, Eaton and Francis reported their experience with this technology in a day surgical unit setting in the United Kingdom.[27] Forty men underwent plasma kinetic prostate vaporization treatment by one surgeon using a dedicated continuous flow 27F Sheath resectoscope and saline irrigant, with an intent for same-day discharge, which was achieved in 85%. Mean prostate volume and operative time were 34.9 cc and 33 minutes, respectively. All voided successfully at 48 hours, but 2 required attention for blocked catheters. At 4 months,

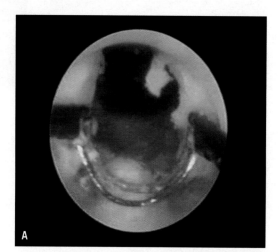

A

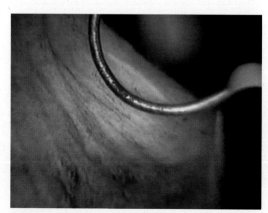

Figure 71B-20 Endoscopic view of orange glow of activated sodium plasma around Coblation (ACMI Corp., Southborough, MA) double loop as it comes into contact with the tissue.

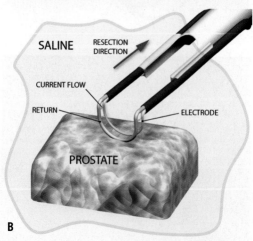

B

Figure 71B-21 Voltage outputs in cut and coagulation mode settings for Vista Coblation bipolar generator (ACMI Corp., Southborough, MA) at low frequencies. Note low voltage of coagulation.

IPSS and quality of life improved by 64 and 83%, respectively, and flow rate improved by a mean 200% (though no baseline data were reported in any of these categories). In another small prospective randomized trial from Australia reported in abstract form, McFarlane and colleagues[28] compared outcomes between 12 men treated with PK vaporization and 10 men treated with regular TURP. At 3 months, American Urological Association symptom scores improved by 19.6 for PK vaporization and by 13.6 for TURP, while flow rates improved by 9 mL/sec. in the PK group compared to 14 mL/sec in the TURP group. Operative time was longer in the PK vaporization group (30 vs 22 minutes), as was recatheterization rate (30% vs 5% for TURP), but clot evacuation rates were higher at 19% in the TURP group. Though these early data tell us that PK bipolar vaporization has sparked the interest of a few urologists and that it is associated with reasonable early clinical outcomes, mature outcomes data in a large cohort of patients treated at many different centers is still lacking for this modality, and there are still no peer-reviewed published data from any prospectively randomized trials comparing monopolar electrovaporization with bipolar plasma kinetic vaporization. Watson[29] used this technology to try to emulate the holmium laser enucleation technique developed by Gilling and Fraundorfer. In this small study of 22 men, a Plasma-Cise electrode was tested, but the duration of postoperative catheterization was 29.8 hours, compared to 17.8 hours after holmium laser resection. Furthermore, there is no peer-reviewed published data to date on either the Plasma-Sect single small bipolar loop from the same manufacturer.

Dunsmuir and colleagues reported a prospective single-blind study of 51 patients randomized to bipolar vaporization (*n* = 30) or monopolar TURP (*n* = 21), of whom 40 (20 in each group) attended for follow-up at 1 year.[30] There was no subjective or objective difference between the groups in clinical outcomes, amount of irrigant used, hematocrit of effluent, or hospital stay. However, recatheterization rate was significantly higher in the bipolar vaporization group (30%) compared to 5% in the TURP group. Of course, one does not know whether those who did not attend for 1 year follow-up (10 PK vaporization and 1 TURP) had an unsatisfactory outcome as the reason for nonattendance.

Though these early data tell us that PK bipolar vaporization has sparked the interest of some urologists, and that it is associated with reasonable early clinical outcomes, mature outcomes data in a large multicenter cohort of patients is still lacking and there are still no peer-reviewed published data from any prospectively randomized controlled trials comparing completeness and rates of tissue removal, as well as clinical outcomes and morbidity after the best of monopolar electrovaporization, with that of bipolar plasma kinetic vaporization. The optimal technique for bipolar Gyrus PK electrovaporization has also not been described in detail yet, specifically whether the active electrode should be moved unidirectionally from bladder neck to apex, or whether this movement should be bidirectional to get the best combination of vaporization and coagulation.

Certainly, one theoretical concern would be of a possible higher urethral stricture rate with the use of a 27F Bipolar PK Gyrus resectoscope, but only time and longer follow-up in such clinical series in the future can give us useful information in this regard. Further, use of these systems in future may be made more attractive by the manufacture of appropriately sized working elements that fit resectoscopes of all common manufacturers.

Recently, Vista Bipolar loop resection was compared to standard monopolar loop resection with regard to cutting qualities, ablation rate, blood loss, and depth of coagulation using an isolated blood perfused porcine kidney model.[31] The Vista system and active electrode used with saline were compared to a 5-mm diameter monopolar loop (Storz, Tuttlingen, Germany) in standard mannitol/sorbitol solution (Fresenius, Bad Homburg, Germany). The Vista bipolar loop ablation rate (determined by the loop diameter and drag rate through the tissue) was similar to the ablation rate reached with the monopolar loop, indicating that the loops moved through the tissue at similar speeds. At Vista cut setting 7 (265 V) and 8 (292 V), blood loss was significantly lower ($p < .05$) than monopolar resection at a power setting of 160 W (Autocon, Karl Storz, Tuttlingen). The bleeding rate was 13.16 ± 5.47 g/min (setting 7) and 10.43 ± 4.76 g/min (setting 8), compared to 17.08 ± 4.57 g/min for the monopolar loop. The bleeding rates (g/min) in cut modes and coagulation depths (μm) in coagulation modes, respectively, are shown in Figures 71B-22 and 71B-23.

These data confirm that coagulation zones were smaller with bipolar resection compared to monopolar equivalents, as expected from the lower voltages in the bipolar system. The limited bipolar surface coagulation at the resected tissue interface whilst avoiding deep tissue heating, should in theory avoid delayed tissue sloughing and prolonged irritative symptoms. On the flip side of this coin, the theoretical disadvantages could be a higher incidence of delayed hemorrhage in fibrous prostates or when the patient strains heavily in the early postoperative period (either at stool or from vomiting caused by anesthetic or opiate analgesic agents). Furthermore, there is no firm evidence of efficacy in reducing bleeding complications in the anticoagulated patient, as yet. These issues must be studied further and proven in the context of multicenter randomized controlled trials in future.

With regard to bipolar loop resection in humans, Issa and colleagues reported a subgroup of 5 patients from an institutional cohort of 58 patients treated with PK bipolar TURP between 2001 and 2003.[32] This subgroup had large prostate resection weights (greater than 35 g) and significant comorbidity as determined by ASA risk category 3 or more. Of this subgroup, mean resected weight was 49.6 g (32–67 g), achieved during a mean operating time of

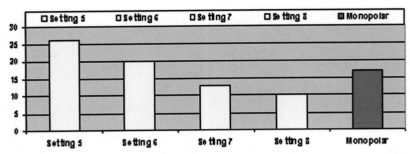

Figure 71B-22 Bleeding rates in cut modes.

2 hours and 22 minutes (98 to 175 minutes) giving a tissue removal rate of 0.35 g/min. In these long operations, which would have carried a high risk of developing TUR syndrome with monopolar resection, the mean serum sodium concentration decreased by only 1.6 mg/dL, while mean hematocrit dropped by 5.6%. These findings were consistent with the range expected for procedures of this duration. None of these patients required transfusion and all voided spontaneously before discharge.

Our own series of 32 patients were treated with the Vista continuous flow resection system which, contrary to the other systems (all 27F Gyrus or 26F Olympus), had a smaller 25F resectoscope.[33] The theoretical advantage of the smaller instrument size would be a lower incidence of urethral stricturing, especially with a predilated urethra, which was our routine. For the Vista Coblation system, there was a double loop electrode (see Figure 71B-18D) with a thin leading active loop (0.35 mm) and a thicker (0.5 mm) trailing return loop held in parallel with a gap between the two of 1.52 mm. The working elements will take existing lenses from the same manufacturer, limiting expenditure somewhat. Of our patients, 12 had prostates larger than 50 cc on transrectal ultrasonography, with the largest resection weight of 62 g in a 126 cc^3 prostate measured. Median operation time (defined as the interval between the commencement of resection to the placement of the final Foley catheter) in this cohort of large glands was 73 minutes (25 to 120 minutes) and median dry resection weight was 36 g (20 to 62 g), giving a median tissue removal rate in these large glands of 0.49 g/min. Preliminary feasibility trials in our center have shown that the gap between the loops is better seen with a 30° lens, but the extremes of the electrode excursion are better seen with a 12° lens

(Figure 71B-24). Cutting was immediate, only occurring when the loop made contact with the tissue and was "felt" by the operators to be smoother than with monopolar loop TURP. There was excellent visualization of the capsule and other endoscopic landmarks, such as the bladder neck and apex. The cut setting could be increased by the surgeon from a white button on the foot pedal in a cyclical fashion from the preset starting value of 6 on the generator. Coagulation required accurate placement of the bleeding vessel in the gap between the loops, but slightly closer to the thicker back loop, followed by gentle downward pressure to permit the current to flow tangentially through the mouth of the open vessel. Coagulation was best when there was no movement of the loops across the vessel during activation of the foot pedal. A longer activation time (approximately 5 seconds) for the coagulation mode (coupled with a slightly lower flow of irrigant, if possible, without compromising visual control) also appeared to improve the coagulation effect in our experience. As length of resection increased beyond 30 minutes, tissue debris accumulated on the rear of the two loops and required cleaning with a gauze swab, later replaced by a soft brush provided by the manufacturers.

Although there should be no problem with TUR syndrome with bipolar resection, we adhered to the principle that there should be no place for complacency as far as surgical technique was concerned. Hypervolemia and hypothermia from cold saline absorption through the resection fossa can still occur, leading to heart failure in elderly patients with cardiac comorbidity, so we recommend that irrigant fluid should still be warmed before use and that the operator should empty the bladder of accumulated irrigant from time to time (since inflow is usually greater than outflow, even with continuous flow resectoscope

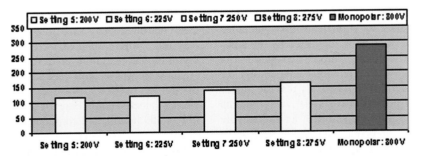

Figure 71B-23 Coagulation depths in coagulation modes.

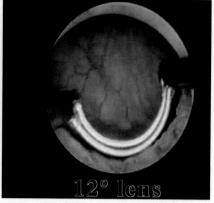

Figure 71B-24 Difference in view of gap between Vista double loop (ACMI Corp., Southborough, MA) using a 30° or 12° lens.

systems). Furthermore, regular emptying of the bladder helped to better reveal bleeding points so they could be controlled in a timely fashion. We also took advantage of the gap between the double loops, and devised a "wedging" coagulation technique around the bladder neck by trapping the cut edge in the gap between the two loops and activating the coagulating current for better hemostasis at this important site.

In 2005, Tefekli and colleagues from Turkey published the results of a prospective randomized comparison of monopolar TURP versus a hybrid of bipolar Gyrus PK vaporization and loop resection in a total of 101 men with either symptomatic LUTS from benign prostatic obstruction or urinary retention with indwelling catheters, with complete data on 96 men.[34] As with previous studies, there seemed to be significant advantages of shorter operating time (40.3 vs 57.8 minutes), less irrigant volume requirement, and shorter catheterization times (2.3 vs 3.8 days), in favor of the PK hybrid treatment. Although completeness of tissue removal was not quantified, there was no difference in overall subjective and objective improvement between the two groups and no difference in blood transfusion requirement postoperatively (low at 2%). Early postoperative problems, however, occurred in 16.3% of the PK hybrid group versus only 8.5% of the monopolar TURP group ($p = .0014$), early severe irritative symptoms were more common, at 12.2% versus 4.3%, respectively, and long-term complications for the PK hybrid group were higher, at 10.2% versus 6.3%, respectively (not significant). The urethral stricture rate was also significantly higher, at 6.1% versus 2.1% in the PK hybrid group. These data tell us that the shorter catheter time of the hybrid PK technique in this study was offset by significant disadvantages postoperatively. If, as is suggested by the studies of Wendt Nordahl,[11] bipolar coagulation is less deep than with monopolar coagulation for the Vista system, then it is likely that the higher incidence of postoperative irritative symptoms (which are usually the result of an excessively coagulated tissue bed and delayed sloughing of this tissue, as was seen with Nd:YAG laser therapies in the past) in this particular study was due to the primary use of the larger surface area bipolar vaporization electrode before the bipolar loop was deployed at the end to tidy up the apex. These irritative symptoms could potentially have been avoided by using the bipolar loop throughout, rather than an expensive hybrid technique predominantly with a larger surface area vaporization electrode. This mistake was compounded by reuse of the electrodes to save cost (especially as either design of bipolar active electrodes are not labeled for reuse, despite the local practice in this particular institution). Evidence to support this contention is provided by the study of Singh and colleagues from India, who also performed a randomized controlled trial in 60 men comparing the Vista bipolar resection system versus a regular monopolar loop.[35] Here, there was no difference in clinical-outcome parameters, and in particular, irritative symptoms of postoperative dysuria were less common with a thin-wire bipolar resection loop. Furthermore, their data indicated a significantly lower fall in serum sodium (1.2 milliequivalents per liter [meq/L] for bipolar vs 4.6 meq/L for monopolar) in exchange for a slightly slower tissue removal rate (0.61 g/min vs 0.74 g/min), and no difference in any other clinical or laboratory parameter studied. Additional studies on a larger scale will be needed to specifically address this issue for each of the various bipolar devices, comparing them to their monopolar equivalents (ie, bipolar loop vs monopolar loop and bipolar vaporization electrode vs monopolar vaporization electrode used predominantly in the cut mode with the right generator), because not all bipolar prostate resection systems are alike in quality or mode of function.

The most recently published clinical randomized controlled study was from de Sio and colleagues,[36] where 70 men were randomized to Gyrus bipolar resection versus monopolar TURP. Again there was a significant advantage in favor of shorter need for postoperative irrigation, shorter catheterization time for the bipolar group (72 vs 100 hours), and consequently, for shorter hospital stay. No other differences were found between the groups either perioperatively or at 1 year follow-up.

There is no clinical or basic scientific information in the peer-reviewed literature on the Surgmaster system from Olympus. This system uses loops of design principles similar to those developed by Gyrus for their loops, but they are of a slightly smaller diameter, thin-wire design separated by yellow insulating material from a thicker more bulbous return end (see Figure 71B-18E). The resectoscope itself is 26F in size and has a working length of 194 mm. As with the older two systems, this design permits current crowding at the thinner active loop to allow the plasma pockets to be formed. The current reaches the active portion of the loop from the generator through the white plastic housing in the bottom of the working element, while the return current flows through the return portion of the electrode in contact with the working element and then back to earth through a lead connected to the working element handle as shown in Figure 71B-25. Hence, part of the telescope housing of the working element is specially insulated to make it fit for this purpose without compromising patient or operator safety by return current leakage. At the resectoscope tip, the electrode and telescope are separated from the metallic outer sheath by insulating material (Figure 71B-26). The Surgmaster generator in the "TURis" mode allows saline resection through two cutting modes (pure and blend with maximum power output of 320 W) and coagulation through two modes designated Coag 1 (maximum 200 W) and Coag 2 (maximum 80 W), though only in combination with the Surgmaster resectoscope. It also has a capability to produce a monopolar output for standard surgical and endosurgical use. In a limited personal clinical experience with this device, cutting seems to be reliable.

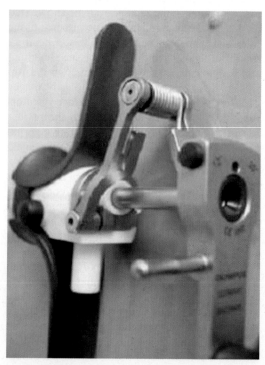

Figure 71B-25 Surgmaster resecting bipolar working element design.

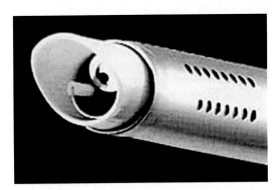

Figure 71B-26 White insulating material between active loop and outer sheath for Surgmaster resectoscope.

The Storz bipolar resection system is the newest of the four commercially available systems and was introduced only in the past year. Again, to date, there are no clinical data, but Wendt-Nordahl and colleagues tested this device against a standard monopolar loop under laboratory conditions similar to the ones they previously reported on for the Vista system using an isolated porcine blood-perfused kidney model.[37] The Storz system loop design is shown in Figure 71B-27. It consists of a double loop with a 5-mm diameter thin-wire active component and a flat thick bow loop bent in the opposite direction, which is the return component, with both loops mounted on the same axis of a dedicated resectoscope. In their study, however, both the monopolar and the bipolar loops were activated by the same electrosurgical generator, an Autocon 400 II (Storz) using an output power of 240 W and coagulation degree 2 for the ex vivo, and an output power of 350 W and coagulation degree 4 for the in vivo experiments. They found that bipolar cutting with this device was impossible ex vivo at low power 80 W (compared to monopolar loop cutting), but became easier as power increased to above 240 W, whereas 300 W was needed for in vivo cutting. Furthermore, there was a delay of almost 1 second until the loop became submerged in the tissue before reliable cutting occurred. When cutting did take place at the higher power, bleeding was reduced from the monopolar device rate of 20.78 ± 1.52 g/min to 15.16 ± 3.3 g/min for the bipolar device ($p < .05$) as shown in Figures 71B-28A and 71B-28B, though the exact incident set power for the monopolar and bipolar modes for these measurements is not stated in the paper. The coagulation zone was slightly deeper for the bipolar device, but the difference with monopolar was not significant (Figure 71B-29). Electrical recordings by

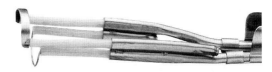

Figure 71B-27 Storz bipolar resection system loop design with thin active loop and flat band return component (Karl Storz, Tuttlingen, Germany).

these authors suggested that using the standard generator, the 0.8-second delay in onset of bipolar cutting, and consistency of cutting quality (as with many of its predecessors) is due to the time taken for the high current output at low impedance to produce the vapor pocket, and this, in turn, is critically dependent on electrode configuration, and generator design and function. To my mind, the electrical measurements in Figure 71B-30 taken during a single bipolar cut, showing the delay to actual cutting, followed by voltages of up to 450 V and power of up to 475 W under varying impedance conditions during actual cutting support the need for dedicated generator design with such devices, for it is likely that systems that do have difficulty initiating fire-up will have greater thermal spread in tissue at the point RF initiation because the surgeon cannot move the loop until the vapor pocket and plasma have been (slowly) established.

TRAINING AND MORBIDITY

Bipolar TURP should allow more time for teaching and training urology residents how to resect prostatic adenomatous tissue without compromising patient safety, for all preliminary studies have shown the risk of hyponatremia to be uniformly low. This is a welcome advantage for the novice trainee, freed of the shackles of time constraint to a large degree, both for the resection phase and also for the coagulation phase of the operation. This is particularly important when the use of TURP has been declining, and a large proportion of patients requiring surgery are either in acute or chronic retention or have large vascular glands. With regard to the technique, only minor changes are needed, and for urologists already proficient in performing monopolar TURP, as bipolar systems

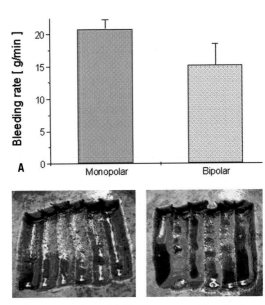

Figure 71B-28 *A*, Bleeding rate comparison for Storz bipolar resection loop (Karl Storz, Tuttlingen, Germany) to standard monopolar loop ($n = 5$) using Autocon Generator (Karl Storz) ($p < .05$, Sig.). *B*, Bleeding kidney surfaces after ablation with the bipolar resection device (left) and the conventional monopolar resectoscope (right).

are almost identical with regard to equipment, the learning curve should be almost negligible. At this time, it is not known whether the risk of capsular perforation and subsequent impotence will be reduced until this issue is formally studied.[38,39] Hemostasis seems to be slightly improved at the resected tissue surface, but deep coagulation is limited, and care must still be taken to avoid opening large venous sinusoids.

One of the concerns that exist for many transurethral bipolar resection systems, as with monopolar electrosurgery, is the potential for urethral and bladder neck stricture formation postoperatively. Although reports on bladder neck strictures for the bipolar systems are sparse, the incidence of urethral strictures in the study by Tefekli and colleagues at 6.1% (versus 2.1% for the monopolar TURP arm) is of concern.[34] Etiologically, there are many possible reasons for the higher stricture rate in these two studies. These include larger resectoscope diameter (27F), especially if the urethra is not adequately pre-dilated before passage of the resectoscope, higher incident power (even if in short bursts), and if a larger prostate is tackled, or one is tackled by a relative novice, resulting in a long operating time. The higher recatheterization rates reported by Dunsmuir and colleagues [30] and Tefekli and colleagues [34] in the PK vaporization studies may be a consequence of residual tissue edema, but may also contribute to urethral stricture formation and may be an indication that bipolar loop resection may be preferable to the vaporization option. Of interest is the paper from Morishita and colleagues which, in 1992, indicated that urethral stricture formation post-TURP may be closely related to electrical resistance and current leakage of appliances.[40] They investigated old and new monopolar and bipolar loops. They found that the new unused bipolar loops had low electrical resistance of 0.5 to 0.6 Ω, increasing with multiple use (for at least 60 minute durations) to 1 to 115 Ω (mean 26.4 Ω), while none showed current leakage. In comparison, all monopolar loops exhibited current leakage after first use and showed relatively high resistance. These data indicate the superior durability of bipolar loops compared to their monopolar counterparts, and if reproduced in currently available bipolar loops, confirms their

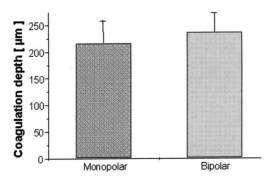

Figure 71B-29 Coagulation depth comparison for Storz Bipolar resection loop (Karl Storz, Tuttlingen, Germany) to standard monopolar loop ($n = 5$) using Autocon Generator (Karl Storz) ($p > .05$, NS).

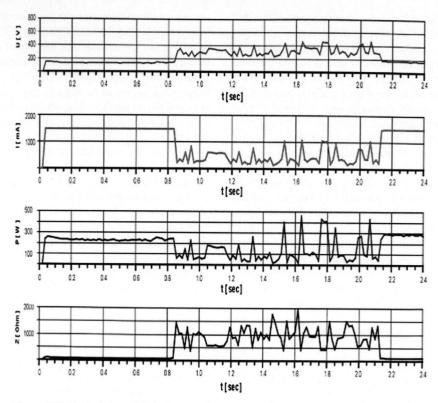

Figure 71B-30 Real-time electrical measurements during single cut with Storz bipolar resection loop (Karl Storz, Tuttlingen, Germany) showing delayed onset of cutting action of 0.85 seconds, voltage, current, power, and impedance, respectively. Note that current was high while impedance was low during the delay before cutting started.

technologies that have failed to endure, will depend on mass acceptance of the technique in the established urological workplace and particularly in training centers that will nurture the urological surgeon of tomorrow. In order to achieve this, the cost comparisons and outcomes in appropriately designed larger multicenter studies, where bipolar loop resection is pitted against the enduring gold standard of monopolar resection, must be forthcoming as a high-quality solid evidence base that will ultimately drive registration and reimbursement, without which no new technology can endure.

ACKNOWLEDGEMENTS

I am grateful to Robert H. Quint for his teaching on electrosurgical engineering principles and for igniting my interest in this field, to Gerhard J. Fuchs and Jorge Gutierrez-Aceves for their support in my clinical work in this area of urology, to Aesculap for information on their generator design, to Francis Amoah for information on the Gyrus PK systems generators, and to Gunnar Wendt-Nordahl for the figures on the Storz bipolar device.

TRANSITIONAL CELL TUMOR RESECTION

No doubt, there will soon be a growing impetus to use bipolar systems to resect transitional cell tumors in the bladder (and possibly in the renal pelvis). Less char will mean better potential histologic analysis, but use of an isotonic solution means that loose cancer cells from higher grade bladder tumors would not be lysed as they would in a bladder full of hypotonic irrigant such as sterile water, leaving greater theoretical possibility of seeding viable cancer cells. One must stress, however, that these are theoretical concerns, and none have been studied in detail at this time. Safety with regard to systemic fluid absorption and its sequelae would certainly be increased with saline irrigant when resecting renal pelvis tumors (though, in the overall spectrum of TCC treatment, this represents only a small number of cases).

COST

This issue has not been studied in detail. A financial analysis study by Ruiz-Deya and colleagues showed the cost of bipolar saline TURP to be 10.56% less than for conventional monopolar TURP.[41] This translated into a cost saving of $1,138 per patient in their institution, but they did not take into account the cost of purchasing a new dedicated generator, a new resectoscope, or at least a new working element, active electrodes that are more than 8 to 10 times the cost of a regular loop, not to mention a longer possible operating room time (which could be offset by lower morbidity). Furthermore, one does not yet have a good sense of loop durability in long resections, and cost will increase if more than one loop has to be used in larger glands. Thinner loops may also be damaged or deformed by repeated contact with prostatic concretions of the variety that are sometimes encountered at the junction between transition and peripheral zones. On the other hand, costs may be lowered in future through multi-specialty use of the generator (in dermatologic, ENT, orthopedic and gynecologic procedures),[42–44] as well as its use in laparoscopic surgery, and will certainly go a long way to improving both its attractiveness and affordability throughout the developed world.

CONCLUSIONS

Transurethral bipolar electrosurgical vaporization and resection systems undoubtedly have future potential for a variety of reasons outlined in this chapter, particularly at a time when urologists may be tackling more large prostates endoscopically. In the face of stiff competition from higher powered lasers (both holmium and KTP), whether this potential is bright, making it an indispensable tool in the prostate kitchen of tomorrow, or just a passing fad like so many other

REFERENCES

1. Iglesias J, Sporer A, Gellmon A. New Iglesias resectoscope with continuous irrigation: simultaneous suction and low intravesical pressure. J Urol 1975;114:929–33.
2. Kirwin TJ. The treatment of prostatic hypertrophy by a new "shrinkage" method. J Urol 1934;32:481.
3. Bush IM, Malters E, Bush J. Transurethral vaporization of the prostate (TVP): new horizons [Abstract]. Soc Minim Invas Ther 1993;2 Suppl:98.
4. Meade WM, Mcloughlin MG. Endoscopic rollerball electrovaporization of the prostate—the sandwich technique: evaluation of the initial efficacy and morbidity in the treatment of benign prostatic obstruction. Br J Urol 1996; 77:696–700.
5. Okada T, Terai A, Terachi T et al. Transurethral electrovaporization of the prostate: preliminary clinical results with pressure-flow analysis. Int J Urol 1998;5:55–9.
6. Dineen MK, Brown BT, Cantwell AL et al. Outpatient transurethral resection of the prostate with vaporization assistance: a two year experience in a free standing ambulatory surgery center [Abstract]. J Urol 1997;157 Suppl:314.
7. Kaplan SA, Laor E, Fatal M et al. Reply by Authors Re: Transurethral resection of the prostate versus transurethral electro-vaporization of the prostate: a blinded prospective comparative study with 1 year follow-up. J Urol 1998; 160(3 Part 1):839.
8. Narayan P, Tewari A, Coker B, et al. Factors affecting size and configuration of electrovaporization lesions in the prostate. Urology 1996;47:679–88.
9. Lim LM, Patel A, Ryan TP, et al. Quantitative assessment of variables that influence soft-tissue electrovaporization in a fluid environment. Urology 1997;49:851–6.
10. Van Swol CFP, van Vliet RJ, Verdaasdonk RM, et al. Electrovaporization as a treatment modality for transurethral resection of the prostate: influence of generator type. Urology 1999;53:317–21.
11. Perlmutter AP, Muschter R, Razvi, HA. Electrosurgical vaporization of the prostate in the canine model. Urology 1995;46:518–23.
12. Wolf JS Jr, Rayala HJ, Humphrey PA, et al. In vivo comparison of electrosurgical vaporization electrodes. J.Endourol 1997;11:83–7.
13. Reis RR, Cologna AJ, Suaid HJ, et al. Electrovaporization of the prostate (VAP): a comparison of roller electrode configurations for resecting prostate tissue [Abstract]. J Urol 1996;155 Suppl:406.
14. Eggleston JL, Kennedy JS, Platt RC, et al. "Instant Response™" electrosurgery generator for laparoscopy and endoscopy. Minim Invasive Ther Allied Technol 1997;5/6:491–5.
15. Larsen TR, Religo WM, Collins JM, et al. Detailed prostatic

superior safety over their monopolar counterparts. But clearly, there is a need to develop bipolar continuous flow resectoscopes smaller than 27F diameter in the not-too-distant future.

interstitial thermal mapping during transurethral grooved rollerball electrovaporization and loop electrosurgery for benign prostatic hyperplasia. Urology 1996;48:501–7.

16. Patel A, Fuchs GJ, Gutiérrez-Aceves J, et al. Prostate heating patterns comparing electrosurgical transurethral resection and vaporization: a prospective randomized study. J Urol 1997;157:169–72.

17. Patel A, Fuchs GJ, Gutiérrez-Aceves J, et al. Completeness and efficiency of prostate tissue removal : loop resection compared with a new operative technique of transurethral resection of the prostate. Br J Urol 1999;84:43–9.

18. Patel A, Quint RH. Electrovaporization of the prostate at low power settings below 100 watts. J Endourol 2001;15:619–23.

19. McAllister WJ, Karim O, Plail R, et al. Transurethral electrovaporization of the prostate: is it any better than conventional transurethral resection of the prostate? Br J Urol 2003;91:211–4.

20. Perk H, Serel TA, Kosar A, Hoscan MB. Comparative early results of the sandwich technique and transurethral electroresection in benign prostatic hyperplasia. Prostate Cancer Prostatic Dis 2001;4:242–4.

21. Jennings SB, Karafin LJ, Rukstalis DB. High-frequency electrosurgery using the microcomputer-controlled Erbe ICC 350 unit. J Endourol 1998;12:67–9.

22. Kupeli S, Sotgur T, Yilmaz E, Budak M. Combined transurethral resection and vaporization of the prostate using newly designed electrode: a promising treatment alternative for benign prostatic hyperplasia. J Endourol 1999;13:225–8.

23. Talic RF, El Tiraifi A, El Faquih SR, et al. Prospective randomized study of transurethral vaporization resection of the prostate using the thick loop and standard transurethral prostatectomy. Urology 2000;55:886–90.

24. Netto NR Jr, Matheus WE, Ferreira U, et al. Transurethral electrovaporization of the prostate: use of a new device [Abstract]. J Endourol 2002;16 Suppl 1:14–5.

25. Hartung R, Leyh H, Liapi C, et al. Coagulating intermittent cutting: improved high-frequency surgery in transurethral prostatectomy. Eur Urol 2001;39:676–81.

26. Stadler KR, Woloszko J, Brown IG, Smith CD. Repetitive plasma discharges in saline solutions. Appl Phys Lett 2001;79:4503–5.

27. Eaton AC, Francis RN. The provision of transurethral prostatectomy on a day-case basis using bipolar plasma kinetic technology. BJU Int 2002;89:534–7.

28. McFarlane JP, Tan AF, Kourambas J, et al. Gyrus electrovaporization and TURP; preliminary results of a prospective randomised trial [Abstract]. J Endourol 2001;15 Suppl 1: A91, C5-P10.

29. Watson G. A randomized study comparing Holmium laser enucleation with bipolar plasma enucleation of the prostate. J Endourol 2002;16 Suppl 1:P11–19, A51.

30. Dunsmuir WD, McFarlane JP, Tan A, et al. Gyrus bipolar electrovaporization versus transurethral resection of the prostate: a randomized prospective single blind trial with 1 year follow-up. Prostate Cancer Prostatic Dis 2003;6: 182–6.

31. Wendt-Nordahl G, Häcker A, Reich O, et al. The Vista system: a new bipolar resection device for endourological procedures: comparison with conventional resectoscope. Eur Urol 2004;46:586–90.

32. Issa MM, Young MR, Bullock AR, et al. Dilutional hyponatremia of TURP syndrome: a historical event in the 21st century. Urology 2004;64:298–301.

33. Patel A, Adshead J. First clinical experience of a new transurethral bipolar prostate electrosurgery resection system: controlled tissue ablation (Coblation technology®). J Endourol 2004;18:967–72.

34. Tefekli A, Muslumanoglu AY, Baykal M, et al. A hybrid technique using bipolar energy in transurethral prostate surgery: a prospective randomized comparison J Urol 2005; 174 (4 Pt 1):1339–43.

35. Singh H, Desai MR, Shrivastav P, et al. Bipolar versus monopolar transurethral resection of prostate: randomized controlled study J Endourol 2005;19:333–8.

36. de Sio M, Autorino R, Quarto G, et al. Gyrus bipolar versus standard monopolar transurethral resection of the prostate: a randomized prospective trial. Urology 2006;67:69–72.

37. Hanbury DC, Sethia KK. Erectile function following transurethral prostatectomy. Br J Urol 1995;75:12–3.

38. Bieri S, Iselin CE, Rohner S. Capsular perforation localization and adenoma size as prognostic indicators of erectile dysfunction after transurethral prostatectomy. Scand J Urol Nephrol 1997;31:545–8.

39. Wendt-Nordahl G, Hacker A, Fastenmeier K, et al. New bipolar resection device for transurethral resection of the prostate: first ex-vivo and in-vivo evaluation. J Endourol 2005;19:1203–9.

40. Morishita H, Nakajima Y, Chen X, et al. Electrical resistance and current leakage of appliances for transurethral resection. Hinyokika Kiyo 1992;38:413–7.

41. Ruiz-Deya G, Hellstrom W, Thomas R. Minimally invasive treatment of BPH using a novel electrocautery system (Gyrus): a retrospective financial analysis versus standard monopolar resection. J Endourol 2002;16 (Suppl 1):A25.

42. Mancini PF. Coblation: a new technology and technique for skin resurfacing and other aesthetic surgical procedures. Aesthetic Plast Surg 2001;25:372–7.

43. Timms MS, Temple RH. Coblation tonsillectomy: a double blind randomized controlled study. J Laryngol Otol 2002; 116:450–2.

44. Fernandez H, Gervaise A, de Tayrac R. Operative hysteroscopy for infertility using normal saline solution and a coaxial bipolar electrode: a pilot study. Hum Reprod 2000;15:1773–5.

45. Hammadeh MY, Fowlis GA, Singh M, et al. Transurethral electrovaporization of the prostate—a possible alternative to transurethral resection: a one-year follow-up of a prospective randomized trial. Br J Urol 1998;81:721–5.

46. Gallucci M, Pupo P, Perachino M, et al. Transurethral electrovaporization of the prostate vs. transurethral resection. Eur Urol 1998;33:359–64.

47. Kupeli S, Baltaci S, Soygur T, et al. A prospective randomized study of transurethral resection of the prostate and transurethral vaporization of the prostate as a therapeutic alternative in the management of men with BPH. Eur Urol 1998;34:15–8.

48. Shokeir AA, Al-Sisi H, Farage YM, et al. Transurethral prostatectomy: a prospective randomized study of conventional resection and electrovaporization in benign prostatic hyperplasia. Br J Urol 1997;80:570–4.

49. Patel A, Fuchs GJ, Gutierrez-Aceves J, et al. A prospective randomized double blind study of transurethral resection (TURP) vs. electrovaporization (TUEVAP) of the prostate. SIU Proceedings [Abstract]. Br J Urol 1997;80 Suppl 2:190.

50. McAllister WJ, Karim O, Plail R et al. A prospective randomized multicentre trial of transurethral electrovaporization of the prostate against TURP: preliminary results [Abstract]. Br J Urol 1998;81 Suppl 4:81.

51. Hammadeh MY, Madaan S, Hines J, et al. 5 year outcome of a prospective randomized trial to compare transurethral electrovaporization of the prostate and standard transurethral resection. Urology 2003;61:1166–71.

The Rotoresect System for Bloodless Transurethral Resection of the Prostate

Maurice Stephan Michel, MD, PhD

Peter Alken, MD

INDICATIONS

The indications for transurethral rotoresection of the prostate correspond to those of the conventional TURP. The inclusion and exclusion criteria of the study in Mannheim are shown in Table 71C-1.

PATIENT PREPARATION

Same as for conventional TURP.

INFORMED CONSENT

Same as for conventional TURP.

PREOPERATIVE PREPARATION

Same as for conventional TURP.

INSTRUMENTATION

The Rotoresect (Karl Storz, Tuttlingen, Germany) system is designed for transurethral application. Instead of a loop electrode, an axially adjustable, actively rotating crank with a milling head electrode is fitted into a specially designed working element of the resectoscope. This crank is driven by an easy-to-handle, infinitely variable micromotor. The rotation of this micromotor is transmitted to the electrode by an angle drill handle. The micromotor is regulated by a foot switch connected to a multidrive control unit. The high-frequency current is conducted to the rotating crank in the working element of the rectoscope by a sliding contact. A common 24 French (F) resectoscope shaft and standard 0° optics were used for clinical application (Table 71C-2 and Figure 71C-1). The rotating crank conducting the high-frequency current is insulated up to the electrode by a Teflon coating. The milling head electrode is provided with spikes. An Autocon 350 (Karl Storz, Tuttlingen, Germany) high-frequency current generator was used in clinical application; the maximum power output can be restricted by the digital setting on the generator. The generator is equipped with an electronic spark control that adjusts the power output according to tissue resistancy. The device is operated by a dual-control foot switch for separate regulation of cutting and coagulation.[1-3]

STEP-BY-STEP DESCRIPTION OF OPERATIVE PROCEDURE

The following parameters were chosen in accordance with the results gained from prior clinical studies with the Rotoresect device: cutting current output 220 watt and rotation speed 2,900 to 6,100 rpm. The working and physical principles of this new resection procedure for clinical application are described as follows: (1) the active rotation without the conduction of HF current induces only very slight bleeding of the tissue; (2) the activation of HF current without rotation of the milling head enables vaporization and coagulation of the tissue, but coagulated tissue sticks to the electrode; (3) with rotation, the electrode remains clean and the tissue is mechanically ablated; and (4) the coagulation layer is diminished. In contrast to the standard loop resection, where the electrode is guided from the bladder neck to the apex, during rotoresection the active rotating electrode is guided in a transversal mode beginning at the bladder neck. The electrode is then beltwise moved to the apex area. The procedure commenced as follows: (1) resection of the bladder neck or middle lobe and paracollicular sections; (2) after that, resection of the right and left side lobes; and (3) finally, resection of the ventral surface and apex area (Figure 71C-2).

Table 71C-1 Inclusion and Exclusion Criteria of the Study in Mannheim
Inclusion Criteria:
Patient age > 45 years.
Maximum urine flow rate ≤ 15 mL/s or residual urine > 100 mL or urine retention.
Life expectancy ≥ 2 years and willingness to participate.
Exclusion Criteria:
Prostate volume in TRUS ≤ 15 mL or ≥ 80 mL.
Suspected or histologically confirmed prostate or bladder carcinoma.
Urethral stenosis or abdominal radiation therapy.
Therapy resistent urinary tract infection.
Previous instrumental BPH therapy.
Suspected or urodynamically confirmed neurogenic bladder instability.

Table 71C-2 Technical Details of the Rotoresect System	
Manufacturer	Karl Storz GmbH, Tuttlingen, Germany
Micromotor	
Revolution	2,900–6,100 rpm
Weight	300 g
Electrode	
Length	5 mm
Diameter	3 mm
Profile	Roller with spikes
Resectoscope Shaft	
Diameter	24F
Irrigation	High or low pressure
Optic	
0° or 12°	Hopkins (diameter 4 mm)

POSTOPERATIVE CARE

Same as for conventional TURP.

RESULTS

A total number of 84 patients (age 68.7 ± 7.9 years) were recruited for a clinical study in Mannheim in accordance with the inclusion and exclusion criteria given in Table 71C-1. Preoperative transrectal ultrasound examination revealed a prostate volume of 46.0 ± 18.4 mL. Intraoperative, as well as postoperative and follow-up, evaluations were completed to determine the effectivity and any possible side effects.

INTRAOPERATIVE FINDINGS During resection without high-frequency current, the milling head electrode did not ablate prostatic tissue, but achieved only a slight erosion of the mucosa. Activation of the coagulation current without simultaneous rotation resulted in slight surface vaporization and extensive coagulation. Activation of rotation enabled additional mechanical tissue ablation under maintenance of minimum blood loss. Postoperatively, no significant changes in hemoglobin ($\Delta 1.2 \pm 0.7$ g/dL) and sodium concentration ($\Delta 2.4 \pm 2.7$ mmol/L) could be detected. No reduced efficacy was observed at deeper depths during the course of the procedure. The capsule layer was always reliably revealed.

Compared with the conventional resection loop, there was a distinct decline in bleeding during and at the end of rotorsection. There was no demand for a blood transfusion. In 1 patient, a TUR syndrome was observed. No other side effects than the typical TUR ones were observed. The complete rotoresection of the prostate was possible in all patients. The resection time was 57.2 ± 16.6 minutes. In the initial phase of the study, the following technical problems occurred:

- In three cases the distal isolation of the electrode was damaged.
- In two cases the rotation was blocked during the resection.

Theses problems were intraoperative managed by the replacement of the system. Because of this problem, the system was modified, which increased the robustness of the system.

POSTOPERATIVE RESULTS AND FOLLOW-UP Pale, flesh-coloured irrigation liquid was observed in the majority of patients and the catheter was removed on either the first or second postoperative day. The average catheter indwelling time was 1.4 ± 1.1 days. After removal of the catheter, the mentioned evaluation of properties was made at the time of discharge. Residual urine and maximum flow were distinctly improved (see Figure 71C-2, and Figure 71C-3). During the first 6 months after rotoresection, the IPSS score as well as the LQI decreases significantly (Figures 71C-4 and 71C-5). In further follow-ups, the residual urine, peak flow rate, as well as the IPSS and the LQI, remained stable (see Figures 71C-2, 71C-4, 71C-5, and Figure 71C-6).[3]

COMPLICATIONS

After catheter removal on the first postoperative day, persisting macrohematuria in 2 patients demanded recatheterization for 1 further day. On the second postoperative day, 1 patient suffered from hydronephrosis on the left side. Cystoscopy revealed an edamatous swelling reaching up as far as the ureteral orifice. The insertion of a ureteric stent relieved the obstruction. Examination after 6 weeks revealed normal findings, so no further treatment was required. Two patients developed postoperative subfibrile temperatures that were successfully managed by antibiotics. During the postoperative period, 26% of the patients complained of dysuric disorders and/or urge symptoms after removal of the catheter ranging from 3 days to 8 weeks (median 2.5 weeks). One patient developed a bladder neck stricture 1 year after resection, which required incision, and 2 patients required a re-TURP during the follow-up period. No persisting impotency or stress incontinence and no urethral stricture were observed during the follow-up.

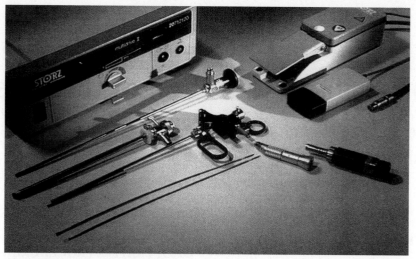

Figure 71C-1 Rotoresect system with working element, micromotor, shaft, optic, electrode, and the multidrive unit with foot pedal.

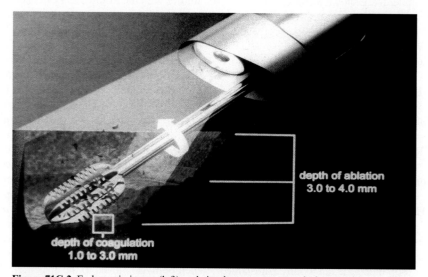

Figure 71C-2 Endoscopic image (left) and simultaneous transrectal ultrasound image (transversal plane) (right) at the beginning (up) and at the end (down) of the rotoresection.

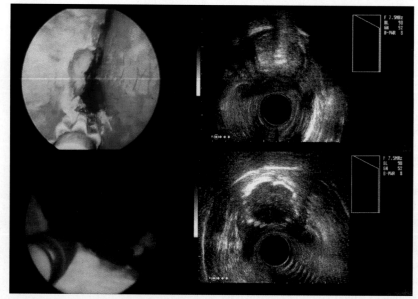

Figure 71C-3 Working principle of the Rotoresect system: vaporization, coagulation, and simultaneous mechanichal removal of the coagulated tissue.

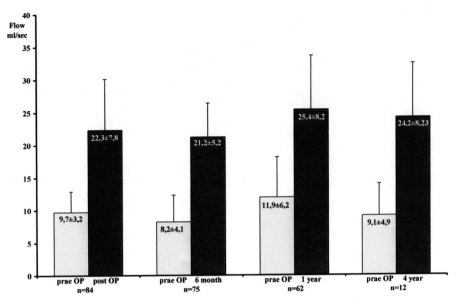

Figure 71C-4 Urine peak flow prior to and after transurethral rotoresection of the prostate.

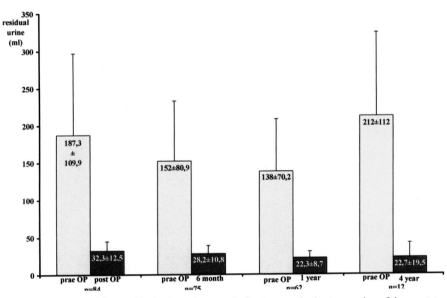

Figure 7C-5 Post voiding residual urine prior to and after transurethral rotoresection of the prostate.

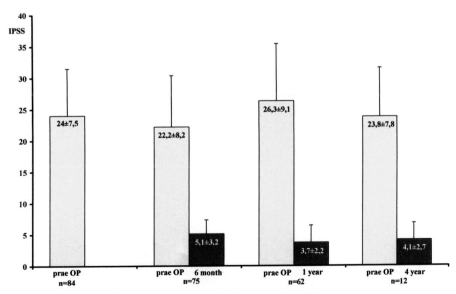

Figure 71C-6 IPSS prior to and after transurethral rotoresection of the prostate.

REFERENCES

1. Michel MS, Köhrmann KU, Weber A, et al. Rotoresect: new technique for resection of the prostate: experimental phase. J Endourol 1996;10:473–8.
2. Michel MS, Koehrmann KU, Knoll T, et al. Clinical evaluation of a newly developed endoscopic resection device (Rotoresect): physical principle and first clinical results. Surg Endosc 2001;15:1395–400.
3. Michel MS, Knoll T, Trojan L, et al. Rotoresect for bloodless transurethral resection of the prostate: a 4-year follow-up. BJU Int 2003;91:65–8.

Transurethral Incision of the Prostate Revisited

Atul A. Thakre, MD
Robert M. Moldwin, MD

Transurethral resection of the prostate (TURP) has been the gold standard for the treatment of obstructive benign prostatic hyperplasia (BPH) for over 30 years. However, the morbidity rate (18%)[1] combined with the demand for minimally invasive, cost-effective treatment has fueled the search for other treatment modalities. Transurethral incision of the prostate (TUIP), a procedure initially described by Orandi in 1969, has been "rediscovered" and may even replace TURP as the treatment of choice for select populations of men with BPH.[2] Since its introduction, TUIP has slowly gained favor among clinicians, most notably because of its simplicity, relatively few complications, and satisfactory long-term results. In addition, most authors report that the procedure is easy to teach and to learn.[2–7]

ORANDI'S PROCEDURE

In 1964 Aboulker and Steg[8] performed "divulsion of the prostate." They used an expandable sound to rupture the prostatic urethra in 218 patients with obstructive symptoms. Although satisfactory results were achieved in 75% of the patients, there were significant complications, most notably profuse bleeding, incontinence, and phlegmon in the space of Retzius. Orandi[9] expanded on this idea and theorized that endoscopic incision in certain locations could achieve a similar efficacy with fewer complications. He first performed his procedure in 1969 on a 36-year-old diabetic patient with urinary retention. Orandi gained access to the bladder through a perineal urethrotomy. A continuous-flow resectoscope fitted with a knife electrode was inserted, and the bladder filled to a pressure under 40 to 50 cm H_2O.

Incisions were created at the 5- and 7-o'clock positions from the ureteral orifices down to the bladder neck and prostatic urethra to either side of the verumontanum. The incisions were gradually deepened to include the full thickness of the bladder neck and prostate until the capsule was reached. In larger glands Orandi found it necessary to split the bladder neck and capsule of the prostate, which caused bleeding and extravasation. For younger patients who wished to avoid retrograde ejaculation, he modified the procedure by creating shallower incisions and limiting these to the prostatic urethra without extension into the bladder neck. Extensive fulguration in the depth of the incisions was also avoided. Later

Orandi further modified these incisions and included only the prostatic urethra without manipulation of the bladder neck to avoid damaging the internal sphincter mechanism. Histopathologic specimens were obtained with a single pass of the cutting loop or the resectoscope biopsy needle (Greenwald Surgical, Lake Station, IN). The procedure had the additional effect of opening the obstructed prostatic duct, draining trapped prostatic secretions, and releasing stones.

Postoperatively a 22 French (F) three-way Foley catheter was inserted to drain the bladder with continuous irrigation for 24 hours. Traction was applied if bleeding persisted.[2] The catheter was removed in 1 to 3 days.

MODIFICATIONS Modifications made by later investigators are variations on Orandi's original procedure. Different instruments have been used, including the Collings knife, Sachs knife, Orandi knife, and the standard resectoscope. Ruzic and colleagues[10] modified the TUIP technique by short and shallow incision of the prostate at the 5 and 7 o clock position. The incisions were made, limited to the prostatic urethra and reaching to the fibrous capsule. There was significant increase in the peak flow rates and International Prostate Symptom Score (IPSS) decreased significantly. All 28 patients sexually active before surgery retained their sexual activity after surgery; only one developed retrograde ejaculation. This technique is an effective method for long-term relief of bladder outlet obstruction in patients with small, benign prostates. It has an equally good long-term outcome as the classic long and deep TUIP. Recently the free-beam and the contact Nd:YAG lasers have been used for TUIP as well as TURP.[11,12] Johnson and colleagues[13] have evaluated the holmium:YAG laser on dogs with good results. No definitive studies have been completed to document whether certain modifications are superior to others.

Double vs Single Incision TUIP, as originally described by Orandi, involved two incisions. The technique has been modified by several investigators who describe using single incisions for TUIP.[14–17] The single incisions were typically performed at the 5-, 6-, or 7-o'clock positions. Turner-Warwick[18] reported a significantly reduced incidence of retrograde ejaculation (15–5%) and comparable clinical results using a single full-thickness incision and bilateral

incisions. Other investigators reported similar findings.[15,19,20] No differences in treatment outcome were observed using single or double incisions. The most popular unilateral incision is located at the 6-o'clock position (Figure 71D–1). The most commonly performed bilateral incisions are at the 5- and 7-o'clock positions.[21]

TUIP Plus Prostatic Resection Lin[22] added a posterior resection to 4- and 8-o'clock incisions. He claimed this avoided the adhesions encountered between the incised portions of the prostate, making it easier to create deeper incisions through the prostatic capsule and to eliminate the ball valving that occurs from both posterior incisions interfering with urine flow. Simsek and colleagues[23] reported on the technique of grooving prostate tissue at the 5- and 7-o'clock positions as an alternative to TUIP. They claimed similar results with the added benefit of being able to obtain prostatic tissue for histopathologic diagnosis. Although they reported that efficacy was similar to TUIP, they also reported a higher reoperation rate.

Yeni and colleagues[24] evaluated the effectiveness and complications of combination of minimal transurethral resection of prostate and bladder neck incision in comparison with those of the standard TURP. The results showed the bladder neck incision group fared better than the TURP group by preventing the difficulty of urethral catheter positioning at the end of the operation,

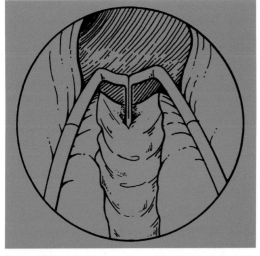

Figure 71D-1 Cystocopic view of the 6-o'clock incision in TUIP. A Collings knife is being used.

decreasing bladder neck contracture and lowering the incidence of retrograde ejaculation.

INDICATIONS

The original intention was for TUIP to be a new surgical procedure for treating patients with small but obstructing prostates who were not candidates for either TURP or open surgery.[2] This population of patients consisted of young men who had obstructive symptoms but who did not have markedly enlarged glands. Since the understanding at that time was that BPH occurred only in older men with large prostates, the symptoms were attributed to prostatitis. In later years, propelled by the early excellent results, the indications were extended to men of all ages (19–98 years) who had bladder outlet obstruction and prostates of various sizes (estimated weight from 3–40 g). Dorflinger and colleagues[25] examined the urodynamic findings in men with prostatism and correlated these with their histologic profiles. They demonstrated that men with smaller glands predominantly had stromal hyperplasia and responded less favorably to TURP than men with glandular hyperplasia. This led Kelly and colleagues[26] to presume that men with small prostates who had obstructive symptoms could be helped more by an incision than a resection.

Currently most investigators agree that the ideal candidates for TUIP are patients who would have a resected weight of < 30 g.[11,20,27,28] Orandi[29] believed that larger glands required deep incisions into the capsule. This invariably led to the opening of venous sinuses and perforation of the capsule, causing extravasation and uncontrolled venous bleeding. Frequently extensive fulguration was necessary, which significantly increased the incidence of postoperative complications. Mebust and colleagues,[1] in their study of 3,885 TURP patients, reported an average resected prostatic weight of 22 g, suggesting the potential for TUIP in the treatment of these patients.

Jocius and Sukyas[30] described another indication of TUIP where they used TUIP as an effective method in treating the cases of postopen prostatectomy or TURP bladder neck obstruction. Fuse and colleagues[31] reported TUIP for hematospermia in cases with midline cyst in the prostatic urethra. Tan and colleagues[32] described of 79 patients, 1 patient underwent TUIP for bladder neck contracture following high-power holmium laser vaporization. Klijer and colleagues[33] achieved good results by treating 16 of 19 women with bladder outlet obstruction by bladder neck incision through 5- and 7-o' clock position and 2 patients having distal urethral incision at 12-o'clock position.

RESULTS

The first cited review of TUIP was by Orandi in 1973.[9] He presented excellent initial results in the treatment of 40 patients. Later, after 646 procedures, he published a chronologic appraisal spanning 15 years.[29] He achieved good symptomatic relief in 79% of patients, fair relief in 11%, and a poor outcome in 10%. In 84% of 38 consecutive patients, a better postoperative maximum flow rate was achieved. Drago[7] performed TUIP on 100 men with outflow obstruction who had a prostatic weight of 30 g. Incisions were made at 5 and 7 o'clock from 1 mm inside the bladder neck to 1 mm proximal to the verumontanum. Mean peak urinary flow improved from 7.6 mL/s preoperatively to 12.6 mL/s postoperatively, and 80% of these patients experienced an improvement in symptom scores after 1 year. Twelve patients required TURP, 1 required hospitalization for clot retention, and 3% experienced retrograde ejaculation. Drago found that costs were significantly lower because patients in his study were treated in an outpatient setting using local anesthesia and a periprostatic block.

Kelly and colleagues[26] evaluated 26 men in whom TUIP was performed from 1 cm distal to the ureteral orifices to the proximal area of the verumontanum at the 4- and 8-o'clock positions, exposing periprostatic fat. They documented a significant decrease in symptom scores (9.6–2.8) and a significant improvement in urodynamic parameters such as peak flow (5.1–10.8 mL/s), detrusor pressure at peak flow (102.5–58.3 cm H_2O), and incidence of detrusor instability (46–27%). They reported 1 complication (clot retention) and no patient required transfusion or further surgical intervention.

Sirls and colleagues[4] evaluated the long-term efficacy of TUIP using various objective (urodynamic) and subjective (symptom score and assessment of sexual function) parameters. They reviewed 41 men at a mean follow-up of 53 months and compared pre- and postoperative symptom scores (Madsen-Iversen), urodynamic evaluation, and interview responses. Men selected for this study had bladder outlet obstruction confirmed by pressure-flow analysis and an estimated prostatic weight of 30 g. TUIP was performed from 1 cm distal to the ureteral orifices to the proximal area of the verumontanum at the 4- and 8-o'clock positions, exposing periprostatic fat.

Mean symptom scores decreased from 12.5 to 6.9, mean detrusor pressure at peak flow decreased from 85 to 44 cm H_2O, and flow rates increased from 10 to 15 mL/s. There was an 11% incidence of new-onset retrograde ejaculation, but no significant difference in subjective assessment of potency or sensation of orgasm. One patient required prolonged hospitalization for hematuria (3 days) and 1 patient had an episode of epididymitis that responded to antibiotic therapy. Of the 4 patients who underwent TURP, 2 experienced symptomatic improvement, 1 had persistent irritative symptoms, and 1 remained on intermittent catheterization. This study supports TUIP as an effective long-term therapy for selected men with outlet obstruction.

COMPARATIVE STUDIES Orandi[34] performed a prospective study of 132 patients with bladder outlet obstruction who were managed either by TUIP or TURP. These patients all had uniform characteristics, including symptoms of bladder outlet obstruction and small prostates, and all could have been managed by either incision or resection of the prostate. Of the 42 patients who underwent TUIP, the mean peak flow increased from 8.2 to 13.7 mL/s. Of the 39 patients who underwent TURP, mean peak flow increased from 7.6 to 12.7 mL/s. Dorflinger and colleagues[5] randomized 38 patients with an estimated prostatic weight of 20 g into a group that underwent TUIP with a single incision at 7 o'clock (17 patients) and a group that underwent TURP (21 patients). In the TUIP group, they found a significant reduction in both blood loss requiring transfusion (19% for TURP and 0% for TUIP) and operative time (30 minutes for TURP and 15 minutes for TUIP). They found no significant difference in postoperative parameters such as length of hospitalization, incidence of sepsis, or time with an indwelling catheter. At 3 months of follow-up there was a similar improvement in symptom score and maximum flow rates in both groups. There was a major difference in the incidence of retrograde ejaculation (45% for TURP and 0% for TUIP). Dorflinger and colleagues concluded that TUIP was as effective as TURP in relieving bladder outlet obstruction in small prostates and resulted in significantly fewer complications.

Christensen and colleagues[35] compared the results of 49 men who underwent TUIP and 44 men who underwent TURP in a prospective, randomized study. They selected men with outlet obstruction who had an estimated prostatic weight of 20 g. In the TUIP group, patients had a single, deep incision at 6 o'clock, extending from the interureteric ridge to the verumontanum. Long-term follow-up was recorded for 38 men in each group. In the TURP group, 95% of patients showed significant improvement at 3 months and 64% at 3 to 4 years. In the TUIP group 81% of patients showed improvement at 3 months and 78% at 3 to 4 years. At 4-year follow-up the peak flow rate was significantly higher than the preoperative peak flow rate in the TUIP group (10.9 vs 7.8 mL/s). This change was similar to the TURP group (14.6 vs 9.7 mL/s). There was 1 complication in each treatment group. In the TURP group, 1 patient died as a result of a pulmonary embolus, and in the TUIP group 1 patient had significant urinary extravasation, necessitating an exploratory laparotomy. Christensen and colleagues[35] concluded that in men with small prostates, TUIP was equivalent to TURP with regard to efficacy and that TUIP was favored when cost and the number of adverse effects were taken into consideration.

Soonawalla and Pardanani[6] conducted a prospective study of 220 patients with urinary obstruction caused by a small prostate. The patients were randomized into either a TURP or TUIP group. In the TUIP group, a single, deep incision was made in either the 5- or the 7-o'clock position from just below the ureteral orifice up to the verumontanum, exposing periprostatic fat. Follow-up ranged from a minimum of 3 months to 2 years. A comparison of the results revealed no significant difference between the two procedures.

Peak flow rates increased from 7.91 to 19.38 mL/s after TUIP compared with 8.04 to 20.69 mL/s after TURP. Postvoid residuals decreased in 90% of TUIP patients and 88% of TURP patients.

TUIP initially failed in 7 patients. Of these, 4 required a repeat procedure for cure. Three had protruding lateral lobes on cystoscopy that required resection. TURP initially failed in 4 patients. Two required a repeat resection and 2 underwent TUIP. In the TUIP group, 1 patient died from a myocardial infarction and 2 died after resection as a result of sepsis and myocardial infarction. Blood transfusion was required in 38% of the TURP patients and none of the TUIP patients. TUR syndrome was experienced in 6.4% of TURP patients and in none of the TUIP patients. Overall, Soonawalla and Pardanani noted a higher incidence of major complications following TURP.

A variety of studies have used different parameters to measure treatment outcome. The Benign Prostatic Hyperplasia Guideline Panel[29] was formed to identify the most effective methods for diagnosing and treating BPH. The panel did an extensive review of the literature on BPH, surveying over 1,200 abstracts and 200 articles published in peer-reviewed journals. The panel concluded that TUIP is currently an underutilized procedure. It also concluded that for patients with prostate glands of 30 g of resectable weight, TUIP has a long-term effectiveness equivalent to TURP, but with less cost and less morbidity. Other groups have also reported remarkably promising long-term results with TUIP similar to those with TURP but associated with significantly reduced morbidity, mortality, hospitalization, and costs (Table 71D-1).[4,29,36] In comparing the overall results of TURP and TUIP, the panel found that TURP had a 75 to 96% chance of improving a patient's urinary symptoms, whereas TUIP patients had a 78 to 83% chance of symptom improvement. It found that TURP may have a slightly better outcome than TUIP in urinary symptoms. It reports that the cumulative failure rate is 9% for TUIP and 10% for TURP. Taking into account the low overall morbidity of TUIP, these findings confirm that TUIP is an excellent treatment modality. Tkocz and Prajsner[37] in their long-term comparison of TUIP with TURP showed TUIP as an effective and safe procedure for patients with a small number of complications. Yang and colleagues[38,45] concluded TUIP appeared to be underused and prostate size plays an important role in determining the role of TUIP.

COMPLICATIONS

For any procedure to be considered a viable alternative to the established standard of care, it must not only equal the advantages of the standard treatment, but also have fewer potential risks.[28] It is beyond the scope of this discussion to include all of the complications associated with TURP; however, understanding its pitfalls will help us to assess the value of TUIP as a treatment modality. In a review by Mebust and colleagues,[1] TURP was associated with an astounding 18% morbidity

rate in a survey of 3,885 patients undergoing TURP at 13 institutions. The most common urologic complications were failure to void and bleeding that required blood transfusions. A study by Evans and colleagues,[39] showed that significant, unexpected hemodynamic responses occurred during TURP. These included a significant increase in the left ventricular afterload, resulting in increased myocardial work and oxygen demand. They concluded that this may contribute to the increase in cardiovascular morbidity and mortality associated with TURP. They reported that the hemodynamic changes were unrelated to the individual surgeon, age of the patient, cardiac risk index, weight resected, length of surgery, hemorrhage, or irrigation fluid load. Despite the lack of a valid explanation, the fluid shifts that occur during TURP and bleeding remain the two major drawbacks of TURP and indicate areas where other therapies without these drawbacks have a potential advantage over TURP.

Sexual dysfunction following TURP includes impotence and retrograde ejaculation. Impotence has been reported in approximately 5% of cases in most series.[1,28,38] The incidence of retrograde ejaculation can vary from 30 to 100%.[42,43]

Permanent urinary incontinence in patients who had TURP/TUIP following prostate brachytherapy is common. It is considered multifactorial and may include the degree of physical damage to the urinary sphincter and the radiation dose to the urethral region.[45]

Intraoperative Because operating time for TUIP is relatively short, fluid shifts and serum electrolyte abnormalities are not likely, and indeed are not mentioned in any major study reviewed. Soonawalla and Pardanani[6] found that TUIP could be performed much faster than TURP (20.4 and 59.3 minutes, respectively) and that the amount of irrigation fluid needed was significantly less (4.7 and 15.9 L, respectively). Hemorrhage severe enough to require blood transfusions in patients undergoing TUIP occurred extremely rarely, if at all. Dorflinger and colleagues[5] found that blood transfusions were required by 4 of 31 (13%) TURP patients and none of 29 TUIP patients. Edwards and colleagues[16] reported a transfusion rate of 1.6% in TUIP patients and 19.6% in TURP patients. In Orandi's series of 646 patients treated with TUIP, 30 six patients (1%) required transfusion. Christiansen and colleagues[35] showed that the estimated blood loss in TUIP patients was 25 mL compared with 150 mL

in TURP patients. Soonawalla and Pardanani[6] noted that 38 of 110 TURP patients required blood transfusion, with an average of 0.44 units of blood for each patient. In contrast, none of 110 TUIP patients required transfusion. This series revealed a significantly higher transfusion rate for TURP than previously reported.

Postoperative Edwards and colleagues[16] noted a 1.3% incidence of clot retention in the TUIP group and a 2.3% rate in the TURP group. Dorflinger and colleagues[5] reviewed 43 sexually active patients randomized into a TUIP or TURP group. At 1-year follow-up they noted that 1 of 19 TUIP patients experienced retrograde ejaculation compared with 12 of 24 TURP patients.

Larsen and colleagues[43] reported that 2 of 7 TUIP patients experienced retrograde ejaculation, whereas 8 of 8 TURP patients experienced this problem. Dorflinger and colleagues[5] reported that none of their 7 TUIP patients experienced retrograde ejaculation, whereas 5 of 11 of their TURP patients experienced this problem. Christensen and colleagues[35] reported a 13% incidence of retrograde ejaculation in the TUIP group and a 37% incidence in the TURP group. Soonawalla and Pardanani[6] found a similar rate of retrograde ejaculation in their series. Of 60 sexually active patients who underwent TUIP and 49 who underwent TURP, 33% of TUIP patients and 36% of TURP patients had retrograde ejaculation. The incidence of this complication in the TUIP series by Soonawalla and Pardanani[6] was much higher than in the studies by other investigators.

Dorflinger and colleagues[5] evaluated randomized patients and found that 2 of 17 incision patients had urinary retention within the first week. These patients were treated with TURP. One of 21 TURP patients had urinary retention.

CONCLUSION

Since its introduction over 20 years ago, TUIP has been established as an excellent treatment modality for relieving urinary outflow obstruction caused by a prostate gland weighing 30 g or less. Based on the findings in the numerous studies presented, several conclusions can be reached. TUIP is an excellent choice for patients who are interested in maintaining sexual function. TUIP can be performed using local anesthesia, making it possible for patients with significant medical problems to be candidates for this procedure.

Table 71D-1 Comparison of Hospital Stays by Patients Undergoing BPH Treatment				
Treatment Modalities	No. of Patients	Average Stay (days)	Shortest Reported Stay (days)	Longest Reported Stay (days)
Retropubic prostatectomy	4,699	12.8	9.0	19.1
Suprapubic prostatectomy	2,796	12.0	11.0	12.0
Open prostatectomy, any method	251	17.0	18.0	18.0
Open surgery (average)	7,746	13.2	9.9	18.0
TUIP	438	4.1	3.0	6.2
TURP	3,696	6.2	3.2	8.0
Transurethral surgery (average)	4,134	5.3	3.0	8.0

Long-term results with TUIP are almost equal to those with TURP, but TUIP is associated with significantly lower morbidity, lower cost, and decreased hospital stay. Hugosson and colleagues[3] estimated that in Sweden the cost of TURP was six times the cost of TUIP performed in an outpatient setting using local anesthesia. On the other hand, TUIP is not an effective procedure for patients with an enlarged median lobe or with a prostate that weighs greater than 30 g. Furthermore, with TURP, no tissue is retrieved for pathologic analysis.

As newer therapies for BPH have arrived, such as laser therapy, microwave thermotherapy, transurethral needle ablation of the prostate, and the intraprostatic injection of various agents, the surgeon is faced with the dilemma of choosing the most appropriate and efficacious treatment for the patient. After many years of clinical use, TUIP has become an established treatment modality that is clearly minimally invasive and has good long-term efficacy that compares favorably with the more recent "advancements" in therapy.

REFERENCES

1. Mebust WK, Holtgrewe HL, Cockett AT, Peters PC. Transurethral prostatectomy: immediate and postoperative complications. A cooperative study of 13 participating institutions evaluating 3,885 patients. J Urol 1989;141:243–7.
2. Orandi A. Transurethral resection versus transurethral incision of the prostate. Urol Clin North Am 1990;17:601–12.
3. Hugosson J, Bergdahl S, Norlen L, Ortengren T. Outpatient transurethral incision of the prostate under local anesthesia: operative results, patient security and cost effectiveness. Scand J Urol Nephrol 1993;27:381–5.
4. Sirls LT, Ganabathi K, Zimmern PE, et al. Transurethral incision of the prostate: an objective and subjective evaluation of long-term efficacy. J Urol 1993;150(5 Pt 2):1615–21.
5. Dorflinger T, Jensen FS, Krarup T, Walter S. Transurethral prostatectomy compared with incision of the prostate in the treatment of prostatism caused by small benign prostate glands. Scand J Urol Nephrol 1992;26:333–8.
6. Soonawalla PF, Pardanani DS. Transurethral incision versus transurethral resection of the prostate. A subjective and objective analysis. Br J Urol 1992;70:174–7.
7. Drago JR. Transurethral incision of the prostate. Urology 1991;38:305–6.
8. Aboulker P, Steg A. La divulsion de la prostate d'après 218 observations personnelles. J Urol Nephrol 1964;70:337.
9. Orandi A. Transurethral incision of the prostate. J Urol 1973;110:229–31.
10. Ruzic B, Trnski D, Kraus O, et al. New modification of transurethral incision of the prostate in surgical treatment of bladder outlet obstruction: prospective study. Croat Med J. 2002;43:610–4.
11. Jonler M, Bruskewitz RC. Transurethral incision of the prostate. Curr Opin Urol 1994;4:29–31.
12. Riehmann M, Bruskewitz RC. Transurethral incision of the prostate and bladder neck. J Androl 1991;12:415–22.
13. Johnson DE, Cromeens DM, Price RE. Transurethral incision of the prostate using the holmium:YAG laser. Lasers Surg Med 1992;12:364–9.
14. Edwards L, Powell C. An objective comparison of transurethral resection and bladder neck incision in the treatment of prostatic hypertrophy. J Urol 1982;128:325–7.
15. Moisey CU, Stephenson TP, Evans CA. A subjective and urodynamic assessment of unilateral bladder neck incision for bladder neck obstruction. Br J Urol 1982;54:114–7.
16. Edwards LE, Bucknall TE, Pittam MR, et al. TUR of the prostate and bladder neck incision: a review of 700 cases. Br J Urol 1985;57:168–71.
17. Hellstrom P, Lukkarinen O, Kontturi M. Bladder neck incision or transurethral electroresection for the treatment of urinary obstruction caused by a small, benign prostate. Scand J Urol Nephrol 1986;20:187–92.
18. Turner-Warwick RT. A urodynamic review of bladder outlet obstruction in the male and its clinical implications. Urol Clin North Am 1979;6:171–92.
19. Nielson HO. Transurethral prostatotomy versus transurethral resection of prostate in benign prostatic hyperplasia. A prospective randomized study. Br J Urol 1988;61:435–8.
20. Delaere KPJ, Debruyne FMJ, Moonen WA. Extended bladder neck incision for outflow obstruction in male patients. Br J Urol 1983;55:225–8.
21. Jonler M, Bruskewitz RC. Transurethral incision of the prostate for the treatment of benign prostatic hyperplasia. Semin Urol 1994;12:156–60.
22. Lin CT. Transurethral incision and posterior resection of prostate (TUI-PRP) for selected patients with benign obstructive prostatic disease. Urology 1992;39:508–11.
23. Simsek F, Turkeri N, Ilker YN, Akdas A. Transurethral grooving of the prostate in the treatment of patients with benign prostatic hyperplasia. An alternative to transurethral incision. Br J Urol 1993;72:84–7.
24. Yeni E, Unal D, Verit A, Gulum M. Minimal transurethral prostatectomy plus bladder neck incision versus standard transurethral transurethral prostatectomy in patients with benign prostatic hyperplasia: a randomized prospective study. Urol Int 2002;69:283–6.
25. Dorflinger T, England DM, Madsen PO, Bruskewitz RC. Urodynamic and histological correlates of benign prostatic hyperplasia. J Urol 1988;140:1487–90.
26. Kelly MJ, Roskamp D, Leach, GE. Transurethral incision of the prostate: a preoperative and postoperative analysis of symptoms and urodynamic findings. J Urol 1989;142:1507–9.
27. Kletscher BA, Oesterling JE. Transurethral incision of the prostate: a viable alternative to transurethral resection. Semin Urol 1992;10:265–72.
28. McConnell JD, Barry MJ, Bruskewitz RC. Benign prostatic hyperplasia: diagnosis and treatment. Clinical Practice Guideline Number 8. Agency for Health Care Policy and Research publication AHCPR 94-0582. Rockville, MD: US Department of Health and Human Services; 1994.
29. Orandi A. Transurethral incision of the prostate (TUIP): 646 cases in 15 years—a chronological appraisal. Br J Urol 1985;57:703–7.
30. Jocius KK, Sukyas D. [Treatment of bladder neck obstruction (sclerosis): personal experience and literature review]. Medicina (Kaunas) 2002;38 Suppl 1;48–55.
31. Fuse H, Nishio R, Murakami K, Okumura A. Transurethral incision for hematospermia caused by ejaculatory duct obstruction. Arch Androl 2003;49:433–8.
32. Tan AH, Gilling PJ, Kennett KM, et al. Long-term results of high-power holmium laser vaporization (ablation) of prostate. BJU Int 2003;92:707–9.
33. Klijer R, Bar K, Bialek W. Bladder outlet obstruction in women: difficulties in the diagnosis. Urol Int 2004;73:6–10.
34. Orandi A. Transurethral incision of prostate compared with transurethral resection of prostate in 132 matching cases. J Urol 1987;138:810–5.
35. Christensen MM, Aagaard J, Madsen PO. Transurethral resection versus transurethral incision of the prostate. A prospective randomized study. Urol Clin North Am 1990;17:621–30.
36. Katz PG, Greenstein A, Ratliff JE, et al. Transurethral incision of the bladder neck and prostate. J Urol 1990;144:694–6.
37. Tkocz M, Prajsner A. Comparison of long-term results of transurethral incision of the prostate with transurethral resection of the prostate, in patients with benign prostatic hypertrophy. Neurourol Urodyn 2002;21:112–6.
38. Yang Q, Abrams P, Donovan J, et al. Transurethral resection or incision of the prostate and other therapies: a survey of treatments for benign prostatic obstruction in the UK. BJU Int 1999;84:640–5.
39. Evans JWH, Singer M, Chapple CR, et al. Hemodynamic evidence for preoperative cardiac stress during transurethral resection of prostate: preliminary communication. Br J Urol 1991;67:376–80.
40. Finkle AL, Prian DV. Sexual potency in elderly men before and after prostatectomy. JAMA 1966;196:139–43.
41. Caine M. The late results and sequelae of prostatectomy. Br J Urol 1954;26:205–26.
42. Melkior J, Valk WL, Foret JD, Mebust WK. Transurethral prostatectomy: computerized analysis of 2,223 consecutive cases. J Urol 1974;112:634–42.
43. Larsen EH, Dorflinger T, Gasser TC, et al. Transurethral incision versus transurethral resection of the prostate for the treatment of benign prostatic hypertrophy. A preliminary report. Scand J Urol Nephrol 1987;104:83–6.
44. Hu K, Wallner K. Urinary incontinence in patients who have a TURP/TUIP following prostate brachytherapy. Int J Radiat Oncol Biol Phys 1998;40:783–6.
45. Yang Q, Peters TJ, Donvan JL, et al. Transurethral incision compared with transurethral resection of the prostate for bladder outlet obstruction:a systematic review and meta-analysis of randomized controlled trials. J Urol 2001;165:1526–32.

Thermotherapy of the Prostate: Principles and Experimental Data Overview

Stavros Gravas, MD, FEBU

Pilar Laguna, MD, PhD

Jean de la Rosette, MD, PhD

The application of heat for the management of numerous complaints and diseases is a well-known and old attitude in medicine. However, it was not until the late '80s that modern treatment of the prostate included microwaves and radio waves to produce heat, delivered either rectally or transurethrally.[1] Hyperthermia, defined as a temporary heating of the body, or parts thereof, at temperatures ($> 40°C$ to $45°C$) not resulting in denaturation of proteins, was the first technique that was developed. This later advanced into thermotherapy, in which temperatures range from 45 to $60°C$, resulting in effective necrosis.[1] Many different energy sources are used to produce heat, but application of microwave technology, solely through the transurethral route, has gained a firm position between the currently ablative methods due to the excellent clinical results from the treatment of symptomatic benign prostatic hyperplasia (BPH). The most recent EAU guidelines on BPH have identified transurethral microwave thermotherapy (TUMT) as the most attractive interventional modality alternative to TURP for patients who want to avoid surgery or who do not respond favorably to medication.[2]

PRINCIPLES

The concept of microwave thermotherapy of the prostate is to emit microwave radiation through an intraurethral antenna in order to deliver heat within the prostate with the eventual goal of destroying tissue by achieving temperatures that exceed the cytotoxic threshold, and includes cell death. The extent of the necrosis is governed by two physical variables: intraprostatic temperature and duration of heat exposure.[3] If the intraprostatic temperatures don't get high enough, one must treat for a longer time, and vice versa (Figure 72A-1).

Microwaves are electromagnetic radiation with an oscillating electrical and magnetic field in the range of 300 to 3,000 megahertz (MHz). These waves propagate in free space or in a medium and are reflected or scattered at the interfaces of two media with different impedances. The heat is produced when the microwaves are absorbed by the tissue, and arises mainly by two processes: electric dipoles (eg, water molecules) oscillating in the field, and electric charge carriers (eg, ions) moving

back and forth in the field. These movements transfer energy to the tissue in the form of heat.

Penetration of microwaves is usually defined as the depth in tissue at which the strength of the microwave field has decreased to 37% of its origin value.[4] Penetration is deeper in low–water-content tissue (fat) than in high–water-content tissue (muscle, prostate) because the water molecule is a primary absorption target.[5] It also depends on the wave frequency: the higher the frequency, the shorter the wavelength, and the less penetration depth in the tissue. Ideally, the penetration in water-rich tissues is approximately 100 mm at 100 MHz, while at a frequency of 2,450 MHz, the penetration is about 10 mm. Another important physical principle of microwave-induced heat distribution is that it is distance-dependent: the farther the target from the microwave applicator, the lower the temperature. This temperature decrease is due to the declining microwave penetration and the cooling effect of blood flow. Based on this principle, it is obvious that the peak temperature will occur at the mucosa adjacent to the applicator. In order to move the peak of the heat distribution into the prostate and avoid adjacent tissue injuries, a surface coolant was introduced to reduce the temperature in the vicinity of the applicator.

The TUMT devices, used for the management of symptomatic BPH, comprise a power oscillator, urethral cooling system, temperature monitoring system, and control console. The energy is delivered to the target tissue by the microwave antenna through a transurethral catheter, while the treatment is controlled by a computer software system. The transrectal route was abandoned after it met a lot of criticism, including heating the periphery and not the transition zone of the prostate, difficulty in appropriate and firm positioning of the probe, and disappointing long-term results.

EXPERIMENTAL STUDIES

Historically, microwave delivery systems designed to heat prostatic tissue were initially tested in vivo in a dog model. Magin and colleagues were the first to conduct an animal study on the application of microwave-induced heat in the prostate.[6] Eight canine prostates were treated with 2,450 MHz microwaves in order to achieve a $60°C$ tempera-

ture for 15 minutes. Four animals were sacrificed at 1 week and the remaining 4 at 6 months. The prostate volume of the first 4 dogs was unchanged, but complete devitalization was found. In the other 4 dogs, the prostate had been replaced by fibrous scar tissue. In addition, there was no temperature increase in the rectal wall of the 8 dogs. In another preliminary animal study by Harada and colleagues, transurethral application of microwave radiation in 20 dogs resulted in central necrosis of the prostate and fibrous tissue at the periphery of the heated area, suggestive of the ablative properties of heat generated through the absorption of microwave energy by the canine prostate.[7]

The histopathologic alterations in the canine prostate after hyperthermia (intraprostatic temperatures between 40 and $47°C$) were evaluated by Leib and colleagues, who found a mononuclear inflammatory infiltration in the interstitium and polymorphonuclear infiltration in the glandular elements of all the prostates. Furthermore, permanent tissue damage was time- and temperature-dependent.[8] Later, Bostwick and Larson examined the prostates of 13 sacrificed dogs after transurethral microwave thermotherapy (intraprostatic temperatures $> 45°C$).[9] The pathologic findings included coagulative necrosis with hemorrhage, cystically dilated urethra due to sloughed necrotic tissue, and inflammation depending on the elapsed time between treatment and sacrifice. In all cases, the prostatic capsule was intact and the urethral mucosa preserved.[9]

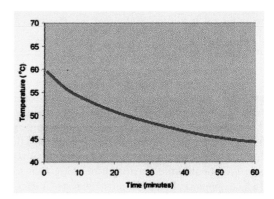

Figure 72A-1 Time versus temperature. When the temperature/time threshold represented by the continuous line is exceeded, tissue necrosis is obtained. The area above the line expresses dead cells.

All these pioneering animal studies provided the experimental basis for many of the principles applied in the treatment of humans and showed that the method is feasible and safe. The studies in humans on the application of thermotherapy (temperature > 45°C) started in the early 1990s by Devonec and colleagues, who treated patients with symptomatic BPH during 50-minute sessions with mild relief.[10] Histologic sections of human prostates after TUMT revealed symmetric bi-lobar destruction that extended 15 to 20 mm from the urethra. Acinar and smooth muscle cells were totally destroyed.[10] Since then, an impressive and steadily increasing number of studies have been performed providing evidence for the clinical efficacy and safety of the method. The most recent experimental studies have focused on the understanding of the mechanism of microwave thermotherapy and the factors that can influence the treatment outcome in order to eventually individualize the therapy and optimise the clinical result.

MECHANISM OF ACTION   It has been shown that heating in excess of 45°C results in coagulation necrosis,[11] following the general pattern of burn wounds that is characterised by inflammatory reactions, which lead to a rapidly developed necrosis and edema.[12] Microthrombi will occlude vessels, and the blood flow will not be adequate for cell survival, even less so for repair. On the cellular level, heat causes thermal inactivation of enzymes and structural proteins, and rupturing of cell membranes. Cell death occurs when the thermal damage is so severe that repair mechanisms (replacement of enzyme proteins and synthesis of new membranes) are insufficient, or when DNA and RNA transcription enzymes that mediate repair mechanisms are destroyed.[13–15]

In one of the earliest studies, Moritz and Henriques showed that 7 hours at 45°C caused approximately the same thermal damage on pig skin as 5 minutes at 50°C.[16] Cell survival studies on mammalian cells confirm the relationship in the temperature range used for microwave thermotherapy: 43 to 57°C.[13] However, different cell types and tissues may have different heat sensitivity. This observation reflects differences on the sub-cellular level: a change of only a few amino acids in proteins can make them more or less heat resistant.[13] A significant finding is that, in order to maintain the same biological isoeffect for a given cell line, the duration of heating should be increased by a factor of about 2 (R value) if the temperature is decreased by 1°C.[13]

In addition, it was reported that apoptosis was observed in a variety of cell systems and actually in temperatures lower than those inducing necrosis.[17] In the periphery (where the thermal exposure is lower), apoptosis may be the contributing cell kill mechanism.[12,18] Furthermore, Brehmer and Svensson investigated the feasibility of using heat to induce apoptosis in human prostatic stromal cells. Cell cultures were exposed to 47°C for 1 hour, and the most extensive apoptosis (in 76% of the cells) was noted 24 hours after heat treatment.[18]

It has also been proposed that induced necrosis disrupts periurethral α-adrenergic receptors, reflecting in denervation of the smooth muscle cells.[19] These findings may be responsible for the increased urinary flow after TUMT. It was demonstrated that TUMT increased the sensory threshold (evoked by electrical stimulation) in the posterior urethra by ≥ 30%, resulting in the alleviation of irritative symptoms.[20]

FACTORS AFFECTING THERMOTHERAPY OF THE PROSTATE   Thermotherapy of the prostate is mainly affected by those factors that control the whole course of the treatment. There are three main steps in the course of heating the prostate: (1) the generation of microwave power, delivery of the energy to the tissue, and generation of heat through absorption of the applied microwave energy, (2) the dispersion of heat by conduction in the tissue, and (3) the loss of heat through blood flow. The first step depends on the operating characteristics of the TUMT device and the antenna used to deliver the energy; the second is determined by the tissue composition; and the third is affected by the spatial and temporal variations of blood flow.[21]

Generation-Delivery-Absorption of Microwave Energy   Several TUMT devices are available, and they differ in frequency of the generator and design of the antenna. It seems, however, that the antenna design affects the heating pattern more than the wave frequency.[21] It is known that microwave penetration depends on the wave frequency (ie, at 900 to 1,300 MHz, the penetration in water-rich tissue is estimated to be about 15 mm; while at 2,450 MHz, it is about 10 mm). It has been demonstrated that the heating of the prostate occurs in the vicinity of the antenna where the electromagnetic field is disturbed, thus the penetration depth of the microwave or heat is independent of the frequency within the broad interval from 680 to 2,450 MHz.[22] Therefore, the range of coagulation necrosis achieved by standard TUMT with an applicator emitting 900 MHz microwaves would be similar to that obtained with a 2,450 MHz microwave frequency. Since the vast majority of the thermotherapy devices use 915 or 1,296 MHz, on a conceptual basis, these TUMT devices do not substantially differ and should therefore be evaluated as one group.

Knowledge of the spatial distribution of the heat in the prostate is of paramount importance in order to achieve ablation of the transition zone and to avoid undesired tissue injuries due to uncontrolled radiation. Therefore, the delineation of the radial and axial emission characteristics of antennas used to deliver energy to the prostate plays a main role in the choice of the appropriate antenna for a specific patient. Bolmsjö and colleagues performed an excellent study comparing the heat characteristics of three microwave antennas in a tissue-equivalent phantom prostate.[21] The monopole antenna is made of a coaxial cable with an exposed inner conductor at the tip and creates long back-heating tails along the feeding cable. In contrast, the dipole and helical coil antennas prevent microwave currents from flowing backwards along the antenna cable, resulting in well-focused heating. Using the dipole antenna, the maximum heat will be generated around the antenna junction point and will extend axially about 2 cm in each direction. The helical coil antenna provides a shorter and more focused heating pattern compared to the dipole antenna. It was also calculated that the energy absorbed in the phantom model was only a part of the emitted energy, and varied from 13 to 21% depending on the type of antenna.[21]

In an attempt to quantify the heating characteristics of microwave antennas, the concept of specific absorption rate (SAR) is used. SAR describes the spatial distribution of the power deposition and is expressed as watts per kilogram of tissue weight (W/Kg).

Experiments were performed on the basis of measured temperature elevations in a volume of phantom gel in order to obtain a three-dimensional SAR distribution following microwave thermotherapy-induced heating.[23]

Another operating characteristic of TUMT devices is the software protocol used to emit energy. Initial lower-energy thermotherapy (LE-TUMT) protocols were clinically evaluated confirming safety and efficacy.[24–26] High-energy thermotherapy (HE-TUMT) was developed following the hypothesis that more energy would create higher temperatures and eventually achieve better clinical outcomes. The higher-energy protocols result in a mean increase of 40% in the total energy delivered to the prostate and in intraprostatic temperatures ranging between 45 to 80°C that lead to coagulative necrosis that can create a prostatic cavity. The contribution of the total amount of energy to the response rate sounds logical since it is obvious that, if more energy is delivered, the result is a more pronounced thermo-ablative effect.[27] Data from HE-TUMT studies confirmed that the clinical outcomes achieved by the high-energy protocols were more improved and durable than those by earlier lower-energy treatment programs. The indication to use microwave treatment gradually changed from application to patients with solely irritative symptoms to include patients with evident obstructive elements and patients in chronic urinary retention.

The next step was to introduce the heat-shock strategy in order to overpass the adaptation of the vessels to the slow increase of intraprostatic temperature, leading to resistance to heat effects. Heat-shock strategy is characterized by a rapid build-up in power/temperatures that causes immediate vascular thromboses resulting theoretically in similar or better clinical outcome in a shorter duration of treatment.[28]

Dispersion of Heat by Conduction in the Tissue   Study of the thermophysical properties of prostatic tissue in animal and experimental models, including thermal conductivity, diffusivity, density, and specific heat sensitivity, provides useful information that may explain variations in treatment outcome, despite the differences between the canine and the human prostate. The canine prostate has a much higher gland-to-stroma ratio compared to the human prostate, and is less resistant to heat.[29] The proportion of the various components of the prostate (epithelium/stromal ratio, E/S) differs for each individual and depends on the size and location in the prostate. This heterogeneity of the prostate histopathology has been suggested as the intrinsic factor responsible for the variability in clinical outcome owing to the different reaction of each component to microwaves. Microscopic examination showed that acinar cells seem to be more resistant to heat than smooth muscle cells when exposed to the same temperature level.[29] Arai and colleagues found a poor interaction of microwave thermotherapy and prostate with an artificial lack of glandular tissue due to previous medication, suggesting that prostates with larger percentages of glandular tissue tend to respond better to treatment.[30] d'Ancona and colleagues correlated histologic findings from biopsy material with the therapeutic response to TUMT. No significant difference could be demonstrated for the tissue ratio between good and poor responders despite the observation of a trend towards a lower E/S ratio in poor responders.[31] Furthermore, a large prostate is reported to be a favourable predictive factor for TUMT because it seems that large prostatic volume serves as a physical barrier to temperature distribution outside the gland, mainly the rectal wall.[27] This can prevent temporary treatment interruptions from excessive elevations of rectal temperatures.

In one study, Bhowmick and colleagues provided basic data for a better understanding of thermotherapy.[32] The investigators assessed the heat sensitivity of human prostatic tissue for various temperature-time combinations. After heat treatment, the tissue slices were cultured and viability was assessed using histologic examination and dye uptake. They found a progressive histologic increase in irreversible injury with increasing temperature-time severity. The dye uptake and histology results for stromal viability were similar for all temperature-time combinations. Ninety-percent stromal destruction was identified after 60 minutes at 45°C, 5 minutes at 55°C, 2 minutes at 60°C and 1 minute at 70°C. After heat treatment at 50°C for 15 minutes and 55°C for 5 minutes, over 80% of both layers of glandular epithelium (basal and luminal) were sloughed off. Apoptosis was also identified in the control and milder-treated tissues with the degree of glandular apoptosis ($\approx 20\%$) more than that seen in the stromal regions ($< 5\%$). These experimental data can be used to assess how much tissue is actually being destroyed during treatment, and indicate that the use of higher temperatures could shorten treatment duration.

Blood Flow Blood flow has been identified as a decisive factor affecting the thermotherapy outcomes and contributing to the lack of uniformity in clinical results. Prostatic blood flow acts as a natural coolant, resulting in a decrease of intraprostatic temperature and delay of the coagulation mechanism.[33] Blood perfusion rates were measured in different regions of the canine prostate under normal and hyperthermal conditions.[34] Results showed an approximate 3.5-fold increase in perfusion from the baseline measurements when the local tissue temperature was increased above 41.5°C. It seemed that the increased blood perfusion was a function of tissue temperature and its temporal gradient.[33] Other studies on thermoregulation in the canine prostate during transurethral thermal therapy have focused on both temperature and blood flow response to the microwave heating.[35,36] Characteristic temperatures and time associated with different types of temperature responses.[35] It has also been found that the canine prostate blood perfusion is strongly linked to the geometric location within the gland, the local tissue temperature, and the imposed thermal dose. More specifically, higher values of blood perfusion were reported by Xu and colleagues in the periurethral zone than in the parenchyma of the gland.[36]

Studies have shown that blood flow varies greatly among individuals, with the blood flow being 17.7 ± 5.2 mL/min/100 g (range from 10.8 to 24.2 mL/min/100 g) in BPH patients, 15.7 ± 7.5 mL/min/100 g in normal controls, and 29.4 ± 7.8 mL/min/100 g in cancer patients.[37] Blood flow changes dynamically as treatment continues. In the beginning of the treatment, an increase of blood flow is usually seen, probably reflecting the vasodilation caused by the elevated temperature. Wagrell and colleagues, using positron emission tomography to measure the intraprostatic blood flow, noted a rapid increase in blood flow up to 100% during the first 25 to 30 minutes of the treatment.[38] Toward the end of the treatment, blood flow decreases, most probably due to occurred microthrombosis, with the consequent capture of heat in the exposed tissue causing a faster development of coagulation necrosis.

The removal of thermal energy through the circulating blood (the theory of "heat sink") affects the local effective temperature. Floratos and colleagues studied the baseline intraprostatic vascularization using (at baseline) three-dimensional contrast enhanced power-flow-Doppler (3D-CE-PFD) prostate ultrasonography in a group of 22 patients treated with TUMT.[39] Assuming that percentage of perfused area (PPA) is a realistic measure of blood flow, PPA was used to quantify intraprostatic vasculature. It was concluded that the baseline intraprostatic vascularization, documented by CE-PFD studies, has no predictive value for the efficacy of TUMT. It seems that static baseline blood flow does not reflect the dynamic thermoregulatory role of blood flow during treatment.[39]

OPTIMAL THERMAL TREATMENT BY TEMPERATURE MONITORING AND USE OF PREDICTIVE MODELS It is well understood now that the response to the heat treatment differs among patients and is dependent on all the previously analysed factors, emphasizing the need for individualization of the therapy. It is also known that there is a relationship between intraprostatic temperatures and clinical results.[40] The availability of continuous monitoring of spatiotemporal intraprostatic temperature distribution would contribute to a better understanding of the basic mechanism of thermotherapy and tailoring of the treatment as well. Experimental studies have been conducted in order to evaluate the thermal mapping of the prostate, with the ultimate goal to teach us how to heat the prostate. Several intraprostatic thermometry techniques have been proposed, including invasive and non-invasive methods. Interstitial thermal mapping in canine and human prostates using thermocouple arrays has been reported but the invasive nature of the method makes it less attractive.[10,41,42] A less invasive method was introduced and is commercially available (ProstaLund Feedback Treatment [PLFT]).[43] PLFT continuously monitors the intraprostatic temperature using three sensors in a row on a needle-like temperature probe that protrudes through the catheter into one of the lateral prostatic lobes. Temperatures from the tip, middle and apex of the prostate are recorded, allowing the operator to manually adjust the microwave power according to the actual measurements. The measured temperature is used for calculation of the amount of necrotized tissue by using a combination of the bioheat equation and cell survival data of thermal exposure.[33,44] Figure 72A-2 presents a diagrammatic view of the temperature distribution.

Microwave radiometry thermometry is based on thermal noise power, which is the electromagnetic radiation emitted by a given body whose temperature is raised. It has been clinically evaluated, but it appears the disadvantage of limited spatial resolution.[45] Magnetic resonance imaging (MRI) allows thermal mapping at the time of the treatment due to its temperature sensitivity. There are different techniques of magnetic resonance (MR) that have been used, including water diffusion, coefficient, T1 relaxation time, proton resonance frequency, and MR spectroscopic imaging.[46] Results suggest that MRI is a promising method because it offers good spatial localization and sufficient temperature sensitivity.[47] Ultrasound thermometry is another promising modality that is based on temperature-dependent, acoustic tissue parameters such as sound velocity, attenuation, backscattered power and thermal expansion.[48,49]

The extent of tissue debulking due to coagulation necrosis may play a significant role for clinical TUMT outcome in terms of response and durability, which are likely TURP aims to the resection of prostatic adenoma for the alleviation of lower urinary tract symptoms. Quantification in real time of the amount of ablated tissue will result in the adjustment of treatment for every patient individually and will indicate the termination of thermotherapy when the desired volume has been destroyed. Bolmsjö and colleagues developed a cell-kill (tissue death) model to estimate the amount of the necrotized tissue using both Henrique's damage integral and Jung's compartment model, which were implemented in a

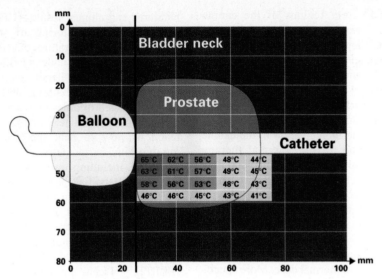

Figure 72A-2 Temperature distribution. A diagrammatic view of the temperature distribution. A schematic treatment catheter and a medium-sized prostate have been inserted for clarity. The *red and blue boxes* show the mean maximum temperatures at each location. The red elements represent locations where therapeutic temperatures are reached during typical treatment times of 15 to 30 minutes.

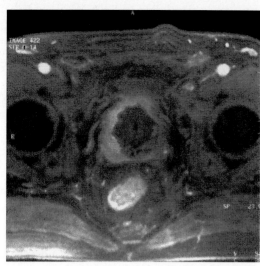

Figure 72A-3 Magnetic resonance image (MRI) one week after transurethral microwave thermotherapy (TUMT). Tissue necrosis is visualized with MRI one week after TUMT using ProstaLund Feedback Treatment. The perfusion defect is seen as a large dark area caused by low uptake of GaD in the necrotic region.

computer program.[44] The authors used data from 22 patients treated with microwave thermotherapy and found that cell-kill was calculated during TUMT with reasonable accuracy compared to transrectal ultrasound (TRUS)-determined volume reduction 3 months after TUMT. This cell-kill model was integrated in the ProstaLund treatment software. In a prospective study, Hoffmann and colleagues compared the calculated cell-kill from 33 patients treated with ProstaLund PLFT to the post-TUMT prostate shrinkage as measured by three-dimensional transrectal ultrasound (3D-TRUS) step-section planimetry.[50] It was found that the predicted cell-kill quantity is proportional to the 3D-TRUS prostate shrinkage by a factor of 0.5 and with a precision of approximately ± 10 cm³ for 90% of the patients. The advantage seems to be the ability to individually tune treatment. In addition, Nordling and colleagues concluded in a prospective randomized multicenter study on 100 patients treated with PLFT that the calculated cell-kill was a valid and good predictor to determine when to stop treatment.[51]

Theoretical models may also provide a way for predicting temperature fields in heated tissue. Xu and colleagues developed a model for prediction of the temperature distribution in the prostate.[52] The predictions of the model were compared to temperature distributions measured in a non-perfused, tissue-equivalent phantom gel and in canine prostates. In 1995, Yuan and colleagues presented a two-dimensional, finite difference model and compared its predictions exclusively to experimental data obtained in a non-perfused, tissue-equivalent phantom heated with a Urologix T3 catheter and not to any data measured in vivo.[53] Larson and colleagues compared the recorded interstitial temperatures in 22 patients treated with

the Urologix Targis TUMT device to the model predictions and they were found to be in accord. Continuous temperature measurements were achieved by placement of fiberoptic thermosensors using a stereotactic method.[42]

A new mathematical model for predicting intraprostatic temperatures and necrosis zone during TUMT treatment with Urologix Targis was developed (S. Ramadhyani, E.N. Rudie, personnal communication). This model includes better representations of variations of thermal conductivity, and of blood perfusion as functions of the local tissue temperature and the extent of thermal damage, based on experimental data obtained from the canine model and interstitial temperature-mapping studies in human prostates. First comparisons between model predictions and measurements in human patients seem to provide the clinician with the ability to adjust the treatment duration on an individual basis.

Gadolinium-enhanced MRI has been used to determine the extent and pattern of coagulation necrosis caused by TUMT. Osman and colleagues treated 13 patients using the Urologix Targis device and performed a post-treatment MRI.[54] Necrotic tissue presented as perfusion defect that was accurately correlated with prostatic tissue exposed to temperatures ≥ 45°C for at least 45 minutes. Huidoro and colleagues investigated the intraprostatic heat distribution and the relation to histopathology, MRI imaging, and cell-kill calculations using the ProstaLund Coretherm TUMT device. Microwave treatment causes necrosis of the prostate, bladder neck, and urethral mucosa; in addition, tissue necrosis assessed by pathology, MRI, and cell-kill calculation was comparable.[55] Figure 72A-3 shows how tissue necrosis is visualized with MRI one week after PLFT.

CONCLUSIONS

Thorough evaluation of microwave technology led to the application of several principles of microwave radiation in clinical use for thermotherapy of the prostate. During the last 15 years, experimental studies have come a long way. The start was the demonstration of the efficacy and safety of the method in animal and human experimental models with the generation of high intraprostatic temperatures and consequent thermal ablation of the prostatic tissue without the risk of injury of the adjacent tissues. After the basic steps that allowed the use of microwave thermotherapy, experimental studies focused on the investigation of potential mechanisms of heat action. The next reasonable step was to identify all those parameters, including differences in generators, thermophysical properties of the prostate, and blood flow, that may affect the response to the thermal therapy, and to conduct studies in order to optimize the clinical outcome. Efforts to obtain feedback information on intraprostatic temperature, which seems to be the key factor for good response, have also been made. All these experimental data have been integrated in the development of mathematical models that could predict the intraprostatic temperature and quantify the amount of the destroyed tissue, with the ultimate goal being to tune the thermotherapy on an individual basis.

REFERENCES

1. Laguna MP, Muschter R, Debruyne FMJ. Microwave thermotherapy: historical overview. J Endourol 2000;14: 603–10.
2. de la Rosette JJ, Alivizatos G, Madersbacher S, et al. EAU guidelines on benign prostatic hyperplasia (BPH). Eur Urol 2001;40:256–63.

3. Wagrell L, Schelin S, Bolmsjo MB, Mattiasson A. Aspects on transurethral microwave thermotherapy of benign prostatic hyperplasia. Techniques in Urology 2000;6:251–5.

4. Bolmsjö MB, Vrba J. Microwave applicators for thermotherapy of benign prostatic hyperplasia: a primer. Tech Urol 2000;6:245–50.

5. Johnson C, Guy AW. Nonionizing electromagnetic wave effects in biological materials and systems. Proc IEEE 1972;60:692.

6. Magin RL, Fridd CW, Bonfiglio TA, Linke CA. Thermal destruction of the canine prostate by high intensity microwaves. J Surg Res 1980;29:265–75.

7. Harada T, Etori K, Kumazaki T, et al. Microwave surgical treatment of diseases of the prostate. Urology 1985;26:572–6.

8. Leib Z, Rothem A, Lev A, Servadio C. Histopathological observations in the canine prostate treated by local microwave hyperthermia. Prostate 1986;8:93–102.

9. Bostwick DG, Larson TR. Transurethral microwave thermotherapy: pathologic findings in the canine prostate. Prostate 1995;26:116–22.

10. Devonec M, Berger N, Perrin P. Transurethral microwave heating of the prostate: from hyperthermia to thermotherapy. J Endourol 1991;5:129–35.

11. Brehmer M, Baba S. Transurethral microwave thermotherapy: how does it work? J Endourol 2000;14:611–5.

12. Arturson G. Pathophysiology of the burn wound. Ann Chir Gynaecol 1980;69:178–90.

13. Dewey WC. Arrhenius relationships from the molecule and cell to the clinic. Int J Hyperthermia 1994;10:457–83.

14. Pearce JA, Thomsen SL. Rate process analysis of thermal damage. In: Welsh AJ, van Gemert MJE, editors. Optical-thermal response of laser irradiated tissue. New York: Plenum; 1995.

15. Corry PM, Robinson S, Getz S. Hyperthermic effects on DNA repair mechanisms. Radiology 1977;123:475–82.

16. Moritz AR, Henriques FC. Studies of thermal injury—the relative importance of time and surface temperature in the causation of cutaneous burns. Am J Path 1947;23:695–720.

17. Brehmer M. Morphological changes in prostatic adenomas after transurethral microwave thermotherapy. Br J Urol 1997;80:123–7.

18. Brehmer M, Svensson I. Heat-induced apoptosis in human prostatic stromal cells. BJU Int 2000;85:535–41.

19. Brehmer M, Hilliges M, Kinn AC. Denervation of periurethral prostatic tissue by transurethral microwave thermotherapy. Scand J Urol Nephrol 2000;34:42–5.

20. Brehmer M, Nilsson BY. Elevation of sensory thresholds in the prostatic urethra after microwave thermotherapy. BJU Int 2000;86:427–31.

21. Bolmsjö M, Wagrell L, Hallin A, et al. The heat is on—but how? A comparison of TUMT devices. Br J Urol 1996;78:564–72.

22. Roos D, Hamnerius Y, Alpsten M. Two microwave applicators for intracavitary hyperthermia treatment of cancer colli uteri. Phys Med Biol 1989;34:1917–21.

23. Zhu L, Xu LX, Chencinski N. Quantification of the 3-D electromagnetic power absorption rate in tissue during transurethral prostatic microwave thermotherapy using heat transfer model. IEEE Trans Biomed Eng 1998;45:1163–72.

24. Blute ML, Tomera KM, Hellerstein DK, et al. Transurethral microwave thermotherapy for management of benign prostatic hyperplasia: results of the United States Prostatron cooperative study. J Urol 1993;150:1591–6.

25. Dahlstrand C, Walden M, Geirsson G, Pettersson S. Transurethral microwave thermotherapy versus transurethral resection for symptomatic benign prostatic obstruction: a prospective randomized study with a 2-year follow-up. Br J Urol 1995;76:614–8.

26. de Wildt MJAM, d'Ancona FCH, Hubregtse M, et al. 3 Years follow-up in patients treated with lower energy thermotherapy (Prostasoft version 2.0). J Urol 1996;156:1959–63.

27. d'Ancona FCH, Francisca EAE, Debruyne FMJ, de la Rosette JJMCH. High-energy transurethral microwave thermotherapy in men with lower urinary tract symptoms. J Endourol 1997;11:285–9

28. Eliasson T, Damber JE. Temperature controlled high energy transurethral microwave thermotherapy for benign prostatic hyperplasia using a heat shock strategy. J Urol 1998;160:777–81.

29. Devonec M, Berger N, Fedler JP, et al. Thermoregulation during transurethral microwave thermotherapy: experimental and clinical fundamentals. Eur Urol 1993;23 Suppl 1:63–7.

30. Arai Y, Fukuzawa S, Terai A, Yoshida O. Transurethral microwave thermotherapy for benign prostatic hyperplasia: relation between clinical response and prostate histology. Prostate 1996;28:84–8.

31. d'Ancona, Albers YH, Kiemeney LA, et al. Can histopathology predict treatment outcome following high energy transurethral microwave thermotherapy of the prostate? Results of a biopsy study. Prostate 1999;40:28–36.

32. Bhowmick P, Coad JE, Bhowmick S, et al. In vitro assessment of the efficacy of thermal therapy in human benign prostatic hyperplasia. Int J Hyperthermia 2004;20:421–39.

33. Bolmsjö M, Sturesson C, Wagrell L, et al. Optimizing transurethral microwave thermotherapy a model for studying power, blood flow, temperature variations and tissue destruction. Br J Urol 1998;81:811–6.

34. Xu LX, Zhu L, Holmes KR. Blood perfusion measurements in the canine prostate during transurethral hyperthermia. Ann N Y Acad Sci 1998;858:21–9.

35. Xu LX, Zhu L, Holmes KR. Thermoregulation in the canine prostate during transurethral microwave hyperthermia, part I: temperature response. Int J Hyperthermia 1998;14:29–37.

36. Xu LX, Zhu L, Holmes KR. Thermoregulation in the canine prostate during trans urethral microwave hyperthermia, part II: blood flow response. Int J Hyperthermia 1998;14:65–73.

37. Inaba T. Quantitative measurements of prostatic blood flow and blood volume by positron emission tomography. J Urol 1992;148:1457–60.

38. Wagrell L, Sundin A, Norlén BJ. Intra-prostatic blood flow changes during feedback microwave thermotherapy measured by positron emission tomography. In: Feedback thermotherapy for benign prostatic enlargement: a clinical and methodological evaluation [PhD thesis]. Uppsala, Sweden: Uppsala University; 1999.

39. Floratos DL, Sedelaar JPM, Kortmann BBM, et al. Intraprostatic vasculature studies: can they predict the outcome of transurethral microwave thermotherapy for the management of bladder outflow obstruction? Prostate 2001;46:200–6.

40. Carter S, Tubaro A. Relation between intraprostatic temperature and clinical outcome in microwave thermotherapy. J Endourol. 2000;14:617–25.

41. Astrahan MA, Ameye F, Oyen R, et al. Interstitial temperature measurements during transurethral microwave hyperthermia. J Urol 1991;145:304–8.

42. Larson TR, Collins JM, Corica A. Detailed interstitial temperature mapping during treatment with a novel transurethral microwave thermoablation system in patients with benign prostatic hyperplasia. J Urol 1998;159:258–64.

43. Wagrell L, Schelin S, Bolmsjö M, Brudin L. Intraprostatic temperature monitoring during transurethral microwave thermotherapy for the treatment of benign prostatic hyperplasia. J Urol 1998;159:1583–87.

44. Bolmsjö M, Schelin S, Wagrell L, et al. Cell-kill modeling of microwave thermotherapy for treatment of benign prostatic hyperplasia. J Endourology 2000;14:627–35.

45. Mauroy B, Chive M, Stefaniak X, et al. Study on the effects of thermotherapy in benign prostatic hyperplasia. Eur Urol 1997;32:198–208.

46. Germain D, Chevallier P, Laurent A, Saint-Jame H. MR monitoring of tumour thermal therapy. MAGMA 2001;13:47–59.

47. Chen JC, Moriarty JA, Derbyshire JA, et al. Prostate cancer: MR imaging and thermometry during microwave thermal ablation—initial experience. Radiology 2000;214:290–7.

48. Nasoni RL, Bowen T. Ultrasonic speed as a parameter for non-invasive thermometry. Automedica 1987;8:269.

49. Simon C, van Baren P, Ebbini ES. Two-dimensional temperature estimation using diagnostic ultrasound. IEEE Trans Ultrason Ferroelectr Freq Contr 1998;45:1088.

50. Hoffmann AL, Laguna MP, de la Rosette JJMCH, Wijkstra H. Quantification of prostate shrinkage after microwave thermotherapy: a comparison of calculated cell-kill versus 3D transrectal ultrasound planimetry. Eur Urol 2003;43:181–7.

51. Nordling J, Schelin S, Mattiasson A, et al. Intraprostatic temperature measurement during microwave treatment provides online control of tissue necrosis volume using ProstaLund microwave feedback treatment. J Endourol 2001;15:A89.

52. Xu LX, Rudie EN, Holmes KR. Transurethral thermal therapy (T3) for the treatment of benign prostatic hyperplasia (BPH) in the canine: analysis using the Pennes Bioheat equation. In: Advances in bioheat and mass transfer: microscale analysis of thermal injury processes, instrumentation, modelling, and clinical applications, Proc Am Soc Mech Eng 1993;268:31–5.

53. Yuan DY, Valvano JW, Rudie EN, Xu LX. 2-D finite difference modeling of microwave heating in the prostate. Proc Am Soc Mech Eng 1995;322:107–15.

54. Osman YM, Larson TR, El-Diasty T, Ghoneim MA. Correlation between central zone perfusion defects on gadolinium-enhanced MRI and intraprostatic temperatures during transurethral microwave thermotherapy. J Endourol 2000;14:761–6.

55. Huidobro C, Bolmsjö M, Larson T, et al. Evaluation of microwave thermotherapy with histopathology, magnetic resonance imaging and temperature mapping. J Urol 2004;171:672–8.

Transurethral Microwave Heat Treatments for Benign Prostatic Hypertrophy

Lance A. Mynderse, MD

Michael L. Blute, MD

MICROWAVE PHYSICS AND TISSUE INTERACTION

Microwaves are part of the electromagnetic spectrum and have wave frequencies from 30 to 3,000 megahertz (MHz). Microwaves follow the basic physical properties of electromagnetic radiation transmission in free space or in a medium and are reflected, deflected, or scattered at the interfaces of two media with different impedance. Microwaves interact with biologic tissues to create an alternating electrical field that produces heat through excitation and oscillation of ions and dipole molecules. As electromagnetic waves penetrate tissue, molecular kinetic energy dissipates and is transformed to heat. This thermal energy is dissipated by the blood supply.[1] Propagation of heat within a prostate follows a curve that rapidly decreases with the distance from the urethra. The curves in Figure 72B-1 represent heat distribution as a function of distance from the urethra, and the heat distribution with surface cooling. A maximum temperature can be reached at a point distant from the treatment applicator. The depth of penetration depends on the frequency of the microwave and type of tissue interaction. Penetration of microwaves is greater in low–water-content (fat) than in high–water-content (muscle) tissue.[2] The penetration depth of microwaves decreases with increasing frequency. The microwave antenna design also seems to affect the depth or range of tissue heating. Therefore, the heating pattern obtained by these devices depends on the distribution of energy in the target tissue (Figure 72B-2). Energy is delivered by convective and absorptive mechanisms. The biologic effect of heat depends on the intensity, duration, and mode of application. In addition, there are a number of factors that affect radiative heating, which are not easily measured, such as water composition of tissue (ie, glandular vs. stromal elements), tissue vascularity, size of prostate, prostate shape, and glandular symmetry.

The microwave devices used for heating the prostate include a computer system that modulates feedback and power output, a power oscillator that is responsible for the microwave emission at the antenna, and a thermometry system that measures urethral and rectal temperatures. Servo control mechanisms sensitive to urethral and rectal temperatures control the power output. The thermal sensors are protective mechanisms that ensure therapeutic temperatures remain within a narrow range and do not exceed safe tissue levels.

HISTORICAL PERSPECTIVES— MICROWAVE HEAT THERAPY BY TRANSRECTAL DEVICE

The application of heat to treat prostatic disease has been advocated for more than a century.[3] In 1982, microwave hyperthermia was first used in the treatment of prostate adenocarcinoma by Yerushalmi and colleagues.[4] The differential effect of heat on normal versus tumor cells was estimated to be between a temperature of 40 and 43°C. Heat therapy of tumor cells is thought to be related to the heat sensitivity of cells in the S phase of the cell cycle. At temperatures below 40°C, neither cell type was affected to an appreciable extent. Both malignant and normal cells were affected at temperatures above 45°C. Yerushalmi and colleagues and Sevadio and colleagues reported results on the use of transrectal, water-cooled, microwave thermotherapy.[5,6] Early results suggested some efficacy, but the varied results reported with transrectal hyperthermia can be related to improper study design, uncontrolled studies, variations in microwave frequency, differences in device design, deposition of maximum energy to the periphery of the prostate gland and not to the target transition zone adenoma, and the variability in the natural history of benign prostatic hyperplasia (BPH) (Table 72B-1). Testing against sham controls by Zerbig and colleagues did not support the continued use of this technology.[7]

EARLY TRANSURETHRAL MICROWAVE DEVICES IN ANIMAL STUDIES

The histologic changes that occur in canine prostates following heat treatment were studied before initiating human trials. The first article on the use of microwave hyperthermia in an animal

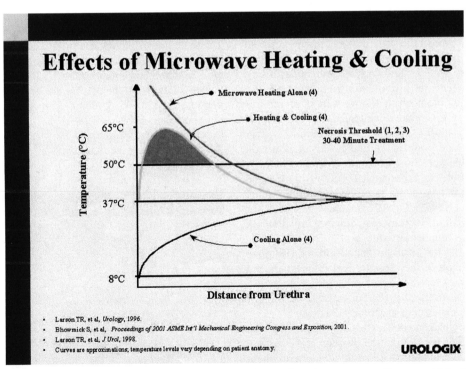

Figure 72B-1 Heating patterns in tissue as a function of distance from the treatment applicator as obtained from interstitial temperature mapping. Additive effect of heating and cooling produces higher intraprostatic, transition zone temperatures. Reproduced with permission from Larson TR, et al.[17]

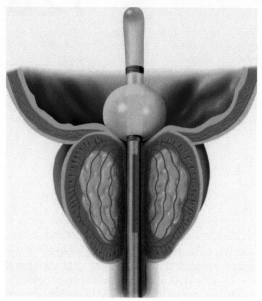

Figure 72B-2 Diagram of transurethral microwave thermotherapy catheter (Prostatron) with cooling, placed in the prostatic urethra delivering thermal energy into the transition zone of the prostate. Urethra is protected by circulating coolant. Photograph courtesy of Urologix, Inc., Minneapolis, MN.

study was published by Magin and colleagues in 1980.[8] Twenty dogs were treated by a water-cooled probe to determine tissue-tolerable temperatures. Each animal had six sequential treatments, with time intervals between treatments varying from 48 to 72 hours. The authors concluded that heating to temperatures up to 42.5°C (± 0.5°C) for 90 minutes was safe with this water-cooled device. This was a complicated study in eight urinary-diverted dogs. Four animals were sacrificed at 1 week and four animals at 6 months. Experiments were directed to total thermal destruction of the canine prostate with 60°C temperatures for 15 minutes. A complicated shielding device was used to protect the structures and tissues adjacent to the prostate. Lieb and colleagues found that time as well as temperature were controlling parameters in microwave treatments of the prostate.[9] No necrotic lesions were observed following a 15-minute treatment at 47°C. Prolonged therapy at 40°C appeared to be well tolerated by the canine population, and no histopathologic changes were noted. Canine prostates demonstrated diffuse mononuclear cell infiltration and edema but no necrosis following six 90-minute sessions at 42.5°C.[8] Any treatment at 44.5°C for longer than 30 minutes, however, resulted in necrosis and hemorrhage.

This treatment produced almost complete destruction of the prostate. In 1985, Harada and colleagues reported a preliminary study on the use of a transurethral probe for prostate microwave radiation thermodestruction in 20 dogs.[10] Astrahan and colleagues in 1989 described an applicator for heating the prostate gland using a transurethral approach in a 38-kg German Shepherd dog.[11] They studied the longitudinal temperature distributions measured in situ at the applicator-urethral interface and the longitudinal

radial temperature distribution measured in a normal canine prostate. They described a technique capable of elevating temperatures to 42°C in a cylindrically symmetric volume up to 5 cm in length and 0.5 cm in radial penetration around the applicator. Roehrborn and colleagues reported temperatures of 42°C in periurethral tissue of dogs treated with a transurethral catheter.[12] There was, however, a 1°C decrease in temperature per 3-mm distance from the treatment applicator. These canine studies served as a foundation for many of the microwave principles that are applied to studies of transurethral hyperthermia or thermotherapy in humans.

BIOPHYSICS OF HUMAN PROSTATE MICROWAVE HYPERTHERMIA

Thermal-based therapies use high temperature to achieve coagulation necrosis of the prostate adenoma. Microwaves have been a primary means to heat the prostate tissue. Intraprostatic temperatures in excess of 45°C (thermotherapy) are known to produce necrosis, but temperatures below 45°C (hyperthermia) have no clear demonstrable effect on prostate tissue.[13]

In both animal and human studies, there is substantial evidence that transurethral microwave heat treatment does produce significant pathologic effect on the prostate. Interstitial temperature mapping of canine and human subjects have all shown relative sparing of the periurethral and urethral tissues, with varying temperatures throughout the prostate adenoma.[14] Larson and Collins described the use of biplanar ultrasound imaging to accurately place thermistors throughout the prostate. Using this technique, temperature mapping was carried out using the (Targis) device. At an average power of 31.4 watts (W), prostate tissue temperature at 5 mL radial distance from the urethra reached 62.4°C within 7 minutes of achieving maximum power. Temperatures remained within a range of 60.9 to 68.7°C throughout treatment. At 1.0 cm of distance radially from the urethra, the average temperature was 50.5°C. Urethral temperatures varied between 38.7 and 41.1°C, and rectal temperature was maintained between 37.7 and 39.1°C throughout the treatment.[15,16]

Histopathologic changes have correlated well with temperatures in different parts of the prostate. Tissues exposed to a minimum of 45°C for 60 minutes (Targis, T3 device) suffered hemorrhagic necrosis with a clear border between necrotic and viable tissue (Figure 72B-3).[17] Using a different high-energy device (Prostasoft 2.5 -Prostatron), d'Ancona and colleagues found similar histologic findings that were predictive of clinical response.[18] Those prostates with higher epithelial, stromal ratio and larger volume glands did better with high-energy microwave therapy.

Blood-flow properties of the prostate appeared to play a significant role in the variability of treatment outcome and also appeared to be linked to changes in histology of the gland. In the canine model, Xu and colleagues demonstrated five different types of temperature responses to different microwave power levels during microwave therapy.[19] Larson and Collins used color Doppler ultrasonography to evaluate blood-flow changes during treatment.[20] This study described an increase in blood flow in the peripheral zone and the posterior half of the transition zone as microwave heat was generated. Floratos and colleagues conducted three-dimensional, contrast-enhanced, power-flow Doppler prostate ultrasonography to quantify the percentage of perfused area of the prostate in 25 patients during high-energy microwave therapy.[21] This study showed no predictive value of the static, baseline, intraprostatic vasculature for the efficacy of the microwave therapy, although high intraprostatic vascularization and blood flow during treatment had a negative influence on the therapeutic efficacy. Additionally, d'Ancona and colleagues had shown a clear trend of lower blood vessel density on histologic biopsy analysis among good responders with microwave therapy.[18] Furthermore, Schelin demonstrated diminished energy requirements, shorter treatment time, and lower calculated intraprostatic blood flow in 15 patients pretreated with intraprostatic injection of mepivacaine-epinephrine prior to microwave therapy.[22] Current efforts to improve the efficacy of microwave thermotherapy are centered on improving the ability of treatment devices to tailor therapy to individual prostatic blood flows, vessel density, epithelial stromal

Series	Instrument	Length (h)	No.	Temperature (°C)	No. of patients	Improvement (%)	Improvement (%)	Follow-up (mo)
Yerushalmi (1985)	Prototype	1	1–18	43	18	57	—	23
Servadio (1987)	Prostathermer	1	5–10	43	16	48	48	24
Saranga (1990)	Prostathermer	1	4–7	42.5	11	19	28	12
Servadio (1990)	Prostathermer	1	8	42	140		47	12
Watson (1992)	Prostathermer	1	6	44.5	19	50	55	12
Watson (1991)	Primus	1	6	44	17	38	32	6
Stawarz (1991)	Prototype	0.5	6	43	16	51	189	3
Strohmaier (1990)	Prostathermer	1	8	42.5	23	24	10	4
Yerushalmi (1992)	Prostathermer	1	8–20	43	89	80	27	96
Montorsi (1992)	Prostathermer	1	5–10	43	118	n/a	n/a	24
Kaplan (1993)	Primus	1	10	43.5	30	65	33	6

Table 72B-1   Efficacy of Transrectal Hyperthermia in Non-randomized Studies

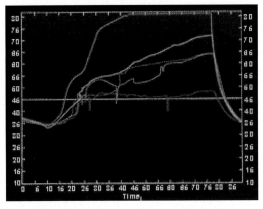

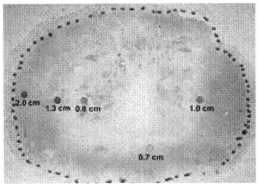

Figure 72B-3 Relationship between anatomic temperature, location from interstitial thermometry, and pathologic findings in whole mount transverse section of prostate following microwave thermotherapy. Location of interstitial thermosensors are shown as open circles on pathologic specimen along with corresponding distance of each from the urethra. The continuous temperature measurements made throughout treatment are shown below. Reproduced with permission from Larson TR, et al.[17]

ratios, and prostate volumes using various cell-kill models and calculations.[23]

MICROWAVE ANTENNA DESIGN

The delivery device for the transfer of energy by microwave is the antenna. There are two major parts to the antenna applicator: (1) a transmission line (typically a coaxial cable) transmits microwave energy from a generator to the, (2) antenna, which radiates the microwaves to the tissue. There are three basic types of microwave antennas: (1) monopole, (2) dipole, and (3) helical coil. A coaxial cable with exposed interconductor (monopole) has a high degree of "back heating" along the transmission line toward the power source and has less accurate targeting of energy to the prostate. By using coaxial and dipole antennas, better focusing of microwave energy and prevention of back-scatter along the transmission line is accomplished. In 1998, Larson and colleagues used tissue-equivalent phantom models to compare Prostatron and Targis microwave machines and noted structural differences in antenna design, correlated with different radiation patterns, in the phantom models.[24] The Prostatron antenna is a monopole design consisting of a coaxial cable with a 3.3-cm length of innerconductor exposed at the tip, whereas the

Targis antenna consists of a dipole design with a 2.8-cm helical coil attached through a ground connection and a tap point to a coaxial cable. The heating pattern of the Targis antenna was shown to be symmetrical, while the Prostatron heating pattern was asymmetrical, and demonstrated substantial back-heating along the catheter axis in the direction of the microwave power source (Figure 72B-4). As a result of these design differences, the Targis antenna theoretically provided more targeted and symmetrical heating, more efficient thermal energy delivery as evidenced by a more than 20-fold lower percentage of reflected power, and less back-heating than the Prostatron catheter. The significant back-heating of the Prostatron catheter may account for clinically significant pain with high-energy Prostasoft 2.5 software and also for the frequent occurrence of automatic power shutdowns due to heating of the urethra and rectum above allowable thresholds. Similarly, Bolmsjo and colleagues compared several other devices, noting subtle differences in heating patterns that may affect clinical outcomes (Prostatron, Prostcare, and Prostalund machines).[25]

It is important for the clinician to understand each of the unique antenna qualities to deliver the best thermal dose and heat configuration to match the prostate anatomy and optimize efficacy.

MICROWAVE EFFECTS ON URETHRAL AND PERIURETHRAL INNERVATION

As part of its efficacy, microwave thermotherapy has been thought to induce denervation which, in turn, diminishes the α-adrenergic tone in smooth muscle cells of the prostate similar to medicinal α-adrenergic blockade. In 1993, Perachino and colleagues analyzed 10 patients who underwent microwave thermotherapy prior to open prostatectomy.[26] Periurethral tissue to a depth of 2.5 cm was examined, with histologic special stains (S100, neuron-specific enolase, and vimentin) and was compared with controls. Nerve axons were nearly absent, and those present showed disruption in the treatment area. In a Swedish study, immunohistochemical stains for PGP 9.5 (a nonspecific neuro marker) were used in patients treated by microwave therapy who subsequently underwent transurethral resection of the prostate (TURP).[27] Again, nerve fibers were absent or nearly absent in the smooth muscle of the biopsy specimens. Nerve fibers were still seen in the superficial layer of the lamina propria and epithelium not exposed to higher temperatures. Support for this concept using human prostatic α_1-adrenoceptor density was shown by Bdesha and colleagues in 1996.[28] A statistically significant difference was found comparing controls to microwave-treated patients when analyzing radio-labeled ^{3}H-prazosin assays for receptor density. This study suggested a significant reduction in α_1-adrenergic receptors in the region of the prostate exposed to maximum heat. Brehmer and Nilsson found a change in the sensory nerve thresholds of the human prostatic urethra using

evoked sensory nerve thresholds measured by a bipolar electrode molded on a urethral catheter in 13 men following microwave thermotherapy.[29] Specifically, the microwave therapy increased sensory nerve thresholds in the posterior urethra by ≥ 30%, and the effect correlated with the alleviation of irritative voiding symptoms.

These findings suggested a mechanism of positive effect on irritative symptoms and supported the previous data on relief of obstructive symptoms by denervation of the α_1-adrenergic receptors of the smooth muscle.

PATHOLOGY/APOPTOSIS CREATED BY MICROWAVE THERMOTHERAPY

Bostwick and Larson studied the effect of thermotherapy on 13 dogs treated with the Urologix T3 catheter using 16 to 45 W of power, creating temperatures greater than 45°C and noted sharply circumscribed, periurethral, coagulative necrosis with hemorrhage in the acute phase of tissue change.[30] In the subacute phase (17 days), the hemorrhagic necrosis was resolving. The periphery of the prostate and the urethra remained intact. In 1997, Mauroy and associates reported the pathologic appearance of suprapubic prostatectomy specimens (at 10 minutes; 24, 48, and 72 hours; and 1, 6, and 12 weeks) following microwave thermotherapy.[31] In this study, coagulative necrosis extended 30 mm from the urethra and peaked at 8 days from treatment.

In another study using human suprapubic prostatectomy specimens previously subjected to microwave thermotherapy, a limited area of necrosis extending 20 to 25 mm from the urethra was observed.[32] A smaller zone surrounding this showed devitalization and a region of non-inflammatory tissue where it is postulated that apoptotic cell death had occurred. Apoptosis was verified by terminal deoxy-nucleotidyl and nick end labeling (TUNEL) technique. Necrotic areas by this technique were seen to a depth of 4 to 5 cm. The apoptosis may have been caused by heat, ischemia, toxins released by necrotic cells or a combination of these factors.

Heat treatments to temperatures below necrosis threshold were investigated using cell cultures of human prostate stromal cells.[33] Exposure to 47°C induced apoptosis in 76% of cells as measured by caspase-3 like activity. Only 14% of cells were necrotic. This study postulated that the application of moderate heat for longer periods led to more apoptosis. In vivo, these effects are likely modified by a number of factors, including blood flow variations and stromal epithelial interactions.

RADIOLOGIC IMAGING OF MICROWAVE THERMOTHERAPY EFFECTS

The importance of developing real-time or delayed-imaging techniques to demonstrate the defects created by microwave therapy is two-fold: (1) treatment time and energy delivered to the

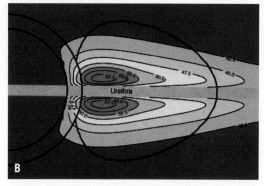
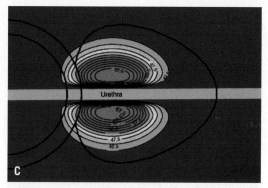

Figure 72B-4 Contrasting heating patterns and efficiency created by each of three generations of microwave technology antennas. Isotherms from generations 2 and 3 were developed from data collected during interstitial mapping studies. Computer simulation with Pennes bio-heat equation was used to create numerical solutions shown. *A*, Generation 1 thermal profile: low-energy, non cooled system with lack of temperatures to cause tissue necrosis. *B*, Generation 2 thermal profile: high-energy, limited cooling creating substantial intraprostatic temperatures with sub optimal urethral cooling - Prostatron antenna. *C*, Generation 3 thermal profile: high-energy, enhanced cooling resulting in focused high intraprostatic temperatures and improved urethral cooling—Cooled Thermocath. Adapted from Larson TR, et al.[24]

prostate could be modified and tailored to the unique qualities of each subject, and (2) different therapy devices could be compared with a standard imaging protocol to assess efficacy and safety.

Using the Prostatron equipment (Prostasoft 2.0) at 60 W of power, Nordenstam and colleagues used magnetic resonance imaging (MRI) to study 20 patients before, 24 hours after, and six months following microwave therapy.[34] Using a Helmholtz body coil and T2 spin echo sequences, the authors were unable to demonstrate significant image differences in the microwave-treated patients. They concluded that their MRI protocol was not sufficiently sensitive or the necrotic effect of treatment was inconsistent. Newhall and colleagues used real-time ultrasonography during microwave thermotherapy while using the Dornier Urowave machine and monitored prostate anatomic changes.[35] D'Angelo and colleagues studied 9 patients with MRI using endorectal and pelvic-phased array coils 4 to 14 days following microwave therapy with Targis and Prostatron machines.[36] Fast spin echo, T2-weighted, gadolinium-enhanced, T1-weighted pulse sequences were used to calculate areas of

non-perfusion, termed the "Gad-defect" (Figure72B-5). The Targis microwave system demonstrated an average of 60% non-perfusion areas within the central zone, while the Prostasoft 2.0 Prostatron equipment demonstrated an average 41% defect.

Hutchinson and colleagues proposed an experimental protocol that would use MRI in real time to monitor changes during thermotherapy of the prostate.[37]

MICROWAVE DEVICES

The results of historically significant clinical series in which transurethral heating devices were used are summarized in Table 72B-2. In 1985, Harada and colleagues reported on transurethral microwave radiation treatment (2,450 MHz) in six patients with prostate obstruction.[10] It was not clear from this early report how many of the patients had obstruction from BPH and how many had prostate cancer. Patients were treated with 100 W of output for 60 seconds, which was repeated two to three times for several minutes in each patient. A catheter was left in place for 7 to

14 days following treatment. Five of the six patients voided after the catheter was removed. All five had urinary retention previously.

Harada and colleagues in 1987 reported on microwave surgery using a transurethral probe as a tool for improving prostate electroresection.[38] A comparative study was made of 16 patients with bladder neck obstruction treated with microwave coagulation and 19 patients who had conventional TURP. Blood loss, irrigant absorption, and frequency of complications were analyzed in both groups. The hyperthermia group had significantly less blood loss and no complications. The authors concluded that the combined microwave coagulation procedure resulted in fewer complications than TURP and was of value in treating patients with both prostatic obstruction and hemorrhagic diathesis as well as high-risk patients.

Astrahan and colleagues tested two prototype transurethral antennae on tissue equivalent.[14] In the first design, a three-dipole applicator was incorporated into a modified Foley catheter, whereas a later design consisted of a flexible helical coil antenna surrounding a modified Foley catheter. Both applicators had similar heating

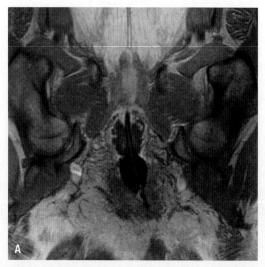
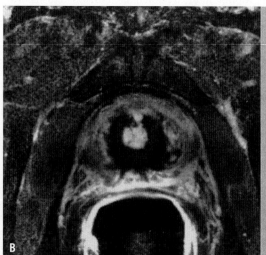
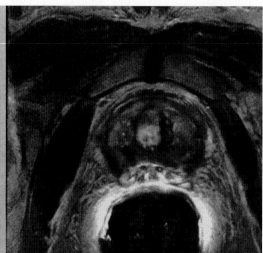

Figure 72B-5 "Gad-defect" *A*, Gadolinium-enhanced, transverse, T1-weighted images of a patient one week following treatment with Cooled Thermocath microwave thermotherapy system. Large area of non-perfusion with centrally enhancing urethral mucosa. *B*, Coronal, T1-weighted image one week following treatment with Prostatron (2.5) system, with a Foley catheter in place. Apical sparing and large area of mid and base region necrosis.

Table 72B-2 Historically Significant Transurethral Hyperthermia Clinical Studies

Series	Device	No. of Sessions	Time (h)	No. of Patients	% Objective Improvement	% Subjective Improvement	Follow-up (mo)
Sapozink et al (1990)	BSD	10	1	21	45	43	12
Baert et al (1990)	BSD	5–10	1	12	98	65	12
Stawarz (1991)	BSD	3–6	1/2	14	79	77	12
Baert et al (1992)	BSD	5	1	79	30	49	12
Watson (1992)	Thermex II	1	3	68	NS	40	1
Vanden Bosscheet al (1993)	Thermex II	1	1	191	45	65	—
Viguier et al	Thermex II	1	1	50	NS	68	12
Bdesha et al	LEO Microthermer	1	1	40	NS	63	3

NS = not significant

characteristics. The helical coil design, however, produced a more cylindrical heating pattern with a broader and more consistent hot spot. The authors demonstrated that the applicator was well suited for heating a cylindrical volume of approximately 4 cm in length and 0.5 cm in radial depth around the applicator.[11] Ameye and Baert then performed temperature interstitial thermometry in canine prostates during transurethral microwave hyperthermia (915 MHz).[39] The selective cylindrical heating produced by phantom studies was confirmed in the dog model. The radial heat penetration produced a hot spot near the longitudinal of the applicator at about 0.5 cm from the applicator, with a dissipation gradient of approximately 27°C/cm.[14] Histologic examination of the canine prostates revealed dilated glands surrounded by interstitial edema. The lumen of the glands was filled with sludged, epithelial material, and necrosis of glandular elements was evident.[44] Tissue obtained during TURP in patients who failed transurethral microwave hyperthermia showed interstitial hemorrhage, blood vessel thrombosis and coagulation, and hemorrhagic necrosis in the periurethral prostate.[39] The depth of penetration of these lesions correlates well with the heating profile of the helical coil applicator. It was believed that selective shrinking or retraction of the prostate tissue dilated the urethra and reduced or eliminated outflow obstruction.[40]

A report by Sapozink and colleagues in 1990 included 21 patients with biopsy-documented BPH who underwent treatment with a pilot protocol involving intracavitary transurethral radiation microwave hyperthermia without extrinsic cooling (630 MHz in 12 patients, and 915 MHz in 9 patients).[41] Interstitial thermometry demonstrated a mean temperature of 44.1°C, mean maximal temperature of 47.7°C, and a maximum temperature of 49°C. There were highly significant increases in urinary flow rate (44% improvement in peak flow) and a decrease in postvoid residual urine of 49%. A decrease in frequency (30%) and nocturia (44%) was also observed. Median follow-up in these patients was 12.5 months, and only three of the patients required subsequent prostatic resection. Complications included bladder spasms in 26% of the patients, hematuria in 23%, and dysuria in 9%.[41] Baert and colleagues demonstrated a doubling of flow rate in patients treated with 5 to 10 sessions of transurethral microwave

hyperthermia (915 MHz) without cooling.[42] This same group subsequently reported the results in 31 patients after at least a 12-month follow-up and an additional 7 patients who failed hyperthermia and underwent surgical therapy.[43] This group was taken from a total of 79 patients (7 patients discontinued treatment) who were scheduled to receive five 60-minute sessions with temperature controlled on the urethral surface at 45.5°C (915 MHz). The mean FDA and recommended symptom score in the 61 patients decreased from 15.1 to 7.7, mostly in the obstructive categories. Mean peak flow rate increased from 8.8 to 11.5 mL/sec. Significant improvement occurred in 73% of patients with lateral lobe hyperplasia but in only 30% with median lobe hyperplasia.[43] Of the seven patients who failed surgery, five had median lobe enlargement and one had median bar enlargement. While many variables, not all known at the present time, influence the delivery of thermal energy to the prostate, catheter design and characteristics of the

thermotherapy machine are significant factors in heat delivery. The early transurethral hyperthermia systems were designed to operate without urethral cooling. Without urethral cooling, urethral tissue closest to the applicator received the highest energy output. A steep gradient of decreasing temperatures ensued a short distance from the applicator. To accommodate these limitations, multiple treatment sessions were necessary . To improve outcomes, contemporary high energy thermotherapy devices with intraprostatic temperatures > 70°C have required urethral cooling systems for patient comfort and to enhance the treatment of the transition zone.

HIGH-ENERGY, COOLED TRANSURETHRAL MICROWAVE DEVICES

There are currently four microwave treatment machines commercially available in the United States and no less than seven additional systems available internationally (Table 72B-3, Figure 72B-6).Furthermore, different catheter delivery systems can be used for different prostate sizes. For example, Prostatron currently has two different catheters (Figure 72B-7): (1) The black Prostaprobe-TUMT 2.0 for prostate lengths between 35 and 50 mm in axial dimension, with maximum power delivery of 60 W, one hour duration, and a maximum energy delivery of 213 kilojoules (Kj) and (2) the blue Prostaprobe for TUMT 2.5 or 30-minute transurethral microwave thermotherapy (TUMT) for axial lengths 25 to 50 mm and to preferentially treat the bladder neck (Figure 72B-8). The blue Prostaprobe can deliver 70 to 80 W of power and up to 240 Kj of energy.

Table 72B-3 Transurethral Heating Devices

Device and Series	Frequency (MHz)	Time (h)/Sessions (No.)
BSD (BSD Medical, Salt Lake City, Utah) 　Baert et al 　Sapozink et al 　Astrahan et al	915	0.3/10
LEO Microthermer(Laser Optics, London, England) 　Bdesha et al	915	1.0/1
Thermex II (Direx, Israel) 　Vanden Bossche et al 　Corica et al 　Nissenkorn et al	915	0.2/10
Prostatron (Urologix Inc, Minneapolis, MN) 　Devonec et al. (Prostasoft 2.0) 　Carter et al. (Prostasoft 2.0) 　Blute et al. (Prostasoft 2.0)	1,296	1.0/1
Targis (Urologix Inc, Minneapolis, MN) 　Larson et al 　Mulvin et al 　Ramsey et al 　Javle et al	915	1.0/1 0.5/1
Other Microwave devices: 　Prostalund/CoreTherm (Lund Inst, Sweden) 　Prostcare (Bruker, Wissembourg, France) 　Urowave (Dornier MedTech, USA) 　Primus U + R (Tecnomatix, Germany)		

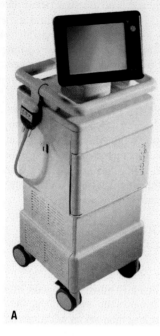 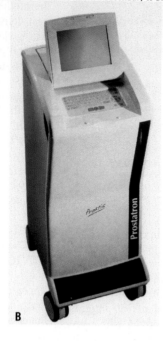 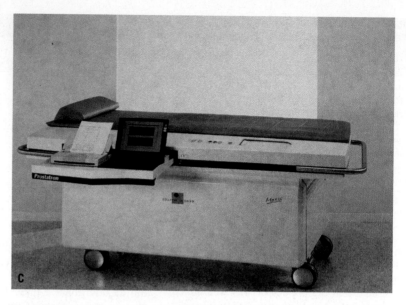

Figure 72B-6 *A*, Targis, cooled thermotherapy console. *B*, Prostatron Praktis transurethral microwave thermotherapy (TUMT) console. *C*, Prostatron Maxis, TUMT console. Photograph courtesy of Urologix, Inc., Minneapolis, MN.

The second most commonly used microwave delivery device in the United States is the Targis device (see Figure 72B-7). This microwave delivery device also has three different treatment schemes. The standard 60-minute treatment uses a maximum power output of 60 W with a frequency between 902 and 928 MHz. The Express treatment protocol uses a 28.5-minute treatment at a maximum power output of 60 W in a similar frequency range. The United States Food and Drug Administration (FDA) approved Cooled Thermocath, which operates at a similar frequency range but up to 75 W of power (see Figure 72B-7). A typical treatment runs 28.5 minutes and accommodates this increased power by an expanded cooling chamber design and enhanced power delivery capability (Figure 72B-9).

It is important for the clinician to understand that each of these devices delivers a different thermal dose and heat configuration. To date, no well-designed, head-to-head trial has been conducted comparing one microwave device to another. Conclusions on efficacy of one device versus another should be made very carefully because results may be simply owing to the differences in microwave technology and study design.

MICROWAVE THERMOTHERAPY RESULTS

Numerous clinical studies in multiple European and North American centers have demonstrated the efficacy of microwave thermotherapy. Subjective improvement in symptom scores have been commonplace, but objective data such as maximum flow rates and decreased bladder outlet pressures often have been more dependent on the type of technology used. Table 72B-4 lists the studies with at least 6 to 12 months follow-up and demonstrates these trends. A number of authors

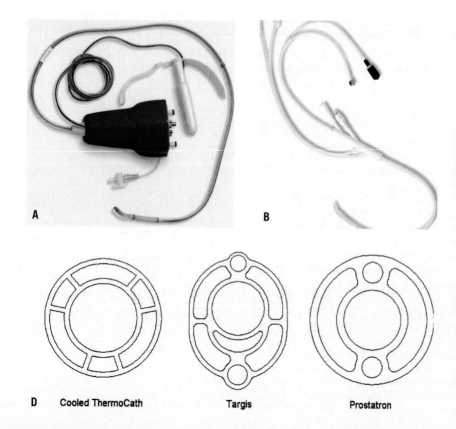 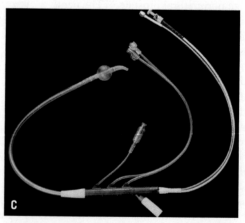

D   Cooled ThermoCath   Targis   Prostatron

Figure 72B-7 *A*, Blue Prostaprobe microwave delivery device with attached rectal thermometry probe. *B*, Targis microwave delivery device (MDS) with connectors for power, fiberoptic thermometry, coolant, Foley balloon and urine drainage ports. *C*, Cooled Thermo-Cath microwave delivery device with enhanced cooling chambers behind inflated Foley balloon. *D*, Cross-sectional profile of each generation of microwave device catheters demonstrating enhanced cooling chamber configuration in third-generation Cooled ThermoCath. (Photographs courtesy of Urologix, Inc., Minneapolis, MN.

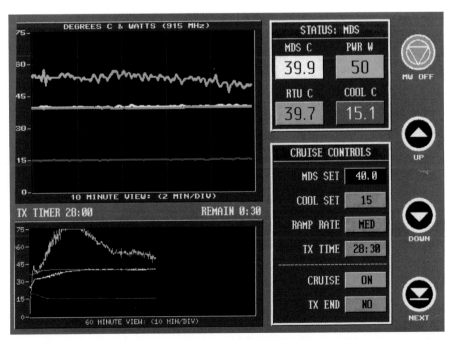

Figure 72B-8 Prostatron transurethral microwave thermotherapy treatment profile. Note continuous cooling (5°C) and urethral temperatures on bottom profile. The rectal temperature curves and power level are seen on top profile. Photograph courtesy of Urologix, Inc., Minneapolis, MN.

are now reporting long-term follow-up for microwave thermotherapy (Table 72B-5). Not all studies can substantiate claims for durability. It is important to note that few studies report long-term data on substantial numbers of patients. Caution is urged when interpreting this data. Devices that can deliver more thermal energy to the prostate appear to show the largest improvement in peak urinary flow rates and reproducible, objective data.

RANDOMIZED-SHAM STUDIES

The placebo response is well documented in all drug trials investigating alternatives for the management of BPH.[44] In device trials, randomized double-blinded studies are necessary to show a meaningful response to therapy that is greater than the placebo, or sham, effect.[45] A sham trial assesses the effect of instrumentation. Several randomized sham studies have been performed to determine the placebo effect of transurethral microwave thermotherapy (Table 72B-6). Ogden and colleagues reported a randomized study of 43 patients with unequivocal benign prostatic obstruction indicated by a Madsen symptom score > 8 and a peak flow rate < 15 mL/sec.[46] Sham treatments were identical to normal transurethral microwave thermotherapy sessions except for the absence of microwave heating. If a patient still met the entry criteria at 3 months, he was offered transurethral microwave thermotherapy. Twenty-one men underwent sham treatment, and 22 underwent transurethral microwave thermotherapy. Baseline symptom scoring and peak flow rates were similar for the two groups. The results showed a significant improvement in all parameters after transurethral microwave thermotherapy but failed to show an instrumentation

effect. In a similar manner, Debruyne and colleagues randomized 46 patients with symptoms of BPH to receive transurethral microwave thermotherapy vs. sham treatment.[47] The preliminary results after a three-month follow-up showed an improvement in the peak flow rate of 3.6 mL/sec in the thermotherapy group but no change in the placebo group. After six months, the results were 13.4 mL/sec in the transurethral microwave thermotherapy group and 11.9 mL/sec in the placebo group. There was clear improvement in Madsen

symptom scores in both groups. The score decreased from an average of 13 and 12.3 before treatment to 5.6 and 6.5 at 12 weeks after treatment. At six-month follow-up, the symptom score improvement persisted in the transurethral microwave thermotherapy group. However, the sham-treated group deteriorated. A prospective double-blind randomized study of transurethral microwave thermotherapy vs. sham treatment was conducted at the Mayo Clinic Jacksonville and Rochester sites.[48] One hundred twenty patients entered the protocol, and 111 reached unblinding at 3 months. Patients were randomized in a 2:1 fashion to receive transurethral microwave thermotherapy or a sham treatment. Blinding verification was performed by questionnaire, which indicated the patient's perception of treatment received. Fifty percent of patients in the transurethral microwave thermotherapy group believed they were treated, and 44% of the patients in the sham group believed they had not received treatment. The results of peak flow rates and mean Madsen symptom score are listed in Table 72B-7. Serum PSA increased 536% 1 week after treatment in the transurethral microwave thermotherapy group (mean 3.3 ng/mL baseline, to mean 18.8 ng/mL at 1 week), whereas there was no change in the sham patients (mean 2.9 ng/mL baseline, to mean 3.7 ng/mL at 1 week). The groups in these studies apparently had similar baseline findings in parameters commonly used to measure outlet obstruction symptoms. Results of the studies appear to show a statistically significant improvement that is greater than the sham effect for patients who underwent transurethral microwave thermotherapy. Furthermore, PSA changes in the transurethral microwave thermotherapy group indicate destruction of prostate

Figure 72B-9 Targis microwave thermotherapy treatment profile. Upper graph demonstrates coolant temperature, power level, rectal thermal unit (RTU) and microwave delivery device (MDS) temperatures over 10 min period. Numerical values of each component and set points for therapy are seen on right side of treatment profile screen. Photograph courtesy of Urologix, Inc., Minneapolis, MN.

Table 72B-4   Improvement in Peak Flow Rate (Q max) and Symptom Score in Series with 6- to 12-Month Follow-Up After Transurethral Microwave Thermotherapy

Reference	Device	No. of Patients	Baseline Qmax (mL/s)	Baseline Symptom Score	3 Mo Qmax (mL/s)	3 Mo Symptom Score	6 Mo Qmax (mL/s)	6 Mo Symptom Score	1 Yr Qmax (mL/s)	1 Yr Symptom Score
Ramsey et al	T3*	154	9.3	20.1A	NA	NA	NA	NA	13.4	8.8A
Roos and Pedersen	Prostalund†	177	8.4	15.1	9.5	9.9	NA	NA	9.9	10.5
Goldfarb et al	Urowave‡	62	8.3 ± 0.6	22.6 ± 0.6	11.3 ± 1.0	10.8 ± 0.81	11.5 ± 0.6	11.4 ± 1.0	11.6 ± 0.6	11.2± 0.8/1
Eliasson et al	Prostcare§	172	9.8 ± 3.4	12.7 ± 4.6	10.3± 3.9	7± 4.1	10.7 ± 4.1	6.9 ± 4.8	10.9 ± 4.2	6.6± 4.4
De la Rosette et al	Prostatron 2.0	130	9.9 ± 3	12.7 ± 3.3M	NA	NA	NA	NA	11.6± 4.9	6.8 ± 4.6M
Devonec et al	Prostatron 2.0	818	8.8	13.3M, 12.9B	13.0	5.7M, 6.5B	12.8	3.5M, 4.5B	12.6	3.5M, 4.3B
Terai et al	Prostatron 2.0	63	6.6 ± 2.4	22.0 ± 7	NA	NA	NA	NA	11.4 ± 7.4	13.1± 6.6/1
Blute et al	Prostatron 2.0	150	8.5 ± 0.3	13.7 ± 0.3M	NA	NA	NA	NA	11.3 ± 0.4	5.4± 0.4M
Kirby et al	Prostatron 2.0	140	10.1± 4.7	23.7 ± 4.4B	12.3 ± 3.2	10.6± 27B	12.9± 2.1	10.4± 3.4	12.4 ± 3.4	11.6 ± 3.3B
Marteinsson and Due	Prostatron 2.0	115	9.8	15.7	13.3	3.8	13.3	3.2	13.7	2.6
de la Rosette et al	Prostatron 2.5	116	9.6 ± 3.3	3.6± 3.6M	15.2 ±6.5	6.0 ± 4.5M	14.1	5.5	14.5±5.9	4.9±4.4M
Roehrborn et al	Urowave‡	220 (2:1 sham)	7.7	23.6A	NA	NA	10.7	12.7A	NA	NA
Nawrocki et al	Prostatron 2.0	120 (38 TUMT)	8.8	19A	NA	NA	9.9	9.5A	NA	NA
Javle et al	T3*	50	9.1	19.9A	14.9	7.4A	14.6	6.8A	14.0	6.7A
Brehmer and Kinn	ECP‖	66	8.8	19.0D	NA	NA	NA	NA	14.2	8.4D
Larson et al	T3*	169 (44 sham)	7.8	20.8A	11.7	9.6A	11.8	10.5A	NA	NA
De Wildt et al	Prostatron 2.5	85	9.4 ± 3.3	13.9 ± 3.6M	15.8 ± 7.0	6.7 ± 4.6M	14.4 ± 6.7	5.7 ± 4.6M	14.9 ± 6.7	5.8 ± 4.7M

Adapted from Simopoulos DN, Blute ML. Transurethral microwave thermotherapy. In: Lepor H. editor. Prostate diseases. Philadelphia: W.B. Saunders; 2001. p. 277–91.

A = AUA symptom score; B = Boyarsky symptom Score; D = DAN-PSS-1 symptom score (Danish Prostatic Symptom Score); I = International Prostatic Symptom Score; M = Madsen score; NA = not available; Qmax = peak urinary flow rate.

*Urologix, Minneapolis, MN.

†Dantec Medical AIS, Denmark.

‡Dornier Medical Systems, Marietta, GA.

§Bruker Spectospin, Wissembourg, France

‖Comair, Sweden

tissue as the physiologic basis of response, as opposed to no change in PSA levels in sham-treated patients. These results suggest that the efficacy observed after transurethral microwave thermotherapy is not related to a sham effect or instrumentation.

Several additional studies using high-energy protocols further reinforced the meaningful response to therapy being greater than sham effect of instrumentation. Two specific studies involving sham versus microwave heat therapy deserve special note. Nawrocki and colleagues using the Prostasoft 2.0 software suggested placebo impact only.[49] Specifically, no differences were noted in the degree of improvement in peak flow rates, whether microwave energy was present or absent. Furthermore, symptomatic improvement was greater when the patients had no therapy. In another study showing substantial sham effect, Mulvin and colleagues used a microwave delivery device and compared it to ureteral catheterization alone.[50] This study showed no change in peak flow rates or symptom score improvement at three months.

TRANSURETHRAL MICROWAVE THERMOTHERAPY VERSUS TURP

In the evaluation of new treatments for BPH, the results of each new therapy should be compared with those obtained with conventional surgical procedures. It is unlikely that microwave heat treatments will compete realistically with TURP in terms of flow rate improvement. Symptom relief and post-treatment morbidity, however, may define the exact role of microwave heat ther-

apies in the management of BPH. There have been several trials comparing microwave thermotherapy and TURP (Table 72B-8). These studies have shown microwave to be an effective modality, but in no way capable of duplicating the objective and subjective results of TURP.

Dahlstrand and colleagues compared TURP (39 patients) and transurethral microwave thermotherapy (40 patients-Prostasoft 2.0) in a prospective randomized study.[51] Patients were observed for 12 months following treatment. The baseline objective and subjective parameters appeared to be similar in both groups. There was a statistically and clinically significant improvement in peak flow rate at 12 months after therapy for both transurethral microwave thermotherapy and TURP groups. Although peak flow rate improvement was 4.3 mL/sec (54%) in the thermotherapy group, there was a statistically significant greater improvement in the TURP group of 9.8 mL/sec (124% improvement at 12 months, $p < .01$). In addition, there was a statistically and clinically significant improvement in both groups in Madsen symptom scores. The patients treated with transurethral microwave thermotherapy improved 76% in symptom scores versus a 93% in the TURP group. This, although statistically significant, clinically represents only a slight difference. Dahlstrand also found postvoid residual volumes statistically unchanged after transurethral microwave thermotherapy at one year. However, there was a marked statistically significant improvement in postvoid residuals at 12 months for the TURP group.

d'Ancona and colleagues also compared microwave thermotherapy with TURP using high

energy Prostasoft 2.5 software and noted an improvement in symptom score of 74% for TURP versus 56% for microwave.[52] Of significance, however, is that mean peak urinary flow rates, while not surpassing TURP (mean of 19.1 mL/sec) increased substantially from a baseline for microwave (9.3 to 15.1 mL/sec) and were maintained through 30 months of follow-up.

Floratos and colleagues showed that these differences became more pronounced with time, as patients undergoing TURP continued to improve in both objective and subjective parameters after 1, 2, and 3 years.[53] This was not the case for the microwave group. Additional procedures were required in 19.8% of the microwave thermotherapy group compared to 12.9% of the TURP group at 33 months.

Adverse events of the two methods of therapy vary. In general, TURP required secondary procedures as a result of complications, while therapy failure was generally the cause of adverse events in microwave treatment. The complication rates of TURP in these series were generally due to bleeding, clot retention, urinary retention, urinary tract infections, urethral strictures, and retrograde ejaculation, whereas patients undergoing microwave heat treatment were at a higher risk of urinary urgency, urinary retention, and prolonged catheterization

Francisca and colleagues performed a full quality-of-life study on 147 patients randomized to TURP or Prostasoft 2.5 therapy. It was determined that daily activities and perception of urinary difficulties were improved in both groups, but TURP generated greater improvement and overall quality of life and clinical outcome.[54]

Table 72B-5 Durability of Data: Transurethral Microwave Thermotherapy (TUMT) Studies With at Least 2 Years' Follow-up

Reference	Device	No. of Patients	Duration	Retreatment Rate	Baseline Symptom Score	Symptom Score at Follow-up	Baseline Mean Qmax (mL/s)	Follow-up Mean Qmax (mL/s)	Patient Satisfaction
Ramsey et al	Targis (T3)*	152	3 yr	0.83 Kaplan-Meyer No retreatment	20.2A (N = 152)	8.4A (N = 44)	8.5 (N = 147)	12.7 (N = 41)	91.4% satisfied
d'Ancona et al	Prostatron 2.5	301	2 yr	7% retreated (N = 22); 9 TURP 1 open prostatectomy 3 TUIVN 2 laser prostatectomy 7 medical therapy	14.1M 18.9I	5.0M 7.9I	9.7 (N = 301)	13.8 (N = 74)	93% "durable outcome"
Hallin and Berlin	Prostatron 2.0	187	4 yr	51.9% retreated (N = 97); 26 TURP 2 TUMT 69 medical therapy	12.2M (N = 56	7.7M (N = 54)	10.1 (N = 55)	8.2 (N = 45)	23% satisfied
Glass et al	Leo Microthermer†	67	> 4 yr	31% retreated (N = 16); 11 TURP 2 TUMT 3 medical therapy	10.28 10.5W (N = 67)	6.28 10.0W (N = 29)	7.9 (N = 67)	11.5 (N = 29)	58% satisfied
Blute et al	Prostatron 2.0	216	4 yr	39.8% retreated (N = 86); 24 TURP 62 medical therapy	14.0M (N = 216)	7.0M (N = 88)	NA	NA	63% subjective improvement
Robinette et al	Prostatron 2.0 and 2.5	320	3 yr	30% retreated (N = 96); 8 TURP 2 open prostatectomy 86 TUMT	11M 17I (N = 320)	6M 4/‡	11 (N = 320)	16‡	NA
Keijzers et al	Prostatron 2.0	231	5 yr	57% retreated (N = 124); 39 TURP 7 open prostatectomy 28 "other invasive" therapy 3 TUMT 47 medical therapy	12.1M (N = 231)	7.6M (N = 29)	9.0 (N = 23)	NA	NA
Ohigashi et al	Prostatron 2.0	102	5 yr	67% estimated	17.6I	NA	8.8	NA	NA
Daehlin et al	Primus U & R	91	5 yr	59% 41 surgery 17 medical therapy	22.4I	12.9I	9.9	9.4	NA
Francisca	Prostatron 2.0	1094	5 yr	5\7% 26% surgery 31% medical therapy	15.2M	8.6M	8.7	11.1	NA

Adapted from Simopoulos DN, Blute ML. Transurethral Microwave Thermotherapy. In: Lepor H. editor. Prostate diseases. Philadelphia: W.B. Saunders 2001; p. 277–91.

A = AUA Symptom score; B = Boyarsky symptom score; I = International Prostatic Symptom Score; M = Madsen symptom score; NA = not available; Qmax = peak urinary flow rate; TURP = transurethral resection of prostate; TUIVN = transurethral incision of the vesical neck; TUMT = transurethral microwave thermotherapy; W = WHO Symptom score.

*Urologix, Minneapolis.
†Laser Electro Optics Ltd., London, U.K.
‡Dornier Medical Systems, Marietta, GA.

In another study addressing sexual function, Arai and colleagues reported an 18.2% rate of erectile dysfunction in the microwave thermotherapy group treated with a high-energy machine.[55] This was in contrast to a 26.5% rate in those undergoing TURP. Overall, satisfaction with sexual function seems higher in patients who have had microwave thermotherapy than in those having had TURP; those undergoing microwave thermotherapy reported being "very satisfied" (55%), versus 21% of those having had TURP. However, 74% of this TURP population were satisfied with their urinary flow rates compared to 27% after microwave thermotherapy.

PATIENT SELECTION FOR MICROWAVE HEAT TREATMENT

Many urologists have a high regard for the efficacy of transurethral microwave thermotherapy in treating patients with lower urinary tract symptoms. Others feel it has no place in the therapeutic options for BPH. The ideal patient for this modality has yet to be fully characterized. Initially, microwave thermotherapy was stressed as an alternative treatment for obstructive BPH in patients at high surgical risk. With the advantage of low morbidity and the ambulatory nature of the treatment, it is an alternative therapy for an increasing population of men. Whether or not

Table 72B-6 Randomized Transurethral Hyperthermia Sham Studies

Series	No. of Patients	Baseline Qmax (mL/sec)	Baseline Symptom Score	3 Months Qmax (mL/sec)	3 Months Symptom Score
Ogden et al					
TUMT	21	8.5	14.5	13.5	3.6
Sham	19	8.6			
Debruyne et al					
TUMT	25	NA	13	+3.6	5.6
Sham	25	NA	12.3	NC	6.5
Blute et al					
TUMT	75	7.3	13.9	11.5*	6.3†
Sham	36	7.4	14.9	9.5	10.7
Mulvin et al					
Targis	20	12.8	24.2	14.6	14.1
Sham	20	10.0	21.0	12.4	9.6
Larson et al					
Targis	125	7.8	20.8	11.8 (6 mos)	10.5 (6 mos)
Sham	44	7.8	21.3	9.8 (6 mos)	14.3 (6 mos)
deWildt et al					
Prostatron 2.5	47	9.2	13.7	13.4 (1 yr)	4.2 (1 yr)
Sham	46	9.6	12.9	10.6 (1 yr)	8.2 (1 yr)
Nawrocki et al					
Prostatron 2.0	38	8.83	19	9.94 (6 mos)	9.5
Sham	40	9.44	18	9.49 (6 mos)	9.5

Adapted from Blute ML. Microwave thermotherapy for the treatment of benign prostatic hyperplasia. Sem Urol 1994;7:181–92.
NA = not applicable; NC = no change; Qmax = peak urinary flow rate; TUMT = transurethral microwave thermotherapy.
*P < 0.01.
†P < 0.001.

these variable, and at times contradictory, results may simply reflect differences in microwave delivery-device technology. Additional study is necessary to fully characterize the ideal microwave thermotherapy patient.

CONTRAINDICATIONS

As with other transurethral urologic procedures, all patients must have a documented sterile urine and be cleared of prostate or urothelial malignancy. Bladder calculi or evidence of bacterial prostatitis are also exclusionary. Neurogenic bladder dysfunction should have the underlying neurologic problem evaluated and treated. The safety and effectiveness of microwave heat therapy has not been established in patients with disorders of coagulation, an interest in preservation of fertility, or large intravesical median lobes.

As microwave thermotherapy technology evolves, specific contraindications are being amended and altered. Patients with penile prostheses, artificial genitourinary sphincters, severe peripheral vascular disease, and severe urethral stricture disease are to be excluded from treatment. Those patients having had previous radiation therapy to the pelvic region or having undergone previous pelvic or rectal surgery (other than hemorrhoidectomy) should also not be treated. Those patients with pacemakers and defibrillators need direction from their cardiologist on deactivation of these devices during therapy. Hip arthroplasty is no longer a contraindication to microwave thermotherapy of the prostate. In the past, urinary retention was considered a contraindication. Patients presenting with urinary retention, however, are generally at an increased anesthetic risk and have larger prostate volumes, and this therapy has been offered as a less invasive and sometimes successful therapy. Djavan and colleagues reported a 94% success rate after 4 months in treating 31 patients who presented with urinary retention.[61] Robinette and colleagues reported that 44 of 60 patients in retention were able to void at 6 months, and 32 of 35 patients followed for 12 months were also voiding without catheters.[62]

prostate size, or the severity of symptoms, can predict clinical outcome of microwave heat therapy is a source of disagreement among authors. In 116 patients treated with a high-energy protocol, de la Rosette and colleagues demonstrated that patients with moderate to severe outlet obstruction were best responders to microwave therapy.[56] Similarly, de Wildt and colleagues showed that prostates larger than 40 cc and severe outlet obstruction responded best to the high-energy Prostasoft 2.5 software.[57] Contrasting these findings, Walden and colleagues found patients with low to moderate obstruction (as graded by detrusor-adjusted mean pressure urethral resistance relative factor [PURR]

responded better than those with high-grade obstruction.[58] Javle and colleagues also reported similar findings of the best response in mild to moderate obstructive symptoms.[59] Tubaro and coworkers demonstrated a significantly better outcome for patients with predominantly constrictive obstruction as defined by PURR, as opposed to compressive obstructive symptoms.[60] The patients with constrictive obstruction had an equivalent improvement in symptom score but a significantly better increase in the peak flow rates at 6 months. Similarly, a significantly greater fall in residual urine volume was seen in this constrictive group of patients. It is again important to note that

Table 72B-7 Outcomes of Minimally Invasive Therapies: Estimates of Change in Efficacy Scores/Rates

Thermal-based therapies	AUA/IPSS 3–9 Months	AUA/IPSS 10–16 Months	AUA/IPSS >16 Months	Peak Flow Rate (Qmax) 3–9 Months	Peak Flow Rate (Qmax) 10–16 Months	Peak Flow Rate (Qmax) >16 Months	QoL Question Score 3–9 Months	QoL Question Score 10–16 Months	QoL Question Score >16 Months	BPH Impact Index 3–9 Months	BPH Impact Index 10–16 Months
Thermal-based therapies											
TUMT Prostatron Version 2.0	−10.93*	−10.47*	−9.27*	3.39*	2.81*	2.26*	−1.95*	−1.75*	−1.70*		
TUMT Prostatron Version 2.5	−8.83*	−10.72*	−10.73*	4.51*	4.54*	4.42*	−1.25*				
Targis TUMT	−10.14‡	−9.44	−10.76*	2.64‡	5.29	3.28*	−2.20‡	−2.44	−2.31*		
Watchful Waiting	−1.00*	−0.50*		−0.03*		2.16					
Sham (control)	−6.37*			1.03*			−1.04*				−2.30*
TURP (control)	−14.65*	−14.80*	−13.54*	10.54	10.77*	8.06*	−3.44*	−3.34*	−3.03*		

Adapted from AUA Practice Guidelines Committee.[65]
Cells without asterisks are RCT comparisons to TURP.
*These numbers are based on single-arm analyses—no RCT data available. Note that single-arm analyses are the same for TURP comparisons.
†Single-arm numbers used here because the RCT results were deemed unreasonable due most likely to technique, patient selection or other problems.
‡RCT comparison to sham.

SAFETY AND MORBIDITY

Reports of complications following microwave thermotherapy of the prostate vary in range from 0 to 38% based on the investigator's cited criteria for complications and the study cited (Table 72B-9). In an FDA trial, regional and general anesthesia was required in 32% of patients; oral sedation was used in 19% of men, and 12% required parenteral sedation.[63] Adverse events were minimal. The most prominent side effect was a minor degree of procedural hematuria (40%). Urinary tract infections were documented in 7.4%, and 6.7% had ejaculatory disturbances including hematospermia, dry ejaculate, and reduced ejaculate volume. Twenty-eight percent experienced urinary retention with a mean catheterization time of 9.6 days. Men with larger prostates and high treatment energies had significantly higher rates of retention.

It is important to note that significant differences in morbidity have been reported when comparing the Prostatron and Targis microwave delivery systems (Table 72B-10),[64] whereas 69% and 26% of patients in the Prostatron group experienced hematuria and urinary retention requiring catheterization, respectively. In patients treated with the Targis catheter, these numbers were 4% and 3%, respectively. In published American Urological Association Practice Guidelines for the Management of BPH, the Guidelines Committee reviewed the status of microwave heat therapy as it related to morbidity. Findings are presented in Table 72B-11.[65]

A variety of other rare but reported complications following transurethral microwave thermotherapy occur. This includes, but is not limited to, bladder perforation, urethrovesical fistula, and emphysematous, prostatic abscess. The FDA published safety recommendations for the use of transurethral microwave heat treatment devices.[66] This FDA notice was released because of unex-

Table 72B-8 Trials Comparing Transurethral Microwave Thermotherapy (TUMT) with Transurethral Resection of the Prostate (TURP)

Reference	Treatment	Duration of Follow-Up	Baseline Symptom Score	Baseline Qmax (mL/s)	Follow-Up Symptom Score	Follow-Up Qmax (mL/s)
Dahlstrand et al	TURP (N = 32)	2 yr	13.6M	8.6	1.2M	17.6
	TUMT, Prostatron 2.0 (N = 37)		12.1M	8.6	2.3M	12.3
d'Ancona et al	TURP (N = 21)	30 mo	13.8M	9.3	3.6M	19.1
	TUMT, Prostatron 2.5 (N = 31)		13.3M	9.3	5.8M	15.1
Ahmed et al	TURP (N = 30)	6 mo	18.4A	9.5	5.2A	14.6
	TUMT, Prostatron 2.5 (N = 30)		18.5A	10.1	5.3A	9.1
Floratos et al	TURP (N = 66)	3 yr	20.0I	7.8	5.0I	24.7
	TUMT, Prostatron 2.5 (N = 78)		20.0I	9.2	12.0I	11.9
Wagrell et al	TURP (N = 46)	12 mo	20.0I	7.9	7.1I	15.2
	Prostalund (N=100)		21.0I	7.6	7.2I	13.3

A = AUA symptom score; I = IPSS; M = Madsen symptom score; Qmax = peak urinary flow rate.

Table 72B-9 Morbidity After Transurethral Microwave Thermotherapy

Reference	No. of Patients	Catheterization	Retention (%)	Hematuria (%)	UTI (%)	Erectile Dysfunction (%)	Ejaculatory Problem (%)	Stricture (%)	Incontinence (%)	Retreatment (%)
Miller et al	103	—	—	—	—	—	—	—	—	—
Roos and Pedersen	177	—	3.3	2.2	2.3	—	—	0.0	0.0	9.0
Goldfarb et al	62	—	4.8	12.9	0.0	0.0	3.2	0.0	0.0	—
Eliasson et al	172	—	6.0	62.0	2.3	—	0.0	—	0.0	1.1
Bdesha et al	22	—	—	31.8	—	0.0	0.0	—	—	—
van Cawelaert et al	128	3.1 days	33.0	2.6	—	0.0	0.0	—	—	0.6
de la Rosette et al	130	—	26.0	4.5	—	—	0.8	0.0	0.0	10.7
Ogden et al	22	—	22.0	—	—	—	—	—	—	4.5
Devonec et al	818	—	10–40	—	—	0.0	0.0	—	—	7.0
Terai et al	63	3.9 days	36.0	1.5	1.5	—	1.5	—	—	—
Blute et al	150	—	36.0	40.0	—	—	0.6	—	—	—
Hofner et al	32	—	—	—	—	—	—	—	—	—
Kirby et al	140	—	25.0	*	15.0*	5.0	—	—	—	3.0
Dahlstrand et al	37	1–7 days	13.5	0.0	13.5	—	—	—	—	10.8
Marteinsson and Due	115	14.8 days	28.6	—	6.9	0.8	1.7	—	—	—
Netto et al	100	—	—	—	—	—	0.0	11.0	—	—
Perrin et al	72	> 2 wk	80.0	—	—	—	—	—	—	—
de la Rosette et al	116	16 days	100	76.0	7.0	0.0	44.0	0.0	0.0	5.9
de Wildt et al	85	14.3 days	100	—	—	—	33.0	—	—	2.6

Adapted from Simopoulos DN, Blute ML. Transurethral microwave thermotherapy. In: Lepor H. editor. Prostate diseases. Philadelphia: W.B. Saunders; 2001. p. 277–91.

*Hematuria and infections.

UTI = urinary tract infection.

Table 72B-10   Morbidity of Prostatron Compared With Targis Transurethral Microwave Thermotherapy

	Prostatron (N = 78)		Sham (N = 37)		Targis (N = 74)		Sham (N = 20)	
Event	n	%	n	%	n	%	n	%
Hematuria	54	69	19	51	3	4	0	—
Urethral bleeding	16	21	5	14	3	4	0	—
Urethral discharge	2	3	0	—	0	—	0	—
Urinary retention necessitating catheterization	20	26	0	—	2	3	0	—
Urinary tract infection	11	14	0	—	2	3	1	5
Epididymitis	0	—	0	—	1	1	0	—
Incontinence	0	—	0	—	1	1	0	—
Ejaculatory dysfunction	0	—	0	—	0	—	0	—

Table 72B-11   Outcomes of Minimally Invasive Therapies: Estimates of Rates of Occurrence of Adverse Events

	Median (95% CI)							
	Aborted Procedure/ Device Failure	Acute Urinary Retention	BNC/Stricture	Cardiovascular	Cardiovascular Serious	Cardiovascular Thromboembolic	Hematuria Significant	Incontinence
Thermal-based therapies								
Prostatron Version 2.0 TUMT	1% (0–3)	23% (18–29)	1% (0–2)	—	—	—	2% (1–4)	2% (1–4)
Prostatron Version 2.5 TUMT	—	15% (4–33)	2% (0–9)	—	—	—	—	—
Targis TUMT	1% (0–4)	6% (1–17)	3% (1–6)	—	—	—	—	—
Watchful Waiting	—	3% (2–6)	—	—	—	0% (0–1)	—	2% (1–3)
Sham (control)	1% (0–6)	3% (1–5)	1% (0–6)	0% (0–3)	—	—	—	1% (0–6)
TURP (control)	—	5% (4–8)	7% (5–8)	1% (0–2)	2% (0–6)	2% (0–8)	6% (5–8)	3% (2–5)

	Median (95% CI)						
	Infection/UTI	Intraoperative	Post-procedure Irritative	Secondary Procedure	Sexual-Ejaculation	Sexual-Erectile Problems	Transfusion
Thermal-based therapies							
Prostatron Version 2.0 TUMT	9% (5–15)		28% (0–2)	10% (6–16)	5% (4–8)	3% (1–5)	1% (0–4)
Prostatron Version 2.5 TUMT	9% (3–19)		74% (0–9)	10% (5–18)	16% (2–49)	1% (0–8)	2% (0–9)
Targis TUMT	9% (5–15)	3% (1–6)		16% (11–20)	5% (2–10)		0% (0–2)
Watchful waiting	0% (0–1)	0% (0–1)		55% (49–61)		21% (17–26)	0% (0–1)
Sham (control)	5% (2–11)	1% (0–6)	70% (0–6)	24% (10–42)	2% (0–5)	2% (1–6)	1% (0–6)
TURP (control	6% (5–9)	3% (3–4)	15% (4–8)	5% (4–6)	65% (56–72)	10% (7–13)	8% (5–11)

Adapted from AUA Practice Guidelines Committee.[65]

pected procedure-related injuries to patients. This notice further reinforces appropriate patient selection, need for continual physician supervision during the treatment, and specific recommendations on monitoring the patient and treatment device. Additionally, added direction is given to aid in the informed consent of patients.

CONCLUSIONS

Transurethral microwave heat therapy is established as a safe and effective minimally invasive alternative to treat symptomatic benign prostatic hyperplasia. It is not as effective as TURP in improving objective signs of outflow obstruction as measured by either peak urinary flow rates or detrusor pressures at maximum flow. Pathologically, there is a known reproducible change in the prostate adenoma after microwave heat therapy of the prostate. A subjective improvement in symptom score is nearly univer-

sal and seems to be energy-related (high energy > low energy therapy).

It may be argued that no one area of urology has experienced as much innovation and evolution as has been seen in the management of patients with benign prostatic hyperplasia. It is a certainty that new technology and new approaches will continue. As technology develops and more long-term follow-up is completed, the role of transurethral microwave heat therapies will be further defined. Additional multicenter studies using standardized treatment protocols and patient selection will provide data to continue to challenge TURP and other established BPH treatment modalities in terms of safety, efficacy, and patient comfort.

REFERENCES

1. Devonec M, Berger MD, Perrin P. Transurethral microwave heating of the prostate—or from hyperthermia to thermotherapy. J Endourol 1991;5:129–33.

2. Devonec M, Berger N, Fendler, JP. Thermoregulation during transurethral microwave thermotherapy: experimental and clinical fundamentals. Eur Urol 1993;23 Suppl:63.

3. Edwards, LE. History of non-surgical treatment. In: Hinman F, Boyarsky S editors. Benign prostatic hypertrophy. New York: Springer Verlag; 1983. p. 30.

4. Yerushalmi A, Servadio C, Leib Z, et al. Local hyperthermia treatment of carcinoma of the prostate: a preliminary report. Prostate 1982;3:623–30.

5. Yerulshalmi A, Fishelovitz Y, Singer D, et al. Localized microwave hyperthermia in the treatment of poor operative risk patients with benign prostatic hyperplasia. J Urol 133: 1985;87–91.

6. Servadio C, Leib Z, Lev A. Diseases of prostate treated by local microwave hyperthermia. Urology 1987;30:97–9.

7. Zerbib M, Steg A, Conquy S, et al. Localized hyperthermia versus sham procedure in obstructive benign prostatic hyperplasia of the prostate: a prospective randomized study. J Urol 1992;147:1048–53.

8. Magin RL, Fridd CW, Bonfiglio TA, et al. Thermal destruction of the canine prostate by high intensity microwaves. J Surg Res 1980;29:265–75.

9. Lieb Z, Rothern A, Lev A, et al. Histopathological observations in the canine prostate treated by local hyperthermia. Prostate 1986;8:93–102.

10. Harada T, Etori K, Kumazaki T, et al. Microwave surgical treatment of diseases of prostate. Urology 1985;26:572B–6.

11. Astrahan MA, Sapozink MD, Cohen D, et al. Microwave applicator for transurethral hyperthermia of benign prostatic hyperplasia. Int J Hyperthermia 1989;5:283–96.

12. Roehrborn CG, Krongrad A, McConnell JD. Temperature mapping in the canine prostate during transurethrally applied local microwave hyperthermia. Prostate 1992;20: 97–101.

13. Matzkin H. Hyperthermia as a treatment modality in benign prostatic hyperplasia. Urology 1994;43:17–21.

14. Astrahan MA, Ameye F, Oyen R, et al. Interstitial temperature measurements during transurethral microwave hyperthermia of benign prostatic hyperplasia. J Urol 1991;145: 304–8.

15. Larson TR, Collins JM. An accurate technique for detailed prostatic interstitial temperature-mapping in patients receiving microwave thermal treatment. J Endourol 1995;9:339–47.

16. Larson TR, Collins JM, Corica A. Detailed interstitial temperature mapping during treatment with a novel transurethral microwave thermoablation system in patients with benign prostatic hyperplasia. J Urol 1998;159:258–64.

17. Larson TR, Bostwick DG, Corica A. Temperature-correlated histopathologic changes following microwave thermoablation of obstructive tissue in patients with benign prostatic hyperplasia. Urology 1996;47:463–9.

18. d'Ancona FC, Albers YH, Kiemeney LA, et al. Can histopathology predict outcome following high-energy transurethral microwave thermotherapy of the prostate? Results of a biopsy study. Prostate 1999;40:28–36.

19. Xu LX, Shu L, Holmes KR. Thermoregulation in the canine prostate during transurethral microwave hyperthermia, part I: temperature response. Int J Hyperthermia 1998;14:29–37.

20. Larson TR, Collins JM. Increased prostatic blood flow in response to microwave thermal treatment: preliminary findings in two patients with benign prostatic hyperplasia. Urology 1995;46:584–90.

21. Floratos DL, Sedelaar JPM, Kortmann RG, et al. Intra-prostatic vasculature studies: can they predict the outcome of transurethral microwave thermotherapy for the management of bladder outflow obstruction? Prostate 2001;46:200–6.

22. Schelin S. Mediating transurethral microwave thermotherapy by intraprostatic and periprostatic injection of mepivacaine epinephrine: effects on treatment time, energy consumption, and patient comfort. J Endourol 2002;16:117–21.

23. Bolmsjo M, Schelin S, Wagrell L, et al. Cell kill modeling of microwave thermotherapy for treatment of benign prostatic hyperplasia. J Endourol 2000;14:627–35.

24. Larson TR, Blute ML, Tri JL, et al. Contrasting heating patterns and efficiency of the Prostatron and Targis microwave antenna for thermal treatment of benign prostatic hyperplasia. Urology 1998;51:908–15.

25. Bolmsjo M, Wagrell L, Hallin A, et al. The heat is on – but how? A comparison of TUMT devices. Br J Urol 1996; 78:564–72.

26. Perachino M, Bozzo W, Puppo P, et al. Does transurethral thermotherapy induce a long-term alpha blockade? Eur Urol 1993;23:299–301.

27. Brehmer M, Hilliges M, Kinn AC. Denervation of periurethral prostatic tissue by transurethral microwave thermotherapy. Scan J Urol Nephrol 2000;34:42–5.

28. Bdesha AS, Schachter M, Sever P, et al. Radioligand-binding analysis of human prostatic alpha-1 adrenoreceptor density following transurethral microwave therapy. Br J Urol 1996;78:886–92.

29. Brehmer M, Nilsson BY. Elevation of sensory thresholds in the prostatic urethra after microwave thermotherapy. BJU Intl 2000;86:427–31.

30. Bostwick DG, Larson TR. Transurethral microwave thermotherapy: pathologic findings in canine prostate. Prostate 1995;26:111–22.

31. Mauroy B, Chive M, Stefaniak X, et al. Study of the effects of thermotherapy in benign prostatic hypertrophy. Eur Urol 1997;32:198–208.

32. Brehmer M. Morphological changes in prostatic adenomas after transurethral microwave thermotherapy. Br J Urol 1997;80:123–7.

33. Brehmer M, Svensson I. Heat-induced apoptosis in human prostatic stromal cells. BJU Int 2000;85:535–41.

34. Nordenstam G, Aspelin P, Isberg B, et al. Effect of transurethral microwave thermotherapy. an evaluation with MR imaging. Acta Radiol 1996;37:933–6.

35. Newhall PM, Burdette EC, Ferraro R, et al. Real-time non-invasive prostatic temperature imaging during microwave thermotherapy [abstract]. J Urol 1997;157:434.

36. D'Angelo MF, Hanson KA, King BF, et al. Prospective, comparative analysis of MRI gadolinium enhanced central zone perfusion effects using Prostatron 2.0 and Targis thermotherapy devices [abstract]. J Urol 1998;159:304.

37. Hutchinson E, Dahleh M, Hynynen K. The feasibility of MRI feedback control for intracavitary phased array hyperthermia treatments. Int J Hyperthermia 1988;14:39–56.

38. Harada T, Tsuchida S, Nishizawa O, et al. Microwave surgical treatment of the prostate: clinical application of microwave surgery as a tool for improved prostatic electroresection. Urol Int 1987;42:127–31.

39. Ameye F, Baert L. Urological effects of local microwave hyperthermia of prostatic tissues. In: Petrovich Z, Baert L, editors. Innovations in the management of benign prostatic hyperplasia. Berlin: Springer-Verlag; 1994. p. 239–74.

40. Lauweryns J, Baert L, Vandenhove J, et al. Histopathology of prostatic tissue after transurethral hyperthermia. Int J Hyperthermia 1991;7:221–30.

41. Sapozink MD, Boyd SD, Astrahan MA, et al. Transurethral hyperthermia for benign prostatic hyperplasia: preliminary clinical results. J Urol 1990;143:944–50.

42. Baert L, Ameye F, Willemen P, et al. Transurethral microwave hyperthermia for benign prostatic hyperplasia: preliminary clinical and pathological results. J Urol 1990;144: 1383–8.

43. Baert L, Willemen P, Ameye F, et al. Treatment response with transurethral microwave hyperthermia in different forms of benign prostatic hyperplasia: a preliminary report. Prostate 1992;18:315–20.

44. Issacs JT. Importance of the natural history of benign prostatic hyperplasia and the evaluation of pharmacologic intervention. Prostate 1990;3 Suppl:1.

45. Lepor H, Sypherd D, Machi G, et al. Randomized double-blind study comparing the effectiveness of balloon dilation of the prostate and cystoscopy for the treatment of symptomatic benign prostatic hyperplasia. J Urol 1992; 147:639–44.

46. Ogden CW, Reddy P, Johnson H, et al. Sham versus transurethral microwave thermotherapy in patients with symptoms of benign prostatic outflow obstruction. Lancet 1993;341:14–7.

47. Debruyne FMJ, Bloem FAG, de la Rosette JOMCH, et al. Transurethral microwave thermotherapy (TUMT) in benign prostatic hyperplasia: placebo versus TUMT. J Urol 1993;149:146.

48. Blute ML, Patterson DE, Segura JW, et al. Transurethral microwave thermotherapy versus sham: a prospective double blind randomized study. J Urol 1994;151:752A.

49. Nawrocki JD, Bell TJ, Lawrence WT, et al. A randomized controlled trial of transurethral microwave therapy. Br J Urol 1997;79:389–93.

50. Mulvin D, Creagh T, Kelly D, et al. Transurethral microwave therapy versus transurethral catheter therapy for benign prostatic hyperplasia. Eur Urol 1994;26:6–9.

51. Dahlstrand C, Walden M, Geirsson G, et al. Transurethral microwave thermotherapy versus transurethral resection for symptomatic benign prostatic obstruction: a prospective randomized study with a 2 year follow up. Br J Urol 1995;76:614–8.

52. d'Ancona FC, Francisca EA, Witjes WP, et al. Transurethral resection of the prostate versus high-energy thermotherapy of the prostate in patients with benign prostatic hyperplasia: long-term results. Br J Urol 1998;81:259–64.

53. Floratos DL, Sonke GS, Francisca EA. High energy transurethral microwave thermotherapy for the treatment of patients in urinary retention. J Urol 2000;163:1457–60.

54. Francisca EA, Kortmann BB, Floratos DL, et al. Tolerability of 3.5 versus 2.5 high-energy transurethral microwave thermotherapy. Eur Urol 2000;38:59–63.

55. Arai Y, Aoki Y, Okubo K. Impact of interventional therapy for benign prostatic hyperplasia on quality of life and sexual function: a prospective study. J Urol 2000;164:1206–11.

56. de la Rosette JJMCH, de Wildt MJAM, Hofner K, et al. High-energy thermotherapy in the treatment of benign prostatic hyperplasia: results of European BPH study group. J Urol 1996;156:97–102.

57. de Wildt MJAM, Debruyne FMJ, de la Rosette JJMCH. High-energy transurethral microwave thermotherapy: a thermoablative treatment for benign prostatic obstruction. Urology 1996;48:416–23.

58. Walden M, Dahlstrand C, Schafer W, et al. How to select patients suitable for transurethral microwave thermotherapy: a systematic evaluation of potentially predictive variables. Br J Urol 1998;81:817–22.

59. Javle P, Blair M, Palmer M, et al. The role of an advance thermotherapy device in prostatic voiding dysfunction. Br J Urol 78:391–7.

60. Tubaro A, Carter SS, de la Rosette J, et al. The prediction of clinical outcome from transurethral thermotherapy by pressure flow analysis: a European multicenter study. J Urol 1995;153:1526–30.

61. Djavan B, Seitz C, Ghawidel K, et al. High-energy randomized transurethral microwave thermotherapy in patients with acute urinary retention due to benign prostatic hypertrophy. Urology 1999;54:18–22.

62. Robinette MA, Honey JD, Buckley RJ, et al. Results of transurethral microwave thermotherapy (TUMT) in patients presenting with: 1. symptomatic BPH or 2. urinary retention. J Urol 1997;157:375A.

63. Blute ML, Tomera KM, Hellerstein DK, et al. Transurethral microwave thermotherapy for the management of benign prostatic hyperplasia: results of the United States Prostatron cooperative study. J Urol 1993;150:1591–6.

64. Blute ML, Larson TR, Hanson KA, et al. Current status of transurethral thermotherapy at the Mayo Clinic. Mayo Clin Proc 1998;73:597–602.

65. AUA Practice Guidelines Committee. AUA guidelines on management of benign prostatic hyperplasia (2003). Chapter 1: diagnosis and treatment recommendations. J Urol 2003;170:530–47.

66. FDA/Center for Devices and Radiological Health (CDRH) Public Health Notification. Serious injuries from microwave thermotherapy for benign prostatic hyperplasia. October 1, 2000. U.S. Food and Drug Administration Website. Available at: http://www.fda.gov/cdrh/safety/bph.pdf (accessed January, 25, 2003).

ProstaLund Feedback Treatment

Lennart Wagrell, MD

PHYSICAL CHARACTERISTICS OF MICROWAVES

Microwaves are electromagnetic radiation with an oscillating electrical and magnetic field in the range of 300 to 30,000 megahertz (MHz). Heat is produced when the microwaves are absorbed by the tissue and arises mainly by two processes: electric dipoles (eg, water molecules) oscillate in the field and electric charge carriers (eg, ions) move back and forth in the field. These movements transfer energy to the tissue in the form of heat. The ProstaLund device (ProstaLund, Sweden) uses 915 MHz. Higher frequency means shorter wavelength, and thus less penetration depth in the tissue. The tissue temperature during transurethral microwave thermotherapy is mainly determined by three processes: (1) generation of heat through absorption of microwave energy (2) the dispersion of heat by conduction in the tissue and (3) loss of heat through blood flow. The first factor is related to the treatment catheter being used; the second depends on tissue composition, and the third depends on the blood flow.

THERMOTHERAPY PATHOLOGY

The goal of the treatment is to achieve a coagulation necrosis of prostatic tissue in the transition zone. There is a correlation between time and temperature to achieve coagulation necrosis. This was shown in the late 1940s by Henriques who did his observations on the skin of pigs. More recently, Bischof and colleagues showed the correlation for human prostate tissue (Figure 72C-1). There is a difference between stroma and glandular tissue. This can explain the observation made some years ago that stroma epithelial ratio has something to do with outcome after microwave treatment. Microscopic examination post-treatment shows coagulation necrosis of the treated area within the transition zone. Acinar and smooth muscle cells are totally destroyed. Although small vessels are thrombosed, large blood vessels are preserved.

THE PROSTALUND DEVICE

The ProstaLund device consists of a unit in which a microwave generator is located (Figure 72C-2). The treatment is performed and monitored from a laptop computer on top of the unit. The microwave antenna and an intraprostatic temperature probe are introduced in a treatment catheter. Inside the catheter there is a channel for the intraprostatic temperature probe that will go into one of the lateral lobes of the enlarged prostate. The probe holds three thermosensors spaced at 1 cm intervals. To prevent the risk of damage to the penile urethra, the treatment catheter has a cooling system that takes care of the transmission losses in the antenna cable. The ProstaLund treatment catheter does not have a cooling system for the prostatic urethra. A rectal probe, withholding three thermosensors, is used for safety reasons and will not guide the treatment. With the ProstaLund device, there is one little gadget that is not available on other microwave devices, although it is very important for safety reasons—a penile safety sensor. It is placed at the penoscrotal angle and will shut down the treatment at a preset safety limit protecting the penis if there should be any mechanical problems, making the catheter slide in a distal direction (Figure 72C-3).

PROSTALUND FEEDBACK TREATMENT

During standard microwave treatment, rectal and urethral temperatures are used to monitor the treatment. However, our group and Wenn and colleagues has shown that there is no correlation between the intraprostatic, the rectal, or the urethral temperature. Thus, the urethral and the rectal temperatures don't say anything about the actual temperature in the targeted area in the prostate. Based on this fact, our group started to measure the intraprostatic temperature during treatment in the late 1990s. Later, we also described a model to assess the amount of tissue that was destroyed during treatment, trying to get more consistent results after microwave treatment of the prostate. In this section, we will deal with these questions and try to explain them.

Intraprostatic measurements during treatment are performed by means of an intraprostatic temperature probe that is introduced into the catheter and then inserted into one of the lateral lobes of the prostate (Figure 72C-4). From the intraprostatic temperatures achieved, it is possible to tailor the treatment and apply sufficient microwave power. There are three different things that affect the intraprostatic temperature: (1) microwaves that supply heat, (2) blood flow that removes heat, and (3) heat conduction (Figure 72C-5). Intrapro-

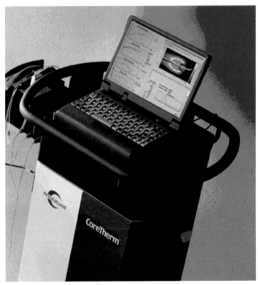

Figure 72C-2 The ProstaLund device.

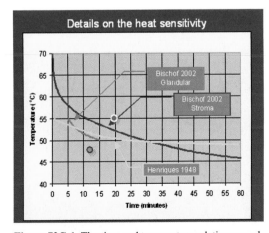

Figure 72C-1 The time and temperature relation according to Henriques and Bischof. Bischof has used human prostate tissue and shows the difference between glandular and stroma cells.

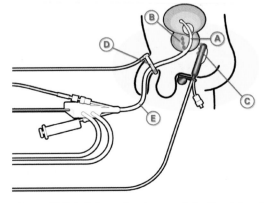

Figure 72C-3 Schematic picture of the ProstaLund setup.

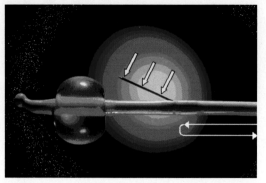

Fig 72C-4 The ProstaLund treatment catheter with the balloon and the intraprostatic thermosensor. The *white arrow* shows were the cooling water returns. The ProstaLund device has no cooling of the prostatic urethra.

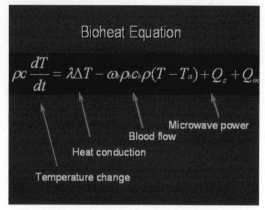

Figure 72C-6 Bioheat equation by Pennes.

static blood flow varies between individuals, and the difference is significant, as shown by a positron emission tomography (PET) study performed during microwave treatment. In some cases, the intraprostatic blood flow increased more than 100% during treatment. Back in the late 1940s, it was shown by Penne that there is a correlation between energy, blood flow and heat conduction, and he described it in the bio heat equation (Figure 72C-6). By using this equation, it is possible to calculate the intraprostatic blood flow, and it is shown to be very accurate. Using the PET scan, we found a correlation factor of 0.88 between the calculated intraprostatic blood flow and the actual blood flow measured by the PET scan. When the intraprostatic blood flow is known, it is easy to do a temperature map over the targeted volume in the prostate. In the late 1940s, Henriques postulated a cell kill model, saying that cells starts in a normal state, heat alters bio molecules, and the cells will come into an intermediate activated state from where some are repaired while others are permanently damaged and end up in a denatured state. Henriques also described this in an equation (Figure 72C-7). Using this equation and putting in all the different temperatures from the bioheat equation, it is possible to get a good estimation of the amount of tissue that has been destroyed during the treatment.

PATIENT PREPARATION

Patients eligible for transurethral prostatic resection (TURP), or open prostatic surgery, are good candidates for ProstaLund treatment. The size of the prostate should be at least 30 cc (the upper limit is not yet determined; the biggest that the author has treated is 250 cc). Patients in retention are also good candidates (see "Clinical Results"). To reveal the prostate size and shape, transrectal ultrasonography is necessary. In cases with a lot of irritative symptoms, a cystoscopy could be of value.

There are different ways of giving anesthesia to patients. In our department, we currently use prostatic block given by means of the Schelin Catheter. We don't give any sedation at all, meaning all patients can leave the department almost immediately after treatment. Prior to the introduction of prostatic block, we used IV sedation and analgesia. Some centers just use oral medication for sedation and analgesia.

TREATMENT STRATEGY

Using the ProstaLund device, it is always the operator who decides the amount of microwave power and the treatment time. The intraprostatic temperature is displayed on the computer screen online during the treatment session. Depending on the development of the intraprostatic tempera-

ture, the power can be raised or lowered. The calculated amount of the coagulation necrosis is also displayed during treatment. The operator finalizes the treatment once optimal necrosis is achieved.

It is shown in studies that shrinkage of 30% of the prostate volume is sufficient to give results comparable with TURP (see "Clinical Results"). The goal is to achieve temperatures of about 55° to 60°C in the prostatic tissue during the treatment session. Coagulation necrosis is initiated already at temperatures of 45°C, but it will take almost 3 hours reach the treatment goal at this temperature, compared to only minutes at 55° to 60°C.

One way of performing the treatment would be as follows: Start at 40 W; after 2 minutes, raise by 10 W; if the raise in intraprostatic temperature is less than 1°C/30 s, then raise the microwave power in steps of 10 W every 2 minutes until the goal of 55° to 60°C is reached. The computer will show on the screen online the percentage of the prostate volume destroyed.

CLINICAL RESULTS

There are several studies supporting the good results seen after ProstaLund Feedback Treatment. In Table 72C-1, three studies are presented, one prospective randomized multicenter, one single-center prospective and randomized, and one single-center open without reference group. All three studies have the same protocol for inclusion and exclusion and have 12-month follow up. TURP was used as reference in the two randomized studies. The total number of patients in these studies was 258; out of these, 186 were treated by means of microwaves (see Tables 72C-1, 72C-2, and 72C-3).

In one study, ProstaLund Feedback Treatment was compared to TURP or open surgery in patients in chronic retention. This study shows that 8 out of 10 patients were relieved from the catheter in the ProstaLund Feedback group, and the corresponding figure in the operated group was 9 out of 10.

The conclusion is that microwaves now have a place in the armamentarium when treating benign prostatic hyperplasia and have matured to be the gold standard in some centers.

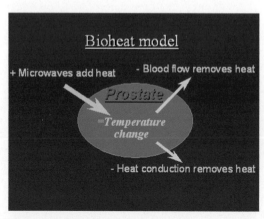

Figure 72C-5 Bioheat model.

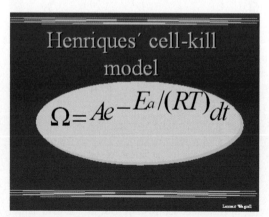

Figure 72C-7 The cell kill equation.

Table 72C-1 Pooled Analysis from Three Studies, Showing Patient Distribution.

| | Pooled Analysis | | |
| | Patients Included (*n*) | | |
Study	PLFT	TURP	Total
Study A	100	46	154
Study B	42	19	62
Study C	41	*	42
Total	183	65	258

*Study C had no control group

PLFT = ProstaLund feedback treatment; TURP = transurethral prostate resection.

Table 72C-2 Outcome for the ProstaLund Feedback Treated Patients in the Pooled Analysis

| Parameter | Outcome 12 mo after PLFT (n = 163) | | |
	Before PLFT	12 month After PLFT	Change
IPSS	20.9 (± 5.1)	6.4 (± 5.7)	−69 %
Bother Score	4.2 (± 0.9)	1.2 (± 1.2)	−71 %
Qmax (mL/s)	7.7 (± 2.7)	16.1 (± 9.3)	109 %
Prostate volume (mL)	51.9 (± 18)	34.1 (± 15)	−35 %

PLFT = ProstaLund feedback treatment.

Table 72C-3 Number of Responders in the Two Compared Groups

| Responders | Percentage of Responders | |
	PLFT	TURP
Study A	82	87
Study B	92	79
Study C	88	—
Pooled Data	85	86

PLFT = ProstaLund feedback treatment; TURP = transurethral prostate resection.

Prostatic Stents

Atul A. Thakre, MD

Samuel A. Amukele, MD

Gopal H. Badlani, MD

Benign prostatic hyperplasia (BPH) is a frequent disease in men and a major cause of lower urinary tract symptoms (LUTS). Transurethral resection of the prostate (TURP) or open surgery remains the gold standard of treatment of symptomatic BPH. However, 10 to 15% of patients with BPH cannot undergo surgery because of grave comorbidities. For patients with contraindications to surgery or anesthesia, several minimally invasive alternate treatments are available. One such therapeutic option is prostatic stenting, which can serve as a temporary or permanent solution for bladder outlet obstruction (BOO) caused by BPH.

The concept of stenting for relieving BOO secondary to BPH was first described by Fabian.[1] The evolution of this concept has led to development of various types of stents. Broadly, these stents are designed for either permanent or temporary placement. Characteristic of permanent stents is that they allow ingrowth with eventual complete epithelialization. Temporary stent design prevents epithelial ingrowth, and thus these devices are removable. The duration of use in temporary stents varies from just a few weeks to up to 6 months. The very nature of programmed dissolution of the group of biodegradable stents renders them temporary.

The ideal prostatic stent should be easy to insert and position under topical anesthesia. The stent should not extend beyond the prostatic urethra into the bladder. It should not cause any local reaction or promote encrustation. Endoscopy through the stent should be feasible. Finally, it should be easy to remove if necessary. During the Third International Consultation on BPH in 1995,[2] three other criteria were added: stents should be malleable in order to conform to the shape of prostatic urethra; they should not migrate; and they should be relatively inexpensive.[2] Available stents differ in their properties on the basis of material, lumen, size, radial strength, and surface characteristics, and therefore their retention in situ and the tissue response is varied.

TEMPORARY STENTS

An emerging strategy for management of BOO is placement of a short-term temporary stent in conjunction with various thermotherapy treatments designed to relieve the obstruction. Temporary stents can effectively decrease the incidence of postoperative retention, which is a common side effect after such therapies. After conventional low-energy transurethral microwave therapy (TUMT), 12 to 36% of patients have been reported to require catheterization from 1 to 4 weeks.[3]. With the use of high-energy TUMT, which is designed to provide enhanced treatment efficacy, all the patients had transient retention, requiring indwelling catheter or intermittent self-catheterization. The average reported duration of catheterization was 14 to 16 days. Catheterization for more than 1 month was needed in 10%. Prolonged urinary catheterization was required in 38% of patients after laser ablation of prostate.[4]

The use of short-term or long-term temporary stents has also been introduced into the management of patients with spontaneous urinary retention owing to BPH, who are not suitable candidates for surgery, who refuse proposed surgical treatment, or who are awaiting surgical therapy.[5] In such situations, stents need replacement at a 6- to 12-month interval. Temporary stents in combination with androgen ablation or irradiation have also been advocated for the relief of BOO owing to carcinoma of the prostate. Whether the toxicity, both acute and chronic, of pelvic irradiation is influenced by the presence of a metallic stent is an issue for further research and evaluation.[6]

The currently used temporary stents reported in the literature include a spiral stent made of biodegradable material,[7] an intraurethral prostatic bridge catheter (Trestle) made of silicone,[3] the ContiCath catheter,[8] and the Prostacoil catheter.[9] The main advantage of these stents is ease of application and removal under local anesthesia.

The Trestle stent or prostatic bridge is made up of polyurethane. It consists of two tubes and an interconnecting thread. The tube that lies in the prostate has a diameter of 22 French (F) and has a 30-degree angulation. The length is 75 mm and it has a smooth tip. It is to be used in prostates with a volume of less than 80 mL. The connecting thread is 25 mm, which passes through the distal sphincteric mechanism. The second tube lies in the bulbar urethra and is 35 mm long. It is inserted with the patient under topical anesthesia using a delivery system comprising a positioning stylet, an inflatable balloon with injection cannula, and an outer pusher tube. In a report by Djavan and colleagues, 54 patients with BPH underwent high-energy TUMT under topical urethral anesthesia, followed by placement of a prostatic bridge catheter.[3] Immediate significant percentage improvements ($p < .0005$) were observed in mean peak flow rate, International Prostate Symptom Score (IPSS), and quality of life score of 59.3%, 33.5%, and 23.6%, respectively, compared with baseline values. Further improvement was observed at 1 month, when the percentage improvement in peak flow rate, IPSS, and quality of life score had reached 79.0%, 54.9%, and 56.5%, respectively, versus baseline ($p < .0005$). At 14-day follow-up evaluation in the prostatic bridge catheter group, mean peak flow rate was 101.8% higher, and IPSS and quality of life score were 47.9% and 51.1% lower, respectively, than the corresponding values in the standard catheterization group ($p < .0005$). The prostatic bridge catheter was well tolerated and remained indwelling throughout the entire 1-month follow-up in 48 of 54 patients (88.9%). Early prostatic bridge catheter removal was required in 3 patients (5.6%) because of urinary retention, and in 3 (5.6%) because of catheter migration. Also, the magnitude of the improvement in peak flow rate, IPSS, and quality of life score at 14 days in this study were markedly greater than those recently observed in terazosin recipients.[10]

In a similar study of 47 men with symptomatic BPH, Trestle stents were inserted after high-energy TUMT.[11] Patients were evaluated at 2, 7, and 14 days. The stent was removed on day 14. All patients showed an improvement in IPSS, quality of life, uroflowmetery, and postvoid residue from the baseline values. Complications such as stent migration or secondary retention were not observed.

Cecchi and colleagues[5] used Trestle stents in 5 patients aged 65 to 78 years, who were suffering from urinary retention because of BPH. Micturition resumed immediately.[5]

ContiCath is another temporary stent made of polyurethane and consists of four segments: a proximal curl (17F) that prevents distal migration; a prostatic segment (20F), either 4.3 or 6.0 cm in length, that maintains a patent prostaic urethra; a narrow sphincteric segment that passes through the membranous urethra ending with a small plastic "cage" that prevents proximal migration into bladder; and a bulbous urethral segment that ends with a small rolene catheter that comes out of the urethral meatus.

Corujo and colleagues described their initial experience of a newly designed temporary catheter, ContiCath, as an aid in the management of postoperative or temporary outflow obstruction.[8] In patients with supposedly normal detrusor and sphincter function, this catheter allows volitional voiding, while maintaining an open prostatic urethra. The ContiCath was placed in the office setting. Patients were assessed at 3 hours and at 7, 14, 21, and 28 days, at which time the device was removed. Among patients with a neuropathic cause for their retention (5 patients) and those with non-neuropathic causes of retention for longer than 1 week (19 patients), only 3 patients were able to void after the catheter was placed. Of the 37 patients with a non-neuropathic cause and retention lasting 1 week or less, controlled voiding was seen in 33 patients (89%).

Prostacoil temporary stent[9] has been used as a temporary stent in the treatment of recurrent anastomotic stenosis after radical prostatectomy in 9 patients, and in 1 patient with stricture between orthotopic bladder and urethra. The stent was left in situ for 6 to 13 months (mean 11 months), and could subsequently be easily removed. In 7 patients, stenosis disappeared, and they had excellent continence. Three patients at the last follow-up were voiding through the stent and were awaiting removal.

In a recent report Knutson [14] used temporary prostate stents to evaluate patients with prostatic obstruction marked by severe overactive bladders. The study was based on the concept that, a prostatic stent relieves outflow obstruction and simulates transurethral resection of the prostate. The test identifies that patients who do not leak and experience improvement in symptoms after a stent placement. Such patients can subsequently be advised to have a transurethral resection of the prostate. The application of this test can also be made in the work up of neurogenic overactive bladder patients with bladder outlet obstruction.

Biodegradable stents disappear by biodegradation and hence do not require removal. This idea was introduced in urology when Kemppainenain in 1993 used a degradable stent in rabbits after urethrotomy.

In a randomized study of biodegradable polyglycolic acid stents,[4] significant improvements in peak flow rate and symptom score were observed as soon as 1 month after visual laser ablation of prostate. Some patients had diminished stream force and increased obstructive symptoms 3 weeks after stent placement, which was attributed to fragments resulting from biodegradation of the stent. A biodegradable poly d-lactic acid spiral stent was compared with a suprapubic catheter after visual laser ablation of the prostate.[7] Significant flow rate improvement was demonstrable by 1 month, and symptom improvement by 3 months. Urinary tract infection occurred in 41% of spiral stent recipients, however, which was managed by antibiotics. The chief advantage of biodegradable stents as temporary endoprostheses is that they obviate subsequent removal.

In a recent report by Devonec and Dahlstrand,[12] two types of stents were used at two sites after high-energy TUMT; at one site a silicone transurethral prostatic bridge was used ($n = 42$), and at the second site a self-reinforced polyglycolic acid biodegradable spiral was used ($n = 16$). Patients were assessed at 1 week as well as at 1, 3, 6, and 12 months. Significant improvements were observed in the symptom score, peak flow rate, and voided volume. Improvement was seen at first visit and was sustained during the follow-up period. Indeed, in the patients receiving the silicone tubes, improvement was significant as early as during the first week for flow and 1 month for symptoms, whereas in those receiving the spiral stents, significant improvement was not observed until 3 months for symptoms and 1 to 3 months for flow. A comparison of stents with various diameters was also performed; there was no clear relationship between the diameter of the stent and improvement in flow rate in patients with a comparable flow before insertion.

There are several potential uses of temporary prostatic stents, although none of these stents are presently being used in America. The main problem faced in their use is regarding the irritative voiding symptoms.

PERMANENT STENTS

Permanent stents are intended as treatment, rather than as management, which is the goal of temporary stents. Endoprostheses made of steel superalloy, titanium, and nitinol allow epithelial ingrowth, and thus significantly reduce the chances of infection and encrustation. The advantages of permanent stents include procedural speed and simplicity, immediate improvement in voiding dysfunction, rapid patient recovery, and use in patients who are not suitable candidates for surgery. The main concern about the use of such stents was the potential for high explantation rate, hyperplastic tissue response, encrustation, and a theoretic concern regarding carcinogenicity.

Badlani and colleagues reported on a 7-year follow-up of a cohort of 27 patients enrolled in a postlong-term study of UroLume patients. These were from the 126 patients reported in the multicenter North American trial.[26] The 27 patients showed sustained statistical improvement in the symptom score over the 7 years. Comparison of flow rates with baseline values showed statistically significant improvement at 3, 6, 12, 24, and 48 months, and also at the 5-year and 7-year marks, although it was not statistically significant. Age (mean age at implant 70.2 years) or reobstruction may play a role. Of the original 126 patients, 28 were explanted and 35 expired owing to various medical problems unrelated to stent placement. Anjum and colleagues[16] presented similar data at the end of 5 years of follow-up, when 22 of 62 patients with stents were doing reasonably well. Fifteen patients died owing to unrelated causes and 5 were lost to follow-up. Their explantation rate was highest in the first year, and was mainly related to poor placement and its related complications. Gesen-berg and Sintermann[17] also obtained similar results in their study. Forty-four out of 126 patients died during follow-up. Their average follow-up was 12.2 months. Because of a drastically reduced number of cases (4 patients at 4 years) at long-term follow-up, the authors made projections regarding outcomes.

Complete epithelialization of the endoprosthesis was seen between at 6 and 12 months in all series. Badlani and colleagues at 7 years follow-up on 27 patients reported that 25 had mild or no tissue response, whereas 2 had moderate to marked hyperplasic tissue response.[26] The observation of the other groups was similar. The hyperplastic epithelium when clinically indicated was managed by fulguration and rarely warranted stent removal.

Complications related to UroLume placement reported include transient dysuria, urge symptom, and hematuria, which often abate after 2 to 3 weeks. Improper placement of stent can lead to encrustation, and reobstruction at proximal or distal end. The 7-year follow-up of urinary incontinence that was present before placement of stent[18] indicated that it had worsened in 3 patients, improved in 10, and remained the same in 11. The type of incontinence was most commonly postvoid dribble caused by pooling of urine in the large lumen of the UroLume.[19]

Ellis and colleagues[13] reported implantation of Memokath prostatic stent in 124 patients (mean age 79.3 years) with severe BOO in last 5 years. These men were unfit for surgery. Stent placement was simple and undertaken under local anesthesia. Fifty-eight patients are alive with functioning stent. Twenty-six stents were explanted, 23 owing to failure, and in 3 patients, stent was no longer needed. Forty-four patients died with functioning stent. UTI was seen in 13 patients. Urethral discomfort was present in 5 patients for a period of 3 weeks postinsertion.

Ricciotti and colleagues[19] used Memokath stents in 37 BPH patients, 28 urethral stricture patients, and 5 patients with sphincterotomies. The age ranged between 24 and 84 years. Patients were discharged 1 to 5 days after stent placement. Forty-six patients (65.7%) had pain and dysuria lasting 1 to 4 weeks, and 3 patients had severe mucosal hyperplasia during long-term follow-up.

EXPLANTATION

Most explantations of the UroLume stent are done within year 1 and are largely the result of incorrect placement or migration.[21,22] Stents placed for urethral stricture were least likely to require removal after 1 year. A similar experience was reported from Europe.[23] Higher risk is associated with urethroplasty, a history of traumatic stricture of greater than 10 years or urethral irradiation. Why stents placed for detrusor-external sphincter dyssynergia and BPH are more likely to require removal than those placed for stricture is a matter for further study.

Properly positioned permanent stents provide significant advantage over temporary stents because they become incorporated into the mucosa, precluding displacement and exposure to the urine, which can lead to encrustation and infection. However, the stents are cylindrical, whereas the prostatic urethra is not. Moreover, the urethra exits obliquely from the bladder and the prostate lobes may be asymmetrically enlarged. As a consequence, stent attachment to the urethral wall may not be uniform, increasing the chance of poor epithelialization.[24] The high incidence of migration in cases of detrusor-external sphincter dyssynergia could reflect urethral configuration and variations in radial forces at different levels during external sphincter contraction. The bulbar urethra has uniform radial forces, leading to better stent fixation and epithelialization.[25]

Clinical trials of the UroLume have defined several factors that affect its success.[24–26] As noted, correct placement is imperative. To ensure complete contact with the prostate and bladder neck epithelium, the stent should be deployed more distal, even at the risk of inadequate bladder neck stenting or subsequent ventral tissue growth, resulting in ball valve obstruction. In detrusor-external sphincter dyssynergia cases, stent geometry, elastic properties, and radial forces allow it to maintain its position and prevent obstruction by the external sphincter. It is essential that the distal end of the stent should extend at least 5 mm into the bulbar urethra. The proximal half should cover the caudal half of the verumontanum. An overlapping stent may be needed to ensure that the external sphincter is completely bridged. Too small or improperly placed stents migrate because of the vigorous reflex sphincter contraction.[27] Tissue quality also is important for success. Stents have been recommended only for bulbar urethral strictures because this tissue has a rich spongiofibrous structure that makes it less susceptible to erosion than other areas of the urethra. The stent ends should be at least 5 mm beyond the strictured area. If multiple stents are needed, their ends should overlap at least 0.5 cm to prevent overgrowth of tissue with repeat stenosis in the junctional area. Stenting should be avoided in irradiated urethras because epithelialization is likely to be poor. Previous urethroplasty is a relative contraindication. Stents should not be placed across the external sphincter after traumatic rupture of the membranous urethra in neurologically intact patients since they cause pain.

Further treatment after UroLume stent removal has been successful in patients with all types of pathological conditions. For example, Chancellor and colleagues reported on 4 patients with spinal cord injuries in whom the device was easily explanted 6 months or more after insertion without damage to the external sphincter or urethra.[28] Mean voiding pressure remained unchanged and no patient had stress urinary incontinence or endoscopically apparent urethral stricture. When reporting on the removal of UroLume endoprostheses in detrusor-external sphincter dyssynergia cases, Gajewski and colleagues commented that there is a potential for

urethral injury or bleeding, but extraction is generally easy with minimal complications and no lasting consequences.[20]

Rehabilitation after stent explantation is a serious concern. Patients with BPH and detrusor-external sphincter dyssynergia can be treated in the same way as those with the same disease who have not had stents. However, if the indication for placement was stricture and the lesion is beyond repair, substitution urethroplasty or continent diversion may be done depending on the length, severity, and site of the stricture.

EXPLANTATION TECHNIQUE

Several techniques have been described for removing the UroLume prosthesis after it becomes epithelialized. Stents implanted for BPH and detrusor-external sphincter dyssynergia are usually removed endoscopically in one piece, whereas stents placed for bulbar urethral stricture may require removal piece by piece endoscopically or intact removal by open surgery with urethrectomy. For intact endoscopic removal the overlying urothelium is resected with a low cutting monopolar current using a standard resectoscope loop and sheath (Figures 73-1 to 73-4). Pure cut frequency current should be used in a smooth motion with care not to pause while removing tissue from within the prosthesis. The stent is then extracted from its bed with alligator forceps and pulled gently to lengthen and narrow it, so that it can be pulled inside the sheath and removed without further trauma. An alternative is resection of the overlying mucosa and passage of a 0.038-inch guidewire through the stent lumen into the bladder. The stent is then pushed into the bladder over the guidewire and drawn into the resectoscope sheath by pulling each end of the wire. Stents in the bulbous urethra are denuded, cut into pieces, and removed piece by piece through the endoscope sheath. The holmium:YAG laser has been used for this purpose without injury to the urethra. In our series, in a patient with continent diversion and a nonfunctioning urethra, the stent and urethra were removed together. In a few cases wire-by-wire extraction of the stent has proved necessary.

CONCLUSION

The short-term temporary stents of various biostable and biodegradable polymers are needed after minimally invasive therapy of the prostate with heat. Transient urinary retention and voiding difficulty resulting from these procedures is better managed with stents than with the indwelling catheter or intermittent catheterization, based on early trials. Most studies do not report or evaluate detrusor function, hence failures could be secondary to stent design, placement technique or detrusor dysfunction.

Temporary stents are a management option, whereas the permanent stents are a treatment option, thus their results should be compared with other modalities of treatment for BPH. When looked at as a treatment option, they offer imme-

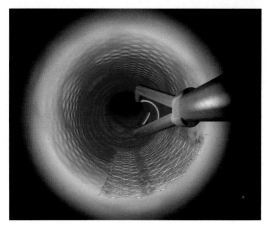

Figure 73-1 Thoroughly resect the overlying tissue from the inner surfaces of the stent using a 24F electrosurgical loop. Use the lowest possible current settings. Using smooth, even cutting motions, completely remove all tissue within the stent and tissue overlying the proximal and distal stent edges.

diate relief. Sustained results for 4 to 7 years make them ideally suited for medically compromised patients. Placement procedure needs to be more exact for permanent stents when compared with temporary stents. Prostatic size and shape (median lobe) are factors under consideration in permanent stents, whereas they do not matter for temporary stents. The reasons for higher explantation rate of permanent (UroLume) stents in patients with BPH, when compared with that in patients with urethral stricture and detrusor sphincter dyssynergia, needs further analysis.

The learning curve for placement of permanent stents is steeper than that for the temporary stents. Stents are likely to have an increasing role in the treatment and management of BOO secondary to BPH.

With 11 years of follow-up, one can say that the initial concern about the frequency and difficulty of UroLume permanent urethral stent explantation and the local tissue effect appears to be excessive. The device benefits the majority of patients. When removal is required, it can be done with minimal complications and no lasting consequences.[30,31]

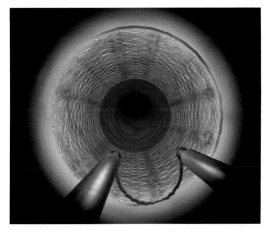

Figure 73-2 Create a circular trench, or loop access space, in the urethral wall. This is done at each edge of the stent.

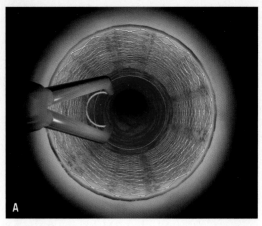

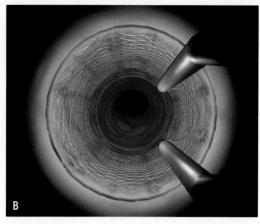

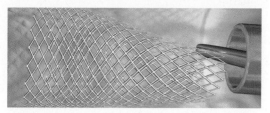

Figure 73-4 Use a cystoscope with a long firm grasping forceps to hold 3 or 4 rows of stent diamonds and pull the stent through the sheath. Inspect the stent to ensure complete removal of all the stent wires.

Figure 73-3 *A,* Keep electrosurgical loop in the "off" position. Engage the proximal edge of the stent in the loop and pull toward you. Do this at 3-, 6-, 9-, and 12-o' clock positions. *B,* Keep electrosurgical loop in the "off" position. Engage the distal edge of the stent in the loop and push toward the bladder neck. Do this at 3-, 6-, 9-, and 12-o' clock positions.

REFERENCES

1. Fabain KM. Der intraprostatische 'Partielle Katheter' (Urologische Spirale). Urologe (A) 1992;19:21–8.
2. Crockett AT, Aso Y, Denis L, et al. Recommendation of the International Consensus Committee concerning: 4. Treatment recommendations for benign prostatic hyperplasia (BPH). Proceedings of the 3rd International Consultation on Benign Prostatic Hyperplasia, Monaco, 26–28 June, 1995. p. 625–40.
3. Djavan B, Fakhari M, Shariat S, et al. A novel intraurethral prostatic bridge catheter for prevention of temporary prostatic obstruction following high energy transurethral microwave thermotherapy in patients with benign prostatic hyperplasia. J Urol 1999;161:144–51.
4. Petas A, Talja M, Tamella T, et al. A randomized study to compare biodegradable self-reinforced polyglycolic acid spiral stents to suprapubic and indwelling catheters after laser ablation of the prostate. J Urol 1997;157:173–6.
5. Cecchi M, Sepich CA, Pagni GL, et al. Prostatic endoprosthesis for prostatic obustruction treatment: preliminary experience with Trestle new device. Chir Ital 1998;50–1:37–40.
6. Gez E, Cederbaum M. External irradiation for prostate cancer in patients with urethral stents. In: Yachia D, editor. Stenting the urinary system. 1st ed. Oxford: ISIS Medical Media; 1998. p. 359–63.
7. Petas A, Talja M, Tamella T, et al. The biodegradable self inforced poly-DL-lactic acid spiral stent compared with a suprapubic catheter in the treatment of post-operative urinary retention after visual laser abalation of the prostate. Br J Urol 1997;80:439.
8. Corujo M, Badlani GM, Regan JB, et al. A new temporary catheter (ContiCath) for the treatment of temporary, reversible, postoperative urinary retention. Urology 1999; 53:1104–7.
9. Yachia D. Treatment of recurrent anastomotic stenosis after radical prostatectomy or radical cystoprostatectomy and orthotopic bladder replacement with temporary Prostacoil stent [abstract]. J Endourol 1998;P6–4:144.
10. Djavan B, Roehrborn CG, Shariat S, et al. Prospective randomized comparison of high energy transurethral microwave thermotherapy versus alpha blocker treatment in patients with benign prostatic hyperplasia. J Urol 1999;161:139–43.
11. Djavan B, Devonec M, Shariat S, Marberger M. Trestle self retaining intraurethral catheter for treatment of temporary prostatic obstruction: safety, efficacy and early clinical results [abstract]. Thirteenth congress of the EAU, Barcelona. Eur Urol 1998;33:76.
12. Devonec M, Dahlstrand C. Temporary urethral stenting after high-energy transurethral microwave thermotherapy of the prostate. World J Urol 1998;16:120–3.
13. Ellis BW, Gidlow AB, Roodhouse A, Gill T. Nickel-titanium prostatic stents in frail or unfit men, a risk free and worthwhile option [abstract]. J Endourol 1998;P6–8:S145.
14. Knutson T. Can prostate stents be used to predict the outcome of transurethral resection of the prostate in difficult cases? Curr Urol Rep 2004;14:35–9.
15. Osterling JE, Defaalco AJ, Kaplan SA, et al. The North American experience with the UroLume endoprosthesis as a treatment for benign prostatic hyperplasia: long-term results. The North American UroLume Study Group. Urology 1994;44:353–62.
16. Anjum MI, Chari R, Shetty A, et al. Long-term clinical results and quality of life after insertion of a self-expanding flexible endourethral prosthesis. Br J Urol 1997; 80:885–8.
17. Gesenberg A, Sintermann R. Management of benign prostatic hyperplasia in high risk patients: long-term experience with the Memotherm stent. J Urol 1998;160:72–6.
18. Marinkovic S, Badlani G. Seven year outcome analysis of the UroLume stent for benign prostatic hyperplasia [abstract]. J Endourol 1999;PS7–12:A79.
19. Ricciotti E, Bozzo W, Perachino M, et al. Heat-expandable permanent intraurethral stents for benign prostatic hyperplasia and urethral strictures. J Endourol 1995;9:417–22.
20. Gajewski JB, Chancellor MB, Ackman CF, et al. Removal of UroLume endoprosthesis: experience of the North American Study Group for detrusor-sphincter dyssynergia application. J Urol 2000;163:773–6.
21. Anjum MI, Chari R, Shetty A, et al. Long-term clinical results and quality of life after insertion of a self-expanding flexible endourethral prosthesis. Br J Urol 1997;80:885–8.
22. Milroy E, Allen A. Long-term results of UroLume urethral stent for recurrent urethral strictures. J Urol 1996;155:904–8.
23. Milroy EJ, Rickards D. Anatomic limitations of prostatic urethra in using cylindrical stents. J Endourol 1997;11:455–8.
24. Curujo M, Badlani GH. Epithelialization of permanent stents. J Endourol 1997;11:477–80.
25. Marinkovic S, Badlani G. Seven-year outcome analysis of the UroLume stent for benign prostatic hyperplasia. J Endourol 1999;14:A79.
26. Badlani GH, Press SM, Defalco A, et al. UroLume endourethral prosthesis for the treatment of urethral stricture disease: long-term results of the North American Multicenter UroLume Trial. Urology 1995;45:846–56.
27. Chancellor MB, Rivas DA, Watanabe T, et al. Reversible clinical outcome after sphincter stent removal. J Urol 1996;155:1992–4.
28. Chancellor MB, Gajewski J, Ackman CF, et al. Long-term followup of the North American Multicenter UroLume Trial for the treatment of external detrusor-sphincter dyssynergia. J Urol 1999;161:1545–50.
29. Osterling JE, Kaplan SA, Epstein HB, et al. The North American experience with the UroLume endoprosthesis as a treatment for benign prostatic hyperplasia: long-term results. The North American UroLume Study Group. Urology 1994;44:353–62.
30. Badlani GH. Role of permanent stents. J Endourol 1997; 11:473–5.
31. Shah DK, Paul EM, Badlani GH. 11-year outcome analysis of UroLume endourethral prosthesis for the treatment of recurrent bulbar urethral stricture. J Urol 2003;170(4 Pt 1):1255–8.

Transurethral Needle Ablation of the Prostate

Ralph C. Benson Jr, MD
Emanuel E. Gottenger, MD

Endoscopic surgical treatment for benign prostatic hyperplasia (BPH) has evolved during the last decade from the conventional and gold standard transurethral resection of the prostate (TURP) to several minimally invasive techniques. All of these relatively new procedures have been developed with the primary goal of obtaining comparable results, while minimizing the morbidities and potential complications associated with TURP, or even open prostatectomy.

Transurethral needle ablation of the prostate (TUNA) is one of these minimally invasive techniques that utilizes radiofrequency energy to generate heat and produce thermal ablation of the prostatic tissues. The present chapter will review and discuss this technology, including its clinical results.

DEFINITIONS

THERMAL ABLATION THERAPY Treatment modality that is based on the principle of heating the target tissue to temperatures above 45°C. This raise in temperature will eventually produce tissue necrosis.

Low-level thermal therapy, when temperature ranges between 45° and 55°C, usually results in limited tissue ablation with minimal clinical improvement. When temperatures are raised to more than 55°C, particularly between 60°C and 100°C, then significant tissue ablation occurs (thermoablation).[1]

RADIOFREQUENCY Radiofrequency (RF) is a form of energy that can be used for thermal ablation therapy. RF is applied by direct contact of the device that transmits the RF signal and the target tissue. As a consequence, there is precise thermal tissue ablation of the target tissue with protection of the adjacent tissues from thermal injury (there is limited space heat dissipation).[2,3] Once the RF energy reaches the tissue, thermal energy is generated through inductive heating of water molecules and by friction.[1] The end result is tissue necrosis.

TUNA An endoscopic monopolar thermal ablation therapy for BPH that uses low RF energy waves (460–490 kHz) to generate heat within the prostatic tissue that subsequently will produce prostatic tissue necrosis. The thermal ablation will produce devascularization and denervation of prostatic tissue, which may produce relief of

BPH symptoms and improved urinary flow. The RF signal is delivered into the prostate via two needle electrodes. The degree of thermal ablation that is obtained depends on the length of the needles (amount of tissue in contact with the needles), the magnitude of the energy delivered (wattage), and the duration of treatment.

HISTORY

RF for tissue ablation has been used previously in other fields such as cardiology and neurosurgery. The first studies in the use of RF for tissue ablation of the prostate were done on animals in the early 1990s.

In 1993 Goldwasser and colleagues[4] performed a study on canine prostates. They found that necrotic lesions of approximately 1 cm in diameter and conical in shape were created by inserting a specially designed catheter through which needle antennas were advanced into the dog prostatic tissue. RF energy was then transmitted through these needles. The size of the lesion was directly related to power level used, time of ablation, and length of needle deployment. Subsequent macroscopic and histopathological evaluation of the dog's urethra, prostate, bladder neck, and anterior rectal wall revealed that the urethral temperature rose to 46.1°C, while the rectal wall temperature did not increase. They also found that there were no changes on the distal prostatic urethra, bladder neck, or anterior rectal wall similar to the necrosis that occurred within the target prostatic tissue, and thus concluded that this was a safe procedure that could be tried in humans.

Ramon and colleagues[5] performed RF thermal ablation in human ex vivo prostatic models and found that tissue temperature was the fundamental lesion parameter. Lesions were created when the temperature rose above 45°C and their size correlated with the RF power delivered and the electrode length. They suggested that the "ideal" setting to treat prostatic adenomas was

with an RF power of 5 to 7.5 W for a period of 3 minutes and a needle length of 7 to 10 mm. Shorter needle length and treatment duration will decrease the amount of tissue ablation. Also, an increase in the energy delivered (higher wattage) will decrease the amount of tissue ablation, since at temperatures above 100°C water evaporation will occur with subsequent tissue charring. The charring produces a barrier that will not conduct the energy any further, limiting thermal tissue ablation.

That same year Rasor and colleagues[6] using a turkey breast model and the TUNA device demonstrated that central lesion temperatures with the device were approximately 80° to 100°C.

Another study done on 20 patients treated with TUNA prior to a scheduled retropubic prostatectomy also showed that proximal lesion temperature was about 40° to 50°C with central lesion temperatures of about 80° to 100°C. Urethral temperature averaged 37° to 42°C and rectal temperature remained unchanged. Macroscopic examination of the specimens demonstrated localized lesions averaging 12 × 7 mm and microscopic examination showed lesions of extensive coagulative necrosis averaging 30 × 15 mm.[7]

MECHANISM OF ACTION

The exact mechanism of action of TUNA is unknown. Based on different studies as described herein, it has been shown to produce tissue ablation as well as devascularization and denervation of prostatic tissue.

HISTOPATHOLOGIC Macroscopic Macroscopic changes in prostate glands treated with TUNA are evident in the transitional zone and they correspond to the areas where needles were deployed. The gross appearance varies depending on the length of time that has past from the time of treatment until the specimen is recovered for evaluation (for in vivo prostates). Table 74-1 describes these changes. The gross appearance of

Table 74-1 Macroscopic Changes of In Vivo Prostates after TUNA Treatment

Time of Specimen Recovery after TUNA Treatment	Macroscopic Appearance
3 hours	Minimally hemorrhagic lesion with diffuse edges
1 week	Larger hemorrhagic lesions with more pronounced edges
2 weeks and later	Dark brown lesions well demarcated

TUNA = transurethral needle ablation.

in vitro prostates after being treated with TUNA differs from the in vivo model since they are pale, have a firm texture, and are devascularized.

Microscopic Initially there are significant inflammatory changes and edema that is followed by a coagulative and hemorrhagic necrosis of epithelial and smooth muscle cells. The microscopic extension of the lesions can be twice as large as their gross counterpart.[7]

Immunohistochemical Following TUNA, the treated prostatic tissue shows significant decrease or absence of staining for prostate-specific antigen (PSA), smooth muscle actin, alpha-adrenergic and nitrogen receptors, and neural tissue.[1] Zlota and colleagues[8] performed a neurohistochemical study on open prostatectomies specimens recovered 1 to 46 days after TUNA. They found that there was no staining of any axon or isolated nerve cell on the treated specimens as opposed to predominant staining of nerve fibers in the urethral submucosal layer and in the stroma surrounding the epithelial nodules in the untreated or control specimens. There was a sharp and clear demarcation between treated and untreated parenchyma. They concluded that there is severe thermal damage to intraprostatic nerve fibers after TUNA and that the long-term denervation of alpha-receptors and/or sensory nerves could explain the clinical effects of TUNA of the prostate.

ULTRASONOGRAPHIC Schulman and colleagues performed transrectal ultrasounds 30 and 90 days after the TUNA procedure and found that there was no significant decrease in the prostatic size after treatment. They also found that in some patients there was a modification of the echogenicity of the gland with creation of hypoechoic areas or cystic cavities in the transitional zone, although this finding did not correlate with the clinical outcome.[9]

Another study by Murai and colleagues did show that there was a significant decrease in prostatic volume 6 months after the treatment but not at 1 year.[10] However Namike and colleagues found a significant reduction in prostatic volume 12 months after the procedure.[11]

Our own experience is that in the majority of patients there is no significant change in overall prostatic size, and when noted, it is small and does not correlate with the treatment result.

CYSTOSCOPIC Shulman and colleagues also did not find any significant lesions or changes on urethroscopy except for inflammatory zones at the level of the needle entry point seen during the first 3 weeks after treatment.[9]

We noted that during a 6-month postoperative cystoscopy, the prostatic urethra does appear to have a lesser degree of obstruction from the lateral prostatic lobes, although not to the same degree as the cavitation seen after a transurethral resection of the prostate.

Although it has been well documented that all of these changes take effect after TUNA, it is still unclear which is mainly responsible for the clinical effects and benefits obtained with this mode of therapy.

INSTRUMENTATION

The TUNA device consists of a low-level radio frequency generator and a special handpiece. Both of these have evolved over the last decade, and at the present time, the third generation device is available (Figures 74-1 and 74-2).

MEDTRONIC TUNA PRECISION GENERATOR Medtronic TUNA precision generator (Medtronic, Inc., Minneapolis, MN) is a portable Windows-based computer that incorporates a dual RF energy generator that produces a 465 kHz RF signal that can deliver up to 15 watts of energy (see Figure 74-2). The handpiece is connected to the generator, and via the thermocouples located on the handpiece, the system can monitor the intraprostatic and urethral temperatures during treatment and use this information to adjust its power output to maintain an intraprostatic temperature of 100° to 110°C. The system also monitors the tissue impedance. The generator also can selectively deliver RF to a single needle, which is useful for treatment of large median prostatic lobes. The current software allows the therapeutic temperature of 110°C to be reached in less than 1 minute and maintains it for a total of 3 minutes per treated lesion. The generator has a shut-off safety mechanism that will be activated if the impedance of the tissue increases to more than 400 ohms. This will prevent the tissue from being overheated and becoming charred, which will limit thermal propagation. This mechanism will also be activated if the urethral temperatures rise above 46°C, thus preventing thermal injury to the urethra.

The current generator measures $21 \times 15 \times 8$ in and weights 27.5 lb. It is supplied with a foot pedal control used to initiate the energy deliver. Previous generators were slightly smaller ($11 \times 11 \times 9$ in) and did not have a computer screen, but rather a multiple digital display panel for monitoring the different treatment parameters.

MEDTRONIC TUNA HANDPIECE The Medtronic TUNA Handpiece (Medtronic, Inc.,) is a special 18.5 French (F) cystoscopic instrument that has

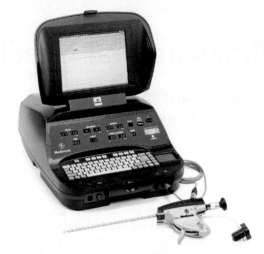

Figure 74-2 Current TUNA Generator and Handpiece. Reprinted with permission of Medtronic, Inc. ©2003.

three pieces: a zero-degree fiberoptic lens, a TUNA cartridge, and a reusable handle (Figure 74-3). The cartridge is disposable, but both the lens and the handle are resterilizable. Each disposable cartridge kit contains one sterile TUNA cartridge, one sterile TUNA tubing system, and one TUNA return electrode.

The cartridge measures 24.7 cm long and has 1 cm incremental markings. The two treatment needles are located at the tip of the cartridge and they can be deployed for a maximal distance of 22 mm. An insulating shield that protects the prostatic urethra from being heated covers each one. The thermocouples are located at the tip of each of the insulating shields and also at the tip of the TUNA cartridge. These will monitor the temperature within the prostatic tissue and in the urethra respectively. When the needles are deployed, they will diverge out at an angle of 90 degrees posteriorly from the cartridge tip and at 40 degrees from each other.

The reusable handle has an outflow port that will allow for continuous irrigation and bladder emptying. It also has a dial with preset needle length options (ranging from 12–22 mm). The trigger mechanism allows simultaneous deployment and retraction of the needles and shields. The preset shield length is 6 mm.

The telescope is a 2.8 mm rigid zero-degree lens that is compatible with light cords from Karl Storz, Wolf, CIRCOM/ACMI, and Olympus endoscopes.

PATIENT SELECTION AND PREOPERATIVE EVALUATION

The TUNA system product label indication is for the treatment of symptomatic urinary outflow obstruction secondary to BPH in men over the age of 50 and prostate sizes between 20 and 50 cc. The recent updated American Urological Association (AUA) guidelines on benign prostatic hyperplasia recommended TUNA as an option for minimally invasive treatment of symptomatic BPH.[12]

The contraindications of the TUNA procedure as per the manufacturer, Medtronic, Inc., are

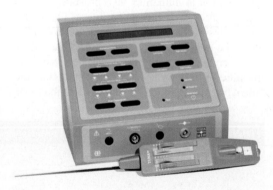

Figure 74-1 First Generation TUNA Generator and Handpiece. Reprinted with permission of Medtronic, Inc. ©2003.

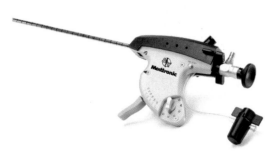

Figure 74-3 Medtronic TUNA® Handpiece. Reprinted with permission of Medtronic, Inc. ©2003.

listed on Table 74-2. Even though bleeding disorders or patients taking anticoagulation medication are listed as contraindications, we have performed the procedure successfully on these patients since the prostatic urethra is preserved and there is no debulking of prostatic tissue with subsequent minimal intra- and postoperative bleeding. Also, we have performed the procedure successfully on prostate cancer patients before or after undergoing radiotherapy (brachytherapy and/or external beam therapy) for treatment of prostate cancer. In addition, we and others[13] have performed TUNA on patients with prostates larger than 50 cc.

Although it is a published contraindication, we have also performed the procedure successfully in patients with cardiac pacemakers or implantable defibrillators that are implanted in the patient's thorax. In patients with defibrillators, we have routinely deactivated the device during the procedure. We would recommend a cardiology evaluation and clearance in this regard for this particular group of patients prior to the procedure.

In our personal experience, the only limit to perform the procedure in patients with a malleable penile implant is the adequacy of the length of the TUNA cartridge to reach the prostatic urethra.

Preoperative evaluation should follow the AUA guidelines for evaluation and treatment of patients with BPH.[12] A urinalysis and urine culture should be obtained in every patient, and if an infection is detected it should be treated appropriately before the procedure. In addition, a transrectal ultrasound of the prostate (TRUSP) must be done prior to the procedure to determine the maximal prostatic transverse diameter.

This measurement is needed to determine the optimal needle length required for the treatment. The area of heating extends approximately 6 mm beyond the needle tip, thus the measured width in millimeters is divided by 2, and then 6 is subtracted from that value. The result is a needle length in millimeters required to appropriately treat a particular prostate, preventing at the same time tissue necrosis extending beyond the prostatic capsule.[14] Additional benefits of pretreatment TRUSP include the ascertainment of prostatic size and the identification of any abnormalities that might require a guided biopsy. Moreover, the presence of asymmetry necessitating the possible tailoring of needle length for each lobe and the presence of a median lobe can be identified.

Finally, the presence of intraprostatic calculi can also be determined. This might be useful since placing the needle near these areas may increase the tissue impedance, thus decreasing the degree of heating and the therapeutic effect.

Cystoscopy, although not mandatory, is recommended in order to identify any bladder pathology as well as to visualize the internal prostate anatomy and to measure the length of the prostatic urethra. This will allow accurate preprocedure planning and estimation of procedure duration. If local anesthesia is anticipated for the procedure, then either flexible or rigid cystoscopy will help the physician judge the patient's pain tolerance and determine in advance the possible adequacy of local anesthesia.

Patients are instructed to discontinue any anticoagulants, nonsteroidal anti-inflammatory drugs, vitamin E, or aspirin at least 10 days before the procedure if this is not contraindicated, otherwise the procedure might still be performed while taking these medications, as explained above. There is no need for a bowel preparation preoperatively. Similarly, there is no need for overnight fasting unless general anesthesia or intravenous sedation will be administered.

ANESTHESIA

The procedure can be done under local anesthesia, local anesthesia with supplemental sedation and/or analgesia, or under general or regional anesthesia. Various authors have developed different anesthetic protocols, but almost invariably 2% lidocaine jelly is injected intraurethrally and left in place for at least 10 minutes prior to the procedure. Adjuvant sedation and/or analgesia can be administered intravenously, intramuscularly, or orally. Different agents have been used, including meperidine, diazepam, midazolam, propofol, fentanyl, and nonsteroidal anti-inflammatory drugs.

Transperineal and transrectal prostatic blocks have been used with success. An anesthetic solu-

Table 74-2 Contraindications for the Use of the TUNA System

Active urinary tract infection
Neurogenic bladder
Urethral stricture
Bleeding disorders or patients taking anticoagulation medication unless it has been discontinued for at least 10 days
ASA class group V patients
Presence of active prostate cancer or bladder cancer
A prostate that measured < 34 mm or > 80 mm in transverse diameter
Presence of any prosthetic device in the region that may interfere with the procedure
Previous endoscopic treatment (such as TUMT, laser prostatectomy, TURP)
Presence of cardiac pacemaker, implantable defibrillator or malleable penile implants
Patients with any component(s) of an implantable neurostimulator

tion is injected between the prostate and the rectum in the region of the prostatic nerves. Issa and colleagues[15,16] showed the feasibility and effectiveness of the use of transperineal prostatic blocks (TPPB) by instilling a mixture of 1% lidocaine and 0.25% bupivacaine, each with epinephrine (1:100,000 concentration ratio). The mean pain score on these patients using this protocol was between 3.3 and 3.4, and the use of supplemental conscious sedation did not increase the patient comfort level. They concluded that TUNA could be done safely in an outpatient or office setting using intraurethral lidocaine and TPPB without the need of an anesthesia team.

Because the necessity to perform a TRUSP to measure the transverse diameter of the prostate, if this is done immediately prior to the procedure, then at the same time a transrectal prostatic block can be performed by injecting 5 to 10 cc of 1% lidocaine at the prostatic base bilaterally.

Benson demonstrated that the TUNA procedure could be done successfully under local anesthesia alone in the office setting. He proved that with the use of a combination of oral meperidine, valium, and intravesical and intraurethral cold 2% lidocaine, the mean pain score on a scale of 1 to 10 was 4.08, and overall patient satisfaction was high.[17]

At the present time we are using the above protocol with the substitution of meperidine by acetaminophen with oxycodone.

SURGICAL PROCEDURE

The patient is brought to the operative room or cysto room and placed in the dorsal lithotomy position on the cysto table. The return electrode is placed on the patient's lower back. All patients received one dose of a broad-spectrum antibiotic, usually a first generation cephalosporin. If supplemental sedation or anesthesia will be used, it is applied at this time. At this point, a TRUSP is done to measure the transverse prostatic diameter if this was not done preoperatively. This value in mm is entered into the Medtronic TUNA generator software and will determine the needle length to be used during this treatment.

A treatment plane is defined as placement of both needles in a particular area of the prostate resulting in a lesion created around each individual needle (ie, one treatment plane = two lesions). With the current software, each plane is treated adequately for a total of 3 minutes.

The dial on the Medtronic TUNA handpiece handle is now set to the predetermined needle length and the device is inserted under direct vision and placed at approximately 0.5 to 1 cm distal to the bladder neck. Treatment is begun on either lateral lobe. The needles are deployed at approximately the 8- to 10-o'clock position on the right lobe and at the 2- to 4-o'clock position on the left lobe, although this could change based on the prostate anatomy. Additional treatment planes are created in an identical fashion by retracting the device distally in 1 cm increments and redeploying the needles. The last treatment plane should be no less than 1 cm proximal to the verumontanum to avoid damage to the genitourinary sphincter. In patients with large median lobes, successful treatment by direct placement of the needles within the median lobe has been performed.[18] Depending on the size of the prostate, between two and four treatment planes may be needed on each lateral lobe and one on the median lobe as needed. This results in an approximate average treatment time of 15 minutes.

Patients may experience a vague feeling of discomfort during the procedure as well as urgency or feeling of bladder fullness. Probably because of increased neural inervation, treatment close to the bladder neck results in the most patient discomfort. If a patient complains of fullness, they can be encouraged to void around the instrument during the procedure. In addition, the bladder can be easily emptied using the provided tubing system. Care should be taken to minimize the amount of irrigant instilled during the procedure.

If after the start of treatment of one plane the temperature rise in one or both needles is not adequate, this could be due to positioning of the needle(s) against a prostatic calculus, inside the bladder, or even outside the prostate. In these cases we will generally stop the treatment, retract the needles, reposition them, redeploy them, and then restart the treatment.

If the urethral temperature rises above 43°C, the generator will emit an alarm. At that point, manual irrigation of the handpiece should be done with saline or water to cool the urethra using the minimal amount of fluid as necessary. If large volumes of irrigant are used, the bladder should then be emptied periodically as needed to prevent overdistention. If the urethral temperature rises above 46°C, then a shut-off mechanism will be activated and the treatment of that lesion will stop.

POSTOP CARE

At the end of the procedure and based on the surgeons preference, an indwelling catheter can be left in place or the patient may be given a chance to void spontaneously before discharge. In the latter case, if the patient is unable to void, then a Foley catheter is inserted upon discharge. If the patient is discharged with a catheter, it usually is removed 24 to 72 hours later.

The urine may be pink or light red, and patients are instructed that they may see blood in the urine for the first week after treatment and then intermittently. They are also told about the possibility of hematospermia, frequency, dysuria, and urgency after treatment.

An oral antibiotic is given for 3 days, usually a quinolone, as well as an analgesic (acetaminophen with codeine or oxycodone). If they were taking an alpha-blocker, they should continue it until further notice. Anticholinergics and anti-inflammatory drugs are prescribed by some physicians after the procedure.

Patients are also instructed to drink adequate fluid volumes and avoid vigorous exercise for 2 weeks. However, they are encouraged to resume their normal work activities within 24 to 48 hours.

Finally, the patient needs to be counseled that he may not see any improvement of his BPH symptomatology for at least 2 to 6 weeks after the procedure, and even on occasion, for several months.

CLINICAL RESULTS

TUNA has proved to be an efficacious treatment modality for BPH. Multiple studies have evaluated different objective and subjective parameters that measure treatment effectiveness. These include: International Prostate Symptom Score (IPSS), peak urinary flow rate (Qmax), post void residual (PVR), and quality of life (QOL) scores. Unfortunately there is a diversity of studies that do not include all the parameters or that report limited follow-up data. Nevertheless, there has been a significant number of patients reported to allow evaluation of the procedure and its efficacy.

There are also only a few randomized prospective studies comparing TUNA versus the gold standard of TURP.

Table 74-3 shows baseline and changes in IPSS scores in 13 studies. As noted, all studies have shown individually and as a group a significant decrease in the IPSS scores from baseline to 1 year. In four studies 5-year data are available showing a sustained improvement. Overall, the mean baseline IPSS score was 21.54 with a mean score of 8.83 at 1 year and 8.9 at 5 years.

Table 74-4 shows baseline and changes in Qmax scores in 13 studies. Again, all these studies show that there was an average 53% improvement of the maximal flow rate that was sustained at 5 years in those studies with that length of follow-up. The mean baseline Qmax was 8.15 mL/s with a mean increase in the flow rate to 13.07 mL/s at 1 year and 12.53 mL/s at 5 years.

Table 74-5 shows baseline and changes in PVR scores in nine studies. There was a statistically significant decrease in the residual volume in each individual study and in all studies as a group. The mean baseline PVR was 83.68 mL, and that decreased to a mean of 41.27 mL after 1 year.

Quality of life outcomes were assessed at baseline and at 1 year in 10 studies. All of these have shown a significant improvement in the quality of life, with a mean decrease of the QOL score in all the studies of 62% at 1 year. (Baseline mean score 5.35, 12 months mean score 2.04).

At least seven authors have addressed the subject of pressure flow studies pre- and post-TUNA procedure.[19–25] In all studies, maximal detrusor pressures were decreased after the procedure, and this difference was statistically significant in all but the smallest two studies[24,25] (Table 74-6). Abrams-Griffiths numbers were given in three studies and at 12 months. Rosario and colleagues[20] reported 78% to be obstructed, and Campo and colleagues[19] reported 16% obstructed and 41.7% to be equivocal. Roehrborn and colleagues[21] showed the mean Abrams-Griffiths number for their 65 patients to decrease from 61.2 to an unobstructed 37.2. It appears that pressure-flow studies, although improved after TUNA, do not predict the degree of symptomatic improvement observed and may not be helpful in patient selection for transurethral needle ablation.

There are currently four randomized studies comparing TUNA versus TURP. Schatzl and colleagues[26] demonstrated that both groups had a significant improvement in the IPSS 24 months after treatment and that there was no statistically significant difference between the two groups. Similarly, the PVR was significantly decreased after both procedures. Qmax also increased significantly after both procedures, but patients who underwent TURP had a significantly better improvement (19.7 mL/s) than patients undergoing TUNA (11.6 mL/s) at 24 months. The improvement in Qmax after TUNA diminished with time and was lower at 24 months than at 6 to 18 months.

Chandrasekar and Virdi[27] showed that 3 years after treatment, the IPSS decreased by 11.2 points and the Qmax increased by 6.6 mL/s for TUNA patients compared with 14.8 points and 10.9 mL/s, respectively, for TURP. Overall results from both treatments were comparable.

Hill and colleagues[28] showed that the IPSS decreased to similar levels in both groups of

Table 74-3 IPSS Score Changes in 13 Studies of Transurethral Needle Ablation of the Prostate				
Study	Number of Patients	Baseline	1 Year	5 Years
Bergamaschi et al[35]	204	20.4	6.2	10.9
Chandrasekar and Virdi[27]	76	19.1	7.8	5.3
Cimentepe et al[29]	26	22.9	8.5 (18 months)	N/A
Hill et al[28]	65	24	11.7	10.7
Kahn et al[41]	45	20.9	9.9	N/A
Murai et al[10]	98	21.9	10	N/A
Namiki et al[11]	33	20.7	11.2	N/A
Naslund et al[18]	48	21.6	6	N/A
Rosario et al[20]	71	23	10.6	N/A
Rotman et al[36]	100	24.6	10.6	N/A
Schatzl et al[26]	15	17.7	6.5	N/A
Steele and Sleep[22]	47	22.4	7	N/A
Zlotta et al[30]	188	20.9	N/A	8.7
Mean	—	21.54	8.83	8.9

IPSS = International Prostate Symptom Score; N/A = not applicable.

Table 74-4 Peak Urinary Flow Rate Changes in 13 Studies of Transurethral Needle Ablation of the Prostate

Study	Number of Patients	Baseline (mL/s)	1 Year (mL/s)	5 Years (mL/s)
Bergamaschi et al[35]	204	8.2	14.8	11.8
Chandrasekar and Virdi[27]	76	7.5	15	13.1
Cimentepe et al[29]	26	9.8	17.7 (18 months)	N/A
Hill et al[28]	65	8.8	14.6	13.1
Kahn et al[41]	45	8.3	14.9	N/A
Murai et al[10]	98	7.6	11.5	N/A
Namiki et al[11]	33	8	11	N/A
Naslund et al[18]	48	8	10.4	N/A
Rosario et al[20]	71	9	11.3	N/A
Rotman et al[36]	100	6.4	13.6	N/A
Schatzl et al[26]	15	9.3	11.9	N/A
Steele and Sleep[22]	47	6.6	10.2	N/A
Zlotta et al[30]	188	8.6	N/A	12.1
Mean	–	8.15	13.07	12.53

N/A = not applicable.

patients after 5 years (11 points after TUNA and 10.6 points after TURP). PVR and Qmax improved significantly more after TURP than TUNA.

Finally, Cimentepe and colleagues[29] randomized 59 patients to undergo TUNA or TURP. Similarly, they found that improvements in Qmax, PVR, IPSS, and QOL scores were statistically significant for both groups at 18 months follow-up. Although the increase in the mean Qmax for the TURP group was higher than that in the TUNA group, there was no difference between the groups regarding the improvements in IPSS and QOL scores.

We can conclude that TUNA is comparable with TURP for treatment of BPH, and despite showing less favorable objective improvement after treatment (mainly less improvement in Qmax), the subjective results are very similar for both procedures.

TUNA AND PSA

Although significant zonal areas of tissue destruction have been demonstrated, no authors have reported a significant change in PSA after TUNA treatment of men with either BPH[23,30] or prostatitis.[31,32]

COMPLICATIONS

HEMATURIA Mild hematuria is usually present during the first 48 hours after the procedure and is self-limited. The incidence has been reported to be approximately 21%.[3] No blood transfusions were required for TUNA patients as compared with 10.5% for TURP patients as reported by Chandrasekar and colleagues.[33]

URINARY RETENTION Retention is common and has been reported between as low as 13.3% and as high as 41%.[2,3,9,11] Usually is transient and is of short duration (< 48 h).

IRRITATIVE VOIDING SYMPTOMS As mentioned earlier, dysuria, frequency, and urgency may occur after the procedure with a reported inci-

dence as high as 40%[2] and is also transient, lasting rarely more than 1 week and usually between 24 to 96 hours. Prescribing an anti-inflammatory drug may help with these symptoms.

URINARY TRACT INFECTION The incidence of postoperative urinary infection is low (up to 7%).[2,3] Verification of a sterile urine before the procedure and the use of intraoperative and prophylactic short course of postoperative antibiotics will minimize the risk of post-treatment infection.

RETROGRADE EJACULATION AND ERECTILE DYSFUNCTION The incidence of retrograde ejaculation is extremely uncommon (< 1%)[28,34–36] as is the incidence of erectile dysfunction (< 2%) after the TUNA procedure.[2,3,18,28,36] Recently the long-term results (more than 5 years of follow-up) of a prospective, randomized study were presented by Chandrasekar and colleagues[33] and showed no ejaculatory dysfunction in patients who underwent TUNA compared with 57% of patients after a TURP.

URETHRAL STRICTURE The incidence of urethral stricture after TUNA procedure is significantly lower (1.5%) when compared with TURP (7.3%).[2,3]

URINARY INCONTINENCE There have been no reports of urinary incontinence after the TUNA procedure.

MORTALITY There have been no reports of mortality associated to the TUNA procedure.

NON-FDA–APPROVED USES

TUNA IN URINARY RETENTION PATIENTS Traditionally, patients with acute urinary retention related to BPH who failed medical treatments are treated with prostatic surgery (TURP or open prostatectomy based on prostate size), or if they are not surgical candidates, with intermittent or long-term catheterization. We have performed

TUNA of the prostate in this scenario with good results. Most of the patients are able to void spontaneously and are catheter-free by 8 weeks after the procedure. Similar results have been described by others.[37]

TUNA IN PROSTATE CANCER PATIENTS There is no literature available regarding the use of TUNA in patients with prostate cancer. Frequently, patients who are being treated with radiation therapy (brachytherapy, external beam radiation, or a combination of both) may develop significant obstructive and irritative symptoms post-treatment, and are often difficult to manage and do not respond to medical and pharmacological therapies. It is well known also that these patients are at a higher risk to develop urinary incontinence if they undergo a transurethral resection of the prostate. Since TUNA produces thermoablation of prostatic tissue without the need to resect the tissue itself, the risk of incontinence should be minimal. Moreover, since PSA levels do not change after TUNA on patients with BPH or prostatitis,[23,30–32] the same may occur in prostate cancer patients. In that case, PSA could still be used as a tumor marker post-treatment. We have successfully treated several postbrachytherapy patients with urinary retention or significant urinary obstructive symptoms without any significant adverse events. Consideration may also be given to preradiation TUNA therapy in patients with severe obstructive symptoms. Clearly, clinical and histopathological studies are needed to determine the safety and efficacy of TUNA on these patients before definitive recommendations can be made.

TUNA IN PROSTATITIS Chronic pelvic pain syndrome/chronic prostatitis is a major health care burden of uncertain etiology. Successful treatment is difficult, and most of the treatments used are empirically targeted to relieve symptoms. Because of its efficacy for the treatment of benign prostatic hyperplasia and the assumption that all or a portion of the effect may be based on heat-induced alpha blockade, TUNA therapy has been investigated for the treatment of patients

Table 74-5 PVR Changes in 9 Studies of Transurethral Needle Ablation of the Prostate

Study	Number of Patients	Baseline (mL)	1 Year (mL)
Cimentepe et al[29]	26	67.4	46.4
Hill et al[28]	65	91	66
Kahn et al[41]	45	97	35
Murai et al[10]	98	80.6	48.8
Naslund et al[18]	48	73	33
Rosario et al[20]	71	70	37
Rotman et al[36]	100	113	23.3
Schatzl et al[26]	15	85	30
Steele and Sleep[22]	47	76.1	51.9
Mean	–	83.68	41.27

PVR = post void residual.

Table 74-6 Changes in Maximal Detrusor Pressure Following TUNA

Study	Number of Patients	Baseline (cm H$_2$0)	3 Months Post-TUNA (cm H$_2$0)	6 Months Post-TUNA (cm H$_2$0)	12 Months Post-TUNA (cm H$_2$0)	24 Months Post-TUNA (cm H$_2$0)	p Value
Campo et al[19]	108	85.3	53.1	61.3	63.7	67.8	< .01
Rosario et al[20]	71	97	79	N/A	82	N/A	< .001
Roehrborn et al[21]	65	78.7	N/A	64.5	N/A	N/A	< .036
Steele and Sleep[22]	41	92.4	68.5	54.8	72.9	58.9	< .05
Minardi et al[23]	24	64.9	N/A	42.3	40.0	36.3	< .05
Millard et al[24]	20	70.7	N/A	59.9	N/A	N/A	.09
Issa[25]	12	91.8	N/A	70.9	N/A	N/A	.09

N/A = not applicable; TUNA = transurethral needle ablation.

with recalcitrant chronic pelvic pain syndrome/chronic prostatitis.

In an uncontrolled study of 7 patients, Chiang and colleagues demonstrated complete resolution of symptoms in 4 patients and partial response in the remaining 3.[38] In a larger prospective uncontrolled study of 42 patients with nonbacterial prostatitis, 30 (71%) had normalization of express prostatic secretion at 3 months of follow-up.[39] Symptoms scores and quality of life scores also improved significantly. In both of these studies there was no change in semen quality after TUNA in the men assessed.

There are two sham-controlled studies that have been published that present somewhat conflicting results. In a controlled study involving 27 patients, a small but statistically significant improvement in prostatitis symptoms was achieved in the TUNA group compared with the sham group.[32] A slightly larger (33 patients) sham-controlled study reported improvement in symptoms scores and in quality of life scores in both groups, but no statistically significant difference was detected between them.[31]

It is clear that in order to determine the possible usefulness of TUNA for the treatment of chronic nonbacterial prostatitis, larger, randomized, long-term studies must be performed.

TUNA IN LARGE PROSTATES Although the approved prostate size for TUNA treatment is 20 to 50 grams, most published studies included patients with prostatic sizes larger than 50 grams, but results for these larger glands cannot be dissected out of the global published results.[14] One study does specifically address this issue. Sullivan and colleagues evaluated the effectiveness of TUNA in 10 patients with benign hyperplastic prostates greater than 60 grams.[13] The mean prostatic weight was 76.9 grams (range 62–98 grams). Symptoms scores, quality of life, and maximal and average flow rates were measured before and at 1, 3, and 6 months post-treatment, and statistically significant improvement in all outcome measurements was noted. Therefore, it appears that one can expect improvements of the same magnitude in patients with glands larger than 60 grams as observed in those with glands smaller than 60 grams, although treatment time will be proportionally longer.

COST-EFFECTIVENESS

TUNA has proved to be a cost-effective minimally invasive treatment alternative for BPH. A study by Campo and colleagues[19] calculated that the approximate cost to perform a TUNA procedure in Italy was $1,700 (US) compared with $2,700 (US) for a TURP. Since TUNA can be performed in an office setting without the added cost of anesthesiology or operating room fees, the overall savings may be even greater.

Another study by Naslund calculated the cost-effectiveness of TUNA, TURP, and microwave therapy (TUMT) using Medicare reimbursement data from the year 2001 to estimate the costs of these procedures. He defined cost-effectiveness as the dollars per unit of IPSS improvement and the dollars per cc/s of improvement in peak flow rates after each treatment. He demonstrated that TUNA was the most cost-effective treatment modality in improving IPSS. It was the least expensive treatment for achieving improvement in IPSS ($49.10 [US]/unit IPSS) when compared with the other two treatment modalities. TURP was the most cost-effective treatment for improving Qmax ($44.50 [US]/cc/s), but TUNA was close behind it ($49.10 [US]/cc/s).[40]

CONCLUSIONS

Based on the previously described histopathological and clinical studies performed on human and animal prostates, we can conclude that TUNA offers the following advantages (Table 74-7):

PRESERVATION OF PROSTATIC URETHRA Since there is selective tissue ablation without excessive heating of nontarget surrounding tissues,

Table 74-7

Advantages of the TUNA Procedure

Preservation of prostatic urethra
Protection of adjacent organs
Preservation of antegrade ejaculation
Performed under local anesthesia
Performed on anticoagulated patients

TUNA = transurethral needle ablation.

TUNA of the prostate protects the prostatic urothelium from thermal injury. This urothelium is very sensitive to pain, thus preservation of the prostatic urethra allows TUNA to be performed under topical anesthesia. Urethral preservation also minimizes postoperative hematuria, urinary retention, and irritative voiding symptoms.[1]

PROTECTION OF ADJACENT ORGANS Based on the same principle of selective tissue ablation, there is minimal heat dissipation beyond the target tissue, which prevents injury to adjacent tissues such as the prostatic capsule, neurovascular bundles, urinary sphincter, or the rectum. This prevents the occurrence of erectile dysfunction, urinary incontinence, or rectal injury/fistulas.

PRESERVATION OF ANTEGRADE EJACULATION Since there is no significant anatomical debulking of prostatic tissue during the TUNA procedure, the bladder neck is preserved and so is antegrade ejaculation. This factor may be of importance to younger patients or those concerned about their fertility potential after a surgical intervention for the prostate.

NO NEED FOR GENERAL OR REGIONAL ANESTHESIA Since the prostatic urethra is preserved, the procedure can be done and is well tolerated under local (topical) anesthesia.

CAN BE PERFORMED ON ANTICOAGULATED PATIENTS Since the prostatic urethra is preserved and there is no debulking of prostatic tissue, there is minimal intra- and postoperative bleeding, making this procedure ideal for patients with BPH who are anticoagulated. There is no need to discontinue anticoagulation preoperatively on these patients.

Long-term data are still needed to determine if the satisfactory results obtained with this treatment will remain for more than 5 or 6 years. Also, new studies should be developed to prove the safety and efficacy of this technique when used to treat other prostatic conditions such as prostatitis, urinary retention related to prostatic hyperplasia, and obstruction in prostate cancer patients after radiation therapy.

Because of the demonstrated efficacy, durability, low adverse effects profile, and apparent cost-effectiveness of TUNA, we believe that this minimally invasive therapy should be included in the urologist's therapeutic armamentarium and should be offered to most patients with symptomatic benign prostatic hyperplasia.

REFERENCES

1. Issa MM, Myrick SE, Symbas NP. The TUNA procedure for BPH: review of the technology. Infect Urol 1998;11:104–11.
2. Issa MM, Oesterling JE. Radiofrequency thermal therapy for benign prostatic hyperplasia by transurethral needle ablation of the prostate. In: Narayan P, editor. Benign prostatic hyperplasia. London: Churchill Livingstone; 2000. p. 269–80.

3. Bruskewitz R, Issa MM, Roehrborn,CG, et al. A prospective, randomized 1-year clinical trial comparing transurethral needle ablation to transurethral resection of the prostate for the treatment of symptomatic benign prostatic hyperplasia. J Urol 1998;159:1588–93.

4. Goldwasser B, Ramon J, Engelberg S, et al. Transurethral needle ablation (TUNA) of the prostate using low-level radiofrequency energy: an animal experimental study. Eur Urol 1993;24:400–5.

5. Ramon J, Goldwasser B, Shenfeld O, et al. Needle ablation using radio frequency current as a treatment for benign prostatic hyperplasia: experimental results in ex vivo human prostate. Eur Urol 1993;24:406–10.

6. Rasor JS, Zlotta AR, Edwards SD, Schulman CC. Transurethral needle ablation (TUNA): thermal gradient mapping and comparison of lesion size in a tissue model and in patients with benign prostatic hyperplasia. Eur Urol 1993;24:411–14.

7. Schulman CC, Zlotta AR, Rasor JS, et al. Transurethral needle ablation (TUNA): safety, feasibility, and tolerance of a new office procedure for treatment of benign prostatic hyperplasia. Eur Urol 1993;24:415–23.

8. Zlotta AR, Raviv G, Peny MO, et al. Possible mechanisms of action of transurethral needle ablation of the prostate on benign prostatic hyperplasia symptoms: a neurohistochemical study. J Urol 1997;157:894–9.

9. Schulman CC, Zlotta AR. Transurethral needle ablation of the prostate for treatment of benign prostatic hyperplasia: early clinical experience. Urology 1995;45:28–33.

10. Murai M, Tachibana M, Miki M, et al. Transurethral needle ablation of the prostate: an initial Japanese clinical trial. Int J Urol 2001;8:99–105.

11. Namiki K, Shiozawa H, Tsuzuki M, et al. Efficacy of transurethral needle ablation of the prostate for the treatment of benign prostatic hyperplasia. Int J Urol 1999;6:341–5.

12. AUA Practice Guideline Committee. AUA guidelines on management of benign prostatic hyperplasia (2003). Chapter 1: Diagnosis and treatment recommendations. J Urol 2003;170(2 Pt 1):530–47.

13. Sullivan LD, Paterson RF, Gleave M E, et al. Early experience with transurethral needle ablation of large prostates. Can J Urol 1999;6:686–91.

14. Naslund MJ. Transurethral needle ablation of the prostate. Urology 1997;50:167–72.

15. Issa MM, Stein B, Benson R, et al. Prospective multicenter study of transperineal prostatic block for transurethral needle ablation of the prostate. Urology 2000;56:1052–5.

16. Issa MM, Perez-Brayfield M, Petros JA, et al. A prospective study of transperineal prostatic block for transurethral needle ablation for benign prostatic hyperplasia: the Emory University experience. J Urol 1999;162:1636–9.

17. Benson RC. Efficacy of local anesthesia for the transurethral needle ablation of the prostate (TUNA) procedure performed in the office—a prospective trial. J Endourol 2001;15 Suppl 1:A90.

18. Naslund MJ, Benson RC, Cohen ES, et al. Transurethral needle ablation (TUNA) for BPH in patients with median lobe enlargement. Report of a prospective multi-center study. J Urol 2000;163:270.

19. Campo B, Bergamaschi F, Corrada P, Ordesi G. Transurethral needle ablation (TUNA) of the prostate: a clinical and urodynamic evaluation. Urology 1997;49:847–50.

20. Rosario DJ, Woo H, Potts KL, et al. Safety and efficacy of transurethral needle ablation of the prostate for symptomatic outlet obstruction. Br J Urol 1997;80:579–86.

21. Roehrborn CG, Burkhard FC, Bruskewitz RC, et al. The effects of transurethral needle ablation and resection of the prostate on pressure flow urodynamic parameters: analysis of the United States randomized study. J Urol 1999;162:92–7.

22. Steele GS, Sleep DJ. Transurethral needle ablation of the prostate: a urodynamic based study with 2-year followup. J Urol 1997;158:1834–8.

23. Minardi D, Garofalo F, Yehia M, et al. Pressure-flow studies in man with benign prostatic hypertrophy before and after treatment with transurethral needle ablation. Urol Int 2001;66:89–93.

24. Millard RJ, Harewood LM, Tamaddon K. A study of the efficacy and safety of transurethral needle ablation (TUNA) for benign prostatic hyperplasia. Neurourol Urodyn 1996;15:619–29.

25. Issa MM. Transurethral needle ablation of the prostate: report of initial United States clinical trial. J Urol 1996;156 (2 Pt 1):413–9.

26. Schatzl G, Madersbacher S, Djavan B, et al. Two-year results of transurethral resection of the prostate versus four "less invasive" treatment options. Eur Urol 2000;37:695–701.

27. Chandrasekar P, Virdi JS. Transurethral needle ablation of the prostate (TUNA)—a prospective study, six-year follow-up. J Urol 2001;165:294.

28. Hill B, Belville W, Bruskewitz R, et al. Five year results of a prospective randomized trial comparing transurethral needle ablation (TUNA) to TURP for treatment of symptomatic BPH. J Urol 2002;167:294.

29. Cimentepe E, Unsal A, Saglam R. Randomized clinical trial comparing transurethral needle ablation with transurethral resection of the prostate for the treatment of benign prostatic hyperplasia: results at 18 months. J Endourol 2003;17:103–7.

30. Zlotta AR, Giannakopoulos X, Maehlun O, et al. Long-term evaluation of transurethral needle ablation of the prostate (TUNA) for treatment of symptomatic benign prostatic hyperplasia: clinical outcome up to five years from three centers. Eur Urol 2003;44:89–93.

31. Leskinen MJ, Kilponen A, Lukkarinen O, Tammela T. Transurethral needle ablation for the treatment of chronic pelvic pain syndrome (category III prostatitis): a randomized sham-controlled study. Urology 2002;60:300–4.

32. Aaltomaa S, Ala-Opas M. The effect of transurethral needle ablation on symptoms of chronic pelvic pain syndrome—a pilot study. Scand J Urol Nephrol 2001;35:127–31.

33. Chandrasekar P, Virdi JS, Kapasi F. Transurethral needle ablation of the prostate (TUNA) in the treatment of benign prostatic hyperplasia; a prospective, randomized study, long-term results. J Urol 2003;169:1754.

34. Issa MM, Myrick SE, Symbas NP. The TUNA procedure for BPH: basic procedure and clinical results. Infect Urol 1998 11:148–54.

35. Bergamaschi F, Manzo M, Autieri G, et al. Five year experience using transurethral needle ablation (TUNA) in 204 BPH patients. J Urol 2000;163:333–4.

36. Rotman M, Salant R, Nagler HM. A comparative analysis of transurethral needle ablation and interstitial laser thermal therapy of the prostate. J Urol 2002;167:294.

37. Meyer J. Use of transurethral needle ablation of the prostate for acute urinary retention. J Urol 2002;168:1107.

38. Chiang PH, Tsai E M, Chiang CP. Pilot study of transurethral needle ablation (TUNA) in treatment of nonbacterial prostatitis. J Endourol 1997;11:367–70.

39. Lee KC, Jung PB, Park HS, et al. Transurethral needle ablation for chronic nonbacterial prostatitis. BJU Int 2002;89:226–9.

40. Naslund MJ. Cost-effectiveness of minimally invasive treatments and transurethral resection (TURP) in benign prostatic hyperplasia (BPH). J Urol 2001;165:295.

41. Kahn SA, Alphonse P, Tewari A, Narayan P. An open study on the efficacy and safety of transurethral needle ablation of the prostate in treating symptomatic benign prostatic hyperplasia: the University of Florida experience. J Urol 1998;160:1695–700.

Prostate Brachytherapy Radioactive Seed Implantation

Jed Pollack, MD

Prostate cancer is the second most common noncutaneous malignancy in men, and, if localized at the time of diagnosis, carries a generally good to excellent prognosis, depending on Gleason score and PSA, as well as T stage. Brachytherapy, defined as the permanent or temporary implantation of radioactive sources directly into the prostate, is one standard treatment approach. Surgery or external beam radiation therapy with or without brachytherapy are also considered standard treatment.

HISTORY

Initially, prostate implants were done with an open retropubic technique, with the prostate being exposed via a laparotomy incision pioneered by Hilaris and colleagues at Memorial Sloan Kettering.[1] It should be noted, however, that implantation of radium into the prostate was actually first described by Barringer in 1917.[2]

From 1970 to 1985, about 1,000 patients were treated with open retropubic technique, which involved arbitrary seed placement into the prostate with roughly 1 cm spacing using a free-hand technique, one or two fingers in the rectum to find the posterior aspect of the prostate. Dose was defined a MPD (matched peripheral dose), which corresponded to an ellipsoid about the same size and shape as the prostate. It was determined with crude measurements without ultrasonography or any other sophisticated imaging. Not surprisingly, this technique led to variable and generally suboptimal results owing to great variation of dosimetric coverage of the prostate. If the MPD was at least 15,000 cGy, local recurrence was about 10%. If coverage was worse, local recurrences were at least 30%.[3] By T stage, local failure was 15% for T1 lesions and 40 to 50% for T2 and T3 lesions. It should be noted that this early work was done in the pre-PSA era, therefore, patient selection and definition of

treatment failure was based on much less accurate clinical criteria in what is now used. Blasko and colleagues[4] and Holm and colleagues[5] pioneered the use of ultrasound-guided transperineal implantation, and the technique is now well established as a standard therapy for localized prostate cancer alone or in combination with external beam radiation. Data from CaPSURE showed that the use of brachytherapy in low-risk patients has increased from 4% in 1993 through 1995 to 22% in 1999 to 2001.[6]

INDICATIONS AND PATIENT SELECTION

Patients with stage T1c-T2b, N0 M0 are generally candidates for implant, with or without external beam radiation therapy, depending on Gleason score and PSA. Implant for stage T3 is somewhat more controversial. "Standard" staging work-up for localized prostate cancer is somewhat variable.

CT scan and bone scan are no longer necessary for low-risk group patients, but MRI with endorectal coil may help to more accurately define areas of the prostate involved with cancer as well as possible unsuspected extracapsular extension that could affect the proposed method of treatment. Bone scan and CT scan are standard for staging intermediate-risk and high-risk patients.

PROSTATE SIZE Prostate size (greater than or equal to 60 cc) may be a relative contraindication to permanent seed implant due to several factors:

1. A large size decreases the ability to accurately image the anterior prostate.
2. Larger prostates, especially if combined with a narrow pubic arch, may preclude a good implant if the pubic bone prevents the introduction of seeds into the anterior aspect of the prostate. Extended lithotomy position can often overcome this problem.
3. Controversy exists as to whether or not patients with larger prostates are more likely to have obstructive problems after an implant, including acute urinary retention. Merrick and colleagues,[7] using the EPIC (Expanded Prostate Center Index Composite) did not find long-term urinary morbidity was related to size. Locke and colleagues,[15] Crooke and colleagues,[14] and Lee and colleagues[12] also found large size to be a factor in acute obstruction. Crook and colleagues[14] found that patients with large prostates requiring androgen ablation for downsizing had a fourfold increased risk of acute retention compared with those with smaller glands. The American Brachytherapy Society (ABS),[20] however, does recommend hormonal cytoreduction for 2 to 3 months prior to implant in patients with prostate volumes greater than 60 cc.

PRIOR TURP (TRANSURETHRAL PROSTATECTOMY) Prior TURP was considered by many early on to be an absolute contraindication to implant in the mid- to late 1980s and early to mid-1990s. Although American Brachytherapy Society considers prior TURP to be at least a caution in a patient being considered for implant, it is not an absolute contraindication unless it was done recently, or there is a large TURP defect making it impossible to adequately implant the anterior prostate. Moran and colleagues,[8] Wallner and colleagues,[9] and Merrick and colleagues[10] have shown that if there is at least 2 months interval from the time of TURP to implant to allow for re-epithelization of the TURP defect, implant can be done. The caution is that the dose to the TURP defect, and therefore the urethra, should be minimized as much as possible, especially in the apex where there will not be much tissue between the TURP defect and the rectal mucosa. The smaller the prostate, the harder it will be to obtain satisfactorily low doses to the urethra and the TURP defect.

AMERICAN UROLOGICAL ASSOCIATION SCORE AND INTERNATIONAL PROSTATE SYMPTOMS SCORE

There is conflicting evidence as to whether or not high American Urological Association Score (AUA) score or high International Prostate Symptoms Score (IPSS) may be a relative contraindication to implant in that the risk of long-term urinary retention and dysuria may be higher. It is accepted that the vast majority of patients implanted will have at least 2 to 4 months of obstructive and irritative symptoms. Acute retention will occur in 5 to 30% of patients after implant.[7,9,12,14–16] Locke and colleagues[15] and Bucci and colleagues[16] found high AUA and IPSS increased the risk of acute retention as well as need for more prolonged catheterization. Catheterization was required in 10% of patients with IPSS of 0 to 5, 70% with IPSS of 6 to 15, and 33% with IPSS of greater than 15. McElveen and colleagues[17] found high IPSS (and urethral dose) to be predictive of a higher risk of urinary incontinence (all grade 1 or 2). Patients without incontinence had an IPSS of 6.6, plus or minus 4.5 compared with IPSS of 10, plus or minus 6.4 for those with incontinence. At Long Island Jewish Medical Center, we recommend a urodynamic study for patients with high AUA or IPSS and do not usually recommend implant if the study shows unsatisfactory results. Landis and colleagues,[18] in a perspective study, did not find preimplant urodynamic studies or IPSS to correlate with acute or long-term urinary morbidity; however, we feel it best to approach implant in such patients with caution.

MEDIAN LOBE HYPERPLASIA

Although the median lobe may present technical difficulties in achieving adequate dosimetry, the main concern is possible increased urinary morbidity owing to the necessarily high doses to the urethra that must be given to achieve adequate coverage near the base. Wallner and colleagues[19] found 25% of patients with significant medial lobe hyperplasia developed prolonged dysuria and retention; therefore, it is best to be cautious when considering such patients for implant. Some have recommended preimplant resection of some hyperplastic tissue a few months prior to implant.

DISEASE FACTORS

The American Brachytherapy Society[20] recommends implant monotherapy with either I-125 or palladium-103 for patients with T1-T2a lesions with Gleason score of 6 or less and a PSA of less than or equal to 10 ng/mL. For stage T2b, T2c, or Gleason score equal to or greater than 7 or PSA greater than 10, the recommendation is to add external beam radiation. ABS has no specific recommendation on hormonal therapy in such settings. Davis and colleagues[21] found that the vast majority of extracapsular extension is within 5 mm of the prostate capsule, so brachytherapy may still be acceptable in such patients with the recommendation to expand the coverage around the prostate capsule covered by the implant, and to add external beam radiation as well.

OTHER FACTORS

If the patient's general medical condition is good, neither age, weight, nor inflammatory bowel disease is a contraindication to implant. The use of supplementary external beam radiation in patients with inflammatory bowel disease is controversial.

PATIENT PREPARATION

We recommend an enema the night before the implant. Antibacterial prophylaxis started 2 days prior to the implant. Anticoagulants, depending on the medication used, should be stopped 1 week to 10 days prior to the implant. The patient should be NPO from midnight on, the evening before the implant. We feel that Decadron, 8 to 10 mg administered during the implant may decrease the risk of acute postimplant urinary morbidity and retention, though this is also not proven. It is also common to use alpha-blockers starting a week or two before the implant, which may also minimize urinary morbidity.

ISOTOPE CHOICE

The two isotopes used in permanent implants are iodine-125 and palladium-103. The American Brachytherapy Society[20] does not specifically favor either one regardless of Gleason score, T stage, or PSA. Cha and colleagues[22] and Wallner and colleagues[23] found no difference in outcomes regardless of isotope used. (Wallner evaluated low-risk group patients only).

TECHNIQUE

PLANNING In the 1980s and early 1990s, most implants were done using a nomogram for operative planning technique, in which the prostate dimensions (height, width, length) were determined at the start of the procedure,[24] and the total amount of radioactivity millicuries was determined, with approximately 50 to 75% being placed arbitrarily in the periphery, depending on the isotope used. Radioactive seed spacing was arbitrarily 1 cm apart. The technique was developed before the advent of powerful and fast software that can now give almost instantaneous real-time dosimetry and allow for real-time interactive planning or very detailed preplanning. The nomogram technique, while still in use, is justifiably being abandoned because of inability to actually conform dose to the shape of the prostate with any real accuracy, as well as inability to calculate and minimize dose to the urethra and rectum in an accurate way. The technique used at many institutions, including Long Island Jewish (LIJ) Medical Center, is a preplanning technique in which a detailed ultrasound study of the prostate is done with 5 mm axial slice intervals with catheter in the urethra. This is done about 2 weeks ahead of the scheduled implant date. Figure 75-1 shows the ultrasound-generated planning images at 5 mm intervals. Figure 75-2 shows the schematic diagram of the needles used with customized preloading. It allows for fairly good and detailed planning; however, the disadvantages are that in addition to the extra time taken to do the ultrasound study, in the OR, the patient may not be exactly in the same position relative to the ultrasound probe and the probe itself may be at a different angle and position relative to the prostate. Figure 75-3 shows the preplanning results in geographical form, expressed as a dose-volume histogram (DVH). Note the peripheral seed placement. In addition, patient movement and prostate movement during the preplanning ultrasound may also contribute to some

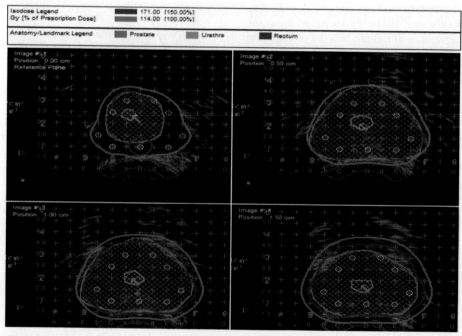

Figure 75-1 Either preplanning or intraoperative planning will use 5 mm axial slices from the base of the prostate to the apex. Each axial planning slice will have isodose curves illustrating prescription dose and any other dose levels desired. Blue circles indicate a "hot" seed; red circles indicate a nonradioactive spacer.

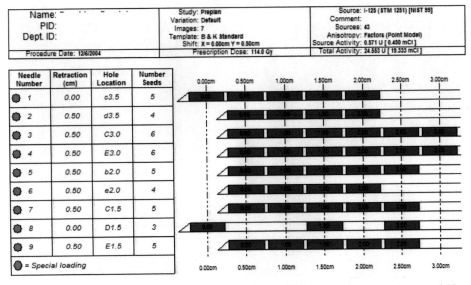

LIJ Medical Center · 1 · 1 · 1/24/2005 2:13:40 PM

| Name:
PID:
Dept. ID: | | Study: Preplan
Variation: Default
Images: 7
Template: B & K Standard
Shift: X = 0.00cm Y = 0.50cm | | Source: I-125 (STM 1251) [NIST 99]
Comment:
Sources: 43
Anisotropy: Factors (Point Model)
Source Activity: 0.571 U [0.450 mCi] |
| Procedure Date: 12/6/2004 | | Prescription Dose: 114.0 Gy | | Total Activity: 24.553 U [19.333 mCi] |

Needle Number	Retraction (cm)	Hole Location	Number Seeds
● 1	0.00	c3.5	5
● 2	0.50	d3.5	4
● 3	0.50	C3.0	6
● 4	0.50	E3.0	6
● 5	0.50	b2.0	5
● 6	0.50	e2.0	4
● 7	0.50	C1.5	5
● 8	0.00	D1.5	3
● 9	0.50	E1.5	5
● = Special loading			

Figure 75-2 Schematic plan using nine preloaded needles. Each blue rectangle represents one seed. Needle #8 has several nonradioactive spacers between seeds.

(usually small) degree of inaccuracy translating the preplan exactly to the actual procedure. Nevertheless, we have found good to excellent implant quality in over 700 patients implanted since 1994. We have now changed to a real-time intraoperative planning technique, in which ultrasound images are sent directly to our planning program and the target volume digitized in at the time of implant. The contours of the urethra are digitized in as well. This is done in 5 mm axial slices. Real-time planning takes approximately 10 to 15 minutes. Whatever method of planning is used, a 3 to 5 mm margin anteriorly and laterally around the prostate is recommended.[26] Some practitioners will also obtain real-time dosimetry as each seed or several seeds in one needle are deposited into the prostate, thus achieving instant feedback on the adequacy of the implant and making dosimetry and planning adjustments accordingly. It is, however, very difficult to visualize all of the seeds adequately on ultrasound. It is important to note that the vast majority of seeds will be placed peripherally, as the center of the prostate (and the urethra) always receive substantially more than the prescription dose, often by a factor of two or three.

IMPLANT EQUIPMENT Equipment involved in the actual implant includes presterilized iodine-125 or palladium-103 seeds; presterilized hollow needles (with an inner trocar), which will introduce the seeds through the perineum into the prostate; the sterile template, which will be mounted on the probe through which needles will pass; and the probe itself with ancillary equipment. A Mick applicator may be used and will be brought sterilized into the operating room. We prefer to use preloaded needles that are shipped to LIJ as per our preplan, or the needles may be preloaded in the OR if intraoperative planning is going to be carried out. We have not used the Mick applicator in about 8 years and find that

preloaded needles are easier and faster to use. Needles contain an inner plastic tube crimped at the distal end (isosleeve) that minimizes the chance of seed bunching in the prostate.

PROCEDURE Spinal, general, or laryngeal mask anesthesia may be used. After induction, the patient is placed in the lithotomy or extended lithotomy position. A Foley catheter is inserted under sterile conditions into the bladder. The scrotum is pulled up out of the perineal field either by a stitch, tape, or a wet towel rolled under the scrotum. The ultrasound probe is inserted into the rectum and satisfactory images of the prostate are obtained. Figure 75-4 illustrates the patient position with the rectal probe in place. The long axis to the probe should be parallel to the long axis of the prostate. The perineal area is then sterilized and the legs draped. The template is

mounted on the probe flush against the perineum. Needle insertion into the prostate is then begun (Figure 75-5). Some practitioners like to insert "stabilization" needles in the posterolateral aspect of the prostate on either side. We have not really found this necessary. Needle insertion and seed deposition can be done in a variety of ways. The most important principle is to start anteriorly and laterally and work posteriorly. We usually prefer to put the first needles in the anterolateral position to determine right away if there is going to be any problem with pubic arch interference. If so, then the extended lithotomy position will be used and the probe adjusted as well to try to get the anterior needles under the pubic bone and into the anterior aspect of the prostate. The other reason to start anteriorly is that visualization of the anterior prostate will become progressively poorer in the latter part of the implant as intraprostatic bleeding and edema occur. Needles can be placed either all at once as per a preplan and seeds then deposited, or each needle can then be placed sequentially and the seeds deposited with removal of each needle prior to going onto the next. Generally, needle tips are referenced to the base and the deposition of seeds starts at the base and moves toward the apex with the needle tip gradually being withdrawn from the base to the apex as each seed is deposited. We employ fluoroscopy during the implant procedure to assure us that there is no seed bunching, although this is certainly optional. For the implantation of the apex, we will often have several needles individually loaded with one or two seeds apiece, in which case the needle tips will not be referenced from the base. It is important to use ultrasound imaging both axially and sagittally (to confirm needle tip position at the base). This should be done throughout the case for each needle. After all the seeds planned for are deposited in the prostate, the probe and Foley catheter are removed and a cystoscopy is performed in order to find and remove any seeds or blood clots that

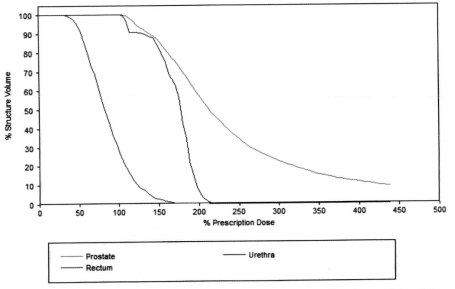

Figure 75-3 This planning dose-volume histogram allows precise information about anticipated dose to any volume of urethra, bladder, prostate, and anterior rectal wall.

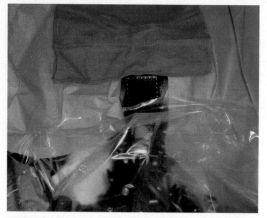

Figure 75-4 Note the template with grid in place against the perineum. The transrectal ultrasound probe is just beneath the template and is covered by a sterile plastic drape so that the probe can be manipulated without contamination. The hollow steel needles containing the radioactive seeds will be inserted through the template at the appropriate positions on the grid, and then into the prostate, where the seeds will be deposited.

may have gotten into the bladder or urethra. Plain film images are taken to document seed position and to confirm the number of seeds in place. This will also help to achieve accurate dosimetry when combined with the postimplant CT. We usually discharge the patient the same day with a Foley catheter in place and CT dosimetry is done the next morning (Figure 75-6). CT dosimetry is mandatory and is recommended by the American Brachytherapy Society. Figure 75-7 shows a postimplant DVH. We prefer to do it in the morning after the implant, although many prefer to do anywhere from 1 to 4 weeks later to allow for acute postimplant prostate edema to subside. The American Brachytherapy Society[25] takes no position on the ideal time to do postimplant CT dosimetry. We recommend that all patients have

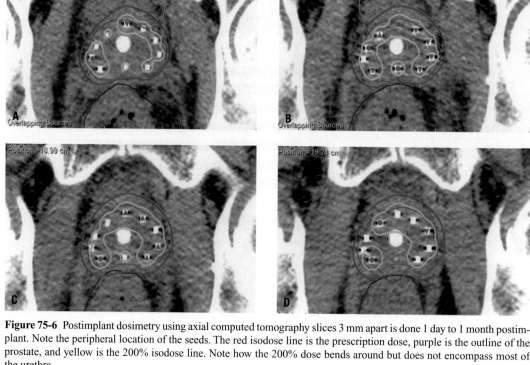

Figure 75-6 Postimplant dosimetry using axial computed tomography slices 3 mm apart is done 1 day to 1 month postimplant. Note the peripheral location of the seeds. The red isodose line is the prescription dose, purple is the outline of the prostate, and yellow is the 200% isodose line. Note how the 200% dose bends around but does not encompass most of the urethra.

antibiotic coverage during the implant, and for 1 week postimplant, we routinely use alpha-blockers pre- and postimplant.

RESULTS OF PROSTATE BRACHYTHERAPY

Prostate brachytherapy alone was shown in the early work from Memorial Sloan Kettering[3] to be less effective in more advanced (T2, T3) lesions. Using T stage, PSA, and Gleason score, many

authors have stratified prostate cancer patients into three risk groups (Table 75-1), which vary slightly in definition. Using these risk factors, it is clear that for low-risk prostate cancer, implant alone has yielded very good results, comparable with surgery or external beam radiation (Table 75-2). In patients with intermediate-risk disease, the results with implant only are good, but may be less satisfactory than the results for low-risk patients (Table 75-3) with greater result variability. For high-risk patients, the results with implant only

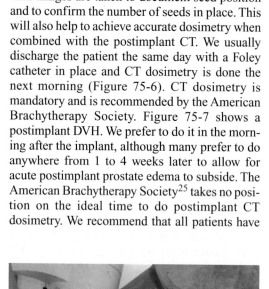

Figure 75-5 The hollow steel needle containing the radioactive seeds is now being inserted through the template into the prostate. Note the fluoroscopic imaging head just above the sterile field. Fluoroscopy is optional in prostate implantation, but we have found that it provides a useful adjunct to ultrasound imaging, especially toward the end of the procedure, when image degradation owing to intraprostatic bleeding, swelling, and artifact from the seeds and air can occur.

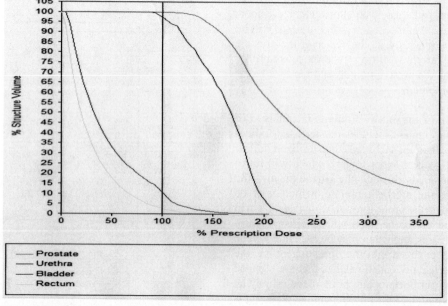

Figure 75-7 Postimplant dose volume histogram illustrating excellent coverage of the prostate by the prescription dose. Note the very low rectal dose (yellow curve) and the bladder dose (blue curve).

Table 75-1

Risk Group	T Stage	Gleason Score	PSA
Low	T_1–T_{2a}	≤ 6	≤ 10 ng/mL
Intermediate	T_{2b}–T_{2c}	7	10–20 ng/mL
High	≥ T_3	≥ 8	≥ 20 ng/mL

Note: Any single intermediate- or high-risk criteria will place a patient in that risk group.

MSKCC/Seattle Risk Grouping			
Risk Group	Disease State	Gleason Score	PSA
Low	≤ T_{2a}	≤ 6	≤ 10
Intermediate			
High		More than one intermediate- or high-risk factor	

Adapted from Quantara et al.[27]

Table 75-3 Implant Alone: Results for Intermediate-Risk Patients

Author	bNED (%)	Follow-Up (yr)
Blasko et al[28]	82	5
Zelefsky et al[29]	72	5
Stock & Stone[33]	60	5
Stokes[35]	64	5
Kollmeier et al[36]	65	8
Brachman et al[37]	51	5

bNED = biochemical no evidence of disease.

are even less gratifying (Table 75-4). Decreasing results for implant monotherapy with increasing risk group has been shown graphically by Peter Grimm (Figure 75-8). Although not proven in randomized studies, there appears to be improved results using a combination of external beam radiation, 4,500 cGy to 5,000 cGy, combined with implant (Table 75-5). Not all findings have supported the hypothesis of external beam radiation as necessary to improve implant outcomes in intermediate- and high-risk patients.[48] Current practice trends support combined therapy in such patients as opposed to implant only. Hormonal therapy has also been widely used in combination with external beam radiation in the treatment of prostate cancer with unfavorable disease parameters[49–51] showing a real benefit in local (pelvic) control as well as biochemical freedom from failure, cause-specific survival, and possibly overall survival. Therefore, it seems logical to add hormonal therapy for high- and possibly intermediate-risk patients being treated with implant with or without external beam radiation. Nevertheless the data for this are controversial. Lee and colleagues,[52] evaluated 201 patients with intermediate- to high-risk disease treated in a nonrandomized fashion with implant with or without hormonal ablation 3 months before implant and 2 to 3 months after (no external beam radiation). At 5 years, the hormonal group had 79% bNED versus 54% bNED with implant only. Potters and colleagues[53] did not find an advantage to short-course hormonal therapy prior to implant only, nor did Galalae and colleagues[45] in patients receiving external radiation, followed by high-dose-rate temporary implant, with or without a short course of neoadjuvant/concurrent hormonal therapy. At this time, although hormonal therapy is often used for patients with high-risk disease (and sometimes for intermediate-risk patients) undergoing implant, the data to support its use are controversial. Its use in patients with high-risk disease receiving external beam radiation only is standard.

IMPORTANCE OF GOOD TECHNIQUE

It has been shown by numerous authors[36,54–56] that good quality implants, not surprisingly, lead to better results than suboptimal implants. A good implant is generally accepted to be one in which the D90 (minimum dose received by 90% of the target volume) is at least 90% of the prescribed dose. Another definition used is the V100, the percentage of target volume receiving 100% of the prescribed dose. Table 75-6 illustrates results from two series showing different outcomes for patients receiving optimal and suboptimal implants.

COMPARISON WITH OTHER MODALITIES

There is no randomized data comparing implant with external beam radiation or surgery. There is also no randomized data comparing implant with implant plus external beam radiation. The Radiation Therapy Oncology Group (RTOG) activated protocol 0232 in June of 2003. This compares external beam radiation plus implant with implant only in patients with T1c through T2b disease, Gleason score less than or equal to 7, and PSA less than or equal to 20 with or without hormonal therapy. The RTOG has also activated a single arm study (RTOG 0321) for external beam radiation plus high-dose-rate temporary implant, as well as a similar study (RTOG P0019) for intermediate-risk patients treated with external beam radiation and I-125 implant. A single arm study with implant only (RTOG 9805) is closed. Hopefully, results should be available in the near future. Quantara and colleagues,[27] comparing surgery with brachytherapy in low-risk patients concluded that results with either modality were equally good. For intermediate-risk patients, the bNED at 5 years was roughly similar with per-

haps a slight edge to implant and radiation. Poorer results were seen in high-risk patients. Potters and colleagues[57] analyzed 1,819 patients treated with radiation, surgery, or implant at Memorial Sloan Kettering at Mercy Medical Center and at the Cleveland Clinic and found equivalent results with all three methods with bNED above 90% at 5 years and bNED of 74 to 79% at 7 years. The conclusion was that any of the three modalities was appropriate and probably equivalent in efficacy. Results will be more determined by risk group factors rather than modality of treatment.

SIDE EFFECTS AND COMPLICATIONS

It is important that clinicians adequately inform prospective patients that permanent prostate radioactive seed implant is likely to produce at least 2 to 6 months of some mild to significant urinary side effects and morbidity, which can include dysuria, weak stream, urgency, frequency, and nocturia. In some cases, symptoms may be prolonged for up to a year. Kang and colleagues[58] evaluated 139 patients and found acute urinary toxicity in 88%, 23% of whom had grade I, 45% grade II, and 20% grade III (RTOG GU toxicity scale[58]) and 14% did require at least 1 week of catheterization. The isotope used (I-125 or Pd-103) made no difference. Higher toxicity correlated with larger prostate volume and more seeds implanted. Locke and colleagues[15] also found size and high AUA score to be risk factors predictive of obstruction. Lee and colleagues[12] evaluated 91 patients and had a 12% incidence of acute obstruction mostly related to prostate volume and number of needles used. Incidence of urethral stricture was 2 to 3%. Merrick and colleagues[59] evaluated 581 patients, some of whom had supplemental external beam radiation and all of whom were started on alpha-blockers 2 weeks before implant and continued until the IPSS returned to baseline. The conclusion was that the use of prophylactic alpha-blockers did decrease the incidence of acute urinary obstruction. Merrick and colleagues[60] also found that return to preimplant IPSS occurred a mean of 3.5 months, although Kang and colleagues[58] reported complete resolution of symptoms could take up to 1 year in some patients. Brown and colleagues[61] found that only 6% of patients had grade 3 GU morbidity at 6 months postimplant. Long-term urinary complications, especially incontinence, may be correlated with

Table 75-2 Implant Alone: Results for Low-Risk Patients

Author	bNED (%)	Follow-Up (yr)
Blasko et al[28]	94	5
Zelefsky et al[29]	88	5
Grimm et al[30]	85	10
Ragde et al[31]	66	10
D'Amico et al[32]	85	5
Stock & Stone[33]	88	5
Potters et al[34]	92	5

bNED = biochemical no evidence of disease.

Table 75-4 Implant Alone: Results for High-Risk Patients

Author	bNED (%)	Follow-Up (yr)
Beyer et al[38]	65	5
Sharkey et al[39]	59	3
Kwok et al[40]	24	7
D'Amico et al[32]	5	5
Zelefsky et al[29]	38	5

bNED = biochemical no evidence of disease.

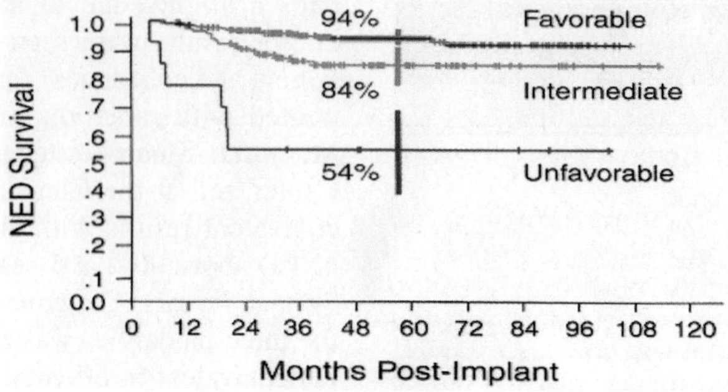

Figure 75-8 Biochemical freedom from recurrence after implant for 403 patients treated with monotherapy. Adapted from Grimm et al.[30]

high urethral dose,[17] which also is a risk factor for prolonged dysuria.[59] Others[61] have suggested that with the use of a peripheral loading technique, the urethral dose may be less an issue in long-term urinary problems. Nevertheless, it is recommended to keep urethral doses as low as possible. This can be achieved by using predominantly a peripheral loading technique, which is now standard. Urinary incontinence is most likely to develop in patients who require a transurethral prostatectomy for obstructive problems. Gelblum, and colleagues[62] found 4% of patients required a TURP for obstructive problems. Hu and Wallner[63] found 10 of 109 implanted patients required a TURP and 7 of those 10 patients had some degree of incontinence. Potters[54] cites a risk of 17% incontinence in patients undergoing a TURP, while Quantara and colleagues[27] cite a risk of 25 to 48% incontinence in TURP patients and emphasizes as do others[54] that surgical intervention should be avoided or delayed as long as possible. We certainly agree with this recommendation. Urinary symptoms should be managed aggressively with alpha-blockers and nonsteroidal anti-inflammatory agents. We have also found that some patients may benefit from brief courses of steroids for exacerbation of symptoms in the postimplant period.

RECTAL TOXICITY

Rectal toxicity with implant only is uncommon. The incidence of radiation proctitis is reported at less than 10% by Snyder and colleagues[65] in 212 patients. Most of the toxicity was grade 2 (RTOG toxicity scale), mostly occurring between the first and second year postimplant, and was related to rectal volume receiving the prescription dose or higher. If greater than 1.3 cc of rectum received the prescription dose or higher, the risk of grade 2 or greater toxicity was 18% versus only 5% if less than 1.3 cc of rectum received the prescription dose. Waterman and Dicker[66] had similar findings, with late GI morbidity of 0.4% if the maximal rectal dose was 150 Gy and 1.2% if the maximal rectal dose was 200 Gy. In neither series was any grade 4 (fistula) or grade 5 (death) toxicity reported. We have found virtually no rectal morbidity with implant only. Merrick and colleagues[67] felt that the addition of supplemental

external beam radiation may have increased rectal toxicity as did Kang and colleagues[68] but again, neither series had any incidence of fistula or death owing to rectal toxicity. Fistula can occur, and the risk is probably increased if areas of radiation proctitis are biopsied; therefore, biopsy of radiation proctitis is contraindicated in most cases. Theodorescu and colleagues[69] reviewed 765 patients treated with prostate brachytherapy, 7 of whom developed fistula between 9 and 12 months postimplant, all of whom had previous biopsies of radiation proctitis, but no risk difference was found whether or not external beam radiation was used. Conservative management and proctitis with rectal steroid enemas, Proctofoam cream, and lasering for bleeding are commonly used for proctitis.

IMPOTENCY

There is a wide range of claims regarding sexual potency after surgery, external beam radiation, and implant. Stock and colleagues[70] found a 6-year potency rate of 59%, Potters and colleagues[74] reported a 52.7% potency rate of 5 years with external beam radiation plus implant, and 76%

Table 75-5 External Beam Radiation and Implant Results for Intermediate- and High-Risk Patients

Intermediate Risk		
Author	bNED (%)	Follow-Up(yr)
Critz et al[41]	75	4
Dattoli et al[42]	79	7
Sylvester et al[44]	77	10
Ragde et al[31]	79	10
Galalae et al[45]	87	5[†]
High Risk		
Author	bNED (%)	Follow-Up (yr)
Stock et al[43]	86	5[*]
Sylvester et al[44]	45	10
Martinez et al[46]	63	5[†]
Critz et al[41]	69	4
Galalae et al[45]	69	5[†]

bNED = biochemical no evidence of disease.
*Patients received 9 months of hormonal therapy.
[†]Brachytherapy was given as high-dose-rate temporary implant.

with implant only. Not surprisingly, the patients receiving adjuvant hormonal therapy plus external beam radiation and implant had only 29% 5-year potency. Merrick and colleagues[75] reported on 209 patients with a 6-year potency rate of only 39% and found preservation to be directly correlated with the degree of preimplant potency and inversely correlated with external beam radiation and diabetes. He noted that Sildenafil seemed to help in most patients with pretreatment potency; 92% of patients who were potent prior to implant who had Sildenafil postimplant were potent or regained potency. Zelefsky and colleagues[71] also reported similar good results after external beam radiation. There are no data yet on newer medications such as Levitra or Cialis.

SAFETY PRECAUTIONS

Michalski and colleagues[72] measured radiation exposures in 44 patients implanted with I-125 or Pd-103 for 3 weeks postimplant. The findings showed that the average spouse would receive 0.2 mSv over 1 year of exposure. The average dose equivalent received in the United States. to the general population owing to environmental and cosmic radiation exposure is 3.6 mSv. Thus, implants give only an additional 5% exposure. Palladium-103, with a lower radiation energy of only 21 KeV versus 28 KeV for iodine-125, gave even less exposure. Smathers and colleagues[73] determined that based on NRC regulations, at 3 feet, it would take a minimum of 1,429 hours to reach the annual exposure limit for I-125 and even longer for a palladium-103. Therefore, general safety to the public and even people in close contact with postimplant patients is not a major concern. However, following the principle of ALARA (as low as reasonably achievable), it is recommended that pregnant women and young children not have prolonged *close* contact with the patient on a daily basis for 2 isotope half-lives (4 months for iodine, 5 weeks for palladium). In general, there is no reason to wear lead shields, though garments providing pelvic shielding are commercially available.

CONCLUSIONS

Prostate brachytherapy, either as monotherapy for low- to intermediate-risk disease or as part of multimodality treatment for intermediate- to

Table 76-6 Implant Quality vs bNED Results

Author		bNED (8 Years) (%)
Kollmeier et al[36]	Optimal implant	82
	Suboptimal implant	68
		bNED (4 Years) (%)
Potters[54]	Optimal implant	95.4
	Suboptimal implant	88

bNED = biochemical no evidence of disease.

high-risk disease, is now well established. Curative results are equivalent to surgery or external beam radiation therapy. With appropriate technique and patient selection, morbidity and complication rates are acceptably low. Investigations for the future will include comparison with temporary high-dose-rate iridium implants, the role of hormonal therapy in combination with seed implant for high-risk patients, and the possible addition of other imaging modalities, such as MRI, to further refine the implant technique.

REFERENCES

1. Hilaris B, Whitmore W, Batata M, Barzell W. Behavioral patterns or prostate adenocarcinoma following I-125 implant and pelvis node dissection. Int J Radiat Oncol Biol Phys 1997;2:631–7.
2. Barringer B. Radium in the treatment of carcinoma of the bladder and prostate. JAMA 1917;68:1227–30.
3. Batata MA, Hilaris BS, Whitmore WF. Factors affecting tumor control. In: Hilaris BS, Batata MA, editors. Brachytherapy oncology: advances in prostate and other cancers. New York: Memorial Sloan Kettering Cancer Center; 1983; p. 65–73.
4. Blasko J, Ragde H, Schumacher D. Transperineal percutaneous iodine-125 implantation of prostatic adenocarcinoma using transrectal ultrasound and template guidance. Endocuriether Hyperthermia Oncol 1987;3:131–9.
5. Holm HH, Juul N, Pedersen JF, et al. Transperineal 125iodine seed implantation in prostatic cancer guided by transrectal ultrasonography. J Urol 1983;130:283–6.
6. Cooperberg M, Lubeck D, Meng M, et al. The changing face of low-risk prostate cancer: trends in clinical presentation and primary management. J Clin Oncol 2004;22:2141–9.
7. Merrick GS, Butler WM, Wallner KE, et al. Long-term quality of life after permanent prostate brachytherapy. Int J Radiat Oncol Biol Phys 2003;56:454–61.
8. Moran BJ, Stutz MA, Gurel MH. Prostate brachytherapy can be performed in selected patients after transurethral resection of the prostate. Int J Radiat Oncol Biol Phys 2004;59:392–6.
9. Wallner K, Lee H, Wasserman S, Dattoli M. Low risk of urinary incontinence following prostate brachytherapy in patients with a prior TURP. Int J Radiat Oncol Biol Phys 1997;37:565–9.
10. Merrick GS, Butler WM, Wallner KE, Galbreath RW. Effect of transurethral resection on urinary quality of life after permanent prostate brachytherapy. Int J Radiat Oncol Biol Phys 2004;58:81–8.
11. Sherertz T, Wallner K, Wang H, et al. Long-term urinary function after transperineal brachytherapy for patient with large glands. Int J Radiat Oncol Biol Phys 2001;51:1241–5.
12. Lee N, Wuu CS, Brody R, et al. Factors predicting for postimplantation urinary retention after permanent prostate brachytherapy. Int J Radiat Oncol Biol Phys 2000;48: 1457–60.
13. Merrick GS, Butler WM, Lief JH, Dorsey AT. Temporal resolution of urinary morbidity following prostate brachytherapy. Int J Radiat Oncol Biol Phys 2000;47:121–8.
14. Crook J, McLean M, Catton C, et al. Factors influencing risk of acute urinary retention after TRUS-guided permanent prostate seed implantation. Int J Radiat Oncol Biol Phys 2002;52:453–60.
15. Locke J, Ellis W, Wallner K, et al. Risk factors for acute urinary retention requiring temporary intermittent catheterization after prostate brachytherapy: a prospective study. Int J Radiat Oncol Biol Phys 2002;52:712–9.
16. Bucci J, Morris WJ, Keyes M, et al. Predictive factor of urinary retention following prostate brachytherapy. Int J Radiat Oncol Biol Phys 2002;53:91–8.
17. McElveen TL, Waterman FM, Kim H, Dicker AP. Factors predicting for urinary incontinence after prostate brachytherapy. Int J Radiat Oncol Biol Phys 2004;59:1395–404.
18. Landis D, Wallner K, Locke J, et al. Late urinary function after prostate brachytherapy. Brachytherapy 2002;1:21–6.
19. Wallner K, Smathers S, Sutlief S, et al. Prostate brachytherapy in patients with median lobe hyperplasia. Int J Cancer 2000;90:152–6.
20. Nag S, Beyer D, Friedland J, et al. American Brachytherapy Society (ABS) recommendations for transperineal permanent brachytherapy of prostate cancer. Int J Radiat Biol Phys 1999;44:789–99.
21. Davis BJ, Pisansky TM, Wilson TM, et al. The radial distance of extraprostatic extension of prostate carcinoma: implications for prostate brachytherapy. Cancer 1999;85:2630–7.
22. Cha CM, Potters L, Ashley R, et al. Isotope selection for patient undergoing prostate brachytherapy. Int J Radiat Biol Phys 1999;45:391–5.
23. Wallner K, Merrick G, True L, et al. 125I versus 103Pd for low-risk prostate cancer: preliminary PSA outcomes from a prospective randomized multicenter trial. Int J Radiat Biol Phys 2003;57:1297–303.
24. Stone NN, Stock RG. Real-time interactive seed implantation. In: Smith AD, Badlani GH, Bagley DH, et al, editors. Smith's textbook of endourology. St. Louis, MO: Quality Medical Publishing; 1996. p.
25. Nag S, Bice W, DeWyngaert K, et al. The American Brachytherapy Society recommendations for permanent prostate brachytherapy postimplant dosimetric analysis. Int J Radiat Biol Phys 2000;46:221–30.
26. Gray JR, Merrick GS, Beyer DC, et al. Comparative analysis of prostate brachytherapy pre-planning. Radiother Oncol 2000;55:42–3.
27. Quantara BP, Marks LB, Anscher MS. Comparing radical prostatectomy and brachytherapy for localized prostate cancer. Oncology 2004;18:1289–302.
28. Blasko JC, Grimm PD, Sylvester JE, et al. Palladium-103 brachytherapy for prostate carcinoma. Int J Radiat Biol Phys 2000;46:839–50.
29. Zelefsky MJ, Hollister T, Raben A, et al. Five-year biochemical outcome and toxicity with transperineal CT-planned permanent I-125 prostate implantation for patients with localized prostate cancer. Int J Radiat Biol Phys 2000;47:1261–6.
30. Grimm P, Blasko J, Sylvester JE, et al. 10-year biochemical (prostate-specific antigen) control of prostate cancer with I-125 brachytherapy. Int J Radiat Biol Phys 2001;51:31–40.
31. Ragde H, Korb LJ, Elgamal AA, et al. Modern prostate brachytherapy. Prostate-specific antigen results in 219 patients with up to 12 years of follow-up. Cancer 2000; 89:135–41.
32. D'Amico AV, Whittington R, Malkowicz SB, et al. Biochemical outcome after radical prostatectomy, external beam radiation therapy, or interstitial radiation therapy for clinically localized prostate cancer. JAMA 1998;280:969–74.
33. Stock RG, Stone NN. The effect of prognostic factors in therapeutic outcome following transperineal prostate brachytherapy. Semin Surg Oncol 1997;13:454–60.
34. Potters L, Cha C, Oshinsky G, et al. Risk profiles to predict PSA relapse-free survival for patients undergoing prostate brachytherapy. Cancer J Sci Am 1999;5:301–6.
35. Stokes SH. Comparison of biochemical disease-free survival of patients with localized carcinoma of the prostate undergoing radical prostatectomy, transperineal ultrasound-guided radioactive seed implantation, or definitive external beam irradiation. Int J Radiat Biol Phys 2000;47: 129–36.
36. Kollmeier MA, Stock RG, Stone N. Biochemical outcomes after prostate brachytherapy with 5 year minimum follow-up: importance of patient selection and implant quality. Int J Radiat Biol Phys 2003;57:645–53.
37. Brachman DG, Thomas T, Hilbe J, Beyer DC, et al. Failure-free survival following brachytherapy alone or with external beam irradiation alone for T1-2 prostate tumors in 2222 patients: results from a single practice. Int J Radiat Biol Phys 2000;48:111–7.
38. Beyer D. Permanent prostate brachytherapy: the Arizona experience. Radiother Oncol 2000;55:13–4.
39. Sharkey J, Cantor A, Solc Z, et al. Brachytherapy versus radical prostatectomy in patients with clinically localized prostate cancer. Curr Urol Rep 2002;3:250–7.
40. Kwok Y, DiBiase SJ, Amin P, et al. Risk group stratification in patients undergoing permanent I-125 prostate brachytherapy as monotherapy. Int J Radiat Biol Phys 2002:53:588–94.
41. Critz FA, Williams WH, Levinson AK, et al. Simultaneous irradiation for prostate cancer: intermediate results with medial techniques. J Urol 2000;164(3 Pt 1):738–41.
42. Dattoli M, Wallner K, True L, et al. Long-term outcomes after treatment with external beam radiation therapy and palladium 103 for patients with high-risk prostate carcinoma: influence of prostatic acid phosphatase. Cancer 2003;97: 979–83.
43. Stock RG, Cahlon O, Cesaretti JA, et al. Combined modality treatment in the management of high-risk prostate cancer. Int J Radiat Biol Phys 2004;59:1352–9.
44. Sylvester JE, Blasko JC, Grimm PD, et al. Ten-year biochemical relapse-free survival after external beam radiation and brachytherapy for localized prostate cancer: the Seattle experience. Int J Radiat Biol Phys 2003;57:944–52.
45. Galalae RM, Martinez A, Mate T, et al. Long-term outcome by risk factors using conformal high-dose-rate brachytherapy (HDR-BT) boost with or without neoadjuvant androgen suppression for localized prostate cancer. Int J Radiat Biol Phys 2004;58:1048–55.
46. Martinez AA, Kestin LL, Stromberg JS, et al. Interim report of image-guided conformal high-dose-rate brachytherapy for patients with unfavorable prostate cancer: the William Beamont phase II dose-escalating trial. Int J Radiat Biol Phys 2000;47:343–52.
47. Kestin LL., Martinez AA, Stromberg JS, et al. Matched-pair analysis of conformal high-dose-rate brachytherapy boost versus external-beam radiation therapy alone for locally advanced prostate cancer. J Clin Oncol 2000;18:2869–80.
48. Potters L, Cha C, Oshinsky G, et al. Risk profiles to predict PSA relapse-free survival for patients undergoing permanent prostate brachytherapy. Cancer J Sci Am 1999;5:301–6.
49. Lawton CA, Winter K, Murray K, et al. Updated results of the phase III radiation therapy oncology group (RTOG) trial 85-31 evaluating the potential benefit of androgen suppression following standard radiation therapy for unfavorable prognosis carcinoma of the prostate. Int J Radiat Biol Phys 2001;49:937–46.
50. Pilepich MV, Winter K, John MJ, et al. Phase III radiation therapy oncology group (RTOG) trial 86-10 of androgen deprivation before and during radiotherapy in locally advanced prostate cancer. Int J Radiat Biol Phys 2001;50: 1243–52.
51. Bolla M, Collette C, Blank L, et al. Long-term results with immediate androgen suppression and external irradiation in patients with locally advanced prostate cancer (an EORTC study): a phase III randomised trial. Lancet 2002;360:103–6.
52. Lee LN, Stock RG, Stone NN. Role of hormonal therapy in the management of intermediate- to high-risk prostate cancer treated with permanent seed implantation. Int J Radiat Biol Phys 2002;52:444–52.
53. Potters L, Torre T, Ashley R, Leibel S. Examining the role of neoadjuvant androgen deprivation in patient undergoing prostate brachytherapy. J Clin Oncol 2000;18:1187–92.
54. Potters L. Permanent prostate brachytherapy: lessons learned, lessons to learn. Oncology 2000;14:981–91.
55. Stock RG, Stone NN, Talbert A, et al. A dose-response study for I-125 prostate implants. Int J Radiat Biol Phys 1998;41:101–8.
56. Merrick GS, Butler WM, Galbreath RW, Lief JH. Five-year biochemical outcome following permanent interstitial brachytherapy for clinical T1-T3 prostate cancer. Int J Radiat Biol Phys 2001;51:41–8.
57. Potters L, Klein EA, Kattan MW, et al. Monotherapy for stage T1-T2 prostate cancer: radical prostatectomy, external beam radiotherapy, or permanent seed implantation. Radiother Oncol 2004;71:29–33.
58. Kang SK, Chou RH, Dodge RK, et al. Acute urinary toxicity following transperineal prostate brachytherapy using a modified Quimby loading method. Int J Radiat Biol Phys 2001;50:937–45.
59. Merrick GS, Butler WM, Wallner KE, et al. Dysuria after permanent prostate brachytherapy. Int J Radiat Biol Phys 2003;55:979–85.
60. Merrick GS, Butler WM, Lief JH, Dorsey AT. Temporal resolution of urinary morbidity following prostate brachytherapy. Int J Radiat Biol Phys 2000;47:121–8.
61. Brown D, Colonias A, Miller R, et al. Urinary morbidity with a modified peripheral loading technique of transperineal (125)i prostate implantation. Int J Radiat Biol Phys 2000;47:353–60.
62. Gelblum DY, Potters L, Ashley R, et al. Urinary morbidity following ultrasound-guided transperineal prostate seed implantation. Int J Radiat Biol Phys 1999;45:59–67.
63. Hu K, Wallner K. Urinary incontinence in patients who had a TURP/TUIP following prostate brachytherapy. Int J Radiat Biol Phys 1998;40:783–6.
64. Beyer DC. Complications and late toxicity following permanent prostate brachytherapy. Int J Radiat Biol Phys 1998; 42:309.
65. Snyder KM, Stock RG, Hong SM, et al. Defining the risk of developing grade 2 proctitis following 125I prostate brachytherapy using a rectal dose-volume histogram analysis. Int J Radiat Biol Phys 2001;50:335–41.
66. Waterman FM, Dicker AP. Probability of late rectal morbidity in 125I prostate brachytherapy. Int J Radiat Biol Phys 2003;55:342–53.

67. Merrick GS, Butler WM, Wallner KE, et al. Late rectal function after prostate brachytherapy. Int J Radiat Biol Phys 2003;57:42–8.

68. Kang SK, Chou RH, Dodge RK, et al. Gastrointestinal toxicity of transperineal interstitial prostate brachytherapy. Int J Radiat Biol Phys 2002;53:99–103.

69. Theodorescu D, Gillenwater JY, Koutrouvelis PG. Prostate-urethral fistula after prostate brachytherapy. Cancer 2000;89:2085–91.

70. Stock RG, Kao A, Stone NN. Penile erectile function after permanent radioactive seed implantation for treatment of prostate cancer. J Urol 2001;165:436–9.

71. Zelefsky MJ, McKee AB, Lee H, Leibel SA. Efficacy of oral sildenafil in patients with erectile dysfunction after radiotherapy for carcinoma of the prostate. Urology 1999; 53:775–8.

72. Michalski J, Mutic S, Eichling J, Ahmed SN. Radiation exposure to family and household members after prostate brachytherapy. Int J Radiat Biol Phys 2003;56:764–8.

73. Smathers S, Wallner K, Korssjoen T, et al. Radiation safety parameters following prostate brachytherapy. Int J Radiat Biol Phys 1999;45:397–9.

74. Potters L, Torre T, Fearn PA, et al. Potency after permanent prostate brachytherapy for localized prostate cancer. Int J Radiat Biol Phys 2001;50:1235–42.

75. Merrick GS, Butler WM, Lief JH, et al. Efficacy of sildenafil citrate in prostate brachytherapy patients with erectile dysfunction. Urology 1999;53:1112–6.

76

Cryoablation of the Prostate: Minimally Invasive and Minimally Morbid Management of Prostate Cancer

Aaron E. Katz, MD

John C. Rewcastle, PhD

The American Cancer Society estimates that each year there will be approximately 200,000 new cases of prostate cancer diagnosed and that the disease will claim 30,000 lives in the United States alone. After skin cancer, prostate cancer has become the most commonly diagnosed cancer in North American men and is the second most common cause of cancer death in males, following lung cancer.[1] Since the introduction of widespread prostate-specific antigen (PSA) screening for prostate cancer, proportionally more men are now being diagnosed in the early stages of the disease when local cure is possible. Although the optimal treatment for localized disease is unclear, there has been a recent strong movement within urologic oncology toward minimally invasive therapies. Three prime examples of this for prostate cancer are laparoscopic radical prostatectomy, brachytherapy, and cryoablation. The goals of minimally invasive therapies for a malignancy of a solid organ are to eradicate the local disease, shorten hospital stay, limit postoperative morbidities, quicken return to daily functions and work, and to reduce the overall cost of the procedure. Although some of these therapies are relatively new, they are gaining popularity rather quickly, and several worldwide experiences have demonstrated that they are quite effective at achieving most of all these goals.[2]

The interest among urologists in prostate cryoablation is both as a primary therapy as well as a salvage therapy following failed radiation therapy. Cryoablation is defined as the in situ freezing of a tissue. The goals of cryoablation for prostate cancer are to ablate the entire gland, rendering the patient free of disease while preventing the freezing of surrounding structures such as the bladder, rectum, and external striated sphincter. Currently the procedure is performed percutaneously, introducing small cryoprobes through the perineal skin into the gland. The ideal probe locations within the prostate are determined using an intraoperative treatment planning system, and placement of the cryoprobes is performed using ultrasound guidance. Modern techniques of cryoablation include the use of an argon-based cryoablation system (as opposed to liquid nitrogen) and thermocouples to measure temperature at strategic locations in and around the prostate.

HISTORY OF CRYOABLATION

Cryoablation has been used for the treatment of many benign and malignant conditions. The use of freezing techniques in the treatment of carcinoma began in London during the 1850s when "iced" (–18°C to –22°C) saline solutions were used to treat advanced carcinoma of the breast, uterus, and cervix.[3] In 1907 cryoablation was used in dermatologic patients, with the reported cure rate for skin cancer equal to that obtained by surgical excision. In recent years, cryoablation has been used in the treatment of a wide variety of diseases, including liver, kidney, lung, and prostate malignancies.[4] The first use of transurethral cryoablation of the prostate in humans was reported in 1966.[5] However, several problems became apparent. Gross urethral sloughing, severe bladder outlet obstruction, and prolonged hospitalizations were observed.[5–7] Flocks modified the technique in 1969 to involve the open perineal exposure of the posterior prostate surface with direct application of the cryoprobes.[8] This approach produced much less urethral sloughing than the transurethral approach.[9] However, effective monitoring of the iceball in both techniques was inadequate or absent. This caused freezing of the surrounding structures and complications such as fistulas as well as urinary and fecal incontinence to be observed in a significant number of patients undergoing this operation.[10,11]

In 1993, after the development of transrectal ultrasound (TRUS), which allows for real-time imaging of the prostate, Onik and colleagues described a modification of the technique in which cryoprobes were guided into the prostate using TRUS visualization via a percutaneous transperineal approach.[12] TRUS was also used to visualize the propagation of the iceball.

Although TRUS allowed for unprecedented visualization during prostate cryoablation, it was not without limitation. Incident sonographic waves are reflected almost completely at the interface between frozen and unfrozen tissue. This allows for accurate visualization of the proximal iceball edge, which is seen as a hyperechoic rim, but renders the user blind to all distal tissues frozen or unfrozen.

Thermocouple monitoring was introduced as a means of determining temperatures within the iceball. Thermocouples can also be placed transperineally under TRUS guidance and will read the temperature of the tissue into which their tips have been placed long after TRUS visualization of that location is no longer possible. This allows the physician to ensure sufficient cold temperatures are reached within and at the margin of the prostate, while maintaining nonablative temperatures in sensitive adjacent anatomy (ie, the striated external sphincter and the rectum).

Treatment planning algorithms have also recently become available that, based on individual patient anatomy, determine the most efficient number of cryoprobes to be used and their optimal placement. This has resulted in a significant reduction of the learning curve associated with the procedure.

MECHANISMS OF TISSUE INJURY DURING CRYOABLATION

Freezing and thawing tissue results in necrosis. It is important to note that cryoablation injures not only individual cells at the time of therapy (direct damage), but also the tissue as a whole by impairing the microvasculature (indirect damage).[13] Unlike radiation, the ability of cryoablation to eradicate a tumor is not dependent on the nuclear characteristics of individual cells, but rather on the ability to expose the entire tumor volume to a lethal freezing process. Cellular survival during cryoablation not only depends on the freezing and thawing rates, but, most importantly, also on the lowest temperature reached and the hold time at subzero temperatures.[14] During cryoablation, ice, which is essentially pure water, initially forms outside the cell, increasing the extracellular concentration. It does not form initially inside the cells because the lipid membrane blocks ice crystal growth, resulting in an osmotic imbalance. Direct cellular injury can result and is due to two damage mechanisms: intracellular ice formation (IIF) and solution effects.

Freezing rates are high enough only within a few millimeters of the cryoprobe to induce IIF.[15,16] Although IIF is usually a lethal event associated with irreversible membrane damage, it is not known if cell death is a cause or a result of IIF, and several mechanistic theories exist.[17–23]

Most of the iceball experiences lower freezing rates that lead to cellular dehydration resulting from the osmotic imbalance.[15,16] This mechanism has been termed "solution effects," and there exist several hypotheses, but no consensus, as to its physical basis. Resulting solute concentration alone has been held responsible for the damage,[24] as has attainment of a critical minimum volume shrinking beyond which damages the membrane.[25,26] Recently, Muldrew and colleagues speculated that proteins with salt bridges within the cytoplasm (salt into) solution are due to exposure to high salt concentrations.[27,28] This lowers the intracellular salt concentration, causing salt to move through the cation channels into the cytoplasm. On thawing, the proteins will reform their salt bridges and release the salt owing to the dilution of the cytoplasm with water influx.

Direct injury does not completely destroy all cells. In the hours and days following cryoablation, indirect damage occurs. Microvasculature endothelial cells are also damaged by the direct injury mechanisms, resulting in platelet aggregation, leading to vascular stasis, resulting in ischemic necrosis. This greatly enhances cell kill within the iceball and may be the dominant killing mechanism during cryosurgery.[29,30] In vitro studies have shown that induced apoptosis may also play a role.[30] Enhancing apoptosis with adjuvant chemotherapy may indeed lead to a significant increase in in vivo cryoinjury, and investigations are ongoing.[31] There also exists some evidence of an immunologic response to cryoablation, but experimental results have been inconsistent, and its existence, let alone significance, remains controversial.[13]

CLINICAL ENDPOINTS

Temperature is the easiest parameter to measure during cryoablation and defines the clinical endpoints. The goal of cryoablation is to decrease the target volume temperature to or below a critical temperature that correlates with cancer control as verified by thermocouple readings. This is a tissue-dependent temperature and, for double freeze-thaw cycle prostate cryoablation the critical temperature is between –20° and –40°C. The lower end of this range was determined in multiple in vitro cryobiology studies[15,32] and in an in vivo human clinical trial.[33] It was shown that achievement of –40°C during two separate freeze-thaw cycles leads to confluent necrosis, and further decreasing the tissue temperature will not result in further biologic damage. This is juxtaposed by excellent published clinical results obtained using a target temperature of –20°C.

Although at least –20°C is required to achieve confluent necrosis sufficient for cancer control, warmer subzero temperatures are sufficient to lead to complications. As such, sensitive adjacent structures must remain unfrozen during the procedure.

The increase in thawing rate resulting from an active thaw is minimal insofar as cellular effect is concerned, and use of an active thaw to optimize procedural time will not compromise clinical outcome.[34]

Cryoablation should be performed with the intent of reaching at least –20°C throughout the entire target tissue volume, and colder if possible, recognizing that no further biologic damage occurs below –40°C. This needs to be done while not exposing the rectum and the striated external sphincter to subfreezing temperatures.

The injury sustained by tissues exposed to subzero temperatures results in damage to the tissue as a whole and is independent of the characteristics of the individual cells. If the cancer is completely contained within the volume that reaches sufficiently cold temperatures, it will be completely ablated regardless of Gleason score and ploidy status.

PATIENT SELECTION

Cryoablation is a definitive local therapy aimed at the complete ablation of the prostate. Any patient with biopsy-proven adenocarcinoma of the prostate can be considered for prostate cryoablation provided the disease is localized (T1-3, N0, M0). This includes patients who have not had any previous definitive prostate cancer therapy and those with a local recurrence following any form of radiation therapy, including brachytherapy.

The anatomic characteristics of the prostate must be considered. The ideal gland volume for cryoablation is between 20 and 35 cc as determined with transrectal ultrasound (TRUS). Although it is certainly possible to treat larger glands, they are more clinically challenging and, generally, a volume greater than 65 cc is considered a contraindication. However, a 3- to 6-month trial of hormone therapy often results in a sufficient volume decrease to allow for effective therapy. Prior transurethral resection of the prostate (TURP) is considered a contraindication as it does not allow for sufficient contact between the urethral warmer and the urethra to avoid urinary complications. It is advised that if cryosurgery is to be performed in a patient with a history of a prior TURP, a transrectal ultrasound be performed in the office prior to cryoablation. If there is a persistent TUR defect on TRUS, cryoablation could result in an increased risk of urethral sloughing and urinary incontinence.

TECHNIQUE

PREPARATION OF THE PATIENT Patients are given a Fleet enema on the morning of the procedure and Flagyl 500 mg IV at the start of the procedure. Cryosurgical ablation of the prostate can be performed under spinal or general anesthesia. The patient is placed in a standard lithotomy position, and the external genitalia, lower abdominal wall, and perineum are draped and prepped in the usual sterile manner. Initially, an 18 French (F) Foley catheter is placed into the bladder and the bladder is distended with 300 cc of sterile water.

The Foley is left indwelling and clamped to allow the bladder to remain distended, and so that the urethra can be visualized under ultrasound. The scrotal skin is then tacked up to the anterior abdominal wall with two small towel clips, allowing the surgeon to have exposure to the perineum. At this point a transrectal ultrasound is introduced into the rectum and connected to a brachytherapy-like stand. This allows for accurate measurements of the gland to be performed using both the transverse and longitudinal planes. At our institution, we have used a B & K 7.5 mHz probe and a Barzell-Whitmore stand.

TREATMENT PLANNING AND CRYOPROBE PLACEMENT Prostate cryoablation is performed with the goal of enclosing the prostate within a temperature thought to ensure confluent necrosis while minimizing collateral damage. Given that cryoprobe placement has been characterized and accurately modeled, the determination of an optimal probe placement becomes a mathematical problem.[35] Optimization algorithms based on objective functions have been used, but the computational time is on the order of hours, and is therefore not practical intraoperatively.[36] Fortunately, consistent cryoprobe performance allows for geometric optimization that can be performed on the order of seconds. Commercially available treatment planning systems use algorithms based on four accepted "rules" of cryoprobe placement as reported by Ellis[61]:

1. Cryoprobes of 2.4 mm should not be placed more than 2.0 cm apart
2. Cryoprobes should not be placed more than 1.0 cm from the margin of the prostate
3. The distance between the urethra and any cryoprobe should not be less than 0.8 cm
4. The posterior cryoprobes should be placed such that their separation is less than twice the distance to the posterior capsule of the prostate

The prostate is imaged using real-time TRUS. Further, the transducer is fixed in space using an arm fixed to the operating table and a stepper similar to those used during prostate brachytherapy. These images are transferred to a treatment planning system hardwired to the ultrasound. Image recognition software is used with the aid of anatomic reference points defined by the user to determine the geometric anatomy of the prostate, urethra, and rectum. Using this information, a geometric probe optimization is performed that recommends to the user the number of cryoprobes (typically 6–8) as well as their individual locations in the transverse plane.

The recommended cryoprobe locations correlate to the holes in a brachytherapy-like grid that is fixed to the ultrasound stepper and placed as close as possible to the perineum. Trocar-tipped 2.4 mm diameter cryoprobes with insulated shafts are guided into the prostate by first passing through the appropriate holes in the grid then passing transperineally into the prostate. Probe depth is guided in the sagittal plane and cryoprobe tips are advanced to the base of the gland.

The grid can be removed from the platform and the stepper, and then the ultrasound probe can be used freehand, unobstructed by the stepper or grid. The platform has release levers so that the grid is detached with little effort and no disturbance to probe placements. Because the grid is lightweight plastic, it will not pull the probes out of the body when released from the platform.

The grid is almost 2 cm thick to provide stable, parallel probe placement. Note that the 2.4 mm probes are rigid enough that they are not deflected as they pass through the body, even in the presence of calcifications. If angling is desired or in the uncommon but possible case where additional probe length is needed, the grid can be reduced to only 3 mm thick. By unclipping the front panel of the grid and removing it, only one thin side of the grid remains. This side is also labeled with grid coordinates to help in placement. The panel removal must be done prior to placing any probes, but may be done after the grid is assembled to the platform and stepper.

Thermocouple placement is also aided by the treatment planning system. Each thermocouple is mapped on the system and the computer determines the correlating hole on the grid through which the thermocouple should be placed. As with the placement of the cryoprobes, the guidance of the thermocouple to the desired depth is monitored in the sagittal plane.

PROCEDURAL CYSTOSCOPY, EXTERNAL SPHINCTER THERMOCOUPLE PLACEMENT, AND URETHRAL WARMER PLACEMENT   Once all cryoprobes and thermocouples are inserted, the indwelling Foley catheter is removed and a flexible cystoscope is preformed. The flexile scope is passed into the prostatic urethra where inspection of this area is carefully performed. If one or more cryoprobes are seen in the urethra, it must be removed and re-inserted under ultrasound guidance. The cystoscope is then advanced into the bladder, and a punch suprapubic cystostomy tube can be placed under direct visualization. The scope is then brought back to the area of the external sphincter and a thermocouple device can be guided via the grid and passed through perineal skin and into the sphincter. The placement of the temperature probe can be checked using both the cystoscope and TRUS. Use of the external sphincter temperature probe has dramatically reduced the incidence of urinary incontinence following cryoablation. Finally, the cystoscope can be passed into the bladder again and a glide (or guide) wire is inserted through the scope. The scope is removed, and over the wire, a councill-tipped urethral warming device is inserted and left in the urethra. The warmer continuously circulates, in a closed loop, saline warmed to and maintained at 39°C throughout the procedure. This allows the inner lumen of the urethra to remain unfrozen, thus preserving its integrity. The warmer is left in place until after the conclusion as well as for 2 hours in the recovery room.

FREEZING OF THE PROSTATE

Prior to the initiation of the freezing process, the surgeon must make sure that the tip of each probe is positioned such that it lies at the base of the prostate. The freezing is conducted in an anterior to posterior manner. Sonographically, only the near edge of the iceball can be visualized because near complete reflection of the incident sound waves at the frozen/unfrozen interface renders the user blind to all beyond the proximal ice margin. Activation of the probes results in the circulation of argon gas through the probes. When the gas reaches the tip it undergoes a rapid expansion from high to low pressure. Argon gas decreases in temperature during this expansion known as the Joule-Thompson effect and results in a temperature of –186°C inside the cryoprobe tip. Convective energy transfer results in the decreasing tissue temperatures around the cryoprobe and the formation of ice inside the tissue. The power of the cryoprobes can be controlled in 5% increments from 5 to 100%, allowing for different speeds of freezing that may be desired based on anatomic considerations and physician preferences.

Once in position, the anterior probes are initiated first. This will generate a core of central ice within the gland. The lateral probes can then be turned on, resulting in ice formation to and beyond the lateral margins of the prostate. Freezing should continue until a reading of –40°C is observed in both lateral thermocouples placed near the neurovascular bundles. Once achieved, the posterior medial probes are activated. Temperature as measured by the temperature probe in the Denonvilliers' fascia will decrease and should continue until sufficiently cold temperatures are achieved. The hyperechoic rim of the iceball is used to monitor the progression of the ice as it nears the anterior rectal wall. Once lethal temperatures are confirmed in this region, the argon gas can be turned off. The primary endpoint in this region is the safety of the rectal wall. If the iceball appears to be encroaching on the rectal wall, the probes should be turned off, regardless of the thermocouple reading, to avoid injury.

At this point, the gland is completely engulfed in ice and no visible prostate tissue should be seen. Once this is achieved, all cryoprobes are warmed by allowing helium gas to flow through them. Helium warms when undergoing the Joule-Thompson effect. Active warming continues until the gland is completely thawed as indicated by positive temperature readings from all temperature probes and no visual ice on TRUS. A second freeze-thaw cycle is initiated after checking that none of the cryoprobes or thermocouples have moved. Following completion of the second freeze-thaw cycle, cryoprobes and temperature probes are removed and compression is held on the perineum for several minutes. Suturing the puncture sites is not often done, as digital pressure is usually sufficient to stop bleeding. The patient is then transferred to the recovery room. It is the authors' preference to continue the urethral warming catheter for 2 hours.

There now exists an alterative to manual control of the cryoprobes. Autofreeze is a commercially available software that allows targeted temperatures to be inputted by the user for each thermocouple placed. Typically, these are –40°C for the thermocouples placed in zones to ensure ablation and +10°C for those placed in sensitive structures to ensure their preservation. Once the values have been set, the user double-checks the cryoprobe and thermocouple locations, and when satisfied initiates the freeze process. All cryoprobes are controlled by the computer that determines optimal settings and powers based on temperature recorded at the thermocouple tips. Freezing commences in an anterior to posterior manner to maximize transrectal ultrasound visualization. Once the anterior iceballs coalesce, the later cryoprobes are operated. On reaching the target temperature of the anterior thermocouple, the anterior cryoprobes are operated to maintain that temperature within 5°C of the target. In a similar fashion, the lateral probes are operated until the target temperatures are reached in each neurovascular bundle. These temperatures are then maintained by the computer.

Overly aggressive posterior cryoprobe operation can lead to rectal complications. As such, these probes are initiated at no more than 25% power and are terminated once the target temperatures are reached. Also, if the temperature reading of the thermocouple located in the external sphincter decreases below the target temperature, all the cryoprobes are simultaneously warmed to ensure viable functionality of the external sphincter. Clinical validation of this software is ongoing.

POSTOPERATIVE CARE

Patients are routinely discharged home the following morning with oral antibiotics (ciprofloxacin 500 mg bid) for 5 days. The suprapubic tube is left open for several days. Patients are instructed to clamp the tube on postoperative day 4. If the patient is voiding well with minimal postvoid residual urine (< 100 cc), the tube can be removed. It is the author's experience (AEK) that 90% of the patients can have the tube removed 1 week following cryoablation.

For salvage cryoablation patients, the use of anticholinergic medications may be useful to prevent or decrease the amount of urinary urgency. Although there is no prospective trial to date that has investigated the prophylactic use of anticholinergic medications, it is the authors' opinion that these medications may be used empirically following salvage cryoablation, and continued for several weeks. The follow-up schedule used is identical to that used following any definitive local therapy for prostate cancer. The nadir PSA value after cryosurgery is around 6 to 8 weeks after the procedure.

RESULTS AND COMPARISON WITH OTHER TREATMENT ALTERNATIVES

Over the past decade, several institutions have published cryoablation results. Many of the published series from the early to mid-1990s report significant complication rates. Despite the inability to adequately control ice formation and treat only the prostate without compromising proximal anatomic structures in this "early" cryoablation period, follow-up PSA and biopsy data indicate that cryoablation could eradicate both radioresistant and previously untreated prostate cancer.

The high morbidity presented in these reports can be attributed to several factors. For one, the use of thermocouples was not universal at the time of these reports. In addition, there was a period when the urethral warming device was banned by the United States Food and Drug Administration. Without proper warming, urethral sloughing was prevalent and patients developed pain, urinary retention, urinary sloughing, and urinary incontinence. Furthermore, several of theses studies were performed using a liquid-nitrogen-based system. Although the delivery of cold temperatures into the gland was rapid, the ability to control the growth of the iceball was limited, especially in the absence of temperature monitoring. Lastly, suboptimal placement of the cryoprobes was a major contributing factor to the development or rectal fistulas. The second generation of cryosurgical devices has led to significant advances in the technology that cannot be understated. The modern cryoablation procedure consists of an argon-based system in which the urethra is maintained at nonablative temperatures with an FDA-approved warming device, and temperatures are monitored at strategic locations with thermocouples. The following analysis of published results is limited to those series in which, at least, the latter two standards were used.

ROLE OF CRYOABLATION AS A PRIMARY PROSTATE CANCER THERAPY

EFFICACY The comparative analysis that follows is based on all studies of primary prostate cancer therapies reporting 5-year biochemical disease-free survival (BDFS) that have been published as full manuscripts in the peer-reviewed literature in the past 10 years (1992–2002) and stratified by risk groups generally defined as the following:

1. Low risk: Stage T1-T2a, Gleason $\leq$ 6 and PSA < 10
2. Moderate risk: one of the following: stage > T2a, Gleason > 6, or PSA > 10
3. High risk: two or more of the following: stage > T2a, Gleason > 6, or PSA > 10

Although there is no consistency in BDFS definitions, there certainly is merit in this analysis, which is intended to look for trends and is not designed to conclusively compare the different therapies.

Figure 76-1, A to C shows the published range of BDFS for each therapy observed 5 years following therapy. Note that high-intensity-focused ultrasound does not appear in this comparison, as there are no 5-year reports of its efficacy.

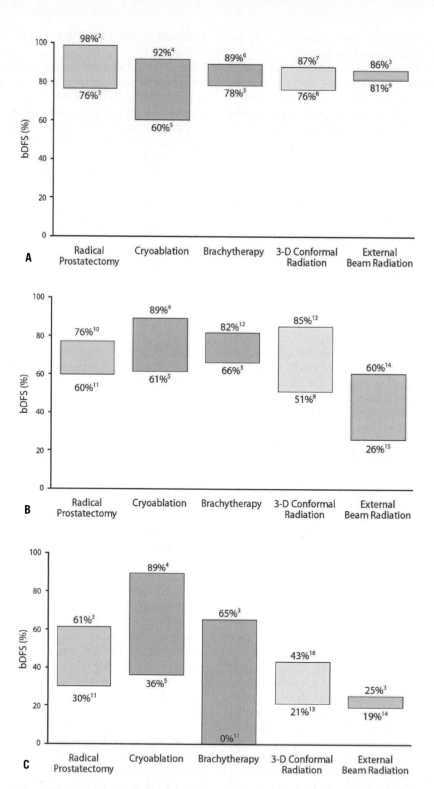

Figure 76-1 *A*, The range biochemical disease-free rates reported in the last 10 years for a low-risk disease; *B*, for a moderate-risk disease; and *C*, for a high-risk disease.

For low-risk disease, all the currently available treatment modalities (radical prostatectomy, cryoablation, brachytherapy, 3-D conformational radiation, and external beam radiation) achieve excellent local and systemic control (see Figure 76-1).[37–44] Given the relative equivalence in efficacy, the treatment decisions for patients with low-risk disease are based more on morbidity and quality of life factors rather than the ability to cure the cancer. Notably, the durable long-term results (> 15-year follow-up) available for radi-

cal prostatectomy reinforce its role as the gold-standard therapy for localized prostate cancer.

More uncertainty arises in determining the optimal approach for patients with moderate- and high-risk disease. Figures 76-1B[38–40,43,45–49] and 76-1-C[38–40,43,45,48] compare the range of reported BDFS for patients with moderate- and high-risk disease. Compared with Figure 76-1A, a drop in efficacy is observed for all therapies with increasing disease risk. However, the drop is not as substantial for cryoablation as it is for both surgical and radiation series. Based on this comparison, the efficacy of cryosurgery appears to be at least equivalent, if not superior, to all forms of radiation therapy and surgery for moderate- and high-risk patients.

Further, among the recent cryoablation studies, biopsy results were reported by Bahn and colleagues[39] and Donnelly and colleagues.[51] Bahn, with a mean follow-up of 5.72 years, found an overall rate of positive biopsy of 13%, while Donnelly observed 72 of the 73 patients in his study to be negative for local malignancy. The biopsy outcomes found in the literature for brachytherapy, conformal beam radiation, and external beam radiation are less compelling. Percentages of positive biopsy findings in brachytherapy studies ranged from 5 to 26%,[41,52,53] with mean follow-up periods of 18 months to 10 years. It should be noted that the study that produced the 5% positive biopsy finding[41] consisted of a highly selected study population composed solely of patients with low pretreatment PSA levels and with disease characterized by slow-growing, mildly aggressive tumor in the early clinical stages. Percentage of positive biopsy findings in conformal beam radiation was 48% at a mean follow-up of > 30 months,[54] and the percentage of positive biopsy results in studies of external beam radiation therapy ranged from 20 to 71%, with mean follow-up of 2 to 6.8 years.[55–59] These results are summarized in Table 76-1.[41,52–61]

MORBIDITY

The ability of cryoablation to effectively ablate tissue has never been questioned. Akin to radiation, the question has been whether a sufficient dose of cold could be delivered to effectively treat the cancer without an unacceptable morbidity. The morbidity associated with prostate cryoablation has steadily declined with advances in technology, refinements in clinical protocol, and greater understanding of cryobiology.[60] The latest studies illustrate the very low rates of morbidity associated with the current practice of cryoablation in comparison with other prostate cancer therapies.

It is well known that the lives of prostate cancer patients who have received treatment for localized cancer are impacted greatest by adverse changes in bowel, bladder, and sexual functioning. Of the three latest cryoablation studies,[39,51,61] only one found rectal complications (Bahn and colleagues[39] with fistula < 0.1%), while rates of incontinence in the three studies ranged from 1.3 to 5.4% and rates of postoperative impotence ranged from 82.4 to 100%. In contrast to the low morbidity exhibited in the latest cryoablation studies are the bowel, bladder, and potency data taken from several studies involving radical surgery and beam radiation.

Among radical surgery studies, rates of bowel urgency ranged from 6 to 16%,[62,63] rectal bleeding ranged from 1 to 3%,[63,64] and diarrhea ranged from 6 to 19%.[62,64] Among recipients of beam radiation, bowel urgency ranged from 19 to 43%,[62,63] rectal bleeding from 13 to 17%,[63,64] and diarrhea from 12 to 42%.[62,64] Urinary morbidity among radical surgery patients included permanent incontinence in 7 to 52%,[63,65] while urinary morbidity among beam radiation patients included incontinence in 0 to 15%.[63,64] Incontinence in all studies was defined as the use of at least one pad per day.

Impotence occurred at a rate of 51 to 96% in radical surgery studies,[64,66] and at a rate of 50 to 61% in beam radiation studies.[63,67] All studies reviewed used patient-derived, rather than physician-derived information. There is wide variation in the reporting of morbidity data in studies of treatment of primary prostate cancer. It is believed that patient-derived information is more accurate than physician-derived information on treatment morbidity. An example of this discrepancy is the study performed by McCammon and colleagues,[68] who reviewed the complications that resulted from "nerve-sparing" radical surgery, an approach that is intended to retain presurgical potency. They found that the physician-reported studies arrived at 1-year potency rates of 54 to 71%, while the patient-reported studies arrived at 1-year potency rates of 2 to 32%.

QUALITY OF LIFE

The impact on quality of life (QOL) has recently been recognized as a vitally important dimension in evaluating a prostate cancer treatment. The results of a new long-term study on the impact of cryoablation on QOL provides strong evidence that the postcryoablation QOL is comparable, if not superior, with that of other treatments.[69] The authors administered two scales, the FACT-P, and the SNQ. At 1-year outcome, the results indicated a return to presurgical functioning in all areas, with the exception of sexual functioning. At 3-year outcome, close to 50% of impotent men who were previously potent prior to the procedure regained the ability to have erections sufficient for intercourse. All other areas of functioning remained high. There was no delayed-onset morbidity associated with cryoablation.

In sharp contrast to the gradual regeneration of sexual functioning in a large proportion of patients and absence of late-onset morbidity associated with cryoablation, several studies have documented a decline in sexual function, protracted morbidity, and the emergence of late-onset morbidity among brachytherapy patients. Lee and colleagues[70] found a significant decline that persisted at 3 months in urinary symptoms, physical side-effects, and overall QOL associated with brachytherapy; van der Hoeven and colleagues[71] found that 48% of their sample developed erectile dysfunction at 3 months, which persisted at 12 months; Ben-Josef and colleagues[72] reported that 71% of their sample was able to have intercourse at 36 months, which declined to 50% at 60 months; Zelefsky and colleagues[73] observed that 79% of their sample was able to engage in intercourse at 24 months, which declined to 47% at 60 months; and Hollenbeck and colleagues[74] found at 24 month follow-up, 33% of patients under the age of 69 and 26% of patients over 69 were able to achieve intercourse, compared with 78% and 61%, respectively, of age-matched controls.

Late onset morbidity associated with brachytherapy has been documented by Zelefsky and colleagues,[75] who found that protracted grade 2 urinary toxicity, which manifested after the implant and persisted more than 1 year, occurred in 31%, with a median duration of 23 months. Five-year actuarial likelihood of developing a urethral stricture (grade 3 toxicity) was 12%, with a likelihood of resolution or improvement 36 months from onset of 59%. The 5-year likelihood of grade 2 rectal toxicity was 11%. Merrick and colleagues[75] found that 19.2% of patients receiving brachytherapy reported worsening bowel function following implantation.

Collectively, these results indicate that brachytherapy can lead to persistent morbidity following the treatment, delayed onset, and progressive morbidity that persist over time, including gradual long-term erosion in sexual function-

Table 76-1	Positive Biopsy Results Observed Following Radiation Therapy and Cryoablation						
Study	Tx	n	Pretreatment PSA (ng/mL)	Gleason	Clinical T Stage	Median Follow-Up	% Positive Biopsy
Stock et al 1996[53]	Brachy	97	75% < 20	82% < 7	T1–T2	18 mos	26%
Ragde et al 1997[41]	Brachy	126	78.7% < 10; Median 5.0	2–6	T1–T2	7 yrs	5%*
Ragde et al 1998[52]	Brachy	152	Median 11.0	91% < 8	98% < T3	10 yrs	15%
Zelefsky et al 1998[54]	3D-CRT	743	Median 15	81 < 8	T1–T3	> 30 mos	48%
Dinges et al 1998[55]	XRT	82	Median 14.0	–	T2–T3	24 mos	27%
Crook and Bunting 1998[56]	XRT	102	–	–	T1–T3	40 mos	20%†
Babaian et al 1995[57]	XRT	31	70% > 10	–	T1–T3	51 mos	71%
Laverdiere et al 1997[58]	XRT	120	Median 11.2	24.3% > 6	T1–T3	24 mos	62%
Ljung et al 1995[59]	XRT	55	–	35% > 6	T1–T3	6.8 yrs	67%
Bahn et al 2002[39]	TCAP	590	24.5% > 10	58.4% > 6	T1–T4	5.72 yrs	13%
Donnelly et al 2002[51]	TCAP	76	38% > 10	56% > 6	T1–T3	5.1 yrs	15%

3D-CRT = three-dimensional conformal radiation therapy; brachy = brachytherapy; TCAP = targeted cryoablation of the prostate; XRT = external beam radiation therapy.
*13% indeterminate.
†15% indeterminate.

ing. In sharp contrast, cryoablation results in substantially less bowel and bladder morbidity, no delayed-onset morbidity, and the reversal of erectile dysfunction in many patients over time.

Regarding more global measures of QOL, the Robinson results compare favorably with the results of Litwin and colleagues,[76] who measured the 5-year QOL outcomes of radical surgery, radiation, and observation, and with Krupski and colleagues,[77] who performed a 9-month QOL follow-up study on brachytherapy patients (Table 76-2).[76,77] All authors used the FACT-P, which has a maximum score of 30 for each domain, with the higher score indicating higher QOL. The QOL following cryoablation was comparable, if not superior, with that of conventional prostate cancer therapies. The following are noted in Table 76-2: Compared with cryoablation, brachytherapy patients manifested significantly worse scores on the Social/Family Well-Being scale; cryoablation patients manifested higher scores on the Functional Well-Being scale than patients who received radical surgery and radiation; and cryoablation patients produced somewhat higher scores on the Relationship with Doctor scale than patients receiving all other treatments (scores on this scale unavailable for brachytherapy patients). In summary, the quality of life among cryoablation patients is comparable with that of patients receiving surgery, radiation treatment, brachytherapy, and observation, and superior along some QOL outcome dimensions.

The newly published long-term results of prostate cryoablation demonstrate durable efficacy equivalent to other therapies for low-risk disease and possibly, but not conclusively, superior efficacy for moderate- and high-risk prostate cancer. Is there a scientific foundation to explain this clinical observation? There are two fundamental shortcomings to the standard therapies that can limit their ability to effectively treat all prostate cancer: positive margins observed after radical prostatectomy and the preferential ablation of lower Gleason grade cancer by radiation therapy. The ability of radical prostatectomy to remove all the cancer is limited if there is extension of the cancer beyond the surgical margin. Positive margins occur in up to 40% of patients

undergoing radical prostatectomy.[78] During cryosurgery, one can and usually does freeze beyond the margins of the gland, which will minimize the chances of yielding positive margins. If the patient is at high risk for extracapsular extension, the operator can freeze aggressively beyond the capsule of the gland.

Radiation therapy damages the nucleus of individual cells, and the more aggressive the cancer is, the harder the cells are to kill. Although any cell will be irreversibly damaged if exposed to enough radiation, the sensitivity of the anatomic neighborhood of the prostate limits the lifetime dose of radiation that can be delivered to the gland. Clinical results indicate that efficacy of radiation therapy declines significantly if a patient's Gleason score is greater than 7. In fact, if cancer recurs following a trial of radiation therapy, it is often a more aggressive form, which indicates a preferential killing of less aggressive cells only to leave those that are more radioresistant.[79]

Also, the technical, procedural, and scientific evolution of targeted cryoablation of the prostate in the past decade has led to a significant reduction in the morbidity profile associated with the procedure. The postprocedure morbidity profile is mild in comparison with other therapies with the exception of sexual function impairment. However, sexual function returns in time in a large proportion of patients and no late-onset morbidities are observed. This is in contrast with radiation therapy, specifically brachytherapy, where several recent studies have documented a decline in sexual function, protracted morbidity, and the emergence of late-onset morbidity.

CRYOABLATION AS A SALVAGE THERAPY FOLLOWING FAILED RADIATION THERAPY

Of the 200,000 men who are diagnosed with prostate cancer each year, roughly 60,000 of them will choose some form of radiation therapy as their treatment. Unfortunately, approximately 30% of them will not be cured of their disease as exhibited by biochemical failure.[80] Recurrent prostate cancer following definitive radiation therapy, regardless of modality, is an aggressive disease associated with an often increased Glea-

son score in comparison with the primary diagnosis and has a poor prognosis.[38] The 5-year cancer-specific mortality rate following observation of a rising PSA is at least 27%.[81] The traditional treatment options for radioresistant prostate cancer are limited and include salvage radical prostatectomy, which is associated with a significant morbidity profile, and hormone therapy, which can delay the progression of the disease but will not stop it.[82] Prostate cryoablation has been investigated as a definitive local therapy for those men believed to have a local recurrence.

As with primary prostate cryoablation, the early experience yielded mixed results, notably in terms of morbidity. The following is a review of efficacy and morbidity of prostate cryoablation in comparison with salvage radical prostatectomy. Cryoablation series are limited to those obtained using the modern technique as defined earlier and those in which hormone therapy was discontinued at the time of cryoablation.

Table 76-3[83–86] is a survey of the outcomes as published for both salvage cryoablation and salvage radical prostatectomy. It is difficult to compare different modalities as the follow-up periods and definitions of biochemical failure vary. There does not appear to be a discernible difference between the efficacies of the two therapies. This is not surprising as both are definitive local therapies and should cure the patient of their disease, provided it is truly localized. The difference between salvage cryoablation and salvage radical prostatectomy arises as one investigates their associated morbidity profiles. A review of the published incontinence and rectal injury rates is presented in Table 76-4,[87–97] along with a weighted average for each. Salvage radical prostatectomy is associated with an approximate 41.6% incontinence rate and a 7.7% rectal injury rate compared with 0.8% and 5.3%, respectively, for salvage cryoablation.

Both salvage radical prostatectomy and salvage cryoablation have the ability to cure localized disease. However, the frequent and often significant complications associated with salvage radical prostatectomy often render the therapy unpalatable for both patients and their physicians. Salvage cryoablation as a definitive local therapy for localized radioresistant prostate cancer seems to be an acceptable balance between the efficacy and morbidity, offering new hope for many men.

CONCLUSION

There has been a revolution in the way that cryosurgery is currently being performed. This has led to a renewed enthusiasm for this approach for curing patients with localized disease, as well as those patients with recurrent cancers following radiation. Medicare and insurance carriers now recognize cryosurgery as a reimbursable option for patients with prostate cancer. Currently, with the use of transrectal ultrasound, temperature monitoring, smaller probes, and

Table 76-2 Quality of Life of Men Treated with Cryosurgery Compared with Men Treated with Radical Prostatectomy, Radiation, Brachytherapy, or Observation

Variables	Cryosurgery* (n = 64)	Surgery* (n = 98)	Radiation* (n = 60)	Brachytherapy† (n = 41)	Observation* (n = 60)
	Mean	Mean	Mean	Mean	Mean
FACT-P Scales					
Physical Well-Being	26.1	25.4	24.9	25.4	25.2
Social/Family Well-Being	21.9	21.6	21.6	14.9	21.1
Emotional Well-Being	18.1	16.6	17.3	21.3	16.6
Functional Well-Being	24.6	20.9	21.2	23.6	20.7
Relationship with Doctor	7.5	6.5	6.5	N/A	6.3

N/A = not available.
*Litwin et al 1996,[76] average follow-up 5 years.
†Krupski et al 2000,[77] 9-months follow-up.

Table 76-3

Study	Year	BDFS Definition	Biochemical Disease-free Rate Follow-up (yr)					
			2	3	4	5	6	7
Salvage Cryoablation								
Saliken (Calgary)	2003	PSA < 0.3	44%					
		PSA < 1.0	58%					
Katz (Columbia)	2002	PSA < 0.3		65%				
Bahn (PCA)	2003	PSA < 0.5						59%
		PSA < 1.0						69%
Salvage Radical Prostatectomy								
Rogers (Baylor)	1995	Progression				55%		
Zincke (Mayo)	1992	Progression				82%		
Brenner (Memorial SK)	1995	Progression				30%		

Table 76-4

	No. Pts.	Rectal Injury (%)	Incontinence (%)
Salvage Cryoablation			
Saliken et al[82]	46	2	4.3
Katz and Ghafar[83]	38	0	7.9
Bahn et al[39]	59	0.4	4.3
Weighted average (Cryo)		0.8	5.3
Salvage Radical Prostatectomy			
Mador et al[87]	4	50	0
Thompson et al[88]	5	0	80
Neerhut et al[89]	16	19	25
Rainwater and Zincke[90]	13	0	10
Moul and Paulson[91]	22	10	0
Link and Freiha[92]	14	0	55
Stein et al[93]	13	8	64
Ahlering et al	34	0	63
Pontes et al[94]	43	9	46
Rogers et al[95]	40	15	58
Lerner et al[96]	79	6.3	42
Vaidya and Soloway[97]	6	0	17
Weighted average (Surgery)		7.7	41.6

computer-guided systems that plan the treatment intraoperatively, cryoablation can be performed safely and effectively.

REFERENCES

1. American Cancer Society. Cancer facts & figures 2002. Atlanta: American Cancer Society; 2002.
2. Corral DA, Pisters LL, von Eschenbach AC. Treatment options for localized recurrence of prostate cancer following radiation therapy. Urol Clin North Am 1996;23:677–84.
3. Gage AA. History of cryosurgery. Semin Surg Oncol 1998; 14:99–109.
4. Gage AA. Cryosurgery in the treatment of cancer. Surg Gynecol Obstet 1992;174:73–92.
5. Chang Z, Finkelstein JJ, Ma H, Baust J. Development of a high-performance multiprobe cryosurgical device. Biomed Instrum Technol 1994;28:383–90.
6. Green NA. Cryosurgery of the prostate gland in the unfit subject. Br J Urol 1970;42:10–20.
7. Jordan WP Jr, Walker D, Miller GH Jr, Drylie DM. Cryotherapy of benign and neoplastic tumors of the prostate. Surg Gynecol Obstet 1967;125:1265–8.
8. Addonizio JC. Another look at cryoprostatectomy. Cryobiology 1982;19:223–7.
9. Loening S, Lubaroff D. Cryosurgery and immunotherapy for prostatic cancer. Urol Clin North Am 1984;11:327–36.
10. Wieder J, Schmidt JD, Casola G, et al. Transrectal ultrasound-guided transperineal cryoablation in the treatment of prostate carcinoma: preliminary results. J Urol 1995; 154(2 Pt 1):435–41.
11. Onik G, Porterfield B, Rubinsky B, Cohen J. Percutaneous transperineal prostate cryosurgery using transrectal ultrasound guidance: animal model. Urology 1991;37:277–81.
12. Onik GM, Cohen JK, Reyes GD, et al. Transrectal ultrasound-guided percutaneous radical cryosurgical ablation of the prostate. Cancer 1993;72:1291–9.
13. Hoffman NE, Bischof JC. The cryobiology of cryosurgical injury. Urology 2002;60(2 Suppl 1):40–9.
14. Smith DJ, Fahssi WM, Swanlund DJ, Bischof JC. A parametric study of freezing injury in AT-1 rat prostate tumor cells. Cryobiology 1999;39:13–28.
15. Bischof JC, Smith D, Pazhayannur PV, et al. Cryosurgery of dunning AT-1 rat prostate tumor: thermal, biophysical, and viability response at the cellular and tissue level. Cryobiology 1997;34:42–69.
16. Rewcastle JC, Muldrew, Sandison GA. In vitro injury mapping for single cryoprobe cryosurgery. Cryobiology 2001; 43:322.
17. Mazur P. Freezing of living cells: mechanisms and implications. Am J Physiol 1984;247(3 Pt 1):C125–42.
18. Toner M, Cravalho EG, Armant DR. Water transport and estimated transmembrane potential during freezing of mouse oocytes. J Membr Biol 1990;115:261–72.
19. Toner M, Cravalho E. Kinetics and likelihood of membrane rupture during electroporation. Phys Lett 1990;143A: 409–12.
20. Toner M, Karel M, Cravalho E. Cellular response of mouse oocytes of freezing stress: prediction of intracellular ice formation. J Biochem Eng 1993;115:169–74.
21. Toner M, Karel M, Cravalho E, et al. Thermodynamic and kinetics of intracellular ice formation during freezing of biological cells. J Appl Phys 1990;67:1582–93.
22. Muldrew K, McGann LE. Mechanisms of intracellular ice formation. Biophys J 1990;57:525–32.
23. Muldrew K, McGann LE. The osmotic rupture hypothesis of intracellular freezing injury. Biophys J 1994;66(2 Pt 1): 532–41.
24. Lovelock JE. The haemolysis of human red blood cells by freezing and thawing. Biochem Biophys Acta 1953;10:414–6.
25. Meryman HT. Modified model for the mechanism of freezing injury in erythrocytes. Nature 1968;218:333–6.
26. Meryman HT. Osmotic stress as a mechanism of freezing injury. Cryobiology 1971;8:489–500.
27. Muldrew K, Wan R. A quantitative model of posthypertonic lysis [abstract]. Cryobiology 1999;39:298.
28. Muldrew K, Acker J, McGann LE. A mechanistic approach to understanding cryoprotective intracellular freezing. Cryobiology 2001;43:343–4.
29. Gage AA, Baust J. Mechanism of tissue injury in cryosurgery. Cryobiology 1998;37:171–86.
30. Baust JM, Van B, Baust JG. Cell viability improves following inhibition of cryopreservation-induced apoptosis. In Vitro Cell Dev Biol Anim 2000;36:262–70.
31. Clarke DM, Baust JM, Van Buskirk RG, Baust JG. Chemo-cryo combination therapy: an adjunctive model for the treatment of prostate cancer. Cryobiology 2001;42:274–85.
32. Tatsutani K, Rubinsky B, Onik G, Dahiya R. Effect of thermal variables on frozen human primary prostatic adenocarcinoma cells. Urology 1996;48:441–7.
33. Larson TR, Robertson DW, Corica A, Bostwick DG. In vivo interstitial temperature mapping of the human prostate during cryosurgery with correlation to histopathologic outcomes. Urology 2000;55:547–52.
34. Finelli T, Rewcastle JC, Jewett ASJ. Cryotherapy and radiofrequency ablation: pathophysiologic basis and laboratory studies. Curr Opin Urol 2003;13:187–91.
35. Rewcastle JC, Sandison GA, Muldrew K, et al. A model for the time dependent three-dimensional thermal distribution within iceballs surrounding multiple cryoprobes. Med Phys 2001;28:1125–37.
36. Baissalov R, Sandison GA, Saliken JC, et al. A semi-empirical treatment planning model for optimization of multiprobe cryosurgery. Phys Med Biol 2000;45:1085–98.
37. Polascik TJ, Pound CR, deWeese TL, Walsh PC. Comparison of radical prostatectomy and iodine 125 interstitial radiotherapy for the treatment of clinically localized prostate cancer: a 7-year biochemical (PSA) progression analysis. Urology 1998;51:884–90.
38. Stokes SH. Comparison of biochemical disease-free survival of patients with localized carcinoma of the prostate undergoing radical prostatectomy, transperineal ultrasound-guided radioactive seed implantation, or definitive external beam irradiation. Int J Radiat Oncol Biol Phys 2000;47:129–36.
39. Bahn DK, Lee F, Badalament R, et al. Targeted cryoablation of the prostate: 7-year outcomes in the primary treatment of prostate cancer. Urology 2002;60(2 Suppl 1): 3–11.
40. Long JP, Bahn D, Lee S, et al. Five-year retrospective, multi-institutional pooled analysis of cancer-related outcomes after cryosurgical ablation of the prostate. Urology 2001;57:518–23.
41. Radge H, Blasko JC, Grimm PD, et al. Interstitial iodine-125 radiation without adjuvant therapy in the treatment of clinically localized prostate carcinoma. Cancer 1997;80: 442–53.
42. Rossi CJ. Conformal proton beam therapy of prostate cancer—update on the Loma Linda University medical center experience. Strahlenther Onknol 1999;175 Suppl 2:82–4.
43. Hanlon AL, Hanks GE. Failure pattern implications following external beam irradiation of prostate cancer: long term follow-up and indications of cure. Cancer J 2000;6 Suppl 2: S193–7.
44. Martinez AA, Gonzalez JA, Chung AK, et al. A comparison of external beam radiation therapy versus radical prostatectomy for patients stages with low risk prostate carcinoma diagnosed, stages, and treated at a single institution. Cancer 2000;88:425–32.
45. D'Amico AV, Whittington R, Malkowicz SB, et al. Biochemical outcome after radical prostatectomy, external beam radiation therapy, or interstitial radiation therapy for clinically localized prostate cancer. JAMA 1998;280:969–74.
46. Blasko JC, Grimm PD, Sylvester JE, et al. Palladium-103 brachytherapy for prostate carcinoma. Int J Radiat Oncol Biol Phys 2000;46:839–50.
47. Hanks GE, Hanlon AL, Schultheiss TE, et al. Conformal external beam treatment of prostate cancer. Urology 1997;50:87–92.
48. Zagars GK, Pollack A, von Eschenbach AC. Prognostic factors for clinically localized prostate cancer. Cancer 1997;79:1370–80.
49. Perez CA, Michalski JM, Purdy JA, et al. Three-dimensional conformal therapy or standard irradiation in localized carcinoma of prostate: preliminary results of a nonrandomized study. Int J Radiat Oncol Biol Phys 2000;47: 629–37.
50. Fiveash JR, Hanks C, Roach M, et al. 3D conformal radiation therapy (3DCRT) for high grade prostate cancer: a multi-institutional review. Int Radiat Oncol Biol Phys 2000;47: 335–42.
51. Donnelly BJ, Saliken JC, Ernst DS, et al. A prospective trial of cryosurgical ablation of the prostate: five-year results. Urology 2002;60:645–9.
52. Radge H, Elgamal AA, Snow PB, et al. Ten-year disease free survival after transperineal sonography-guided Iodine-125 brachytherapy with or without 45-gray external beam irradiation in the treatment of patients with clinically localized, low to high Gleason grade prostate carcinoma. Cancer 1998;83:989–1001.

53. Stock RG, Stone NN, DeWyngaert JK, et al. Prostate specific antigen findings and biopsy results following interactive ultrasound guided transperineal brachytherapy for early stage prostate carcinoma. Cancer 1996;77:2386–92.

54. Zelefsky MJ, Leibel SA, Gaudin PB, et al. Dose escalation with three-dimensional conformal radiation therapy affects the outcome of prostate cancer. Int Radiat Oncol Biol Phys 1998;41:491–500.

55. Dinges S, Deger S, Koswig S, et al. High-dose rate interstitial with external beam irradiation for localized prostate cancer-results of a prospective trial. Radiother Oncol 1998;48:197–202.

56. Crook JM, Bunting PS. Percent free prostate-specific antigen after radiotherapy for prostate cancer. Urology 1998;52:100–5.

57. Babaiain RJ, Kojima M, Saitoh M, et al. Detection of residual prostate cancer after external radiotherapy. Cancer 1995;75:2153–8.

58. Laverdiere J, Gomez JL, Cusan L, et al. Beneficial effect of combining hormonal therapy administered prior and following external beam radiation therapy for localized prostate cancer. Int J Radiat Oncol Biol Phys 1997;37:247–52.

59. Ljung G, Norberg M, Hansson H, et al. Transrectal ultrasonically guided core biopsies in the assessment of local cure of prostatic cancer after radical external beam radiotherapy. Acta Oncologica 1995;34:945–52.

60. Hoffman NE, Chao BH, Bischof JC. The cryobiology of cryosurgical injury. Urology 2002;60(2 Suppl 1):40–9.

61. Ellis DS. Cryosurgery as primary treatment for localized prostate cancer: a community hospital experience. Urology 2002;60(2 Suppl 1):34–9.

62. Talcott JA, Rieker P, Clark JA, et al. Patient-reported symptoms after primary therapy for early prostate cancer: results of a prospective cohort study. J Clin Oncol 1998;16:275–83.

63. Shrader-Bogen CL, Kjellberg JL, McPherson CP, Murray CL. Quality of life and treatment outcomes. Cancer 1997;79:1977–86.

64. Lim AJ, Brandon AH, Fiedler J, et al. Quality of life: radical prostatectomy versus radiation therapy for prostate cancer. J Urol 1995;154:1420–5.

65. Walsh PC, Catalona WL, Litwin MS. Radical prostatectomy for localized prostate cancer provides durable cancer control with excellent quality of life: a structured debate. J Urol 2000;163:1802–7.

66. Jonler M, Messing EM, Rhodes PR, Bruskewitz RC. Sequelae of radical prostatectomy. Br J Urol 1994;74:352–8.

67. Fossa SD, Woehre H, Kurth KH, et al. Influence of urological morbidity on quality of life in patients with prostate cancer. Eur Urol 1997;31 Suppl 3:3–8.

68. McCammon KA, Kolm P, Main B, Schellhammer PF. Comparative quality-of-life analysis after radical prostatectomy or external beam radiation for localized prostate cancer. Urology 1999;54:509–16.

69. Robinson JW, Donnelly BJ, Saliken LC, et al. Quality of life and sexuality of men with prostate cancer 3 years after cryosurgery. Urology 2002;60(2 Suppl 1):12–8.

70. Lee WR, McQuellon RP, McCullough DL. A prospective analysis of patient-reported quality of life after prostate brachytherapy. Sem Urologic Oncol 2000;18:147–51.

71. Van den Hoeven J, Bevers RFM, van Mosselaar JRA, et al. A prospective study of erectile function following transperineal I-125 seed implantation for localized prostate cancer. J Urol 2002;167:340.

72. Ben-Josef E, Forman JD, Cher ML, et al. Erectile function following permanent prostate brachytherapy. J Urol 2002;167:391.

73. Zelefsky MJ, Wallner KE, Ling CC, et al. Comparison of the 5-year outcome and morbidity of three-dimensional conformal radiotherapy versus transperineal permanent iodine-125 implantation for early-stage prostatic cancer. J Clin Oncol 1999;17:517–22.

74. Hollenbeck BK, Dunn RL, Wei JT, et al. Neoadjuvant hormonal therapy and older age are associated with adverse sexual health-related quality-of-life outcome after prostate brachytherapy. Urology 2002;59:480–4.

75. Merrick GS, Butler WM, Dorsey AT, et al. Rectal function following prostate brachytherapy. Int J Radiat Oncol Biol Phys 2000;48:667–74.

76. Litwin MS, Hays RD, Fink A, et al. Quality-of-life outcomes in men treated for localized prostate cancer. JAMA 1995;273:129–35.

77. Krupski T, Petroni GR, Bissonette EA, et al. Out-of-life comparison of radical prostatectomy and interstitial brachytherapy in the treatment of clinically localized prostate cancer. Urology 2000;55:736–42.

78. Bonney WW, Fallon B, Gerber WL, et al. Cryosurgery in prostatic cancer survival. Urology 1982;14:37–42.

79. Cumes DM, Goffinet DR, Martinez A, et al. Complications of 125 iodine implantation and pelvic lymphadenectomy for prostatic cancer with special reference to patients who had failed external beam therapy as their initial mode of therapy. J Urol 1981;126:620–2.

80. Brawer MK. Radiation therapy failure in prostate cancer patients: risk factors and methods of detection. Rev Urol 2002;4 Suppl 2:S2–11.

81. Rukstalis DB. Treatment options after failure of radiation therapy—a review. Rev Urol 2002;4 Suppl 2:S24–9.

82. Saliken JC, Donnelly BJ, Brasher P, et al. Outcome and safety of transrectal US-guided percutaneous cryotherapy for localized prostate cancer. J Vasc Interv Radiol 1999;10:199–208.

83. Katz AE, Ghafar M. Selection of salvage cryotherapy patients. Rev Urol 2002;4 Suppl 2:18–23.

84. Rogers E, Ohori M, Kassabian VS, et al. Salvage radical prostatectomy: outcome measured by serum prostate specific antigen levels. J Urol 1995;153:104–10.

85. Zincke H. Radical prostatectomy and exenterative procedures for local failure after radiotherapy with curative intent: comparison of outcomes. J Urol 1992;147(3 Pt 2):894–9.

86. Brenner PC, Russo P, Wood DP, et al. Salvage radical prostatectomy in the management of locally recurrent prostate cancer after 125I implantation. Br J Urol 1995;75:44–7.

87. Mador DR, Huben RP, Wajsman Z, Pontes JE. Salvage surgery following radical radiotherapy for adenocarcinoma of the prostate. J Urol 1985;133:58–60.

88. Thompson IM, Rounder JB, Spence CR, Rodriguez FR. Salvage radical prostatectomy for adenocarcinoma of the prostate. Cancer 1988;61:1464–6.

89. Neerhut GJ, Wheeler T, Cantini M, Scardino PT. Salvage radical prostatectomy for radiorecurrent adenocarcinoma of the prostate. J Urol 1988;40:544–9.

90. Rainwater LM, Zincke H. Radical prostatectomy after radiation therapy for cancer of the prostate: feasibility and prognosis. J Urol 1988;140:1455–9.

91. Moul JW, Paulson DF. The role of radical surgery in the management of radiation recurrent and large volume prostate cancer. Cancer 1991;68:1265–71.

92. Link P, Freiha FS. Radical prostatectomy after definitive radiation therapy for prostate cancer. Urology 1991;37:189–92.

93. Stein A, Smith RB, deKernion JB. Salvage radical prostatectomy after failure of curative radiotherapy for adenocarcinoma of prostate. Urology 1992;40:197–200.

94. Pontes JE, Montie J, Klein E, Huben R. Salvage surgery for radiation failure in prostate cancer. Cancer 1993;71:976–80.

95. Rogers E, Ohori M, Kassabian VS, et al. Salvage radical prostatectomy: outcome measured by serum prostate specific antigen levels. J Urol 1995;153:104–10.

96. Lerner SE, Blute ML, Zincke H. Critical evaluation of salvage surgery for radio-recurrent/resistant prostate cancer. J Urol 1995;154:1103–9.

97. Vaidya A, Soloway MS. Salvage radical prostatectomy for radiorecurrent prostate cancer: morbidity revisited. J Urol 2000;164:1998–2001.

77

Transvesical Access

Gary C. Bellman, MD
Andrew I. Shpall, MD

Hippocrates declared, "Cuy vesica persecta … lethale" ("to cut through the bladder is lethal"). In modern urologic practice, percutaneous access to the bladder has proved effective for both bladder drainage and endourologic procedures.

PERCUTANEOUS CYSTOSTOMY

ANATOMIC CONSIDERATIONS The indications for percutaneous cystostomy are numerous, as are the variety of suprapubic catheters available. Percutaneous cystostomy is an excellent means of providing short- or long-term urinary diversion as well as access for antegrade procedures. Certain anatomic considerations must be kept in mind when inserting a suprapubic catheter. The infant bladder is an abdominal organ whether empty or full. The bladder descends into the pelvis to become a truly pelvic organ as the child matures. As the adult bladder fills, it gradually rises into the abdomen, displacing the peritoneal contents superiorly. Peritoneal contents can be injured when attempting to access an incompletely filled bladder (Figure 77-1).

TECHNIQUE Douenias and colleagues described two methods for percutaneous access to the bladder: an endoscopic and a fluoroscopic approach.[1] The method used depends on whether urethral access is possible and whether fluoroscopy is available. For bladder drainage, the percutaneous site for cystostomy should be two fingerbreadths above the superior border of the pubic symphysis in the midline. If, however, the tract will be used to perform an antegrade procedure, the puncture should be made higher, toward the dome, to avoid acute angulation of the bladder outlet.

ENDOSCOPIC APPROACH The patient is placed in the lithotomy position. The lower abdominal wall and genitals are prepared and draped (endourologic drape with drainage pack) in a sterile fashion. The urethra is anesthetized with 2% lidocaine

jelly. The skin, subcutaneous tissue, and fascia at the proposed site of suprapubic access (two to three fingerbreadths above the pubic symphysis) is infiltrated generously with 1% lidocaine solution. A small (1.5 cm) skin incision is made. A flexible or rigid cystoscope is then introduced through the urethra into the bladder and the bladder is distended. An 18-gauge needle is introduced percutaneously into the bladder under direct cystoscopic evaluation. A 0.038-inch guidewire is passed through this needle and retrieved cystoscopically using a grasping forceps or an open stone basket. The sheath of the cystoscope should be left in situ and the wire brought out through the sheath. The wire now extends from the suprapubic puncture site to the urethral meatus. The tract is sequentially dilated over the guidewire using the Amplatz dilating system. The sheath of the cystoscope at the bladder neck prevents the dilator from entering the urethra and defines the limit to which the dilator should be pushed. Dilation is limited to 24 French (F) if a long-term cystostomy tube is being placed (reentry tube without the ureteral tail) and is limited to 34F for an intravesical procedure.

FLUOROSCOPIC APPROACH If urethral access is not possible, the bladder is distended and opacified with diuresis using intravenous contrast material. Intravesical instillation of contrast material with a small 22-gauge needle may also be used to achieve distension. The patient is placed supine on the fluoroscopy table. The lower abdominal wall and genital areas are prepared and draped (with the endourologic drape) in a sterile fashion. The skin, subcutaneous tissue, and fascia are infiltrated with 1% lidocaine solution. A 1.5 cm skin incision is made three fingerbreadths above the pubic symphysis in a nonscarred area. An 18-gauge needle is introduced into the bladder. Once fluid is freely obtained from the adequately distended bladder, a 0.038-inch J-tipped guidewire is introduced. The tract is sequentially

dilated until a safety guidewire introducer can be inserted. After introducing a safety guidewire, the working guidewire is used to dilate the tract under fluoroscopic guidance using the Amplatz dilating system. Once the bladder neck is visualized endoscopically, a Bentson guidewire can be threaded down the urethra, if necessary, and retrieved at the meatus. This may be accomplished fluoroscopically using a Cobra catheter to manipulate the guidewire antegrade down the urethra or by asking the patient to attempt to void, thus directing the wire down the outlet.

There are several factors to consider when selecting a suprapubic catheter or insertion kit. The type of retaining device, anticipated duration of drainage, size of the catheter desired, unique anatomic variations in a given patient (obesity and previous lower abdominal surgery), and consistency or flexibility of the catheter are all important issues. When the bladder cannot be distended or if the patient is extremely obese, a curved perforated sound (Lowsley, van Buren, or Turner-Warwick sound) can be used for retrograde guidance of the catheter (Figure 77-2).

OBLITERATED URETHRA

Posterior urethral truama can occur in 4 to 14% of pelvic fractures, especially with bilateral pubic rami fractures (straddle fracture) and sacroiliac diathesis. Urethra trauma occurs mostly in males but can occur in females. Urethral trauma should be suspected with the presence of blood at the meatus, high-riding prostate, inability to urinate, inability to place urethral catheter, and/or rare presence of perineal hematoma. Retrograde urethrography is used to confirm the diagnosis. Primary open realignment is not recommended since it has higher incidence of impotence, incontinence, stricture formation, and potential for significant blood loss. Therefore, primary endoscopic realignment is recommended. With primary endoscopic realignment, 50 to 65% of

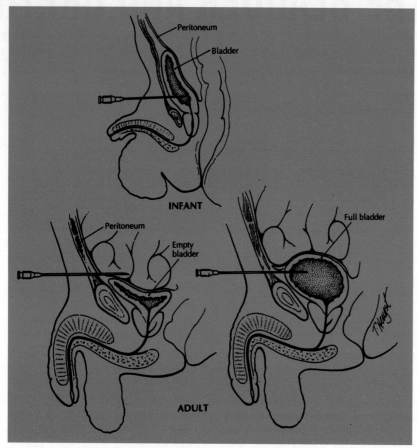

Figure 77-1 Two anatomic considerations relevant to percutaneous cystostomy are illustrated. The abdominal position of the pediatric bladder compared with the pelvic position in the adult and the relative positions of the filled and unfilled adult bladder.

patients heal without stricture, and most with stricture have mild stricture. As few as 7% will require urethroplasty. Urethral disruptions secondary to pelvic trauma have been successfully managed by endourologic techniques.[2,3]

Combined antegrade and retrograde endoscopy is used to manage the ruptured urethra. The light visible across the scarred area indicates the region that can safely be incised to restore continuity.

The suprapubic tube is removed over a guidewire and the tract is dilated with the Amplatz dilating system to 24F and a working sheath is passed. A flexible cystoscope is then passed through the working sheath and the bladder neck identified. Following visualization of the bladder neck, prostatic urethra, and verumontanum, a rigid cystoscope is passed into the urethral meatus and anterior urethra. The flexible cystoscope and the rigid cystoscope are alternately dimmed so that the light from the other scope can be seen. Fluoroscopy is used to maintain the instruments on the same cephalocaudal axis. Once the scopes are aligned, a 0.038-inch guidewire is passed from the flexible scope into the rigid scope. A Councill catheter is then passed over the guidewire into the bladder.

A case was reported in which complete disruption of the bulbous urethra was managed by endoscopic realignment with a thin trocar needle.

The procedure consisted of direct observation of the proximal end of the obliterated urethra by an antegrade flexible cystoscope and the adjustment of the trocar penetration direction under fluoroscopy and direct vision. The precise trocar position and penetration was then confirmed by antegrade flexible cystoscope. Guidewire was then placed following the trocar penetration as guidance for urethrotomy followed by the placement of a Foley catheter.[4]

PERCUTANEOUS CYSTOLITHOLAPAXY

Bladder stones in adults are usually associated with bladder outlet obstruction (BOO) caused by benign prostatic hypertrophy (BPH). Treatment consists of removing the bladder calculus and alleviating the BOO. An open procedure can be chosen for managing patients with BOO and bladder stones as well. If the prostate is large, a retropubic or suprapubic prostatectomy can be performed at the same time as stone removal. The endoscopic management of BOO commonly involves transurethral resection of the prostate (TURP). Vesical calculi can be managed simultaneously and endoscopically either by the transurethral or suprapubic percutaneous approach.

Endoscopic management, either percutaneous or transurethral route, involves fragmentation of the stone with an intracorporeal lithotripsy device.

Lithoclast, electrohydraulic (EHL), ultrasonic probe, or laser can be used. Primary extracorporeal shock wave lithotripsy (ESWL) in managing a large bladder calculus followed by secondary cystolithopaxy and evacuation of fragments can be utilized as well.[5] Transurethral management of bladder stones is possible if the prostate and stones are small. However, the disadvantage of transurethral cystolithotripsy, especially for large bladder stones, is that a large-caliber scope needs to be kept in the urethra for a prolonged period. This predisposes to the formation of urethral stricture and exposes the bladder neck to unnecessary trauma. Percutaneous removal of large stones can be carried out with minimal trauma, and the suprapubic removal of calculi through a large-caliber Amplatz sheath is much faster than tranurethral removal. An advantage of suprapubic drainage at the time of TURP is that the prostate resection is quicker. Furthermore, presence of a freely draining suprapubic tube allows uninterrupted resection of the prostate under low intravesical pressure with excellent vision.[6] This reduces fluid absorption, fluid overload, and hyponatremia, especially in patients with compromised renal and cardiac functions. Combined TURP and percutaneous cystolithotripsy should be used in patients with large calculi and/or large prostates since it allows rapid stone fragmentation and removal, faster resection of the prostate, excellent visualization, reduced fluid absorption, and minimal trauma to the urethra and bladder neck.

CONTINENT URINARY DIVERSIONS WITH STONES

Continent urinary diversion is the primary option for bladder substitution in patients who undergo cystectomy for invasive bladder cancer and severe neurogenic bladder. The increased use of bowel segments to augment as well as to completely replace the bladder has improved the quality of life for many patients. However, the improvement has been accompanied by various complications. The Incidence of calculus formation in the intestinal bladder substitute has been reported to be around 18 to 30%.[7,8] The incidence varies, depending on the type of reservoir. Studies have implicated intestinal mucus as the lithogenic agent in augmented or neobladder. In some cases, lack of or increased levels of stone inhibitors may play a significant role in the stone formation. Exposed staples, mesh, or suture alone can serve as a nidus for stone formation as well. There are multiple hypotheses of stone formation and inhibition that imply the stone formation involves multiple factors.

New instruments and novel techniques have minimized the need to perform open bladder surgery to remove bladder calculi. Ingenious techniques for removing calculi from augmented or neobladder have been developed, since access to the bladder may not be safe or possible through the native urethra, but only through a stoma in some patients. Therefore, the caliber and type of continence mechanism as well as the status of the urethra and bladder neck are important limiting factors in selecting treatment.

The adult patient with a simple augmented bladder with normal urethra and bladder neck is best suited for endoscopic removal of calculi. The large size of the urethra allows the use of large-caliber instruments to remove small stones and fragments. ESWL can be used to manage calculi in the neobladder and in augmented bladders of adults and children. The technique is best suited for the small solitary calculus in male children and adults. The Food and Drug Administration (FDA) limits its use in women of child-bearing age and young girls for the possiblity of damage to reproductive organs.

Many continent cutaneous diversions such as Kock pouches are best managed transtomally. Overly aggressive manipulation with large rigid instruments can traumatize the stoma, rendering it incompetent or resulting in a stricture. An alternative approach is to access the pouch percutaneously, avoiding the continence mechanism entirely. Percutaneous cystolithotomy is ideally suited for patients with an augmented bladder and an impassable or ligated bladder neck, or those with a neobladder with a small-caliber efferent channel. Percutaneous approach is less invasive than an open method and can provide excellent visualization for removing multiple calculi as well as for removing large calculi. This technique involves making a puncture in the augmented bladder or neobladder and progressively dilating the tract with Amplatz dilators so that a nephroscope can be passed via a 24F sheath. The increased flow and visualization is achieved when a nephroscope is used. This allows entry into the small pockets and corners of the pouch that are difficult to access even with use of a flexible cystoscope. This technique has been used effectively, but there are inherent complications to this procedure. The initial puncture into the intestinal bladder is blind and the bowel can be perforated. If dilation of the tract occurs over the mesentery of the intestinal bladder, ischemic damage can occur. The best site for placement of a percutaneous puncture is at the original suprapubic tube site. Ultrasound can be used during the procedure to aid in determining a puncture site in which bowel is not interposed.

Because the majority of pouch stones are infected, it is imperative to render the patient stone free to prevent recurrence. All exposed foreign bodies such as staples and sutures should be removed. Endoscopic scissors as well as the Nd:YAG laser have been used to remove pieces of eroded mesh from Kock pouches. There are other reports of percutaneous management of stones in continent urinary diversions. Hollensbe and colleagues[9] described the percutaneous removal of stones from a pouch with a Mitrofanoff valve, and Seaman and colleagues[10] reported percutaneous extraction of large stones from an Indiana pouch.

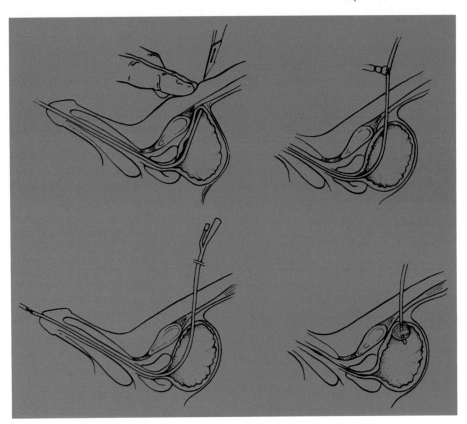

Figure 77-2 Technique of suprapubic cystostomy using the Lowsley sound showing the advantage of a curved, perforated sound in retrograde guidance of the catheter.

Initially urologists were reluctant to perform percutaneous stone extraction on continent diversions. Our experiences and those of other authors reinforce the view that such manipulation is safe and well tolerated. One group of researchers created a percutaneous tract and allowed it to mature for a month prior to stone extraction,[9] but we have found such a delay unnecessary. There was concern about injuring the vascular pedicle, and consequently CT scans were used when placing the percutaneous tube to avoid the pedicle. We have also found this to be unnecessary. If the pouch is distended and the access is anterior, injury to the vascular pedicle is unlikely, and the percutaneous site heals quickly with no sequelae to the pouch.

When managing patients with large stone burdens in continent urinary diversions, it is important to consider the particular continence mechanism. We have found the ultrasonic lithotriptor to be the most effective power lithotripsy device for large stone burdens, but all types are useful. Perforation of the intestinal bladder can occur intraperitoneally with lithotripsy devices. Fluid extravasation into the peritoneal cavity can lead to serious morbidity. Thus, extreme caution should be taken when using a lithotripsy device in the bladder.

The best treatment for bladder calculi in intestinal bladders is to prevent them from forming. Measurement of urine citrate levels with appropriate supplementation will keep many patients from forming stones. A more cost-effective and simple prevention is daily routine irrigation of the bladder.

INTERNAL DRAINAGE OF A BULBOURETHRAL ABSCESS

A percutaneous approach can be particularly helpful in the management of a bulbourethral abscess, which is often associated with a proximal urethral abscess. A suprapubic tract high on the dome is established as previously described. A rectoscope is passed to unroof the abscess. A suprapubic tube is then left for drainage.

ACCESS TO THE PEDIATRIC BLADDER

Antegrade procedures can be applied to children as well. They are particularly useful because the urethra is bypassed entirely, thus reducing the risk of strictures. Zaontz and Firlit reported two cases of ablation of posterior ureteral valves in premature neonates.[11] A 12F suprapubic cystocatheter was cut to a length of 5 cm. The 12F sheath was positioned midway between the symphysis and umbilicus to allow passage of the 9.5F resectoscope. The straight 0-angle lens was used to visualize the posterior urethra, bladder neck, and the valve leaflets. A 90-degree hook electrode was used with a monophasic cutting current. The procedure was successful in both children.

COMPLICATIONS

Complications following suprapubic cystostomy include hemorrhage, intestinal injury, injury to nonintestinal organs, and infection and extravasation.

HEMORRHAGE   Bleeding following suprapubic cytostomy is usually mild and resolves spontaneously. A puncture directed too inferior and caudal may injure a vessel in the space of Retzius. An approach directed lateral to the midline risks injuring the inferior epigastric vessels. Significant injury may result secondary to injury of adjacent organs such as the median lobe of the prostate or trigone and will be discussed further.

INTESTINAL INJURY   An important relative contraindication to percutaneous suprapubic cystostomy is previous lower abdominal or pelvic surgery. Loops of small or large bowel may be trapped by adhesions immediately beneath the anterior abdominal wall. Bowel or peritoneal perforation is a dreaded complication and can result in enterovesical or enterocutaneous fistulas. Bowel injury may initially go undetected, with peritoneal signs developing only after several hours. Sonography is helpful to identify a bowel-free path in patients who have had previous surgery. If there is doubt, an open suprapubic cystostomy should be performed.

INJURY TO NONINTESTINAL ORGANS   If the trocar is angled or oriented too caudad, the median lobe of the prostate can be injured. Significant hemorrhage may result, requiring transurethral fulguration. Injuries to the vagina, uterus, and rectum have been reported.

If the trocar is inserted too aggressively, the opposite wall of the bladder can be injured and result in transfixion of the bladder. Injuries of the trigone, ureter, and ureteral orifice have all been reported. The catheter tip can be inadvertently advanced into the ureteral orifice, causing flank pain and ureteral obstruction. The catheter can also be advanced into the urethra, causing urgency or incontinence.

INFECTION   Any manipulation of the urinary tract can result in urosepsis. Cellulitis can occur at the catheter site. Obstruction of the catheter from debris or stones predisposes to infection. Rarely, perivesical extravasation and urinoma can occur. In an obese patient, the use of a perforated sound is useful to push the dome of the bladder up beneath the anterior abdominal wall.

CONCLUSION

Percutaneous access to the bladder is a safe procedure and can be used to perform many therapeutic maneuvers. It can be safely performed on patients with continent urinary diversions.

In the young child, the urethra cannot accommodate cystoscopic manipulation, and even in the older child, ureteral stricture is a potential and unfortunate complication. A transvesical approach can be safely performed to manage posterior ureteral valves.

REFERENCES

1. Douenias R, Smith AD, Badlani GH. Endourology of lower urinary tract. Urology 1991;37:545–8.
2. Cohen JK, Berg G, Carl GH, Diamond DD. Primary endoscopic realignment following posterior urethral disruption. J Urol 1991;146:1548–50.
3. Gupta NP, Gill IS. Core-through optical internal urethrotomy in management of impassable traumatic posterior urethral stricture. J Urol 1986;136:1018–21.
4. Nakajima K, Deguchi M, Ishii MN, et al. Endoscopic management of a traumatic disruption of the bulbous urethra using a thin trocar puncture. Int J Urol 2001;8:202–4.
5. Husain I, el-Faqih SR, Shamsuddin AB, Atassi R. Primary extracorporeal shockwave lithotripsy in management of large bladder calculi. J Endourol. 1994;8:183–6.
6. Holmquist BG, Holm B, Ohlin P. Comparative study of the Iglesias technique and the suprapubic drainage technique for transurethral resection. Br J Urol 1979;51:378–81.
7. Blyth B, Ewalt DH, Duckett JW, Snyder HM 3rd. Lithogenic properties of enterocystoplasty. J Urol 1992;148(2 Pt 2):575–9.
8. Hendren WH, Hendren RB. Bladder augmentation: experience with 129 children and young adults. J Urol 1990;144(2 Pt 2):445–53.
9. Hollensbe DW, Foster RS, Brito CG, Kopecky K. Percutaneous access to a continent urinary reservoir for removal of intravesical calculi: a case report. J Urol 1993;149:1546–7.
10. Seaman EK, Benson MC, Shabsigh R. Percutaneous approach to treatment of Indiana pouch stones. J Urol 1994;151:690–2.
11. Zaontz MR, Firlit CF. Percutaneous antegrade ablation of posterior urethral valves in premature or underweight neonates: an alternative to primary vesicostomy. J Urol 1985;134:139–41.

78

Urethral Stents

Samuel A. Amukele, MD

Atul Thakre, MD

Gopal H. Badlani, MD

ANATOMY OF URETHRAL STRICTURES

For purposes of discussion, the urethra can be divided conceptually into five divisions: (1) The prostatic urethra lies proximal to the verumontanum and is surrounded by the prostatic glandular tissue. (2) The membranous urethra is a short segment of urethra surrounded in its entirety by the external urethral sphincter. (3) The bulbar urethra lies distal to the external sphincter and proximal to the suspensory ligaments of the penis; it is covered by the bulbospongiosus muscles and is centrally located in the bulbospongiosum. (4) The penile urethra is also located centrally in the bulbospongiosum, but lies distal to the suspensory ligaments of the penis. The fossa navicularis portion of the urethra lies within the glans penis and terminates at the junction of the urethral epithelium and the skin of the glans. (5) The prostatic and membranous portions of the urethra are sometimes referred to together as the posterior urethra, whereas the bulbar and penile urethra, are sometimes called the anterior urethra. Posterior urethral injuries resulting in stricture are generally the result of prior external trauma such as pelvic fracture (95%), in which the membranous urethral segment is torn away with a piece of the pelvic bone. Anterior urethral injuries resulting in stricture are usually caused by straddle-type injuries, inflammation (eg, from sexually transmitted diseases or catheter placement), prior use of instrumentation, or they may be idiopathic.

A urethral stricture is composed of inelastic scar tissue that forms in response to an insult to the urothelium. The resultant stricture will vary in length and depth of involvement. An evaluation of the depth of the urethral stricture may be made with real-time ultrasound with the urethra filled with lubricating jelly.[1] Devine and colleagues classified urethral strictures into categories on the basis of depth of invasion into the surrounding spongiosum.[2] Stage A is a mucosal fold, stage B is a small iris constriction not involving the spongiosum, stage C is a full-thickness involvement of the urethra without any underlying spongiosum inflammation, stage D is a full-thickness stricture with spongiofibrosis, stage E involves inflammation and fibrosis outside of the spongiosum itself, and stage F is a complex stricture complicated by a fistula.

OPTIONS FOR TREATMENT OF URETHRAL STRICTURES

Until recently there have been three ways of treating urethral strictures: dilation, internal urethrotomy, and urethroplasty. The purpose of dilation is to slowly stretch the stricture to a size at which urine flow is not diminished. The danger of this procedure is that overzealous dilation can result in tearing of the scar tissue, with subsequent refibrosis and possible worsening of the stricture. This technique is indicated only for patients with stage A strictures.[2] Patients treated with dilation must return for dilation procedures every 6 to 12 months. Dilation is not a curative procedure.

The goal of optical internal urethrotomy is to incise the stricture under direct vision and open up the urethral caliber for subsequent epithelialization. An optical urethrotome is used to cut the stricture at the 12-o'clock position. Optical internal urethrotomy is useful for strictures classified as stages A through C and can be curative; however, more often than not, the stricture recurs. Sometimes inflammation from the urethrotomy causes the recurrent stricture to be more extensive.

Urethroplasty has traditionally been the last line of therapy for strictures failing internal urethrotomy and/or dilation. It is first-line therapy for strictures classified as stages D through F.[2] Repeated failed urethroplasties following multiple failed internal urethrotomies leave the patient with the remaining alternative of lifelong self-catheterization or a perineal urethrostomy. This is psychologically unacceptable to most patients and not feasible for others. The results of recent investigations of urethral stenting as a possible treatment for these difficult recurrent bulbar urethral strictures have been encouraging.

The concept of using a stent to maintain patency of a lumen was first described in the vascular literature by Wallsten for the prevention of restenosis after balloon angioplasty.[3] Since these initial experiments with dogs, many studies performed in human patients have demonstrated the efficacy of stenting in large-diameter vessels with rapid arterial flow.[4–8] Fabian was the first to describe using a stent or spiral in the lower urinary tract as a natural extension of endovascular stenting.[9] He used a spiral coil to maintain patency of the prostatic urethra in patients with urinary retention secondary to benign prostatic

hyertrophy (BPH). The work of Fabian[9] and Flier and Suppelt[10] led to the acceptance of lower urinary tract stenting as a possible therapy for bladder outlet obstruction. Milroy and colleagues[11,12] were the first to use a urethral stent for the treatment of recurrent bulbar urethral strictures. In their initial study, 12 patients with recurrent bulbar urethral strictures were treated with insertion of the UroLume Wallstent after dilation of the stricture to 30 French (F). No patient had a recurrent stricture. Postoperative urine flow rates were significantly improved in all patients. This study stimulated interest in the use of a urethral stent for treatment of urethral stricture disease.

The main urethral stent available today is the UroLume endourethral prosthesis (American Medical Systems, Inc., Minetonka, MN) (Figure 78-1) and it was Food and Drug Administration (FDA) approved in 1996. Several investigational reports of other urethral stents have been described.[13–16] Some of the urethral stents such as the UroLume are designed as a permanent prosthesis, while some others such as the Urocoil are designed as a temporary prosthesis.

UROLUME ENDOURETHRAL PROSTHESIS   At our institution we have been involved with the multicenter North American UroLume trial and have previously reported on the 2-year results with the UroLume.[17] In this chapter we will also present

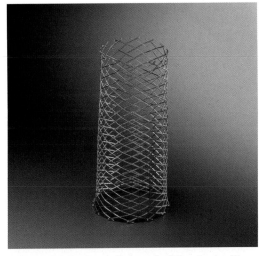

Figure 78-1 UroLume Endourethral Prosthesis. (Courtesy of American Medical Systems.)

our recently published report on our 11-year follow-up data. Therefore, most of the data we present here regard results and complications pertaining to the UroLume. First developed by Hans Wallsten in Switzerland, the UroLume is a biocompatible, inert endoprosthesis made from a nonmagnetic superalloy and woven into a tubular mesh.[18] The stent is flexible and self-expanding, with an internal diameter of 42F. One advantage of the stent is that urothelium can grow through the interstices in its wires, completely covering it. This helps to prevent any exposure to urine, which can cause the subsequent encrustation, infection, and migration that compromised earlier attempts at permanent urethral stenting.[11] Endothelialization has been shown to begin by 6 weeks and is complete by 6 to 12 months.[11,12,18,19] The elastic properties of the stent keep the device in place until epithelialization is sufficient to anchor it. The fully deployed stent is shown in Figure 78-2.

INDICATIONS

There are no concrete indications for urethral stenting. However, currently the relative indications are the following:

1. Patients who have failed multiple urethroplasties
2. Patients who have failed multiple internal urethrotomies and are poor surgical candidates for urethroplasty
3. Patients who have failed both internal urethrotomy and urethroplasty multiple times

Relative contraindications include:

1. Meatal strictures
2. Coexisting urologic pathology that may cause false failures (eg, prostate cancer, bladder tumor, hydronephrosis, neurogenic bladder dysfunction, and active urinary tract infection)
3. Patients under the age of 21
4. Strictures extending beyond the bulbar-scrotal junction
5. Strictures > 6 cm
6. Inability to dilate to 26F

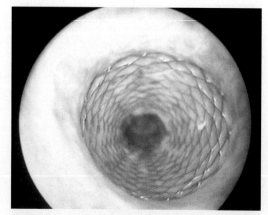

Figure 78-2 Final stent position across the stricture When stent is properly positioned, second safety lock is removed, and sheath is slowly retracted. Stent will detach from insertion tool to lie free across stricture. (Courtesy of American Medical Systems.)

PATIENT AND PREOPERATIVE PREPARATION

Patients should be informed that they will be undergoing a surgical procedure, albeit a minor one. We inform patients of the three most common postoperative complaints: postvoid dribbling, perineal discomfort, and light bleeding. Patients should be informed that they may feel some dysuria and perineal discomfort for the first week after surgery, that this is normal, and that this improves over time. The reasons for postvoid dribbling are reviewed and explained. They are informed of the possibility of urethral restenosis requiring subsequent retreatment, although the incidence of this following insertion of the urethral stent is much lower than without any treatment. Pain on erection has been noted, but this usually resolves within 6 months of surgery. Patients with prior urethroplasties are told that they are at higher risk for restenosis than are patients with strictures from all other causes.

Stent placement is performed as an ambulatory procedure, and some baseline office testing is done beforehand. Tests include urethroscopy or urethrography for visualization of the bladder and urethra to identify the site, length, and number of urethral strictures. Depending on the length of the stricture, one or more stents may be needed to overlap. Regrowth of tissue between two consecutive stents can lead to restenosis if overlap of the two stents is not adequate. Additionally, urine flow parameters are measured and an AUA symptom score is determined.

INSTRUMENTATION

Cystoscopy table with fluoroscope (optional)
50% Hypaque solution (optional)
20 and 17F cystoscopes
Optical urethrotome with semicircular blade
30- and 0-degree lenses
0.038-gauge Bentson guidewire
6F open-ended ureteral catheter (optional)
Amplatz dilator system to 28F
UroLume endoscopic insertion tool

TECHNIQUE

The wire mesh stent comes preloaded in a disposable endoscopic insertion tool (Figure 78-3). This tool houses the stent and the lens, provides a port for irrigant, and permits complete observation and control of device deployment. The device may be retracted into the sheath and repositioned if necessary before release.

Ideal candidates for UroLume placement should have a bulbar urethral stricture ≤ 3 cm long and have at least 5 mm of healthy urethra distal to the external sphincter. This should be determined by urethrogram before the procedure. Our preference is to begin prophylactic administration of ciprofloxacin 48 hours before the insertion procedure.

The procedure requires suitable analgesia, but may be performed without anesthesia in a relaxed patient.

We use 2% lidocaine jelly as an anesthetic lubricant in the urethra before endoscopy. Most patients benefit from some mild sedation as well. A cystoscope is inserted into the urethra and a 6F open-ended catheter with a guidewire is passed across the stricture. The catheter is removed and the guidewire remains in place. It is helpful to have a fluoroscope available to check the position of the guidewire if necessary. Once the guidewire is bridging the stricture, a cold-knife internal urethrotomy may be performed at the 12-o'clock position. Alternatively, dilation is carried out sequentially over the guidewire over an 8F Teflon catheter and an Amplatz dilator to a final diameter of 28F. In either case the urethral stricture should be dilated to 28F before insertion of the stent.

The appropriate stent for insertion should be at least 0.5 cm longer than the stricture itself. The 2 or 3 cm insertion tool is selected on this basis. We tend to overestimate the stricture length slightly to compensate for the tool's less-than-ideal accuracy: 5 mm is added to each end of the estimated stricture length. This obviates the occasional need for a second procedure to overlap an additional stent to the device already in place.

A 0-degree lens is then inserted into the tool. The outer sheath of the tool is heavily lubricated and the entire assembly is gently advanced to the site of the bulbar stricture under direct vision (Figure 78-4). The sheath is then moved through the stricture so that its length and the external sphincter beyond can be visualized (see Figure 78-4). One must be careful not to overdistend the bladder during this procedure. The lens is moved back and forth within the insertion tool until the proximal portion of the stent is visualized at the end of the lens. At this point the outer safety stop that prevents premature deployment is removed, and the second safety stop is rotated to a vertical position for easy reach. It is important to note that the thumb ring of the device maintains the position in the urethra, while the forefinger grip of the device pulls the sheath back to release the stent;

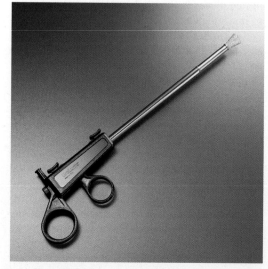

Figure 78-3 Disposable endoscopic insertion tool. (Courtesy of American Medical Systems.)

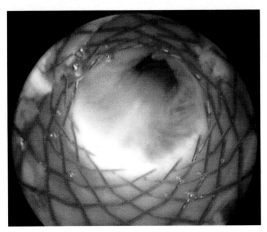

Figure 78-4 Stent is placed under direct vision. (Courtesy of American Medical Systems.)

the thumb grip remains stationary during deployment for correct device positioning.

The stent is slowly deployed 5 mm distal to the external sphincter. We have found that it is easier to have the device positioned a few millimeters distal to the sphincter and to pull the stent down in a more distal direction than to move the stent to a more proximal position once deployed. Moving the stent proximally requires retracting the stent into the sheath and redeploying it. A number of tries with the deploy-retract maneuver will quickly reassure the operator that he or she can easily control the device during this early positioning phase (Figure 78-5). It must be kept in mind that the stent will shorten over time as the device expands to full diameter. Once the surgeon is comfortable with the stent position, the outer sheath is retracted with the forefinger while holding the thumb fixed. The 0-degree lens must be pulled back during this process to observe the progress of the deploying stent as the sheath is moved back. The lens is advanced to confirm the position of the external sphincter and the proximal position of the stent. If the stent is not positioned correctly, it may be retracted into the sheath again and repositioned.

Once the positioning of the stent is deemed adequate, the second safety lock, which prevents

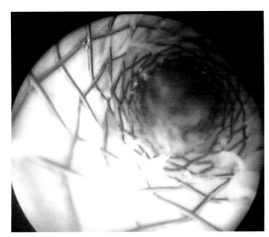

Figure 78-5 Deploying and retracting of device confirms easy control. (Courtesy of American Medical Systems.)

final release of the stent, is removed. The sheath is then slowly retracted and the stent pops off the insertion tool and lies free across the stricture (see Figure 78-2). If the stent gets hung up on the end of the deployment tool, a gentle rotation of the assembly should release the stent from the end. If the stent does not release, the sheath is not fully retracted. Once the stent is deployed, the finger grips of the deployment tool are then extended apart again to withdraw the stent-holding prongs back into the sheath and prevent urethral injury during sheath removal. At this point the sheath should not be passed back into the expanded stent because of the risk of dislodging it. It is much better to inspect the stent with a small cystoscope of 17F or smaller using a 0-degree lens. Care is taken not to strike the end of the wires during this maneuver. Once insertion is completed, a urethrogram will confirm that the stent is patent (Figures 78-6 and 78-7). A uroflow assessment may be attempted in patients who are not too sedated.

Strategic stent placement is very important in patients who have had prior prostate surgery. One must be vigilant when placing the stent into the urethra of such a patient. If the stricture is very close to the external sphincter, the stent must be placed so as to avoid causing incontinence. Since the internal sphincter has been destroyed, the patient will become incontinent if the stent extends into the external sphincter.

POSTOPERATIVE CARE

No urinary catheter is required postoperatively. We advise patients to drink adequate fluids for 48 hours to flush the urethra. We instruct our patients to avoid sexual activity for 2 weeks and to continue taking ciprofloxacin for 2 weeks. For postoperative dysuria and perineal discomfort, we prescribe a mild analgesic such as ibuprofen. A postdeployment lateral x-ray examination is performed immediately after the procedure and again in 24 hours to confirm the position and full expansion of the device. We advise patients that they may have some postvoid dribbling from urine remaining in the distended portion of the urethra. Several weeks after the procedure we allow patients to milk the urethra to get rid of this urine. Earlier attempts at this may dislodge the stent.

We follow two precautions to prevent inadvertent displacement of the stent in the early postoperative period. If at all possible, we do not catheterize the patient. If this is unavoidable, we insert a catheter using a Councill tip catheter over a guidewire placed with a flexible cystoscope. Second, when endoscopy is necessary, we do not let the scope touch the stent.

Postinsertion follow-up is required at 6 weeks, 6 months, 12 months, and annually thereafter. At 6 weeks a uroflow reassessment and retrograde urethrography are performed. At this first follow-up visit some distance may be noted between the wall of the stent and the dye column on urethrography. This is caused by some hyperplastic tissue reaction, but it is our experience that this settles down with time.

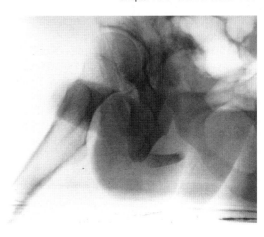

Figure 78-6 X-ray film of the UroLume stent in position in the bulbar urethra. (Courtesy of American Medical Systems.)

RESULTS

EARLY EXPERIENCE Our experience with the UroLume stent stems from our involvement in the FDA-sponsored North American UroLume trial. The trial was designed as a multicenter, prospective, controlled trial of the UroLume endourethral prosthesis for the treatment of recurrent urethral strictures. A total of 22 investigators at 12 investigational sites in the United States and 3 sites in Canada enrolled 175 patients for participation in this study. Follow-up was over 2 years.

All 175 patients had strictures in the bulbar urethra and had undergone prior procedures to relieve the obstruction. Most of the patients had been treated for stricture disease for more than 5 years and had undergone five or more dilation procedures or urethrotomies. Exclusion criteria were as listed in the indications.

The stent was inserted endoscopically after internal urethrotomy and/or sequential dilation of the stricture over a guidewire to 30F. One hundred fifty-eight of 175 patients (90%) underwent one insertion procedure, 16 of 175 patients (9%) underwent two insertion procedures, and 3 patients (1%) underwent multiple insertion procedures.[17]

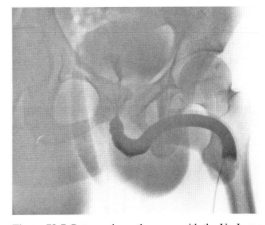

Figure 78-7 Retrograde urethrogram with the UroLume in place in the bulbar urethra. (Courtesy of American Medical Systems.)

Patients' follow-up compliance rate through the follow-up period was 79% at 2 years.

Table 78-1 summarizes the results. Overall, the mean symptom score decreased after placement of the device from 12.5 to 3.7 at the 6-week follow-up and was sustained at the 2-year follow-up.

The peak urine flow rate increased after placement of the device from a mean of 9.9 to 24.6 mL/s at the 6-week follow-up and was sustained at the 2-year follow-up.

The mean flow rate increased after placement of the device—6.5 to 15.9 mL/s at the 6-week follow-up—and was sustained at the 2-year follow-up.

A total of 27 of 175 patients (15%) required re-treatment for urethral narrowing either within or adjacent to the UroLume; 12 of 27 (44%) required removal of tissue from the lumen of the stent, and the remaining 15 patients (55%) received an additional stent to maintain a patent urethra. Eighteen of 175 patients (10%) required subsequent treatment for urethral strictures that occurred separate from the stented region. Only 7 of the 175 patients (4%) required removal of the stent since the beginning of the study. Re-treatment rates before insertion (by internal urethrotomy, dilation, or urethroplasty) versus postinsertion (by transurethral resection, stent removal, repeat stenting, or dilation) at 2 years are noted in Table 78-2. Insertion of the UroLume endourethral prosthesis decreased re-treatment rates for urethral strictures at 1 year and was sustained at 2 years. Re-treatment fell from 75.3% before insertion to 14.3% following insertion in 105 patients with the UroLume for at least 1 year.[17] In addition, since no urethroplasties were required in the postinsertion group, the morbidity of re-treatment was significantly less in the UroLume-treated patients.

Epithelialization of the stent was determined by endoscopy at each follow-up interval. Based on these data, epithelialization generally began within the first 6 weeks after stent placement. The extent of urothelial tissue coverage was quite variable at 6 weeks. Coverage progressively increased with time. At 2 years, 93% of the stents examined were 90 to 100% covered by urothelial tissue.[17] In only 1 patient in the study a stone formed on an exposed surface of stent. This was found 3 years after insertion and was easily treated with a stone crusher forceps and removed with no complications or recurrence. No patient developed encrustation of the stent within the 2-year follow-up period regardless of the per-

centage of epithelialization over the stent. The data demonstrate that those few patients with inadequate epithelialization at 2 years after insertion are not at increased risk for encrustation. Additionally, other postoperative complications (eg, urine infections, restenosis, pain, and incontinence) are not increased in these patients. The complications that these patients experienced were not any more severe than those in patients with adequately epithelialized stents. It is possible that with extended follow-up more patients with exposed stents will develop encrustation; however, to date this has not been demonstrated.

LATE EXPERIENCE Eleven-year data were recently made available on 24 patients with bulbar urethral strictures enrolled in a postapproval long-term follow-up study of UroLume stent implantation.[19] At the time of recruitment, follow-up study time points were at 6 weeks, 6 months, 1 year, and then annually for the first 5 years after stent insertion. Evaluations were then performed biannually for an additional 5 years as an optional postapproval study phase. All patients in the initial study group were given the option of enrolling in this postapproval phase, and 24 of 179 patients consented to continue after the completion of the initial study reported by the North American Study Group. All of these patients were followed for a total of 11 years after implantation.

All 24 patients in the postapproval phase of the study had been enrolled before 1992 and completed 11 years of study follow-up. Follow-up examinations included uroflowmetry, assessment of current Madsen-Iverson symptom scores, cystoscopy to estimate the percentage of the stent covered by epithelium, and a rating of any tissue change within the stent (none, mild, moderate, or marked).

Analyses were performed for device exposure at 1, 2, 3, 4, 5, 7, 9, and 11 years after stent insertion. At final analysis 9 of the original 179 patients (5%) had undergone permanent stent removal. Information was available for 24 patients who consented to follow-up for a total of 11 years. The remaining patients discontinued follow-up because of early exit from the study or opted not to participate in the postapproval study beyond 5 years. The etiologies of stricture disease and average number of treatments before UroLume placement in the 24 patients are listed in Table 78-3.

Valid urinary flow rate (valid uroflow indicating more than 125 mL of voided volume) data

Table 78-2 Comparison of the Number of Stricture Treatments 2 Years Before and After UroLume Insertion

No of Treatments	Before		After	
	No.	%	No.	%
0	10	16	45	74
1	9	15	13	21
2–5	23	38	3	5
5+	19	31	0	0
	61	100	61	100

p value < .001

before and after stent were available for 19 of the 24 study patients. Before stent placement, the mean peak urinary flow rate for these 19 patients was 9.5 mL/s (range 4.0–16.0). At 11 years after insertion, the mean peak urinary flow rate had improved to 20.8 mL/s (range 7.6–46.0). Table 78-4 lists comparative data for peak flow rates before and after insertion for all patients who underwent uroflowmetry. Improvement noted at 1 year of follow-up was maintained throughout the study.

Paired before and after current symptom score data were available for 23 of the 24 study patients at 11 years of follow-up. Comparative data for mean current symptom scores before and after insertion of the UroLume stent are presented in Table 78-5. Improvement was evident at 1 year after implantation and this improvement was maintained throughout the study. At 11 years, mean symptom score had improved from 11.3 before insertion to 3.0 after insertion. Results indicated clinically significant improvement at all 8 follow-up evaluation time points during the 11-year period.

Urethroscopy was performed to document site-specific tissue changes in the stented region at all follow-up visits. Figure 78-5 illustrates the incidence and rating of stent site-specific tissue change. At 11 years, 16 (72.7%) had mild or no tissue change, 5 (22.7%) had moderate, and 1 (4.6%) had marked tissue change. Complete epithelialization (90% or more coverage) of the endoprosthesis was seen at 1 year of follow-up in more than 90% of patients, and was persistent throughout the 11 years. Urethral biopsies were taken from the stented area in patients identified with moderate or severe tissue changes. Microscopically, a consistent pattern of nonspecific acute and/or chronic inflammatory change was observed. Benign hyperplastic squamous epithelium was identified in 2 patients. There have been no stent-specific malignant tissue changes.

A total of 9 re-treatment procedures were performed on 8 of 24 patients (33.3%) within the stented areas owing to reasons such as hyperplastic tissue overgrowth, or restricture formation at the proximal or distal ends of the stented area. Of these re-treatments, 5 were performed in the first year following stent insertion (4 hyperplastic tissue resections and 1 additional stent placement). For the remaining 4 patients the time to re-treatment ranged from less than 6 to 11.2 years

Table 78-1 Comparison of Preinsertion Patient Parameters with Postinsertion Results at 2 Years

Two-Year	Symptom Score		Peak Flow Rate (%)		Mean Flow Rate (%)	
	Before	After	Before	After	Before	After
Mean	12.53	2.55	8.98	23.56	5.82	14.89
SD	4.87	3.87	5.76	11.87	3.59	7.59
Valid N	75		62		57	
t value	14.13		–9.54		–9.08	
p value	< .001		< .001		< .001	
Mean change (%)	–76.1		265.0		236.8	

Table 78-3 Stricture Etiologies and Prior Interventions

Etiology	No. Pts	No. Urethroplasty	Average No. Internal Urethrotomies Before Stent Placement	Average No. Dilations Before Stent Placement
Traumatic	6	3	1.3 ± 0.58	22.3 ± 24.01
Inflammatory	5	0	2.0 ± 0.0	30.0 ± 19.09
Congenital	2	1	2.0 ± 2.83	5.0 ± 7.07
Catheterization	3	0	1.3 ± 0.58	15.0 ± 5.86
Unknown	7	1	2.2 ± 2.61	33.8 ± 45.83

and all were in the form of urethral dilations. There were 3 patients (12.5%) who had 2 Uro-Lume stents placed as the primary procedure owing to longer strictures. All of these patients required an additional treatment after stent insertion (2 dilations and 1 additional stent insertion).

In 1996 Milroy and Allen reported on the long-term results of 52 patients enrolled between 1987 and 1989 with up to 6 years of follow-up.[20] The mean peak flow rate was 19.7 mL/s at the last evaluation, with 91% of patients reporting being moderately to very satisfied with the outcome owing to improved flow rates and fewer symptoms, thus obviating the need for further treatment. Stent coverage was complete in most patients by 3 months after insertion. Complications included initial postvoid dribbling and transient discomfort. Patients with stricture recurrence included a subgroup of patients (2) with previous traumatic etiologies or previous urethroplasties (4). When this subgroup was excluded from the analyses, the failure rate decreased from 16 to 5.4%.

In comparison with Milroy and Allen's data, 43 of 179 patients (24.2%) in the North American Study Group treated with the UroLume had undergone prior urethroplasties. Of these 43 patients, 17 (40%) required secondary treatment for restenosis after insertion of the device. Only 14 of the remaining 136 patients (10%) who had not undergone previous urethroplasties required secondary treatment ($p < .001$), and 8 of the 17 patients (47%) requiring secondary treatment underwent transurethral resection of tissue within the stent. The incidence of resection among patients who had urethroplasty compared with those who did not was 8 of 43 (18%) versus 3 of 136 (2%), respectively ($p < .001$). Of our 24 patients followed for 11 years, 5 had been previously treated with urethroplasty. The outcome for these patients was similar to that of the remaining 19 patients in our cohort. However, prior urethroplasty still remains a relative contraindication for UroLume placement.

Stents have been recommended only for bulbar urethral strictures because this tissue has a rich spongiofibrous structure that makes it less susceptible to erosion than other areas of the urethra. The ends of the stent should be at least 5 mm beyond the strictured area, and if multiple stents are needed, their ends should overlap at least 5 mm to prevent overgrowth of tissue with restenosis in the junctional area. Stenting should be avoided in the irradiated urethra because epithelialization is likely to be poor.

The incidence of hypertrophic tissue growth (HTG) associated with the use of the UroLume has been widely discussed in the literature of late. Numerous case reports have documented HTG occurring between the wires of the UroLume stent. Although the incidence of HTG is relatively high, the incidence of clinically significant HTG is low. Many investigators believe that it occurs more frequently in post-traumatic strictures.[21,22] In our cohort of patients with long-term follow-up, 72.7% had no to minimal HTG.

Of the 179 patients in the multicenter trial, 9 stent removal procedures were required during the 11-year follow-up period. Explant data are reported to American Medical Systems, thereby confirming that no other explants were performed at other institutions. Of the 9 explants, 7 (77.7%) were performed during the first year after stent placement. Of the remaining 2 stent removal procedures, 1 occurred 4 years after stent placement, and the other at 5 years and 3 months after stent insertion.[23] Our 11-year follow-up establishes that explantation is an uncommon event.

Ashken and colleagues reported on 71 patients with up to 3 years of follow-up at four European sites.[24] Mean peak flow rates increased from 6 mL/s before insertion to 22 mL/s at 15 months of follow-up. Of the 71 patients, 68 were satisfied with the result. Three patients with traumatic stricture etiologies experienced stricture recurrence. Complications included postvoid dribbling and transient urethral or perineal discomfort.

Our 11-year follow-up of 24 patients further confirms the safety and effectiveness of the UroLume endoprosthesis. Improvements in mean peak flow rates and in mean symptom scores as observed during the first year were maintained during 11 years of follow-up and were statistically significant at all time points. Epithelialization of the stent was 90% or greater in at least 90% of patients at all time points, with minimal tissue change observed. Endoscopy through the stent lumen was feasible and allowed for ease of ongoing urological care. Re-treatment and stent removal rates were low.

CONCLUSIONS

The UroLume stent is a safe and effective minimally invasive approach for the management of recurrent bulbar urethral stricture disease, with few complications, low re-treatment rates, and the uncommon need for explantation. Its advantages include short operating time, minimal blood loss, ease of insertion, short hospitalization, and, most notably, minimal anesthesia, which renders it suitable even for the medically compromised patient. Based on our experience, we advocate its use for patients with less than 3 cm bulbar urethral strictures after at least 2 recurrences, with a minimum distance of 7 to 10 mm from the external sphincter. It is contraindicated in patients with a ruptured membranous urethra. Patients with strictures longer than 3 cm or with prior urethroplasties should be made aware of the higher re-treatment rates. At 11 years of follow-up, symptomatic and objective improvement persisted with endoscopic evidence of a good epithelial lining with little tissue change.

STENTS AND DETRUSOR-EXTERNAL SPHINCTER DYSSENERGIA (DESD)

The mainstay of treatment for DESD is external sphincterotomy. Even though many patients achieve a successful outcome, a significant number continue to have problems as a result of persistent hydronephrosis, vesicoureteric reflux, febrile UTI, or autonomic dysreflexia.[25] A search for alternative therapies has led to an examination of the use of urethral stents for this indication.

In a recent review, Chancellor and colleagues reported the long-term efficacy and safety of the UroLume stent in the treatment of 160 men with spinal cord injury with DESD at 15 centers in North America.[26] The mean voiding pressure was 75.1 cm H_2O before treatment and decreased to 37.4 cm H_2O at 1 year. This decrease was durable and held up until 5 years in 41 patients. The residual volume decreased after stent placement and

Table 78-4 Peak Flow Rates

Follow-Up (yr)	Mean mL/s Peak Flow Rate ± SD (range)	No. Valid Uroflow (> 125 mL voided volume)
Pre-evaluation	9.5 ± 3.5 (4.0–16.0)	20
1	24.9 ± 12.6 (12.5–63.0)	20
2	27.1 ± 12.5 (13.5–62.0)	20
3	23.6 ± 14.2 (6.0–63.2)	19
4	23.4 ± 14.2 (8.6–62.0)	19
5	22.8 ± 10.6 (8.7–45.2)	12
7	24.6 ± 12.5 (8.0–58.0)	16
9	21.2 ± 13.2 (6.9–44.8)	11
11	20.8 ± 11.0 (7.6–46.0)	19

Table 78-5 Current Symptom Scores

Follow-Up (yr)	Mean Symptom Score ± SD (range)	No. Complete Score Data
Pre-evaluation	11.26 ± 34.8 (4–25)	23
1	1.78 ± 2.15 (0–8)	23
2	1.26 ± 1.48 (0–4)	19
3	2.09 ± 2.50 (0–8)	23
4	2.10 ± 2.45 (0–8)	20
5	2.73 ± 2.84 (0–9)	15
7	3.08 ± 2.39 (0–8)	12
9	3.69 ± 3.82 (0–15)	16
11	3.04 ± 3.64 (0–15)	23

remained stable throughout the 5-year follow-up. The mean cystometric capacity was unchanged during the follow-up period and hydronephrosis and autonomic dysreflexia improved or stabilized in most patients with functioning stents. In the 24 patients (15%) in whom an explant was necessary, mostly owing to stent migration, the process was relatively easy to learn. In fact, 4 (16.7%) of these patients had a new stent reinserted.

In a separate prospective, multicenter trial, 57 men with spinal cord injury with urodynamically diagnosed DESD underwent randomization to either treatment with an external sphincterotomy or placement of a UroLume stent.[27] The primary endpoint was maximum detrusor pressure and secondary measures of bladder capacity and postvoid residual taken preoperatively and 3, 6, 12, and 24 months postoperatively. At 12 months, the outcomes did not significantly differ for both groups. By 24 months, the maximum detrusor pressure had decreased from 90.6 to 41.6 for the sphincterotomy group and from 101.9 to 71.6 for the stent group. The mean bladder capacity did not change significantly for either sphincterotomy or stent groups from preoperative values of 245 mL and 251 mL, respectively. The preoperative postvoid residuals were 212 mL and 168 mL for both sphincterotomy and stent groups, and although these values decreased at various follow-up points, the trend was not stable. Six (19%) patients with a stent required explantation owing to migration with no adverse sequelae. In conclusion, the authors note that the urethral stent not only is effective, but is also potentially reversible.

OVERALL EXPLANT EXPERIENCE

The early experience with the UroLume showed an increased rate of explantation during years 1 and 2, leading to the perception among urologists that this device was not durable. This has not borne out as shown in a recent study of the experience of patients in the North American Study Group.[23,28]

In a UroLume explant study by Shah and colleagues, 465 patients had UroLume placed for diverse diagnoses such as benign prostatic hyertrophy (BPH) (126), bulbar urethral stricture (179), and DESD (160). Of these patients, 69 (14.8% of the series) required removal of a total of 73 stents (15.6% of stents) in 7 years. This low incidence of failure is consistent with use of the UroLume appropriately. The breakdown of the explants showed that for patients treated for bladder outlet obstruction secondary to benign prostatic hyperplasia, 23% of the stents were removed, 5% in patients with bulbar urethral strictures, and 22% of patients with DESD (see Figure 78-6). Most of the explants were done in the first 2 years (Table 78-6) and the most common cause for explant was migration and/or inappropriate placement (Table 78-7). At the time of explant, the most common tissue finding was focal inflammation with a hyperplastic tissue response (Table 78-8).

Stent explant is technically feasible and several techniques have been described for removing the UroLume prosthesis. Stents implanted for BPH and DESD are usually removed endoscopically in one piece, whereas stents placed for bulbar urethral stricture may require removal piece by piece endoscopically or intact removal by open surgery with urethrectomy. For intact endoscopic removal, the overlying urothelium is resected with a low cutting monopolar current using a standard resectoscope loop and sheath. Pure cut frequency current should be used in a smooth motion with care not to pause while removing tissue from within the prosthesis. The stent is then extracted from its bed with alligator forceps; the gentle pulling motion lengthens and narrows it, allowing the stent to be pulled inside the sheath and removed without further trauma. An alternative is resection of the overlying mucosa and passage of a 0.038-inch guidewire through the stent lumen into the bladder. The stent is then pushed into the bladder over the guidewire and drawn into the resectoscope sheath by pulling each end of the wire. Stents in the bulbous urethra are denuded, cut into pieces, and removed piece by piece through the endoscope sheath. The holmium:YAG laser has been used for this purpose without injury to the urethra. In our series in a patient with continent diversion and a nonfunctioning urethra, the stent and urethra were removed together. In a few cases wire-by-wire extraction of the stent has proved necessary.

BIODEGRADABLE STENTS

The last decade has seen remarkable progress in the development of biodegradable urethral stent.[29] Polymers of hydroxyl acids have good biocompatibility properties, and stents with different expansion rates and degradation times can be made. In 1993, the first biodegradable, self-reinforced poly-L-lactic acid (SR-PLLA) urethral stent was introduced.[30] An ideal biodegradable stent would support the urethral wall during and after the healing process, and be absorbed completely.[30] It would be rigid enough for the urethra, have degradation products that are biocompatible, and break down at a rate that allows adequate tissue regeneration.

At present, several reports of the various uses of the biodegradable stent have been reported.[29-41] To explore the possibility of an endoscopic urethroplasty with a free graft on a biodegradable, self-reinforced polyglycolic acid spiral stent, a preliminary study was designed.[31] Ten patients with bulbar strictures from 2 to 4 cm in length and failed previous urethrotomies were treated and follow-up was from 3 to 39 months (mean 21 months). At 2 years, 1 stricture had recurred in a man who underwent regular endoscopies for recurrent bladder tumors. All other patients were successful. One stent got lost in the bladder during the procedure, but could be brought at the right place. Other complications were 1 hematuria, 1 urosepsis, 1 perineal pain, 1 painful evacuation of a part of the stent 16 days after operation, and 1 difficult micturition. The authors conclude that preliminary experiences indicate that this technique is a possible treatment of short bulbar strictures after failure of endoscopic treatment.

The application of the biodegradable stent to the treatment of recurrent urethral strictures has been reported as both an early series and recently with the long-term follow-up.[32,33] Isotalo and colleagues studied whether a new bioabsorbable self-expandable, self-retaining, and self-reinforced poly-L-lactic acid double spiral stent was able to prevent the edges of a cut recurrent urethral stricture from adhering together and the scar from shrinking, thus obviating stricture recurrence in 22 patients with recurrent urethral stricture.[32] They performed uroflowmetry, measurement of residual urine volume, urine culture, and urethroscopy before and 1, 3, 6, and 12 months after optical urethrotomy. One hundred percent of the patients voided by postoperative day 2. All 22 patients voided freely on day 1 or 2 after urethrotomy. The stent slipped partially proximal to the stricture and had to be changed in only 1 patient. The stent was totally epithelialized in all but 1 patient at 6 months and had degraded in all at 12 months. The improvement in flow rate was maintained during follow-up in 54.5% of the patients. Ten patients had a stricture recurrence, which was outside the stent area usually close to the external sphincter in 7 and in the stent area in 3. All recurrences were treated with repeat optical urethrotomy and a new stent was inserted. Urinary infections developed in 2 patients and were successfully treated with oral antibiotics. The authors appeared to be optimistic about potential application of this new stent, although they called for longer follow-up and controlled studies.

The long-term follow-up of biodegradable stents for recurrent urethral stents revealed at a mean follow-up of 46 months that the treatment was successful in 8 of the 22 patients (36%).[33] Six recurrences were found within the stented

Table 78-6 Frequency of Explantation According to Dwell Time

Years	No. BPH	No. Stricture	No. Detrusor-Sphincter Dyssynergia	Total No. (% removed)
0–1	11	7	14	32 (43.8)
1–2	6	0	4	10 (13.6)
2–3	2	0	6	8 (10.9)
3–4	1	0	6	7 (9.5)
4–5	5	2	3	10 (13.6)
5–6	2	0	0	2 (2.7)
6–7	2	0	2	4 (5.4)
Total (% placed)	29 (6.2)	9 (1.9)	35 (7.4)	73 (15.6)

Table 78-7   Major Reasons for Explantation According to Indication for Stent Placement

	No. BPH	No. Detrusor-Sphincter Dyssynergia	No. Stricture	Total (% removed)*
Migration/misplacement on cystoscopy	7	19	2	28 (38.4)
Migration/misplacement on cystoscopy + associated autonomic dysreflexia	0	2	0	
Encrustation	4	4	0	8 (10.9)
Patient-reported symptoms:	13	2	7	22 (30.1)
Worse voiding symptoms	13	2	5	
Recurrent stricture	0	0	2	
Malignancy:	5	0	1	6 (8.2)
Prostate cancer	5	0	0	
Urethral squamous cell cancer	0	0	1	
Penile skin lesion:	0	4	0	4 (5.4)
Prosthesis infection	0	1	0	
Urethral fistula	0	2	0	
Skin breakdown	0	1	0	
Incomplete epithelialization on cystoscopy	1	7	0	8 (10.9)
Squamous metaplasia	0	2	0	2 (2.7)
Urinary tract infection	1	4	1	6 (8.2)
Other	5	9	2	16 (21.9)

*More than 1 cause in some patients.

area and 15 outside. Patients with failure have since been treated with several urethrotomies and repeat self-dilatations or free skin urethroplasties. In conclusion, they note that the results of the use of a bioabsorbable SR-PLLA urethral stent for the treatment of recurrent strictures were encouraging. They argue that without this therapy, the recurrence rate of strictures might have been much higher. They note that the main problem was sudden collapse of the stent, possibly induced by outer compression, and that a new generation of bioabsorbable stents is already under development.[34]

Biodegradable stents have also been used for acute urinary retention after minimally invasive therapy of the prostate.[35–39] Petas and colleagues[38] in two randomized controlled studies examined the utility of two different polymers for the prevention of acute urinary retention after visual laser ablation of the prostate (VLAP).[35,36] In the first study,[35] 72 men with BPH who underwent placement of a suprapubic catheter and visual laser ablation of the prostate were separated into three groups. In group 1 (27), the self-reinforced polyglycolic acid spiral stent was inserted into the prostatic urethra after treatment, while 23 in group 2 received no other devices. In 22 men in group 3, an indwelling catheter was left in situ for an average of 6.5 days. They found that the self-reinforced polyglycolic acid spiral stent is superior to the suprapubic catheter alone and to combined indwelling and suprapubic catheters for the treatment of postoperative urinary retention after laser therapy, offering possibilities for shorter catheterization time. The second polymer catheter examined the self-reinforced poly-DL-lactic acid (SR-PLA) spiral stent was compared with a suprapubic catheter after VLAP in a randomized study.[36] Here 45 patients received either a SR-PLA stent (22 patients) and a suprapubic catheter, or a suprapubic catheter only (23 patients) after undergoing VLAP. The suprapubic

catheter was removed when voiding started. The results showed that improvements in patient-weighted symptom score, mean Qmax, and PVR were significant in both groups at the 6-month follow-up. The mean stent degradation time was 6 months. The infection rate increased with the duration of suprapubic catheterization, from 25% (0–3 days) to 44% (> 3 days). Stones were seen in 2 stented patients during the follow-up. They conclude that the SR-PLA spiral stent is safe and effective for the treatment of postoperative urinary retention after laser therapy. Also the stent degradation time was unnecessarily long compared with the duration of prostatic edema and tissue sloughing after laser therapy. The infection rate depends on the duration of suprapubic catheterization.

The experience of the use of a biodegradable stent with that of a urethral Foley catheter after transurethral microwave thermotherapy (TUMT) was reported by Dahlstrand and colleagues.[37] The study comprised 30 men scheduled for prostatectomy for symptomatic BPH. The patients were treated using the Prostatron (EDAP-Technorned, France) TUMT system; the software used provided a maximum power of 70 W. Patients were catheterized after treatment with either a Foley catheter or a biodegradable stent. The effective follow-up period was 3 months. In the entire group, the mean (SD) free flow increased from 7.7 (2.4) to 14.0 (3.3) mL/s, the residual urine decreased from 125 (86) to 23 (25) mL, and the symptom score decreased from 16 (8) to 5 (4). The biodegradable stent completely avoided post-treatment retention. They conclude that the biodegradable stent is useful in relieving the problems of catheterization after treatment.

Petas and colleagues[38] performed a randomized study to investigate the feasibility and efficacy of a biodegradable self-reinforced polyglycolic acid (SR-PGA) stent in preventing postoperative urinary retention and the need for prolonged

catheterization after interstitial laser coagulation (ILC) treatment. In the study, 35 males with benign prostatic enlargement (BPE) entered the study: 21 in the ILC + stent group, and 14 in the ILC group without a stent. All patients had a suprapubic catheter inserted, and ILC was performed. In the ILC + stent group, voiding started on the first postoperative day in 17 patients and on the second day in 2 patients. Voiding was delayed in 2 cases: in 1 case owing to inadequate length of the stent, and in the other as a result of the stent placement being too proximal. There was 1 case of urinary retention owing to early degradation of the stent. In the ILC-only group, voiding started on average 6.1 days postoperatively. They conclude that the use of a SR-PGA stent enabled early voiding and is safe and effective in the treatment of postoperative urinary retention after ILC. The 3- to 4-week degradation time of the SR-PGA stent was too short for some patients. They call for further development work to improve the stents and larger controlled studies to show the true value of biodegradable stents in the treatment of BPE

In a follow-up to the previous study, a different configuration of the stent was tested in 50 patients.[39] They tested a new self-expandable self-reinforced (SR) PLGA copolymer (lactic:glycolic ratio 80/20) spiral stent inserted after interstitial laser coagulation of prostate procedure to promote voiding. The SR-PLGA stent has a degradation time of 2 to 2.5 months. As in the previous study, a suprapubic catheter was placed in all patients and was removed when voiding commenced. All except 3 patients started to void on the first postoperative day. In 2 of the 3 cases, the stent had moved proximally and had to be relocated, whereafter voiding succeeded. The mean maximum and average flow rates increased, while DAN-PSS-1 symptom score and postvoiding residual urine volume decreased statistically significantly. At 2 months, the stent was still intact in the urethra in all except 3 patients. At 4 months, it had been degraded into small fragments, and at 6 months, it had been completely eliminated. The only exceptions were 3 patients with an uncalcified piece of the stent in the bladder. They concluded that the self-expandable SR-PLGA copolymer stent was safe and highly biocompati-

Table 78-8   Tissue Reaction at Stent Site

	No. BPH	No. Stricture	No. Detrusor-Sphincter Dyssynergia
Nodular hyperplasia	12	0	1
Focal acute inflammation	2	2	0
Squamoous metaplasia	1	0	2
De novo malignancy:	5	1	0
Prostate cancer	5	0	0
Urethral squamous cell cancer	0	1	0
Unknown*	9	6	32

*Tissue resected during prosthesis removal was not examined in all patients.

ble. It ensured voiding in the case of temporary obstruction caused by prostatic edema, and the degradation time covers all patients in need of postprocedure urinary drainage.

Two studies assessed whether patients with acute urinary retention from benign prostatic enlargement can be treated with a combined therapy comprising a bioabsorbable SR-PLLA urethral stent and finasteride.[40,41] The patients had a suprapubic catheter inserted and the SR-PLLA stent placed cystoscopically. The patients were allowed to attempt to void spontaneously after 2 days. After 2 weeks the patients were randomized to receive either finasteride 5 mg daily or placebo. In the preliminary study, they showed that all patients started to void spontaneously within 2 weeks. They conclude that the bioabsorbable SR-PLLA stent combined with finasteride therapy provides a promising new alternative in the treatment of acute urinary retention, especially in patients unfit for surgical therapy. The second larger study had 55 patients.[41] They were assessed at baseline and at 6, 12, and 18 months for maximum urinary flow rate, prostate volume, and serum prostate-specific antigen (PSA). Nineteen patients completed the study, while 36 discontinued. There was a statistically significant increase in the mean maximum flow rate, and a statistically significant decrease in the prostatic volume and serum PSA in the finasteride group. The same number of patients discontinued in both groups; the major reason for discontinuation was insufficient therapeutic response. They conclude that the major problems were discontinuation of treatment because the response to therapy was insufficient, and uncontrolled breakdown of the spiral stent.

The arena of biodegradable stents is an exciting and promising addition to the therapeutic armamentarium. For now, the failure rate in recurrent strictures is still too high, and the cost of the stent might make it not cost-effective for use in postoperative urinary retention.[29] The polymers of the alpha-hydroxyl acids have a good biocompatibility, and its use in urology has advantages.[30]

REFERENCES

1. McAninch JW, Laing FC, Jeffrey RB Jr. Sonourethrography in the evaluation of urethral strictures: a preliminary report. J Urol 1988;139:294–7.
2. Devine CJ Jr, Jordan GH, Sclossberg SM. Surgery of the penis and urethra. In Walsh PC, Retik AB, Stamey TA, et al, editors. Campbell's urology. 6th ed. Philadelphia: WB Saunders; 1992. p. 2957.
3. Dotter CT. Transluminally placed coil spring endarterial tube grafts: long-term patency in canine popliteal artery. Invest Radiol 1969;4:329–32.
4. Maass D, Kropf L, Egloff L, et al. Transluminal implantation of intravascular "double helix" spiral prostheses: technical, biological considerations. Proc Eur Soc Artif Organs 1982;9:252–7.
5. Dotter CT, Buschmann RW, McKinney MK, Rosch J. Transluminal expandable nitinol coil stent grafting: preliminary report. Radiology 1983;147:259–60.
6. Wright KC, Wallace S, Charnsangavej C, et al. Percutaneous endovascular stents: an experimental evaluation. Radiology 1985;156:69–72.
7. Palmaz PC, Kopp DT, Hayashi H, et al. Normal and stenotic renal arteries: experimental balloon expandable intraluminal stenting. Radiology 1987;164:705–8.
8. Sigwart U, Puel J, Mirkovitch V, et al. Intravascular stents to prevent occlusion and restenosis after transluminal angioplasty. N Engl J Med 1987;316:701–6.
9. Fabian KM. Per intraprostatische "Partielle Katheter" (Urologische Spirale). Urologe A 1980;19:236.
10. Flier G, Suppelt U. Einfahrungen mit der urologischen spiral. Urologe B 1987;27:304.
11. Milroy EJ, Chapple CR, Cooper JE, Eldin A. A new treatment for urethral strictures. Lancet 1988;1:1424–7.
12. Milroy EJ, Chapple CR, Eldin A, Wallsten H. A new stent for the treatment of urethral strictures. Br J Urol 1989;63:392–6.
13. Yachia D, Beyar M. Temporarily implanted urethral coil stent for the treatment of recurrent urethral strictures: a preliminary report. J Urol 1991;146:1001–4.
14. Corica AP, Larson BT, Sagaz A, et al. A novel temporary prostatic stent for the relief of prostatic urethral obstruction. BJU Int 2004;93:346–8.
15. Parra RO. Treatment of posterior urethral strictures with a titanium urethral stent. J Urol 1991;146:997–1000.
16. Kemppainen E, Talja M, Riihela M, et al. A bioresorbable urethral stent: an experimental study. Urol Res 1993;21:235–8.
17. Badlani GH, Press SM, Defalco A, et al. UroLume endourethral prosthesis for the treatment of urethral stricture disease: long-term results of the North American Multicenter UroLume Trial. Urology 1995;45:846–56.
18. Oesterling JE. Urologic applications of a permanent epithelializing urethral endoprosthesis. Urology 1993;41:10–8.
19. Shah DK, Paul EM, Badlani GH, et al. 11-year outcome analysis of endourethral prosthesis for the treatment of recurrent bulbar urethral stricture. J Urol 2003;170(4 Pt 1):1255–8.
20. Milroy E, Allen A. Long-term results of UroLume urethral stent for recurrent urethral strictures. J Urol 1996;155:904–8.
21. Sneller ZW, Bosch RJ. Restenosis of the urethra despite indwelling Wallstent. J Urol 1992;148:145–6.
22. Verhamme L, Van Poppel H, Van deVoorde W, Baert L. Total fibrotic obliteration of urethral stent. Br J Urol 1993;72:389–90.
23. Shah DK, Kapoor R, Badlani GH, et al. Experience with urethral stent explantation. J Urol 2003;169:1398–400.
24. Ashken MH, Coulange C, Milroy EJ, Sarramon JP. European experience with the urethral Wallstent for urethral strictures. Eur Urol 1991;19:181–5.
25. Reynard JM, Vass J, Sullivan ME, Mamas M. Sphincterotomy and the treatment of detrusor-sphincter dyssynergia: current status, future prospects. Spinal Cord 2003;41:1–11.
26. Chancellor MB, Gajewski J, Ackman CF, et al. Long-term followup of the North American Multicenter UroLume trial for the treatment of external detrusor-sphincter dyssynergia. J Urol 1999;161:1545–50.
27. Chancellor MB, Bennett C, Simoneau AR, et al. Sphincteric stent versus external sphincterotomy in spinal cord injured men: prospective randomized multicenter trial. J Urol 1999;161:1893–8.
28. Gajewski JB, Chancellor MB, Ackman CF, et al. Removal of UroLume endoprosthesis: experience of the North American Study Group for detrusor-sphincter dyssynergia application. J Urol 2000;163:773–6.
29. Azuma H, Chancellor MB. Overview of biodegradable urethral stents. Rev Urol 2004;6: 98–9.
30. Tammela TL, Talja M. Biodegradable urethral stents. BJU Int 2003;92:843–50.
31. Oosterlinck W, Talja M. Endoscopic urethroplasty with a free graft on a biodegradable polyglycolic acid spiral stent. A new technique. Eur Urol 2000;37:112–5.
32. Isotalo T, Tammela TL, Talja M, et al. A bioabsorbable self-expandable, self-reinforced poly-l-lactic acid urethral stent for recurrent urethral strictures: a preliminary report. J Urol 1998;160(6 Pt 1):2033–6.
33. Isotalo T, Talja M, Valimaa T, et al. A bioabsorbable self-expandable, self-reinforced poly-L-lactic acid urethral stent for recurrent urethral strictures: long-term results. J Endourol 2002;16:759–62.
34. Vaajanen A, Nuutinen JP, Isotalo T, et al. Expansion and fixation properties of a new braided biodegradable urethral stent: an experimental study in the rabbit. J Urol 2003;169:1171–4.
35. Petas A, Talja M, Tammela T, et al. A randomized study to compare biodegradable self-reinforced polyglycolic acid spiral stents to suprapubic and indwelling catheters after visual laser ablation of the prostate. J Urol 1997;157:173–6.
36. Petas A, Talja M, Tammela TL, et al. The biodegradable self-reinforced poly-DL-lactic acid spiral stent compared with a suprapubic catheter in the treatment of post-operative urinary retention after visual laser ablation of the prostate. Br J Urol 1997;80:439–43.
37. Dahlstrand C, Grundtman S, Pettersson S. High-energy transurethral microwave thermotherapy for large severely obstructing prostates and the use of biodegradable stents to avoid catheterization after treatment. Br J Urol 1997;79:907–9.
38. Petas A, Isotalo T, Talja M, et al. A randomised study to evaluate the efficacy of a biodegradable stent in the prevention of postoperative urinary retention after interstitial laser coagulation of the prostate. Scan J Urol Nephrol 2000;34:262–6.
39. Laaksovirta S, Isotalo T, Talja M, et al. Interstitial laser coagulation and biodegradable self-expandable, self-reinforced poly-L-lactic and poly-L-glycolic copolymer spiral stent in the treatment of benign prostatic enlargement. J Endourol 2002;16:311–5.
40. Isotalo T, Talja M, Valimaa T, et al. A pilot study of a bioabsorbable self-reinforced poly L-lactic acid urethral stent combined with finasteride in the treatment of acute urinary retention from benign prostatic enlargement. BJU Int 2000;85:83–6.
41. Isotalo T, Talja M, Hellstrom P, et al. A double-blind, randomized, placebo-controlled pilot study to investigate the effects of finasteride combined with a biodegradable self-reinforced poly L-lactic acid spiral stent in patients with urinary retention caused by bladder outlet obstruction from benign prostatic hyperplasia. BJU Int 2001;88:30–4.

Bioinjectables

Rodney A. Appell, MD, FACS

F. Brantley Scott

In the treatment of patients with urinary incontinence it is essential to identify the etiology of incontinence before injectables can be recommended as appropriate therapy. Urinary incontinence may originate at the level of the bladder or the urethra and injectable treatment exists for both. While bulking agents are available for the underactive urethra, chemical denervation is gaining importance in the treatment of the intractable overactive bladder and sphincter. Incontinence originating at the level of the urethra occurs as a result of intrinsic incompetence of the urethral closure mechanism (intrinsic sphincteric dysfunction or ISD). Patients with ISD are candidates for slings, the artificial sphincter, and intraurethral injectables. Reimbursement trends have also placed an emphasis on interventions which require minimal hospitalization, or, more optimally, can be performed entirely in the ambulatory office location without requirements for general or regional anesthesia and attendant recuperative facilities. Injection therapy certainly falls into this category, and has been used sparingly for the management of stress urinary incontinence (SUI) for nearly two decades, but has been limited by durability and antigenicity issues associated with bovine collagen. Relatively recent Food and Drug Administration (FDA) approval of carbon particulate technology (Durasphere) has provided another option for bulking, but one that is somewhat limited by difficulty with injection (because of carrier extrusion resulting in injection needle obstruction). Because of these concerns, many physicians would use Durasphere only in the controlled setting of the operative suite, thus detracting from the financial benefit associated with in-office bulking therapy. This was addressed by the manufacturer, and an improved formulation (Durasphere EXP) was introduced following FDA approval in October 2003, making its injection as easy as collagen. Therefore, the use of bulking therapy had been less than optimal to that

date. However, the advent of several new bulking agents, each with unique tissue interaction characteristics and holding the promise of greater durability, with fewer actual injection sessions, and no antigenicity, promises to dramatically alter the role of bulking therapy in the overall management schemata for SUI.

INDICATIONS AND PATIENT SELECTION

Selection of patients appears crucial to the outcome of the intraurethral injection of bulking agents. The ideal candidate for this procedure is one who has good anatomical support; a compliant, stable bladder; and a malfunctioning urethra evidenced by a low leak point pressure. Other subsets of patients who may benefit from the procedure are patients with high leak point pressure and minimal hypermobility and elderly women with bladder base mobility who are less active and are a poor surgical risk for other interventions. Contraindications include an active urinary tract infection, untreated detrusor overactivity, and hypersensitivity to the injected agent, relatively unknown with the newer inert, synthetic agents, but affecting around 3% of those undergoing collagen injection.[1] For this reason, patients contemplating collagen injection for incontinence must have a skin test 1 month prior to the procedure to determine if they have a hypersensitivity to bovine collagen.

INJECTABLE MATERIAL

The successful use of periurethral bulking agents is dependent on several factors inclusive of the composition of the material, facility of agent use (ease of preparation and implantation), and a receptive host environment (optimized hormonal environment, integrity of urethral anatomic components, and intact periurethral fascia). Three categories of materials have been investigated for

intraurethral bulking: human (autologous or allograft), xenograft, and synthetic.

The optimal attributes for bulking materials are: biocompatibility, minimal or no immunogenicity (hypoallergenic), integrity of the material formulation (there should be little or no separation of agent subcomponents [carrier and particulate solid]), rheologic (deformation within tissue) characteristics of the agent should also be positively affected by adequate material viscosity, surface tension, and tissue response (wound healing). These attributes for any specific agent should also be reproducible. Tissue response characteristics should further demonstrate minimal fibrotic ingrowth, little extracapsular inflammatory response (if encapsulation occurs at all), and agent volume after injection should be retained with minimal resorption. The most ideal scenario for any soft tissue bulking agent would be a single injection with permanent tissue residence of the agent (and partial or total incorporation into the host tissues). However, the current reality for the available agents is that they do not fulfill the above criteria either owing to isolated or combined agent and host factors (eg, lack of resorption, agent admixture separation).

The goal of endoscopic injection therapy for SUI is to provide a minimally invasive, effective, and safe alternative to open surgery. Although the technique has been available for decades, the ideal injectable has yet to be developed. In addition to safety issues by being biocompatible, nonantigenic, noninfectious, and noncarcinogenic, any material must demonstrate "anatomic integrity." This implies that the material conserves its volume over time. Despite the safety of using bovine collagen as a material for injection treatment for SUI, it lacks this anatomic integrity. This reduces the ability of collagen to be cost-effective.[2] A significant volume is required at each injection session and multiple injection sessions are the rule, not the exception, thus reducing not only the cost effectiveness of this material, but also translating into first, patient inconvenience and ultimately, to patient dissatisfaction with collagen and, perhaps, injectable therapy in general. Information on collagen has been well documented.[3]

Durasphere pyrolytic carbon-coated zirconium oxide beads, was approved by the FDA in 1999. The bead are suspended in a water-soluble beta-glucan vehicle. The randomized, multicenter, double-blind study accepted by the FDA compared collagen with Durasphere and showed similar outcomes, the original Durasphere offering a slight benefit. Durasphere is more viscous than collagen and, as mentioned above, its injection was more technically demanding until the introduction of Durasphere EXP. Recently, renewed concern has been expressed about material migration after injection.[4] Microcrystalline components of the bulking agent should be composed of uniform spheroidal particles with sizes above 80 microns (approximate size required to avoid migration, determined in studies involving polytetrafluorethylene [Teflon]). Migration is clearly influenced by the ability of host macrophages to phagocytize particles, and smaller particle sizes have been shown to migrate to distant locations with Teflon injection. However, direct embolization of material is caused by high-pressure injection, resulting in material displacement into vascular or lymphatic spaces. Injection technique should therefore rely on larger particle sizes administered with low-pressure injection instrumentation. This should not become a problem with Durasphere EXP, as its smallest particle is 95 microns and ranges up to 200 microns, significantly smaller than the original Durasphere (200–550 microns), but still in the size greater than the 80-micron minimum needed for safety.

SPECIFIC AGENTS IN DEVELOPMENT Synthetic calcium hydoxylapatite is identical to the same material found in human teeth and bones. The agent is composed of hydroxylapatite spheres (which are extremely uniform in shape, smooth, and 75–125 microns in size) in an aqueous gel composed of sodium carboxylmethylcellulose (Coaptite). Plain film radiography or ultrasonography may be used localize this material and can be useful adjuncts to assessing implantation. In fact, the first FDA-approved indication for this material has been obtained, specifically for soft tissue marking (as an adjunct to radiographic focusing for radiotherapeutics). Agent injection is carried out with a small-bore (21-gauge) needle, with standard cystoscopic instruments. A large-scale North American pivotal trial is nearly completed, accruing more than 250 women. Thus far, 21 women have received Coaptite and 18 have received collagen and have been followed for 1 year since last injection.[5] The average number of injections was 2.0 for Coaptite and 2.3 for collagen. The total volume injected was 3.7 cc for Coaptite and 7.4 cc for collagen. Eighty-six percent of Coaptite patients improved by at least 1 Stamey grade, 67% improved by 2 grades, and

38 % were completely continent (compared with women who received collagen with 66%, 55%, and 44%, respectively). Overall pad weight reduction in the 1-hour stress pad test was at least 75% in 77% of Coaptite patients, but in only 55% of collagen patients, and was 90% or greater in 46% (Coaptite) and 33% (collagen), respectively. No prolonged retention, urgency, or periurethral erosion or abscess was seen in either group. This agent has similar injection characteristics to collagen, and thus far appears to require less injected volume for somewhat more durable effect than collagen.

Another biologic agent, Zuidex consists of dextranomer microspheres in a cross-linked hyaluronic acid (HA) vehicle. HA is a water-insoluble, complex glycosaminoglycan composed of disaccharide units, which form molecules of 23 million molecular weight and is dissolved in normal saline for urethral bulking purposes. This composite gel has significant elasticity and high viscosity. These biologic characteristics have led to the use of hylan gels for soft tissue bulking purposes. It is completely biodegradable and nonimmunogenic. Hyaluronic acid functions as the transport compound and is resorbed within 2 weeks after injection. The dextranomer microspheres actually function as the bulking agent, and are 80 to 200 microns in size and do not show fragility with insertion, remaining in the injection site for about 4 years. Injection is performed using standard cystoscopic equipment, with minimal injection pressure. A clinical trial has just begun in the United States to evaluate this agent for SUI. Of interest is that the technique requires no endoscopy. A small device is placed into the urethra and the needles direct the injected material in 1 mL aliquots at the midurethra. However, substantive data exist for the efficacy and safety of this agent, allowing FDA approval in the United States for the indication of vesico-ureteral reflux and for pediatric incontinence, although the incontinence injections are at the bladder neck, as has been the convention for SUI until the new trial in adult women with SUI.

Results of dextranomer injection for pediatric incontinence show no associated adverse events, and substantial improvement at 12 months postinjection.[6] Sixteen patients (with a variety of underlying etiologies for their incontinence) underwent a mean of 2.3 injections with a mean volume of 2.8 mL with subsequent annual follow-up. Seventy-five percent were improved at 6 months and 50% at 12 months as determined by 1-hour pad tests and diary data. Further follow-up at 2 years indicated relative stability of incontinence parameters as compared with the 1-year data. No local injection site complications or immunologic sequelae resulted. Similar durability and safety findings have been identified with this material when used for the reflux indication.

Synthetic agents pose a potential benefit as bulking agents owing to their stability (non-biodegradability). Silicone is a hydrogel suspension composed of polyvinylpyrrolidone (povi-

done) as the carrier (which also acts as a lubricant for the injection system), while the bulking agent is solid polydimethylsiloxane elastomer (vulcanized silicone). The elastomer is a particulate of varying shapes and conformal configurations. Particle size is markedly variable with 25% of particles less than 50 microns in size, and some greater than 400 microns in largest dimension. Silicone delivery also requires high-pressure administration, but with newer equipment, this material is more easily delivered. Although well established in Europe, concerns regarding silicone stimulation of the immunologic response have limited evaluation of this agent in the United States. However, a clinical trial evaluating this agent (Macroplastique) for this indication now is in progress in North America. A recent Scandinavian report followed 22 women long term (2 years postinjection) who had received this agent.[7] Subjective and objective criteria showed stability and persistent benefit for those patients. Overall pad test data showed dramatic reduction (147 g mean pretreatment reduced to 9 g posttreatment). No long-term local or systemic complications were noted.

Ethylene vinyl alcohol copolymer suspended in dimethyl sulfoxide (DMSO) or Uryx solution is being evaluated as an embolic agent and a bulking agent. Upon injection and exposure to solution (blood or extracellular space) at physiologic temperatures, the DMSO diffuses from the copolymer and causes the ethylene vinyl alcohol to precipitate into a complex spongiform mass. This phase change requires diligent separation of agent and body temperature fluids until implantation occurs. Early experience with this agent suggested that optimal results were obtained with injection in a slightly more distal urethral location within the urethra (approximately 1.5 cm distal to the bladder neck), with a slower rate of injection (at least 30 seconds/mL/injection site), and without the need to observe visual coaptation at the completion of injection, as the volume injected is limited to 2.5 mL on each side of the urethra. Using these end-point criteria, results with this agent have been intriguingly good. An interesting difference with this material is that injection is this set volume and not an end point of coaptation of the urethra/bladder neck at the time of injection. A large-scale North American trial is in progress. The trial incorporates 237 women with genuine stress urinary incontinence (GSUI), and used a prospective, randomized (2:1 Uryx to bovine collagen) schema.[8] The study has now finished accrual, and all treated patients will be followed for 1 year post-last injection. At 6 months, 40 patients in the Uryx arm and 23 in the collagen arm have been evaluated (currently at 12 months, 21, and 13, respectively, have been evaluated). Thus far, mean total volume of material required for injection has been less for Uryx (4.4 cc compared with 6.9 cc for collagen). At 6 months, 63% of Uryx patients are dry (no incontinent episodes) as compared with 48% of the collagen patients. Interestingly, at 12 months, 74% of the Uryx patients are dry as compared with 40% of the collagen patients. Rates of postimplantation urgency and dysuria were essentially the same between the two arms. This result suggests that, unlike collagen, Uryx maintains a durability of response not noted with biologic agents and may provide the first synthetic material to do this without substantive complication issues.

A requirement for FDA trials with these agents is active comparison with bovine collagen. No current head-to-head data exist between these evolving agents at the time of this writing.

INJECTION TECHNIQUES

One will have to pay attention to the individual injectable material in the future for agent-specific techniques, as alluded to in the above segment on Uryx and Zuidex. The methods of injection are not difficult but do require precision to ensure an optimal therapeutic response. The intraurethral injection is primarily submucosal, but should also include the superficial muscle fibers of the proximal urethra (or, for Zuidex, the midurethra). Standard injection techniques are to position the needle into the space from within the urethral lumen or through the urethral wall from a peri-urethral entrance. Men are injected either retrograde via the transurethral technique or antegrade by a transvesical method. Women are injected either transurethrally or via the periurethral method, that is, the spinal needle inserted in the periurethral sinus at the level of the meatus and positioned in the tissues adjacent to the urethra whole, observing the manipulation cystoscopically.[9] The etiology of the problem leading to the incontinence, the tissue condition at the injection site, and the place of delivery of the material affect the treatment results. Those preferring the periurethral technique in women list these advantages: elimination of extrusion of the injected material through the injection site and bleeding complications that can hamper visualization, while admitting that material placement requires a longer learning curve than the transurethal, direct-vision technique via cystourethroscopy.[10]

INJECTIONS IN MEN After an appropriate level of anesthesia is achieved, the man is positioned in a semilithotomy position. If a local anesthetic is to be used, 2% lidocaine jelly is placed intraurethrally and left in place at least 10 minutes prior to instrumentation. Local anesthesia may be augmented by the use of 5 to 10 mL of 1% plain lidocaine injected with a 22-gauge spinal needle through the perineum under finger guidance per rectum in the fashion of perineal prostate biopsies.

Cystourethroscopy is then performed with a zero-degree lens and the material is delivered under direct vision until the urethral mucosa protrudes in the midline. This requires several needle placements in a circumferential manner (Figure 79-1). If the ISD has followed prostatic resection, a short segment of urethra remains below the verumontanum and proximal to the external sphincter. If visualization of this level is difficult, the needle may be inserted at the level of the external sphincter and advanced proxi-

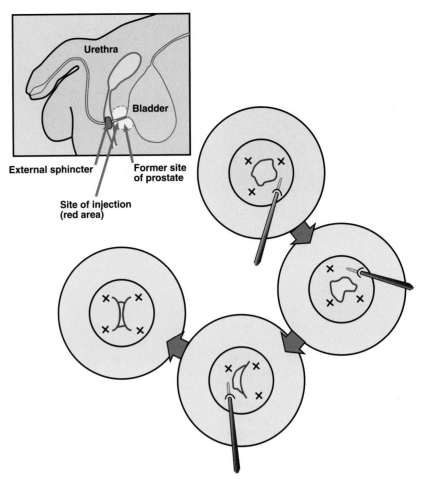

Figure 79-1 Stepwise collagen injections in the male patient. Note that the injection is made proximal to the urinary sphincter. (From McGuire EJ and Appell RA.[27])

mally to ensure deposition of the material proximal to the sphincter.[11]

Injection is more difficult in patients with postradical prostatectomny incontinence. Considerable practice is needed to reach the correct tissue depth for the needle. Extrusion of material into the lumen from the needle hole during its withdrawal may occur and can be minimized by preventing passage of the cystoscope beyond the injection area.

Antegrade injection directly at the bladder neck through a suprapubic percutaneous cystotomy allows placement of a pediatric urethroscope that contains a 5 French (F) working port for the needle.[12]

INJECTIONS IN WOMEN Injections can be given painlessly under local anesthesia alone. Women are placed in the lithotomy position and the introitus is coated in 20% benzocaine ointment and the urethral lumen is anesthesized with 2% lidocaine jelly. After waiting for 10 minutes, 2 to 4 mL of 1% plain lidocaine is injected peri-urethrally at the 3- and 9-o'clock positions. Transcystoscopic techniques are available with needles through an ordinary cystoscope and with specialty devices on the market. Periurethral needles are available, although in most instances a 20-gauge spinal needle can be advanced with the bevel of the needle directed toward the lumen.

The needle is advanced through the urethral muscle into the lamina propria and can then be advanced to the proper position for injection and verified by wiggling the needle while observing through the cystoscope. When the needle tip is observed to be positioned to 0.5 cm below the vesical neck, material is injected until swelling is visible on the ipsilateral side of the urethra. When the urethra appears approximately 50% occluded, the needle is removed and reinserted on the opposite side of the urethra and material is injected until the urethral mucosa is reapposed in the midline (Figure 79-2).

POSTPROCEDURAL CARE Perioperative antibiotic coverage is continued for 2 days following the procedure. If transient retention develops, clean intermittent catheterization is preferable to an indwelling catheter, as an indwelling catheter promotes molding of the material around the catheter and results in certain failure.[13] Patients are contacted within 2 weeks of injection and their continence status assessed, with repeat injections scheduled 1 month later, if necessary.

RESULTS

Patients are considered improved if social continence is obtained (wetting controlled with the use of tissues or a small minipad). Social continence or

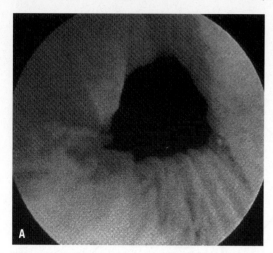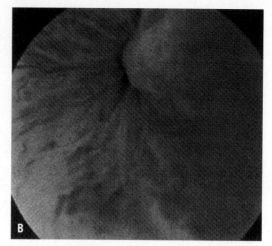

Figure 79-2 Endoscopic view of bladder neck in a female patient during collagen injection. *A,* The urethral lumen gradually occludes as collagen is injected into the lamina propria. *B,* Occlusion following completion of procedure. (From Appell RA.[28])

dryness is considered a successful result in the evaluation of the procedure. Success rates are just below that of slings and sphincters, but are the least invasive manner to treat ISD. However, injectables have not gained universal acceptance owing to (1) the inability to quantify the amount of material needed for injection in a particular patient and (2) the lack of durability of the result, requiring booster injections. Another problem is that the surgeon has to do enough procedures on a regular basis to attain the best possible results for the patient. The treatment response in women to injectable procedures for ISD is close to that obtained with surgical techniques with markedly fewer complications and adverse sequelae. In men, however, the results do not approach the results attained by the use of the artificial urinary sphincter, and have limited utility at this point in time.

SAFETY AND COMPLICATIONS

The currently available materials, if nothing else, are safe with no concerns of real note arising. Likewise, postprocedural complications are quite uncommon. The rate of transient urinary retention has been less than 20% with all substances. Associated urinary tract infections remain at < 2%. The number of periurethral abscesses is so rare that they remain reportable case reports at this point in time. Repeat injections are frequently necessary, yet are safely performed under local anesthesia.

INJECTABLES FOR DETRUSOR OR SPHINCTER OVERACTIVITY

Attempts at this treatment modality were first reported in 1969 with subtrigonal injections of 6% (aqueous) phenol.[14] Injection of phenol causes neurolysis of terminal pelvic nerve branches as they enter the trigone. Approximately 10 to 20 mL of the material is injected through a cystoscope in the submucosal level, bilaterally halfway between the bladder neck and each ureteral orifice. The procedure requires either general or regional anesthesia. This treatment modality has yielded mixed results with some investigators reporting success rates as high as 82 to 90%,[15,16] while others report poor success rates of < 20%.[17] Some studies attempted to identify subcategories of patients who were most likely to benefit from this procedure. Blackford and colleagues reported a success rate of 82% in women with multiple sclerosis over the age of 55 years and less than 14% in women younger than that.[15] In order to improve patient selection Madjar and colleagues used a transvaginal bupivacaine injection (0.25%) on the assumption that patients who respond to the local anesthetic will later respond to the subtrigonal phenol injection.[18] In their study, 23 out of 42 patients (54.7%) responded to the bupivacaine injection. Of all the patients who responded to the phenol injections, 26% had symptomatic relief that lasted more than 3 months. In most cases relief of symptoms is temporary and lasts from a few weeks to several months. Severe complications, such as vesico-vaginal fistulas, excoriation of the vaginal wall, and even the need for urinary diversion, were reported in 25 to 40% in 2 series.[16,19] However, in these patients the phenol was mixed in a nonaqueous, glycerol solution, which retained the phenol in the perivesical fat for a longer period of time. Because of the high complication rate, many physicians consider previous pelvic surgery or pelvic irradiation to be contraindications for this treatment.

Botulinum toxin (Botox) has proven to be a safe and effective therapy for a variety of somatic and autonomic motor disorders and appears to have some clinical efficacy in the treatment of detrusor-external sphincter-dyssynergia (DESD), pelvic floor spasticity, and overactive bladder. It is interesting that the most potent and lethal biological toxin known can be transformed into a health benefit. The toxin acts by inhibiting acetylcholine release at the presynaptic cholinergic junction. Clinically, Botox has been used successfully to treat spinal cord-injured patients who suffer from DESD[20] and neurogenic detrusor

overactivity,[21] resulting in a significant reduction in maximum detrusor voiding pressure. In a longer-term study of detrusor overactivity by these same investigators, 87 patients reported that the clinical response lasted only 4 to 14 months, but there were no adverse events.[22] Thus, although safe, the maintenance of clinical results requires repeated transcystoscopic injections. An added problem is that the Botox is expensive and currently not reimbursed for urological injection, as it is not FDA approved for this or any indication involving the urinary tract. Costs can be reduced by doing the procedure under local anesthesia in the office.

APPELL'S TECHNIQUE FOR BOTOX INJECTION INTO THE BLADDER UNDER LOCAL ANESTHESIA

Anesthetize the urethra with 2% lidocaine jelly, empty the bladder and instill 50 mL of 1% plain lidocaine solution and let that remain for 10 minutes before placing the cystoscope and beginning the injections. I inject the first 100 units in 0.5 mL (5 units of Botox) aliquots across the back of the trigone. Therefore, that is 20 small injections. I then inject another 100 units in radial fashion from the trigone up the posterior wall toward the dome of the bladder. In this portion I inject in 4 radial positions with 5 injections in each radial (Figure 79-3). There are other techniques for the injection, as well as the concentration of the Botox to be used, and none have been reported more effective than another.

It is only natural that the technique would be extended beyond the neurogenic bladder patient to the idiopathic overactive bladder (OAB) patient. Radziszewski and colleagues reported favorably

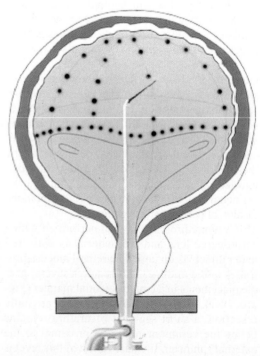

Figure 79-3 Technique of Botox injection for detrusor overactivity.

on intravesical Botox A injection in a pilot study with either OAB or functional outlet obstruction.[23] Following intravesical or sphincteric injections there was resolution of incontinence and improved voiding efficiency, respectively, but again, with only short duration.

Chemical denervation of the external sphincter begins within 2 to 3 days, and is reversed within 3 to 6 months, as terminal nerve sprouting occurs.[24] Dykstra and Sidi published the only double-blind, placebo-controlled study of Botox A.[25] In the Botox-injected patients the urethral pressure decreased an average of 25 cm H_2O, postvoid residual (PVR) decreased an average of 125 mL, and detrusor pressure during voiding decreased an average of 30 cm H_2O, whereas the patients on placebo (normal saline injection) were unchanged. Phelan and colleagues confirmed this with results at between 3 and 16 months postinjection, demonstrating a reduction in voiding pressures during that time of 38%.[26]

CONCLUSIONS

It is clear that injectable treatment for SUI and UI can be effective and safe; however, it is clear that durability of the positive result remains a primary concern when implementing these minimally invasive techniques. With time and further research, improvements in the use of injectables for SUI are inevitable. However, chemical denervation for detrusor and sphincter overactivity is in its infancy. Clearly the dose and the volume injected would appear to play an important role in inducing results and probably relates to possible systemic toxicity also. There is no question that targets for future chemical denervation go beyond DESD and detrusor motor overactivity, involving various forms of bladder neck obstruction, including benign prostatic hyperplasia, and

perhaps moving into the sensory/urgency realm, which might include interstitial cystitis.

REFERENCES

1. Appell R. Collagen injection therapy for urinary incontinence. Urol Clin N Am 1994;21:177–82.
2. Culligan PJ, Rackley R, Koduri S, et al. Is it safe to reuse a syringe of glutaraldehyde cross-linked collagen? A microbiological study. J Urol 2000;164:1275–6.
3. Kershen RT, Dmochowski RR, Appell RA. Beyond collagen: injectable therapies for the treatment of female stress urinary incontinence in the new millennium. Urol Clin N Am 2002;29:559–74.
4. Ritts RE. Particle migration after transurethral injection of carbon coated beads for stress urinary incontinence. J Urol 2002;167:1804–5.
5. Dmochowski R, Appell RA, Klimberg I, et al. Initial clinical results from coaptite injection for stress urinary incontinence, comparative clinical study [poster presentation 282]. Annual meeting of the Program of the International Continence Society; 2002 Aug; Heidelberg, Germany.
6. Caione P, Capozza N. Endoscopic treatment of urinary incontinence in pediatric patients: 2-year experience with dextranomer/hyaluronic acid copolymer. J Urol 2002;168(4 Pt 2):1868–71.
7. Peeker R, Edlund C, Wennberg AL, Fall M. The treatment of sphincter incontinence with periurethral silicone implant (Macroplastique). Scand J Urol Nephrol 2002;36: 194–8.
8. Dmochowski RR, Herschorn S, Corcos J, et al. Multicenter randomized controlled study to evaluate Uryx urethral bulking agent in treating female stress urinary incontinence. J Urol 2002;167:LB–10.
9. Appell R. The artificial urinary sphincter and periurethral injections: role in the treatment of female urinary incontinence. Obstet Gynecol Rep 1990;2:334–42.
10. Winters J, Appell R. Periurethral injections in the treatment of intrinsic sphincteric dysfunction. In: Marshall F, editor. Textbook of operative urology. Philadelphia: WB Saunders; 1996. p. 720–8.
11. Appell R. Injectables for urethral incompetence. World J Urol 1990;8:208–11.
12. Winters JC, Appell RA. Collagen injection therapy in the treatment of urinary incontinence. Tech Urol 1996;2: 59–64.
13. Winters J, Appell R. Complications of the use of injectables in the treatment of incontinence and reflux. In: Carson C, editor. Complications of interventional procedures in urology. Topics in urology. New York: Igaku-Shoin; 1995. p. 95–105.
14. Susset JG, Pinheiro J, Otton P, et al. [Selective phenolization and neurotomy in the treatment of neurogenic bladder dysfunction due to an incomplete central lesion.] J Urol Nephrol (Paris) 1969;75:502.
15. Blackford HN, Murray K, Stephenson TP, Mundy AR. Results of transvesical infiltration of the pelvic plexuses with phenol in 116 patients. Br J Urol 1984;56:647–9.
16. Harris RG, Constantinou CE, Stamey TA. Extravesical subtrigonal injection of 50% ethanol for detrusor instability. J Urol 1988;140:111–6.
17. Ramsey IN, Clancy S, Hilton P. Subtrigonal phenol injections in the treatment of idiopathic detrusor instability in the female—a long-term urodynamic follow-up. Br J Urol 1992;69:363–5.
18. Madjar S, Smith ND, Balzarro M, et al. Bupivacaine injections prior to subtrigonal phenolization: preliminary results. In: Proceedings of the 22nd Annual Meeting of the Society for Urodynamics and Female Urology. Anaheim, CA; 2001.
19. Bennani S. [Evaluation of sub-trigonal injections in the treatment of the hyperactive bladder.] Ann Urol (Paris) 1994;28:13–9.
20. Petit H, Wiart E, Gaujard E, et al. Botulinum A toxin treatment for detrosr-sphincter-dyssynergia in spinal cord disease. Spinal Cord 1998;36:91–4.
21. Schurch B, Stohrer M, Kramer, et al. Botulinum-A toxin for treating detrusor hyperreflexia in spinal cord injured patients: a new alternative to anticholinergic drugs? Preliminary results. J Urol 2000;164(3 Pt 1):692–7.
22. Schurch B, Stohrer M, Kramer G, et al. Botulinum toxin A to treat detrusor hyper-reflexia in spinal cord injured patients. Neurourol Urodyn 2001;20:521–2.
23. Radziszewski P, Dobronski P, Borkowski A. Treatment of the non-neurogenic storage and voiding disorders with the chemical denervation caused by botulinum toxin A. A pilot study. Neuroruol Urodyn 2001;20:410–2.
24. de Paiva A, Meunier FA, Molgo J, et al. Functional repair of motor endplates after botulinum neurotoxin type A poisoning: biphasic switch of synaptic activity between nerve sprouts and their parent terminals. Proc Natl Acad Sci U S A 1999;96:3200–5.
25. Dykstra DD, Sidi A. Treatment of detrusor-sphincter dyssynergia with botulinum A toxin: a double blind study. Arch Phys Med Rehabil 1990;71:24–6.
26. Phelan MW, Franks M, Smogyi GT, et al. Botulinum toxin urethral sphincter injection to restore bladder emptying in men and women with voiding dysfunction. J Urol 2001;165:1107–10.
27. McGuire EJ, Appell RA. Collagen injection for the dysfunctional urethra. Contemp Urol 1991;3:11–9.
28. Appell RA. Periurethral collagen injection for female incontinence. Probl Urol 1991;5:134–40.

80

Management of Male Stress Urinary Incontinence: Male Slings

R. Clay McDonough 3rd, MD

R. Duane Cespedes, MD

The opinions contained herein are those of the authors and are not to be construed as reflecting the views of the Air Force or the Department of Defense.

Multiple options exist for treating incontinence in male patients. This chapter will describe novel, minimally invasive methods for managing postprostatectomy incontinence using a male sling. Three methods of performing a male sling will be discussed, as well as their indications, patient evaluation and preparation, complications, and results. In addition, a brief history of the evolution of the different male slings will be discussed.

HISTORICAL BACKGROUND

Postprostatectomy incontinence (PPI) after a radical prostatectomy can be a debilitating problem with a reported incidence of 5 to 20%.[1,2] Early therapy for PPI includes Kegel exercises and medical therapy. However, after 9 to 12 months, surgical therapies should be considered if the patient has persistent stress urinary incontinence. In cases of mild to moderate incontinence, some patients can be significantly improved or cured with collagen injections.[3] More recently, with the innovations in performing radical prostatectomy, many PPI cases are mild, and because collagen injections are a minimally invasive procedure, some patients will be candidates for collagen or other injectable agents.[4,5] For more severe cases of PPI, the artificial urinary sphincter (AUS) has been quite successful and remains the gold standard therapy for PPI. Nevertheless, revisions may be necessary owing to infections, erosions, or mechanical problems. In addition, some patients are reluctant to have the AUS placed for a variety of reasons, including the desire to "void normally" without having to manipulate a device. While many patients will be cured or have substantial improvement with an AUS, 20 to 50% will require surgical revision or a double-cuff procedure in some cases to treat recurrent stress incontinence.[6–8]

More recently, the male sling has had a resurgence of popularity in the search for a minimally invasive, efficacious, "natural voiding" alternative to treat PPI. Currently, there are two main methods of performing the male sling with multiple variations. Like many "novel" procedures, male slings and the concept of using urethral compression to achieve continence is not new. The concept of urethral compression was originally used in female patients with stress or neurogenic incontinence, while male slings were introduced later for PPI. Player and Callander reported the first successful series in 1927 using a gracilis muscle flap around the bulbar urethra to provide compression.[9] Decades later, two separate male sling series were described using a combined abdominal and perineal approach to place fascial strips around the bulbar urethra or bladder neck.[10,11] A review of the results of multiple male sling series from the 1940s to 1960s found the overall cure rates to be between 32 and 50%, with significant improvement in an additional 19 to 21%.[12] Two series of male slings in the 1970s by Servadio[13] and Pettersson and Bratt[14] showed similar results. While other procedures for achieving continence (including a "urethral twist") were described during this period, the most popular method for treating male incontinence in the 1970s was urethral compression using the penile crura or perineally placed prosthetic devices.[15,16] The Kaufman procedure and later the Kaufman prosthesis would undergo many modifications in the 1970s, and good results were reported; however, these procedures were eventually abandoned owing to problems with erosions, infections, and the introduction of the AUS.[17,18] In 1979, Kaufman and Raz reported their long-term results using urethral compression: 61% were cured or significantly improved; however, 11% of patients suffered major complications and 24% had minor complications.[19] This series, along with previous series, demonstrated that urethral compression did indeed cure or improve PPI in many cases; however, the surgical approach, instrumentation, and patient selection would require additional modifications to further improve results and reduce morbidity.

Since the late 1970s, compressive-type procedures have rarely been used for PPI; however, in the mid-1990s, O'Donnell began using autologous fascial slings using a combined abdominal and perineal approach to treat PPI.[20] Sutures were attached to an autologous rectus fascia sling and then transferred to the abdominal incision using a ligature passer, similar to the female procedures performed. The sling was then tied over the rectus fascia under substantial tension. His initial experience has not yet been published; however, the procedure was subsequently adopted, modified, and performed by others. Many names have been used for this procedure, including the bladder neck sling, modified bulbar sling, needle suspension male sling, and others. Autologous fascia was originally used and acceptable results were obtained; however, the use of allografts, xenografts, and mesh grafts have greatly reduced patient morbidity and improved cure rates since that time.[21–24] The original procedure called for detachment of the bulb from the central tendon with placement of the sling directly under the membranous urethra. This dissection is somewhat difficult and may increase the erosion risk; therefore, more recently, the sling has been placed over the bulb with a limited bulb dissection to allow urethral compression.

Another variation of the male sling is the bulbourethral male sling using multiple Gore-Tex grafts as reported by Schaeffer, Clemens, and colleagues.[25,26] Using a combined abdominal and perineal approach, three Gore-Tex vascular grafts are used to compress the bulbar urethra with the suture ends tied over the rectus muscle similar to the pubovaginal sling in a female. Following a single procedure, 56% of 36 patients were dry and 8% were significantly improved with a median follow-up on 18 months. In 17 patients, retightening procedures were performed, increasing the success rate to 75%. They also reported a 27% revision rate, 6% erosion rate, and 3% infection rate. A later report noted that of 61 evaluable patients, 53% did not wear pads and 85% wore 2 pads or less; however, 52% had persistent perineal numbness or discomfort.[26]

Slings have also been used in male patients with neurogenic bladders and incompetent sphincters. Daneshmand and colleagues described placing an autologous puboprostatic fascial sling distal to the prostatic urethra in 12 patients using an abdominal approach.[27] Eight patients were completely dry and 2 had significant improvement, for an overall success rate of 83%. All patients voided by clean intermittent catheterization. Although these slings are relatively efficacious, it is difficult to perform after a radical prostatectomy and is relatively invasive; therefore, it will not be described in this chapter.

The most recent and least invasive version of the male sling involves placement of an allograft, xenograft, or mesh sling between the inferior pubic rami using bone anchoring techniques.[28–31]

The perineal male sling uses an entirely perineal approach, with the sling compressing the urethra just distal to the membranous urethra by placing bone screws into the inferior pubic rami to provide strong permanent fixation points. A 4 by 7 cm sling made of an allograft, xenograft, or polypropylene mesh has been most commonly used; however, mesh is quickly becoming the material of choice as other materials have not been as durable owing to the extreme amount of pressure placed on the sling.

It is important to note that as with any "new" procedure, multiple methods and materials will be used and reported as the male sling is continuously improved, eventually yielding a more effective and less morbid procedure. This is not unlike the AUS or pubovaginal slings, which both evolved over many years and continue to be updated.

PREOPERATIVE EVALUATION

Almost all patients with PPI have minimal urethral hypermobility; therefore, stress urinary incontinence (SUI) after radical prostatectomy is essentially the male equivalent of intrinsic sphincter deficiency (ISD). Incontinence after a radical prostatectomy can also be urgency related, and therefore it is important to determine the exact pattern and nature of the incontinence. If the patient describes a significant urge component and no evidence of obstruction or urinary tract infection is found, it is possible that a dysfunctional bladder could be the source of the patient's incontinence. In many cases, these patients will have had similar symptoms prior to the prostatectomy. Some investigators have reported that up to 60% of patients are incontinent after a prostatectomy owing to bladder overactivity as a sole or contributing factor; however, in the authors' experience and others, it is rarely the sole cause, and most patients are found to have mixed incontinence.[32,33]

In some patients, however, it is unclear if incontinence is due to sphincteric incompetence, detrusor instability, or both. Multichannel urodynamic testing with fluoroscopy can be helpful in determining if the incontinence is due to detrusor instability or ISD. To help guide in the decision making, Sanchez-Ortiz and colleagues demonstrated that those with a Valsalva leak point pressure (VLPP) of greater than 60 cm of H_2O have a 70% chance of cure with collagen injections, whereas those with a lower VLPP have a cure rate of only 19%.[34] Unfortunately, many patients have narrowing at the vesicourethral anastomosis and the patient cannot be made to leak, even with vigorous coughing, until the urodynamic catheter is removed. In these cases, determining a VLPP with the rectal catheter alone may be helpful.

Voiding studies in PPI patients are often performed, but are difficult to correlate with surgical outcomes. It is difficult to predict preoperatively who will have difficulty voiding after an incontinence procedure, as PPI patients have an extremely low voiding pressure after the obstructive properties of the prostate are removed. From prior urodynamics performed on patients with a male sling, most patients will void in the 25 to 35 cm H_2O range after a male sling. Clinically, there have been rare cases of retention after a male sling, and all have resolved with time. Therefore, the clinical usefulness of a preoperative voiding pressure is unclear.

Cystoscopy can be helpful in ruling out other etiologies that can cause incontinence, as well as providing some basic urodynamic information. Cystoscopy can determine whether anastomotic strictures, occult bladder cancer, retained sutures, or bladder stones are present. A postvoid residual can also be obtained at the time of the procedure. Demonstration of incontinence with straining or cough after filling the bladder during cystoscopy is presumptive evidence that ISD exists. This is really all that is necessary in the PPI patient with pure SUI.

SELECTING AND CONSENTING PATIENTS FOR A MALE SLING

Perhaps the most important determinant of surgical success when using the male sling is patient selection. Originally, we used male slings on any patient desiring them, including those who had multiple previous AUS revisions or failures. It became clear that in patients with severe incontinence, the results were worse than in those with milder incontinence. Although no strict guidelines can be given because patient activity levels and habits are different, we prefer to use male slings only in those patients who use less than 6 pads per day. If the patient still desires a sling procedure, it is still probable that he will be improved; however, cure is less likely. In the more severe cases, we generally recommend an AUS. We have not found any difference in outcomes in patients with detrusor instability or radiation therapy; however, Clemens and colleagues reported a dramatic decrease in the cure rate after radiation therapy.[26]

As experience has been gained performing slings in patients with a coexisting penile prosthesis, it is clear that these cases are more difficult because the proximal cylinders generally overlie where the bone anchors are placed. In most cases, the crura have to be mobilized to place the bone anchors, potentially causing damage to the inflatable cylinders or causing perineal numbness because of the extensive dissection required. In one case in which a penile prosthesis was placed after a male sling, the corporal dilation was extremely difficult; however, the procedure was successfully performed and no degradation in continence was noted. In another case, the continence was severely degraded after prosthesis placement, presumably owing to dislodgement of the sling or the bone anchors. Therefore, if a penile prosthesis is also desired, a simultaneous sling and prosthesis placement should be considered.

When consenting a patient for a male sling, they should understand that other alternatives do exist and include injection therapies, AUS, or not having surgery at all. They should also understand the risks of male sling placement, which include infection, bleeding, sling infection or erosion, osteitis pubis, nerve paresthesias from patient positioning in stirrups, perineal nerve injury causing genital numbness or persistent discomfort, potential for infections from cadaveric sling material (if used), urinary retention, and failure to improve incontinence, as well as the normal risks of anesthesia and open surgery. In patients with normal erectile function, there should not be any change in status because the dissection is lateral to the nerve bundles. Lastly, they should be aware of the expected success rates as described later in this chapter.

DESCRIPTION OF PROCEDURES

BLADDER NECK SLING The fascial bladder neck sling is performed through a combined abdominal and perineal approach using allograft or xenograft materials (a modification of this procedure using a mesh sling will be described below). An autograft can be effectively used but is not recommended to minimize patient morbidity. A 4 to 5 cm midline incision is made in the perineum and the bulbous urethra is dissected free from the central tendon using cautery. This must be done carefully so as not to injure the underlying urethra. Once the bulb has been dissected free, the proximal urethra at the site of the previous anastomosis can be visualized (Figure 80-1A). Because all these patients have had prior prostatic surgery, retropubic dissection adjacent to the bladder neck and proximal urethra can be difficult. Using Metzenbaum scissors, the retropubic space is entered just lateral to the membranous urethra. Using careful dissection and keeping the tips of the scissors directly on the pubic periosteum at all times, the proximal urethra and the bladder neck can be dissected free from the underside of the pubis to allow a 6 to 8 cm sling to be placed behind the pubis. Practically, this means that retropubic tunnels of approximately 3 to 4 cm on each side are required. It is not necessary to be able to pass a finger all the way to the rectus muscle as in a female pubovaginal sling.

Once this dissection is completed, attention is directed to the abdominal incision. The incision for passage of the sling sutures is generally 2 to 3 cm long and should be made approximately 1 cm cranial to the pubis and is carried down to the rectus fascia.

The fascial sling is then prepared. The sling should be at least 2 cm wide and 6 to 8 cm long with the ends oversewn with No. 1 polypropylene suture. A Pereyra needle or other ligature passer is passed from the abdominal incision down to the perineal incision, ensuring that the tip of the needle maintains constant contact with the pubic periosteum. The sling suture from one end of the sling is then pulled up into the abdominal incision. This is repeated for the other side. The sling is fixated in position beneath the urethra with two midline sutures. The completed sling procedure can be seen in Figure 80-1B. As most of these patients will have some difficulty voiding postoperatively because of the considerable pressure

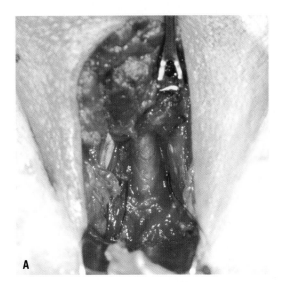

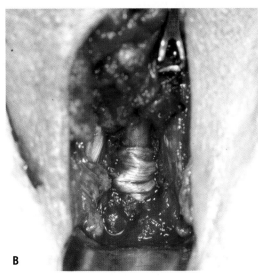

Figure 80-1 Intraoperative photographs of a bladder neck sling procedure. *A*, A Babcock clamp is retracting the dissected urethral bulb with the sling visible in the foreground. The sling sutures can be seen entering the retropubic space lateral to the exposed proximal urethra. *B*, The fascial sling in place around the urethra. More recent modifications include using a polypropylene mesh sling that is placed over the bulb with minimal dissection to reduce erosion risk.

placed on the urethra, a suprapubic tube is usually placed. This is accomplished using either a Lowsley retractor or preferably one of the standard punch suprapubic catheter kits. Cystoscopy is then performed to determine that there are no bladder or urethral injuries present.

If the patient is awake and able to cough, the sling is tightened until no leakage occurs with a full bladder and vigorous cough. If the patient cannot perform a Valsalva test or cough, the sling is tightened until 60 to 90 cm H_2O is obtained using retrograde perfusion and then tied down over the rectus.[35] To perform this test, a Foley catheter is advanced into the fossa navicularis and the balloon is inflated with 1 to 3 cc to form a seal and hold the catheter in place. A saline infusion bag is connected to the Foley and the "zero point" at the bladder level is noted. Starting at the zero point, the clamp on the

saline bag is opened and the saline bag slowly raised until a brisk retrograde flow is noted in the drip chamber. This is the retrograde perfusion pressure. If urethral compression is inadequate (less than 60 cm H_2O), the sling pressure should be increased.

Once the sling is tied in place, the abdominal and perineal wounds are closed in standard fashion. A small Foley catheter can be used overnight, but is generally not left in for more than 24 hours for fear of erosion. Voiding trials can be initiated within a few days and the suprapubic tube used to measure postvoid residuals.

MESH BLADDER NECK SLING More recently, these slings have become my male sling of choice for more severe degrees of incontinence or where cost is a concern because they allow a substantial amount of compression at the bladder neck, and yet have little chance of erosion owing to the bulk of tissue between the sling and the urethra. For this reason, it is an especially useful option for patients with neurogenic bladders who must perform intermittent catheterization. The use of mesh also prevents the late failures owing to suture "pull through" that sometimes occur when using natural materials.

In this modification, the perineal dissection is simpler in that all of the midline structures are initially left intact. After incising the perineal skin and subcutaneous tissues, the dissection is directed laterally to expose the inferior pubic rami at the level of the pubic symphysis leaving the urethra and all of its overlying structures intact. The retropubic space is dissected and entered as previously described using sharp dissection. A 2 to 3 cm Pfannenstiel incision is made 1 cm above the pubis and dissected down to the fascia. A polypropylene (Prolene) mesh sling approximately 3 cm at the center and tapering to 1.5 cm at the ends is oversewn using 1-0 Prolene sutures. A Pereyra needle is then passed and the sling pulled up as previously described. Of note, some authors describe using a wider sling and placing two sutures on each end of the sling, much like a vaginal wall sling in the female.[23] The sling is placed on tension and then secured in place to the bulbocavernosus fascia directly under the bladder neck region using several small nonabsorbable sutures. When the sling is placed on significant tension, in most cases, urethral compression will be limited by the bulbar attachments to the central tendon. With the sling on constant tension, the bulbar attachments to the central tendon are carefully dissected free using cautery until the bulb "pops" loose. Thereafter, tensioning is similar to the previous discussion; however, ensure that a small Foley can be passed since a suprapubic catheter is not used. The mesh is irrigated copiously with dilute Betadine solution and the incisions closed in a standard fashion. The Foley can be removed within 24 hours, with most patients voiding spontaneously.

PERINEAL MALE SLING The perineal male sling uses an entirely perineal approach, with the

sling compressing the urethra just distal to the membranous urethra by placing bone screws into the inferior pubic rami to provide strong permanent fixation points. Originally, we used a 4 by 7 cm sling of cadaveric fascia or dermis; however, more recently it has become clear that these materials have a higher incidence of suture "pull through" owing to the considerable amount of tension placed on these slings. More recently, we have used polypropylene mesh as the sling with fewer late failures. Broad-spectrum intravenous antibiotics are given preoperatively since bone anchors are used, and regional anesthesia is preferred as it allows the patient to cough or strain during the case to test the efficacy of sling compression. The patient is placed in standard lithotomy position and the skin prepped and draped to exclude the anus. A large Foley catheter or Van Buren sound is placed to assist in identifying the urethra during dissection.

A 4 to 5 cm midline perineal incision is made starting at the inferior edge of the scrotum and ending 1 to 2 cm away from the anus. After penetrating the subcutaneous tissues, the dissection is directed laterally to expose the inferior pubic rami from the pubic symphysis to the ischial tuberosity bilaterally. To minimize bleeding, enhance the compressive effect of the sling, and to minimize the risk of sling erosion, the urethra and all of its overlying structures are avoided. A Scott or Lone Star-type retractor can be used to maintain exposure. Excessive dissection on the periosteum of the rami, especially electrocautery, may damage the perineal branch of the pudendal nerve, resulting in perineal numbness. In patients with penile prostheses, the crura must be mobilized medially (in most cases) in order to correctly place the bone anchors.

A series of two, or preferably three, bone screws with a permanently attached No. 1 polypropylene suture is placed into the inner aspect of the inferior pubic rami bilaterally. These bone anchors can be difficult to place owing to the thickness of the periosteum in this region and the thin area of exposed bone available, as seen in Figure 80-2. It is extremely important that the most superior bone anchor on each side is placed well above where the urethra exits below the pubic symphysis. The caudal bone anchor is placed after carefully measuring the width of the sling, but it should be well above the ischial tuberosity to minimize pain when the patient is sitting. If the caudal bone anchor measurement places it near the ischial tuberosity, it is likely that the cephalad anchor needs to be moved higher. A third bone anchor is then placed at the midpoint between the other two screws. The same procedure is repeated on the other side (Figure 80-3).

A 4 by 7 cm graft is generally sufficient to reach both ischial rami and provide good urethral compression. The ends of the suture from each of the bone screws on one side are placed through one side of the mesh or graft material. A free needle is the easiest method to pass the sutures if graft material is used. The sutures are then sequentially tied down, fixating one end of the

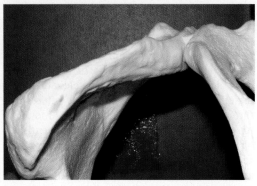

Figure 80-2 A pelvic inlet view of the inferior pubic rami. Bone screw or anchor placement for the perineal sling is on the inner aspect of the pubic rami. Placement of these screws can be difficult because the bone here is rounded and quite thick.

sling to the pubis (Figure 80-4). The tension will be set when the other side of the sling is tied down. The Foley is removed and the free end of the sling grasped and pulled to the opposite pubic ramus. As the sling is usually tied down under maximal tension, the sutures are placed through the sling where they overlie the bone anchors with the sling on maximum stretch. The sling can then be tied down to the bone anchors (Figures 80-5 and 80-6).

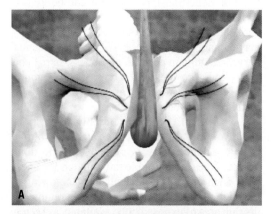

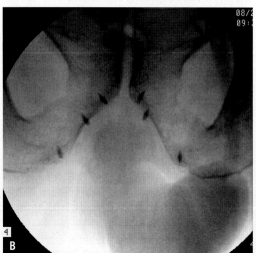

Figure 80-3 *A*, Diagrammatic representation of the placement of the 6 bone anchors typically used in placing a perineal sling. *B*, Radiographic view of the correct placement of the bone anchors.

In most cases, maximal tension will yield a retrograde perfusion pressure over 60 cm H_2O; however, to test the compression achieved, retrograde perfusion can be performed as previously described. If the urethral compression is less than 60, a series of 2 to 3 imbricating sutures can be placed to further tighten the sling (Figure 80-7). The Foley catheter is then advanced to the bladder neck to ensure that it freely passes. The surgical site is irrigated with antibiotic solution and then closed in several layers.

POSTOPERATIVE CARE In all cases, a regular diet can be resumed on the day of surgery. Patients can be discharged to home on the same day providing they have adequate pain control and are able to tolerate a regular diet. Strenuous activity should be avoided for 6 weeks postoperatively to allow proper healing of the sling. Oral antibiotics, generally a fluoroquinolone, are prescribed for 5 to 7 days after surgery.

If a Foley catheter is placed with a suburethral bladder neck sling, this is removed by the first postoperative day and the bladder is thereafter drained via the suprapubic tube. If the patient has significant complaints of bladder spasm, anticholinergic medications can be initiated. Voiding trials can be initiated 2 to 3 weeks postoperatively to allow the sling to heal in place, and the suprapubic tube is discontinued after the patient has a consistent postvoid residual of less than 100 mL. In patients with neurogenic bladder for which voiding is not expected, clean intermittent catheterization can begin at this time.

With the modified mesh bladder neck sling and perineal sling, the urethral catheter can be removed prior to discharge if the patient can pass a voiding trial. The authors prefer to bring the patient back to the clinic on the first postoperative day, at which time a fill and pull is performed. Pain control with nonsteroidal analgesics is generally sufficient. Having the patient sit on an inflatable "donut" cushion can also minimize perineal pain.

RESULTS

BLADDER NECK SLINGS In long-term followup of patients who have had a graft sling placed under the membranous urethra, 60% of patients were dry, 1 patient was improved, and 2 have failed. All patients were able to void postoperatively, although 1 patient had intermittently elevated postvoid residuals (> 100 mL) for over a year. Some patients did require 2 to 3 months before normal voiding occurred. With the more recent modification using mesh and leaving the bulb intact, the results have been slightly better, with a 75% cure or significantly improved rate with qualitatively decreased pain and morbidity. Although we have not adequately evaluated this procedure in patients with a neurogenic bladder or in pediatric myelodysplasia patients, similar results can be anticipated.

Other recent male sling series have confirmed these results. Migliari and colleagues,

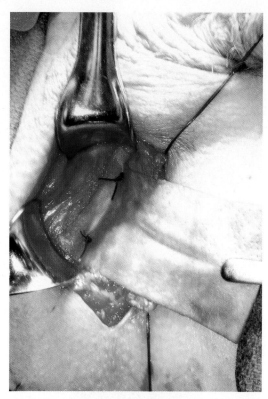

Figure 80-4 Intraoperative photograph with one end of a dermal sling tied down to the inferior ramus. Typically, 3 bone anchors are placed per side.

using a similar procedure and polypropylene sling, reported a 78% cure or significantly improved rate in their PPI patients.[22] Kapoor and colleagues performed a similar procedure in their patients; however, a Dacron graft was used.[23] They reported that "all patients were continent" postprocedure, although some used 1 or 2 pads. One patient required removal of the graft for infectious reasons. Lastly, Shoukry and el-Salmy used a modified version of this procedure in patients with both PPI and neurogenic incontinence. In long-term follow-up, 83% of patients were dry and 1 patient required removal of the graft for an infection.[24]

While the authors of these three series confirmed the relative simplicity of this procedure, they also pointed out another beneficial feature of

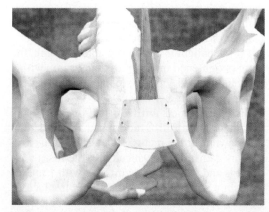

Figure 80-5 This diagram depicts the final result when all of the sling sutures are tied down.

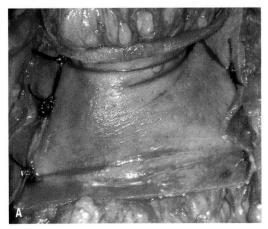 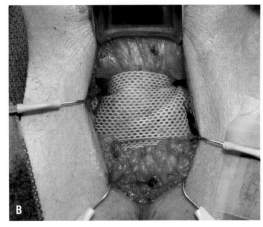

Figure 80-6 *A*, An intraoperative photograph of a perineal male sling after all the sutures have been secured to the pubic rami. In this case, a dermal graft was used and the tension placed on the graft can easily be seen. *B*, An intraoperative photograph of a polypropylene mesh sling after all the sutures are tied down.

this type of male sling: its low cost. The AUS remains an excellent choice for PPI; however, it is relatively expensive and may be beyond the reach of patients in some countries. This type of male sling would certainly be useful in these situations.

PERINEAL MALE SLING The first published data for the bone-anchored perineal sling were tabulated from a multi-institutional series of 58 patients.[28] The majority of patients had prior failed incontinence procedures and the median number of pads used per day was 4.5, with a range of 1 to 25. With moderate term follow-up, 26 of 58 patients (45%) were completely dry, and overall, 47 of 58 (81%) were significantly improved or were dry. A recent update of the authors' results using either cadaveric or xenograft materials for the sling confirmed these early results. At a mean 13 months postoperatively (range 4–29 months), 19 of 28 patients (65%) were dry (0–1 pads per day), and overall, 20 of 26 patients (77%) showed significant improvement (greater than 75%) or were dry. In 2 of these patients, an AUS was placed without difficulty, demonstrating that the perineal sling does not limit future surgical options.

Subsequently, Ghoneim and Bryan also reported a series of 10 patients using a cadaveric fascia bone-anchored sling.[31] In short-term follow-up they reported that 70% were dry, 10% were improved, and that 20% had failed after a brief period of dryness. These latter failures are consistent with our own experience in that a small percentage will fail after an early cure, presumably due to "suture pull through" when using natural materials. In some cases, it may also be due to dislodgement of a bone screw; however, this can also occur when using mesh slings.

Two recent series using mesh as the sling have also been reported. Madjar and colleagues reported a 75% cure rate and overall 100% cure or improved rate in their series of 16 patients using a Dacron mesh sling.[29] No mesh or osseus complications occurred, all patients were able to void postoperatively, and the authors recom-

mended its routine use. More recently, Comiter reported a prospective series of 21 male sling patients using a polypropylene sling.[30] With a mean 12-month follow-up, 76% of patients were dry, 14% were substantially improved, and only 5% showed no improvement at all. An incontinence survey was also performed that demonstrated significant improvement in all queried parameters. No erosions, infections, or urinary retention were noted.

The last two series using mesh materials show that results can be improved by using mesh materials with no increase in complications. For this reason, mesh materials and in particular, polypropylene mesh, is considered to be the material of choice. More importantly, the combined results of these three series demonstrate that a perineal male sling can produce results similar to an AUS, yet with minimal morbidity, decreased cost, and the allowance of normal voiding postoperatively. The implications, especially where cost is an issue, are enormous.

Certain technical aspects of these procedures are paramount to ensure a successful and safe outcome. With the bladder neck slings, it is important to keep the needle passer in contact with the pubis at all times to minimize potential damage to local structures. Also, the area of dissection just lateral to the bladder neck and at the bulb must be complete in order to allow sufficient compression of the urethra.

For the perineal (bone-anchored) xenograft slings, it appears that proper tension is also paramount to success. A sling compression of 60 cm H_2O was hypothesized to be optimal in the early patients, and the sling was routinely tied down at that pressure, in some cases leaving an air knot. With experience, the procedure was modified such that both ends of the sling are in direct contact with the pubic periosteum and the sling is tied down as tightly as possible. Since that time, the results have improved somewhat. Conversely, Comiter, using a polypropylene sling, routinely used 60 cm H_2O as the standard sling tension and obtained good results.[30] Therefore, the exact ten-

sion to place on the sling is not yet standardized, but a minimum of 60 cm H_2O appears to be safe and effective in most cases. Sling placement is also important, the urethra must be compressed where it egresses from underneath the symphysis pubis. If the sling is placed proximally to this point, inadequate urethral compression will occur, while placement distally will simply cause urethral obstruction.

One of the great mysteries of this procedure is the mechanism by which it functions. Some investigators have postulated that the sling acts by compressing and elevating the urethra, thereby increasing urethral resistance.[25] It has been demonstrated using fluorourodynamic studies that minimal if any mobility of the bladder neck region is present after a radical retropubic prostatectomy.[33] Therefore, the sling must improve continence by compressing the urethra and not by simply providing urethral support, as in treating hypermobility-related stress incontinence in females. If the urethra is compressed against something immobile, then we would expect significant obstruction to occur during voiding. This is likely the reason for the higher incidence of obstruction using the bladder neck sling, since the isolated urethra is compressed behind the pubis. In the perineal sling, however, all of the periurethral tissues are maintained, which should allow both compression and voiding to occur, since the compressed fatty and muscular tissue can be displaced during voiding. Fluorourodynamic evaluation of patients after a perineal sling procedure demonstrates that the sling is usually within 1 to 2 cm of the external sphincter (Figures 80-8 and 80-9). It is likely that the male sling improves continence by increasing the functional length of the sphincteric unit since it

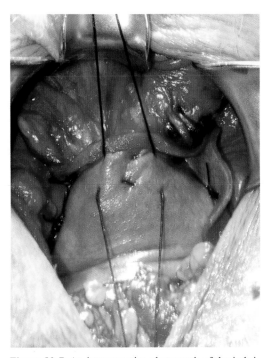

Figure 80-7 An intraoperative photograph of the imbricating suture placement (before tying) typically used to tighten a perineal sling used when sling compression is below 60 cm H_2O.

is placed at the distal edge of the sphincter. This may be why perineal male slings don't appear to work as well in severe incontinence, as there is no sphincteric function to augment. It is possible that the sling may also function through a primarily obstructive mechanism; however, it is well known that simple bulbar urethral strictures do not significantly improve postprostatectomy incontinence. Clearly, further studies will be necessary to further define the mechanism of action of a compressive device such as the male sling.

COMPLICATIONS

Significant complications of male sling procedures are rare. The most significant complications—sling erosion or infection—can be devastating and usually require removal of the sling. Fortunately, these complications are extremely uncommon, as demonstrated in most of the series. This low rate may be due to leaving the bulk of muscular and fatty tissue in place around the urethra even though significant tension is usually placed on the sling. The use of cadaveric tissues for sling material does carry an extremely small theoretical risk for transmission of viral disease from the donor; however, cadaveric materials are not recommended because of the significant tension required for these slings.

Osteitis pubis or even osteomyelitis can occur with the use of bone screws or anchors, although these complications have not been reported in any series.

Neural injury is another possible complication, although this is uncommon and usually temporary. Peroneal nerve damage is avoided by proper leg positioning and padding prior to initiating the procedure. Perineal nerve injury is limited by careful dissection on the inferior pubic ramus and limiting the use of electrocautery.

Scrotal numbness is still possible, but is usually transient, and generally resolves within the first few postoperative months. One version of the male sling, the Gore-Tex bulbourethral sling, does appear to have a higher incidence of this complication, however.[26]

Significant loss of blood has not been reported; however, 1 patient developed a symptomatic scrotal hematoma.

No patient has developed permanent retention with either the bladder neck or perineal sling. However, some of the patients in the bladder neck sling population do develop high postvoid residuals that can take months to resolve. As previously stated, this is anticipated at the time of surgery with the placement of a suprapubic tube. Of course, retention can be the goal in the neuropathic population and can usually be achieved if the sling is pulled tight enough.

When pressure flow studies are performed after perineal male slings, voiding pressures are generally in the area of 25 to 35 cm H_2O, and the storage pressures have been normal. Therefore, despite high retrograde urethral compression pressures (> 100 cm H_2O) having been achieved in many of these cases, it is highly unlikely that upper tract changes will ever occur as voiding and storage pressures are within normal limits.

Lastly, failure of the procedure is always a possibility. Fortunately, if the patient desires, an AUS can be placed after a sling procedure without significant difficulty. For patients with mild residual incontinence, injectable agents placed at the proximal edge of the sling have worked well in the few cases that have been performed.

CONCLUSIONS

The male sling can be used in almost all patients with postprostatectomy incontinence who do not desire an AUS or have failed injection therapies. The procedures themselves are not difficult; however, proper patient selection and attention to detail when performing the procedure are important factors for achieving success. It is our opinion that the bladder neck mesh sling is ideally suited for those patients who have moderate to severe PPI or neurogenic incontinence with proximal

sphincter dysfunction and are not expected to void after the procedure. The perineal mesh sling, although less invasive and simpler to perform, appears to be most effective in those patients with mild to moderate incontinence. As the early results of male slings are similar to the AUS, it is unlikely that male slings will ever challenge the role of the AUS for PPI; however, the male sling now offers an additional choice for these patients. Additionally, if the male sling fails, an AUS can subsequently be placed without difficulty.

Currently, the AUS remains the gold standard for treatment of significant postprostatectomy incontinence; however, if these new sling procedures continue to be efficacious and durable in long-term studies, the male sling will become an important option in the management of PPI owing to its simplicity, low cost, early return of continence, and low incidence of morbidity.

REFERENCES

1. Donnellan SM, Duncan HJ, MacGregor RJ, Russell JM. Prospective assessment of incontinence after radical retropubic prostatectomy: objective and subjective analysis. Urology 1997;49:225–30.
2. Goluboff ET, Saidi JA, Mazer S, et al. Urinary continence after radical prostatectomy: the Columbia experience. J Urol 1998;159:1276–80.
3. Bevan-Thomas R, Westney OL, Cespedes RD, McGuire EJ. Long-term follow-up of periurethral collagen injections for male intrinsic deficiency [abstract 992]. J Urol 1999;161:257.
4. Cespedes RD, Leng WW, McGuire EJ. Collagen injection therapy for post prostatectomy incontinence. Urology 1999;54:597–602.
5. Smith DN, Appell RA, Rackley RR, Winters JC. Collagen injection therapy for post-prostatectomy incontinence. J Urol 1998;160:364–7.
6. Elliott DS, Barrett DM. Mayo Clinic long-term analysis of the functional durability of the AMS 800 artificial urinary sphincter: a review of 323 cases. J Urol 1998;159: 1206–8.
7. Litwiller SE, Kim KB, Fone PD, et al. Post-prostatectomy incontinence and the artificial urinary sphincter: a long-term study of patient satisfaction and criteria for success. J Urol 1996;156:1975–80.
8. Brito CG, Mulcahy JJ, Mitchell MM, Adams MC. Use of a double cuff AMS-800 urinary sphincter for severe stress incontinence. J Urol 1993;149:283–5.
9. Player LP, Callander CL. A method for the cure of urinary incontinence in the male: preliminary report. JAMA 1927;88:989.
10. Cooney CJ, Horton GR. An operation of the cure of urinary incontinence in the male. J Urol 1951;66:586–92.
11. Millin T. Discussion of stress urinary incontinence in micturition. Proc Royal Soc Med 1947;40:361–70.
12. Matos-Ferreira A. Male urinary incontinence after prostatic surgery. In: Steg A, editor. Urinary incontinence. London: Churchill-Livingstone; 1992. p. 170.
13. Servadio C. The use of fascial sling for correction of post prostatectomy incontinence. Israel J Med Sci 1974;10:612–6.
14. Pettersson S, Bratt CG. Selection of patients for surgical correction of urinary incontinence after prostatic surgery. Scan J Urol Nephrol 1976;10:205–8.
15. Beneventi FA. A new operation of the correction of postoperative urinary incontinence in the male patient. J Urol 1966;96:740–2.
16. Kaufmann JJ. Surgical treatment of post-prostatectomy incontinence. Use of the penile crura to compress the bulbous urethra. J Urol 1972;107:293–7.
17. Kaufman JJ. Treatment of post-prostatectomy incontinence using a silicone gel prosthesis. Br J Urol 1973;45:646–53.
18. Raz S, Kaufman JJ. Pathophysiology of the urethral compression operation. The use of silicone gel prosthesis. J Urol 1976;115:435–8.
19. Kaufman JJ, Raz S. Urethral compression procedure for the treatment of male urinary incontinence. J Urol 1979;121:605–8.
20. Crowley JD, Cespedes RD. Male slings for post prostatectomy incontinence. 79th Annual Meeting of the South Central

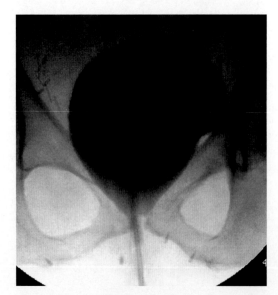

Figure 80-8 A voiding shot taken during a pressure-flow study performed for urgency after placement of a perineal sling. An impression of the sling's compressive effects on the proximal urethra can be seen. Of note, dislodgement of the right medial bone screw can be seen; however, the patient did not have recurrent stress incontinence.

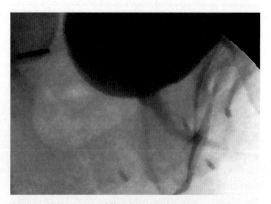

Figure 80-9 A magnified lateral view taken during the voiding phase of a voiding cystourethrogram (VCUG). The bone screws are in place and the compressive effect of the sling is easily seen on the urethra.

Section of the American Urologic Association, Inc.; 2000 Sep 20; Montreal, Canada.

21. Carpio FG, Cespedes RD. Urethral diverticulectomy and cadaveric pubourethral sling after artificial urinary sphincter erosion and prostatectomy. J Urol 1999;162:1379–80.

22. Migliari R, Pistolesi D, De Angelis M. Polypropilene sling of the bulbar urethra for post-radical prostatectomy incontinence. Eur Urol 2003;43:152–7.

23. Kapoor R, Dubey D, Kumar A, Zaman W. Modified bulbar urethral sling procedure for the treatment of male sphincteric incontinence. J Endourol 2001;15:545–9.

24. Shoukry MS, el-Salmy S. Urethral needle suspension for male urinary incontinence. Scand J Urol Nephrol 1997; 31:267–70.

25. Schaeffer AJ, Clemens JQ, Ferrari M, Stamey TA. The male bulbourethral sling procedure for post-radical prostatectomy incontinence. J Urol 1998;159:1510–5.

26. Clemens JQ, Bushman W, Schaeffer AJ. Questionnaire based results of the bulbourethral sling procedure. J Urol 1999;162:1972–6.

27. Daneshmand S, Ginsberg DA, Bennet JK, et al. Puboprostatic sling repair for treatment of urethral incompetence in adult neurogenic incontinence. J Urol 2003;169:199–202.

28. Cespedes RD, Jacoby K. Male slings for postprostatectomy incontinence. Tech Urol 2001;7:176–83.

29. Madjar S, Jacoby K, Giberti C, et al. Bone anchored sling for the treatment of post-prostatectomy incontinence. J Urol 2001;165:72–6.

30. Comiter CV. The male sling for stress urinary incontinence: a prospective study. J Urol 2001;167(2 Pt 1):597–602.

31. Ghoneim GM, Bryan W. Male perineal sling. Tech Urol 2001;7:229–32.

32. Leach GE, Yun SK. Post-prostatectomy incontinence: part 1, the urodynamic findings in 107 men. Neurourol Urodyn 1992;11:91–105.

33. Gudziak MR, McGuire EJ, Gormley EA. Urodynamic assessment of urethral sphincter function in post-prostatectomy incontinence. J Urol 1996;156:1131–5.

34. Sanchez-Ortiz RF, Broderick GA, Chaikin DC, et al. Collagen injection therapy for post-radical retropubic prostatectomy incontinence: role of Valsalva leak point pressure. J Urol 1997;158:2132–6.

35. Leach GE. Incontinence after artificial urinary sphincter placement: the role of perfusion sphincterometry. J Urol 1987;138:529–32.

81

Transurethral Ultrasound in the Diagnosis and Treatment of Ejaculatory Dysfunction

Sarah K. Girardi, MD

Ejaculatory dysfunction is defined as any disorder of the seminal vesicles and ejaculatory apparatus that may cause symptoms or lead to infertility. Transrectal ultrasound (TRUS) is the imaging modality of choice to evaluate this group of disorders. This chapter will discuss the normal anatomy of the ejaculatory apparatus and its appearance on TRUS, the different disorders that may result in ejaculatory dysfunction and their appearance on TRUS, and the growing use of TRUS as a therapeutic tool in treating some of these disorders.

NORMAL ANATOMY AND TRUS APPEARANCE

The increasing use of TRUS in the evaluation of disorders of the prostate has enabled us to gain a much more detailed understanding of the anatomy of the seminal vesicles, vasa deferentia, and ejaculatory ducts. The normal anatomy of the prostate and seminal vesicles was reviewed in Chapter 65; however, some of the important points will be reviewed here.

The vas deferens emerges from the scrotal compartment to traverse the inguinal canal and enter the extraperitoneal space of the pelvis at the internal inguinal ring. There it curves inferiomedially toward the base of the bladder where it terminates as a dilated and convoluted segment known as the ampulla of the vas.

The ampulla of the vas lies medial to the seminal vesicles. The ampulla of the vas and the seminal vesicles fuse within the base of the prostate to form the ejaculatory duct. The ejaculatory duct penetrates the glandular portion of the prostate, and the prostatic capsule invaginates to surround the ejaculatory ducts as they traverse the verumontanum. The capsular invagination forms a longitudinal sheath of smooth muscle bundles that are in continuity with the muscle fibers of Denonvilliers' fascia.[1] The cylindrical sheath envelops the ejacu-

latory ducts with a well-vascularized stroma that proceeds through the central zone of the prostate to terminate in the posterior urethra, just proximal and lateral to the verumontanum.

The smooth muscle bundles and muscular fibers of Denonvilliers' fascia enable the ejaculatory apparatus to serve a peristaltic and sphincteric function. During ejaculation the muscular wall of the duct, which is composed of an inner longitudinal and an outer circular layer, actively propels seminal fluid into the posterior urethra. At all other times the basal muscular tone allows the ejaculatory duct wall to coapt. In this way, leakage of seminal fluid into the posterior urethra, as well as reflux of urine into the ejaculatory duct are prevented.

The ejaculatory apparatus is best imaged with a multiplane sagittal scanner ultrasound probe with frequencies of 7 to 10 megahertz. Sagittal scanning allows alignment of the probe with the ejaculatory ducts. Transaxial images are useful for determining the symmetry of the seminal vesicles and for calculating seminal vesicle volume. One limitation is reaching the superior aspect of the seminal vesicle with the axial probe. When visualization is limited, a full bladder can help, providing contrast to the echogenic fat surrounding the seminal vesicles.[2]

The seminal vesicles are paired structures lying posterior to the base of the bladder. They have a characteristic bow-tie appearance when imaged transversely on ultrasound. Their outline is usually smooth, but the saccular nature of the gland is evident. The glands are relatively hypoechoic, but thin septations can often be seen that correspond to the folds of the glandular epithelium.[2] The intraprostatic portion of the seminal vesicle is also relatively hypoechoic and has been referred to by Lee and colleagues[3] as the "beak sign." Carter and colleagues[2] suggest that the most effective way to measure the seminal vesicles is the greatest length and anteroposterior

diameter. The length usually exceeds 2.5 cm, and the normal anteroposterior dimension is usually between 0.7 and 1.5 cm. Although TRUS measurements are not precise, these numbers provide a guideline for comparison when considering the diagnosis of ejaculatory disorders. Hernandez and colleagues[4] reported that it is not necessary to standardize abstinence intervals prior to these measurements, as the seminal vesicle length and anteroposterior dimensions do not change significantly after ejaculation.

The ampulla of the vas can usually be visualized behind the bladder, but nearer to the prostate it is not easily distinguished from the seminal vesicles. Villers and colleagues[1] reported on the anatomic variation seen in this area. In their study of pathological specimens, 18% demonstrated fusion of the ampulla of the vas and seminal vesicles. On TRUS this fusion appears as a central zone basilar hypoechoic area. The ejaculatory duct lumen is normally 2 mm in diameter, and is not usually visualized on TRUS. It can be visualized in pathological conditions such as obstruction of the ejaculatory duct when it becomes dilated as the result of distal obstruction.[1] The ejaculatory ducts are best visualized in the sagittal plane, where they appear as a linear echogenic focus coursing to the verumontanum. Small echogenic foci are often seen at the junction of the ejaculatory ducts and the prostatic urethra and can provide a landmark for orientation.[2]

EJACULATORY DISORDERS

The most common ejaculatory disorders are hematospermia, complete and partial obstruction of the ejaculatory ducts, and congenital absence of the vas deferens. Hematospermia is usually a benign condition that warrants limited investigation. It is defined as blood in the seminal fluid and can be isolated or persistent. In younger men, it is usually inflammatory or idiopathic, self-limited, and requires no more than a digital rectal examination and a urine cytology for evaluation. In older patients, however, a more aggressive evaluation is necessary because of the increased likelihood of malignancy.

Transrectal ultrasound findings associated with chronic hematospermia include dilated seminal vesicles with or without increased echogenicity as a result of hemorrhage into the vesicles. Other findings include ejaculatory duct cysts, ejaculatory or seminal vesicle calculi, and prostatic cysts. Worischeck and Parra performed TRUS on 26 men ages 25 to 77 with chronic hematospermia.[5] Ultrasound abnormalities were detected in 24 of 26 men. The most common abnormalities were dilated seminal vesicles, ejaculatory duct cysts, ejaculatory duct or seminal vesicle calculi, and ejaculatory duct and seminal vesicle dilatation. Two patients were discovered to have unilateral seminal vesicle cysts with ipsilateral renal agenesis and absence of the vas deferens.

Another common ejaculatory disorder is complete or partial obstruction of the ejaculatory ducts. The normal semen volume is between 1 and 5 mL with an alkaline pH. A semen analysis showing less than 1 mL of fluid with an acidic pH should raise suspicion of an ejaculatory duct blockage. Ejaculatory duct obstruction can be due to extrinsic compression of the ejaculatory ducts or intrinsic obstruction. Extrinsic factors include müllerian cysts, müllerian remnants, and seminal vesicle or ejaculatory duct cysts that can compress the ejaculatory ducts extrinsically. Intrinsic factors include ejaculatory duct stones, hemorrhage, or benign inflammation. Partial ejaculatory duct blockage has been associated with a variety of disturbances in sperm quality. Sperm density ranges from azoospermia to normospermia, and ejaculate volume may be low to normal. Sperm motility is consistently impaired as a result of delay in transit through the excurrent duct system, and sperm viability can be impaired for the same reason.[6] The physical examination is normal, although a cystic structure can sometimes be palpated in the midline of the prostate gland, representing cystic dilation of the ejaculatory duct or ducts.

Congenital bilateral absence of the vas deferens (CBAVD) is a rare but important abnormality of the ejaculatory apparatus that is found in 1 to 2% of infertile men.[7] In this disorder, there is a failure of the development of derivatives of the mesonephric duct. Therefore, all or a portion of the vas deferens, epididymis, seminal vesicle, or ejaculatory duct may be absent. In unilateral absence, there may be agenesis of the ipsilateral kidney. The diagnosis of CBAVD is made on physical examination with the failure to palpate vasa in the spermatic cords bilaterally. Invariably the caput epididymis is present, and sometimes the body and tail are also present. Transrectal ultrasound is the diagnostic tool of choice as it will detect any associated absence or abnormality of the seminal vesicles, as well as evaluate for any

other abnormalities of the ejaculatory ducts or seminal vesicles that might explain azoospermia.

Congenital absence of the vas is associated with mutations in the gene responsible for cystic fibrosis. Whereas almost all men with cystic fibrosis have absent vasa, up to 82% of men with CBAVD will be heterozygous for a cystic fibrosis gene mutation.[8] Because healthy sperm can be retrieved from the epididymis is men with CBAVD and used successfully in in vitro fertilization (IVF), it is imperative that the patient and his wife be evaluated for CF mutations to establish the risk of the couple conceiving a child with cystic fibrosis.

INDICATIONS

The indications for TRUS to diagnose ejaculatory dysfunction include chronic hematospermia, ejaculatory pain, and infertility when the semen volume is low and sperm concentration and motility are impaired. Also, in any patient in whom complete or partial absence of the vas deferens is diagnosed, TRUS in conjunction with renal ultrasound will evaluate for any other missing portions of the mesonephric duct derivatives (Table 81-1).

PATIENT PREPARATION

When TRUS is performed without any other interventions, such as biopsy or needle aspiration, no preparation is necessary. Some practitioners recommend an enema the morning of the procedure, but this is not necessary. If a biopsy or needle aspiration is planned, an enema and antibiotics are recommended. The enema is recommended the night before or morning of the procedure, and the antibiotic should be started 24 hours before the procedure. The bladder should be somewhat full to provide contrast to the perivesical fat. A standard informed consent should be obtained.

Frequencies of 7 to 10 MHz are ideal for imaging the male excurrent duct system. Bipolar probes are best to allow for sagittal and transverse imaging. End-fire probes are ideal for reaching the superior aspect of the seminal vesicles for transverse images. If seminal vesicle aspiration or seminal vesiculography is planned, the probe should be equipped with a needle guide, as for prostate biopsy.

The patient should be positioned in the left lateral decubitus position. A digital rectal examination is performed and findings are recorded. The ultrasound probe is then inserted under sagittal imaging. A short distance into the rec-

tum, the apex of the prostate is encountered. The bladder can then be identified as a large cystic structure lacking internal echoes. The seminal vesicles are then imaged by simply rotating the probe clockwise and counterclockwise at the level of the bladder base. The anteroposterior measurements can be taken at the greatest dimension. Attention should be paid to the junction of the seminal vesicles and prostate. If the linear ejaculatory duct can be visualized, it is likely significantly dilated, and this suggests either partial or complete ejaculatory duct obstruction. The ejaculatory duct diameter should be measured when obstruction is present.

ULTRASOUND APPEARANCE OF EJACULATORY DISORDERS

The easiest ejaculatory disorder to diagnose on TRUS is complete obstruction of the ejaculatory ducts. Figure 81-1 shows the ultrasound appearance of complete obstruction of the ejaculatory duct. In this figure, the seminal vesicles are normal. What is abnormal is the increased anteroposterior dimension of the seminal vesicles, up to 0.15 mm. Also the cystic appearance of the ampulla of the vas is abnormal and suggestive of obstruction. In Figure 81-2 the dilated ejaculatory duct is visualized. This image is a sagittal view. The dilation can then be confirmed with transverse imaging. In Figure 81-3 ejaculatory duct obstruction is again visualized, this time with adjacent hyperechoic areas representing calcifications. Figure 81-4 shows a müllerian duct cyst in the transverse plane. The cyst can cause extrinsic compression of the distal ejaculatory duct and result in proximal obstruction. The origin of the cyst is best confirmed with a sagittal image that confirms the location of the seminal vesicle, vas deferens, ampulla of the vas, and ejaculatory ducts.

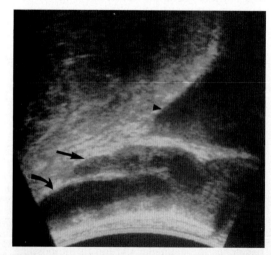

Figure 81-1 Sagittal image of patient with complete ejaculatory duct obstruction. The bladder (arrowhead) is seen above the ampulla of the vas (arrow), which lies superior to the seminal vesicle (curved arrow). Note the cystic appearance of the ampulla near the junction with the prostate.

Table 81-1	Indications for TRUS

Ejaculatory pain
Chronic hematospermia
Infertility: azoospermia, low volume, low sperm
  motility, low sperm viability

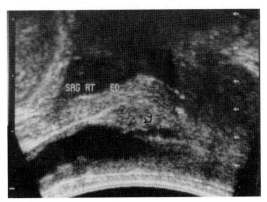

Figure 81-2 Sagittal image of patient with complete ejaculatory duct obstruction. The dilated ejaculatory duct (open arrow) is measured at 1.9 mm. Normally the lumen is not measurable unless obstruction is present.

TECHNIQUE

The therapeutic uses of TRUS include seminal vesicle aspiration for cytological examination, seminal vesiculography to evaluate partial vasal and seminal vesicle agenesis, dye administration for localization of the ejaculatory ducts in transurethral resection of obstructed ejaculatory ducts, and aspiration of müllerian cysts. The presence of sperm in a seminal vesicle aspirate is both diagnostic and therapeutic, in that those sperm have been used successfully in conjunction with in vitro fertilization efforts.[9]

Patient preparation for TRUS-guided therapeutic procedures is as described. The patient is in a left lateral decubitus position or lithotomy position if cystoscopy is going to be performed. A TRUS-guided seminal vesicle cyst aspiration can be performed with a 5 French (F), 23-gauge Williams cystoscopic injection needle (Cook Urological, Spence, IN). The needle should fit through most biopsy guides used with the endorectal probe. The needle is prefilled with sterile normal saline and connected to a 10 mL syringe with a Luer-lock top, leaving 1 to 2 mL of saline in the syringe. The seminal vesicle is visualized in the sagittal plane, and the needle is advanced through the rectal wall and into the seminal vesicle. One or 2 mL of saline is instilled to facilitate aspiration of the seminal vesicle contents, which are then examined under a microscope to check for the presence of sperm. Alternatively, the seminal vesicle aspirate may be sent directly to pathology to examine for bacteria and leukocytes. The procedure is repeated for the contralateral seminal vesicle.

For seminal vesiculography, the procedure for seminal vesicle aspiration is followed. After aspiration, the seminal vesicle is immediately instilled with a 50% contrast/methylene blue mixture. The mixture is instilled slowly under fluoroscopic guidance. The procedure is performed with a Foley catheter draining the bladder. The absence of methylene blue in the bladder confirms a high-grade obstruction of both ejaculatory ducts. Figure 81-5 shows the seminal vesiculogram from a patient with complete ejaculatory duct obstruction. A ureteral catheter balloon dilator has been left in the ejaculatory duct in preparation for relieving the obstruction.

Transurethral resection of the ejaculatory ducts is the treatment of choice for symptomatic ejaculatory duct obstruction. After seminal vesiculography with a contrast/dye mixture, the location of the ejaculatory ducts within the posterior urethra is easily recognized. The smallest available resectoscope can be used to resect the ejaculatory duct openings. The verumontanum can be resected to aid in identifying the ejaculatory duct openings.[10] To confirm that the ejaculatory ducts were completely resected, a 3F probe can be advanced into the ejaculatory duct opening. Seminal vesicle filling will confirm ejaculatory duct patency.

The success of transurethral resection of the ejaculatory ducts has been reported. Up to 55% of patients have experienced an improvement in semen parameters, and up to 33% reported a pregnancy after the relief of the obstruction.[11] Approximately half of the patients reported no improvement in semen parameters. This may have been due to early restenosis. One small series of

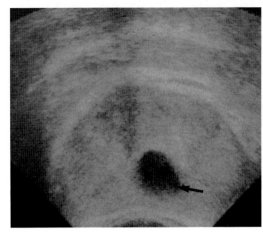

Figure 81-4 Transverse image of patient presenting with severe oligoasthenospermia. A midline prostatic cyst (arrow) usually represents a müllerian duct remnant.

patients who underwent balloon dilation of the ejaculatory duct obstruction reported improvement in semen parameters in 7 of 7 patients studied with either complete or partial blockage of the ejaculatory ducts. In this series, pregnancies were not reported.[12]

COMPLICATIONS

There are no known complications from TRUS. Complications do, however, occur when TRUS is combined with needle aspiration and instillation procedures. The complications include bleeding, infection, bacteremia, sepsis, hematuria, hematospermia, and rectal injury. Transurethral resection of the ejaculatory ducts is associated with reflux of urine into the resected ducts. This can result in recurrent epididymitis or a watery, yellow semen with low pH. Urinary incontinence after transurethral resection of the ejaculatory ducts has also been reported.

CONCLUSIONS

Transrectal ultrasound of the seminal vesicles, prostate, and ejaculatory apparatus is the imaging modality of choice for investigation of ejaculatory disorders. Ejaculatory disorders diagnosed with TRUS include complete and partial ejaculatory duct obstruction, disorders that lead to hematospermia, and infertility associated with the absence of portions or all of the excurrent duct system. The indications and uses for TRUS-guided interventions have been described, and the list continues to grow as the miniaturization of instruments continues and the quality of ultrasound images improves (Table 81-2).

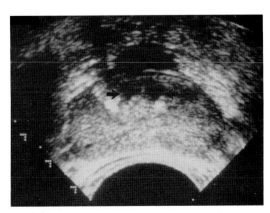

Figure 81-3 Transverse image of patient with partial ejaculatory duct obstruction. Dilated ejaculatory ducts (arrows) are readily identified; adjacent hyperechoic lesions with acoustic shadowing indicate calcification.

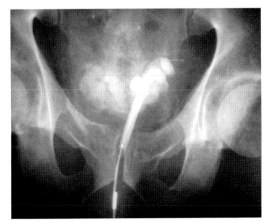

Figure 81-5 Radiograph following TRUS-guided seminal vesiculography in the same patient as seen in Figure 81-1. Note the ureteral balloon catheter in the left ejaculatory duct for dilation. In complete obstruction, contrast should not be seen in the bladder.

Table 81-2 TRUS-Guided Interventions
Seminal aspiration: sperm, cytology, bacteriology
Seminal vesiculography
Transurethral resection of ejaculatory ducts
Balloon dilation of ejaculatory ducts

REFERENCES

1. Villers A, Terris MK, McNeal JE, Stamey TA. Ultrasound anatomy of the prostate: the normal gland and anatomical variations. J Urol 1990;143:732–8.
2. Carter SS, Shinohara K, Lipshultz LI. Transrectal ultrasonography in disorders of the seminal vesicles and ejaculatory ducts. Urol Clin North Am 1989;16:773–90.
3. Lee F, Torp-Pedersen ST, McLeary RD. Diagnosis of prostate cancer by transrectal ultrasound. Urol Clin North Am 1989;16:663–73.
4. Hernandez AD, Urry RI, Smith JA Jr. Ultrasonographic characteristics of the seminal vesicles after ejaculation. J Urol 1990;144:1380–2.
5. Worischeck JH, Parra RO. Chronic hematospermia: assessment by transrectal ultrasound. Urology 1994;43:515–20.
6. Hellerstein DK, Meacham RB, Lipshultz LI. Transrectal ultrasound and partial ejaculatory duct obstruction in male infertility. Urology 1992;39:449–52.
7. Jequier AM, Ansell ID, Bullimore MJ. Congenital absence of the vas deferens presenting with infertility. J Androl 1985;6:15–9.
8. Oates RD, Amos JA. The genetic basis of congenital bilateral absence of the vas deferens and cystic fibrosis. J Androl 1994;15:1–8.
9. Jarow JP. Seminal vesicle aspiration in the management of patients with ejaculatory duct obstruction. J Urol 1994;152:899–901.
10. Meacham RB, Hellerstein DK, Lipshultz LI. Evaluation and treatment of ejaculatory duct obstruction in the infertile male. Fertil Steril 1993;59:393–7.
11. Vasquez-Levin MH, Dressler KP, Nagler HM. Urine contamination of seminal fluid after transurethral resection of the ejaculatory ducts. J Urol 1994;152(6 Pt 1):2049–52.
12. Schlegel PN, Sosa RE. Balloon dilation of ejaculatory duct obstruction: minimally invasive adjunctive treatment for obstructive male infertility [abstract]. Presented at the American Fertility Society Meeting; 1994 Nov 5–10; San Antonio.

82

Diagnosis and Treatment of Disorders of the Ejaculatory Ducts and Seminal Vesicles

Assaad El-Hakim, MD, FRCS (C)

The seminal vesicles are believed to play a major, but not yet fully understood, role in male fertility. They are part of a complex of accessory sex glands and structures including the prostate, the bulbourethral glands (Cowper's glands) and vassal ampullae. Seminal vesicles, unlike the prostate, are not universal in all mammalians and vary in size and shape among species. Human and rat glands are large; the cat and the dog, however, do not have seminal vesicles.[1] The seminal vesicles and other accessory sex tissues are well positioned to intercept pathogens or invading substances from reaching the gonads. They also produce biologically active secretions that travel in the urethra.

In order to have a better understanding of seminal vesicles' anatomy and pathology, a brief description of the embryology of the male genital tract and lower urinary tract is mandatory, for the two systems are integrally related.

EMBRYOLOGY

Between 10 and 13 weeks of gestation, the seminal vesicles develop as outpouchings from the distal end of the wolffian ducts (mesonephric ducts).[2] The latter form, in addition to the seminal vesicles, the epididymis, vas deferens, vassal ampullae, and ejaculatory ducts. The portion of the vas deferens distal to the developing seminal vesicle is called the ejaculatory duct, which opens in the urethra. The development of these accessory sex tissues is stimulated by testosterone, unlike the prostate gland, which is stimulated by dihydrotestosterone (DHT).[3] It is notable that the prostate and bulbourethral glands sprout off the urethra, whereas the seminal vesicles derive from the mesonephric duct. This embryologic difference between the prostate and the seminal vesicle may explain in part the difference in pathologies of these structures, and the very high incidence of both benign and malignant diseases affecting the prostate, compared to a relatively low rate in the seminal vesicle. Paradoxically, the bulbourethral glands, like the seminal vesicles, are essentially protected from malignancy.

At 4 weeks gestation, before the seminal vesicle development, the ureteral bud originates, also from the distal end of the mesonephric duct where it connects to the urogenital sinus. The ureter elongates on one end to join the metanephric blastema (primitive kidney), and on the other end, gets resorbed cephalad into the uro-genital sinus until the ureteral orifice reaches its final position in the bladder. Normally, by the time the seminal vesicle starts developing, the ureter is already separated from the mesonephric duct and connected directly to the bladder. If the ureter buds too much cranial on the mesonephric duct, it will be absorbed late into the urogenital sinus and will end in an ectopic position anywhere from the posterior urethra to the seminal vesicles and vas deferens.[4] It is believed that, according to this embryologic timetable, insults to the mesonephric duct before the seventh week of gestation result in both renal and genital tract abnormalities. If the event occurs after the seventh week, renal development is normally not altered (see congenital disorders).

ANATOMY

The seminal vesicles are paired glands measuring 3 to 5 cm in length, and 1 cm in diameter, with a capacity of 3.4 to 4.5 mL. Located on either side of the midline, each gland lies lateral to the ampulla of the vas deferens, posterior to the bladder and superior to the prostate. They are separated from the rectum by Denonvilliers' fascia. The ureter enters the bladder medial to the tip of the seminal vesicle. The seminal vesicle and the ampulla of the vas join at the base of the prostate and form the ejaculatory duct. At this level, they are separated from the posterior bladder neck by a thin fibromuscular layer that we identified and termed the sub-detrusor, pre-seminal vesicle fascia.[5] The ejaculatory ducts are narrow tubes (2 mm in diameter) that enter the prostate obliquely at its base, course medially and anteriorly through the central zone for 2 to 2.5 cm, and enter the prostatic urethra at the verumontanum on each side of the utricle (distal remnant of the müllerian ducts) (Figure 82-1 and 82-2). The utricle does not communicate with any other structure. Histologically, the seminal vesicle is composed of a single coiled tube with minimal side branches covered by a columnar epithelium with few apocrine cells. A thin layer of smooth muscle covers the central canal, and an adventitial layer invests the whole gland. The smooth muscle and connective tissue around the seminal vesicle and the ampulla of the vas blend with the prostatic capsule at the point where these structures meet.[6]

The blood supply for the seminal vesicle is derived from the vesiculodeferential artery, a branch of the superior vesical artery, or the umbilical artery. Other collateral branches from the inferior vesical artery and the superior and middle rectal arteries may also supply the gland. The venous drainage is via the vesiculodeferential veins and the inferior vesical plexus. Lymphatic drainage passes to the external and internal iliac nodes. Innervation comes from the hypogastric nerves and the pelvic plexus. Major sympathetic excitatory efferent fibers to the seminal vesicle and vas deferens are contributed by the hypogastric nerves.[7] Damage to the latter during retroperitoneal surgery results in anejaculation.

PHYSIOLOGY

Despite its name, the seminal vesicle does not store sperm, but it contributes the major fraction of the seminal fluid (2 to 2.5 mL). Seminal vesicle secretions enrich the final fraction of the ejaculate and are responsible for its rapid coagulation.[8] Beyond semen coagulation, the physiologic role of the seminal vesicle is not entirely known, although the seminal vesicle fluid is believed to be important in fertility and uterine sperm motility.[9] It primarily contains fructose, prostaglandins, and important proteins and enzymes involved in the clotting of the ejaculate. Semenogelin I, a 52-kDa protein, has been identified as the major clotting protein.[8] Afterwards, ejaculate liquefaction ensues. Plasminogen activators and prostate-specific antigen (PSA), two proteolytic enzymes, play a predominant role in the liquefaction reaction, by cleaving semenogelin.[10]

PATHOLOGY

CONGENITAL DISORDERS Congenital anomalies of the seminal vesicles can be categorized as abnormalities of number (agenesis, fusion, duplication), maturation (hypoplasia), and canalization (cysts).[11] Isolated seminal vesicle anomalies are unlikely to cause infertility unless the ductal system is also compromised. In the section on midline cysts, we focus on utricle and müllerian duct cysts, and wolffian or ejaculatory duct cysts (see "Midline Cysts and Ejaculatory Ducts Obstruction"). An in-depth discussion of ejaculatory duct obstruction will also be presented under this topic.

Seminal Vesicle Agenesis Unilateral agenesis of the seminal vesicles is not uncommon, with an incidence of 0.6% to 1%. It may be associated with unilateral absence of the vas deferens, as well as ipsilateral renal anomalies in over 80%

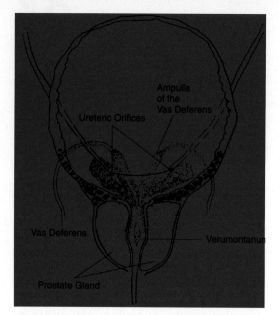

Figure 82-1 Anteroposterior view of the anatomy of the lower urinary tract and reproductive ductal system.

of cases.[12] An aberration in the proper sequence of mesonephric embryological development may partly explain this constellation of abnormalities. The frequency of associated renal anomalies varies from as low as 30% up to 90%.[13] In one series, 22 of 25 patients with absence of a seminal vesicle and/or vas deferens were missing the ipsilateral renal unit, and contralateral abnormalities also occurred in seven of these 22 patients (33%).[14] Bilateral absence of the seminal vesicles will result in a low-volume, acidic, fructose-negative ejaculate. Affected individuals present with infertility or symptoms of cystic fibrosis. Seminal vesicles are often, but not always, absent or hypoplastic in patients with congenital bilateral absence of the vas deferens (CBAVD).[15] This is commonly associated with a mutation of the

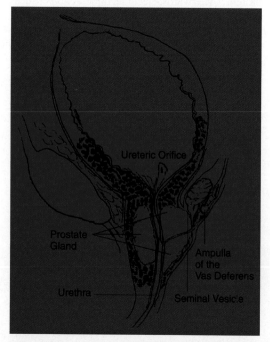

Figure 82-2 Sagittal view of the anatomy illustrated in Figure 82-1.

cystic fibrosis transmembrane receptor (CFTR).[16] Unilateral renal agenesis has also been noted in patients with CBAVD, but not in patients with CFTR.[17] Treatment should be directed at harvesting sperm for intracytoplasmic sperm injection, but couples with infertility due to this condition should be counseled regarding the risk of cystic fibrosis. No other specific treatment of seminal vesicle agenesis is required because it only affects fertility. Incidental findings of absent seminal vesicle should prompt renal imaging and genetic studies for CFTR gene mutation if the patient desires to have a family.

Seminal Vesicle Fusion and Duplication Both of these entities are extremely rare, and there are few case reports in the literature that document them. Clinical presentation of seminal vesicle fusion may include perineal discomfort or infertility. If distal obstruction is present, the semen analysis will reveal azoospermia with low-volume, acidic ejaculate. This anomaly can be detected by transrectal ultrasonography (TRUS) or computed tomography (CT), and aspiration provides sperm for assisted reproduction. On vasography, seminal vesicle fusion appears as a midline single rounded cavity with contrast material passing retrograde into the contralateral vas.[18] An incidental isolated unilateral seminal vesicle duplication was described at the time of radical prostatectomy.[19] The patient did not have a history of infertility or other urologic complaints. Postoperative intravenous pyelogram confirmed normal ipsilateral renal function. Bilateral seminal vesicle duplication was also reported in a man with multiple mesonephric duct abnormalities, including unilateral vasal duplication, epididymal and renal dysplasia, and a dysgenetic prostatic cyst.[20]

Seminal Vesicle Hypoplasia Hypoplasia of the seminal vesicle follows a similar clinical pattern as agenesis. The condition is normally associated with other mesonephric duct abnormalities. Hypoplasia is seldom recognized on TRUS performed for other reasons. Although hypoplasia alone should not cause infertility, it may contribute to low-volume ejaculate in affected patients. More severe abnormalities, such as seminal vesicle aplasia and atrophy, are commonly associated with infertility in up to 2.5% of infertile men.[21]

Seminal Vesicle Cysts Seminal vesicle cysts may be congenital, or acquired as a result of obstruction after transurethral prostatectomy. The majority of patients with acquired cysts are asymptomatic. We will discuss congenital cysts because of their possible association with renal anomalies. Incomplete differentiation of the mesonephric duct may give rise to congenital seminal vesicle cyst. Cysts can be associated with an ipsilateral ectopic ureter,[22] and approximately two-thirds are associated with ipsilateral renal agenesis.[23] This is explained by the proximity of the origin of the ureteral bud on the mesonephric duct, as explained earlier in the embryology section. An association between seminal vesicle cysts and adult polycystic kidney disease has also been

reported.[24] Some authors feel that the pathogenesis of these cysts associated with polycystic kidney disease is due to a general defect in the basement membrane of multiple organs, including the seminal vesicles, but most cysts diagnosed by TRUS are now incidental findings. These cysts should be differentiated from midline cysts (see "Midline Cysts and Ejaculatory Ducts Obstruction") and from simple dilatation of the seminal vesicles due to obstruction (see "Ultrasonography"). When symptomatic, clinical presentation includes perineal discomfort, dysuria, painful ejaculation, hematospermia, or recurrent epididymitis. Cysts that become a source of infection should be drained. On aspiration, fluid from a seminal vesicle cyst will contain no sperm and will test positive for fructose. Open or laparoscopic surgical excision may be necessary in cases associated with an ectopic ureter or renal agenesis.[25]

Midline Cysts and Ejaculatory Ducts Obstruction Midline cysts can be classified into two general categories: those that contain sperm and those that do not.[26] The latter are generally called utricle or müllerian duct cysts. The difference between utricle and müllerian cysts is based on several distinctions. The utricle cyst has an endodermal origin (it originates from the urethra), whereas the müllerian cyst has a mesodermal origin (it originates from the müllerian ducts). The utricle cyst is located near the verumontanum, and the müllerian duct cyst nearer the prostate base. On the other hand, midline cysts that contain sperm have been called wolffian or ejaculatory duct cysts, or diverticula. These cysts are less common than non–sperm-containing cysts.[27] Confusion as to whether a cyst is müllerian or wolffian in origin can result from secondary epididymal obstruction in wolffian cysts, therefore rendering Wolffian duct cysts non-sperm harboring. In any case, both types of cysts cause ejaculatory duct obstruction. Besides infertility, midline cysts can manifest with lower urinary tract irritative symptoms or urinary retention.[28] Usually, patients develop symptoms in the third or forth decade of life.

Ejaculatory duct (ED) obstruction is a clinical entity that manifests with infertility, decreased force of ejaculate, pain during or after ejaculation, decreased ejaculate volume, hematospermia, perineal or testicular pain, history of prostatitis or epididymitis, low back pain, urinary obstruction, or it can be asymptomatic.[29] The etiology of obstruction can be congenital or acquired. Congenital causes are most common and include all types of midline cysts, in addition to congenital atresia or stenos of the ejaculatory ducts. Congenital atresia represents the opposite end of the spectrum of ductal system anomalies that begin with congenital complete absence of the vas deferens and most of the epididymis. When the aplastic segment occurs at the terminal end of the vas, where the ejaculatory duct enters the urethra, it is potentially correctable by transurethral resection. Acquired causes may be secondary to trauma, infections, or inflammation, with scarring of the ejaculatory duct openings.[30] Semen analysis findings with complete ED obstruction are similar to bilateral seminal vesicle agenesis. Partial obstruction may present with oligospermia or azoospermia, decreased motility, and decreased ejaculate volume.[31] In some men with only mild partial obstruction, semen analyses can approach normal parameters, although motility may remain low.[31] TRUS findings suggestive of ejaculatory duct obstruction include midline cysts, dilated seminal vesicles or ejaculatory ducts, and hyperechoic regions suggestive of calcification along the course of the ejaculatory ducts.[32] However, none of these findings is pathognomonic for obstruction. Treatment of presumed ejaculatory duct obstruction is accomplished with transurethral resection of the ejaculatory ducts (TURED) after excluding other correctable causes of infertility.

ACQUIRED DISORDERS Acquired disorders of the seminal vesicles and ejaculatory ducts include infections, calculi, cyst formation and diverticula of the ejaculatory ducts. Acquired cysts of the seminal vesicles are usually asymptomatic and are secondary to obstruction or trauma. Congenital cysts of the seminal vesicle constitute a more interesting entity and are discussed above (see "Seminal Vesicle Cysts"). Diverticula of the ejaculatory ducts and ampulla of the vas deferens are controversial in terms of etiology and nomenclature. We believe that these entities are actually Wolffian duct dilatations, and therefore are discussed under the congenital disorders' section (see "Midline Cysts and Ejaculatory Ducts Obstruction").

Infections Overt symptomatic seminal vesiculitis is a rare problem in developed countries. Undiagnosed bacterial and viral infections of the seminal vesicles and genital ducts, however, may be important etiologic factors for male infertility. Infectious processes may lead to deterioration of spermatogenesis, impairment of sperm function and/or obstruction of the seminal tract.[33] Chronic bacterial vesiculitis is thought to be secondary to prostatitis. Treatment is essentially similar to chronic bacterial prostatitis. A prolonged course of systemic antibiotics is usually curative, obviating the need for surgery.[34] Occasionally, chronic bacterial seminal vesiculitis may require surgical excision to eliminate symptoms and to prevent recurrent septicemia. In developing countries, tuberculosis and schistosomiasis remain common causes of seminal vesicle masses, abscesses, and calcification. *Schistosoma haematobium* oviposition in seminal vesicles has long been recognized. Egg burdens of seminal vesicles and ejaculatory ducts are high and correlate well with infection intensity.[35] Oviposition in these structures commonly results in asymptomatic hematospermia and ovispermia but, paradoxically, rarely causes male infertility.[36] Hematospermia and ovispermia may manifest before eggs appear in the urine.

There are fewer than 30 cases of seminal vesicle abscesses reported in the literature.[37] The exact pathogenesis of seminal vesicle abscess remains unknown, but acute bacterial prostatitis and urinary tract infections seem to be the main predisposing factors.[38] Symptoms consist of high-grade fever, chills, irritative urinary symptoms, incontinence, and possibly, hematuria and testicular pain. Rectal examination usually reveals a palpable, tender mass above the prostate, or an enlarged prostate gland. TRUS or CT scan confirms diagnosis. Magnetic resonance imaging (MRI) is rarely indicated. Specimen cultures usually demonstrate enterobacteria, with *Escherichia coli* being the most prevalent microorganism. Traditionally, treatment has been with open surgical drainage,[39] although transurethral unroofing or percutaneous transperineal drainage are adequate alternatives if the abscess is not multiloculated.[40] Conservative management of seminal vesicle abscess, using systemic antibiotics, has also been reported, obviating the need for drainage.[41]

Seminal Vesicle Calculi Stones in the seminal vesicles are extremely rare. The nucleus is composed of epithelial cells and a mucoid substance that is covered with lime salts. The stones are smooth and hard and range in size from 1 mm to 1 cm in diameter.[42] They are usually related to obstruction, infection, or both.[43] Patients usually present with either pain or infection related to the stone, although hematospermia or infertility can be the presenting complaint. If symptomatic, removal of the stone is required, usually through an open or laparoscopic vesiculectomy. Antibiotic coverage is necessary in cases of systemic infection.

NEOPLASMS Tumors of the seminal vesicles are exceedingly rare. These neoplasms are often difficult to diagnose and can be confused with other primary adenocarcinomas. Epithelial and mesenchymal tumors can arise in the seminal vesicles, while fibromas, myomas, and sarcomas are extremely rare.[44] Of all seminal vesicle tumors, carcinoma is the most prevalent

Benign Tumors Papillary adenoma or cystadenoma and amyloid are the most common benign tumors of the seminal vesicle. Cystadenomas mimic simple seminal vesicle cysts in their presentation and imaging. They generally occur in middle-aged men and involve one side only. The histologic features are characterized by cystically dilated glandular spaces admixed with spindle-shaped stromal cells.[45] Cystadenomas fall under the category of mixed epithelial-stromal tumors of the seminal vesicle. If a solid lesion identified in the seminal vesicle shows no evidence of local spread and is benign on biopsy, treatment depends on symptoms. If the patient is asymptomatic, close follow-up consisting of repeat rectal examination and TRUS to determine subsequent growth of the tumor is reasonable. If in doubt, surgical excision is the treatment of choice because preoperative diagnosis is rarely made.

Subepithelial deposits of amyloid in the seminal vesicles have been reported in 4% to 17% of male autopsies, with an incidence up to 20% in men older than 76 years.[46] Because of increased incidence in the older population, it is frequently present concomitant with other conditions, such as bladder or prostate cancer. Misinterpreting enlargement of the seminal vesicles from senile amyloidosis as carcinomatous invasion is unlikely.[47] If patients are asymptomatic, no treatment is necessary.

Malignant Tumors Although 51 documented cases of seminal vesicle carcinoma had been reported in the current literature,[48] many more had been reported but did not qualify as primary seminal vesicle carcinoma when strict diagnostic criteria were applied. Acceptable case criteria now include a primary focus of adenocarcinoma in the seminal vesicles with no concomitant primary tumor in the prostate. The tumor should preferably be a papillary adenocarcinoma resembling the mucosa of the normal seminal vesicles. In case of anaplastic carcinoma, mucous production is required to distinguish it from anaplastic prostate carcinoma. In addition, tumors of seminal vesicle origin must be negative for PSA, prostatic acid phosphatase (PAP), and preferably, carcinoembryonic antigen (CEA) to be distinguishable from prostatic and colorectal carcinomas.[49,50] The majority of cases of primary seminal vesicle carcinoma have been diagnosed at later stages of disease. Unfortunately, differentiation of this disease entity from secondary invasion of the seminal vesicles by tumors of adjacent organs has been difficult. Late diagnosis contributes to the poor prognosis that has traditionally been associated with seminal vesicle carcinoma, and there is no optimal therapeutic protocol for managing this disease. General symptoms that may occur include urinary retention, dysuria, hematuria, or hematospermia. A mass is often palpable above the prostate and is usually not tender. TRUS is usually the next step in diagnosis and may be accompanied by needle aspiration or biopsy for diagnosis. CT or MRI would then be appropriate to stage the patient. Patients with a suspected seminal vesicle abnormality or mass felt on rectal examination should first have TRUS. If the mass is solid and non-cystic, a transperineal or TRUS-guided biopsy is a reasonable next step. If the tumor is confirmed, a CT scan should be done next for staging purposes; MRI is necessary only to confirm the hemorrhagic nature of the mass or to better define the extent of the mass to contiguous organs within the pelvis. Because fewer than 10 cases of primary tumors of the seminal vesicles have been treated at any one institution, it is difficult to define optimal treatment with any degree of certainty. Treatment strategies have primarily concentrated on attempts to excise the tumor surgically. Approaches have ranged from local excision of a seminal vesicle to more aggressive surgery, including retropubic prostaticovesiculectomy, cysto-prostaticovesiculectomy with urinary diversion, and even pelvic exenteration. The extent of resection was dependent on the degree of involvement of adjacent organs by the seminal vesicle tumor, as well as patient age. Radiotherapy has been used as a treatment modality in seminal vesicle carcinoma, especially when the tumor has reached or penetrated the surgical margins,[51] but the available data relating to its effectiveness are scarce. Hormonal manipulation may play a role in the treatment algorithm. The rationale for antiandrogenic therapy is derived from the androgen-dependent development and function of the seminal vesicles. Six patients have been treated with adjuvant androgen ablation with recurrence-free survival over 18 months.[48] Radical surgery with pelvic lymphadenectomy appears to offer the best chance for cure. Hormonal manipulation and radiotherapy may be effective as adjuvant treatment modalities. No chemotherapeutic regimen has demonstrated efficacy.

The majority of malignant involvement of the seminal vesicles represents invasion from primary prostate cancer. Seminal-vesicle invasion (pT3bN0M0) is found in 5 to 10% of men undergoing radical prostatectomy for prostate cancer. Numerous studies indicate that a majority of these patients will experience biochemical failure rapidly after surgery. If untreated, the five-year disease-free survival of such patients ranges between 10 to 40%, and the median disease-free survival is 10 to 30 months. Patients with seminal vesicle invasion usually have positive surgical margins (45 to 63%) and poorly differentiated tumors (Gleason ≥ 7). The risk of metastatic disease and death from prostate cancer is higher in patients with short disease-free intervals after surgery. While little data exist regarding the optimal therapeutic approach, adjuvant versus salvage therapies, including radiation, androgen blockade, or a combination of both, should be considered. We favor early salvage therapy with androgen blockade (with or without radiation), depending on the recurrence profile.

DIAGNOSTIC MODALITIES

HISTORY, PHYSICAL EXAMINATION, AND LABORATORY TESTS
Seminal vesicles and ejaculatory duct pathologies have a variety of presenting signs and symptoms, including lower urinary tract symptoms, perineal pain, painful ejaculation, infertility, recurrent epididymitis, and hematospermia. Although isolated hematospermia is common, generally benign, and self-limiting, it can be associated with significant pathologies of the seminal vesicles or other genital tract tissues (Table 82-1).[52,53] Hematospermia has also been reported as a presenting sign of ductal adenocarcinoma of the prostate, non-seminomatous germ cell testicular tumor and metastatic melanoma.[54–56] When hematospermia is associated with gross hematuria, infertility, lower urinary tract symptoms or painful ejaculation, a work-up is indicated.

Physical examination of the seminal vesicles is difficult. Normal seminal vesicles are not pal-

pable on rectal examination. The area above the base of the prostate is usually soft and non-tender. Seminal vesicle cysts may be felt as a relatively compressible enlargement cranial to the prostate. Primary or secondary tumors are firm indurated areas on rectal exam, but may not have absolutely definable borders. These lesions may compress the bladder base anteriorly instead, and thus, may not be readily palpable.

Laboratory examination of seminal vesicle fluid requires a semen sample. Fructose levels provide a direct measure of seminal vesicle function. If absent, bilateral seminal vesicle agenesis or obstruction is suspected. Semen volume and coagulation reaction are useful indirect measurements. Split ejaculate bacterial cultures are not useful in localizing infection, although the terminal portion of the ejaculate originates from the seminal vesicles.[57] Urinalysis usually shows leukocyturia and microscopic hematuria in all cases of seminal vesicle masses, except those with an asymptomatic cyst or edema.[58] Urine leukocytes are significantly higher for seminal vesicle empyema than for simple utricle and seminal vesicle cyst.

VASOGRAPHY AND VESICULOGRAPHY
Once considered the mainstay of seminal vesicle diagnosis, vasography is no more the preferred method of imaging. It is associated with potentially serious complications and does not provide accurate details in patients with vesiculitis, cysts, or tumors.[59,60] Vasography is most useful in documenting ejaculatory duct obstruction in patients with azoospermia and normal testicular biopsy. It can be performed either retrogradely by transurethral contrast injection at the seminal colliculus, or anterograde by surgical exposure of the scrotal vas. The transurethral route of injection was often unsuccessful owing to the lack of small endoscopes and the difficulty in identifying the ejaculatory duct orifices, in addition to the possible complication of ejaculatory duct obstruction.

Anterograde Technique The vas is identified through a scrotal incision and isolated at the junction of the straight and convoluted portions. Incisional technique or fine needle vasography can be used. The former entails using an operating microscope and hemitransection of the vas until the lumen is revealed. Fine needle vasography obviates the need for hemitransection of the vas. A 30-gauge lymphangiogram needle attached to Silastic tubing is used. Contrast medium is injected to confirm patency radiographically.[61] Any fluid is placed on a slide for microscopic examination. Ejaculatory duct obstruction is associated with copious vasal fluid containing many sperm. In these cases, the vas is usually markedly dilated. If motile sperm are found, sperm cryopreservation for potential future use should be done before injection with indigo carmine or radiographic contrast material. A Foley catheter is inserted and the air-filled balloon is placed on gentle traction to prevent reflux of contrast medium into the bladder, which can obscure visualization of the underlying seminal vesicles.

Injection of water-soluble contrast media is performed. If vasography reveals obstruction at the site of the ejaculatory ducts, indigo carmine is injected into both vasa to facilitate a transurethral resection of the ejaculatory ducts (see "Endoscopic Techniques"). Complications include stricture of the vas, injury to the vasal blood supply, hematoma formation and sperm granuloma.[62]

Transrectal or transperineal seminal vesiculography obviates the need for formal open scrotal vasography in men with documented dilatation of the seminal vesicles (Figure 82-3).[63] The technique is similar to TRUS-guided biopsy of the prostate. Findings suggestive of obstruction include anteroposterior diameter more than 15 mm and length more than 35 mm,[64] but this has not been universally accepted. If sperm are found in the aspirate fluid, transurethral resection (TUR) may immediately be undertaken. If no sperm are found in the aspirated fluid, it suggests that secondary epididymal obstruction exists. These abnormalities are associated with a poor outcome for combined vasoepididymostomy and TUR of the ejaculatory ducts. In the presence of both ejaculatory duct obstruction and bilateral epididymal obstruction, the best option would be epididymal sperm aspiration for future in vitro fertilization.[65]

ULTRASONOGRAPHY
Transabdominal or transrectal ultrasonography has been increasingly popular for the diagnosis of seminal vesicle and ejaculatory ducts pathologies. When ultrasonography is well documented, primary versus secondary lesions of the seminal vesicle can be readily characterized. Nevertheless, ultrasonography is operator- and equipment-dependent. On TRUS, seminal vesicles are paired tubular structures about 3 cm long and 1.5 cm wide. They lie above the base of the prostate and behind the bladder.

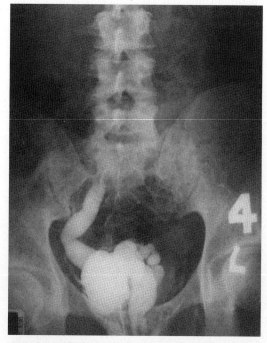

Figure 82-3 Transperineal seminal vesiculogram of a patient with a large seminal vesicle cyst. Note the dilated right ureter.

Table 82-1 Causes of hematospermia
Seminal vesicle / ejaculatory duct dilatation
Seminal vesicle / prostate stones
Cystic müllerian remnants
Ectopic prostatic tissue
Prostate ducts / ejaculatory ducts sloughing

The seminal vesicles are routinely imaged during prostatic ultrasonography and in the investigation of male infertility. The seminal vesicle appears predominantly symmetrical, smooth, and saccular. The center of the seminal vesicle is echopenic, with occasional areas of increased echogenicity relating to luminal folds within the vesicle itself.[66] The ampulla of the vas can usually be seen, particularly near the prostate, as a tortuous tube on sagittal scans. The ejaculatory duct may also be seen within the substance of the prostate. The verumontanum is characteristically seen as a more densely echoic structure in the midline at the termination of the ejaculatory ducts. Although sagittal images are best for examining the length of seminal vesicles and adjacent ductal anatomy, transaxial scans are best for detecting symmetry and volume. TRUS of the seminal vesicles does not require any special preparation, although a half-full bladder allows easier differentiation of the vesicles and adjacent structures.

Cysts Ultrasonography will easily differentiate between müllerian and seminal vesicle cysts, a distinction which is sometimes difficult on clinical examination. Müllerian duct cysts are seen as echo-free midline cystic structures located in the posterior portion of the prostate gland superior to the verumontanum. Seminal vesicle cysts are within the substance of the seminal vesicle or may rise out of the pelvis and displace the bladder and other pelvic structures (Figure 82-4).[67] Ultrasonography can be used to guide needle placement for drainage or contrast studies to more fully delineate the lesion. Dahms and colleagues proposed a diagnostic guideline for cystic retrovesical masses according to clinical symptoms and relation to bladder neck on ultrasonography.[58] Lateral cysts with non-inflammatory symptoms are diagnostic of seminal vesicle cyst, edema, ectopic ureter, or ectopic ureterocele. Inflammatory symptoms indicate infection, such as seminal vesicle empyema. Medial cysts with acute inflammatory symptoms are diagnostic of prostatic utricle empyema or prostatic abscess; the absence of inflammatory symptoms favors a non-infected utricle cyst.

Infections Ultrasonography has also been used to attempt to differentiate inflammatory

conditions of the seminal vesicle, although TRUS findings are relatively nonspecific, other than for calcifications with chronic schistosomiasis.[68]

Tumors Ultrasonography cannot differentiate reliably between benign and malignant tumors. Primary tumors, however, are usually unilateral, whereas secondary tumors more likely involve both seminal vesicles and usually originate from the rectum, bladder, or prostate. The TRUS image of a solid tumor is hyperechoic compared to the normal seminal vesicle and isoechoic to the prostate. Ultrasound-guided biopsies provide pathologic diagnose of seminal vesicle tumors.

CT SCAN CT has proved somewhat disappointing for evaluation of the seminal vesicles. The seminal vesicles are medium-density structures with Hounsfield units similar to muscle. They are seen directly below the bladder and measure 3.1 cm in length and 1.5 cm in width.[69]

Cysts Congenital abnormalities can be detected on CT scan if they alter the size or contour of the seminal vesicle, and/or if they displace surrounding structures. This indication may be the best use of CT in seminal vesicle diagnosis (Figure 82-5). Uncomplicated cysts, if sufficiently large, are seen as low-density areas with smooth margins and Hounsfield units from 0 to 10 like most clear–fluid-filled structures. If the cysts become infected or hemorrhagic, the intraluminal density may change. A seminal vesicle cyst containing hemorrhagic fluid with spermatozoa may be misinterpreted as malignant tumor.[70] The prostatic utricle may contain a calculus, which can be seen on CT images.

Infections Inflammatory masses in the seminal vesicles, such as tuberculosis or old bacterial abscesses, can be calcified and thus distinguished from tumors,[71] although a history of infection and related symptoms can usually be elicited. A long-term history of diabetes mellitus has also been associated with seminal vesicle calcification.[72]

Tumors CT scan cannot distinguish between benign and malignant tumors. Primary seminal vesicle tumors are readily seen as a unilateral enlarged gland with higher CT attenuation values in the area of the tumor than in the normal seminal vesicle. Tissue planes are usually obliterated by secondary tumors invading from the prostate or rectum,[73] but CT cannot routinely distinguish between primary and secondary tumors.

MRI MRI offers the advantage of clearly defining the anatomic relationships of pelvic organs because of its multiplanar imaging capacity. Normally, the anatomic location of the seminal vesicles is similar to that shown on CT except that, on T1-weighted images, seminal vesicles are of low signal intensity, which increases substantially on T2-weighted images.[74] Magnetic resonance, unlike other imaging modalities, can visualize the surrounding Denonvilliers' fascia. The latter is of low intensity on both T1- and T2-weighted images.

Cysts Due to its excellent display of anatomy, multiplanar MRI is useful in demonstrating the size and location of seminal vesicle

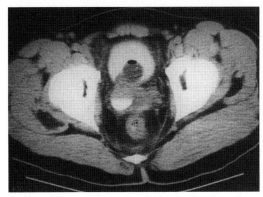

Figure 82-5 CT scan showing a seminal vesicle cyst with pooling of radiocontrast agent that was injected during prior seminal vesiculography.

cysts as well as the typical midline location of müllerian cysts. The signal intensity of the cysts depends on the fluid content. Serous fluid similar to urine will have a low-intensity signal on T1-weighted images and an increased signal intensity on T2-weighted images. These cysts often become infected or hemorrhagic, however, and will then show a variety of signal intensities on either T1- or T2-weighted images.[75]

Infections Seminal vesiculitis appears as decreased signal intensity on T1-weighted images. On T2-weighted images, seminal vesiculitis has an intensity higher than that of normal seminal vesicle or fat.[76]

Tumors MRI cannot distinguish between benign and malignant solid masses within the seminal vesicle. Tumors on MRI are usually heterogeneous with a medium intensity on T1-weighted images and a mixed intensity on T2-weighted images. Definitive treatment for most seminal vesicle lesions can be appropriately determined only with CT scan. MRI is necessary to confirm the hemorrhagic nature of the mass or to further stage the extent of the mass within the pelvis.

MINIMALLY INVASIVE TREATMENT MODALITIES

Today, seminal vesiculectomy is rarely necessary in developed countries. Large series of seminal vesiculectomy were described for the treatment of tuberculosis. Most surgeries on seminal vesicles nowadays are in conjunction with radical surgical treatment of pelvic neoplasms such as bladder, prostate, urethral, or rectal cancer. Several open approaches to the seminal vesicle have been described, including transperineal, transvesical, perivesical, retrovesical, and transcoccygeal. These procedures carry with them potential morbidity associated with pelvic surgery. We are going to focus on the minimally invasive treatment modalities of the seminal vesicle and ejaculatory duct pathologies.

Indications include: (1) drainage of symptomatic seminal vesicle cysts or en-bloc excision, along with nephroureterectomy if associated with ipsilateral renal dysplasia and ectopic ureter, (2) drainage of seminal vesicle abscess,

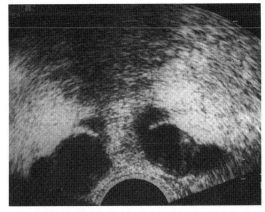

Figure 82-4 Bilateral seminal vesicle cysts seen on transrectal ultrasonography.

(3) transurethral unroofing of obstructive midline cysts, (4) excision of chronically infected seminal vesicles, and (5) biopsy and extirpative surgery for solid masses.

PERCUTANEOUS TECHNIQUES Percutaneous approaches to the seminal vesicles are limited to the transperineal and transrectal routes. Indications are usually diagnostic with ultrasound guidance. Fluid can be aspirated from symptomatic cystic structures and sent for analysis. Midline cysts with normal seminal vesicles that contain sperm are wolffian or ejaculatory duct cysts. Those that do not harbor sperm are müllerian duct cysts. Cysts in the region of the seminal vesicle with normal contralateral glands are seminal vesicle cysts and usually do not contain sperm and test positively for fructose.[77] Fluid can also be sent for cytologic analysis and culture when indicated. The same accesses can be used to inject antibiotics or contrast medium. TRUS-guided biopsy of solid seminal vesicle mass and seminal vesiculography are described above (see "Diagnostic Modalities").

ENDOSCOPIC TECHNIQUES Endoscopic approaches to the seminal vesicles and ejaculatory ducts include transurethral resection of the ejaculatory ducts, transvesical aspiration of seminal cyst, and seminal vesiculoscopy.

TURED should be performed only in azoospermic men or in severely oligoasthenospermic men who fully understand the risks of the procedure. In addition, the infertile couple should be unwilling to undergo in vitro fertilization. The surgical setup is similar to that of transurethral resection of the prostate. An O'Connor drape is used. A prophylactic antibiotic with gram-negative coverage is administered. Urethroscopy is performed to rule out strictures in the anterior and bulbar urethra, as well as for evaluation of the posterior urethra. Endoscopic findings include distorted verumontanum, splaying of the ejaculatory ducts, bulbous or bi-lobed verumontanum, midline cysts, and inflammatory calcifications.[78] The proximal verumontanum is resected in the midline. Resection is performed using pure cutting current. Commonly, one or two chips are resected, removing the proximal verumontanum only (Figure 82-6). Although, lateral cold knife incisions were historically performed, resection lateral to the verumontanum is not necessary because the ejaculatory ducts open in the midline. With the bladder filled with irrigation fluid, palpation of the seminal vesicles is made easier. Mild pressure is exerted on the seminal vesicles, resulting in fluid expressed from the respective ejaculatory ducts. Alternatively, efflux of previously injected indigo carmine in the dilated seminal vesicles can be demonstrated. If no fluid is expressed, another small bite can be taken from the verumontanum, and seminal vesicle pressure applied again. Care should be exerted to avoid the bladder neck and the external sphincter. A Foley catheter is left overnight. The patient is asked to refrain from sexual activity for 7 to 10 days. When

sexual activity is resumed, hematospermia may be evident but is self-limited. A semen analysis is obtained 1 month following the resection.

Complications include retrograde ejaculation and reflux of urine into the ejaculatory ducts, vas and seminal vesicles. Contamination of semen by urine impairs sperm quality. Reflux can lead to acute and chronic epididymitis. Recurrent epididymitis often results in epididymal obstruction. Symptomatic chemical epididymitis may also occur from refluxing urine. Chronic low-dose antimicrobials may be used until pregnancy is achieved.

TURED results in increased semen volume about two-thirds of the time and appearance of sperm in the ejaculate in about 50% of previously azoospermic men. Meacham and colleagues reported on 24 patients with ejaculatory duct obstruction treated with TURED.[79] Fifty percent had an increase in sperm density or motility and 29% had an increase in ejaculate volume only. Seven of 24 (29%) were able to impregnate their wives. Turek and colleagues showed a greater than 50% improvement in semen parameters in 65% of patients after TURED.[80] Twenty percent were able to initiate a pregnancy. There was a 20% overall complication rate, with the most common being a watery ejaculate. The etiology of the ejaculatory duct obstruction is a significant predictor of success after TURED.[81] In those patients with a congenital cause to the obstruction, success rates are excellent, with 100% improvement in semen parameters (motility, volume), 83% improvement in sperm count, and 66% pregnancy rate. In those patients with an acquired cause to the obstruction, only 37.5% have improved semen parameters and 12.5% improved pregnancy rate. Furthermore, although 33% of each group had complications, those in the congenital group were more minor in nature. Response to TURED depends as well on the degree of obstruction.[82] Improvements in semen parameters are significantly better in patients

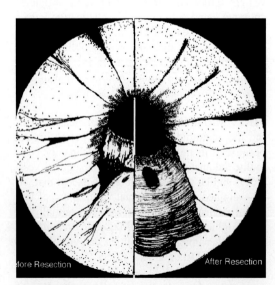

Figure 82-6 Representation of the prostatic urethra as it appears normally (left) and after transurethral resection with unroofing of the ejaculatory duct (right).

with partial obstruction (94%) than those with complete obstruction (59%).

Seminal vesiculoscopy, or direct-vision endoscopy of the seminal vesicles, has been reported. Razvi and Denstedt described a case in which a semirigid 6.9 French ureteroscope was used to access and drain a seminal vesicle cyst transurethrally, obviating the need for open surgery.[83] More recently, Yang and colleagues successfully scoped the ejaculatory ducts and seminal vesicles in 37 patients with refractory hemospermia exceeding 3 months, and 2 patients with prostate cancer, using 6 and 9F semirigid ureteroscopes.[84] In hemospermic patients, hemorrhage was found in the seminal vesicles or the ejaculatory ducts in 23 (62.2%) and 3 (8.1%), respectively. Calculi were present in the seminal vesicles or ejaculatory ducts in 6 (16.2%) and 2 (5.4%), respectively. No complications were observed. The follow-up of this study was rather short, with a minimum of 3 months. Although feasibility and safety of vesiculoscopy has been demonstrated, its clinical applicability is not yet well determined. This possible diagnostic/therapeutic modality is only investigational at the time of writing.

LAPAROSCOPIC APPROACH Laparoscopy has been advocated as an optimal minimally invasive technique for the surgical treatment of seminal vesicle pathology.[85] The transperitoneal laparoscopic approach provides straightforward access and excellent visualization of the retrovesical seminal vesicles. The blood supply can be meticulously controlled, and the seminal vesicles can be cleanly dissected free of the bladder, prostate, and overlying peritoneum, without entering the bladder or rectum. The primary application of laparoscopic seminal vesicle dissection is in the context of laparoscopic radical prostatectomy. Other indications include symptomatic seminal vesicle cysts, especially those associated with ipsilateral renal dysplasia, chronic seminal vesiculitis refractory to conservative treatment, and primary seminal vesicle tumor.

Preoperative preparation for laparoscopic seminal vesicle surgery depends on the extent of the pathology. An enema or mechanical bowel preparation may be administered according to surgeon preference. We prefer a mechanical bowel preparation administered orally the evening before surgery. A prophylactic systemic antibiotic is administered preoperatively. Deep vein thrombosis prophylaxis, such as use of intermittent compression stockings during and immediately after surgery, is advisable. A cross-match is performed, or alternatively, autologous blood can be obtained because these operations are rarely emergencies.

The patient is positioned supine in Trendelenburg's position. A Foley catheter is inserted, and pneumoperitoneum is achieved. In general, four or five trocars are used in a diamond configuration as for laparoscopic prostatectomy. A transverse incision of the peritoneum overlying the rectovesical pouch is made (Figure 82-7). The peritoneum is dissected off the ampulla of the vas deferens in the midline. Each ampulla is dis-

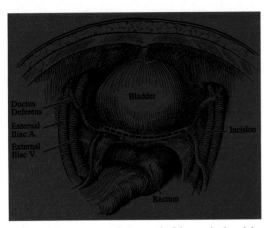

Figure 82-7 Laparoscopic removal of the seminal vesicle. The incision (3 cm) is made 2 cm from the rectovesical cul-de-sac on the anterior peritoneal surface. Reproduced with permission from Kavoussi LA, et al.[85]

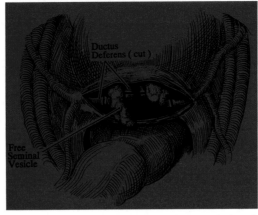

Figure 82-9 Laparoscopic removal of the seminal vesicle. Following transaction of the vas, traction on the lateral portion will expose the seminal vesicles. Reproduced with permission from Kavoussi LA, et al.[85]

sected away from the underlying seminal vesicle and gently retracted superiorly. The vas deferens may be transected at this point to allow further mobilization. The seminal vesicle is then dissected circumferentially staying close to its margins in order to prevent adjacent organ injury (Figure 82-8). The vascular supply to the seminal vesicle is secured and divided. Dissection off the neurovascular bundle can be achieved with gentle medial traction. Blunt dissection is then used to push the rectum away from the base of the prostate. At this point, the seminal vesicle can be clipped distally and removed (Figure 82-9). The technique for laparoscopic transperitoneal en bloc excision of the ipsilateral seminal vesicle, cyst, ectopic ureter, and dysplastic renal tissue is similar. The cystic and dilated seminal vesicle is dissected down to its junction with the prostate gland, where it is clipped and divided with the vas deferens. The tubular dilated ureteral stump extends from the seminal vesicle to above the iliac vessels, where it may terminate blindly or be associated with a small dysplastic kidney. Dissection of this stump requires mobilization of the colon. The whole specimen is removed en bloc.[86] Laparoscopic approach affords excellent visibility to the pelvic structures and significantly

improves the access to the plan between the bladder and rectum compared to open surgery. All advantages of laparoscopic surgery are evidenced postoperatively, including decreased blood loss and analgesic requirements, shorter hospital stay, improved cosmists, and quicker return to normal activities and work.[87–89]

ROBOTIC APPROACH The robotic approach to the seminal vesicles is similar to the laparoscopic approach. This technique has been primarily applied to the surgical management of localized prostate cancer.[90,91] Since its inception, robotic radical prostatectomy has been performed at many institutions in the United States and Europe, and the caseload is rising exponentially year after year. The robotic approach offers advantages over standard laparoscopy, particularly in terms of three-dimensional stereoscopic vision, wrist action of the robotic arms providing 6° of freedom, compared with 4° of freedom for standard laparoscopic instruments, and tremor elimination filters with optional motion scaling, which maximize dexterity and precision. In addition, physical separation of the surgeon from the patient improves ergonomics and promotes telesurgery. Also of note is the ability to transform the surgical act into digitized data, which facilitates surgical simulation and training, and real-time interfacing of preoperative imaging.[92]

REFERENCES

1. Aumuller G, Seitz J, Lilja H, et al. Species- and organ-specificity of secretory proteins derived from human prostate and seminal vesicles. Prostate 1990;17:31–40.
2. Aumuller G, Riva A. Morphology and functions of the human seminal vesicle. Andrologia 1992;24:183–96.
3. Small EJ, Prins GS. Physiology and endocrinology of the prostate. In: Vogelzang NJ, Scardino PT, Shipley WU, Coffey DS editors. Comprehensive textbook of genitourinary oncology. Baltimore: Williams & Wilkins; 1995. p. 600–20.
4. Mackie GG, Stephens FD. Duplex kidneys: a correlation of renal dysplasia with position of the ureteral orifice. J Urol 1975;114:274.
5. El-Hakim A, Gonzalez R, Beneck D, Tewari AK. Sub-detrusor, pre-seminal vesicle fascia: characterization and composition [Abstract]. J Endourol 2005;19 Suppl:281.
6. Aboul-Azm TE. Anatomy of the human seminal vesicles and ejaculatory ducts. Arch Androl 1979;3:287–92.
7. Kolbeck SC, Steers WD. Origin of neurons supplying the vas deferens of the rat. J Urol 1993;149:918–21.
8. Lilja H, Oldbring J, Rannevik G, Laurell CB. Seminal-secreted proteins and their reactions during gelation and liquefaction of human semen. J Clin Invest 1987;80:281–5.
9. Peitz B, Olds-Clarke P. Effects of seminal vesicle removal on fertility and uterine sperm motility in the house mouse. Biol Reprod 1986;35:608–17.
10. Robert M, Gagnon C. Semenogelin I: a coagulum forming, multifunctional seminal vesicle protein. Cell Mol Life Sci 1999;55:944–60.
11. Vohra S, Morgentaler A. Congenital anomalies of the vas deferens, epididymis, and seminal vesicles. Urology 1997; 49:313–21.
12. Schlegel PN, Shin D, Goldstein M. Urogenital anomalies in men with congenital absence of the vas deferens. J Urol 1996;155:1644–8.
13. Hall S, Oates RD. Unilateral absence of the scrotal vas deferens associated with contralateral mesonephric duct anomalies resulting in infertility: laboratory, physical and radiographic findings, and therapeutic alternatives. J Urol 1993;150:1161–4.
14. Donohue RE, Fauver HE. Unilateral absence of the vas deferens. A useful clinical sign. JAMA 1989;261:1180–2.
15. Goldstein M, Schlossberg S. Men with congenital absence of the vas deferens often have seminal vesicles. J Urol 1988; 140:85–7.
16. Chillón M, Casals T, Mercier B, et al. Mutations in the cystic fibrosis gene in patients with congenital absence of the vas deferens. N Engl J Med 1995;332:1475–80.
17. Mickle J, Milunsky A, Amos JA, Oates RD. Congenital unilateral absence of the vas deferens: a heterogeneous disorder with two distinct subpopulations based upon aetiology and mutational status of the cystic fibrosis gene. Hum Reprod 1995;10:1728–35.
18. Malatinsky E, Labady F, Lepies P, et al. Congenital anomalies of the seminal ducts. Int Urol Nephrol 1987;19:189–94.
19. Christiano AP, Palmer JS, Chekmareva MA, Brendler CB. Duplicated seminal vesicle. Urology 1999;54:162.
20. Hublet D, Kaeckenbeeck B, De Backer E, Schmitz. Dysgenetic prostatic cyst and bilateral duplication of seminal vesicles with unilateral duplication of vas deferens, epididymis and renal dysplasia. One case and review of the literature. Acta Urol Belg 1980;48:424–9.
21. Carter SS, Shinohara K, Lipshultz LI. Transrectal ultrasonography in disorders of the seminal vesicles and ejaculatory ducts. Urol Clin North Am 1989;16:773–90.
22. Giglio M, Medica M, Germinale F, Carmignani G. Renal dysplasia associated with ureteral ectopia and ipsilateral seminal vesicle cyst. Int J Urol 2002;9:63–6.
23. Heaney JA, Pfister RC, Meares EM Jr. Giant cyst of the seminal vesicle with renal agenesis. AJR Am J Roentgenol 1987;149:139–40.
24. Hendry WF, Rickards D, Pryor JP, Baker LR. Seminal megavesicles with adult polycystic kidney disease. Hum Reprod 1998;13:1567–9.
25. van den Ouden D, Blom JH, Bangma C, de Spiegeleer AH. Diagnosis and management of seminal vesicle cysts associated with ipsilateral renal agenesis: a pooled analysis of 52 cases. Eur Urol 1998;33:433–40.
26. Goluboff ET, Stifelman MD, Fisch H. Ejaculatory duct obstruction in the infertile male. Urology 1995;45:925–31.
27. Kirkali Z, Yigitbasi O, Diren B, et al. Cysts of the prostate, seminal vesicles and diverticulum of the ejaculatory ducts. Eur Urol 1991;20:77–80.
28. Aragona F, Spinelli C, Campatelli A, D'Elia F. Urinary retention due to a müllerian duct cyst: role of ultrasonically guided fine needle aspiration in the diagnosis and treatment. J Urol 1985;134:364–6.
29. Meacham RB, Hellerstein DK, Lipshultz LI. Evaluation and treatment of ejaculatory duct obstruction in the infertile male. Fertil Steril 1993;59:393–7.
30. Pryor JP, Hendry WF. Ejaculatory duct obstruction in subfertile males: analysis of 87 patients. Fertil Steril 1991;56:725–30.
31. Hellerstein DK, Meacham RB, Lipshultz LI. Transrectal ultrasound and partial ejaculatory duct obstruction in male infertility. Urology 1992;39:449–52.
32. Worischeck JH, Parra RO. Transrectal ultrasound in the evaluation of men with low volume azoospermia. J Urol 1993;149:1341–4.
33. Keck C, Gerber-Schafer C, Clad A, et al. Seminal tract infections: impact on male fertility and treatment options. Hum Reprod Update 1998;4:891–903.
34. Gutierrez R, Carrere W, Llopis J, et al. Seminal vesicle abscess: two case reports and a review of the literature. Urol Int 1994;52:45–7.
35. Smith JH, Christie JD. The pathobiology of *Schistosoma haematobium* infection in humans. Hum Pathol 1986;17:333.
36. Cheever AW, Kamel IA, Elwi AM, Mosimann JE, Danner R. *Schistosoma mansoni* and *Schistosoma haematobium* infections in Egypt: II. Quantitative parasitological findings at necropsy. Am J Trop Med Hyg 1977;26:702.

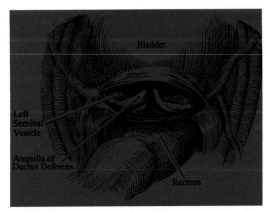

Figure 82-8 Laparoscopic removal of the seminal vesicle. The seminal vesicles can be identified by blunt dissection under the vas deferens. Reproduced with permission from Kavoussi LA, et al.[85]

37. Pandey P, Peters J, Shingleton WB. Seminal vesicle abscess: a case report and review of literature. Scand J Urol Nephrol 1995;29:521–4.

38. Kennelly MJ, Oesterling JE. Conservative management of a seminal vesicle abscess. J Urol 1989;141:1432–3.

39. Lee SB, Lee F, Solomon MH, et al. Seminal vesicle abscess: diagnosis by transrectal ultrasound. J Clin Ultrasound 1986;14:546–9.

40. Fox CW Jr, Vaccaro JA, Kiesling VJ Jr, Belville WD. Seminal vesicle abscess: the use of computerized coaxial tomography for diagnosis and therapy. J Urol 1988;139:384–5.

41. Nicolas TJA, Banon PV, Valdelvira NP, et al. Abscess of seminal vesicle: conservative treatment. Arch Esp Urol 2001;54:445–6.

42. White JL. Stones in prostate and seminal vesicles. Texas J Med 1928;23:581.

43. Li YK. Diagnosis and management of large seminal vesicle stones. Br J Urol 1991;68:322–3.

44. Hajdu SI, Faraque AA. Adenocarcinoma of the seminal vesicle. J Urol 1968;99:798.

45. Baschinsky DY, Niemann TH, Maximo CB, Bahnson RR. Seminal vesicle cystadenoma: a case report and literature review. Urology 1998;51:840–5.

46. Pitkanen P, Westermark P, Cornwell GG 3rd, Murdoch W. Amyloid of the seminal vesicles. A distinctive and common localized form of senile amyloidosis. Am J Pathol 1983;110:64–9.

47. Kaji Y, Sugimura K, Nagaoka S, Ishida T. Amyloid deposition in seminal vesicles mimicking tumor invasion from bladder cancer: MR findings. J Comput Assist Tomogr 1992; 16:989–91.

48. Thiel R, Effert P. Primary adenocarcinoma of the seminal vesicles. J Urol 2002;168:1891–6.

49. Benson RC, Clark WR, Farrow GM. Carcinoma of the seminal vesicle. J Urol 1984;132:483.

50. Dalgaard JB, Giertsen JC. Primary carcinoma of the seminal vesicle; case and survey. Acta Pathol Microbiol Scand 1956;39:255.

51. Oxley JD, Brett MT, Gillatt DA. and Burton, P.: Seminal vesicle carcinoma. Histopathology 1999;34:562.

52. Furuya S, Ogura H, Saitoh N, et al. Hematospermia: an investigation of the bleeding site and underlying lesions. Int J Urol 1999;6:539–47.

53. Lencioni R, Ortori S, Cioni D, et al. Endorectal coil MR imaging findings in hemospermia. MAGMA 1999;8:91–7.

54. Rubinowicz DM, Soloway MS, Lief M, Civantos F. Hemospermia and expressed tumor in the urethra: an unusual presentation of ductal carcinoma of the prostate. J Urol 2000;163:915.

55. Maheshkumar P, Otite U, Gordon S, et al.Testicular tumor presenting as hematospermia. J Urol 2001;165:188.

56. Meng MV, Werboff LH. Hematospermia as the presenting symptom of metastatic malignant melanoma of unknown primary origin. Urology 2000 1;56:330.

57. Comhaire F, Verschraegen G, Vermeulen L. Diagnosis of accessory gland infection and its possible role in male infertility. Int J Androl 1980;3:32–45.

58. Dahms SE, Hohenfellner M, Linn JF, et al. Retrovesical mass in men: pitfalls of differential diagnosis. J Urol 1999;161: 1244–8.

59. Dunnick NR, Ford K, Osborne D, et al. Seminal vesiculography: limited value in vesiculitis. Urology 1982;20:454–7.

60. King BF, Hattery RR, Lieber MM, et al. Seminal vesicle imaging. Radiographics 1989;9:653–76.

61. Dewire DM, Thomas AV. Microsurgical end-to-side vasoepididymostomy. In: Goldstein M, editor. Surgery of male infertility. Philadelphia: WB Saunders; 1995. p. 128–134.

62. Howards SS, Jesse S, Johnson A. Micropuncture and microanalytic studies of the effect of vasectomy on the rat testis and epididymis. Fertil Steril 1975;26:20–7.

63. Kim ED, Lipshultz LI. Role of ultrasound in the assessment of male infertility. J Clin Ultrasound 1996;24:437–53.

64. Jones TR, Zagoria RJ, Jarow JP. Transrectal US-guided seminal vesiculography. Radiology 1997;205:276–8.

65. Jarvi K, Zini A, Buckspan MB, et al. Adverse effects on vasoepididymostomy outcomes for men with concomitant abnormalities in the prostate and seminal vesicle. J Urol 1998;160:1410–2.

66. Carter SS, Shinohara K, Lipshultz LI. Transrectal ultrasonography in disorders of the seminal vesicles and ejaculatory ducts. Urol Clin North Am 1989;16:773–90.

67. Steers WD, Corriere JN Jr. Case profile: seminal vesicle cyst. Urology 1986;27:177–8.

68. Littrup PJ, Lee F, McLeary RD, et al. Transrectal US of the seminal vesicles and ejaculatory ducts: clinical correlation. Radiology 1988;168:625–8.

69. Silverman PM, Dunnick NR, Ford KK. Computed tomography of the normal seminal vesicles. Comput Radiol 1985; 9:379–85.

70. Kneeland JB, Auh YH, McCarron JP, et al. Computed tomography, sonography, vesiculography, and MR imaging of a seminal vesicle cyst. J Comput Assist Tomogr 1985;9: 964–946.

71. Birnbaum BA, Friedman JP, Lubat E, et al. Extrarenal genitourinary tuberculosis: CT appearance of calcified pipestem ureter and seminal vesicle abscess. J Comput Assist Tomogr 1990;14:653–5.

72. Hricak H. Noninvasive imaging for staging of prostate cancer: magnetic resonance imaging, computed tomography, and ultrasound. NCI Monogr 1988;(7):31–5.

73. Sussman SK, Dunnick NR, Silverman PM, Cohan RH. Case report: carcinoma of the seminal vesicle: CT appearance. J Comput Assist Tomogr 1986;10:519–20.

74. David V. MR imaging of the prostate and seminal vesicles. Magn Reson Imaging Clin N Am 1996;4:497–518.

75. Thurnher S, Hricak H, Tanagho E. Müllerian duct cyst: diagnosis with MR imaging. Radiology 1988;168:25–8.

76. Ramchandani P, Banner MP, Pollack HM. Imaging of the seminal vesicles. Semin Roentgenol 1993;28:83–91.

77. Shabsigh R, Lerner S, Fishman IJ, Kadmon D. The role of transrectal ultrasonography in the diagnosis and management of prostatic and seminal vesicle cysts. J Urol 1989;141:1206–9.

78. Fisch H, Kang YM, Johnson CW, Goluboff ET. Ejaculatory duct obstruction. Curr Opin Urol 2002;12:509–15.

79. Meacham RB, Hellerstein DK, Lipshultz LI. Evaluation and treatment of ejaculatory duct obstruction in the infertile male. Fertil Steril 1993;59:393–7.

80. Turek PJ, Magana JO, Lipshultz LI. Semen parameters before and after transurethral surgery for ejaculatory duct obstruction. J Urol 1996;155:1291–3.

81. Netto NR, Esteves SC, Neves PA. Transurethral resection of partially obstructed ejaculatory ducts: seminal parameters and pregnancy outcomes according to the etiology of obstruction. J Urol 1998;159:2048–53.

82. Schroeder-Printzen I, Ludwig M, Kohn F, Weidner W. Surgical therapy in infertile men with ejaculatory duct obstruction: technique and outcome of a standardized surgical approach. Hum Reprod 2000;15:1364–8.

83. Razvi HA, Denstedt JD. Endourologic management of seminal vesicle cyst. J Endourol 1994;8:429–31.

84. Yang SC, Rha KH, Byon SK, Kim JH. Transutricular seminal vesiculoscopy. J Endourol 2002;16:343–5.

85. Kavoussi LR, Schuessler WW, Vancaillie TG, Clayman RV. Laparoscopic approach to the seminal vesicles. J Urol 1993;150:417.

86. Cherullo EE, Meraney AM, Bernstein LH, et al. Laparoscopic management of congenital seminal vesicle cysts associated with ipsilateral renal agenesis. J Urol 2002;167: 1263–7.

87. McDougall EM, Afane JS, Dunn MD, et al. Laparoscopic management of retrovesical cystic disease: Washington University experience and review of the literature. J Endourol 2001;15:815–9.

88. Carmignani G, Gallucci M, Puppo P, et al. Video laparoscopic excision of a seminal vesicle cyst associated with ipsilateral renal agenesis. J Urol 1995;153:437–9.

89. Ikari O, Castilho LN, Lucena R, et al. Laparoscopic excision of seminal vesicle cysts. J Urol 1999;162:498–9.

90. El-Hakim A, Leung RA, Tewari A. Robotic prostatectomy: a pooled analysis of published literature. Expert Rev Anticancer Ther 2006;6:11–20.

91. El-Hakim A, Tewari A. Robotic prostatectomy—a review. MedGenMed 2004;6:20.

92. El-Hakim A, Tewari A. Robotic laparoscopic radical prostatectomy. State of the art. Hosp Physician 2005:37–43.

Part VII

Pediatric Procedures

83

Pediatric Endoscopic Instrumentation

R. Guy Hudson, MD
Steven J. Skoog, MD, FAAP, FACS

Endoscopy of the urinary tract originated with the introduction of the cystoscope by Max Nitze over 100 years ago. Endoscopic evaluation of the upper urinary tract was first performed with a pediatric endoscope in 1929 in a male with posterior urethral valves.[1] Since that time, advances in optics, radiographic techniques, energy sources, and endoscopic equipment have resulted in new and advanced endoscopic operations and applications in the urinary tract. The uses of these new technologies in the pediatric patient improved and expanded the field of pediatric endoscopy. The entire spectrum of endoscopy, including cystourethroscopy, ureterorenoscopy, percutaneous nephroscopy, and laparoscopy, is currently utilized in the care of the pediatric patient.

Significant modifications of adult endoscopes have been made, which have decreased the size of both rigid and flexible cystoscopes. The integrated cystoscope and interchangeable rod-lens cystoscopes allow excellent visualization of small urethras. Image quality continues to improve with the advent of the charged coupling device chip camera and digital video capability.[2] In addition, the introduction of needlescopic instruments in laparoscopy improved the minimally invasive focus in pediatric urologic laparoscopic surgery. Hence, the improvements in size, optical clarity, maneuverability, and ease of use of endoscopic equipment expanded the procedures performed in the pediatric patient.

The essential instrumentation for the performance of pediatric endoscopic procedures will be discussed. The equipment common to all endoscopy will also be reviewed and the equipment particular to each type of pediatric endoscopic procedures will be presented in the relevant sections.

SPECIAL CONSIDERATIONS IN THE PEDIATRIC PATIENT

Patient size and age are of particular importance when the male urethra or ureter is the point of interest. In general, the smallest instruments are generally best. Unlike some procedures in adults, pediatric endoscopy inevitably requires a general anesthetic, and this must be factored into the decision when catheters or stents must be retrieved or multiple endoscopic procedures performed. Irrigation fluids must be heated to body temperature and the infant and small child must be kept out of a wet environment to preserve body temperature. Hypothermia can have severe consequences.[3] The irrigation fluid should be isotonic since extravasation of fluid is always a risk during upper tract endoscopy. Extravasation of fluid and systemic absorption can result in hyponatremia and fluid overload.

Positioning of the pediatric patient is related to patient size. In the infant, a small towel roll under the knees held with 1-inch tape may be all that is necessary. We have found that the child Allen universal stirrup provides the best lithotomy position for cystoscopy and ureteroscopy in the young child and adolescent (Figure 83-1).

With an increase in laparoscopic technology and equipment, the applications of laparoscopy in pediatric urology surgery are expanding. The urologic laparoscopic surgeon should be aware of the physiologic implications of the laparoscopic procedure in infants and children in order to avoid potential morbidity. In children, CO_2 uptake is more efficient than in adults owing to the decreased distance between capillaries and peritoneum and the greater absorptive area of peritoneum in relation to patient body-weight.[4] The resulting hypercarbia in prolonged procedures (> 1 hr) can lead to increased sympathomimetic activity. Increased heart rate and blood pressure, as well as cardiac irritability, can result, leading to cardiac arrhythmias and potential cardiovascular compromise.[4]

During laparoscopy, intra-abdominal pressure and patient position are critical determinants of cardiovascular function. As a general rule, intra-abdominal pressure should be maintained below 15 mm Hg in the pediatric patient.[4,5] At higher pressures, venous return is decreased as the inferior vena cava is compressed. A reduction in cardiac output and arterial blood pressure can result.[4] Trendelenburg's position, often used during pelvic laparoscopic procedures, potentiates venous return and can consequently affect blood pressure. In addition, cardiovascular compromise in an otherwise healthy child can result from the increased vasovagal reflex response to peritoneal stimulation from insufflation and/or trocar placement leading to pronounced bradycardia and asystole.[4] Furthermore, severe complications, such as a venous gas embolism in laparoscopy, can lead to rapid cardiovascular collapse. Anticipating potential physiologic problems in laparoscopy is essential to avoid patient morbidity and mortality.

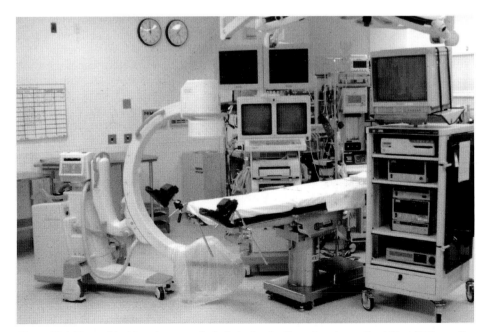

Figure 83-1 Pictured in this endoscopy suite is the hydraulically equipped operating table with C-arm fluoroscopy and affiliated monitors. Child Allen stirrups are in position on the table. The videoendoscopy cart is available for video monitoring of the procedure. In addition, with a centralized computer video system, the room monitors project the procedure to provide the greatest convenience for the endoscopist.

ENDOSCOPIC EQUIPMENT

All endoscopic procedures require fluoroscopic imaging (usually a C-arm), an electrosurgical unit, video camera, video monitor, light source, appropriate endoscopes, and working instruments.

Fluoroscopy is an integral part of ureteroscopy, percutaneous nephrostomy, and cystourethroscopy with retrograde ureteropyelograms. It provides vital guidance to assess location and proper course of action during the performance of pediatric endoscopy. An operating room table with adequate clearance for the fluoroscopic unit to fit underneath with good mobility is essential (see Figure 83-1). Fluoroscopy must be available to any surgeon who performs upper tract endoscopic procedures.[6]

A video camera that attaches to the endoscopic eyepiece has become an integral part of pediatric endoscopy. The clarity and magnification provided by a variety of products on the market have improved surgical results, provided an excellent method of documentation, and improved teaching to all who participate in the operative procedure. The output of the camera can be formatted to VHS, S-VHS, slide makers, color printers, or digital image capture devices for documentation and teaching.

Advances in imaging technology have greatly improved visualization during laparoscopic procedures.[2] Recent endoscopes have incorporated a charged coupling device chip camera, which provides superior image quality. Digital imaging technology is emerging to replace conventional analogue systems. The digital signal prevents image quality degradation and improves color, contrast, sharpness, and depth of field when compared to conventional systems.[7,8] The emergence of three-dimensional video imaging systems incorporates a stereoendoscope to mimic normal three-dimensional vision and to facilitate precise laparoscopic maneuvers and training.[9,10] Video advances such as high-definition television produce an extremely high resolution image in a wide screen format, which provides superior image quality and visualization during endoscopy.

The high-intensity xenon light source provides the illumination necessary to accomplish all of the endoscopic procedures. An additional flash lamp allows through-the-lens metering and flash for 35-mm endoscopic photographic applications. Care must be taken to avoid thermal injury resulting from heat transfer to the patient when using the xenon light source fiberoptic cord. Appropriate adapters must be purchased when the cable and endoscope are from different manufacturers than the light source. Some light sources come with multiple ports to accommodate a variety of fiberoptic cables. Recent modifications in laparoscopic instrumentation have combined the camera and light source into a single working instrument. This integrated laparoscope is available in 5- and 10-mm sizes (Figure 83-2).

An electrosurgical unit should be an integral part of the endoscopic equipment. This is standard equipment in any operating room suite. The operating surgeon should be familiar with the function of the electrosurgical unit. Prior to laparoscopic procedures, which require CO_2 insufflation in most cases, the CO_2 tank should be inspected to ensure an adequate quantity is available for the procedure. As a general rule, a full, spare CO_2 tank should be kept available during laparoscopic procedures in case an immediate replacement is required. All of the essential hardware can be efficiently and conveniently located in a mobile cart, which has an isolation transformer to supply the power to the several outlets located within the cart (Figure 83-3).

CYSTOURETHROSCOPY

The most common indications for cystourethroscopy in pediatric patients include treatment of obstructive lesions of the male urethra, evaluation of gross hematuria, defining the anatomy of genitourinary congenital anomalies, assessment and diagnosis of genitourinary malignancies, and treatment of calculi. Noticeably absent from the indications for cystourethroscopy are the assessment of urinary infections, evaluation of vesicoureteral reflux, and microscopic hematuria.[11,12] The majority of children with these disorders can be thoroughly evaluated with noninvasive radiologic imaging.[13] Most urologists who primarily treat children do not advocate cystoscopy or urethral dilation in female children with urinary infection and/or vesicoureteral reflux.[14]

Pediatric cystourethroscopes are available as integrated instruments, or with a number of variable-sized sheaths with interchangeable telescopic lenses. The integrated cystourethroscopes are the smallest in diameter, least prone to lens injury, and have an adequate working channel. The telescope is not available for other instruments, such as the optical urethrotome, since the telescope and sheath are all one piece. The 0° or direct-vision lens can be used with the infant or child resectoscope and urethrotome, while 30° and 70° lenses are available to fully assess the bladder architecture, ureteral orifices, bladder neck, and urethra. The 7.5 French infant integrated cystourethroscope with fixed 5° lens and 3F working channel is our preferred cystoscope because it permits access to small male and female urethras. The working channel is adequate for retrograde ureteral catheterization, guidewire passage, and laser fiber passage (Figure 83-4).

The general and critical features of a pediatric cystoscope are small size, adequate flow of irrigation fluid, optical clarity, and a working channel of 2.4F or greater. The products of a number of companies with these characteristics are shown in Table 83-1.

In general, the rod lens system provides better optics and various angles of view not available with a fiberoptic rigid cystoscope. The size of the cystourethroscope needs to be assessed at the tip, mid, and proximal shaft of the instrument as it changes in the different manufactured instruments. Depending on the specifications of the manufacturer, circular versus ellipsoid tip sizes are measured. The size and number of working channels will determine the adequacy of flow of irrigation and types of instruments that can be passed. The offset lens cystoscope with a straight working channel allows passage of small rigid instruments such as an ultrasonic lithotrite or subureteric injection needle, which are difficult to pass via curved working channels (Figure 83-5).

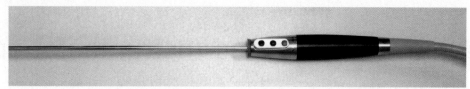

Figure 83-2 The 5-mm "integrated" laparoscope combines the light source and camera into a single working instrument whose cable exits through the end and attaches to the videoendoscopy cart. It eliminates the need for an additional light cord, which would exit at a right angle to the laparoscope, requiring frequent manipulation. It is available in 5- and 10-mm sizes.

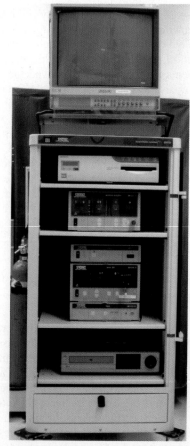

Figure 83-3 The videoendoscopy cart contains the video monitor, video camera, xenon light source, laparoscopic insufflator, and slide maker for endoscopic photography.

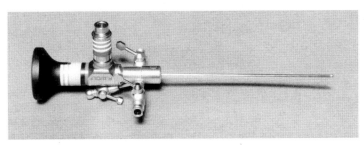

Figure 83-4 The 7.5 French infant integrated cystourethroscope with fixed 5° lens and 3F working channel.

The 10.5F offset lens cystourethroscope with a 5F working channel and 0° lens is our preferred choice for endoscopic subureteric injection of dextranomer/hyaluronic acid copolymer (Deflux) for the treatment of vesicoureteral reflux.

Operative instrumentation includes the pediatric infant and child resectoscopes and optical urethrotome (Table 83-2). The 8.5F optical urethrotome with sickle-shaped knife blade is our instrument of choice for the incision of posterior urethral valves. This instrument is used without electrocautery, avoiding potential thermal injury and stricture formation in the neonate. A potential disadvantage of this instrument is that the urethrotome and resectoscope require separate sheaths and working elements (Figure 83-6). The resectoscope (9 to 13.5F) has a larger outer diameter than the urethrotome (8.5 to 10.5F), which differs according to the manufacturer, accommodates the rod-lens telescope, provides electrocautery and is a vital part of the armamentarium. As the size of the child increases, larger instruments that provide better irrigation and illumination are available. Each manufacturer has a wide variety of accessory instruments, including bridges, grasping forceps, biopsy forceps, coagulation electrodes, cold knives, ureteral catheters, and loop electrodes.

Flexible pediatric cystoscopes are made by all of the major manufacturers. There are actively and passively deflectable scopes in sizes that are not significantly smaller than the rigid systems. The working channel in the rigid and flexible pediatric cystoscope is similar in size. The flexible cystoscope is more maneuverable, but has decreased illumination and clarity given the fiberoptic lens vs. the rod-lens system. In adults, flexible cystoscopes can be used for office procedures, with the patient given a topical anesthetic. This benefit of flexible cystoscopy is not applicable to the majority of pediatric patients, who require a general anesthetic to perform the procedure.

URETERORENOSCOPY

The primary indications for ureterorenoscopy in children are treatment of calculi, evaluation of hematuria and filling defects, and treatment of secondary strictures at the ureteropelvic junction.[6,15,16]

Ureterorenoscopy can be performed with rigid and flexible ureterorenoscopes. The rigid ureterorenoscopes have combined the fiberoptic image bundle and rod-lens system to achieve a smaller size (Table 83-3). The tip size begins at 4.5F to a maximum of 9.4F. The shaft body size is graduated and increases in size up to 12.4F. The lens is fiberoptic with a viewing angle from 0° to 8° (Figure 83-7). The endoscopes have one or two working channels (2.3 to 5.4F) with access for a variety of accessories including stone baskets, forceps, graspers, laser fibers, and electrohydraulic lithotripsy probes. The Hulbert knife (Cook) and Rite Cut (Circon) electrodes have made incision of ureteral strictures with rigid or flexible ureterorenoscopes easier. In a large series of pediatric patients undergoing ureteroscopic procedures, dilation of the ureteral orifice was usually not necessary with the smaller rigid scope.[17]

The majority of the rigid instruments have graduated shafts that progressively dilate the ureteral orifice. The semi-rigid mini-ureteroscopes are easily introduced into the ureter with minimal risk of ureteral injury and seem well adapted to the pediatric patient.[18,19] Rigid instruments, however, are often difficult to pass above the iliac vessels in children, and the entire renal collecting system cannot be visualized. These disadvantages are avoided with the actively deflectable flexible ureteroscopes.

Flexible endoscopes all contain a fiberoptic imaging bundle, fibers for illumination, a deflecting mechanism, and a working channel (Figure 83-8). Actively deflectable, small-diameter, flexible ureterorenoscopes allow access and treatment of the ureter and kidney (Table 83-4). Improvement in ureteroscopic design, accessories, and techniques has led to a significant increase in the success of diagnostic and therapeutic ureteroscopy in the pediatric patient.[20,21] Active tip deflection combined with secondary passive deflection allows the tip of the endoscope to be positioned into all

Company	Model	Tip Diameter (F)	Midshaft Diameter (F)	Proximal Diameter (F)	Working Channel(s) (F)	Viewing Angle (degrees)	Comments
ACMI	MR-PC	6.9	8.3	10.2	2.3/3.4	12	Smallest two-channel scope
	MR-915	6.9	8.3	10.2	2.1/5.4	12	Fiberoptic, two-channel scope
Olympus	A37026A	7.9	–	–	4.2	7	Angled ocular
	A37027A	7.9	–	–	4.2	7	Straight ocular
	A37025A	11.0	–	–	7.5	7	Angled ocular
Storz	27030K	7.5	–	8.5	3.5	0	Fiberoptic, offset lens
	27030AN	10.0	–	10.5	5.5	0	Fiberoptic, offset lens
	27030KS	12			7.5	0	Fiberoptic, offset lens
Wolf	4615.401	4.5	–	6.0	2.4	0	Smallest operating cystoscope
	8616.411	6.0	–	7.5	4.0	0	Steel shaft
	8626.431	9.5	–	–	5.0	5	Offset lens, straight working channel
	8616.401	10.5	–	–	5.0	25	Steel shaft
	8642.403	14	–	–	5.0	25	Steel shaft

Table 83-1   Pediatric Integrated Cystourethroscopes (Smallest Size with Working Channel)

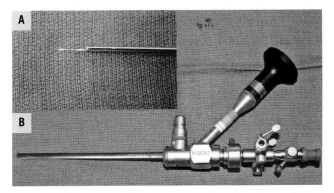

Figure 83-5 *A*, Rigid subureteric injection needle with bevel-up position. Two markings on the needle at 5 mm and 8 mm guide the depth and orientation of the bevel for accurate injection. *B*, The 10.5 French offset 0° lens cystourethroscope with 5F working channel. A straight working channel allows placement of a rigid subureteric injection needle.

Table 83-2   Pediatric Urethrotomes/Resectoscopes

Company	Model	Shaft Diameter (F)	Lens (Degrees)	Comments
Optical Urethrotomes				
ACMI	—	10.5	12/30	Wide angle view, no working element
Olympus	A3764A A37028A A37014A	9.5	0	Same working element as resectoscope
Storz	27145EK 27047B	10	0	Working element also used with resectoscope sheath
Wolf	8616.014	8.5	0	Sickle blade for PUV, separate sheath and working element, no electrocautery
Resectoscopes				
ACMI	PRSO-13	13.5	0/30/70	Electrocautery, cold knife attachment with working element, autoclavable telescopes
Olympus	A3764A A37004A A37014A	10.0	0	Same working element as urethrotome
Storz	27145EA 27047E/C	11/13	0	Requires different sheath than urethrotome with same working element
Wolf	8688.014	9.0	0	Different sheath and working element from optical urethrotome
	8677.014	11.5	0	HF electrodes or cold cutting elements

portions of the collecting system. The new generation ureterorenoscopes have a distal tip diameter of 7.5F or less, a 3.6F working channel, and a two-way active endoscopic tip deflector with a minimum of 160° of deflection in one direction. Logical deflection of the tip occurs when downward rotation of the thumb lever produces downward tip movement. Passive secondary deflection results from an inherent weakness in the endoscope durometer. This allows flexion off the upper collecting system, which effectively lengthens the deflected segment of the ureteroscope, allowing positioning of the tip into the dependent portion of the lower-pole caliceal system.[22]

Ureteroscopic access with smaller flexible instrumentation has required less frequent dilation of the ureteral orifice.[22] Usually, a single 0.018- to 0.038-inch guidewire placed cystoscopically under fluoroscopic guidance is all that is necessary for diagnostic ureteroscopy with flexible instrumentation. The small-diameter flexible endoscope is passed in monorail fashion over the guidewire to the renal pelvis. When dilation of the intramural ureter is required, it should be done only to the smallest size that will allow introduction of the ureteroscope. Graduated dilators (Not-tingham dilator), and ureteral dilating balloons are available. In general, dilation of the ureter up to 12F in children did not result in vesicoureteral reflux.[17] Close follow-up of these children is needed, however, to detect any renal damage as a result of either reflux or obstruction.[23] After ureteroscopy, the majority of pediatric patients require postoperative ureteral stenting. Stents are available with attached strings to facilitate removal without anesthesia. Sizes of 4 to 5F and 10 to 20 cm in length are commonly utilized and left in place for 72 hours.

Commonly used working instruments are now available in sizes of 3F or less, permitting their use with flexible ureteroscopes. These include many varieties of stone baskets, graspers, cup biopsy forceps, and cutting and fulgurating electrodes. We prefer the 3F Teflon–sheathed, three-pronged graspers for stone manipulation through the flexible ureteroscope. The Teflon sheath allows maximal deflection of the ureteroscope, which permits access to stones in the lower-pole calix in the majority of cases. Furthermore, because the flexible ureteroscopes have only one working channel, engaging a stone too large to remove in a basket can be a potentially dangerous situation. This can be avoided by using a three-pronged grasper, which allows easy release of the stone when necessary.

Energy sources available for stone destruction include the electrohydraulic lithotriptor, pulsed-dye laser lithotriptor, electromechanical impactor, Lithoclast mechanical lithotriptor, and holmium laser. The ultrasonic probes, pulsed-dye laser lithotrite, and electrohydraulic lithotrite have all been successfully used in the pediatric population.[15,17,24] A major advance in the energy sources

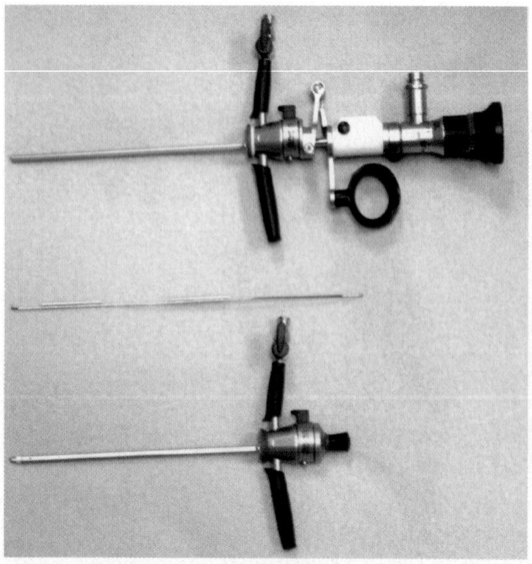

Figure 83-6 The optical urethrotome with 9.5 French sheath and accompanying angled knife blade.

Table 83-3   Rigid Ureterorenoscopes

Company	Model	Tip Size (F)	Midshaft Diameter (F)	Proximal Diameter (F)	Length (cm)	Working Channel(s) (F)	Lens (degrees)	Comments
ACMI	MR-PC	6.9	8.3	8.3	15.5	3.4/2.3	5	Graduated shaft
	MRO-715	7.7	9.2	10.8	15	5.4	5	Self dilating tip, offset lens
	MR-915	9.4	10.2	12.4	15	5.4/2.1	5	
	MR-6	6.9	8.3	10.2	33/42	3.4/2.3	5	
	MRO-633 MRO-642	6.9	8.3	10.2	33/42	3.4/2.3	5	Offset lens
Olympus	A2940A A2941A	6.4	—	7.8	43/33	4.2	7	Graduated shaft Autoclavable, offset lens
	WA02944A WA02946A	7.5	—	9.0	43/33	2.4/3.4	7	Autoclavable, straight lens
	WA02943A	7.5	—	9.0	43	2.4/3.4	7	Offset lens
Storz	27830A	7.5	9.0	10.5	25	2.5/3.6	8	Autoclavable
	27410SK 27410SL	7.5	9.0	10.5	34/43	2.5/3.6	8	Autoclavable
	27430K 27430L	8.0	10.5	11.5	34/43	5.0	8	Autoclavable
Wolf	4721.402	4.5	—	6.0	31	2.5	0	Not autoclavable
	8702.402	6.0	—	7.5	31	4.0	0	Autoclavable
	8712.402	6.0	—	7.5	42.5	2.4/2.4	0	
	8707.402	8.0	—	9.8	31	5.0	10	
	8703.402	8.0	—	9.8	42.5	3.0/3.0	10	
		7.0	—	8.5	31	3.3	10	Offset lens
	8708.401	7.0	—	8.5	42.5	2.4/2.4	10	Offset lens
	8702.533	6.0	7.5/8.5	11.0	31.5/43	5.0	0	Autoclavable, offset lens

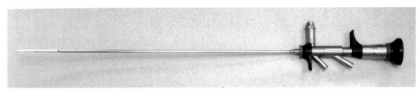

Figure 83-7 The 7.5 French rigid ureterorenoscope with two working channels, 2.4 and 3.4F, which will accommodate a variety of working instruments. The shaft is graduated to 9.0F proximally and contains a fixed 7° fiberoptic lens.

available for use with the flexible ureteroscope has been the holmium laser (Figure 83-9). The majority of ureteral and renal calculi have been successfully treated with the holmium laser.[25] The small 200- to 400-micron fibers easily pass through the working channel of the flexible ureteroscope and calculi in all areas of the ureter and kidney have been successfully fragmented in the pediatric population.[20,25] The high water absorption of the holmium laser limits tissue penetration to 0.4 mm and allows clean tissue incisions with minimal coagulation beyond the level of the cut. Its uses include incision of ureteral strictures and secondary strictures of the ureteropelvic junction, as well as ablation of urothelial lesions in the pediatric population. The holmium laser is our instrument of choice for stone destruction and incision of secondary ureteropelvic junction strictures.

Although technological advances have resulted in ureteroscopic equipment that can be used in the urinary tract of children, caution must be exercised. The margin for error is small, and the urologic surgeon must be familiar with the equipment, ureteroscopic techniques, and their limitations. The long-term consequences of ureteral endoscopic manipulations in the pediatric population remain undefined.

PERCUTANEOUS NEPHROSCOPY

Percutaneous access to the kidney in infants and children is a well-established procedure used primarily to drain the obstructed upper urinary tract.[26] Percutaneous surgical techniques in the pediatric population are frequently used for a number of urologic indications. The most common pediatric percutaneous endoscopic proce-

dures performed are nephrostolithotomy and endopyelotomy.[27,28] Major concerns regarding the percutaneous approach have been the size of the instruments, patient size, blood loss, and mobile, smaller kidneys. The advent of extracorporeal shock wave lithotripsy and improved retrograde access to renal calculi has decreased the indications for percutaneous renal surgery. In some instances, however, there are still pediatric patients who benefit from this approach to the kidney.[29] The instrumentation necessary for percutaneous procedures is no different than in the adult population. Both rigid and flexible nephroscopes are available. The rigid nephroscopes range in size from 17 to 24F (Table 83-5). These large nephroscopes have an offset lens with a straight working channel allowing passage of rigid probes and instruments (Figure 83-10). These tips are rounded, not beveled like a cystoscope, decreasing the risk of perforation. At our institution, the smaller 10 to 12F pediatric cystoscopes with offset lens and 5F straight working channel are valuable for both cystoscopy and percutaneous nephroscopy. Flexible instrumentation is often necessary to access the entire intrarenal collecting system. The flexible nephroscope has a tighter turning radius than the flexible cystoscope, facilitating inspection of the collecting system. Currently available flexible nephroscopes are 14 to 15F in diameter and contain a 6F working channel. The tip will deflect more than 160°. In certain cases, due to size restrictions, a flexible ureteroscope is necessary for entry into the small caliceal infundibulum. Hence, the operating surgeon must have a variety of endoscopes available for use during percutaneous procedures.

Instrumentation for accessing the kidney is similar to that used in adults, but the tract size is

smaller. Access to the kidney is under fluoroscopic control. A cystoscopically placed ureteral catheter allows filling of the collecting system for the fluoroscopic puncture. The percutaneous tract is established with either sequential dilators (Amplatz) or a balloon dilator. The size of the working sheath will depend upon patient size, pathology, and instrument size. An 11F peelaway access sheath for percutaneous nephrostolithotomy in infants and preschool children has been developed and used in children as young as age 2 with success.[30] When using a smaller sheath, free egress of the irrigation fluid must be monitored to avoid high-pressure fluid extravasation.[31] If an adult size sheath is required, it can be trimmed to an appropriate length to accommodate the pediatric scope and working instruments.

Percutaneous stone manipulation involves use of instruments, such as the tri-radiate grasper, forceps, and baskets, to entrap the smaller stone particles. Energy sources for fragmentation of the stones include ultrasound, electrohydraulic lithotripsy and the holmium laser. Endoscopic holmium laser lithotripsy has been successful in children as young as one year. The use of the holmium laser is believed to have an increased margin of safety and efficacy in children when compared with other intracorporeal lithotrites.[20]

Percutaneous endopyelotomy has generally been performed in infants and children with secondary ureteropelvic junction obstruction resulting from failed surgery.[32,34] The incision through the strictured segment can be made with a hooked knife, electrocautery or a holmium laser (200 or 400 micron) fiber. At the conclusion of the procedure, a stent is left in place. Endopyelotomy stents sized for children, double pigtail stents, and infant feeding tubes have been employed for this purpose.

LAPAROSCOPY

Pediatric urologic laparoscopic surgical procedures continue to expand with increases in surgeon experience and advances in technology. Initially, diagnostic laparoscopy for evaluation of the undescended non-palpable testis was the primary urologic indication. Presently, laparoscopic orchiopexy for the intra-abdominal testis appears to have better results than the open approach.[35]

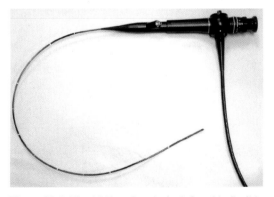

Figure 83-8 The 6.9 French actively deflectable flexible ureterorenoscope with a 3.6F working channel and 180° of deflection in two directions. The shaft is graduated to 8.4F proximally and has a 70-cm working length.

Table 83-4	Actively Deflectable Flexible Ureterorenoscopes						
Company	Model	Tip Size (F)	Midshaft Diameter (F)	Proximal Diameter (F)	Length (cm)	Working Channel Size (F)	Deflection (Up/Down Degrees)
ACMI	AUR 7	7.2	7.4	11.0	65	3.6	170/180
	AUR 735	7.4	—	8.2	35	3.6	120/160
Olympus	URF-P3	6.9	—	8.4	70	3.6	180/180
Storz	11278AU1	6.7	7.5	8.4	70	3.6	270/270
	11278AC1	6.7	7.5	8.4	40	3.6	270/270
	11274AC	7.5	—	8.0	40	3.6	120/170
Wolf	7325.122	7.5	—	—	20	3.6	130/160
	7325.152	7.5	—	—	45	3.6	130/160
	7325.172	7.5	—	—	70	3.6	130/160
	7305.071	6.0	—	8.8	70	3.6	270/270

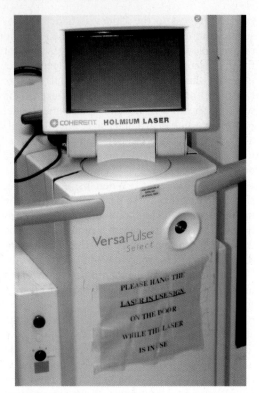

Figure 83-9 Holmium Laser.

Table 83-5	Rigid Nephroscopes					
Company	Model	Shaft Size, Sheath Size (F)	Working Channel (F)	Length (cm)	Lens (Degrees)	Comments
ACMI	MRO-2004	19.5 22.5	12	30	9	Reticulating irrigation port Angled eyepiece
	MRO-2005	19.5	15	30	9	Reticulating irrigation port Angled eyepiece
Olympus	A37025A	11.0	7.5	22	7	
	A37022A	15.9				Continuous flow, stainless steel offset, rotating sheath
Storz	27095AA	11.0	5.5	14	6	Rod lens, angled eyepiece, 30-cm working instruments
	27095B	17.0				
Wolf	8964.401	—	10.5	20.5	12	Rod lens, 35-cm instruments
	8964.021	20.8				

The pediatric urologic experience with laparoscopic nephrectomy, intersex evaluation and gonadectomy, pyeloplasty, orchiopexy, extravesical ureteral reimplantation, varicocelectomy, and laparoscopic-assisted procedures are a partial list of the procedures presently performed.[36]

Pediatric laparoscopes are smaller in diameter than their adult counterparts (Figure 83-11). They typically measure 1.9 to 5.5 mm in width and ≤ 33 cm in length (Figure 83-12). Variable degrees of view from 0° to 70° are available. The smaller 1.9 mm scope used via 2-mm trocar designed for diagnostic laparoscopy can be utilized with improved cosmesis and decreased convalescence.[37] Recent advances in laparoscopic technology have combined the light source and camera capabilities into a single system that is user friendly. It eliminates the need for an extra cable connection and allows photographic capabilities accessible on the instrument handle (see Figure 83-2). Compared to the 2-mm laparoscopes, the ≥ 3 mm laparoscopes provide better abdominal cavity illumination, optical resolution, and image clarity, but the 2 mm laparoscopes are steadily improving in quality (Table 83-6).

Laparoscopic instruments can be divided into insufflation needles, trocars, graspers, dissectors, scissors, retractors, needle holders, knot pushers, clips, staplers, and tissue removal devices. These instruments are available in disposable or non-disposable forms. The operative instruments used with electrocautery are insulated to the tip of the instrument. A variety of blades, hooks, and spatulas are available for use (Figure 83-13). In addition, the instrument handle can lock the jaws of the grasper with a spring or ratchet mechanism. A reticulating device in the handle allows movement of the tip of the instrument while minimizing movement of the arm and hand. Handles can have an electrocautery connection and/or locking mechanism, depending on desired use and surgeon preference (Figure 83-14). Shorter instruments of 10 to 20 cm in length for the pediatric patient are available. Most instruments are 2 mm to 12 mm in diameter. The diameters of instruments, including the laparoscope and trocars, have decreased to 2 to 5 mm, allowing operative needlescopic orchiopexy and retroperitoneal procedures.[37] This further refinement in size is a step forward in minimally invasive procedures in infants and children.

Laparoscopic instruments used to apply clips and staples are both disposable and non-disposable and can be used in a single- or multiple-loaded device. The multi-loaded clip applier is available as a 5-mm instrument with a rotating shaft. The laparoscopic staplers, linear cutters, and large clip applicators can require a port size up to 35 mm. In addition to Endoclips, the Endoloop (U.S. Surgical, Norwalk, CT) is available for intracorporeal ligature. A variety of suture material on an ST-3 needle can be passed intracorporeally for reconstructive procedures, such as pediatric pyeloplasty. Laparoscopic needle holders are specifically designed for this purpose.

In addition to the instruments necessary for all endoscopic procedures, two additional pieces of hardware are necessary for pediatric laparoscopy: the insufflation system and the aspiration/irrigation system. The insufflation system allows the surgeon to obtain and maintain the pneumoperitoneum at a specific abdominal pressure. Laparoscopic insufflation is accomplished with CO_2. The insufflator should monitor the rate of CO_2 inflow, total CO_2 used, and intra-abdominal pressure. The insufflation rate can be varied and should shut off automatically when the peak preset intra-abdominal pressure is reached. As little as 300 cc of CO_2 may be necessary for an adequate pneumoperitoneum in the infant. As mentioned previously, intra-abdominal pressure should be kept below 15 mm Hg in the pediatric patient to avoid potentially severe physiologic consequences.[4,5]

Access to the pediatric abdominal cavity with a Veress needle and blind trocar insertion can be associated with trocar-induced vascular and viscus injury.[38] Hence, an open periumbilical cutdown technique is utilized with a threaded fascial screw trocar sheath for placement under direct vision.[39] All secondary trocars are placed under direct vision. Trocars are available in sizes from 2 mm to 12 mm in diameter with a shorter length for pediatric patients. In addition, trocars are made of nonconductive material and can be used safely with electrocautery. The disposable trocar offers a spring-loaded safety shield that retracts as the trocar enters the abdomen and slides over the sharp obturator after abdominal penetration. Trocars are available with reducer caps and adjustable stability threads to facilitate insertion of variable-size instruments and creation of the abdominal wall seal to preserve pneumoperitoneum.

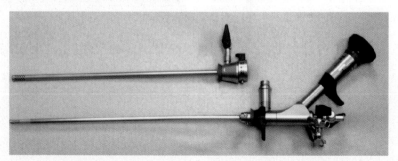

Figure 83-10 The rigid nephroscope with a 15.9 French rotating sheath, 7.5F straight working channel, stainless steel construction, and 7° angled ocular system.

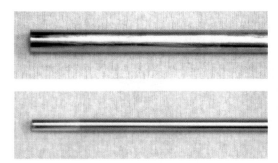

Figure 83-11 The comparison in size between the 10-, 5- and 3-mm laparoscopes is demonstrated. With advances in optics, the smaller laparoscopes provide similar image quality and video capability.

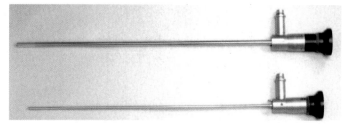

Figure 83-12 This 5-mm laparoscope is 33 cm in length and provides full screen optic capability with a 0°, 30°, or 45° lens. The 3-mm laparoscope is 28 cm in length with a 0° or 30° lens. Both are autoclavable.

The Step Access System (U.S. Surgical) for laparoscopic entry utilizes a radially expanding sleeve and needle to initiate the port entry. Regardless of the desired port size, a needle sleeve assembly establishes a dilating tract with a narrow cross-sectional profile (2.1 mm). The initial needle tract is radially expanded by insertion of the port through the sleeve. The resulting width of the fascial defect is approximately half the size of the wound left by direct penetrating trocars.[40] The sleeve/port system generates radial traction which helps prevent cannula displacement during laparoscopy.[41–43]

Aspiration and irrigation are necessary with operative laparoscopic procedures. The aspiration equipment can be connected directly to the vacuum system in the operating room. A dual trumpet valve connected to a straight metal tube allows for both suction and pressurized irrigation. Pressurized irrigation can be accomplished with either a pressurized cuff around the irrigant bag or a CO_2-driven device (Nezhat CO_2 pressurized aspiration/irrigation system).

The harmonic scalpel system, consisting of a generator, hand piece with cable, blade system, and foot piece, provides less lateral thermal damage, decreased smoke production, and no electrical energy transmission to the patient (Figure 83-15). This system is a useful adjunct during laparoscopic nephrectomy or heminephrectomy and fits via a 5-mm port. Both disposable and nondisposable harmonic scalpels are available for use. Laparoscopic coagulation shears can be used for dissection, cutting, and coagulation with improved safety compared to electrocautery or laser.

A useful tool in pediatric urologic laparoscopic procedures is the LigaSure vessel sealing system (Valleylab). Designed for a 5mm working port, the LigaSure permanently fuses vessels and tissue with a combination of pressure and energy. The device has a feedback controlled response which discontinues energy delivery to the tissue/vessel when the seal cycle is complete. Thermal spread with the use of this device is between 1 and 2 mm. The entire working element can be controlled on the handheld device. The design minimizes lateral thermal tissue damage and reduces the need for instrument exchange. Vessels can be sealed and controlled up to 7mm in diameter with this device. This instrument is useful in application of clipless first stage orchiopexy, as well as ligating the vessels in laparoscopic heminephrectomy.

Two other laparoscopic devices are the specimen retrieval bag and the tissue morcellator. They are used when solid organs such as the kidney are removed laparoscopically. The organ is placed in the retrieval bag and reduced in size into small pieces by the morcellator to facilitate removal via the laparoscopic port.

Modifications of adult instruments continue to be made for appropriate application in the pediatric patient. Smaller-sized endoscopes, clip appliers, and trocars are now available specifically for the pediatric patient. These adaptations have improved the safety of laparoscopic procedures in infants and children.

CONCLUSION

The miniaturization of equipment, improvements in illumination and fiberoptics, and applications of new energy sources, combined with the inventiveness of urologic surgeons, have expanded the applications of endoscopic procedures in the pediatric patient. The pediatric endoscopic surgeon should be well-informed regarding the variety of instrumentation and equipment available for all endoscopic procedures. A list of endoscopic equipment/instrument manufacturers with appropriate contact information is provided in Appendix 1.

Table 83-6 Pediatric Laparoscopes					
Company	Model	Diameter (mm)	Length (cm)	Lens (Degrees)	Comments
ACMI	LAP27-0	2.7	30	0	Wide angle image, fiberoptic
	LAP5-0MA	5	30.6	0	Autoclavable
	LAP5-30MA	5	30.6	30	Autoclavable
	LAP5-45MA	5	30.6	45	Autoclavable
	LAP5-70MA	5	30.6	70	Autoclavable
	L5-0A	5	30.6	0	High image brightness, high resolution, increased depth of focus
	L5-30A	5	30.6	30	High image brightness, high resolution, increased depth of focus
Olympus	A4672A	3	28	0	Autoclavable
	WA50372B	5	33	0	Full-screen optics
	WA50373B	5	33	30	
	WA50374B	5	33	45	
	A50021A	5	33	0	Integrated camera and light source
	A50023A	5	33	30	
Storz	7218AA	2.7	18	0	Autoclavable
	7218BA	2.7	18	30	
	7218FA	2.7	18	45	
	26006BA	5	29	0/30/45	Autoclavable
Wolf	8754.401	2	27	0	Full instrumentation available, straight ocular system
	8754.501	2	19	0	
	8974.401	2.7	31.6	25	
	8660.411	3.3	30	0	
	8660.412	3.3	30	70	
	8930.401	3.5	30	0	
	8930.402	3.5	30	25	
	8746.401	3.8	30	12	Offset lens, 5 French straight working channel
	8935.411	5.0	30	0	
	8935.412	5.0	30	25	
	8935.413	5.0	30	50	
	8920.401	5.5	21.6	0	Offset lens, 3.5-mm, straight working channel

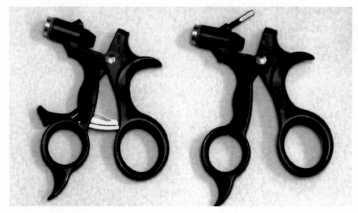

Figure 83-13 Rachet-type hand laparoscopic instruments available through a 5-mm port include claw grasping forceps, atraumatic wave-type grasping forceps, hook scissors, spiked biopsy forceps, atraumatic grasping forceps, and mini-Metzenbaum scissors. Many laparoscopic instruments are available in 1.9- to 5-mm pediatric sizes.

Figure 83-14 Hand instruments are available in a variety of designs to fit the surgeon's hand without causing fatigue. Locking handles with an easy release mechanism and handles with electrocautery capability are designed for surgeon preference and ease of use.

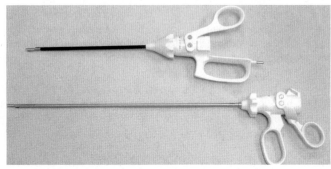

Figure 83-15 The harmonic scalpel system provides cutting and cauterization capabilities. The reusable 5-mm scalpels have a 360° rotating shaft with compatibility to an electrosurgical unit.

REFERENCES

1. Young HH, McKay RW. Congenital valvular obstruction of the prostatic urethra. Surg Gynecol Obstet 1929;48:509.
2. Kourambas J, Preminger GM. Advances in camera, video, and imaging technology in laparoscopy. Urol Clin North Am 2001;28:5–14.
3. Meyers MB, Oh TH. Prevention of hypothermia during cystoscopy in infants. Anesth Analg 1976;55:592.
4. Pennant JH. Anesthesia for laparoscopy in the pediatric patient. Anesthesiol Clin North America 2001;19:69–88.
5. Kavoussi LR. Pediatric applications in laparoscopy. In: Clayman RV, McDougall EM, editors. Laparoscopic urology. St. Louis: Quality Medical Publishing; 1993. p. 209–24.
6. Eshghi M, Reda EF, Franco I. Endoscopic surgery in the upper tract in children. In: Kelalis PP, King LR, Belman AB, editors. Clinical pediatric urology. Philadelphia: WB Saunders; 1992. p. 726–72.
7. Aslan P, Kuo RL, Hazel K, et al. Advances in digital imaging during endoscopic surgery. J Endourol 1999;13:251.
8. Berci G, Wren SM, Stain SC, et al. Individual assessment of visual perception by surgeons observing the same laparoscopic organs with various imaging systems. Surg Endoscopy 1995;9:967.
9. Babayan RK, Chiu AW. The comparison between 2-dimensional and 3-dimensional laparoscopic video systems in a pelvic trainer. J Endourol 1993;7:S195.
10. Durrani AF, Preminger GM. Three dimensional video imaging for endoscopic surgery. Comput Biol Med 1995;25:237.
11. Kroovand RL. Endoscopy. In: Kelalis PP, King LR, Belman AB, editors. Clinical pediatric urology. Philadelphia: WB Saunders; 1992. p. 166–85.
12. Johnson DK, Kroovand RL, Perlmutter AD. The changing role of cystoscopy in the pediatric patient. J Urol 1980; 123:232.
13. Walther PC, Kaplan GW. Cystoscopy in children: indications for its use in common urologic problems. J Urol 1979; 122:717.
14. Kaplan GW, Sammons TH, King LR. A blind comparison of dilation, urethrotomy, and medication alone in treatment of urinary tract infections in girls. J Urol 1973;109:917.
15. Hill DE, Segura JW, Patterson DE, Kramer SA. Ureteroscopy in children. J Urol 1990;144:481.
16. Docimo SG, Peters CA. Pediatric endourology and laparoscopy. In: Campbell's urology. 8th ed. Philadelphia: WB Saunders; 2002.72:2564.
17. Thomas R, Ortenberg J, Harmon EP. Safety and efficacy of pediatric ureteroscopy for management of calculous disease. J Urol 1993;149:1082.
18. Watson GM, Landers B, Nauth-Misir R, Wickham JE. Developments in the ureteroscopes, techniques, and accessories associated with laser lithotripsy. World J Urol 1993;11:19.
19. Minevich E, Rousseau MB, Wacksman J et al. Pediatric ureteroscopy: technique and preliminary results. J Ped Surg 1997;32:571.
20. Wollin TA, Teichman JMH, Rogenes VJ, et al. Holmium:YAG lithotripsy in children. J Urol 1999;162:1717.
21. Shroff S, Watson GM. Experience with ureteroscopy in children. Br J Urol 1995;75:395.
22. Grasso M, Bagley D. Small diameter, actively deflectable, flexible ureteropyeloscopy. J Urol 1998;160:1648.
23. Hill DE, Segura JW, Patterson DE, et al. Ureteroscopy in children. J Urol 1990;144:481.
24. Caione P, DeGennavo M, Capozza N, Zaccara A. Endoscopic manipulation of ureteral calculi in children by rigid operative ureterorenoscopy. J Urol 1990;144:484.
25. Reddy PP, Barrieras DJ, Bagli DJ, et al. Initial experience with endoscopic holmium laser lithotripsy for pediatric urolithiasis. J Urol 1999;162:1714.
26. O'Brien WM, Matsumoto AH, Grant EG, Gibbons MD. Percutaneous nephrostomy in infants. Urology 1990;36:269.
27. Callaway TW, Lingardh G, Basata S, Sylvan M. Percutaneous nephrolithotomy in children. J Urol 1992;148:1067.
28. Figenshau RS, Clayman RV, Colberg JW, et al. Pediatric endopyelotomy: the Washington University experience. J Urol 1966;156:2025.
29. Badawy H, Salama A, Eissa M, et al. Percutaneous management of renal calculi: experience with percutaneous nephrolithotomy in 60 children. J Urol 1999;162:1710.
30. Jackman SV, Hedican SP, Peters CA, et al. Percutaneous nephrostolithotomy in infants and preschool age children: experience with a new technique. Urology 1998;52:697.
31. Pugach JL, Moore RG, Parra RO, et al. Massive hydrothorax and hydro-abdomen complicating percutaneous nephrolithotomy. J Urol 1999;162:2110.
32. Kavoussi LR, Meretyk S, Dierks SM, et al. Endopyelotomy for secondary ureteropelvic junction obstruction in children. J Urol 1991;145:345.
33. Mor Y, Elmasry YET, Kellert M, et al. The role of percutaneous nephrolithotomy in the management of pediatric renal calculi. J Urol 1997;158:1319.
34. Capolicchio G, Homsy YL, Houle AM, et al. Long-term results of percutaneous endopyelotomy in the treatment of children with failed open pyeloplasty. J Urol 1997;158:1534.
35. Docimo SG. The results of surgical therapy for cryptorchidism: a literature review and analysis. J Urol 1995;154:1148.
36. Duel BP. Laparoscopy in pediatric urology: where do we stand? Dial Ped Urol 1999;22:1.
37. Soble JJ, Gill IS. Needlescopic urology: incorporating 2-mm instruments in laparoscopic surgery. Urology 1998;52:187.
38. Esposito C, Ascione G, Garipoli V, et al. Complications of pediatric laparoscopic surgery. Surg Endoscopy 1997;11:655.
39. Conlin MJ, Skoog SJ. Safe laparoscopic access in pediatric patients. Urology 1994;44:579.
40. Bhoyrul S, Mori T, Way LW. Radially expanding dilation: a superior method for laparoscopic trocar access. Surg Endose 1996;10:775–8.
41. Baggish MS, Lovins CM. Randomized prospective study of radial expanding trocar and conventional trocar/sleeve for operative laparoscopy. Abstract for International Congress of Gynecologic Endoscopy (AAGL), 1996.
42. Rothenberg S. The use of radially expandable laparoscopic access in pediatric patients. Abstract submitted to the V International Congress for Endosurgery in Children, 1996.
43. Turner DJ. A novel radially expanding access system for laparoscopic procedures versus conventional trocars: a prospective, self-controlled clinical study. J Am Assoc Gynecol Laparosc 1996;3:609.

84

Endoscopic Approaches to Anterior and Posterior Urethral Valves

Stephen A. Zderic, MD, FACS, FAAP

INDICATIONS

The clinical presentation of posterior urethral valves in the neonate is characterized by a weak stream, urinary retention, or a palpable abdominal mass (due to a distended bladder, hydroureteronephrosis, or urinary extravasation). Less severe cases may go undetected until the child develops a urinary tract infection or fails to attain continence of urine. Today, with the widespread use of screening antenatal ultrasonography, the majority of these cases will be detected in utero. Unilateral or bilateral hydroureteronephrosis and a thick-walled bladder that empties poorly in a male fetus suggest a likely diagnosis of posterior urethral valves.[1] This becomes even more likely if oligohydramnios is present. It is important to emphasize that posterior urethral valves is the most likely diagnosis. However, on occasion, fetal ultrasonographic findings consistent with posterior urethral valves have proven to be prune belly syndrome. It is clear that posterior valves present with a broad spectrum. For the most severe cases as shown in Figure 84-1, severe oligohydramnios is associated with pulmonary hypoplasia, which proves fatal. Associated with these findings are the presence of a hypertrophied and thick-walled bladder, bilateral hydroureter, and renal cortical cysts. The issue of fetal intervention for hydronephrosis and urethral valves will be discussed in Chapter 91, "Antenatal Surgical Intervention for Urinary Obstruction". An assessment of postnatal outcomes after prenatal intervention suggests that pulmonary function (the major cause of neonatal demise in severe cases) will improve, but renal function will not.[2,3]

There is ample clinical evidence that vesical dysfunction in patients with posterior urethral valves is a major source of long-term morbidity.[4,5] This manifests itself as either an atonic bladder with poor emptying, uninhibited contractions, or a small, stiff, noncompliant bladder. The noncompliant valve bladder places the upper urinary tract at risk of significant deterioration secondary to the elevated storage pressures. This increases the likelihood that these patients will progress to end-stage renal disease, and can also place the transplanted kidney at greater risk for deterioration.[6] Experimentally, Peters has accumulated evidence in the fetal lamb that outlet obstruction is associated with an increase in bladder mass due to smooth muscle hypertrophy and

the deposition of extracellular matrix.[7] This matrix accumulation may result from alterations in gene expression or diminished matrix breakdown due to an increase in the inhibitor of the matrix metalloproteinases (tissue inhibitor of metalloproteinases [TIMP]).[7,8] Fetal bladder

obstruction results in thick-walled bladders with an especially prominent deposition of collagen fibers in fetal lambs, which correlates with similar findings in human fetal specimens.[9,10] A great deal of effort has been focused on research on the molecular pathways that lead to bladder wall

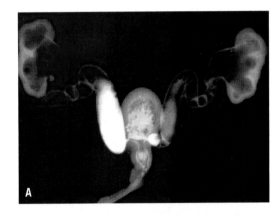
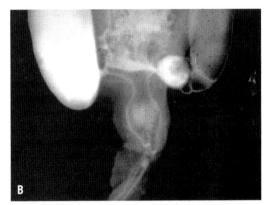
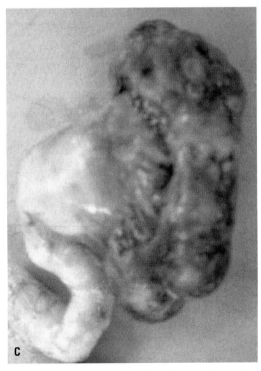
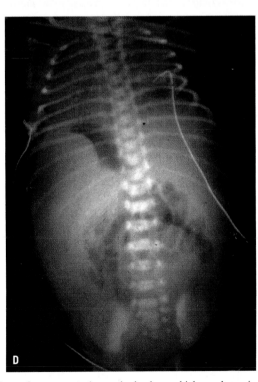

Figure 84-1 This panel shows the primary and secondary effects of severe posterior urethral valves, which are shown in this double air contrast study in a postmortem specimen. *A, B,* The valve cusps are highlighted prominently and should be compared with the radiographic image in Figure 84-2. *A,* the thick-walled bladder and associated high-grade reflux in this severe case are apparent. Associated with this valve are *C,* the superimposed findings of renal dysplasia with cortical cysts and *D,* a chest film showing severe pulmonary hypoplasia, which ultimately proved fatal in this case. *A, B,* and *C* courtesy of Christopher Austin, MD, and Dale Huff, MD.

hypertrophy. These changes in matrix deposition can be reversed by surgical relief of outlet obstruction, which produces dramatic improvements in bladder function; still, persisting voiding dysfunction is noted in up to 30% of cases.[11] Fetal intervention of posterior urethral valves, however, has been reported to carry a 50% rate of fetal demise.[3] Hopefully, with a better understanding of the pathways responsible for smooth muscle hypertrophy and wall fibrosis, medical management might be instituted in utero to optimize bladder function.

Increased labor on the part of the bladder in response to increased voiding pressure is a major trigger that initiates the process of bladder wall hypertrophy. Early on, the bladder may be able to generate enough pressure such that low residual urine is maintained. With time, this compensatory response fails, and the post-void residual urine increases sharply. Evidence suggests that during this decompensatory phase, stretch on the smooth muscle elements leads to additional scarring and fibrosis. The importance of providing intravesical pressure relief is provided by an experiment of nature. In those patients with pop-off mechanisms (such as massive unilateral reflux), which serve to lower bladder pressures, Kaefer and colleagues demonstrated improved bladder compliance when compared to a cohort in whom no such venting mechanism was present.[12] The renal prognosis is also more favorable when these venting mechanisms are present.[13]

These clinical and experimental observations all lead to the conclusion that it is imperative for urethral valves to be treated promptly once a diagnosis is made. The goals of such early intervention are to optimize renal and bladder function and to minimize the chances for urosepsis to develop. A primary valve ablation eliminates high pressure voiding and allows the bladder to continue cycling. Today, endoscopy in the neonate is greatly simplified by an array of endoscopes ranging from 7 to 9 French in size, with excellent image quality. Instrument size is still a significant concern in the premature neonate, and forcing an endoscope into a fragile newborn urethra invites stricture formation, which becomes a significant complication. A temporizing vesicostomy is an excellent option in patients with posterior urethral valves whose small size precludes safe urethral instrumentation.[14] A vesicostomy might also be considered for a neonate with severe renal dysfunction or urinary extravasation. Today most authors agree that primary valve ablation is preferable to diversion, because many believe it is important for the bladder to experience the filling and emptying cycle. A vesicostomy allows for bladder cycling, in contrast to high urinary diversion where the bladder is fully defunctionalized.[15–17]

This chapter emphasizes the diagnosis and management of posterior urethral valves, which account for 90% of all cases, but on occasion, anterior valves are seen. Anterior urethral valves also present with wide variations in severity; the most severe cases also produce outlet obstruction, secondary bladder changes, and associated renal insufficiency. They are often associated with a urethral diverticulum, which may fill during voiding; the bulge or subsequent dribbling may prompt the parents to seek clinical evaluation. If the obstruction is severe enough, the diagnosis of hydronephrosis may be made prenatally.

PATIENT PREPARATION

Irrespective of whether one is evaluating a neonate in whom the diagnosis was suspected based on prenatal ultrasonography, or an older patient who is symptomatic, a renal bladder ultrasound and a voiding cystourethrogram (VCUG) are essential to establishing a diagnosis and prognosis. Classic ultrasound findings will include a thick-walled bladder, dilated posterior urethra, and in most instances, the presence of hydroureteronephrosis. The presence of well-defined corticomedullary junctions in the renal parenchyma is a favorable prognostic sign with regard to future function.[18] Unilateral dysplasia (which is often associated with reflux), a retroperitoneal urinoma, or urinary ascites seen on sonograms are indicators of a more favorable renal prognosis.[13]

The gold standard for diagnosis remains the VCUG. On occasion, it may be necessary for the urologist to assist with catheter placement, which is readily accomplished with an 8F coude tip catheter. The demonstration of a dilated posterior urethra with a classic valve cusp is made in the voiding phase and is most readily seen as the catheter is withdrawn (Figure 84-2). The VCUG will also demonstrate whether reflux is present (unilateral or bilateral), the bladder capacity, and the presence of diverticula (Figure 84-3). All of these findings provide some important clues as to the potential for future bladder and renal function. Imaging the entire urethra on a VCUG is necessary given the fact that an anterior urethral valve may be seen at any point, including the fossa navicularis. The VCUG may reveal a diverticulum that fills to a point and then creates a lip or flap valve that balloons out to occlude antegrade flow. Retrograde studies may demonstrate the anatomy of valves, but they are not physiologic and can actually miss the diagnosis if the diverticulum is not filled. A well-performed VCUG offers the best means of diagnosing either kind of urethral valve. Intravenous broad-spectrum antibiotics (ie, ampicillin and carefully dosed gentamicin) should be started prior to obtaining such a VCUG in the newborn period. Many pediatric urologists have begun using oral antibiotics. However, this probably can not be declared to be standard of care.

After the VCUG, a catheter should be left in place until the time of valve ablation. The timing of valve resection is primarily determined by an assessment of the child's metabolic state and renal function. A neonate should be monitored closely in the intensive care nursery for any signs of postobstructive diuresis. This is extremely important because dehydration can occur quite rapidly in this setting and can induce prerenal azotemia. Superimposed dehydration may result

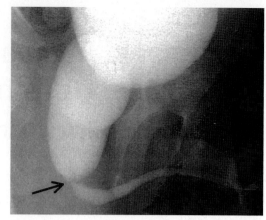

Figure 84-2 A fluoroscopic view of a classic posterior urethral valve cusp (arrow) from a type I valve.

in an elevated creatinine until the diuresis subsides and intravascular volume is stabilized. A serum creatinine that remains persistently elevated despite several days of catheter drainage is always cause for concern. Several studies have shown that a child whose creatinine at 1 year of age drops below 0.8 to 1 mg/dL has a good renal prognosis.[19] For stable, term infants whose creatinine levels are below 2 mg/dL and/or who have good renal parenchyma, it is appropriate to proceed with valve resection as soon as possible. In situations where the creatinine is rising despite catheter drainage, or diuresis requiring hourly fluid replacements is present, it is best to wait until the infant's medical condition is stable.

The patient whose VCUG is shown in Figure 84-3 was an ideal candidate for valve resection. His diagnosis was suspected prenatally as a result of unilateral hydroureteronephrosis with a bladder that was always full, yet no oligohydramnios was noted on serial sonograms. Following delivery, he was transferred to the neonatal intensive care unit. Sonography revealed a normal right kidney with sharply defined corticomedullary differentiation, and a severely hydronephrotic left kidney. Intravenous antibiotics were started, and a VCUG confirmed the diagnosis of posterior urethral valves with significant reflux into the left ureter and collecting system. His creatinine in the neonatal intensive care unit was 1.2 mg/dL. The following day, endoscopic valve ablation and circumcision were performed. A renal scan performed at follow-up demonstrated that the left kidney contributed 5% of total glomerular filtration rate. Eleven years later, his renal function was stable, with a creatinine of 0.8 mg/dL.

Families must understand that the child with urethral valves will require lifetime follow-up. The complications from incision of urethral valves are minimal compared with the resulting loss of bladder and renal function. Potential complications of the actual valve resection consist primarily of urethral strictures. A noncompliant or poorly contractile bladder, urinary incontinence, and poor renal function may become apparent after valve resection,[4,19] but these should not be considered complications of the surgical procedure. These conditions reflect the response of bladder smooth

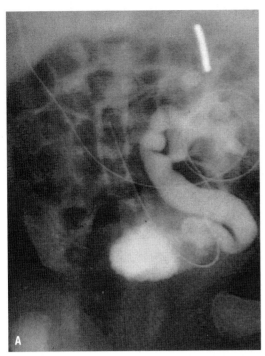

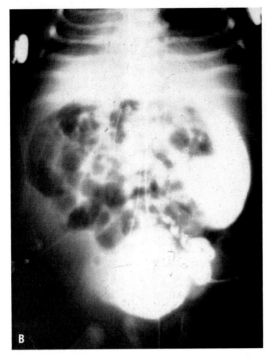

Figure 84-3 Two types of pop-off mechanisms are demonstrated in these radiographs, and are associated with a better renal prognosis as well as improved bladder function. *A*, There is unilateral reflux associated with poor renal function in this left kidney. *B*, There is unilateral reflux and fornical extravasation. In both instances, the contralateral right kidney underwent compensatory hypertrophy, and the children were left with an excellent renal prognosis.

muscle to long-term obstruction and may not even become apparent for several years. It is important that, early on, families understand exactly what benefits endoscopic decompression may provide and what long-term sequelae may be seen. The issue of circumcision should always be discussed in advance with the family. Wiswell and Geshke provided strong evidence that lack of circumcision is associated with an increased risk of urinary tract infection in the first year of life.[20] In this high-risk population, the consequences of a breakthrough infection are much greater, whereas the complications of circumcision in the operating room are minimal and consist primarily of bleeding. The significant risks of infection outweigh this small risk for this subset of patients with compromised renal function.

INSTRUMENTATION

Posterior urethral valves may be treated using several methods, but the technique chosen must be guided, first and foremost, by the size of the patient. It is imperative that the urethra readily accept whichever instrument is chosen, and if in doubt, the urethra should be calibrated using bougies to help in this choice. For term infants, a 9F neonatal cystoscope with a side port through which a Bugbee electrode may be passed is easy to use (Figure 84-4), and the electrodes come in a variety of configurations that can be selected according to individual preference. Rotating an angled electrode will allow the surgeon to "hook" the valve leaflets under direct vision (Figure 84-5). Smaller rigid cystoscopes are also avail-

able, with 6.9F and 7.7F outer diameters that will allow for passage of the Bugbee electrode. Flexible endoscopes with a 7.4F diameter are also available, depending upon the surgeon's preference. For the older patient, there is the option of using a pediatric resectoscope; several manufacturers offer these, and sheath sizes range from 10 to 13.5F (Figure 84-6). A surgeon can choose from several types of cutting elements, including the traditional loop for electrocautery or a cold knife urethrotome. The major criteria for selection should be the size of the urethra. It is imperative that any lubricated instrument pass gently into the bladder; any undue exertion of force can induce urethral stricture formation.

A number of other alternatives for valve ablation have been mentioned over the years, which include: Fogarty catheter disruption,[21,22] laser-assisted ablation,[23] and antegrade valve resection via suprapubic cystostomy.[24] Whitacker developed a hook that is insulated everywhere except within the inner aspect of the curve. This hook may be passed blindly into the urethra, and the valve leaflet is engaged by "feel." Upon attaching the hook to the cutting current, the valve is incised. Such a device represents an option that might be used in situations where advanced miniaturized fiberoptics are not available. Cromie and colleagues describe using a venous valvulotome under fluoroscopic guidance with good results.[25]

TECHNIQUE

At our center, the patient is positioned in the standard dorsal lithotomy position using Allen universal stirrups, which come in pediatric sizes. For newborns, the legs may be placed over intravenous fluid bags and taped into proper position. Sterile precautions are observed, with drapes, gowns, and gloves, and a Betadine skin prep is applied. Intravenous antibiotics should be administered prior to instrumentation. The cystoscope is attached to the camera and all images are displayed on the color monitor, which allows for video recording and photography. An initial

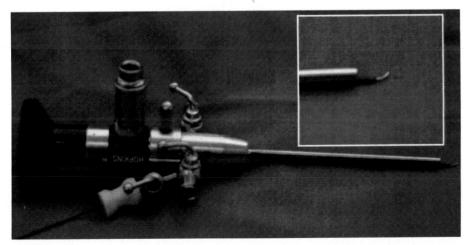

Figure 84-4 The 9 French neonatal cystoscope with side port offers an opportunity to pass the curved Bugbee electrode (inset) under direct vision with a good flow of irrigant, which facilitates the procedure.

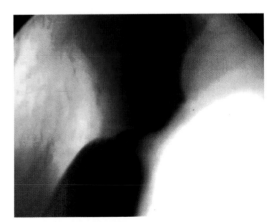

Figure 84-5 The curved Bugbee electrode may be hooked around the valve leaflet and stabilized prior to activating the cutting current and simultaneously pulling back the electrode.

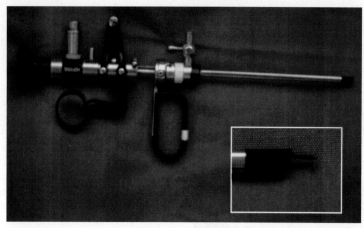

Figure 84-6 A 13 French pediatric resectoscope is also available for use and is often preferred by some surgeons for valve ablation in an older boy. Shown in the inset is a cutting loop, although in its place some surgeons may prefer to use a cold knife urethrotome.

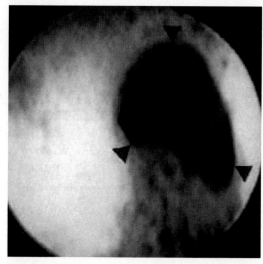

Figure 84-9 Valves may be incised at the 5- and 7-o'clock positions, the 12-o'clock position, or all three, depending upon the surgeon's preference. The importance of applying suprapubic pressure and eliciting antegrade flow from the bladder is that this allows the surgeon to better identify any residual obstructing leaflets (see Figure 84-8).

endoscopic examination is carried out to document the urethral anatomy and location of the external sphincter. Once the external sphincter is passed, the valve leaflet will appear (Figure 84-7). The typical valve (type I) will consist of cusps that start out at the verumontanum and fan out laterally and distally, at which point, they fuse in a membrane at the 12-o'clock position. On occasion, these valves may not be so apparent; in such a situation, the cystoscope should be withdrawn to just inside the external sphincter and manual pressure applied to a full bladder (Figure 84-8). This maneuver will result in urinary flow and cause the valves to balloon out and thus mimic the in vivo physiology. This maneuver helps define the portion of the valve that is most obstructing. Having identified the valve, it is essential to complete the endoscopic examination of the bladder, taking note of the degree of trabeculation, presence of diverticula, capacity, and presence and location of ureteral orifices.

One option is to incise the valves at the 5- and 7-o'clock positions (Figure 84-9) and see how the valve performs following manual compression of the bladder. There will almost always be residual ballooning of the leaflet at the 12-o'clock position, which will be incised (Figure 84-10). The lowest settings of cutting currents are preferable, and the use of the coagulation current should be kept to an absolute minimum and only to achieve hemostasis. The effect of valve ablation may be roughly assessed by comparing the expressed streams before and after. Great care must be taken not to incise the bladder neck or external sphincter; the current quality of optic systems—even for small cystoscopes—makes this less likely today.

Type III valves will appear as circumferential strictures distal to the verumontanum and proximal to the external sphincter. They may not be perfectly symmetric and have a proportionately greater share of leaflet area at the 12-o'clock position. They do not have cusps attached to the distal

verumontanum as do type I valves. Again, manual expression will help determine the most significant portion of the valve where incision will produce the greatest increase in flow. For anterior urethral valves, the cystoscope is advanced up to the valve leaflet and any associated diverticulum is noted. By pushing on the full bladder, it is possible to assess the area of the valve that is the most urodynamically compromised.

POSTOPERATIVE CARE

A catheter is not necessary postoperatively, and final urine culture results should be checked prior to discontinuation of parenteral antibiotics. Once a sterile urine is documented, oral prophylaxis should be started with an agent appropriate for the patient's age. Amoxicillin prophylaxis is used for the first 2 months of life; thereafter trimethoprim-sulfamethoxazole is an ideal agent

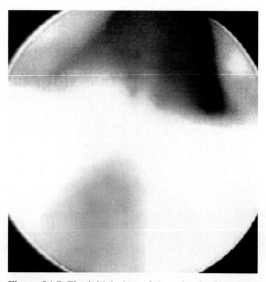

Figure 84-7 The initial view of the valve leaflet as one advances passed the striated external sphincter with retrograde flow of irrigation fluid pushing the valve leaflets out of the way.

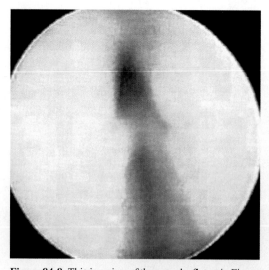

Figure 84-8 This is a view of the same leaflet as in Figure 84-7, except that the irrigation flow has been shut off, and the bladder is being manually expressed. With this antegrade flow from the bladder, the valve leaflets are clearly demonstrated as they balloon out into the field of view.

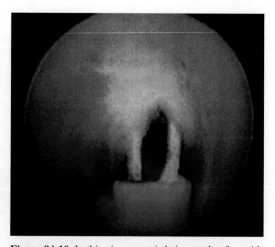

Figure 84-10 In this view, a cut is being made of a residual obstructing leaflet that is quite prominent at the 12-o'clock position. The instrument used in this older boy was a 13 French pediatric resectoscope with a cutting loop.

for prophylaxis. It is essential to monitor the serum creatinine in the postoperative period, and the frequency of this will be determined by the severity of renal compromise.

Long-term follow-up visits are set up with a frequency determined by the renal status. For cases in which the serum creatinine rapidly returns to normal values, a follow-up creatinine determination and renal ultrasound scan every 6 months for 1 to 2 years will ensure that the renal function remains stable. Thereafter, annual examinations are sufficient. For more severe cases (Cr > 0.7 mg/dL), children should be followed by both a urologist and a nephrologist on a more regular basis. Setting up a day so that both specialists can see these patients simultaneously will minimize the social disruption for the family and allow for a multidisciplinary approach to care. In this kind of setting, general issues such as growth and development may be assessed in addition to preparing the child and family for dialysis and/or renal transplantation.

Since a substantial portion of patients (50%) with posterior urethral valves have reflux, antibiotic prophylaxis must be maintained over the long term until the reflux resolves.[19] In many of these patients, the reflux will resolve, and at that point, antibiotics may be discontinued if the child shows signs of a normal voiding pattern. In the past, high-grade reflux was managed with reimplantation (if there was salvageable function) or a nephroureterectomy. Recent data suggest, however, that the loss of the pressure pop-off may have subtle effects on serum creatinine.[19] With the success of ureteral augmentation, avoiding nephroureterectomy for poorly functioning kidneys seems very reasonable, especially if the patient is free of infection.[26,27]

Even when these issues are resolved, these patients should be closely followed for any signs of lower urinary tract or voiding dysfunction. Studies have suggested that, with adolescence, bladder function changes to a large overdistended bladder with poor emptying ability.[28] Parkhouse and Woodhouse noted that the failure to achieve urinary continence in boys with a history of posterior urethral valves was an adverse prognostic sign with regard to renal function.[29] Two major factors contribute to this incontinence: (1) poor concentrating ability resulting in diuresis, and (2) a bladder that may be stiff and noncompliant or with poor contractile ability. There is good evidence to support the contention that a stiff and noncompliant valve bladder may place compromised kidneys at an even greater risk. There are no known pharmacologic measures to induce renal growth, but one may prevent, or at least delay further renal deterioration, by optimizing bladder function. Maintaining or achieving optimal bladder function is essential, even when the renal function is deteriorating and transplantation is inevitable because a noncompliant bladder can compromise a transplant. A proactive video-urodynamic reassessment of bladder function should be undertaken well before renal transplantation is anticipated, such that bladder augmentation may be performed. The

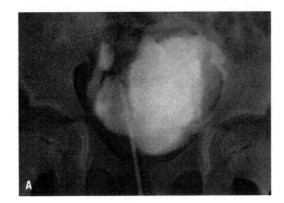
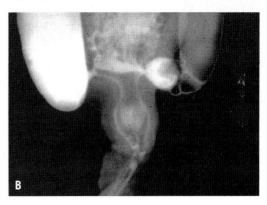
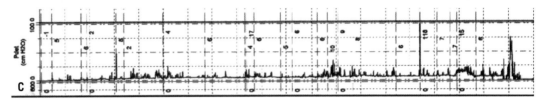

Figure 84-11 Video-urodynamics is an important means of assessing the long-term functional outcomes following valve ablation. This is especially important prior to transplantation because a bladder with poor compliance characteristics places the engrafted kidney at risk. If standard urodynamics were done in this patient, the CMG curve (C) would look quite compliant. By monitoring the filling with fluoroscopy, however, it becomes apparent that much of the "compliance" in this system comes not from the bladder (A) (early filling phase), but the reflux into this massively dilated upper urinary tract (B) (late filling phase).

importance of using video-urodynamics in such an assessment is shown in Figure 84-11. If one looked only at the cystometrogram, one might interpret the data as showing a very compliant bladder. When one correlates the cystometrogram with the video component, however, one sees that the high-grade reflux begins early on in filling, and much of the compliance of the system may be attributed to the dilated upper tracts. Given the potentially poor compliance of this bladder, it is imperative that these native kidneys and ureters be preserved so that, if augmentation is required pre- or post-transplant, the use of bowel may be avoided.

RESULTS

The results of primary endoscopic valve ablation have been encouraging. In a recent review of the series of patients with posterior urethral valves at Children's Hospital of Philadelphia, Smith and colleagues reported that over 70% of the patients achieved and maintained stable renal function.[19] No urethral strictures were seen after 1985, although 15% of these patients underwent vesicostomy (for reasons of size or renal function). None of the patients in this series who underwent a vesicostomy subsequently required bladder augmentation. The percentage of patients achieving full urinary continence was 19% at 5 years, 46% at 10 years, and 99% at 20 years. This delay in attaining continence is similar for all major series.

COMPLICATIONS

The ability to ablate valves endoscopically with low morbidity has improved dramatically over the past 20 years due to major advances in fiberoptic technology. Smaller instruments with

better visualization have lowered the urethral stricture rate from 12% in an earlier review[30] to a rate that is negligible today.[19,31] In part, this reflects new instrumentation, and in part, a willingness to carry out vesicostomy in the smallest of patients. The major surgical complication of valve ablation is urethral stricture, and it may be prevented by careful choice of instrumentation and minimizing resection times. In earlier series, some patients were left with residual incontinence following bladder–neck-plasty; today, it is recognized that bladder neck procedures have no role in the management of urethral valves. Although other reviews about urethral valves have discussed renal and bladder function as complications of this operative procedure, these are really determined by the obstruction itself and are not directly related to the endoscopic surgery.

REFERENCES

1. Cendron M, Elder JS. Perinatal urology. In: Gillenwater JY, Grayhack JT, Howards SS, Mitchell ME, editors. Adult and pediatric urology. Philadelphia: Lippincott Williams & Wilkins; 2002. p. 2041–128.
2. Coplen DE, Hare JV, Zderic SA, et al. A 10 year experience with antenatal intervention. J Urol 1996;156:1142–5.
3. Holmes N, Harrison MR, Baskin LS. Fetal surgery for posterior urethral valves: long-term postnatal outcomes. Pediatrics 2001;108:E7.
4. Peters CA, Bolkier M, Bauer SB, et al. The urodynamic consequences of posterior urethral valves. J Urol 1990;140:122.
5. Nguyen HT, Peters CA. The long-term complications of posterior urethral valves. BJU Int 1999;83:23–8.
6. Reinberg Y, Gonzalez R, Fryd D, et al. The outcome of renal transplantation in children with posterior urethral valves. J Urol 1988;140:1491.
7. Peters CA. Lower urinary tract obstruction: clinical and experimental aspects. Br J Urol 1998;81 Suppl 2:22–32.
8. Peters CA, Freeman MR, Fernandez CA, et al. Dysregulated proteolytic balance as the basis of excess extracellular matrix in fibrotic disease. Am J Physiol 1997;272(6 Pt 2):R1960–5.

9. Kim KM, Kogan BA, Massad CA, Huang YC. Collagen and elastin in the obstructed fetal bladder. J Urol 1991;146: 528.

10. Shapiro E, Becich MJ, Perlman E, Lepor H. Bladder wall abnormalities in myelodysplastic bladders: a computer assisted morphometric analysis. J Urol 1991;145:1024.

11. Stein R, Hutcheson JC, Krasnopolsky L, et al. The decompensated detrusor V: molecular correlates of bladder function following reversal of experimental outlet obstruction. J Urol 2001;166:651–7.

12. Kaefer M, Keating MA, Adams MC, Rink RC. Posterior urethral valves, pressure pop-offs and bladder function. J Urol 1995;154:708–11.

13. Rittenberg MH, Hulbert WC, Snyder HM, Duckett JW. Protective factors in posterior urethral valves. J Urol 1988; 140:993.

14. Duckett JW, Zhilyan O. Uses and abuses of vesicostomy. AUA Update Series 1995;14:16.

15. Podesta M, Ruarte AC, Gargiulo C, et al. Bladder function associated with posterior urethral valves after primary valve ablation or proximal urinary diversion in children and adolescents. J Urol 2002;168(4 Pt 2):1830–5.

16. Close CE, Carr MC, Burns MW, Mitchell ME. Lower urinary tract changes after early valve ablation in neonates and infants: is early diversion warranted? J Urol 1997;157: 984–8.

17. Glassberg KI. The valve bladder syndrome: 20 years later. J Urol 2001;166:1406–14.

18. Hulbert WC, Rosenberg HK, Cartwright PC, et al. The predictive value of ultrasonography in evaluation of infants with posterior urethral valves. J Urol 1998;148:122–4.

19. Smith GH, Canning DA, Schulman SL, et al. The long-term outcome of posterior urethral valves treated with primary valve ablation and observation. J Urol 1996;155:1730–4.

20. Wiswell TE, Geshke DW. Risks from circumcision in the first month of life compared with those for uncircumcised boys. Pediatrics 1989;83:1011.

21. Diamond DA, Ransley PG. Fogarty balloon catheter ablation of neonatal posterior urethral valves. J Urol 1987;137:1209.

22. Chertin B, Cozzi D, Puri P. Long-term results of primary avulsion of posterior urethral valves using a Fogarty balloon catheter. J Urol 2002;168:1841–3.

23. Ehrlich RM, Shanberg A, Fine RN. Neodynium:YAG laser ablation of posterior urethral valves. J Urol 1987;138:959.

24. Zaontz MR, Firliet CF. Percutaneous antegrade ablation of posterior urethral valves in underweight or premature infants: an alternative to primary vesicostomy. J Urol 1985;134:139.

25. Cromie WJ, Cain MP, Bellinger MF, et al. Urethral valve incision using a modified venous valvulotome. J Urol 1994;151:1053–5.

26. Carr MC, Docimo SG, Mitchell ME. Bladder augmentation with urothelial preservation. J Urol 1999;162:1133–7.

27. Churchill BM, Aliabadi H, Landau EH, et al. Ureteral bladder augmentation. J Urol 1993;150:716.

28. Holmdahl G, Sillen U, Hanson E, et al. Bladder dysfunction in boys with posterior urethral valves before and after puberty. J Urol 1996;155:694–8.

29. Parkhouse HF, Woodhouse CRJ. Long-term status of patients with posterior urethral valves. Urol Clin North Am 1990;17:373.

30. Churchill BM, Krueger RP, Fleischer MH, Hardy BE. Complications of urethral valve surgery and their prevention. Urol Clin North Am 1983;10:519.

31. Mitchell ME. Complications of urethral valve surgery. In: Marshall FF, editor. Urologic complications: medical, surgical, adult and pediatric. 2nd ed. Chicago: Mosby-Year Book; 1990. p. 511–25.

85

Endoscopic Treatment of Strictures

Agana Filipas
Margit Fisch

Urethral strictures are uncommon in children and can be classified according to etiology (traumatic, iatrogenic, inflammatory, or congenital) (Figure 85-1).[1] Traumatic strictures result from external force to the urethra (eg, pelvic fracture and straddle injury). Iatrogenic injury, unfortunately, continues to be a common cause of childhood stricture. Iatrogenic stricture can follow open surgery (eg, for hypospadias), endoscopy, and catheterization. The incidence of iatrogenic stricture is high following posterior valve resection performed in the neonate or small infant. This sequela can be prevented by performing primary vesicostomy and delaying valve resection until after the first year of age.[2] Iatrogenic strictures following open surgery typically develop during the year following the initial procedure; iatrogenic strictures resulting from endoscopic manipulations, however, may not become symptomatic for several years.[1] Strictures in children rarely occur secondary to urethral inflammation, and those that do are a result of urethritis secondary to a non-traumatic indwelling catheter.[1]

The so-called congenital stricture (eg, Cobb's collar[3] and Moorman's ring[4]) located at the site of fusion of the membranous and bulbar urethra with incomplete canalization of the urogenital membrane remains controversial. A new designation for these congenital urethral lesions is the congenital obstructing posterior urethral membrane (COPUM), postulated by Dewan.[5] The clinical significance of these lesions, however, and their treatment still remains obscure. In some patients, a relationship to syringoceles is described, rarely requiring endoscopic deroofing.[6] Other authors believe that congenital childhood

strictures are a urologic myth and suggest using the term "strictures of unknown origin."[7,8] A congenital origin can be accepted in patients without a history of antecedent injury, instrumentation, inflammation, or surgery. However, "congenital strictures" do not always occur at the site of the embryologic junction of posterior and anterior urethra.[1] We have seen two patients with distal penile congenital strictures who had a positive family history (the father and grandfather). Congenital strictures will present in either the neonatal or postpubertal period.[3] In the group of patients in the neonatal period, there are significant signs of infravesical obstruction associated with upper urinary tract abnormalities. In contrast, boys after puberty will present with localized irritative symptoms (urinary tract infection, hematuria) and decreased flow rates.

On voiding or retrograde urethrography, a bulbar spasm or contraction of the compressor nuda muscle with subsequent indentation of the urethra can mimic a urethral stricture, as noted in the uroradiology literature.[9] Consequently, congenital childhood strictures may be grossly overdiagnosed.[7] Unnecessary intervention can be avoided if one remains alert to this radiographic misinterpretation.

The etiology of strictures in children differs from that in adults. In children, most strictures are the result of trauma, primarily iatrogenic, rather than inflammation. External and iatrogenic trauma accounts for approximately 80% of all cases,[1] suggesting that most childhood strictures are preventable. The best prophylaxis against strictures following pelvic injury appears to be surgical pelvic fixation.

Pelvic injuries and associated ruptures of the prepubertal urethra will cause strictures in the membranous urethra as well as close to the bladder neck, whereas straddle injuries will most frequently cause bulbar strictures (Table 85-1). Strictures following hypospadias repair occur at the site of the urethral anastomosis. Strictures following endoscopic manipulation, however, occur predominantly in the non-distensible penile and distal bulbous urethra. Because iatrogenic strictures are frequently related to inappropriate dilatation or cystoscopy, extreme care should be exercised in performing these procedures. Instruments that are too large should be avoided, and cystoscopy for hematuria in children should be limited to clear and well-defined indications. Urethrorrhagia idiopathica or posterior urethritis frequently occurs in prepubertal and pubertal boys and is a benign condition, which disappears spontaneously. Development of a urethral stricture is extremely rare and occurs mainly in patients with prolonged urethrorrhagia.[10]

INDICATIONS

Ideally, the method of treatment selected for strictures in children should have documented efficacy in a high percentage of cases, cause minimal morbidity, and involve a single operation. Achieving a definitive result with the first therapeutic intervention is especially important in children. Thus, any so-called "minimally invasive" method has to be evaluated carefully because it may result in an extremely invasive modality, if multiple procedures become necessary. We believe that open urethroplasty remains the treatment of choice in most childhood strictures, especially iatrogenic and traumatic strictures. Endoscopic management is contraindicated in longer, more complex strictures, particularly those associated with fistulas, extensive scarring, or persistent inflammation. Such strictures should

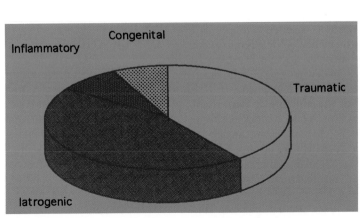

Figure 85-1 Etiology and distribution of childhood urethral strictures.

Table 85-1 Location and Etiology of Urethral Strictures	
Etiology	Location
Congenital	Bulbar
Trauma: straddle injury	Bulbar
Trauma: pelvic injury	Membranous and prostatic
Infections	Anterior up to bulbar

be treated by urethroplasty. Since its initial description, the buccal mucosa graft technique has proved extremely successful.[11] This graft is superior to all other urethral substitute materials, particularly when used in an onlay-patch fashion. In children with posterior urethral strictures following distraction injuries, anastomotic urethroplasty via perineal or perineal-abdominal approach shows a high success rate.[12–14]

Since the first pediatric endourologic stricture repair was described in 1974 by Sachse[15] several endoscopic procedures (dilation, internal urethrotomy, and internal electroresection/fulguration) have been proposed for strictures in children. These techniques are adaptations of procedures done in adults, and it is important to know that approximately 50% of adult patients eventually need repeat endoscopic or even open interventions. Long-term follow-up studies of patients who had endoscopic urethrotomy of childhood strictures indicate a similar need for repeat treatment in pediatric patients.[16,17]

Proper patient selection for endoscopic management of childhood urethral stricture is therefore of the greatest importance and remains crucial to the success of any therapeutic intervention. Endoscopic treatment appears ideal for short, localized strictures. In selected cases multiple short strictures may be managed endoscopically. Of the three endoscopic procedures, only internal urethrotomy and electroresection will be described here. Some authors favor the use of neodymium:yttrium-aluminum-garnet (Nd:YAG) laser urethrotomy in recurrent post-traumatic strictures. Experience in children is limited, but the high rate (up to 26%) of postoperative dilatation to prevent recurrent strictures casts doubts on this procedure.[18,19] Dilatation appears to be unsuccessful as a long-term therapy because it is clearly deleterious and results in secondary stricture formation or perpetuation of fibrosis, especially in the vulnerable growing urethra of the child. Long-term results of dilatation were reviewed by Devereux and Burfield, who noted that routine dilatation placed younger patients at an increased risk of lower urinary tract complications.[20] Similarly, Blandy and colleagues reported that 30% of patients had complications after routine dilatation.[21] Some complications even occurred years following the procedure. Thus, other more definitive modalities appear preferable to avoid both complications and having the patient undergo multiple anesthesias.

Endoscopic reconstitution of severe post-traumatic posterior urethral obliteration by simultaneous antegrade and retrograde instrumentation in conjunction with internal urethrotomy has been reported with good success rates.[22]

To summarize, the child with a short, localized stricture who has had no prior manipulation or surgery appears to be the best candidate for endoscopic management (internal urethrotomy and electroresection) with the option of achieving a definitive solution later with open urethroplasty should the stricture recur. A long, complicated, or recurrent stricture should be treated by open urethroplasty.

PATIENT AND PREOPERATIVE PREPARATION

Endoscopic management is generally performed as an outpatient procedure. No special patient preparation is required. Urinalysis and urine culture are necessary to rule out urinary tract infection. The diagnosis of stricture requires a thorough history and physical examination and should be documented during voiding cystourethrography, either after intravenous pyelography (indirect) or by suprapubic puncture (direct). Retrograde urethrography is difficult to perform in children and places them at risk for severe urinary tract infection and, in some cases, sepsis caused by bacterial invasion during injection of the contrast agent. In some cases, however, a combined retrograde and antegrade investigation is needed for estimation of exact stricture localization and length. The workup should also include a sonogram (to determine if hydronephrosis is present and to evaluate bladder wall thickness) as well as residual urine and uroflow studies. Although flow rates are a helpful noninvasive evaluation, their value as an initial diagnostic tool is limited because the length and severity of the stricture are not addressed. Therefore urethrography and/or urethroscopy is crucial in planning therapeutic intervention, in that it is the first step for treatment.

Information about the risks of recurrent stricture, infection, sepsis, incontinence, and postoperative urethral bleeding must be included in the informed consent.

The procedure is performed using a general anesthetic. Prophylactic antibiotics are administered intraoperatively and postoperatively.

INSTRUMENTATION

The technical aspects of this treatment method have improved considerably with the development of pediatric instrumentation. We recommend a small caliber endoscope such as the Wolf 9.5 French pediatric resectoscope (0 or 30° lens) as it allows direct-vision urethrotomy (using a mounted knife blade) and resection, and provides adequate visualization.

TECHNIQUE

Sterile lubricating jelly is introduced into the urethra. The resectoscope is inserted carefully and advanced gently with meticulous inspection of the urethra up to the point of the stricture. In extremely narrow strictures a guidewire may be introduced for easier advancement of the instrument.

Urethrotomy of the stricture is performed using the cold knife at the 12 o'clock position. The 5 o'clock and 7 o'clock positions can also be added if necessary. Alternatively, electroresection or fulguration of the circular membrane or stricture can be carried out. Endoscopic treatment is especially successful in short post-traumatic strictures localized close to the external sphincter. This is an area where open repairs are extremely difficult to perform. The half–moon-shaped, slightly

laterally dislocated stricture/membrane is easily resected after internal urethrotomy with a weak cutting cautery between either the 11 o'clock and 7 o'clock or 1 o'clock and 5 o'clock positions. Urethrotomy may be aided by antegrade transvesical endoscopy and a "cutting to the light" technique.

Injection of triamcinolone diacetate into the stricture at two or three different sites (2 to 5 mL) either before or after the urethrotomy reportedly increases the success rate.[15] The integrity of the external sphincter is inspected, and the resectoscope advanced into the bladder for the final cystoscopy. The instrument is removed and an 8F to 12F silicone Foley catheter inserted. An 8F feeding tube may also be used. The feeding tube lumen is somewhat larger, which makes drainage more efficient; it may be passed more easily without the attached balloon and has to be secured at the glans.

POSTOPERATIVE CARE

The catheter should be left in place for approximately 1 to 3 days. Antibiotics are continued during this time. After removal of the catheter, ultrasonography should be performed to check for possible residual urine and the uroflow rates compared with the preoperative findings. If a suprapubic catheter is placed intraoperatively, a postoperative voiding cystogram can be performed, but it is not mandatory. Sequential measurements of flow rates have proven a useful noninvasive diagnostic tool in the follow-up of stricture patients.

RESULTS

Long-term follow-up studies of endoscopically managed childhood strictures show an average success rate of approximately 90%, although 30% of patients will need repeat procedures.[16] Transurethral incision by a cold knife seems to be superior to that by knife electrode from the point of view of reoperation (78 vs. 92% success rates).[5] The knife electrode seems to have the risk of submucosal burning, which results in de novo urethral stricture thereafter. Conversely, with the cold knife, it is relatively easy to control the depth, and there are rarely sequelae after cutting. Additionally, success is strongly related to proper patient selection.

COMPLICATIONS

The most frequent complication of internal urethrotomy is recurrent stricture formation. Although an initial success rate of approximately 90% can be achieved, approximately one-third of patients require further treatment. Other complications include urinary tract infection and urosepsis following endoscopic manipulation. When the stricture is close to the external sphincter, the parents must be informed that the possible complications include sphincter lesions with subsequent incontinence. Incontinence following pelvic trauma and posterior urethral disruption sometimes improves when the patient reaches puberty, and prostatic growth results in increased intrinsic urethral resistance. Impotence can also result from posterior urethral injuries, but this has not been reported after endoscopic intervention.

REFERENCES

1. Kaplan GW, Brock WA. Urethral strictures in children. J Urol 1983;129:1200–3.
2. Mayers DA, Walker RD. Prevention of urethral strictures in the management of posterior urethral valves. J Urol 1981;126:655–7.
3. Cobb BG, Wolf JA, Ansell JS. Congenital stricture of the proximal urethral bulb. J Urol 1968;99:629–31.
4. Moorman JG. Congenital bulbar urethral stenosis as cause of diseases of the urogenital junction. Urologe A 1972;11:157–60.
5. Katsuya N, Takayuki K, Hidehiro K, et al. Impact of congenital narrowing of the bulbar urethra (Cobb`s collar) and ist transurethral incision in children. Eur Urol 1999;36:144–9.
6. Dewan PA. A study of the relationship between syringoceles and Cobb`s collar. Eur Urol 1996;30:119–24.
7. Harshman MW, Cromie WJ, Wein AJW, Duckett JW. Urethral stricture disease in children. J Urol 1981;126:650–4.
8. Currarino G, Stephens FD. An uncommon type of bulbar urethral stricture, sometimes familial, of unknown cause: congenital versus acquired. J Urol 1981;126:658–60.
9. Currarino G. Narrowings of the male urethra caused by contractions or spasm of the bulbocavernosus muscle: cysto-urethrographic observations. Am J Roentgenol 1976;108:641–4.
10. Walker BR, Ellison ED, Snow BW, Cartwright PC. The natural history of idiopathic urethrorrhagia in boys. J Urol 2001;166:231–2.
11. Bürger RA, Müller SC, El-Damanhoury H, et al. Buccal mucosal graft: a preliminary report. J Urol 1992;147:662–4.
12. Santucci RA, Mario LA, McAninch JW. Anastomotic urethroplasty for bulbar urethral stricture: analysis of 168 patients. J Urol 2002;167:1715–9.
13. Basiri A, Shadpour P, Moradi MR, et al. Symphysiotomy: a viable approach for delayed management of posterior urethral injuries in children. J Urol 2002;168:2166–9.
14. Podesta ML. Use of perneal and perineal-abdominal (transpubic) approach for delayed management of pelvic fracture urethra obliterative strictures in children: long-trem outcome. J Urol 1998;160:160–4.
15. Sachse H. Zur Behandlung der Harnröhrenstriktur: die transurethrale Schlitzung unter Sicht mit scharfem Schnitt. Fortschr Med 1974;92:12–6.
16. Noe HN. Long-term follow-up of endoscopic management of urethral strictures in children. J Urol 1987;137:951–3.
17. Noe NH. Endoscopic management of urethral strictures in children. J Urol 1981;125:712–4.
18. Dogra PN, Nabi G. Core-through urethrotomy using neodymium:YAG laser for obliterative urethral strictures after traumatic urethral disruption and/or distraction defects: long-term outcome. J Urol 2002;167:543–6.
19. Dogra PN, Nabi G. Neodymium:YAG laser core-through urethrotomy in obliterative posttraumatic urethral strictures after failed initial urethroplasty. Urol Int 2002;68:265–7.
20. Devereux MH, Burfield GD. Prolonged followup of urethral strictures treated by intermittent dilation. Br J Urol 1970;42:321–4.
21. Blandy JP, Wadhwa S, Singh M, Tresidder GC. Urethroplasty in context. Br J Urol 1976;48:697–700.
22. Spirnak JP, Smith EM, Elder JS. Posterior urethral obliteration treated by endoscopic reconstitution, internal urethrotomy and temporary self-dilation. J Urol 1993;149:766–8.

86

Endoscopic Treatment of Incontinence in Pediatric Patients

Caleb P. Nelson, MD

John M. Park, MD

Humans depend on continence for the convenience of everyday life as well as for social acceptance, and urinary continence is a developmental milestone necessary for the successful integration of growing children into their peer group and society. The management of incontinence in children, however, differs from that of adults. The most obvious difference lies in the etiology of incontinence. Most childhood incontinence is functional in nature and resolves with time. However, incontinence secondary to anatomic abnormalities, such as congenital neuropathic conditions (spina bifida, sacral agenesis), exstrophy-epispadias complex, and bilateral ectopic ureters, will not improve typically without intervention. The management of pediatric incontinence must also be tailored to the physical, psychological, and social needs of a growing child and family. Every effort should be made not only to increase the efficacy of the treatment, but also to minimize the adverse impact on the child's overall well-being.

Although many surgical procedures have been developed to treat incontinence over the past century, our abilities as surgeons to reconstruct a physiological bladder and its outlet remain far from complete. The Young-Dees bladder neck reconstruction has been improved only incrementally since its popularization in 1920s.[1–3] Slings offer a more satisfactory outcome for stress incontinence in women, but this approach has been met with variable degree of success in children with congenital anomalies. Surgical obliteration of the bladder neck in favor of continent catheterizable conduit (Mitrofanoff)[4] is an alternative of last resort. It was not until recently that advances in instrumentation and materials science made a minimally invasive endoscopic treatment feasible.

Endoscopic implantation of bulking agents is a simple and logical attempt to increase an outlet resistance with minimal morbidity. The morbidity and physiological impact of endoscopic injection are low and well tolerated. The first reports of endoscopic treatment of incontinence involved the injection of sclerosing agents (sodium morrhuate, Dondren) into the anterior vaginal wall or peri-urethral tissues.[5,6] The resultant scarring produced a compression of the urethra and temporary continence, but also induced significant damage to the tissues. Subsequently, less reactive substances have been injected to coapt the urethral lumen and thereby increase the outlet resistance, and this technique has formed the basis of endoscopic treatment of incontinence. A variety of new injectable agents have become available in the last decade, and the ever-advancing biomedical materials science will undoubtedly bring other substances into our armamentarium. In this chapter we will discuss the current indications for and results of endoscopic treatment of incontinence in children.

THE IMPORTANCE OF DEFINING THE MECHANISM OF INCONTINENCE

The endoscopic treatment strategy for incontinence must be developed within the physiological framework of *normal* bladder function. The hallmarks of a normal lower urinary tract include safe storage pressures, ample storage volumes (capacity), effective outlet resistance that can withstand increased intra-abdominal pressures, and finally, complete emptying of urine during a short duration with modest increase in intravesical pressure. In this context, urinary incontinence is rarely an isolated matter of inadequate outlet resistance alone. Bladder capacity, detrusor function (ie, compliance), and the detrusor-sphincter interactions are all important elements that demand attention in the management of urinary incontinence. There are anatomic afflictions in pediatric patients, such as exstrophy-epispadias complex, spina bifida, and bilateral ectopic ureters, which disable the outlet mechanism primarily, and thus call for an outlet remedy. However, most of these patients also have an abnormal detrusor function that must be evaluated and addressed. The importance of clearly defining the mechanism of incontinence cannot be overemphasized, since any therapeutic strategy addressing the outlet resistance alone without ensuring adequate detrusor function will inevitably lead to an unsatisfactory outcome.

Conceptually, incontinence reflects a urinary storage failure, an emptying failure, or combination of both (Figure 86-1). The urinary storage failure can be further categorized into either inadequate reservoir function (ie, elevated storage pressure and/or small capacity) or incompetent outlet. The emptying failure can result in incontinence owing to high residual urine volume and urinary overflow. Most endoscopic treatment strategies for incontinence have focused on improving the quality of bladder outlet closure mechanism by implanting various bulking agents. In order to ensure the successful outcome of such endoscopic intervention, however, other aspects of bladder function must be evaluated carefully. Underlying diagnoses of exstrophy-epispadias, spina bifida, or bilateral ectopic ureters must trigger a suspicion of abnormal detrusor function. A history of constant urinary leakage or urge incontinence, rather than stress incontinence, should also suggest dysfunction of the bladder urine storage.

Radiographic and urodynamic evaluation is critical in delineating the mechanism of incontinence. On sonography or cystography, a thickened bladder wall and trabeculation usually indicate a possible detrusor problem (Figure 86-2). The most complete information regarding detrusor function can be obtained via urodynamic study. If the child does not have a significant, high-grade vesicoureteral reflux, a simple, single-channel cystometrogram (CMG) will provide the necessary information regarding bladder capacity and compliance. If the urodynamic parameters are abnormal (Figure 86-3), then initial therapy should be aimed at improving bladder compliance and capacity using pharmacological agents such as oxybutynin chloride. In some cases, this will lead to an acceptable level of continence, obviating the need for any intervention on the outlet mechanism. If the etiology of uri-

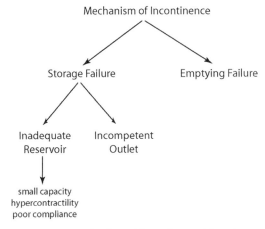

Figure 86-1 Mechanism of incontinence. The primary goal of endoscopic treatment of pediatric incontinence is aimed at improving outlet mechanism by injecting bulking agents, but other mechanism of incontinence must be evaluated and addressed to improve the outcome and avoid complication.

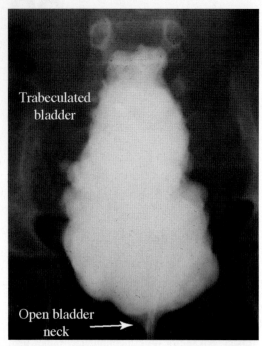

Figure 86-2 Cystogram of a 6-year-old boy with imperforate anus and sacral agenesis presenting with incontinence. Trabeculated bladder suggests poor bladder compliance, along with incompetent outlet mechanism caused by open bladder neck.

nary storage failure is not clearly definable using a single-channel CMG, as in children with a severe bladder neck problem and high-grade vesicoureteral reflux, one may gain additional information with a multichannel urodynamic study under fluoroscopy (Figure 86-4).

As for assessing the adequacy of outlet mechanism, an open bladder neck on cystogram generally implies an intrinsic sphincter deficiency, as commonly seen in children with spina bifida and exstrophy-epispadias (Figure 86-5). The role of Valsalva leak point pressure and urethral pressure profile (UPP) has not been clearly established in children as a reliable and systematic technique of evaluating the competency of outlet mechanism. One must also assess the functional length of the bladder neck and proximal urethra to determine whether there is adequate space for endoscopic injection. A wide-open bladder neck, associated with multiple previous surgeries, makes it unlikely that endoscopic implantation will provide any meaningful benefit.

INDICATIONS

IMPROVE OUTLET RESISTANCE The majority of pediatric incontinence amenable to endoscopic treatment results from congenital anatomic and neuropathic conditions associated with inadequate outlet resistance. Specifically, intrinsic sphincter deficiency, in which the bladder neck and proximal urethra fail to close during bladder filling, is the primary culprit in stress urinary incontinence. One must not confuse the significance of high outlet resistance offered by external urethral sphincter, with the continence mechanism offered by the functional bladder neck and proximal urethra. Some patients with myelodysplasia, for example, will demonstrate an elevated passive leak point pressure (which is a reflection of the fixed outlet resistance offered by the external urethral sphincter), and yet suffer significant stress incontinence. The endoscopic implantation of bulking agents, therefore, should be aimed at improving the luminal closure of bladder neck and proximal urethra.

IMPROVE BLADDER FUNCTIONAL CAPACITY AND COMPLIANCE Recently, endoscopic treatment has been used in selected patients in whom the primary abnormality is one of detrusor dysfunction. In these techniques, therapy is aimed at modification of detrusor function to improve bladder storage.

Botulinum-A toxin induces a flaccid muscle paralysis by blocking the fusion of acetylcholine-containing vesicles with the cell membrane, thereby impeding the release of acetylcholine into the synaptic space.[7] This agent has been widely used for a variety of spastic neuromuscular conditions as well as for cosmetic purposes. The most common urologic indication has been the injection of botulinum-A toxin into the external urethral sphincter for the treatment of detrusor-sphincter dyssynergia, primarily in patients with spinal cord injury.[8-11] More recently, several investigators have used botulinum-A toxin injected directly into the detrusor muscle to decrease contractility and increase functional capacity.[12-14] The largest reported pediatric series evaluated 17 children with myelodysplasia and other types of neurogenic bladder.[12] They found that urodynamic parameters including compliance and functional capacity improved significantly after botulinum-A toxin injection (Figure 86-6). Incontinence scores tended to improve as well, although the dif-

ference was not significant. At the present time, the primary issues with botulinum-A toxin injection are durability, safety, and cost. Many reports have suggested that benefits may persist for 9 months or more, but long-term studies are needed to define its role. As the understanding of detrusor-sphincter physiology evolves, new endoscopically delivered agents may become available that can impact bladder compliance and capacity.

Another endoscopic approach to improve bladder storage function is the modulation of external urethral sphincter activity. In select myelodysplasia patients with a markedly elevated passive leak point pressure and poor detrusor compliance, aggressive dilation of external urethral sphincter lowers the outlet resistance and subsequently improves bladder capacity and compliance. Many of these patients experience long-term improvement of continence as a result of increased bladder capacity.[15]

Occasionally, patients can also present with detrusor instability and incontinence associated with severe external urethral sphincter instability. This may manifest itself as urge incontinence or, rarely, as severe giggle incontinence. In these patients, injection of bulking agents into the region of external urethral sphincter may stabilize the external sphincter closure and improve continence (Figure 86-7).

Finally, some have attempted to surgically improve bladder reservoir function through minimally invasive techniques such as laparoscopic bladder autoaugmentation (detrusor myectomy)[16-18] and laparoscopic enterocystoplasty.[19,20]

The remainder of this chapter, however, will focus on the most common endoscopic technique for treatment of pediatric incontinence—the injection of bulking agents to improve outlet resistance.

ENDOSCOPIC INSTRUMENTATION

The instruments required for endoscopic treatment of incontinence are the standard operative

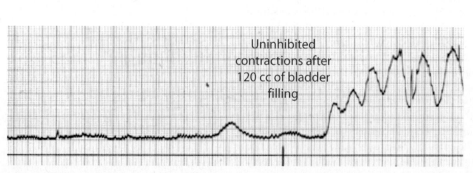

Figure 86-3 A single-channel cystometrogram (CMG) tracing of an 8-year-old female with tethered spinal cord and incontinence. Detrusor hypercontractility is evident during filling, and her incontinence improved with anticholinergic therapy.

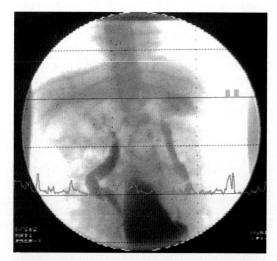

Figure 86-4 A simultaneous urodynamic study and fluoroscopy (cystogram) in a 4-year-old boy with prune-belly syndrome. A decent bladder compliance is noted, but it must be interpreted in conjunction with high-grade vesicoureteral reflux.

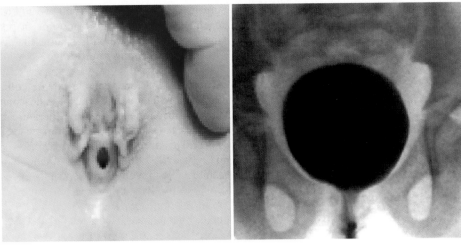

Figure 86-5 A 12-year-old girl presented with stress incontinence. Genital exam reveals a bifid clitoris consistent with epispadias. Cystogram reveals pubic diastasis along with wide open bladder neck.

cystoscope and an injection needle, which can be inserted through the operating channel of the scope. For most pediatric cases (other than infants), a 10 to 14 French (F) cystoscope is adequate, using a 0-degree or 30-degree lens. The 30-degree lens may be preferable in most cases for easy visualization of the needle tip.

For bovine collagen injection in children over 5 years old, a 25-gauge Williams needle can be attached to a 3.5F catheter, which is then passed through an 11F cystoscope working channel. The injection is performed under direct vision. For adolescents and adults, the Contigen system (Bard, Covington, GA) consists of a collagen-filled syringe attached to a flexible 5F catheter with a 23-gauge needle. A stabilizing cannula with a working channel cap at the proximal end provides steady needle control for precise placement. The cannula is passed through a 17F or 21F cystoscope and the cap secured onto the working channel port. The needle is then passed through the cannula and injection is performed transurethrally.

For Teflon paste injection, special reinforced devices are needed to withstand the high pressures required to inject thick paste through tubing. Wolf and Storz companies both make instruments for this purpose. The Wolf device is an 11F cystoscope with an offset lens and a straight steel needle attached to a reinforced glass syringe with finger grips. The Storz device is shaped like a traditional caulking gun, and it also allows measured-dose injection.[21,22]

INJECTION TECHNIQUE

Injection of a bulking substance into the submucosal space of the urethra and bladder neck can be accomplished via either of two approaches. In the *transurethral* approach, the injection needle is passed through the working channel of the cystoscope and the needle is positioned into the submucosa of the bladder neck and proximal urethra under direct vision. The substance is then injected slowly, while observing the bulging of the mucosa into the lumen (Figure 86-8). In females, the bulking agent may be placed either

transurethrally or periurethrally. In the *periurethral* approach, the injection needle (typically a long 25-gauge) is passed through the anterior vaginal wall to the appropriate submucosal location at the bladder neck, and the injection is performed under direct vision (Figure 86-9). Visualization of the bladder neck and proximal urethra can be accomplished with the cystoscope or, in older females, by gently spreading open the urethral meatus with a nasal speculum.

The choice of transurethral versus periurethral approach is based on the surgeon's experience and preference. It has been recommended that the periurethral approach be used in patients with short urethra and relatively normal anatomy—for example, females with neurogenic incontinence. For males and the patients of both sexes with exstrophy-epispadias and prior bladder neck reconstruction, the transurethral approach may be preferable since it may be difficult to properly position the injection needle through the perineal or perimeatal skin.[23]

For most pediatric patients, general anesthesia is preferred, although some patients with neuropathic conditions (such as spina bifida) may tolerate the procedure without anesthesia. After induction of anesthesia and patient positioning in dorsal lithotomy, standard skin preparation and draping are performed. After performing diagnostic cystourethroscopy, the needle is positioned at bladder neck and proximal urethra. The injection is performed circumferentially at any location around the region of bladder neck to accomplish luminal coaptation and mucosal bulging (Figure 86-10), but the suppleness of the mucosal epithelium and the potential submucosal space must be assessed visually before administering the bulking agent. One must be also careful not to advance the needle too far into the bladder lumen. Care must be taken to avoid unnecessary punctures, since needle puncture holes may lead to leakage of the injected substance. Assessing the bladder neck competency can be difficult endoscopically, but the general principle is that the closer the injection occurs to the bladder neck and proximal urethra, the more effective the outlet mechanism becomes against stress urinary incontinence.

Postoperative care is straightforward in most cases. Patients on clean intermittent catheterization (CIC) may resume cathing using a small-

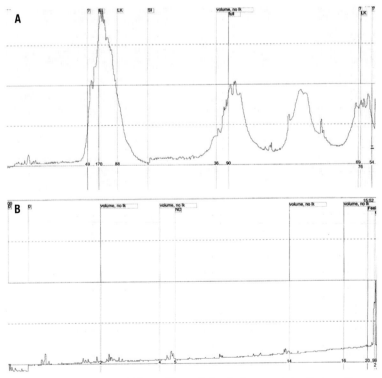

Figure 86-6 An 11-year-old boy with myelodysplasia presented with incontinence refractory to anticholinergic therapy and clean intermittent catheterizations. *A,* Multiple uninhibited bladder contractions are seen on CMG. *B,* Cystoscopic injection of botulinum-A toxin into the bladder wall (200 units) resulted in a complete silencing of bladder contractions and total continence.

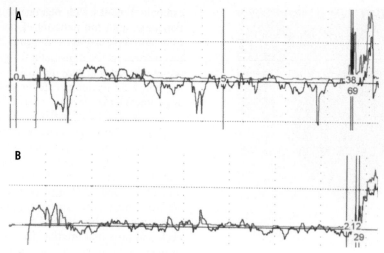

Figure 86-7 A 14-year-old girl presented with severe giggle incontinence. *A*, Urodynamic study indicated that external urethral sphincter coaptation was unstable (blue line.) Bladder pressure remained low during filling (purple line). *B*, After endoscopic injection of bovine collagen into the external urethral sphincter, its coaptation became stable, along with cessation of incontinence.

caliber catheter. Use of an indwelling catheter should be avoided to prevent volume loss and molding of the injected substance. A temporary percutaneous cystostomy tube may be preferable to an indwelling urethral catheterization. Most patients who are able to void continue to do so after the procedure. Postoperative medications commonly include prophylactic antibiotics for 2 to 3 days after the procedure. In addition, anticholinergic medications (eg, oxybutynin chloride) may used to reduce the incidence of detrusor instability, which may develop following the increase in bladder outlet resistance.[24]

INJECTABLE AGENTS AND RESULTS OF TREATMENT

There are no randomized, controlled trials of endoscopic treatment of incontinence in children. Most of the reported series include a small number of patients with a variable mixture of diagnoses and genders, thus making the comparative analysis even more difficult. Many studies have not addressed the issue of bladder reservoir function. Moreover, each series has used different methods of evaluating the outcome. Most investigators have used some sort of grading system to estimate the degree of incontinence pre- and postinjection. However, none of these instruments have been validated for accuracy or reproducibility. Although validated instruments for the assessment of urinary incontinence are now becoming available in adult incontinence arena, they have not been evaluated in children. For these reasons, the results of endoscopic treatments must be interpreted with some caution.

In the last decade, a variety of new agents have joined the old standbys of Teflon and bovine collagen for the endoscopic treatment of incontinence. Some of these agents are still experimental, while others are becoming increasingly popular and common. The ideal agent for injection therapy should be easy to sterilize and implant, stable in the body, inert, and free of immunogenic, mutagenic, and carcinogenic potential. It should also be inexpensive. At the current time, none of the substances fulfills all of these criteria, but newer agents may continue to provide additional benefit.

The previous chapter by Dr. Rodney Appell addressed the biology of injectable substances in greater detail. In our discussion, we will focus on each bulking agent as it pertains to pediatric incontinence, and we will examine the available studies documenting its efficacy.

COLLAGEN Biodegradable bovine collagen is the most widely used agent for endoscopic therapy for incontinence, and the literature for this agent is far and away the most extensive (Table 86-1). This agent is a mixture of 95% Type I and 5% Type III collagen, cross-linked with glutaraldehyde to reduce breakdown by endogenous collagenase. It is easily injected and provokes a mild inflammatory response. Histologically, the collagen implant is neovascularized, infiltrated by fibroblasts, and replaced by endogenous collagen.[25] The primary disadvantage of collagen appears to be volume loss over time and the reduction of bulking effect. Incontinence may recur, resulting in high re-treatment rates. Frey and Mangold reported that a next-generation collagen substance—GAX 65 (Collagen Corp, Palo Alto, CA), with a higher concentration of collagen—may retains its volume better over time.[26]

In addition, concerns have been raised regarding the potential for immunologic reactions to bovine collagen antigens. A small percentage of patients will develop antibovine collagen antibodies after the treatment, but the clinical significance of this is unknown.[27,28] Although few data exist to imply a direct causality, there are case reports of patients developing lupus erythematosis, dermatomyositis, and polymyositis following collagen injection.[29]

Patients scheduled to receive collagen injection should undergo skin testing for hypersensitivity reactions 4 weeks prior to the planned procedure. The test is generally performed by injecting 0.1 cc of glutaraldehyde cross-linked bovine collagen subcutaneously. A control injection of saline is generally performed at the same time. Erythema and induration at the injection site lasting more than 6 hours represents a positive response. The allergic response may be delayed more than 24 hours, and this too represents a positive test. It is believed that a positive response represents preformed antibodies to bovine collagen owing to prior exposure. In patients with a positive collagen skin test, other agents should be used. It is reported that positive skin tests are observed in about 2.5% of patients.[30]

The initial experience in 8 children (a mixed group of spina bifida, exstrophy-epispadias, and other diagnoses) was reported by Wan and colleagues,[31] and this series was later updated to 40 patients by Bomalaski and colleagues.[32] Although the first article reported that 88% were dry or improved on a short-term follow-up (63% and 25%, respectively), with longer follow-up and more subjects, this fell to 76% being dry or improved (22% and 54%, respectively). Exstrophy-epispadias patients appeared to do better, with 92% being "satisfied" compared with only 50% of the spina bifida patients. Other series of collagen injection have reported success (dry or improved) rates ranging between 30 and

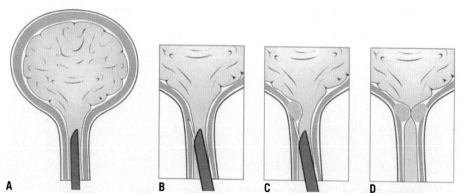

Figure 86-8 A schematic principle of transurethral injection of bulking agent. *A*, Bladder neck and proximal urethra are visualized with a cystoscope. *B*, Submucosal space is engaged with an injection delivery needle. *C*, Under direct visualization, bulking agent is implanted. *D*, Mucosal bulging and coaptation are achieved following injection.

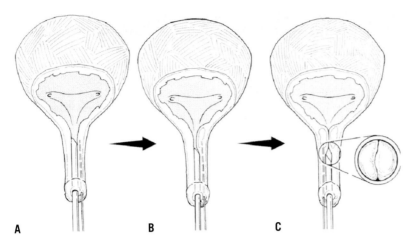

Figure 86-9 A schematic principle of periurethral injection of bulking agent. *A*, While the cystoscope is in visualizing the bladder neck and proximal urethra, a delivery needle is advanced through the periurethral tissue. *B*, Bulking agent is delivered into the submucosal space. *C*, Mucosal bulging and coaptation are achieved following injection.

90%. Most studies suggest that approximately 50% of patients will report recurrent incontinence after collagen injection. In most cases, initial results are better, but the effect seems to deteriorate after 6 months. Patients who have partial or minor improvement with the initial injection may have further improvement with additional injections. Few significant complications or side effects were reported.

TEFLON Polytetrafluoroethylene paste (Teflon, polytef) was initially used by otolaryngologists for vocal cord augmentation,[33] and by the early 1970s, urologists were injecting it for the treatment of incontinence in adults.[34,35] Although initial short-term results were generally encouraging, concern developed over potential morbidity related to Teflon particle migration. Teflon particles are 4 to 40 microns in diameter, small enough to enter and pass through the circulation.[36] Pulmonary Teflon granulomas have been identified in a 76-year-old male at autopsy 4 years after periurethral injection, and Malizia and colleagues. demonstrated Teflon particle migration to lymph nodes, lungs, kidneys, spleen, and brain in dogs and monkeys.[37] There has not been a confirmed case of Teflon particle migration causing the actual morbidity or mortality. In fact, a large European series of subureteric injections of Teflon for vesicoureteral reflux in children reported no negative effects.[38] Because of this potential concern, however, most urologists have abandoned the use of Teflon injection for incontinence, particularly in children.

DEFLUX Developed by Stenberg and Lackgren, Deflux consists of dextranomer microspheres (cross-linked dextran polysaccharide molecules) suspended in sodium hyaluronan.[39] Although the hyaluronan is absorbed by the tissue within 1 week of injection, the 80- to 120-micron microspheres persist, degrading slowly by hydrolysis. They are eventually replaced by fibrous tissue that retains approximately 75% of the original injected volume. Immunogenicity and particle migration appear to be minimal.

Two clinical series have been reported on the use of Deflux in treatment of incontinence in children. Caione and Capozza reported a mixed group of 16 patients who underwent 37 injections, all with follow-up of at least 1 year.[40] Seventy-five percent were either dry or improved (19% and 56%, respectively) after 1 year. This contrasts with a report by Lottmann and colleagues, who found that in their series of 33 patients, only 46% were dry or improved (25% and 21%, respectively).[41] Initial results at 1 month were better: 46% dry, 27% improved. Although there was little difference in success rates between spina bifida and exstrophy-epispadias patients, they noted that 65% of males were dry or improved compared with only 38% of females. Treatments were generally well tolerated, although Lottmann and colleagues reported a 30% rate of urinary tract infection. Repeat injections were helpful in the Caione and Capozza study, while the effect of repeat treatments was not reported in the Lottmann and colleagues study.

PARTICULATE SILICONE MICROIMPLANTS (POLYDIMETHYLSILOXANE, MACROPLASTIQUE) This agent consists of 200-micron solid polydimethylsiloxane particles suspended in a polypyrrolidone carrier gel. The gel is reabsorbed, leaving the particles to be encapsulated in fibrin and collagen. Studies in dogs have demonstrated migration of silicone particles less than 70 microns, although they do not appear to provoke the same granulomatous response as Teflon.[42]

Macroplastique injection in children with incontinence has been reported in two series. Duffy and Ransley reported a series of 12 boys with exstrophy-epispadias complex with mean follow-up of 10.3 months (range: 3–22).[43] Of these, 75% were dry or improved (25% and 50%, respectively). In a follow-up of a previous study,[44] Guys and colleagues reported on 44 patients, most of whom had spina bifida.[45] At a median follow-up of 28 months, 59% of patients were dry or improved (34% and 25%, respectively). Although overall success rates (dry or improved) were equivalent for boys and girls, the girls were more likely to be "dry" (44% vs 21%). No significant complications were reported in either series.

OTHER BULKING AGENTS A variety of injectable agents are in various stages of development, but have not yet been reported regarding their clinical efficacy for the treatment of incontinence in children. Injectable bioglass and polyvinyl alcohol foam are inert substances that maintain volume well after injection in vivo, but have not been pursued further because of difficulties with injection and mutagenesis concerns, respectively. Small intestinal submucosa (SIS) is purified extracellular matrix derived from porcine small intestine. It has been used for a variety of tissue engineering and reconstructive surgical applications. An injectable form of SIS has been studied in the dog, wherein SIS injected into bladder submuscosal tissue appeared to induce smooth muscle regeneration.[46] It was easily injected and no complications were noted. This agent has not yet been tried in humans.

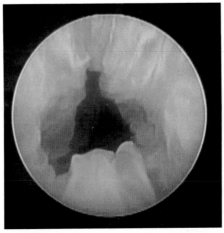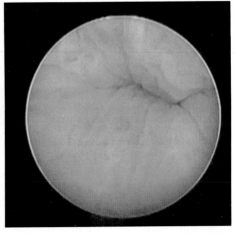

Figure 86-10 Bladder neck and proximal urethra are open prior to injection of bovine collagen in a 10-year-old girl with myelodysplasia and incontinence (*left*). After injection of 2.5 cc of collagen, the lumen is coapted by mucosal bulging (*right*).

Table 86-1   Results of Endoscopic Injection of Collagen for Treatment of Incontinence in Children

Study	No. of Patients	Diagnostic Mix	Follow-Up	Success Rate	Comments
Caione et al[52]	16	7 exstrophy 9 epispadias	1.5–4 years	14/16 (88%) "improved"	measured outcomes differently before and after BNR (see text)
Ben Chaim et al[56]	19	14 exstrophy 3 epispadias 2 CE	26 months, range: 9–84	10/19 (53%) dry or improved	
Bomalaski et al[32]	40	25 spina bifida 12 EEC 3 other	2.1 years, range: 0.25–6.3	22% dry 54% improved	EEC more satisfied with outcome than spina bifida
Leonard et al	18	10 NGB 6 EEC 2 other	15 months, range: 5–21	5/18 (28%) dry, 4/18 (22%) improved	–
Perez et al[55]	32	24 spina bifida 7 EEC 1 other	10 months, range: 3–19	8/32 (25%) dry, 8/32 (25%) "good"	–
Chernoff et al[57]	11	7 spina bifida 2 EEC 2 other	14.4 months, range: 4–20	6/11 (55%) improved	if preop VLPP < 45 cm H_2O, 6/8 improved; if VLPP > 45, 0/3 improved
Kim et al	8	8 NGB	>15 weeks in only 3 subjects	1/3 (33%) improved	100% "initial improvement" up to 15 weeks – 5 subjects lost to further follow-up
Sundaram et al[54]	20	12 spina bifida 4 EEC 4 other	15.2 months, range: 9–23	6/20 (30%) dry or improved	–
Silveri et al[59]	23	23 spina bifida	19.2 months, range: 6–54	13/23 (56%) improved	–
Kassouf et al	20	20 spina bifida	4.2 years, range: 1–6	4/20 (20%) improved	14 subjects had transient improvement lasting < 3 months
Block et al[53]	19	19 spina bifida	2.9 years	7/19 (37%) improved (none dry)	–

BNR = bladder neck reconstruction; CE = cloacal exstrophy; EEC = exstrophy/epispadias complex; NGB = neurogenic bladder; VLPP = Valsalva leak point pressure.

In addition to these exogenous agents, several autologous tissue sources have been investigated as injectable bulking agents. Autologous injectable fat has been used by several investigators for treatment of incontinence in women, but results have been disappointing compared with collagen,[47,48] likely owing to the significant volume loss in these grafts.[36] Autologous collagen and bladder muscle have also been used in the laboratory setting. Also reported are autologous chondrocytes, harvested from the patient's ear, expanded in culture, and injected as a calcium alginate gel. This agent appears to maintain volume over time and does not migrate.[49] In one study, 81% of women injected with this agent were dry or improved after a single injection.[50] Another series reported moderately durable success in treatment of vesicoureteral reflux in children.[51] Investigations into the use of this agent for incontinence in children reportedly are ongoing.

TIMING OF BLADDER NECK RECONSTRUCTION

Many incontinent children have an incompetent bladder neck, whether because of neuropathic or anatomic abnormalities. In some cases these children undergo injection prior to bladder neck reconstruction (BNR) in an attempt to increase outlet resistance and improve bladder cycling and capacity, in addition to improving continence. Other children undergo injection after BNR as a supplement to the level of continence already achieved with an open surgery. The evidence regarding the timing of endoscopic injection with respect to BNR is mixed and controversial. We have summarized the data from the series, which stratified outcomes by timing of BNR (Table 86-2). By pooling these data we noted that the results appear to be comparable for the two groups. These patients represent a mixture of diagnoses and injection agents, but there does not appear to be a major difference in the eventual success based on BNR timing. It should be noted that although Caione and colleagues did not find a major difference between prior BNR and no prior BNR, they defined success differently in the two groups (improved continence vs increased capacity, respectively).[52]

COMPLICATIONS

In general, endoscopic treatment of incontinence is well tolerated. Side effects can be divided into two general categories: complications of the procedure itself, and side effects related to the injected substance. Direct operative complications tend to be mild and infrequent. In the series reviewed, complications included urinary tract infection,[41] cellulitis of percutaneous cystostomy tube site,[53] gluteal hematoma,[54] urinary retention,[55] and bladder perforation.[56] Most series reported one or fewer complications.

One potential hazard of injection therapy is the risk of urodynamic deterioration of bladder after treatment. Chernoff and colleagues performed postinjection urodynamics on 11 patients in their collagen series, 3 of whom were found to have increased detrusor leak point pressure along with significantly decreased bladder compliance after injection.[57] Similarly, Lottmann and colleagues reported 3 patients who had bladder "deterioration" after injection of dextranomer/hyaluronic acid (Deflux).[41] These patients eventually required bladder augmentation. In these cases, it is impossible to know if the bladder decompensation was due to the injection itself, or represented the evolving natural history of abnormal bladder pathology existing prior to injection therapy. In any event, these cases illustrate the need to urodynamically monitor these children, especially in the setting of changing symptoms, such as delayed recurrence of leakage after endoscopic treatment.

CONCLUSIONS

It is doubtful that we will ever find the perfect injectable material with a durable 100% continence rate. In fact, the failure to achieve a perfect continence with endoscopic injection treatment may not be a fault of the materials science but rather a reflection of complex etiology involving outlet dysfunction as well as detrusor abnormality. Nevertheless, injectable implants, delivered endoscopically, have an important, albeit imperfect, role in the management of incontinence in children. Although straight forward in concept, endoscopic implantation for continence is not a casual exercise through a cystoscopic needle. Experience, precise technique, and reliable equipment, along with ever-improving materials science, all combine to increase the chance for success. The endoscopic treatment will likely remain an important arsenal in our armamentarium in solving pediatric urinary incontinence.

Table 86-2   Patients Dry or Improved after Endoscopic Treatment of Incontinence, Stratified by Timing of Bladder Neck Reconstruction (Sling, Young Dees, etc)

	Agent	Pior BNR	No Prior BNR
Chernoff et al[57]	Collagen	2/3	4/8
Diamond et al[58]	Detachable balloon	0/2	6/9
Caione et al[52]	Collagen	9/10	5/6
Silveri et al[59]	Collagen	–	13/23
Lottmann et al[41]	Deflux	7/12	10/19
Guys et al[45]	Macroplastique	13/24	13/20
Total		31/51 (60.8%)	51/85 (60%)

BNR = bladder neck reconstruction.

REFERENCES

1. Young HH. An operation for the cure of incontinence associated with epispadias. J Urol 1922;7:1.
2. Dees JE. Congenital epispadias with incontinence. J Urol 1949;62:513–22.
3. Leadbetter GW Jr. Surgical correction of total urinary incontinence. J Urol 1964;91:261–6.
4. Liard A, Seguier-Lipszyc E, Mathiot A, Mitrofanoff P. The Mitrofanoff procedure: 20 years later. J Urol 2001;165 (6 Pt 2):2394–8
5. Murless BC. The injection treatment of stress incontinence. Br J Obstet Gynecol Br Emp 1938;45:67–73.
6. Sachse H. Treatment of urinary incontinence with sclerosing solutions: indications, results, complications. Urol Int 1963;15:225–44.
7. Jankovic J, Brin MF. Botulinum toxin: historical perspective and potential new indications. Muscle Nerve Suppl 1997;6:S129–45.
8. Dykstra DD, Sidi AA, Scott AB, et al. Effects of botulinum A toxin on detrusor-sphincter dyssynergia in spinal cord injury patients. J Urol 1988;139:919–22.
9. Schurch B, Hauri D, Rodic B, et al. Botulinum-A toxin as a treatment of detrusor-sphincter dyssynergia: a prospective study in 24 spinal cord injury patients. J Urol 1996; 155:1023–9.
10. Petit H, Wiart L, Gaujard E, et al. Botulinum A toxin treatment for detrusor-sphincter dyssynergia in spinal cord disease. Spinal Cord 1998;36:91–4.
11. de Seze M, Petit H, Gallien P, et al. Botulinum a toxin and detrusor sphincter dyssynergia: a double-blind lidocaine-controlled study in 13 patients with spinal cord disease. Eur Urol 2002;42:56–62.
12. Schulte-Baukloh H, Michael T, Schobert J, et al. Efficacy of botulinum-a toxin in children with detrusor hyperreflexia due to myelomeningocele: preliminary results. Urology 2002;59:325–7.
13. Schurch B, Stohrer M, Kramer G, et al. Botulinum-A toxin for treating detrusor hyperreflexia in spinal cord injured patients: a new alternative to anticholinergic drugs? Preliminary results. J Urol 2000;164(3 Pt 1):692–7.
14. Mall V, Glocker FX, Frankenschmidt A, et al. Treatment of neuropathic bladder using botulinum toxin A in a 1-year-old child with myelomeningocele. Pediatr Nephrol 2001;16:1161–2.
15. Park JM, McGuire EJ, Koo HP, et al. External urethral sphincter dilation for the management of high risk myelomeningocele: 15-year experience. J Urol 2001;165(6 Pt 2):2383–8.
16. McDougall EM, Clayman RV, Figenshau RS, Pearle MS. Laparoscopic retropubic auto-augmentation of the bladder. J Urol 1995;153:123–6.
17. Siracusano S, Trombetta C, Liguori G, et al. Laparoscopic bladder auto-augmentation in an incomplete traumatic spinal cord injury. Spinal Cord 2000;38:59–61.
18. Braren V, Bishop MR. Laparoscopic bladder autoaugmentation in children. Urol Clin North Am 1998;25:533–40.
19. Hedican SP, Schulam PG, Docimo SG. Laparoscopic assisted reconstructive surgery. J Urol 1999;161:267–70.
20. Elliott SP, Meng MV, Anwar HP, Stoller ML. Complete laparoscopic ileal cystoplasty. Urology 2002;59:939–43.
21. O'Donnell B, Puri P. Endoscopic correction of primary vesicoureteric reflux. Br J Urol 1986;58:601–4.
22. Franco I, Reda EF, Kaplan WE. Injectable prosthetic materials for the management of reflux and urinary incontinence in children. Semin Urol 1992;10:184–93.
23. Capozza N, Caione P, De Gennaro M, et al. Endoscopic treatment of vesico-ureteric reflux and urinary incontinence: technical problems in the paediatric patient. Br J Urol 1995;75:538–42.
24. Kasabian NG, Bauer SB, Dyro FM, et al. The prophylactic value of clean intermittent catheterization and anticholinergic medication in newborns and infants with myelodysplasia at risk of developing urinary tract deterioration. Am J Dis Child 1992;146:840–3.
25. Frey P, Lutz N, Berger D, Herzog B. Histological behavior of glutaraldehyde cross-linked bovine collagen injected into the human bladder for the treatment of vesicoureteral reflux. J Urol 1994;152(2 Pt 2):632–5.
26. Frey P, Mangold S. Physical and histological behavior of a new injectable collagen (GAX 65) implanted into the submucosal space of the mini-pig bladder. J Urol 1995;154 (2 Pt 2):812–5.
27. Shortliffe L M, Freiha FS, Kessler R, et al. Treatment of urinary incontinence by the periurethral implantation of glutaraldehyde cross-linked collagen. J Urol 1989;141:538–41.
28. Frank DH, Vakassian L, Fisher JC. Ozkan N. Human antibody response following injection of bovine collagen. Plast Reconstr Surg 1991;87:1080–8.
29. Cukier J, Beauchamp RA, Spindler JS, et al. Association between bovine collagen dermal implants and a dermatomyositis or a polymyositis-like syndrome. Ann Intern Med 1993;118:920–8.
30. Appell R. Collagen injection therapy for urinary incontinence. Urol Clin North Am 1994;21:177–82.
31. Wan J, McGuire EJ, Bloom DA, Ritchey ML. The treatment of urinary incontinence in children using glutaraldehyde cross-linked collagen. J Urol 1992;148:127–30.
32. Bomalaski MD, Bloom DA, McGuire EJ, Panzl A. Glutaraldehyde cross-linked collagen in the treatment of urinary incontinence in children. J Urol 1996;155:699–702.
33. Arnold GE. Vocal cord rehabilitation of paralytic dysphonia. IX. Technique of intracordal injection. Arch Otolaryngol 1962;76:358–68.
34. Berg S. Polytef augmentation urethroplasty. Correction of surgically incurable urinary incontinence by injection technique. Arch Surg 1973;107:379–81.
35. Politano VA, Small MP, Harper JM, Lynn CM. Periurethral Teflon injection for urinary incontinence. J Urol 1974; 111:180–3.
36. Kershen RT, Atala A. New advances in injectable therapies for the treatment of incontinence and vesicoureteral reflux. Urol Clin North Am 1999;26:81–94.
37. Malizia AA Jr, Reiman HM, Myers RP, et al. Migration and granulomatous reaction after periurethral injection of polytef (Teflon). JAMA 1984;251:3277–81.
38. Puri P. Ten year experience with subureteric Teflon (polytetrafluoroethylene) injection (STING) in the treatment of vesico-ureteric reflux. Br J Urol 1995;75:126–31.
39. Stenberg A, Lackgren G. A new bioimplant for the endoscopic treatment of vesicoureteral reflux: experimental and short-term clinical results. J Urol 1995;154(2 Pt 2):800–3.
40. Caione P, Capozza N. Endoscopic treatment of urinary incontinence in pediatric patients: 2-year experience with dextranomer/hyaluronic acid copolymer. J Urol 2002; 168(4 Pt 2):1868–71.
41. Lottmann HB, Margaryan M, Bernuy M, et al. The effect of endoscopic injections of dextranomer based implants on continence and bladder capacity: a prospective study of 31 patients. J Urol 2002;168(4 Pt 2):1863–7.
42. Henly DR, Barrett DM, Weiland TL, et al. Particulate silicone for use in periurethral injections: local tissue effects and search for migration. J Urol 1995;153:2039–43.
43. Duffy PG, Ransley PG. Endoscopic treatment of urinary incontinence in children with primary epispadias. Br J Urol 1998;81:309–11.
44. Guys J M, Simeoni-Alias J, Fakhro A, Delarue A. Use of polydimethylsiloxane for endoscopic treatment of neurogenic urinary incontinence in children. J Urol 1999;162:2133–5.
45. Guys JM, Fakhro A, Louis-Borrione C, et al. Endoscopic treatment of urinary incontinence: long-term evaluation of the results. J Urol 2001;165(6 Pt 2):2389–91.
46. Furness PD 3rd, Kolligian ME, Lang SJ, et al. Injectable small intestinal submucosa: preliminary evaluation for use in endoscopic urological surgery. J Urol 2000;164:1680–5.
47. Palma PC, Riccetto CL, Herrmann V, Netto NR Jr. Repeated lipoinjections for stress urinary incontinence. J Endourol 1997;11:67–70.
48. Haab F, Zimmern PE, Leach GE. Urinary stress incontinence due to intrinsic sphincteric deficiency: experience with fat and collagen periurethral injections. J Urol 1997;157:1283–6.
49. Cozzolino DJ, Cendron M, DeVore DP, Hoopes PJ. The biological behavior of autologous collagen-based extracellular matrix injected into the rabbit bladder wall. Neurourol Urodyn 1999;18:487–95.
50. Bent AE, Tutrone RT, McLennan MT, et al. Treatment of intrinsic sphincter deficiency using autologous ear chondrocytes as a bulking agent. Neurourol Urodyn 2001;20:157–65.
51. Caldamone AA, Diamond DA. Long-term results of the endoscopic correction of vesicoureteral reflux in children using autologous chondrocytes. J Urol 2001;165(6 Pt 2):2224–7.
52. Caione P, Lais A, de Gennaro M, Capozza N. Glutaraldehyde cross-linked bovine collagen in exstrophy/epispadias complex. J Urol 1993;150(2 Pt 2):631–3.
53. Block CA, Cooper CS, Hawtrey CE. Long-term efficacy of periurethral collagen injection for the treatment of urinary incontinence secondary to myelomeningocele. J Urol 2003;169:327–9.
54. Sundaram CP, Reinberg Y, Aliabadi HA. Failure to obtain durable results with collagen implantation in children with urinary incontinence. J Urol 1997;157:2306–7.
55. Perez LM, Smith EA. Parrott TS, et al. Submucosal bladder neck injection of bovine dermal collagen for stress urinary incontinence in the pediatric population. J Urol 1996;156(2 Pt 2):633–6.
56. Ben Chaim J, Jeffs RD, Peppas DS, Gearhart JP. Submucosal bladder neck injections of glutaraldehyde cross-linked bovine collagen for the treatment of urinary incontinence in patients with the exstrophy/epispadias complex. J Urol 1995;154(2 Pt 2):862–4.
57. Chernoff A, Horowitz M, Combs A, et al. Periurethral collagen injection for the treatment of urinary incontinence in children. J Urol 1997;157:2303–5.
58. Diamond DA, Bauer SB, Retik AB, Atala A. Initial experience with the transurethral self-detachable balloon system for urinary incontinence in pediatric patients. J Urol 2000; 164(3 Pt 2):942–5.
59. Silveri M, Capitanucci ML, Mosiello G, et al. Endoscopic treatment for urinary incontinence in children with a congenital neuropathic bladder. Br J Urol 1998;82:694–7.

87

Endoscopic Approaches to the Treatment of Vesicoureteral Reflux

Andy Y. Chang, MD
Jennifer Kirk, MSN, CPNP
Douglas A. Canning, MD

Endoscopic treatment of vesicoureteral reflux (VUR) dates back to 1983 when Matouschek[1] first described injection of the ureteral orifice in an attempt to correct VUR. Working independently, Politano and colleagues[2] and McDonald and McDonald[3] described successful correction of reflux using endoscopic techniques. It was not until the first reported results in pigs[4] and humans,[5,6] however, that the subureteral Teflon injection (STING) came to be appreciated as a viable new way to less invasively correct one of the most common pediatric urologic problems.

The technique is straightforward and is usually performed as an outpatient procedure. It does require general anesthesia in children and may require repeat injections, particularly in patients with high-grade reflux. Up until 2001, the endoscopic injection to correct VUR had failed to gain popularity in North America. Two main problems existed. First, no implant substance provided the safety and durability to make it attractive for use in children. Second, success in children with high-grade reflux was less than reported for open reimplant techniques. In the past 5 years, however, newer products have become available that are changing the indications for endoscopic correction. We are now experiencing a resurgence of interest in endoscopic surgery to correct VUR in children.

INDICATIONS

VUR is common, occurring in 0.4% of the general population.[7] In children with urinary tract infection, the incidence is as high as 29% to 50%.[8] When reflux coexists with urinary tract infection and intrarenal reflux, the child is at significant risk of renal scarring,[7] which can lead to end-stage renal disease. The current management of VUR has evolved in response to several observations that have changed over the past 40 years.[9]

1. *Low-grade reflux frequently resolves, whereas high-grade VUR usually persists.* The resolution rate for VUR is dependent on the initial grade. Approximately 80% of low-grade reflux resolves with medical management. Often, however, this takes considerable time. Higher grades of reflux resolve much less frequently. In a recent review of patients from the

Children's Hospital of Philadelphia, we found that resolution of VUR grades I to III was identical to historically reported rates, with 50% of children showing resolution at 3.59 years after diagnosis. Grade IV VUR resolved much less frequently, with resolution in 50% of children projected to be 11.59 years. Moreover, grades I to III VUR resolved at 13% yearly for the first 5 years and dropped to 3.5% for the last 10 years. Grade IV and V reflux resolved at 5% yearly.[10] With an 80% overall resolution rate for low-grade reflux compared with a 20% overall resolution for high-grade reflux, the decision as to who requires surgery becomes more straightforward.

2. *Sterile reflux does not cause renal damage, but persistent reflux of infected urine may cause renal damage.* Ransley and colleagues have taught us the importance of the anatomy of the renal papilla in preventing or promoting intrarenal VUR.[11–13] Scarring following bacterial infection occurs most commonly at the polar regions of the kidney where the renal papillae are often confluent, allowing intrarenal reflux. In the absence of infection, when voiding pressures are low, scarring does not occur. Medical management is generally safe and effective in the absence of high voiding pressures. The International Reflux Study (IRS) in children, a multinational prospective study, compared medical and surgical management in children with grades III and IV VUR. No advantage of surgical over medical treatment could be found with regard to renal scarring or renal function at the conclusion of the study.[14] More recently, Smellie and colleagues conducted a randomized prospective trial of medical versus surgical treatment for children with bilateral grades III to V VUR with bilateral renal scarring. After four years, no significant change in glomerular filtration rate was observed between the two groups.[15] A 10-year follow-up study using patients from the European subset of the IRS showed that medical management of grades III to IV VUR is safe.[16]

3. *Ureteroneocystostomy in the hands of the pediatric urologist is safe and effective.* Of 87 patients in the IRS undergoing surgery for grades III and IV VUR, five (5.7%) had per-

sistent low-volume reflux after surgery. In four of the five patients, VUR resolved spontaneously over an average of 20 months follow-up, leaving 1 of 154 (0.6%) reimplanted ureters that required reoperation. No patients in the American arm of the study developed obstruction.[17] Thus, management of children with VUR can be divided between medical and surgical therapy, with medical therapy usually offered initially, and surgery reserved for patients in whom medical management is unsuccessful. Most patients "fail" medical management because of persistent reflux into adolescence, breakthrough urinary tract infections, or failure to comply with maintenance prophylactic regimens.

SURGICAL CONSIDERATIONS

After a diagnosis of VUR, all children are placed on antibiotic prophylaxis and carefully followed (Figure 87-1). We recommend the more aggressive surgical approach to families who are considered unreliable with regard to follow-up or

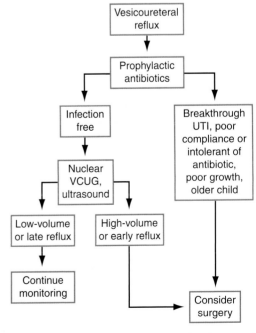

Figure 87-1 Algorithm for treatment of vesicoureteral reflux.

administration of prophylactic antibiotics and to all patients in whom infection develops despite antibiotic prophylaxis (breakthrough infection).

In general, patients presenting to Children's Hospital of Philadelphia with VUR are nearly always followed for at least 1 year, regardless of reflux grade. In many of these children, the grade of reflux will be lowered as the infection is controlled and the children begin to void more comfortably. Infants with high grades of reflux will benefit from a period of monitoring, since reflux improves most dramatically within the first year.[18] At the same time, the infant bladder increases in volume most rapidly within the first 18 months.[19] Infants with pronounced VUR have been shown to void with high pressures,[20] a phenomenon that may become less evident as they age. As a result of reduced severity of reflux and increased bladder volume, antireflux surgery is safer and more effective in older infants.

After the first year, the child undergoes follow-up nuclear cystography, which measures the bladder volume when the bladder is filled to capacity, the bladder volume at which reflux is first noted, and the volume of urine refluxing into either ureter. We have noted improved resolution rates in patients in whom reflux occurs only after the bladder is more than 60% full or if the volume of urine refluxing into either ureter is 2.6% of the bladder volume at capacity.[21] If the child still has high-volume reflux early in bladder filling, he or she is considered for correction (Figure 87-2).

We carefully ask about the child's voiding pattern. Hesitancy, urgency, or infrequent voiding, all of which can be suggestive of dysfunctional voiding, must be identified prior to surgery. If symptoms of dysfunctional voiding can be elicited, care should be taken to improve the coordination of voiding before proceeding to surgical treatment of reflux, since the failure rate following antireflux surgery in these children is greater.[22,23] We have established a center for assessment and treatment of voiding dysfunction at Children's Hospital of Philadelphia. Many children with a history of urinary tract infections will have some degree of voiding dysfunction, which must be controlled before surgery. With careful treatment of voiding dysfunction, many patients with reflux and recurrent infections will show a reduction in both the predisposition to infection and the grade of reflux volume.

If high-volume reflux persists at the second study and the patient is not a dysfunctional voider, surgical correction should be considered. We reemphasize that medical management in the absence of infection is safe but may not be the most effective way to manage the patient with high-volume VUR. Even if symptoms of dysfunctional voiding do not exist in the patient with high-volume VUR, a prolonged period of medical management may be necessary before resolution can be expected. Surgical correction of VUR, if it becomes necessary later on, may be emotionally more difficult for the older child. Faced with the prospect of numerous radiologic studies and years of antibiotic prophylaxis without good odds of spontaneous resolution of VUR,

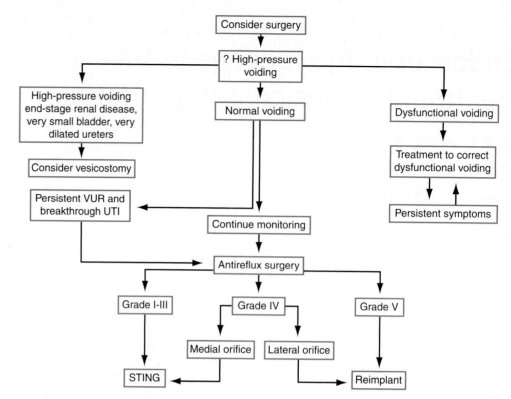

Figure 87-2 Considerations prior to surgery in patients with vesicoureteral reflux. Prior to surgery, the bladder must empty with low pressure. If the ureteral orifice is lateral, traditional ureteral reimplantation should be considered rather than endoscopic correction.

many families elect to proceed with surgery, particularly if a relatively less morbid (ie, endoscopic) approach is available.

Endoscopic treatment of VUR has obvious advantages over conventional approaches. Endoscopic correction is usually done on an outpatient basis. In an adult, it can be done with conscious sedation or with local anesthesia. The hospital stay is short, and there is no surgical scar. As a result, overall hospital charges are decreased.

Because of the lower morbidity of endoscopic surgery and lower costs compared to open procedures, one could argue that additional patients should be offered surgery rather than prophylaxis as the initial treatment. Alternatively, Stenberg and colleagues recently recommended that most children with VUR managed conservatively with antibiotics for longer than 1 year be offered endoscopic treatment, specifically with dextranomer/hyaluronic acid copolymer, as an alternative to long-term antibiotic prophylaxis or open surgery.[24] Data presented by Capozza and Caione[25] lends further support for this new treatment algorithm. Sixty-one children with grades II to IV reflux were randomized to endoscopic treatment with dextranomer/hyaluronic acid copolymer (40 patients) or antibiotic prophylaxis. At 12 months follow-up, 69% of the endoscopically treated children had grade I or less VUR, versus 38% of the medically treated patients ($p = .029$).[25] With success rates approaching 90%, even in series with considerable numbers of patients with high volume VUR,[26] one can begin to substitute endoscopic correction for antibiotic prophylaxis in some cases (Figure 87-3).[24,25,27]

Unfortunately, because endoscopic repair is less successful in patients with high-grade primary VUR, multiple procedures are frequently necessary. This translates into additional costs and hospital stays for repeat surgery. In addition, even after successful endoscopic correction, reflux can recur. As a result, there is a risk that the child who is removed from antibiotic prophylaxis and suffers a recurrence may return with pyelonephritis and a new scar, the very thing we try to prevent with antireflux surgery. For these reasons, we tend to offer endoscopic correction only to the few with low-grade primary VUR in whom medical management has failed or to the few who have persistent VUR after ureteroneocystostomy.

On the other hand, endoscopic correction is an attractive alternative for some more complicated cases in which ureteroneocystostomy is probably unnecessary. Adults,[28,29] renal transplant recipients with reflux into the native kidneys,[30–32] or transplant recipients with recurrent urinary tract infection associated with reflux into the allograft ureter,[33] and patients with neuropathic bladder[34,35] have all been successfully treated endoscopically. Ureteroneocystostomy is more complicated and less successful in these patients. In these cases, endoscopic correction may be indicated even if multiple attempts are necessary to correct reflux.

PATIENT PREPARATION

Nearly all patients undergo ultrasonography as the initial study to assess the shape of the kidney and

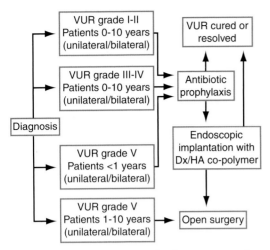

Figure 87-3 New vesicoureteral reflux treatment algorithm as proposed by Lackgren et al.[27]

the presence of scarring. The potential for renal failure is estimated using the echo texture of the renal parenchyma relative to the liver or spleen and the presence or absence of corticomedullary junctions. These criteria have been shown to correlate with future renal function.[36] If significant scarring exists, the volume of renal parenchyma is small, the kidney looks echo dense, or the corticomedullary junctions are obscure, a renal scan is obtained to further assess preoperative function and drainage. If function is poor (< 10%), consideration should be given to removal of the kidney and ureter rather than correction of the VUR. Rarely, a secondary ureteropelvic junction (UPJ) obstruction exists. If a UPJ obstruction is suspected to coexist with reflux, correction should be made prior to, or at the time of, antireflux surgery if the obstruction appears to be primary. Otherwise, UPJ obstruction suspected to be secondary to high-grade VUR should be carefully monitored following antireflux surgery.[37]

Patients with posterior urethral valves, neuropathic bladder, or severe dysfunctional voiding should be considered for antireflux surgery only after very careful deliberation (see Figure 87-2).[38] Vesicostomy is usually a better option. In many cases, high-volume VUR effectively improves capacity in the valve bladder and should be allowed to remain as long as the patient has no upper urinary tract infection.

Whether attempting endoscopic or open repair of VUR, the bladder volume must be adequate to allow for low-pressure storage following voiding. If the bladder empties poorly or is poorly compliant, recurrent infections, progressive upper tract dilation, or renal scarring may result. If bladder capacity is suspect, attempts to correct reflux by any means usually fail.

Because successful subureteral injection requires at least some type of submucosal ureteral tunnel in which to place the implant, lower grades of reflux are more easily corrected than higher grades of reflux. If subureteral correction is planned in a patient with high-grade VUR, the patient and his or her family must be cautioned that additional attempts may be necessary to cor-

rect the problem. Primary ureteroneocystostomy is usually a better option in these patients.

Prior to scheduling, the plan for preoperative, intraoperative, and short- and long-term follow-up care should be made clear to the patient and his family. Specifically, the risks of persistent reflux and the possible need for additional surgery should be outlined and compared with the risks of open surgical repair. The risk of obstruction of the ureter, both transient and long term, should also be outlined, along with the steps needed to correct such an eventuality. Urinary tract infection, bleeding, obstruction, and persistent reflux can occur following endoscopic or open surgery. Risks specific to the implant material are particularly important considerations prior to planning endoscopic surgery. The relative risks and benefits of each substance are considered under the description of each substance.

PREOPERATIVE PREPARATION

No special preoperative studies are necessary. In children, general anesthesia is administered via endotracheal intubation or laryngeal mask airway with no additional special requirements. The patient is placed in the dorsal lithotomy position. The legs should be separated enough to provide easy access even to a very lateral ureteral orifice. Special imaging equipment is not necessary. Endoscopic camera equipment is helpful because it allows the assistant and the surgeon to coordinate their efforts during the injection.

INSTRUMENTATION AND IMPLANTS

CYSTOSCOPES AND NEEDLES Cystoscopic equipment varies with the implant. The two most widely used substances, Deflux (QMed, Uppsala, Sweden) and Polytef (Mentor, Hingham, MA) require little in the way of extensive equipment. Deflux can be injected through a needle as small as 3.7 French without too much difficulty with a hand-held conventional syringe. No special equipment other than conventional endoscopic equipment is needed. Some practitioners, however, prefer to use a 10F pediatric cystoscope with an offset lens to allow the needle to be inserted without bending.[26,39]

For Polytef, a cystoscope large enough to accommodate a 4 or 5F ureteral catheter is an advantage since the thick Polytef suspension requires considerable force to propel it through the needle—the larger the needle the easier the injection. Using a hand-held gun to increase the force of injection can help push the Polytef through a smaller needle.

The Stinger endoscope (Richard Wolf Medical Instruments, Vernon Hills, IL) is ideal for injection of Polytef paste. The Stinger combines an offset lens endoscope with a stiff 5F cannula onto which is swaged a 21-gauge needle. The stiff needle is easily introduced and passed through the working channel without difficulty. A modification of the Stinger has been manufactured (Karl Storz Endoscopy-America, Culver City, CA). The Storz system uses a fiberoptic lens with

an offset ocular lens. It has a 9.5F sheath with a 5F lumen, which is ideal for use in smaller children. Many practitioners are using conventional endoscopes with a flexible needle (Puri 5F cannula, Karl Storz). If the flexible needle is used, an offset lens is not needed and no special endoscopic equipment other than a working port of 4 to 5F is necessary.

IMPLANT SUBSTANCES Over the years, endoscopic enthusiasts have researched many substances, but only one or two materials are widely used. The following are a few of the more commonly used materials and substances of historical and experimental interests.

ACTIVELY USED IMPLANTS **Deflux** One of the greatest advances made for the endoscopic correction of vesicoureteral reflux was developed by Stenberg and Läckgren[40] and is now the most widely used implant. Deflux is a suspension of dextranomer microspheres (80 to 120 μm) in sodium hyaluronate solution (NaHa). The dextranomer particles are cross-linked dextran polymers, and the NaHa is an endogenous polysaccharide. No particles exist freely in solution.

Deflux is easily injected through a 23-gauge needle because of the "pseudo-plastic properties" of the microspheres that seem to allow expansion and compression of the implant during injection. This property allows injection through a small needle but seems to prevent extrusion even in ureters with high-grade reflux where little room exists for placement of the implant. A 10F cystoscope, with or without an offset lens, and an ordinary syringe are used. In most cases, implant volume of 0.5 to 1.5 mL is effective in correcting VUR.[26]

Deflux maintained 80% of the injected volume for at least 12 months when injected subcutaneously in rats. Ingrowth of native fibroblasts has been noted as early as 2 weeks after injection. Multinucleated giant cells are present but appear to be sparse. As with collagen, the ingrowth of native fibroblasts appears to result in minimal volume replacement and may stabilize the implant somewhat (Figure 87-4). Although skin testing is not done prior to injection, Stenberg and Läckgren did not note an allergic reaction in any patient.[40]

Deflux was approved for use in the United States in 2002. Since that time, its use in North America has exploded, and now, nearly all pediatric urologists have some experience with it.

Polytef Although Matouschek,[1] Politano and colleagues,[2] and McDonald and McDonald[3] each experimented with Polytef before O'Donnell's original report, O'Donnell and associates developed the technique and popularized it.[4–6,41–43] By 1991, O'Donnell estimated that more than 3,000 ureters had been treated in Europe and the United States. More recently, Puri and colleagues[44] reported results on 12,251 ureters in 8,332 children worldwide, which included their previous reports of 6,216 ureters in 4,166 children from 18 European centers.[45]

Polytef is readily available and easy to use. Its injection characteristics allow relatively easy

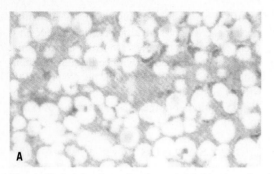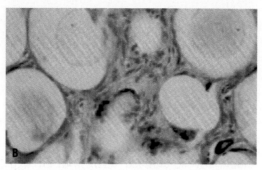

Figure 87-4 *A,* Implant taken from pig bladder 2 weeks after injection of Deflux. Collagen and fibroblasts are present between microspheres. *B,* Three and a half months after injection in-growth has progressed to surround the microspheres. This effect may stabilize the implant. Native fibroblasts and production of native collagen may replace the implant to minimal degree.[40]

implantation even in laterally placed ureters. The major concern with Polytef stems from two articles by Malizia and colleagues[46,47] that examined the effects of Teflon in dogs and subsequently in pigs. Nearly simultaneously with the initial report of O'Donnell and Puri,[6] Malizia and colleagues demonstrated profound local inflammatory tissue reaction to Polytef injected into the urethra in dogs.

Polytef is a 50% suspension of Teflon particles in glycerol. The Teflon particle size ranges from 4 to 100 μm, with more than 90% smaller than 40 μm (Figure 87-5). Histiocytic infiltration with foreign body giant cell reaction was noted in all animals that had been exposed to the particles for longer than 10.5 months in Malizia's study (see Figure 87-5). Perhaps more disturbing, migrated particles as large as 80 μm were found in the pelvic lymph nodes, kidneys, spleen, and lung and in the subarachnoid space of the brain stem and cerebral hemispheres. The tissue reaction associated with the migrated particles was variable. Multinucleated giant cells were found in lymph nodes and lung tissue but were not associated with particles that migrated to the kidney or brain.[47,48]

A similar study performed with smaller injection volumes placed beneath the trigone in monkeys appeared to confirm these earlier reports.[49]

Longer term follow-up in this group of monkeys demonstrated persistent masses identifiable on radiographic images.[50]

Information regarding migration in humans is less clear. Spencer and colleagues[51] carefully followed 10 patients treated with subureteral injections for up to 3 years with computed tomography scans and ultrasonography. They found no evidence of enlargement of the granuloma implant over time. Although a Teflon granuloma has been noted surrounding a particle that had migrated to the lung in patients treated with periurethral injections of Polytef paste,[52,53] no symptoms or long-term morbidity has been associated to date with the use of this substance in the urinary tract, despite widespread experience in more than 4,000 patients described in published reports.[1–3,38,51,54–57]

North American pediatric urologists have always been concerned about the potential for migration of the Teflon particles, despite its wide acceptance throughout the world. Nevertheless, Polytef has always been the gold standard with which we have measured any new substance, because Polytef seemed so superior in durability and implantability. No substance had been as easy to use up until 2002 when the US Food and Drug

Administration (FDA) approved Deflux for use in the United States. At that time, even those with large experiences using Polytef paste migrated over to the use of Deflux.

HISTORICAL AND EXPERIMENTAL IMPLANTS
With the advent of Deflux, discussions of the following substances are for historical and experimental purposes.

Collagen Because of the uncertainty surrounding the long-term effects of particle migration and local tissue reaction to Polytef paste and recognizing the efficacy of the STING, Peters and Jeffs began experimenting with a glutaraldehyde cross-linked bovine collagen preparation (Zyplast, INAMED Aesthetics, Santa Barbara, CA) as an alternative.[58]

Cross-linked bovine collagen had been widely used for years in cardiac valves as a hemostatic agent and, in the injectable form, as a soft tissue substitute.[59] Zyplast is bovine corium collagen, which is solubilized by exposure to pepsin in acetic acid and purified by ultrafiltration and ion-exchange chromatography. Following purification, the collagen is reconstituted in a pH-neutral solution, harvested, and re-suspended in saline solution to provide non–cross-linked collagen. To this substance is added purified glutaraldehyde in a final concentration of 0.0075% to cross link the reconstituted collagen fibrils.[60,61] The added glutaraldehyde binds adjacent collagen fibrils to improve the integrity of the implant after injection. Zyplast demonstrates 90% to 100% wet weight persistence as a stable implant in subdermal[62] and suburothelial[63] injections in animals. Zyplast elicits little local tissue reaction and no granuloma formation when injected beneath the urothelium. There is variable fibroblast ingrowth and partial replacement of the implant with small amounts of native collagen.[64–66]

Zyplast is more fluid than Polytef, which allows injection through a 23- or 25-gauge needle without difficulty.[51] However, placing the implant with precision is more difficult. As a result, injec-

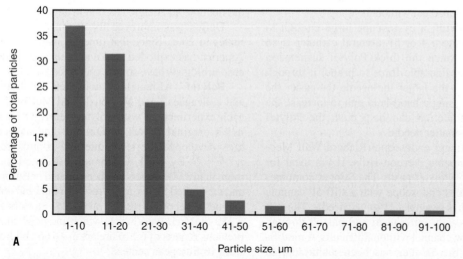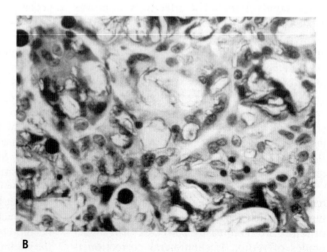

Figure 87-5 *A,* Distribution of particles by size in Polytef paste. Note more than 90% are smaller than 40 μm.[47] *B,* Local tissue reaction to injected Polytef paste in periurethral injection site. Note multinucleated giant cell (upper left) surrounding Teflon particle.[46]

tion with collagen for high-grade VUR has not been as effective as injection with Polytef. But because of widespread resistance to the use of Polytef in the United States and the FDA approval of collagen for incontinence (Contigen) in 1993, collagen began to gain popularity for endoscopic treatment of reflux in North America.

Despite a relatively rapid increase in popularity in collagen in the late 1980s and early 1990s, by the end of the 1990s, most centers that were initial enthusiasts of collagen injections began to perceive that the implant was breaking down relatively quickly after 24 months following initial and repeat injections.[67,68] That, along with the approval for the use of Deflux, has made collagen a less commonly used bulking agent for correction of vesicoureteral reflux today.

Particulate Silicone Microimplants In an effort to reduce migration of implant particles while maintaining a durable implant, Schulman began to experiment with particulate silicone macroparticles (Macroplastique, Bioplasty, Minneapolis, MN).[69] Macroplastique is 40% vulcanized polydimethylsiloxane particles in a 60% water-soluble carrier medium composed of low–molecular-weight polyvinylpyrrolidone. The advantage of this substance over Polytef is that it contains few small particles. Since the largest macrophages are approximately 80 μm, particles smaller than 80 μm can migrate via the macrophage to distant organs. Macroplastique implant particles range in size from 16 to 409 μm (average 171 μm). This results in fewer particles small enough to migrate.

Despite the larger average particle size, limited migration of a few smaller particles to the lung in rabbits[69] and to the spleen in dogs[70] has been reported. A single migrated particle was found in 1 of 6 dogs and 2 of 12 rabbits. Despite the small number of migrated particles, even minimal migration is cause for concern and prevented Macroplastique from gaining popularity in the United States, although it has been used in Europe and Canada[71] with success that approaches that of Deflux.

AUTOLOGOUS TRANSPLANTS **Fat** Since 1890, fat transplantation has been used to correct soft tissue defects.[72] In 1983, surgeons transplanted fat via small syringes following liposuction surgery to increase breast size.[73] Small quantities of fat harvested from the abdomen or thigh under local anesthesia maintain 50% to 75% of the original volume when transplanted to other fat-bearing areas.[74]

In a preliminary study in rabbits, we tested the persistence and local tissue response to fat transplanted from the abdomen or retroperitoneum to the bladder. Twenty-one immature rabbits received transplanted fat taken from the abdomen. We injected 1 mL of fat through a standard hypodermic needle (19 to 23 gauge) beneath the urothelium at the dome of the bladder.

Autopsies were performed at intervals ranging from 1 day to 11 months after injection. The diameter of the implant was measured after sectioning and compared with the size immediately after injection. Microscopic examination of stained sections assessed nuclear integrity and local tissue response.

Nineteen animals survived the surgery. Two had complete loss of the injected fat. Volume loss of 25% to 50% occurred in seven. The implant was stable in seven and grew to as large as twice the original size in three long-term survivors. The integrity of the fat-cell nucleus, an indicator of fat-cell viability in injected cells, was preserved in each case when fat was present at autopsy. Implants initially showed areas of central necrosis, but vascular ingrowth to the center of the implant developed by 8 weeks. There was no significant inflammatory reaction within or at the periphery.[75] The absence of a local tissue response suggests that fat is a truly benign injectable substance with little local tissue reaction. More information must be obtained regarding its long-term persistence in humans, however, before its effectiveness can be determined. Variations in the harvesting technique, origin of the transplanted fat,[75] and volume of the implant may have dramatic effects on the durability of the implant.[76,77] Because fat survival depends on ingrowth of vessels from the periphery, the smaller the implant, the better the survival. The fat must be harvested carefully to prevent injury to the adipose cell and injected through as large a needle as possible. When successfully transplanted in small quantities, fat has been shown to remain in place for long periods and maintain functional integrity at the injection site,[78] but implants larger than 1 cc fail to persist. This along with the difficulty in delivering viable fat cells through small-gauge needles has made their approach impractical for clinical treatment of vesicoureteral reflux.

Autologous Collagen Despite the apparent effectiveness and safety of cross-linked bovine collagen, Cendron and colleagues (recognizing the potential for hypersensitivity from foreign collagen) began experimenting with processed autologous collagen as a substitute for bovine cross-linked collagen.[79] Autologous collagen injected within the urinary tract should, like fat, be recognized as self by the body and, therefore, should not elicit an immune response.

Autologous collagen can be extracted by removal of a small segment of skin from which the dermis is isolated. The dermis is minced and pulverized into a dispersion of collagen fibers that are washed and then concentrated by centrifugation. The concentration of injectable collagen is dependent on the centrifuge speed.[80]

Cendron and colleagues showed that collagen implants harvested from rabbits and injected into the anterior bladder wall maintained their integrity and elicited little immune response for as long as 50 days.[79] Comparison of autologous collagen-based extracellular matrix versus bovine collagen injected into rabbit bladder walls showed similar stability (6 of 12 autologous, and 7 of 12 bovine, collagen blebs found during necropsy at 12 weeks), but the autologous group showed increased focal fibroblastic and vascular infiltration. More significant was the fourfold decrease in inflammatory response associated with the autologous animals, which led the authors to hypothesize that the autologous collagen-based extracellular matrix may have increased lifespan than the bovine collagen implant.[81] Studies are needed to test long-term durability and effectiveness in correcting VUR.

Cultured Human Fibroblasts To improve the durability of bovine collagen preparations, tissue culture specialists joined with collagen chemistry experts to integrate cultured cells with reconstituted collagen strands. One forthcoming development is the introduction of cultured human fibroblasts to a collagen matrix.

In one study, fragments of freshly discarded facial skin were harvested from healthy patients and grown in culture media.[82] After a period of growth on the culture plate, the cells were washed and injected beneath the dermis in athymic mice. Additional cells were mixed with non–cross-linked collagen prior to injection. For comparison, a third group of mice received pure collagen injections.

Three weeks later, the pure fibroblast implants had a necrotic center with active cells at the periphery. Necrosis was missing in the collagen-fibroblast suspension. Between 3 and 9 weeks, the numbers of human fibroblasts decreased markedly in both the pure fibroblasts and the fibroblast-collagen implants. By 9 weeks, mice in both the pure fibroblast and fibroblast-collagen groups lost more than two-thirds of the injected volume. In contrast, the pure collagen implant maintained complete integrity.

This study shows that viable human fibroblasts with sufficient volume to correct VUR can be transferred easily through small-gauge needles. Additional study of the factors responsible for persistent growth of implanted cultured human fibroblast suspensions is needed before they assume a role as injectable substances in the urinary system.

Chondrocyte-Alginate Suspension Chondrocytes can be grown and expanded in culture media[83] and combined with synthetic polymers to preserve viability for up to 6 months.[84] Atala and colleagues at Children's Hospital in Boston initially used these techniques to combine chondrocytes harvested from calf articular cartilage with alginate, an injectable organic copolymer.[85] The chondrocyte-alginate suspension was then injected into the dorsum of athymic mice. The implant maintained integrity, laying down a matrix of native cartilage as the alginate particles were absorbed.[86] Atala and colleagues then used the technique in minipigs in which reflux had been induced by unroofing the ureteral tunnel. Chondrocytes were harvested from the auricular cartilage, expanded in vitro, suspended with alginate, and then endoscopically injected using a 22-gauge needle through a 15.5F cystoscope. Each implant was successfully placed beneath the ureteral orifice. Reflux was successfully corrected in all four minipigs. No evidence of ureteral obstruction was noted for as long as 6 months, and no inflammation was present. The implant maintained its integrity in the form of a firm, rubbery prosthesis beneath the trigone.

This novel approach using tissue-engineering techniques has been employed in humans as reported by Caldamone and Diamond.[87] Twenty-nine children with 47 refluxing ureters ranging from grades II to IV VUR underwent posterior auricular cartilage harvest. The procured chondrocytes were cultured for 6 weeks prior to autologous injection into the affected vesicoureteral junction. Reflux was corrected in 55% of the ureters treated with 1 injection and 62% of those requiring a second injection for a total of 86% success at 3 months. Seventy percent of the ureters remained free of reflux at 1 year.[87] Further trials are needed before this technology is developed as an alternative substance to what is currently used successfully. Even with results that equal or surpass those of Deflux, the need for a minimum of two anesthetics (chondrocyte procurement and initial injection) may impede the wide acceptance of this system.

Nonautologous Transplants **Detachable Balloon Membrane System** In an effort to control migration of the injectable substance, Atala and colleagues developed a detachable silicone membrane system.[88] This system uses a detachable balloon attached to a catheter, both of which can be passed through a 19-gauge cystoscopic needle. The needle is introduced at the appropriate site beneath the ureteral orifice. The catheter with the membrane is then introduced, and the needle is removed, leaving the catheter in place. The membrane is then injected with hydroxy-ethylmethacrylate (HEMA). The catheter is then removed, leaving the HEMA-filled silicone membrane behind.

Using the minipig model, reflux was corrected in all 6 pigs with uniformly excellent results. No obstruction occurred and no loss or gain of implant volume was noted in short follow-up. Implant migration and granuloma formation were not observed. Minimal tissue response was noted. Although potentially promising, work on this technology has yielded to other materials.

Injectable Bioglass Another substance, injectable Bioglass (University of Florida, Gainesville, FL), has been evaluated by Walker and colleagues.[89] Bioglass is a glass ceramic that has the ability to bond to soft tissue, thereby preventing particle displacement. Bioglass is prepared by mechanically rounding small glass particles and suspending them in sodium hyaluronate. The glass particles do not elicit a local tissue reaction. Mechanical rounding allows more of the particles to be placed in suspension.

To determine the durability, local tissue reaction, and risk of migration, Walker's group injected rabbits. Each injection was placed beneath the urothelium in the bladder using a 17-gauge needle. After 2, 4, 6, 8, 10, and 12 weeks, no evidence of Bioglass was noted in the kidneys, lungs, liver, or lymph nodes in these rabbits. Nodules were present at 8 of 12 injection sites. No inflammatory reaction was noted. The implant seems to bind to the tissues by attachment of collagen fibers to the Bioglass surface, which prevents movement of the implant.[90] Pigs injected to increase resistance at the bladder neck as a test of the integrity of the implant all had persistent increased resistance for at least 6 months. No migration of particles could be detected.[89]

Particle size ranges from 125 to 355 μm. The suspension can be passed through a 16- to 17-gauge needle. Smaller needle sizes result in passage of the sodium hyaluronate past the Bioglass, leaving the Bioglass particles behind packed in the syringe. This problem may make injection in small children more difficult and thus less attractive than Deflux, which has similar desirable properties without the delivery problems.

Polyvinyl Foam Sponge Ivalon (GE Healthcare, Waukesha, WI) is a polyvinyl alcohol converted to sponge by foaming agents. Like collagen, it is injectable or can be shaped into discrete sponges of fixed size. Rather than losing mass over time as do collagen products, Ivalon remains for as long as 20 years after implantation.[91] It produces considerable fibrotic reaction, a feature surgeons use to advantage when Ivalon is sewn along the rectal wall to induce scarring in the correction of rectal prolapse.

Merguerian and colleagues[92] used an 18-gauge needle to inject this substance beneath the urothelium in rabbits to measure its persistence in the bladder and to view the inflammatory reaction. Implant volume remained constant over 3 months. Local tissue response was similar to that seen with Teflon paste—that is, a giant cell reaction with granulomata formation. In a previous animal study Walter and Charamonte reported similar findings in subcutaneous implants.[93] Nineteen albino mice received surgically implanted Ivalon sponges, resulting in a persistent giant cell reaction that surrounded the implant beginning on the fifth day. Granulomas gradually matured to scarring in all animals and the implants maintained their volume. There have been no reports of migration of Ivalon sponges.

Unfortunately, cancer cells grew at a few of the Ivalon implant sites. One animal in Walter's study developed a prominent bulge with areas of fibroblastic proliferation at the site of implant at 29 months. Two other animals also developed tumors. One was an obvious sarcoma, the other a fibroma or low-grade fibrosarcoma. Many resist using Ivalon based on these results alone. Alternately, the size and shape of the implant influence tumor development and may be more important in tumor growth than the type of material implanted, particularly in rats.[94] No reports exist of Ivalon-related tumors in humans.

TECHNIQUE

O'Donnell and Puri The principle of the STING is identical to that of open ureteroneocystostomy—to create a solid support behind the refluxing intravesical ureter.[6] With the STING, this support is created by injection of the implant beneath the affected ureteral orifice.

The patient is placed in the dorsal lithotomy position and cystoscopy is performed. The patient's legs should be wide enough apart to provide good visualization and access to each ureter. The location and configuration of the ureteral orifice are carefully evaluated. Lateral or gaping ureteral orifices are more difficult to treat, particularly with less viscous substances such as collagen or fat.

After cystoscopic examination, the bladder is drained to provide just enough distention to allow inspection of the trigone. With the bladder less full, the ureteral tunnels are easier to inject (Figure 87-6A). The appropriate needle is primed to prevent injection of air or irrigant at the implant site and advanced into the orifice at the 6-o'clock position. The needle is then advanced the appropriate distance to support the trigone but not so far as to result in injection outside Waldeyer's sheath into the detrusor or extravesical space. The needle must be just under the urothelium. The initial injection should be made very gently to assess the location of the implant (Figure 87-6B). If an immediate hump is not identified, the needle is either buried too deep in the trigone or advanced too far into Waldeyer's sheath and should be repositioned. The injection is then continued to raise an implant appropriate to close the ureteral orifice and provide significant backing to the ureter (Figure 87-6C). As the injection proceeds, the distal ureter flattens and the orifice closes, assuming a slit-like configuration near the top of the implant mound at the conclusion of the procedure. Depending on the substance, the implant should slightly overcorrect (or over-close) the ureteral orifice. The delivery agent (glycerine, saline solution, or sodium hyaluronate) is absorbed within the first month, leaving the implant behind. This may reduce the precision of the injection somewhat, but this phenomenon is readily overcome as one becomes familiar with the technique. Most refluxing ureters require 1.0 mL of implant, and many need as little as 0.05 to 0.2 mL. The needle should be kept in position for 30 to 60 seconds after injection to prevent extrusion of the implant.[95] A ureteral catheter can be helpful in laterally placed ureters or in those with gaping orifices. The catheter is used to elevate the ureteral orifice to allow more precise placement of the needle just beneath the urothelium.

Duplex systems can be injected without difficulty. The injection is placed just superficial to the wall of the upper-pole ureter. Care must be taken to prevent perforation of the upper-pole ureter, which will not always be apparent. Placement of a ureteral catheter is particularly helpful in duplex systems. The injection is identical to that for single-system ureters and a similar appearance at the end of the injection is desirable.

Repeat injections may be necessary. If reflux recurs or if, despite several attempts to correct it, reflux still exists, a second or even a third or fourth injection may be necessary.[96] At the time of repeat injection, the previous implant is often seen lateral or proximal to the ureteral orifice. The same injection technique can then be used to correct the reflux. In some cases, the second injection may be more satisfactory than the first since scar-

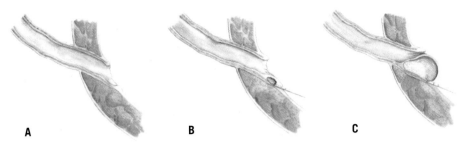

Figure 87-6 After cystoscopic examination, the bladder is drained to provide just enough distention to allow inspection of the trigone. *A,* With the bladder less full, the ureteral tunnels are easier to inject. *B,* The initial injection should be made very gently to assess the location of the implant. *C,* The injection is then continued to raise an implant appropriate to close the ureteral orifice and provide significant backing to the ureter. (Image provide by Q-Med, Uppsala, Sweden.)

ring beneath the ureteral orifice may tend to stabilize the implant site and make extravasation outside Waldeyer's sheath less likely.

Patients with persistent VUR following ureteroneocystostomy may also be treated. Following unsuccessful ureteral advancement procedures, the implant should be placed as previously described, just beneath the ureteral orifice. Following an unsuccessful cross-trigonal reimplantation, the injection should be at right angles to the path of the ureter at or near the ureteral orifice.

KIRSCH AND COLLEAGUES The technique employed by Kirsh and colleagues for implantation of dextranomer/hyaluronic acid copolymer is so similar to the STING procedure described above that they named their technique the "modified STING."[26] A 9.5 or 10F pediatric cystoscope with an offset lens allowing for direct pas-

sage of the 3.7F needle is preferred. The needle is thus inserted unbent and can then be properly manipulated without inadvertent damage to the mucosa of the bladder and bladder neck, causing bothersome bleeding. The bladder is filled to half or three-quarters volume, permitting visualization of the ureteral orifice and intraluminal ureter (Figure 87-7A). This volume will prevent distortion and tension of the ureteral submucosa caused by overdistention. Hydrodistention of the ureter is performed by directing a pressurized jet of irrigant at the ureteral orifice to open it before injection (Figure 87-7B). This maneuver allows for identification of the ureteral submucosal injection site.

With hydrodistention, the needle is inserted (with the bevel up) approximately 4 mm into the submucosa of the mid to distal ureteral tunnel at the 6-o'clock position (Figure 87-7C). The needle

used has been modified to have a black mark 4 mm proximal from the bevel. A small amount of implant (less than 0.1 mL) is injected to confirm location (Figure 87-7D). To avoid leakage of material and ensure good visualization, continued irrigation is avoided. The cystoscope is then brought back to the bladder neck with care not to dislodge the needle. This cystoscope position allows for observation of ineffective caudal, medial, or lateral tracking of the implant that might not otherwise be noticed if only the ureteral orifice and tunnel are in the visual field. The needle tip can be repositioned for another injection if optimal implantation is not achieved, but multiple needle holes can lead to leakage of material.

A fully coapted ureter is the end result of a proper implantation (Figure 87-7E). Kirsch and colleagues emphasize that the most critical part of the procedure is to place the needle in the submucosal plane so that material can travel cephalad within the ureteral submucosa, maximizing the length of ureteral coaptation. Volume of injected material ranges from 0.5 to 1.5 mL per ureter. Hydrodistention of the ureter after injection should reveal a properly coapted ureter. Observation for efflux from the ureteral orifice to confirm antegrade flow of urine is not necessary because Kirsch and his colleagues have not had any incidents of hydronephrosis from this modified STING technique. The modified STING had significantly improved the reflux-free rate to 92% from 79% for the standard STING.[26]

A learning curve was observed by Kirsch and colleagues with their previous injection technique. The initial success rate for the first 20

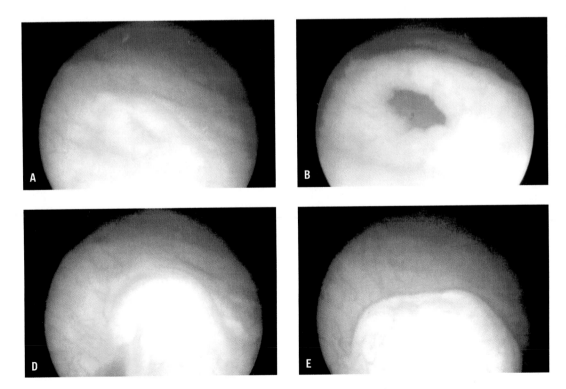

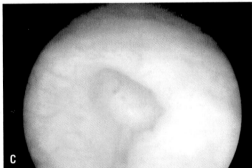

Figure 87-7 Demonstration of endoscopic injection of implant. *A,* Ureteral orifice prior to injection. *B,* Hydrodistention of the ureter by directing pressurized irrigant at the ureteral orifice. This dilates the ureter and allows for localization of the ureteral submucosa area in which to place the needle. *C,* Placement of the needle into the mid to distal ureteral tunnel. Hydrodistention of the ureter prior to needle insertion has allowed for optimal visualization. *D,* Preliminarily injecting a small volume to confirm the location of the implant. Once location is confirmed, the cystoscope is pulled back to the bladder neck with care not to dislodge or manipulate the needle. The remainder of the implant is injected while looking for caudal, medial, or lateral tracking of implant. *E,* Appearance at completion of injection. Note the raised mound with a crescent opening at the top, indicating a well coapted ureter. (Reprinted with permission from A. Kirsch.)

patients was 60%, which improved to 80% for the last 20 patients.[39] Hence, patient outcomes should improve with greater technical experience.

POSTOPERATIVE CARE

Patients are continued on antibiotic prophylaxis for 3 months, at which time a voiding cystogram is obtained. If reflux is no longer present, antibiotic prophylaxis is discontinued, and the patient is followed closely for signs of infection. It is essential that the patient and his or her family be aware that reflux may return if migration or breakdown of the implant occurs. The child's family is instructed to return if the child shows signs of febrile urinary tract infection. No subsequent voiding cystograms are obtained unless signs of upper urinary tract infection are present. Ultrasound imaging of the kidneys and bladder is performed annually to assess the position, size, and location of the implant.

RESULTS

Despite the array of substances emerging for correction of VUR, only four—Deflux, Polytef, collagen, and Macroplastique—have been used in humans in large enough numbers to enable assessment of effectiveness.

DEFLUX In the first-ever human trial with Deflux, Stenberg and Läckgren[40] noted excellent success in both low and high grades of reflux. Their initial report involved patients with primarily grade III and IV reflux. Overall success in 62.7% of ureters with a single injection was reported in this initial series. These results are comparable to or better than those reported with both collagen and Polytef when compared grade for grade.[40,45,97] All patients tolerated the injection well. Kirsch and colleagues recently reported a 76% reflux-free rate for 137 cases treated with a single injection with at least 3 months of follow-up.[26] Puri and colleagues had even better results, with 86% cure rate after a single injection with median follow-up of 6 months. They were able to render all 166 ureters reflux-free after a second or third injection.[98] A long-term follow-up by Läckgren and colleagues reported a 68% response rate (grade I or less) after 1 to 3 treatments in patients who mainly had grades III and IV reflux.[99]

As of this writing, no reports exist of problems at the time of ureteroneocystotomy after failed Deflux implant. In a recent study, Stenberg and colleagues excised the Deflux implant and surrounding tissue at the time of ureteral reimplant. Histologically, giant–cell-type granulomatous reaction, inflammatory cell infiltration, and implant pseudo-encapsulation commonly associated with foreign bodies were observed. Also present were calcifications (Figure 87-8).[100] These findings suggest that Deflux is safe for use in children with vesicoureteral reflux.

Because of its organic composite, large particle size, and minimal local tissue reaction, Deflux may be a more attractive choice for injection than Polytef or Macroplastique. If follow-up continues to show good long-term success, Deflux should gain even more popularity as the implant for the treatment of VUR in the United States.

POLYTEF Polytef was the most widely used substance. Puri and colleagues[96] reported treatment in 12,251 ureters in 8,332 children from 53 pediatric urologists and pediatric surgeons at 41 centers worldwide. This study included patients with all grades of VUR, but 61% of the ureters were grade III or IV. Collectively, 89% of ureters were rendered reflux-free with up to four injections.[96] Nearly all (93%) patients underwent STING as an outpatient procedure. These figures are similar to those reported earlier by Puri and O'Donnell[101] for high-grade reflux. The large number of patients in this series demonstrates how popular this procedure had become throughout the world. That numerous centers can duplicate the success of Puri and O'Donnell underscored the effectiveness of the technique in various hands.

Polytef injection has been particularly effective in adults[29] and in patients with primary VUR prior to renal transplantation.[30,31] It has also been used in the refluxing allograft ureter in transplant recipients with recurrent urinary tract infection.[33]

Most centers have obtained cystograms at 3 months, 1 year, and 3 years after implantation. Seventy percent of all patients treated have remained cured after 1 year.[102] Puri and colleagues[95] report a 93% persistent cure rate in infants followed from 1 to 9 years.

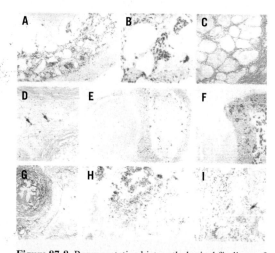

Figure 87-8 Representative histopathological findings of dissected distal ureter, including dextranomer-hyaluronic acid copolymer implant. *A*, Granulomatous reaction with multinucleated giant cells within implant, which is surrounded by fibrotic pseudocapsule. *B*, Typical giant cells at high magnification. *C*, Fibrotic bands (red areas) surround pseudocapsule and extend between individual dextranomer pearls (yellow areas). *D*, Section of fibrotic ureteral wall shows mast cells (arrows). *E*, Cross-section of distal ureter (left side) and implant (right side) reveals central degeneration of dextranomer pearls. *F*, Cross-section of distal ureter and implant demonstrates persistent dextranomer pearls. *G*, Accumulation of fibrotic tissue around muscle fibers in ureter and within pseudocapsule surrounding implant. *H*, Calcification (dark brown and black areas) within implant. *I*, Isolated eosinophils (arrows) between dextranomer pearls.[100]

Forty-one ureters (0.33%) in this study developed vesicoureteral junction obstruction following STING and required reimplantation. The follow-up status was not indicated, but the previously reported subset of 20 reimplanted ureters from the European centers indicated that all those patients did well and underwent uneventful ureteroneocystotomy.[45] Puri and associates reported no untoward side effects from the implant technique or the Teflon. Nevertheless, the animal data on migration of the smaller particles[47–49,103] and isolated reports of migration in humans[53,104] make widespread acceptance of this material for use in children in the United States unlikely.

COLLAGEN Results following collagen injection have not been as favorable as those with Deflux or Polytef. Leonard and colleagues[105] reported 75% of ureters corrected at 1 month. Of that group, 79% had a persistent cure at 1 year, for an overall success rate of 61% in primary nonduplicated ureters (Figure 87-9). Success was not as good for higher grades of reflux. A few patients were cured at 1 month and had recurrent reflux at 1 year. Leonard's series included a child in whom collagen injection had been unsuccessful; that patient returned with pyelonephritis and was hospitalized. Recurrence becomes a serious problem if antibiotic prophylaxis is stopped and pyelonephritis occurs. Although certainly possible, this occurrence is probably uncommon. Frey and colleagues reported recurrence rates of up to 50% following collagen injection with many late recurrences, but not one episode of pyelonephritis was noted in their large series.[97] More recently, Haferkamp and colleagues reported 91% recurrence rate at 37 months follow-up for their cohort of 58 ureters treated with a single injection.[67] They did find a statistically significant prolongation of reflux-free period for ureters injected a second time compared to those that

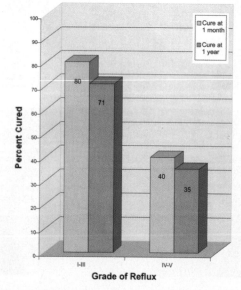

Figure 87-9 Collagen injection success rate in primary non-duplicated ureters. Note injection was not as effective for high-grade reflux and both groups had some recurrences within the first year.[105]

only had one injection. Still, 62% of the ureters that underwent a repeat injection had VUR at a mean follow-up of 10 months.[68]

Morbidity from endoscopic injection of collagen is minimal. Irritative voiding symptoms have occurred but these, too, are minimal. One patient in Leonard's series required readmission for catheterization and overnight hospitalization to monitor an episode of clot retention. In patients who have a failed injection or a recurrence, the implant is often displaced or considerably decreased in size. Neither Frey nor Leonard noted difficulty in reimplanting previously injected ureters in patients who opted for open repair after unsuccessful endoscopic treatment.

A few patients have developed minor reactions to the collagen skin test, generally a self-limited rash or raised wheal at the site of injection. One patient in the series of Lipsky and Wurn-schimmel developed anaphylactic shock following injection.[106] It is unclear whether this patient reacted to the collagen or to the lidocaine added to the implant. The theoretical risk of an autoimmune response is probably unfounded. Patients with positive skin tests following intradermal injection of bovine collagen have not demonstrated cross-reactivity to native collagens.[107,108]

MACROPLASTIQUE Macroplastique has been injected in 114 children with grade II to IV reflux. An initial report quoted a cure rate higher than 90% with follow-up between 6 and 30 months.[69] More recently, Abontaleb and colleagues reported a similar cure rate of 92% using a single injection with an average follow-up of 12 months.[71] Like Polytef, however, concerns of particle migration will likely prevent widespread popularity in the United States.

COMPARISON OF ENDOSCOPIC AND STANDARD TECHNIQUES

A recent meta-analysis of randomized controlled trials concluded that little benefit from additional surgery over antibiotics alone is measurable.[109] Although successful correction of reflux was associated with fewer febrile urinary tract infections, it was difficult to measure a surgical benefit in terms of fewer renal scars, even with long-term follow-up.

Nevertheless, the current standard of care is to operatively correct VUR in children who fail a trial of prophylactic antibiotics. With this in mind, surgeons must continue to compare the value of endoscopic VUR correction to that of the standard open reimplant. Until we have a technique and a substance that equals or surpasses the 95% success rate following open surgical repair, endoscopic correction will continue to be considered an alternative to ureteroneocystostomy, despite the increased pain, hospital stay, and scarring following an open repair.

Even with widespread experience, the success rate in high-grade reflux with a single injection of any of the available substances still fails to equal that following open ureteroneocystostomy.

The initial results following a single injection (and a single anesthetic) for each of the current substances are still too low for many parents. A meta-analysis conducted by Elder and colleagues showed success rates of 57% to 77% for a single injection of the four most widely used substances (Figure 87-10). The overall resolution rate was 72%, which included results from chondrocyte and blood studies (not depicted in Figure 87-10).[110] Success rates with one injection for a high grade of reflux is 51% to 63% regardless of the substance used (Figure 87-11). Elder and associates also reported the probability of recurrent reflux after treatment to be 9.25%.[110] Combining these data, about 50% of children with a high grade of reflux will not be cured without multiple injections. Additional treatments, however, improve the success rates. Elder's meta-analysis reports a success rate of 85% with multiple treatments. With these results, despite the need for additional anesthetics, many families elect an endoscopic treatment approach to avoid the trauma of open surgery.

Even if the cure rate does not equal that of open surgical correction, additional protection may be provided from ascending infection while awaiting spontaneous resolution of reflux. By offering Deflux as an alternative to ureteroneocystostomy for patients who fail conservative medical management, Kobelt and colleagues calculated a savings of $1,118 (16.8%) per patient for similar cure rates over a treatment course of 6 years.[111] Adults with recurrent infections and pyelonephritis are candidates for primary endoscopic treatment, as are transplant recipients with infections associated with the native or allograft ureter. Open surgery in these patients is less–well-tolerated and not as successful. Children with persistent reflux following ureteroneocystostomy are usually successfully treated endoscopically, with minimal morbidity, and should be given this option prior to consideration of "redo" ureteroneocystostomy.

When one considers the multiple factors resulting in renal scarring along with Wheeler's study[109] suggesting minimal benefit of open surgery over prophylactic antibiotics, it becomes more and more difficult to recommend ureteroneocystostomy as an alternative for those families wishing to discontinue antibiotic prophylaxis. The substantial increase in pain and duration of hospitalization may not be worth the convenience afforded by the open approach of being off prophylactic antibiotics. In a study from Italy conducted by Capozza and colleagues, 80% of the parents with children diagnosed with grade III VUR chose endoscopic treatment over prophylactic antibiotics (5%) or open reimplant (2%).[112] The parents were given detailed information (including expected risks, benefits, cure rates, and mechanisms of action) on all three treatment options prior to completing a treatment preference questionnaire. It is very conceivable that parents in North America will similarly select endoscopy overwhelmingly over antibiotic prophylaxis or open surgery if given the choice.

CONCLUSION

More than two decades have passed since the initial report by O'Donnell and Puri[6] of the use of STING in their first 13 patients. The technique is sound. The debate over optimal implant material appears to be over, as previously differing camps and proponents of other substances have adopted the use of dextranomer/hyaluronic acid copolymer throughout the world. Use of other materials has become less common as the use of Deflux gains momentum, but more experience and long-term follow-up are needed before Deflux is declared the "ideal substance." With continued acceptance, success, and minimal to no side effects from Deflux, endoscopy will gain a permanent and prominent place in the treatment of vesicoureteral reflux.

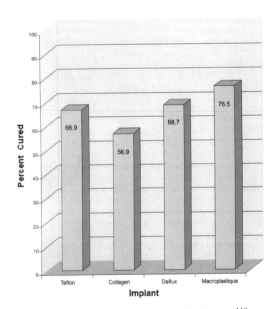

Figure 87-10 Success rate with a single injection.[110]

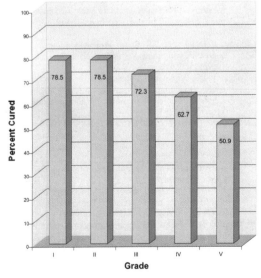

Figure 87-11 Results according to vesicoureteral reflux grade after a single injection of implant.[110]

REFERENCES

1. Matouschek E. Treatment of vesicoureteral reflux by transurethral Teflon injection. Urologe 1981;20:263.
2. Politano V, Molina L, Lynne C. Endoscopic correction of vesicoureteral reflux with Polytef paste. Presented at the American Urological Association 83rd Annual Meeting, Boston, MA, 1988.
3. McDonald H Jr, McDonald H Sr. Treatment of vesicoureteral reflux using endoscopic Teflon paste injection. Presented at the American Urological Association, Abstract 446, Las Vegas, NV, 1983.
4. Puri P, O'Donnell B. Correction of experimentally produced vesicoureteric reflux in the piglet by intravesical injection of Teflon. Br Med J 1984;289:5.
5. O'Donnell B, Puri P. Endoscopic correction of primary vesicoureteric reflux: results in 94 ureters. Br Med J 1986; 293:1404.
6. O'Donnell B, Puri P. Treatment of vesicoureteric reflux by endoscopic injection of Teflon. Br Med J 1984;289:7.
7. Bailey R. Vesicoureteral reflux and reflux nephropathy. In: Schrier R, Gottschalk C, editors. Diseases of the kidney; 1988. p. 747–83.
8. Walker R, Duckett J, Bartone F, et al. Screening school children for urologic disease. Birth Defects 1977;13:399.
9. Walker R. Vesicoureteral reflux. In: Gillenwater J, Grayhack J, Howards S, et al, editors. Adult and pediatric urology. Vol 2. 2nd ed. Chicago: Year Book Medical Publishers; 1992. p. 1889–920.
10. Schwab CW Jr, Wu HY, Selman H, et al. Spontaneous resolution of vesicoureteral reflux: a 15-year perspective. J Urol 2002;168:2594.
11. Ransley P, Risdon R. Renal papillae and intra-renal reflux in the pig. Lancet 1974;2:1114.
12. Ransley P, Risdon R. Reflux nephropathy: effects of antimicrobial therapy on the evolution of the early pyelonephritic scar. Kidney Int 1981;20:733.
13. Ransley P, Risdon R, Godley M. High pressure sterile vesicoureteral reflux and renal scarring: an experimental study in the pig and minipig. Contrib Nephrol 1984;39:320.
14. Weiss R, Duckett J, Spitzer A. Results of a randomized clinical trial of medical versus surgical management of infants and children with grades III and IV primary vesicoureteral reflux (United States). The International Reflux Study in Children. J Urol 1992;148:1667.
15. Smellie JM, Barratt TM, Chantler C, et al. Medical versus surgical treatment in children with severe bilateral vesicoureteric reflux and bilateral nephropathy: a randomised trial.[see comment]. Lancet 2001;357:1329.
16. Smellie JM, Jodal U, Lax H. et al. Outcome at 10 years of severe vesicoureteric reflux managed medically: Report of the International Reflux Study in Children [see comment]. Journal of Pediatrics 2001;139:656.
17. Duckett JW, Walker RD, Weiss R. Surgical results: International Reflux Study in Children—United States branch. J Urol 1992;148:1674.
18. Skoog SJ, Belman AB, Majd M. A nonsurgical approach to the management of primary vesicoureteral reflux. J Urol 1987;138:941.
19. Zerin JM, Chen E, Ritchey ML, et al. Bladder capacity as measured at voiding cystourethrography in children: relationship to toilet training and frequency of micturition. Radiology 1993;187:803.
20. Sillen U, Hjalmas K, Aili M, et al. Pronounced detrusor hypercontractility in infants with gross bilateral reflux. J Urol 1992;148:598.
21. Mozley PD, Heyman S, Duckett JW, et al. Direct vesicoureteral scintigraphy: quantifying early outcome predictors in children with primary reflux [see comments]. J Nucl Med 1994;35:1602.
22. Hinman F Jr, Baumann FW. Complications of vesicoureteral operations from incoordination of micturition. J Urol 1976;116:638.
23. Noe HN. The role of dysfunctional voiding in failure or complication of ureteral reimplantation for primary reflux. J Urol 1985;134:1172.
24. Stenberg A, Hensle TW, Lackgren G. Vesicoureteral reflux: a new treatment algorithm. Current Urology Reports 2002; 3:107.
25. Capozza N, Caione P. Dextranomer/hyaluronic acid copolymer implantation for vesico-ureteral reflux: a randomized comparison with antibiotic prophylaxis. J Pediatr 2002; 140:230.
26. Kirsch AJ, Perez-Brayfield M, Smith EA, et al. The modified sting procedure to correct vesicoureteral reflux: improved results with submucosal implantation within the intramural ureter. J Urol 2004;171:2413.
27. Lackgren G, Lottmann H, Hensle TW, et al. Endoscopic treatment of vesicoureteral reflux and urinary incontinence in children. AUA Update Series 2003;22:294.
28. Yachia D. Submeatal injection of polytetrafluoroethylene paste for the endoscopic treatment of vesicoureteric reflux in adults. Br J Urol 1989;64:552.
29. Giannotti P, Pistolesi D, Murzi P, et al. Treatment of vesicorenal reflux in adults by endoscopic injection of Teflon. Acta Urol Belg 1986;54:168.
30. Sironvalle MS, Gelet A, Martin X, et al. Endoscopic treatment of vesicoureteral reflux prior to renal transplantation. Transpl Int 1992;5:231.
31. Oza UG, Punjani HM, Thatte SW, et al. Management of vesicoureteral reflux in renal transplant recipients by endoscopic Teflon injection. Transplant Proc 1992;24.
32. Jackson CL, Kay R, Bretan P, et al. Endoscopic correction of vesicoureteral reflux in the renal transplant candidate. J Urol 1989;142:710.
33. Cloix P, Gelet A, Desmettre O, et al. Endoscopic treatment of vesicoureteric reflux in transplanted kidneys. Br J Urol 1993;72:20.
34. Puri P, Guiney EJ. Endoscopic correction of vesicoureteric reflux secondary to neuropathic bladder. Br J Urol 1986; 58:504.
35. Quinn FM, Diamond T, Boston VE. Endoscopic management of vesico-ureteric reflux in children with neuropathic bladder secondary to myelomeningocoele. Z Kinderchir 1988;2:43.
36. Hulbert WC, Rosenberg HK, Cartwright PC, et al. The predictive value of ultrasonography in evaluation of infants with posterior urethral valves. J Urol 1992;148:122.
37. Hollowell JG, Altman HG, Snyder HD, et al. Coexisting ureteropelvic junction obstruction and vesicoureteral reflux: diagnostic and therapeutic implications. J Urol 1989;142:490.
38. Johnston JH. Vesicoureteric reflux with urethral valves. Br J Urol 1979;51:100.
39. Kirsch AJ, Perez-Brayfield MR, Scherz HC. Minimally invasive treatment of vesicoureteral reflux with endoscopic injection of dextranomer/hyaluronic acid copolymer: the Children's Hospitals of Atlanta experience. J Urol 2003; 170:211.
40. Stenberg A, Lackgren G. A new bioimplant for the endoscopic treatment of vesicoureteral reflux: experimental and short-term clinical results. J Urol 1995;154:800.
41. O'Donnell B, Puri P. Technical refinements in endoscopic correction of vesicoureteral reflux. Presented at the 56th Annual Meeting of the American Academy of Pediatrics, New Orleans, Louisiana, 1987.
42. O'Donnell B, Puri P. Technical refinements in endoscopic correction of vesicoureteral reflux. J Urol 1988;140:1101.
43. O'Donnell B. Progress in the management of vesicoureteric reflux. Postgrad Med J 1990;66:S44.
44. Puri P, Granata C. Multicenter survey of endoscopic treatment of vesicoureteral reflux using polytetrafluoroethylene. J Urol 1998;160:1007.
45. Puri P, Ninan GK, Surana R. Subureteric Teflon injection (STING). Results of a European survey. Eur Urol 1995; 27:71.
46. Malizia A, Dewanjee M, Reiman H, et al. Polytef (Teflon) migration after periurethral injection: tracer and x-ray microanalysis techniques in experimental study. Trans Am Soc Artif Intern Organs 1983;30:330.
47. Malizia A, Reiman H, Myers R, et al. Migration and granulomatous reaction after periurethral injection of Polytef (Teflon). JAMA 1984;251:3277.
48. Aaronson IA, Rames RA, Greene WB, et al. Endoscopic treatment of reflux: migration of Teflon to the lungs and brain. European Urology 1993;23:394.
49. Malizia A, Rushton H, Woodard J, et al. Migration and granulomatous reaction after intravesical-subureteric injection of Polytef [Abstract]. J Urol. Presented at the 82nd annual meeting of the American Urological Association, Anaheim, CA, 1987.
50. Malizia A, Woodard J, Rushton H, et al. Intravesical subureteric injection of Polytef: serial radiologic imaging [Abstract]. J Urol. Presented at the 83rd annual meeting of the American Urological Association, Boston, Massachusetts, 1988.
51. Spencer J, Donaldson J, Zaontz M, et al. The sting: postoperative evaluation for granuloma development in the pediatric patient. J. Urol, Abstract 93, presented at the 83rd annual meeting of the American Urological Association, Boston, Massachusetts, 1988.
52. Mittleman R, Marracini J. Pulmonary Teflon granulomas following periurethral Teflon injection for urinary incontinence. Arch Path Lab Med 1983;107:611.
53. Claes H, Stroobants D, Van Meerbeek J, et al. Pulmonary migration following periurethral polytetrafluoroethylene injection for urinary incontinence [see comments]. J Urol 1989;142:821.
54. Gelet A, Salas M, Martin X. et al. [Vesico-ureteral-renal reflux in the adult. Preliminary results of endoscopic treatment]. Presse Med 1988;17:373.
55. Kaplan WE. Endoscopic injection of polytetrafluoroethylene for treatment of vesicoureteral reflux. Urol Clin North Am 1988;15:777.
56. Lynne C, Politano V. Periureteral Teflon injection for vesicoureteral reflux. Presented at the 78th annual meeting of the American Urological Association, Las Vegas, Nevada, 1983.
57. Schulman C, Simon J, Pamart D, et al. Endoscopic treatment of vesicoureteral reflux in children. J Urol 1987;138:950.
58. Peters C, Jeffs R. Endoscopic correction of vesicoureteral reflux with bovine collagen injected submucosally at the ureteral orifice. J Urol, Abstract 76, presented at the 82nd annual meeting of the American Urological Association, Anaheim, California, 1987.
59. McPherson J, Sawamura S, Conti A. Preparation of (3H) collagen for studies of the biologic fat of xenogenic collagen implants in vivo. J Invest Derm 1986;66:673.
60. McPherson J, Wallace D, Sawamura S, Conti A, et al. Collagen fibrillogenesis in vitro: a characterization of fibrell quantity as a function of assembly conditions. Collagen Rel Res 1985;5:119.
61. McPherson J, Ledger P, Sawamura S, et al. The preparation in physicochemical characterization of an injectable form of reconstituted, glutaraldehyde cross-linked bovine collagen. J Biomed Mat Res 1986;20:79.
62. McPherson J, Sawamura S, Armstrong R. An examination of the biologic response to injectable, cross-linked collagen implants. J Biomed Mat Res 1986;20:93.
63. Canning D, Peters C, Gearhart J, et al. Local tissue response to glutaraldehyde cross-linked collagen in the rabbit bladder. J Urol Abstract 381, presented at the 83rd annual meeting of the American Urological Association, Boston, Massachusetts, 1988.
64. Frey P, Berger D, Jenny P, et al. Subureteral collagen injection for the endoscopic treatment of vesicoureteral reflux in children. Follow-up study of 97 treated ureters and histological analysis of collagen implants. J Urol 1992;148:718.
65. Frey P, Lutz N, Berger D, et al. Histological behavior of glutaraldehyde cross-linked bovine collagen injected into the human bladder for the treatment of vesicoureteral reflux. J Urol 1994;152:632.
66. Leonard MP, Canning DA, Epstein JI, et al. Local tissue reaction to the subureteral injection of glutaraldehyde cross-linked bovine collagen in humans. J Urol 1990;143:1209.
67. Haferkamp A, Contractor H, Mohring K, et al. Failure of subureteral bovine collagen injection for the endoscopic treatment of primary vesicoureteral reflux in long-term follow-up. Urology 2000;55:759.
68. Haferkamp A, Mohring K, Staehler G, et al. Pitfalls of repeat subureteral bovine collagen injections for the endoscopic treatment of vesicoureteral reflux. J Urol 2000;163:1919.
69. Schulman C. Use of particulate silicone microimplants for the endoscopic correction of vesicoureteric reflux in children. Dialogues in Pediatric Urology 1994;17:6.
70. Smith DP, Kaplan WE, Oyasu R. Evaluation of polydimethylsiloxane as an alternative in the endoscopic treatment of vesicoureteral reflux [see comments] [published erratum appears in J Urol 1994 Dec;152(6 Pt 1):2108]. J Urol 1994;152:1221.
71. Aboutaleb H, Bolduc S, Upadhyay J, et al. Subureteral polydimethylsiloxane injection versus extravesical reimplantation for primary low grade vesicoureteral reflux in children: a comparative study. J Urol 2003;169:313.
72. Newman J, Ftaiha Z. The biographical history of fat transplant surgery. Am J Cosmetic Surgery 1987;4:85.
73. Johnson G. Body contouring by macroinjection of autologous fat. Am J Cosmetic Surgery 1987;4:103.
74. Wetmore S. Injection of fat for soft tissue augmentation. Laryngoscope 1989;99:50.
75. Matthews RD, Christensen JP, Canning DA. Persistence of autologous free fat transplant in bladder submucosa of rats. J Urol 1994;152:819.
76. Billings E, May J. Historical review and present status of free fat graft autotransplantation in plastic and reconstructive surgery. Plast Reconstr Surg1989;83:368.
77. Santiago Gonzalez de Garibay AM, Castillo Jimeno JM, Villanueva Perez I, et al. [Injection of autologous fatty tissue in the bladder submucosa: experimental study in swine]. Arch Esp Urol 1992;45:985.
78. Canning D, Seibold J, Saito M, et al. Use of injectable fat to

obstruct the urethra in rabbits. Neurourol Urodyn 1995; 14:259.

79. Cendron M, Devore D, Connolly R, et al. The biological behavior of autologous collagen injected into the rabbit bladder. J Urol 1995;154:808.

80. DeVore D, Kelman C, Fagien S, et al. Autologen: autologous, injectable dermal collagen. In: Basniak S, editor. Principles and practices in ophthalmic, plastic and reconstructive surgery. New York: W.B. Saunders; 1995. p. 492–499.

81. Cozzolino DJ, Cendron M, DeVore DP, et al. The biological behavior of autologous collagen-based extracellular matrix injected into the rabbit bladder wall. Neurourol Urodyn 1999;18:487.

82. Remmler D, Thomas J, Mazoujian G, et al. Use of injectable cultured human fibroblasts for percutaneous tissue implantation and experimental study. Arch Otolaryngol Head Neck Surg 1989;115:837.

83. Klagsburn M. Large-scale preparation of chondrocytes. Meth Enzymol 1979;58:560.

84. Vacanti C, Langer R, Schloo B, et al. Synthetic polymers seeded with chondrocytes provide a template for new cartilage formation. Plast Reconst Surg 1991;88:753.

85. Atala A, Kim W, Paige KT, et al. Endoscopic treatment of vesicoureteral reflux with a chondrocyte-alginate suspension. J Urol 1994;152:641.

86. Atala A, Cima LG, Kim W, et al. Injectable alginate seeded with chondrocytes as a potential treatment for vesicoureteral reflux. J Urol 1993;150:745.

87. Caldamone AA, Diamond DA. Long-term results of the endoscopic correction of vesicoureteral reflux in children using autologous chondrocytes. J Urol 2001;165:2224.

88. Atala A, Peters CA, Retik AB, et al. Endoscopic treatment of vesicoureteral reflux with a self-detachable balloon system. J Urol 1992;148:724.

89. Walker RD, Wilson J, Clark AE. Injectable bioglass as a potential substitute for injectable polytetrafluoroethylene. J Urol 1992;148:645.

90. Wilson J, Noletti D. Bonding of soft tissues to Bioglass. In: Yamamuro T, Hench L, Wilson J, editors. Handbook of bioactive ceramics. Vol. I. Boca Raton: CRC Press; 1990. p. 283.

91. Hulman G, Kirkham J. Ivalon (polyvinyl alcohol) sponge presenting as an extrarectal mass. Histopathology 1990; 16:502.

92. Merguerian P, McLorie G, Khoury A, et al. Submucosal injection of polyvinyl alcohol foam in rabbit bladder. J Urol 1990;144:531.

93. Walter J, Charamonte L. The tissue responses of the rat to implanted Ivalon, Etheron, and polyfoam plastic sponges. Br J Surg 1965;52:49.

94. Oppenheimer B, Oppenheimer E, Stout A, et al. Studies of the mechanism of carcinogenesis by plastic films. Acta Int Cancer 1959;15:659.

95. Puri P, Palanimuthu M, Dass L. Endoscopic treatment of primary vesicoureteral reflux in infants by subureteric injection of polytetrafluoroethylene: a 9 year follow-up. Eur Uol 1995;27:67.

96. Puri P, Ninan G, Surana R. Subureteric Teflon injection (STING). Eur Urol 1995;27:71.

97. Frey P, Lutz N, Jenny P, et al. Endoscopic subureteral collagen injection for the treatment of vesicoureteral reflux in infants and children. J Urol 1995;154:804.

98. Puri P, Chertin B, Velayudham M, et al. Treatment of vesicoureteral reflux by endoscopic injection of dextranomer/hyaluronic acid copolymer: preliminary results. J Urol 2003;170:1541.

99. Lackgren G, Wahlin N, Skoldenberg E, et al. Long-term followup of children treated with dextranomer/hyaluronic acid copolymer for vesicoureteral reflux. J Urol 2001;166:1887.

100. Stenberg A, Larsson E, Lackgren G. Endoscopic treatment with dextranomer-hyaluronic acid for vesicoureteral reflux: histological findings. J Urol 2003;169:1109.

101. Puri P, O'Donnell B. Endoscopic correction of grades IV and V primary vesicoureteric reflux: six to 30 month follow-up in 42 ureters. J Pediatr Surg 1987;22:1087.

102. Vereecken R, Proesmans W. Results of endoscopic treatment for vesico-ureteric reflux. Eur Urol 1995;27:76.

103. Kossovsky N, Millett D, Juma S, et al. In vivo characterization of the inflammatory properties of poly(tetrafluoroethylene) particulates [published erratum appears in J Biomed Mater Res 1992;26:269]. J Biomed Mater Res 1991;25:1287.

104. Leth PM. [Spread of teflon particles from periurethrally injected teflon paste to pulmonary tissue]. Ugeskr Laeger 1994;156:981.

105. Leonard MP, Canning DA, Peters CA. et al. Endoscopic injection of glutaraldehyde cross-linked bovine dermal collagen for correction of vesicoureteral reflux [comment]. J Urol 1991;145:115.

106. Lipsky H, Wurnschimmel E. Endoscopic treatment of vesicoureteric reflux with collagen. Five years' experience. Br J Urol 1993;72:965.

107. Cooperman L, Michaeli D. The immunigenicity of injectable collagen II. A retrospective review of seventy-two tested and treated patients. J Am Acad Derm 1984;10:647.

108. Ellingsworth L, Delustro F, Breiman J, et al. The human immune response to reconstituted bovine collagen. J Immunol 1986;136:877.

109. Wheeler D, Vimalachandra D, Hodson EM, et al. Antibiotics and surgery for vesicoureteric reflux: a meta-analysis of randomised controlled trials. Arch Dis Child 2003;88:688.

110. Elder JS, Diaz M, Caldamone AA, et al. Endoscopic therapy for vesicoureteral reflux: a meta-analysis. Reflux resolution and urinary tract infection. J Urol 2006;175:716.

111. Kobelt G, Canning DA, Hensle TW, et al. The cost-effectiveness of endoscopic injection of dextranomer/hyaluronic acid copolymer for vesicoureteral reflux. J Urol 2003; 169:1480.

112. Capozza N, Lais A, Matarazzo E, et al. Treatment of vesicoureteric reflux: a new algorithm based on parental preference. BJU Int 2003;92:285.

88

Endoscopic Treatment of Ureteroceles

Douglas E. Coplen, MD
Howard M. Snyder III, MD

Ureterocele is a cystic dilatation of the intravesical submucosal segment of the ureter. Earlier terminology concerning ureteroceles was a bit confusing, so guidelines were issued by the Committee on Terminology, Nomenclature and Classification of the Urology Section of the American Academy of Pediatrics.[1] The current recommended nomenclature classifies ureteroceles as either intravesical (entirely within the bladder) or ectopic (some portion is situated permanently at the bladder neck or in the urethra). The position of the orifice is not important in the classification. A single-system ureterocele is one associated with a kidney with a single ureter, whereas a duplex-system ureterocele is associated with the upper-pole ureter in a kidney with a complete ureteral duplication.

The embryology of ureteroceles is not entirely clear.[2–6] Historically, Chwalla suggested that ureteroceles arise after incomplete breakdown of a ureteral membrane that exists between the ureteral bud and mesonephric duct.[2] This theory would explain the majority of ureteroceles but does not explain the development of ureteroceles with patulous ureteral orifices in the urethra, ureteroceles associated with multicystic dysplasia and atretic ureteral segments, or the presence of ectopic ureters without ureterocele formation. Another theory is that the same forces that cause expansion of the urogenital sinus to form the bladder act on the distal ureteral segment.[3,5] With this theory, one would expect any ectopic ureter to be associated with a ureterocele—but this is clearly not the case. It is likely that a ureterocele is the result of an abnormal induction of the trigone and distal ureter by many of the genes and growth factors that are important in renal and ureteral growth and development. Stephens's histologic studies support this concept. Histologic analysis of the intravesical portion of ureteroceles shows deficiencies in the trigonal musculature of patients with ureteroceles that were not present in ectopic ureters without ureterocele formation.[5] This field defect results in pseudodiverticulum (ureterocele eversion) and reflux into laterally displaced, poorly supported ureters.

Campbell reported the incidence of ureteroceles to be 1 in 4,000 autopsies of children,[7] while Uson and colleagues reported an incidence of 1 in 500.[8] Ureteroceles are seen most commonly in whites and are unusual in blacks. Ureteroceles occur in females four to seven times more commonly than in males.[9] Although some series have demonstrated a slight left-sided predominance, about 10% occur bilaterally.[10] Sixty to 80% of ureteroceles are ectopic,[3,11,12] and about 80% are associated with the upper-pole ureter in a duplex kidney.[13] Single-system ectopic ureteroceles are unusual and occur most frequently in males; they may also be associated with cardiac and genital anomalies.[14] Rarely, ureteroceles have been reported with blind-ending ureters.[15] Associated urologic anomalies, particularly the renal anomalies of fusion and ectopia, are also seen with ureteroceles. When the ureterocele is associated with a duplex kidney, the upper pole exhibits dysplasia in about one-third of cases.[16,17]

Most ureteroceles are now detected with antenatal ultrasonography, although presentation with a urinary tract infection is still common.[18–20] Prolapse of a ureterocele in females may lead to bladder outlet obstruction; this is the most common urethral obstruction seen in girls.[21] Although less common, ureteroceles rarely obstruct the urethra in boys.[22] The ureteroceles that obstruct tend to "ball valve" into the bladder neck and are tense. Most ureteroceles are compressible during voiding and do not cause urethral obstruction even when they are ectopic. Rarely, a ureterocele may present with abdominal or flank pain. Incontinence is not a frequent presenting symptom, although occasionally a large ureterocele with an abnormally lax distorted bladder neck may lead to incontinence before or after the ureterocele is treated.[23,24] Husmann and colleagues reported a 5% post-pubertal incontinence rate in ectopic ureteroceles that had been treated solely with a partial nephrectomy.[19]

Ultrasound typically reveals a well-defined cystic intravesical mass that is associated with the posterior bladder wall (Figures 88-1 and 88-2).[25–27] This can be followed into a dilated ureter in the bony pelvis. A duplex renal unit with upper-pole hydroureteronephrosis is also commonly present. The thickness and echogenicity of the renal parenchyma should be evaluated since ureteroceles are often associated with dysplasia and poor function. An experienced pediatric radiologist is important because a full bladder may compress the ureterocele, and the mucosal irregularity of the bladder base might be missed. The dilated ureter behind the bladder may be mistaken for an ectopic ureter or a primary obstructive megaureter. The use of intravenous pyelography and the large spectrum of findings in patients with ureteroceles have been well reviewed (see Figure 88-1).[28] A well-executed voiding cystourethrogram is critically important to the evaluation of ureteroceles. There is ipsilateral lower-pole reflux in approximately 50% of patients with ureteroceles.[20,29] In approximately 25%, there is contralateral reflux, and in about 10%, there is reflux into the ureterocele itself.[29,30] Less frequently, reflux can occur into single-system ureteroceles.[29] This is generally into a wide-mouth ureterocele, a ruptured one, or a cecoureterocele.

Cystoscopic evaluation of ureteroceles can be challenging because the findings can be quite variable and frequently confusing. When a ureterocele is small, it may not be seen until a peristaltic wave or flank compression causes it to fill. With very large ureteroceles, cystoscopic identification of any ureteral orifice in the bladder may be impossible. With a large ureterocele and bilateral obstruction produced by the ureterocele, it can be difficult to tell from which system the ureterocele originated. In this situation, the use of a small needle wedged into the end of a fine ureteral catheter can be used to puncture the ureterocele under direct vision at cystoscopy, and injection of contrast medium may then permit an intraoperative radiograph that can define the anatomy. An alternative approach is to use a spinal needle passed transabdominally into the bladder and then into the ureterocele under cystoscopic control with an intraoperative x-ray examination. Because ureteroceles are compressible, it is important to examine the bladder carefully when it is nearly empty as well as when full. When a ureterocele has poor detrusor support and prolapses through the ureteral hiatus, the cystoscopic view may lead to misdiagnosis of the ureterocele as a bladder diverticulum.[31] When the bladder is emptied and the flank compressed, the ureterocele may be observed to refill, permitting a correct diagnosis. Trigonal cysts are very rare, but can at times be confused with a ureterocele when viewed cystoscopically.[32] Upper tract imaging should be used to distinguish these. Occasionally, the dilated lower end of an ectopic ureter may elevate the trigone, causing a pseudoureterocele, as demonstrated on ultrasonography, voiding cystourethrography, or even cystoscopy.[33] Because contralateral duplications are frequent with ureteroceles, one must make every effort to evaluate contralateral ureteral anatomy during cystoscopy to avoid possible damage to a ureteral orifice that was not readily apparent.

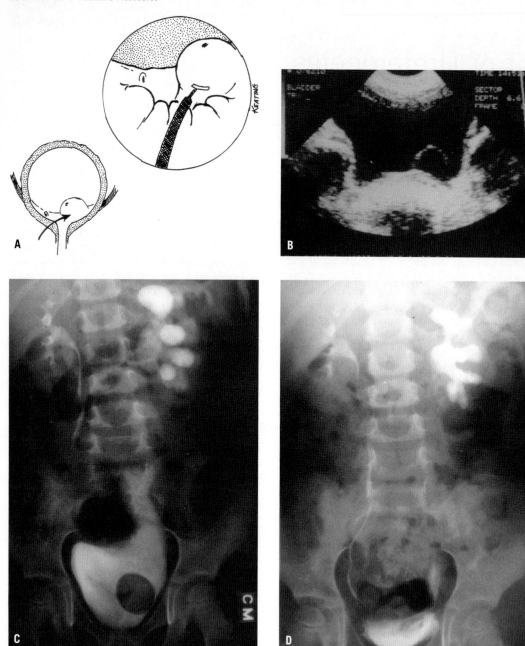

Figure 88-1 *A*, Low puncture incision of intravesical ureterocele. A short, low incision just above the bladder wall is made by an initial puncture and a minimal side movement of the Bugbee electrode. Keeping the bladder near empty preserves maximal ureterocele distention to facilitate the procedure. The incision should include the ureteral orifice only if it is low. *B*, Ultrasonographic scan of a single-system intravesical ureterocele. *C*, Intravenous pyelogram shows the hydroureteronephrotic left kidney with negative filling defect in the bladder produced by the ureterocele. *D*, Three months after ureterocele incision, an intravenous pyelogram shows good decompression. A voiding cystourethrogram also showed no reflux.

CHOICE OF TREATMENT STRATEGY

The goals of ureterocele treatment include control of infection, preservation of renal function, protection of normal ipsilateral and contralateral units, and maintaining continence. Several approaches including endoscopic decompression, staged reconstruction (upper-pole partial nephrectomy and bladder level surgery), or ureterocele excision and complete reconstruction have been used to accomplish these goals.

Historically, ureterocele incision was not popular because it often failed as a definitive procedure in relieving obstruction and avoiding

iatrogenic reflux. It is now apparent, however, that endoscopic incision is a useful alternative in the treatment of ureteroceles (see Figure 88-1). The management algorithm for ureteroceles is complex and is one of the areas of greatest sophistication in pediatric urologic management. A number of factors are worth careful consideration in determining how to treat a ureterocele. From the following discussion, it will become evident that, while endoscopic incision is attractive, it is not the solution for all children.

The age of the patient is an important consideration. It is clear that antenatal diagnosis decreases the overall incidence of infection in

these children since they are started on prophylaxis at birth. One non-randomized study, however, showed no difference in the incidence of infection in infants treated with early incision when compared to those managed on antibiotic prophylaxis.[34] When a ureterocele is detected antenatally, endoscopic incision provides simple and direct decompression of the obstructive uropathy. The procedure is also less morbid in older children in whom bladder-level surgery (ureterocele excision and bladder neck reconstruction) causes a considerable degree of voiding symptomatology and postoperative discomfort. An upper-pole partial nephrectomy can be safely performed at any age and reproducibly decompresses the ureterocele. It may be a better option than incision in some cases.[19,20]

The amount of functioning parenchyma must also be considered. If a child has never had pyelonephritis, salvage of functional renal parenchyma is theoretically possible. The upper-pole system serving a ureterocele, however, typically makes up only the parenchyma subserved by the upper-pole infundibulum.[17,35] Histologic evaluation of upper-pole nephrectomy specimens shows predominantly chronic inflammation and dysplasia regardless of antenatal diagnosis or detection after infection. Usually less than one-third of the renal function of one kidney is represented by the parenchyma, and preservation of function is not a major issue in decision making. There is little or no indication, however, for removing a poorly functioning renal unit that is serving a decompressed ureterocele with no reflux.

Single-system and duplex ureteroceles are entirely different clinical entities. The single system usually has excellent function, less hydronephrosis, is almost always intravesical, and may have indeterminate obstruction on lasix scintigraphy. Some can be managed expectantly in a fashion similar to the non-obstructed megaureter. If obstruction is present, the single-system ureterocele is best managed endoscopically with relief of obstruction without causing reflux nearly 100% of the time.[36–38] Open reconstruction is rarely required in this group of patients, but after endoscopic incision, the decompressed ureter is easier to reimplant if clinically significant reflux develops. When the renal unit is duplex, however, previously and subsequently discussed issues are more critical in deciding the appropriateness of a primary endoscopic approach.

The location of the ureterocele intravesically or ectopically is important because of the differences in endoscopic success and the need for subsequent open surgical procedures. Blyth and colleagues found that 82% of intravesical ureteroceles could be managed definitively with endoscopic incision (Table 88-1, and see Figure 88-2).[36] With ectopic ureteroceles, however, the success rate is much lower. Iatrogenic reflux occurs in 40% of children, and 60 to 70% eventually have bladder-level surgery to manage symptomatic vesicoureteral reflux (Table 88-2).

Detrusor backing is an important consideration because a poorly supported ureterocele that

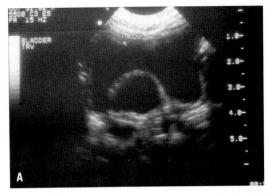 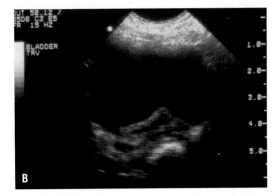

Figure 88-2 Intravesical ureterocele before and after incision. *A,* Intravesical ureterocele in ultrasound profile. *B,* Ultrasound scan of ureterocele after endoscopic incision showing collapsed ureterocele preserving a flap valve mechanism to prevent reflux.

everts with voiding and mimics a bladder diverticulum may be more likely to require secondary reconstruction of the ureteral hiatus than one that is well supported. Occasionally, however, after a ureterocele is decompressed, the support appears to improve, thus making it impossible to say that poor detrusor backing of a ureterocele is a predictor of a need for subsequent open bladder surgery.

The degree of ureteral dilatation is also important. Occasionally, one finds a small ureter running to a small intravesical ureterocele during an operation for what was thought to be primary reflux. The reimplantation of this small ureter from a poorly functioning upper pole serves as good definitive treatment.[39] But if a ureter subserving the ureterocele is massively dilated, as is more frequently the case, then attempts at tapered reimplantation of such a dilated system will carry a greater complication rate than an ablative procedure in the upper pole of the kidney.

It is becoming increasingly clear that the most important predictor of the need for open ureterocele surgery is associated vesicoureteral reflux. If high-grade reflux is present at diagnosis, a primary endoscopic incision is logical because subsequent surgery at the bladder level is likely and will be facilitated by a decompressed ureterocele. On the other hand, if there is no vesicoureteral reflux, the simplified approach of an upper-pole partial nephrectomy in a duplex system is appropriate. A review by Husmann and colleagues showed that reflux was clearly the major factor leading to the need for subsequent surgery after upper-pole partial nephrectomy to decompress a ureterocele.[19] Among patients in whom the ureterocele was not associated with reflux on either side, none required additional bladder-level surgery. If reflux was less than grade III and into only one ureter, it resolved slowly in 60% of the patients, and they required no further surgery. By contrast, a higher grade of reflux into one or more renal moieties almost invariably led to the need for further surgery (96%). A careful assessment of the voiding cystourethrogram performed at presentation is a critical factor in decision making.

It can be readily seen that there will not be one simple solution to all ureterocele problems. The challenge to the pediatric urologist is to minimize

the number of anesthetics and surgical procedures as well as postoperative discomfort for the child.

TECHNIQUE

Endoscopic decompression of ureteroceles was initially suggested by Zielinski and then Hutch and Chisholm.[40,41] Tank popularized this idea by advocating the unroofing of ureteroceles without regard for reflux and found that 50% of his patients had improved function and subsequent upper tract surgery was not thought necessary.[42] He carried out lower tract reconstructive surgery for recurrent infection; this was needed in only 10% of patients.

The current approach to endoscopic incision of ureteroceles is to create a small incision or puncture to decompress the ureterocele, with placement sufficiently low on the ureterocele so that a flap valve of collapsed ureterocele is present to prevent subsequent vesicoureteral reflux (Figure 88-3). This was suggested by Blyth and colleagues and Monfort and colleagues.[36,43]

There are several technical points worth mentioning concerning the endoscopic treatment of ureteroceles in general. Since most ureteroceles are compressible with bladder filling, it is useful to keep the bladder rather empty and to massage the flank to distend the ureterocele to ensure that the incision is as low as possible on the front wall of the ureterocele, just above the bladder neck. A 3 French Bugbee electrode with the cutting current set at a level high enough to ensure a clean incision is important. If a clean cut is not achieved primarily, one may end up pushing the inner mucosal layer of the ureterocele away from the outer layer and thus not achieving decompression. A perpendicular approach to the surface of the ureterocele is also important to avoid a skiving incision that may likewise miss the lumen of the ureterocele. Also, although a low incision is preferred to create an effective flap valve mechanism of decompressed ureterocele, if the incision is too low, it may be below the level of the ureterocele floor. A very small 2- or 3-mm incision or puncture is adequate because the thermal effect of the incision will lead to an enlargement of the hole with healing. Only if the ureterocele appears to be thick-walled would an incision any larger than this be appropriate. It is more prudent to make as small an incision as possible, accepting the fact that, occasionally, an endoscopic re-incision will be necessary. Adequate decompression of the ureter can usually be confirmed when a jet of urine emerges from the incision site in the ureterocele. Massage of the ipsilateral flank can make this more prominent.

A number of technical points in the endoscopic incision of an ectopic ureterocele differ from those for an intravesical ureterocele (Figure 88-4). Achieving decompression of the ureterocele requires a good clean puncture with maintenance of a flap valve to prevent reflux. Thus a low

Table 88-1 Clinical Outcomes after Endoscopic Incision of Intravesical Ureteroceles

Series	No. of Ureteroceles	Successful Decompression	Iatrogenic Reflux	Subsequent Reconstruction	Duration of Follow-up
Cooper et al[38]	22	13 (92%)	7 (32%)	4 (18%)	84 months
Hagg et al[37]	26	21 (95%)	4 (18%)	5 (23%)	20 months
Husmann et al[51]	22	24 (92%)	1 (4%)	1 (4%)	24 months
Pfister et al[52]	16	15 (94%)	1 (6%)	1(6%)	60 months
	86	85%	15%	13%	

Table 88-2 Clinical Outcomes after Endoscopic Incision of Ectopic Ureteroceles

Series	No. of Ureteroceles	Successful Decompression	Iatrogenic Reflux	Subsequent Reconstruction	Duration of Follow-up
Cooper et al[38]	22	18 (82%)	7 (32%)	14 (64%)	84 months
Smith et al[45]	11	10 (91%)	3 (27%)	8 (80%)	22 months
Sperling et al[53]	24	16 (67%)	5 (21%)	13 (54%)	36 months
Pfister et al[52]	21	17 (81%)	8 (39%)	18 (86%)	60 months
Pesce et al[54]	45	37 (82%)	25 (56%)	28 (62%)	30 months
Husmann et al[51]	75	72 (96%)	34 (45%)	55 (73%)	24 months
Jayanthi and Koff[55]	21	17 (81%)	10 (48%)	15 (71%)	34 months
Hagg et al[37]	29	27(93%)	11 (38%)	14 (48%)	20 months
	248	86%	42%	66%	

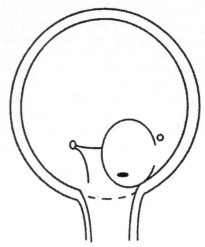

Figure 88-3 Endoscopic incision of intravesical uterocele. A low incision of the ureterocele will lead to decompression with the preservation of a flap valve mechanism to prevent vesicoureteral reflux. A 3 French Bugbee electrode is used with a high cutting current to ensure a clean incision into the ureterocele. The incision should be done with the bladder reasonably empty to preserve ureterocele distention.

puncture on the wall of the ureterocele is important and commonly accepted.[18,44,45] The treatment of the urethral extension of an ectopic ureterocele into the urethra has raised concern that an obstructing distal tongue might remain following decompression. This was the rationale for Blyth and colleagues[36] suggesting an incision of the

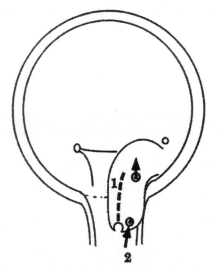

Figure 88-4 Endoscopic incision of extravesical (ectopic) ureterocele. *1*, An incision is carried from the ureterocele orifice upward to above the bladder neck to decompress an ectopic ureterocele. NOTE: The opening of the bladder neck with voiding may facilitate reflux into the ureterocele if this technique is performed; therefore this approach is no longer advocated. The proper technique is direct incision of the ureterocele where it presents just inside the bladder neck. This point can be determined by sliding a cystoscope laterally to medially and incising the ureterocele perpendicularly just above the bladder neck. One clean incision at this point suffices to decompress the ureterocele and is less likely to result in reflux. A second puncture point, *2*, is used to decompress the intraurethral extension but is not necessary in most cases.

ureterocele from the urethral extension up into the bladder. Schlussel and colleagues and Smith and colleagues, however, reported no difficulties resulting from the urethral extension of the ureterocele after successful decompression through puncture at the intravesical level alone.[44,45] Care was taken to perform a low transverse small incision within the bladder with the bladder neck closed. Technically, this can be accomplished by sweeping the cystoscope along the bladder wall from a lateral to a medial position and picking up the edge of the ureterocele just inside the bladder neck. If the bladder is kept fairly empty so that the ureterocele remains fairly distended, a clean puncture in the wall should be possible using a technique similar to that described earlier for the treatment of an intravesical ureterocele.

The technique described by Blyth and colleagues of incising the intraurethral extension of the ureterocele upward into the bladder (see Figure 88-4) may create a physiologic situation in which the opening of the bladder neck opens the orifice of the ureterocele, resulting in a greater likelihood of reflux.[36] This may be the reason for the higher reflux rate following puncture seen in the Blyth and colleagues series[36] versus the Schlussel and colleagues series.[45] Concern about the distal extension of the ureterocele may be more appropriate for open ureterocele excision; the urethral extension of the ureterocele could remain as a valve cusp, catching urine during voiding and thus obstructing the urethra.[46] If the ectopic ureterocele is satisfactorily decompressed by intravesical puncture, it is likely that the urethral extension will also be adequately decompressed and thus will be unlikely to cause any difficulty.

At follow-up after an endoscopic incision, we usually examine the patient with ultrasonography 1 month after the outpatient procedure. Typically, there will still be residual hydroureteronephrosis, but a diminution of some degree indicates that decompression has been achieved. We then wait 6 months before carrying out a voiding cystourethrogram and follow-up upper tract imaging.

INTRAVESICAL URETEROCELES

Intravesical ureteroceles of a single ureter are more commonly seen in adults than in children and may be an acquired lesion.[47] Typically, obstruction and hydroureteronephrosis are more severe in children than in adults.[48] Although Snyder and Johnston wrote that the endoscopic incision of single-system ureteroceles was contraindicated because of the frequency with which secondary ureteral reimplant surgery for reflux was needed,[31] their 1978 review was published well before the era of better and more precise endoscopic techniques. It is important to remember that, even in cases with iatrogenic reflux, reimplantation of the decompressed ureter is technically easier. Thus, for single-system ureteroceles, a primary endoscopic approach appears to be advisable in almost all cases.

For intravesical ureteroceles, it has become clear that up to 90% of patients may be ade-

quately treated by this endoscopic incision approach (see Table 88-1). For an intravesical ureterocele, whether associated with a single or duplex unit, a primary endoscopic approach would be our recommendation, although an upper-pole partial nephrectomy may be considered in the absence of vesicoureteral reflux. While intravesical ureteroceles are less common in the presence of a ureteral duplication, the outcomes with endoscopic incision are nearly as good as those found in single systems. The ureterocele is reproducibly decompressed, and the incidence of post-incision reflux into the upper pole is 10 to 20%. Consequently, as long as reflux into other moieties is not present at diagnosis, the need for subsequent bladder-level surgery after incision is unlikely in these children.

ECTOPIC URETEROCELES

Many question the benefit of incision in ectopic ureteroceles, since it is a definitive procedure in a minority of patients.[49] Ectopic ureteroceles are most commonly associated with the upper moiety of a duplex kidney. Most series show a reduced rate of partial nephrectomy and facilitated lower tract reconstruction after endoscopic incision.[36,37,50] The ureter decreases in caliber, and tapering or imbrication is rarely required if bladder level reconstruction is indicated. The indications for an upper-pole partial nephrectomy decrease if it is accepted that a nonfunctioning, non-dilated renal pole with no reflux can safely be left in situ.

A retrospective comparison of partial nephrectomy and endoscopic decompression showed that, in patients with an ectopic ureterocele and no vesicoureteral reflux, partial nephrectomy was a definitive procedure 85% of the time.[51] In this subset of patients, endoscopic decompression was definitive only 36% of the time. If reflux was present preoperatively, bladder level surgery was required 85% of the time regardless of the initial approach. Most infants with an ectopic ureterocele have reflux,[29] but in the small subset without reflux, an upper tract operation is the preferred treatment. In general, endoscopic treatment of ectopic ureteroceles has not been as successful as for intravesical ones.

Despite the higher secondary surgery rate, the endoscopic approach would appear to be the preferred treatment for a neonate in need of relief of an obstructive uropathy. Subsequent definitive bladder and bladder neck surgery can be carried out electively when the child is between 1 and 2 years of age. At this age, complicated reconstructive procedures are more safely accomplished, and yet it is well before the age of toilet training, after which bladder discomfort following surgery at the bladder neck becomes more difficult for the child to tolerate.

The advent of new and refined endoscopic equipment and techniques has materially improved our ability to manage ureteroceles. From the discussion above, it is readily evident why this new option presents an exciting new approach to the treatment of this often complex urologic problem.

REFERENCES

1. Glassberg KI, Braren V, Duckett JW, et al. Suggested terminology for duplex systems, ectopic ureters and ureteroceles. Report of the Committee on Terminology, Nomenclature and Classification, American Academy of Pediatrics. J Urol 1984;132:1153.

2. Chwalla R. The process of formation of cystic dilatations of the vesical end of the ureter and of diverticula at the ureteral ostium. Urol Cutan Rev 1927;31:499.

3. Stephens FD, Smith ED, Hutson JM. Congenital anomalies of the urinary and genital tracts. Oxford: Isis Medical Media; 1996. p. 243–62.

4. Stephens FD. Caecoureterocele and concepts on the embryology and aetiology of ureteroceles. Aust N Z J Surg 1971; 40:239.

5. Tanagho EA. Embryologic basis for lower ureteral anomalies: a hypothesis. Urology 1976;7:451.

6. Tanagho EA. Ureteroceles: embryogenesis, pathogenesis and management. J Contin Educ Urol 1979;18:13.

7. Campbell M. Ureterocele: a study of 94 instances in 80 infants and children. Surg Gynecol Obstet 1951;93:705.

8. Uson AC, Lattimer JK, Melicow MM. Ureteroceles in infants and children: a report based on 44 cases. Pediatrics 1961;27:971.

9. Eklof O, Lohr G, Ringertz H, et al. Ectopic ureterocele in the male infant. Acta Radiol [Diagn] 1978;19:145.

10. Royle MG, Goodwin WE. The management of ureteroceles. J Urol 1971;106:42.

11. Ericsson NO. Ectopic ureterocele in infants and children. Acta Chir Scand 1954;197 Suppl:8.

12. Mandell J, Colodny AH, Lebowitz R, et al. Ureteroceles in infants and children. J Urol 1980;123:921.

13. Brock WA, Kaplan WG. Ectopic ureteroceles in children. J Urol 1978;119:800.

14. Johnson DK, Perlmutter AD. Single system ectopic ureteroceles with anomalies of the heart, testis and vas deferens. J Urol 1980;123:81.

15. Amar AD. Simple ureterocele at the distal end of a blind-ending ureter. J Urol 1971;106:423.

16. Perrin EV, Persky L, Tucker A, et al. Renal duplication and dysplasia. Urology 1974;4:660.

17. Bolduc S, Upadhyay J, Sherman C, et al. Histology of upper pole is unaffected by prenatal diagnosis in duplex system ureteroceles. J Urol 2002;168:1126.

18. Coplen D, Duckett J. The modern approach to ureteroceles. J Urol 1995;153:166.

19. Husmann DA, Ewalt DH, Glenski WJ, et al. Ureterocele associated with ureteral duplication and nonfunctioning upper pole segment: management by partial nephroureterectomy alone. J Urol 1995;154:723.

20. Caldamone AA, Snyder HM, Duckett JW. Ureteroceles in children: follow-up of management with upper tract approach. J Urol 1984;131:1130.

21. Klauber GT, Crawford DB. Prolapse of ectopic ureterocele and bladder trigone. Urology 1980;15:164.

22. Diard F, Eklof O, Lebowitz R, et al. Urethral obstruction in boys caused by prolapse of simple ureterocele. Pediatr Radiol 1981;11:139.

23. Leadbetter GW Jr. Ectopic ureterocele as a cause of urinary incontinence. J Urol 1970;103:222.

24. Holmes NM, Coplen DE, Strand W, et al. Is bladder dysfunction and incontinence associated with ureteroceles congenital or acquired? J Urol 2002;168:718.

25. Athey PA, Carpenter RJ, Hadlock FP, et al. Ultrasonic demonstration of ectopic ureterocele. Pediatrics 1983;71:568.

26. Summer TE, Crowe JE, Resnick MI. Diagnosis of ectopic ureterocele using ultrasound. Urology 1980;15:82.

27. Nussbaum A, Dorst J, Jeffs R, et al. Ectopic ureter and ureterocele: their varied sonographic manifestations. Radiology 1986;159:227.

28. Cooper CS, Snyder HM. Ureteral anomalies. In: Gillenwater JY, Grayhack JT, Howards SS, et al, editors. Adult and pediatric urology. 4th ed. Philadelphia: Lippincott Williams & Wilkins; 2002.

29. Sen S, Beasley SW, Amed S, et al. Renal function and vesicoureteric reflux in children with ureteroceles. Pediatr Surg Int 1992;7:192.

30. Leong J, Mikhael B, Schillinger JF. Refluxing ureteroceles. J Urol 1980;124:136.

31. Snyder HM, Johnston JH. Orthotopic ureteroceles in children. J Urol 1978;119:543.

32. Tacciuoli M, Laurenti C, Racheli T. Trigonal cyst in childhood. Br J Urol 1976;48:323.

33. Sumfest JM, Burns MW, Mitchell ME. Pseudoureterocele: potential for misdiagnosis of an ectopic ureter as a ureterocele. Br J Urol 1995;75:401.

34. Husmann DA, Strand WR, Ewalt DH, et al. Is endoscopic decompression of the neonatal extravesical upper pole ureterocele necessary for prevention of urinary tract infections or bladder neck obstruction? J Urol 2002;167:1440.

35. Privett JTJ, Jeans WD, Roylance J. The incidence and importance of renal duplication. Clin Radiol 1976;27:521.

36. Blyth B, Passerini-Glazel G, Camuffo C, et al. Endoscopic incision of ureteroceles: intravesical versus ectopic. J Urol 1993;149:556.

37. Hagg MJ, Mourachov PV, Snyder HM, et al. The modern endoscopic approach to ureterocele. J Urol 2000;163:940.

38. Cooper CS, Passerini-Glazel G, Hutcheson JC, et al. Long-term followup of endoscopic incision of ureteroceles: intravesical versus extravesical. J Urol 2000;164:1097.

39. Bauer SB, Retik AB. The non-obstructive ectopic ureterocele. J Urol 1978;119:804.

40. Zielinski J. Avoidance of vesicoureteral reflux after transurethral ureteral meatotomy for ureterocele. J Urol 1962;88:386.

41. Hutch JA, Chisholm ER. Surgical repair of ureterocele. J Urol 1966;96:445.

42. Tank ES. Experience with endoscopic incision and open unroofing of ureteroceles. J Urol 1986;136:241.

43. Monfort G, Morisson-Lacombe G, Coquet M. Endoscopic treatment of ureteroceles revisited. J Urol 1985;133:1031.

44. Schlussel R, Peters C, McClintock J, et al. Efficacy of transurethral incision of ureteroceles [Abstract]. Presented at the American Academy of Pediatrics Section on Urology Meeting, Dallas, TX, October 1994.

45. Smith C, Gosalbez R, Parrott T, et al. Transurethral puncture of ectopic ureteroceles in neonates and infants. J Urol 1994;152:2110.

46. Ashcraft K, Hendren W. Bladder outlet obstruction after operation for ureterocele. J Pediatr Surg 1979;14:819.

47. Thompson GJ, Kelalis PP. Ureterocele: clinical appraisal of 176 cases. J Urol 1964;91:488.

48. Rabinowitz R, Barkin M, Schillinger JF, et al. Bilateral orthotopic ureteroceles causing massive ureteral dilatation in children. J Urol 1978;119:839.

49. Shekarriz B, Upadhyay J, Fleming P, et al. Long-term outcome based on the initial surgical approach to ureterocele. J Urol 1999;162:1072.

50. Petit T, Ravasse P, Delmas P. Does the endoscopic incision of ureteroceles reduce the indications for partial nephrectomy? BJU Int 1999;83:675.

51. Husmann D, Strand B, Ewalt D, et al. Management of ectopic ureterocele associated with renal duplication: a comparison of partial nephrectomy and endoscopic decompression. J Urol 1999;162:1406.

52. Pfister C, Ravasse P, Barret E, et al. The value of endoscopic treatment for ureteroceles during the neonatal period. J Urol 1998;159:1006.

53. Sperling H, Kropfl D, Rubben H. [Endoscopic therapy of ectopic ureterocele]. Urologe A 1996;35:57.

54. Pesce C, Musi L, Campobasso P, Belloli G. Endoscopic and minimal open surgical incision of ureteroceles. Pediatr Surg Int 1998;13:277.

55. Jayanthi VR, Koff SA. Long-term outcome of transurethral puncture of ectopic ureteroceles: initial success and late problems. J Urol 1999;162:1077.

89

Laparoscopic Pyeloplasty in Children

Steven G. Docimo, MD

Ureteropelvic junction (UPJ) obstruction usually presents as either prenatal hydronephrosis or later in children or adults as a cause of abdominal pain. In adults, the management of UPJ obstruction has been revolutionized by the introduction of endoscopic endopyelotomy, Accucise endopyelotomy (Applied Medical, Irvine, CA), and laparoscopic pyeloplasty. There are several reasons why these procedures have been more slowly evaluated in pediatric urology, including smaller patient and ureteral size, a perception of compromise in terms of outcomes, and the more rapid recovery seen after open surgery in small children.[1] The success of open pyeloplasty in children is so high, and the morbidity so low, that it would be irresponsible for the pediatric urological community to embrace these new technologies without a thorough review.

Endopyelotomy has not been widely applied in children. The Accusize device is not applicable to small children, and both retrograde and antegrade visual endopyelotomy have yielded success rates much lower than standard open management.[2] Most pediatric urologists have not seen the advantages of these procedures, which are often associated with long-term stenting and/or nephrostomy tubes. This is especially true when compared to open pyeloplasty through a fairly small anterior or posterior incision. Thus, this chapter will not attempt to deal with endopyelotomy as a primary therapy for pediatric UPJ obstruction.

Laparoscopic pyeloplasty has generated more interest in the pediatric urological community. First, laparoscopic pyeloplasty was initially described in adults as a transperitoneal operation.[3,4] Many pediatric practitioners have been uncomfortable converting an extraperitoneal operation to a transperitoneal procedure.[5] It is important to realize, however, that there is little evidence to suggest a morbidity difference related to transperitoneal versus retroperitoneal endoscopic surgery in children. For example, it has been established that the incidence of post-laparoscopic adhesions is almost negligible.[6] Second, in adults, the operation is often done with the assistance of the Endo-Stitch (U.S. Surgical, Norwalk, CT),[7] a suture aid device that is not suitable for reconstruction of the pediatric ureter. Pediatric pyeloplasty, therefore, is a technically challenging procedure owing to the need for hand suturing and knot-tying in a small space. The first reported pediatric pyeloplasty involved an interrupted anastomosis with nephrostomy drainage, 36 hours in the hospital, and a good outcome

radiographically.[8] After that initial attempt, a few pioneers published expanded series of pediatric procedures, including procedures performed in young infants.[9–11] Since then, a number of centers have adopted and modified the technique, using both retroperitoneal and transperitoneal approaches.

INDICATIONS FOR SURGICAL MANAGEMENT OF UPJ OBSTRUCTION

Ureteropelvic junction obstruction can be a difficult diagnosis to establish with certainty, especially in the infant with prenatally detected hydronephrosis. There has been a gradual evolution to observation of even the significantly dilated infant kidney as long as function is preserved as measured by diuretic renal scan.[12] It is beyond the scope of this chapter to address the controversies regarding surgical correction of prenatally detected hydronephrosis. In general, the initial diagnosis is established with pre- and post-natal ultrasonography. Mild degrees of hydronephrosis can be observed with serial sonograms, but children with more severe hydronephrosis should be evaluated functionally. The most commonly used study in this situation is the diuretic renogram, preferably using MAG-3 as the radionuclide of choice (Figure 89-1). Indications for repair include an obstructive pattern on the diuretic phase of the study, and decreased function of the affected kidney. Other indications might include worsening hydronephrosis and/or febrile urinary infections in the absence of vesicoureteral reflux.

In older children and adults, UPJ obstruction is more likely to present with symptoms of pain and vomiting. The sine qua non of the diagnosis of intermittent UPJ obstruction is worsening hydronephrosis by ultrasonography or computed tomography scan during an episode of pain. Repair of symptomatic UPJ obstruction is indicated regardless of preserved ipsilateral function or effective drainage between symptomatic episodes.

PATIENT PREPARATION

No specific preoperative preparation is used for pediatric pyeloplasty. Preoperative labs are rarely obtained, and then only if there is a family history of bleeding diathesis, or the child has an underlying medical condition. Some advocate a minimal preoperative bowel cleanout, although this is not routinely necessary.

INFORMED CONSENT

It is important for parents to understand that laparoscopic pyeloplasty is a newer approach than open pyeloplasty, and the experience of the surgeon should be disclosed. The possibility of open conversion must be discussed. Risks including, but not limited to, bleeding, infection, per-

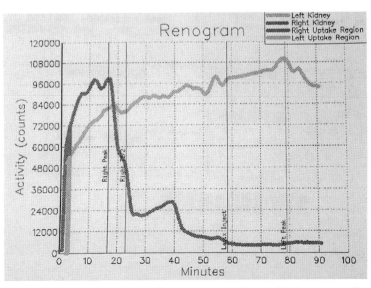

Figure 89-1 A diuretic renogram demonstrates no evidence of drainage even after the administration of furosemide, suggesting high-grade obstruction.

sistent or recurrent obstruction, urinary leakage, and decreased ipsilateral kidney function should be discussed. If a stent is to be used, the need for eventual removal and the consequences of a retained stent should be clear. The potential for intra-abdominal injury, as in any laparoscopic procedure, should be discussed.

PREOPERATIVE PREPARATION

Prior to the laparoscopic portion of the procedure, perform cystoscopy and a retrograde pyelogram to confirm the diagnosis and define the anatomy (Figure 89-2), and place a guidewire to, or through, the UPJ. The guidewire is placed in a sterile plastic bag so that it can be prepped into the field during the laparoscopic procedure, or place a stent at this juncture, rather than the guidewire. If a transmesenteric approach is being contemplated, a guidewire is helpful, as it allows manipulation of the ureter for identification through the mesentery. A guidewire can be left alongside the stent, if this advantage is desired. The patient is secured to the table in a 45° flank position. Appropriate padding must be used; a flat gel pad is recommended instead of an axillary roll, as one patient in this position developed a latissimus injury with elevated creatine phosphokinase levels. Rolling the table from side to side allows the patient to be positioned supine to full flank. The skin preparation must be done with the planned open incision in mind, in case of the need for conversion.

INSTRUMENTATION

Standard laparoscopic instruments are all that is required for this procedure. For infants and tod-

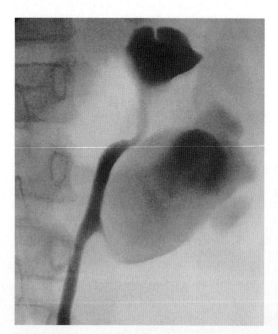

Figure 89-2 Retrograde pyelogram reveals an unexpected bifid pelvis with lower pole ureteropelvic junction obstruction. A pyeloureterostomy was performed in this situation.

dlers, 3-mm instruments are used. The 3-mm scissors is also useful in older children and adolescents for spatulating the narrow ureter. Two good laparoscopic needle drivers are essential, and the surgeon should have the opportunity to try various styles to pick the one that is most ergonomic for him or her. The harmonic scalpel can be useful for dissection with minimal blood loss and less risk of injury due to heat transmission. A Carter-Thomason closure device is useful for passing the renal pelvic hitch stitch through the anterior abdominal wall in larger children and adults. Non-traumatic graspers (DeBakey type) are indispensable for manipulation of the ureter and renal pelvis.

THE OPERATIVE PROCEDURE

Use a transperitoneal approach to the ureteropelvic junction. With the patient supine, open access is obtained using a radially dilating trocar at the umbilicus.[13] Either 3- or 5-mm accessory trocars are placed, depending on the size of the patient. The accessory ports are in the midepigastrium and in the lower abdomen in the midclavicular line ipsilateral to the affected kidney (Figure 89-3). For a right kidney, the cecum is mobilized as necessary to expose the UPJ. On the left, access to the UPJ is most commonly obtained through a small incision in the mesentery, thus avoiding colon mobilization and creating minimal raw surface within the peritoneal cavity.[14] Often, movement of a guidewire placed cystoscopically at the beginning of the procedure will aid in identification of the UPJ through the mesentery. Occasionally, a mesenteric vessel needs to be divided, which is safe as long as the marginal vasculature exists and remains intact.

The ureter is dissected and mobilized taking care to maintain its adventitial blood supply. Dissection is carried out posteriorly as the UPJ is approached, since there should not be any significant structures in this plane. If there is not a crossing vessel, the pelvis can be divided just

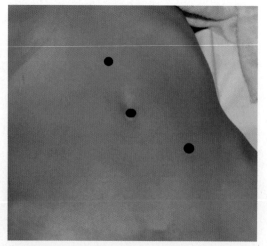

Figure 89-3 Port placement for a left pyeloplasty. For a right-sided procedure, the mirror image configuration is used.

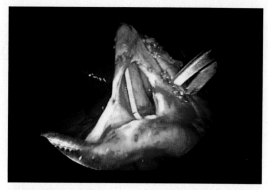

Figure 89-4 Division of the pelvis just proximal to the ureteropelvic junction, leaving a tag of anterior pelvis on the ureter to use as a handle during the anastomosis. This is removed just prior to completing the repair.

above the UPJ to leave a "handle" of distal pelvis on the ureter (Figure 89-4). It is not necessary to attempt to remove the UPJ or to reduce the pelvis. In fact, spatulating the pelvis through the UPJ leaves a rounded apex, which visually suggests a wider opening at the dependant anastomosis. If crossing vessels are encountered (Figure 89-5), the pelvis is exposed above the vessels by opening the investing layers sharply, and the space between the vessels and the UPJ is developed. If the vessels are tightly apposed to the UPJ, the ureter can be divided just below the UPJ. The UPJ is then pulled anterior to the vessels for the anastomosis. The ureter is spatulated laterally to match the length of the defect in the pelvis. A "hitch stitch"[15] is placed in the anterior pelvis and brought through the anterior abdominal wall using a Carter-Thomason device in older children, or a Keith, or gently curved, needle in infants. This stabilizes the pelvis for anastomosis, but is often placed during dissection because it can be helpful during exposure as well (Figure 89-6). The first anastomotic stitch is placed at the distal apex of the pelvis and ureter and tied using standard intracorporeal technique. Depending on the size of the patient, 5-0 or 6-0 absorbable suture is used. The back wall is then closed using a simple running stitch. This can be done with the same apical suture, or a second stitch can be placed at the cephalad end of the back wall and run down. At this point in the procedure, a double-pigtail stent is placed either antegrade or retrograde over the previously positioned guidewire, if it was not placed at the beginning of the case. It is useful to have fluoroscopy in the room to verify stent placement, and to allow appropriate manipulation if the stent is not easy to introduce. The anterior wall is then closed using a running suture (Figure 89-7). A perianastomotic drain is not necessary unless there is some concern about the integrity of the anastomosis. For transmesenteric procedures, the defect in the mesentery does not need to be closed. Likewise, if the colon is mobilized, do not reattach it.

Robotic assistance has been used to make the potentially difficult task of suturing easier. Robotic assistance is not necessary, nor perhaps

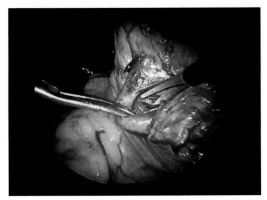

Figure 89-5 Crossing vessels are seen below the ureteropelvic junction (UPJ) at this point of the operation. The vessels have been freed so that the UPJ and proximal ureter can be pulled above the vessels prior to division of the UPJ.

particularly helpful, for the skilled laparoscopist, but could have two significant advantages. First, it may decrease operative time and/or improve the accuracy of suture placement for those with experience. Second, by flattening the learning curve, robotics might increase the number of practitioners who adopt minimally invasive reconstruction, and thus increase the availability of complex laparoscopic procedures.[16] In infants, however, 3-mm instruments can be used with essentially no visible postoperative scars for the standard procedure—this cannot yet be said for the robotic procedure.

POSTOPERATIVE MANAGEMENT

A Foley catheter is generally left overnight, but this may not be necessary. In our series of more than 45 children, the average hospital stay has been 1.4 days, with most patients home in under 24 hours. The stent is removed two weeks postoperatively.

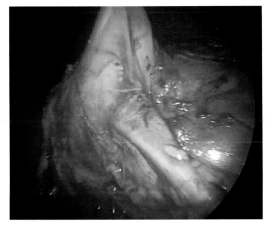

Figure 89-6 In this transmesenteric exposure of the left renal pelvis, the hitch stitch is placed early in the dissection. This helps to bring the ureteroplvic junction into a more advantageous position for dissection, as well as for anastomosis later in the procedure.

RESULTS

Since the initial report of laparoscopic pyeloplasty in a child,[8] few series have been reported in the literature. Early series by Yeung and colleagues, and by Tan demonstrated good outcomes for both retroperitoneal and transperitoneal approaches, with the transperitoneal failures occurring in young infants.[5,15] This has caused most practitioners to be hesitant about applying this technique in infants, although at our institution we have gradually reduced our acceptable age, which is now 6 months. More recent series have looked at specific questions, such as dismembered versus non-dismembered pyeloplasty, with success of the former being 94%, and the latter, 43%.[17] Despite the small numbers in this series, most pediatric urologists feel that dismembered techniques are likely to be more successful, as this was established decades ago in open pyeloplasty. In the author's personal series when last tabulated, mean patient age was 10.6 years (range, 1 to 19 years), and follow-up was available on 19 of 21 patients with a mean duration of 8.3 months (range 1 to 26 months). Procedures performed included 18 laparoscopic Anderson-Hynes pyeloplasties, 2 laparoscopic Heineke-Mikulicz pyeloplasties, and 1 laparoscopic pyeloureterostomy. All 21 cases were completed laparoscopically. Twelve patients had lower-pole crossing vessels. Average length of stay was 1.5 days (range 1 to 3 days), and no intraoperative or postoperative complications occurred. Postoperative ultrasonography had been performed in 19 patients, of which 18 (94.7%) demonstrated significant improvement. One patient (5.3%) continued to have symptomatic and radiographic evidence of obstruction with the need for additional adjunctive procedures. As noted previously, our group now has more than 45 procedures with only one documented failure (98%).

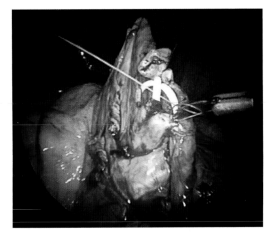

Figure 89-7 The anterior wall anastomosis is completed using a simple running absorbable suture. The stent has already been placed.

COMPLICATIONS

Complications of laparoscopic pyeloplasty would be expected to be identical to those for the open procedure, and include urine leakage and recurrent obstruction. As for any laparoscopic procedure, the possibility of open conversion must be discussed with the patient and family. In either the trans- or retroperitoneal approach, bowel injury can occur as in any open or laparoscopic procedure. The limited field of view may be a factor in laparoscopic bowel injury, and special care should be used when applying cautery, or when manipulating instruments that are not in the visual field.

CONCLUSIONS

Pediatric laparoscopic pyeloplasty is in its infancy, although it is being adopted by more centers. Although not necessary for success, robotic assistance may allow more practitioners to attempt the technique. The benefit may be largely cosmetic, but the importance of this in children should not be underestimated. Success rates in experienced hands appear to be identical to the open operation. This is a procedure that will have a prominent place in the repertoire of all pediatric urologists in the future.

REFERENCES

1. Docimo SG, Kavoussi LR. The role of endourological techniques in the treatment of the pediatric ureteropelvic junction. J Urol 1997;158:1538.
2. Tan HL, Najmaldin A, Webb DR. Endopyelotomy for pelvi-ureteric junction obstruction in children. Eur Urol 1993;24:84.
3. Schuessler WW, Grune MT, Tecuanhuey LV, et al. Laparoscopic dismembered pyeloplasty. J Urol 1993;150:1795.
4. Kavoussi LR, Peters CA. Laparoscopic pyeloplasty. J Urol 1993;150:1891.
5. Yeung CK, Tam YH, Sihoe JD, et al. Retroperitoneoscopic dismembered pyeloplasty for pelvi-ureteric junction obstruction in infants and children. BJU Int 2001;87:509.
6. Pattaras JG, Moore RG, Landman J, et al. Incidence of postoperative adhesion formation after transperitoneal genitourinary laparoscopic surgery. Urology 2002;59:37.
7. Jarrett TW, Chan DY, Charambura TC, et al. Laparoscopic pyeloplasty: the first 100 cases. J Urol 2002;167:1253.
8. Peters CA, Schlussel RN, Retik AB. Pediatric laparoscopic dismembered pyeloplasty. J Urol 1995;153:1962.
9. Tan HL. Laparoscopic Anderson-Hynes dismembered pyeloplasty in children using needlescopic instrumentation. Urol Clin North Am 2001;28:43.
10. El-Ghoneimi A, Farhat W, Bolduc S, et al. Laparoscopic dismembered pyeloplasty by a retroperitoneal approach in children. BJU Int 2003;92:104.
11. Yeung CK, Tam YH, Sihoe JD, et al. Retroperitoneoscopic dismembered pyeloplasty for pelvi-ureteric junction obstruction in infants and children. BJU Int 2001;87:509.
12. Koff SA. Postnatal management of antenatal hydronephrosis using an observational approach. Urology 2000;55:609.
13. Cuellar DC, Kavoussi PK, Baker LA, et al. Open laparoscopic access using a radially dilating trocar: experience and indications in 50 consecutive cases. J Endourol 2000;14:755.
14. Docimo SG. Trans-mesenteric approach to left laparoscopic pyeloplasty. J Endourol 2003;17:A321.
15. Tan HL. Laparoscopic Anderson-Hynes pyeloplasty in children [Letter; Comment]. Pediatr Surg Int 1999;15:597.
16. El-Ghoneimi A. Paediatric laparoscopic surgery. Curr Opin Urol 2003;13:329.
17. Casale P, Grady RW, Joyner BD, et al. Comparison of dismembered and nondismembered laparoscopic pyeloplasty in the pediatric patient. J Endourol 2004;18:875.

90

Pediatric Ureteroscopy/Nephroscopy and Percutaneous Stone Procedures

Matthew E. Rutter, MD

Bradley P. Kropp, MD

Urolithiasis is a rare condition in pediatric age groups in developed countries. Third world nations have a much greater incidence of pediatric stone disease, often attributed to malnutrition. These patients have historically been treated with open procedures that can result in considerable morbidity and lengthy convalescence. In the modern era, treatment of urolithiasis has been revolutionized with the advent of endoscopic techniques and improved technology. Until the last several years, most of the technology has benefitted the adult population. Initial concerns for extending the procedures to children arose from potential morbidity related to the size of the instruments. Furthermore, because of the rarity of urolithiasis in this population, little data has been available. Recently, with the development of smaller instrumentation, pediatric patients have begun to profit from skilled endoscopists.

Initially, extracorporeal shockwave lithotripsy (ESWL) was extended to the pediatric population. Certainly, this offers tremendous advantages over open stone procedures. However, not all stones are amenable to the treatment. Ureteroscopy and percutaneous renal surgery present safe and effective alternatives to open stone surgery and ESWL, and have virtually eliminated open procedures for calculi. In fact, open stone procedures should be the "exception rather than the rule."[1]

This chapter reviews current technology for ureteroscopy and percutaneous nephrolithotomy and their use in children. In addition, technique for each of the procedures will be outlined. Finally, a review of the literature with results and complications will be discussed.

URETEROSCOPY

The first ureteroscopy was described by Dr. Young in 1929. He had performed the procedure in 1912 on a child with a pediatric cystoscope. The patient had a dilated system secondary to posterior urethral valves, and Dr. Young was able to advance the scope to the level of the kidney and inspect the pelvis. Modern ureteroscopy stemmed from the late 1970s when Dr. Lyon and Dr. Goodman independently reported their experiences using pediatric cystoscopes to evaluate the distal portions of adult ureters.[2–4] These efforts opened the door for the development of smaller, longer scopes; fiberoptics; and new instrumentation and energy

sources for ureteroscopic interventions. Quickly ureteroscopy became commonplace in adult evaluation and treatment, and it was accepted as first-line therapy for distal ureteral stones. The urologic community has been slow to accept ureteroscopy for the pediatric population. Concerns for trauma of the urethra and ureter have been the root of the hesitation. However, in the hands of a skilled endoscopist, ureteroscopy is safe and effective in children.

INDICATIONS Ureteroscopy has become the mainstay of therapy for small distal ureteral stones in the adult population. Since the advent of smaller endoscopes, and as the literature supports the success in children, ureteroscopy has also become first-line therapy for distal stones in accomplished hands[5] (Figure 90-1). Initial concerns revolved around the possibility of damaging the small, delicate, pediatric urethra and ureter. However, multiple reports of pediatric ureteroscopy have put these concerns to rest. Another indication includes the use in those patients in whom extracorporeal shockwave lithotripsy was unsuccessful. For instance, if the lithotriptor cannot be focused on a ureteral calculus and appears to be too large to be passed spontaneously, endoscopic removal is indicated. It can also be beneficial in the event that a Steinstrasse develops. Some urologists have even used it in combination with shock wave lithotripsy.[6–8] Certainly, it can also be used safely in the middle and proximal ureter. In addition to traditional retrograde techniques, it can be performed safely in an antegrade fashion through a nephrostomy tract.[9] However, this is rarely indicated. Also, new percutaneous techniques have been described to access distal stones in patients who have had cross trigonal ureteral reimplantations.[10] Furthermore, ureteroscopy can be used in children for reasons other than stones. It has been reported in the evaluation of hematuria and ureteral polyps.[9,11] Finally, ureteroscopy has been used in children for retrograde endopyelotomy techniques with lasers.[12]

PATIENT PREPARATION Prior to any intervention, appropriate preoperative evaluation is essential. Other than proper radiologic assessment, examination of the urine is crucial. Endoscopic manipulation with infected urine could

result in life-threatening septicemia; therefore, urine should be cultured and treated with culture-specific antibiotics prior to ureteral manipulation. If the system is obstructed and infection is suspected, a retrograde stent or percutaneous nephrostomy tube should be placed to establish drainage. Manipulation is performed only after the urine culture has become sterile and the clinical signs of infection have resolved.

Expectations of the procedure must be addressed when obtaining consent from the child's parents. It must be made clear that complete stone removal may not be achieved. The stone may be flushed back to the kidney and may require secondary ESWL. In narrow ureters it may be impossible to reach the stone. In this situation, retrograde stent insertion may be useful to relieve obstruction and passively dilate the ureter. Ureteroscopy is usually possible 2 to 3 days later without further problems. On occasion, retrograde ureteroscopy may not be possible, and a percutaneous approach may be the most appropriate therapy. As with all surgery, there is risk of iatrogenic trauma. The child's parents must be

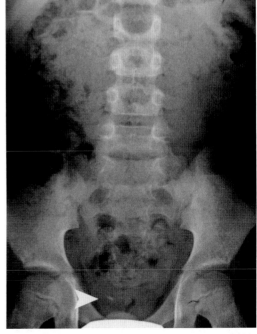

Figure 90-1 A 10-year-old boy with a right intramural ureteral stone measuring 8 mm × 4 mm requiring ureteroscopy.

aware of the possibilities, including urethral, bladder, and ureteral injuries, and the rare potential need for immediate repair. Furthermore, parents must comprehend the use of ureteral catheters or stents following the procedure and the possibility that a second, short anesthetic may be required for stent removal.

PREOPERATIVE PREPARATION Following general endotracheal anesthesia, the child is placed in a modified dorsal lithotomy position at the end of a standard operating table. Larger children may be positioned with well-padded standard stirrups. The contralateral leg should be flexed higher at the hip to allow for maneuverability of the scope. Smaller children and infants can be positioned at the end of a table with padded towel rolls under their knees and their thighs supported with tape to the table. All pressure points must be adequately padded and the patient must be secured. After adequate positioning, the patient is prepped and draped with standard cystoscopy drapes. A C-arm fluoroscopy unit is then draped in the usual manner for imaging throughout the case. A standard fluoroscopic cystoscopy table can be used for larger children. Leaded protection gowns should be strategically used to protect the child and allow for appropriate imaging.

INSTRUMENTATION In the last 20 years there has been an explosion of new technology facilitating the extension of ureteroscopy into the diagnostic and therapeutic armamentarium of a pediatric urologist. In addition to miniaturization of the standard rod lens, fiberoptic technology has permitted the development of small flexible endoscopes to better visualize and treat stones in the proximal collecting system. Following the advances in endoscope technology has been a complement of baskets, graspers, small hydrophilic wires, and energy sources to facilitate treatment of urinary stones.

Semirigid scopes are available at varying French (F) sizes and lengths. These scopes typically have a small French distal tip with a gradual increase in the diameter proximally. Many of these scopes are also slightly beveled at the tip. This feature allows for ease of manipulation of the scope into the ureteral orifice (Figure 90-2). Smaller (4.5F) "needle" scopes may not be so useful for the treatment of stone disease because of limited working port size. However, most pediatric ureters will accommodate 6.9F to 8F semirigid scopes with or without ureteral orifice dilation. The newer semirigid scopes provide excellent visualization of the distal and middle ureter, and they have two channels for instrumentation and flow of irrigation. Most will accommodate up to or larger than 3F baskets, graspers, and energy sources for lithotripsy, and still allow excellent irrigation flow. Scopes with an offset lens can be particularly useful if planning to use a pneumatic lithotriptor. In addition to the semirigid scopes, newer generations of flexible scopes have been introduced that may increase the indications for retrograde ureteral access for proxi-

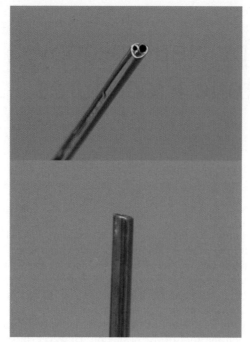

Figure 90-2 A semirigid 6.9 French ureteroscope with beveled distal tip. Note the configuration of the channels and lens (ACMI Corp, Southborough, MA).

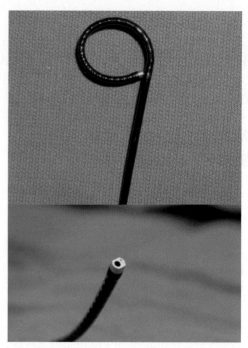

Figure 90-3 Flex-X 7.5 French flexible ureteroscope. Note the degree of flexion (Karl Storz, Culver City, CA).

mal stone treatment. These scopes have significantly improved optics compared with earlier generations and are smaller at the distal tip (6.7–8.5F) (Figure 90-3). The degree of flexion and durability of the scopes are superior, and the flexion is better preserved when a device is in the working channel.[13] Retrograde access to lower-pole renal stones and complete visualization of the proximal collecting system is possible, and improved active flexion decreases the reliance of passive flexion for lower-pole access. The newer scopes offer a greater field of view than the older versions.[13] Similar to the semirigid scopes, the flexible scopes will accommodate up to 3F instruments, but the flow of irrigation is limited in comparison. In fact, the flow rate is less than the earlier flexible scopes when the working channel is in use.[13]

Ureteroscopic lithotripsy can be managed safely in the pediatric population with a laser, electrohydraulic lithotripsy, or pneumatic lithotripsy. Ultrasonic lithotripsy has also been employed.[5,14–17] However, this technique requires a larger-caliber scope. With the advent of the holmium laser, the use of pulsed-dye lasers and electrohydraulic lithotripsy has become relatively extinct. In fact, according to Scarpa and colleagues, electrohydraulic lithotripsy should be avoided.[6] Both 200-micron and 365-micron holmium laser fibers are easily accommodated by the semirigid and flexible scopes and are safe to use in the pediatric ureter.[18] The laser should be used to vaporize the calculus. However, if small fragments are created, 2.4F or 3.0F nitinol tipless baskets can safely extract the stones (Figure 90-4). If a stone is impacted or large, basket extraction without fragmentation is discouraged for concern of possible ureteral dam-

age. Additional items necessary for ureteroscopy include a complement of guidewires, ureteral catheters, and Double-J stents. Rarely necessary, serial ureteral dilators or a small ureteral balloon dilator may be useful. Last, but not least, low-pressure irrigation devices are useful to improve visibility during ureteroscopy (Figure 90-5). This may be required because resistance of a long narrow channel in the ureteroscope reduces the flow of irrigation, hindering visibility. Several bulb- or syringe-based systems are available to combat this problem.

TECHNIQUE Cystoscopy is initially performed with an age-appropriate cystoscope. A ureteral catheter and contrast should be used to gently perform a retrograde study to confirm the location of the stone and outline the anatomy. Next, a safety hydrophilic guidewire (0.025–0.038) should be placed retrograde through the cystoscope with fluoroscopic guidance and confirmed coiling in the renal pelvis. If necessary, a ureteral

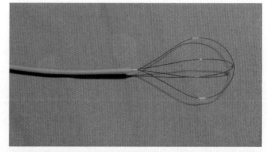

Figure 90-4 Tipless nitinol stone basket, safe for use in both the kidney and ureter. Tipped baskets may increase the risk of ureteral perforation or renal trauma (Cook Urological, Spencer, IN).

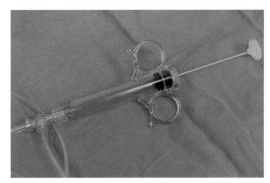

Figure 90-5 An example of a low-pressure irrigation device for ureteroscopy. Syringe and bulb-type irrigators are available (Boston Scientific/Microvasive, Spencer, IN).

catheter can be used to assist wire placement. Sometimes, particularly if instrumenting a reimplanted ureter, a torquable ureteral catheter or angled wire is helpful. On occasion, a small ureteroscope can be used to "look" a wire into the ureter. This may be necessary if false passages have been created. After wire placement, the orifice should be closely inspected to see if it will accommodate a ureteroscope. If necessary, gentle dilation can be performed. The authors' preference is to use hydrophilic serial dilators with fluoroscopic guidance (Figure 90-6). A balloon dilator can be used as an alternative to the serial dilators. Dilation greater than 8F is rarely necessary and should not be performed alongside a stone as it could traumatize the ureter. Scarpa and colleagues. suggest that dilation is never necessary, and smaller instruments should be chosen if the orifice is small.[6] If the orifice is very stenotic or if the caliber of the ureter is too narrow to accommodate the scope, ureteral stent placement for passive dilation is preferred. Ureteroscopy can typically be approached safely in a few days.

Depending on stone location, a semirigid or flexible ureteroscope may be chosen. A semirigid scope is preferable in the distal ureter. The scope should be placed into the bladder under direct vision with saline irrigation. Once the orifice is identified, the scope can be used to displace the guidewire, allowing the orifice to be tented open. Negotiating the orifice should be performed by carefully rotating the scope to allow the beveled tip to slide in first. Inspection of the tip of the instrument prior to use is critical. The scope should have a large working channel, a smaller working/irrigation channel, and a smaller lens. Knowing the detail of the tip of your scope will make intubation of the ureteral orifice easier. Despite rotating maneuvers, sometimes additional assistance is necessary. A second wire, a basket, or a small ureteral catheter can be placed through the scope and into the ureteral orifice alongside the safety wire. Rotation of the scope approximately 180 degrees will cause the wires to "split." The scope should then be easily negotiated between the wires. Once in the intramural portion of the ureter, the second wire should be removed to allow for better irrigation flow. Maneuvering through the distal ureter can be

complicated at times, and knowledge of the tip of the scope is crucial. Gentle rotation will often position the lens in the center of the lumen, and advancement under direct vision can usually be achieved easily. Wide side-to-side or up-and-down maneuvers should be avoided to minimize trauma. The previous retrograde study can serve as a road map, and fluoroscopy can be used to assist in the position of the scope. Care must be taken at all times to visualize the lumen; mild syringe or bulb pressure irrigation is useful. Sometimes, tortuous passages or kinks in the ureter may be encountered. Passing a guidewire through the scope may be helpful to straighten the ureter and make passage of the scope easier. This may be particularly helpful when trying to advance the scope at the level of the iliac vessels. At times, the scope catches the mucosa, and with advancement, the scope actually kinks the ureter. Simply pulling back the scope will straighten the ureter. This may occur if the lumen is too narrow to accommodate the scope. In this situation, gentle mechanical dilation over a wire or passive dilation with a stent is recommended. Forcing the scope will risk the possibility of stricture, perforation, or telescoping and avulsion. In the event a perforation is suspected, placement of a Double-J stent over the safety wire is recommended. Alternatively, nephrostomy drainage can be used. Avulsion warrants immediate open repair.

Flexible scopes are very useful for more proximal stones or if endoscopy is being performed in a reimplanted or tortuous ureter. Flexible scopes can be introduced in a similar manner as the rigid scopes under direct vision. Often, it is simpler to place a second guidewire to assist placement of the ureteroscope into the ureter. After the second wire is in position, the scope can be advanced over the wire using both direct vision and fluoroscopic guidance. Upon reaching the ureteral orifice, rotation of the scope in a similar manner as noted above will allow the wires to "split," and the orifice will open generously. Once inside the ureter, the guidewire can be removed and the scope can be advanced to the appropriate level under direct vision. A tortuous ureter is typically easy to navigate with the flexible scope because of its deflecting capabilities. Rotation of the distal end of a flexible scope is most effective when holding the scope between the index finger and thumb at the level of the urethral meatus. Because of this, an assistant may be useful for other manipulations as both of the scope operator's hands are in use.

Once the level of the stone has been reached, lithotripsy can commence. It is our preference to leave a safety wire in position during the entire procedure. Care must be taken to completely visualize the stone and the tip of energy source, otherwise damage may occur to the ureter or safety wire. A holmium laser fiber has an aiming beam that helps identify its end. This should be in direct contact with the stone for maximum effectiveness. When using the laser, the surface of the stone should be "painted," rather than drilling multiple holes. Painting the surface

maximizes vaporization of the stone and minimizes a collection of fragments. Care must be taken to prevent proximal migration of the stone, which can be a particular problem with the pneumatic lithotripsy. A device is commercially available to prevent proximal migration of fragments. However, the caliber of the Stone Cone (Boston Scientific/Microvasive, Natick, MA) is rather large (7–10 mm) in diameter, and to our knowledge has not been investigated for use in small children (Figure 90-7).

Following adequate lithotripsy, a Double-J stent may or may not be placed. Stenting is often used at the discretion of the surgeon's judgment of trauma during a case. Concern of postoperative edema often is the basis for stenting. However, current trends in adult urology are investigating stentless ureteroscopy in selective patients.[19,20] Pediatric cases may be no different. Eliminating stent placement would reduce the need for a secondary anesthesia and stent-related discomfort. Some advocate the placement of a ureteral catheter that is externalized or a Double-J stent with a string externalized that can be removed in 24 to 48 hours. This also eliminates the need for further anesthesia; unfortunately, in these cases the patients likely require admission.

RESULTS AND COMPLICATIONS Ureteroscopy in children renders excellent stone-free results with successes from 86 to 100% (Table 90-1). Some authors have noted that it is easier to perform in girls compared with boys.[5,16] Repeat procedures have been required to become stone free, and some stones were pushed back into the kidney requiring ESWL.[5,9,16] In addition, failures were noted resulting in some open surgery.[5] However, for the most part, ureteroscopy is quite efficacious for the treatment of pediatric ureteral stones. Novel techniques have been performed to access the previously reimplanted ureters. Santarosa and colleagues performed percutaneous

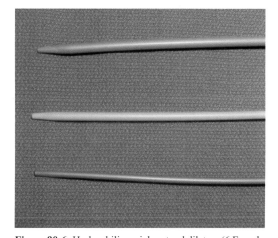

Figure 90-6 Hydrophilic serial ureteral dilators (6 French, 8F, and 10F). These should be passed gently over a guidewire with both fluoroscopic guidance and direct vision. The dilators may not fit through a cystoscope and should be passed along side the scope. Care must be taken not to dilate past the stone as ureteral trauma could occur (Boston Scientific/Microvasive, Spencer IN).

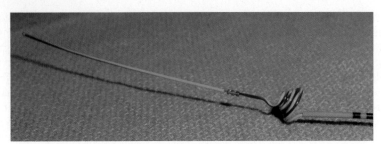

Figure 90-7 Seven-millimeter Stone Cone. This device was developed to prevent proximal migration of fragments during ureteral lithotripsy.

transvesical ureteroscopy for a distal stone in a cross trigonal reimplanted ureter.[10] A larger scope was used in this case, and the ureteral orifice was cut to retrieve the stone. No long-term complications were reported.[10] Shroff and colleagues also described a unique approach via an established vesicostomy in a 13-month-old boy, showing that it was safe and effective.[21]

Concerns of both short-term and long-term complications have been relatively unfounded.

Initially there was concern about potential urethral and ureteral trauma resulting in stricture, incontinence, and vesicoureteral reflux. However, this has not been widely demonstrated. Few reports of transient vesicoureteral reflux have been noted.[14,17] Esen and colleagues suggested that large-caliber scopes would more likely result in reflux.[22] In fact, al Busaidy and colleagues noted that only 1 of the patients who required mechanical dilation resulted in low-grade

reflux.[14] Postoperative voiding cystourethrograms have demonstrated that reflux is unlikely as a long-term complication.[6,14] Ureteral stricture is also uncommon. One case has been reported in a 6-year-old girl when fragments from a previous ureteroscopy failed to pass. A holmium laser was used to open the stricture, and the stone proximal to the stricture was treated. A stent was left for 4 weeks, and no recurrence of the stricture was noted.[9] Ureteral perforation has been reported and conservatively treated with indwelling stents or nephrostomy drainage.[14,23] More common complications include transient renal colic, hematuria, fever, and pyelonephritis (see Table 90-1).

Patients should be followed closely following ureteroscopy to evaluate for the redevelopment of stones or complications. Intravenous urograms are very useful to evaluate for stones and strictures. Alternatively, a plain abdominal film and renal ultrasound may be used to limit radiation exposure. Helical computed tomography is an excellent way to evaluate for recurrent or residual stones, but its expense and radiation exposure

Table 90-1 Ureteroscopy

	n	Age (yrs)	Procedures	Location	Size	Scope Size (F)	Dilation	Lithotriptor	Success (%)	Complications	Indications	Stent
Al Busaidy et al[14]	43	6–12	50	9 proximal 7 middle 30 distal	1.26 cm	8.5 9.5 11.5	19	EHL Ultrasonic	93	1 ureteral perforation 5 hematuria 2 renal colic 6 fever	Stones	46
Bassiri et al[5]	66	2–15	66	2 proximal 5 middle 59 distal	5–15 mm	8 8.5 9 11.5	25	EHL Ultrasonic Lithoclast	88	3 pyelonephritis 1 renal colic 11 hematuria	Stones	66
Caione et al[15]	7	3–8	8	2 middle 5 distal	1.1–2.7 cm	11.5	0	Ultrasonic	100	0	Stones	8
Delakas et al[16]	4	3.5–14	6	1 middle 3 distal	6–13 mm	9	0	EHL Ultrasonic	100	1 renal colic 2 hematuria	Stones	4
Fraser et al[7]	16		16	2 middle 14 distal		6.9	0	EHL Pulsed-dye	87.50	1 perirenal urinoma	Stones	
Hill et al[11]	4	4–10	4	3 distal		8.5	0	Pulsed-dye	100	0	Stones Fibroepithelial polyps	3
Kurzrock et al[8]	17	1.5–16	17	2 renal 1 proximal 3 middle 13 distal	10.5 mm	7.2 6.9	1	Candela	100	1 renal colic	Stones	5
Minevich et al[46]	10	7–16	11	All distal		6.9 7 9.5	5	EHL	86	0	Stones Evaluation for obstruction	8
Ritchey et al[47]	1	4	1	Distal		8.5	0	Pulsed-dye	100	0	Stones	1
Santarosa et al[10]	1	17	1	Distal		11	Cut orifice		100	0	Stones	1
Scarpa et al[6]	7	3.5–10	7	1 proximal 6 distal 1 Steinstrasse	6 mm – 3 cm	4.8 7	0	Lithoclast Pulsed-dye	100	0	Stones	7
Shroff and Watson[9]	14	1–14	20	4 proximal 3 middle 14 distal	4 mm – 3.5 cm	7.2 9.5	1	Holmium Pulsed-dye EHL Lithoclast	93	1 stricture 1 urinary retention 1 hematuria 1 migrated stent 1 aspiration	Stones Hematuria Migrated stent	5
Thomas et al[17]	16	1.3–15	18	5 middle 13 distal		7.2 8.5 11.5	8	EHL Ultrasonic Laser	100	1 transient reflux	Stones	18
Van Savage et al[23]	17		17		1–15 mm	4.5 7	0	Pulsed-dye Holmium Lithoclast	88	1 ureteral perforation	Stones	17

may limit its use. Routine voiding cystourethrogram is not necessary and should be reserved for those cases where reflux is suspected.

PERCUTANEOUS MANAGEMENT OF RENAL CALCULI

Staghorn and large renal calculi have historically been managed with open surgery. The introduction of percutaneous renal techniques in the 1970s offered a new approach for these difficult stones, and now percutaneous nephrolilthotomy is the preferential treatment. Unfortunately, minimally invasive techniques have been relatively limited to the adult population. Esen and colleagues reported that percutaneous nephrolilthotomy is efficacious, less invasive than open surgery, and it should be performed more often in the pediatric population.[22] Surgeons have been slow to accept these procedures for use in children because of concerns for renal trauma. The most common concern is that the size of sheath traditionally used in adult surgery can pose a risk of injury to the smaller pediatric kidney. For instance, Jackman and colleagues noted that a 24F sheath in a small child would be the equivalent of a 72F sheath in an adult.[24] The concern that permanent renal damage may result from such a procedure has not been proven. Studies have shown that even with adult-sized instruments, renal function is not significantly altered.[8,25] Another reason that percutaneous surgery has been slow to gain popularity in children is that the etiology of their stone burden can be related to an anatomic abnormality. Some would argue that open surgery is most appropriate in this situation to remove the stone and correct the abnormality. However, even some anatomic variants contributing to the etiology of stones can be corrected with percutaneous endoscopic procedures.

The advent of newer technology, including smaller scopes with better optics, miniaturized energy sources, and revised techniques, allows most pediatric renal stones to be safely managed with percutaneous nephrolilthotomy in skilled hands. The advantages of this approach to stone treatment are reduced morbidity, decreased hospital stay, and, overall, the recovery is much quicker than when compared with open surgery. In addition, children who are at risk of recurrent stone disease benefit from the minimally invasive techniques, as it ultimately may reduce the risk of repeat open procedures.

INDICATIONS One of the more common noted reasons for percutaneous management of pediatric renal stones is the failure of extracorporeal shockwave lithotripsy. Nazli and colleagues recommended that large stones that may require multiple ESWL treatments would best be managed with percutaneous nephrolilthotomy.[26] It is certainly indicated for large stone burdens, staghorn calculi, and multiple renal stones (Figure 90-8). Another indication involves the treatment of poorly functioning renal units with obstructed or infected dilated systems. The

stones should be approached percutaneously following a period of drainage.[27,28] In the event that the dilated system was related to ureteropelvic junction obstruction, this can be treated at the same time with an antegrade endopyelotomy. Initially, percutaneous renal surgery was recommended for only children over the ages of 5 to 8 years for fear of increased complications in younger children.[27,29–31] However, others have suggested that complications encountered are not age dependent, and several major complications have been reported in the older children. It appears that these complications are more likely related to the size of the stone burden and not the age of the patient.[32] Finally, results have clearly shown that younger children can safely undergo percutaneous nephrolilthotomy by experienced endourologists.[8,24,25,27,28,33,34]

PATIENT PREPARATION Prior to intervention, it is imperative to have precise knowledge of the anatomy of the urinary tract and the position of the stones. An intravenous urogram with oblique films is very useful to delineate the caliceal anatomy and the location/size of the stone. If dealing with a caliceal diverticulum, a computed tomography scan is also often beneficial to assess an anterior or posterior position. These studies will serve as road maps to plan location of access prior to the operation. If the function of the renal unit is in question, a nuclear scan may be valuable. Certainly a complicated percutaneous approach would not be advised if the kidney was not worth preserving. A lasix renogram may help in the decision-making process in the event a ureteral pelvic junction obstruction is entertained and concominant endopyelotomy is planned.

Preoperative urine cultures are advised. Positive urine cultures should be treated prior to

manipulation with culture-specific antibiotics. Suspicion of an infected obstructing stone warrants preoperative drainage and treatment with culture-specific antibiotics prior to definitive stone management. If these measures are not observed, there may be an increased risk of life-threatening sepsis.

Informed consent is important to outline the surgical plan and to help the parents of the child have a clear understanding of the goals and expectations of the procedure. Parents must understand that multiple procedures may be necessary in order to become stone free. They should have a clear understanding of the purpose of a nephrostomy tube for drainage. A thorough discussion of the associated risks is required, and they must also understand the possibility of recurrence and need for intervention in the future.

INSTRUMENTATION Many of the same instruments and techniques used in adult nephrolilthotomy can be used in children. However, in recent years, smaller scopes and sheaths have become available for use in pediatric nephrolilthotomy. Minimal tract dilation can be achieved with excellent results using today's technology. Disposable Amplatz sheaths from 14F to 16F are available that accommodate pediatric offset rigid nephroscopes (14F) and flexible cystoscopes.[33] Furthermore, with the advent of mini-percutaneous (mini-perc) techniques, smaller 11F peel-away sheaths or 13F ureteral access sheaths can be used with pediatric flexible cystoscopes (7.5F), flexible ureteroscopes (6.9F, 7.5F, 9.5F), and offset rigid pediatric cystoscopes (7.5F)[24,35,36] (Figure 90-9).

An ultrasonic lithotriptor is ideal for fragmentation and evacuation of stone with the larger scopes (Figure 90-10). In addition, a newer device combining pneumatic and ultrasonic lithotripsy

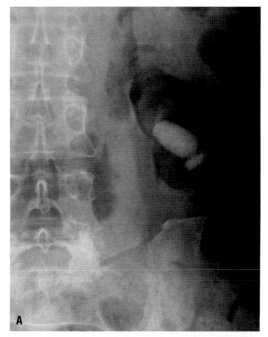
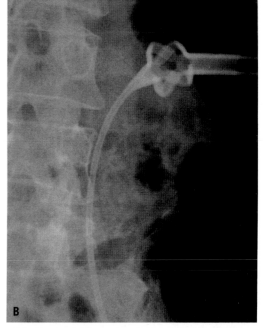

Figure 90-8 *A*, Large left renal pelvic stones in a teenage girl. She required a percutaneous nephrolithotomy. *B*, Postopative day 1 from percutaneous nephrolithotomy. She was stone free with one procedure. Note the re-entry nephrostomy tube in place.

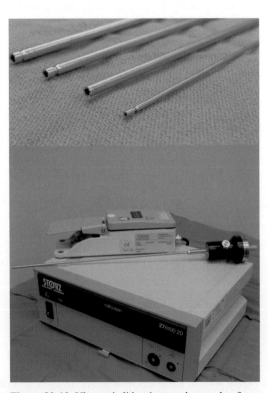

Figure 90-9 Pediatric offset cystoscope is excellent for percutaneous nephrolithotomy with minimal tract dilation or "mini-perc" technique (ACMI Corp, Southborough, MA).

has become available that efficiently fragments and removes stone.[37] These devices, however, are too large for the mini-perc techniques. Small probes for the ultrasonic and pneumatic lithotriptors do exist, but they are less effective in evacuating large stone burden. Since the mid-1990s, the holmium laser has become a priceless addition to the management of urinary calculi with the smaller scopes. It precisely fragments and vaporizes the stone, and if used appropriately, minimal fragment extraction is necessary.[18] Furthermore, it can treat all variants of stone, unlike the other energy sources that cannot fragment harder calculi. Because of the holmium laser's effectiveness, the electrohydraulic lithotriptor has virtually become obsolete. In addition to the improvements in lithotriptors and scopes, multiple small grasping devices and tipless baskets (2.4–3.0F) have been developed for the smaller working channels, facilitating stone extraction.

TECHNIQUE Techniques for percutaneous access and nephrolithotomy in children are very similar to the adult. Detailed instructions of access techniques are discussed elsewhere. The following is an overview of the authors' approach and description of the options for the mini-perc technique.[33]

The child is administered a general endotracheal anesthesia on a bed that will accommodate a C-arm fluoroscope. The patient is placed in lithotomy and cystoscopy is performed. Next, a 3F to 5F open-tip ureteral catheter or an occlusion balloon catheter (5F or 8F) is placed (Figure 90-11). The catheter should be advanced to the level of the ureteropelvic junction. If using an occlusion balloon, care should be taken to ensure that the tip of the catheter is well into the renal pelvis prior to inflating the device to prevent ureteral injury. Fluoroscopy is recommended to confirm this position with the assistance of contrast, then inflate the balloon and pull it back to the ureteropelvic junction. After this is complete, a Foley catheter should be placed. The Foley and ureteral catheters can be secured together or separately. The child is now repositioned prone with the head facing the ipsilateral side. The ipsilateral arm is place in the swimmer's position and the contralateral arm is tucked. The affected side is elevated approximately 30 degrees on a foam wedge or towel roll. All pressure points are appropriately padded.

Following positioning, the child should be prepped in a sterile manner and drapes applied. A standard nephrolithotomy drape can be used. Alternatively, a disposable laparotomy drape can be used. Sterile adhesive cellophane or iodinated cellophane drapes and drainage pouches should be applied strategically to collect irrigation. Careful attention to the draping is important to prevent the patient from getting "soaking wet," which can lead to hypothermia.

Once the patient is properly draped, contrast is injected into the ureteral catheter, illuminating the collecting system, and using biplaner fluoroscopy, the end of the chosen calix is entered with an 18-gauge renal access needle. Once in the calix, the stylet is removed. Return of urine or contrast material confirms position in the collecting system. Next, a guidewire (0.035) is placed via the needle into the collecting system and negotiated across the ureteropelvic junction and down the ureter. If the wire cannot be manipulated down the ureter, it may be coiled within the pelvis. A small incision is made with an 11-blade scalpel, and

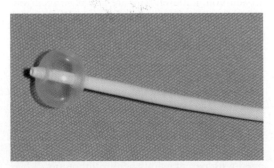

Figure 90-10 Ultrasonic lithotriptor and example of various probe tips (Karl Storz, Culver City, CA).

the needle is removed. Serial dilation over the wire is carried out with fascial dilators 6F to 10F under fluoroscopic guidance. An 8F/10F coaxial catheter is then placed over the wire into the system, and the 10F sheath is placed over the 8F catheter. With the 10F sheath in place, a second wire can be placed. If there is difficulty negotiating the ureteropelvic junction with the wire, it can be repositioned under direct vision with a scope once the tract has been created. In difficult cases, a wire may be placed retrograde through the ureteral catheter and grasped within the renal pelvis establishing "through and through" access. Usually, an Amplatz superstiff wire is used as a working wire for tract dilation. However, depending on experience, nearly any wire can suffice. After two wires are in place, serial dilation with Amplatz dilators using fluoroscopic guidance can commence up to 14F or 16F. Some advise using a small (4.5F) fascial incising needle prior to tract dilation.[35] Care must be taken with all dilation to proceed in the same path as the original needle access to minimize renal trauma. It is also important to keep in mind that a child's kidney is much closer to the skin than an adult's. Therefore, the depth of dilation is much less.[1] Also, it must be remembered that the child's kidney is much more mobile in the retroperitoneum, thereby making dilation more difficult. An alternative approach is minimal dilation using a mini-perc technique with an 11F sheath/trocar set, or even a 13F ureteral access catheter[24,35,36] (Figure 90-12). Following the placement of a safety and working guidewire, the peel-away sheath and trocar are placed over the working wire with fluoroscopic guidance. Once in position, the inner trocar and wire can be removed to accommodate a small flexible cystoscope (7.5F), offset rigid pediatric cystoscope, or a similar-sized semirigid or flexible ureteroscope.

Now that access is established, the stone may be treated. Smaller stone burdens are effectively treated with the mini-perc access using a holmium laser and small tipless baskets. However, if there is a considerable burden of stone, larger tract dilation (up to 22F) is recommended so a 14F pediatric nephroscope with an ultrasonic or pneumatic lithotriptor can be used. This approach efficiently fragments stone, and still

Figure 90-11 Ureteral occlusion balloon catheter. This catheter allows gentle distention of the collecting system facilitating access, and prevents premature drainage of contrast. During the nephrolithotomy, fragments will not migrate distally into the ureter with proper balloon placement (Boston Scientific/Microvasive, Spencer IN).

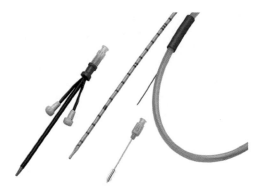

Figure 90-12 The "mini-perc" access set with peel-away sheath (upper) (Cook Urological, Spencer, IN). A ureteral access sheath (lower), which can be used as an alternative to the peel-away sheath. This sheath can be cut to the appropriate length after placement (Boston Scientific/Microvasive, Spencer, IN).

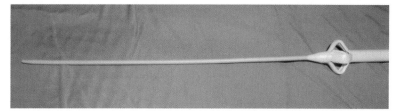

Figure 90-13 An example of a malecot re-entry nephrostomy tube. This facilitates ureteral access in the event a relook procedure is necessary (Boston Scientific/Microvasive, Spencer, IN).

minimizes trauma with limited tract dilation. Stones in difficult locations can usually be accessed with a small flexible scope, and this usually obviates the need for secondary access. In fact, in smaller pediatric kidneys, it has been recommended to limit the procedure to one access to minimize trauma.[28] All calices should be systematically inspected to evaluate for residual fragments. If it is suspected that fragments passed into the ureter, antegrade flexible ureteroscopy is a simple and effective way to evaluate and even retrieve small fragments. In the event that visibility is poor, the procedure should be terminated with plans to perform a second-look procedure in 2 to 3 days. Also, nephroscopy time and irrigation should be limited to prevent fluid absorption and hypothermia.[27,38] Keep in mind that large stone burdens may need to be staged for these reasons.

On completion of the procedure, a nephrostomy tube should be placed. The size and type of tube placed is age dependent. Sahin and colleagues recommend the use of a small 14F or 16F malecot re-entry nephrostomy tube in older children[39] (Figure 90-13). This is particularly useful when planning a second-look procedure. Often a small Foley catheter or red rubber catheter is sufficient. In the case of the mini-perc procedure, a small 8F or 10F pigtail nephrostomy tube may be useful. Once the tube is secured to the skin, contrast injection confirms the tube is in the appropriate position.

RESULTS AND COMPLICATIONS Percutaneous nephrolithotomy in children has been proven to be quite successful, achieving strict stone-free rates of 67 to 100% prior to discharge. Multiple reports have been compiled into Table 90-2. Many have required relook procedures to achieve these results. Few complications have been reported overall. Hemorrhage has been one of the most common complications reported.[30,32,34,39,40] Rizvi and colleagues reported intraoperative bleeding requiring transfusion in 17 patients, and an additional 21% required transfusion after the procedure owing to hematuria.[40] Zeren and colleagues also reported need for transfusion in several patients, but noted that the incidence of bleeding was less with more experience.[34] Desai

and colleagues have suggested that bleeding and renal trauma is less likely when tract size is limited.[27] Helal and colleagues introduced a novel technique for minimal tract dilation, paving the way for the mini-perc techniques. The initial description utilized a 15F Hickman vascular access sheath.[41] Following this description, Jackman and colleagues introduced the mini-percutaneous nephrolilthotomy with small-caliber (11F) sheaths that are commercially available. The great advantages are less trauma and bleeding, and possibly less pain associated with minimal manipulation.[24] In addition to the 11F peel-away sheaths, 13F ureteral access sheaths that accommodate larger instruments have also been used with similar success.[35,36] Although the benefits of the mini-perc techniques appear obvious, some have argued that longer operative times may be necessary with larger stone burdens, which could contribute to further complications.[33] Hypothermia is a consideration, particularly if operative times are long. Al-Shammari and colleagues noted 2 patients developed significant hypothermia when the procedures lasted longer than 150 minutes.[42] Prevention of hypothermia is recommended by decreasing operative times,

proper draping, using warm saline irrigation, warming the operating room temperature, and using a brief anesthesia induction.[33] Only 1 case of urosepsis has been reported as a complication in the pediatric population.[32] However, transient fever has been reported commonly following percutaneous nephrolilthotomy. Most of the patients are covered with culture-specific or broad-spectrum antibiotics, and the fever resolves spontaneously. Another rarely reported complication is hydrothorax. Rizvi and colleagues reported 1 incidence treated with chest tube drainage without further complication.[40] Uncommon complications include colonic fistula, renal pelvis perforation, disruption of the ureter at the ureteropelvic junction, and broken instrumentation.[27,28,34,43,44]

Routine follow-up is recommended to evaluate for recurrent or residual calculi. Similar to the evaluation after ureteroscopy, intravenous urogram is useful. However, renal ultrasound and plain abdominal x-ray is usually sufficient, unless radiolucent calculi are suspected. Helical computed tomography would be best utilized in this situation. Metabolic evaluation is recommended for all children to identify an etiology and outline a regimen for prevention.

Table 90-2 Percutaneous Nephrolithotomy						
	Patients (*N*)	Age	Stone Burden (cm)	Sheath Size (F)	Hospital Stay (days)	Complications	Stone Free (%)
Al-Shammari et al[42]	10	4–11	0.8–4	24		Hypothermia	87.50
Badawy et al[28]	60	3–13	0.8–3.7	26–28	5.9	Fever, colonic fistula	83.30
Boddy et al[30]	10	5–16		24–26	3–8	Bleeding	90.00
Callaway et al[32]	18	19 mo – 16 yr				Bleeding, sepsis	67.00
Desai et al[27]	40	11 mo – 15 yr	0.9–4.5	21–24	4–13	Fever, nephrostomy leak, pelvic perforation	91.00
Fraser et al[7]	3	11–14		22		None	100.00
Helal et al[41]	1	2	0.5–0.7	15		None	100.00
Hulbert et al[29]	6	11–16	0.6–2.3		3–8		100.00
Jackman et al[24]	11	2–6	1.2	11	6	None	85.00
Jayanthi et al[43]	2	4, 10	1–1.5	> 24		Disrupted ureter	100.00
Kurzrock et al[8]	8	3–16	1–6.5	24	5	None	100.00
Mor et al[25]	25	3–16		24–26	2–13	Fever, lost access	92.00
Papanicolaou et al[31]	2	8–13	0.9–2	28	4		100.00
Rizvi et al[40]	62	4–14	2.5–5	22	3–9	Bleeding, fever, hydrothorax, extravasation	67.70
Rutter and Kropp[33]	9	16 mo – 18 yr		11–16		None	100.00
Sahin et al[39]	14	8–17	301 mm²	24–30	3–10	Bleeding, fever	69.00
Woodside et al[45]	7	5–18			3–6	Fever	100.00
Zattoni et al[44]	6	9–14		20		Broke ultrasound probe in kidney	100.00
Zeren et al[34]	53	10 mo – 14 yr	283 mm²	18–30	3–8	Bleeding, fever, broken guidewire	86.90

CONCLUSION

Although stone disease is rare in this population, children should be treated with the same techniques available to the adult population. During the last decade numerous reports of minimally invasive techniques for pediatric stone management have confirmed their safety. Despite concerns for trauma and long-term complications, ureteroscopy and percutaneous nephrolilthotomy have been proven efficacious for the selected pediatric patient. Advancements in technology and experience have essentially made open stone surgery obsolete. Certainly, it is recommended for endourologists with significant skill and experience.

REFERENCES

1. Harmon EP, Neal DE, Thomas R. Pediatric urolithiasis: review of research and current management. Pediatr Nephrol 1994;8:508–12.
2. Lyon ES, Banno JJ, Schoenberg HW. Transurethral ureteroscopy in men using juvenile cystoscopy equipment. J Urol 1979;122:152–3.
3. Lyon ES, Kyker JS, Schoenberg HW. Transurethral ureteroscopy in women: a ready addition to the urological armamentarium. J Urol 1978;119:35–6.
4. Goodman TM. Ureteroscopy with pediatric cystoscope in adults. Urology 1977;9:394.
5. Bassiri A, Ahmadnia H, Darabi MR, Yonessi M. Transureteral lithotripsy in pediatric practice. J Endourol 2002;16:257–60.
6. Scarpa RM, De Lisa A, Porru D, et al. Ureterolithotripsy in children. Urology 1995;46:859–62.
7. Fraser M, Joyce AD, Thomas DF, et al. Minimally invasive treatment of urinary tract calculi in children. BJU Int 1999;84:339–42.
8. Kurzrock EA, Huffman JL, Hardy BE, Fugelso P. Endoscopic treatment of pediatric urolithiasis. J Pediatr Surg 1996;31:1413–6.
9. Shroff S, Watson GM. Experience with ureteroscopy in children. Br J Urol 1995;75:395–400.
10. Santarosa RP, Hensle TW, Shabsigh R. Percutaneous transvesical ureteroscopy for removal of distal ureteral stone in reimplanted ureter. Urology 1993;42:313–6.
11. Hill DE, Segura JW, Patterson DE, Kramer SA. Ureteroscopy in children. J Urol 1990;144(2 Pt 2):481–93.
12. Gerber GS, Kim J, Nold S, Cromie WJ. Retrograde ureteroscopic endopyelotomy for the treatment of primary and secondary ureteropelvic junction obstruction in children. Tech Urol 2000;6:46–9.
13. Chiu KY, Cai Y, Marcovich R, et al. Are new-generation flexible ureteroscopes better than their predecessors? BJU Int 2004;93:115–9.
14. al Busaidy SS, Prem AR, Medhat M. Paediatric ureteroscopy for ureteric calculi: a 4-year experience. Br J Urol 1997;80:797–801.
15. Caione P, De Gennaro M, Capozza N, et al. Endoscopic manipulation of ureteral calculi in children by rigid operative ureterorenoscopy. J Urol 1990;144(2 Pt 2):484–93.
16. Delakas D, Daskalopoulos G, Metaxari M, et al. Management of ureteral stones in pediatric patients. J Endourol 2001;15:675–80.
17. Thomas R, Ortenberg J, Lee BR, Harmon EP. Safety and efficacy of pediatric ureteroscopy for management of calculous disease. J Urol 1993;149:1082–4.
18. Reddy PP, Barrieras DJ, Bagli DJ, et al. Initial experience with endoscopic holmium laser lithotripsy for pediatric urolithiasis. J Urol 1999;162:1714–6.
19. Hollenbeck BK, Schuster TG, Faerber GJ, Wolf JS Jr. Routine placement of ureteral stents is unnecessary after ureteroscopy for urinary calculi. Urology 2001;57:639–43.
20. Hollenbeck BK, Schuster TG, Seifman BD, et al. Identifying patients who are suitable for stentless ureteroscopy following treatment of urolithiasis. J Urol 2003;170:103–6.
21. Shroff S, Rushton MA, Watson GM, et al. Ureteroscopy through vesicostomy. Br J Urol 1995;75:420–1.
22. Esen T, Krautschick A, Alken P. Treatment update on pediatric urolithiasis. World J Urol 1997;15:195–202.
23. Van Savage JG, Palanca LG, Andersen RD, et al. Treatment of distal ureteral stones in children: similarities to the american urological association guidelines in adults. J Urol 2000;164(3 Pt 2):1089–93.
24. Jackman SV, Hedican SP, Peters CA, Docimo SG. Percutaneous nephrolithotomy in infants and preschool age children: experience with a new technique. Urology 1998;52:697–701.
25. Mor Y, Elmasry YE, Kellett MJ, Duffy PG. The role of percutaneous nephrolithotomy in the management of pediatric renal calculi. J Urol 1997;158(3 Pt 2):1319–21.
26. Nazli O, Cal C, Ozyurt C, et al. Results of extracorporeal shock wave lithotripsy in the pediatric age group. Eur Urol 1998;33:333–6.
27. Desai M, Ridhorkar V, Patel S, et al. Pediatric percutaneous nephrolithotomy: assessing impact of technical innovations on safety and efficacy. J Endourol 1999;13:359–64.
28. Badawy H, Salama A, Eissa M, et al. Percutaneous management of renal calculi: experience with percutaneous nephrolithotomy in 60 children. J Urol 1999;162:1710–3.
29. Hulbert JC, Reddy PK, Gonzalez R, et al. Percutaneous nephrostolithotomy: an alternative approach to the management of pediatric calculus disease. Pediatrics 1985;76:610–2.
30. Boddy SA, Kellett MJ, Fletcher MS, et al. Extracorporeal shock wave lithotripsy and percutaneous nephrolithotomy in children. J Pediatr Surg 1987;22:223–7.
31. Papanicolaou N, Pfister RC, Young HA 2nd, et al. Percutaneous ultrasonic lithotripsy of symptomatic renal calculi in children. Pediatr Radiol 1986;16:13–6.
32. Callaway TW, Lingardh G, Basata S, Sylven M. Percutaneous nephrolithotomy in children. J Urol 1992;148(3 Pt 2):1067–8.
33. Rutter ME, Kropp BP. Pediatric percutaneous urologic surgery. AUA Update Series 2002;21:274–9.
34. Zeren S, Satar N, Bayazit Y, et al. Percutaneous nephrolithotomy in the management of pediatric renal calculi. J Endourol 2002;16:75–8.
35. Jackman SV, Docimo SG, Cadeddu JA, et al. The "mini-perc" technique: a less invasive alternative to percutaneous nephrolithotomy. World J Urol 1998;16:371–4.
36. Chan DY, Jarrett TW. Mini-percutaneous nephrolithotomy. J Endourol 2000;14:269–73.
37. Olbert P, Weber J, Hegele A, et al. Combining Lithoclast and ultrasound power in one device for percutaneous nephrolithotomy: in vitro results of a novel and highly effective technology. Urology 2003;61:55–9.
38. Kukreja RA, Desai MR, Sabnis RB, Patel SH. Fluid absorption during percutaneous nephrolithotomy: does it matter? J Endourol 2002;16:221–4.
39. Sahin A, Tekgul S, Erdem E, et al. Percutaneous nephrolithotomy in older children. J Pediatr Surg 2000;35:1336–8.
40. Rizvi SA, Naqvi SA, Hussain Z, et al. Management of pediatric urolithiasis in pakistan: experience with 1,440 children. J Urol 2003;169:634–7.
41. Helal M, Black T, Lockhart J, Figueroa TE. The Hickman peel-away sheath: alternative for pediatric percutaneous nephrolithotomy. J Endourol 1997;11:171–2.
42. Al-Shammari AM, Al-Otaibi K, Leonard MP, Hosking DH. Percutaneous nephrolithotomy in the pediatric population. J Urol 1999;162:1721–4.
43. Jayanthi VR, Arnold PM, Koff SA. Strategies for managing upper tract calculi in young children. J Urol 1999;162(3 Pt 2):1234–7.
44. Zattoni F, Passerini-Glanzel G, Tasca A, et al. Pediatric nephroscope for percutaneous renal stone removal. Urology 1989;33:404–6.
45. Woodside JR, Stevens GF, Stark GL, et al. Percutaneous stone removal in children. J Urol 1985;134:1166–7.
46. Minevich E, Rousseau MB, Wacksman J, et al. Pediatric ureteroscopy: technique and preliminary results. J Pediatr Surg 1997;32:571–4.
47. Ritchey M, Patterson DE, Kelalis PP, Segura JW. A case of pediatric ureteroscopic lasertripsy. J Urol 1988;139:1272–4.

91

Lithotripsy

Ezekiel H. Landau, MD

Since Chaussy and colleagues pioneered extracorporeal shock wave lithotripsy (ESWL) for the management of renal calculi in adults,[1] the technique was soon expanded to ureteral calculi[2,3] and then was applied successfully to a child by Eisenberger and colleagues 5 years later.[4] Within 2 years of the introduction of ESWL in the United States, numerous additional presentations and publications described the increased use and wider application of the technique in children.[5–10] The technical experience accumulated enabled the application of ESWL in children with large renal[11–18] and ureteral calculi.[19–21] ESWL has since been proven to be efficient and safe in infants less than 1 year of age.[14,18,22–25] The management of bladder calculi by ESWL in children has been promising, though experience has been limited.[26–28]

Indications for ESWL in the treatment of pediatric stones have been established that are similar to those in adults: pain, hematuria, infection, obstruction, or potential of obstruction.[29] Obstruction may be silent, or may be symptomatic, with pain, anuria, or urinary retention. Previously, many children were referred for ESWL only after a failed open surgery.[30–32] Currently, ESWL is the first-line treatment for most renal and ureteral stones.

The incidence of urinary tract stones in children is very low. From a total of 14,498 patients who were treated with ESWL at our institution from 1986 to 2006, 225 were younger than 14 years (1.55%).

It is mandatory to evaluate every child with urolithiasis prior to ESWL with complete metabolic workup for underlying abnormalities and urinary tract imaging.[33] Though ESWL has a major role in the management of urolithiasis in children, pre- and postoperative management is even more important. This includes hydration, urinary pH alteration, and medications (as in cases of calcium, cystine, or uric acid stones). Some congenital anomalies complicated by stones (ureteropelvic junction obstruction, obstructive megaureter) may be treated by open, percutaneous, or laparoscopic extraction of the stone combined with definitive reconstruction.

Initial concerns regarding complications of ESWL in children were unfounded. Improvements in anesthesia enabled the treatment of infants without increased risk. Long-term follow-up is available now regarding renal growth, function, injury, and the potential development of hypertension.[16,34] These issues will be discussed in this chapter.

TECHNICAL CONSIDERATIONS

ANESTHESIA Most prepubertal patients require general anesthesia during treatment with ESWL regardless of the type of lithotriptor. That is true for the Dornier Human Machine 3 (HM3) lithotriptor[14,19,21] and the MPL 9000 (Dornier Medical Systems),[17] the Sonolith 3000 (14 kV, Technomed Corp, Lyon, France), the Nova (14-20 kV, Direx Medical Systems, Paris, France),[22] the Wolf Piezolith 2300, and the Dornier Compact Delta (Dornier Medical Systems).[35] The Lithostar Plus, however, requires anesthesia for children younger than 3 years of age, whereas older patients can be managed with sedation only.[16] Demirkesen and colleagues[36] treated 7 children (13% of his patient population) with the Lithostar, using general anesthesia, whereas the rest (87%) were managed with sedation (with midazolam and alfentanil). All patients were less than 16 years of age. In Ather and Noor's study[17] using the Dornier MPL 9000 for 105 children, 85% were treated under general anesthesia. All his patients were 14 years of age or younger. Of these, 31 were under 5 years, 47 were between 6 and 10 years, and 27 were 11 to 14 years old. In both series, the distribution of treatment type by age, within this group, was not specified. Elsobky and colleagues used two second-generation lithotriptors, the Dornier MPL 5000 (Dornier MedTech GmBH Germany) a spark gap, low-pressure generator lithotriptor, and the Ecolith, a piezoelectric machine.[37] Of the 148 patients, 52% (all aged less than 12 years) required general anesthesia, while 48% received sedation and analgesia only. The same lithotriptor was used by Tan and colleagues in 100 patients aged 16 years or less.[38] General anesthesia was required by 74.8% of them, while sedation was used in 24.4%. Children with neurological deficit, such as myelodysplasia, sacral agenesis, and trauma to the cord do not require anesthesia.

A gradual increase of shock energy, with peak energy mainly during the second half of the procedure, has been shown to reduce anesthetic requirements.[39,40]

High-frequency general anesthesia reduced renal movement during ESWL, thus improving targeting of the stone.[41–43] Our initial experience supported these findings, but we realized that standard general anesthesia was equally effective.[44] A summary of the types of anesthesia used in children for ESWL is presented in Table 91-1. Commonly, general anesthesia is required for first-generation lithotriptors, whereas intravenous sedation combined with topical analgesia with EMLA cream suffices with the use of most second- and third-generation machines.[45]

It should be emphasized that ESWL is contraindicated with urinary infection, non-functioning kid-

Table 91-1 Types of Anesthesia for ESWL in Children

Reference	Year	Lithotriptor	No. of Patients	Age (yr)	Anesthesia
Rodrigues Netto[16]	2002	Lithostar P	86	3	SED
Rodrigues Netto[16]	2002	Lithostar P	86	>3	no anesthesia
Landau[21]	2001	HM3	38	8m–14	GA
Gofrit[14]	2001	HM3	38	<6	GA
Jayanthi[19]	1999	HM3	24	<14	GA
Vilanyi[61]	2001	Compact	16	6–14	GA
Lottmann[15]	2001	Sonolith	14	5m–12	GA
Lottmann[15]	2001	Nova	9	5m–12	GA
Cass[54]	1996	HM3	38	11–18	GA
Cass[54]	1996	Medstone	107	0–18	GA
Lifshitz[55]	1998	HM3	29	1–17	GA
Demirkesen[36]	1999	Lithostar	56	0–16	GA/SED
Ather[17]	2003	MPL 9000	105	0–14	GA/SED
Tan[38]	2004	MPL 5000/ Lithotron	100	10m–16	GA
Aldridge[35]	2006	Piezolith/	69	10m–13	GA
	2006	Compact Delta			
DeFoor[62]	2005	Compact Delta	88	6m–10	GA
Rhee[83]	2006	Not specified	8	3.5–17	GA
Demirkesen[75]	2006	Lithostar	131	1–16	SED/GA
Tan[73]	2006	Lithostar	85	2–16	SED
Onal[72]	2004	Lithostar	33	2–16	SED

GA = general anesthesia; SED = sedation.

ney, uncontrolled hypertension, coagulopathy, obstruction distal to the stone (ureteropelvic junction obstruction, obstructive megaureter, a second distal stone), and urethral stricture.

Routine administration of prophylactic antibacterial treatment is unnecessary for patients with proven sterile urine undergoing ESWL.[46] We do, however, recommend administration of pretreatment antibiotics in cases with history of recurrent infection and suspected struvite calculi, as will be discussed later.

INSTRUMENTATION Most lithotriptors were used successfully in children, with good results and few complications.[13–22,24,25,28,32,36,37,47–54] The most common lithotriptors are the HM3,[14,19,21,25,54–56] EDAP LT02 (EDAP Technomed),[28] Lithostar Plus [16,57,58] Sonolith 3000 (EDAP Technomed),[15,22,50] Nova (Direx Medical Systems),[15,22] Lithostar (Siemenns Medical Systems),[20,24,36,56,59] MPL 9000[13,32,52,60] DL 50[13] MPL 9000X[48,49] MPL 5000,[37] Echolith (Toshiba Medical Systems, Japan),[37] Compact Moblie Lithotriptor,[61] Piezolith 2501 (Richard Wolf GmBH, Knittlingen, Germany),[18] and the STS (Medstone International).[54] The first-generation HM3 lithotriptor required modifications of the gantry, depending on the age and size of the patients. Jayanthi and colleagues[19] used a modified car seat for small children and infants (Figure 91-1). The back of the seat was cut in order to allow the shock access to the child's back. This modification enabled treatment of renal and upper ureteral calculi, but not stones located in the mid- or distal ureter. We placed the children in a hammock made of gauze straps tied to the HM3 gantry (Figure 91-2). This simple modification enabled us to treat all renal and ureteral calculi. Stones in the kidney, proximal ureter, and distal ureter necessitated the supine position, whereas mid-ureteral calculi (the part of the ureter anterior to the sacroilium) required the patients to be placed in the prone position. The straps used in both systems kept the patients from floating in the tub. Orsola and colleagues[12] used the prone position for their patients, with the reflector of the Lithostar-Ultra lithotriptor helping with immobilization (Figure 91-3). Silver developed a gantry for the Sonolith 3000 lithotriptor.[50] This gantry is made of a nylon "knotless" fishnet that enables safe positioning of a small child in the small tub of this lithotriptor (Figure 91-4). The fishnet is hooked to the bottom edge of the lithotriptor with elastic bungee cords (Figure 91-5), and the patient is safely positioned on the fishnet, with underwater ultrasonography (Figure 91-6). Silver stated that this fishnet could also be used in other lithotriptors with a tub. Lottmann and colleagues treated 19 infants under 2 years old with the Sonolith 3000 and Nova lithotriptors.[22] They reduced the size of the opening above the generator for a safe positioning of the patients (Figure 91-7). McLorie and colleagues[25] positioned infants on a transparent sling in order to achieve better coupling while using the MPL 5000 lithotriptor. Most second- and third-generation lithotriptors do not

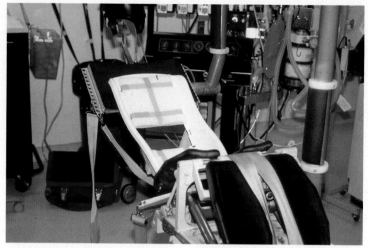

Figure 91-1 Infant car seat with hole cut in back allows small children to be safely treated I adult gantry. Reproduced with permission from Jayanthi VR, et al.[19]

require modifications for positioning children. Mobile lithotriptors, such as the Dornier Compact Delta, are currently used successfully in combination with a universal urologic table.[62]

When using the HM3 lithotriptor, the water level must be reduced to avoid submerging the patient. In these circumstances, the anterior exit site of the shock wave from the body may remain uncovered by water, thus increasing the likelihood of exit site hematoma. This can be obviated by placing ultrasound gel and a 1-L bag of saline solution over the exit site.[8] In our experience with the HM3 lithotriptor, no exit-site hematoma was noted in any of our more than 200 pediatric patients, regardless of whether the exit site was covered or not. With the Lithostar, gel and a bag of fluids may be required for the treatment in cases when the bellows cannot be adjusted. In these circumstances the bag of fluids is positioned between the shock head and the patient, allowing continued propagation of the shock wave.[63]

Duration of the procedure and average number of shock waves with either first-, second-, or third-generation lithotriptors have generally been similar for children and adults. Shock wave intensity, however, has been significantly lower in chil-

dren compared with adults. The range of shock wave intensity with the HM3 has been 18 to 25 kV in adults, whereas for children we have used a significantly lower range, 14 to 20 kV. For infants younger than 2 years of age we used an even lower range, 12 to 18 kV, with the same outcome.

The danger of pulmonary blast injury caused by the shock wave during ESWL is well known, necessitating protection. We used a rat model for demonstration of pulmonary blast injury using the unmodified HM3 lithotriptor.[64] Lethal blast injuries caused bilateral pneumothorax and hemothorax in the rats. Nonlethal doses of shock waves caused intra-alveolar and intrabronchial hemorrhage with an immediate two- to threefold increase in the lung weight. Additional increase in lung weight started 12 to 24 hours later. Pulmonary blast injury was completely prevented by using an air-containing vest on the rat's chest during shock waves. Lung protection is of particular importance in infants and small children, where lower lung segments are very close to the kidneys. The barrier between the lungs and the generator can be metal or foam in order to impede the forward propagation of the shock waves. Prior to initiating shock waves, one must

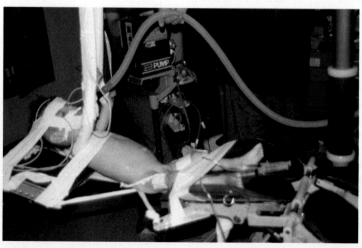

Figure 91-2 Child placed in hammock constructed of banditos tied to HM3 gantry. Reproduced with permission from Gofrit ON, et al.[14]

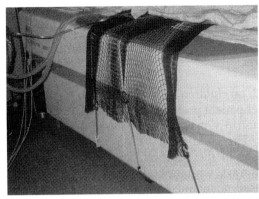

Figure 91-5 Fishnet gantry held in position with a set of six bungee cords, three on each side of the lithotripsy machine. For each bungee cord, the upper hook passes through a hole in the net and the lower hook catches the bottom edge of the table. Tension of the fishnet gantry is easily adjusted by repositioning the upper bungee cord hooks on the hole in the fishnet. Reproduced with permission from Silver RI, et al.[50]

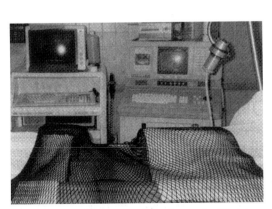

Figure 92-3 Child positioned prone coaxially to wave reflector. Note how shock head with gel disk helps to immobilize the child. Reproduced with permission from Orsola A, et al.[12]

be certain that the lung is not visible (by fluoroscopy or ultrasonography) along the course of the shock waves. The back of the car seat used by Jayanthi and colleagues for the HM3 lithotriptor[19] protected the patient's lungs very effectively. None of their patients had hemoptysis. The modification of the HM3 gantry in our unit positioned the lungs above the upper part of the gantry, thus isolating them from the shock wave.[14] The likelihood of pulmonary blast injury is significantly reduced when using second-generation [36] (Lithostar) and third-generation lithotriptors for ESWL. When the MPL 9000 was used, Nazli and colleagues did apply pulmonary protection,[52] while others did not.[65] No patient in either series developed lung contusion.

The use of adjunctive procedures in preparation for ESWL in children, or postoperatively, has been well established. Our initial experience with intravenous pyelography during lithotripsy for radiolucent stone localization was poor. Dilution of the contrast by relative over-hydration of the

patient during anesthesia, and the long duration until the contrast accumulated in the renal collecting system limited effectiveness. Therefore, we insert a retrograde ureteral catheter and inject contrast for stone enhancement when using the HM3 lithotriptor. In second- and third-generation lithotriptors, ultrasound can localize most any renal stones, eliminating the need for ureteral stents for localization of radiolucent calculi.

We and others have found that internal stents were useful in cases of stones larger than 2.5 cm or of staghorn calculi, in order to avoid ureteral obstruction by stone fragments ("Steinstrasse").[21,47] Retrograde insertion of a ureteral catheter was efficient for manipulation, which was popular in the early days of ESWL for ureteral calculi. Currently, most ureteral stones are managed in-situ, and therefore manipulation is unnecessary. Ureteral catheters may still be useful in lithotriptors in which fluoroscopy is used for stone localization, as a ureteral calculus may be hidden from the contralateral camera by the spine or the sacrum.[21] Currently they are seldom used. [27,29,49,57]

Kroovand[10] noted that the urethra of most boys over the age of 9 months will atraumatically

accept an 8 French pediatric panendoscope. A 7.5F panendoscope with a 3F working channel can easily allow a 3F ureteral catheter to be safely introduced into the ureter of a male neonate. Percutaneous nephrostomy should be reserved for the drainage of septic and/or obstructed kidneys, and should be combined with antibacterial therapy. Lithotripsy is performed following recovery of the renal unit.

RESULTS The review of initial results of ESWL for the treatment of urinary calculi in children included a number of reporting variables. The differences were in treatment parameters, duration of follow-up, and the definition of success. Variations also included differences in definition of "children". In some series, only patients younger than 12 years were considered children,[15,19,21,51,58] whereas other patients are considered "children" at up to 18 years of age.[37,56] The youngest patients treated were reported to be 4 months of age.[66] Variability existed in reporting the location of stones treated. Most studies included the treatment of renal calculi only, whereas others, particularly those reporting results with second-generation lithotriptors, included both renal and ureteral calculi. Unfortunately, some publications are confusing because of these variables.[13,19,24,37] In later years, there were more reports discussing the management of ureteral calculi in situ,[20,21,49,51,57] and several reports discussed the outcome of ESWL monotherapy for staghorn stones. [12,15,18,40]

Extracorporeal shock wave lithotripsy for vesical calculi had been rarely reported initially.[26,67] In 2003, Rizvi and colleagues[28] reported on children with bladder calculi less than 1 cm in size who were treated with ESWL. In 39 of them (45.5%) the treatment was successful after one session. Muslumannoglu and colleagues[48] treated 16 bladder calculi in children; 8 stones were smaller than 1 cm and 8 stones were larger than 2 cm. They used the Lithostar Plus lithotriptor and achieved a 100% stone-free state, including a re-treatment rate of 25% in the former group, and 50% in the latter.

Newman and colleagues reported one of the earliest results of ESWL in children using the HM3

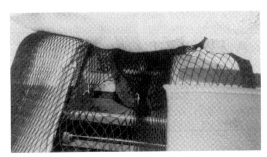

Figure 91-6 Patient positioned on the fishnet gantry on the Sonolith 3000 lithotriptor at the time of lithotripsy. The head, neck, and back are well-supported and the positioning is secured and reliable. Adjustments are quick and easy to perform. Note the hole in the net to allow passage of the ultrasound imaging probe into the water. Reproduced with permission from Silver RI, et al.[50]

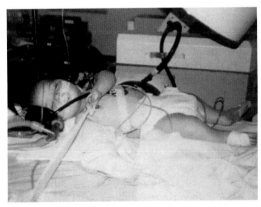

Figure 91-7 The positioning of the patient during treatment with the Nova lithotriptor. Reproduced with permission from Lottmann HB, et al.[22]

Figure 91-4 Fishnet gantry draped over the lithotripsy table to cover waterbath window. Reproduced with permission from Silver RI, et al.[50]

lithotriptor.[6] Their initial report in 1986 included 28 children aged 1 to 17 years (mean, 11 years). They updated their results in another report of 44 patients in 1989.[68] Their work was summarized, together with an additional 24 studies, in the first edition of Smith's textbook in 1996.[69] The experience accumulated since then is presented in Table 91-1 for renal calculi and in Table 91-2 for renal and ureteral calculi.

The relatively low stone-free rate for lower-pole calculi is a well-known problem that is related to low clearance of fragments rather than stone disintegration. An acute lower infundibulopelvic angle (less than 90°), small lower infundibulum diameter, complex caliceal anatomy, and a long caliceal length all have adverse effects on lower-pole stone clearance in adults,[70] as well as in pediatric patients.[6,71] Onal and colleagues contradicted this conclusion by showing that caliceal pelvic anatomy has no significant impact on fragment clearance following ESWL for lower caliceal calculi in children.[72] The calculation of either ureteropelvic axis or the pelvic axis reliably predicted stone clearance following ESWL.[73] Interestingly, stone burden and infundibulum diameter were not found to affect the occurrence of retained fragments in children.[74] In a more recent study, however, Demirkesen and colleagues studied the efficacy of ESWL for isolated lower caliceal calculi in a pediatric age group and compared it with that for isolated upper/middle caliceal and renal pelvic calculi.[75] They concluded that ESWL was equally effective for stones in all renal locations.

Cass found a statistically significant difference between the stone-free rate using the first-generation lithotriptor HM3 (68%) when compared with the second-generation lithotriptor Medstone STS (93%) in the treatment of single renal calculi.[54] No such difference was found when two second-generation lithotriptors, the MPL 5000 and the Echolith were compared.[37] The initial enthusiasm for the first-generation lithotriptors (ie, the Dornier HM3) was supplanted by the smaller, less powerful ultrasound-guided lithotriptors (second-generation), which usually required sedation only and eliminated the need for a tub. The results were poorer than those associated with the HM3, necessitating more sessions in order to achieve a stone-free state. Disappointment with the second-generation machine led to the evolution of the third-generation lithotriptors, which have a more powerful generator and have versatile ultrasound and fluoroscopy imaging facilities.[76,77] Postoperative complications, including perinephric hematoma, and the need for blood transfusions, however, was still higher in second- and third-generation lithotriptors than in the HM3 due to higher power density created by the some of the newer machines.

The treatment of cystine stones with ESWL requires special attention. Cystine stones that have smooth surfaces were reported to be harder to break than brushite and calcium oxalate monohydrate stones.[78] ESWL for children with cystine stones was successful in only 50% of cases.[79] We, however, have not found any difference between cystine and other calculi regarding success and complication rates associated with ESWL in children.[14,21]

ESWL was successfully used in anomalous kidneys. Semerci and colleagues treated adults and children with calculi in duplex, horseshoe, and pelvic ectopic kidneys.[60] They used the standard supine position and concluded that stone-bearing anomalous kidneys might be treated by ESWL as the primary option of treatment. Slavkovic and colleagues used the prone position for successful ESWL of a horseshoe kidney.[59] Tan and colleagues successfully treated 4 patients with serious anomalies including complete ureteral duplication (2), malrotated kidney, and a horseshoe kidney (1 each).[73] We have successfully managed ureteral calculi in crossed-fused renal ectopia in two children.[21] Ureteral catheters assisted in stone localization.

ESWL was successful in the management of a "stoned" ureteral stent that was left indwelling for 2 years.[80] The child became stone-free following four lithotripsy sessions.

COMPLICATIONS AND CONCERNS

GENERAL   Marberger and colleagues stated in 1989 that the ideal treatment of stones in the upper urinary tract should be removal of all calculus material with minimal morbidity and minimal damage to the surrounding structures, along with elimination of the cause of stone formation.[66] This statement is still valid today. Theoretically, ESWL is associated with increased risks in the pediatric population compared with adults. The reasons include exposure of pediatric kidneys and soft tissues to a high-pressure zone, the more detrimental effect of a high-energy shock wave to the growing kidney than to the mature one, the smaller caliber of the ureter and urethra with regard to stone fragment passage and endourologic stone manipulation, and the possibility of greater susceptibility to radiation exposure.

In recent reports, most post-lithotripsy complications were minor, and major complications occurred rarely.[12–16,18,19,21,22,24,25,28,32,36,38,54,62,71,73,75,81] The different types of complications were those that occurred during the lithotripsy per se, those

Table 91-2 Results of ESWL in Children

Author	No. of Patients	ESWL	Lithotriptor Type	Average No. of Shocks per Session	No. Stone-Free	% Stone-Free
Jayanthi[19]	24		HM3	≤ 2,500	17p	70
Landau[21]	38	ureter	HM3	1,884	37p	97
Gofrit[14]	38		HM3	2,012	35p	95
Lottmann[15]	23	staghorn	Sonolith 3000/Nova	< 3,000	19p	82
Sukla[23]	8	infants	HM3	2,100	8p	100
Orsola[12]	15	staghorn	Lithostar Ultra	3,025	11p	73
Al Busaidy[18]	47	ureter	Wolf 2500 piezolith	4,825	40p	63
Nazli[52]	67		MPL 9000	3.180	60p	70
Demirkesen[36]	54		Lithostar	1.619	38p	64
Tekin[32]	59		MPL 9000	1.235	42p	71
Cass[54]	38		HM3	1,152–1,459	26p	68
Cass[54]	107		Medstone STS	1,669–2,233	99p	93
Brinkmann[24]	64		Lithostar	2,996	53p	83
Delakas[49]	25	ureter	MPL 9000x	1,880	21p	84
Lottmann[22]	19	infants	Sonolith 3000/Nova	2,100	18p	95
Choong[13]	23		MPL 9000 & Dornier DL 50	ns	21p	93
Rodrigues Netto[16]	86		Lithostrar Plus	4,000-6,000	82p	97
Elsobky[37]	106		MPL 5000	5,348	90p	85
Elsobky[37]	42		Echolith	15,336	37p	84
Lifshitz[55]	29		HM3	1,323	20p	68
Goel[58]	50		Lithostar Plus	2,652	40p	76
McLorie[25]	24	infants	HM3	900–2,400	24p	100
McLorie[25]	10		MPL 5000	2,210	10p	100
Ozgur-Tan[57]	38		Lithostar Plus	2,827	31p	82
Al-Busaidy[51]	42	staghorn	Piezolith 2501	10,279	33p	79
Ather[71]	101		MPL 9000	2,327	96p	95
Rizvi[28]	177		EDAP LT02	ns	149p	84
Rizvi[28]	85	ureter	EDAP LT02	ns	46p	54
Rizvi[28]	63	bladder	EDAP LT02	ns	30p	48
Aksoy[47]	129		MPL 9000	1,850	114p	89
Ather[71]	21		MPL 9000	1,567	17p	81
Tan[38]	100		MPL 5000	2,455	68p	68
DeFoor[62]	88		Compact Delta	1,600	65p	74
Rhee[83]	8		ns	3,000	7p	90
Demirkesen[75]	126		Lithostar	1,500	90p	71
Tan[73]	85		Lithostar Plus	2,500	72p	85
Onal[72]	33		Lithostar	1,600	22p	61
Afshar[89]	83		Lithostar, Philips	ns	40p	46

ns = not specified

noted during the immediate postoperative period, and long-term complications.

ACUTE SHOCK WAVE SEQUELAE Pretreatment simulation was advocated by Newman and colleagues[6] and Shepherd and colleagues.[82] We used simulation only in very rare circumstances, such as in severe skeletal deformities or in cases with faintly opaque renal stones that were difficult to locate by fluoroscopy using the HM3 lithotriptor. As second- and third-generation lithotriptors locate the stones by ultrasound, fluoroscopic imaging is not a problem. Also, no difficulties were noted in our series in treating children with Harrington rods or other spine hardware, as opposed to others.[82] The use of "dry" treatment (without tubs for immersion) in second- and third-generation machines eliminated such problems almost entirely. Protection of all organs from pressure-related complications is mandatory in all lithotriptors.

Premature ventricular contractions were described in the early days of pediatric ESWL.[11,31] This potential high risk was eliminated with appropriate cardiac gating and has not been described in more recent publications. Recent experience with ungated ESWL demonstrated its safety and efficacy in the pediatric population.[83]

The use of fluoroscopy during ESWL is, obviously, associated with exposure of the patient to x-rays. Kroovand and colleagues[10] carefully monitored radiation exposure during ESWL treatment and estimated an average exposure of 14.4 roentgens per kidney treated (range, 1.8 to 46.1), indicating that such exposure was typical of pediatric diagnostic abdominal radiographic procedures such as voiding cystourethrography or barium enema. They also noted that, in view of the extremely small field of radiation, the actual exposure during ESWL is probably considerably less than estimated and can be further minimized by reducing fluoroscopic time, number of spot films, and x-ray field.[10] The gonads should be shielded in boys, which is easier to achieve in tubless second- and third-generation lithotriptors. The female gonads are always exposed to x-rays during ESWL, especially when treating lower ureteral calculi. The use of ultrasonography for stone localization obviously eliminates this risk.

Ecchymoses and hematuria have been recognized universally during ESWL treatment or in the immediate postoperative period in children managed with the Dornier HM3 lithotriptor. An entrance-site bruise is seen in all patients,[21,68] and an exit-site bruise is seen in many.[8] Ecchymoses have been reported also when second- or third-generation lithotriptors have been used.[22,24,36,51,58] Many recent publications do not mention the occurrence of post-ESWL ecchymoses, probably because they do not consider this as a complication.[13,14,16,24,51] Transient hematuria is also extremely common after ESWL. It happens in up to 100% of children who undergo ESWL.[24,36,49,52] Hemoptysis, secondary to pulmonary contusion, which was described in the early days of ESWL,[9,10] is currently eliminated by lung protec-

tion, and has been reported recently only in infants.[15] Mahboubi and colleagues reported on blood in the stool following ESWL in pelvic kidneys.[84] Laryngeal spasm,[14] hematemesis,[15] and perirenal hematoma[58] were reported in one patient each. Pancreatitis and gastric/duodenal erosions were noted in children in 1989 and in 1991, respectively,[68,85] and never since.

The management of renal calculi in children with hyperoxaluria is controversial, and should be addressed. ESWL was reported to be safely and successfully executed by Grateau and colleagues[86] and Kamoun and colleagues.[87] In contradiction to this experience, ESWL was found to provoke oxalosis leading to deterioration of renal function.[88] Our experience with ESWL for renal calculi in a hyperoxaluric patient was dismal. One child we treated lost the entire function of the treated kidney within a month. His sister, who also had hyperoxaluria, underwent percutaneous nephrolithotomy (PCNL) in another hospital with similar results. Another brother from the same family presented to us with multiple small renal calculi that periodically moved to the distal ureter, causing partial obstruction. Having the experience of the detrimental damage caused by ESWL and PCNL to the kidneys of his siblings, we performed ESWL to the distal ureteral stones only, avoiding the kidneys entirely. We repeated this procedure several times when new calculi reached the distal ureters. Liver transplantation subsequently solved the problem of recurrent nephrolithiasis in this child.

COLIC, OBSTRUCTION, AND INFECTION Renal colic secondary to stone fragments has been reported in 3% to 5%[17,49,51,52,71] of children undergoing ESWL. Most of these fragments pass spontaneously with no further sequelae. Ureteral obstruction by steinstrasse is generally uncommon, and was reported only in 1–6.5% of patients undergoing ESWL.[16,17,28,54,75] Stone fragments were found to pass faster in children than in adults.[66,68] Gofrit and colleagues compared a group of[40] children aged less than 6 years with 38 adults. Both groups had renal calculi that were identical in number, size (larger than 10 mm), and localization.[14] The pediatric ureter was found to be as efficient as the adult ureter in transporting stone fragments. Small (< 4 mm) residual stone fragments, however, were found to increase the chance of adverse clinical outcome by Afshar and colleagues.[89] The result in growth or symptoms in 69% of the cases, and thefore, should be followed closely, especially in the presence of metabolic or anatomical disorder.

The need for ureteral stenting during lithotripsy is controversial. Unstented lithotripsy procedures were more successful than stented, both in terms of success after one ESWL session (74%) and in overall success rate (93%).[25] Most of these infants were treated with the HM3 lithotriptor. Al-Busaidy, on the other hand, used a piezoelectric lithotriptor (Piezolith 2501, Richard Wolf GmbH, Knittlingen, Germany), and found a 21% complication rate in the unstented group of

children with staghorn calculi, compared to none in the stented group.[18] This difference may be explained by the use of different lithotriptors in the two groups, the high-energy HM3 versus the low-energy Piezolith. Also, all stones in the latter study were staghorn, whereas in the former they had variance in all size. DeFoor and colleagues stented 31% of their patient prior to ESWL with the mobile Dornier Compact Delta lithotriptor.[62] The average stone size was 6.1 mm. Indications for pre-ESWL stent insertion were not specified. Similar policy (25% stented patients) was executed by Tan and colleagues.[38] Postoperative insertion of percutaneous nephrostomy[17,18,22] or a Double J stent[52] can solve the problem of steinstrasse without any additional procedure.

Ureteroscopy is required uncommonly as an adjunctive procedure following ureteral obstruction, including one patient in our series.[13,18,21,26,32,49,51,52,57,73] Interestingly, open ureterolithotomy is still used for clearance of steinstrasse.[32,36,51,52,57] None of our patients, however, required open ureterolithotomy for the clearance of post-lithotripsy steinstrasse.[14,21,25] In my opinion, the new development of smallcaliber ureteroscopes should suffice to extract most fragments, eliminating the need for open ureterolithotomy.

Urinary infection is rare following ESWL in children.[18,24,38,75] Inappropriate preoperative antibacterial treatment and postoperative obstruction were the main precipitators of infection. Such obstruction should be managed as soon as it is diagnosed, either by percutaneous nephrostomy or by a retrograde insertion of a ureteral stent, followed by adequate stone management. In the adult setting, post-ESWL urinary tract infection, including pyelonephritis and urinary sepsis, may occur in cases with pretreatment negative cultures. A possible explanation for this is that struvite stones incorporate bacteria that are not expressed in the urine, resulting in negative preoperative urine culture. The lithotripsy process releases bacteria from the stone fragments, causing infection. We, therefore, recommend administration of pre-lithotripsy antibacterial treatment in every case with a history of recurrent urinary infection and suspected struvite calculi even though the pre-lithotripsy urine culture is sterile.

EXPERIMENTAL STUDIES AND CHRONIC EFFECTS

Imaging and biochemical studies have evaluated the quality and quantity of renal sequelae caused by ESWL. There have been numerous biochemical and imaging studies suggesting changes secondary to ESWL. They include studies using magnetic resonance imaging (MRI), computerized tomography (CT), and nuclear imaging.

Villanyi and colleagues evaluated the metabolic effects of ESWL on pediatric kidneys. Urinary levels of sodium, potassium, urea, creatinine, and β_2-microglobulin were examined.[61] Urinary activity of aspartate transferase, alanine transferase, alkaline phosphatase, and lactate dehydrogenase were assessed, as well as serum parameters of sodium, potassium, urea, and creatinine. Serum and urine electrolyte levels, as well as C-reactive protein, remained unchanged after lithotripsy. Urine activity of all enzymes, however, increased significantly by day 1 (except that of alanine transferase), suggesting acute cellular renal and liver injury. The activities of all enzymes returned to pre-ESWL levels by day fourteen.

Mostafavi and colleagues[90] demonstrated decrease in renal cortical blood flow and simultaneous increase in medullary flow in patients undergoing ESWL, as measured by Gd-DTPA-enhanced MRI, suggesting that renal hemodynamics are modified acutely by ESWL on a regional basis. These changes were avoided when intravenous aminophylline was administered prior to ESWL,[91] suggesting that aminophylline is a competitive antagonist of adenosine, which is a vasoconstrictor of the afferent arteriole in the glomerulus.

Animal studies have demonstrated the gross morphologic and microscopic changes in the kidney secondary to ESWL. Evan and colleagues[92] used the HM3 lithotriptor in a minipig model. They stated that the minipig was an ideal model for such studies because of its size, the size of the kidneys compared to human kidneys, the number of nephrons contained within each kidney, and the general characteristics of renal function that can be measured with studies similar to those performed in humans. Evan and another group[93] also found that renal disease potentiates acute injury caused by ESWL in a juvenile pig model. They created bilateral vesicoureteral reflux and then infected the bladder with one of two types of *Escherichia coli*, a virulent and a less virulent type (groups 1 and 2, respectively). The lower calix of one kidney in each animal was then exposed to 2,000 shock waves at 24 kV, at 7 days, with no antibacterial treatment (group 1), and at 7 weeks, with antibiotics (group 2). The study showed that, when kidneys compromised by reflux pyelonephritis are challenged by ESWL, there is an exaggerated impairment of renal blood flow and glomerular filtration rate. The severity of these changes mimics the injury observed after a high dose of shock waves (8,000 at 24 kV). The changes in group 2 were milder than those observed in group 1, suggesting that acute untreated pyelonephritis enhances the damage more than chronic treated pyelonephritis. The same group evaluated the macroscopic and microscopic injury to the kidney of juvenile pigs undergoing ESWL with the HM3 lithotriptor.[94] They demonstrated subcapsular hematoma in the anterior or posterior aspect of the affected kidneys. Microscopic changes in these kidneys included intraparenchymal hemorrhage compressing the cortex and the tip of renal papillae located in F2 of the lithotriptor. Regions of cortical bleeding were connected to subcapsular hematomas via lacerations of the renal parenchyma. Transmission electron microscopy revealed sites of intraparenchymal hemorrhage correlated with damaged vasa recta, which showed focal regions of endothelial and base-

ment membrane injury that were always associated with inflammatory reaction. ESWL was also shown to cause cell lysis in vivo.[95]

Several interventions were undertaken in an effort to reduce renal damage following ESWL. When a pressure release reflector, which suppressed cavitation, replaced the standard rigid reflector in the Dornier HM3 for ESWL in juvenile pigs, the above-mentioned macroscopic and microscopic damage was almost eliminated.[95] Pre-lithotripsy administration of allopurinol, using a microdialysis system, reduced the free radical activity during ESWL in the juvenile pig.[96] Yaman and colleagues[97] reported on the protective effect of verapamil on rabbit renal tissue during ESWL. They used the Dornier MPL 9000 for this purpose, and delivered different numbers of shock waves (1,000, 1,500, or 2,000) at a constant 18 kV in the control group. The study group was fed with verapamil for 3 days before lithotripsy application. MRI scans, performed at 24 hours revealed in the control group intrarenal hematomas at the corticomedullary junction, loss of corticomedullary differentiation, and diffuse radially oriented hemorrhages in the parenchyma. Evaluation of kidneys 3 months after ESWL treatment revealed disappearance of the acute pathologic findings in almost all animals. Loss of corticomedullary junction, however, and shrinkage of the parenchyma persisted in 6 and 3 animals, respectively. Almost none of these pathologic alterations could be demonstrated in the study group. Histologic studies performed 24 hours post-ESWL demonstrated tubular dilation with vacuolar and hydrophobic degeneration, protein deposition, and free erythrocytes in the tubuli. Only limited histopathologic findings were observed in the verapamil group. These limited changes comprised few alterations at the tubular and interstitial levels, but not in the glomeruli. Similar differences were noted in the animals sacrificed 3 months following ESWL.

ESWL was found to cause cell lysis in in vitro experiments.[98,99] Air bubbles significantly enhanced this effect. It has been postulated that fluid near air bubbles, within a vial, would be agitated and/or enriched with cavitation nuclei, such that cell damage was increased in that local region of the vial.[98,100] In vitro cell lysis caused by ESWL was significantly lower with the pressure release reflector than with the rigid reflector.[95]

Rassweiler and colleagues[101] used the Modulith SL20 electromagnetic shock wave generator to induce renal trauma in a canine model. They concluded that the degree of trauma increased proportionately with increasing generator voltage and was not related to the number of shock waves. Adrenomedullin is a reno-protective peptide with potent vaso-relaxing, natriuretic, and cell–growth-modulating properties. Sarica and colleagues[102] evaluated renal damage by measuring serum adrenomedullin levels in rabbits undergoing ESWL. They, unlike Rassweiler and colleagues, have clearly shown that renal damage was directly related to the number of shock waves while the energy was kept constant at 14 kV.

The type of lithotriptor, and especially the size of the focal point, has an important impact on the outcome of ESWL. The second- and third-generation lithotriptors have high-pressure focal zones that are significantly smaller than those of the Dornier HM3.[63,66] The power of the lithotriptor is proportional to peak pressure at the focal point and the size of the focal point.[103] The larger the focal point is, the more powerful the lithotriptor. Renal injury, however, is also proportional to the size of the focal point. It has been postulated that more precise focusing results in lower parenchymal injury.[63,66] In the pediatric patient, the smaller focal zone potentially causes damage to a significantly lower proportion of the kidney than a large focal zone which may, in fact, cover most of the kidney because of its small size. It should be emphasized, however, that renal injury can occur with any type of lithotriptor and has been induced experimentally with all of the lithotriptors currently in clinical use. Regardless of the type of lithotriptor, it is quite clear from the animal studies that acute renal damage does occur. The experimental data further lead to the conclusion that the treatment of children should be limited to the lowest number of shock waves and the lowest energy level that adequately produces fragmentation. Furthermore, the data suggest that repeated treatment with a lesser number of shock waves is preferable to a single excessive dose of shock waves. With these parameters in mind, all lithotriptors that are clinically available can be used to safely treat stones in pediatric patients.

Sokolov and colleagues used a dual-pulse lithotriptor modified from the classic Dornier HM3.[104] This lithotriptor consisted of two opposing, confocal, and simultaneously triggered electrohydraulic sources. The pulses superimposed at the common focus, resulted in pressure doubling and enhanced cavitation growth in the localized 1-cm-wide volume. Model gypsum stones were exposed in vitro to dual pulses and single pulses. At the focus, model stones treated with 100 dual pulses at 15 kV broke into 8 times the number of fragments as stones treated with 200 single pulses at 18 kV in half the time. At axial positions 2 cm and 4 cm away from the focus, lysis of erythrocytes was reduced or equivalent for dual pulses versus single pulses. Similar modification of second- or third-generation lithotriptors may improve the outcome of ESWL in children, reducing risk of renal injury. Sheir and colleagues[105] designed a synchronous twin-pulse lithotriptor. The effects of utilization of one shock wave reflector and the simultaneous use of two shock wave reflectors (twin head) were compared in several ways. A sheet of aluminum was used to test the cavitation effect. Ceramic blocks were used to test the quality of disintegration, shape of focal zone, and the ideal position of second focus of the lithotriptor. The efficiency of disintegration was tested by using balls made of dental cement. They concluded that the synchronous twin-pulse technique improves the quality and the rate of stone disintegration during ESWL.

The best results were obtained when the angle between the axes of the two reflectors was 90°. They recommended an in-vivo test that will be followed by clinical trials to test the efficacy and the safety of this procedure.

Clinical and experimental studies have looked at the chronic renal effects of ESWL, especially those related to renal growth and function. Lottmann and colleagues evaluated the long-term effect of ESWL on kidneys of 15 children aged 9 months to 15 years.[106] Technetium (Tc) 99m dimercaptosuccinic acid renal scan performed 6 months following lithotripsy did not reveal any significant changes compared with a pre-lithotripsy scan. The same group had similar results in infants less than 2 years of age.[22] Ultrasonography did not show any evidence of parenchymal injuries in these patients.[106] Ultrasonography, however, did demonstrate reduction in renal growth, compared with predictive values, 9 years after ESWL with the Dornier HM3.[55] Interestingly enough, in this study, both treated and untreated kidneys were affected. Vlajkovic and colleagues[34] evaluated pre- and post-ESWL Tc 99m diethylenetriamine pentaacetic acid (DTPA) clearance studies in 84 children aged 2 to 14 years. They found that total DTPA clearance and individual renal clearance 3 months after lithotripsy were higher than before the treatment regardless of acute or chronic renal disease, with or without partial stasis. Goel and colleagues reported similar findings.[58] They found a decrease in post-lithotripsy renal function, measured by DTPA scan, occurring in two refluxing renal units only. Thomas and colleagues[107] measured effective renal plasma flow by quantitative iodine 131 radionucleotide scanning immediately preceding ESWL, and a follow-up between 74 and 238 weeks. They found no statistically significant differences between the outcome of these patients and the expected changes in renal plasma flow according to age.

New onset of hypertension after ESWL is a well known sequelae in adults and in pediatric patients. The changes within the kidney following ESWL were found to be similar to those seen in blunt renal trauma.[85] A post-lithotripsy atrophic kidney caused hypertension secondary to hyperreninemia.[108] Janetschek and colleagues[109] evaluated pre- and post-ESWL blood pressure, and resistive index levels in adults. They found an increase in resistive index levels in 75% of patients older than 60 years. During a 26-month follow-up, these values continued to increase in 45% of the patients in this age group, and it was these patients who had new onset hypertension. There was a strong correlation between elevated resistive index levels and blood pressure, suggesting underlying renovascular disease. Of all the series mentioned in Table 91-1, only 7 reported on the measurement of post-lithotripsy blood pressure in children; and of these, only 1 case or hypertension was documented.[53] Despite the rarity of this phenomenon, Bataille and colleagues, in an extensive review of 55 articles, strongly recommended that blood pressure

should be monitored in every patient treated by ESWL.[110] Furthermore, in elderly or uremic patients (plasma creatinine > 3 mg/dL) and in children, ESWL should be used cautiously, and post-procedure follow-up of renal function and blood pressure is advised.

Linear body and bone growth following ESWL were evaluated. No effect of ESWL on total growth was found in the rabbit model,[111] and on body growth in children.[107] Conflicting results were found on the effect of ESWL on bone growth. Yeaman and colleagues showed that 8 of 18 rat epiphyses that were treated were affected by ESWL.[112] Van Arsdalen and colleagues[113] however, found no adverse effect on epiphyseal growth in the rabbit.

Concern has been raised regarding the adverse effects of shock waves on the ovaries of pediatric patients during treatment of distal ureteral stones. McCullough and colleagues evaluated the effects of shock waves on the rat ovary.[114] Rats underwent unilateral oophorectomy, while the contralateral ovary received shock waves. There was no difference between the control and study groups in the number of pregnancies, fetal numbers and weights, and spontaneous abortions. Although microscopic hemorrhages were seen in the ovaries examined immediately following shock wave treatment, the number of follicles did not change between the shocked versus the control ovaries taken from the same animal. Vieweg and colleagues conducted a clinical study of 84 women aged 17 to 43 years who underwent ESWL for distal ureteral calculi.[115] No adverse effect on their fertility potential or on their offspring was found, although a spontaneous abortion resulted during treatment of one woman who was not aware of her pregnancy. Long-term effects on ovaries of girls following shock wave lithotripsy to the distal ureter are currently unknown, but short-term complications are negligible.

CONCLUSIONS

More than two decades have passed since the introduction of ESWL, and the indications for the use of this modality in the treatment of renal and ureteral calculi in children are still valid. Preoperative evaluation should be targeted to the anatomic and metabolic abnormalities specific to this age group, and to those that may refer the child to a different treatment modality (open procedure or PCNL). Postoperative medical treatment in order to prevent stone recurrence is of equal importance.

The treating pediatric urologist should be aware of the concerns related to ESWL in children. These include the exposure of a relatively larger portion of the pediatric kidney as opposed to the adult kidney to the high-pressure shock waves, higher potential of radiation exposure in the pediatric age group, and acute macroscopic and microscopic changes occurring within and around the growing kidney as a result of the trauma caused by the shock waves. Furthermore,

the physician should consider the chronic adverse effects of ESWL on renal growth and function, and the potential for new onset of hypertension. All these issues should be thoroughly discussed with the parents prior to the treatment. The operator should pay particular attention to details related to positioning, shielding of the lungs and gonads, and technical treatment parameters to limit the potential for adverse side effects.

The outcome of ESWL in children is excellent, as shown by numerous studies. The stone-free rates are equal or superior to those achieved in adults,[16] and are generally achieved more rapidly.[115] Stones less than 2.5 cm in size can efficiently be negotiated by ESWL, with an equal or more rapid passage of fragments through the pediatric ureter than via the adult ureter[14] due to the shorter presence of the stone within the pediatric urinary tract, smaller size of the patient, greater physical activity of children, and greater distensibility of their urinary tracts.[66] Staghorn calculi can be managed by ESWL very efficiently,[15,18] even in the infant age group.[22,25] Calculi 2.5 cm or larger can be managed either by ESWL or by PCNL or, even better, by a combination of the two, as in adults. Stones associated with congenital obstructive anatomic anomalies should generally be treated by open surgery in conjunction with reconstruction of these anomalies. ESWL is still the first-line treatment for ureteral calculi, even in the current era of small-caliber flexible ureteroscopes.

Finally, in addition to the clinical efficacy of ESWL, it is important to emphasize its clinical safety, as proven by numerous studies cited in this chapter. Despite the theoretical concerns elucidated above, very few major complications have actually been reported in the clinical setting.[116] Those reported appear less frequently and require fewer adjunctive procedures than in adults. When weighing potential risks and complications versus benefits, it is most important to compare the potential adverse effects that may occur to untreated kidneys, as well as to compare potential injuries and other risks associated with alternative surgical procedures including PCNL, ureteroscopy, and even open surgery.

The experience gathered in more than 20 years shows that ESWL is the treatment of choice for renal and ureteral calculi in children, even at the beginning of the twenty-first century, and is associated with minimal short- and long-term sequelae.

REFERENCES

1. Chaussy C, Brendel W, Schmiedt E. Extracorporally induced destruction of kidney stones by shock waves. Lancet 1980;2:1265–8.
2. Schmiedt E, Chaussy C. Extracorporeal shock-wave lithotripsy of kidney and ureteric stones. Urol Int 1984;39:193–8.
3. Rassweiler J, Lutz K, Gumpinger R, Eisenberger F. Efficacy of in situ extracorporeal shock wave lithotripsy for upper ureteral calculi. Eur Urol 1986;12:377–386.
4. Eisenberger F, Fuchs G, Miller K, et al. Extracorporeal shock-wave lithotripsy (ESWL) and endourology: an ideal combination for the treatment of kidney stones. World J Urol 1985;3:41–7.
5. Bub P, Clayman RV, Fuchs G, Eisenberger F. Change of indications in the treatment of urinary stones in children. Pre-

sented at the Second Symposium on Shock Wave Lithotripsy, March 1, 1986. 1986.
6. Newman DM, Coury T, Lingeman JE, et al. Extracorporeal shock wave lithotripsy experience in children. J Urol 1986;136:238–40.
7. Boddy SAM, Kelett MJ, Fletcher MS, et al. Extracorporeal shock wave lithotripsy and percutaneous nephrolithotomy in children. J Pediatr Surg 1987;22:223–7.
8. Kramolowsky EV, Willoughby BL, Loening SA. Extracorporeal shock wave lithotripsy in children. J Urol 1987:939–41.
9. Sigman M, Laudone VP, Jenkins AD, et al. Initial experience with extracorporeal shock wave lithotripsy in children. J Urol 1987;138:839–41.
10. Kroovand RL, Harrison LH, McCullough DL. Extracorporeal shock wave lithotripsy in childhood. J Urol 1987;138: 1106–8.
11. Abara E, M.P, McLorie GA, et al. Lithostar extracorporeal shock wave lithotripsy in children. J Urol 1990;144(2 pt 2): 489–91.
12. Orsola A, Diaz I, Caffaratti J, et al. Staghorn calculi in children: treatment with monotherapy extracorporeal shock wave lithotripsy. J Urol 1999;162(3 pt 2):1229–33.
13. Choong S, Whitfield H, Duffy P, et al. The management of paediatric urolithiasis. BJU Int 2000;86:857–60.
14. Gofrit ON, Pode D, Meretyk S, et al. Is the pediatric ureter as efficient as the adult ureter in transporting fragments following extracorporeal shock wave lithotripsy for renal calculi larger than 10 mm? J Urol 2001;166:1862–4.
15. Lottmann HB, Traxer O, Archambaud F, Mercier-Pageyral B. Monotherapy extracorporeal shock wave lithotripsy for the treatment of staghorn calculi in children. J Urol 2001; 165(6 pt 2):2324–7.
16. Rodrigues Netto NJ, Longo JA, Ikonomidis JK, Rodrigues Netto M. Extracorporeal shock wave lithotripsy in children. J Urol 2002;167:2164–6.
17. Ather MH, Noor MA. Does size and site matter for renal stones up to 30-mm in size in children treated by extracorporeal lithotripsy? Urology 2003;61:212–5.
18. Al-Busaidy SS, Prem AR, Medhat M. Pediatric staghorn calculi: the role of extracorporeal shock wave lithotripsy monotherapy with special reference to ureteral stenting. J Urol 2003;169:629–33.
19. Jayanthi VR, Arnold PM, Koff SA. Strategies for managing upper tract calculi in young children. J Urol 1999;162 (3 pt 2):1229–33.
20. Van Savage JG, Palanca LG, Andersen RD, et al. Treatment of distal ureteral stones in children: similarities to the American Urological Association guidelines in adults. J Urol 2000;164(3 pt 2):1089–93.
21. Landau EH, Gofrit ON, Shapiro A, et al. Extracorporeal shock wave lithotripsy is highly effective for ureteral calculi in children. J Urol 2001;165(6 pt 2):2316–9.
22. Lottmann HB, Archambaud F, Traxer O, et al. The efficacy and parenchymal consequences of extracorporeal shock wave lithotripsy in infants. BJU Int 2000;85:311–5.
23. Shukla AR, Hoover DL, Homsy YL, et al. Urolithiasis in the low birth weight infant: the role and efficacy of extracorporeal shock wave lithotripsy. J Urol 2001;165(6 pt 2): 2320–3.
24. Brinkmann OA, Griehl A, Kuwertz-Broking E, et al. Extracorporeal shock wave lithotripsy in children. Efficacy, complications and long-term follow-up. Eur Urol 2001;39:591–7.
25. McLorie GA, Pugach J, Pode D, et al. Safety and efficacy of extracorporeal shock wave lithotripsy in infants. Can J Urol 2003;10:2051–5.
26. Husain I, el-Faqih SR, Shamsuddin AB, Atassi R. Primary extracorporeal shockwave lithotripsy in management of large bladder calculi. J Endourol 1994;8:183–6.
27. Al-Rasheed SA, el-Faqih SR, Husain I, et al. The aetiological and clinical pattern of childhood urolithiasis in Saudi Arabia. Int Urol Nephrol 1995;27:349–55.
28. Rizvi SA, Naqvi SA, Hussain Z, et al. Management of pediatric urolithiasis in Pakistan: experience with 1440 children. J Urol 2003;169:634–7.
29. Wehle MJ, Segura JW. Pediatric urolithiasis. In: Belman AB, King LR, Kramer SA, editors. Clinical pediatric urology. London: Martin Dunitz; 2002. p. 1223–45.
30. Wilbert DM, Schofer O, Riedmiller H. Treatment of paediatric urolithiasis by extracorporeal shock-wave lithotripsy. Eur J Pediatr 1988;147:579–81.
31. Thornhill JA, Moran K, Mooney EE, et al. Extracorporeal shockwave lithotripsy monotherapy for paediatric urinary tract calculi. Br J Urol 1990;65:638–40.
32. Tekin I, Tekgul S, Bakkaloglu M, Kendi S. Results of extracorporeal shock wave lithotripsy in children using the Dornier MPL 9000 lithotriptor. J Pediatr Surg 1998;33:1257–9.
33. Lottmann HB, Gagnadoux MF, Daudon M. Urolithiasis in children. In: Gearhart JG, Rink RC, Mouriquand PDE, editors. Pediatric urology. Philadelphia: W.B. Saunders Company; 2001. p. 828–59.
34. Vlajkovic M, Slavkovic A, Radovanovic M, et al. Long-term functional outcome of kidneys in children with urolithiasis after ESWL treatment. Eur J Pediatr Surg 2002;12:118–23.
35. Aldridge RD, Aldridge RC, Aldridge LM. Anesthesia for pediatric lithotripsy. Paediatric Anesth 2006;16:236–41.
36. Demirkesen O, Tansu N, Yaycioglu O, et al. Extracorporeal shockwave lithotripsy in the pediatric population. J Endourol 1999;13:147–50.
37. Elsobky E, Sheir KZ, Madbouly K, Mokhtar AA. Extracorporeal shock wave lithotripsy in children: experience using two second-generation lithotripters. BJU Int 2000; 86:851–6.
38. Tan AN, Al-Omar M, Waterson JD, et al. Results of shock-wave lithotripsy for pediatric urolithiasis. J Endourol 2004;18:527–30.
39. Mishriki SF, Wills M, Mukherjee A, et al. Extracorporeal shock wave lithotripsy for renal calculi in children. Br J Urol 1992;69:303.
40. Esen AA, Kirkali Z, Guler C. Open stone surgery: is it still a preferable procedure in the management of staghorn calculi? Int Urol Nephrol 1994;26:247.
41. Zeitlin G, Roth RA. Effect of three anesthetic techniques on the success of extracorporeal shock wave lithotripsy in nephrolithiasis. Anesthesiology 1988;68:272–6.
42. Harries A, Bagley G, Lim M. Anaesthesia for extracorporeal shock-wave lithotripsy. A comparison of propofol and methohexitone infusions during high frequency jet ventilation. Anaesthesia 1988;43(1 Suppl):100–5.
43. Warner MA, Warner ME, Buck CF, Segura JW. Clinical efficacy of high frequency jet ventilation during extracorporeal shock wave lithotripsy of renal and ureteral calculi: a comparison with conventional mechanical ventilation. J Urol 1988;139:486–7.
44. Perel A, Segal E, Pizov R, et al. QRS-activated ventilation during general anesthesia for extracorporeal shock wave lithotripsy. J Clin Anesth 1989;1:268–71.
45. Tiselius HG. Cutaneous anesthesia with lidocaine-prilocaine cream: a useful adjunct during shock wave lithotripsy with analgesic sedation. J Urol 1993;149:8–11.
46. Bierkens AF, Hendrikx AJ, Ezz el Din KE, et al. The value of antibiotic prophylaxis during extracorporeal shock wave lithotripsy in the prevention of urinary tract infections in patients with urine proven sterile prior to treatment. Eur Urol 1997;31:30–5.
47. Aksoy Y, Ozbey I, Atmaca AF, Polat O. Extracorporeal shock wave lithotripsy in children: experience using a MPL-9000 lithotriptor. World J Urol 2004;23.
48 Muslumanoglu AY, Tefekeli A, Sarilar O, et al. Extracorporeal shock wave lithotripsy as first line treatment alternative for urinary tract stones in children: a large scale retrospective analysis. J Urol 2003;170:2405–8.
49. Delakas D, Dakalopoulos G, Metaxari M, et al. Management of ureteral stones in pediatric patients. J Endourol 2001; 15:675–80.
50. Silver RI. A fishnet gantry for pediatric extracorporeal shock wave lithotripsy on the Sonolith 3000. Urology 2001; 57:795–7.
51. Al Busaidy SS, Prem AR, Medhat M, et al. Paediatric ureteric calculi: efficacy of primary in situ extracorporeal shock wave lithotripsy. Br J Urol 1998;82:90–6.
52. Nazli O, Cal C, Ozyurt C, et al. Results of extracorporeal shock wave lithotripsy in the pediatric age group. Eur Urol 1998;33:33–336.
53. Kroovand RL. Pediatric urolithiasis. Urol Clin North Am 1997;24:173–84.
54. Cass AS. Comparison of first-generation (Dornier HM3) and second-generation (Medstone STS) lithotriptors: treatment results with 145 renal and ureteral calculi in children. J Endourol 1996;10:493–9.
55. Lifshitz DA, Lingeman JE, Zafar FS, et al. Alternations in predicted growth rates of pediatric kidneys treated with extracorporeal shockwave lithotripsy. J Endourol 1998; 12:469–75.
56. Lim DJ, Walker DR, Ellsworth PI, et al. Treatment of pediatric urolithiasis between 1984 and 1994. J Urol 1996;156 (2 Suppl):702–5.
57. Ozgur Tan M, Karaoglan U, Sozen S, Bozkirli I. Extracorporeal shock-wave lithotripsy for treatment of ureteral calculi in paediatric patients. Pediatr Surg Int 2003;8.
58. Goel MCB, N.S, Babu RV, et al. Pediatric kidney: functional outcome after extracorporeal shock wave lithotripsy. J Urol 1996;155:2044–6.
59. Slavkovic A, Vlajkovic M, Radovanovic M, et al. ESWL in the treatment of a stone in a child with horseshoe kidney. Int Urol Nephrol 2001;32:327–9.
60. Semerci B, Verit A, Nazli O, et al. The role of ESWL in the treatment of calculi with anomalous kidneys. Eur Urol 1997;31:302–4.
61. Villanyi KK, Szekely JG, Farkas LM, et al. Short-term changes in renal function after extracorporeal shock wave lithotripsy in children. J Urol 2001;166:222–4.
62. DeFoor W, Dharamsi N, Smith P, et al. Use of mobile extracorporeal shock wave lithotriptor: experience in a pediatric institution. Urology 2005;65:778–81.
63. Myers DA, Mobley TB, Jenkins JM, et al. Pediatric low energy lithotripsy with the Lithostar. J Urol 1995;153:453–7.
64. Pode D, Landau EH, Lijovetzky G, Shapiro A. Isolated pulmonary blast injury in rats—a new model using the extracorporeal shock-wave lithotriptor. Mil Med 1990;154: 288–93.
65. Tekin A, Tekgul S, Astu N, et al. Cystine calculi in children: the results of a metabolic evaluation and response to medical therapy. J Urol 2001;165(6 pt 2):2328–30.
66. Marberger M, Turk C, Steinkogler I. Piezoelectric extracorporeal shock wave lithotripsy in children. J Urol 1989; 142:349–52.
67. Mozam F, Nazir Z, Jafarey AM. Pediatric urolithiasis. To cut or not to cut. J Pediatr Surg 1994;29:761–4.
68. Adams MC, Newman DM, Lingeman JE. Pediatric ESWL: long-term results and effects on renal growth. J Endourol 1989;3:245–54.
69. Van Arsdalen KN. Lithotripsy. In: Smith AD, Badlani GH, Bagley DH, et al, editors. Smith's textbook of endourology. Vol 2. 1st ed. St. Louis: Quality Medical Publishing, Inc.; 1996. p. 1430.
70. Sampaio FJB, Aragao AHM. Inferior pole collecting system anatomy: its probable role in extracorporeal shock wave lithotripsy. J Urol 1992;147:322–4.
71 Ather MH, Noor MA, Akhtar S. The effect of intracalyceal distribution on the clearence of renal stones of > 20 mm in children after extracorporeal lithotripsy. BJU Int 2004;93:827–9.
72 Onal B, Demirkesen O, Tansu N, et al. The impact of calyceal pelvic anatomy on stone clearance after shock wave lithotripsy for pediatric lower pole stones. J Urol 2004; 172:1082–6.
73 Tan MO, Kirac M, Onaran M, et al. Factors affecting the success rate of extracorporeal shock wave lithotripsy for renal calculi in children. Urol Res 2006;Mar 4.
74. Ozgur Tan M, Karaoglan U, Sen I, et al. The impact of radiological anatomy in clearance of lower calyceal stones after shock wave lithotripsy in paediatric patients. Eur Urol 2003;43:188–93.
75 Demirkesen O, Onal B, Tansu N, et al. Efficacy of extracorporeal shock wave lithotripsy for isolated lower calyceal stones in children compared with stones in other renal locations. Urology 2006;67:170–5.
76. Kim SC, Nadler RB. ESWL: Quo vadis? AUA update series 2001 (Lesson 17);XX:130–5.
77. Preminger GM, Assimos DG, Lingeman JE, et al. Chapter 1: AUA guideline on management of staghorn calculi: diagnosis and treatment recommendations. J Urol 2005;713: 1991–2000.
78. Bhatta KM, Prien EL Jr, Dretler SP. Cystine calculi—rough and smooth: a new clinical distinction. J Urol 1989; 142:937–40.
79. Slavkovic A, Radovanovic M, Siric Z, et al. Extracorporeal shock wave lithotripsy for cystine urolithiasis in children: outcome and complications. Int Urol Nephrol 2002–2003; 34:457–61.
80. Slavkovic A, Vlajkovic M, Siric Z, Stefanovic V. Extracorporeal shock wave lithotripsy monotherapy of 'stoned' ureteral stent in children. Case report. Urol Int 2000;64:33–5.
81. Downey P, McNeill A, Smith G, et al. Shockwave lithotripsy in children [Abstract]. BJU Int 2000;85(Suppl 5):46–7.
82. Shepherd P, Thomas R, Harmon EP. Urolithiasis in children. J Urol 1988;140:790–2.
83 Rhee K, Palmer JS. Ungated extracorporeal shock wave lithotripsy in children: an initial series. Urology 2006;67: 392–3.
84. Mahboubi S, Smith JE, Van Arsdalen KN, et al. Extracorporeal shock wave lithotripsy in children. IPR abstract 1987.
85. Bregg K, Vaughan ED Jr. Acute and chronic cellular, tissue and systemic effects of ESWL. AUA Update Series 1991; 10:26–31.
86. Grateau G, Grunfeld JP, Beurton D, et al. Post-surgical deterioration of renal function in primary hyperoxaluria. Nephrol Dial Transplant 1987;1:261–4.
87. Kamoun A, Daudon M, Zghal A, et al [Primary hyperoxaluria: Tunisian experience apropos of 24 pediatric cases]. Nephrologie 1997;18:59–64.
88. Tan IL, Zonderland HM, Boeve ER. Oxalosis provoked by extracorporeal shock wave lithotripsy. Lancet 1994;344: 757–8.

89 Ashfar K, McLorie GA, Papanikolau F, et al. Outcome of small residual stone fragments following shock wave lithotripsy in children. J Urol 2004;172:1600–3.

90. Mostafavi MR, Chavez DR, Cannillo J, et al. Redistribution of renal blood flow after SWL evaluated by Gd-DTPA-enhanced magnetic resonance imaging. J Endourol 1998; 12:9–12.

91. Chan AJ, Prasad PV, Priatna A, et al. Protective effect of aminophylline on renal perfusion changes induced by high-energy shockwaves identified by Gd-DTPA-enhanced first-pass perfusion MRI. J Endourol 2000; 14:117–21.

92. Evan AP, Willis LR, Connors B, et al. Shock wave lithotripsy-induced renal injury. Am J Kidney Dis 1991;17:445–50.

93. Evan AP, Connors BA, Pennington DJ, et al. Renal disease potentiates the injury caused by SWL. J Endourol 1999; 13:619–28.

94. Shao Y, Connors BA, Evan AP, et al. Morphological changes induced in the pig kidney by extracorporeal shock wave lithotripsy: nephron injury. Anat Res 2003;275A:979–89.

95. Evan AP, Willis LR, McAteer JA, et al. Kidney damage and renal functional changes are minimized by waveform control that suppresses cavitation in shock wave lithotripsy. J Urol 2002;168(4 pt 1):1556–62.

96. Munver R, Delvecchio FC, Kuo RL, et al. In vivo assessment of free radical activity during shock wave lithotripsy using a microdialysis system: the renoprotective action of allopurinol. J Urol 2002;167:327–34.

97. Yaman O, Sarica K, Ozer G, et al. Protective effect of vera-pamil on renal tissue during shockwave application in rabbit model. J Endourol 1996;10:329–33.

98. Williams JC Jr, Stonehill MA, Colmenares K, et al. Effect of macroscopic air bubbles on cell lysis by shock wave lithotripsy in vitro. Ultrasound Med Biol 1999;25:473–9.

99. Lokhandwalla M, McAteer JA, Williams JC Jr, Sturtevant B. Mechanical haemolysis in shock wave lithotripsy (SWL): II. in vitro cell lysis due to shear. Phys Med Biol 2001; 46:1245–64.

100. Miller MW, Miller DL, Brayman AA. A review of in vitro bioeffects of interial ultrasonic cavitation from a mechanistic perspective. Ultrasound Med Biol 1996;22:1131–54.

101. Rassweiler J, Kohrmann KU, Back W, et al. Experimental basis of shockwave-induced renal trauma in the model of the canine kidney. World J Urol;1993;11:43–53.

102. Sarica K, Sari I, Balat A, et al. Evaluation of adrenomedullin levels in renal parenchyma subjected to extracorporeal shockwave lithotripsy. Urol Res 2003;31:267–71.

103. Lingeman JE. Extracorporeal shock wave lthotripsy. Development, instrumentation, and current status. Urol Clin North Am 1997;24:185–211.

104. Sokolov DL, Bailey MR, Crum LA. Dual-pulse lithotripter accelerates stone fragmentation and reduces cell lysis in vitro. Ultrasound Med Biol 2003;29:1045–52.

105. Sheir KH, El-sheikh AM, Ghoneim MA. Synchronous twin-pulse technique to improve efficacy of SWL: preliminary of an experimental study. J Endourol 2001;15: 965–74.

106. Lottmann HB, Archambaud F, Hellal B, et al. 99m Tech-necium-dimercapto-succinic acid renal scan in the evaluation of potential long-term renal parenchymal damage associated with extracorporeal shock wave lithotripsy in children. J Urol 1998;159:521–4.

107. Thomas R, Frentz HM, Harmon E, Frentz GD. Effect of extracorporeal shock wave lithotripsy on renal function and body height in pediatric patients. J Urol 1992;148.

108. Sasaguri M, Noda K, Mastumoto T, et al. A case of hyper-reninemic hypertension after extracorporeal shock wave lithotripsy. Hypertens Res 2000;23:709–12.

109. Janetschek G, Frauscher F, Knapp R, et al. New onset hypertension after extracorporeal shock wave lithotripsy: age related incidence and prediction by intrarenal resistive index. J Urol 1997;158:346–51.

110. Bataille P, Cardon G, Bouzernidj M, et al. Renal and hypertensive complications of extracorporeal shock wave lithotripsy: who is at risk? Urol Int 1999;62:195–200.

111. Kaji DM, Xie HW, Hardy BE, et al. The effects of extracorporeal shock wave lithotripsy on renal growth, function and arterial blood pressure in an animal model. J Urol 1991;146:544–7.

112. Yeaman LD, Jerome CP, McCullough DL. Effects of shock waves on the growth of the immature rat epiphysis. J Urol 1989;141:670–4.

113. Van Arsdalen KN, Kurzweil SJ, Smith JE, Levin RM. Effects of lithotripsy on immature rabbit bone and kidney developement. J Urol 1991;146:213–6.

114. McCullough DL, Yeaman LD, Bo W, et al. Effects of shock waves on the rat ovary. J Urol 1989;141:666.

115. Vieweg J, Weber HM, Miller K, Hautmann R. Female fertility following extracorporeal shock wave lithotripsy of distal ureteral calculi. J Urol 1992;148:1007–10.

116. Nijman RJM, Ackaer K, Scholtmeijer RJ, et al. Long-term results of extracorporeal shock wave lithotripsy in children. J Urol 1989;142:609–11.

92

Antenatal Intervention for Urinary Obstruction and Myelomeningocele

Hubert S. Swana, MD

Ronald S. Sutherland, MD

Laurence Baskin, MD

BACKGROUND

During the past two decades pediatric urologists have begun acquiring many patients from a new referral source, the womb. With the widespread use of antenatal maternal ultrasound, fetal hydronephrosis has become increasingly detected, and it comprises the most common prenatally diagnosed malformation. This dilation of the urinary tract was initially suspected to arise solely from obstruction, and efforts were made to ameliorate this without a clear understanding of the multiple etiologies, pathophysiology, and natural history of the "obstructed" urinary tract. Techniques were devised to restore normal urinary drainage with the intent of preventing renal failure, and the sequelae of oligohydramnios and pulmonary hypoplasia. Attempts at alleviating fetal hydronephrosis became the signature procedure during the early phases of prenatal intervention. The concept of the unborn child as a surgical patient has become firmly established. Fetal medicine has rapidly evolved since those early experiences with the management of fetal hydronephrosis. The variety and complexity of fetal interventions has increased. Nonlethal, but devastating, anomalies such as myelomeningocele can also be treated antenatally. With time, the natural history and pathophysiology of urinary tract obstruction has become better understood. Improvements in diagnostic imaging tools, advances in fetal urine sampling, enhanced interventional techniques and equipment, and a better understanding of the risks and outcomes in these babies have helped to develop rational intervention and observation strategies. Nevertheless, the management of the fetus with hydronephrosis has remained controversial.

This chapter reviews antenatal intervention and its history. The basics of normal fetal development will be integrated with the techniques used to diagnose disorders of the urinary tract. Particular attention will be devoted to the diagnostic techniques of ultrasound, fetal urine sampling, and amniocentesis. Newer modalities such as fetal MRI will be described. Methods of intervention will be described along with their indications, contraindications, and complications.

EMBRYOLOGY Perturbation of the developing ureteral bud and its intended target, the metanephric blastema, by distal obstruction will affect normal renal development.[1–6] By the fifth week of gestation, the ureteral bud has arisen from the mesonephric duct and begins to lengthen and subsequently undergo canalization. Induction of the adjacent metanephric blastema occurs by the end of the seventh week. Primitive renal function is established between the seventh and ninth weeks, and by the twentieth week, about one-third of the total number of nephrons are present (Figure 92-1). Branching of the collecting system is nearly complete by this time as well. Nephrogenesis is complete by the thirty-second week of fetal life, after which no demonstrable increase in the number of glomeruli is noted.[7–10] The most active phase of nephrogenesis is between the twentieth and thirtieth weeks,[7,11] and it is during this period of greatest growth that pathology of the developing kidney is first detected and where intervention most often takes place. Unfortunately, insult to the kidney prior to this period is difficult to detect and most likely causes irreversible damage.

Spinal cord and subsequent vertebral formation begins at day 18 of gestation. Neural tube infolding (neurulation) occurs between 18 and 27 days of gestation and is normally followed by migration of mesodermal tissue around the developing spinal cord. Neurulation begins centrally at the level of the neck, proceeds rostrally, which eventually gives rise to the brain and then proceeds in a caudal direction. The mesoderm gives rise to the vertebral arches, as well as the spinal and back musculature. The location and extent of the abnormal closure leads to the varying degrees and levels of neural tube defects. Lesions can vary in severity and location to include spina bifida occulta (a closed tube defect), meningocele (a protruding meningeal sac without neural elements), myelomeningocele (a menigeal sac with neural elements), and lipomeningocele (a meningeal sac with neural elements and fatty tissue). Myelomeningocele is the most common neural tube defect. Lumbar vertebrae are most commonly involved, followed by sacral, thoracic, and cervical vertebrae in decreasing frequency. Failure to close at the cau-

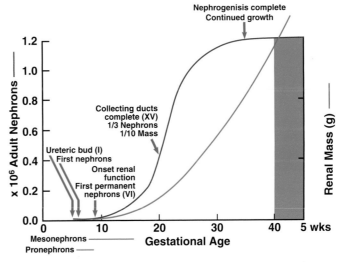

Figure 92-1 Fetal renal development. The branching of the collecting system is complete by 20 weeks, but the majority of nephrons and most of the functional mass form in the renal cortex after 20 weeks. (Reproduced with permission from Harrison MR, et al.[73])

dal end results in a distal defect with resultant lower limb paralysis and bladder dysfunction.[12] An Arnold-Chiari type II malformation occurs in up to 85% of children with myelomeningocele (MMC). There can be herniation of the cerebellar tonsils through the foramen magnum. This can result in obstruction of the fourth ventricle and necessitates ventriculoperitoneal shunting.

SPECTRUM OF ANTENATAL DISORDERS The spectrum of deleterious changes seen in antenatal urinary obstruction is the result of many different factors (Figure 92-2). They include the time of onset, duration, and degree of urinary obstruction. The timing of the obstruction is undoubtedly the most important determinant of severity: The earlier the obstruction occurs, the more disturbed the development of the fetal kidneys.[7] The most severe form of renal injury and maldevelopment, renal dysplasia, has been attributed to a very early effect of elevated pressures in the urinary tract[1] or possibly by ureteral bud malposition with subsequent misconnection between the bud and the metanephric blastema.[3,13] Without the inducing effect of the ureteral bud, the blastema fails to develop.

Pathologically, conglomerates of disorganized metanephric structures are surrounded by abundant fibrous tissue. Cortical cysts are often but are not always present. Ninety percent of cases of renal dysplasia are associated with urinary obstruction during nephrogenesis. Sonography is highly specific when diagnosing dysplasia. The demonstration of renal cysts in a fetus with known obstructive uropathy effectively indicates the presence of dysplasia. They can be seen as early as the twentieth week of gestation.[14] The absence of cortical cysts, however, does not exclude renal dysplasia.

Other entities commonly associated with hydronephrosis and arising from the upper urinary tract include physiological hydronephrosis, ureteropelvic junction obstruction (UPJO), congenital obstructed and nonobstructed megaureter, multicystic kidney, duplication anomalies with upper-pole ectopia or obstructing ureterocele, and vesicoureteral reflex (VUR).[15] Obstruction

of the upper urinary tract as it results from physiologic ureterectasis or from UPJO is rarely complete.[16] The most common entity in the differential diagnosis is physiological hydronephrosis, which usually spontaneously resolves prior to delivery or within the first year of life.[15] More distal causes of obstruction include posterior urethral valves, urethral atresia, cloacal anomalies, and prolapsing, obstructing ureteroceles. These entities can result in marked distortion of both ureters and kidneys as well as pathological changes to the bladder. Often confused as being associated with obstruction is the prune-belly syndrome, which has rarely been associated with renal obstruction, although the urinary tract is massively dilated.[17] Some argue, however, that prune-belly syndrome is a consequence of transient fetal urethral obstruction, causing the characteristic urinary tract dilation.

Urologic morbidity in patients with MMC is significant. Myelodysplasia can result in a poorly compliant bladder, sphincteric dysfunction, secondary vesicoureteral reflux, a predisposition to urinary tract infections, possible renal scarring, and renal failure.[18] Urologic morbidity is the sequela of neurologic injury. The neurologic deficit seen in MMC is believed to be due to several factors, the first to defective development. Evidence supporting a secondary insult to the exposed spinal cord has resulted in a "two-hit hypothesis." Histologic findings support the idea that the exposed spinal cord is vulnerable to damage by physical trauma as the cord contacts the uterine wall. Pressure necrosis, erosions, and abrasions of the spinal cord have been described in fetuses with MMC.[19] The changing chemical composition of amniotic fluid has also been found to be toxic to cultured spinal cords. During the last 3 months of gestation, amniotic fluid consists largely of fetal urine. There is an increase over time in the concentration of urea and creatinine. Drewek and colleagues showed that amniotic fluid at 34 weeks gestation was more toxic to cultured spinal cord cells than earlier in gestation.[20] Human meconium has also been found to cause spinal cord necrosis in a rat model.[21] Fetal lower limb movements were described in fetuses

with MMC at 16 to 17 weeks.[22] Animal studies, in which laminectomy was performed at midgestation, compared in utero repair to no treatment. The animals that underwent fetal intervention were spared flaccid paralysis and incontinence of urine and stool.[23] Histologic specimens of bladder tissue from children with spina bifida reveal increased intracellular matrix between muscle bundles, decreased muscarinic receptor density, abnormal smooth muscle growth, and decreased innervation.[24–26] These factors likely contribute to bladder dysfunction in human spina bifida patients.

HISTORY OF ANTENATAL INTERVENTION The first attempts at fetal intervention were targeted at treating fetal hydrops associated with maternal Rh sensitization by intra-abdominal fetal transfusion of blood.[27] The correction of fetal anatomic defects detected by sonography relies on the presence of a compelling physiological rationale for prenatal correction. In addition to congenital hydronephrosis, diaphragmatic hernia and congenital cystic adenomatoid malformation of the lung associated with hydrops are examples of malformations in which a simple anatomic lesion may interfere with fetal organ development and, if corrected, fetal development may proceed normally. Early animal experiments showed that vesicoamniotic shunts could be placed antenatally and were successful at restoring amniotic fluid volume. Human fetal intervention then followed in the early 1980s.[27] The recognition of fetal therapy as a viable medical specialty came about as a result of a meeting in 1982 hosted by the Kroc Foundation. The following year the International Fetal Medicine and Surgery Society (IFMSS) was founded. In 1988, the Society for Fetal Urology was founded to study, by registry, the postnatal evolution and management of prenatally detected hydronephrosis.

The first repair of myelomeningocele occurred in a primate model in 1984.[29] Subsequent animal studies and fetal observations led to the rational consideration of fetal intervention. This led to the first human fetal myelomeningocele repair in 1997.[30] Since these early interventions, the techniques and technologies have been refined. With fetal surgery the challenge has remained the same, to improve diagnostic modalities so that one may identify fetuses that can potentially benefit from relatively high-risk procedures.

DIAGNOSIS OF OBSTRUCTION

OBSTRUCTION DEFINED (EXPERIMENTAL STUDIES) The definition of urinary obstruction is far from precise. Unfortunately it is not feasible to use the same measurements or diagnostic tools for measuring obstruction in the fetus that one uses for the postpartum infant, child, or adult. Further, there is a broad spectrum of anatomic types of obstruction that occur with an equally broad effect on renal development. Animal studies have helped to improve our understanding of the pathophysiology and natural history of fetal urinary tract obstruction. It has become clear

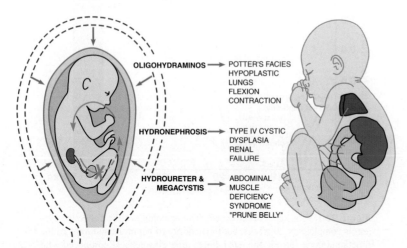

Figure 92-2 Consequences of urethral obstruction.

that congenital obstruction differs from postnatal obstruction. Early studies with fetal sheep showed that complete ureteral obstruction occurring late in gestation results in simple hydronephrosis. When unilateral or bilateral ligation was carried out during the first half of gestation, the resultant kidneys were small, contracted, and resembled human renal dysplasia.[1] Creation of lower tract obstruction in the sheep model was initially performed by ligation of the urachus followed by graded ligation of the urethra, mimicking the features of human urethral obstruction.[2] These experiments demonstrated that lung development is dependent on urine production, and that reversal of urinary obstruction by placement a vesicoamniotic shunt allowed resumption of pulmonary growth if decompression took place during the last trimester. Urinary tract obstruction during the last trimester produced progressive distortion of the urinary tract with bladder dilation and hypertrophy, megaureters, and bilateral hydronephrosis. In fetal lambs, decompression of the obstructed bladder into the amniotic sac reversed all of these effects.

Subsequent studies using similar models have attempted to better define the physiologic changes in obstructed fetal kidneys. Bogaert and colleagues[30] studied renal blood flow and fetal urine production in third trimester sheep with and without partial urethral ligation. They found that fetal renal blood flow increases and renal function (as measured by glomerular filtration rate, filtration fraction, fractional excretion of sodium, and total sodium excretion) progressively deteriorates in response to partial bladder outlet obstruction over a period of 10 days.[30] Subsequent studies in second trimester sheep obstructed for longer periods (> 30 days) have shown that significant partial bladder outlet obstruction resulted in no deterioration in renal blood flow or function despite 35 days of obstruction. There was a trend toward an increase in both parameters. Histologically the investigators found only parenchymal thinning with preservation of the cytoarchitecture.[31] The same laboratory also studied the effects of endothelin, a potent vasoconstrictor, and found that endothelin-1 acts primarily as a vasodilator in the fetal lamb renal circulation. Studies of endothelin-1 in the postnatal renal circulation demonstrate that it acts primarily as a vasoconstrictor. They postulate that the endothelin receptors in the fetus are different from those seen in the adult. Therefore, if endothelin plays a role in the renal response to obstruction, the consequences of obstruction on the fetal kidney will be markedly different from those observed after birth.[30]

At the cellular level, antenatal obstruction has been shown to alter the expression of genes responsible for normal cellular differentiation.[32] Increased activity of the renin-angiotensin system can allow for some tolerance to fetal urinary obstruction, but if severe enough, decompensation can occur.[33] This can result in the injury pattern seen in dysplastic kidneys.

These studies underscore the fact that the responses to obstruction by the fetal urinary tract differ significantly from postnatal obstruction and can lead to vastly different results. These data also suggest that intervention may not be necessary in some of the cases that presently are recommended for such therapy.

ULTRASOUND The evolution of fetal intervention has paralleled the advancements in ultrasound technology. The development of high-resolution, real-time scanners with the ability to choose the depth of the focal zone has been a significant advantage.[2] Some important considerations in the performance of fetal ultrasound include the impact that developmental stage has on visualization of the target organ and fetal positioning that pathologic structures are frequently more visible than their normal counterparts and normal physiologic function. For example, the fetal bladder is difficult or impossible to visualize in a term fetus that has recently voided. Fetal positioning plays a critical role in the interpretation and understanding of the fetal anatomy. The prone fetus is in the optimal position for imaging the kidneys.[27] Early identification of normal kidneys can be made by the fifteenth week of gestation, but reliable and reproducible imaging is not possible until the eighteenth week.[34]

Hydronephrosis is the most common cause of an abdominal mass in the neonate, and antenatal sonography readily detects fetal urinary tract dilation.[27] Pelviectasis is found in 18% of normal fetuses.[35] The criteria for pathological renal pelvic distention has been suggested to be an anteroposterior renal pelvic diameter of 10 mm or more or a ratio of the pelvic diameter to the AP renal diameter greater than 50%.[36] Harrison and Filly have refined this definition by taking into account caliectasis as a sign of hydronephrosis, and a more reliable dysmorphic feature for predicting hydronephrosis than pelviectasis.[27] Cendron and colleagues confirmed Filly's finding that the presence of caliectasis or abnormal cortical echogenicity identifies fetuses in need of postnatal urologic evaluation.[37] The Society of Fetal Urology has adopted a grading system for hydronephosis that is widely used by pediatric urologists (Figure 92-3).

Prenatal sonography is very sensitve in detecting the level of obstruction as well. The diagnosis of UPJO is the most common cause of neonatal hydronephrosis.[38] Ultrasonographic criteria to diagnose UPJO antenatally include the aforementioned parameters and lack of evidence of ureterectasis, vesicomegaly, ectopic ureterocele, or posterior urethral dilation.[39] Flake and colleagues evaluated 44 cases from UCSF in which the prenatal diagnosis of UPJO coincided with postnatal findings in every case.

While ultrasonography remains the primary imaging modality for the screening and evaluation of congenital abnormalities, it is not without limitations. Maternal obesity, oligohydramnios, and suboptimal fetal position can make accurate imaging difficult.

Early use of MRI was limited by slow acquisition times, which were hampered by fetal motion. Fetal sedation or paralysis was required for imaging. Newer methods have been developed that can reduce acquisition times and provide excellent image quality.[41]

MRI can provide images unaffected by fetal position, maternal obesity, oligohydramnios, or overlying bowel, and possibly could provide a definitive diagnosis of obstructive uropathy.

Coakley and colleagues compared MR with ultrasonography and found that in 24 complex cases MR provided additional information that directly affected treatment in only 17% of cases, and none involved the genitourinary tract.[42] Aaronson and colleagues compared transabdominal ultrasonography with fetal MR imaging and found that they were equally accurate in determining the lesion level in fetuses with myelomeningocele.[43] MRI does seem to be superior in identifying the intracranial lesions, such as agenesis of the corpus callosum, cerebellar dysplasia, and holoprosencephaly, that can accompany myelomeningocele.[44] Presently, MR is a useful adjunct to ultrasonography. MR provides additional information in myelomeningocele, other complex fetal cases, and cases of hydronephrosis with indeterminate ultrasound (US) studies. Future studies in molecular imaging in which MR can be used to study cellular and molecular events could further refine diagnostic accuracy and improve selection of intervention candidates.[45]

FETAL URINE AND AMNIOTIC FLUID TESTING Invasive acquisition of fetal urine for analysis has become one of the most important measures of

Grade	Central Renal Complex	Renal Parenchymal Thickness
0	Intact	Normal
1	Slight splitting	Normal
2	Evident splitting confined within renal border	Normal
3	Wide splitting pelvis outside renal border (calices uniformly dilated)	Normal
4	Further dilation of renal pelvis and calices	Thin

Figure 92-3 Society of Fetal Urology Grading Scale.

assessing fetal renal function. Measurement of fetal urine electrolytes and urinary proteins is a useful guide to the clinician in deciding whether prenatal intervention is indicated. Additional methods of assessing the overall status of the fetus include amniocentesis, chorionic villus sampling, percutaneous umbilical blood sampling (all for karyotyping), as well as amniotic fluid volume and its biochemical constituent measurement. Fetal urine is normally hypotonic, reflecting developing glomerular and tubular function.[29] Glick and colleagues,[11] in their work with human fetuses with obstructive uropathy and renal dysplasia, have shown a production of almost isotonic urine, suggesting obstructed-related defects in tubular function resulting in inability to reabsorb sodium and chloride. The amniotic fluid, in comparison, is somewhat hypertonic, and is not as reliable an index of renal function as the fetal urine. Amniotic fluid volume is useful only in the extremes (ie, oligohydramnios), and biochemical analysis of amniotic fluid has not proven useful. Studies of glomerular filtration rate (GFR) as an index of fetal renal function were done using iothalamate and endogenous creatinine clearance in fetal sheep with a single ureter ligated.[46] They demonstrated severe decrease in the GFR of the obstructed kidney compared with the normal control side, as well as diminished tubular function as assessed by fractional excretion of sodium and urinary electrolyte concentration.

Determination of human fetal renal function is limited to simple concentration of specific urinary constituents. More physiologic measurements of glomerular function are more difficult. Clearance of iothalamate has been done and shown to be nonpredictive of renal outcome.[11] Assessment by endogenous creatinine clearance is more difficult and has not been carried out. Retrospective analysis of individual urine constituents have shown that a sodium of less than 100 mEq/L, osmolality less than 210 mOsm/L, and chloride less than 90 mEq/L, if accompanied by lack of ultrasonographic evidence of dysplasia, are helpful in predicting residual fetal renal function. By categorizing patients according prognosis, assessment of the potential efficacy of intervention can be made.[47] Evans suggested that a single evaluation of urinary constituents may incorrectly reflect current fetal or long-term renal function. Elder and colleagues reported several false-positive and negative fetal urine electrolyte panels.[48] Evans proposed providing transient relief of obstruction by vesicocentesis followed by sequential sampling (3 or 4 samples over several days) of urinary electrolytes. This was felt to provide an assessment of the severity of the renal injury and potential for reversibility of renal injury. Those fetuses that experienced an improvement in their biochemical parameters following decompression may benefit most from interventional therapy.[49] Others have suggested that sampling of fetal urine electrolytes and osmolarity is not an optimal method to evaluate fetal renal function and recommend continued search for a better substance.[50–52] A serum

marker which has provided some clinical utility is beta-2 microglobilin. It is excreted by the kidney without placental crossover so that fetal levels represent fetal renal function. One can see an elevation in renal dysplasia.[53]

Other urinary constituents commonly associated with the presence of renal disease include proteins such as albumin, retinol-binding protein, and N-acetyl-b-glucosaminidase.[53] These constituents are rarely found in the urine except in the presence of glomerular or tubulointerstitial disease and may be more reliable indicators of reversible renal damage. More recently, researchers have identified certain extracellular matrix (ECM) metalloproteinases (MMP) and their inhibitors, namely, the tissue inhibitors of metalloproteinases (TIMP). When expressed, these may be sensitive indicators for magnitude of renal injury. These ubiquitous proteins are expressed during tissue remodeling, whether during normal development or senescence or in pathological states. These are released along with oxygen free radicals in response to the presence of Tamm-Horsfall protein and phagocytosis by mononuclear cell activity.

Unfortunately, human fetal urine sampling lacks known control normals at different stages

of development. Further limitation includes the inability to accurately and physiologically measure renal function by fractional excretion of biochemical constituents and glomerular filtration without risky invasive fetal and maternal testing.

INTERVENTIONAL TECHNIQUES

CURRENT INDICATIONS AND CONTRAINDICATIONS For most fetuses with obstructive uropathy, intervention is not necessary[56] (Figure 92-4). The selection criteria for fetal therapy of obstructive uropathy has been evolving such that presently patient selection is good enough to avoid intervention in patients who are either too well (no benefit) or too ill to recover. It has been conclusively shown that decompression in utero will restore amniotic fluid, which can prevent the development of fatal pulmonary hypoplasia. What seems less clear is whether or not in utero decompression can arrest or reverse cystic dysplastic changes caused by obstruction.[57]

Spontaneous resolution of hydronephrosis is common, which has led to a more cautious approach to fetal intervention.[1,58] In most cases with normal amniotic fluid volume, the mother should be followed by serial ultrasound examina-

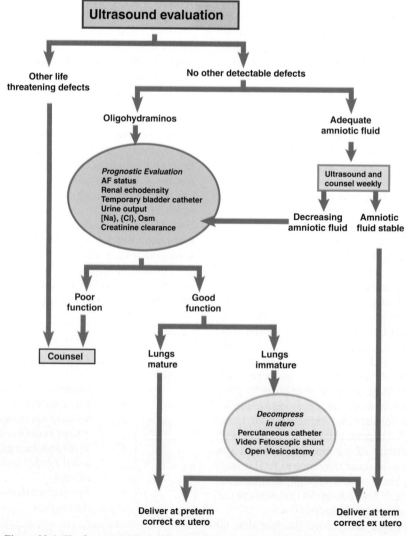

Figure 92-4 The fetus with bilateral hydonephosis. Treatment algorithm.

tions, and the fetus should be evaluated and treated postnatally. If moderate to severe oligohydramnios develops, the fetus should undergo complete prognostic evaluation to assess the potential for normal renal and pulmonary function at birth. If the ultrasound demonstrates presence of dysplasia, aggressive obstetrical care or prenatal decompression is not indicated. When preserved renal function is predicted, early delivery for postnatal decompression is indicated if the lungs are mature. Early delivery usually does not compromise pulmonary function as long as amniotic fluid volume has been maintained.[1] If the lungs are immature, however, in utero decompression can be considered.

METHODS OF INTERVENTION   Early interventional techniques in the late 1970s and early 1980s attempted the Seldinger-type procedure, but without success. A tight-fitting double-pigtail catheter placed over a puncture needle using a pusher worked; although it was far from ideal (the Harrison catheter) owing to the difficulties in catheter placement, migration, and plugging. A Malecot-type catheter was subsequently developed that fitted over an introducer needle and was used with some success. More recently, the Rocket catheter, developed in England, has the advantage of being able to be placed through a trocar needle, and with a right angle external coil set flush against the skin to avoid disruption by fetal movements. It is this catheter that is currently most frequently placed percutaneously under ultrasound guidance.

Open fetal surgery was begun in the early 1980s and was performed on only 8 highly selected cases of obstructive uropathy from 18 to 24 weeks gestation. Unfortunately, this method of treatment carried significant morbidity, predominantly from preterm labor.[59] As a result, open fetal surgery to correct urinary tract obstruction has not since been performed. In those early patients, open decompression procedures included cutaneous vesicostomy in 7, and bilateral ureterostomies in 1. Only 4 had prolonged return of normal amniotic fluid and had adequate pulmonary function at birth. Of these, only 2 have normal renal function at ages 5 and 8 years.[60]

With advances in endoscopic equipment, the technique of transuterine endoscopy was developed at the University of California, San Francisco.[61] This was used in the fetal sheep model to create a vesicocutaneous fistula through which an expandable wall stent is placed (Figure 92-5). This procedure was successful in maintaining patency and has a reduced risk of dislodgment and migration. MacMahon and colleagues reported a similar fetoscopic approach in a human fetus with prune-belly syndrome and oligohydramnios at 17+ weeks. They used a neodymium-YAG laser to create a vesicoamniotic shunt that was successful at restoration of the amniotic fluid volume. The fistula closed by 33 weeks and the child was delivered early with normally developed lungs.[62]

Fetal cystoscopy and valve ablation have been reported. Both antegrade and retrograde tech-

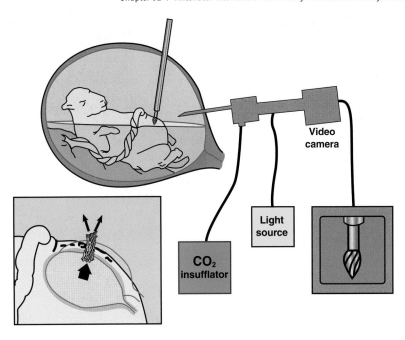

Figure 92-5   Endoscopic treatment of obstruction in a sheep fetus with a vesicoamniotic shunt using a expandable mesh stent that has less risk of occlusion, displacement, and abdominal wall disruption. (From Estes JM, et al.[61])

niques have been reported. Flexible and rigid instruments were used as well. Significant fetal mortality was reported.[63]

Repair of MMC has been attempted both endoscopically and through open surgery via a hysterotomy. While technically possible, surgery for MMC is not presently being performed via a fetoscopic approach. Fetoscopy is limited by the need for multiple port sites, which can lead to membrane fixation and rupture as the uterus enlarges. In addition, it is difficult to visualize large spinal defects and requires prolonged operative times.[64]

Open fetal surgery requires careful planning (Figure 92-6). Attempts at enhancing fetal lung maturity are made through the use of preoperative glucocorticosteroid administration to the mother. Broad-spectrum antibiotics and balanced anesthesia allow the procedure to take place. The amniotic fluid is removed and kept in sterile warm syringes. A standard neurosurgical closure is performed through an approximately 8 cm hysterotomy. The neural placode is dissected from the adjacent arachnoid tissue and placed in the spinal canal. The dura is then dissected off for another layer of coverage. The skin then is freed for a final layer of closure. The amniotic fluid and added antibiotics are replaced and the uterus closed. Prophylactic tocolytics are then used.[65]

RESULTS AND COMPLICATIONS   The results of intervention were difficult to assess because of a poor understanding of the natural history of the variety of fetal uropathies and the inherent inability to study a normal control population. Early results reassured the interventionists that the procedures could be performed safely and that catheter drainage was well tolerated in most cases. Whether prenatal shunting improves outcome

remains a different matter. The issues of patient selection centered on finding the dilated urinary tract with severe enough obstruction to compromise renal and pulmonary function at birth, and yet not so severe that renal function, could not be salvaged even with decompression.[27]

In a review of the San Francisco experience in 1990, Crombleholme and colleagues[47] recounted 40 fetuses that underwent invasive testing, and 19 of which had fetal intervention for obstructive uropathy. They concluded from this retrospective study that by assessing urine electrolyte levels and ultrasonographic appearance, that residual fetal renal function and neonatal outcome could be accurately predicted, and that prenatal intervention could be selectively performed to prevent the development of pulmonary hypoplasia.[47]

Seven years later, Copleri reviewed prenatal intervention for hydronephrosis. His review revealed that obstruction and dysplasia were difficult to predict. In addition, although technically feasible, fetal interventions were associated with only a 47% survival rate. In addition, 45% of fetuses had complications.[65]

A recent review by McLorie and colleagues,[66] outcomes in patients who underwent vesicoamniotic shunting and who had bilateral hydronephrosis, oligohydramnios, and evidence of bladder outlet obstruction revealed that even though oligohydramnios could be reversed, the ability to sustain good renal function was variable. In addition they could not identify specific prenatal parameters that were effective in predicting good renal function.[66]

A longer-term review of the University of California at San Francisco experience in patients undergoing fetal surgery for posterior urethral valves revealed similar results. A fetal mortality rate of 43% was demonstrated. Despite favorable

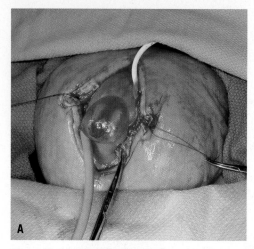 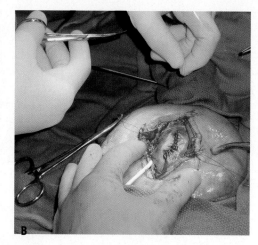 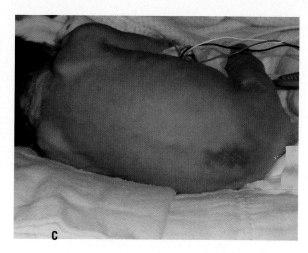

Figure 92-6 Fetal surgery for myelomenigocele preoperative (A), after intraoperative closure (B), and postoperative result (C). (Courtesy of Nalin Gupta, MD, Dept. Neurosurgery UCSF.)

urinary electrolytes, no positive predictive factor for postnatal renal function could be identified.[67]

The most common complication arising from open in utero fetal intervention is the instigation of preterm labor, requiring tocolytic therapy in most mothers to arrest it.[59] Although still a threat, preterm labor has not been a substantial issue for percutaneous procedures. Premature delivery of some of the severely afflicted babies can lead to a catastrophic outcome. Problems also frequently arise from the catheters that fail either by plugging or migrating, thus limiting this procedure to short-term therapy. Percutaneous transabdominal placement of these catheters under ultrasound guidance can be malpositioned, causing fetal injury and death.[68] Frequent displacerment and obstruction often require multiple reinsertions, thus increasing the risks of fetal injury and infections. Indeed chorioamnionitis occurred in 3 patients in Crombleholme and colleague's review resulting in pregnancy termination.[60] All 3 of these patients had externalized catheters over many hours for renal function assessment. Prenatal surgery for myelomeningocele has yielded some unexpected outcomes.

Tubbs and colleagues[69] were not able to show improved lower extremity function in patients who underwent intrauterine intervention. They compared 37 fetuses that underwent intrauterine repair between 20 and 28 weeks gestation with 40 fetuses that underwent postgestational repair. They were unable to find statistically significant differences between the level of lower extremity function and the vertebral level of the defect between the two groups.[64]

Bruner and colleagues[70] compared 29 fetal surgery patients with 23 controls matched for level of defect, diagnosis, calendar time, and practice parameters. They reported a statistically significant ($p = .01$) decrease in the need for ventriculoperitoneal shunt placement and a lower incidence of hindbrain herniation ($p = .001$). Patients who underwent fetal surgery did, however, have a higher risk of oligohydramnios (48% vs 4%; $p = .001$), and admissions for preterm contractions (50% vs 9%; $p = .002$). They were

also more susceptible to prematurity. Age at delivery was earlier (33 vs 37 weeks; $p < .001$) and birth weights were lower (2,171 vs 3,075 gm; $p = .001$).[65]

The effect of fetal intervention for myelomeningocele on postnatal bladder function has been studied.[66,67] Despite the early repair, patterns of abnormal bladder function were exhibited. One still sees poor compliance, poor detrusor contractility, detrusor-sphincter dysynergia, hydronephrosis, and vesicoureteral reflux. The previously described global defect in bladder development makes success of fetal surgery to preserve or improve bladder function unlikely.

Presently a multicenter trial is underway. Two hundred mothers and their fetuses will be randomized to either standard postdelivery repair or fetal intervention.

CONCLUSIONS

The field of fetal medicine has grown over the past 2 decades. Well-defined animal studies have yielded clues to the natural history and pathogenesis of obstructive uropathy and the efficacy of interventional techniques to ameliorate the sequelae of such obstruction. With advances in technology, the complexity of anomalies that can be treated has increased, as evidenced by the growing experience with fetal myelomeningocele repair. In addition, these new scenarios provide new ethical challenges. Carrying out procedures in human fetuses must continue to be appropriately cautious and circumspect. The uncertainties and true pathologic processes surrounding urinary tract obstruction must continue to be explored. More reliable methods of determining fetal renal function lie on the horizon. Interventional techniques continue to evolve and improve. Because of the potential risks of preterm labor and maternal compromise, fetal surgery should continue to be performed only for carefully selected cases at centers that are equipped with a multidisciplinary health care team committed to ongoing, well-designed research protocols.

REFERENCES

1. Beck AD. The effect of intra-uterine urinary obstruction upon the development of the fetal kidney. J Urol 1971;105:784–9.
2. Berman DJ, Maizels M. The role of urinary obstruction in the genesis of renal dysplasia. J Urol 1983;128:1091–6.
3. Barrett DM, Wineland RE. Renal cell carcinoma in multicystic dysplastic kidney. Urology 1980;15:152–4.
4. Longino LA, Martin LW. Abdominal masses in the newborn infant. Pediatrics 1958;21:596–604.
5. Glick PL, Harrison MR, Noall RA, Villa RL. Correction of congenital hydronephrosis in utero. III. Early midtrimester ureteral obstruction produces renal dysplasia. J Pediatr Surg 1983;18:681–7.
6. Bellinger MF, Comstock CH, Grosso D, Zaino R. Fetal posterior urethral valves and renal dysplasia at 15 weeks gestational age. J Urol 1983;129:1238–9.
7. Gasser B, Mauss Y, Ghnassia JP, et al. A quantitative study of normal nephrogenesis in the human fetus: its implication in the natural history of kidney changes due to low obstructive uropathies. Fetal Diagn Ther 1993;8:371–84.
8. Bernstein J. Developmental abnormalities of the renal parenchyma—renal hypoplasia and dysplasia. Pathol Annu 1968;3:213–23.
9. McGrory WW. Developmental nephrology. Cambridge: Harvard University Press; 1972. p. 48.
10. Potter E. Normal and abnormal development of the kidney. Chicago: Year Book Medical; 1972.
11. Glick PL, Harrison MR, Golbus MS, et al. Management of the fetus with congenital hydronephrosis II: prognostic criteria selection for treatment. J Pediatr Surg 1985;20:376–87.
12. Moore KL, Persaud TVN. The developing human: clinically oriented embryology. Philadelphia: W. B. Saunders; 2003. p. 428–33.
13. King LR. The management of multicystic kidney and ureteropelvic junction obstruction. In: King LR, editor. Urologic surgery in neonates and young infants. Philadelphia: W. B. Saunder; 1988. p. 140–54.
14. Mahony HS, Filly RA, Callen PW, et al. Fetal renal dysplasia: sonographic evaluation. Radiology 1984;152:143–6.
15. Gordon AC, Thomas DFM, Arthur RJ, et al. Prenatally diagnosed reflux: a follow-up study. Br J Urol 1990;65:407–12.
16. Anderson PA, Rickwood AM. Features of primary vesicoureteric reflux detected by prenatal sonography. Br J Urol 1991;67:267–71.
17. Snow BW, Duckett JW. Prune-belly syndrome. In: Gillenwater JY, editor. Adult and pediatric urology, 2nd ed. St. Louis: Mosby; 1991. p. 1921.
18. Muller T, Arbeiter K, Aufricht C. Renal function in myelomeningocele: risk factors, chronic renal failure, renal replacement therapy and transplantation. Curr Opin Urol 2002;12:479–84.
19. Meuli M, Meuli-Simmeti C, Hutchins GM, et al. The spinal cord lesion in human fetuses with myelomeningocele: implications for fetal surgery. J Pediatr Surg 1997;32:448–52.
20. Drewek MJ, Bruner JP, Whetsell WO, Tulipan N. Quantitative analysis of the toxicity of human amniotic fluid to cultured rat spinal cord. Pediatr Neurosurg 1997;27:190–3.
21. Correia-Pinto J, Reis JL, Hutchins GM, et al. In utero meconium exposure increases spinal cord necrosis in a rat model of myelomeningocele. J Pediatr Surg 2002;37:488–92.

22. Korenromp MJ, Van Good JD, Bruinese HW, Kriek R. Early fetal movements in myelomeningocele. Lancet 1986;1:917–8.

23. Meuli M, Meuli-Simmen C, Hutchins GM, et al. In utero surgery rescues neurologic function at birth in sheep with spina bifida. Nat Med 1995;1:342–7.

24. Shapiro E, Becich MJ, Perlman E, Lepor H. Bladder wall abnormalities in myelodysplastic children: a computer assisted morphometric analysis. J Urol 1991;145:1024–9.

25. Gup DI, Baumann M, Lepor H, Shapiro E. Muscarinic cholinergic receptors in normal pediatric and myelodysplastic bladders. J Urol 1989;142(2 Pt 2):595–9.

26. Shapiro E, Seller MJ, Lepor H, et al. Altered smooth muscle development in the lower genitourinary and gastrointestinal tract of the male fetus with myelomeningocele. J Urol 1998;160(3 Pt 2):1047–53.

27. Harrison M, Filly R. The unborn patient, 2nd ed. Philadelphia: W.B. Saunders; 1991.

28. Harrison MR, Ross N, de Lorimier AA. Correction of congenital hydronephrosis in utero. I. The model: fetal urethral obstruction produces hydronephrosis and pulmonary hypoplasia in fetal lambs. J Pediatr Surg 1983;18:247–56.

29. Adzick NS, Sutton LN, Crombelhome TM, Flake AW. Successful fetal surgery for spina bifida. Lancet 1998;352:1675–6.

30. Bogaert GA, Kogan BA, Mevorach RA, et al. Endothelin-1 causes renal vasodilation in the fetal lamb. J Urol 1996;156(2 Pt 2):847–53.

31. Gluckman GR, Bogaert GA, Mevorach RA, et al. Partial bladder obstruction in second-trimester sheep: preservation of renal blood flow and function [abstract 58]. Dallas, TX: American Academy of Pediatrics, Pediatric Urology Section: 1994.

32. Chevalier RL, Kim A, Thornhill BA, Wolstenholme JT. Recovery following relief of unilateral ureteral obstruction in the neonatal rat. Kidney Int 1999;55:793–807.

33. Attar R, Quinn F, Winyard PJ, et al. Short-term urinary flow impairment deregulates PAX 2 and PCNA expression and cell survival in fetal sheep kidneys. Am J Pathol 1998;152:1225–35.

34. Merguuerian P. The evaluation of prenatally detected hydronephrosis. Monograph Urol 1995;16:1–5.

35. Hoddick WK, Filly RA, Mahony BS, Callen PW. Minimal fetal renal pyelectasis. J Ultrasound Med 1985;4:85–9.

36.

37. Cendron M, Morin L, Crombleholme T, et al. Early minimal fetal hydronephrosis: clinical outcomes and implications for management [abstract 30]. Dallas, TX: American Academy of Pediatrics, Pediatric Urology Section; 1994.

38. Birken G, King D, Vane D, Lloyd T. Adenocarcinoma arising in a multicystic dysplastic kidney. J Pediatr Surg 1985;20:619–21.

39. Kleiner B, Callen PW, Filly RA. Sonographic analysis of the fetus with ureteropelvic junction obstruction. AJR Am J Roentgenol 1987;148:359–63.

40. Manning FA, Harrison MR, Rodeck C. Catheter shunts for fetal hydronephrosis and hydrocephalus. N Engl J Med 1986;315:336–40.

41. Yamashita Y, Namimoto T, Abe Y, et al. MR imaging of the fetus by a HASTE sequence. AJR Am J Roentgenol 1997;168:513–9.

42. Coakley FV, Hricak H, Filly RA, et al. Complex fetal disorders: effect of MR imaging on management-preliminary clinical experience. Radiology 1999;213:691–6.

43. Aaronson OS, Hernanz-Schulman M, Bruner JP, et al. Myelomeningocele: prenatal evaluation—comparison between transabdominal US and MR imaging. Radiology 2003;227:839–43.

44. Levine D, Barnes PD, Madsen JR, et al. Central nervous system abnormalities assessed with prenatal magnetic resonance imaging. Obstet Gynecol 1999;94:1011–9.

45. Tempany CM, McNeil BJ. Advances in biomedical imaging. JAMA 2001;285:562–7.

46. Woodard JR. Neonatal and perinatal emergencies. In: Harrison JH, Gittes RF, Perlmutter AD, et al, editors. Campbell's urology. 4th ed. Philadelphia: W. B. Saunders; 1979. p. 1855.

47. Crombleholme T, Harrison MR, Golbus MS, et al. Fetal intervention in obstructive uropathy: prognostic indicators and efficacy of intervention. Am J Obstet Gynecol 1990;162:1239–44.

48. Elder JS, O Grady JP, Ashmead G, et al. Evaluation of fetal renal function: unreliability of fetal urinary electrolytes. J Urol 1990;144(2 Pt 2):574–8.

49. Johnson MP, Corsi P, Bradfield W, et al. Sequential analysis improves evaluation of fetal renal function in obstructive uropathy. Am J Obstet Gynecol 1995;173:59–65.

50. Johnson MP, Bukowski TP, Reitleman C, et al. In utero surgical treatment of fetal obstructive uropathy: a new comprehensive approach to identify appropriate candidates for vesicoamniotic shunt therapy. Am J Obstet Gynecol 1994;170:1770–6.

51. Elder JS, Duckett JW Jr, Snyder HM. Intervention for fetal obstructive uropathy: has it been effective? Lancet 1987;2:1007–10.

52. Wilkins IA, Chitkara U, Lynch L, et al. The nonpredictive value of fetal urinary electrolytes: preliminary report of outcomes and correlations with pathologic diagnosis. Am J Obstet Gynecol 1987;157:694–8.

53. Mandell J, Blyth BR, Peters CA, et al. Structural genitourinary defects detected in utero. Radiology 1991;178:193–6.

54. Dommergues M, Muller F, Ngo S, et al. Fetal serum beta-2-microglobulin predicts postnatal renal function in bilateral uropathies. Kidney Int 2000;58:312–6.

55. Longaker MT, Golbus MD, Filly RA, et al. Maternal outcome after open fetal surgery. JAMA 1991;265:737–41.

56. Adzick NS, Harrison MR. Fetal surgical therapy. Lancet 1994;343:897–902.

57. Adzick NS, Harrison MR. The unborn surgical patient. Curr Probl Surg 1994;31:1–68.

58. Onen A, Jayanthi VR, Koff SA. Long-term follow-up of prenatally detected severe bilateral newborn hydronephrosis initially managed nonoperatively. J Urol 2002;168:1118–20.

59. Harrison MR, Adzick NS. The fetus as a patient. Surgical considerations. Ann Surg 1991;213:279–91.

60. Crombleholme TM, Harrison MR, Golbus MS, et al. Fetal intervention in obstructive uropathy: prognostic indicators and efficacy of intervention. Am J Obstet Gynecol 1990;162:1239–44.

61. Estes JM, MacGillivray TE, Hedrick MH, et al. Fetoscopic surgery for the treatment of congenital anomalies. J Pediatr Surg 1992;27:950–4.

62. Najmaldin A, Burge DM, Atwell JD. Fetal vesicoureteric reflux. Br J Urol 1990;65:403–6.

63. Quentero RA, Hume R, Smith C, et al. Percutaneous fetal cystoscopy and endoscopic fulguration of posterior urethral valves. Am J Obstet Gynecol 1995;172(1 Pt 1):206–9.

64. Olutoye OO, Adzick NS. Fetal surgery for myelomeningocele. Semin Perinatol 1999;23:462–73.

65. Coplen DE. Prenatal intervention for hydronephrosis. J Urol 1997;157:2270–7.

66. McLorie G, Farhat W, Khoury A, et al. Outcome analysis of vesicoamniotic shunting in a comprehensive population. J Urol 2001;166:1036–40.

67. Holmes N, Harrison MR, Baskin LS. Fetal surgery for posterior urethral valves: long-term postnatal outcomes. Pediatrics 2001;108:E7.

68. Harrison MR, Golbus MS, Filly RA, et al. Fetal hydronephrosis: selection and surgical repair. J Pediatr Surg 1987;22:556–8.

69. Tubbs RS, Chambers MR, Smyth MD, et al. Late gestational myelomeningocele repair does not improve lower extremity function. Pediatr Neurosurg 2003;38:128–32.

70. Bruner JP, Tulipan N, Paschall RL, et al. Fetal surgery for myelomeningocele and the incidence of shunt-dependent hydrocephalus. JAMA 1999;282:1819–25.

71. Holzeberelin J, Pope JC, Adams MA, et al. The urodynamic profile of myelodysplasia in childhood with spinal closure during gestation. J Urol 2000;164:1336–9.

72. Holmes NM, Nyguen HT, Harrison MR, et al. Fetal Intervention for myelomeningocele: effect on postnatal bladder function. J Urol 2001;166:2383–6.

73. Harrison MR, Golbus MS, Filly RA, et al. Management of the fetus with congenital hydronephrosis. J Pediatr Surg 1982;17:728–42.

93

Laparoscopic and Endoscopic Ureteral Reimplantation in Children

Jason S. Lai, MD
Patrick C. Cartwright, MD
Brent W. Snow, MD

Vesicoureteral reflux is the most common radiologic abnormality found in children undergoing evaluation for urinary tract infections (UTI). In this circumstance, one of three children will demonstrate reflux by voiding cystourethrography. Vesicoureteral reflux warrants close attention from urologists because of the potential morbidity to the patient. Major long-term sequelae of reflux with UTI include renal scarring, hypertension, and renal insufficiency or failure.

The management of reflux traditionally involves one of two strategies: prophylatic antibiotics and observation or ureteral reimplantation. In general, grades IV to V reflux are managed with ureteral reimplantation, whereas grades I and II (and probably III) are managed with observation owing to the higher likelihood of spontaneous resolution. During the observation period, annual radiologic follow-up is required to assess the degree of reflux and check for appropriate renal growth.

As always, there are benefits and drawbacks to both observation and surgical management of vesicoureteral reflux. Surgical reimplantation of the ureters incurs a high one-time cost, has associated postoperative discomfort, involves the risks of anesthesia and in a very small percentage of patients may result in persistent reflux or ureteral obstruction. Observation, on the other hand, involves the expense, discomfort and radiation exposure of sequential x-rays, the risks and side effects of prophylactic antibiotics, and the possibility for breakthrough UTI with renal scarring. As well, some portion of these patients will eventually require reimplantation for failure of the reflux to resolve.

In an attempt to combine advantages of both medical and surgical treatments for vesicoureteral reflux, several investigators have developed minimally invasive techniques to correct reflux. Minimally invasive reimplantation, along with laparoscopy and endourology, is relatively new, having its beginnings in the early 1990's. The three main approaches are: (1) a combined transvesical and endoscopic technique, (2) laparoscopic or robotic extravesical reimplantation, and (3) endoscopic treatment with subureteric injection of bulking agent, which will not be discussed in this chapter.

EXTRAVESICAL URETERAL REIMPLANTATION

Initial descriptions were of an extravesical approach (transperitoneal) with a modified Lich-Gregoir reimplantation technique.[1]

In 1993 and 1994, several groups reported experimental efforts with extravesical laparoscopic reimplantation in the porcine model. Animals first had reflux created by incision of the submucosal tunnel performed endoscopically. Reimplantation technique was fairly similar among these studies because they all used either a Lich-Gregoir or a detrusorrhaphy procedure. Trocars were placed in a transperitoneal fashion to access the posterior bladder wall. To achieve reimplantation, a detrusor incision was created proximal to the ureteral hiatus, the ureter was positioned within the trough, and the detrusor closed over it with either staples or absorbable sutures.

With short-term follow-up (3 weeks to 6 months), 13 of 15 laparoscopically reimplanted ureters were free of reflux, whereas one ureter became obstructed. Average surgical times were 132 and 141 minutes in two of the studies.[2–4] More prolonged follow-up was not reported.

Ehrlich and associates reported (1994) the use of this technique in two patients, with successful outcomes and minimal perioperative discomfort.[5] Janetschek and colleagues in 1995 described their experience in six children.[6] One required postoperative ureteral stenting for 6 weeks. Although technically achievable, the authors felt that the procedure was quite complex and offered no significant advantage to the patient.

In a larger series, Lakshmanan and Fung performed the extravesical laparoscopic reimplant in 99 ureters in 66 children aged 4 to 18 years.[7] In their technique, four trocars are used, with the three working ports placed along a Pfannenstiel incision. The peritoneum is incised transversely over the ureter, and the ureter is isolated with a 5-mm Babcock clamp. A percutaneous suture is placed for traction anterior to the end of the detrusor tunnel. Detrusor myotomy is then made with electrocautery and scissors in an inverted-Y configuration, preserving the distal trigonal attachments to the ureter. The ureter is placed in

this tunnel, and the detrusor muscle is approximated with interrupted sutures.

All procedures were completed with no conversions to open surgery. Average operative time for each ureter was 84 minutes, and average blood loss was < 10 cc. Average hospitalization was 1.6 days, and the majority of their recent cases were discharged within 24 hours. Postoperative analgesic requirement averaged 3.8 days, and convalescence ranged from 5 to 7 days. With the first 13 cases (the initial learning curve) of their series excluded, they reported a success rate of 97.8% with a mean follow-up of 34 months. One patient developed ureterovesical junction obstruction, and one had persistent vesicoureteral reflux. In their initial 13 patients, two required stenting for obstruction, and three required open reimplantation for persistent reflux.

Roth and colleagues incorporated a similar technique to that of Lakshmanan and Fung. Although their experience has not yet been published, they have stated that the laparoscopic extravesical approach offers an advantage in older patients who may experience greater morbidity with open reimplantation.

The extravesical approach has also been attempted using robotic technology. Advantages of robotic surgery over classic laparoscopy include greater degrees of freedom and dexterity, improved three-dimensional visualization, elimination of surgeon tremor, and the ability to scale movements. Sung and Gill reported their experience with remote, robotic extravesical reimplantation in the canine model.[8] Compared with the conventional laparoscopic group done by the same surgeons, the robotic group required more operative time (395.3 versus 318.5 minutes). There was one ureteral obstruction in each group. The authors concluded that the robotic procedure, while technically feasible, has yet to prove its usefulness in humans due to its drawbacks, such as lack of tactile feedback and limited selection in instrumentation.

Although Lakshmanan and Fung remain enthusiastic, many authors have felt that the difficulty of the technique puts it in disfavor when compared to fairly prompt recovery seen following open reimplantation surgery. Difficult visualization in the deep retropubic space along with a protracted operative time has caused the extravesical approach to laparoscopic reimplantation to have limited applications thus far.

TRANSVESICAL URETERAL REIMPLANTATION

Shortly after the initial reports of extravesical ureteral reimplantation, experience with a combined transvesical and transurethral endoscopic approach to ureteral reimplantation was reported by two groups.[9,10] The initial attempt by each group was to use the Gil-Vernet or trigonoplasty technique. The procedure has been termed endoscopic trigonoplasty, or the percutaneous endoscopic trigonoplasty (PET) procedure.

TRANSVESICAL TECHNIQUE

The patient first undergoes cystourethroscopy for assessment of the bladder. If the ureteral orifices appear to be at least 2 cm apart and the bladder is otherwise normal, the percutaneous endoscopic trigonoplasty may be performed.

Two transvesical trocars are placed, one 5-mm and one 2-mm port (Figure 93-1). The 5-mm port is used for the telescope, and the 2-mm port for working instruments. The incisions for these ports are made 1 to 2 cm superior to the pubic ramus, lateral to the midline on each side in a skin crease.

Looking into the bladder with a cystoscope placed from below, puncture is made into the bladder with the first trocar. A suture-passing needle places a 2-0 polyglactin 910 suture alongside the trocar through the rectus fascia, muscle, and bladder wall into the intravesical space (Figure 93-2). This suture is grasped with a flexible grasper passed through the cystoscope. The empty passing needle is placed again on the opposite side of the trocar, and then the suture is passed intravesically into the jaw, and the needle is withdrawn. The suture can then be pulled anteriorly during the procedure to keep the bladder wall fixed against the posterior rectus and prevent

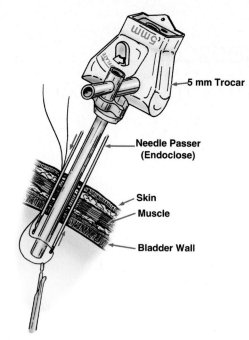

Figure 93–2 Transvesical trocar insertion during percutaneous endoscopic trigonoplasty.

the bladder from slipping off the trocar. The suture placement is repeated for the 2-mm trocar on the opposite side.

At this point, the bladder is drained via the cystoscope and CO_2 insufflation is begun. The role of the cystoscope from this point on is to suction the operative field and evacuate smoke to improve visualization.

For the trigonoplasty, mucosa over the interureteric ridge is cauterized from orifice to orifice to minimize bleeding. The miniature scissor is used to open the line between the orifices. The mucosa is then dissected away proximal and distal to this line of dissection for 1 cm (Figure 93-3). Two 3-0 polyglactin 910 horizontal mattress sutures are placed on the medial edge of both orifices. Knots are tied extracorporeally using the knot pusher. This maneuver advances both ureteral orifices to the midline along the previously de-epithelialized trough and lengthens the submucosal tunnels. Four interrupted sutures of 4-0 polyglactin 910 are then used to re-approximate the bladder mucosa in the midline.

Catheter drainage is used postoperatively. Either a urethral catheter is left in place or a small

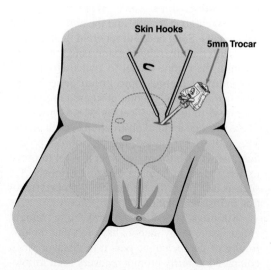

Figure 93-1 Trocar placement during percutaneous endoscopic trigonoplasty.

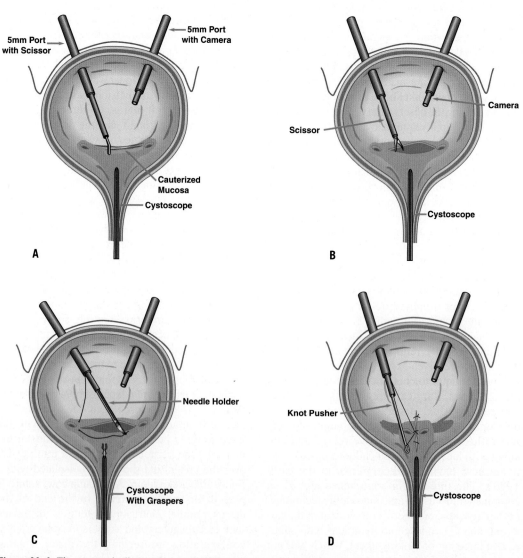

Figure 93–3 The mucosa is dissected away during percutaneous endoscopic trigonoplasty.

piece of 8 French Silastic tubing is slipped through one of the trocars to the intravesical space before it is removed. This small tubing remains in place temporarily to decompress the bladder. The two trocar site sutures are tied once the trocars are removed. This results in a suture that closes bladder wall, rectus muscle, and anterior rectus fascia simultaneously.

TRANSVESICAL REIMPLANTATION RESULTS

In 1995, Okamura and associates detailed outcomes in 12 adult patients, mostly with low or moderate grade vesicoureteral reflux.[9] Their technique involved two suprapubically placed trocars in the midline and a cystoscope via the urethra. A trough between the ureters was created after bladder insufflation with CO_2, and the suturing was done via SKI-type needle placed via the urethral cystoscope rather than via suprapubic port. A single horizontal mattress suture was used to draw the orifices toward the midline (Gil-Vernet). Early follow-up cystograms showed resolution of reflux in all patients.

In 1996, Cartwright and colleagues reported their experience in 22 children undergoing percutaneous endoscopic trigonoplasty.[10] Reflux was of moderate grade in most, and high grade in a few. Although no ureteral obstruction was created with the Gil-Vernet trigonoplasty procedure, reflux resolved in 20 of 32 ureters at six months, for a resolution rate (by ureter) of 62.5%. Success was not dependent on patient age, laterality of reflux, initial reflux grade, operative sequence, or presence of preoperative bladder instability. Three complications were encountered, including vesicovaginal fistula, significant hyponatremia, and a perivesical urinoma requiring drainage. The authors concluded that this technique was technically feasible but involved a distinct learning curve. Additionally, with only a modest success rate, technical modifications were needed before consideration could be given to this as an alternative for the management of reflux.

Following this initial disappointing resolution rate with trigonoplasty, members of the same group performed transvesical mobilization of the ureters again using two suprapubic transvesical ports and a cystoscope.[11] Using similar instru-

mentation and a stent within the ureteral orifice, the ureteral orifices were dissected from their detrusor attachments using miniature laparoscopic scissors. Dissection gained approximately 2.5 cm of ureteral mobility into the intravesical space. No further mobilization was attempted owing to concern of rapid escape of CO_2 into the retroperitoneal space and subsequent pneumoretroperitoneum and bladder collapse. The ureters were then reimplanted in a cross-trigonal fashion after the detrusor hiatus had been reapproximated with interrupted polyglactin 910 sutures. The length of the submucosal tunnel was limited, and the procedure probably achieved a 2- to 2.5-cm ureteral reimplantation on each side. The orifice was matured with polyglactin 910 suture, and the submucosal tunnel was closed with the same material as well. At 1 year follow-up, 10 of 12 ureters managed in this fashion showed no reflux, but this corresponded to resolution of reflux in only 5 of 7 patients.

Gill and associates in 2001[12] reported their series utilizing the laparoscopic technique described by Cartwright and associates (Figure 93-4). Of three patients, reflux resolved in two

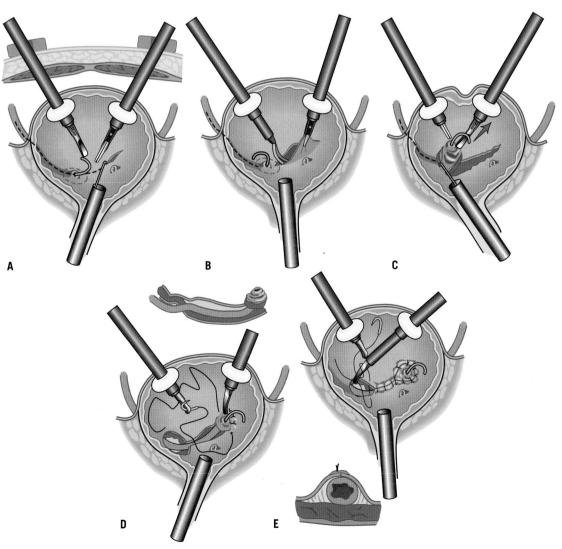

Figure 93–4 Laparoscopic Cohen cross-trigonal –technique developed in 2001.

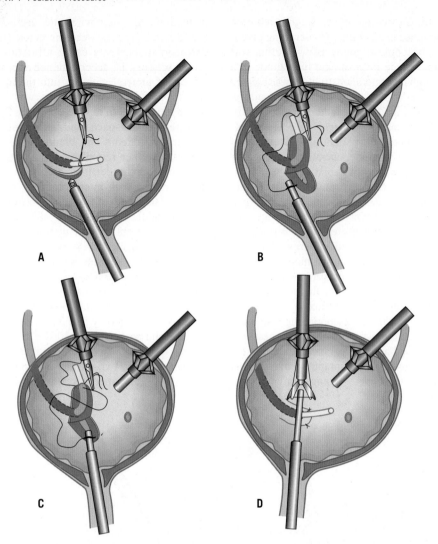

Figure 93–5 The endoscopic trigonoplasty II –technique creates a U-shaped flap.

and persisted as grade II in one patient at 6-month follow-up.

In 1997, Okamura and associates published a study with longer follow-up of 28 patients (many children) undergoing endoscopic trigonoplasty.[13] Whereas at 1 to 3 months postoperatively, reflux resolved in 95%, this had decreased to 79% when evaluated at 12 months. A select group of 13 patients underwent cystoscopy to evaluate the appearance of their surgical repair. Five were noted to have trigonal splitting, and three of these were noted to have postoperative recurrence of reflux. Three further patients were noted to have retreating ureteral orifices, with 1 of 3 demonstrating reflux.

In an effort to improve on their results, Okamura and associates developed a new procedure called endoscopic trigonoplasty II,[14] which is based on the open antireflux procedure reported by Orikasa.[15] Using the same approach (cystoscope

and trocar placement) as the endoscopic trigonoplasty I, this procedure created a U-shaped flap including the ureter, tightened the muscular backing and then elongated the intramural ureter (Figure 93-5). In their initial experience with 14 refluxing ureters in 8 patients, mean operative time was 245 minutes, with reflux resolution in 11 of the 14 ureters (86%) at a follow-up of 12 months. In two of the three failures, the cause was noted to be a ureterovesical fistula in one case and insufficient U-flap fixation in the other. There was no ureteral obstruction reported, and analgesic use in most patients consisted of a once daily medication for 4 days. Although this initial report seems promising in terms of a similar resolution rate to open surgery, longer-term follow-up and experience will reveal if these results are durable and if the learning curve is too steep for this procedure to be widely used for primary reflux.

CONCLUSION

The current practice of open ureteral reimplantation often requires only a 24-hour hospital stay. We have, in fact, managed a good number of unilateral, extravesical reimplant cases on an outpatient basis over 6 months. As such, shortening the hospital stay with laparoscopic approaches in most children does not hold great promise. It may prove that older children (and probably adults) are the ones who benefit the most from a more prompt discharge and recovery than would occur with open techniques. For all patients, there is the cosmetic benefit of having only two small trocar scars. The future of transvesical and extravesical minimally invasive procedures in children is undetermined and should be most interesting to follow over the next 5 to 10 years. It is likely that progress in the area of transvesical and extravesical surgery in children will be made through future innovations in equipment and the ensuing changes in operative techniques.

REFERENCES

1. Lich R, Howerton LW, Davis LA. Recurrent urosepsis in children. J Urol 1961;86:851.
2. Atala A, Kavoussi L, Goldstein D, et al. Laparoscopic correction of vesicoureteral reflux. J Urol 1993;150(2 Pt 2):748–51.
3. Schimberg W, Wacksman J, Rudd R, et al. Laparoscopic correction of vesicoureteral reflux in the pig. J Urol 1994;151:1664–7.
4. McDougall EM, Urban DA, et al. Laparoscopic repair of vesicoureteral reflux utilizing the Lich-Gregoir technique in the pig model. J Urol 1995;153:497–500.
5. Ehrlich RM, Gershman A, Fuchs S. Laparoscopic vesicoureteroplasty in children: initial case reports. Urology 1994;43:255.
6. Janetschek G, Radmayr C, Bartsch G. Laparoscopic ureteral ant-reflux plasty reimplantation: first clinical experience. Annales d'Urologie 1995;29:101.
7. Lakshmanan Y, Fung LC. Laparoscopic extravesicular ureteral reimplantation for vesicoureteral reflux: recent technical advances. J Endourol 2000;14:589–93.
8. Sung GT, Gill IS. Remote, robotic laparoscopic extravesical ureteral reimplantation with ureteral advancement technique. Dial Ped Urol 2001;24(10).
9. Okamura K, Ono Y, Yamada Y, et al. Endoscopic trigonoplasty for primary vesicoureteric reflux. Br J Urol 1995;75:390–4.
10. Cartwright PC, Snow BW, Mansfield J, et al. Percutaneous endoscopic trigonoplasty: a minimally invasive approach to correct vesicoureteric reflux. J Urol 1996;156(2 Pt 2):661–4.
11. Gatti J, Cartwright P, Hamilton B, Snow B. Percutaneous endoscopic trigonoplasty in children: long-term outcomes and modifications in technique. J Endourol 1999;13(b):581–4.
12. Gill IS, Ponsky LE, et al. Laparoscopic cross-trigonal Cohen ureteroneocystostomy: novel technique. J Urol 2001;166:1811–4.
13. Okamura K, Kato N, Takamura S, et al. Trigonal splitting is a major complication of endoscopic trigonoplasty at 1-year follow-up. J Urol 1997;157:1423–5.
14. Tsuji Y, Okamura K, et al. A new endoscopic ureteral reimplantation for primary vesicoureteral reflux (endoscopic trignoplasty II). J Urol 2003;169:1020–2.
15. Orikasa S. A new antireflux procedure. Eur Urol 1990;17:330.

94

Laparoscopic Management of the Non-palpable Testicle

Linda Baker, MD

Gerald H. Jordan, MD

The absence of a testicle in the scrotum is termed cryptorchidism. The testis differentiates adjacent to the mesonephric kidneys during embryonic life, normally descending via the inguinal canal to its scrotal position; but in 0.8 to 1.8% of boys aged 1 year,[1,2] this process of descent is flawed, resulting in cryptorchidism. A testicle is palpable in the groin in most cryptorchid boys; in approximately 20%, it is non-palpable.[3] When the testicle is non-palpable, the gonad might be absent, intra-abdominal (ie, along the normal path of descent or ectopic), or within the inguinal canal (ie, canalicular).[4,5]

Clinical consequences of cryptorchidism include decreased fertility and an increased risk of developing testicular cancer. Fertility is impaired in approximately 50 to 70% of boys born with one undescended testicle and up to 75% of those born with two undescended testicles, even after surgical correction (ie, orchiopexy).[6] Histologic deterioration is believed to be worse with higher testicles; therefore, it was thought that fertility varies in association with this finding. One study, however, indicated that paternity (which does not necessarily correlate with histology of an unilateral undescended testicle) may be similar in both abdominal and extra-abdominal unilateral undescended testicles.[7] Because the serum level of inhibin B is believed to reflect Sertoli's cell function and seminiferous tubule integrity, lower levels of circulating inhibin B in boys with a history of cryptorchidism may be a better predictor of impaired spermatogenesis later in life.[8]

A man with a history of cryptorchidism is at a 9.7 times increased risk of developing testicular cancer over the general population (overall risk ≤ 1 in 2,000). Unfortunately, early orchiopexy does not necessarily reduce the risk of testicular cancer,[9] and relocation of an undescended testicle is not generally warranted for this reason alone. Treatment is recommended, however, to relocate the testicle to the scrotum for easier examination, correct the associated inguinal hernia, prevent testicular torsion, or alleviate possible psychological trauma resulting from the empty hemiscrotum.[10] In addition, it may improve fertility or diminish the potential for malignant transformation.

MANAGEMENT

Management of a non-palpable testicle can be medical (ie, hormonal therapy) or surgical. Surgical options include laparoscopic or open techniques, both of which are associated with significant advantages and disadvantages.

HORMONAL CHALLENGE Hormonal therapy using human chorionic gonadotropin-β subunit (hCG-β) or testosterone preparations has been used under a number of proposed protocols. Although rarely therapeutic, in some cases of non-palpable testicles, hormonal therapy can initiate testicular descent, rendering the testicle palpable. Occasionally, it results in a fully descended testicle.[11] This therapy is felt to be best applied to the patient with bilateral non-palpable testicles. To date, there is no evidence that use of hormonal therapy complicates the outcome of either laparoscopic or open orchiopexy.

SURGICAL MANAGEMENT Before 1976, surgical management of a non-palpable testicle consisted of inguinal exploration. If the testicle, nubbin, or blind-ending vessels were not identified, exploration was extended into the retroperitoneum. The testicle was then either identified as absent or was removed or scrotally positioned. Rarely, the surgeon was unable to locate the testicle. In 1976, Cortesi and colleagues described a method of diagnostic laparoscopy to locate the non-palpable testicle.[12] Soon thereafter, therapeutic laparoscopy was performed by Bloom,[13] Jordan and colleagues,[14] and Bogaert and colleagues.[15] Although the introduction of these techniques initially caused debate among pediatric urologists regarding appropriate management of a non-palpable testicle,[16–18] today laparoscopic approaches to the non-palpable testicle have gained worldwide acceptance and incorporation into daily practice by pediatric urologists

SURGICAL TIMING At birth and into the first year of life, undescended testicles have been shown to have normal histology, including a normal population of germ cells. Beyond age 18 months, both light and electron microscopy demonstrate histologic changes suggesting deterioration of the testicular germ cell population,[19,20] with testicular histology correlating with position (ie, greater pathology occurs in higher testicles). Although some reports have noted testicular damage as early as age 6 months in the human cryptorchid testicle, spontaneous

testicular descent has been reported as late as age 4 to 6 months. Considering these factors and that anesthesia risks in a healthy infant aged 6 months are similar to those in a healthy adult, the current recommended timing for orchiopexy is between ages 6 and 12 months.

Although there may also be anatomic and technical advantages to orchiopexy within the first 6 months—especially in patients with high undescended testicles and prune belly syndrome, where eventual descensus is highly unlikely—orchiopexy at about 1 year maximizes the opportunity for those few testicles that will descend later during the first year of life, while preventing the histologic changes that occur in those testicles that remain undescended beyond the first year of life. Data supporting the recommendation for early orchiopexy is being reported: testicular growth is more common in children operated on before age 18 months compared with that performed in older children[21]; and early orchiopexy appears to benefit Leydig's cell function in adults, potentially enhancing fertility.[22] Elder's recent analysis would suggest that orchiopexy at six months is optimal because it capitalizes on the anatomic advantages conferred by the child's small size, yet optimizes the real chance of spontaneous descent.[23]

Decisions regarding orchiopexy after age 2 years are based on the risks and benefits of the testicle to the individual patient. Although an undescended testicle may have poor fertility function, its usefulness for androgen production should be considered, especially in cases of a solitary testicle. In contrast, in occasional postpubertal males found to have a palpable or non-palpable undescended testicle, sperm production is rare,[24] and they are at significant risk for malignant change. An updated analysis of the anesthetic risks of orchiectomy versus the lifetime risk of germ cell cancer was performed by Oh and colleagues,[25] who advocate orchiectomy in all healthy, cryptorchid males (ASA I and II) until age 50, although, for some patients with comorbid conditions, the risks of surgery can be significant even before age 50. If the undescended testicle is not palpable, diagnostic laparoscopy with laparoscopic orchiectomy (especially if combined with another surgical procedure) is an optimal means of management that minimizes pain, time away from work, and scarring. Further, while sperm production is rare in the undescended testicle addressed later in life, the availability of assisted fertilization techniques may significantly alter the mix of recommendations for these patients.

PREOPERATIVE ASSESSMENT The initial evaluation of an undescended testicle includes a detailed patient history of the gonadal descensus pattern at birth, palpable gonads, hypospadias, genital surgery, or inguinal herniorrhaphy. Physical exam of the groin—important to identification of a difficult-to-feel testicle—should be carefully performed in a warm, non-threatening environment with warm lubricant. If the contralateral testicle is descended, its size should be noted. A contralateral descended testicle that manifests compensatory hypertrophy (as judged by growth comparison to standard nomograms) may indicate lack of functioning testicular tissue on the non-palpable side.[26,27] This finding is not always accurate, however, and the non-palpable side must be further evaluated. Bilateral non-palpable testicles represent a distinct subgroup; the considerations of hormonal therapy or earlier orchiopexy were addressed earlier (see "Surgical Timing").

Preoperative diagnostic modalities used in the evaluation of patients with a non-palpable testicle include hormonal challenge (see "Hormonal Challenge" above), radiological tests, and laparoscopy. A diagnostic test for a non-palpable testicle should uniformly and unequivocally determine the presence or absence and locality of gonadal tissue. Only laparoscopy uniformly accomplishes these goals.[5,28–30]

Radiologic Evaluation Radiologic techniques that have been used to locate the non-palpable testicle include ultrasonography, venography, computed tomography (CT), and magnetic resonance imaging (MRI); in most cases, however, none of these modalities are sufficiently sensitive to be definitive.[2,31–34] Furthermore, although herniography, venography, or arteriography can give indirect evidence of the presence of an undescended testicle, none can unequivocally define the gonad. Because radiographic localizing studies cannot rule out the presence of an intra-abdominal testicle,[31] they cannot preclude surgery in a child with a non-palpable testicle. Although ultrasonography does image the non-palpable undescended testicle in some cases, many inguinal orchiopexies have been performed based on a sonogram indicating an inguinal gonad that was actually a lymph node. While MRI or gadolinium-enhanced magnetic resonance angiography (MRA) have better sensitivity,[35] they do not have the same accuracy as laparoscopy. Furthermore, cost issues and anesthetic requirements negate the utility of MRI or MRA, while surgical exploration is still required.

In select cases, radiographic imaging studies can be useful. In patients who have been identified as likely to derive maximal benefit from laparoscopy,[33] inguinal ultrasonography can help locate non-palpable inguinal and abdominal testicles, although examination under anesthesia at the time

of orchiopexy is probably equally helpful.[5] Imaging can also be useful in unusual cases (eg, overweight boys with non-palpable inguinal testicles) or in follow-up of adolescents who are not surgical candidates because of comorbid conditions.

Laparoscopy Evaluation Laparoscopy is an excellent diagnostic tool to verify the existence and location of the non-palpable testicle.[36–39] It has been found useful for the diagnosis of both the unilateral and bilateral non-palpable testicle. The principal goal of diagnostic laparoscopy is to identify non-palpable testicular tissue. When non-palpable testicular tissue is found, the surgeon should decide whether orchiopexy or testicular removal is indicated. In addition, mobility of the testicle, its vas deferens, and its vascular supply are assessed—crucial features in planning the therapeutic surgical approach.

Diagnostic Laparoscopic Procedure After administration of adequate anesthesia, the patient is secured to the bed in a supine, frog leg position, with arms tucked. Preparation and draping should be suitable for an open abdominal procedure. A urethral Foley catheter and an orogastric tube are passed, and all laparoscopic equipment is assembled and verified.

A supra- or infraumbilical skin incision is made, and the peritoneum is accessed. Abdominal access can be achieved using a Veress needle, Hasson technique, or open access. Because most patients are aged between 6 and 24 months, safety concerns have led most surgeons to prefer open versus blind access techniques (ie, Veress needle). Holding sutures are placed in the fascia to assist elevation for the peritoneotomy. The authors use a radially dilating access sheath, the InnerDyne Step introducer system,[40,41] to achieve 5- or 10-mm access. Alternatively, needlescopic 2-mm access (and working ports), as reported by Ferrer and colleagues,[40] Gill and colleagues,[42] and Ross and colleagues[43] can be used, but they provide less light and a smaller visual field. After insufflation to 14 to 15 cm of water, a 5-mm, 0° camera is used to inspect the abdomen for injury.

The patient is then placed in Trendelenburg's position and each internal ring bilaterally inspected. The testicular vessels and vas are easily identified, and the closed internal ring noted on the unaffected side (Figure 94-1). Caudal traction on the descended testicle can help visualization of its cord structures. On the affected side, the internal ring is noted and the testicle, vas, and testicular vessels are sought. Possible findings on the affected side include the following:

1. The vas and testicular vessels appear normal and exit a closed internal ring (see Figure 94-1). The groin is explored for the testicle or nubbin via laparoscopic or open approach. Removal of any remaining testicular nubbin has been controversial, but 10% of nubbins may contain viable germ cells,[44–46] which ostensibly could undergo malignant change.
2. The vas and testicular vessels appear normal and exit an open internal ring (Figure 94-2).

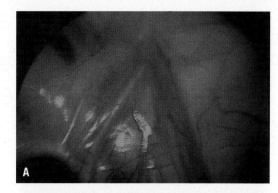
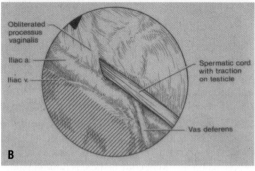

Figure 94-1 Diagram of the appearance of the normal right internal ring.

Retrograde milking of the inguinal canal may push a canalicular (peeping) testicle or nubbin into the abdomen (Figures 94-3). If the gonad is not located, the groin must be explored[47] either by a laparoscopic or an open technique.

3. The blind-ending vessels are clearly identified ending in a 'horse tail' appearance, often within proximity to a blind-ending vas, indicating that the testicle is not viable. The procedure is terminated, although some surgeons

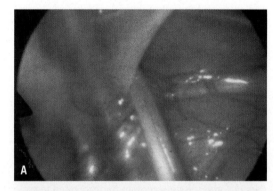
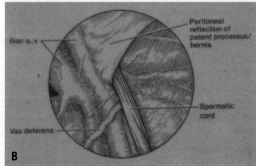

Figure 94-2 Diagram of the appearance of the right internal ring with a patent processus vaginalis.

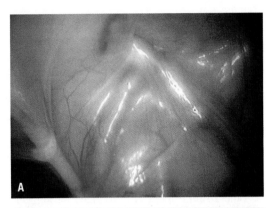

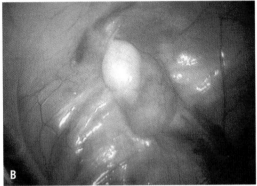

Figure 94-3 The appearance of the right internal ring in a patient with a peeping testicle. With external pressure on the inguinal canal, the peeping testicle is pushed back into the abdominal cavity.

still remove any intervening tissue identified (Figure 94-4).

4. An intra-abdominal testicle is located (Figures 94-5, and 94-6).

5. A blind-ending vas is seen without testicular vessels in the vicinity, a finding termed gonadal disjunction. The laparoscopic exploration is not complete and should be continued rostrally toward the aortic origin of the testicular vessels until the gonad is located.

Among cases of non-palpable testicle, 50 to 60% are identified as an intra-abdominal testicle or peeping testicle, 30% as an atrophic nubbin, and 20% as an absent testicle. If a testicle is located within 2 cm of the internal ring (30.6%) or peeping (17.4%), it is usually a normal size with a normal appearing epididymis, vas, and vessels. Alternatively, the testicle can be located > 2 cm from the internal ring, either along the normal path of descent (44.8%) or in an ectopic site (eg, beside the bladder, rectum, kidney, liver, spleen, or crossed ectopia) (7.1%).[48]

In some cases, the testicle and testicular vessels are not clearly identified with the camera alone. If loops of bowel are blocking the view, a manipulating instrument is a useful aid to visualize the testicular vessels. The Veress needle or other small probes have been used for this purpose, and 2 to 3 mm instruments are ideal. In these cases, however, therapeutic maneuvers will be eventually necessary 89 to 90% of the time, and cannula placement may be the most expedient way of proceeding.

If therapeutic laparoscopy is indicated, insufflation is temporarily increased up to 20 cm of water, while two 2- or 5-mm ports are secured at the level of the umbilicus just lateral to the inferior epigastric vessels (Figure 94-7). The testicle is then located using a grasper and laparoscopic scissors with cautery. Either laparoscopic orchiectomy, single-stage laparoscopic orchiopexy (primary or one-stage Fowler-Stephens), or two-stage laparoscopic orchiopexy is chosen.

THERAPEUTIC LAPAROSCOPY Laparoscopic Surgery for a Unilateral Non-palpable Testicle Laparoscopic management of a non-palpable testicle is referred to as therapeutic laparoscopy. The goal of therapeutic laparoscopy for a unilateral

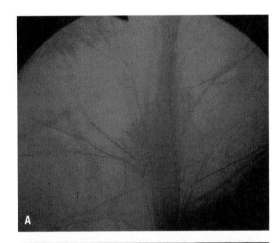

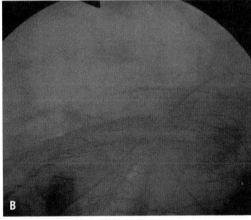

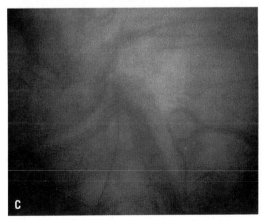

Figure 94-4 The classic appearance of blind-ending vessels. The classic appearance of a blind-ending vas deferens. The classic appearance of blind-ending spermatic vessels ending in proximity to the blind-ending vas deferens.

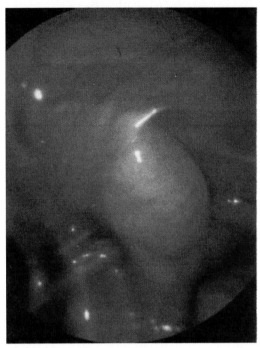

Figure 94-5 Photograph of the right groin in a child with low abdominal undescended testicle.

undescended testicle is either removal of the poor testicle or permanent fixation of the testicle in the scrotum. Therapeutic laparoscopic procedures include laparoscopic orchiectomy, primary laparoscopic orchiopexy, laparoscopic one-stage Fowler-Stephens orchiopexy, and laparoscopic two-stage Fowler-Stephens orchiopexy. Preoperatively, the family is counseled concerning the possibilities of an absent testicle, small atrophic testicle, or an intra-abdominal testicle, with the choice of surgical procedure determined by the algorithm presented in Figure 94-8.

Risks of surgery include bleeding, infection, anesthesia risks, injury to intra-abdominal or retroperitoneal organs necessitating emergent laparotomy, loss of a testicle (acute atrophy), mechanical injury to the vas, epididymis, testicular vessels or testicle, poor testicular position, or need for a two-stage procedure.

Primary Laparoscopic Orchiopexy The patient is placed in Trendelenburg's position with the side of the bed tilted contralateral to the undescended testicle. Cannulas are placed as illustrated in Figure 94-7. A peritoneotomy is made just lateral to the testicular vessels, carried over the top of the internal ring, and continued laterally and superior to the vas, taking care to not injure the inferior epigastric vessels or the bladder (Figure 94-9). Some urologists make a mirror peritoneotomy medial to the vessels and vas, while others (including the authors) leave both the peritoneal area medial to the testicular vessels and the vas undisturbed.

After completing the peritoneotomy, the testicular vessels, testicle, and vas are elevated on the peritoneal pedicle which is then dissected in the plane between these structures and the external iliac vessels, taking care not to harm the external iliac vessels, inferior epigastric vessels,

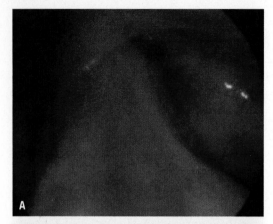

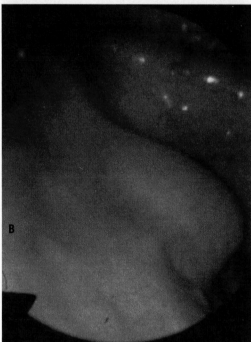

Figure 94-6 The appearance of the right groin in a child with a high abdominal undescended testicle. Note the patent processus and the disassociation of the vas deferens and epididymis from the testicle. The appearance of the testicle high in the abdomen.

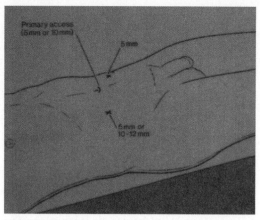

Figure 94-7 Diagram of the cannula placement for a right laparoscopic orchiopexy.

could prevent testicular mobility are carefully dissected, and once adequate length is assured, the testicle is transferred to the scrotum.

In some cases, the length is inadequate. An effective next step is to incise the peritoneum parallel to the testicular vessels as far proximal as safely possible, and then extend the peritoneal incision perpendicular over the testicular vessels to join the line of incision adjacent to the vas deferens. This relaxing incision may significantly lengthen the vessels, allowing scrotal positioning. If length still remains an issue, and the peritoneum in the triangle between the vas and vessels is intact, the spermatic vessels can be divided (see Fowler-Stephens approach below). It is the authors' opinion, however, that it is best to avoid this scenario whenever possible by performing a staged orchiopexy.

Several techniques to deliver the testicle into the scrotum have been described, including retrograde placement of a clamp or port. Placing a port assures that the pneumoperitoneum can be maintained in the event the testicle is "fumbled."

The authors currently use the 10-mm InnerDyne Step Cannula for the transfer.[40,41] Lucent cannulas can be helpful, however, and prototype reusable lucent cannulas are currently under development. The grasper in the ipsilateral abdominal port is passed medial to the inferior epigastric vessels just over the top of the superior pubic ramus, and a scrotal skin incision is made in the ipsilateral hemiscrotum, generating a subdartos pouch. The laparoscopic grasper is then guided out through the scrotal incision, the 10-mm Step introducer is passed on the grasper, and the 10-mm trocar is introduced through the Step introducer (Figure 94-13A). The graspers are then transferred to the scrotal port, the gubernaculum of the testicle is grasped (Figure 94-13B), and the testicle is delivered via the port (Figure 94-13C and 94-13D) into the scrotum (Figure 94-13E). The testicle is secured intrascrotally in the subdartos pouch by the surgeon's preferred fixation technique, the intra-abdominal pressure is lowered to 4 mm Hg, and the surgical field assessed for bleeding (Figure 94-14). In children, the fascia of all 5- or 10-mm port sites is closed to avoid development of hernias. All CO_2 is evacuated, and skin wounds are closed and dressed. Adjuvant caudal anesthesia and local injection of cannula sites using bupivacaine hydrochloride (Marcaine) is beneficial in these patients.

The children are awakened, recover from anesthesia, and are discharged. In most cases, diet is rapidly advanced, and no physical restrictions are imposed, except avoidance of straddle implements. Most parents report that the child exhibits a low activity level on the day of surgery or, when surgery is performed in the afternoon, the next day. In both cases, however, they report that the child rapidly returns to normal activity level within 24 hours and remains seemingly unimpeded by his laparoscopic procedure from that time forward.

or a long looping vas. The testicle is rostrally retracted, inverting the processus vaginalis and the gubernaculum. The gubernaculum is thinned and cut across with monopolar cautery, watching for a long looping vas (Figure 94-10). Cautery is necessary because of the vascularity of the gubernacular attachments (Figure 94-11). Other modalities such as the Ligasure (Valleylab) or Harmonic Scalpel (Ethicon Endoscopic-Surgery, Inc.) could be used, but the authors believe that, because cautery is so sparingly used, the added expense of these instruments is not justified.

The testicle is then retracted towards the contralateral internal ring to assess length. If the testicle can reach the contralateral internal ring, in most cases, the length is sufficient to place the testicle well dependent in the respective hemiscrotum (Figure 94-12). To avoid testicular atrophy, the vas should not be vigorously mobilized; it should, however, be sufficiently mobilized to prevent ureteral kinking from the paravasal attachments. Any remaining attachments that

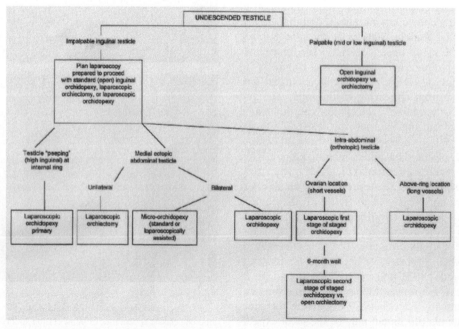

Figure 94-8 Algorithm outlining management of the impalpable undescended testicle.

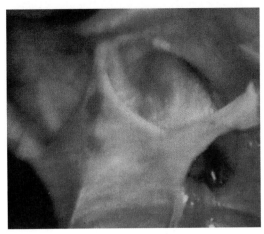

Figure 94-9 Child with a peeping testicle, the appearance of the right groin as the peritoneum is opened around the patent processus vaginalis.

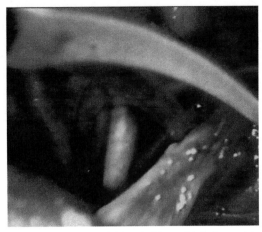

Figure 94-11 Same child as in Figure 94-9, the testicle has been freed; the gubernaculums is exposed and is divided with cautery.

Single-Stage Fowler-Stephens Laparoscopic Orchiopexy If the procedure outlined above (under primary laparoscopic orchiopexy) results in testicular vessel length that is inadequate for desirable scrotal positioning, a single-stage Fowler-Stephens procedure can be performed. In this procedure, the testicular artery and vein are clipped and transected via contralateral 5-mm port, preserving the vasal blood supply to the testicle. This technique allows the testicle to be placed in the scrotum with a single laparoscopic procedure. Division of the testicular vessels with single-stage transfer, however, is clearly associated with higher atrophy rates than the single-stage orchiopexy without vessel division or staged orchiopexy, described below.

Two-Stage Fowler-Stephens Laparoscopic Orchiopexy If diagnostic laparoscopy reveals a high testicle that cannot reach the scrotum without transection of the testicular vessels, a two-stage Fowler-Stephens laparoscopic orchiopexy can be used. In the first-stage, a contralateral 5-mm port is placed and a parallel peritoneotomy is performed immediately medial to the testicular vessels, a safe distance proximal to the iliac vessels. The peritoneotomy encircles the vessels, which are

then ligated using a 5-mm vascular clip applier. The vessel transection completes the first-stage.

During the ensuing 6-month interval, collateral blood supply is enhanced via the paravasal arteries. Six months after the initial spermatic vessel ligation, the testicle is brought to the scrotum, based on the paravasal vascular supply, using either the laparoscopic technique outlined above for a primary laparoscopic orchiopexy or an open technique.

Some authors have suggested that testicles managed with staged division of the spermatic vessels should be evaluated with color Doppler to evaluate the viability of the testicle before undertaking the second stage. Realistically, however, even if the testicle does not appear to be viable by Doppler, the remaining gonadal tissue should be removed, as atrophy by ultrasound criteria should not be considered pathognomonic of complete atrophy of the gonadal tubular structures, and these structures could continue to carry the risk of malignant transformation.

As early as 1903, Bevan advocated division of the spermatic vessels to "aid" with orchiopexy.[49] The staged approach of Fowler and Stephens based on collateralization along the long loop of the vas deferens is an extension of Bevan's technique. Originally, a long looping vas was believed to be a prerequisite for the Fowler-Stephens procedure, but intra-abdominal testicles without a long looping vas deferens have also been successfully treated with this technique.

The staged approach has been compared to other forms of flap delay. Delay is a term in the reconstructive literature that implies a first-stage tissue transposition followed by a second-stage axial blood supply division, with the transfer tissue surviving on random collateralization that occurred between the first and second stages. This principle does not exactly apply to a staged orchiopexy because part of the axial blood supply is divided during the first stage. Further, it is assumed that the second blood supply enhances during the period between the first and second stages, but whether this actually occurs has been called into question by Koff and Sethi.[50] Most

agree, however, that the paravasal blood supply appears to become "prominent" after division of the spermatic vessel leash and the waiting period.

Intraoperative Scenarios **Normal Vessels Enter an Open or Closed Ring** In most of these cases, a laparoscopic inguinal exploration can be performed. For a high canalicular testicle (peeping testicle) and most low abdominal testicles (< 2 cm from the internal ring), primary laparoscopic orchiopexy is the best laparoscopic technique. In our opinion, staged orchiopexy should be considered for testicles > 2 cm from the internal ring.

Blind-Ending Vas and Medially Ectopic Testicle Undescended testicles are occasionally found proximate to blind-ending vessels with dissociation from the blind vas. If a blind-ending vas deferens is found in the pelvis, the testicle should not be considered "vanished" without further exploration to locate blind-ending vessels.

A medial ectopic abdominal testicle descends to a point medial to its respective medial umbilical artery. These testicles appear to be ovarian, often with a prominent peritoneal fold reminiscent of the broad ligament, and a horizontal (as opposed to vertical) orientation. Prominent gubernacular vessels that appear similar to a round ligament, and vascular gubernacular structures that extend to the location of a normal internal ring—usually closed (ie, no patent processus vaginalis)—are associated with these testicles. The vas deferens is short; most of these testicles do not have looping vas or dissociation of the paratesticular tubular structures, and the spermatic vessel leash is short. Laparoscopic techniques can be used to place these testicles in the scrotum, although correct placement is difficult. In addition, the advantages of medial transposition are negated because they are already medial to the obliterated umbilical artery, and the advantages of either primary or staged spermatic vessel division are negated because the testicles are not associated with looping of the vas. Orchiectomy should be considered in cases of a unilateral undescended testicle. In cases of bilateral maldescensus, staged orchiopexy, aggressive mobilization, or microvascular reanastomosis of the free transferred testicles are options.

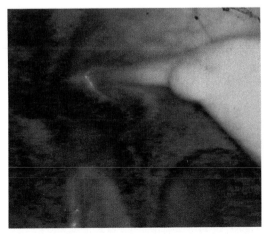

Figure 94-10 The appearance of a long looping vas deferens, the testicle is being retracted into the abdomen; the vas is noted coursing along the path of the gubernaculums.

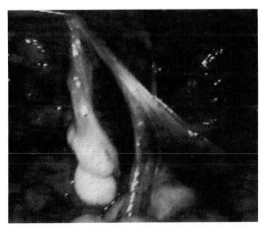

Figure 94-12 The appearance of the testicle, with the spermatic vessels dissected and the vas dissected.

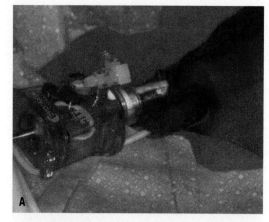

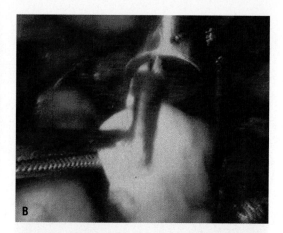

Figure 94-13 *A*, The appearance after a cannula has been placed through the scrotum and the canal of nook into the abdomen, the course of the cannula is lateral to the bladder and medial to the ipsilateral medial umbilical ligament. *B*, The gubernaculum of the testicle is grasped. *C*, The testicle is drawn into the cannula. *D*, The appearance of the testicle as it is brought down into the scrotum within the cannula. *E*, The testicle is released and fixed into the scrotum, in this case by a subdartos pouch.

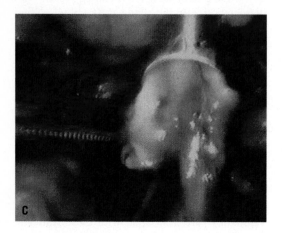

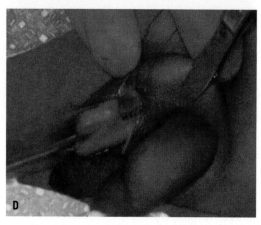

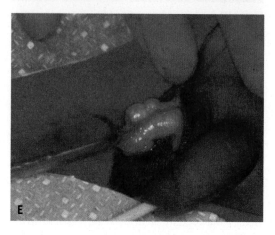

Laparoscopic Surgery for Bilateral Non-palpable Testicles Approximately 1 of every 600 males has bilateral undescended testicles at birth, representing 10% to 25% of patients with cryptorchidism. Because normal testicular descent is an event of the third trimester of pregnancy, cryptorchidism may be a common physical finding in premature male neonates. It is further estimated that an endocrine disorder is the etiology in at least 6% of patients with bilateral undescended testicles.[51,52]

When both are palpable, bilateral undescended testicles are managed using the techniques described for unilateral palpable undescended testicles. Bilateral non-palpable testicles, however, can have life-threatening implications in the neonatal period, especially in association with severe hypospadias. The differential diagnosis of bilateral non-palpable cryptorchidism includes anorchism, ambiguous genitalia caused by female pseudohermaphroditism, or another intersex condition. The possibility of female pseudohermaphroditism should trigger an immediate and thorough evaluation to rule-out life-threatening congenital adrenal hyperplasia (CAH). A normal-appearing virilized phallus does not rule-out CAH, but a karyotype, endocrine testing, radiographic studies, and if indicated, laparoscopy usually provide sufficient information to diagnose an intersex condition.

After excluding an intersex disorder, endocrine studies (ie, human chorionic gonadotropin [HCG] stimulation test, serum müllerian-inhibiting substance [MIS] level, or serum inhibin B level) can be useful to differentiate bilateral cryptorchidism from anorchia.[53] HCG administration can be used to biochemically detect testicular tissue by stimulating testosterone production and can also stimulate the gonads to become palpable by physical examination. Unresponsive Leydig's cells, however, can yield false-negative HCG stimulation testing, and no consensus has been reached concerning dosing and frequency of HCG; therefore, HCG stimulation testing is combined with gonadotropin measurement to diagnose anorchism. Markedly elevated gonadotropins before puberty are indicative of anorchism,[53] but all boys with normal serum gonadotropin levels should undergo exploration regardless of the HCG stimulation test outcome.

Measurement of serum MIS can be used to provide additional evidence that testicular tissue is present, but this test is not widely available. In prepubertal cryptorchid children, serum inhibin B level has been shown to negatively correlate with serum follicle-stimulating hormone (FSH) levels (basal or HCG-stimulated)[54] and positively correlates with a negative testosterone response to HCG stimulation.[55] Serum inhibin B levels can also be low in children with gonadal dysgenesis or a history of testicular trauma. If clinical experience with this serum marker continues to demonstrate its reliability, it may eliminate the need for the HCG stimulation test.

Thus, with a male genotype, a diagnosis of anorchism can be made with a low serum testosterone, negative HCG stimulation test, increased serum gonadotropins, negative serum MIS, a low basal serum inhibin B level, normal levels of adrenal steroid precursors, and radiographic studies demonstrating the absence of müllerian structures. In equivocal cases, diagnostic laparoscopy or open surgical exploration with gonadal biopsy may be required to confirm the diagnosis of anorchism. Some pediatric urologists, however, contend that, regardless of the laboratory results after HCG stimulation or serum MIS sampling, laparoscopic management is imperative for a child with bilateral non-palpable testicles.

Intraoperative decision-making for bilateral disease is impacted by the location of the testicles. In patients with high bilateral intra-abdominal tes-

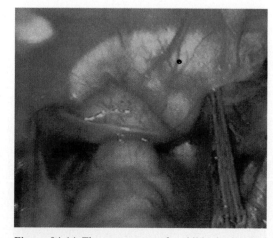

Figure 94-14 The appearance of a child who has had simultaneous bilateral laparoscopic orchiopexies. Notice the cord structures coursing medial to their respective ipsilateral medial umbilical ligament.

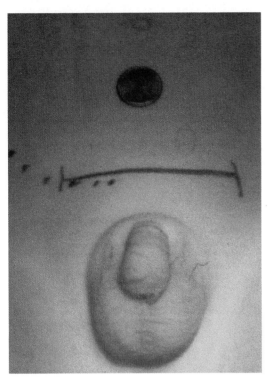

Figure 94-15 Postoperative appearance at 6 months showing a patient following laparoscopic right orchiopexy for a right intra-abdominal testicle. Notice the complete normal appearance of the right hemiscrotum. A penny is placed on the child's abdomen for reference. Notice that the laparoscopic cannula sites are virtually invisible. The abdominal incision/s for an open abdominal orchiopexy are drawn on the child's abdomen.

ticles, most pediatric urologists will perform staged reconstruction, with surgery completed on one side to confirm unilateral testicle survival before embarking on the contralateral side. A Fowler-Stephens approach is the most useful in many of these complex cases.

Micro-orchiopexy Micro-orchiopexy is the term applied to the procedure in which an abdominal undescended testicle is autotransplanted to the scrotum. As originally described by Silber and Kelly, the abdominal testicle is dissected using an open incision.[56] The spermatic vessels are then divided, followed by microanastomosis to the recipient vessels, and the testicle is placed in the scrotum.

Wacksman and associates,[57] who modified the procedure, have accumulated the greatest experience with this procedure. Their modification involves elevation, harvest, and transposition of the abdominal testicle using laparoscopic techniques; therefore, an open incision is only required for dissection and microanastomosis of the recipient vessels.[58] The authors have had excellent results using this procedure in a small series of difficult cases, although they recognize that their success is related to significant experience with the procedure.

Laparoscopic Orchiopexy for Intersex States Diagnostic laparoscopy for intersex evaluation was first described by Gans and Berci in 1973.[59] Advancements in the laboratory diagnosis of intersex states mean most cases are

clearly diagnosed before surgery; exceptions include differentiating between true hermaphroditism and the XX male with genital ambiguity and non-palpable gonads.[60] Therapeutic laparoscopic techniques include laparoscopic gonadal biopsy, gonadectomy (for dysgenetic gonads or when contrary to sex assignment), and orchiopexy. Removal of ductal structures is also used in management of some intersex children (primarily male pseudohermaphrodites). Minimizing surgical scarring is critical in these patients, who often suffer from poor body image and low sexual self-esteem.

Advantages of Diagnostic and Therapeutic Laparoscopy Diagnostic laparoscopy is considered a highly effective and safe procedure for localization and diagnosis of the non-palpable testicle. In most series, procedures have been performed with > 95% accuracy.[5] Although the numbers vary among studies, advocates of laparoscopy for non-palpable testicles report that it is useful in 43 to 51% of unilateral cases for identification of either an absence (27%) or an intra-abdominal testicle (16 to 21%), and in 75% of bilateral cases (ie, blind-ending vessels [17%] or intra-abdominal testicles [58%]).[61] Thus, unnecessary inguinal exploration with subsequent extended open abdominal exploration in the "vanishing testicle" syndrome and testicular aplasia is prevented. Others report identifying up to 52% of laparoscopically identified intra-abdominal testicles as viable,[5,62] thereby improving surgical planning. In addition, several rare conditions, including absent vasa and vessels with a retroperitoneal testicle,[28] persistent müllerian ducts,[63] and other intersex states (ie, transverse testicular ectopia, polyorchidism, and gonadal disjunction from the wolffian ducts),[60] can best be simultaneously identified and treated laparoscopically.

Careful intra-abdominal mobilization can be extensive with therapeutic laparoscopy, allowing orchiopexy with or without testicular vessel division. In addition, laparoscopic orchiopexy is associated with less access trauma, rapid recovery, minimal adhesion formation,[64] and potentially less psychological burden from surgery and scarring. In skillful hands, the operating time for laparoscopic orchiopexy is equivalent to open abdominal orchiopexy, with a reasonable expectation of < 90 minutes for a bilateral orchiopexy for abdominal testicles, in most cases.

Disadvantages of Diagnostic and Therapeutic Laparoscopy As with any surgical approach, laparoscopic orchiopexy can be associated with complications,[48] although many of the complications are due to blind cannula placement and Veress needle insufflation, which is discouraged by the authors. Major complications reported include acute testicular atrophy, bowel perforation,[65] cecal volvulus, bladder perforation,[15] ileus, minor vas laceration, bowel incarceration at the site of the parietal peritoneal closure, and spermatic vessel avulsion necessitating a single-stage Fowler-Stephens orchiopexy.[48] While these complications are significant, it is likely that they can be limited with experience.

In addition, opponents of therapeutic laparoscopic orchiopexy have voiced concerns that the procedure subjects patients with an inguinal testicle or nubbin to an unnecessary laparoscopic procedure in 37 to 64% of cases,[16,17,28,66] a long incision in the peritoneum, lengthy operation, higher operating room costs, potential injury to intra-abdominal or retroperitoneal organs, and the long-term risk of adhesions.[67] Operating room costs can be diminished by the use of reusable equipment[68] and countered by shorter and simpler hospitalization,[69] and the incidence of adhesion formation from pediatric urological laparoscopic procedures is lower than that expected with open exploration.[64]

OPEN SURGERY An alternative to laparoscopic orchiopexy is open inguinal exploration with a proximal extension of the inguinal incision to explore the abdomen or primary open abdominal approach (Figure 94-15). Investigators have raised serious concerns regarding the reliability of open inguinal exploration to rule out an intra-abdominal testicle. Pooled data from five series[38,48,70–73] revealed that 40 testicles were identified via laparoscopy after 78 negative open explorations for a non-palpable testicle. Although a large sampling bias is expected in such reports, the fact that testicles missed by open inguinal exploration are found by laparoscopy should not be ignored considering intra-abdominal testicles are at highest risk for malignant degeneration. Furthermore, a critical assessment of the surgical outcomes of open orchiopexy for the intra-abdominal testicle reveals the need for improvement,[74,75] with therapeutic laparoscopy presently offering the highest success rate for orchiopexy for management of the intra-abdominal testicle.[48]

CASE REPORT

Laparoscopic exploration revealed a normal appearing vas deferens passing through an open internal ring, with structures that appeared to be normal spermatic vessels merging with the vas deferens. The hernia sac, vessels, and vas deferens were dissected, but instead of a true undescended gonad, what appeared to be viable gonadal tissue was only a prominence associated with the vas deferens/epididymis. Fortunately, the orchiopexy was continued and a testicle was found beneath the cecum as these structures were released. Although it was clear that the true spermatic vessels went to the testicle, the prominence of the vessels extending to the open ring (ie, gubernacular attachments) and ending proximate to an epididymis could easily cause confusion. Further, an extended inguinal approach to exploration could have led to a misdiagnosis—emphasizing the potential superiority of laparoscopy versus open exploration.

OUTCOMES

Orchiopexy allows repair of the often-associated inguinal hernia, fixes the testicle in the scrotum,

Table 94-1 Comparison of open versus Laparoscopic Orchiopexy Success Rates* from Two Large Published Series

	Primary Orchiopexy		Single-Stage Fowler-Stephens		Two-Stage Fowler-Stephens	
	n	%	n	%	n	%
Open orchiopexy [Docimo 1995]	80	81.3	321	66.7	56	76.8
Laparoscopic orchiopexy [Baker 2001]	178	97.2	27	74.1	58	87.9

*Success was defined as scrotal position and lack of atrophy.

n = number of testicles

thereby preventing torsion, and prevents psychological issues associated with an empty hemiscrotum. Outcomes analysis always compares to a gold standard. In the case of orchiopexy, open surgical techniques have been the gold standard, with the early postoperative outcome variables being testicular position (ie, scrotal) and lack of testicular atrophy. In 1995, Docimo assembled a meta-analysis of open surgical results,[74] reporting that open orchiopexy for the intra-abdominal testicle yielded an overall success rate of 76.1%. Success rates for individual procedures were as follows: open single-stage Fowler-Stephens orchiopexy, 67%; two-stage Fowler-Stephens orchiopexy, 73%; transabdominal orchiopexy, 81%; and microvascular orchiopexy, 84%. In comparison, a 2001 multi-institutional analysis of laparoscopic orchiopexy from 10 US centers collated results from 310 laparoscopic orchiopexies in 252 patients during a 9-year period.[48] In this study, 15.2% were lost to follow-up; primary laparoscopic orchiopexy succeeded in 97.2% of 178 testicles, single-stage Fowler-Stephens laparoscopic orchiopexy succeeded in 74.1% of 27 testicles, and two-stage Fowler-Stephens laparoscopic orchiopexy in 87.9% of 58 testicles. Comparison of these two meta-analyses reveals that laparoscopic orchiopexy yielded higher success rates than the same approach performed with an open technique (Table 94-1). In addition, both analyses demonstrated significantly higher rates of atrophy with single-stage Fowler-Stephens versus the two-stage repair. Early experience with needlescopic orchiopexy suggests excellent safety, speed, cosmetic results and testicular outcomes,[42,76] and laparoscopic orchiopexy has been found effective for the management of all testicles, from high canalicular (associated with hernias) to high abdominal.

Without treatment, bilateral cryptorchidism eventually results in infertility. Whether early orchiopexy ultimately improves fertility remains to be seen because antisperm antibodies, abnormalities of the epididymis and vas deferens, and surgical injury to the vas deferens during orchiopexy may also contribute to infertility in patients with a history of cryptorchidism. It is also known that anatomic aberrances are more profound the higher the testicle resides in the abdomen, and there have been reports of carcinoma in situ in postpubertal cryptorchid patients[77] and numerous cases of malignancy in retained intra-abdominal testicles.[78] Although the long-term function of these testicles with respect to

malignant degenerative potential is unknown, leaving the advocacy of performing orchiopexy for the severely dysmorphic abdominal testicle a debated issue, the development of sperm aspiration techniques associated with various applications of assisted fertilization favors orchiopexy

SUMMARY

Laparoscopy for the non-palpable testicle has become the standard approach at many US and European centers. While laparoscopy is invasive and requires general anesthesia, the advantages are felt by most to far outweigh the disadvantages, particularly now that the laparoscopy can be part of management as well as diagnosis. Using laparoscopic versus open techniques, the experienced surgeon can accomplish identical or even improved surgical results with similar operative time and diminished surgical morbidity. It is clear that laparoscopic orchiopexy provides higher retroperitoneal mobilization of the testicular vessels and vas than can be achieved via inguinal open approaches. Given several reports of testicles found laparoscopically after false-negative inguinal explorations, the reports of carcinoma in situ in postpubertal cryptorchid patients, and numerous cases of malignancy in retained intra-abdominal testicles, a consistent definitive diagnosis by laparoscopy is imperative and outweighs the risk of its invasiveness. Although critiques have argued it is technology seeking application,[79] there is strong evidence that this procedure is associated with the highest success rate (ie, scrotal position without testicular atrophy) for the intra-abdominal testicle. If not the procedure of choice, laparoscopic orchiopexy is an acceptable and very successful approach to the non-palpable testicle.

REFERENCES

1. Berkowitz GS, Lapinski RH, Dolgin SE, et al. Prevalence and natural history of cryptorchidism. Pediatrics 1993;92:44–9.
2. Rajfer J. Congenital anomalies of the testicle and scrotum. In: Walsh, et al, eds. Campbell's urology. Philadelphia: WB Saunders Company; 1998. p. 2172–92.
3. Levitt SB, Kogan SJ, Engel RM, et al. The impalpable testicle: a rational approach to management. J Urol 1978;120:515–20.
4. Jordan GH. Children's genitourinary laparoscopic surgery: the pro side [Editorial]. Urology 1994;44:812–14.
5. Cisek LJ, Peters CA, Atala A, et al. Current findings in diagnostic laparoscopic evaluation of the non-palpable testicle. J Urol 1998;160:1145–50.
6. Cendron M, Keating MA, Huff DS, et al. Cryptorchidism, orchiopexy and infertility: a critical long-term retrospective analysis. J Urol 1989;142:559–62.
7. Lee PA, Coughlin MT, Bellinger MF. Paternity and hormone

levels after unilateral cryptorchidism: association with pre-treatment testicular location. J Urol 2000;164:1697–701.
8. Tomboc M, Lee PA, Mitwally MF, et al. Insulin-like 3/relaxin-like factor gene mutations are associated with cryptorchidism. J Clin Endocrinal Metab 2000;85:4013–8.
9. Pike MC, Chilvers C, Peckham MJ. Effect of age at orchidopexy on risk of testicular cancer. Lancet 1986;1:1246–8.
10. Bell AI. Psychologic implications of scrotal sac and testicles for the male child. Clin Pediatr 1974;13:838–47.
11. Polascik TJ, Chan-Tack KM, Jeffs RD, Gearhart JP. Reappraisal of the role of human chorionic gonadotropin in the diagnosis and treatment of the non-palpable testicle: a 10-year experience. J Urol 1996;156:804–6.
12. Cortesi N, Ferrari P, Zambarda E, et al. Diagnosis of bilateral abdominal cryptorchidism by laparoscopy. Endoscopy 1976;8:33–4.
13. Bloom DA. Two-step orchiopexy with pelviscopic clip ligation of the spermatic vessels. J Urol 1991;145:1303–33.
14. Jordan GH, Winslow BH, Robey EL. Laparoendoscopic surgical management of the abdominal/transinguinal undescended testicle. J Endourol 1992;6:157.
15. Bogaert GA, Kogan BA, Mevorach RA. Therapeutic laparoscopy for intra-abdominal testicles. Urology 1993;42:182–8.
16. Duckett JW. Pediatric laparoscopy: prudence, please [Editorial]. J Urol 1994;151:742–3.
17. Molenaar JC, Hazebroek FW. Diagnostic laparoscopy should not be routinely done in non-palpable testicles. Neder Tijdschr Geneesk 1993;137:582.
18. Jordan GH, Winslow BH. Laparoscopic single stage and staged orchiopexy. J Urol 1994;152:1249–52.
19. Huff DS, Hadziselimovic F, Duckett JW, et al. Germ cell counts in semithin sections of biopsies of 115 unilaterally cryptorchid testicles. The experience from the Children's Hospital of Philadelphia. Eur J Pediatr 1987;146 Suppl 2:25–7.
20. Huff DS, Hadziselimovic F, Snyder HM 3rd, et al. Histologic maldevelopment of unilaterally cryptorchid testicles and their descended partners. Eur J Pediatr 1993;152 Suppl 2:11–4.
21. Nagar H, Haddad R. Impact of early orchidopexy on testicular growth. Br J Urol 1997;80:334–5.
22. Lee PA, Coughlin MT. Leydig cell function after cryptorchidism: evidence of the beneficial result of early surgery. J Urol 2002;167:1824–7.
23. Elder JS. Management of the abdominal undescended testicle. Presented at the American Association of Genitourinary Surgeons. Amelia Island FL, April 2004.
24. Rogers E, Teahan S, Gallagher H, et al. The role of orchiectomy in the management of postpubertal cryptorchidism. J Urol 1998;159: 851–4.
25. Oh J, Landman J, Evers A, et al. Management of the postpubertal patient with cryptorchidism: an updated analysis. J Urol 2002;167:1329–33.
26. Koff SA. Does compensatory testicular enlargement predict monorchism? J Urol 1991;146:632–3.
27. Huff DS, Snyder HM 3rd, Hadziselimovic F, et al. An absent testicle is associated with contralateral testicular hypertrophy. J Urol 1992;148:627–8.
28. Moore RG, Peters CA, Bauer SB, et al. Laparoscopic evaluation of the non-palpable testicle: a prospective assessment of accuracy. J Urol 1994;151:728–31.
29. Tennenbaum SY, Lerner SE, McAleer IM, et al. Preoperative laparoscopic localization of the non-palpable testicle: a critical analysis of a 10-year experience. J Urol 1994;151:732–4.
30. Barqawi AZ, Blyth B, Jordan GH, et al. Role of laparoscopy in patients with previous negative exploration for impalpable testicle. Urology 2003;61:1234–7.
31. Hrebinko RL, Bellinger MF. The limited role of imaging techniques in managing children with undescended testicles. J Urol 1993;150:458–60.
32. Wolverson MK, Houttuin E, Heiberg E, et al. Comparison of computed tomography with high-resolution real-time ultrasound in the localization of the impalpable undescended testicle. Radiology 1983;146:133–6.
33. Cain MP, Garra B, Gibbons MD. Scrotal-inguinal ultrasonography: a technique for identifying the non-palpable inguinal testicle without laparoscopy. J Urol 1996;156:791–4.
34. Maghnie M, Vanzulli A, Paesano P, et al. The accuracy of magnetic resonance imaging and ultrasonography compared with surgical findings in the localization of the undescended testicle. Arch Pediatr Adolesc Med 1994;148:699–703.
35. Yeung CK, Tam YH, Chan YL, et al. A new management algorithm for impalpable undescended testicle with gadolinium enhanced magnetic resonance angiography. J Urol 1999;162:998–1002.

36. Castilho LN, Ferreira U. Laparoscopy in adults and children with non-palpable testicles. Andrologia 1987;19:539–43.

37. Froeling FM, Sorber MJ, de la Rosette JJ, de Vries JD. The non-palpable testicle and the changing role of laparoscopy. Urology 1994;43:222–7.

38. Perovic S, Janic N. Laparoscopy in the diagnosis of non-palpable testicles. Br J Urol 1994;73:310–3.

39. Milad MF, Haddad MJ, Zein TA, et al. Laparoscopy for the impalpable testicles. Initial experience of one center. Int Surg 1994;79:163–5.

40. Ferrer FA, Cadeddu JA, Schulam P, et al. Orchiopexy using 2 mm. laparoscopic instruments: 2 techniques for delivering the testicle into the scrotum. J Urol 2000;164:160–1.

41. Schulam PG, Hedican SP, Docimo SG. Radially dilating trocar system for open laparoscopic access. Urology 1999;54:727–9.

42. Gill IS, Ross JH, Sung GT, Kay R. Needlescopic surgery for crytorchidism: the initial series. J Pediatr Surg 2000; 35:1426–30.

43. Ross JH, Gill IS, Kay R. Needlescopic surgery for cryptorchidism. Dialogues Pediatr Urol 1999;22.

44. Rozanski TA, Wojno KJ, Bloom DA. The remnant orchiectomy. J Urol 1996;155:712–4.

45. Merry C, Sweeney B, Puri P. The vanishing testicle: anatomical and histological findings. Eur Urol 1997;31:65–7.

46. Grady RW, Mitchell ME, Carr MC. Laparoscopic and histologic evaluation of the inguinal vanishing testicle. Urology 1998;52:866–9.

47. Elder JS. Laparoscopy for impalpable testicles: significance of the patent processus vaginalis. J Urol 1994;152: 776–8.

48. Baker LA, Docimo SG, Surer I, et al. A multi-institutional analysis of laparoscopic orchidopexy. BJU Int 2001; 87:484–9.

49. Bevan A. The surgical treatment of undescended testicle: a further contribution. JAMA 1903;41:718.

50. Koff SA, Sethi PS. Treatment of high undescended testicles by low spermatic vessel ligation: an alternative to the Fowler-Stephens technique. J Urol 1996;156:799–803.

51. Hortling H, Chapelle A, Johansson CJ, et al. An endocrinologic follow-up study of operated cases of cryptorchism. J Clin Endocrinol Metab 1967;27:120–9.

52. Snyder HM 3rd. Bilateral undescended testicles. Eur J Pediatr 1993;152 Suppl 2:45–6.

53. Jarow JP, Berkovitz GD, Migeon CJ, et al. Elevation of serum gonadotropins establishes the diagnosis of anorchism in prepubertal boys with bilateral cryptorchidism. J Urol 1986;136:277–9.

54. Raivio T, Dunkel L. Inverse relationship between serum inhibin B and FSH levels in prepubertal boys with cryptorchidism. Pediatr Res 1999;46:496–500.

55. Kubini K, Zachmann M, Albers N, et al. Basal inhibin B and the testosterone response to human chorionic gonadotropin correlate in prepubertal boys. J Clin Endocrinol Metab 2000;85:134–8.

56. Silber SJ, Kelly J. Successful autotransplantation of an intra-abdominal testicle to the scrotum by microvascular technique. J Urol 1976;115:452–4.

57. Wacksman J, Dinner M, Handler M. Results of testicular autotransplantation using the microvascular technique: experience with 8 intra-abdominal testicles. J Urol 1982;128:1319–21.

58. Wacksman J, Billmire DA, Lewis AG, Sheldon CA. Laparoscopically assisted testicular autotransplantation for management of the intraabdominal undescended testicle. J Urol 1996;156:772–4.

59. Gans SL, Berci G. Peritoneoscopy in infants and children. J Pediatr Surg 1973;8:399–405.

60. Denes FT, Mendonca BB, Arap S. Laparopscopic management of intersexual states. Urol Clin North Am 2001; 28:31–42.

61. Diamond DA, Caldamone AA. The value of laparoscopy for 106 impalpable testicles relative to clinical presentation. J Urol 1992;148:632–4.

62. Guiney EJ, Corbally M, Malone PS. Laparoscopy and the management of the impalpable testicle. Br J Urol 1989; 63:313–6.

63. Wiener JS, Jordan GH, Gonzales ET Jr. Laparoscopic management of persistent Mullerian duct remnants associated with an abdominal testicle. J Endourol 1997;11:357–9.

64. Moore RG, Kavoussi LR, Bloom DA, et al. Postoperative adhesion formation after urological laparoscopy in the pediatric population. J Urol 1995;153:792–5.

65. Caldamone AA, Amaral JF. Laparoscopic stage 2 Fowler-Stephens orchiopexy. J Urol 1994;152:1253–6.

66. Carr MC. The non-palpable testicle. AUA Update Series 2001;20:226–31.

67. Lindgren BW, Darby EC, Faiella L, et al. Laparoscopic orchiopexy: procedure of choice for the non-palpable testicle? J Urol 1998;159:2132–5.

68. Fahlenkamp D, Winfield HN, Schonberger B, et al. Role of laparoscopic surgery in pediatric urology. Eur Urol 1997;32:75–84.

69. Poppas DP, Lemack GE, Mininberg DT. Laparoscopic orchiopexy: clinical experience and description of technique. J Urol 1996;155:708–11.

70. Lakhoo K, Thomas DF, Najmaldin AS. Is inguinal exploration for the impalpable testicle an outdated operation? Br J Urol 1996;77:452–4.

71. Boddy SA, Corkery JJ, Gornall P. The place of laparoscopy in the management of the impalpable testicle. Br J Surg 1985;72:918–9.

72. Koyle MA, et al. The role of laparoscopy in the patient with previous negative inguinal exploration for impalpable testicle [Abstract]. J Urol 1994;151:236.

73. Koyle MA, Rajfer J, Ehrlich RM. The undescended testicle. Pediatr Ann 1988;17:39–46.

74. Docimo SG. The results of surgical therapy for cryptorchidism: a literature review and analysis. J Urol 1995; 154:1148–52.

75. Gibbons MD, Cromie WJ, Duckett JW Jr. Management of the abdominal undescended testicle. J Urol 1979;122:76–9.

76. Gill IS. Needlescopic urology: current status. Urol Clin North Am 2001;28:71–83.

77. Sexton WJ, Assimos DG. Diagnostic and therapeutic laparoscopy for the adult cryptorchid testicle. Tech Urol 1999;5:24–8.

78. Ford TF, Parkinson MC, Pryor JP. The undescended testicle in adult life. Br J Urol 1985;57:181–4.

79. Ferro F, Lais A, Bagolan P et al. Impact of primary surgical approach in the management of the impalpable testicle. Eur Urol 1992;22:142–6.

95

Laparoscopic Renal Surgery

Alaa El-Ghoneimi, MD, PhD

Laparoscopic procedures in pediatric urology are gaining popularity with an increasing number of centers performing advanced surgery. In the early experience, the indications for laparoscopy in pediatric urology were unclear and unproven compared with the advantages of open procedures. Gradually, indications are expanding from diagnostic to ablative surgery and more recently to reconstructive procedures. Currently, nephrectomy and partial nephrectomy are accepted laparoscopic procedures in children and are included in the routine practice of many pediatric centers.[1]

INDICATIONS FOR PEDIATRIC RENAL SURGERY

Upper urinary tract surgery in children includes two main categories: ablative and reconstructive. The most frequent ablative surgeries are the total and the partial nephrectomy. Other rare indications are stone removal, renal cyst, and caliceal diverticulum. In this chapter we will deal with the main two indications: total and partial nephrectomy.

Extracorporal shock wave lithotripsy or percutaneous and endoscopic techniques can be used to manage most pediatric kidney stones. Open surgery may be required in rare cases when these techniques are not applicable, such as in young children with bulky cystine lithiasis. For these exceptions, laparoscopic pyelolithotomy is a suitable alternative to open surgery, and may avoid parietal scarring in these children, who usually need repeat surgery later in life. The procedure can be achieved either through transperitoneal or extraperitoneal access.[2–4]

LAPAROSCOPIC NEPHRECTOMY   The first laparoscopic nephrectomy in adults was reported in 1991 by Clayman and colleagues.[5] One year later, Ehrlich and colleagues reported their first series of pediatric cases.[6] Since then many authors have reported successful results of nephrectomy and nephroureterectomy in pediatrics, all advocating the transperitoneal approach.[7,8] Roberts suggested the extraperitoneal approach to the kidney in 1976, reporting his experience with extraperitoneal endoscopy with gas insufflation in animals.[9] Retroperitoneal operative laparoscopy was described by Gaur in 1992,[10] and then by others in both adult and pediatric urology.[11–13] Despite the expanding application of retroperitoneal laparoscopic renal surgery in adults,[14,15] this technique was adapted later by pediatric urologists and is progressively expanding in the different centers.[3,13,16–18]

Currently, malignant renal tumors in children are not considered suitable for laparoscopic exposure. The most common renal tumor in children is nephroblastoma. These tumors are of large size, frequently extending outside the kidney, and with high risk of rupture during dissection.

Most nephrectomies in children are done for nonfunctioning kidneys secondary to obstructive uropathy, reflux, or ectopic implantation of the ureter. The laparoscopic approach is excellent for most of these cases.[3,19] Although, laparoscopic nephrectomy for multicystic dysplastic kidney (MCDK) is an easy and safe procedure, the indication for nephrectomy is still debatable. The acceptable indications for these are the increase in size of cysts or complications by hypertension or infection, all of which are rare.

Nephrectomy may be indicated in children with end-stage renal disease before transplantation, when the primary renal disease is associated with hypertension, severe nephrotic syndrome, or severe hemolytic uremic syndrome. During open surgery in these children, a large incision is necessary to control the renal pedicle and to extract a large kidney, and therefore, the laparoscopic approach is particularly advantageous for this population.[20] In a few cases of severe congenital nephrotic syndrome, simultaneous bilateral nephrectomy is indicated early in life. In our experience with 13 simultaneous bilateral nephrectomies through a lateral retroperitoneal approach, 7 were under 1 year of age.[21] To avoid positioning the patient twice for bilateral nephrectomy, the procedure can also be performed through a posterior retroperitoneal approach with the child positioned prone.[22] In this specific group of pretransplant nephrectomy, it is recommended to use a bag to retrieve the kidney to reduce postoperative retroperineal adhesions. These adhesions were noted during renal transplantation in children who underwent kidney fragmentation during extraction without a bag.[21] Recently, Zuniga and colleagues reported the first case of transperitoneal bilateral nephrectomy in a young child aged 6 months, this option has the advantage of limiting the number of trocars, and also being able to deal with large-size kidneys in small children.[23]

Nephrectomy for xanthogranulomatous pyelonephritis is a challenging procedure because of the perirenal adhesions to the great vessels and to the surrounding viscera. Halachmi and colleagues suggested the subcapsular dissection of the upper part of the kidney to avoid lesions to the duodenum and the adrenals on the right side.[24]

LAPAROSCOPIC PARTIAL NEPHRECTOMY   Partial nephrectomy is usually done in children to remove a nonfunctioning upper or lower pole secondary to complicated duplex anomalies of the kidney. The usual pathology of the upper pole is obstruction associated with a ureterocele or incontinence secondary to an ectopic ureter. The usual pathology in the lower pole is reflux. Laparoscopic partial nephrectomy is technically more demanding than total nephrectomy. Jordan and Winslow described the first case of upper pole partial nephrectomy in a child by transperitoneal laparoscopy.[25] Janetschek and colleatgues reported their series of 14 cases of successful partial nephrectomies in children.[26] Currently, this procedure is performed using a retroperitoneal[27] or transperitoneal approach.[28] Laparoscopic techniques are well suited to this procedure, with the benefits of perfect global exposure to the anatomy of the full kidney and its vascularization without the need to mobilize the remaining part of the kidney. Our preference goes to the retroperitoneal approach, as it provides a posterior access to the kidney, avoiding the dissection of the renal pedicle of the conserved moiety, which is obligatory during the transperitoneal anterior approach. The retroperitoneal access can be achieved either posteriorly in a prone position or in a lateral decubitus position. Borzi has compared the two approaches and found that the lateral approach creates more inferomedial space, and gives better access to ectopic kidneys and allows for a complete ureterectomy in all cases.[29]

PATIENT PREPARATION

Patient preparation for laparoscopic renal surgery is not different from conventional surgery preparation. We do not prescribe any specific diet measures before surgery. We follow the usual recommendations for general anesthesia preparations. The child is on a strict diet for a period between 4 and 8 hours, depending on age, and premedicated before going to the operating theater. Some surgeons recommend a liquid diet and enema on the night preceding surgery.[30]

An indwelling bladder catheter is recommended in cases of high-grade reflux or in cases for which ureterectomy is indicated to facilitate the dissection of the ureter as close as possible to its junction with the bladder. Usually a catheter is recommended in the transperitoneal approach to avoid bladder injury during trocar insertion. A perioperative catheter is also needed when urine output monitoring is mandatory for the anesthesia management in certain associated cardiac or renal diseases.

A nasogastric tube is placed after induction of general endotracheal anesthesia. Noninvasive hemodynamic and ventilatory monitoring is needed during the laparoscopic nephrectomy in either a trans- or retroperitoneal approach.

We administer a cephalosporin intravenously in the operating room in all cases of partial nephrectomy, and some cases of total nephrectomy with a past history of infected kidney. No ureteral catheters are inserted. All patients are screened for blood type. Serum electrolytes, creatinine, and coagulation studies are performed, and all patients should have preoperative sterile urine cultures.

INFORMED CONSENT

The surgery is thoroughly explained to the child, adapted to age, and his parents. The possibility of conversion to open surgery has to be mentioned in the consent along with a discussion of options and potential complications.

INSTRUMENTATION

Standard laparoscopic instruments are suitable for total or partial nephrectomy without the requirement for special instruments or equipment. We recommend the following set as a routine for any laparoscopic renal surgery:

Conventional surgical instruments for access:

1. Sterile marker to identify the major landmarks and optimal trocar placement
2. Stab scalpel, No. 11, to achieve stab incision adapted for trocar insertion
3. Blunt dissection scissors, helpful for muscle dissociation
4. Needle driver
5. Nontoothed forceps
6. Nonresorbable monofilament suture for the purse-string suture
7. Two artery forceps
8. Pair of retractors, narrow and long blades
9. Sutures necessary for wound closure
10. Drains, at surgeon's preference, with or without suction
11. A complete conventional open-surgery set, to be available in the operating room in case of conversion to open surgery

Laparoscopic instruments for renal surgery:

The choice of single use or reusable instruments is a matter of surgeon's preference and the economic constraints of the institution. Currently most of the instruments are available in the two categories. The laparoscopic instruments are the same for general pediatric surgery, and the common pool of instruments can be of great help, especially in the initial phase during the learning curve. We mostly use reusable instruments, and for the few unavailable instruments, we use single-use instruments. A full set of single-use instruments is a necessary backup for reusable instruments.

1. Laparoscope: 5 mm, 0°, is the standard laparoscope for pediatric nephrectomy

2. Trocars: 3 trocars of 5 mm, 1 of them should be blunt for the placement of first trocar. Self-retaining trocars are useful especially in young children to avoid the slipping of the trocars outside the abdominal wall
3. Atraumatic grasping forceps
4. Curved dissecting forceps for vascular dissection
5. Scissors
6. Monopolar diathermy (should be used sparingly in retroperitoneal surgery)
7. Bipolar diathermy or Harmonic scalpel (especially for partial nephrectomy, difficult nephrectomy)
8. Needle driver
9. Toothed grasping forceps for organ retrieval
10. Resorbable ligature for endocorporeal vascular or ureteral ligation when needed. A ready-made laparoscopic loop suture can be used for ureteral ligature
11. Resorbale suture, with round 3/8-curved needle, for transfixing ligature when needed for repair of vascular tear
12. Vascular clips, reusable or single-use
13. Laparoscopic bag for organ retrieval, the currently available bags are at least 10 mm diameter and if the kidney is of large size, the first trocar and the laparoscope should be of 10 mm from the beginning to avoid trocar replacement at organ retrieval
14. Irrigation-suction device

STEP-BY-STEP DESCRIPTION OF OPERATIVE PROCEDURE

RENAL ACCESS   The kidney can be approached and exposed by either extraperitoneal or transperitoneal approach.

Retroperitoneal Access   *Lateral Approach*
The patient is placed in the lateral oblique position, with sufficient flexion of the operating table to allow exposure adequate for trocar placement between the last rib and the iliac crest (Figure 95-1). In infants and young children (under 6 years), our preference is to put a lumbar padding to laterally flex the patient without flexing the operating table. Retroperitoneal access is achieved through the first incision, 10 to 15 mm in length, and one finger width from the lower border of the tip of the twelfth rib (Figure 95-2A). The use of narrow retractors with long blades allows a deep dissection with a short incision. The Gerota's fascia is approached by a muscle-splitting blunt dissection, then it is opened under direct vision and the first blunt trocar (5 or 10 mm) is introduced directly inside the opened Gerota's fascia (Figure 95-2B). A working space is created by gas insufflation dissection, and the first trocar is fixed with a purse-string suture that is applied around the deep fascia to ensure an airtight seal and to allow traction on the main trocar if needed to increase the working space. We prefer this type of fixation to single-use self-retaining trocars, as we find that these trocars interfere with the mobility of instruments because of their size and design. The second trocar (5 mm) is inserted posteriorly in the cos-

tovertebral angle, anterior to the lumbosacral muscle. The third trocar (5 mm) is inserted, in the anterior axillary line, a finger width from the top of the iliac crest. To avoid transperitoneal insertion of this trocar, the working space is fully developed and the deep surface of the anterior abdominal wall musculature is identified before the trocar insertion. Insufflation pressure does not exceed 12 mm, and the CO_2 flow rate is progressively increased from 1 liter to 3 liters/min. Access to the retroperitoneum and creation of the working space are the keys to success in retroperitoneal renal surgery. Age is not a limiting factor for this approach. Young children have less fat and the access is easier; our youngest child was 3 weeks old.

Prone Posterior Approach   The access begins with an incision in the costovertebral angle at the lateral edge of the paraspinous muscles. The secondary trocars are placed just above the iliac crest, one medially at the edge of the paraspinous muscles, and one laterally at the posterior clavicular line.[30] Borzi compared the lateral with the posterior retroperitoneal approach in children in a randomized prospective study on 36 complete and 19 partial nephrectomies.[29] There was no significant difference in the operative time. We prefer the lateral approach as it permits a wide diversity of renal surgery, at any age, with good exposure to the distal ureter.

Another Technique to Access the Retroperitoneal Space   Since the description by Gaur,[10] balloon dissection of the retroperitoneal tissues has been the method applied by most urologists. The disadvantages of the balloon are the cost of the disposable material and the possible complications with rupture of the balloon.[31] On the other hand, balloon dissection does allow the creation of a working space without opening Gerota's fascia, which is important for radical nephrectomy.

Capolicchio and colleagues described a modification of lateral access.[32] They recommended insertion of the first trocar through the costovertebral angle. This modification helped the authors to avoid accidental peritoneal tear during the access through the first lateral incision, and also allowed a smaller incision for the laparoscope.

Micali and colleagues reported the use of the Visiport visual trocar to access the retroperitoneal space directly.[4] The advantage of this method is the possibility to use a small incision for the first trocar, which may be advantageous in reconstructive surgery, but not in ablative surgery, as the first incision is needed for organ retrieval.

Transperitoneal Access   Several options exist regarding patient positioning. The most frequently described is the flank position.[30] The pneumoperitoneum is created through an open umbilical approach. The child is positioned with the surgeon standing in front of the abdomen (opposite side of nephrectomy). The most frequent configuration has been with the umbilical port and two ipsilateral ports in the midclavicular line above and below the umbilicus (Figure 95-3). A fourth trocar may be placed in the midaxillary line if needed for exposure to retract the liver or spleen. The kidney is exposed by medial mobilization of

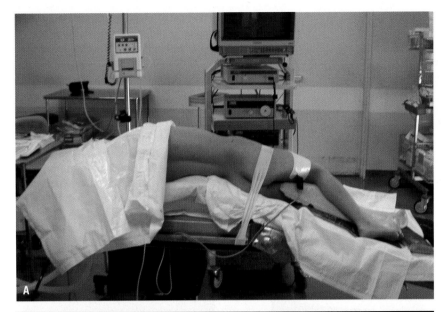

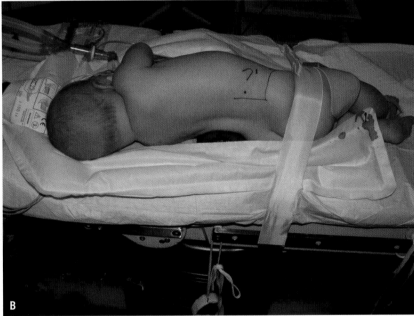

Figure 95-1 Patient positioning for right retroperitoneal laparoscopic renal surgery. The patient is placed lateral, with sufficient flexion of the operating table so as to expose the area of trocar placement (A), between the last rib and the ileac crest, for younger children as shown, a lumbar support is sufficient for the exposure (B). The child is secured by two adhesive bands, one on the greater trocanter level and a second on the chest to keep the child on a perpendicular angle with the table. The surgeon, assistant, and scrub nurse are all on the back side of the child. The front side of the child is left free for the monitor, which is placed cranial while doing the kidney dissection and caudal to proceed with the distal ureterectomy.

length of the clip, the vein is first ligated by resorbable intracorporeal knot. The diameter is thus reduced and the ligature is secured by juxtaposed clips. The use of staples, as described in adult nephrectomy, requires a 12 mm port and is not needed in pediatric patients. The ureter is then identified and dissected as far distally as necessary. In the absence of reflux, the ureter is coagulated and sectioned at the level of the lumbar ureter (especially in pretransplant nephrectomy, the native ureter might be used for the transplantation). In the presence of reflux, the dissection is followed distally, the vas deferens is identified in males, and the ureter is ligated as close as possible to the ureterovesical junction. During this distal dissection, the surgeon moves toward the head of the child, and the screen goes toward the feet of the child. In the beginning of our experience, we were using a fourth trocar to dissect and ligate the distal ureter.[3] Currently, we use an endoloop or, if the ureter is large, a transparietal suture to fix the ureter to the abdominal wall to facilitate its distal

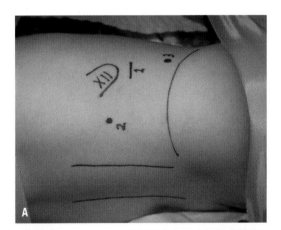

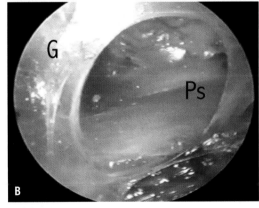

Figure 95-2 Trocar placement and retroperitoneal access for renal surgery. *A,* Area of trocar placement, between the last rib and the iliac crest. Retroperitoneal access is achieved through the first incision (1), 10–15 mm in length, and one finger width from the lower border of the tip of the twelfth rib. Second trocar (2) is inserted posteriorly in the costovertebral angle. Third trocar (3) is inserted, in the anterior axillary line, one finger width from the top of the ileac crest. *B,* The Gerota's fascia (G) is approached by a muscle-splitting blunt dissection, then it is opened under direct vision and the first blunt trocar is introduced directly inside the opened Gerota's fascia to start insufflation. Psoas muscle (Ps) is the landmark after opening the Gerota's facia; it must remain on the bottom of the screen during surgery.

the colon. In case of bilateral nephrectomy, accessory 5 mm trocars are placed halfway between the xiphoid process and the umbilicus, and just above the dome of the bladder in the midline.[23]

NEPHRECTOMY BY LATERAL RETROPERITONEAL APPROACH The landmarks of the retroperitoneal space are first identified. The psoas muscle is the posterior landmark and should remain in the bottom of the screen. The kidney remains attached anteriorly to the peritoneum, and should remain upward on the screen. The renal pedicle is identified and approached posteriorly (Figure 95-4), and dissected close to the junction with the aorta and vena cava, to avoid multiple ligations of

branches of the renal vessels. On the left side the vein is ligated distal to the genital and adrenal branches. On the right side the vein is short and a careful dissection at its junction with the vena cava is necessary to avoid mistaking the vena cava for the renal vein. After dissecting the renal artery and then the vein, the vessels are clipped, ligated, or coagulated. The choice of method depends on the vessel diameter and the surgeon's experience. In general, small arteries of MCDK can be coagulated by bipolar cautery or harmonic scalpel, while the most common method is to double ligate the artery proximally by two clips and distally by one. The vein is generally clipped in the same way; if the diameter is bigger than the

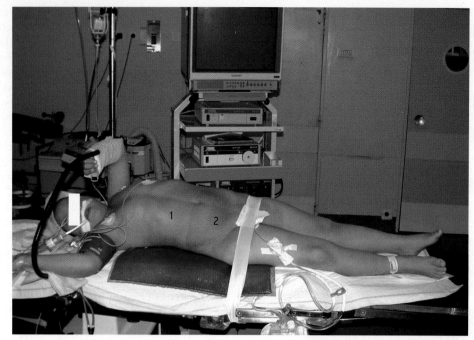

Figure 95-3 Patient positioning and trocar placement for left transperitoneal laparoscopic renal surgery. The child is positioned with the surgeon standing in front of the abdomen (opposite side of nephrectomy). The most frequent configuration has been with the umbilical port and two ipsilateral ports (1 and 2) in the midclavicular line above and below the umbilicus. A fourth trocar can be placed in the midaxillary line if needed for exposure to retract the liver or spleen.

dissection and ligation. A fourth trocar is still used if the dissection is not sufficiently close to the bladder, and it is inserted at the edge of the lumbosacral muscle close to the iliac crest. As the peritoneum is very close to the ureter in this distal part, its dissection is left to the end of the procedure to avoid any peritoneal tear.

The last part of dissection is the anterior surface of the kidney. The kidney is dissected from the peritoneum very close to its capsule in the cleavage plane of areolar tissue. Usually no hemostasis is necessary in this plane, whereas, in inflammatory adherent kidneys, a sharp dissection with bipolar coagulation may be necessary. In the rare cases of xanthogranulamatous pyelonephritis, we do the dissection of the adherent kidney through the subcapsular plane to avoid injury of intraperitoneal structures.[24]

Kidney Retrieval The kidney is usually retrieved by the main incision. A 5 mm telescope is inserted through the accessory port, and a toothed grasping forceps is introduced through the first port to extract the kidney. The kidney is grasped at one of the poles, and pulled in this axis, to pull on the smallest diameter of the kidney. In most cases, the kidney can be divided under vision during extraction through the muscle wall. In cases of severe pyelocaliceal dilatation or MCDK, direct evacuation by puncture helps in organ retrieval. An extraction bag is used for infected or large kidneys, and the kidney is morcellated inside the bag (Figure 95-5). Our current preference is for using the bag routinely for extraction to avoid extending the incision and spilling the parenchyma in the retroperitoneum, which might produce more postoperative inflammation. This is particularly important in the pre-

transplant group where we have to minimize all the factors that might increase the postoperative retroperitoneal adhesions. In our experience, these adhesions can render the vascular dissection during transplantation more difficult. If nephectomy is done at the time of another lower urinary tract procedure, nephrectomy is done first and the kidney is placed near the bladder without transecting the ureter. Retrieval is done through the Pfannenstiel incision.

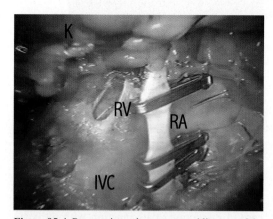

Figure 95-4 Retroperitoneal exposure and ligature of the renal pedicle. The landmarks of the retroperitoneal space are first identified in order to be oriented with the retroperitoneal exposure. The psoas muscle (Ps) is the posterior landmark and should remain in the bottom of the screen. The kidney (K) remains attached anteriorly to the peritoneum, and should remain upward on the screen. The renal pedicle is identified and approached posteriorly. In this picture, the artery is already ligated by clips and dissected close to the junction with the aorta and vena cava. On the right side, the renal vein (RV) is short and a careful dissection at its junction with the vena cava (IVC) will allow a safe exposure of its full length.

PARTIAL NEPHRECTOMY *Retroperitoneal Upper-Pole Nephroureterectomy* The upper-pole ureter is identified at the lower pole of the kidney and dissected very close to its wall to avoid injury to the vascular supply of the lower-pole ureter. We find it helpful to ligate the proximal ureter before cutting it, so the proximal ureter remains dilated, facilitating the dissection of the upper pole (Figure 95-6). Because the exposure is posterior, contrary to the transperitoneal anterior approach, the upper-pole ureter is lifted off the vessels by blunt dissection superiorly. The upper-pole ureter is used as a handle to facilitate this part of dissection. The plane between the dilated upper-pole pelvis and the lower-pole parenchyma is easily identifiable by blunt dissection until the

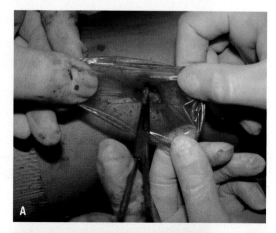

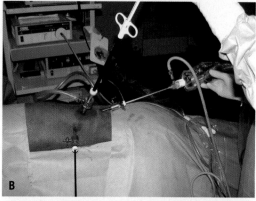

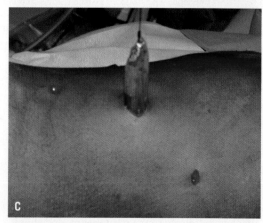

Figure 95-5 The endobag is introduced through the first trocar, and the kidney is placed inside the bag (A). Morcellation of the kidney by an artery forceps under direct vision allows kidney retrieval without the need to extend the incision (B, C).

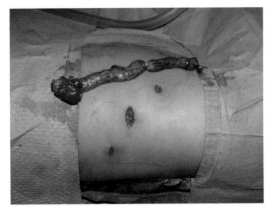

Figure 95-6 Right retroperitoneal upper-pole nephrectomy. The upper pole is retrieved easily through the main incision. Note that the ureter was ligated at the beginning of dissection to keep the upper-pole system dilated and make the dissection easier.

edges of the thin parenchyma of the upper moiety are recognized. At this step, the upper-pole vessels are identified, running from the aorta or the renal vessels to the upper-pole parenchyma. They are either clipped or coagulated, depending on

their size. The upper pole is identified by color changes after vessel ligation and by the difference in appearance between the normal lower pole and the dilated dysplastic upper pole. The duplex system anomalies have a well-defined vascular line of demarcation between the upper and lower poles of the kidney. However, sometimes it is difficult to individualize upper-pole vessels, and the parenchymal transection is started before vascular control of the upper pole. Transection can be done by electrocautery, but we prefer the Harmonic scalpel with the curved jaws, as it provides a clean cut at the junction between the upper and lower poles.

To minimize mobilization of the lower pole, and consequently the risk of indirect vascular trauma of the renal pedicle, the lower pole remains attached to the peritoneum during all the steps of the procedure. The upper pole is completely freed from peritoneal attachment before transecting the parenchyma to avoid transperitoneal bowel injury.

If upper-pole partial nephrectomy is done using a transperitoneal approach, the proximal ureter must be passed behind the renal hilum and delivered under the vessels from above after

mobilization of the upper-pole ureter. This step is technically the most difficult part of the procedure and requires dissection of the lower-pole vessels.[28] Identification of the upper-pole vessels and parenchymal transection are identical to the retroperitoneal approach.

Retroperitoneal Lower-Pole Nephroureterectomy Access is the same as for the upper pole. The lower-pole ureter is identified and followed to the lower-pole pelvis to be sure of its identity. Contrary to the upper-pole nephrectomy, full dissection of the lower-pole vessels is necessary before transecting the parenchyma (Figure 95-7). As the main pathology is reflux with repeated infections, the lower pole is usually retracted and easily identified from the healthy upper-pole parenchyma. Meanwhile, the transection is usually very close to the upper-pole vessels and makes it difficult to identify this line of demarcation. Currently, we routinely do cystoscopy and we insert a ureteral catheter in the upper-pole ureter. This catheter is connected to a syringe of methylene blue. At the time of transection, the circulating nurse injects the methylene blue, and any doubt about the line of demarcation

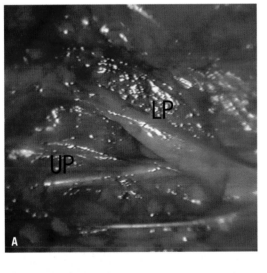
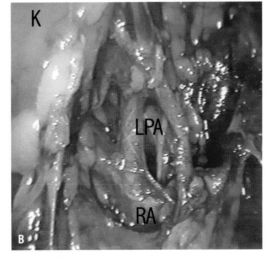
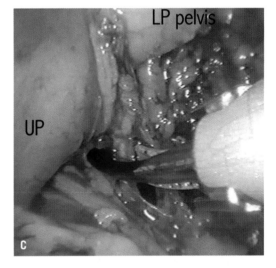
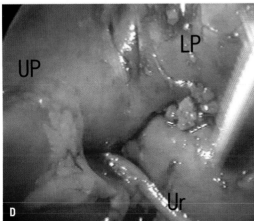
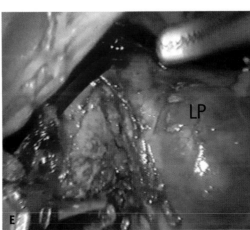
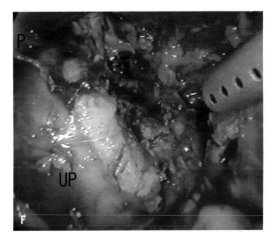

Figure 95-7 Right retroperitoneal lower-pole nephrectomy. *A*, The upper-pole (UP) and lower-pole (LP) ureters are identified easily and the lower-pole ureter is dissected and isolated. *B*, Renal artery (RA) is dissected and branches to the lower pole (LPA) and the upper pole are identified. Note that the kidney (K) is kept in the top of the screen and remains attached to the peritoneum. *C*, Artery to the lower pole is sectioned by Harmonic scalpel. Lower-pole pelvis and upper-pole parenchyma (UP) are exposed. *D*, The vascular limit is well demonstrated between the upper pole (UP) and the lower pole (LP), after section of the lower-pole renal pedicle. Note that the ureter to the upper pole (Ur) is identified before any structure section. *E*, The parenchyma between the upper and the lower pole (LP) is sectioned by Harmonic scalpel. *F*, The cut section is irrigated to rule out any bleeding, and at this moment, methylene blue is injected in the ureteral catheter to rule out any injury to the upper-pole calice. Note that the upper pole (UP) remains attached to the peritoneum (P).

or upper-pole caliceal tear can be ruled out immediately. The ureter should be ligated close to the bladder to avoid postoperative reflux into a long ureteral stump using the same technique as for simple nephrectomy with refluxing ureter.

POSTOPERATIVE CARE

Postoperative care is identical after transperitoneal or retroperitoneal laparoscopy. The nasogastric tube is removed at the end of surgery. Analgesics are given according to the child's comfort and adapted pain scores. In a few cases, especially after a difficult procedure or perioperative bleeding, postoperative ileus may develop, requiring prolonged nasogastric suction until bowel motility returns. In the case of postoperative abdominal distension, or discomfort, repeated abdominal examination is mandatory and completed by imaging if needed to exclude intraperitoneal organ injury. Even in the retroperitoneal approach, the surgeon should keep in mind the possibility of such complications, especially if monopolar diathermy was used.

RESULTS

NEPHRECTOMY In the exclusively pediatric laparoscopic nephrectomy series, results are consistent with the feasibility of the procedure and a very low rate of conversion to open surgery, ranging from 0 to 3%.[3,18,33–35]

The operative time is variable in the different series according to the approach, indications, and the experience of the surgeon. In the retroperitoneal series, the mean operative time for nephrectomy or nephroureterectomy ranges from 47 to 110 minutes,[3,18,29] with longer times observed in the pretransplant group of children with a mean operative time of 2 hours.[20] In the transperitoneal pediatric nephrectomy series, the mean operative time is relatively longer, around 160 minutes.[34,35] As each group of surgeons does one of the two approaches, it is difficult to take into consideration this difference of operative time as a comparison between the two approaches. Guilloneau and colleagues reported in a retrospective study of adults and children that retroperitoneal and transperitoneal approaches were equivalent in morbidity and postoperative stay, but operating time was shorter with the retroperitoneal approach.[12]

The hospital stay after laparoscopic nephrectomy depends on the indication for the surgery. Most children operated for urologic indications are discharged in less than 24 hours after surgery.[3,18,35] Meanwhile, with nephrectomy in the pretransplant population, the hospital stay is longer with a mean of 4 days.[20]

The effects of retroperitoneal CO_2 insufflation during renal surgery have been studied in children.[20,36] These studies demonstrated a significant increase in systolic blood pressure and end-tidal carbon dioxide, while there was no modification of the other hemodynamic or ventilatory parameters. These changes do not need any special modification of the ventilatory parameters, whereas special care with hypertensive patients is required.

LAPAROSCOPIC VERSUS OPEN NEPHRECTOMY The evaluation of pain and discomfort is difficult and should not be undertaken in a nonrandomized series. To our knowledge, such a study on laparoscopic nephrectomy has not yet been published. The general impression is that consumption of analgesics, especially morphine painkillers, is less in the laparoscopic group. The shorter postoperative hospital stay may suggest that children are more comfortable and discharged earlier; here again, prudence is required in the analysis of retrospective nonrandomized series.[20]

We have retrospectively studied a comparable group of children who underwent pretransplant nephrectomy in our department before beginning our experience with retroperitoneal laparoscopic nephrectomy.[20] In this specific group of patients with end-stage renal disease, the hospital stay was significantly shorter after laparoscopic versus open nephrectomy (5.2 vs 8.4 days). Even when the operating time for laparoscopic versus open nephrectomy was longer (120 vs 104 minutes), the difference was not statistically significant. Hamilton and colleagues found comparable results with transperitoneal laparoscopic nephrectomy with significant decrease in hospital stay after laparoscopic compared with open nephrectomy (22.5 vs 41.3 hours).[33] Operative time was significantly longer in the laparoscopic group (175.6 vs 120.2 minutes). Other studies on mixed groups of adults and children had comparable results, with significant briefer postoperative course in the laparoscopic group.[37]

Even though there is no comparative study on the cosmetic results, it is obvious that the cosmetic results are excellent after laparoscopic nephrectomy, especially if the 3 or 5 mm trocars are used and the kidney retrieval is done through a laparoscopic bag when needed, without extension of the incision.

Although there are more publications dealing with the outcomes and not only the feasibility, efforts are still needed to validate the benefits of laparoscopic procedures over open surgery.[1]

PARTIAL NEPHRECTOMY We have shown, in a retrospective comparative study, that retroperitoneal laparoscopic partial nephrectomy can be performed in a comparable operative time with that of an open procedure.[27] The mean operative time was 146 minutes (50–180) and 152 minutes (75–240) for the open surgery and the laparoscopy groups, respectively. The main advantage to the laparoscopic approach is that it shortens significantly the hospital stay compared with that of an open procedure. The mean hospital stay was 1.4 days (1–3) and 3.9 days (3–5) for the laparoscopy and the open surgery groups, respectively ($p < .0001$). Eight of 13 children were discharged on the day following that of the laparoscopic procedure. The hospital stay was significantly shorter in the laparoscopic group compared with the open surgery group.[27]

Robinson and colleagues compared, in a prospective nonrandomized study, costs and outcome of laparoscopic partial nephrectomy with open surgery in children.[38] Mean operative time in the laparoscopic and open groups was 200.4 and 113.5 minutes, mean hospital stay was 25.5 and 32.6 hours, respectively ($p < .0005$). Patients in the laparoscopic group required fewer doses of analgesics than those who underwent open surgery. The main disadvantage that was reported in this series is the long operative time. The operative time in this series was relatively longer than the other pediatric series and probably it will be shortened with experience.[27,29]

COMPLICATIONS

Complications of abdominal laparoscopy for urologic procedures, such as bowel and great-vessel injury, have been documented in both the adult and pediatric populations.[39–41] In a multicentric survey of 5,400 pediatric urologic laparoscopy procedures, Peters showed that the clearest predictor of complication rate was laparoscopic experience.[39] Soulie and colleagues have reported a decrease of complication rate from 9% for the first 100 to 4% for the subsequent 250 procedures.[41] Most intraoperative complications (2.6%) were vascular and visceral injuries, while postoperative complications (2.8%) were predominantly thromboembolism and wound infection at trocar sites. Complications of retroperitoneal renal surgery are rare and consist mainly of vascular or colonic injury. Kumar and colleagues reported a major complication rate of 3.5% of 316 patients (aged 4–88 years) who underwent retroperitoneoscopic urologic surgery.[42] Vascular injuries occurred in 7, 5 of which required immediate conversion to open surgery. Four patients (1.2%) had other major complications, including colonic injury, retroperitoneal collections, and incisional hernia. The strict respect of safety rules in pediatric patients, which are the routine use of open laparoscopy and the limitation of monopolar cautery can avoid most of these complications.[43]

In our experience with 105 retroperitoneal nephrectomies, we had 1 vascular tear, during a teaching session, at the origin of a lumbar vein, in a case of xanthogranulomatous pyelonephritis.[24] A clip without the need to convert to open surgery successfully closed the tear. In retroperitoneal procedures, traction on the kidney toward the top of the screen stretches the renal vessels, reducing bleeding while evaluating the feasibility of the hemostasis by laparoscopic measures. The only postoperative complication we had was a postoperative hematoma after pretransplant bilateral nephrectomy; this hematoma was drained percutaneously. In pretransplant kidney, we recommend leaving an indwelling drainage tube for 24 hours.

The most common complication of the retroperitoneal approach is the pneumoperitoneum secondary to peritoneal tear.[3,42] This occurred in nearly 30 % of our cases early in the experience, then could be avoided by careful preparation of the retroperitoneal space for insertion of the anterior working ports. When this occurs in the beginning of the procedure, the retroperitoneal working space is reduced by the effect of the pneumoperitoneum. This can be managed either by laparoscopic suturing of the tear or, if not possible, by inserting a Veress needle in the peritoneal cavity to evacuate the gas during the procedure. If the tear occurs after the ligature of the renal vessels, during dissection of the anterior surface of the kidney or the ureter, the procedure can usually be accomplished without special management of the pneumoperitoneum.

A specific complication of partial nephrectomy is the vascular lesion of the pedicle of the remaining part of the kidney. We have already reported this accident during our first experience with retroperitoneal partial nephrectomy.[3]

We strongly recommend mentored laparoscopic teaching as a safe way to introduce advanced urologic laparoscopic procedures in a pediatric urology department.[44] Moreover, it may improve the results of the initial experience with laparoscopy and encourage its development among a larger number of pediatric urologists.

CONCLUSION

Minimally invasive procedures emphasize our goals of improving patient comfort and safety, while adapting the laparoscopic procedures as closely as possible to conventional surgical techniques with respect to the operative time, cost, and surgical principles. Currently, laparoscopic nephrectomy and partial nephrectomy are procedures that achieve these goals. Indications for laparoscopy in pediatric urology are expanding with more centers being involved in the evolution of the different procedures. To avoid a discouraging learning curve, we recommend pediatric urologists acquire their experience in a progressive pattern. Nephrectomy for MCDK or hydronephrosis is a relatively safe and easy procedure, getting the surgeon accustomed to laparoscopic exposure of the upper tract. When the surgeon is familiar with the exposure he can proceed to more difficult nephrectomies, pretransplant, and partial nephrectomy.

REFERENCES

1. El-Ghoneimi A. Paediatric laparoscopic surgery. Curr Opin Urol 2003;13:329–35.
2. Jordan GH, McCammon KA, Robey EL. Laparoscopic pyelolithotomy. Urology 1997;49:131–4.
3. El-Ghoneimi A, Valla JS, Steyaert H, Aigrain Y. Laparoscopic renal surgery via a retroperitoneal approach in children. J Urol 1998;160(3 Pt 2):1138–41.
4. Micali S, Caione P, Virgili G, et al. Retroperitoneal laparoscopic access in children using a direct vision technique. J Urol 2001;165:229–32.
5. Clayman RV, Kavoussi LR, Soper NJ, et al. Laparoscopic nephrectomy: initial case report. J Urol 1991;146:278–82.
6. Ehrlich RM, Gershman A, Mee S, Fuchs G. Laparoscopic nephrectomy in a child: expanding horizons for laparoscopy in pediatric urology. J Endourol 1992;6:463–5.
7. Das S, Keizur JJ, Tashima M. Laparoscopic nephroureterectomy for end-stage reflux nephropathy in a child. Surg Laparosc Endosc 1993;3:462–5.
8. Ehrlich RM, Gershman A, Fuchs G. Laparoscopic renal surgery in children. J Urol 1994;151:735–9.
9. Roberts J. Retroperitoneal endoscopy. J Med Primatol 1976;5:124–7.
10. Gaur D. Laparoscopic operative retroperitoneoscopy: use of a new devise. J Urol 1992;148:1137–9.
11. Doublet JD, Barreto HS, Degremont AC, et al. Retroperitoneal nephrectomy: comparison of laparoscopy with open surgery. World J Surg 1996;20:713–6.
12. Guilloneau B, Ballanger P, Lugagne PM, et al. Laparoscopic versus lumboscopic nephrectomy. Eur Urol 1996;29:288–91.
13. Valla JS, Guilloneau B, Montupet P, et al. Retroperitoneal laparoscopic nephrectomy in children. Preliminary report of 18 cases. Eur Urol 1996;30:490–3.
14. Abbou C, Cicco A, Gasman D, et al. Retroperitoneal laparoscopic versus open radical nephrectomy. J Urol 1999;161:1776–80.
15. Hemal AK, Gupta NP, Wadhwa SN, et al. Retroperitoneoscopic nephrectomy and nephroureterectomy for benign nonfunctioning kidneys: a single-center experience. Urology 2001;57:644–9.
16. Borer JG, Cisek LJ, Atala A, et al. Pediatric retroperitoneoscopic nephrectomy using 2 mm. instrumentation. J Urol 1999;162:1725–9.
17. Kobashi KC, Chamberlin DA, Rajpoot D, Shanberg AM. Retroperitoneal laparoscopic nephrectomy in children. J Urol 1998;160(3 Pt 2):1142–4.
18. Shanberg AM, Sanderson K, Rajpoot D, Duel B. Laparoscopic retroperitoneal renal and adrenal surgery in children. BJU Int 2001;87:521–4.
19. Kim HH, Kang J, Kwak C, et al. Laparoscopy for definite localization and simultaneous treatment of ectopic ureter draining a dysplastic kidney in children. J Endourol 2002;16:363–6.
20. El-Ghoneimi A, Sauty L, Maintenant J, et al. Laparoscopic retroperitoneal nephrectomy in high risk children. J Urol 2000;164(3 Pt 2):1076–9.
21. El-Ghoneimi A, Farhat W, Beckers G, et al. Feasibility and outcomes of pediatric simultaneous retroperitoneal laparoscopic bilateral pretransplant nephrectomy. BJU Int 2003;91:74.
22. Fujisawa M, Kawabata G, Gotoh A, et al. Posterior approach for retroperitoneal laparoscopic bilateral nephrectomy in a child. Urology 2002;59:444–6.
23. Zuniga ZV, Ellis D, Moritz ML, Docimo SG. Bilateral laparoscopic transperitoneal nephrectomy with early peritoneal dialysis in an infant with the nephrotic syndrome. J Urol 2003;170:1962.
24. Halachmi S, El-Ghoneimi A, Farhat W. Successful subcapsular laparoscopic nephrectomy in a child with xanthogranulomatous pyelonephritis. J Pediatr Endosurg Inn Tech 2002;6:269–72.
25. Jordan GH, Winslow BH. Laparoendoscopic upper pole partial nephrectomy with ureterectomy. J Urol 1993;150:940–3.
26. Janetschek G, Seibold J, Radamayr C, Barsch G. Laparoscopic heminephroureterectomy in pediatric patients. J Urol 1997;158:1928–30.
27. El-Ghoneimi A, Farhat W, Bolduc S, et al. Retroperitoneal laparoscopic versus open partial nephroureterectomy in children. BJU Int 2003;91:532–5.
28. Horowitz M, Shah SM, Ferzli G, et al. Laparoscopic partial upper pole nephrectomy in infants and children. BJU Int 2001;87:514–6.
29. Borzi P. A comparison of the lateral and posterior retroperitoneoscopic approach for complete and partial nephroureterectomy in children. BJU Int 2001;87:517–20.
30. Peters C. Laparoendoscopic renal surgery in children. J Endourol 2000;14:841–7.
31. Adams JB 2nd, Micali S, Moore RG, et al. Complications of extraperitoneal balloon dilation. J Endourol 1996;10:375–8.
32. Capolicchio JP, Jednak R, Anidjar M, Pippi-Salle JL. A modified access technique for retroperitoneoscopic renal surgery in children. J Urol 2003;170:204–6.
33. Hamilton BD, Gatti JM, Cartwright PC, Snow BW. Comparison of laparoscopic versus open nephrectomy in the pediatric population. J Urol 2000;163:937–9.
34. York GB, Robertson FM, Cofer BR, et al. Laparoscopic nephrectomy in children. Surg Endosc 2000;14:469–72.
35. Yao D, Poppas DP. A clinical series of laparoscopic nephrectomy, nephroureterectomy and heminephroureterectomy in the pediatric population. J Urol 2000;163:1531–5.
36. Halachmi S, El-Ghoneimi A, Bissonnette B, et al. Hemodynamic and respiratory effect of pediatric urological laparoscopic surgery: a retrospective study. J Urol 2003;170(4 Pt 2):1651–4.
37. Fornara P, Doehn C, Friedrich HJ, Jocham D. Nonrandomized comparison of open flank versus laparoscopic nephrectomy in 249 patients with benign renal disease. Eur Urol 2001;40:24–31.
38. Robinson BC, Snow BW, Cartwright PC, et al. Comparison of laparoscopic versus open partial nephrectomy in a pediatric series. J Urol 2003;169:638–40.
39. Peters CA. Complications in pediatric urological laparoscopy: results of a survey. J Urol 1996;155:1070–3.
40. Rassweiler J, Fornara P, Weber M, et al. Laparoscopic nephrectomy: the experience of the laparoscopy working group of the German Urologic Association. J Urol 1998;160:18–21.
41. Soulie M, Seguin P, Richeux L, et al. Urological complications of laparoscopic surgery: experience with 350 procedures at a single center. J Urol 2001;165(6 Pt 1):1960–3.
42. Kumar M, Kumar R, Hemal AK, Gupta NP. Complications of retroperitoneoscopic surgery at one centre. BJU Int 2001;87:607–12.
43. Esposito C, Lima M, Mattioli G, et al. Complications of pediatric urological laparoscopy: mistakes and risks. J Urol 2003;169:1490–2.
44. Farhat W, Khoury A, Bagli D, et al. Mentored retroperitoneal laparoscopic renal surgery in children: a safe approach to learning. BJU Int 2003;92:617–20.

96

Laparoscopic Bladder Reconstruction

Rajen P. Patel, MD

Steven G. Docimo, MD

Over the last decade, advances in the field of pediatric endourology have allowed minimally invasive approaches to challenging surgical problems. Indications for pediatric laparoscopy have expanded from the simple diagnosis of a nonpalpable testis to the challenging reconstruction of the upper and lower urinary tract. Laparoscopic reconstruction adheres to the tenets of conventional open reconstructive surgery, while minimizing the associated morbidities.[1,2]

This chapter will review the fundamentals of laparoscopic bladder reconstruction, including experience with various bowel segments, as well as the creation of catheterizable bowel and bladder stomas.

HISTORY

The search for the ideal replacement for bladder began as early as 1855, when Tuffier reported his first experience with the ureterosigmoidostomy.[3] The application of isolated bowel segments, such as stomach, ileum, and colon, was not investigated until the 1950s. Unlike the ileum and colon, which are now routinely used for urinary reconstruction, the gastric reservoir has been technically more demanding, and as a result has been performed at fewer centers.

In 1976, laparoscopy was introduced into urology as a diagnostic procedure for a nonpalpable testis by Cortesi and colleagues.[4] Following a period of stagnation, a resurgence in interest occurred in the past 2 decades with the application of laparoscopy for adult pelvic lymph node dissections and nephrectomies.[5] The complexity of lower tract reconstruction delayed the introduction of laparoscopy into this area. The first laparoscopic bladder augmentation, a gastrocystoplasty, was not published by Docimo and colleagues until 1995.[6] Since then, a number of investigators have performed laparoscopic and laparoscopic-assisted reconstructive procedures with similar success.[7,8]

INDICATIONS AND CONTRAINDICATIONS

The objective of performing a lower urinary tract reconstruction is to create a system that will protect existing renal function, reduce the occurrence of significant urinary tract infections, and improve urinary continence. In general, patients who are ideal candidates for a laparoscopic enterocystoplasty or autoaugmentation should fulfill the following criteria: (1) a significantly reduced bladder volume, and/or (2) the lack of adequate detrusor compliance ($\Delta V/\Delta P < 10$ mL/cm H_2O, and/or (3) the presence of intractable uninhibited involuntary detrusor contractions.[9]

Contraindications to laparoscopic reconstructive procedures include severe inflammatory processes involving the bladder or bowel (eg, inflammatory bowel disease, bacterial cystitis); uncorrectable coagulopathy; short-gut syndrome; multiple prior open abdominal procedures or previous radiation therapy leading to the formation of significant adhesions or scar tissue; and poor patient compliance with, or the inability to perform, chronic intermittent self-catheterization. Prior abdominal surgery and the presence of a ventriculoperitoneal shunt do not represent contraindications to laparoscopic surgery.[10]

ADVANTAGES AND DISADVANTAGES

The benefits of decreased morbidity and improved cosmesis remain the principle arguments in favor of laparoscopy and other minimally invasive procedures over similar open procedures. Pediatric patients with myelodysplasia often have abnormal fixation or malrotation of the cecum, requiring the open surgeon to make a large, cosmetically unappealing midline scar.[11,12] Current laparoscopic technique allows the surgeon to harvest either gastric, appendiceal, small bowel, or colonic segments, while limiting incisions to less morbid lower abdominal approaches or mere port site scars.

Open procedures have been associated with the formation of significant intra-abdominal adhesions. These adhesions create a lifelong risk for bowel obstruction as well as a hindrance to future abdominal surgical procedures. Laparoscopy decreases the incidence of adhesion formation, thus decreasing the lifetime morbidity associated with reconstructive surgery.[13] Minimally invasive procedures have been reported to reduce postoperative analgesia requirements as well as the time to full convalescence.[15]

Perhaps the greatest barrier to laparoscopy or other minimally invasive procedures is the steep learning curve associated with the more challenging reconstructive procedures. Longer operative times have raised cost concerns for minimally invasive procedures. However, experience can lead to shorter operating times, and shorter hospital stays may also result in overall reduced costs.

PRINCIPLES OF RECONSTRUCTIONS

Bladder enlargement can be achieved with or without the use of bowel segments.[3,6,7] All of these procedures adhere to the same basic principle of creating a large-capacity, low-pressure reservoir. The goals are to preserve renal function, minimize infection, and permit easy emptying of the reservoir. The latter is commonly achieved by performing clean intermittent catheterization, either via a patent urethra or a catheterizable channel such a Mitrofanoff[16] or a Monti[17] continent stoma. Patients with inadequate bladder outlet resistance may be treated with bladder neck reconstruction, artificial urinary sphincter, urethral sling, or bladder neck division.

For those patients requiring bladder augmentation with bowel segments, Hinman has described four basic principles: (1) geometric capacity, (2) accommodation, (3) compliance, and (4) contractility.[18] Geometric capacity of a bowel segment relies on whether it is used intact (as a cylinder) or detubularized and refashioned into a more desirable configuration (a sphere). Reconfiguring the bowel by detubularizing it theoretically yields twice the volume of the original segment. In theory, the capacity of the reservoir will be the highest for any given bowel segment if reconfigured into a sphere.[19] According to Laplace's law, a reservoir having a larger radius will accommodate a greater volume at the same pressure and a higher wall tension.[19] Dividing the bowel longitudinally disrupts the circular muscle fibers that are responsible for the generation and propagation of high-pressure peristaltic waves.[19]

PREOPERATIVE EVALUATION

A urodynamic study is carried out to characterize the bladder. Indications for bladder augmentation include low volume, poor bladder wall compliance, or intractable uninhibited detrusor contractions. Prior to bladder augmentation, most patients will have failed anticholinergic therapy, and perhaps other treatments, including injection of botulinum toxin. If incontinence is the indication for repair, bladder neck resistance will determine the need for reconstruction at this level. Associated concerns should be addressed at the same time, including vesicoureteral reflux or ureterovesical junction obstruction. Bowel continence and function should also be addressed, as surgery for bowel continence can often be carried out simultaneously with bladder reconstruction, and the use of intestinal segments for urinary reconstruction might affect bowel function. Baseline laboratory studies may be necessary to document preoperative renal function, in addition to any electrolyte abnormalities.

Most importantly, it is imperative that the patient is willing and able to perform clean intermittent catheterization before pursuing lower urinary tract reconstruction. It is a disaster to reconstruct the lower urinary tract, especially incorporating enterocystoplasty and/or bladder neck division, only to find that the patient or the family is not able to adhere to a catheterization regimen. It is generally wise to demand weeks to months of catheterization on a consistent basis prior to proceeding to reconstruction.

OPTIONS FOR MINIMALLY INVASIVE LOWER URINARY TRACT RECONSTRUCTION

The first laparoscopic bladder augmentation was a gastrocystoplasty described by Docimo and colleagues.[6] A 12 mm trocar was placed through a subumbilical incision. The second and third 12 mm ports were placed under direct vision at the anterior axillary line bilaterally at the level of the umbilicus, allowing work in the epigastrium and in the pelvis (Figure 96-1).

The bladder was freed from the anterior abdominal wall to the level of the urethra. The greater omentum was divided distal to the gastroepiploic arcade. The right gastroepiploic vessels were separated from the distal stomach and pylorus, using an endoscopic clip applier, to create a pedicle that would reach the pelvis. A 20 cm wedge of stomach was measured and an additional 12 mm cannula was placed in the midepigastrium. An EndoGIA stapler (Auto Suture Company, Norwalk, CT) was serially fired to separate the gastric segment from the rest of the stomach. The stomach

was oversewn with a continuous 3-0 Vicryl suture using the Endo Stitch (Figure 96-2).

The bladder was opened from the anterior bladder neck to the level of the trigone, and the Endo Stitch was used to suture the gastric segment to the bladder. The closure was started on the posterior wall and carried anteriorly on both sides. A Malecot catheter was introduced into the bladder, and a suction drain was placed in the perivesical space. The procedure took nearly 11 hours, and there was a period of postoperative urinary drainage. The patient did well. As far as we are aware, this procedure has not been performed again. Other minimally invasive forms of bladder augmentation have been developed and will be outlined below.

LAPAROSCOPIC BLADDER AUTOAUGMENTATION (LBAA): TRANSPERITONEAL APPROACH[21]

PORT SITE PLACEMENT A 5 mm trocar is placed at the level of the umbilicus using open or closed technique. Two additional 5 mm ports are placed under direct vision in the left and right lower quadrants just lateral to the epigastric vessels (Figure 96-3).

SURGICAL TECHNIQUE Using either the Harmonic scalpel or the endoshears, the peritoneal reflection over the dome is incised, creating a plane between the muscularis and mucosa. An elliptical incision is made into the detrusor muscle and the muscularis is extracted through the port sites. The bladder is distended with normal saline to evaluate the size of the diverticulum and to check for leaks (Figure 96-4).

RESULTS In one series, 7 girls 7 to 15 years of age with uncontrollable day and nighttime wetting

underwent this procedure. Follow-up ranged from 10 months to 4 years. Bladder capacity increase ranged from 55 to 95% of preoperative volume. Six children developed complete dryness; time to dryness varied from immediate to 6 weeks (mean 3.5 weeks). The remaining child who was not completely dry was reported to have a significant improvement in her incidence of wetting from several times a day to twice a week. Two patients suffered an intraoperative bladder perforation, which was immediately recognized and repaired without any short- or long-term effect. Operative times varied from 55 to 93 minutes.[21]

PREPERITONEAL LBAA[22]

PORT SITE PLACEMENT A skin incision and fasciotomy are made in the midline midway between the umbilicus and the symphysis pubis. Blunt finger and balloon dissection create a working area in the retroperitoneal space. A 10 mm port is placed into this incision and the space is insufflated to 15 mm Hg. A 12 mm and a 5 mm port are placed to the left and right of the first port lateral to the abdominus rectus. A fourth 5 mm port is placed 2 cm above the symphysis pubis at the lateral border of the left abdominus rectus muscle.

SURGICAL TECHNIQUE The bladder is mobilized from the surrounding attachments using electrocautery scissors. An intravesical balloon is inflated with normal saline, and the detrusor muscle is scored and incised using a 3 French (F) right-angle Greenwald electrode. The dissection is continued on both sides to free the underlying mucosa from the overlying muscularis. Loose detrusor flaps are created bilaterally and are secured to Cooper's ligament (Figure 96-5).

RESULTS One patient has been reported. She was a 26-year-old woman, s/p MVA, with neurologic deficit at the sacral level. Urodynamics demonstrated a poorly compliant bladder with high leak point pressures. Operating time was 6.5 hours without any intra- or postoperative complications. After 6 months she was completely dry day and night and voided by Valsalva's maneuver every 3 hours.[22]

LAPAROSCOPIC INTESTINAL AUGMENTS: EXTRACORPOREAL BOWEL ANASTOMOSIS[7]

PORT SITE PLACEMENT A 12 mm trocar is placed at the superior umbilical crease. Under direct vision, two 5 mm ports are placed at the level of the umbilicus near the right and left lateral border of the abdominus rectus muscle. A fourth 5 mm trocar is placed at the level of the left anterior superior iliac spine (Figure 96-6).

SURGICAL TECHNIQUE A 15 cm length of bowel (ileum, right colon, or left colon) is chosen based on its arterial supply and the ease of mobilizing it down to the level of the bladder neck. After desufflation, the selected bowel segment is delivered via a 2 cm extension of the umbilical port site.

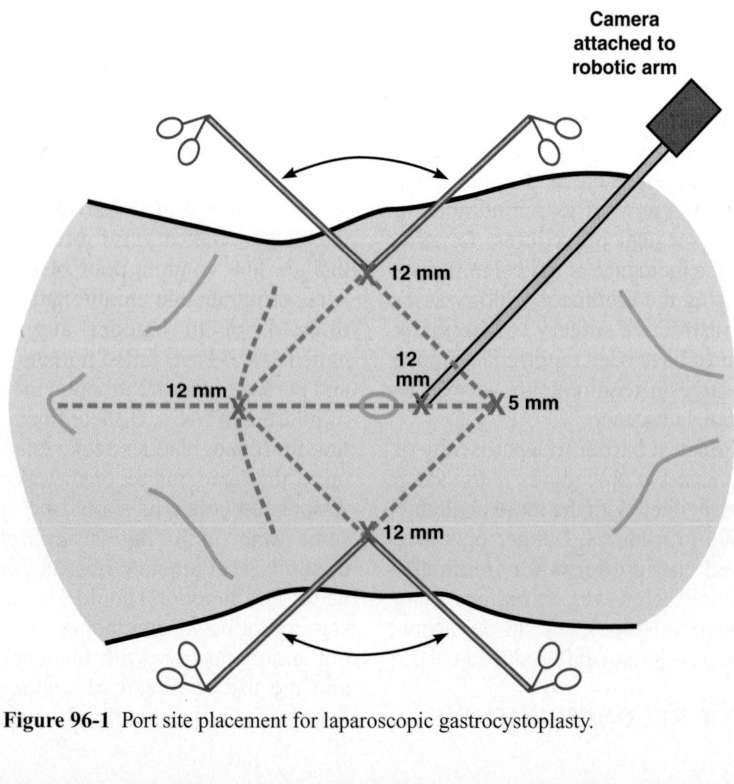

Camera attached to robotic arm

12 mm

12 mm

12 mm

12 mm

5 mm

Figure 96-1 Port site placement for laparoscopic gastrocystoplasty.

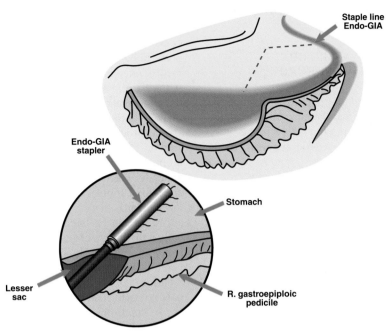

Figure 96-2 The line of division of the stomach is demonstrated using the EndoGIA.

cautery shears to incise the white line of Toldt. A 15 cm segment of ileum is selected and ligated using the EndoGIA stapler. The mesentery is then incised using laparoscopic coagulating shears (LCS) (Ethicon, Cincinnati, OH).

Bowel continuity is reestablished in an isoperistaltic side-to-side anastomosis using the Endo-GIA stapler once enterotomies are created at the ends of both segments using monopolar cautery. The enterotomies are then closed with a silk suture in a single interrupted Lembert fashion.

The perivesical space is entered and dissection is carried down to the endopelvic fascia. A midsagittal incision is made just above the anterior bladder neck and extended posteriorly just above the trigone.

Once the bowel is cleansed with the suction irrigator, it is divided longitudinally along the antimesenteric border. The edges are approximated using a running 3-0 Vicryl suture in order to create a U-shaped plate. The ileal patch is then secured to the bladder using initial interrupted 3-0 Vicryl sutures at the anterior and posterior positions. The remainder of the anastomosis is com-

Using standard open technique, the bowel segment with its associated mesentery is isolated, and bowel continuity is reestablished and the mesentery window is closed (see Figure 96-6).

The isolated bowel is divided longitudinally and cleansed. In the case of an ileal segment, the bowel is reconfigured to a U-shaped plate by a side-to-side anastomosis using continuous 2-0 Vicryl sutures. The bowel is then returned to the abdominal cavity and the enlarged umbilical port is closed around a 12 mm cannula. Continuous, full-thickness anastomosis of the bowel and the bladder mucosa is created by either the Endo Stitch device (U.S Surgical, Norwalk, CT) or freehand laparoscopic suturing. Drains are placed when necessary and the port sites are closed under direct vision.

RESULTS The initial report of this technique consisted of 2 women and 1 man, 32 to 45 years of age with neurogenic bladders secondary to trauma and progressive neuropathology. Total surgical times

varied from 5.3 to 8 hrs. Estimated blood loss varied from 50 to 200 cc. The only intraoperative complication was a trocar-induced rectus sheath hematoma, which was controlled laparoscopically. Postoperative continence or urodymanic status was not reported in the initial publication.

PURE LAPAROSCOPIC ILEOCYSTOPLASTY[9]

PORT SITE PLACEMENT A total of five ports are placed. After obtaining pneumoperitoneum via Veress needle, a 10 mm umbilical port is placed. Two 10 mm ports are placed at the level of either anterior superior iliac spine. An additional 10 mm port is placed at the level of the umbilicus at the lateral margin of the right abdominus rectus muscle. The fifth 12 mm trocar is placed at the level of the umbilicus near the left lateral border of the abdominus rectus muscle (Figure 96-7).

SURGICAL TECHNIQUE The proximal ascending colon and cecum are mobilized using the electro-

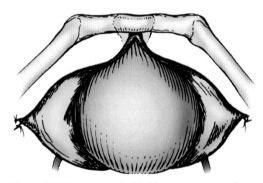

Figure 96-5 Laparoscopic bladder autoaugmentation—preperitoneal approach. Detrusor flaps secured to Cooper's ligament.

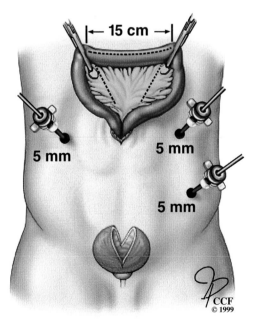

Figure 96-6 Port sites for laparoscopic enterocystoplasty using extracorporeal anastomosis. Selected bowel is exteriorized through an enlarged umbilical incision.

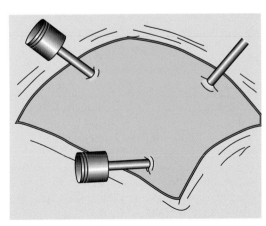

Figure 96-3 Port placement for Laperoscopic bladder autoaugmentation. Upper left is umbilicus. Bilateral lower quadrant ports are lateral to the epigastrics.

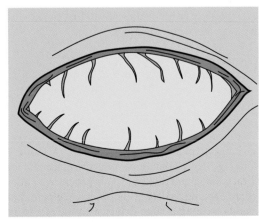

Figure 96-4 Elliptical incision of detrusor muscle creating a plane between muscularis and mucosa.

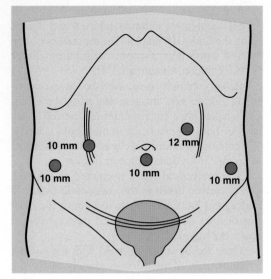

Figure 96-7 Port site placement for pure laparoscopic ilealcystoplasty.

pleted using a running, full-thickness 3-0 Vicryl suture in a single-layer closure. A 10F Blake (Ethicon, Somerville, NJ) drain is placed perivesically and brought out through a lateral port site (Figure 96-8).

RESULTS This represented the first purely laparoscopic ileal cystoplasty. As far as we know, it is the only published case of its kind to date. The patient was a 31-year-old paraplegic women with C6 spinal cord injury on clean intermittent catheterization. Urodynamics demonstrated a small bladder capacity with frequent uninhibited bladder contractions. Total operative time was 9 hours. Follow-up at 4 weeks demonstrated

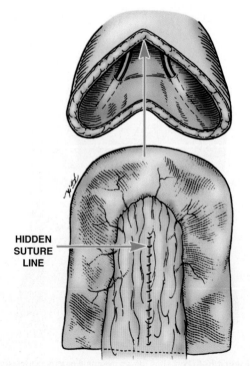

Figure 96-8 Placement of the ileal U-patch onto the bladder.

good bladder capacity with good continence between catheterizations.[9]

LAPAROSCOPIC-ASSISTED RECONSTRUCTIVE SURGERY

Through the evolution of laparoscopic surgery it has become evident that the most beneficial portion of the laparoscopic procedure is the mobilization of the cecum, gastric segment, or the appendix for the creation of a continent stomal channel. If the reconstructive procedure is divided into the following stages (1) abdominal access, (2) dissection and lysis of adhesions, (3) selection and mobilization of augment and stomal tissue, (4) mobilization of bladder and reconstruction of bladder neck, and (5) assembly of parts, then laparoscopy can accomplish the first three tasks, and a small Pfannenstiel incision can be used to create the anterior cystotomy; reconstruct the bladder neck, if necessary; and assemble the bowel, bladder, and stomal segments using standard open technique through a small incision site, which often incorporates the lower abdominal port sites. A compromise between open and laparoscopic technique is created that uses the strengths of each technique, while reducing the morbidity associated with open reconstructive cases and the time and costs associated with a purely laparoscopic approach.[23]

SURGICAL PREPARATION AND POSITIONING
One day prior to laparoscopic-assisted bladder reconstruction, the patient undergoes a mechanical and antibiotic bowel cleansing in preparation for the use of either ileum or colon.

The patient is initially placed in a low lithotomy position in order to perform cystoscopy. In the absence of severe cystitis, the patient is then returned to the standard supine position. The ipsilateral flank is elevated in instances where a nephrectomy is anticipated in preparation for a ureterocystoplasty. Care is taken to pad all pressure points with foam or gel to prevent ulceration. The patient is secured to the operating table to allow steep Trendelenburg's position or lateral rotation.

Following the induction of general anesthesia and endotracheal intubation, a nasogastric tube is placed and antibiotics are administered to cover gram-negative and anaerobic organisms. Epidural anesthesia may be used as an adjunct in patients without spinal abnormalities.

OPERATIVE TECHNIQUE
If a concealed umbilical stoma is anticipated, then the initial access is obtained by developing a U-shaped flap of the lower umbilicus as described by Glassman and Docimo.[24] Once the flap is raised, the midline umbilical fascia is incised sharply and the peritoneum is entered using a hemostat. A radially dilating 10 or 12 mm trocar sleeve is placed under direct vision and dilated.[25] This provides an adequate opening to deliver the stomal segment, but avoids creating a large defect with the attendant risk of a peristomal hernia. Additional ports are placed based on the proposed procedure—if a

Pfannenstiel incision is planned for a bladder augmentation or an MACE (Malone antegrade continent stoma) is expected, then the second port can be placed in a location where it is easily incorporated into either the incision or the stoma. A third 2 or 3 mm port site then can be placed in the midepigastrium. All ports are sutured in place to avoid unintentional removal.

In procedures using the appendix for a catheterizable stoma, the right colon can be mobilized laparoscopically until the base of the appendix reaches the Pfannensteil incision. The appendix can then be divided from the cecum in the standard open fashion. On the other hand, the appendix can be harvested purely laparoscopically with the use of an EndoGIA, taking care not to compromise its blood supply from the mesoappendix. Additionally, procedures requiring the creation of only an appendicovesicostomy can now be performed entirely laparoscopically. The use of small bowel often requires no dissection because it is easily brought down to the low abdominal incision for division and reconstruction. Similarly, mobilizing a redundant sigmoid will require little dissection; however, if necessary, the lateral peritoneal reflection can be incised to provide appropriate length.

Once the bowel segments are mobilized, a 4 to 5 cm Pfannensteil incision is created for the lower urinary tract reconstruction. Bladder procedures, including bladder neck reconstruction or division, ureteral reimplantation, or cystolithalopaxy, can all be performed extraperitoneally in order to reduce unnecessary bowel manipulation. Bladder augmentation is accomplished using standard open techniques once the tissue of interest (ie, stomach, ileum, sigmoid) is acquired. The ports can be left in the stoma sites until the end of the case to facilitate delivery of the stoma segments. All stomas (ie, MACE, appendicovesicostomy, ileal, or sigmoid Monti) are matured to the skin and redundant conduits are shortened in order to prevent any difficulties with catheterization. The dorsal aspect of the bladder stoma is spatulated and secured to the previous U-flap, thereby preventing stenosis and concealing its appearance.[24] Postoperative drains are placed, including a nasogastric tube, a suprapubic catheter, and a 10F Foley catheter for the bladder stoma, which is sutured to the skin to prevent balloon traction on the continence mechanism. Fascial layers and skin are closed in the standard fashion.

RESULTS The largest series of laparoscopic-assisted reconstructive procedures reported by Chung and colleagues included a total of 30 patients with no intraoperative complications.[26] One patient was converted to an open procedure secondary to dense adhesions and was therefore excluded from data analysis. No patient required blood transfusions and median hospital stay was 6 days (range 2–20).

A total of 39 stomas were created in 29 patients, including 26 Mitrofanoff stomas (appendix 17, sigmoid 5, ileum 3, and bladder 1),

13 with or 13 without concurrent bladder augmentations, and 13 MACE stomas (12 appendix and 1 ileum). Additionally, 1 gastrocystoplasty takedown with appendiceal Mitrofanoff and ileal augmentation, as well as 2 laparoscopic-assisted nephrectomies with subsequent ureterocystoplasty were performed. Concurrent MACE (9 appendix and 1 ilieum) and Mitrofanoff (4 appendix, 3 ileum, 2 sigmoid, and 1 tubularized bladder) procedures were performed in 10 patients. Open incisions included 23 Pfannensteil, 6 lower midline (incorporating incisions from previous surgery), and 1 small midline incision. Adjuncts to stoma reconstruction included bladder neck reconstruction (9), fascial sling (3), epispadias revision (2), ureteral reimplant (1), redo orchiopexy (1), and bladder augmentation (4 sigmoid, 9 ileum, and 2 ureter).

Thirty-seven of 39 stomas (95%) were continent of urine or stool and easily catheterizable after a mean follow-up of 32 months (range 3–57). Stomal revision owing to persistent incontinence or difficulty with catheterization was necessary in 3 stomas (7.7%) after a mean follow-up of 19 months (range 8–36). Minor procedures including indwelling catheterization, dilation, collagen injection, and cystoscopy were required in 10 newly constructed stomas (25%).

A total of 5 postoperative complications occurred, 2 requiring abdominal exploration for a spontaneous bladder perforation and a partial small bowel obstruction. The remaining complications included a delayed postoperative ileus, deep venous thrombosis, and a wound infection, all treated nonsurgically.

POSTOPERATIVE COMPLICATIONS The general complications following laparoscopy are well described. These include infection, hemorrhage, bowel or vessel injury during the placement of the Veress needle or trocar insertion, and thromboembolic or air-embolic phenomena. While performing lysis of adhesions or mobilizing bowel or bladder segments, inadvertent injury to surrounding structures may occur, necessitating open conversion if one is unable to gain control or if there is a failure to progress. Port site hernias tend to occur if port sites greater 5 mm are not formally closed.[27] Possibilities of bowel obstruction, stricture formation, or leakage can occur in instances where the bowel has been divided. Bladder calculi have been documented to form along anastomotic suture lines closed with nonabsorbable sutures. However, strict adherence to basic laparoscopic principles should minimize the incidence of complications and yield successes comparable to open approaches.

CONCLUSION

The large unsightly incisions that were once necessary for lower urinary tract reconstructive surgery are now avoided through the laparoscopic mobilization and reconstruction of bowel and bladder. With advancement in technology, newer avenues of laparoscopic reconstructive techniques will be explored. The impact of robotics is only beginning to be evaluated. Although currently only a few specialized centers perform laparoscopic enterocystoplasties, in time more institutions may incorporate these approaches in their arsenal for the management of neurogenic bladder disorder.

REFERENCES

1. Abdullah A, Blakeney P, Hunt R, et al. Visible scars and self-esteem in the pediatric patients with burns. J Burn Care Rehabil 1994;15:164–8.
2. Kerbl K, Clayman RV, Petros J A, et al. Staging pelvic lymphadenectomy for prostate cancer: a comparison of laparoscopic and open techniques. J Urol 1993;150(2 Pt 1):396–8.
3. Goodwin WE. Experiences with intestines as a substitute for the urinary tract. In: King LR, Stone AR, Webster GD, editors. Bladder reconstruction and continent urinary diversion. Chicago: Year Book Medical Publishers; 1987. p. 9–29.
4. Cortesi N, Ferrari P, Zambada E, et al. Diagnosis of bilateral abdominal cryptorchism by laparoscopy. Endoscopy 1976;9:33–4.
5. Clayman R, Kavoussi L, Long S, et al. Laparoscopic nephrectomy: initial report of pelviscopic organ ablation in the pig. J Endourol 1990;4:247–9.
6. Docimo SG, Moore RG, Adams J, Kavousi L. Laparoscopic bladder augmentation using stomach. Urology 1995;46:565–9.
7. Gill I, Rackely R, Meraney A, et al. Laparoscopic enterocystoplasty. Urology 2000;55:178–81.
8. Meng M, Anwar H, Elliott S, Stoller ML. Pure laparoscopic enterocystoplasty. J Urol 2002;167:1386.
9. Elliott SP, Meng MM, Anwar HP, Stoller ML. Complete laparoscopic ileal cystoplasty. Urology 2002;59:939–43.
10. Jackman SV, Weingart JD, Kinsman SL, Docimo SG. Laparoscopic surgery in patients with ventriculoperitoneal shunts: safety and monitoring. J Urol 2000;164:1352–4.
11. Brown SF. Congenital malformations associated with myelomeningocele. J Iowa Med Soc 1975;65:101–4.
12. Baker RH, Sharrard WJ. Correction of lordoscoliosis in spina bifida by multiple osteotomy and fusion with dwyer fixation: a preliminary report. Dev Med Child Neurol Suppl 1973;29:12–23.
13. Garrard CL, Clements RH, Nanney L, et al. Adhesion formation is reduced after laparoscopic surgery. Surg Endosc 1999;13:10–3.
14. Hedican SC, Schula PG, Docimo SG. Laparoscopic assisted reconstructive surgery. J Urol 1999;161:267–70.
15. Lukaszczyk JJ, Pretletz RJ Jr. Laparoscopic resection of benign stromal tumor of the stomach. J Laparoendosc Surg 1992;2:331–4.
16. Liard A, Seguier-Lipszyc E, Mathiot A, Mitrofanoff P. The Mitrofanoff procedure: 20 years later. J Urology 2001;165(6 Pt 2):2394–8.
17. Monti PR, de Carvalho JR, Arap S. The Monti procedure: applications and complications. Urology 2000;55:616–21.
18. Hinman FJ Jr. Selection of intestinal segments for bladder substitution: physical and physiological characteristics. J Urol 1988;139:519–23.
19. Hensle TW, Ring KS. Urinary tract reconstruction in children. Urol Clin North Am 1991;18:701–15.
20. Docimo SG. Improved technique for open laparoscopic access. J Endourol 1998;12 Suppl 1:S185.
21. Braren V, Bishop MR. Laparoscopic bladder autoaugmentation in children. Urol Clin North Am 1998;25:533–40.
22. MacDougall E, Clayman R, Figenshau R, Pearle M. Laparoscopic retropubic auto-augmentation of the bladder. J Urol 1995;153:123–6.
23. Cadeddu JA, Docimo SG. Laparoscopic-assisted continent stoma procedures: our new standard. Urology 1999;54:909–12.
24. Glassman DT, Docimo SG. Concealed umbilical stoma: long-term evaluation of stomal stenosis. J Urol 2001;166:1028–30.
25. Cuellar D, Kavoussi PK, Baker LA, Docimo SG. Open laparoscopic access using a radially dilating trocar: experience and indications in 50 consecutive cases. J Endourol 2000;14:755–6.
26. Chung SY, Meldrum K, Docimo SG. Laparoscopic-assisted reconstruction: a 7-year experience. J Urol 2004;171:372–5.
27. Bloom DA, Erhlich RM. Omental evisceration through small laparoscopic port sites. J Endourol 1993;7:31–2.

Part VIII

State of the Art Endoscopic Technology

97

Outcomes Analysis:
Treatment Options for Stones

Paramjit S. Chandhoke, MD, PhD

COST-EFFECTIVENESS, OUTCOME, AND DECISION ANALYSIS

When at least two different treatment options (with variable efficacy and outcomes) are available for the treatment of a specific diagnosis, one can use the techniques of outcome, cost-effectiveness, and decision analysis to help determine which treatment option may be best suited for the management of a particular medical condition. These analytical tools are especially useful when a new technology is being introduced into the market to determine its benefits and drawbacks to previously established treatments. These analyses may also be used for allocating funds between competing technologies and, in health maintenance organizations, for choosing between alternative services for patients.[1,2]

There are four scenarios when considering the use of cost-effectiveness analysis in adopting a new technology over an existing or competing technology (Table 97-1). From a cost-effectiveness standpoint, if the new technology is less costly and more effective than the existing technology, then the new technology should be readily adopted. On the other hand, if the new technology is more expensive and less effective than the existing alternative, then the new technology should be discarded. Cost-effectiveness analysis is best applied to new technologies if they are either less costly with lower efficacy or more costly with higher efficacy than the existing technology.[3]

Inherent in the technique of cost-effectiveness for assessment of a new technology (eg, a new surgical procedure) is the necessity of a "good estimate" of both the cost of the technology and its outcome or effectiveness. This is the key step that determines the feasibility of such an analysis.[4] The models of cost-effectiveness and outcomes analysis are at best only as good as the data used and the assumptions made in the analysis. The surgical management of kidney stone disease

is suited for a cost-effectiveness analysis for a variety of reasons:

1. The efficacy of stone treatment can be accurately defined. Most investigators will accept success or failure of treatment if the patient is stone free or not, respectively, after a particular treatment.
2. Competing, controversial treatment options are available for a given stone size, stone type, and stone location. Examples are the treatment of staghorn calculi by extracorporeal shock wave lithotripsy (ESWL), percutaneous nephrolithotomy (PNL), or combination therapy (COMBO),[5–7] and the treatment of lower-pole calculi by ESWL monotherapy or PNL.[8]
3. Outcome analysis can be used to allocate resources to the treatment option that is more cost-effective. To be clinically useful, the differences in cost-effectiveness must be significant between the treatment options.
4. If a treatment option has been clinically shown to be more efficacious than another (eg, COMBO vs ESWL monotherapy for staghorn calculi), then showing that it is also the more cost-effective option will strengthen its clinical acceptance.
5. Good outcomes data are available to assess the efficacy of various treatment options for staghorn calculi, lower-pole calculi, and distal ureteral calculi.

Outcome analysis is the evaluation of treatment outcomes that may include cost comparisons, cost-effectiveness measurement, and/or patient morbidity. For kidney stone disease, outcome analyses generally measure the morbidity of alternative treatments when the cost-effectiveness of the treatments is similar. An example would be the comparison of ESWL and ureteroscopy (URS) for distal ureteral stones, which may have similar costs and efficacies.[9] As such, it is of interest to know the morbidity of passing residual fragments, the time to clearance of stone fragments,

the number of return visits after surgery, and the time to return to work.

Decision analyses generally incorporate a hypothetical model with various decision tree points that result in potential outcomes.[10,11] Estimates are often required not only of the cost and efficacies of treatment, but also of the choice of secondary procedures when the initial therapy fails. Sensitivity analyses provide an adjunct to examine the performance or predictions of the model within the range of practical choices made at the branch points of the decision tree. These models can be powerful to guide decisions that may be more cost-effective when initial treatment is not completely successful.[12]

COST AND OUTCOMES MEASUREMENT

Economists consider three types of costs in the assessment of a medical service: direct, indirect, and intangible. Direct medical costs are those necessary to provide medical care, such as personnel, supplies, and facility costs. Often overlooked direct costs are those necessary to accomplish the delivery of medical care outside the facility itself. These include patient's cost of transportation, special clothing or equipment, special housing, etc., which may be necessary to deliver special care. Indirect costs are those that relate to the loss of productivity because of a health care intervention. These costs are sustained by the patients and their employers and are especially relevant when comparing minimally invasive surgery with traditional open surgery. Intangible costs are those owing to pain, suffering, grief, and death from the medical condition itself and/or a particular medical intervention.

Studies of cost-effectiveness of the treatment of stone disease have primarily looked at facility and physician costs or charges in determining cost-effectiveness. When comparing the cost-effectiveness of various alternative treatments, it is often convenient to use charges as an estimate of cost.[13] Although charges do not represent the true costs of delivering a medical service, they do accurately reflect costs for the patient or the medical insurance program that is responsible for paying the bills. As such, billing charges may still be used for evaluating the cost-effectiveness of different treatment options at the same provider facility.[13] The implicit assumption is that the relative costs of the two treatments being compared

Table 97-1 Use of Cost-Effectiveness Analysis in Assessment of New Technology			
Possible Scenario	Expense of New Technology	Efficacy of New Technology	Decision
1	More	Less	Disregard new technology
2	Less	More	Use new technology
3	More	More	Use cost-effectiveness analysis
4	Less	Less	Use cost-effectiveness analysis

are reflected by the billing charges. The most important aspect of cost-effective analysis is that similar cost estimates (be it costs, billing charges, or reimbursements) be used for the treatment options being compared.

Outcome analysis has played a limited role in the management of kidney stone disease partly because of the subjectivity in outcomes measurement. When two alternative techniques may be equally cost-effective, such as ESWL and URS for distal ureteral stones, outcome analysis is especially helpful in evaluating the morbidity and convalescence of the treatment options. The morbidity of passing stone fragments, use of stents, and time missed from work are the usual outcomes measured in the treatment of stones.[14]

MANAGEMENT OF STAGHORN CALCULI

A variety of treatment options are available for the treatment of staghorn calculi. The American Urological Association (AUA) Guidelines Panel made recommendations based on stone surface area and expected efficacies of ESWL, PNL, and COMBO therapies.[5] Not evaluated in these recommendations was the cost comparison of each treatment option, as cost data were unavailable at the time of their recommendations. Open surgical treatment is rarely considered these days for staghorn calculi, but it is likely a good treatment option when extensive branching of the staghorn calculi are present that may require three or more percutaneous tracts to reach all the stone-bearing calices. This option may also be more cost-effective, but limited data are available regarding the cost of open surgery in direct comparison with alternative minimally invasive therapies.

Cost-effectiveness analysis has been used by Chandhoke to evaluate the treatment options for staghorn calculi.[15] This study estimated the cost-effectiveness of various treatment options by defining a cost-effectiveness index (CEI) that estimated the cost incurred for making 1 patient stone free by a particular treatment option.[15] Estimates of cost were determined from billing charges for PNL and ESWL. Efficacy of treatment and the number of primary and secondary procedures were obtained from the American Urological Association (AUA) Guidelines Panel.[5] This study showed that both PNL monotherapy and COMBO therapy were more cost-effective options than ESWL monotherapy for staghorn calculi. Furthermore, computations of CEI for ESWL monotherapy and COMBO therapy showed that when the stone surface area was less than 500 mm[2], these two treatment options were equally cost-effective. However, when the stone surface area exceeded 500 mm[2], COMBO therapy became more cost-effective (Table 97-2).

In a separate analysis using cost and effectiveness data from their own institution, Murray and colleagues also showed that ESWL monotherapy should be discouraged for large renal calculi (> 3 cm), especially if the stone surface area exceeded 500 mm[2], or if the stone was not located within the renal pelvis.[6] These two studies incorporating economic analysis of various treatment options for large renal calculi have significant clinical relevance. They cement the conclusion of the AUA Guidelines Panel that ESWL monotherapy should not be used as primary therapy for kidney stones with surface area greater than 500 mm[2].[15]

TREATMENT OF LOWER-POLE STONES

Clinical controversy also exists regarding the treatment of lower-pole calculi by ESWL, URS, or PNL monotherapy. Not only is the cost analysis of the various treatment options an issue, but also the efficacy of each treatment is dependent on stone size as well as the caliceal anatomy of the lower pole. In comparison to ESWL and PNL, limited data are available on the efficacy of URS for lower-pole stones. Flexible URS requires significant endourologic skills and the appropriate ancillary equipment: smaller laser fibers, dual deflection ureteroscopes, tipless baskets, etc., that determine the ultimate success of URS. As the efficacy of URS for lower-pole stones can vary, dependent on a variety of factors, and it is a relatively new and evolving technique, URS has not yet been the subject of cost-effectiveness analysis for lower-pole stones. Most such studies have compared PNL versus ESWL monotherapy as the alternative treatment options for lower-pole stones.

Whereas PNL monotherapy has better efficacy than ESWL monotherapy for lower-pole stones, a single PNL is costlier than a single ESWL treatment. As outlined in Table 97-1 above, these features qualify the comparison of these techniques by cost-effectiveness analysis. May and Chandhoke have looked at this issue by stratifying lower-pole calculi based on stone size,[16] as the efficacy of ESWL monotherapy declines with an increase in stone size.[8] Using a stone-free status as the desired outcome in their decision analysis model, they assumed that all patients failing primary ESWL would need a secondary PNL to make them stone free. Thus they compared the total treatment costs necessary to render a patient with a lower-pole calculi stone free. Again, effectiveness data were used as established in the literature for lower-pole cal-

culi. The results of their economic analysis showed that ESWL monotherapy was more cost-effective when the stone size was less than 2 cm, but PNL became more cost-effective when the lower-pole stone size was greater than 2 cm. Such a conclusion, which may affect the clinical treatment of lower-pole calculi in the future, would not have been evident without the use of cost-effectiveness analysis.

Currently, randomized trials are being conducted to more accurately determine the efficacy of ESWL (with second-generation machines), PNL, and URS. As such data become available, cost-effectiveness analysis should be revisited to determine which one of these treatment options is superior.

ESWL VERSUS URETEROSCOPY FOR DISTAL URETERAL STONES

Although cost-effectiveness analysis seems to have been applied quite successfully to some of the controversies in the management of stone disease, such analysis is probably inadequate for situations in which the effectiveness and costs of competing treatments are similar. An example of this would be the option of ESWL or ureteroscopy for the management of distal ureteral calculi.[9] Outcomes analysis, which determines the quality of care delivered by the treatment options, seems to be a reasonable approach to resolve this controversy. Until good prospective outcomes data become available, it is likely that this issue will remain unresolved.

A decision analysis approach was initially used by Wolf and colleagues to address the controversy regarding the management of distal ureteral calculi.[10] In addition to comparing the costs and effectiveness of ESWL and ureteroscopy, utility values were also assigned to patient satisfaction for the two procedures. Their study showed that not only was ureteroscopy more cost-effective than ESWL for the management of distal ureteral calculi, but also a significant number of patients preferred ureteroscopy as the initial treatment choice.[10]

Computer software programs are also available commercially to construct decision tree models. As an adjunct, one can use meta-analysis and sensitivity analysis for a range of potential

Table 97-2 Cost-Effectiveness of ESWL vs Combination Therapy (COMBO) for Staghorn Calculi Based on Stone Surface Area*

	Surface Area					
	< 500 mm[2]		500 mm[2] to 1,000 mm[2]		> 1,000 mm[2]	
Outcome Variable	ESWL	COMBO	ESWL	COMBO	ESWL	COMBO
Median stone-free rate (%)**	63	94	46	86	22	82
No. primary procedures**	2.1	2.8	2.1	2.8	2.1	2.8
No. secondary procedures**	0.2	0.02	0.2	0.02	0.2	0.02
Cost-Effective Index (CEI)* (US$)	44,900	41,400	60,200	45,400	118,700	47,400

*Chandhoke PS.[15]
**Lam HS et al.[7]
ESWL = extracorporeal shock wave lithotripsy.

outcomes to compare competing technologies. This strategy has been used by Lotan and colleagues to compare ESWL, URS, and observation for the management of distal ureteral stones with *Data 3.5* software.[11] Observation with secondary intervention for failures was the most cost-effective option. In direct comparison with the reported efficacy of ESWL and URS, Lotan and colleagues found URS to be cheaper and more cost-effective than ESWL.[11]

It should also be recognized that the efficacy of ESWL is likely dependent on the lithotripsy machine used to treat ureteral stones. Second-generation machines do not have the same efficacy as that of the original HM3 lithotriptor, which was reported to have equivalent efficacy as URS.[9] Peschel and colleagues evaluated the outcome of a second-generation ESWL machine with that of URS and found that the definitiveness of URS treatment outweighed the nuisance and morbidity of passing stone fragments after ESWL.[14] This outcome measure was patient satisfaction and based on whether patients would chose ESWL versus URS for future stone episodes.

MEDICAL PREVENTION FOR RECURRENT CALCIUM STONES

With the introduction of minimally invasive procedures such as ESWL and URS, medical prophylaxis has lost some of its clinical emphasis. However, from a patient's perspective, almost 90% of them are interested in finding out why they form kidney stones and are willing to undergo either diet therapy or take medications to prevent future stone episodes.[17] It would seem prudent to promote medical prevention if surgical treatment for recurrent stones would be more costly than prophylaxis. Several studies addressing the cost-effectiveness of medical therapy have been published recently.[18–22]

Based on patient stone episodes prior to and after medical therapy, Parks and Coe estimated that a net saving of $1.62 million to $3.162 million (US) per 1,000 patients could have been made per year with the implementation of medical prevention at their institution.[18] These financial estimates depend significantly on stone recurrence rates with and without medical therapy; the average stone frequency for recurrent stone formation was 1.6 stone episodes/year in their study. They also achieved a 78.6% reduction in stone episodes per patient year in their series. The strength of this study was that actual (rather than estimated) stone recurrence rates were used to compare the costs of medical and surgical intervention.

Tiselius has suggested that stone formers should be stratified to individualize a strategy for metabolic evaluation and medical management.[20,23] He recommends five categories of stone patients based on the severity of their stone recurrence and whether they had residual stone fragments after ESWL.[23] For patients with an annual stone frequency of 0.2 (severe recurrent stone formers and those with residual stone fragments), Tiselius reported that the annual savings of medical management were approximately €1,875 per patient over a 5-year follow-up period.[20] In his calculation, Tiselius assumed that a 50% reduction in stone episodes occurred with selective medical management. He also reported that selective medical management was more cost-effective than nonselective medical management.

Strohmaier conducted a similar economic analysis of the German population.[21] His computations showed that medical management of recurrent stone formers could save DM 333.1 per year for the German health care system. Robertson has conducted an economic analysis of medical prophylaxis in the United Kingdom over a 30-year period.[19] At 1998 prices, the annual savings to the British Health Care System, for a remission rate of 50% in patients with an average annual stone frequency of 0.2, were estimated to be £64,624.

The cost of work cessation is an additional item that would further favor medical prevention of recurrent urolithiasis. However, these cost estimates have not been included in the above studies as they can vary widely among patients and societies. Cost-effectiveness analysis can also be significantly affected by practice patterns. For example, many patients with urolithiasis in Germany are hospitalized for ESWL and ureteroscopic procedures, which are outpatient procedures in most of the other developed countries. Thus, cost-effectiveness analysis should be performed for specific geographic sites and specific practice patterns.[24]

Chandhoke asked the economic question in a slightly different way[25]: In which particular calcium stone former (with a specific stone recurrence rate) is medical prophylaxis cost-effective? Stone recurrence rates, as well as the anticipated remission rates, impact the cost of medical therapy in individual patients. In this study, cost data were obtained for the metabolic evaluation and medical treatment of stone disease, as was the cost of an acute stone episode from 10 countries (Table 97-3). Within the constraints of the necessary assumptions made in his study as to how medical prophylaxis and stone episodes are managed, it appears that in patients who form stones less frequently than once every 3 years, a medical prevention program may not be cost-effective. As shown in Table 97-3, in many countries the stone frequency probably has to be even higher to justify medical prophylaxis for recurrent calcium stones. The cost data in this study also support the view that a metabolic evaluation and a specific medical prevention program are not recommended for the first-time calcium stone former in any country.

REFERENCES

1. Detsky AS, Naglie IG. A clinician's guide to cost-effectiveness analysis. Ann Intern Med 1990;113:147–54.
2. Jewett MA, Bombardier C, Menchions CW. Comparative costs of the various strategies of urinary stone disease management. Urology 1995;46(3 Suppl A):15–22.
3. Phelps CE. The methodologic foundations of studies of the appropriateness of medical care. N Engl J Med 1993; 329:1241–5.
4. Fuchs VR, Garber AM. The new technology assessment. N Engl J Med 1990;323:673–7.
5. Segura JW, Preminger GM, Assimos DG, et al. Nephrolithiasis Clinical Guidelines Panel summary report on the management of staghorn calculi. The American Urological Association Nephrolithiasis Clinical Guidelines Panel. J Urol 1994;151:1648–51.
6. Murray MJ, Chandhoke PS, Berman CJ, Sankey NE. Outcome of extracorporeal shockwave lithotripsy monotherapy for large renal calculi: effect of stone and collecting system surface areas and cost-effectiveness of treatment. J Endourol 1995;9:9–13.
7. Lam HS, Lingeman JE, Mosbaugh PG, et al. Evolution of the technique of combination therapy for staghorn calculi: a decreasing role for extracorporeal shockwave lithotripsy. J Urol 1992;148(3 Pt 2):1058–62.
8. Lingeman JE, Siegal YI, Steele B, et al. Management of lower pole nephrolithiasis: a critical analysis. J Urol 1994; 151:663–7.
9. Anderson KR, Keetch DW, Albala DM, et al. Optimal therapy for the distal ureteral stone: extracorporeal shockwave lithotripsy versus ureteroscopy. J Urol 1994;152:62–5.
10. Wolf JS, Carroll PR, Stoller ML. Cost-effectiveness v patient preference for distal ureteral calculi; a literature-based decision analysis. J Endourol 1995;9:243–8.
11. Lotan Y, Gettman MT, Roehrborn CG, et al. Management of ureteral calculi: a cost comparison and decision making analysis. J Urol 2002;167:1621–9.
12. Chandhoke PS, DeAntoni E. Cost-effectiveness analysis: application to endourology. J Endourol 1998;12:485–91.
13. Finkler SA. The distinction between cost and charges. Ann Intern Med 1982;96:102–9.

Country	Cost Type	Cost of an Acute Stone Episode (US)	5-Year Cost of Medical Prophylaxis (US$)	Stone Recurrence Rate at Which Cost of Medical Prophylaxis and Cost of Recurrent Stone Episodes are Equal
Australia	NHC	575	2,801	1.3
Canada	IC	680	1,400	0.51
Germany	NHC	248	2,519	2.5
Italy	NHC	1,184	3,398	0.72
Japan	IC	1,453	2,390	0.41
Sweden	IC	1,010	4,116	1.0
Switzerland	BC	1,447	2,067	0.36
Turkey	IC	404	1,472	0.91
United Kingdom	NHC	1,706	2,244	0.33
United States	BC	6,355	8,200	0.32

Table 97-3 Cost Comparison of Medical Prophylaxis versus Treatment of Recurrent Stone Episodes*

BC = billing charges; IC = institutional costs; NHC = National Health Care.
*Chandhoke PS.[25]
**Denotes a cost estimate.

14. Peschel R, Janetschek G, Bartsch G. Extracorporeal shock-wave lithotripsy versus ureteroscopy for distal ureteral calculi: a prospective randomized study. J Urol 1999; 162:1909–12.

15. Chandhoke PS. Cost-effectiveness of different treatment options for staghorn calculi. J Urol 1996;156:1567–71.

16. May DJ, Chandhoke PS. Efficacy of cost-effectiveness of extracorporeal shockwave lithotripsy for solitary lower pole renal calculi. J Urol 1998;159:24–7.

17. Grampsas SA, Moore M, Chandhoke PS. 10-year experience with extracorporeal shockwave lithotripsy in the state of Colorado. J Endourol 2000;14:711–4.

18. Parks JH, Coe FL. The financial effects of kidney stone prevention. Kidney Int 1996;50:1706–12.

19. Robertson WG. Medical management of urinary stone disease. EBU Update Series 1998;7:139–44.

20. Tiselius HG. Comprehensive metabolic evaluation of stone formers is cost-effective. In: Rodgers AL, Hibbert BE, Hess B, et al, editors. Urolithiasis 2000: Proceedings 9th International Symposium on Urolithiasis. Cape Town: University of Cape Town Press; 2000. p. 349–55.

21. Strohmaier WL. Economic aspects of urolithiasis and meta-phylaxis in Germany. In: Rodgers AL, Hibbert BE, Hess B, et al, editors. Urolithiasis 2000: Proceedings 9th International Symposium on Urolithiasis. Cape Town: University of Cape Town Press; 2000. p. 406–9.

22. Robertson WG. The economic case for the biochemical screening of stone patients. In: Rodgers AL, Hibbert BE, Hess B, et al, editors. Urolithiasis 2000: Proceedings 9th International Symposium on Urolithiasis. Cape Town: University of Cape Town Press; 2000. p. 403–5.

23. Tiselius HG. Stone incidence and prevention. Braz J Urol 2000;26:452–62.

24. Tiselius HG. Factors influencing the course of calcium oxalate stone disease. Eur Urol 1999;36:363–70.

25. Chandhoke PS. When is medical prophylaxis cost-effective for recurrent calcium stones? J Urol 2002;168:937–40.

98

Endourologic Surgery during Pregnancy

Andrew H. H. Tan, MBChB, FRACS
Darren T. Beiko, MD, FRCSC
Hassan Razvi, MD, FRCSC

The endourologic management of the pregnant patient may pose significant challenges to the urologist. The well-being of 2 patients, both the mother as well as her fetus increases the stress level of all involved. Anatomic and physiologic changes affecting the maternal urinary tract, and the risks associated with anesthesia and radiation have important management implications. Accurate diagnosis and timely intervention are essential in ensuring successful outcomes.

Significant advances in endoscopic instrumentation and intracorporeal lithotripsy devices have expanded the role of diagnostic and therapeutic endourologic procedures in the pregnant patient. This chapter will focus on the contemporary management of urinary tract disease affecting women during pregnancy and the endourologic treatment options available.

PHYSIOLOGIC AND ANATOMIC CHANGES DURING PREGNANCY

Pregnancy is accompanied by a myriad of physiologic and anatomic alterations involving many organ systems. In order to properly manage urologic conditions in the pregnant patient, the urologist should have a general understanding not only of the changes affecting the genitourinary tract, but also those alterations influencing other organ systems. A listing of the most notable changes is presented in Table 98-1.

Various alterations occur involving the urinary system. The increase in kidney size is explained by an increase in renal vascular volume and in the interstitial space, which usually returns to normal by 6 months postpartum. By the third trimester, nearly 90% of women will exhibit some degree of pelvicaliceal and ureteric dilatation.[1] The ureteric dilatation extends down to the sacral promontory, the result of compression of the gravid uterus, although increased levels of maternal estrogen and progesterone leading to ureteric smooth muscle relaxation[2,3] may also play a role. The right ureter is often more dilated, as the left ureter is protected somewhat by the sigmoid colon. The enlarging uterus displaces the bladder anterosuperiorly. The mucosa becomes more congested and hyperemic. The bladder capacity increases and the detrusor is relatively hypotonic with decreased sensation. In the immediate postpartum period, urinary retention may occur, especially if regional anesthesia has been used.[4]

While the levels of creatinine and urea produced during pregnancy are relatively unchanged, the glomerular filtration rate (GFR) may rise up to 50% from the prepregnancy baseline. The serum creatinine and urea values regarded as normal in a nonpregnant woman would therefore represent compromised renal function in a pregnant woman. The increase in GFR is accompanied by an increase in the urinary concentrations of calcium, uric acid, and protein, among other substances. Increased intestinal absorption of calcium owing to placental production of 1,25-dihydroxycholecalciferol further contributes to inducing a relatively hypercalciuric state.[5] Mitigating the tendencies to stone formation, corresponding increases in the filtered load of inhibitors of urolithiasis, such as magnesium, citrate, and glycosaminoglycans[6] are observed. Crystalluria is equally common in pregnancy as it is in nonpregnant women.[7]

A thorough understanding of the changes in homeostasis affecting the pregnant woman as described above is essential to minimize the risks to mother and fetus with any proposed investigation or surgical intervention.

DIFFERENTIAL DIAGNOSIS OF THE ACUTE ABDOMEN IN PREGNANCY

The differential diagnosis of acute abdominal or flank pain in pregnancy is extensive and encompasses various obstetric, general surgical, as well as urologic causes (Table 98-2). The diagnosis may be challenging because of anatomic alterations related to pregnancy, leading to various conditions mimicking one another. Appendicitis, for example, may be confused with pyelonephritis or cholecystitis after the first trimester, when the appendix may be displaced superiorly and away from the abdominal wall.[8]

The overall incidence of nonobstetric surgery during pregnancy is 1:500 deliveries,[9] with appendectomy the most common intervention. (1:1,500–1:6,600 deliveries).[10,11]

SPECIAL CONSIDERATIONS

RADIATION EXPOSURE Discussion about the need to perform radiography imaging during pregnancy is often anxiety- provoking to all parties involved. A thorough discussion outlining the risks involved and the techniques used to mini-

Table 98-1 Physiologic Changes during Pregnancy	
System	Changes during Pregnancy
Respiratory	Hypoxemia[76,77]
	Decreased functional residual capacity
	Hypoventilation
	Increased consumption of oxygen
Cardiovascular	Increased cardiac output[78]
	Increased heart rate and stroke volume
	Decreased systemic vascular resistance[79,80]
	Decreased cardiac output near end of pregnancy[76]
	Decreased venous return
	Decreased hematocrit[81,82]
	Increased blood volume
Hematologic	Hypercoagulable state[83–85]
	Decreased fibrinolytic activity
	Increased factors VII, VIII, and X
	Increased fibrinogen
Gastrointestinal	Decreased gastrointestinal motility[81]
	Relaxation of gastroesophageal sphincter[81]
Genitourinary	
Kidney	Increased size[86]
	Increased renal vascular volume and blood flow
	Hydronephrosis, R > L[87]
	Increased glomerular filtration rate[81]
	Decreased creatinine and blood urea nitrogen[88]
	Increased proteinuria, uricosuria, calciuria, citraturia
Ureter	Hydroureter[83]
	Decreased ureteral peristalsis
Bladder	Displacement superiorly and anteriorly[89]
	Increased bladder capacity[90]
	Decreased sensation/hypotonic bladder[86]
	Mucosal congestion/ hyperemia[86]
Urethra	Squamous metaplasia

Table 98-2 Differential Diagnosis of the Acute Abdomen in Pregnancy

Gynecologic and Obstetric Causes
Ectopic pregnancy
Pelvic Inflammatory disease
Ovarian torsion
Placental abruption
Premature labor
Chorioamnionitis
General Surgical Causes
Appendicitis
Cholecystitis
Intestinal obstruction
Diverticulitis
Gastroenteritis
Hernia (incarcerated internal or inguinal)
Mesenteric lymphadenitis
Pancreatitis
Urologic Causes
Urolithiasis
Pyelonephritis

mize exposure to the fetus is essential. Whenever possible the use of ionizing radiation should be avoided, particularly during the first trimester when fetal tissues are the most susceptible. Clearly, situations exist, however, when use of radiographic imaging is in the best interest of the pregnant patient. The aim of management in these situations should be to deliver the least harmful dose to the mother and fetus while producing an image of useful diagnostic quality.

Ionizing radiation consists of high-energy photons that can generate free radicals and damage cellular DNA when deposited in tissue. The amount of ionizing radiation that is deposited in tissue from radiographs is traditionally measured in rads. The SI unit for ionizing radiation is the gray (Gy), with one Gy equivalent to 100 rads.

Ionizing radiation can produce adverse effects in one of three ways: teratogenesis (malformations of the fetus), carcinogenesis (cancer causing), or mutagenesis (genetic germline alterations). The risk to the fetus depends on both the gestational age and the radiation dose.

Teratogenic damage from ionizing radiation most commonly affects the developing nervous system during the neurologic phase of development in weeks 8 to 17. The recommendation for cumulative exposure is generally set at 5 rads, although the threshold for teratogenesis is believed to be 15 to 20 rads. At over 100 rads, 40% of fetuses will display abnormalities.[12] A summary of teratogenic effects seen at high (> 20 rads) doses of radiation exposure is presented in Table 98-3.

Exposure to doses as small as 1 rad has been linked with a small risk of childhood malignancies, including leukemia. The absolute increase in risk is small: 1 additional case seen per 10,000 patients exposed.[13]

The estimated cumulative doses associated with various radiologic studies are outlined in

Table 98-4. The cumulative exposure of less than 5 rads during pregnancy has not been shown to be associated with an increase in fetal anomalies or miscarriage.

The risks of delaying proper diagnosis and appropriate treatment will almost always outweigh the minor risks posed by low-dose radiation exposure. Proper communication and counseling prior to radiation exposure will do much to alleviate patient anxiety.

ANESTHESIA The potential risks to the fetus from anesthesia for nonobstetric surgery during pregnancy include congenital malformations, spontaneous abortion, and premature labor.[14] It is generally agreed that nonemergency surgery should not be performed during pregnancy, and that the first trimester in particular should be avoided if possible. The most optimal time to perform nonobstetric surgery during pregnancy appears to be in the second trimester, as there is an increased risk of miscarriage in the first trimester,[15] and an increased risk of premature labor in the third trimester.[16]

In general, the drug dosage requirements for locoregional and general anesthesia are decreased during pregnancy. The minimal alveolar concentrations (MAC) for isoflurane and halothane have been found to be reduced during pregnancy in animals,[17] which may be due to the increased level of circulating endogenous opioids and the sedating effect of progesterone,[18,19] Local anesthetic requirements are also reduced during the first trimester of pregnancy.[20] This is probably due to the progesterone-induced enhancement of membrane sensitivity to local anesthetics.[21] As pregnancy progresses, the drug requirements for spinal and epidural anesthesia decrease further owing to the compression of the cerebrospinal space secondary to epidural venous engorgement.

A member of the obstetric team should be present during any surgical intervention to monitor the fetal heart rate and uterine activity. In the postoperative period, fetal monitoring should continue for 24 hours.[22] Nonsteroidal anti-inflammatory drugs should not be used for analgesia owing to their effect on premature closure of the fetal ductus arteriosus.[23]

URINARY TRACT INFECTIONS AND ANTIBIOTIC USE DURING PREGNANCY The prevalence of asymptomatic bacteriuria among pregnant women ranges from 2 to 7%.[24,25] Kass and Zinner report that 20 to 40% of women with bacteriuria will subsequently develop pyelonephritis if untreated,[26,27]

Table 98-4 Estimated Fetal Radiation Doses during Uro-Radiologic Procedures

Examination	Fetal Dose (rads)
Kidneys, ureter, bladder (KUB) radiograph	0.250[92]
Retrograde pyelogram	0.600[93]
Intravenous pyelogram	1.398[94]
Abdominal computed tomogram (CT)	2.600[13]

which has been linked to an increased risk of premature labor and low birth weight.[28,29] As such, screening for asymptomatic bacteriuria is recommended.[30] The incidence of pyelonephritis decreases to 3 to 4% in women who have their bacteriuria treated with antibiotics.[31]

The use of antibiotics in pregnancy must be based on the sensitivities of the target organism, knowledge of the potential for increased drug clearance owing to an increase in maternal GFR, and the risks of fetal toxicity. Table 98-5 outlines the potential toxicity of antibiotics during pregnancy.

In the absence of maternal allergy, a penicillin or cephalosporin is considered safe throughout pregnancy. If either is contraindicated, nitrofurantoin is a reasonably safe substitute, with the main risk being that of hemolytic anemia in women with glucose-6-phosphate dehydrogenase deficiency.

CONDITIONS NECESSITATING ENDOUROLOGIC INTERVENTION

HYDRONEPHROSIS It is often difficult to differentiate between physiologic hydronephrosis in pregnancy and that owing to a pathologic process. Potential etiologies of hydronephrosis during pregnancy are listed in Table 98-6.

Diagnosis of Hydronephrosis Defining the exact cause of hydronephrosis in pregnancy can be challenging. Physiologic hydronephrosis is the most common cause occurring in up to 90% of patients by the end of the third trimester.[32] Physiologic hydronephrosis may result in flank discomfort or mimic renal colic.

Ultrasonography is the most useful initial test in the investigation of acute flank pain in this setting because of the absence of ionizing radiation. However, the accuracy of ultrasound is operator dependent, which may explain some of the inconsistent results reported in the literature. Stothers and Lee reported that ultrasonography for the detection of renal calculi had a false-

Table 98-3 Effects of Significant Radiation Exposure during Pregnancy[91]

Gestational Age	Fetal Effects
2–4 weeks	Dose-related effects are considered all- (lethal) or-nothing (fetus survives, no malformations are present)
4–10 weeks (organogenesis)	Gross malformation, growth retardation, microcephaly
10–17 weeks (neurological development)	Mental retardation, microcephaly; may have sterility and growth retardation as an adult
After 17 weeks gestation	Most dose-related effects rarely, if ever, seen after this time

Table 98-5 Antibiotic Toxicity during Pregnancy[14,29]

Antibiotic	Potential Fetal Toxicity
Penicillins	No known toxicity
Cephalosporins	No known toxicity
Erythromycin	No known toxicity
Sulfonamides	Hyperbilirubinemia
Nitrofurantoin	Possible hemolytic anemia
Aminoglycosides	CNS toxicity, ototoxicity
Tetracycline	Tooth discoloration, inhibition of bone growth
	Maternal hepatic toxicity
Trimethoprim	Interferes with folate metabolism
Quinolones	Damage to developing cartilage
Chloramphenicol	Gray syndrome, aplastic anemia
Isoniazid	Neuropathy, seizures

CNS = central nervous systems.

negative rate of 68%.[33] In a review of 57 pregnant women presenting with renal colic, Butler and colleagues found that ultrasound scanning missed 40% of calculi, which were subsequently confirmed by limited intravenous urography (IVU).[34] In contrast, Parulkar and colleagues reported a sensitivity and specificity of 95.2% and 87%, respectively, for ultrasound scanning as the initial diagnostic modality in 65 pregnant women presenting with renal colic.[35]

In an attempt to distinguish physiologic from pathologic hydronephrosis, MacNeily and colleagues used color-flow Doppler imaging and reported that the ureter distal to the common iliac vessels was found to taper to a normal caliber in patients with physiologic hydronephrosis.[36] The displacement of bowel gas away from the lower ureter by the enlarging uterus, creating an acoustic window, was also found to facilitate visualization of the distal ureter.

Measurement of the mean intrarenal resistive index (RI) and the difference between the affected kidney and the normal contralateral kidney (Δ RI) has also been used to differentiate pathologic versus physiologic hydronephrosis. Hertzberg and colleagues demonstrated that in pregnant women with physiologic hydronephrosis, the RI was the same as in nonpregnant patients without obstruction.[37] The sensitivity and specificity of assessing ureteral obstruction has been reported as 45% and 91%, respectively, using mean RI and 95% and 100% with Δ RI measurement.[38]

The usefulness of transvaginal ultrasound in detecting distal ureteric calculi in pregnant patients where transabdominal ultrasound had failed has also been described.[39]

Table 98-6 Possible Causes of Hydronephrosis during Pregnancy

Physiologic hydronephrosis
Urolithiasis
Sloughed papillae
Blood clot
Polyhydramnios
Postural change
Uterine rotation
Pregnancy with twins

The judicious use of IVU still has a role to play in those clinical situations in which ultrasound has not been helpful. The risks of intravenous contrast and fetal radiation exposure (up to 1.4 rads) need to be weighed against the danger of a delayed or incorrect diagnosis. If an IVU is necessary, a limited 3-shot protocol should be employed, consisting of a scout film, a 15- to 20-minute film, and selected delayed images using appropriate shielding of the fetus.[40]

Although the use of computed tomography (CT) in pregnancy has been described,[41,42] magnetic resonance imaging (MRI) promises to be a more acceptable alternative because of the lack of radiation exposure. To date, no harmful effects have been reported with the use of MR in pregnancy.[43] High-quality images of the urinary tract and adjacent anatomy can be achieved, and image acquisition times have decreased.[44] The MR urogram can be conducted by using heavily weighted T2 pulse sequences to provide static images of the urinary tract, or intravenous gadolinium can be given to produce images comparable to an IVU. Spencer and colleagues prospectively compared MR urography with Doppler ultrasonography and isotope renography in pregnant patients with symptomatic hydronephrosis and found that MRI had the greatest accuracy while also providing additional anatomic information.[45] Limitations of MR urography include the difficulty of detecting ureteral calculi, which appear as flow voids or filling defects on both T2-weighted and contrast-enhanced scans, and relatively poor spatial resolution in comparison with IVU or CT.[46]

UROLITHIASIS Symptomatic renal calculi have been reported in 1 of every 1,500 pregnancies.[47] In 50 to 80% of cases spontaneous stone passage occurs,[48,49] therefore, the initial approach to most patients should be a conservative one, involving adequate pain control and monitoring of uterine contractility.

Indications for intervention in the pregnant patient with a symptomatic stone are the same as in the nonpregnant population. When intervention was indicated, the traditional dogma had been to proceed with temporizing measures, such as ureteral stent or percutaneous nephrostomy tube insertion, with definitive treatment deferred until after delivery. This approach, while minimizing or eliminating the need for anesthesia, is not without drawbacks.

Ureteric Stenting Ureteral stent insertion usually requires some form of anesthesia. Fluoroscopy is ideal; however, exposure must be kept to a minimum by using pulsed imaging and uterine shielding. Ultrasound-guided positioning of ureteral stents has also been described, thus eliminating the need for ionizing radiation entirely.[50,51] Stent discomfort is often heightened in pregnant patients, however, owing to the overactive bladder symptoms that many women experience in the latter stages of pregnancy. The relative hypercalciuria and hyperuricosuria that occurs in pregnancy are associated with an increased risk of stent encrustation. For this reason, stent changes as often as

every 4 to 6 weeks have been advocated by some to avoid this risk.[52–54] One may argue that the risk of repeated exchanges may exceed that of a single definitive procedure.

Percutaneous Nephrostomy Percutaneous nephrostomy (PCN) tube insertion is an option in certain circumstances, such as the septic patient or during the first trimester, eliminating any need for ionizing radiation. A PCN tube can be placed under local anesthetic with ultrasound guidance. PCN tubes are prone, however, to blockage by debris, requiring frequent and inconvenient tube changes. Tube dislodgement can occur, requiring reinsertion. Bacterial colonization is inevitable, increasing the risk of urinary tract infection, although Kavoussi and colleagues found in their series that no patient developed pyelonephritis or lost their pregnancy because of PCN tube drainage.[55]

Ureteroscopy Advances in the design of small-diameter semirigid and flexible ureteroscopes and lithotripsy modalities now permit the option of treating the stone definitively during pregnancy with minimal risk to the mother and fetus. An increasing number of studies have appeared in the literature in recent years advocating the role of ureteroscopy as a safe first-line treatment for urolithiasis in pregnancy (Table 98-7). The use of intravenous sedation using fentanyl and propofol has been reported during ureteroscopy with 7 French (F) endoscopes in pregnant patients.[56] Although the enlarged uterus may distort the course of the ureter, ureteroscopy is not considered to be technically difficult in pregnant women. In most cases, dilatation of the ureteric orifice is not required when using 8F or smaller semirigid or flexible instruments. Moreover, the physiologic dilatation of the ureter seems to aid with the manipulation of flexible ureteroscopes.[57]

Various intracorporeal lithotriptors have been used to treat stones during pregnancy. Despite the lack of documented obstetric complications using these modalities, there are some theoretic concerns that the energies generated by certain intracorporeal lithotripsy devices may pose unrecognized dangers to the fetus.[58] Electrohydraulic lithotripsy, proven to be effective and safe in the nonpregnant patient,[59] generates very high peak pressures[60] and has the least margin of safety of all the intracorporeal devices.[61] Furthermore, the possibility exists that the electrical energy discharged from the probe could precipitate premature labor.[40] Ultrasonic lithotripsy has been shown to be extremely safe to surrounding tissue.[62] The effect of the high-frequency vibratory energy on the fetus is unknown, however, and may pose a risk to the auditory development of the fetus.[63] Although a recent study by Karlsen and colleagues is the first to suggest that the peak pressure of the sound emitted by all modalities of intracorporeal lithotripsy in the ureter during pregnancy is unlikely to be harmful to fetal hearing, the authors recommend caution in extrapolating their in vitro results.[64] Of particular importance, increased distance from the point source resulted in decreased sound intensities for all lithotriptors except ultrasonic lithotripsy.

Table 98-7 Outcome of Ureteroscopic Treatment of Urolithiasis during Pregnancy

Study	No. of Patients	Equipment	Stone-Free Rate	Complicaitons (no. of pts)
Rittenberg and Bagley[95] (1988)	1	7–8F FU, BE	1/1	Nil
Vest and Warden[57] (1990)	2	9F RU, BE	2/2	Nil
Ulvik et al[63] (1995)	13	9.5–11F RU, US, BE	13/13	Fever (3)
				Ureteral perforation (1)
				Premature contractions (1)
Scarpa et al[56] (1996)	13	7–9F RU, BE	10/13	Nil
Carringer et al[96] (1996)	4	7F RU, PDL	4/4	Nil
Shokeir and Mutabagani[97] (1998)	10	9–11.5F RU, BE, forceps, US	7/10	UTI (2)
Lifshitz and Lingeman[98] (2002)	6	6.9 RU, 7.5F FU, BE	6/6	Nil
Watterson et al[70] (2002)	8	6.9 RU, 7.5–8.0F FU, Ho:YAG	6/8	Nil

BE = basket extraction; FU = flexible ureteroscopy; Ho:YAG = holmium laser lithotripsy; PDL = pulsed-dye laser; RU = rigid ureteroscopy; US = ultrasonic lithotripsy; UTI = urinary tract in fection.

Given the aforementioned concerns, devices designed to deliver their energies to a very localized area with minimal or no stray effects, such as the holmium laser, pulsed-dye laser, or pneumatic lithotriptor, are preferred. The safety of all three of these modalities in nonpregnant patients has been well documented.[65–69]

Watterson and colleagues' series of 8 patients treated with holmium laser lithotripsy provides support for its use in pregnancy.[70] They reported an overall stone-free rate of 89% and successful removal of 2 encrusted stents. No maternal or obstetric complications were noted. The safety of holmium laser lithotripsy is a function of its unique wavelength (2,100 nm). The depth of thermal energy is 0.5 to 1 mm from the probe tip, producing very little effect on periureteral tissues.[71] One theoretic risk of holmium laser lithotripsy is related to the production of cyanide as a by-product of laser lithotripsy of uric acid calculi.[72] To date, there have been no reported cases of cyanide toxicity in adults or children.[73] The actual risk of cyanide toxicity is probably minimal given that any cyanide actually produced is likely to be evacuated from the body with the irrigant rather than systemically absorbed.

The risks of ureteroscopy in experienced hands are low, but include perforation and sepsis,[74] both of which have the potential to adversely affect maternal and fetal well-being.

Other Techniques Percutaneous nephrolithotripsy (PCNL) should be deferred until after pregnancy because of the need for prolonged anesthesia in a prone or oblique position, and the greater radiation exposure that is required. Similarly, extracorporeal shock wave lithotripsy (ESWL) is contraindicated because of the potential adverse effects of high-energy shock waves on the fetus. Asgari and colleagues reported on a series of 6 patients who were treated on the Dornier HM3 lithotripter while unknowingly pregnant and found no detectable malformations or chromosomal anomalies in the children.[75]

CONCLUSION

The endourologic management of the pregnant patient requires a sound knowledge of the impor-

tant physiologic and anatomic changes that occur during each stage of pregnancy. Judicious use of diagnostic imaging and adherence to strict indicators for intervention will minimize patient anxiety and increase the chance of a successful outcome for the mother and fetus.

REFERENCES

1. Peake SL, Roxburgh HB, Langlois SL. Ultrasonic assessment of hydronephrosis in pregnancy. Radiology 1983;146:167–70.
2. Harrow BR, Sloane JA, Salhanick L. Etiology of hydronephrosis of pregnancy. Surg Gynecol Obstet 1964;119:1042–8.
3. Robert JA. Hydronephrosis of pregnancy. Urology 1976;8:1–4.
4. Jain S, Arya VK, Gopalan S, Jain V. Analgesic efficacy of intramuscular opioids versus epidural analgesia in labor. Int J Gynaecol Obstet 2003;83:19–27.
5. Gertner JM, Coustan DR, Kliger AS, et al. Pregnancy as a state of physiologic absorptive hypercalciuria. Am J Med 1986;81:451–6.
6. Lindheimer MD, Katz AI. The renal response to pregnancy. In: Brenner BM, Rector RC, editors. The kidney, 2nd ed. Philadelphia: W. B. Saunders; 1981. p. 1762–819.
7. Harris RE, Dunnihoo DR. The incidence and significance of urinary calculi in pregnancy. Am J Obstet Gynecol 1967;99:237–41.
8. Baer JL, Reis RA, Arens RA. Appendicitis in pregnancy with changes in position and axis of the normal appendix in pregnancy. JAMA 1932;98:1359–64..
9. Kammerer WS. Nonobstetric surgery during pregnancy. Med Clin North Am 1979;63:1157–64.
10. Babaknia A, Parsa H, Woodruff JD. Appendicitis during pregnancy. Obstet Gynecol 1977;50:40–4.
11. Horowitz MD, Gomez GA, Santiesteban R, Burkett G. Acute appendicitis during pregnancy: diagnosis and management. Arch Surg 1985;120:1362–7.
12. Hall EJ. Scientific view of low-level radiation risks. Radiographics 1991;11:509–18.
13. Toppenberg KS, Hill DA, Miller DP. Safety of radiographic imaging during pregnancy. Am Fam Physician 1999;59:1813–8.
14. Loughlin KR. Management of urologic problems during pregnancy. Urology 1994;44:159–69.
15. Kammerer WS. Non-obstetric surgery during pregnancy. Med Clin North Am 1979;63:1157–64.
16. Hill LM, Johnson CE, Lee RA. Cholecystectomy in pregnancy. Obstet Gynecol 1975;46:291–3.
17. Palahniuk RJ, Shnider SM, Eger EI 2nd. Pregnancy decreases the requirements for inhaled anesthetic agents. Anesthesiology 1974;41:82–3.
18. Merrymen W, Boiman R, Barnes L, Rothchild I. Progesterone anesthesia in human subjects. J Clin Endocrinol Metab 1954;14:1567–9.
19. Lyrenas S, Nyberg F, Lindberg B, Terenius L. Cerebrospinal fluid activity of dynorphin-converting enzyme at term pregnancy. Obstet Gynecol 1988;72:54–8.
20. Fagraeus L, Urban BJ, Bromage PR. Spread of epidural analgesia in early pregnancy. Anesthesiology 1983;58:184–7.
21. Datta S, Lambert DH, Gregus J, et al. Differential sensitivities of mammalian nerve fibers during pregnancy. Anesth Analg 1983;62:1070–2.
22. Beilin Y. Anesthesia for nonobstetric surgery during pregnancy. Mt Sinai J Med 1998;65:265–70.
23. Heymann MA, Rudolph AM. Effects of acetylsalicylic acid on the ductus arteriosus and circulation in fetal lambs in utero. Circ Res 1976;38:418–22.
24. Krieger JN. Complications and treatment of urinary tract infections during pregnancy. Urol Clin North Am 1986;13:685–93.
25. Lucas MJ, Cunningham FG. Urinary tract infection during pregnancy. Clin Obstet Gynecol 1993;36:855–68.
26. Kass EH. The role of asymptomatic bacteriuria in the pathogenesis of pyelonephritis. In: Quinn EL, Kass EH, editors. Biology of pyelonephritis. Boston: Little, Brown; 1960. p. 399.
27. Zinner SH, Kass EH. Long-term (10 to 14 years) follow-up of bacteriuria of pregnancy. N Engl J Med 1971;285:820–4.
28. Romero R, Oyarzun E, Mazor M, et al. Meta-analysis of the relationship between asymptomatic bacteriuria and preterm delivery/low birth weight. Obstet Gynecol 1989;73:576–82.
29. Schieve LA, Handler A, Hershow R, et al. Urinary tract infection during pregnancy: its association with maternal morbidity and perinatal outcome. Am J Public Health 1994;84:405–10.
30. Gilstrap LC, Ramin SM. Urinary tract infections during pregnancy. Obstet Gynecol Clin North Am 2001;28:581–91.
31. Whalley P. Bacteriuria of pregnancy. Am J Obstet Gynecol 1967;97:732–8.
32. Boridy IC, Maklad N, Sandler CM. Suspected urolithiasis in pregnant women: imaging algorithm and literature review. AJR Am J Roentgenol 1996;167:869–75.
33. Stothers L, Lee LM. Renal colic in pregnancy. J Urol 1992;148:1383–7.
34. Butler EL, Cox SM, Eberts EG, Cunningham FG. Symptomatic nephrolithiasis complicating pregnancy. Obstet Gynecol 2000;96(5 Pt 1):753–6.
35. Parulkar BG, Hopkins TB, Wollin MR, et al. Renal colic during pregnancy: a case for conservative treatment. J Urol 1998;159:365–8.
36. MacNeily AE, Goldenberg SL, Allen GJ, et al. Sonographic visualization of the ureter in pregnancy. J Urol 1991;146:298–301.
37. Hertzberg BS, Carroll BA, Bowie JD, et al. Doppler US assessment of maternal kidneys: analysis of intrarenal resistivity indexes in normal pregnancy and physiologic pelvicaliectasis. Radiology 1993;186:689–92.
38. Shokeir AA, Mahran MR, Abdulmaaboud M. Renal colic in pregnant women: role of renal resistive index. Urology 2000;55:344–7.
39. Laing FC, Benson CB, DiSalvo DN, et al. Distal ureteral calculi: detection with vaginal US. Radiology 1994;192:545–8.
40. Evans HJ, Wollin TA. The management of urinary calculi in pregnancy. Curr Opin Urol 2001;11:379–84.
41. Forsted DH, Kalbhen CL. CT of pregnant women for urinary tract calculi, pulmonary thromboembolism, and acute appendicitis. AJR Am J Roentgenol 2002;178:1285.
42. Ames Castro M, Shipp TD, Castro EE, et al. The use of helical computed tomography in pregnancy for the diagnosis of acute appendicitis. Am J Obstet Gynecol 2001;184:954–7.
43. Grenier N, Pariente JL, Trillaud H, et al. Dilation of the collecting system during pregnancy: physiologic vs obstructive dilation. Eur Radiol 2000;10:271–9.
44. Tang Y, Yamashita Y, Namimoto T. The value of MR urography that uses HASTE sequences to reveal urinary tract disorders. AJR Am J Roentgenol 1996;167:1497–502.
45. Spencer JA, Tomlinson AJ, Weston MJ, Lloyd SN. Early report: comparison of breath-hold MR excretory urography, doppler ultrasound and isotope renography in the evaluation of symptomatic hydronephrosis in pregnancy. Clin Radiol 2000;55:446–53.
46. Hattery RR, King BF. Technique and application of MR urography. Radiology 1995;194:25–7.
47. Drago JR, Rohner TJ Jr, Chez RA. Management of urinary calculi in pregnancy. Urology 1982;20:578–81.
48. Mostwin J. Surgery of the kidney and ureter in pregnancy. In: Marshall F, editor. Operative urology. Philadelphia: W. B. Saunders; 1991. p. 108–13.
49. Lattanzi DR, Cook WA. Urinary calculi in pregnancy. Obstet Gynecol 1980;56:462–6.
50. Wolf MC, Hollander JB, Salisz JA, Kearney DJ. A new technique for ureteral stent placement during pregnancy using endoluminal ultrasound. Surg Gynecol Obstet 1992;175:575–6.
51. Jarrard DJ, Gerber GS, Lyon ES. Management of acute ureteral obstruction in pregnancy utilizing ultrasound-guided placement of ureteral stents. Urology 1993;42:263–8.

52. Denstedt JD, Razvi HA. Management of urinary calculi during pregnancy. J Urol 1992;148(3 Pt 2):1072–5.

53. Borboroglu PG, Kane CJ. Current management of severely encrusted stents associated with a large stone burden. J Urol 2000;164(3 Pt 1):648–50.

54. Goldfarb RA, Neerhut GJ, Lederer E. Management of acute hydronephrosis of pregnancy by ureteral stenting: risk of stone formation. J Urol 1989;141:921–2.

55. Kavoussi LR, Albala DM, Basler JW, et al. Percutaneous management of urolithiasis during pregnancy. J Urol 1992;148(3 Pt 2):1069–71.

56. Scarpa RM, De Lisa AD, Usai E. Diagnosis and treatment of ureteral calculi during pregnancy with rigid ureteroscopes. J Urol 1996;155:875–7.

57. Vest JM, Warden SS. Ureteroscopic diagnosis and treatment of urinary calculi during pregnancy. Urology 1990;35:250–2.

58. Kroovand RL. Stones in pregnancy and children. J Urol 1992;148(3 Pt 2):1076–8.

59. Elashry OM, DiMeglio RB, Nakada SY, et al. Intracorporeal electrohydraulic lithotripsy of ureteral and renal calculi using small caliber (1.9F) electrohydraulic lithotripsy probes. J Urol 1996;156:1581–5.

60. Vorreuther R. New tip design and shock wave pattern of electrohydraulic probes for endoureteral lithotripsy. J Endourol 1993;7:35–43.

61. Knudsen BE, Denstedt JD. Intracorporeal lithotriptors. In: Smith's textbook of endourology 2nd ed. Smith AD, Badlani GH, Bagley DH, et al, editors. St Louis: Quality Medical Publishing. [In print]

62. Howards SS, Merill E, Harris S, Cohn J. Ultrasonic lithotripsy: laboratory evaluations. Invest Urol 1974;11:273–7.

63. Ulvik NM, Bakke A, Hoisaeter PA. Ureteroscopy in pregnancy. J Urol 1995;154:1660–3.

64. Karlsen SJ, Bull-Njaa T, Krokstad A. Measurement of sound emission by endoscopic lithotripters: an in vitro study and theoretical estimation of risk of hearing loss in a fetus. J Endourol 2001;15:821–6.

65. Piergiovanni M, Desgrandchamps F, Cochan-Priollet B, et al. Ureteral and bladder lesions after ballistic, ultrasonic, electrohydraulic, or laser lithotripsy. J Endourol 1994;8:293–9.

66. Grasso M, Chalik Y. Principles and applications of laser lithotripsy: experience with the holmium laser lithotrite. J Clin Laser Med Surg 1998;16:3–7.

67. Watson G, Murray S, Dretler SP, Parrish JA. An assessment of the pulsed dye laser for fragmenting calculi in the pig ureter. J Urol 1987;138:199–202.

68. Denstedt JD, Razvi HA, Rowe E, et al. Investigation of the tissue effects of a new device for intracorporeal lithotripsy—the Swiss Lithoclast. J Urol 1995;153:535–7.

69. Teichman JM, Rao RD, Rogenes VJ, Harris JM. Ureteroscopic management of ureteral calculi: electrohydraulic versus holmium:YAG laser lithotripsy. J Urol 1997;158:1357–61.

70. Watterson JD, Girvan AR, Beiko DT, et al. Ureteroscopy and holmium:YAG laser lithotripsy: an emerging definitive management strategy for symptomatic ureteral calculi in pregnancy. Urology 2002;60:383–7.

71. Johnson DE, Cromeens DM, Price RE. Use of the holmium:YAG laser in urology. Lasers Surg Med 1992;12:353–63.

72. Teichman JM, Vassar GJ, Glickman RD, et al. Holmium:YAG laser lithotripsy: photothermal mechanism converts uric acid calculi to cyanide. J Urol 1998;160:320–4..

73. Teichman JM, Champion PC, Wollin TA, Denstedt JD. Holmium:YAG lithotripsy of uric acid calculi. J Urol 1998;160(6 Pt 1):2130–2.

74. Harmon WJ, Sershon PD, Blute ML, et al. Ureteroscopy: current practice and long-term complications. J Urol 1997;157:28–32.

75. Asgari MA, Safarinejad MR, Hosseini SY, Dadkhah. Extracorporeal shock wave lithotripsy of renal calculi during early pregnancy. BJU Int 1999;84:615–7.

76. Clark SL, Cotton DB, Lee W, et al. Central hemodynamic assessment of normal term pregnancy. Am J Obstet Gynecol 1989;161(6 Pt 1):1439–42.

77. Ueland K, Parer JT. Effects of estrogens on the cardiovascular system of the ewe. Am J Obstet Gynecol 1966;96:400–6.

78. Goodman RP, Killom AP, Brash AR. Prostacyclin production during pregnancy: comparison of production during normal pregnancy and pregnancy complicated by hypertension. Am J Obstet Gynecol 1982;142:817–22.

79. Ueland K, Hansen JM. Maternal cardiovascular hemodynamics. 3. Labor and delivery under local and caudal anesthesia. Am J Obstet Gynecol 1969;103:8–18.

80. Martin C, Varner MW. Physiologic changes in pregnancy: surgical implications. Clin Obstet Gynecol 1994;37:241–55.

81. Lees MM, Taylor SH, Scott DB, Kerr MG. A study of cardiac output at rest throughout pregnancy. J Obstet Gynaecol Br Commonw 1967;74:319–28.

82. Dudley DJ, Cruikshank DP. Trauma and acute surgical emergencies in pregnancy. Semin Perinatol 1990;14:42–51.

83. Hathaway WE, Bonnar J. Perinatal coagulation. New York: Grune & Stratton; 1978. p. 27.

84. Letsky E. The hematological system. In: Hytten F, Chamberlain G, editors. Clinical physiology in obstetrics. Oxford: Blackwell; 1980. p. 43.

85. Barron WM. Medical evaluation of the pregnant patient requiring nonobstetric surgery. Clin Perinatol 1985;12:481–96.

86. Kelton JH, Hirsch J. Venous thromboembolic disorders. In: Burrow GN, Ferris TF, editors. Medical complications during pregnancy, 2nd ed. Philadelphia: W. B. Saunders; 1982.

87. Prowse CM, Gaensler EA. Respiratory and acid-base changes during pregnancy. Anesthesiology 1965;26:381–92.

88. Archer GW Jr, Marx GF. Arterial oxygenation during apnea in parturient women. Br J Anaesth 1974;46:358–60.

89. Hytten FE, Leitch I. The physiology of human pregnancy, 2nd ed. Oxford: Blackwell; 1971.

90. Crabtree EG. Anatomical and functional changes in the urinary tract. In: Crabtree EG. Urological diseases in pregnancy. Boston: Little, Brown; 1942.

91. Harrison BP, Crystal CS. Imaging modalities in obstetrics and gynecology. Emerg Med Clin North Am: 2003;21:711–35.

92. Osei EK, Faulkner K. Fetal doses from radiological examinations. Br J Radiol 1999;72:773–80.

93. Ratnapalan S, Bona N, Koren G; Motherisk Team. Ionizing radiation during pregnancy. Can Fam Physician 2003;49:873–4.

94. Cunningham FG, McDonald PC, Gant NF, et al, editors. Williams obstetrics. 20th ed. Stamford, CT: Appleton and Lange; 1997. p. 1045–57.

95. Rittenberg MH, Bagley DH. Ureteroscopic diagnosis and treatment of urinary calculi during pregnancy. Urology 1988;32:427–8.

96. Carringer M, Swartz R, Johansson JE. Management of ureteric calculi during pregnancy by ureteroscopy and laser lithotripsy. Br J Urol 1996;77:17–20.

97. Shokeir AA, Mutabagani H. Rigid ureteroscopy in pregnant women. Br J Urol 1998;81:678–81.

98. Lifshitz DA, Lingeman JE. Ureteroscopy as a first-line intervention for ureteral calculi in pregnancy. J Endourol 2002;16:19–22.

99

Minimally Invasive Surgical Options for Ureteropelvic Junction Obstruction

Jonathan D. Kaye, MD

Paulos Yohannes, MD

Michael C. Ost, MD

INTRODUCTION

The popularity of minimally invasive surgical techniques has increased markedly among urologists in recent years. The entity of ureteropelvic junction (UPJ) obstruction has benefited spectacularly from these advances. Minimally invasive therapies including laparoscopic and robotic pyeloplasty, percutaneous endopyelotomy, a combination of the two known as endopyeloplasty and retrograde endopyelotomy (which includes laser incision of UPJ as well as Acucise), have all established their rightful place in the treatment of this anatomical problem. The benefits of shorter hospital stays, fewer postoperative pain requirements, and faster convalescence cannot be ignored.

This chapter is meant as a guide to the urologist to direct his or her patients to the most appropriate treatment modality. Technical aspects of each modality are addressed elsewhere in this text.

Although endopyelotomy has been used regularly and effectively for nearly 20 years,[1] sizeable series on laparoscopic—and more recently, robotic—pyeloplasty have amassed over the last decade, demonstrating superb results.[2] Although we will focus mainly on endopyelotomy and laparoscopic pyeloplasty, other treatment modalities will also be considered when appropriate.

Although new minimally invasive technologies such as endopyeloplasty continue to show promise,[3] success rates for endourological procedures will ultimately depend on the absence or presence of definitive clinical variables. A stenotic UPJ segment greater than 2 cm, massive hydronephosis, and poor renal function, for example, have proven to be poor prognostic factors when endopyelotomy has been used.[4] Under these clinical circumstances, patients may be better served with either a laparoscopic or robotic pyeloplasty or laparoscopic nephrectomy if ipsilateral renal function is less than 15 to 20%.

Modern-day laparoscopic pyeloplasty series have demonstrated success rates exceeding 95%.[5] In this regard, prognostic indicators for failure have not been readily identified. Failure has most often been a function of poor technique, especially during earlier cases in larger

series. In view of this, it is surprising that concerns over the influence of crossing vessels on UPJ obstruction repair outcomes have led to an intense focus on preoperative planning with sophisticated imaging.

PATIENT SELECTION AND PROGNOSTIC FACTORS

OVERALL SUCCESS RATES Both primary and secondary cases of UPJ obstruction can be successfully treated endoscopically. Cumulative success rates for endopyelotomy of 62 to 94% for primary obstruction and 67 to 100% for secondary obstruction have been achieved[6-16] (Table 99-1).

Although Desai and colleagues have achieved 93 to 100% success at 20-month follow-up with endopyeloplasty (Figure 99-1A and B), these results have not yet been replicated by other investigators. This may result from the technical demands inherent to percutaneous, endoscopic suturing of the pelvis in Heineke-Mikulicz fashion. Tearing of the mucosa and underlying muscle layers is a common problem.[17]

Initially, retrograde ureteroscopic endopyelotomy gained significant momentum. However, the modest long-term durability of these repairs has quelled urologists' enthusiasm for them in favor of other minimally invasive approaches. Holmium:YAG laser is frequently used to incise the renal pelvis ureteroscopically, with success rates ranging from 55 to 85%.[18-22] The overall success, reoperation, and complication rates of Acucise are similar, though slightly inferior to retrograde laser endopyelotomy. In a recent prospective, randomized, head-to-head comparison of these two technologies, el-Nahas and colleagues found the retrograde holmium laser endopyelotomy to be 85% effective, as compared with 65% for the Acucise, whereas the complication rate was 25% versus 10%, respectively.[18]

Given these data, no urologist should promote retrograde approach to a UJP obstruction as a definitive—or risk-free—proposition. Specific risks and contraindications are outlined below. Additionally, all of the perils of any uretroscopic procedure (ie, ureteral and urethral structure and ureteral avulsion) apply to these techniques.

However, in skilled hands, the risk of any significant urinary tract trauma is acceptable, and the benefits are numerous: Patients have a smaller chance of significant bleed, are left with no hole in their kidney (or its attendant problems), have no skin scar, and undergo the procedure on an ambulatory basis. Thus, it may be reasonable to offer a retrograde approach as a first resort, especially to those patients with mild or asymptomatic UPJ obstructions who understand that reoperation is a real possibility.

Laparoscopic and robotic pyeloplasty are both extremely effective and safe, rivaling and even exceeding open pyeloplasty in virtually every parameter. Rubinstein and Gill have even demonstrated the feasibility of outpatient laparoscopic pyeloplasty.[23] Once these modalities are chosen for a given renal unit, the decision of whether or not to approach the renal pelvis transperitoneally or retroperitoneally should depend on surgeon comfort level and training, the patient's body habitus, and the postsurgical status of the patient's abdomen (Tables 99-2 and 99-3). Minimally invasive pyeloplasty is only slightly less effective for secondary UPJ obstruction (83–95%) than for primary obstruction (92–100%).[16,24–26]

Like its laparoscopic cousin, robotic pyeloplasty has proven extremely safe and effective thus far, though its data are even more nascent. In both pediatric and adult series, success rates approaching perfection have been published, with decreased length of hospital stay, narcotics requirements, and blood loss as compared with open pyeloplasty.[27–33] In one of the largest single-

Table 99-1 Success Rates in Recent Endopyelotomy Series		
Study	Follow-Up (months)	Success Rate (%)
Pardalidis et al, 2002	53.8	92.8
Lam et al,[40] 2003	37	81.3
Albani et al,[21] 2004	22	63.3
Knudsen et al, 2004	55	65 (primary)
		74 (secondary)
Ost et al,[16] 2005	16	92 (primary)
		58 (secondary)

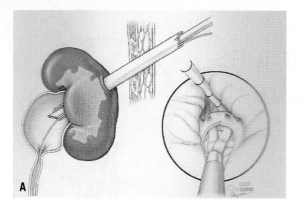

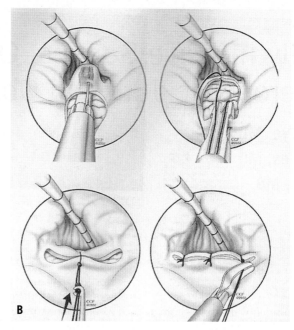

Figure 99-1 *A*, Endopyeloplasty. Standard percutaneous renal access is achieved through upper- or mid-pole renal calix to perform conventional lateral full-thickness endopyelotomy. Inset, 5 mm laparoscopic endoshears are inserted through working channel of 26F nephroscope to mobilize ureteral incision distal edge in preparation for endopyeloplasty suturing.[5] *B*, Endopyeloplasty.

surgeon series to date, Patel reports greater than 96% success with robotic-assisted laparoscopic dismembered pyeloplasty.[33]

An algorithm is proposed below for determining the best treatment modality for a given UPJ obstruction (Figure 99-2). Ost and colleagues recently published a comparison of the treatments for UPJ obstruction regarding morbidity, effectiveness, and cost, as shown in Tables 99-4, 99-5, and 99-6.[16]

It should be noted that the small sample sizes illustrated in Table 4 may have produced sampling error, as authors have historically noted significant differences in outcomes between any given group of 20 or 30 patients. To wit, although Gupta's study of 401 antegrade endopyelotomies reported an overall success rate of 85%, any group of 25 consecutive patients had results varying between 60 and 95%.[4,34]

In patients undergoing reoperation, previous scarring may complicate the determination of the proper depth and length of the incision. In this situation, direct visualization of the incision site is preferable, as it must be sufficiently deep and long to visualize the more distal ureteral segments (Figure 99-3). Acucise, therefore, should not be strongly considered as a therapy for secondary UPJ obstruction, as this modality does not permit direct visualization.

LENGTH OF STRICTURE Long avascular strictures (> 1.5 cm), total obliteration of the UPJ, and severe periureteral fibrosis are clear contraindications to antegrade and retrograde procedures. Overall results in this situation have proven unsatisfactory.[35–37] There is little question that these patients are best served by laparopscopic or robotic pyeloplasty.

CROSSING VESSELS AND HYDRONEPHROSIS The significance of vessels crossing the UPJ remains a matter of debate, and their role in the pathogenesis of obstruction and hydronephrosis, as well as

their influence on the results of various endourologic procedures, are controversial.

The mere presence of a crossing vessel close to the UPJ does not mean that it is the primary cause of the UPJ obstruction. Sampaio and Favorito showed that 71% of kidneys will have a vessel (artery or vein) crossing within 1.5 cm of the UPJ, many of which supply significant renal parenchyma.[38,39]

Whatever the etiology, however, data indicate that a severely dilated renal pelvis has a negative influence on the results of endopyelotomy.[40] The success rate for endopyelotomy decreases from an overall success rate of 81 to 96% for those with mild or moderate hydronephrosis to 39 to 54% when high-grade hydronephrosis was present. This trend may be even more pronounced in the presence of a crossing vessel. Van Cangh and colleagues attained a 95% endopyelotomy success rate when there was no crossing vessel and only a moderate degree of hydronephrosis, as compared with a 39% success rate when a crossing vessel was associated with high-grade hydronephrosis.[4,34,41,42]

On the other hand, Gupta and Smith reported an overall 85% success rate for antegrade endopyelotomy in 401 patients, the largest series reported to date.[4,34] A crossing vessel was found in only 13 of 54 patients during open exploration,

and thus could only possibly be the cause of failed antegrade endopyelotomy in 4% of patients. The most common findings at exploration were severe extrinsic fibrosis at the UPJ, as well as severe hydronephrosis.

Thus, in cases when the crossing vessel is thought to be the primary cause of UPJ obstruction and hydronephrosis, what procedure should be performed? A possible solution is that antegrade and retrograde procedures can address intrinsic factors of obstruction, but cannot correct extrinsic factors or reduce the size of a massively dilated renal pelvis. In such cases, laparoscopic, robotic, or even open dismembered pyeloplasty have yielded success rates exceeding 95%.[43,44] However, the mere presence of a crossing vessel by no means contraindicates an endopyelotomy, as this modality enables visualization—and thereby avoidance—of pulsating vessels. But unlike endopyelotomy, laparoscopic and robotic pyeloplasty enables the surgeon to not only visualize and avoid, but also actually circumvent a crossing vessel. Because of the importance of direct visualization in the case of crossing vessels, Acucise is probably ill advised under this circumstance.

RENAL FUNCTION Renal function is a significant prognostic factor. A high risk of endopyelotomy failure has been reported when the function of the affected kidney is greatly impaired.[4,34,40,45–47] Preoperative high-grade hydronephrosis as well

Table 99-2 Transperitoneal Laparoscopic Pyeloplasty			
Study	Renal Units	Follow-Up (months)	Success Rate (%)
Chen et al, 1998	57	13	100
Janetschek et al, 2000	67	25	98
Jarrett et al,[26] 2002	100	31	96
Turk et al,[44] 2002	49	23.2	97.7
Inaguki et al	147	24	95
Ost et al,[16] 2005	29 (1°)	16	100 (1°)
	21 (2°)	16	95 (2°)
Table courtesy of Dr. Michael C. Ost.[16]			

Table 99-3 Retroperitoneal Laparoscopic Pyeloplasty			
Study	Renal Units	Follow-Up (mo)	Success Rate (%)
Ben Slama et al, 2000	15	16.6	100
Eden et al, 2001	50	18.8	98
Soulie et al, 2001	55	14.4	89
Table courtesy of Dr. Michael C. Ost.[16]			

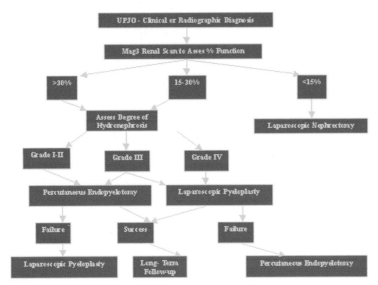

Figure 99-2 Algorithm for electing laparoscopic/robotic pyeloplasty vs endopyelotomy[16]

as poor renal function are significant causes of endopyelotomy failure,[4,34] but anecdotally have only a modest impact on the success of laparoscopic and robotic pyeloplasty. Unfortunately, the isolated impact of this factor is difficult to assess, because no prospective data have been collected. In most series, preoperative function of the involved kidney has been systematically assessed only recently or in selected cases, and its influence cannot be dissociated from that of the degree of hydronephrosis. Nevertheless, Gupta and colleagues reported that of the 205 patients with known renal function who underwent endopyelotomy at a single institution, success rates for endopyelotomy were 92%, 80%, and 54% for good renal function (differential renal function greater than 40%), moderate renal function (differential renal function between 25 and 40%), and poor renal function (differential renal function less than 25%), respectively.[4,34] These data support laparoscopic or robotic pyeloplasty as the modality of choice in renal units with differential function of less than 40%. Nephrectomy is the treatment of choice if the differential renal function falls below 15%, as no treatment modality offers any real chance of functional recovery in this situation.

AGE AND SEX OF THE PATIENT AND THE SIDE OF OBSTRUCTION
Currently, the role of endopyelotomy and other antegrade and retrograde procedures remains unclear in the pediatric population,

as the data are limited for this patient group.[48–56] Many younger children have long proximal ureteral strictures, especially in the proximal one-third of the ureter. In addition, their ureters are of small caliber, requiring small stents. Both these reasons make endopyelotomy challenging in young children. In addition, narrow-lumen stents in young children obstruct easily.

However, the pediatric population may be the most important group to focus on when analyzing the benefits of new technology for the treatment of UPJ obstruction. Similar to adult cohorts, laparoscopic pyeloplasties in three pediatric series have demonstrated success rates from 87 to 100%. The dismembered pyeloplasty has been deemed the ultimate challenge in pediatric urological laparoscopy, as fine suturing with small instrumentation is required. Robotics may aid the pediatric urologist in this demanding operation, serving as a model for the adult urologist wishing to acquire better laparoscopic suturing skills. Future prospective and well-stratified studies in the pediatric population may give us a clearer view of the effect of pneumoperitoneum, pneumoretroperitoneum, and laparoscopy on renal development and functionality over time.

In secondary cases of pediatric UPJ obstruction, such as failures of pyeloplasty, endopyelotomy can be a reasonable option. Furthermore, with further refinements and miniaturization of equipment, it may ultimately become a preferred option, especially in children older than 5 years old.

In elderly patients, endopyelotomy offers results comparable with those in the younger

adult group[57,58] although the indications to address a geriatric UPJ obstruction become fewer and farther between as a patient ages. Not surprisingly, neither the sex of the patient nor the side of the obstruction per se influences the outcome of antegrade endopyelotomy[4,34] endopyeloplasty. However, retrograde endopyelotomy and Acucise are not well suited toward very muscular individuals over whose psoas muscle ureteroscopic navigation can prove difficult and dangerous. On the other hand, the large amount of perirenal fat in obese individuals can complicate laparoscopic access to the kidney, making antegrade or retrograde approach ideal for these patients.

HORSESHOE KIDNEY Many of the tools in the endourologist's armamentarium can be used to treat UPJ obstruction in a horseshoe kidney. Although endopyelotomy is feasible, safe, and effective in a horseshoe kidney, the presence of this anatomic variant, especially when coexisting with other aberrant anatomy, should occasion serious entertainment of a laparoscopic or robotic procedure. Such an approach not only obviates all of the dangers of a blind puncture into uncertain anatomy, but it also enables division of the isthmus, if indicated.

Horseshoe kidney, as well as previous intestinal diverting procedures, may cause aberrant renal-intestinal anatomic relationships. Thus, if these patients are treated with endopyelotomy, they are at higher risk for a transcolonic needle placement. This fact need not preclude endopyelotomy in these patients, but rather necessitates that patients be carefully selected and technique be modified. The access tract is virtually perpendicular to the plane of the back, in a paraspinous, medial position. The surgeon must also consider that a more medial insertion site is uncomfortable for the patient who invariably lies supine after the procedure, and can lead to compression and kinking of the external portion of the nephrostomy tube into the back. A subcostal approach lowers the risk of pneumothorax. Puncture of anterior calices is required only if access to the posterior calices is not possible. Access from an anterior calix to the renal pelvis is very difficult because of the inherent difficulty in directing a wire backward. Direct puncture of the renal pelvis should also be avoided, owing to the significant risk of injury to the posterior branch of the renal artery.

The role of endopyelotomy in cases of horseshoe kidney was first described by Nakamura and colleagues.[58] They reported successful results in 3 patients, including 1 in whom open primary

Table 99-4 Success Rate of Various Minimally Invasive Technologies at a Single Institution[16]

Primary Laparoscopic Pyeloplasty	(29 of 29) 100%
Primary Percutaneous Antegrade Endopyelotomy	(35 of 38) 92%
Secondary Laparoscopic Pyeloplasty	(20 of 21) 95%
Secondary Percutaneous Antegrade Endopyelotomy	(7 of 12) 58%
Endopyeloplasty	(2 of 5) 40%

Table 99-5 Laparoscopic Pyeloplasty vs Percutaneous Endopyelotomy[16]

	Prim Perc Endopyelotomy	Prim Lap Pyeloplasty	Stat Diff (Stud T Test)
Avg Age (yrs)	44.6 ± 15/6	37.9 ± 14.8	
Avg EBL (cc)	152.1 ± 112.8	108.3 ± 109.4	No ($p = 0.80$)
Avg Hospital Stay (days)	2.5 ± 1.0	2.6 ± 0.9	No ($p = 0.60$)
Avg Preop Creatinine	1.2 ± 0.7	1.1 ± 0.4	No ($p = 0.72$)
Avg Postop Creatine	1.2 ± 0.7	1.0 ± 0.4	No ($p = 0.62$)

Tab;e 99-6 Cost of Various UPJ Obstruction Treatment Options	
Procedure	Cost (2003 US $)
Ureteroscopic Endopyelotomy	2,891
Acucise	4,427
Antegrade Endopyelotomy	5,297
Laparoscopic Pyeloplasty	7,026
Open Pyeloplasty	7,119

pyeloplasty and isthmus division failed. In addition, 2 patients had associated renal calculi that were extracted at endopyelotomy. Bellman and Yamaguchi advocated more posterior, medial, and inferior access to the horseshoe kidney and the use of longer instruments.[59] Antegrade percutaneous renal access can also be obtained anteriorly or posteriorly under direct laparoscopic guidance. Jabbour and colleagues reported their experience in 4 patients with horseshoe kidney who underwent percutaneous antegrade endopyelotomy in the standard fashion.[60] At 2 months, endopyelotomy failed in 1 of the 4 patients, and subsequently ileal interposition was performed. The other 3 patients remain symptom-free to this date. Similar successful results were reported by Koikawa and colleagues.[61]

CONCOMITANT STONES Laparoscopic pyeloplasty with concomitant pyelolithotomy has emerged as a popular mode of treatment for instances of nephrolithiasis with a UPJ obstruction. Although series reporting on this approach are few and demonstrate prolonged operative times, the feasibility of this technique has been demonstrated. As more urologists become adept at laparoscopy and robotics, so too will the number of successful procedures performed.

In the largest such series to date, Inagaki performed 22 simultaneous laparoscopic pyeloplasty and lithotomy for concomitant UPJ obstruction and nephrolithiasis. Ninety percent (20 of 22) of these renal units were deemed stone free with intact UPJs.[2] At our institution, we evaluate the extent of edema at the UPJ if repair is anticipated at the time of percutaneous nephrolithotomy. If there is no edema, endopyelotomy is performed. However, the stone should

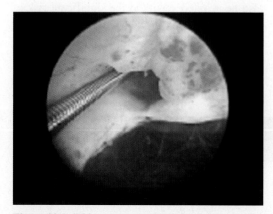

Figure 99-3 Wide open ureter following antegrade incision of UPJ. Note perivesical fat on bottom right.

be removed before the endopyelotomy so that stone fragments, irrigant, and contrast do not migrate into the peripyeloureteral tissue. Conversely, the presence of edema calls for reevaluation of the UPJ with a functional study once all stones have been cleared and the edema has subsided. A UPJ "obstruction" in the presence of nephrolithiasis may be a result of inflammation and edema that will subside following removal of calculus. One must be wary that immediate laparoscopic pyeloplasty with concomitant pyelolithotomy may risk an unnecessary UPJ repair. Similarly, retrograde approach to UPJ obstruction with calculus does not permit the same evaluation, as the approach itself may cause edema. More importantly, retrograde fragmentation and removal of stones will cause retroperitoneal extravasation of fragments at the time of endopyelotomy, which can result in significant retroperitoneal desmoplasia and fibrosis.

PREOPERATIVE EVALUATION

DIAGNOSIS In many patients, the diagnosis is obvious when the patient presents with flank pain, often aggravated by fluid intake, and when urography reveals obstruction at the UPJ. In such circumstances, other diagnostic measures are not indicated. In equivocal cases, such as incidentally discovered hydronephrosis, diuretic renograms, diuretic urograms, or Whitaker pressure-perfusion tests are obtained. The patient's anatomy should be such that the chosen modality is practical and safe. Because of the questionable significance of crossing vessels, the issue of whether to seek them out with preoperative imaging remains a question of debate.

OBTAINING INFORMED CONSENT When counseling a patient, the surgeon may begin by outlining the concept of open pyeloplasty and its goals, and then explain the minimally invasive permutation thereof. The patient should be counseled regarding the risks and benefits of the chosen procedure, including the fact that the success rate of any antegrade and retrograde approach, such as percutaneous or retrograde endopyelotomy, may be less than that of standard open, laparoscopic or robotic pyeloplasty. In advising patients, it is important to consider factors such as age, sex, associated pathology, previous renal surgery, the availability of equipment and resources, whether or not a nephrostomy tube is already in position, the surgeon's experience, and cost. Preoperative expectations undoubtedly bear heavily on a patient's perception of overall postoperative success.

COMPLICATIONS AND CONTRAINDICATIONS

HEMORRHAGE Untreated coagulopathy is contraindicated in all endourologic treatments of UPJ obstruction, especially those requiring percutaneous approach. Bleeding may result from traumatized renal parenchyma or injury to a per-

inephric vessel. However, because the renal parenchyma in patients with UPJ obstruction is generally thinner than that in patients with normal kidneys, and because the collecting system is dilated, this risk seems to be less than in the general population of stone patients undergoing percutaneous manipulation.

Transfusion rates in antegrade endopyelotomy range between 2 and 5%.[51,62–65] While low, they are nonetheless significantly higher than that of other minimally invasive treatment modalities. This difference likely results from the fact that most bleeding comes from the percutaneous, transparanchymal approach to the UPJ, rather than from the actual incision of the UPJ.

A vessel crossing the UPJ can act not only as a contributor to failure of endourologic approaches, but also as a potential source of serious complications.[66,67] Vascular complications of antegrade and retrograde endopyelotomy can be significant, and they remain an important concern to urologists. Careful visual inspection of the operative site to direct the incision away from pulsating vessels is strongly advocated with direct visual endourologic approaches, and is indeed a recognized advantage of endoscopic versus fluoroscopic techniques, such as Acucise.[68]

There is debate as to whether laparoscopic and robotic approaches deal more safely with crossing vessels than other endourologic modalities. Not only can the vessels be pushed aside and transposed, but attempts at repair can be made before ligation, whereas a crossing vessel injured at endopyelotomy will often require selective embolization. However, there is no evidence that laparoscopy or robotics is safer than antegrade endopyelotomy in a solitary kidney.

INFECTION Infection is a risk of any urinary tract manipulation. Regardless of the treatment modality, attempts should be made to sterilize the urinary tract before any procedure is performed, and to avoid instrumentation of an infected system. Active sepsis absolutely contraindicates all procedures other than efforts to expeditiously drain an obstructed system.

Surgeon preference varies significantly with respect to pre- and postoperative antibiotics, and data on this issue are scant. However, common sense dictates the benefit of antibiotics in the immediate pre- and postoperative period, irrespective of the specific procedure performed. Consideration can also be given to the use of prophylactic antibiotics while the endopyelotomy stent or JJ is indwelling for the month following the procedure, especially in women who are more prone to bacteruria.

CONCLUSION

During the past 20 years, the development of new techniques and instrumentation has, in many ways, obviated the need for more invasive surgeries. To be sure, the indications for an open pyeloplasty in this age of antegrade and retrograde, laparoscopic and robotic options are few.

It is of utmost importance to achieve high success rates when treating primary UPJ obstruction. Secondary minimally invasive repairs are technically demanding and with the exception of a few studies, have traditionally demonstrated poorer success rates.[1,2] This reality underscores the importance of subjecting each patient to the treatment modality best suited to his or her particular UPJ obstruction.

Despite the overwhelming success rates of endopyelotomy, laparoscopic pyeloplasty, and even retrograde approaches to UPJ obstruction, it is puzzling that the majority of urologists, when surveyed, are more likely to offer an open pyeloplasty as a first-line therapy in the treatment of UPJ obstruction.[3,4] Perhaps wider distribution of standardized treatment algorithms will emphasize the efficacy of the antegrade and retrograde and laparoscopic modalities available for UPJ obstruction, and thereby popularize them in widespread practice.

Minimally invasive therapies for the management of UPJ obstruction outright challenge the standard open surgical approach to this entity as a new gold standard. In skilled hands, highly successful outcomes can be expected when either antegrade or retrograde endopyelotomy or laparoscopic or robotic pyeloplasty is used to treat a primary UPJ obstruction. In the instance of a UPJ obstruction associated with a high degree of hydronephrosis, patients are better served with a laparoscopic or robotic pyeloplasty. Sophisticated preoperative imaging with CT angiography as an aggressive approach to identify crossing vessels is probably unwarranted, as the influence of this entity on outcome is questionable. To maximize a successful outcome, treatment decisions should be based on patient characteristics, and appropriate referrals should be made based on surgeon comfort level with various procedures.

REFERENCES

1. Karlin G, Badlani G, Smith AD. Endopyelotomy versus open pyeloplasty; comparison in 88 patients. J Urol 1988;140: 476–8.
2. Inagaki T, Rha KH, Ong AM, et al. Laparoscopic pyeloplasty: current status. BJU Int 2005;95 Suppl 2:102–5.
3. Desai MM, Desai MR, Gill IS. Endopyeloplasty versus endopyelotomy versus laparoscopic pyeloplasty for Primary uretopelvic junction obstruction. Urology 2004;64:16–21.
4. Gupta M, Tuncay OL, Smith AD. Open surgical exploration after failed endopyelotomy: a 12-year perspective. J Urol 1997;157:613–8.
5. Jarett TW, Chan DY, Charambura TC, et al. Laparoscopic pyeloplasty: the first 100 cases. J Urol 2002;167:1253–6.
6. Gupta M, Tuncay OL, Smith AD. Open surgical exploration after failed endopyelotomy: a 12-year perspective. J Urol 1997;157:1613–9.
7. Cuzin B, Abbar M, Dawahra M, et al. [100 endopyelotomies percutaneous. Techniques, indication, results.] Prog Urol 1992;2:559–69.
8. Meretyk I, Meretyk S, Clayman RV. Endopyelotomy: comparison of ureteroscopic retrograde and antegrade percutaneous techniques. J Urol 1992;148:775–83.
9. Perez LM, Friedman RM, Carson CC 3rd. Endoureteropyelotomy in adults. Urology 1992;39:71–6.
10. Kletscher BA, Segura JW, LeRoy AJ, Patterson DE. Percutaneous antegrade endoscopic pyelotomy: review of 50 consecutive cases. J Urol 1995;153:701–3.
11. Combe M, Gelet A, Abdelrahim AF, et al. Ureteropelvic

12. Gill HS, Liao JC. Pelvi-ureteric junction obstruction treated with Acucise retrograde endopyelotomy. Br J Urol 1998; 82:8–11.
13. Danuser H, Hochreiter WW, Ackerman DK, Studer UE. Influence of stent size on the success of antegrade endopyelotomy for primary ureteropelvic junction obstruction: results of 2 consecutive series. J Urol 2001;166:902–9.
14. Conlin MJ, Bagley DH. Ureteroscopic endopyelotomy at a single setting. J Urol 1998;159:727–31.
15. Van Cangh PJ, Nesa S, Tombal B. The role of endourology in ureteropelvic junction obstruction. Curr Urol Rep 2001; 2:149–53.
16. Ost MC, Kaye JD, Guttman MJ, et al. Laparoscopic pyeloplasty versus antegrade endopyelotomy: comparison in 100 patients and a new algorithm for the minimally invasive treatment of ureteropelvic junction obstruction. Urology 2005;66:47–51.
17. Desai MM, Desai MR, Gill IS. Endopyeloplasty versus endopyelotomy versus laparoscopic pyeloplasty for primary uretopelvic junction obstruction. Urology 2004; 64:16–21.
18. el-Nahas AR, Shoma AM, Eraky I, et al. Prospective, randomized comparison of ureteroscipic endopyelotomy using holmium:YAG laser and balloon catheter. J Urol 2006;175:614–8.
19. Nakada S. Acucise endopyelotomy. Urology 2000;55:277–82.
20. Mendez-Torez FR, Urena R, Thomas R. Retrograde ureteroscopic endopyelotomy. Urol Clin N Am 2004;31:99–106.
21. Albani JM, Yost AJ, Streem SB. Ureteropelvic junction obstruction: determining durability of endourological intervention. J Urol 2004;171(2 Pt 1):579–82.
22. Matan SF, Yost A, Streem SB. Ureteroscopic laser endopyelotomy: a single center experience. J Endourol 2003;17: 401–4.
23. Rubinstein M, Finelli A, Moinzadeh A, et al. Outpatient laparoscopic pyeloplasty. Urology 2005;66:41–3.
24. Sundaram CP, Grubb RL 3rd, Rehman J, et al. Laparoscopic pyeloplasty for secondary ureteropelvic junction obstruction. J Urol 2003;169:2037–40.
25. Siqueira TM Jr, Nadu A, Kuo RL, et al. Laparoscopic treatment for ureteropelvic junction obstruction. Urology 2002;60:973–8.
26. Jarrett TW, Chan DY, Charambura TC, et al. Laparoscopic pyeloplasty: the first 100 cases. J Urol 2002;167:1253–6.
27. Palese MA, Stifelman MD, Munver M, et al. Robot-assisted laparoscopic dismembered pyeloplasty: a combined experience. J Endourol 2005;19:382–6.
28. Peschel R, Neururer R, Bartsch G, Gettman MT. Robotic pyeloplasty: technique and results. Urol Clin N Am 2004;31:737–41.
29. Gettman MT, Neururer R, Bartsch G, Peschel R. Anderson-Hynes dismembered pyeloplasty performed using the da Vinci robotic system. Urology 2002;60:509–13.
30. Lee RS, Retik AB, Borer JG, Peters CA. Pediatric robot-assisted laparoscopic dismembered pyeloplasty: comparison with a cohort of open surgery. J Urol 2006;175:683–7.
31. Atug F, Woods M, Burgess SV, et al. Robotic assisted laparoscopic pyeloplasty in children. J Urol 2005;174(4 Pt 1): 1440–2.
32. Atug F, Castle EP, Burgess SV, Thomas R. Concomitant management of renal calculi and pelvi-ureteric junction obstruction with robotic laparoscopic surgery. BJU Int 2005;96:1365–8.
33. Patel V. Robotic-assisted laparoscopic dismembered pyeloplasty. Urology 2005;66:45–9.
34. Gupta M, Smith AD. Crossing vessels at the ureteropelvic junction: do they influence endopyelotomy outcome? J Endourol 1996;10:183–7.
35. Motola JA, Badlani GH, Smith AD. Results of 212 consecutive endopyelotomies: an 8-year follow up. J Urol 1993; 149:453–6.
36. Rodrigues Netto N Jr, Ikari O, Esteves SC, D'Ancona CA. Antegrade endopyelotomy for pelvi-ureteric junction obstruction in children. Br J Urol 1996;78:607–12.
37. Preminger GM, Clayman RV, Nakada SY, et al. A multicenter clinical trial investigating the use of a fluoroscopically controlled cutting balloon catheter for the management of ureteral and ureteropelvic junction obstruction. J Urol 1997;157:1625–9.
38. Sampaio FJ. The dilemma of the crossing vessel at the ureteropelvic junction: precise anatomic study. J Endourol 1996;10:411–5.

39. Sampaio FJ, Favorito LA. Ureteropelvic junction stenosis: vascular anatomical background for endopyelotomy. J Urol 1993;150:1787–91.
40. Lam JS, Cooper KL, Greene TD, Gupta M. Impact of hydronephrosis and renal function on treatment outcome: antegrade versus retrograde endopyelotomy. Urology 2003;61:1107–12.
41. Van Cangh PJ, Wilmart JF, Opsomer RJ, et al. Long-term results and late recurrence after endoureteropyelotomy: a critical analysis of prognostic factors. J Urol 1994; 151:934–7.
42. Van Cangh PJ, Nesa S, Galeon M, et al. Vessels around the ureteropelvic junction: significance and imaging by conventional radiology. J Endourol 1996;10:111–9.
43. Parkin J, Evans S, Kumar PV, et al. Endoluminal ultrasonography before retrograde endopyelotomy: can the results match laparoscopic pyeloplasty? BJU Int 2003;91:389–91.
44. Turk IA, Davis JW, Winkelmann B, et al. Laparoscopic dismembered pyeloplasty—the method of choice in the presence of an enlarged renal pelvis and crossing vessels. Eur Urol 2002;42:268–75.
45. Danuser H, Ackermann DK, Bohlen D, Studer UE. Endopyelotomy for primary ureteropelvic junction obstruction: risk factors determine the success rate. J Urol 1998;159:56-61.
46. Kavoussi LR, Albala DM, Clayman R. Outcome of secondary open surgical procedure in patients who failed primary endopyelotomy. Br J Urol 1993;72:157–60.
47. Kapoor R, Zaman W, Kumar A, Srivastava A. Endopyelotomy in poorly functioning kidney: is it worthwhile? J Endourol 2001;15:725–8.
48. Rodrigues Netto N Jr, Ikari O, Esteves SC, D'Ancona CA. Antegrade endopyelotomy for pelvi-ureteric junction obstruction in children. Br J Urol 1996;78:607–12.
49. Figenshau RS, Clayman RV. Endourologic options for management of ureteropelvic junction obstruction in the pediatric patient. Urol Clin N Am 1998;25:199–209.
50. Capolicchio G, Homsy YL, Houle AM, et al. Long-term results of percutaneous endopyelotomy in the treatment of children with failed open pyeloplasty. J Urol 1997;158:1534–7.
51. Tan HL, Najmaldin A, Webb DR. Endopyelotomy for pelvi-ureteric junction obstruction in children. Eur Urol 1993;24:84–8.
52. Nicholls G, Hrouda D, Kellett MJ, Duffy PG. Endopyelotomy in the symptomatic older child. BJU Int 2001;87:525–7.
53. Schenkman EM, Tarry WF. Comparison of percutaneous endopyelotomy with open pyeloplasty for pediatric ureteropelvic junction obstruction. J Urol 1998;159:1013–5.
54. Austin JC, Hawtrey CE. Re: long-term results of percutaneous endopyelotomy in the treatment of children with failed open pyeloplasty. J Urol 1998;159:2101–2.
55. Rodrigues Netto N Jr, Ikari O, Esteves SC, D'Ancona CA. Antegrade endopyelotomy for pelvi-ureteric junction obstruction in children. Br J Urol 1996;78:607–12.
56. Kletscher BA, Segura JW, LeRoy AJ, Patterson et al. Percutaneous antegrade endoscopic pyelotomy: review of 50 consecutive cases. J Urol 1995;153:701–3.
57. Horgan JD, Maidenberg MJ, Smith AD. Endopyelotomy in the elderly. J Urol 1993;150:1107–9.
58. Nakamura K, Baba S, Tazaki H. Endopyelotomy in horseshoe kidney. J Endourol 1994;8:203–6.
59. Bellman GC, Yamaguchi R. Special considerations in endopyelotomy in a horseshoe kidney. Urology 1996;47:582–5.
60. Jabbour ME, Goldfischer ER, Stravodimos KG, et al. Endopyelotomy for horseshoe and ectopic kidneys. J Urol 1998;160(3 Pt 1):694–7.
61. Koikawa Y, Naito S, Uozumi J, et al. Percutaneous endopyelotomy for ureteropelvic junction obstruction in a horseshoe kidney. Scand J Urol Nephrol 1996;30:145–7.
62. Brooks JD, Kavoussi LR, Preminger GM, et al. Comparison of open and endourologic approaches to the obstructed ureteropelvic junction. Urology 1995;46:791–5.
63. Cassis A, Brannen G, Bush W, et al. Endopyelotomy: review of results and complications. J Urol 1991;146:1492–5.
64. Bellman GC. Complications of endopyelotomy. J Endourol 1996;10:177–81.
65. Weiss JN, Badlani GH, Smith AD. Complications of endopyelotomy. Urol Clin North Am 1988;15:449–51.
66. Malden ES, Picus D, Clayman RV. Arteriovenous fistula complicating endopyelotomy. J Urol 1992;148:1520–3.
67. Badlani G, Karlin G, Smith AD. Complications of endopyelotomy: analysis in a series of 64 patients. J Urol 1988; 140:473–5.
68. Motola JA, Badlani GH, Smith AD. Results of 212 consecutive endopyelotomies: an 8-year follow up. J Urol 1993; 149:453–6.

100

Ureteroenteric Anastomotic Strictures

John S. Lam, MD
Mantu Gupta, MD

The incidence of stricture formation at the ureteroenteric anastomosis at the time of urinary diversion is determined by numerous factors. Urinary conduits have the longest follow-up data available, with stricture rates between 4 and 8%, and more common on the left.[1–4] Possible etiologies of stricture formation include tension at the anastomosis, devascularization and ischemia of the ureter, prior radiation therapy, prior leakage, and infection. In most cases, strictures that arise following urinary diversion are due to ischemia and fibrosis, although recurrent malignancy must be considered.[5] In particular, tumor recurrence should be considered when strictures develop more than 6 months postoperatively.[5,6] Stricture of the anastomosis should be considered in any patient with decreased renal function, hydronephrosis, flank pain, decreased urine output, fever, or sepsis.

Factors potentially influencing outcome include the technique used for ureteral dissection, segment of bowel used for the diversion, type of anastomosis performed, and whether antirefluxing techniques of reimplantation are used.[6] Although mobilization of the ureter is necessary to approximate the ureter and bowel and prevent tension on the anastomosis, stripping the ureter of its surrounding adventitia will lead to distal ureteral ischemia and stricture formation. When performing a conduit, the left ureter is brought underneath the sigmoid mesentery just overlying the aorta. The additional length and dissection needed on the left and the possibility of angulation around the inferior mesenteric artery lead to a higher incidence of stricture formation on the left.[7] The likelihood of stricture formation increases with urinary leakage, which is likely to lead to periureteral fibrosis and scarring. The incidence of urinary leakage and subsequent stricture development appears to be reduced with the use of soft stents following urinary diversion.[5] The incidence of ureteroenteric anastomotic strictures appears to be highest when antirefluxing techniques of reimplantation are used.[6]

The issues influencing stricture formation in continent urinary diversion are more complex owing to the variety of bowel segments, reservoir configurations, and types of anastomoses available for reconstruction. The reported rate of ureteroenteric anastomotic stricture following continent diversion is 4 to 25%, with the majority presenting within the first 2 years.[8,9] Controversy exists over the ideal segment of bowel to employ for conduit diversion. A theoretical advantage of the colon is the feasibility of performing a nonrefluxing anasto-

mosis. Although the incidence of renal deterioration with a nonrefluxing versus a refluxing ureterocolonic anastomosis has not been demonstrated to be significantly different, the risk of obstruction with a nonrefluxing anastomosis has been reported to be significantly higher than that of a refluxing anastomosis. Pantuck and colleagues compared 60 nonrefluxing ureteroenteric anastomoses with 56 direct, refluxing anastomoses and found the long-term stricture rate to be 13% and 1.7%, respectively.[10] There was no significant difference in the two groups with respect to hydronephrosis, pyelonephritis, nephrolithiasis, or renal insufficiency at a mean follow-up of 41 months. Roth and colleagues also found a greater than fivefold increase in ureteral strictures in those patients undergoing a nonrefluxing anastomosis.[11] A prospective, randomized study evaluating a nonrefluxing versus a refluxing anastomosis into an isoperistaltic afferent ileal limb by Studer and colleagues found that stricture formation resulted in 13% of nonrefluxing anastomoses compared with 3% of refluxing anastomoses.[12] These and other studies support the use of a refluxing anastomosis in low-pressure continent reservoirs.

The management of nonmalignant lesions has traditionally been open surgical revision of the anastomosis with reimplantation, but this approach is fraught with hazards and potential complications.[13] Minimally invasive techniques for managing these strictures have evolved over the last 2 decades, in part as a response to (1) the technical difficulty associated with open surgical revision because of dense scarring and adhesions, and (2) the morbidity of open procedures in a generally elderly population with comorbid conditions. Initial enthusiasm for balloon dilation has been tempered by subsequent reports of modest long-term success. In this chapter, we will review the indications for endourologic management of ureteroenteric strictures, the methods and results of endoscopic management, and the factors that influence success or failure.

DIAGNOSIS

Patients with ureteroenteric anastomotic strictures usually present with flank pain, pyelonephritis, sepsis, or renal insufficiency. In many cases, strictures develop slowly following urinary diversion, and some patients are likely to be asymptomatic despite the presence of significant obstruction. For this reason, routine radiographic surveillance of the upper urinary tract should be performed

following urinary diversion to identify patients with ureteral obstruction.[6] In addition, patients with renal colic, recurrent urinary tract infections, or loss of renal function should undergo evaluation. The diagnosis can be made with ultrasound (US), computed tomography (CT), intravenous pyelography (IVP), and loopogram.

Renal US is the most common modality used for screening the upper tracts in patients who have undergone any type of urinary diversion. The finding of upper tract dilation in a patient who has had urinary diversion or bladder substitution should raise suspicion that an anastomotic stricture is present, since this is the most common site of obstruction in these patients. Although most strictures occur at the anastomosis, narrowing may also occur more proximally, particularly on the left side, where the ureter crosses the midline. Reflux is also a common cause of chronic upper tract dilation, particularly in patients with ileal conduits. Presence of obstruction can be confirmed by antegrade contrast studies (IVP or nephrostogram) or by the Whitaker test, diuretic renogram, or direct percutaneous endoscopic inspection (nephroureteroscopy) if the diagnosis is still in doubt. Information on the length and location of the stricture can be obtained from an IVP and contrast study of the conduit or reservoir. Hudson and colleagues reported an 81% correlation of loopography with IVP.[14] Reflux on loopogram rules out stenosis; however, its absence does not confirm obstruction. If a stone or recurrent tumor is suspected, a CT scan may be helpful. Diuretic renography is indicated in some patients to assess differential renal function and confirm the presence of functional obstruction. If renal function is insufficient for an IVP, placement of a nephrostomy tube with subsequent nephrostogram is both therapeutic and diagnostic. Newer techniques, including 3-dimensional reconstructed spiral CT scan, CT urogram, and magnetic resonance imaging (MRI) urogram, can also be used if available.

Obstruction following a urinary diversion that occurs shortly after initial stent removal may be secondary to edema and generally will resolve with observation alone. Obstruction that is severe, bilateral, or persistent may necessitate percutaneous nephrostomy drainage. Sometimes an additional period of stenting via antegrade placement allows edema to resolve satisfactorily and obviates the need for a flank drain and bag. We typically use a single-J stent at the time of surgery. For postoperative antegrade stenting, we place a universal stent (Figures 100-1 and 100-2) and a pigtail nephrostomy tube that is capped when the urine is clear or, alternatively, a nephroureteral pigtail stent. If obstruction persists despite observation, nephrostomy drainage, or further stenting, a technical error should be suspected. Endoscopic ureterotomy and/or balloon dilation may prevent progression of the stricture and is usually worth attempting before remanding the patient to a period of waiting for inflammation to resolve prior to open surgical revision.

Strictures that occur weeks to a few months after the operation are often secondary to ureteral ischemia. One must also be concerned with recurrent malignancy as a cause of stenosis because carcinomas usually develop at the ureteroenteric anastomosis.[15] The incidence of upper tract recurrence following radical cystectomy has been reported to be approximately 3%.[16–19] Urine cytology can be obtained as a part of a tumor surveillance protocol following cystectomy.[20] Initially, the conduit should be examined endoscopically to rule out recurrent malignancy. In cases with established percutaneous access, antegrade ureteroscopy can further aid in defining the nature and extent of the stricture. If the stricture is very dense or long (> 2 cm) or if initial endoscopic management fails, ischemia should be suspected and open surgery undertaken.

Strictures that occur many months to years after surgery can be secondary to malignancy or scarring. Malignant strictures are best managed with permanent indwelling stents or temporary stents until chemotherapy, radiation, or local surgery is performed. Double-pigtail stents or other stents that have holes within the conduit or pouch have a tendency to become obstructed with mucus and should be avoided since sepsis and death have been reported.[21]

When the ureteroenteric anastomotic stricture is identified late and the residual renal unit is nonfunctioning, nephroureterectomy is the treatment of choice. This is particularly true in the setting of underlying urothelial malignancy because a nonfunctioning obstructed upper tract moiety is difficult to follow for recurrent malignancy.

INDICATIONS

Not all patients with urinary diversion and hydronephrosis require intervention. Most patients with a long-term urinary conduit will have an element of chronic hydronephrosis that is not secondary to obstruction. In this population, a decrease in renal function or loss of reflux on a routine loopogram should prompt a diuretic renogram to assess the presence of functional obstruction. Indications for intervention in patients with diversions and hydronephrosis include pain, infection, and renal insufficiency associated with functional obstruction. Although recurrence of transitional cell carcinoma at the level of the anastomosis is uncommon, the radiographic picture of an irregular mass at the level of the stricture and the rapid progression of obstruction and loss of renal function should prompt further evaluation and intervention.[22]

Patients undergoing urinary diversion as part of a pelvic exenteration for gynecologic malignancy are a challenging subset. Penalver and colleagues reported on 66 patients, 95% of whom had undergone previous pelvic irradiation.[23] Early and late complications at the ureteroenteric anastomosis were 22% and 10%, respectively. Eighty-five percent of their postoperative complications were managed successfully by conservative measures such as percutaneous nephrostomy.

PATIENT PREPARATION

In general, percutaneous drainage of the obstructed renal unit is the most appropriate initial step for the majority of patients with ureteral strictures detected postoperatively. This allows for preservation of renal function and resolution of infection. It also facilitates radiographic evaluation of the strictured area to help determine the most appropriate treatment approach. Retrograde insertion of a ureteral stent may be possible in selected patients who have undergone orthotopic urinary diversion. However, it is often difficult to identify and cannulate the obstructed ureteral anastomosis.

Before deciding how to manage a patient's stricture(s), several factors must be evaluated. It is important to know the length and degree of narrowing, the number and location of stenoses, the age of the stricture, the original indication for the patient's diversion, and whether the patient has received radiation therapy. Malignancy as a cause of stricturing can be evaluated by abdominal and/or pelvic CT, urine cytology, and endoscopic visualization of the strictured area with biopsy if necessary. Long, fusiform, or severe strictures are less likely to respond to an endoscopic approach, and open repair should be considered. Prior radiation therapy, a history of gynecologic malignancy, and stricture disease secondary to ischemia decrease the chance of endoscopic success.[24] Strictures of less than 3 to 7 months' duration tend to respond better than older strictures.[25–27]

INFORMED CONSENT

Patients being advised to undergo endoscopic treatment of ureteroenteric anastomotic strictures must be made aware of the potential complications of the procedure in order to make an informed decision on whether to undergo surgery. The patient should be informed about available therapeutic solutions and possible complications. Complications include bleeding, with the possible need for a transfusion; urosepsis, extravasation; perforation; vascular injury; adjacent organ injury; loss of access; recurrent strictures; and obstruction of the stent.

PREOPERATIVE PREPARATION

Preoperative evaluation of the patient includes a careful history and physical examination. Laboratory analyses are the same as in other surgical procedures (complete blood count, chemistry profile, coagulation profile, urinalysis, chest radiograph, and electrocardiogram). Urine culture is performed to rule out infection, and a positive preoperative urine culture should be treated. The decision to use spinal or general anesthesia is up to the patient, anesthesiologist, and surgeon. Following administration of anesthesia, the patient is placed in the supine or dorsal lithotomy position with sequential compression devices and careful padding of the pressure points of the legs if a retrograde approach is used. The retrograde approach is usually reserved for patients with ileal

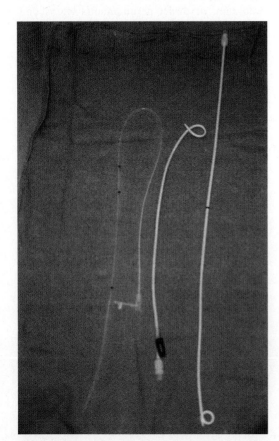

Figure 100-1 Left to right: universal stent; 30 cm, 12F Cope loop catheter; Smith 8/14F endopyelotomy stent.

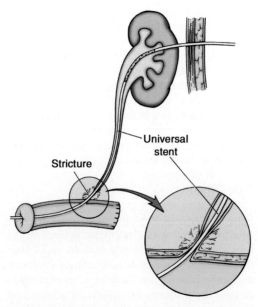

Figure 100-2 Proper positioning of univeral stent for postoperative ureteroenteric strictures.

conduits and neobladders. We have found that retrograde approaches are rarely successful in patients with continent urinary diversions because of the severe angulation necessary to visualize or access the ureteral orifice. We routinely use a nephroscopy drape to help prevent spillage of irrigation fluid onto the operating table when accessing ileal conduits. A blunt 10 to 12 mm laparoscopic trocar is used to help distend the ileal conduit. The patient is placed in a prone position if an antegrade approach is used. The pouch or conduit should be drained with a Foley catheter prior to flipping the patient prone. The authors routinely administer systemic antibiotics prior to the initiation of surgery, usually recommending a first-generation cephalosporin, except in those cases in which a specific drug is indicated.

INSTRUMENTATION

Essential equipment includes a flexible cystoscope to inspect the conduit, pouch, or neobladder and to perform retrograde pyelography. Fluoroscopy is needed for initial ureteral access, monitoring during ureteroscopy, and stent placement. Fluoroscopy can be performed with a mobile C-arm unit or a fixed unit on a table designed for urologic endoscopy. A variety of rigid and flexible nephroscopes and ureteroscopes have been used for balloon dilation and incision of ureteroenteric anastomotic strictures. A standard high-pressure ureteral dilating balloon (usually 6 mm 18 French [F] in the dilated state) can be used. Various methods of endoscopic incision of ureteroenteric anastomotic strictures have been described. A "cold" knife can be used with a rigid ureteroscope. Knife blades are available in straight, half-moon, and hook configurations. Knife blades that pass over a guidewire are also available. If one is to use a smaller-caliber, semirigid, or flexible ureteroscope, flexible fibers must be used to incise the stricture. Electrocautery incision is accomplished with either 2 to 3F ball-tip electrodes or Hulbert electrodes (Cook Urological, Spencer, IN). These are available in straight pencil point, hook, angled, and loop designs. The holmium laser can also be used for incision of ureteroenteric strictures. This energy can be delivered by 200 or 365 μm diameter fibers through rigid or flexible ureteroscopes. High-pressure ureteral dilation balloon catheters are available in inflated diameters of 4 to 8 mm and lengths of 5 to 10 cm. Many of these balloons are designed to withstand pressures of up to 12 to 20 atm. Energy sources such as the holmium:yttrium-aluminum-garnet (holmium:YAG) laser are used to perform endoureterotomy. The Acucise cutting balloon catheter (Applied Medical, Rancho Santa Margarita, CA) is a 6F device incorporating both a monopolar electrocautery cutting wire and a low-pressure balloon, which allows for simultaneous balloon dilation and incision, has also been used but is potentially dangerous because the length and depth of incision are not visually controlled and adjacent vascular structures or organs may be injured, even with appropriate preoperative CT scan imaging.

TECHNIQUE

BALLOON DILATION Dilation of ureteral strictures using a balloon was first reported by Dourmashkin in 1926.[28] In 1979, Grüntzig and colleagues introduced the balloon catheter for dilation of coronary stenoses.[29] The Grüntzig balloon was first reported for the dilation of ureteroenteric strictures by Martin and colleagues in 1982.[30] Numerous series have followed, but initial reports of 40 to 100% success rates have been followed by long-term data indicating poorer results.[24,31]

A nephrostomy tract should be established through an upper-pole or middle-pole posterior calix to allow direct access to the ureter. A 0.035- or 0.038-inch guidewire is negotiated through the tract across the narrowed segment. A glidewire is often helpful in crossing the strictured area if the area is tight or the ureter proximal to it is tortuous. The wire is grasped and pulled through the stoma using a cystoscope, allowing through-and-through access. The initial guidewire is then exchanged for a stiffer wire such as a 0.038-inch super-stiff Amplatz or Lunderquist-Ring torque wire using a 6F open-ended ureteral catheter. A high-pressure reinforced polyethylene balloon catheter that has a balloon 4 cm in length with an inflated diameter of 6 mm is then passed in an antegrade or retrograde fashion and positioned fluoroscopically so that the balloon completely traverses the area of narrowing (Figure 100-3). The balloon is inflated with a pressure-regulating syringe (such as a LeVeen syringe) to 12 to 20 atm and held at this inflation pressure for at least 1 minute or until the waist disappears. Dilation is repeated two or three times if there is inadequate dilation initially. The anastomosis is then stented with a 12F 30 cm Cope loop catheter especially designed for this purpose (see Figure 100-1; Figure 100-4). The end of the catheter traverses the stoma and is left to drain openly into a bag after the loop is fully coiled by pulling the string and securing it. The Luer-Lok hub of the catheter can be irritating to the patient in the prone position, so we usually cut it off distal to

the string exit site. The catheter is left in position for 6 weeks. The nephrostomy tube may be capped when the urine is clear, and antegrade drainage is confirmed by a nephrostogram, although we leave it in situ as a safety valve. Antegrade contrast studies are performed with the nephrostomy tube immediately after removal of the catheter and then 1 week later. Follow-up studies (IVP or US) need to be performed for several weeks after treatment to ensure patency, since late failures (2 to 3 years after initial dilation) have been reported.[31,32]

URETERAL INCISION (ENDOURETEROTOMY) Disappointment with long-term results of balloon dilation of ureteroenteric anastomotic strictures fostered the use of endoscopic incision (endoureterotomy).[33] Through-and-through access is obtained as described earlier for balloon dilation. Endoureterotomy can be performed using a retrograde or an antegrade approach.[34] However, it is generally easiest to use a flexible ureteroscope passed in an antegrade fashion through a nephrostomy tract.[35] It is unnecessary to dilate the tract when using a 7F flexible ureteroscope, which can be simply passed over a guidewire to the level of the stricture. Because it will be necessary to remove the guidewire over which the ureteroscope has been passed, it is always best to have a safety wire in place. If one desires better visualization, the tract can be dilated to 30F using Amplatz semirigid dilators or a balloon device, and a flexible cystoscope can be passed antegrade.

Both percutaneous antegrade and retrograde approaches are feasible, but the retrograde approach by endoscopy of the conduit or reservoir is often frustrating because of difficulty in finding the orifice and cannulating it as a result of acute angulation at the anastomosis. One technique we have found useful for looposcopy is the use of a laparoscopic trocar through the stoma to

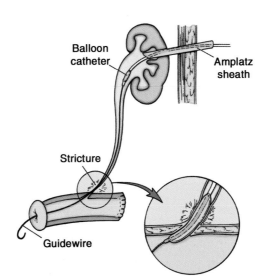

Figure 100-3 Balloon dilation of ureteroenteric anastomotic strictures.

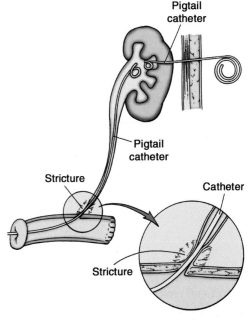

Figure 100-4 Placement of Cope loop catheter to stent anastomosis.

aid in continuous irrigation and conduit disten-sion.[36] A blunt-tip trocar is placed into the stoma after finger dilation. The flexible cystoscope is placed through the one-way valve. The side port of the trocar can be opened for continuous flow. This effectively decreases the mucosal folds of the conduit and allows for easier identification of the ureteral meatus.

Once the strictured area is identified, the inci-sion may be performed using either a small elec-trocautery probe (such as 2F or 3F Greenwald electrode) or the holmium:YAG laser.[37] We have found the laser is a more be precise cutting tool and most commonly use a 200 or 365 μm fiber with power settings of 1.0 to 1.2 joules and a fre-quency of 10 to 15 pulses per second. Bleeding is minimal and a full-thickness incision should be made until periureteral tissues are visualized. Con-firmation that an adequate incision has been made is obtained by injecting contrast material at the level of the stricture. Extravasation of contrast should be seen over the length of the incision. Finally, the strictured area is dilated using a 6 to 7 mm balloon catheter to ensure the adequacy of the incision and to separate the adventitial tis-sues.[38] If the scar tissue of the incised ureteral stricture appears to be particularly dense and no fat is seen, 3 to 5 mL of triamcinolone (40 mg/mL) may be injected into the bed of the incised stricture using a 3F Greenwald needle mounted on a flexi-ble shaft. A LeVeen pressure syringe is used to per-form the injection into the dense scar tissue. Because the risk of injury to adjacent organs and blood vessels is greater with an incision than with balloon dilation, it is important to know the details of the previous urinary diversion operation the patient has undergone. It may be helpful to obtain an abdominal and/or pelvic CT scan before plan-ning endoscopic ureterotomy.

In the antegrade technique, flexible nephrou-reteroscopy is performed from above. The guidewire placed earlier is insulated by passing a 6F open-ended ureteral exchange catheter over it. Using a 3 or 5F Greenwald electrode or a flexible cold-knife ureterotome cold knife, an incision is made starting 1 cm above the area of the stricture and continuing into the bowel segment, in effect marsupializing the stenosis into the conduit or reservoir (Figure 100-5). We currently favor using the holmium:YAG laser to make the inci-sion. The area of intended incision should be inspected carefully to detect any evidence of a pulsating vessel. For left ureteral strictures, endo-luminal ultrasound is helpful in avoiding vascular injury by identifying adjacent vessels.[39] Ante-grade incisions in most cases avoid the iliac ves-sels, but can potentially injure the inferior mesenteric artery or vein as the ureter crosses underneath. The site of incision should vary, depending on the type of diversion and the loca-tion and proximity of surrounding structures. Care should also be taken to avoid injuring the contralateral ureter. The cut should be deepened until it is full thickness and fat can be seen. In our experience, adjunctive balloon dilation is not necessary if the incision is sufficiently deep. A

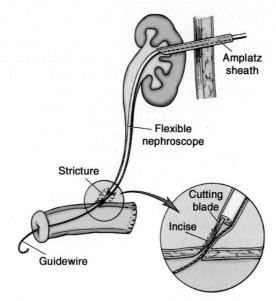

Figure 100-5 Endoscopic incisional ureterotomy.

Smith endopyelotomy catheter (8/14F) is posi-tioned across the anastomosis such that the 14F end is at the incised area and the pigtail lies in the renal pelvis (see Figure 100-1; Figure 100-6). The distal end exits the stoma and is secured to the skin. A catheter is placed into the stoma (12F if the patient has a continent reservoir, 18F if the patient has an ileal conduit) and left draining into a collection bag. A nephrostomy tube is left in the renal pelvis and capped once the urine is clear. At 6 weeks, the endopyelotomy catheter is removed and a nephrostogram is obtained to ensure patency. The nephrostomy tube is left clamped; it is removed if another nephrostogram taken 1 week later demonstrates drainage.

CUTTING BALLOON CATHETER An alternative method of endourologic treatment of ureteroen-teric strictures involves the use of the Acucise bal-loon cutting catheter device.[40,41] It was developed as a less invasive endoscopic approach to ureteral

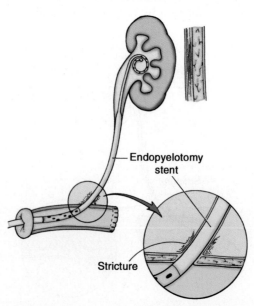

Figure 100-6 Smith endopyelotomy stent placement fol-lowing ureterotomy.

and ureteropelvic junction stenoses.[40] This catheter has a cutting loop external to and along-side a balloon catheter. Simultaneous balloon inflation and loop activation allow incisional ureterotomy. This technique can also be performed using a retrograde or an antegrade approach and does not require direct endoscopic visualization of the strictured area. The use of endoluminal ultra-sonography prior to the activation of the Acucise device may facilitate proper orientation of the instrument and avoid any periureteral vessels.[39,41] Early experience with ureteroenteric strictures resulted in severe hemorrhage in 1 of 3 patients. Others have also reported hemorrhagic complica-tions in patients with ureteroenteric strictures.[42] The advantage of the Acucise catheter is that it is less invasive and in theory it makes a narrower incision because of the stretch of the ureteral wall at the time of the incision. Because of this stretch, it potentially causes less thermal injury than con-ventional cutting electrodes. The major disadvan-tage is lack of visual control over the depth and exact location of the incision.

SPECIAL SITUATIONS Patients who have com-plete obliteration of a ureteroenteric anastomosis pose a challenging problem.[43] This situation is best managed in the healthy or young person by percutaneous nephrostomy drainage and open repair. In the case of malignancy or general debil-ity, a "cut-to-the-light" procedure can be per-formed, but is fraught with risks. This is best approached by combined antegrade and retro-grade fluoroscopy and endoscopy. Injection of methylene blue or contrast dye may help define a small opening through which a glidewire (0.017 or 0.035F) can be passed. If no opening is pres-ent, the light from the retrograde scope should be visualized from above and a guidewire passed through the narrowest area of the stricture. If this also fails, antegrade and retrograde endoscopes can be fluoroscopically aligned and a cold-knife ureterotome can incise the narrowest portion from above toward the light below until an open-ing is created (Figure 100-7). Sequential catheter dilation, balloon dilation, or extension of the incision can then be performed and a single-J diversion stent or endopyelotomy stent (7/14F) placed as described above. This procedure has a high risk of bowel perforation and should be per-formed only by an experienced endourologist under fluoroscopic control.

POSTOPERATIVE CARE

Postoperatively the patient can be discharged if bleeding is minimal and there is no evidence of urosepsis. Otherwise the patient should be admit-ted and placed on intravenous antibiotics. Patients are then maintained on oral antibiotics for 5 to 7 days following discharge, usually a flu-oroquinolone. For patients in whom therapy was definitive and not palliative, the stent bridging the stricture is removed 6 weeks following sur-gery. In patients with percutaneous access, an indwelling nephrostomy should be left but can be

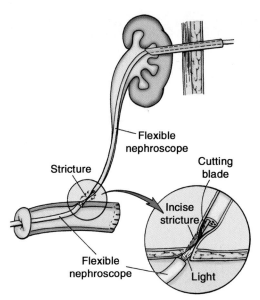

Figure 100-7 Cut-to-the-light technique.

capped if antegrade drainage of contrast into the conduit or pouch can be demonstrated. Since the failure rate is high, this serves as a pop-off mechanism and is highly recommended. For this reason, we prefer the antegrade approach in patients where endoscopic therapy is intended to be definitive. In cases of palliation, the stents should be changed every 2 to 3 months.

RESULTS

BALLOON DILATION Studies with sufficient data on balloon dilation of ureteroenteric strictures are summarized in Table 100-1.[24–27,30–32,44–57] The average success rate in these series was 32% (range 0–100%). Treatment of the strictured area with balloon dilation appears to be associated with a high early success rate.[31,55] Results have been more favorable for short strictures (< 2 cm).[24,26,31,50,52] Likewise, strictures that are acute or recent respond better to balloon dilation. In one series, the success rate for strictures of less than 3 months' duration was 88% as compared with 67% if more than 3 months.[50] In another series, strictures of less than 7 months' duration had 57% success as compared with 0% (0 of 5) for strictures of longer than 7 months' duration.[25]

The degree to which technique affects outcome is unclear. Balloon sizes from 4 to 10 mm have been used without demonstrable differences in long-term success. Likewise, the inflation pressure (5–17 atm), inflation time (30 seconds to 15 minutes), number of inflation repetitions (one to three), and number of inflation sessions (one to six) do not discernibly influence outcome. The type of urinary diversion may have an effect in that ureterocolonic strictures appear to fare worse than ureteroileal strictures.[25]

The optimal stent size is controversial. Some urologists favor large-caliber stents, quoting the principle of the Davis intubated ureterotomy.[25,58] They believe a stent of smaller caliber allows scarring and wound contracture down to the caliber of the stent. Others favor smaller stents because they believe larger stents increase ischemia and therefore promote reformation of strictures. Moon and colleagues recently compared use of a 7F ureteral stent with a 7/14F endopyelotomy stent following incision of induced midureteral strictures in a female minipig model and found no difference in histology or recurrence rate.[59] The small number of animals studied and the short follow-up period (3 months) may account for the lack of effect of stent size on the restricture rate in their study.

The duration of stenting is also controversial (3 days to 3 months). Before 1984, many urologists favored stenting of short duration. This evolved to a majority opinion favoring at least 6 weeks of stenting to allow inflammation to subside. More recently, animal studies have suggested that ureteral stents have a deleterious effect on wound healing that leads to fibrosis.[60,61] To date, no prospective randomized trials have been performed in humans to convincingly argue the optimal duration of ureteral stents.

Stricture recurrence is the rule rather than the exception, even after initial success. Failure may occur up to 2 years from the original dilation, so close radiographic follow-up is imperative. Most recent series indicate that strictures may recur in as many as 50 to 80% of patients treated with balloon dilation alone,[54,55] which is much worse than that for balloon dilation of ureteral strictures in other locations. In addition to the limited likelihood of long-term success, balloon dilation may lead to further ureteral damage and ischemia, thereby increasing the difficulty of subsequent more definitive treatment.

URETERAL INCISION (ENDOURETEROTOMY)
Table 100-2 summarizes the data on endoureterotomy of ureteroenteric anastomotic strictures.[33,53,55,57,63–71] The average success rate in these series was 60% (0–100%). Kramolowsky and colleagues reported on incision of ureteroileal strictures via a flexible endoscope using a 5F Greenwald electrode combined with balloon dilation in 4 patients.[33] Two of their 4 patients had successful outcomes. Meretyk and colleagues extended this series to include 15 patients with 19 ureteroenteric strictures.[62] Chronic indwelling stents were necessary in 5 patients with strictures because of metastatic

Table 100-1	Results of Balloon Dilation for Treatment of Ureteroenteric Anastomotic Strictures									
Series	No. of Strictures	Mean Follow-Up, Range (mo)	Success (%)	Stent Size (F)	Stent Duration	Balloon Size (mm)	Inflation Pressure (atm)	Inflation Time (min)	No. of Inflations per Session	No. of Sessions
Martin et al (1982)[30]	3	Short	100	6	–	8	–	–	–	4
Dixon et al (1982)[44]	1	11	100	6.7	6 wk	4–9	–	–	–	6
Glanz et al (1983)[45]	2	Short, 12	50	9–10	3–10 d	4–6	–	1–15	–	1
Banner and Pollack (1984)[24]	20	< 6	40	7–10	1 wk	4	–	0.5–1	2–3	1
Finnerty et al (1984)[46]	2	9, 6–12	100	6	1 wk	4	–	–	–	1
King et al (1984)[47]	5	–	20	–	6–12 wk	–	–	–	–	1
Johnson et al (1987)[25]	7	> 6	43	5–14	> 2 d	4–10	> 5	0.5–1	3	1
Chang et al (1987)[26]	8	18.2, 4–48	50	8–16	4–6 wk	5–8	–	–	–	1
Kramolowsky et al (1987)[32]	5	17.8, 11–22	0	5–12	4–14 d	1–5	–	–	1–2	1
O'Brien et al (1988)[48]	7	12	14	–	0–4 mo	4–6	6–17	–	1–2	1
Smith (1988)[49]	3	–	66	–	6 wk	6–10	10–17	1–3	1–3	1
Shapiro et al (1988)[31]	37	< 12	16	8.3–10	1–6 wk	4–10	< 17	1–2	–	1
Lang and Glorioso (1988)[27]	–	> 15	–	7–10	3–6 wk	8–10	14–20 lb	0.5–1	> 1	1
Beckman et al (1989)[50]	5	22, 20–25	60	7–10	4–8 wk	4	–	1	1	1
Aliabadi et al (1990)[51]	3	12.3, 7–18	66	–	–	6–8	–	10	–	2
Netto et al (1990)[52]	2	60	50	8.5	15–60 d	4–6	–	10	–	–
Germinale et al (1992)[53]	5	15, 7–30	20	8.5–10	–	–	–	–	variable	variable
Kwak et al (1995)[54]	18	6, 1–9	50	10	4 wk	8	15	0.75	3	1–4
Ravery et al (1998)[55]	14	16, 6–39	61	–	4–20 wk	–	10–20	5–15	–	–
Richter et al (2000)[56]	17	6.3, 2–16	35	7–8	–	8–10	2.5	1.5	–	–
DiMarco et al (2001)[57]	52	24	*15, 15, 5	–	3–6 wk	8–10	–	–	–	variable

*1-, 2-, and 3-year success rate, respectively.

Table 100-2   Results of Ureteral Incision (Endoureterotomy) for Treatment of Ureteroenteric Anastomotic Strictures

Series	No. of Strictures	Mean Follow-Up, Range (mo)	Success (%)	Stent Size (F)	Stent Duration	Method (mm)	Mean Length of Hospital Stay, Range (d)	Mean Stricture Length, Range (cm)
Kramolowsky et al (1987)[33]	5	9.6, 6–14	60	7–18	6–14 d	Electrocautery and balloon dilation	1–2	1.6, 1–2
Meretyk et al (1991)[62]	19	28.6, 9–57	57	12–20	3–6 wk	Electrocautery	3.5, 2–12	1–4
Schneider et al (1991)[63]	2	15, 7–45	100	–	3–6 wk	Cold-knife	–	–
Ahmadzadeh (1992)[64]	5	14	60	7	4 wk	Electrocautery (3F needle electrode)	–	–
Germinale et al (1992)[53]	4	9.75, 4–13	75	8.5–10	–	Electrocautery/cold-knife and balloon dilation	–	–
Bierkens et al (1996)[65]	2	12, 8–16	100	12	6 wk	Cold-knife	–	–
Cornud et al (1996)[66]	33	> 12	71	12–18	8 wk	Electrocautery	–	–
Singal et al (1997)[67]	9	9–18	89	6/12	4–6 wk	Holmium laser and balloon dilation	7.2	–
Wolf et al (1997)[68]	21	2–75	*68, 26	7–16	Variable	Electrocautery, cold-knife, or balloon dilation	–	Variable
Richter et al (2000)[56]	4	–	0	7–8	4 wk	Electrocautery and balloon dilation	–	–
Laven et al (2001)[69]	19	20.5, 9–41	57	7/14	4–6 wk	Holmium laser	1–2	1–1.5
Watterson et al (2002)[70]	24	22	71	6/12	6 wk	Holmium laser	2, 1–4	1.7, 0.5–5
Poulakis et al (2003)[71]	43	38.8, 12–85	60.5	8–12	1–12 wk	Cold-knife	3.6, 2–8	Variable

*1- and 3-year success rate, respectively.

cancer or a complete dense stricture. In the other 14 patients, the success rate was 57% at an average follow-up of 28.6 months. Meretyk and colleagues also reported on endoscopic ureterotomy in 13 patients with benign ureteral strictures, none of which was ureteroenteric.[72] Triamcinolone (120–200 mg) was injected into the strictures of 5 of these patients. Two patients had free bladder urothelial grafts harvested transurethrally, sutured around a ureteral stent, and placed into the bed of the incision. The failure rate was 20% (1 of 5) in patients treated with triamcinolone (19-month follow-up). In both patients with mucosal grafts the strictures (4 and 8 cm in length) had successfully resolved at 21- and 22-month follow-ups, but there is no evidence that the grafts actually adhered. In 1995, Yamada and colleagues reported on 20 ureteral strictures managed by endoscopic incision and balloon dilation, but did not specify whether they were ureteroenteric.[73] They had a "partial" resolution of obstruction in 45% of cases and complete resolution in 40%. Schneider and colleagues performed endoscopic cold-knife incisions on 56 strictures of the ureter with partial or complete success in 75%.[63] Their definition of success was not clear, and the average follow-up was only 15 months. Only two of the stenoses were ureteroenteric strictures (ureterosigmoidostomies), and both remained patent (length of follow-up not reported). Other series have evaluated the efficacy of endoscopic incisional ureterotomy, but have not included patients with ureteroenteric strictures.

The cold-knife technique in general appears to yield better results than hot-knife techniques. This may be attributable to the thermal injury that the latter can cause, leading to more ischemia, fibrosis, and restricture. Triamcinolone or other steriodal agents and mucosal free grafts may improve results, but this has yet to be confirmed. Again, optimal stent size and duration are controversial. Some animal studies indicate that stenting should not be done or should be temporary (less than 2 weeks) following balloon dilation or ureterotomy.[60,61] Other studies indicate that muscle

regeneration requires long-term stents that act as molds or scaffolds.[74] Moon and colleagues found similar histology and restricture rates in pigs with induced and endoscopically incised ureteral strictures when comparing 7 and 7/14F ureteral stents, but their numbers were too small and follow-up too short to draw any firm conclusions.[59]

Wolf and colleagues used a variety of methods to endoscopically incise 30 ureteroenteric strictures in 25 patients.[68] The average operative time was approximately 2 hours and there were 6 major complications, including sepsis, need for blood transfusion, and open repair of a lacerated common iliac artery. At a median follow-up of 15 months, the success rate was 50% (15 of 30). While 4 patients underwent repeat endoureterotomy, only 1 had a successful result. A subset of patients that were identified as likely to have stent-free patency were those with ipsilateral renal function of > 25%, strictures of nonischemic etiology, and strictures < 1 cm in length. Overall, the success rate in patients followed for more than 12 months was 35% (8 of 23).

CUTTING BALLOON CATHETER Table 100-3 summarizes treatment results using a cutting balloon catheter for ureteroenteric anastomotic strictures.[40–42,68,75–79] The average success rate in these series was 53% (range 30–100%). Lin and colleagues used the Acucise device with an antegrade approach in 9 patients with 12 ureteroenteric strictures.[41] Although the procedure was associated with limited morbidity and hospitalization, the success rate after a mean follow-up of 9 months was only 30% among patients without evidence of recurrent malignancy.

OTHER THERAPIES

In 1979, Smith and colleagues first described endoscopic dilation of ureteroenteric strictures using fascial (semirigid) dilators.[80] Rosen and colleagues in 1980 reported on stent placement across the stricture without dilation.[81] Shortly thereafter, balloon dilation became popular.

However, some urologists have continued to use fascial dilation, especially for strictures that have failed balloon dilation because of associated dense scarring, prior radiation therapy, long length, or recurrent malignancy. There have been only scattered individual reports of semirigid fascial dilation of these strictures.[33,82] Therefore, the success or failure rate of this procedure cannot be evaluated, although indications are that the long-term results are poor. Fascial dilation can also be used to increase the diameter of the ureteral lumen sufficiently for a catheter or flexible endoscope to be passed in cases of tight strictures for the purpose of performing balloon dilation or endoureterotomy. Sometimes the sole purpose of fascial dilation is to allow passage of a chronic indwelling ureteral catheter that can be changed periodically.

The use of semirigid fascial dilators is potentially dangerous. Excessive force may result in ureteral perforation or avulsion. Telescoping of the ureteral wall may also occur, and the ureteral mucosa is almost always denuded. A less traumatic method of dilation involves placement of gradually larger catheters over a period of days to weeks. Again, these techniques alone will rarely result in permanent resolution of a stricture, but they are acceptable methods for patients who are to be managed with chronic indwelling catheters.

Chronic indwelling externalized ureteral stents are far from optimal therapy. Lang reported that successful percutaneous stent placement across ureteroileostomy strictures still results in loss of the renal unit in 13 of 28 patients within 6 months.[83] Oshinsky and Smith reported that 7 patients who failed endourologic management had stent changes every 3 months under local anesthesia.[84] Despite careful follow-up, 5 of the 7 had recurrent episodes of stent obstruction, pyelonephritis, and sepsis.

RECURRENT STRICTURES

Treatment options for patients with ureteroenteric anastomotic strictures that recur following

Series	No. of Strictures	Mean Follow-Up, Range (mo)	Success (%)	Stent Size (F)	Stent Duration
Chandhoke et al (1993)[40]	2	3.8, 3–9	100	17/14	4 wk
Babayan (1995)[75]	9	–	33	–	–
Wolf et al (1997)[68]	9	2–75	78, 39	7–16	Variable
Kabalin (1997)[76]	4	22, 11–28	100	10	6 wk
McDougall and Nakada (1997)[77]	1	12	100	10	3 wk
Preminger et al (1997)[42]	6	7.8, 1–17.9	50	7/14	4–6 wk
Lin et al (1999)[41]	10	26, 18–30	30	10	6 wk
Knowles et al (2001)[78]	1	40	100	6	6 wk
Seseke et al (2002)[79]	3	12, 6–16	100	9	4–6 wk

Table 100-3 Results of Cutting Balloon Catheter for Treatment of Ureteroenteric Anastomotic Strictures

*1- and 3-year success rate, respectively.

endoureterotomy are limited. In some patients with a limited life expectancy, the long-term use of a ureteral stent or nephrostomy tube may be the best choice.

UROTHELIAL GRAFT Urban and colleagues used a transurethrally harvested free graft of bladder urothelium placed in the incised ureteral stricture bed in 6 patients with long areas of narrowing (mean, 2.9 cm).[85] Although the average operative time was 5 hours, 4 (66.7%) patients had successful results with follow-up of 22 months or longer.

METALLIC ENDOPROSTHESES The use of an expandable metallic endoprosthesis for ureteroileal stricture disease was first reported in 1990, which involved a 66-year-old man who remained patent at 6-month follow-up.[86] The use of expandable metallic endoprostheses to treat recalcitrant ureteral strictures has been reported in patients with anastomotic benign ureteral strictures.[87,88] Among 15 patients with upper urinary tract obstruction owing to a variety of causes, the placement of a nickel-titanium alloy stent was successful in all cases at a mean follow-up of 10.6 months.[88] Other investigators have reported successful outcomes using alternative metallic stents in smaller groups of patients with difficult ureteral strictures.[87,89] In 1994, Reinberg and colleagues reported on 5 patients with ureteral strictures, including 2 with ureteroileal strictures, who underwent placement of a self-expanding metallic stent (Wallstent, Schneider USA Inc., Minneapolis, MN) after balloon dilation had failed.[87] The 2 patients with ureteroileal strictures did well at 1-year and 13-month follow-ups. One of the 5 patients required removal of the stent for severe vesicoureteral reflux of new onset. At removal the stent was patent, but had epithelial growth. The Palmaz stent (Johnson & Johnson, Interventional Systems, Warren, NJ), which is similar to, but longer than the Wallstent, has also been used for ureteroenteric strictures.[90] The risk involved with these stents is eventual ingrowth of muscle, fibrous tissue, and epithelium, resulting in obstruction. This had occurred with similar stents used for urethral strictures. Should this occur in the ureter, it would require open removal of the prosthesis.

Stent placement has been described using both an antegrade and a retrograde approach. Protrusion of the distal end of the stent into the lumen of the conduit does not seem to be problematic, and the incidence of symptomatic urinary tract infection is no higher in this group of patients.[91]

OPEN SURGICAL REVISION Open surgical resection of an obstructed ureteroenteric anastomosis may be considered if avoidance of a chronic stent or nephrostomy tube is desired. However, these procedures are technically challenging owing to the extensive scarring and limited ureteral length, and they are associated with a longer recovery than endoscopic options. Preoperative placement of a nephrostomy tube and a ureteral stent will aid in the identification of the ureter at the time of exploration. Prior to surgery, it is optimal to sterilize the urine and prepare the bowel. If a cutaneous stoma is present, it should be prepared into the operative field and the conduit or reservoir drained with a Foley catheter during the procedure. Through a midline incision, the conduit or reservoir is identified and preserved, the colon reflected medially, and the proximal ureter is identified and traced down to the area of the previous anastomosis. Care should be taken to preserve the adventitia and associated blood supply. If enough ureter length is available, the ureter can be transected proximal to the stricture, spatulated, and anastomosed to a convenient area of the bowel. Insufficient ureteral length may require an additional segment of bowel to interpose between the ureter and the reservoir. The anastomosis is carried out over a 7F stent and a drain is left in place. The stent remains for 4 to 6 weeks.

COMPLICATIONS

Few complications have been reported for endoscopic balloon dilation of ureteroenteric anastomotic strictures. Earlier balloons made of polyvinylchloride were more likely to rupture, a problem that is rare with newer balloons constructed of reinforced polyethylene. Ureteral disruption as evidenced by extravasation of contrast material outside the ureter has been reported but is also uncommon.[24,25] Fever and sepsis have also been rarely reported.

Endoscopic balloon dilation is a very safe procedure and is still indicated in many situations. The poor long-term results can be substantially improved if patients are carefully selected and the therapeutic goal is kept in mind. Balloon dilation of ureteroenteric anastomotic strictures should be reserved for (1) debilitated patients, patients who cannot tolerate open surgery, and patients with recurrent malignancy with the goal of renal preservation by means of chronic indwelling ureteral stent drainage; and (2) patients with short membraneous strictures that are not very tight and that are recent in origin, with the goal of permanent resolution of obstruction.

The major complications of endoureterotomy include hemorrhage requiring blood transfusion, sepsis, and ureteroenteric fistula.[62,63] Meretyk and colleagues had only one major complication in 19 strictures;[62] Schneider and colleagues had significant complications in 12 of 56 patients.[63] The risk of these complications in patients with ureteroenteric strictures can be minimized by culture-specific antibiotic coverage and preoperative imaging to evaluate adjacent vascular and enteric structures.

CONCLUSIONS

In summary, even with meticulous surgical technique, a nontunneled anastomosis, and the use of soft stents, there will be a 3 to 5% incidence of ureteral obstruction following urinary diversion. Although advances in endourologic equipment and technique have improved our ability to manage these strictures in a minimally invasive fashion, the long-term success rate of endoureterotomy is only 30 to 50%. A variety of minimally invasive methods are available for the management of patients with ureteroenteric strictures. Endourologic management of ureteroenteric strictures is most likely to be successful in short strictures of recent origin. In approximately 20 to 60% of patients, open surgery with its attendant risks and complications can be avoided. In the remainder, the success of eventual open repair does not appear to be impaired by the earlier endoscopic approach. Balloon dilation of these strictures, the simplest approach, has good short-term, but poor long-term results. Endoscopic incision performed under direct vision using either an antegrade or retrograde approach, with or without balloon dilation, appears to have a superior long-term outcome.

REFERENCES

1. Schmidt JD, Hawtrey CE, Flocks RH, Culp DA. Complications, results and problems of ileal conduit diversions. J Urol 1973;109:210–6.
2. Engel RM. Complications of bilateral uretero-ileo cutaneous urinary diversion: a review of 208 cases. J Urol 1969;101:508–12.
3. Frazier HA, Robertson JE, Paulson DF. Complications of radical cystectomy and urinary diversion: a retrospective review of 675 cases in 2 decades. J Urol 1992;148:1401–5.
4. Wilson TG, Moreno JG, Weinberg A, Ahlering TE. Late complications of the modified Indiana pouch. J Urol 1994;151:331–4.
5. Regan JB, Barrett DM. Stented versus nonstented ureteroileal anastomoses: is there a difference with regard to leak and stricture? J Urol 1985;134:1101–3.

6. McDougal WS. Use of intestinal segments and urinary diversion. In: Walsh PC, Retik AB, Vaughan ED Jr, Wein AJ, editors. Campbell's urology. Vol.4. 8th ed. Philadelphia: W. B. Saunders; 2002. p. 3745–88.
7. Mansson W, Ahlgren G, White T. Glomerular filtration rate up to 10 years after urinary diversion of different types. A comparative study of ileal and colonic conduit, refluxing and antirefluxing ureteral anastomosis and continent caecal reservoir. Scand J Urol Nephrol 1989;23:195–200.
8. Lugagne PM, Herve JM, Lebret T, et al. Ureteroileal implantation in orthotopic neobladder with Le Duc-Camey mucosal-through technique: risk of stenosis and long-term follow-up. J Urol 1997;158(3 Pt 1):765–7.
9. Weijerman PC, Schurmans JR, Hop WC, et al. Morbidity and quality of life in patients with orthotopic and heterotopic continent urinary diversion. Urology 1998;51:51–6.
10. Pantuck AJ, Han KR, Perrotti M, et al. Ureteroenteric anastomosis in continent urinary diversion: long-term results and complications of direct versus nonrefluxing techniques. J Urol 2000;163:450–5.
11. Roth S, Weining C, Hertle L. Simplified uretero-intestinal implantation in continent cutaneous urinary diversion using ileovalvular segment as afferent loop and appendix as continent outlet. J Urol 1996;155:1200–5.
12. Studer UE, Danuser H, Merz VW, et al. Experience in 100 patients with an ileal low pressure bladder substitute combined with an afferent tubular isoperistaltic segment. J Urol 1995;154:49–56.
13. Kramolowsky EV, Clayman RV, Weyman PJ. Management of ureterointestinal anastomotic strictures: comparison of open surgical and endourological repair. J Urol 1988;139: 1195–8.
14. Hudson HC, Kramer SA, Anderson EE. Identification of ureteroileal obstruction by retrograde loopography. Urology 1981;17:147–8.
15. Filmer RB, Spencer JR. Malignancies in bladder augmentations and intestinal conduits. J Urol 1990;143:671–8.
16. Balaji KC, McGuire M, Grotas J, et al. Upper tract recurrences following radical cystectomy: an analysis of prognostic factors, recurrence pattern and stage at presentation. J Urol 1999;162:1603–6.
17. Schwartz CB, Bekirov H, Melman A. Urothelial tumors of upper tract following treatment of primary bladder transitional cell carcinoma. Urology 1992;40:509–11.
18. Malkowicz SB, Skinner DG. Development of upper tract carcinoma after cystectomy for bladder carcinoma. Urology 1990;36:20–2.
19. Kenworthy P, Tanguay S, Dinney CPN. The risk of upper tract recurrences following cystectomy in patients with transitional cell carcinoma involving the distal ureter. J Urol 1996;155:501–3.
20. Slaton JW, Swanson DA, Grossman HB, Dinney CPN. A stage specific approach to tumor surveillance after radical cystectomy for transitional cell carcinoma of the bladder. J Urol 1999;162(3 Pt 1):710–4.
21. Walther PJ, Robertson CN, Paulson DF. Lethal complications of standard self-retaining ureteral stents in patients with ileal conduit urinary diversion. J Urol 1985;133:851–3.
22. Tsuji Y, Nakamura H, Ariyoshi A. Upper urinary tract involvement after cystectomy and ileal conduit diversion for primary bladder carcinoma. Eur Urol 1996;29:216–20.
23. Penalver MA, Angioli R, Mirashemi R, Malik R. Management of early and late complications of ileocolonic continent urinary reservoir (Miami pouch). Gynecol Oncol 1998;69:185–91.
24. Banner MP, Pollack HM. Dilatation of ureteral stenoses: techniques and experience in 44 patients. AJR Am J Roentgenol 1984;143:789–93.
25. Johnson CD, Oke EJ, Dunnick NR, et al. Percutaneous balloon dilatation of ureteral strictures. AJR Am J Roentgenol 1987;148:181–4.
26. Chang R, Marshall FF, Mitchell S. Percutaneous management of benign ureteral strictures and fistulas. J Urol 1987;137: 1126–31.
27. Lang EK, Glorioso LW. Antegrade transluminal dilatation of benign ureteral strictures. AJR Am J Roentgenol 1988; 150:131–4.
28. Dourmashkin RL. Dilatation of ureter with rubber bags in the treatment of ureteral calculi. Presentation of a modified cystoscope: a preliminary report. J Urol 1926;15:449–60.
29. Grüntzig AR, Senning A, Siegenthaler WE. Nonoperative dilatation of coronary-artery stenosis: percutaneous transluminal coronary angioplasty. N Engl J Med 1979; 301:61–8.
30. Martin EC, Fankuchen EI, Casarella WJ. Percutaneous dilatation of ureteroenteric strictures or occlusions in ileal conduits. Urol Radiol 1982;4:19–21.
31. Shapiro MJ, Banner MP, Amendola MA, et al. Balloon catheter dilation of ureteroenteric strictures: long-term results. Radiology 1988;168:385–7.
32. Kramolowsky EV, Clayman RV. Advances in endosurgery. Treatment of ureteral-enteric anastomotic strictures. Urol Clin North Am 1988;15:413–8.
33. Kramolowsky EV, Clayman RV, Weyman PJ. Endourological management of ureteroileal anastomotic strictures: is it effective? J Urol 1987;137:390–4.
34. Gerber GS, Kuznetzov D, Leef JA, et al. Holmium:YAG laser endoureterotomy in the treatment of ureteroenteric strictures following orthotopic urinary diversion. Tech Urol 1999;5:45–8.
35. Grasso M, Bagley D. Small diameter, actively deflectable, flexible ureteropyeloscopy. J Urol 1998;160:1648–54.
36. Chang DT, Gupta M. Use of a laparoscopic insufflation port for ileal conduit endoscopy. Urology 1999;53:412–3.
37. Bagley D, Erhard M. Use of the holmium laser in the upper urinary tract. Tech Urol 1995;1:25–30.
38. Conlin MJ, Bagley DH. Ureteroscopic endopyelotomy at a single setting. J Urol 1998;159:727–31.
39. Bagley BH, Liu JB, Goldberg BB, Grasso M. Endopyelotomy: importance of crossing vessels demonstrated by endoluminal ultrasonography. J Endourol 1995;9:465–7.
40. Chandhoke PS, Clayman RV, Stone AM, et al. Endopyelotomy and endoureterotomy with the Acucise ureteral cutting balloon device: preliminary experience. J Endourol 1993; 7:45–51.
41. Lin DW, Bush WH, Mayo ME. Endourological treatment of ureteroenteric strictures: efficacy of Acucise endoureterotomy. J Urol 1999;162(3 Pt 1):696–8.
42. Preminger GM, Clayman RV, Nakada SY, et al. A multicenter clinical trial investigating the use of a fluoroscopically controlled cutting balloon catheter for the management of ureteral and ureteropelvic junction obstruction. J Urol 1997;157:1625–9.
43. Muench PJ, Cates HB, Raney AM, et al. Endoscopic management of the obliterated ureteroileal anastomosis. J Urol 1987;137:277–9.
44. Dixon GD, Moore JD, Stockton R. Successful dilation of ureteroileal anastomotic stenosis using Grüntzig catheter. Urology 1982;19:555–8.
45. Glanz S, Gordon DH, Butt K, et al. Percutaneous transrenal balloon dilatation of the ureter. Radiology 1983;149:101–4.
46. Finnerty DP, Trulock TS, Berkman W, Walton KN. Transluminal balloon dilation of ureteral strictures. J Urol 1984;131:1056–60.
47. King LR, Coughlin PWF, Ford KK, et al. Initial experience with percutaneous and transurethral ablation of postoperative ureteral strictures in children. J Urol 1984;131:1167–70.
48. O'Brien WM, Maxted WC, Pahira JJ. Ureteral stricture: experience with 31 cases. J Urol 1988;140:737–40.
49. Smith AD. Management of iatrogenic ureteral strictures after urological procedures. J Urol 1988;140:1372–4.
50. Beckmann CF, Roth RA, Bihrle W 3rd. Dilation of benign ureteral strictures. Radiology 1989;172:437–41.
51. Aliabadi H, Reinberg Y, Gonzalez R. Percutaneous balloon dilation of ureteral strictures after failed surgical repair in children. J Urol 1990;144(2 Pt 2):486–8.
52. Netto NR Jr, Ferreira U, Lemos GC, Claro JF. Endourological management of ureteral strictures. J Urol 1990;144:631–4.
53. Germinale F, Bottino P, Caviglia C, et al. Endourologic treatment of ureterointestinal strictures. J Endourol 1992;6: 439–43.
54. Kwak S, Leef JA, Rosenblum JD. Percutaneous balloon catheter dilation of benign ureteral strictures: effect of multiple dilation procedures on long-term patency. AJR Am J Roentgenol 1995;165:97–100.
55. Ravery V, de la Taille A, Hoffmann P, et al. Balloon catheter dilation in the treatment of ureteral and ureteroenteric stricture. J Endourol 1998;12:335–40.
56. Richter F, Irwin RJ Jr, Watson RA, Lang EK. Endourologic management of benign ureteral strictures with and without compromised vascular supply. Urology 2000;55:652–7.
57. DiMarco DS, LeRoy AJ, Thieling S, et al. Long-term results of treatment for ureteroenteric strictures. Urology 2001; 58:909–13.
58. Davis DM. Intubated ureterotomy: a new operation for ureteral and ureteropelvic stricture. Surg Gynecol Obstet 1943;76:513–23.
59. Moon YT, Kerbl K, Pearle MS, et al. Evaluation of optimal stent size after endourologic incision of ureteral strictures. J Endourol 1995;9:15–22.
60. Galal H, Lazica A, Lampel A, et al. Management of ureteral strictures by different modalities and effect of stents on upper tract drainage. J Endourol 1993;7:411–7.
61. Kerbl K, Chandhoke PS, Figenshau RS, et al. Effect of stent duration on ureteral healing following endoureterotomy in an animal model. J Urol 1993;150:1302–5.
62. Meretyk S, Clayman RV, Kavoussi LR, et al. Endourologic treatment of ureteroenteric anastomotic strictures: long-term follow-up. J Urol 1991;145:723–7.
63. Schneider AW, Conrad S, Busch R, Otto U. The cold-knife technique for endourological management of stenoses in the upper urinary tract. J Urol 1991;146:961–5.
64. Ahmadzadeh M. Use of a prototype 3-Fr needle electrode with flexible ureteroscopy of antegrade management of stenosed ureteroileal anastomosis. Urol Int 1992;49:215–7.
65. Bierkens AF, Oosterhof GO, Meuleman EJ, Debruyne FM. Anterograde percutaneous treatment of ureterintestinal strictures following urinary diversion. Eur Urol 1996; 30:363–8.
66. Cornud F, Lefebvre JF, Chrétien Y, et al. Percutaneous transrenal electro-incision of ureterointestinal anastomotic strictures: long-term results and comparison of fluoroscopic and endoscopic guidance. J Urol 1996;155:1575–8.
67. Singal RK, Denstedt JD, Razvi HA, Chun SS. Holmium:YAG laser endoureterotomy for treatment of ureteral stricture. Urology 1997;50:875–80.
68. Wolf JS Jr, Elashry OM, Clayman RV. Long-term results of endoureterotomy for benign ureteral and ureteroenteric strictures. J Urol 1997;158(3 Pt 1):759–64.
69. Laven BA, O'Connor RC, Steinberg GD, Gerber GS. Long-term results of antegrade endoureterotomy using the holmium laser in patients with ureterointestinal strictures. Urology 2001;58:924–9.
70. Watterson JD, Sofer M, Wollin TA, et al. Holmium:YAG laser endoureterotomy for ureterointestinal strictures. J Urol 2002;167:1692–5.
71. Poulakis V, Witzsch U, DeVries R, Becht E. Cold-knife endoureterotomy for nonmalignant ureterointestinal anastomotic strictures. Urology 2003;61:512–7.
72. Meretyk S, Albala DM, Clayman RV, et al. Endoureterotomy for treatment of ureteral strictures. J Urol 1992;147:1502–6.
73. Yamada S, Ono Y, Ohshima S, Miyake K. Transurethral ureteroscopic ureterotomy assisted by a prior balloon dilation for relieving ureteral strictures. J Urol 1995;153:1418–21.
74. Oppenheimer R, Hinman F Jr. Ureteral regeneration: contracture vs. hyperplasia of smooth muscle. J Urol 1955;74: 476–84.
75. Babayan RK. Use of the Acucise balloon catheter. In: Smith AD, editor. Controversies in endourology. Philadelphia: W. B. Saunders; 1995. p. 309–14.
76. Kabalin JN. Acucise incision of ureteroenteric strictures after urinary diversion. J Endourol 1997;11:37–40.
77. McDougall EM, Nakada SY. Endourologic management of ureterosigmoidostomy anastomotic stricture. J Endourol 1997;11:135–7.
78. Knowles DR, Staiman VR, Gupta M. Long-term results of the treatment of complete distal ureteral stenosis using a cutting balloon catheter device. J Urol 2001;166:2087–90.
79. Seseke F, Heuser M, Zöller G, et al. Treatment of iatrogenic postoperative ureteral strictures with Acucise endoureterotomy. Eur Urol 2002;42:370–5.
80. Smith AD, Lange PH, Miller RP, Reinke DB. Percutaneous dilation of ureteroileal strictures and insertion of Gibbons ureteral stents. Urology 1979;13:24–6.
81. Rosen RJ, McLean GK, Freiman DB, et al. Obstructed ureteroileal conduits: antegrade catheter drainage. AJR Am J Roentgenol 1980;135:1201–4.
82. Banner MP, Pollack HM, Ring EJ, Wein AJ. Catheter dilation of benign ureteral strictures. Radiology 1983;147:427–33.
83. Lang EK. Antegrade ureteral stenting for dehiscence, strictures, and fistulae. AJR Am J Roentgenol 1984;143:795–801.
84. Oshinsky GS, Smith AD. The failure of endourologic management of ureterointestinal strictures. J Urol 1993;149: 373A.
85. Urban DA, Kerbl K, Clayman RV, et al. Endoureteroplasty with a free urothelial graft. J Urol 1994;152:910–5.
86. Gort HB, Mali WP, van Waes PR, et al. Metallic self-expandable stenting of a ureteroileal stricture. AJR Am J Roentgenol 1990;155:422–3.
87. Reinberg Y, Ferral H, Gonzalez R, et al. Intraureteral metallic self-expanding endoprosthesis (Wallstent) in the treatment of difficult ureteral strictures. J Urol 1994;151:1619–22.
88. Kulkarni RP, Bellamy EA. A new thermoexpandable shape-memory nickel-titanium alloy stent for the management of ureteric strictures. BJU Int 1999;83:755–9.
89. Barbalias GA, Liatsikos EN, Karnabatidis D, et al. Ureteroileal anastomotic strictures. An innovative approach with metallic stents. J Urol 1998;160:1270–3.
90. Sanders R, Bissada NK, Bielsky S. Ureteroenteric anastomotic strictures: treatment with Palmaz permanent indwelling stents. J Urol 1993;150(2 Pt 1):469–70.
91. Barbalias GA, Siablis D, Liatsikos EN, et al. Metal stents: a new treatment of malignant ureteral obstruction. J Urol 1997;158:54–8.

101

Management of Upper Urinary Tract Transitional Cell Carcinoma

Ardeshir Rastinehad, DO

Michael C. Ost, MD

Robert Marcovich, MD

Although nephroureterectomy has been considered the gold standard for the treatment of upper tract transitional cell carcinoma (UTTCC), laparoscopic nephroureterectomy has challenged the open technique as a new standard of care. Along these lines, minimally invasive endoscopic techniques, including percutaneous surgery and ureteroscopy, have emerged as alternative therapies with efficacious oncologic outcomes when appropriately applied. The reservation associated with endoscopic techniques for patients requiring a nephron-sparing approach has proven to be an old adage. Endoscopic approaches have particular advantages when treatment is based on anatomic variation, tumor grade, and tumor location. A percutaneous approach, in particular, has proven to be an effective minimally invasive treatment for large (> 1.5 cm), low-grade, upper tract transitional cell carcinomas, limited to the calices, renal pelvis, and proximal ureter.

The history of percutaneous approaches for the management of UTTCC began in 1985 when Huffman and colleagues reported on a case treated with ureteroscopic resection.[1] Shortly thereafter, Streem and Pontes published the first report of the percutaneous nephroscopic approach to treatment of UTTCC.[2] This technique was subsequently popularized by Smith and colleagues, who were also the first to systematically use topical immunotherapy as an adjunct to tumor resection.[3]

The preliminary rationale for endoscopic management of UTTCC was to preserve renal parenchyma and to decrease the associated morbidity. In this regard, endoscopic management was introduced to treat patients with UTTCC in an anatomic or functional solitary kidney, bilateral disease, or patients who were not candidates for open surgery because of underlying comorbidities. Today, endoscopic management remains the standard of care for such patients, as long as they have noninvasive disease. Some controversy still exists regarding the use of endoscopic management in patients with a normal contralateral kidney, in those who have multiple tumors in the same kidney or ipsilateral collecting system, and in patients with a solitary kidney with high-grade disease. Additionally, it is uncommon to find a patient who is unable to tolerate a laparoscopic procedure for removal of the diseased kidney and ureter, so underlying comorbidity alone has become less an issue.

In evaluating the efficacy of definitive endoscopic management of UTTCC, several outcomes need to be assessed, including tumor recurrence, tumor progression, renal preservation rate, disease-specific survival, and overall survival. Because of the relative rarity of upper tract urothelium cancer, it is difficult to accrue a large pool of patients; this is one reason for the complete paucity of prospective randomized trials in the literature.

GENERAL APPROACH

UTTCC most commonly presents with gross or microscopic hematuria. Patients with a history of recurrent superficial bladder TCC or who have undergone radical cystectomy are more likely to be intensely surveyed for. Work-up with intravenous urography (IVU) or a computed topography (CT) urogram with contrast may reveal a filling defect in the involved kidney or ureter. Positive urine cytology is highly suggestive of the diagnosis in the presence of an upper tract filling defect. In the absence of a visible lesion on urography, positive cytology from the upper tract may be indicative of carcinoma in situ, mandating ureteroscopic inspection of the kidneys and ureters. Figure 101-1 summarizes the management protocol for UTTCC at the North Shore-Long Island Jewish Medical Center.

An abdominal pelvic CT scan, with and without intravenous contrast, is obtained to assess for evidence of parenchymal invasion. CT scans have the added benefit of excluding a radiolucent stone as the cause of the filling defect, as well as ruling out the presence of abdominal metastases. If obvious invasion is noted on CT scan, a metastatic work-up is performed (chest radiograph, liver function tests, bone scintigraphy), and the patient is directed toward laparoscopic nephroureterectomy. If the CT scan fails to demonstrate parenchymal invasion, ureteropyeloscopy should be performed in order to verify the presence of UTTCC and to obtain a specimen for diagnosis, grading, and staging purposes. At the time of ureteroscopy, an attempt is made to completely resect the tumor. If the tumor is deemed unresectable, owing to size or poor visualization from bleeding, the patient undergoes a percutaneous resection. This can be done under the same anesthetic if the patient has been counseled and consented to this approach. If the ureteroscopic resection is adequate, a second-look ureteroscopy and biopsy is performed within 2 to 4 weeks to exclude residual disease. If this is negative, consideration is given to offering the patient topical adjuvant immunotherapy with percutaneous instillation of bacillus Calmette-Guérin (BCG). If tumor is still present on the second-look ureteroscopy, it is resected and a final ureteroscopy is performed to assess the adequacy of treatment. Should tumor persist at this time, the patient undergoes percutaneous resection, followed by a second-look nephroscopy within 1 week. If this is positive, the patient undergoes nephroureterectomy. If negative, the patient is given adjuvant BCG, once per week for 6 weeks. A "third-look" nephroscopy and biopsy is performed 2 weeks after BCG therapy to exclude residual disease. A biopsy is necessary owing to the difficulty of identifying residual tumor because of the inflammatory response induced by BCG and the presence of the nephrostomy tube.

INDICATIONS FOR PERCUTANEOUS APPROACH

Development of endoscopic techniques has enabled urologists to approach superficial UTTCC in a less invasive fashion. The main indication for an endoscopic approach is to preserve functional renal tissue. Patients with bulky and or low-grade (G1-G2) UTTCC, limited to the renal pelvis, whose circumstances do not require a nephron-sparing approach, may choose a percutaneous approach if appropriately counseled on the 25 to 28% recurrence rate and the 5-year disease-specific survival of greater than 95%. Such patients must be motivated and reliable, as they will be subjected to a lifetime of endoscopic and radiographic surveillance. More commonly, conservative surgery for UTTCC is used in patients with bilateral synchronous tumors, cancer in a solitary kidney, and in patients with poor renal function, in whom nephrectomy would result in the need for hemodialysis. Endoscopic surgery for upper tract TCC is also reasonable in those patients with favorable tumor characteristics (Table 101-1).

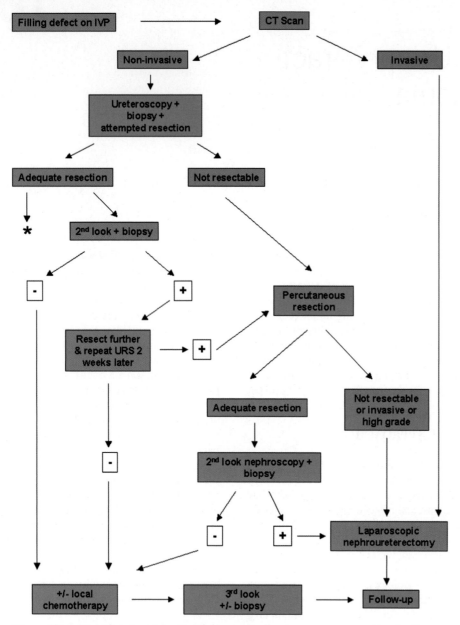

Figure 101-1 Algorithm for minimally invasive approaches to upper tract transitional cell carcinoma. * If high-grade or invasive, proceed to nephroureterectomy.

pelvis and obviates the risk of parenchymal hemorrhage or adjacent organ injury.

The main advantage of the percutaneous approach is that it allows the use of larger endoscopes, which improves visualization. The larger instruments facilitate resection of more extensive lesions and make tumor removal more efficient. Both rigid and flexible endoscopes may be passed through the percutaneous tract so that all calices may be completely inspected. If a single tract is inadequate to reach all portions of the intrarenal collecting system, additional tracts can be created. A percutaneous approach may be the best choice for lower caliceal tumors that may not be accessible by ureteroscopy owing to limitations in scope deflection. In patients with a prior urinary diversion, the percutaneous approach may be the only way to access the collecting system.

An impressive array of instruments can be used percutaneously, including larger resectoscopes and grasping and biopsy forceps, as well as larger-bore laser fibers. All tissue layers can be sampled percutaneously, potentially improving local tumor staging. Second-look nephroscopy, biopsy, and, if necessary, residual tumor resection, are all facilitated by a percutaneous approach, as is the adjuvant instillation of BCG or mitomycin. However, the increased versatility of the percutaneous approach comes at the expense of greater morbidity compared with ureteroscopy, especially with regard to bleeding and the potential for adjacent organ injury.

Because of their distinct advantages, ureteroscopy and percutaneous resection should not be thought of as competing modalities, but complementary methods toward accomplishing the goal of complete tumor removal. Depending on tumor and patient characteristics, the management approach to UTTCC may encompass both treatments in an attempt to provide patients with the best quality of care in diagnosis, therapy, and follow-up.

PATIENT COUNSELING

Patients who are candidates for an endoscopic approach by virtue of their tumor characteristics or because of impaired renal function must still be counseled that nephroureterectomy remains the

CONTRAINDICATIONS TO PERCUTANEOUS APPROACH

Biopsy-proven high-grade (G3-G4) tumors and those appearing to be invasive on radiographic studies or endoscopic inspection should not be treated endoscopically in the presence of a normal contralateral kidney. If disease is unresectable, owing to size, number, or location of tumors, the patient should go on to a laparoscopic nephroureterectomy. If a previously resected lesion progresses to a higher grade or recurs rapidly after resection and topical adjuvant immunotherapy, further attempts at primary endoscopic therapy should be abandoned.

Presence of an active infection, bleeding diathesis or coagulopathy, or uncontrolled hypertension should delay endoscopic resection until remedied. While morbid obesity is not a contraindication to a percutaneous approach, extra-long instruments may be needed to reach the kidney percutaneously; in such cases a ureteroscopic approach, if feasible, might be more effective. Lastly, patients who are unable or unwilling to continue with a strict follow-up protocol should be excluded from definitive endoscopic therapy.

PERCUTANEOUS VERSUS URETEROSCOPIC APPROACH

Both ureteroscopic and percutaneous approaches can be effective in the treatment of superficial TCC of the upper urinary tract, but each has certain advantages and disadvantages. Ureteroscopy is less invasive, relatively easy to perform, and imparts little risk of tumor spillage into the retroperitoneum. It is the best initial method for procuring a tissue sample that is adequate for diagnosis and grading, and it is the most thorough way to survey the whole collecting system during posttreatment follow-up. Ureteroscopy is the best approach for small lesions of the ureter or renal

Table 101-1 Indications for Endoscopic or Percutaneous Surgery for the Treatment of Upper Tract Transitional Cell Carcinoma
Absolute
Bilateral tumors (synchronous/metachronous) Predisposition to form multiple tumors (eg, Balkan nephropathy) Solitary kidney Significant comorbidities
Relative
Renal insufficiency Low-grade/stage lesion
Elective

gold standard treatment for UTTCC. They should understand that although their particular situation may warrant an endoscopic approach in order to spare renal function, at some later date, complete removal of the affected kidney may be required. On the other hand, patients with a solitary kidney or very poor renal function, who are over the age of 65, should know that 5-year survival rates for elderly patients on dialysis are dismal (Table 101-2) and that endoscopic management may afford them several years that are free of dialysis, resulting in a potentially better quality of life.

Patients with a normal contralateral kidney who elect a conservative endoscopic approach must be made especially aware that this course of therapy imparts a higher risk of recurrence than nephroureterectomy, that progression to a higher grade or degree of invasion may occur, and that they may, one day, eventually lose the kidney. They should know that incidence of metachronous bilateral tumors is very low, only 1 to 2%,[4] and that this is less than the incidence of ipsilateral recurrence after percutaneous resection of even well-differentiated tumors.[5] It should also be made clear that there is little risk of developing renal insufficiency or hypertension, even years after removal of the diseased kidney.[6] Finally, patients must be willing to submit to an intense follow-up regimen, which, because it includes frequent ureteroscopy, is more invasive and more expensive than the standard regimen following nephroureterectomy. Despite these potential risks, patients should also understand that with favorable disease, there is a high likelihood of renal preservation.

In addition, the urologist should counsel the patient regarding the risks of the percutaneous approach itself, including bleeding necessitating blood transfusion, infection, failed access, injury to adjacent organs, and pleural injury. This discussion should be balanced by a discussion of the risks of open surgery, as well as laparoscopic nephroureterectomy.

Ultimately, the decision must be made by the well-informed patient, taking into account his or her particular situation and the various risks and benefits associated with the various approaches to treatment.

TECHNIQUE

Percutaneous surgery requires careful patient preparation. Since endoscopic management is indicated only for localized superficial disease, a metastatic work-up should be performed before resection is undertaken. This includes an abdominopelvic CT scan, chest radiography, liver function tests, and serum alkaline phosphatase level. If the last is elevated, bone scintigraphy is warranted.

In order to minimize the risk of bleeding and infection, anticoagulants should be stopped well in advance of surgery. Bleeding diathesis, active infection, and hypertension should be corrected or controlled before bringing the patient to the operating room. A positive urine culture is an absolute contraindication to proceed with percutaneous surgery and prolonged closed upper tract system manipulation.

The patient is given a first- or second-generation cephalosporin intravenously prior to surgery. Patients requiring prophylaxis against spontaneous bacterial endocarditis are given ampicillin and gentamicin, with vancomycin substituted if there is a penicillin allergy. Sequential compression devices are placed on both lower extremities to prevent deep vein thrombosis.

Initially, cystoscopy is performed to rule out the presence of synchronous bladder tumor(s). A 5 or 6F ureteral catheter is advanced into the renal pelvis. The ureteral catheter is fastened to a Foley catheter with a silk tie, and the patient is then carefully transferred to the prone position. The face is padded with foam and chest bolsters are put in place. The head and upper body padding should be adjusted so that the neck is in a neutral position. The elbows and knees are cushioned with foam or gel pads, and the ankles are elevated on a bolster to prevent the toes from touching the table. The shoulders should be abducted to an angle of less than 90 degrees. In morbidly obese patients, chest bolsters can be omitted.

Contrast is injected through the ureteral catheter to outline the pelvocaliceal system (Figure 101-2). To facilitate complete resection, caliceal tumors should be accessed with a puncture directly into the calix, while a pelvic tumor should be accessed through an upper or middle calix. While lower-pole access to renal pelvic tumors has also been recommended,[7] upper-pole or middle caliceal access facilitates complete inspection of the collecting system with rigid endoscopes. By using lower-pole access, it may be impossible to pass a rigid scope into upper calices, as the patient's hip can limit scope mobility.

After the access site is chosen, an 18-gauge diamond-tipped needle is passed into the collecting system under biplanar fluoroscopic guidance. The obturator is removed and efflux of urine confirms correct positioning of the needle. A guidewire is coiled in the collecting system (Figure 101-3) or, preferably, advanced down the ureter. A second (safety) wire should be placed to guard against loss of the tract. The tract is created using a dilating balloon or sequential Amplatz dilators, and a working sheath is appropriately placed. In order to decrease the theoretical risk of tumor seeding, care should be taken to ensure that the sheath never slips out of the collecting system.

After dilation, nephroscopy of the entire system is carried out to identify all areas of the tumor (Figure 101-4). If a guidewire was not able to be manipulated down to the bladder, the tip of the ureteral catheter is grasped, pulled out through the nephrostomy, and intubated with a guidewire. The guidewire is then passed down to provide through-and-through access. The safest way to excise the tumor is by piecemeal removal with cold-cup forceps (Figure 101-5). Biopsies of the tumor base are taken separately, and then the base is resected and cauterized with a resectoscope (Figure 101-6) or laser (Figure 101-7). Deep biopsies or resection into the renal parenchyma will result in a great deal of bleeding and should be avoided. If the operative field is clear enough, a flexible endoscope may be used to inspect the rest of the collecting system or address tumors that cannot be accessed with rigid instrumentation (Figure 101-8). At the conclusion of the operation, a 24F Malecot nephrostomy tube, with a ureteral extension, is appropriately placed (Figure 101-9), and its position is verified under fluoroscopy. Large-bore catheters[5] will tamponade parenchymal bleeding, provide excellent renal drainage, and preserve access to the kidney and ureter for the planned second-look nephroscopy.

Second-look nephroscopy is performed within 1 week of the initial resection, unless permanent section of the tumor reveals high-grade or invasive TCC, in which case nephroureterectomy is indicated. If the tumor is deemed not to be completely resectable through a percutaneous approach, a nephroureterectomy is completed. The second-look provides an opportunity to reinspect the urothelium in a relatively bloodless field, to excise any residual disease, and to biopsy the base of the previously resected tumor. High-grade or invasive disease, apparent during the second-look biopsy, is another indication for nephroureterectomy.

If intracavitary instillation of adjuvant agents is anticipated, the Malecot is exchanged for an 8F pigtail nephrostomy catheter. Instillations may

Table 101-2 Five-Year Survival Rates of Patients with End-Stage Renal Disease[38]	
Age Group (years)	5-Year Survival (%)
0–14	87
15–24	84
25–34	69
35–44	61
45–54	47
55–64	32
65–74	19
75–84	10

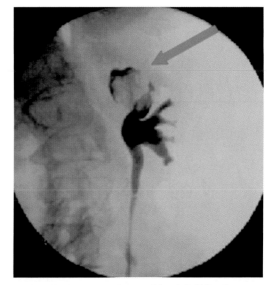

Figure 101-2 Upper Pole Transitional Cell Carcinoma

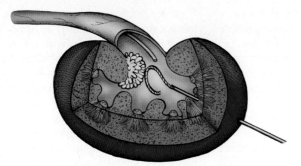

Figure 101-3 Retrograde ureteral catheter is placed and nephrostomy needle is introduced into collecting system through upper calyx. A guide wire is passed into the renal pelvis through the nephrostomy needle.

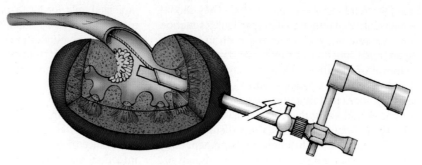

Figure 101-4 After placement of a nephrostomy sheath, the nephroscope is used to inspect the collecting system.

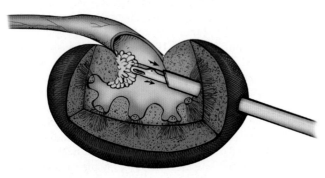

Figure 101-5 Biopsy forceps are used to remove the bulk of the tumor.

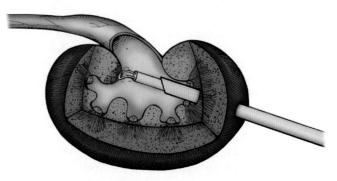

Figure 101-6 The base of the tumor is fulgurated with the cautery loop.

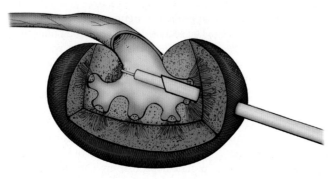

Figure 101-7 The tumor base may also be fulgurated with the neodymium:yttrium-aluminum-garnet (Nd:YAG) laser.

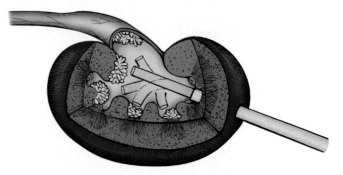

Figure 101-8 A flexible nephroscope may be used to examine all calyces.

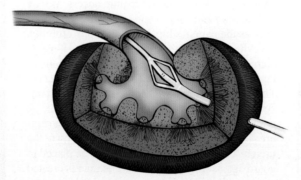

Figure 101-9 After resection and fulguration, a Malecot nephrostomy tube with a ureteral extension is placed through the percutaneous tract for drainage of the collecting system.

begin 2 weeks following the last resection. The authors have used mitomycin and BCG, but have more experience with the latter. The patient is admitted to the hospital for each BCG treatment or, alternatively, therapy may be undertaken in an outpatient chemotherapy infusion unit. Prophylactic intravenous antibiotics are mandatory, as the nephrostomy tubes invariably become colonized, creating a risk of urosepsis. Fluoroquinolones, gentamicin, and doxycycline should *not* be used, as they will inactivate the bacillus,[8] but beta-lactam antibiotics are acceptable. An infusion of normal saline into the nephrostomy tube is started at 10 cc per hour and increased by 10 cc per hour every hour, until the infusion rate reaches 50 cc per hour. The intrarenal pressure is closely monitored to ensure that it remains below 25 cm H_2O (Figure 101-10). If the patient tolerates the saline infusion without difficulty, 50 cc of 1×10^8 colony-forming units of BCG is administered over 1 hour. The patient voids after instillation, and is discharged home the next day. Two weeks after completion of therapy, the patient undergoes a third-look nephroscopy through the existing tract.

RESULTS

There are few studies reporting the results of percutaneous management of UTTCC (Table 101-3), and four are from the same institution.[5,9–11] Most of the patients treated had solitary kidney, bilateral disease, chronic renal failure, or significant comorbid disease, contraindicating open surgery. At present, however, this is representative of the patient population most often considered for a percutaneous approach. Very few institutions have expanded the indications to include motivated, otherwise healthy patients with superficial low-grade disease, who elect a nephron-sparing, minimally invasive approach.[10–14] Recently, Palou and colleagues presented their long-term data of percutaneous nephroscopic management of UTTCC in patients with papillary tumors of low grade and those lesions not amenable to ureteroscopic resection; grade III tumors were considered for resection only in those patients with a solitary kidney or bilateral disease.[13] Almost half of these patients (47.1%, 16 of 34) were treated by a percutaneous route, electively, and all received adjuvant topical therapy with either BCG or mitomycin. Ipsilateral recurrence developed in 41.2% (14 of 34) of patients at a median time of 24 months.

Recurrence is the first measure of the efficacy of therapy, and tumor grade correlates well with recurrence (see Table 101-3). However, Park and colleagues reported that ureteral TCC is associated with a high, local, or distant failure, compared with renal pelvis TCC, even at the same stage and grade.[15] Patients with grade 1 disease have a good prognosis, while outcomes of those with grade 3 tend to have a poorer response to treatment. Grade 1 disease recurs in 5 to 26% of cases,[5,7,10,11,16–18] but progression is less likely, and death from low-grade urothelial carcinoma is rare. There has been only 1 cancer-related death in a patient with grade

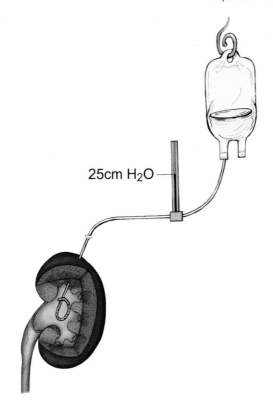

25cm H_2O

Figure 101-10 Schematic diagram of percutaneous infusion of bacillus Calmette-Guerin.

1 disease in 4 different series, and this patient was found to have grade 2 histology on second look.[5,10,17,18] Grade 1 lesions are associated with a good rate of renal preservation. Rastinehad and colleagues reported recurrence in 5 of 19 (26.3%) RU with grade 1 disease, 3 had nephroureterectomies, and 2 others were treated with percutaneous resection.[11] The mean time to recurrence was 27 months for this subset of patients.

The prognosis of grade 2 disease is also good. Recurrence rate in 138 patients from 9 different series is 26.1%.[5,7,9–11,13,16–18] In 5 of the 6 studies where disease-specific survival is reported or can be calculated, patients with grade 2 pathology died of cancer-related causes in less than 5% of cases. Renal retention, however, is a serious consideration. Jarrett and colleagues reported that of 12 patients with grade 2 histology, 6 (50%) had nephroureterectomy, 3 within days of their percutaneous resection, and 3 for recurrence.[5] Jabbour and colleagues published a study that specifically addressed grade 2 disease managed with percutaneous resection. They found that 7 of 24 patients (29%) underwent nephroureterectomy, 4 immediately, and 3 for recurrence.[9]

The prognosis for high-grade upper tract TCC is poor, regardless of management modality. In the second largest published series of grade 3 patients, Liatsikos and colleagues reported 56% recurrence and 64% disease-specific survival.[10] Jarrett and colleagues included 13 grade 3 patients in their series. Eight of them died during follow-up, 6 of disease-related causes (46%), and of those without evidence of disease, only 1 patient had retained the affected kidney.[5] The disparity between the 2 studies may be explained

by the shorter follow-up time in the report by Liatsikos and colleagues. Rastinehad and colleagues reported the largest series of grade 3 patients, 15 of 39 (38%) recurrence rate.[11] Two of the 15 patients developed metastatic disease. It is evident that percutaneous resection should not be offered for high-grade upper tract TCC, except as a last resort in elderly patients with a solitary kidney who would not tolerate hemodialysis.

Tumor stage also affects prognosis in association with grade. Noninvasive (Ta) lesions generally tend to be low grade. In one study, all patients with grade 1 lesions had Ta disease,[5] while in the studies of Plancke and colleagues and Martinez-Pineiro and colleagues, Ta was seen in 86% and 76% of grade 1 tumors, respectively.[17,19] Superficially invasive (T1) tumors tend to be more heterogeneous, with substantial numbers of these lesions occurring as grades 2 and 3 disease.[5,19]

The effect of stage on recurrence and disease-free survival can be seen in a study by Jabbour and Smith, in which 54 patients were followed for a mean of 50 months, after percutaneous resection of upper tract TCC. Stage Ta was associated with 30% recurrence and 93% disease-free survival, while T1 tumors recurred 57% of the time and were associated with 64% disease-free survival. Stage retained its prognostic significance when stratified by grade.[20] The poorer prognosis of higher stage has been confirmed by other investigators. Patel and colleagues found that T1 had a higher recurrence rate than Ta (30% vs 12.5%)[16] and Jarrett and colleagues found lower disease-specific survival (92% vs 57%).[5]

A final consideration is the risk of disease recurrence in the percutaneous tract, which was initially thought to be a significant hazard, owing to the potential of the tumor seeding the tract. Irradiation of the tract was used in two studies[16,21] in order to avoid seeding in patients treated percutaneously. While no cases of tract recurrence occurred in either of these reports, most institutions offering a percutaneous approach have not employed tract irradiation and, in the majority, no cases of tract seeding have been encountered.[5,7,9–11,16–20]

There have been three case reports of tract seeding,[22–24] occurring in situations which were not typical of current treatment protocols. In one case, owing to delay in diagnosis of the etiology of a ureteral obstruction, the percutaneous tract was exposed to high-grade TCC for 1 month prior to resection, while in the other, a second-look procedure to rule out persistence of unresected disease was never undertaken. These two examples highlight the importance of complete tumor resection, second- and third-look nephroscopy, and biopsy to ensure that no disease is left behind and minimize the time that the tract is exposed to unresected cancer. Thirdly, and most recently, Oefelein and MacLennan reported on a TCC nephrostomy tract recurrence following percutaneous resection of a T1 G2 lesion in a patient who had undergone prior radical cystectomy for T2 N0 M0 disease.[24] The patient eventually underwent a nephroureterectomy with upstaging to T2 N1 M0 disease status. Four months postoperatively, a TCC nephrostomy

Table 101-3 Recurrence Rates after Percutaneous Resection of Upper Tract Transitional Cell Carcinoma, Stratified by Tumor Grade (These series included patients treated with adjuvant chemotherapy.)

Series	No. Patients	Mean Follow-Up (mo)	Mean Follow-Up to Recurrence	Grade 1 (%)	Grade 2 (%)	Grade 3 (%)	Total (%)	Disease-Specific Survival (%)
Plancke et al[17] 1995	10	28	7	1/6 (17)	0/3 (0)	0/1 (0)	1/10 (10)	100
Jarrett et al[5] 1995	34	56	N/A	2/11 (18)	3/9 (33)	5/10 (50)	10/30 (33)	87
Patel et al[16] 1996*	26	45	22	2/11 (18)	3/11 (27)	–	6/25* (24)	91
Clark et al[7] 1999	18	21	11	2/6 (13)	2/8 (25)	2/4 (50)	6/18 (33)	–
Lee et al[18] 1999	50	39	N/A	1/20 (5)	1/16 (6)	4/13 (31)	6/49 (12)	–
Jabbour et al[9] 2000	20	48	12	–	5/20 (25)	–	5/20 (25)	84
Liatsikos et al[10] 2001	69	49	N/A	3/15 (20)	7/27 (26)	14/25 (56)	24/67 (36)	84
Palou et al[13] 2004	34	51	24	–	12/28 (43)	3/5 (60)	15/34 (44)	94
Rastinehad et al[11] 2006	125**	61	26	5/19 (26)	9/30 (30)	15/39 (38)	29/88 (33)	–
Total	352	44.2	17	22/102 (21.6)	36/138 (26.1)	43/97 (48.5)	96/337 (30)	–

*One-third of patients with unknown grade recurred.

**39 RU owing to high grade or stage were treated with nephroureterectomy during the immediate treatment phase.

References have overlap in patient data analysis.

tract recurrence presented as an erythematous papule. Despite tract excision, local radiation, and chemotherapy, the patient soon died of metastatic TCC. Although this mortality was associated with a TCC nephrostomy tract recurrence, it is more likely that the patient succumbed to his disease as a result of nodal involvement.

Considerable experience demonstrates that the risk of tumor seeding in appropriately selected patients is negligible. A recent study by Czito and colleagues investigated the role of adjuvant radiotherapy, with and without concurrent chemotherapy, for locally advanced transitional cell carcinoma of the renal pelvis and ureter.[25] Findings in this report suggest that the addition of concurrent cisplatin to adjuvant radiotherapy improves the ultimate outcome in patients with resected, locally advanced upper tract urothelial malignancies. Although this study was in a cohort of patients who underwent extirpative, rather than endoscopic, treatment, perhaps such findings suggest a future role for adjuvant or neoadjuvant treatments involving endoscopic resection for high-grade disease.

COMPLICATIONS OF PERCUTANEOUS RESECTION

Percutaneous resection of upper tract TCC can generally be accomplished safely. Bleeding requiring transfusion occurs in 11 to 37% of cases[7,12,16,20] and can result from injury to a vessel during the creation of the percutaneous tract, or it may be due to the resection itself. If bleeding during establishment of the tract is so brisk as to impair visualization, the procedure should be abandoned. Tamponade of the tract with a large-bore nephrostomy tube or a Kaye balloon catheter will usually limit bleeding in such situations, and the procedure can be resumed in 2 to 3 days. Angiography with super-selective embolization is reserved for those cases in which such conservative measures fail to adequately control hemorrhaging.

Working through a lower-pole caliceal access point may be inhibited by the patient's hip, especially when attempting to angle the nephroscope into the upper-pole calix. In light of this, a direct supracostal approach can offer the best visualization and working angle. Upper-pole access, however, is not without complications. Hemothorax, urothorax, or chylothorax, for example, may complicate percutaneous access if the pleural space is violated. The risk of associated thoracic complications (16–18%), therefore, increases when supracostal or infracostal access is obtained.[26] This patient, for example, incurred a multitude of complications following the treatment of a heavy upper-pole UTTCC tumor burden via supracostal (twelfth rib) percutaneous access (see Figure 101-2). Excessive postoperative hemorrhage coupled with the nephrostomy tube traversing the pleural space and diaphragm (Figure 101-11A and B), resulted in blood tracking around the nephrostomy tube and collecting within the pleural cavity; respiratory failure as a result of hemothorax necessitated intubation and chest tube placement. Selective arterial angiography revealed interlobar artery injuries requiring coil embolization of an amputated lower-pole vessel and dissecting artery in proximity of the nephrostomy tube (Figure 101-12A, B, and C).

In contrast to bleeding from the nephrostomy tract, hemorrhage occurring as a result of tumor resection is effectively controlled only by complete tumor resection or fulguration. Factors influencing the degree of blood loss include the grade and size of the tumor, as well as the depth of resection.[16] It is important to avoid resecting too deeply into parenchyma, as this will greatly increase the risk of bleeding. Complete resection of invasive disease is dangerous and unnecessary, since this situation is best treated by nephroureterectomy. Use of a vaporization electrode or Nd:YAG laser to fulgurate the tumor base may help to reduce the occurrence of significant bleeding.[20]

Perforation of the renal pelvis should be avoided because of the potential for tumor spill into the retroperitoneum, although no such cases have been reported. Since tumor resection cannot be performed with saline irrigation, extravasation of fluid into the retroperitoneum may lead to hyponatremia. Recognition of a significant tear in the collecting system during resection mandates expedient completion of the procedure and placement of a large-bore nephrostomy tube to facilitate drainage and resolution of the defect.

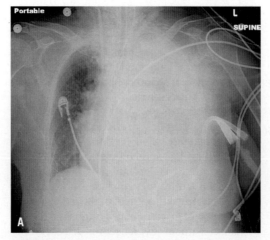
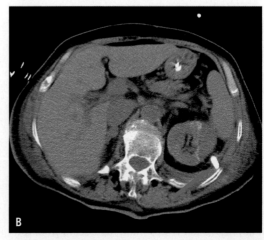

Figure 101-11 *A*, Chest Radiograph: left hemothorax. *B*, CT Scan: left upper pole nephrostomy tube traversing the diaphragm (arrow).

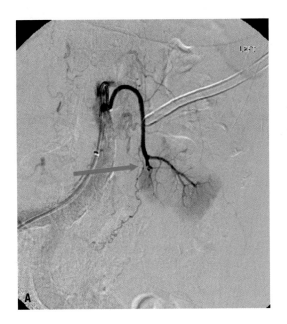
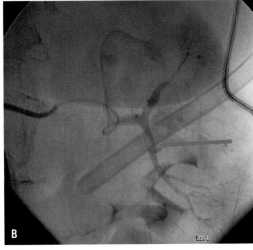
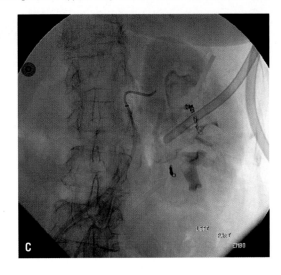

Figure 101-12 *A*, Selective left angiogram: blind ending lower pole vessel (arrow). *B*, Selective left angiogram: dissecting artery in proximity of the nephrostomy tube (arrow). *C*, Selective left angiogram: post coil embolization

Other potential complications are related to percutaneous renal surgery, in general, and include fever, urinary tract infection, failure to obtain access, and injury to adjacent structures, such as pleura or bowel. Fever occurs in 5 to 10% of cases,[7,12] while the others are much less common.

Strictures of the infundibulum or ureteropelvic junction may occur as late complications. These should be investigated by direct visualization through ureteroscopy and possibly biopsy to rule out recurrent tumor as the etiology. Such strictures occurred in 8.7% of cases in one study of 23 patients.[19] They can be managed ureteroscopically or by percutaneous infundibulotomy or endopyelotomy.

SURVEILLANCE FOR PERCUTANEOUS AND URETEROSCOPIC RESECTION

Lifelong surveillance is an absolute requisite for those patients treated primarily with endoscopic resection owing to the potential for recurrence. Since most recurrences appear within 3 years of initial therapy,[27] the follow-up regimen may be tailored to this pattern.

Because of the 30 to 70% risk of recurrent bladder TCC in those with previous upper tract disease, cystoscopy should be performed every 3 months for 1 year, biannually during the second year, and then yearly thereafter. Surveillance ureteroscopy is the modality of choice to follow the upper tracts, owing to the lack of sensitivity of excretory urography and retrograde pyelography. Chen and colleagues found the sensitivity of ureteroscopy with biopsy was 93.4%, compared with 71.7% for retrograde pyelography,[28] while Keeley and colleagues diagnosed only one-fourth of recurrences by retrograde pyelography alone.[29] A reasonable surveillance regimen for the upper tract involves ureteroscopy at 6 month intervals for the first 3 years and then annually thereafter. The contralateral kidney, if present, should be imaged annually, with either retrograde or excretory pyelography.

INSTILLATION THERAPY IN UPPER TRACT UROTHELIAL CARCINOMA

In 1985, Herr reported a case of a patient with a solitary kidney who had been treated for muscle invasive urothelial carcinoma with wide excision of the renal pelvis and entire ureter, followed by creation of a pyelovesical anastomosis. The margins of the resected pelvis and infundibula were positive for carcinoma in situ (CIS), so the patient underwent a 6-week course of BCG instillation, via the bladder. The patient's urinary cytology normalized and remained negative for over 13 months.[30] In 1986, Streem and Pontes reported on a patient with urothelial carcinoma of a solitary kidney treated with percutaneous resection, followed by adjuvant mitomycin C.[2] The following year, Smith and colleagues published results on a series of 9 patients treated with percutaneous resection; 5 of these patients received adjuvant BCG.[3] Since that time, a number of institutions have reported the use of instillation therapy with BCG, mitomycin, epirubicin, or thiotepa, either as primary treatment for CIS or as adjuvant therapy after resection or ablation of papillary tumors. Currently, BCG is the most commonly used agent.

Topical immuno- or chemotherapy delivery may be accomplished by retrograde instillation through a ureteral catheter, via vesicoureteral reflux from an indwelling ureteral stent, or through a pigtail nephrostomy tube. The disadvantage of retrograde catheterization is that cystoscopy must be performed prior to each instillation. To overcome this, Patel and Fuchs passed a single-J ureteral stent through a percutaneous cystotomy and secured it to the skin of the abdomen, obviating the need for endoscopy prior to each instillation.[31] The retrograde techniques may be more expedient when the initial resection is performed ureteroscopically or when instillation is done as primary therapy for CIS situations, in which a nephrostomy tube is not routinely used. Others have advocated a pigtail nephrostomy tube for all

instillations, even those in which percutaneous resection is not required, speculating that contact of the agent with the urothelium is maximized by antegrade administration.[32] A potential disadvantage of the reflux technique is the uncertainty of the amount of agent that actually reaches the renal collecting system. Irie and colleagues performed cystograms to determine the amount of fluid required to induce reflux in each of their patients after placement of a Double-J stent. This volume, which ranged from 80 to 250 cc, was used to guide the subsequent instillation volume of BCG.[33] The main critique of percutaneous instillation is the potential for tumor seeding of the nephrostomy tract during the 6 or more weeks that the tube is in place; however, current protocols emphasize the need for second-look nephroscopy and biopsy to exclude persistence of tumor prior to undertaking instillation therapy. While each method has pros and cons, no evidence in the literature favors any one technique over another.

BCG immunotherapy may be used as a primary treatment for upper tract CIS. Positive initial response rates range from 60 to 100%, with an overall response rate of 86% (Table 101-4). These data, however, are based on normalization of selective urinary cytology, a far less rigorous criterion for success than ureteroscopy and biopsy. Of the initial responders in these studies, one-fourth experienced an upper tract recurrence and almost 10% eventually developed metastatic disease.

A beneficial role for topical adjuvant therapy, following resection of papillary upper tract tumors, has not been proven. No randomized trials of adjuvant therapy have been performed owing to the relative rarity of UTTCC (Table 101-5). Even a multi-institutional effort would take years to reach any conclusions; however, such a trial would be useful in guiding therapy. Currently, seven series specifically assessing adjuvant BCG exist (Table 101-6). Recurrence rates range from 11 to 85%, although they are closer to 33% in the two largest series. Stratification by grade yields recurrence rates of 25% for

Table 101-4 Positive Response and Local Recurrence Rates after Primary Therapy of Upper Tract Carcinoma In Situ with Bacillus Calmette-Guérin

Series	No. Renal Units	Positive Response (%)	Upper Tract Recurrence (%)
Sharpe et al[35] 1993	17	12/17 (71)	0/12 (0)
Yokogi et al[39] 1996	8	5/8 (63)	0/5 (0)
Nishino et al[36] 2000	8	8/8 (100)	0/8 (0)
Nonomura et al[40] 2000	11	9/11 (82)	2/9 (22)
Okubo et al[41] 2001	14	9/14 (64)	2/9 (22)
Irie et al[33] 2002	13	13/13 (100)	1/13 (8)
Thalmann et al[34] 2002	25	22/25 (88)	12/22 (55)
Miyake et al[42] 2002	16	16/16 (100)	3/16 (19)
Hayashida et al[43] 2004	10	10/10 (100)	5/10 (50)
Total	122	105/122 (86)	25/104 (24)

grade 1, 27% for grade 2, and 35% for grade 3, from 110 total patients. These rates do not include the study by Thalmann and colleagues, which had the highest overall recurrence (85%),[34] because this study did not stratify recurrence by grade. To date, there has been only one report comparing outcomes of patients who received postresection BCG versus those who did not, and it failed to show any benefit for grade 2 or 3 disease. However, there was a significantly lower recurrence rate in grade 1 patients receiving BCG compared with those who received no adjuvant therapy; it is necessary to note that the sample size was extremely small.[20] The most recent data from Long Island Jewish Medical Center,[11] regarding 88 RU treated with UTTCC percutaneous resections and 50 of 88 (57%) RU treated with adjuvant BCG immunotherapy, revealed no statistical significance in regard to progression or recurrence when stratified by grade or stage. In addition to not being randomized, this analysis lacked sufficient power to definitively exclude an advantage for any grade/stage of disease.

Our most recent data from the North Shore–Long Island Jewish Medical Center[11] has shown no benefit to using adjuvant topical BCG following UTTCC resection. There is no decrease in recurrence and progression when compared with the untreated groups (Table 101-7). These recent findings, therefore, challenge the use of adjuvant immunotherapy. However, several factors, including the well-known increased risk of recurrence with medium- or high-grade disease in the face of an anatomic or functional solitary kidney, as well as the risk and invasiveness of treating recurrences in patients with normal renal function, are believed to serve as an impetus to do as much as possible with adjuvant therapy.

The major complications of upper tract BCG instillation are BCG dissemination and urosepsis, secondary to gram-negative organisms, with both of these being relatively rare occurrences. Rastinehad and colleagues[11] report 1 death owing to sepsis, a second patient with a testicular granuloma resulting in an orchiectomy, and possibly 1 case of BCG dissemination. The patient developed recurrent febrile episodes of unknown origin. He subsequently died in an automobile accident and no autopsy was performed. In 1 series of 11 patients, there was 1 case of BCG dissemination.[35] Another

study reported 2 patients with sepsis and 1 with BCG dissemination out of 37 patients treated.[34] Minor complications, such as fever without infection and the presence of irritative voiding symptoms throughout the treatment period, are more common. Fever has been reported in up to 67% of patients in 1 series,[36] and colonization of the nephrostomy tube with skin flora is frequent. Biopsies during post-BCG nephroscopy may reveal renal granulomata, but these generally have no clinical significance.[37]

CONCLUSIONS ON PERCUTANEOUS AND URETEROSCOPIC MANAGEMENT

After almost a quarter century, endourologic management of upper tract transitional cell carcinoma is indicated and ideal for addressing bulky low-grade papillary TCC limited to the renal calices, pelvis, or proximal ureter. Ureteroscopy can be used, initially, to treat papillary lesions anywhere along the upper tract urothelium, as long as it is technically feasible. Because of technologic advancements and refinement in endoscopic technique, most patients with UTTCC can now be offered minimally invasive treatment with either single- or multi-modal approaches involving ureteroscopy, percutaneous resection, or laparoscopic nephroureterectomy. A role for BCG in the treatment of upper tract CIS has been demonstrated; however, definitive efficacy of adjuvant topical therapy following endoscopic resection of UTTCC has not been proven. In this regard, multi-institutional studies are necessary. For those motivated patients with noninvasive, low- to medium-grade disease, endourologic therapy provides a reasonable treatment option. In those patients with a functional or solitary kidney, conservative

Table 101-5 TNM Staging System and WHO Grading System for Upper Tract Transitional Cell Carcinoma

TNM Definitions

Primary Tumor (T)

TX: Primary tumor cannot be assessed
T0: No evidence of primary tumor
Ta: Papillary noninvasive carcinoma
Tis: Carcinoma in situ
T1: Tumor invades subepithelial connective tissue
T2: Tumor invades the muscularis
T3: (For renal pelvis only) Tumor invades beyond the kidney into peripelvic fat or the renal parenchyma
T4: Tumor invades adjacent organs or through the kidney into perinephric fat

Regional Lymph Nodes (N)

NX: Regional lymph nodes cannot be assessed
N0: No regional lymph node metastasis
N1: Metastasis in a single lymph node, 2 cm or less in greatest dimension
N2: Metastasis in a single lymph node, more than 2 cm but no more than 5 cm in greatest dimension; or multiple lymph nodes, none more than 5 cm in greatest dimension
N3: Metastasis in a lymph node more than 5 cm in greatest dimension

Distant Metastasis (M)

MX: Distant metastasis cannot be assessed
M0: No distant metastasis
M1: Distant metastasis

Stage Groupings

Stage 0a; Ta, N0, M0
Stage 0is; Tis, N0, M0
Stage I: T1, N0, M0
Stage II: T2, N0, M0
Stage III: T3, N0, M0
Stage IV: T4, N0, M0; Any T, N1, M0; Any T, N2, M0; Any T, N3, M0; Any T; Any N, M0

WHO Grading System

Grade 1: Well differentiated. Slight nuclear enlargement, maintenance of normal cell architecture.
Grade 2: Moderately differentiated. Greater degree of nuclear pleomorphism, prominent nucleoli, disruption of normal cell architecture.
Grade 3: Poorly differentiated. Severe nuclear atypia, frequent mitotic figures, loss of normal cell architecture.

Table 101-6 Local Recurrence Rates for Upper Tract Transitional Cell Carcinoma Treated by Primary Percutaneous or Endoscopic Resection, Followed by Adjuvant Bacillus Calmette-Guérin

Study	Renal Units	Recurrence Grade 1 (%)	Recurrence Grade 2 (%)	Recurrence Grade 3 (%)	Upper Tract Recurrence (%)
Schoenberg et al[44] 1991	9	1/1	0/6	0/2	1/9 (11)
Martinez-Pineiro et al[19] 1996	8	0/1	1/3 (33)	0/2*	1/8 (12.5)
Patel and Fuch[31] 1998	12	0/6	2/5 (40)	0/0	2/12 (16.7)
Clark et al[7] 1999	18	2/6 (33)	2/8 (25)	2/4 (50)	6/18 (33)
Jabbour et al[9] 2000	–	–	3/13 (23)	–	3/13 (23)
Thalmann et al[34] 2002**	14	–	–	–	12/14 (85.7)
Rastinehad et al[11] 2006	50	3/10 (30)	6/17 (35)	9/23 (39.13)	18/50 (36)
Total	141	6/24 (25)	14/52 (27)	11/31 (35)	31/110 (28)

*1 RU with unknown grade.

**Thelmann et al's series is not included in the calculation.

Table 101-7 Rastinehad11: Recurrence and Progression Stratified by Grade in the Patients Treated with Percutaneous Resection of Upper Tract Transitional Cell Carcinoma and the Treated Bacillus Calmette-Guérin and Nontreated Groups

Recurrence	Renal Units	Grade 1 (%)	Grade 2 (%)	Grade 3 (%)
BCG	50	3/10 (30)	6/17 (35)	9/23 (38)
No adjuvant therapy	38	2/9 (22)	3/13 (23)	6/16 (38)
Progression	Renal Units	Grade 1 (%)	Grade 2 (%)	Grade 3 (%)
BCG	50	1/10 (10)	4/17 (24)	3/23 (13)
No adjuvant therapy	38	0/9 (0)	2/13 (15)	2/16 (13)

endourologic management of even high-grade disease may delay the need for nephrectomy and renal replacement therapy. Long-term rigorous follow-up after endourologic treatment, especially with regular surveillance ureteroscopy, is critical to diagnose and treat recurrences in a timely manner, and therefore maintain acceptable cancer-free survival rates.

REFERENCES

1. Huffman JL, Bagley DH, Lyon ES, et al. Endoscopic diagnosis and treatment of upper tract urothelial tumors. A preliminary report. Cancer 1985;55:1422–8.
2. Streem SB, Pontes EJ. Percutaneous management of upper tract transitional cell carcinoma. J Urol 1986;135:773–5.
3. Smith AD, Orihuela E, Crowley AR. Percutaneous management of renal pelvic tumors: treatment option in selected cases. J Urol 1987;137:852–6.
4. Clayman RV, McDougall EM, Nakada SY. Endourology of the upper urinary tract: percutaneous renal and ureteral procedures. In: Walsh PC, Retik AB, Vaughan ED, Wein AJ, editors. Campbell's urology. Vol 3. Philadelphia: W. B. Saunders; 1998. p. 2831–6.
5. Jarrett TW, Sweetser PM, Weiss GH, Smith AD. Percutaneous management of transitional cell carcinoma of the renal collecting system: 9-year experience. J Urol 1995;154:1629–35.
6. Wishnow KI, Johnson DE, Preston D, Tenney D. Long-term serum creatinine values after radical nephrectomy. Urology 1990;35:114–6.
7. Clark PE, Streem SB, Geisinger MA. 13-year experience with percutaneous management of upper tract transitional cell carcinoma. J Urol 1999;161:772–6.
8. Durek C, Rusch-Gerdes S, Jocham D, Bohle A. Sensitivity of BCG to modern antibiotics. Eur Urol 2000;37 Suppl 1:21–5.
9. Jabbour ME, Desgrandchamps F, Cazin S, et al. Percutaneous management of grade II upper urinary tract transitional cell carcinoma: the long-term outcome. J Urol 2000;163:1105–7.
10. Liatsikos EN, Dinlenc CZ, Kapoor RK, Smith AD. Transitional cell carcinoma of the renal pelvis: ureteroscopic and percutaneous approach. J Endourol 2001;15:377–83.
11. Rastinehad AR, Ost MC, Greenberg KL, et al. Percutaneous treatment of upper tract transitional cell carcinoma – 20 year experience. J Urol 2006. [Submitted]
12. Elliot DS, Segura JW, Lightner D, et al. Is nephroureterectomy necessary in all cases of upper tract transitional carcinoma? Long-term results of conservative endourologic management of upper tract transitional cell carcinoma in individuals with a normal contralateral kidney. Urology 2001;58:174–8.
13. Palou J, Piovesan LF, Huguet J, et al. Percutaneous nephroscopic management of upper urinary tract transitional cell carcinoma: recurrence and long-term followup. J Urol 2004;172:66–9.
14. Goel MC, Mahendra V, Roberts JG. Percutaneous management of renal pelvic urothelial tumors: long-term followup. J Urol 2003;169:925–30.
15. Park S, Hong B, Kim C, Ahn H. The impact of tumor location on prognosis of transitional cell carcinoma of the upper urinary tract. J Urol 2004;171(2 Pt 1):621–5.
16. Patel A, Soonawalla P, Shepherd SF, et al. Long-term outcome after percutaneous treatment of transitional cell carcinoma of the renal pelvis. J Urol 1996;155:868–74.
17. Plancke HR, Strijbos WE, Delaere KP. Percutaneous endoscopic treatment of urothelial tumours of the renal pelvis. Br J Urol 1995;75:736–9.
18. Lee BR, Jabbour ME, Marshall FF, et al. 13-year survival comparison of percutaneous and open nephroureterectomy approaches for management of transitional cell carcinoma of renal collecting system: equivalent outcomes. J Endourol 1999;13:289–94.
19. Martinez-Pineiro JA, Garcia Matres MJ, Martinez-Pineiro L. Endourological treatment of upper tract urothelial carcinomas: analysis of a series of 59 tumors. J Urol 1996;156(2 Pt 1):377–85.
20. Jabbour ME, Smith AD. Primary percutaneous approach to upper urinary tract transitional cell carcinoma. Urol Clin North Am 2000;27:739–50.
21. Woodhouse CRJ, Kellett MJ, Bloom JG. Percutaneous renal surgery and local radiotherapy in the management of renal pelvic transitional cell carcinoma. Br J Urol 1986;58:245–9.
22. Sharma NK, Nicol A, Powell CS. Tract infiltration following percutaneous resection of renal pelvic transitional cell carcinoma. Br J Urol 1994;73:597–8.
23. Huang A, Low RK, de Vere White R. Case reports: nephrostomy tract tumor seeding following percutaneous manipulation of a ureteral carcinoma. J Urol 1995;153(3 Pt 2):1041–2.
24. Oefelein MC, MacLennan G. Transitional cell carcinoma recurrence in the nephrostomy tract after percutaneous resection. J Urol 2003;170(2 Pt 1):521.
25. Czito B, Zietman A, Kaufman D, et al. Adjuvant radiotherapy with and without concurrent chemotherapy for locally advanced transitional cell carcinoma of the renal pelvis and ureter. J Urol 2004;172(4 Pt 1):1271–5.
26. Munver R, Delvecchio FC, Newman GE, Preminger GM. Critical analysis of supracostal access for percutaneous renal surgery. J Urol 2001;166:1242–6.
27. Mills IW, Laniado ME, Patel A. The role of endoscopy in the management of patients with upper urinary tract transitional cell carcinoma. BJU Int 2001;87:150–62.
28. Chen GL, El-Gabry EA, Bagley DH. Surveillance of upper urinary tract transitional cell carcinoma: the role of ureteroscopy, retrograde pyelography, cytology, and urinalysis. J Urol 2000;164:1901–4.
29. Keeley FX Jr, Bibbo M, Bagley DH. Ureteroscopic treatment and surveillance of upper urinary tract transitional cell carcinoma. J Urol 1997;157:1560–5.
30. Herr HW. Durable response of a carcinoma in situ of the renal pelvis to topical bacillus Calmette-Guerin. J Urol 1985;134:531–2.
31. Patel A, Fuchs GJ. New techniques for the administration of topical adjuvant therapy after endoscopic ablation of upper urinary tract transitional cell carcinoma. J Urol 1998;159:71–5.
32. Studer UE, Casanova G, Kraft R, Zingg EJ. Percutaneous bacillus Calmette-Guerin perfusion of the upper urinary tract for carcinoma in situ. J Urol 1989;142:975–7.
33. Irie A, Iwamura M, Kadowaki K, et al. Intravesical instillation of bacillus Calmette-Guerin for carcinoma in situ of the urothelium involving the upper urinary tract utilizing vesicoureteral reflux created by a double-pigtail catheter. Urology 2002;59:53–7.
34. Thalmann GN, Markwalder R, Walter B, Studer UE. Long-term experience with bacillus Calmette-Guerin therapy of upper urinary tract transitional cell carcinoma in patients not eligible for surgery. J Urol 2002;168(4 Pt 1):1381–5.
35. Sharpe JR, Duffy G, Chin JL. Intrarenal bacillus Calmette-Guerin therapy for upper urinary tract carcinoma in situ. J Urol 1993;149:457–60.
36. Nishino Y, Yamammoto N, Komeda H, et al. Bacillus Calmette-Guerin instillation treatment for carcinoma in situ of the upper urinary tract. BJU Int 2000;85:799–801.
37. Bellman GC, Sweetser P, Smith AD. Complications of intracavitary bacillus Calmette-Guerin after percutaneous resection of upper tract transitional cell carcinoma. J Urol 1994;151:13–5.
38. Soderdahl D, Fabrizio M, Rahman N, et al. Endoscopic treatment of upper tract transitional cell carcinoma. Urol Oncol 2005;23:114–22.
39. Yokogi H, Wada Y, Mizutani M, et al. Bacillus Calmette Guerin perfusion therapy for carcinoma in situ of the upper urinary tract. Br J Urol 1996;77:676–9.
40. Nonomura N, Ono Y, Nozawa M, et al. Bacillus Calmette-Guerin perfusion therapy for the treatment of transitional cell carcinoma in situ of the upper urinary tract. Eur Urol 2000;38:701–5.
41. Okubo K, Ichioka K, Terada N, et al. Intrarenal bacillus Calmette-Guerin therapy for carcinoma in situ of the upper urinary tract: long-term follow-up and natural course in cases of failure. BJU Int 2001;88:343–7.
42. Miyake H, Eto H, Hara S, et al. Clinical outcome of bacillus Calmette-Guerin perfusion therapy for carcinoma in situ of the upper urinary tract. Int J Urol 2002;9:677–80.
43. Hayashida Y, Nomata K, Noguchi M, et al. Long-term effects of bacille Calmette-Guérin perfusion therapy for treatment of transitional cell carcinoma in situ of upper urinary tract. Urology 2004;63:1084–8.
44. Schoenberg MP, Van Arsdalen KN, Wein AJ. The management of transitional cell carcinoma in solitary renal units. J Urol 1991;146:700–3.

102

Endourology in the Obese Patient

Evangelos N. Liatsikos, MD, PhD

Obesity is a continuously spreading phenomenon among the worldwide population. It has been estimated that approximately a third of the United States population is overweight. The currently high number of overweight children and adolescents further strengthens the increasing trend of obesity within the future generations.[1–6]

The need for a uniform and precise definition of the obese and the morbidly obese patient, has led to the acceptance of a common index that reflects the severity of obesity. Thus, body mass index (BMI) determines the degree of obesity by using a formula dividing weight by height. An overweight male patient presents with a BMI greater than 27.8 and an overweight female patient with a BMI greater than 27.3. BMI greater than 31 suggests severe obesity, and greater than 40 morbid obesity.[3–5]

The main concern is whether obese and morbidly obese patients are considered high-risk patients for operative procedures. Indeed, obesity is related to higher rates of chronic disease (ie, hypertension, diabetes, and/or coronary heart disease). There seems to be a concurrence among investigators suggesting that markedly obese patients have an increased risk of postoperative complications, regardless of the approach or nature of operation.[7–11]

During general anesthesia, and during the immediate postoperative period, morbidly obese patients are more prone to significant impairments of pulmonary gas exchange and respiratory mechanics. When compared with normal patients, functional residual capacity is markedly decreased in morbidly obese patients, the alveolar-arterial oxygenation gradient is increased, and intra-abdominal pressure is higher.[7–8]

In addition, hypoxemia during the induction of general anesthesia for the morbidly obese patient is a major concern for the anesthesiologist. Patient positioning may play an important role in cardiopulmonary physiology in obese patients. Various authors have acknowledged mask ventilation, intubation and/or oxygenation concerns in morbidly obese patients, suggesting that extra time may often be required to secure the airway with an endotracheal tube for general anesthesia.[7–8] Boyce and colleagues showed that the safe apnea period is longest for morbidly obese patients when general anesthesia is induced and patients are intubated in the reverse Trendelenburg's position, and that recovery to safe oxygen saturation levels is shorter when patients are in the reverse Trendelenburg's position.[8]

The main purpose of this chapter is to identify whether obese and morbidly obese patients present any additional perioperative and/or postoperative complications related to their anatomic peculiarity, and whether there are any tips to facilitate the performance of endourologic procedures.

STONE DISEASE

Obese patients do not represent any particular challenges when performing endourology procedures for the management of stone disease. Nevertheless, when treating morbidly obese patients, the urologist has to deal with a variety of technical difficulties. The anesthetic considerations and their related comorbidities were described above and merit attention. In this section, special mention will be addressed to technical difficulties pertaining to endoscopic management of stone disease in morbidly obese patients.

Of all available endoscopic procedures, percutaneous nephrolithotomy represents the most challenging procedure in the morbidly obese patient. A variety of reports have described modifications of technique, positioning, and equipment in percutaneous nephrolithotomy to treat these patients.[12–20]

Extracorporeal shock wave lithotripsy is often not feasible in the morbidly obese patient due to weight limitations of the equipment, failure to aim the stone because of inadequate fluoroscopic or ultrasonographic imaging, and a skin-to-stone distance greater than the 11 to 17 cm distance between the point of shock wave generation and the shock wave focal point. Nevertheless, the use of second-generation lithotriptors has been proposed by some authors with encouraging results. Thomas and Cass used the Medstone STS with a 24.1 cm F1-to-F2 focal point distance and maximal treatment depth of 15 cm to treat 81 patients weighing more than 300 lb. They reported a 78% stone-free rate for renal calculi 1 to 10 mm, and 71% stone-free rate for stones 11 to 20 mm.[21]

In obese patients (BMI > 30) percutaneous nephrolithotomy has a stone-free rate of 43% after one session and 88% after multiple sessions. The transfusion rate is 8.8% with the same rate of complications as for "normal" patients. When BMI is greater than 40, the multi-session stone-free rate is approximately 87%, but the complication rate rises to 14%, and the transfusion rate increases to 21%.[12–20] These results have encouraged various advocates of rigid or flexible ureteroscopic stone extraction, proposing the latter techniques for all upper urinary tract calculi up to 2 cm, as the standard of care in the morbidly obese or super-obese patients.[14,22,23]

Most authors concur that there is no upper limit of BMI above which it is hazardous to perform percutaneous nephrolithotomy. Nevertheless, patients with a BMI greater than 50 present serious problems in terms of positioning, imaging, access and/or transport. In cases of large patients, modification of standard positioning and access have been reported in the literature, facilitating access to the kidney, and thus successful percutaneous nephrolithotomy. Kerbl and colleagues used the flank position in a 328-lb patient in whom the prone position was deemed unsafe by the anesthesiologist.[17] Others have used a cutdown technique by incising the flank musculature to shorten the length of the working sheath needed.[16] Gofrit and colleagues proposed the use of the lateral decubitus position for percutaneous nephrolithotomy in morbidly obese patients.[13]

Pearl and colleagues reviewed their experience with percutaneous nephrolithotomy in patients with a BMI greater than 30 and showed that the stone-free rate in obese patients was comparable to that achieved in an unselected patient population. The complication rate, transfusion rate, and length of hospital stay were also alike.[12]

Equipment consists of rigid nephroscopes with a working length of 17.5 cm and a 30 French, 17-cm Amplatz working sheath. Nevertheless, longer Amplatz sheaths (22 cm or greater) as well as longer rigid nephroscopes with a working length of 20.5 cm are also available for technically demanding cases. Further modifications have been occasionally proposed. Giblin and colleagues used a 32 F Amplatz sheath 18 to 24 cm long and a 30F operating gynecological laparoscope 27 cm long to access stones in 5 patients weighing between 260 and 313 pounds.[18]

An additional technical consideration is the diameter of the needle used for gaining access into the pelviocaliceal system. Many interventional radiologists advocate the use of a 21-gauge needle whereas, in the obese patient, the use of an 18-gauge, 20-cm needle provides extra stiffness and stability as well as length for more efficient and accurate insertion within the kidney.

LAPAROSCOPY

Obese patients in general are expected to have more complications, particularly of wound, pulmonary, and cardiovascular origin (Table 102-1). Nevertheless, obese patients benefit from the lower amount of postoperative pain due to the reduced trauma on the abdominal wall, and the quicker convalescence associated with a laparoscopic approach.[24–28]

The increased risk of complications in obese, compared to non-obese, patients is highlighted by multi-institutional studies of laparoscopic procedures, presenting about 26% of postoperative complications consisting mostly of fever, atelectasis, and subcutaneous emphysema.[25,26] Eichenberger and colleagues showed that, during laparoscopic surgery, morbidly obese patients develop more atelectasis during general anesthesia than non-obese patients, and that 24 hours after the end of the laparoscopic procedure, atelectasis persists in morbidly obese patients, whereas complete resorption occurs in non-obese patients.[7]

Various laparoscopists suggest that obese patients who undergo laparoscopic surgery present with an increased risk for intraoperative complications. Thus, they report that the conversion rate for various laparoscopic operations increases with BMI, due to the presence of abundant intra-abdominal fat masquerading organ visibility. The additional thickness of the abdominal wall often requires an amplified force to maneuver the operating instrument tip, thus diminishing surgeon sensitivity. Furthermore, insufflation of the abdomen with carbon dioxide is cumbersome in the supine obese patient. Modifications of patient positioning have been suggested (ie, the flank position), allowing abdominal subcutaneous fat to move away from the operative field, thus facilitating insufflation.

There have been several studies addressing the laparoscopic management of obese patients. Fazeli-Matin and colleagues compared the outcome of laparoscopic renal-adrenal and standard open surgery when operating on obese patients. They showed that obese patients required less analgesia, presented less blood loss, quicker bowel mobilization, shorter convalescence, and a shorter hospitalization period.[24] Mendoza and colleagues reported that the incidence of complications when performing laparoscopic surgery in morbidly obese patients, was significantly higher than in the general population.[26] Jacobs and colleagues presented their experience with 41 morbidly obese patients who underwent laparoscopic donor nephrectomy, and showed a mean operating time of 40 minutes longer in the obese group than in the normal population. Furthermore, the obese patients required larger laparoscopic ports and presented an increased conversion rate to open nephrectomy.[29] Dublet and Belair reported a similar complication rate for obese and non-obese patients undergoing retroperitoneal laparoscopy.[30] Stifelman and colleagues, who are advocates of hand-assisted laparoscopy, have shown that obese patients undergoing hand-assisted laparoscopic radical nephrectomy required an average of 40 minutes longer operative time but presented blood loss, complication rate, conversion rate, and duration of hospitalization similar to non-obese patients. They suggested that the

---

Table 102-1 Laparoscopic Challenges in Morbidly Obese Patients

Extensive abdominal adiposity
Extra-abdominal fat
  Insufficient trocar, scope and instrument length
  Restricted freedom of movement
  Gas leakage
Intra-abdominal fat
  Fatty viscera, especially liver
  Exposure and/or retraction challenges
  Viscera obscured by fat
Severe obesity and high co morbidity
  Significant cardiopulmonary disease
  ASA III or greater
  Decreased tolerance of CO2 pneumoperitoneum
  Difficult airway requiring advanced intubation
    techniques
Advanced laparoscopic skills

---

hand in the operative field allowed for excellent retraction, maneuverability, and safer dissection with increased vascular control.[31]

There are several considerations that need to be addressed when one decides to perform laparoscopic surgery in a group of patients with such a peculiar body habitus (ie, the obesity).

Before the initiation of the procedure, meticulous mapping of trocar positioning as well as a plan for open conversion, is imperative. Emergency laparotomy should always be expected, and thus, planned beforehand.

Direct placement of the trocars through the pannus should be avoided by moving them laterally or distally according to the procedure (ie kidney-adrenal, or prostate). Thus, mechanical resistance when manipulating the trocars is decreased.

The kidney should be approached with the patient in the flank position to move the pannus medially. This maneuver shortens the distance from the skin to the abdominal cavity, enabling use of normal size laparoscopic ports and instruments. The retroperitoneal flank approach benefits from the gravity effect by shifting most of the overweight tissues anteriorly away of the kidney and adrenal glands. The advocates of the retroperitoneoscopic approach suggest that it offers a shorter and more direct route to the kidney and adrenal gland compared to the transperitoneal laparoscopic approach. Nevertheless, others suggest that the excessive retroperitoneal fat increases the degree of technical difficulty.[24–32]

When the prostate is approached laparoscopically, the trocars should be moved distally to avoid the main bulk of adipose tissue and thus facilitate the initial access and final performance of the procedure. Stolzenburg and colleagues present their experience with endoscopic extraperitoneal prostatectomy, and advocate the positioning of the trocars 1 to 3 cm inferiorly, toward the symphysis, when operating upon obese and super-obese patients.[33]

Obese and super-obese patients may prove to be particularly demanding on equipment (see Table 102-1). A Veress needle is used to establish a pneumoperitoneum in the obese patient, as it is technically cumbersome to perform an open

---

(Hasson) technique due to the presence of abundant subcutaneous fat. A long-length Veress needle of 150 mm is normally required in cases involving morbidly obese patients.

The operating table for laparoscopic surgery in the obese and super-obese patient must have the capacity to support the weight of the patient and provide the necessary rotational movements, allowing adequate exposure.

The use of longer trocars and instrumentation allows optimal access to the region of interest. There is a wide range of instruments that are available in longer editions for the super-obese patient. Laparoscopes are available in various sizes, with a standard length of 32 cm and diameters ranging from 2 to 10 mm. An extra-long laparoscope (45 cm) is very helpful in super-obese patients.

Gas leakage is common problem during laparoscopic surgery in the obese patient and can be very troublesome. Some investigators advocate the use of two insufflators, set at high pressure flow to provide added compensation for gas leakage.[24–32]

Significant laparoscopic experience is recommended, as obese patients offer unique challenges related to organ exposure and visualization. Performance of a laparoscopic procedure safely and effectively is dependent upon the quality of visualization.

CONCLUSION

Reduction in perioperative morbidity is the major advantage of all endoscopic and laparoscopic operations. Morbid obesity presents a significant challenge for the urologist. In addition to the technical challenges of positioning and instrumentation, these patients have a predisposition for postoperative and anesthetic complications. Thus, severely obese patients who are at higher risk for cardiopulmonary, infectious, and wound-related morbidity would benefit from laparoscopic surgery even more than the normal, or non-obese, patient. Technological and instrument-design advancements have allowed the performance of endoscopic and laparoscopic procedures in patients with a challenging body habitus.

Obesity is no longer a relative contraindication to endoscopy and/or laparoscopy for experienced centers, but non-experienced urologists must be cautious when dealing with these technically demanding operations. Acquisition of advanced endoscopic skills is essential for safe and effective performance of these operations in the obese and morbidly obese patient.

REFERENCES

1. Kral JG. Morbidity of severe obesity. Surg Clin North Am 2001;81:1039–1061.
2. Gray DS. Diagnosis and prevalence of obesity. Med Clin North Am 1989;73:1–13.
3. Pi-Sunyer XF, editor. Clinical guidelines on the identification, evaluation, and treatment of overweight and obesity in adults. In: NHLBI Obesity Education Initiative Expert Panel on the identification, evaluation, and treatment of overweight and obesity in adults 98-4083. Bethesda, MD: National Institutes of Health; 1998. p. 228.

4. Kuczmarski RJ, Flegal KM, Campbell SM, Johnson CL. Increasing prevalence of overweight among U.S. adults: the National Health and Nutrition Examination Surveys, 1960 to 1991. JAMA 1994;272:205.

5. Popkin BM, Doak CM. The obesity epidemic is a worldwide phenomenon. Nutr Rev 1998;56:106.

6. Seidell JC, Flegal KM. Assessing obesity: classification and epidemiology. Brit Med Bull 1997;53:238.

7. Eichenberger A, Proietti S, Wicky S, et al. Morbid obesity and postoperative pulmonary atelectasis: an underestimated problem. Anesth Analg 2002;95:1788–92.

8. Boyce JR, Ness T, Castroman P, Gleysteen JJ. A preliminary study of the optimal anesthesia positioning for the morbidly obese patient. Obes Surg 2003;13:4–9.

9. Wilson AT, Reilly CS. Anaesthesia and the obese patient. Int J Obes Relat Metab Disord 1993;18:427.

10. Choban PS, Heckler R, Burge JC, Flancbaum L. Increased incidence of nosocomial infections in obese surgical patients. Amer Surg 1995;61:1001.

11. Alpert MA, Hashimi MW. Obesity and the heart. Amer J Med Sci 1993;306:117.

12. Pearle MS, Nakada SY, Womack JS, Kryger JV. Outcomes of contemporary percutaneous nephrostolithotomy in morbidly obese patients. J Urol 1998;160:669–73.

13. Gofrit ON, Shapiro A, Donchin Y, et al. Lateral decubitus position for percutaneous nephrolithotripsy in the morbidly obese or kyphotic patient. J Endourol 2002;16:383–6.

14. Dash A, Schuster TG, Hollenbeck BK, et al. Ureteroscopic treatment of renal calculi in morbidly obese patients: a stone-matched comparison. Urology 2002;60:393–7.

15. Faerber GJ and Goh M. Percutaneous nephrolithotripsy in the morbidly obese patient. Tech Urol 1997;3:89–95.

16. Curtis R, Thorpe AC, Marsh R. Modification of the technique of percutaneous nephrolithotomy in the morbidly obese patient. Br J Urol 1997;79:138–140.

17. Kerbl K, Clayman RV, Chandhoke PS, et al. Percutaneous stone removal with the patient in a flank position. J Urol 1994;151:686–8.

18. Giblin JG, Lossef S, Pahira JJ. A modification of standard percutaneous nephrolithotripsy technique for the morbidly obese patient. Urology 1995;46:491–3.

19. Carson CC, Danneberger JE, Weinerth JL. Percutaneous lithotripsy in morbid obesity. J Urol 1998;139:243–5.

20. Hofmann R, Stoller ML. Endoscopic and open stone surgery in morbidly obese patients. J Urol 1992;148:1108–11.

21. Thomas R, Cass AS. Extracorporeal shock wave lithotripsy in morbidly obese patients. J Urol 1993;150:30–2.

22. Nguyen TA, Belis JA. Endoscopic management of urolithiasis in the morbidly obese patient. J Endourol 1998;12:33–5.

23. Andreoni C, Afane J, Olweny E, et al. Flexible ureteroscopic lithotripsy: first-line therapy for proximal ureteral and renal calculi in the morbidly obese and superobese patient. J Endourol 2001;15:493–8.

24. Fazeli-Matin S, Gill IS, Hsu TH, et al. Laparoscopic renal and adrenal surgery in obese patients: comparison to open surgery. J Urol 1999;162:665–9.

25. Gill IS, Clayman RV, Albala DM, et al. Retroperitoneal and pelvic extraperitoneal laparoscopy: an international perspective. Urology 1998;52:566.

26. Mendoza D, Newman RC, Albala D, et al. Laparoscopic complications in markedly obese urologic patients (a multi-institutional review). Urology 1996;48:562.

27. Angrisani L, Lorenzo M, De Palma G, et al. Laparoscopic cholecystectomy in obese patients compared with nonobese patients. Surg Lap Endosc 1995;5:197.

28. Loffer FD, Pent D. Laparoscopy in the obese patient. Amer J Obst Gynec 1976;125:104.

29. Jacobs SC, Cho E, Dunkin BJ, et al. Laparoscopic nephrectomy in the markedly obese living renal donor. Urology 2000;56:926–9.

30. Doublet J, Belair G. Retroperitoneal laparoscopic nephrectomy is safe and effective in obese patients: a comparative study of 55 procedures. Urology 2000;56:63–6.

31. Stifelman MD, Handler T, Nieder AM, et al. Hand-assisted laparoscopy for large renal specimens: a multi-institutional study. Urology 2003;61:78–82.

32. Chen R, Moore RG, Micali S, Kavoussi LR. Retroperitoneoscopic renal biopsy in extremely obese patients. Urology 1997;50:195.

33. Stolzenburg JU, Truss MC, Do M, et al. Nerve sparing endoscopic extraperitoneal radical prostatectomy—technique and initial experience after 205 procedures. World J Urol. [In press]

103

Renal Endooncology: Cryotherapy, Radiofrequency Ablation, and Novel Techniques

Steven M. Baughman, MD

Jay T. Bishoff, MD, FACS

The views expressed in this chapter are those of the authors and do not reflect the official policy of the United States Air Force, Department of Defense, or other Departments of the US Government.

Early radiographic identification of small renal masses, with subsequent decreasing stage migration at the time of initial diagnosis, has driven the development of both open nephron-sparing surgery (NSS) and other minimally invasive techniques for the treatment of small renal tumors.[1] Open NSS has proven efficacy in patients with small tumors (less than 4 cm in diameter), despite normal contralateral kidneys.[2,3] In addition, with the low chance (3.7%) of polycentricity of small renal cell cancers, and evidence of increasing rates of renal insufficiency with radical nephrectomy, the argument favoring NSS is strengthened.[4,5]

Progressive development of minimally invasive techniques for urologic malignancies has also revealed multiple therapeutic systems with unique mechanisms and utility. Two well known treatments, cryotherapy and radiofrequency ablation (RFA), produce their respective tissue destruction via cellular freezing or heat production from molecular agitation with overall molecular and cellular destruction. Additional novel ablative techniques harness thermal injury as their respective means of tissue destruction. From the first renal percutaneous cryosurgery by Uchida and colleagues[6] and the well established uses of RFA in aberrant cardiac pathways, hepatic, and other lesions, minimally invasive, energy-based therapy has a developing utility today. In this chapter, we will present the current applications of renal cryotherapy, RFA, and newer ablative technologies, with attention to their respective indications and contraindications, the adjuvant techniques, and results of these new technologies.

INDICATIONS AND CONTRAINDICATIONS FOR ABLATIVE TECHNIQUES:

Although the fundamental mechanisms for various ablative techniques may be dissimilar, they share parallel indications and contraindications (Table 103-1.) Paramount to the use of these alternative surgical therapies is attention to appropriate patient selection. Optimal renal lesions for either cryotherapy or RFA are peripherally based, enhancing, well-circumscribed lesions, distant from the collecting system or other perirenal structures (ie, bowel, vasculature), with dimensions ≤ 4 cm in size.[7–15] Unique patient populations, such as von Hippel-Lindau disease, tuberous sclerosis, hereditary papillary renal cell carcinoma, and even renal carcinomas in transplanted kidneys may be optimal candidates for minimally invasive ablative techniques.[11,14–19] As an alternative to open procedures or observation, patient proclivity for minimally invasive techniques in an effort to obviate or delay symptoms has also been recognized.[14,15,20] Additionally, persistent gross hematuria has also been an indication for radiofrequency ablation in an elderly patient who would not otherwise tolerate an open procedure.[21]

While few animal models have shown that cryotherapy near, and into, the collecting system does not herald a negative outcome, proximity to the collecting system itself is one of the few relative contraindications to all types of treatment.[22,23] Collateral energy from an ablative process can result in significant injury to pararenal structures, but the protected posterior and lateral renal fat layer may decrease these complications. Relative contraindications reported in the current literature also include uncorrected bleeding diatheses, lesions contiguous with bowel, great vessels, or renal sinus (ie, a centrally located renal lesion), and tumor size ≥ 5 cm, although larger tumors may be treated with the use of multiply placed ablative probes.[9,11,13,14,]

CRYOSURGICAL ABLATION

Cryotherapeutic tissue destruction is seen when cryoprobe deployment (typically based on liquid argon or nitrogen [LN_2]) causes extraction of the latent heat of boiling from its immediate environment—with 209 Joules of heat energy extracted from each gram of LN_2 that is converted to gas at the probe tip.[9] The cryoprobe can reach a temperature of −195°C within two to three minutes, which is well below the necessary temperature (−20 to −50°C) needed for tissue destruction.[6,9,24,25] Rapid freezing results in cellular dehydration, intra- and extracellular ice crystallization, cytosolic organelle destruction, uncoupling of oxidative phosphorylation, protein denaturation, osmotic rupturing of cytoplasmic membranes, and endothelial destruction with microvascular thrombosis resulting in local tissue ischemia.[9,24,25,26] Through the exposure of possible tumor antigenic moieties to the immune system and subsequent tumor-antibody formation, cryo-immunologic activity has also been pro-

Table 103-1 Indications and Contraindications to Cryotherapy and Radiofrequency Ablation	
Indications	Contraindications

Lesion Characteristics
  Peripherally based, away from the collecting system
    and hilar vasculature
  Well circumscribed lesion
  Enhancement on computed tomography
  Less than 4 cm; Robson Stage I, AJCC (1997) Stage T1
	Bleeding diatheses
	Centrally located renal lesions (contiguous with
	  bowel, great vessels, renal sinus, or being near
	  [or into] the collecting system)
	Lesion size of 5 cm or greater

Patient Characteristics
  Solitary renal unit
  Bilateral tumors
  Significant renal insufficiency, including compromised
    contralateral renal function and comorbid disease that
    could develop into renal insufficiency.
  Native kidney lesion in a dialysis patient
  Previous renal surgery
  Obesity
  Elderly
  Marked comorbid disease
  Patient's request	

posed as a possible mediator toward inhibition of tumor (re)growth.[6,25,27]

The minimally invasive surgeon can readily gain the basic understanding necessary for the operation of various ablative techniques. Open, laparoscopic, and percutaneous deployment of these energies have been successfully reported.[10,12,24,28,29] Despite a high degree of variability with regard to the techniques used, a number of underlying tenents must be kept in mind when learning and using cryotherapy and RFA. Appropriate patient selection includes complete radiographic and metastatic evaluation. The location of the lesion is of great importance owing to the need to avoid surrounding structures, primarily the bowel, collecting system, and vasculature.

Cryotherapy itself can be delivered with technical simplicity. Adequate tissue destruction with cryotherapy can be seen with multiple "rapid freeze–slow thaw–rapid freeze" cycles.[3,22,24,26] Although the freeze-thaw-freeze method is the most frequently reported technique, single-freeze techniques (for up to 15 minutes) have shown equal efficacy.[16,24]

Cryotherapy lends itself to open or laparoscopic approaches. Steps to cryotherapeutic success include (1) appropriate anatomic approach (where a posterolateral lesion can easily be accessed via posterior percutaneous or retroperitoneoscopic approach, while anterolateral-based lesions may be approached via transperitoneal technique[16,10,24]); (2) mobilization of kidney within Gerota's fascia; (3) excision of overlying perirenal fat; (4) use of in situ ultrasonography; (5) visually and ultrasound-guided needle biopsy; (6) puncture placement of cryoprobe under ultrasound and visual guidance; (7) real-time observation of cryoprobe deployment with ultrasound and thermocouple monitoring; and (8) hemostasis.[3,10,24,25,30]

Cryotherapy in the kidney is easily delivered, both anatomically and technically, when compared to other urologic uses, such as prostate.[10] Each basic step of renal cryosurgery has specific highlights. Prior to actual cryoablation, ideal renal mobilization for direct and ultrasonographic visualization of the lesion is needed, as is evaluating the lesion size, exposing the possibility of satellite lesions, and the proximity to vessels and the collecting system.[3] Minimal hilar dissection is necessary, and typically there is no practical advantage to occluding hilar vessels.[9] In fact, little to no perihilar dissection is necessary in the majority of these lesions using either approach.[3,22] Needle and wire placement for the cryoprobe can be performed either intraoperatively under ultrasound guidance, or as a preoperative percutaneous procedure under similar visualization.[30] Once cryoablation cycling starts, the target tissue temperature must be well below the accepted temperature (–20 to –40°C) needed for cellular destruction.[6,9,24] Gill and Novick noted various temperature gradients seen at the advancing edge of an ablative therapy via the use of thermosensors placed within and at a lesion's edge.[3] A temperature of 0°C at the advancing edge was

observed, with the inner 4 to 6 mm of the cryolesion reaching the needed –20 to –40°C. It is now generally accepted that an advancing edge of a cryolesion needs to be visualized ultrasonographically and extend at least 1 cm beyond the edge of the tumor.[3,10]

Of concern, however, is a recent abstract by Sharp and colleagues.[31] Using 3 mm and 5 mm argon-based cryoprobes, there was considerable nonlinear temperature versus time (or distance between—and even within) each porcine kidney. This intralesional variability showed that mean nadir temperatures at 15 mm from the probe were inadequate for the requisite –20°C needed for tissue desiccation. With some lesions greater than 2 to 3 cm, this variability becomes concerning and will need further investigation.

There appears to be a lack of consensus regarding the timing of the slow-thaw phase of cryoablation, but the current thought is to await the disappearance of the cryolesion on ultrasonography, then refreeze for another 2 to 3 minutes.[3,24] During the second freeze cycle, the advancing ice ball may not be seen via ultrasonography until its advancing edge is seen outside the first cryolesion's perimeter.[3] This stresses the significance of direct visualization because one may see significant subcapsular hemorrhage as a purplish-blue lesion with cryolesion advancement[3,17] either during the primary freeze or during the second freeze, indicating potential stray energy that can lead to perirenal tissue damage.

Finally, forcing an attached or adherent frozen probe from its ablation site can fracture the kidney. The final thaw of the cryolesion will allow the tissue to release the cryoprobe, and due to pressure of gas used during laparoscopy, there may not be any significant bleeding.[3,7] While the probe insertion site is still frozen, hemostatic agents such as Surgicell, Gel Foam, or fibrin sealant can be packed or inserted into the resulting hole to further assist with hemostasis once the region returns to body temperature.[3,7]

Adjuvant technologies for ablative surgery assist with access to renal lesions, assure safe and adequate tissue desiccation, and maintain hemostasis. Cryotherapy and RFA have immediate physical limitations with regard to the volume of local tissue destruction, based on the type and size of probe deployed and the ability of imagining techniques to accurately monitor the size of the lesion created.[30] Intraoperative ultrasound measurements have shown a 13% smaller size compared to computed tomography (CT) images of the same lesion.[10] Therefore, adequate tissue destruction must be regulated in other ways, including the use of temperature sensors, real-time intraoperative imaging (seen primarily with cryoablation) or impedance monitors.[11,26]

Percutaneous access has been reported using both computed tomographic and magnetic resonance guidance.[20,14] While CT or magnetic resonance imaging (MRI) are the primary modalities for preoperative radiographic evaluation, intraoperative ultrasonography is the principal modality for adequate, immediate pre-, intra-, and postop-

erative monitoring for both open and laparoscopic cryotherapy.[9,10,17,24,30] Ultrasonography allows for real-time observation of the biopsy needle, probe placement, margin of frozen tissue, relationship to surrounding structures, monitoring of the actual ablation, and possible identification of synchronous lesions not seen with other preoperative imaging.[9,10,16,24,32]

Steerable, laparoscopic, color-flow Doppler ultrasound, with end-fire probe technology, allows one to see the actual margins of the cryolesion as identified by a hyperechoic advancing crescentic lesion with posterior acoustic shadowing and loss of intra-lesion color-flow, and characteristics indicative of vascular and cellular destruction.[9,10,17,24,33,34]

Uchida and colleagues and Zlotta and colleagues were the pioneers for the clinical application of cryoablation and RFA, respectively.[6,29] Both investigators attempted to define the safety, technical, and early follow-up characteristics of their respective energy system. The work of Uchida and colleagues aided in the understanding of the needed –20°C needed for in vivo tissue desiccation with cryoablation, but their patient selection (two patients with advanced renal cell carcinoma [RCC]) were of little benefit in determining long-term clinical outcomes.[6] Similarly, Zlotta and colleagues showed that extensive tumor and parenchymal necrosis results from the in vivo RFA experience, under both open and percutaneous applications, with the latter performed under local anesthesia.[29]

Outcome studies of minimally invasive technologies are limited to prospective trials using only radiographic follow-up and limited histologic evaluation. Though outcome data are limited, the information currently available is optimistic. Operatively, cryotherapeutic and radiofrequency techniques have proven compatibility with laparoscopic equipment and minimal risk of operative or delayed blood loss.[12,14,15,35] Percutaneous delivery is possible under intravenous sedation and local anesthesia, with many patients having less than 24 hours of hospital stay.[11,15,29,36] To date, no studies report any conversion to an open procedure with either cryoablation or RFA.

Though long-term cancer-free and overall survival data are lacking with both cryoablation and RFA, the current short-term data are encouraging (Table 103-2).[37–40] Gill and colleagues have one of the larger series of cryoablation, with 32 total patients and 23 follow-up CT-guided biopsies at 3 to 6 months, with no radiographic local or port-site recurrence in a mean follow-up time of 16.2 months.[10] Harmon and colleagues showed a 100% post-treatment cancer-specific survival in 76 patients receiving either open or laparoscopic cryoablation (median follow-up of 17 months).[41] Levin and colleagues reported the results of their experience in 39 patients, showing one patient who underwent renal biopsy at 9 months after treatment for a suspicious nodule that was discovered on protocol MRI.[42] The biopsy revealed renal cell carcinoma; the patient underwent laparoscopic radical nephrectomy for

Table 103-2   Summary of Cryoablation Series

First Author/Reference	No. Patients	No. Lesions	Mean Tumor Diameter (cm)	Mean OR Time (min)	Ablation Time	Mean EBL (cc)	Mean Probe Temp	Hospital Stay (d)	Follow-up	Recurrence
Uchida British J Urol 1995	2 (both with advanced disease)	2	NR	NR	Single 22 min	NR	−20°C	NR	CT	Both died of metastatic disease
Delworth J Urol 1996	2	3	4.3	240	NR	450	180°C	5	MRI or CT at 1–3 months	10% enlargement of AML at 3 mo
Gill Urology 1998	10	11	1.9	135	Double freeze 13 min	75	−186°C	< 1	CT or MRI	Biopsy negative
Zegel J Ultrasound Med 1998	6	14	NR	NR	7–15 min	NR	−180°C	NR	CT or MRI	None 3–22 mo postoperative
Bishoff J Endourol 1999	8	8	2.0	210	Single 15 min or double 5 min	140	−180°C	3.5	CT 5 mo	None
Rodriguez Urology 2000	7	7	2.2	234	15 minutes double or single	111	−180°C	4.4	14 months	None
Gill Urology 2000	32	34	2.3	170	15 min	67	−185°C	< 23 hr	MRI/CT guided biopsy	None at 16 mo
Remer Amer J Rad 2000	21	23	< 4 cm	NR	NR	NR	−180°C	NR	MRI	None at 6 mo
Rukstalis Urology 2001	29	29	2.2	NR	Double cycle	150	−140°C – −180°C	3	CT/MRI	1/29
Shingleton J Urol 2001	20	22	3	97	Triple cycle	NR	NR	< 23 hr	MRI	1 patient at 9 mo
Korsandi NAOA 2002	17	17	2.4	180	NR	100 cc (median)	−180°C	2	30 mo	2 via cytology of complex cystic mass at 6 mo
Kim J Urol 2002	12	12	2.2	NR	Double cycle	60	NR	3.25	CT	2/12 biopsy proven at mean 305 days
Bargman J Urol 2003 abstract	23	25	(range)1.5–10 cm	185	NR	303	NR	NR	CT/MRI	1/23 (VHL pt) with radiographic recurrence
Shingleton J Urol 2003 abstract	70	70	NR(< 5 cm inclusion)	NR	Triple cycle	NR	−40°C	NR	MRI or CT at 1, 3, 6, q 6 mos	At avg of 2 yrs: 9 incomplete ablations; 60 pts NED; 5 non-cancer deaths
Harmon J Urol 2003 abstract	76	76	Median = 2.5 cm	NR	Double cycle	100 cc (median)	NR	Median = 2	Radiographic	5 enhancing lesions re-biopsied. 3/5 with recurrent malignancy: one re-ablated, one s/p partial nephrectomy, one on watchful waiting

a 1.3-cm clear cell renal cell carcinoma. Recently, Bargman and colleagues showed that cryo-assisted partial nephrectomy portended negative surgical margins in 23 patients, but one recurrent lesion is noted in a VHL patient with a mean 18-month follow-up.[43] In the initial Johns Hopkins' experience, out of eight patients with small (mean 2.0 cm diameter) renal tumors, one patient (at his 9-month CT follow-up) was found to have an enhancing lesion in the area of cryoablation, although that was after the publication of their initial series. This patient underwent a successful radical nephrectomy.

Shingleton published an abstract on the use of percutaneous cryoablation with MRI guidance in 70 patients. They reported only 9 incomplete ablations, each of which had complete repeat ablation. Furthermore, the series included 60 patients alive without evidence of disease at a 2-year average follow-up. No cancer-specific deaths had been reported as of this writing.[44]

Low complication rates have been reported with cryoablation. Both cryoablation and RFA systems have the risk of direct contact and subse-

quent energy transfer to surrounding structures.[45] Complications specific to cryoablative technique include: mild intraoperative bleeding from a cracked cryolesion (controlled with Gelfoam and hemostatic sutures[16]), poorly understood rising abdominal pressures during the thaw cycle,[7] laparoscopic port-site infection,[14] intra- or post-operative hematoma,[3,26] and the inability to adequately see a primary tumor or the cryolesion on ultrasonography (leading to increased collateral injury and possible incomplete tissue ablation).[15]

The slightest contact to any surrounding tissue by the cryoprobe can have catastrophic effects. For example, cryoprobe contact with the surrounding bowel or collecting system can result in respective bowel obstruction or urine leak and fistulization.[10,26] Savage and Gill and Sung and Gill showed that intentional freezing of the collecting system demonstrated urothelial sloughing to the lamina propria, with complete regrowth, and no leak or extravasation on retrograde pyelography.[22,23] Additionally, Bishoff, and colleagues noted severe adhesions between a cryoablated kidney and overlying bowel in non-

retroperitonealized kidneys in a porcine model, though without any evidence of bowel injury or fistula.[24] There were no complications reported with retroperitonealized kidneys. Gill and colleagues and Campbell and colleagues described the complication of obstructive stricture of the ureteropelvic junction.[9,10,46] No renal complications with renal function or blood pressure had been reported, with Carvalhal and colleagues supporting that fact in 22 patients during a mean follow-up of 20.6 months.[47] Further follow-up by the Cleveland Clinic group revealed urinary biochemical parameters suggesting that cryoablation may have an initial renal injury (as evidenced by elevated β_2-microglobulin levels), but baseline biochemical assays were noted at two months.[48]

Ultrasonography, fluoroscopy, CT, and MRI have all been used for preoperative assessment, patient positioning, intraoperative assessment, and serial follow-up for cryoablation and RFA. Each energy therapy has quite different intra- and post-operative radiographic characteristics. Notwithstanding, preoperative assessment is required, either through adequate enhanced cross-sectional

CT scanning or MRI, with patients having compromised renal function.

Adequate cryoablation requires intraoperative monitoring of the "ice ball." To date, CT and MRI have not proven to be reliable modalities for detecting progression of a cryolesion. Using ultrasonography, however, the cryoablated region appears with a hyperechoic crescentic rim (cryolesion edge), hypoechogenicity within the center of the lesion, and demonstration of a loss of normal color-flow characteristics—characteristics demarcating the size and location of the ice ball (Figure 103-1).[9,17,24,46] Open cryoablation permits the use of standard ultrasound probes and equipment, while laparoscopy requires intraoperative laparoscopic ultrasound (IOLUS), which can be used to monitor the progression of the cryolesion, to ensure a complete rim of normal renal parenchyma, to avoid injury of the collecting system, and to evaluate the kidney for other synchronous lesions not apparent on preoperative imaging.

Serial radiographic evaluation post-ablation is warranted so as to assure no persistent enhancement (a possible sign of persistent tumor) or enlargement. Serially enhanced CT scanning or MRI are adequate in this follow-up. Postoperative CT evaluation of cryolesions at 1 and 3 months revealed persistent hypointense defects in the area of the ice ball, and eventual cortical defects consistent with tissue loss.[24] Follow-up MRI revealed some ambiguity with regard to the signal characteristics of some cryolesions.[3,10,23,25,46] It is otherwise accepted, however, that the "hallmark" is an initial and prolonged "punched-out" avascular lesion with loss of signal with gadolinium-enhanced MRI, which is characteristic of lesion eradication.[3,10,14,25] Decreasing size of the ablation area should be noted. Gill and Novick reported mean percentage decreases in size of 20.5%, 33 to 63.3%[14], and 41% at postoperative day-one, one-month, and three-month CT or MRI evaluations, respectively.[3] Eventual loss of lesion identification and enhancement with either CT or MRI at 6 to 10 months suggests complete eradication.[14]

Immediate and delayed histopathologic changes have been studied following cryoablation and RFA. At one hour, a cryolesion contains a well-demarcated interstitial hemorrhage[9,8,24] with vascular congestion and early coagulative necrosis, primarily in the tubular epithelial cells.[9,49] Electron microscopic studies of these lesions revealed irreversible signs of cellular destruction with partial fragmentation and vacuolization of cytoplasmic membranes, chromatin condensation, nuclear membrane dissipation, and thrombi in glomerular capillaries.[9] At 24 hours, complete coagulative necrosis is seen, with a peripheral zone of partial necrosis (deemed the "zone of sublethal destruction or demarcation[22]), a current topic of concern because this may contain viable, non-desiccated carcinoma.[9,10,49]

The zone of sublethal destruction may correlate with one of the four layers Bishoff and colleagues have described where, at seven days, the histology shows a (1) central necrosis, (2) an inflammatory infiltrative process, (3) residual hemorrhage, and (4) fibrosis with tubular regeneration—the fourth of which may correlate with an incomplete zone of tissue desiccation (Figure 103-2).[8,24] Varying degrees of chronic inflammation, hemosiderosis, fibrosis, necrosis, and regeneration are seen from 3 weeks to 3 months after initial cryoablation [9,24] with ultimate spontaneous resorption of the cryolesion at approximately 3 months.[3] Histologic specimens 3 to 6 months after laparoscopic cryoablation reveal degrees of hemosiderin deposition, fibrosis, inflammation, necrosis, or even recurrence—

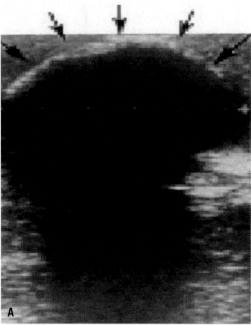

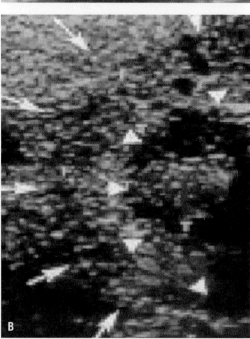

Figure 103-1 *A*, Characteristics of cryoablation on direct ultrasonographic guidance include an advancing hyperechoic crescentic lesion ("ice ball"; *black arrows*), a hypoechogenic central appearance, and loss of color-flow characteristics. *B*, Upon thawing, the extent of the rim is noted with a relative hypoechoic appearance (*white arrows*) when compared to the retreating crescentic edge of the ice ball (*white arrowheads*).

with the recurrence seen after an enhancing renal mass was identified on MRI follow-up.[50]

RADIOFREQUENCY ABLATION

Monopolar low-frequency radiofrequency (RF) energy, generated from alternating current generators, can produce up to 200 watts (current of 1,500 to 1,800 milliamperes) of heat energy and raise tissue temperatures to between 50 and 100°C.[11,13,29] The sustained temperatures produced by the RF energy result in cellular damage through the induction of ionic agitation and molecular frictional heat causing denaturation of proteins, melting of lipid membranes, and resultant coagulative necrosis.[13,15,26]

Radiofrequency ablative therapies have been successfully deployed using open, laparoscopic, and percutaneous approaches (Table 103-3).[12,15,28,29,51] Electrodes of varying configuration are used to produce an ablated area of tissue, with a deployable umbrella configuration (Figure 103-3) being the most commonly used method secondary to its ability to produce a spherical lesion with little intralesional movement (Figure 103-4).

Current RFA technology has proven the ability to successfully ablate a renal volume of up to 5 cm with a single probe with even greater ablative vol-

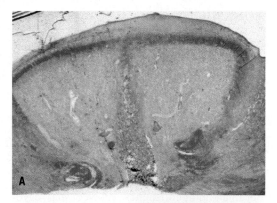

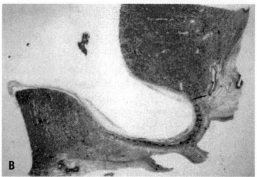

Figure 103-2 Porcine renal tissue one week after cryoablation reveals four distinct zones of histopathologic change: (1) complete necrosis, (2) inflammatory infiltrate, (3) hemorrhage, and (4) fibrosis and regeneration. *A*, Renal parenchyma remains unchanged outside a well-demarcated cryolesion at 13 weeks post-treatment. The lesion, however, will show resorption of the necrotic tissue, with a thickened capsule, marked interstitial fibrosis, and scattered shrunken glomeruli. *B*, 13 weeks post-ablation reveals a complete void of renal parenchyma and a thin rim of fibrous tissue.

umes with the use of concomitant, concentrically placed multi-electrode arrays.[4,11,15,52] Monopolar probes are used typically for the smaller, superficial lesions, while the bipolar technology can be used for larger lesions with larger ovoid, or pillow-shaped ablation zones between the two electrodes.[29]Caution should be used when tumors are ablated in close proximity to the renal collecting system or adjacent structures.[12]

An electrosurgical generator will assist with recording the total energies delivered, the impedance generated, target probe temperatures, and the total time of the procedure.[15,53]Since tissue destruction occurs when temperatures exceed 50°C, using probes that reach, and maintain temperatures of approximately 70°C is recommended. Reports in the literature use ablation-quiescence-ablation cycles up to 10 to 12 minutes (ablation); 5 to 10 minutes (quiescence); 10 to 12 minutes (ablation), with deep medullary tumors undergo-

ing a third ablation.[15] Crowley and colleagues showed that equivalent tissue desiccation was seen with a more limited 3–minute-5–minute-3–minute cycle using 2 cm probes.[53] After ablation, few hemorrhagic problems arise secondary to the local tissue and vascular destruction resulting in acute thrombosis. Gettman and colleagues showed that local intrarenal hemostasis was assured during a post-RFA partial nephrectomy (with a 0.5 to 1.0 cm diameter margin), the assumption being that the RFA adequately coagulated the local tissue, resulting in local hemostasis.[54] But this does not assure probe tract hemostasis and, as a result, some investigators use decreased wattage (15 W) with the RFA probe during its withdrawal to fulgurate the probe tract.[12,15]

Compared to cryotherapy, the use of real-time ultrasonography for RFA is less helpful. Tissue destruction during an RFA cycle can be seen on ultrasonography as an intense echogenicity

spreading from the electrode tip, with little margin identification, leaving an unclear heterogeneous echotexture. This is thought to be secondary to microbubble production from the ablative process itself.[11,28,29,33] The use of ultrasound may be of some utility in the evaluation of the postoperative color-flow Doppler characteristics. With local tissue destruction and disruption of the vascular supply, there is loss of blood flow within a radiolesion. Though the use of intraoperative ultrasound holds little promise for monitoring RFA lesions, the use of a laparoscopic infrared imaging system, correlating with surface temperatures and thermocouple measurements, provides a possible real-time assessment of adequate tumor desiccation.[55]

Thermocouple technology has been used in both cryotherapy and RFA in an attempt to predict adequate tumor destruction. Temperatures associated with tissue cell death can be measured

Table 103-3 Summary of Radiofrequncey Ablation Series

First Author/Reference	No. Pts	Lesions Ablated	Tumor Size (cm)	Mean OR Time	RFA Time	Mean EBL (cc)	Probe Temp	Hospital Stay	Mean/Mode Follow Up	Recurrence
Zlotta J Endourol 1998	3	3	3, 2.5, 5	NR	12 min	NR	NR	NR	1 week CT	NR
Gervis Radiology 2000	8	9	3.3	NR	12 min	NR	NR	NR	10.3 mo	5 lesions have persistent enhancement
Walther J Urol 2000	4	14	NR	NR	Single 5 min or double 5 min	NR	Tissue temp 60°C	NR	NR	No metastatic disease in tumors < 3 cm
Pavlovitch J Urol 2002	21	24	2.4	NR	Double 10–12 min	NR	70°C	< 24 hours	2 mo	None
Rendon J Urol 2001	10	11	2.4	NR	17 min	NR	NR	< 24 hours	Nephrectomy performed after RFA	64% had residual tumor after removal of kidney
Su J Urol 2002 abstract	17	22	2.0	NR	NR	NR	NR	NR	3.2 months	1/22 had enhancement at 3 months
Ogan Urology 2002	12	13	2.4 + 0.6	NR	95 min	NR	105°C (target temp.)	0.9 days	Serial CT at 3, 6, 12 mo, then 6 mos thereafter	None
Jacomides J Urol 2002	13	17	1.9 (range 0.9–3.6)	NR	140 min with in situ RFA 203 min with RFA and partial nephrectomy	NR	NR	NR	Radiographic	1/17 positive operative margin No radiographic recurrences
Matlaga J Urol 2002	10	10	3.2 (range, 1.4–8.0)	NR	NR	NR	NR	NR	Histologic and radiographic	8/10 tumors successfully ablated
Michaels J Urol 2002	15	20	2.4	NR	NR	NR	90–110 °C	NR	Histologic	20/20 specimens with residual tumor
McGovern J Urol 2003 abstract	55	63	Range 1–5.5 cm	NR	NR	NR	NR	NR	Radiographic 6 mo – 5 yr	4/46 (9%) incomplete peripheral ablations 4/17 (24%) incomplete central ablations
Lisson J Urol 2003 abstract	21	21	2.6 (1.0–4.2 cm)	NR	NR	NR	NR	18.6 hr	Radiographic (mean 12.1 mo)	2 with persistent enhancement, one s/p radical nephrectomy
Su Urology 2003 abstract	29	35	2.2 ± 0.7 cm	NR	NR	NR	NR	NR	CT (9 mo mean follow-up)	33/35 with single RFA; 2 with repeat (successful) RFA

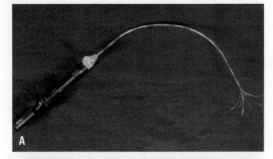

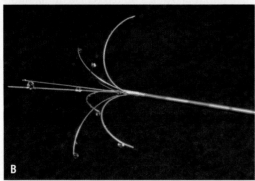

Figure 103-3 RITA Medical Systems probes showing *A*, a valuable characteristic of flexibility (A) and *B*, saline perfusion (note the saline droplets arising from the radiofrequency ablation (FRA) probe tines). Flexible probes assist with placement of various sized probes during computed tomography (CT) guidance, allowing the probe to bend under a tight CT gantry. Saline perfusion augments RFA cycles, creating more efficient radioablation.

with thermocouples immediately within, at the margin, and just outside the margin of a lesion.[7,20,25,26] The kidney's blood supply protects the parenchyma from cooling and heating. Observations during RFA, however, show that temperatures recorded at the edge of the ablation zone can be 20 to 30°C cooler than temperatures recorded at the RFA probe, making sufficient tissue desiccation uncertain with RFA temperature-based monitoring. For this reason, some authors favor an impedance-based system. The higher the electrical impedance, the more the tissue acts as a thermal insulator blocking the flow of RF energy and subsequent tissue destruction. Therefore the intra- and perilesional placement of RF impedance monitors will assist in assuring adequate marginal destruction. Impedance (to approximately 200 ohms) suggests that the tissue is desiccated and that continued lesion growth is unlikely.[29,56] "Dry" renal tissue shows higher impedance versus tissue that is exposed to hypertonic saline at the RFA probe tip, and the use of this local saline (see Figure 103-3) has proven to be of assistance in increasing the size of lesion created.[26,57] Furthermore, there is a known phenomenon of microbubble formation at the site of a radiolesion, which has also been shown to increase local tissue impedance, which only 30 to 60 seconds of RF quiescence seems to alleviate. This is the basis of the radiofrequency-free time between ablative maneuvers. In a porcine model, Rendon and colleagues showed that there may be a "thermal blanketing" phenomenon produced by injected saline (hydrodissection) or CO_2 (gas dis-

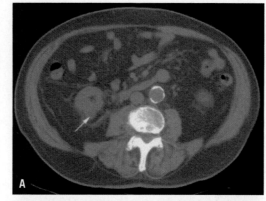

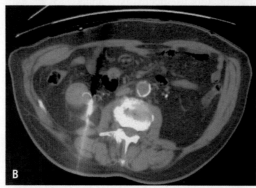

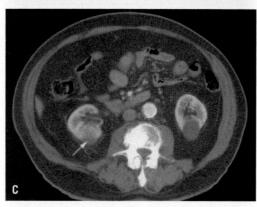

Figure 103-4 *A*, Preoperative computed tomography (CT) assessment reveals a renal mass in the posterior right kidney. Supine patient placement and cutaneous markers have been placed to assist with radiofrequency probe placement. *B*, radiofrequency ablation probe placement within the mass, with umbrella-configured deployed tines, allows for minimal intralesional movement. *C*, CT image immediately post–ablation-cycling shows decreased enhancement in the area of the ablation, but normal enhancing surrounding renal parenchyma.

section) within the perirenal space, resulting in higher temperatures and possibly greater ease of destruction within various peripheral lesions.[35]

There has been histopathologic evidence of incomplete ablation following RFA in certain patient populations. Walther and colleagues explored 14 tumors < 5 cm in diameter in 4 patients with multiple renal lesions and performed RF immediately prior to surgical excision. Complete, immediate treatment effect was noted in 10 of 11 patients; in the final case, only 35% of the tumor was ablated.[36] Rendon and colleagues showed an underestimation of the RFA ablative volume with 7 of 11 lesions (64%) having > 5% tumor residual on gross inspection.[33]

Further results concerning incomplete ablation were seen with a series from the Lahey Clinic where 20 of 20 tumors in 15 patients revealed evidence of persistent residual tumor after only a single ablation cycle.[58]

Gervais and colleagues presented data predicting the size and location of tumors most likely to recur or to have incomplete initial treatment. In their series, central, large tumors (> 5 cm in diameter) recurred with more frequency than the smaller exophytic peripheral lesions (< 3 cm diameter), but statistical significance was not met. This observation is supported by the improved cellular destruction with exophytic, peripherally based tumors secondary to the "oven effect" of the surrounding perirenal fat. Conversely, intraparenchymal tumors may have less destruction secondary to the possible heat dissipation, or heat sink, developed by the surrounding dense vasculature. These phenomena may be obviated through selective arterial embolization of centrally located tumors prior to ablation.[59] Patients who had enhancement on follow-up CT were assumed to have been inadequately treated and were electively re-treated, and followed again with serial imaging.[11]

Despite these data, one Johns Hopkins group shed some optimism on the use of renal RFA.[60] With 35 of 37 ablations performed under intravenous sedation, and 32 of 37 treatments performed on an outpatient basis, 94% of patients (33 of 35) required only a single ablation, while the final two received success with a repeat treatment. Of 13 renal lesions with follow-up over one year, 11 (85%) had no residual tumor growth or enhancement.

Cryoablation has a reported theoretic, but not proven, risk of tumor seeding secondary to probe manipulation during ablation,[26] although a stronger theoretical risk of tumor seeding has been cited with RFA. Through the heat generated with the RF probe, local vasodilatation just outside the ablative zone may become more receptive to possible tumor spillage, resulting in hematogenous metastases.[12,29] Concurrently, both modalities carry the risk of local needle tract, or port-site tumor implantation—again, cited as a potential complication, but not reported.[29] This dilemma may be overcome by low-frequency energy deployment in the needle tract upon withdrawal of the percutaneous apparatus.[61] Additionally, superficial RF probe technology may assist with local cancer and hemorrhage control when deployed during open or laparoscopic partial nephrectomy. Adequate hemostasis with an average of 4 mm of penetrated tissue desiccation, was seen by Coleman and colleagues in 19 renal lesions extirpated from 5 patients via laparoscopic partial nephrectomy.[62] This superficial technique may assist with future open and laparoscopic cellular tumor control.

We have been faced with an isolated generator pad superficial cutaneous burn in an abnormally long cycle (greater than 60 minutes) in one of four pads contralateral to the renal lesion being ablated. Two grounding pad skin burns (in separate patients) were reported in a series by Lisson and colleagues, but the location and relationship to the electrosurgical generator were not described.[63] A conservatively managed hepatic burn was noted in the Johns Hopkins series.[60] In one of the largest series, McGovern and colleagues reported one ureteral stricture, one obstructed ureter secondary to clot, and two significant perinephric hematomas—without a definition of "significant hematoma." Furthermore, their work strengthened the argument that more peripheral tumors are optimal for ablation because they had 4 of 17 (24%) centrally located tumors have incomplete ablations.[64]

Compared to the 10% conversion rate from laparoscopic to open nephrectomy reported in older literature,[7] laparoscopic deployment of cryoprobes or RFA have not been associated with reported conversion to open surgery.

While ultrasonography, fluoroscopy, CT, and MRI have all been used for patient positioning and percutaneous placement of RF probes, none of these modalities has proven reliable for the intraoperative monitoring of the RF lesion. On ultrasonography, there is no immediate change in the echotexture in the area of RF ablation, and color and power Doppler are of no added benefit secondary to the variable and inconsistent findings. Moreover, RF treatment can sometimes disturb ultrasound imaging, creating a marked scatter of the echoes, secondary to microbubble formation as noted previously in this chapter.[11,28,29,33,35] Crowley and colleagues found CT scanning to be an excellent modality for positioning of the patient and probe and for immediate post-treatment imaging, but it was not used for intraoperative monitoring.[53] Lewin and colleagues and Merkle and colleagues used MRI to monitor real-time tissue destruction with RF. These groups demonstrated a zone of decreased signal surrounded by a rim of hyperintensity on T2-weighted and turbo short inversion-time inversion recovery images.[56,65] Confirmatory images obtained after conclusion of the ablation session revealed a propensity for these T2-weighted images to underestimate the size of the RF lesion.[56] Thus, insofar as intraoperative monitoring for RF is concerned, there is no imaging modality that can, in real time, ensure a sufficient extent of tissue ablation while avoiding injury to normal, adjacent parenchyma and structures. The solution may lie in the perfection of what Zlotta and colleagues called "forecast ablation."[29] This is the correlation between the size of the lesion predicted by the diameter of the prongs on the RF electrode and the actual observation of the RF lesion. Both the low frequency of RF energy and its vulnerability to the dissipating effects of blood flow permit the creation of very localized lesions. It is therefore possible to sculpt a lesion with numerous applications of the RF probe. Zlotta and colleagues performed RF ablation in both ex vivo and in vivo human kidneys, comparing probe size to lesion volume. In the in vivo model, the size of the lesion correlated closely with the diameter of the prongs deployed on the electrode

probe: treatment with a 2 cm prong resulting in a lesion measuring 2 by 1.8 cm.[29]

Histologically, RFA-treated lesions are quite different in that they are typically wedge-shaped secondary to their endothelial destruction, and subsequent segmental vascular thrombosis and ischemia. Ischemia likely augments the primary histopathologic destruction from the RF heat energy itself, which results in characteristic hypereosinophilia (unknown mechanism), pyknosis, stromal edema, loss of [or even enhancement of[66]] nuclear and nucleoli architecture, and coagulative necrosis.[15,29] Tissues stained with hematoxylin and eosin (H&E) staining tend to have inconsistent histologies, with the appearance of preserved renal tissue despite attempted ablation. Marcovich and colleagues, however, have shown that nicotinamide adenine dinucleotide (NADH) staining is more helpful in assessing complete tissue desiccation secondary to evaluating the metabolic activity and viability of cells that accept this staining (Figures 103-5).[67] Tissues within saline-cooled RF ablation zones that are completely desiccated do not accept NADH staining, whereas the renal parenchymal transition is easily seen.[66]

HIGH INTENSITY FREQUENCY ULTRASOUND (HIFU)

The biological effects of high intensity focused ultrasound (HIFU) have been known for over 50 years. HIFU has been used in the treatment of glaucoma and as an alternative therapy for benign prostatic hyperplasia and prostate cancer.[68,69]

High-intensity ultrasound fields can be created by focusing ultrasound waves in a very narrow focal zone, akin to the focal targeting with extracorporeal shock wave lithotripsy (ESWL). Temperatures as high as 65°C can be generated by a pulse wave of only 5 seconds. Tissue at the focal point is ablated, while superficial layers are generally spared. An ablative intensity of 1,500 W/cm^2 for one second will produce a lesion roughly 0.5 cm^2 per exposure, creating near-instantaneous tissue destruction, unlike RFA.

HIFU causes tissue destruction by four primary mechanisms: (1) thermal effects, (2) cavitation, (3) mechanical forces, and (4) chemical reactions and accelerations. Thermal effects and cavitation are the predominant forms of tissue ablation in HIFU. Thermal tissue injury was discussed previously in this chapter, but cavitation refers to the development of a shock wave that occurs when a rapidly formed bubble suddenly collapses (the basic principle behind ESWL).

The same physical considerations that are required for diagnostic ultrasound imaging also apply here: a fluid or soft tissue path is necessary for the propagation of the sound wave with the absence of bony or gaseous obstructions. Like ultrasound, the technique is completely noninvasive, obviating the need to access the kidney percutaneously or surgically.

There are three main features of HIFU that make lesion creation unpredictable. First, cavitation itself is a phenomenon in which effects are

difficult to focus and predict. Second, the high acoustic pressures induced by HIFU create nonlinearity of the propagated sound wave. Finally, the preexistence of one thermal lesion may perturb the intended placement of subsequent lesions—the so-called "lesion-lesion interaction." In addition, respiratory movements may move a focused lesion in and out of a small focal zone. This dilemma may be overcome with the use of robotics and the use of image stabilization for adequate targeting.

There are limited reports of clinical use of HIFU for the treatment of renal tumors. Susani and colleagues treated healthy tissue and renal tumors in two patients prior to radical nephrectomy, identifying necrosis of tumor in the ablated areas at the time of harvest.[70] Vallancien and colleagues treated kidney tumors in eight patients, resulting in coagulation necrosis at the site of ablation.[71] No subcapsular or perirenal hematomas were seen, and there was no evidence of renal pelvis or ureteral injury. Several patients, however, suffered second- and third-degree skin burns at the ultrasound's cutaneous operative site. Kohrmann and colleagues reported using HIFU in 24 patients immediately prior to nephrectomy. In 19 of 24 cases, hemorrhage and necrosis was discovered macroscopically.[72] More recently, the same lead investigator reported the use of HIFU to treat three different tumors in a single patient. Each lesion was treated on three different occasions approximately 30 days apart.[73] Three months after the last

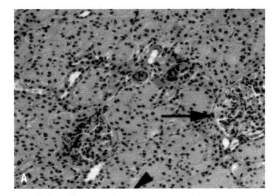

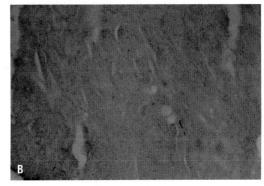

Figure 103-5 *A*, Tissues with hematoxylin and eosin (H&E) staining tend to have inconsistent histologies, with the appearance of preserved renal tissue despite attempted ablation. *B*, Tissues within saline-cooled radiofrequency ablation zones that are completely desiccated do not accept nicotinamide adenine dinucleotide staining, demonstrating the loss of renal metabolic activity. Photographs courtesy of Benjamin Lee, MD.

treatment session, an MRI was obtained, with two tumors showing significant regression, while one tumor in the upper pole of the kidney appeared unaffected. This failure was attributed to absorption of the ultrasound energy by interposed ribs.

Although HIFU by its nature is prepared for real-time monitoring of evolving tissue changes during treatment, the ablative lesion cannot be reproducibly imaged during the actual ablation cycle. Additionally, accurate delivery of HIFU is limited by movement during respiration and blocked by ribs and other bony structures. There are no temperature sensors in the tissue to ensure that all portions of the target lesion reach temperatures sufficient for tissue necrosis. As a minimally invasive technique, HIFU holds great promise, but full realization is currently limited by adequate visualization of the ablated tissue, the potential thermal injury to the skin, and its unpredictable effect on tissues.

MICROWAVE ABLATION

Tissue absorption of microwaves (30 to 3,000 MHz) results in increased temperatures through production of molecular kinetic energy. Probes placed directly into the target tissue increase temperatures according to the frequency used, time of application, and the inherent properties of the tissue being ablated. Urologic applications include the treatment of benign prostatic hyperplasia and renal tumors. In the kidney, microwave tissue coagulation (MTC) has been used clinically to assist with hemostasis during partial nephrectomy. In four patients, Naito and colleagues inserted a MTC needle probe into the kidney during partial nephrectomy without vascular occlusion.[74] Furuya and colleagues and Itoh and colleagues also performed MTC via retroperitoneoscopic approach in 13 and six patients, respectively, again without vascular occlusion.[75,76] Using microwaves generated at 2,450 MHz, 15 to 20 areas around the mass were treated with MTC, and the tumor excised. Tumor extirpation, without significant bleeding was accomplished in all cases. In one case, a positive surgical margin prompted radical nephrectomy.[74]

Murota and colleagues also applied the microwave tissue coagulator in partial nephrectomy procedures performed via retroperitoneoscopy. Their technique in eight patients was using MTC as a hemostatic device rather than a frank tissue desiccator. Despite two frozen-section positive margins prompting further resection with the MTC, no recurrent lesions or urine leaks were seen at a mean follow-up of 10.4 months.[77] With complete negative margins on final pathologic review, in conjunction with no evident recurrences, the MTC may actually destroy a margin that would otherwise have tumor cells. Thus, direct tumor desiccation may augment oncologic outcome for this unique modality.

Hiroya and colleagues have the largest MTC series to date, with 50 patients receiving either open or laparoscopic partial nephrectomies under MTC assistance.[78] Though MTC dissection, with

sharp peripelvic dissection, was with negative surgical margins for malignancy, a number of complications were noted. Caliceal entry was noted in 27 cases (54%), urinoma in 4 (8%), renal vein injury in one patient (2%), and renal pelvic stenosis in one case (2%). Of concern was the postoperative renal infarction in three cases (6%). We support their conclusion that MTC may prove to be a promising future method for dissection and hemostasis, but the infancy of this technology demonstrates the need for study.

Future advances in determining the ideal settings, cycles, temperature monitoring, and ablation times may allow use of microwave coagulation technology to perform extensive resection of renal tissue with minimal blood loss and avoid warm ischemic injury to the kidney.

LASER ABLATION

Laser ablation of target tissue using one or several laser fibers has been described in the treatment of head and neck, liver, brain and kidney tumors, as well as treatment of benign hyperplasia of the prostate and uterine fibroids.

Using magnetic resonance guided interstitial laser thermoablation (ILT), De Jode and colleagues treated kidney tumors in three patients.[79] Laser energy from a neodymium:yttrium-aluminum-garnet (Nd:YAG) source was percutaneously delivered to the tumors under real-time magnetic resonance guidance in an open access scanner. Thermal ablation was monitored with a continuous-subtraction colorization software package with real-time image processing. Serial laser ablation was seen through sequential subtraction imaging with loss of an MR T1 signal with temperature elevations. Follow-up gadolinium-enhanced MRI confirmed necrosis in the target tissue. One patient showed areas of enhancement consistent with viable tumor and underwent an additional ablation of the enhancing areas. Their follow-up evaluation of nine patients revealed a mean tumor volume reduction of only 45%, although viable tumor was noted at a mean follow-up of 16.9 months.[80] Clearly, limits to ILT include assessment of tumor viability post-treatment; additional investigation is needed, however, to determine the ultimate use of lasers in renal (and other) tissue ablation.

INTERSTITIAL PHOTON RADIATION ENERGY

Using radiation as the energy source, this technology also uses the basic mode of thermotherapy to ablate tissue. The photon radiosurgery system (PRS) delivers precise, focused and controllable local radiation therapy without exposing intervening layers of tissue. In contrast to RFA, PRS may not be as sensitive to the dissipating effect of vascular flow and, as such, may be effective in ablating tissue near the renal hilum.

Chan and colleagues report a PRS feasibility trial in a canine model.[81] Through a midline laparotomy, 12 mongrel dogs received photon

radiation to the left lower-pole kidney and right hilum with 15 Gy at a radius of 1.3 cm for 10 minutes, resulting in a 2.5 cm lesion. Histopathologic examination revealed coagulation necrosis, gradually replaced by organizing necrosis and fibrosis. As of this writing, there were no clinical or human trials where renal tumors were ablated with PRS. One would expect this technology, like RF and HIFU, to be similarly limited in its ability for real-time monitoring of the ablative lesion.

CONCLUSION

Open nephron-sparing surgery enjoys the endorsement of numerous clinical trials with sufficient long-term follow-up to document its equivalent safety and efficacy, compared to radical nephrectomy in the treatment of small renal tumors. Prospective clinical trials that would yield a similar endorsement for ablative technologies are ongoing, but have not yet achieved the status of radical nephrectomy or nephron-sparing techniques. Given the uncertain nature of these incidental lesions (benign or malignant), precise pathologic diagnosis is critical for determining appropriate clinical and radiographic follow-up. Most ablative techniques do not permit the collection of tissue specimens after treatment in all patients. Fortunately, most of the clinical trials perform renal biopsy prior to ablation, but renal biopsy can be fraught with inaccuracies. Dechet and colleagues, in their prospective analysis of 110 renal lesions, reported a rate of 26% for non-diagnostic biopsies and 16% for biopsies of actual malignant tumors that were reported as benign.[82] In order to determine the long-term efficacy of new technologies, precise pathologic diagnosis is critical. The primary limit with these treatments lies in the lack of long-term cancer-free and overall-survival data. With further refinements of both energy delivery systems and deployment strategies, one can hopefully witness a new era of progressive, minimally invasive surgery.

New minimally invasive therapies represent exciting advances for patients with small renal lesions, significant comorbidities, or recurrent cancers that would otherwise force one to recommend observation. In the future, it may be possible to use tailored probes that can be conformed to a specific pathologic type, size, and location of renal lesion. Additionally, alternative ablative energy sources such as microwave thermoablation, high-intensity focused ultrasound, and interstitial photon radiation ablation are being studied as future competitors in the arena of minimally-invasive NSS. Overall, cautious optimism is recommended when considering the incorporation of either cryoablation or RFA into one's surgical armamentarium. Excluding any technical and radiographic inconsistencies in any of the short-term results of cryoablation or RFA, early treatment failure needs to be put into the context of long-term, prospective clinical trials. Any new techniques for the treatment of small renal tumors must show clinical and pathologic success compared to open nephron sparing surgery.

REFERENCES

1. Lee CT, Katz J, Shi W, et al. Surgical management of renal tumors 4 cm or less in a contemporary cohort. J Urol 2000;163:730.
2. Clayman RV, Kavoussi LR, Soper NJ, et al. Laparoscopic nephrectomy: Initial case report. J Urol 1991;146:278–82.
3. Gill IS, Novick AC. Renal cryosurgery. Urology 1999;54: 215–9.
4. Nissenkorn I, Burnheim J. Multricentricity in Renal Cell Carcinoma. J Urol 1995;153:620–2.
5. McKiernan J, Simmons R, Katz J, Russo P. Natural history of chronic renal insufficiency after partial and radical nephrectomy. Urology 2002;59:816–20.
6. Uchida M, Sugimoto K, Uehara H, Watanabe H. Percutaneous cryosurgery for renal tumors. Br J Urol 1995;75:132–6.
7. Johnson DB, Nakada SY. Laparoscopic cryoablation for renal-cell cancer. J Endourol 2000;14:873–8.
8. Stephenson RA, King DK, Rohr LR. Renal cryoablation in a canine model. Urology 1996;41:772–6.
9. Gill IS, Novick AC, Soble JJ, et al. Laparoscopic renal cryoablation: initial clinical series. Urology 1998;52:543–51.
10. Gill IS, Novick AC, Meraney AM, et al. Laparoscopic renal cryoablation in 32 patients. Urology 2000;56:748–53.
11. Gervais DA, McGovern FJ, Wood BJ, et al. Radio-frequency ablation of renal cell carcinoma: early clinical experience. Radiology 2000;217:665–72.
12. Yohannes P, Pinto P, Rotariu P, et al. Retroperitoneoscopic radiofrequency ablation of a solid renal mass. J Endourol 2001;15:845–9.
13. Zagoria RJ, Chen MY, Kavanagh PV, Torti FM. Radio frequency ablation of lung metastases from renal cell carcinoma. J Urol 2001;166:1827–8.
14. Shingleton WB, Sewell PE. Percutaneous renal cryoablation of renal tumors in patients with von Hippel-Lindau disease. J Urol 2002;167:1268–70.
15. Pavlovich CP, Walther MM, Choyke PL, et al. Percutaneous radio frequency ablation of small renal tumors: initial results. J Urol 2002;167:10–5.
16. Cozzi PJ, Lynch WJ, Collins S, et al. Renal cryotherapy in a sheep model; a feasibility study. J Urol 1997;157:710–2.
17. Delworth MG, Pisters LL, Fornage BD, von Eschenbach AC. Cryotherapy for renal cell carcinoma and angiomyolipoma. J Urol 1996;155:252–4.
18. Linehan WM. Kidney cancer – a unique opportunity for the development of disease specific therapy [Editorial]. J Urol 2002;168:2411–2.
19. Shingleton WB, Sewell PE. Percutaneous cryoablation of renal cell carcinoma in a transplanted kidney. Br J Urol 2002;90:134–8.
20. Mikus P. Cancer cryosurgery potentially 'hot' for patients, new markets. J Natl Cancer Inst 2000;92:1464.
21. Wood B, Grippo J, Pavlovich CP. Percutaneous radio frequency ablation for hematuria. J Urol 2001;166:2303–4.
22. Savage SJ, Gill IS. Renal tumor ablation: energy-based technologies. World J Urol 2000;18:283–8.
23. Sung GT, Gill IS. Effect of intentional cryoinjury to the renal collecting system [Abstract]. J Endourol 1999;13 Suppl 1:14.
24. Bishoff JT, Chen RB, Lee BR, et al. Laparoscopic renal cryoablation: acute and long-term clinical, radiographic, and pathologic effects in an animal and application in a clinical trial. J Endourol 1999;13:233–9.
25. Chen RN, Novick AC, Gill IS. Laparoscopic cryoablation of renal masses. Urol Clin N Amer 2000;27:813–20.
26. Murphy DP, Gill IS. Energy-based renal tumor ablation: a review. Sem in Urol Onc 2001;19:133–40.
27. Alder AB. Cryosurgery in urology. Br J Urol 1970;42:744.
28. Pautler SE, Pavlovich CP, Mikityansky I, et al. Retroperitoneoscopic-guided radiofrequency ablation of renal tumors. Can J Urol 2001;8(4):1330–3.
29. Zlotta AR, Wildschutz T, Raviv G, et al. Radiofrequency interstitial tumor ablation (RITA) is a possible new modality for treatment of renal cancer: ex vivo and in vivo experience. J Endourol 1998;11:251–8.
30. Feld RI, McGinnis DE, Needleman L, et al. A novel application for the end-fore sonographic probe: guidance during cryoablation of renal masses. Amer J Rad 1999;173: 652–4.
31. Sharp DS, Molina W, Abreu SC, et al. Temperature distribution within developing cryolesions in living perfused porcine kidneys [Abstract]. J Urol 2003;169:202.
32. Zegel HG, Holland GA, Jennings SB, et al. Intraoperative ultrasonography guided cryoablation of renal masses: initial experience. J Ultrasound Med 1998;17:571–6.
33. Rendon RA, Kachura JR, Sweet JM, et al. The uncertainty of radio frequency treatment of renal cell carcinoma: findings at immediate and delayed nephrectomy. J Urol 2002; 167:1587–92.
34. Remer EM, Hale JC, O'Malley CM, et al. Sonographic guidance of laparoscopic renal cryoablation. Am J Roentgen 2000;174:1595–6.
35. Rendon RA, Gertner MR, Sherar MD, et al. Development of a radiofrequency based thermal therapy technique in an in vivo porcine model for the treatment of small renal masses. J Urol 2001;166:292–8.
36. Walther MM, Shawker TH, Libutti SK, et al. A phase 2 study of radio frequency interstitial tissue ablation of localized renal tumors [abstract]. J Urol 2000;163:1424.
37. Rukstalis DB, Khorsandi M, Garcia FU, et al. Clinical experience with open renal cryoablation. Urology 2001;57:34–9.
38. Kim SC, Rubenstein J, Yap RL, et al. Laparoscopic renal cryosurgery: the Northwestern experience [abstract]. J Urol 2002;167:1.
39. Su LM, Jarrett TW, Kavoussi LR, Solomon SB. Percutaneous CT-guided radiofrequency ablation of small renal masses in poor surgical risk patients: preliminary results [abstract]. J Urol 2002;167:1.
40. Rodriguez R, Chan DY, Bishoff JT, et al. Renal ablative cryosurgery in select patients with peripheral renal masses. Urology 2000;55:25–30.
41. Harmon JD, Haleblain G, Stoker ME, et al. Long-term outcomes of renal cryoablation [abstract]. J Urol 2003; 169:229.
42. Levin HS, Meraney AM, Novick AC, Gill IS. Needle biopsy histology of renal tumors 3-6 months after laparoscopic renal cryoablation. J Urol 2000;163(S682):153.
43. Bargman VG, Ghafar MA, Sawczuk IS. Cryotherapeutic assisted partial nephrectomy for localized renal masses [abstract]. J Urol 2003;169:3.
44. Shingleton WB. Long-term follow up of percutaneous renal cryoablation [abstract]. J Urol 2003;169:2.
45. Yohannes P, Rotariu P, Pinto P, et al. Transperitoneal laparoscopic radiofrequency ablation of a solid renal mass: free of complications? J Urol 2002;167:16.
46. Campbell SC, Krishnamurthi V, Chow G, et al. Renal cryosurgery: experimental evaluation of treatment parameters. Urology 1998;52:29–33.
47. Carvalhal EF, Gill IS, Meraney AM, et al. Laparoscopic renal cryoablation: impact on renal function and blood pressure. Urol 2001;58:357–61.
48. Ng CS, Gill IS. Impact of renal cryoablation on urine composition. Urol 2002;59:831–4.
49. Edmunds TB, Schulsinger DA, Durand DB, Waltzer WC. Acute histologic changes in human renal tumors after cryoablation. J Endourol 2000;14:139–4.
50. Levin HS, Meraney AM, Novick AC, Gill IS. Needle biopsy histology of renal tumors 3-6 months after laparoscopic renal cryoablation. J Urol (abstract) 2002;163(4):153.
51. Jacomides L, Ogan K, Watumull L, Cadeddu JA. Laparoscopic application of radio frequency energy enables in situ renal tumor ablation and partial nephrectomy. J Urol 2003;169:49–43.
52. Dupuy DE, Radiofrequency ablation: an outpatient percutaneous treatment. Med Health R I 1999;82:213.
53. Crowley JD, Shelton J, Iverson AJ, et al. Laparoscopic and computed tomography-guided percutaneous radio-frequency ablation of renal tissue: acute and chronic effects in an animal model. Urology 2001;57:976–80.
54. Gettman MT, Bishoff JT, Su LM, et al. Hemostatic laparoscopic partial nephrectomy: initial experience with the radiofrequency coagulation-assisted technique. Urology 2001;58:8–11.
55. Roberts WW, Fugita OE, Ryan BP, et al. Infrared imaging of laparoscopic renal radiofrequency ablation in a porcine model [abstract]. J Urol 2002;167:18.
56. Lewin JS, Connell CF, Duerk JL, et al. Interactive MRI-guided radiofrequency interstitial thermal ablation of abdominal tumors: clinical trial for evaluation of safety and feasibility. J Mag Res Imag 1998;8:40–7.
57. Munver R, Threatt CB, Delvecchio FC, et al. Hypertonic saline-augmented radiofrequency ablation of the VX-2 tumor implanted in the rabbit kidney: a short-term survival pilot study. Urol 2002;60:170–5.
58. Michaels MJ, Rhee HK, Mourtzinos AP, et al. Incomplete renal tumor destruction using radio frequency interstitial ablation. J Urol 2002;168:2406–10.
59. Hall WH, McGahan JP, Link DP, et al. Combined embolization and percutaneous radiofrequency ablation of a solid renal tumor. Am J Roentgenol 2000;174:1592–4.
60. Su LM, Jarrett TW, Chan DY, et al. Percutaneous computed tomography-guided radiofrequency ablation of renal masses in high surgical risk patients: preliminary results. Urology 2003;61:26–33.
61. Ogan K, Jacomides L, Dolmatch BL, et al. Percutaneous radiofrequency ablation of renal tumors: technique, limitations, and morbidity. Urol 2002;60:954–8.
62. Coleman JA, Phillips J, Wood B, et al. Circumferential radiofrequency coagulation for partial nephrectomy and partial adrenalectomy [abstract]. J Urol 2003;169:3.
63. Lisson SW, Paz R, Broderick GA, et al. Treatment of small renal masses with radio-frequency ablation: initial experience [abstract]. J Urol 2003;169:229.
64. McGovern FJ, McDougall S, Gervais D, Mueller P. Percutaneous radiofrequency ablation of human renal cell carcinoma [abstract]. J Urol 2003;169:2.
65. Merkle EM, Shonk JR, Duerk JL, et al. MR-guided RF thermal ablation of the kidney in a porcine model. Amer J Radiology 1999;173:645–51.
66. Matlaga BR, Zagoria RJ, Woodruff RD, et al. Phase II trial of radio frequency ablation of renal cancer: evaluation of the kill zone. J Urol 2002;168:2401–5.
67. Marcovich R, Aldana JPA, Morgenstern N, et al. Radiofrequency ablation of porcine kidney: nicotinamide adenine dinucleotide (NADH) staining as a determinant of cell death – histologic findings. Urology.[Accepted]
68. Hegarty NJ, Fitzpatrick JM. High intensity focused ultrasound in benign prostatic hyperplasia. Eur J Ultrasound 1999;9:55–60.
69. Hill CR, ter Haar GR. Review article: high intensity focused ultrasound – potential for cancer treatment. Br J Radiol 1995;68:1296–1303.
70. Susani M, Madersbacher S, Kratzik C. Morphology of tissue destruction induced by focused ultrasound. Eur Urol 1993;23:34–7.
71. Vallancien G, Harouni M, Veillon B, et al. Preliminary results of a phase I dose escalation clinical trial using focused ultrasound in the treatment of localized tumours. Eur J Ultrasound 1999;9:11–5.
72. Korhmann KU, Michel MS, Back W. Non-invasive thermoablation in the kidney: first results of the clinical feasibility study [abstract]. J Endourol 2000;14 Suppl:34.
73. Kohrmann KU, Michel MS, Gaa J et al. High intensity focused ultrasound as noninvasive therapy for multilocal renal cell carcinoma: case study and review of the literature. J Urol 2002;167:2397–403.
74. Naito S, Nakashima M, Kimoto Y, et al. Application of microwave tissue coagulation in partial nephrectomy for renal cell carcinoma. J Urol 1998;159:960–2.
75. Furuya Y, Tsuchida T, Takihana Y, et al. Retroperitoneoscopic nephron-sparing surgery of renal tumor using a microwave tissue coagulator without renal ischemia: comparison with open procedure. J Endourol 2003;17:.
76. Itoh K, Suzuki Y, Miuru M, et al. Posterior retroperitoneoscopic partial nephrectomy using microwave tissue coagulator for small renal tumors. J Endourol 2002;16:367–71.
77. Murota T, Kawakita M, Oguchi N, et al. Retroperitoneoscopic partial nephrectomy using microwave coagulation for small renal tumors. European Urol 2002;41:540–5.
78. Hiroya O, Yoshiyuku M, Hiroshi I, et al. Partian nephrectomy for renal tumors using microwave tissue coagulator [abstract]. J Urol 2003;169:3.
79. De Jode MG, Vale JA, Gedroyc WM. MR-guided laser thermoablation of inoperable renal tumors in an open-configuration interventional MR scanner: preliminary clinical experience in three cases. J MRI 1999;10:545–9.
80. Dick EA, Joarder R, De Jode MG, et al. Magnetic resonance imaging-guided laser thermal ablation of renal tumours. Br J Urol 2002;90:814–22.
81. Chan DY, Koniaris L, Magee C, et al. Feasibility of ablating normal renal parenchyma by interstitial photon radiation energy: study in a canine model. J Endourol 2000;14:111–6.
82. Dechet CB, Sebo T, Farrow G, et al. Prospective analysis of intraoperative frozen needle biopsy of solid renal masses in adults. J Urol 1999;162:1282–4.

Part IX

Robotics

104

Robotics: Coming of Age

Hyung L. Kim, MD

Peter Schulam, MD

Urology has always been quick to embrace new technology. The benefits of ureteroscopy, lasers and shock wave lithotripsy were readily recognized, and these tools are now an integral part of a modern urology practice. Robotic technology has the potential to expand surgical capabilities and improve clinical outcomes, and urology is taking an active part in developing and evaluating robotic technology.

HISTORY

In our society, the popular conception of robots comes from works of science fiction, such as Blade Runner and Star Wars. In fact, the term "robot" was first coined by Karel Capek, in his 1921 play titled *Rossums Universal Robots*. "Robot" is the Czech word for "industrial worker," and in the play, motorized automatons with artificial intelligence were created to serve humans. Isaac Asimov, another popular science fiction writer, was the first person to use the term "robotics" to refer to the technology of robots. He predicted the rise of a pervasive robotics industry.

Even as robots have become commonplace in science fiction, more practical versions of robots have become an integral part of the manufacturing industry. In manufacturing, robots offer precision and accuracy that cannot be matched by human workers. Robots can work under extreme conditions and for extended durations. For repetitive tasks that require a high degree of consistency, they offer a clear economic advantage. The success of industrial robots has stimulated interest in applying robotics to other areas, including medicine (Figure 104-1).

A robot can be broadly defined as a mechanical device that is controlled using a computer system (Table 104-1). The first medical specialties to use robots were neurosurgery and orthopedics.[1,2] In neurosurgery, robots were well-suited for many of the surgical tasks that require accurate anatomic localization and precise surgical manipulation. Furthermore, the cranial anatomy provides relatively fixed landmarks. Robotic systems were developed for neuro-navigation, stereotactic localization and robotic assistance.[3-6] NeuroMate (Integrated Surgical Systems, Davis, CA) is a commercially available robot, approved by the Food and Drug Administration (FDA), that can help identify and direct the surgeon to neurologic lesions. In orthopedics, the RoboDoc (Integrated Surgical Systems, Inc.,

Sacramento, CA) was developed to assist with placement of prosthetic joints.[7] Using the RoboDoc, bone can be cut for placement of a joint prosthesis with 10 times greater accuracy than is possible manually.

Other specialties have also explored the use of robotics. Cardiac surgery was one of the first specialties to attract the interest of robot manufacturers. Clinical trials using laparoscopic robotic systems for coronary bypass surgery are under way.[8,9] In general surgery, laparoscopic robotic systems have been used in prospective clinical trials to perform cholecystectomies[10] and Nissen fundoplications.[11] The first clinical trials using robots in gynecology were for reversal of tubal ligation.[11,12]

Conventional laparoscopic surgery is now established as the standard for a wide variety of procedures (Figure 104-2). In urology, the decrease in postoperative pain and recovery time for laparoscopic nephrectomy when compared to open surgery is well documented.[13-16] Early mechanical devices designed to facilitate laparoscopy included simple, passive devices for holding the camera during surgery. These devices were cumbersome to use. To move the camera,

the surgeon had to take his hand off the working instruments and position the mechanical device. Therefore, active devices were developed for positioning the camera during laparoscopy.

AESOP, or Automated Endoscopic System for Optimal Positioning (Computer Motion, Goleta, CA), was the first active robotic device approved by the FDA. AESOP is a robotic arm with motorized joints that is controlled by the surgeon through speech recognition.[17] EndoAssist (Armstrong Healthcare Limited, High Wycombe, UK) is a similar device, but the arm is controlled by the surgeon's head movements.[18,19] Both AESOP and the EndoAssist give the operating surgeon full and rapid control of the camera. These devices paved the way for master-slave devices, which not only control the camera but the surgical instruments as well.

ROBOTS IN UROLOGY

IMAGE GUIDANCE Image-guidance robotic systems are able to localize anatomic structures in three-dimensional (3D) space using a series of two-dimensional (2D) images. Both the Neuro-Mate and the RoboDoc mentioned earlier repre-

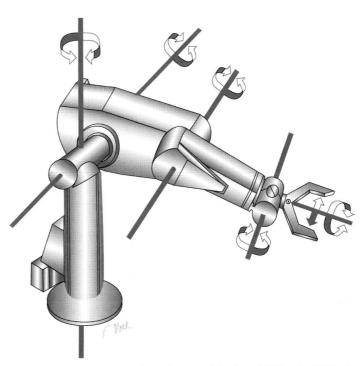

Figure 104-1 Robotic arm with 6 degrees of freedom (DOF). The DOF of a device is the sum of the DOF in all the joints.

Table 104-1 Robotics Terminology

Triangulation	Generation of three-dimensional coordinates from a series of two-dimensional images.
Registration	Use of patient landmarks (fiducial markers) and the robotic coordinate system to determine a transformation matrix. This allows the robot to precisely navigate the target.
Degrees of freedom (DOF)	Number of possible translational or rotational motions at a joint. The DOF of a device is the sum of the DOF in all the joints. (Figures 104-1 and 104-2)
Master-slave devices	A two component system with a control console and a mechanical device that performs the actual task.
Off-line robots	Completely automated and preprogrammed systems that do not require human intervention.
On-line robots	Systems that require continuous human intervention, taking advantage of human perception and judgment.
Robots	Systems that integrate a computer and a mechanical device.
Telesurgery	Use of master-slave devices where the master and slave components are physically separated.

sent robotic systems that use image guidance. Two key concepts for robotic image guidance are triangulation and registration. Triangulation refers to the construction of three-dimensional coordinates using two-dimensional images. Registration refers to the integrating of landmark coordinates on the patient and reference coordinates on the robotic device to construct a transformation matrix. This process allows the robot to calibrate the working space and localize specific anatomic structures.

The first urologic procedure performed with the assistance of a robot was a transurethral resection of the prostate (TURP).[20–22] In 1989, a team at the Imperial College in London developed a device to automate resection of the prostate.[23] The robot had 7° of freedom (DOF). In initial laboratory tests, it was used to core out the inside of a potato. Before use in humans, a safety frame was developed, which restricts the range of motion of the robot to the area of prostate resection. The frame was tested by manually maneuvering the device within the frame and performing a TURP in 30 patients.[24]

After demonstrating the safety of the device, the instrument was connected to a motorized component that automated the resection based on ultrasound images. In the initial clinical trial, the device was successfully used in 5 patients to completely automate prostate resection before hemostasis was achieved manually.[21,22] This was

the first example of off-line robotic surgery. The term off-line describes a robot that is preprogrammed to perform an operation without direct human interaction. This clinical trial identified the need for an alternative to transrectal ultrasonography (TRUS) for accurately imaging the prostate and planning the resection.

A team of investigators at the Politecnico of Milan, Italy, demonstrated the use of a robot to perform a transperineal prostate biopsy.[25–27] TRUS was used to image the prostate, and external video cameras were used to record the patient's anatomy and configuration. The information from the video cameras and the TRUS were integrated to allow positioning of the biopsy needle in 3D space. Using computer software, the surgeon chooses the biopsy site on the TRUS image. The robot then positions the needle in the prostate with an accuracy of 1 to 2 mm. This study was an important demonstration of how internal structures can be localized in 3D space. Given the ease and accuracy of performing standard TRUS-guided prostate biopsies, however, it is unlikely that robots will provide an advantage for performing this procedure.

Similar robots are being investigated for obtaining percutaneous access to the renal collecting system. Again, 2D images are used to navigate in 3D space and target an internal structure, the renal calix. The team at the Imperial College in London developed a robotic system with a passive manipulator to target the renal calix.[28] Sensors on the manipulator record the position of the joints relative to the patient. To target the calix, this information is integrated by a computer with data obtained by fluoroscopy. The trajectory of the needle is shown on the fluoroscopic image. The same group described a system for calibrating the video fluoroscopy to remove distortions and achieve targeting accuracy to within 1.5 mm.[28]

A group at Johns Hopkins Medical Center developed similar robots for obtaining percutaneous renal access.[29–31] The first robot they developed has an active manipulator, a motorized arm that positions and drives the access needle. Information from sensors on the robot is integrated with calibrated images from a biplanar fluoroscopic image to target the calix.[29] In early ex vivo experiments, they were able to access the desired calix in porcine kidneys with an 83% accuracy. In live animal experiments, however, the robot only had a 50% accuracy. The low accuracy

rate was attributed to needle deflection, rib interference and deflection of the kidney by the needle. To reduce cost and complexity, a second robot was developed with a passive manipulator and an active injector system (Figure 104-3).[30,31] This system is currently being evaluated clinically.

MASTER-SLAVE SYSTEMS FOR LAPAROSCOPIC ROBOTIC SURGERY A master-slave device is a two-component system consisting of a control console and a mechanical device that performs the actual task. Robotically assisted surgery can be performed using master-slave devices to overcome some of the limitations of laparoscopy while maintaining the advantages of minimally invasive surgery. Although laparoscopic surgery has clear advantages, there are several important shortcomings as well:

- Many techniques, such as intracorporeal suturing, are more difficult than with open surgery.
- Laparoscopic surgery is performed with a 2D view of the surgical field.
- The surgical ports limit maneuverability and there is a loss of 2 DOF compared to open surgery.
- With laparoscopic surgery, there is loss of tactile sensation.

The FDA approved two master-slave devices for human use: ZEUS (Computer Motion Inc., Goleta, CA) and the da Vinci Surgical System (Intuitive Surgical, Inc., Sunnyvale, CA). Both systems consist of robotic arms and a surgeon's console. The robotic arms are positioned next to the patient in the operating room: two arms control the working instruments, and one arm positions the camera. The surgeon sits at a console, which can be located in the same room or at a distant site. The surgeon has a view of the surgical field from the console. Hand movements at the console are digitized and modified by a computerized system, which then manipulates the robotic arms in real time.

There are several potential advantages afforded by these master-slave systems over conventional laparoscopy:

- The surgeon's console provides an ergonomic environment for performing surgery. The surgeon can also make natural hand movements rather than counterintuitive movements from uncomfortable positions, which is often required by conventional laparoscopy.
- By digitizing the surgeon's hand movements, the robotic system can filter out hand tremors and scale the hand's movements (ie, large hand movements at the surgical console are translated into small and precise movements at the operative site).
- The robotic arms can provide additional degrees of freedom inside the patient's body for enhanced endoscopic dexterity. Compared to the rigid, fixed laparoscopic instruments, the robotic arms have additional joints that can more closely reproduce the movements of the human wrist.

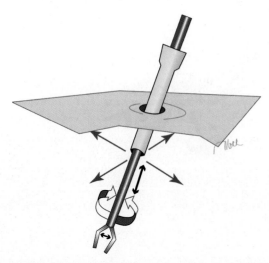

Figure 104-2 A conventional laparoscopic instrument has 5 degrees of freedom.

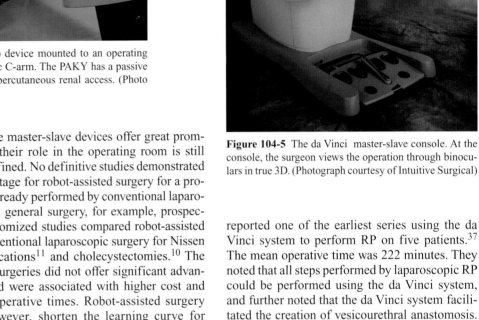

Figure 104-3 Percutaneous Access to the Kidney (PAKY) device mounted to an operating room table with the injector positioned under a fluoroscopic C-arm. The PAKY has a passive arm with 6 degrees of freedom and an active injector for percutaneous renal access. (Photo courtesy of Dr. Dan Stoianovici)

- These systems provide 3D views of the surgical field and, therefore, improve depth perception.

In June 2003, the companies manufacturing the ZEUS and da Vinci systems merged, and the new company maintained the name Intuitive Surgical, Inc. As of 2006, only the da Vinci system remained in clinical use. The da Vinci system was designed using technology first developed at the Stanford Research Institute. The da Vinci system has three to four robotic arms, but they are mounted on a surgical cart that is positioned next to the operating table (Figure 104-4). The tips of the instruments articulate in multiple planes via the EndoWrist (Intuitive Surgical), similar to the human wrist and providing the robotic arm with a total of 7 DOF (Figure 104-5). At the surgical console, the surgeon views the operation through binoculars in true 3D. The stereo images are captured by two parallel cameras with either 0° or 30° lenses. At the console, the images are projected to create the impression that the surgeon's hands are holding the instruments over an open surgical field (Figure 104-6). When a foot pedal is pressed, the surgeon's hand movements control the robotic arm holding the camera.

These master-slave devices offer great promise, and their role in the operating room is still being defined. No definitive studies demonstrated an advantage for robot-assisted surgery for a procedure already performed by conventional laparoscopy. In general surgery, for example, prospective randomized studies compared robot-assisted and conventional laparoscopic surgery for Nissen fundoplications[11] and cholecystectomies.[10] The robotic surgeries did not offer significant advantages and were associated with higher cost and longer operative times. Robot-assisted surgery may, however, shorten the learning curve for surgeons with minimal, previous laparoscopic experience.[32,33] In addition, robotic surgery should be evaluated in the context of ongoing improvements in technology and surgical technique. Force-feedback devices, better video imaging, and improved instrumentation will continue to make robot-assist surgery more effective.

CLINICAL EXPERIENCE In urology, the da Vinci system was approved by the FDA for performing radical prostatectomies (RP) and several series were published.[34–37] Pasticier and colleagues

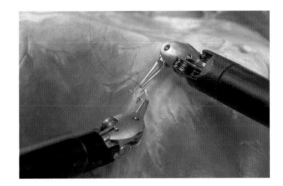

Figure 104-5 The da Vinci master-slave console. At the console, the surgeon views the operation through binoculars in true 3D. (Photograph courtesy of Intuitive Surgical)

reported one of the earliest series using the da Vinci system to perform RP on five patients.[37] The mean operative time was 222 minutes. They noted that all steps performed by laparoscopic RP could be performed using the da Vinci system, and further noted that the da Vinci system facilitated the creation of vesicourethral anastomosis. Another early series was reported by Rassweiler

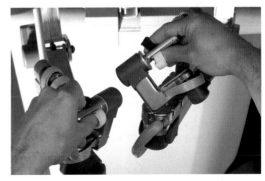

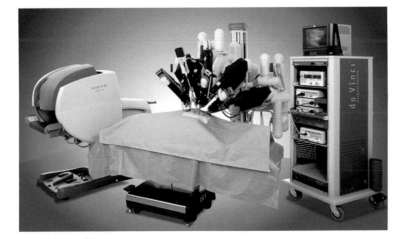

Figure 104-4 The da Vinci surgical cart. The surgical cart is positioned adjacent to the operating room table. (Photograph courtesy of Intuitive Surgical)

Figure 104-6 The da Vinci master-slave controls. At the console, the images are projected to create the illusion that the surgeon's hands are holding the instruments over an open surgical field. The robot arms have 7 degrees of freedom. (Photograph courtesy of Intuitive Surgical)

and colleagues.[36] They used the da Vinci system to perform RP on six patients. The mean operative time was 315 minutes. They stated that the learning curve was steep, but less steep than conventional laparoscopic RP.

Larger series with longer follow-up were published. Bentas and colleagues reported that over 100 da Vinci RP with bilateral pelvic lymphadenectomy had been performed at the University of Frankfurt in Germany.[35] They reported on their first 40 patients with one year follow-up. The mean operative time was 498 minutes. The surgical time decreased by 22 minutes on average with each case. The average intraoperative blood loss was 558 mL, and the transfusion rate was 32.5%. One case was converted to a standard laparoscopic RP, and one case was converted to an open prostatectomy. The positive margin rate was 8% in patients with pT2 tumors and 67% in patients with pT3 tumors. Complications included two pulmonary embolisms, one deep vein thrombosis, one obturator nerve injury and one trocar injury to the epigastric artery. One year following surgery, 68% were completely continent, and 16% used one pad per day for safety. Potency data was not reported.

Patel and colleagues reported their results in the community setting.[38] They performed 200 RPs during an 18-month period. The mean operative time was 141 minutes, and the estimated blood loss was 75 cc. No patients required transfusion or reexploration, and there was no mortality. The positive margin rate was 10.5%, and 98% of patients were continent by 12 months. At a mean follow-up of 9.7 months, 95% of patients were biochemically disease-free. The authors estimate that the learning curve was 20 to 25 cases.

The largest series for RP performed using the da Vinci system is reported by Menon and colleagues from Henry Ford Hospital in Detroit, MI. In a recent description of their surgical technique, they report having performed over 1,100 RPs.[39] They published a detailed report on 200 patients with complete data from their first 250 patients.[34] The mean operative time was 160 minutes, and the average intraoperative blood loss was 153 mL. Complications included three port hernias, three prolonged ileuses, one delayed bleed and one deep vein thrombosis. In this series, the positive margin rate was only 6%, but their definition of positive margins was unconventional. The apical margin was considered positive only if biopsies obtained by the surgeon after the prostate was removed were positive for tumor. The mean hospitalization was 1.2 days, and the mean catheterization time was 7 days. At 6 months, 96% were completely dry or using a pad only for security.

Robotic RP may slightly decrease the postoperative recovery time when compared to open radical retropubic prostatectomy (RRP), but the difference is not likely to be large. In a retrospective review, Menon and colleagues reported that catheterization time, hospital stay, and postoperative pain score favored robotic RP over open RRP.[39] In a prospective comparison of 159 robotic RP and 154 open RRP, there was no difference in patient-reported pain scores and perioperative narcotic use.[40] All patients were managed postoperatively using a clinical pathway. The authors state that patient-reported pain was low regardless of the surgical technique. The same authors report in a separate study that robotic RP is associated with significantly less intraoperative blood loss when compared to open RRP.[41]

The early potency results following robotic RP are promising. Menon and another group of colleagues described a technique for extensive preservation of the prostatic fascia.[42] They reported that, in 35 patients with preservation of the prostatic fascia, 34 (97%) men were able to achieve erections sufficient for intercourse 12 months after surgery. In comparison, 17 of 23 (74%) patients undergoing standard nerve sparing were able to have intercourse 12 months after surgery. Ahlering and colleagues described a cautery-free technique for preservation of the cavernous nerves during robotic prostatectomy. Using this technique, 10 of 23 (43%) patients were able to have intercourse 3 months following surgery; in comparison, 3 of 36 (8%) of patients undergoing traditional nerve sparing were able to have intercourse at 3 months.[43]

These early experiences with robotic RP are encouraging, but large experiences from other institutions are needed. Longer follow-up that documents the oncologic efficacy of robotic RP is also needed. It has been suggested that robotic RP simplifies laparoscopic tasks for surgeons with minimal laparoscopic experience. It is unclear, however, whether robotic RP accomplishes this goal. Therefore, the advantages and disadvantages of robotic RP compared to either open or conventional laparoscopic RP will need to be better documented, especially with regard to the learning curve involved.

Master-slave robotic devices have been used for a variety of other urologic procedures. Guillonneau and colleagues described the first telerobotic nephrectomy in humans using the ZEUS system.[44] The nephrectomy was performed for a nonfunctional right kidney. A larger series of robot-assisted (simple or radical) nephrectomies had not been reported. Donor nephrectomies using the da Vinci system have been described.[45] Robot-assisted adrenalectomies[46,47] and pyeloplasties[48–50] have been performed. Menon and colleagues reported performing da Vinci-assisted radical cystectomies in 14 men and three women.[51] Ileal conduits and orthotopic neobladders were constructed by exteriorizing bowel through a small laparotomy incision. The mean operative times for the radical cystectomies, ileal conduits, and orthotopic neobladders were 140, 120, and 168 minutes, respectively.

TELESURGERY Telesurgery refers to active control of the surgical instruments by a remote surgeon located at a distance from the operative theater with data transmitted over a telecommunication line. Master-slave devices are composed of two separate components, a surgeon's console and robotic arms. Although these two components are usually located in the same room during surgery, the procedure can be performed with the surgical console located in another room, or even another state. Telesurgery has the potential to provide access to surgical expertise anywhere in the world[52,53] or aid in providing surgical care in hazardous locations such as battlefields and disaster sites.

The first international telesurgery was performed in 2001 by surgeons in New York on a patient in France.[52,53] The ZEUS system was used to perform a cholecystectomy. The surgery was successfully completed without complications, but several factors limit widespread implementation of telesurgery. Transmission of data over telecommunication lines requires a large bandwidth. Furthermore, transmission over long distances results in signal latency; there is a delay between the time the surgeon moves his instrument and the movement is seen on the video image of the surgical field. Ideally, the signal delay should be less than 10 milliseconds to prevent overshooting of movements. Surgeons can compensate for delays of 200 to 300 milliseconds, but longer delays may make surgery difficult to perform.[54] Finally, data communications need to be secure to prevent unauthorized viewing and 100% reliability.

Telementoring, which is now feasible, refers to real-time teaching by a mentor who is not physically present at the site of the operation. In 1994, Kavoussi and colleagues demonstrated that the operating surgeon could be guided by a remote surgeon in a separate room.[55] The remote surgeon used the AESOP robotic arm to manipulate the camera during a cholecystectomy, bladder suspension, and varicocele ligation. Others demonstrated that telementoring can be successfully performed between the United States and centers in Austria,[56–58] Italy,[58,59] Singapore,[58,60] and Thailand.[58]

ROBOTIC SURGICAL TRAINING A significant drawback to robot-assisted surgery is the learning curve. It has been proposed that robotic surgery shortens the learning curve for laparoscopic procedures for practitioners with no previous laparoscopic training. Robotic surgery restores 3D visualization and wrist-like flexibility, allowing surgeons experienced in open procedures to operate in a more intuitive environment. This assertion is supported by a report by Yohannes and colleagues.[33] They compared the learning curves for eight physicians in performing a dexterity task and free-hand suturing in a dry-laboratory using robot-assisted or conventional laparoscopy. The participating physicians were classified as novice or experienced laparoscopists. For novice laparoscopists, the learning curves for robot-assisted tasks were significantly shorter when compared to conventional laparoscopy. For experienced laparoscopists, however, robotic surgery did not appear to offer any advantages.

A report by Menon and colleagues describes a structured program for learning to perform robotic RP.[32] Menon had no previous laparoscopy experience, and he was mentored to perform robotic RP by Vallancien and Guillonneau, who at that time had combined laparoscopic RP experience of over 600 cases. They compared the results of 40 robotic RPs performed by Menon with 40 laparoscopic RPs performed by either Vallancien or Guillonneau. The mean operative times for the robotic and laparoscopic RPs were 274 minutes and 258 minutes, respectively. The operative time for robotic RP decreased with experience. After 18 cases, the operative time for robotic RP had decreased to that of laparoscopic RP. The estimated blood loss, change in hemoglobin, positive margin rates, and overall complication rates were similar between the two groups.

Master-slave robots have been promoted as a tool for simplifying laparoscopic tasks that require a high level of dexterity. The cost of master-slave robots, however, is prohibitive at many centers, while conventional laparoscopy is widely available. Furthermore, the increased dexterity of robotic surgery is not necessary for most extirpative urologic procedures. Therefore, it can be argued that conventional laparoscopy serves as a bridge to robotic surgery. Many of the skills required for conventional laparoscopy are readily translated to robotic surgery. Laparoscopy provides experience with tissue handling, recognizing anatomical structures through a laparoscope and operating without tactile feedback. Furthermore, laparoscopic skills may be necessary to complete the surgery without an open conversion in the event of a mechanical failure.

FUTURE DIRECTION

Robotic surgery is on the verge of entering the mainstream of clinical practice. Ongoing advances in technology will continue to make robotic surgery attractive. The greatest impediment to widespread application is cost. As the medical robotics industry grows, the cost of the devices and their reusable components will certainly decrease. Ongoing efforts to develop a force-feedback mechanism will allow surgeons to appreciate the strength and texture of tissues. Smaller and more mobile versions of the robotic devices will be more user-friendly for the surgeon and the operating room staff.

Another exciting prospect is the merger of robotics and virtual reality. Virtual reality trainers will allow surgeons to practice robotic surgery in a virtual 3D environment.[61–63] Surgeries of varying difficulty can be simulated under a variety of conditions. Difficult tissue dissection, complex surgical anatomy and heavy bleeding can be simulated for training purposes. The entire procedure and the surgeon's movements can be recorded and later reviewed by a mentor. This may represent a cost-effective and safe method for training and credentialing surgeons.

Virtual reality technology may also allow physicians to download patient magnetic resonance imaging studies and computed tomography scans into a computer system to create a patient-specific training environment. Physicians can practice an operation in an environment that incorporates patient-specific anatomy and pathology.

The possibilities and potentials for this technology are only limited by our imagination. For example, these 3D images can be superimposed on the actual surgical field during the operation to reveal structures deep within the visualized surface. A mentoring surgeon's movements during a training session may be used to control an off-line robot, guide the operating surgeon, or prevent the surgeon from making an error in surgical technique.

CONCLUSION

In 1965, Gordon Moore, cofounder of Intel Corp., made his famous observation, now known as Moore's Law. He predicted that computing storage capacity would double every 18 to 24 months. Since then, Moore's law has held true; the number of transistors per integrated computer circuit has doubled every couple of years. This relentless advance in computer technology ensures future advances in robotic technology as well. The ultimate goal of robotics is to allow surgeons to perform difficult procedures with a level of precision and improved clinical outcomes not possible by conventional methods. Robotics has the potential to enable surgeons with varying levels of surgical skill to achieve a uniform outcome. Urology has always been ready to embrace new technology. As long as urologists continue to embrace technological advances and incorporate beneficial technology into their practice, the outlook for patients remains bright.

REFERENCES

1. Buckingham RA, Buckingham RO. Robots in operating theatres. BMJ 1995;311:1479.
2. Cadeddu JA, Stoianovici D, Kavoussi LR. Robotic surgery in urology. Urol Clin North Am 1998;25:75.
3. Fankhauser H, Glauser D, Flury P, et al. Robot for CT-guided stereotactic neurosurgery. Stereotact Funct Neurosurg 1994;63:93.
4. Kelly PJ, Kall BA, Goerss SJ. Computer-interactive stereotactic resection of deep-seated and centrally located intraaxial brain lesions. Appl Neurophysiol 1987;50:107.
5. Rousu JS, Kohls PE, Kall B, et al. Computer-assisted image-guided surgery using the Regulus Navigator. Stud Health Technol Inform 1998;50:103.
6. Glauser D, Flury P, Burckhardt CW. Mechanical concept of the neurosurgical robot "Minerva". Robotica 1993;11:567.
7. Paul HA, Bargar WL, Mittlestadt B, et al. Development of a surgical robot for cementless total hip arthroplasty. Clin Orthop 1992;57.
8. Carpentier A, Loulmet D, Aupecle B, et al. Computer-assisted cardiac surgery. Lancet 1999;353:379.
9. Mack MJ. Minimally invasive and robotic surgery. JAMA 2001;285:568.
10. Marescaux J, Smith MK, Folscher D, et al. Telerobotic laparoscopic cholecystectomy: initial clinical experience with 25 patients. Ann Surg 2001;234:1.
11. Cadiere GB, Himpens J, Vertruyen M, et al. Evaluation of telesurgical (robotic) NISSEN fundoplication. Surg Endosc 2001;15:918.
12. Falcone T, Goldberg JM, Margossian H, et al. Robotic-assisted laparoscopic microsurgical tubal anastomosis: a human pilot study. Fertil Steril 2000;73:1040.
13. Dunn MD, Portis AJ, Shalhav AL, et al. Laparoscopic versus open radical nephrectomy: a 9-year experience. J Urol 2000;164:1153.
14. Chan DY, Cadeddu JA, Jarrett TW, et al. Laparoscopic radical nephrectomy: cancer control for renal cell carcinoma. J Urol 2001;166:2095.
15. Kim FJ, Rha KH, Hernandez F, et al. Laparoscopic radical versus partial nephrectomy: assessment of complications. J Urol 2003;170:408.
16. Gill IS, Meraney AM, Schweizer DK, et al. Laparoscopic rad-

17. Unger SW, Unger HM, Bass RT. AESOP robotic arm. Surg Endosc 1994;8:1131.
18. Dagan J, Bat L. Endoassist, a mechanical device to support an endoscope. Gastrointest Endosc 1982;28:97.
19. Aiono S, Gilbert JM, Soin B, et al. Controlled trial of the introduction of a robotic camera assistant (EndoAssist) for laparoscopic cholecystectomy. Surg Endosc 2002;16:1267.
20. Harris SJ, Arambula-Cosio F, Mei Q, et al. The Probot—an active robot for prostate resection. Proc Inst Mech Eng [H] 1997;211:317.
21. Ng WS, Davies BL, Timoney AG, et al. The use of ultrasound in automated prostatectomy. Med Biol Eng Comput 1993;31:349.
22. Nathan MS, Davies BL, Hibberd RD, et al. Devices for automated resection of the prostate. Presented at the Proceedings of the First International Symposium on Medical Robotics and Computer Assisted Surgery, Pittsburgh, Pennsylvania, 1994.
23. Davies BL, Hibberd RD, Coptcoat MJ, et al. A surgeon robot prostatectomy—a laboratory evaluation. J Med Eng Technol 1989;13:273.
24. Davies BL, Hibberd RD, Ng WS, et al. The development of a surgeon robot for prostatectomies. Proc Inst Mech Eng [H] 1991;205:35.
25. Rovetta A, Sala R. Robotics and telerobotics applied to a prostate biopsy on a human patient. Presented at the Proceedings of the Second International Symposium on Medical Robotics and Computer Assisted Surgery, Baltimore, Maryland, 1995.
26. Rovetta A, Sala R, Wen Z, et al. Sensorization of a surgeon robot for prostate biopsy operation. Presented at the Proceedings of the First International Symposium on Medical Robotics and Computer Assisted Surgery, Pittsburgh, Pennsylvania, 1994.
27. Rovetta A, Sala R. Execution of robot-assisted biopsies within the clinical context. J Image Guid Surg 1995;1:280.
28. Potamianos P, Davies BL, Hibberd RD. Intraoperative imaging guidance for keyhole surgery: methodology and calibration. Presented at the Proceedings of the First International Symposium on Medical Robotics and Computer Assisted Surgery, Pittsburgh, Pennsylvania, 1994.
29. Cadeddu JA, Bzostek A, Schreiner S, et al. A robotic system for percutaneous renal access. J Urol 1997;158:1589.
30. Su LM, Stoianovici D, Jarrett TW, et al. Robotic percutaneous access to the kidney: comparison with standard manual access. J Endourol 2002;16:471.
31. Cadeddu JA, Stoianovici D, Chen RN, et al. Stereotactic mechanical percutaneous renal access. J Endourol 1998; 12:121.
32. Menon M, Shrivastava A, Tewari A, et al. Laparoscopic and robot assisted radical prostatectomy: establishment of a structured program and preliminary analysis of outcomes. J Urol 2002;168:945.
33. Yohannes P, Rotariu P, Pinto P, et al. Comparison of robotic versus laparoscopic skills: is there a difference in the learning curve? Urology 2002;60:39.
34. Menon M, Tewari A. Robotic radical prostatectomy and the Vattikuti Urology Institute technique: an interim analysis of results and technical points. Urology 2003;61:15.
35. Bentas W, Wolfram M, Jones J, et al. Robotic technology and the translation of open radical prostatectomy to laparoscopy: the early Frankfurt experience with robotic radical prostatectomy and one year follow-up. Eur Urol 2003;44:175.
36. Rassweiler J, Frede T, Seemann O, et al. Telesurgical laparoscopic radical prostatectomy. Initial experience. Eur Urol 2001;40:75.
37. Pasticier G, Rietbergen JB, Guillonneau B, et al. Robotically assisted laparoscopic radical prostatectomy: feasibility study in men. Eur Urol 2001;40:70.
38. Patel VR, Tully AS, Holmes R, et al. Robotic radical prostatectomy in the community setting—the learning curve and beyond: initial 200 cases. J Urol 2005;174:269.
39. Menon M, Tewari A, Peabody JO, et al. Vattikuti Institute prostatectomy, a technique of robotic radical prostatectomy for management of localized carcinoma of the prostate: experience of over 1100 cases. Urol Clin North Am 2004;31:701.
40. Webster TM, Herrell SD, Chang SS, et al. Robotic assisted laparoscopic radical prostatectomy versus retropubic radical prostatectomy: a prospective assessment of postoperative pain. J Urol 2005;174:912.
41. Farnham SB, Webster TM, Herrell SD, et al. Intraoperative blood loss and transfusion requirements for robotic-assisted radical prostatectomy versus radical retropubic prostatectomy. Urology 2006;67:360.
42. Menon M, Kaul S, Bhandari A, et al. Potency following

robotic radical prostatectomy: a questionnaire based analysis of outcomes after conventional nerve sparing and prostatic fascia sparing techniques. J Urol 2005;174:2291.

43. Ahlering TE, Eichel L, Skarecky D. Rapid communication: early potency outcomes with cautery-free neurovascular bundle preservation with robotic laparoscopic radical prostatectomy. J Endourol 2005;19:715.

44. Guillonneau B, Jayet C, Tewari A, et al. Robot assisted laparoscopic nephrectomy. J Urol 2001;166:200.

45. Talamini MA, Chapman S, Horgan S, et al. A prospective analysis of 211 robotic-assisted surgical procedures. Surg Endosc 2003.

46. Young JA, Chapman WH 3rd, Kim VB, et al. Robotic-assisted adrenalectomy for adrenal incidentaloma: case and review of the technique. Surg Laparosc Endosc Percutan Tech 2002;12:126.

47. Bentas W, Wolfram M, Brautigam R, et al. Laparoscopic transperitoneal adrenalectomy using a remote-controlled robotic surgical system. J Endourol 2002;16:373.

48. Gettman MT, Peschel R, Neururer R, et al. A comparison of laparoscopic pyeloplasty performed with the daVinci robotic system versus standard laparoscopic techniques: initial clinical results. Eur Urol 2002;42:453.

49. Guillonneau B, Jayet C, Cappele O, et al. Robotic-assisted laparoscopic pyeloplasty. J Urol 2001 165(Suppl):V75.

50. Graham RW, Graham SD, Bokinsky GB. Urological upper tract surgery with the daVinci robotic system, pyeloplasty. J Urol 2001 165(Suppl):V74.

51. Menon M, Hemal AK, Tewari A, et al. Nerve-sparing robot-assisted radical cystoprostatectomy and urinary diversion. BJU Int 2003;92:232.

52. Marescaux J, Leroy J, Rubino F, et al. Transcontinental robot-assisted remote telesurgery: feasibility and potential applications. Ann Surg 2002;235:487.

53. Marescaux J, Leroy J, Gagner M, et al. Transatlantic robot-assisted telesurgery. Nature 2001;413:379.

54. Ottensmeyer M, Hu J, Thompson J, et al. Investigations into performance of minimally invasive telesurgery with feedback time delays. Presence Teleoper Virtual Environ 2000;9:369.

55. Kavoussi LR, Moore RG, Partin AW, et al. Telerobotic assisted laparoscopic surgery: initial laboratory and clinical experience. Urology 1994;44:15.

56. Schulam PG, Docimo SG, Saleh W, et al. Telesurgical mentoring. Initial clinical experience. Surg Endosc 1997;11:1001.

57. Janetschek G, Bartsch G, Kavoussi LR. Transcontinental interactive laparoscopic telesurgery between the United States and Europe. J Urol 1998;160:1413.

58. Bauer JJ, Lee BR, Bishoff JT, et al. International surgical tele-mentoring using a robotic arm: our experience. Telemed J 2000;6:25.

59. Micali S, Virgili G, Vannozzi E, et al. Feasibility of telementoring between Baltimore (USA) and Rome (Italy): the first five cases. J Endourol 2000;14:493.

60. Lee BR, Png DJ, Liew L, et al. Laparoscopic telesurgery between the United States and Singapore. Ann Acad Med Singapore 2000;29:665.

61. Chaudhry A, Sutton C, Wood J, et al. Learning rate for laparoscopic surgical skills on MIST VR, a virtual reality simulator: quality of human-computer interface. Ann R Coll Surg Engl 1999;81:281.

62. Haluck RS, Webster RW, Snyder AJ, et al. A virtual reality surgical trainer for navigation in laparoscopic surgery. Stud Health Technol Inform 2001;81:171.

63. Torkington J, Smith SG, Rees BI, et al. Skill transfer from virtual reality to a real laparoscopic task. Surg Endosc,6, 200;15:1071.

105

Robotic-Assisted Urologic Surgery: Setup, Instrumentation, and Troubleshooting

Ravi Munver, MD

Ilya A. Volfson, MD

Recent advancements in minimally invasive surgery have led to the introduction of robotic technology to the field of urology. The expanding role of robotic-assisted laparoscopic surgery has facilitated routine extirpative procedures as well as complex reconstructive procedures by surgeons with minimal laparoscopic experience as well as advanced laparoscopists. Robotic assistance is a novel minimally invasive alternative to conventional laparoscopic surgery and offers significant advantages over traditional open surgery. Similar to conventional laparoscopic procedures, robotic assistance offers benefits of less postoperative pain, reduced blood loss, shorter hospital stay, and faster recovery and return to normal activities. Furthermore, this application may allow for more widespread implementation of complicated reconstructive procedures.

The predominant telerobotic surgical system, the da Vinci Surgical System (Intuitive Surgical, Inc., Sunnyvale, CA), was the result of a culmination of multidisciplinary research efforts to improve upon the current foundations of minimally invasive surgery. Launched in December 1998, this robotic system was created with the intention of offering enhanced surgical capabilities, superior visualization, improved dexterity, greater precision, and ergonomic comfort. As a result of these features, a surgeon would be able to more easily perform both routine and complex laparoscopic procedures.

In 1997, robotic-assistance was utilized to successfully perform a cholecystectomy.[1] Since then, robotics has been implemented in many surgical subspecialties, but nowhere as extensively as in urology. The introduction of the da Vinci Surgical System, and subsequent Food and Drug Administration approval of robotic-assisted radical prostatectomy in 2001, has revolutionized the field of minimally invasive urologic surgery.[2]

In the current telerobotic model, the surgeon sits at a remote console that is located outside the surgical field and looks into a specially designed view piece (stereo viewer), that provides a three-dimensional (3D) view of the operative area. Movements of the surgeon's wrist and fingers are translated to a patient-side surgical arm unit (surgical cart), which controls two or three detachable surgical instruments as well as a camera attached to a binocular laparoscope. EndoWrist® instrumentation allows for six degrees of freedom of movement, with an additional seventh degree of freedom at the instrument tip, an advantage over the four degrees of freedom that limits the performance of conventional laparoscopy. Motion scaling allows movements of a surgeon's arm, hand, and wrist to be scaled and relayed via the surgical arm units to the tips of the robotic instruments. Tremor filtering allows for reduction of hand tremor and increased precision, especially during fine dissection and delicate suturing. These features enable the surgeon to maintain full control of the wristed laparoscopic instruments and improve surgical efficiency.

The advantages of this robotic system for the surgeon include improved visualization and depth perception offered by the three-dimensional view, not widely available to conventional laparoscopy. The ergonomic design of the control console allows the surgeon to operate in a seated position and may potentially reduce muscle strain and fatigue. Through the use of this system, non-laparoscopically trained urologic surgeons are empowered to transfer open surgical skills to the laparoscopic setting.[3]

In order for surgeons to fully benefit from this new and evolving technology, several prerequisites need to be fulfilled. In particular, proper preparation, patient positioning, and trocar placement are of paramount importance. When performed properly, surgeons can take full advantage of the innovation of robotic assistance. On the other hand, poor setup and erroneous trocar placement can preclude a successful surgical outcome.

Despite the increasing enthusiasm of robotic-assisted surgery, important considerations need to be addressed as to the precise application of this novel technology. This chapter addresses the setup and instrumentation for robotic urological surgery, as well as troubleshooting the more common clinical scenarios.

PREOPERATIVE ASSESSMENT AND PREPARATION

INFORMED CONSENT Initial patient preparation is similar to that of conventional laparoscopic procedures and is discussed in detail elsewhere in this text (see Chapter 42, "Patient Preparation and Operating Room Setup"). In general, patients must undergo a comprehensive preoperative evaluation to assure candidacy for a laparoscopic procedure. Informed consent must be obtained from the patient and should involve a discussion of the goals, alternative treatment modalities, and benefits of the individual procedure. The potential risks associated with a robotic-assisted laparoscopic procedure should be explained, including mechanical malfunction of the robotic system and the possibility of conversion to an open surgical procedure in the setting of unexpected bleeding, intra-abdominal injury, or failure to progress.

BOWEL PREPARATION The need for mechanical bowel preparation as well as a type of the preparation used is dependent on an individual surgeon's preferences and on the type of the procedure that is planned. Patients undergoing transperitoneal robotic-assisted procedures typically receive one bottle of magnesium citrate orally in conjunction with a clear liquid diet on the day prior to surgery. Additionally, when a more complicated transperitoneal dissection is anticipated, particularly in patients with a history of prior abdominal surgery, the bowel preparation should include two bottles of magnesium citrate or 4 L of GoLytely orally, followed by three doses of oral antibiotic therapy (erythromycin and neomycin) on the day prior to the procedure. Retroperitoneal or extraperitoneal procedures do not require an extensive bowel preparation because the peritoneal cavity is not traversed and the bowel does not interfere with the surgery. Patients undergoing robotic-assisted radical prostatectomy are also prescribed an enema to be administered on the evening prior to surgery.

BLEEDING RISK AND BLOOD PRODUCT AVAILABILITY All patients undergoing elective procedures must be screened for bleeding diathesis. Aspirin, nonsteroidal anti-inflammatory medications, and other anticoagulant preparations are discontinued 7 to 10 days prior to the procedure. For patients discontinuing warfarin, the International Normalized Ratio (INR) is measured prior to the procedure.

Patients are to be counseled on the potential risk of bleeding and should be offered the opportunity to participate in preoperative autologous blood donation. A type and screen or type and crossmatch should be obtained, depending on the specific procedure.

INTRAOPERATIVE CONSIDERATIONS

Antibiotic prophylaxis with a broad-spectrum formulation is administered on call to the operating suite. A nasogastric or orogastric tube is placed for the duration of the procedure to improve visualization in transperitoneal and upper retroperitoneal procedures by preventing gastrointestinal distention. A Foley catheter is inserted transurethrally to drain the bladder. Sequential pneumatic compression devices are placed on the lower extremities, unless contraindicated, in order to decrease the risk of deep venous thrombosis.

As a general principle, the proper placement of trocars used for robotic-assisted surgery is similar to that in standard laparoscopic procedures. After successful creation of the pneumoperitoneum or pneumoretroperitoneum via closed (Veress needle) or open (Hassan) technique, the initial trocar or port is placed. Secondary trocars are placed under direct videoendoscopic monitoring. Robotic trocars consist of metal reusable cannulas through which sharp or blunt obturators are placed. The trocars are available in standard and long lengths and are inserted perpendicular to the abdominal fascia. Conventional trocars are inserted either perpendicular or at a slight angle toward the operative field. For pelvic procedures, patients are placed in Trendelenburg's position prior to the insertion of secondary ports in order to minimize the risk of visceral injury. A cardinal difference between the conventional laparoscopic and robotic-assisted technique is that the latter minimizes the amount of force that the port applies against the abdominal wall. This is achieved by the fact that each robotic arm rotates around a mechanically fixed point, or "remote center," which is indicated by a thick black line on the outer diameter of the robotic cannula. To ensure adequate placement, these trocars must be inserted until the remote center is visualized at the level of the peritoneum via the laparoscope.

PELVIC SURGERY SETUP

Conventional laparoscopic pelvic surgery has been successfully reported in the literature, but has not gained widespread popularity by urologic surgeons due to the steep learning curve associated with the pure laparoscopic approach. The confined working space of the pelvis and the challenges of intracorporeal suturing have precluded its adoption by many surgeons. The advent of robotic-assistance has facilitated laparoscopic pelvic surgery and has resulted in an increased interest in the minimally invasive approach to surgical procedures.

Patients are placed in a supine position with adequate padding of the back and all pressure points. The patient's torso rests on a gel pad that provides padding and prevents cephalad movement when the patient is placed in Trendelenburg's position. Due to the risk of neural injury, rigid shoulder supports are generally not used. The legs are placed in a low modified lithotomy

position, comfortably supported using Allen stirrups (Allen Medical Systems, Acton, MA) that are lined with additional foam padding to protect the peroneal nerve and also cushion the ankles (Figure 105-1A). Adequate space between the thighs is verified in order to accommodate the robotic surgical cart. The arms are placed and secured on either side of the torso, and thoroughly cushioned with foam padding to protect the ulnar nerve, wrist, and hand (Figure 105-1B). Once the patient is properly positioned, the abdomen is sterilely cleansed from the subcostal margin to the mid-thigh and laterally to the posterior axillary line. Sterile drapes are placed, and a Foley catheter is inserted sterilely on the field.

TRANSPERITONEAL APPROACH Transperitoneal access begins with the creation of a 12-mm transverse supraumbilical incision. The incision is carried to the level of the rectus fascia and a closed or open technique is used to obtain access. In patients with prior history of abdominal surgery and anticipated intraperitoneal adhesions, the Hassan technique is preferred in order to avoid potential injury to intra-abdominal structures.[4]

A pneumoperitoneum (15 mm Hg) is established in the standard fashion via disposable 12-mm trocar. The abdominal cavity is inspected for adhesions as well as to identify familiar anatomic landmarks, such as the contour of the bony pelvis and the medial umbilical ligaments. The patient is placed in a steep Trendelenburg's

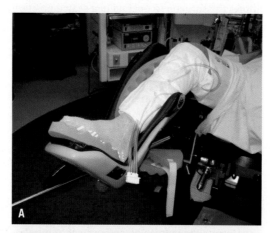

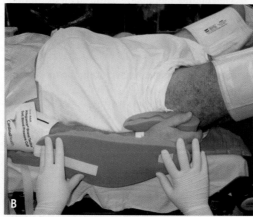

Figure 105-1 Patient positioning for robotic-assisted pelvic surgery. *A*, Padding of the lower extremity in the Allen stirrup. *B*, Padding of the upper extremity.

position in preparation for placement of additional ports (Figure 105-2).

THREE-ARM RADICAL PROSTATECTOMY (TRANSPERITONEAL) In this technique, two 8-mm robotic trocars are placed 8 to 12 cm away from the camera port and approximately 2 cm below the umbilicus (Figure 105-3A). Two additional ports are placed in the right hemiabdomen for a primary patient-side assistant. A 5-mm port used for a suction-irrigation device is placed superior and lateral to the camera port. Care is undertaken to avoid injury to the falciform ligament during the placement of this port. A 12-mm port is placed at the mid-axillary line at the level of the robotic ports. This port is utilized primarily for retraction purposes, introduction and removal of sutures, as well as for larger instruments, such as a clip applier. If a second patient-side assistant is available, an additional 5-mm port is placed at the left mid-axillary line at the level of the robotic ports.[5] In exceptionally tall patients, the camera port may be placed infraumbilically, and the secondary ports may be shifted caudally. After confirmation of a sufficient Trendelenburg's position and placement of all ports, the camera port is docked to the central arm of the robotic surgical cart with a specialized cannula mount clip. Next, the robotic ports are docked to the appropriate robotic arms via cannula holders. The laparoscope is inserted through the camera port and is secured in place with a sterile camera arm adapter. Instruments may then be inserted into the robotic cannulas and are engaged by sterile instrument arm adapters. Once engaged, the instruments are manually advanced into the abdomen under direct vision.

FOUR-ARM RADICAL PROSTATECTOMY (TRANSPERITONEAL) The introduction of the fourth arm for the da Vinci System in 2003 has allowed the primary surgeon to become less dependent on the expertise of a laparoscopic assistant.[6] The secondary port placement for a four-arm approach varies slightly from that of the three-arm approach. The fourth arm can be introduced from either side of the patient. It is important to ensure a minimum distance of 8 cm between adjacent robotic ports in order to avoid collision of the robotic arms with resultant software errors

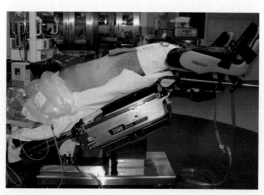

Figure 105-2 Patient positioning for robotic-assisted pelvic surgery: steep Trendelenburg's position.

that can lead to a frustrating operating experience. An optimal trocar configuration consists of each of the three 8-mm robotic trocars placed approximately 2 cm below the umbilicus and one hand breadth away from the adjacent port (Figure 105-3B). If the fourth robotic port is placed on the right, then the 12-mm patient-side assistant port is placed at the left mid-axillary line between the camera port and the left robotic port.

EXTRAPERITONEAL APPROACH The operative space in the extraperitoneal approach is significantly smaller than that in the transperitoneal procedure. With less room for error in port placement, proper and precise positioning of the trocars becomes more important. In this technique, a 12-mm transverse infraumbilical incision is made and dissection is carried through the rectus fascia to the level of the peritoneum. Blunt finger dissection is used to create an extraperitoneal space. A transparent dilating trocar balloon system can be used to expand and dissect the space under direct visualization via laparoscope.[7] After

adequate tissue separation, the balloon is deflated and exchanged for a 12-mm trocar, through which the extraperitoneal space is insufflated. Alternatively, a 12-mm Hassan trocar (Bluntport, U.S. Surgical, Norwalk, CT) can be placed and the space of Retzius is developed by a combination of blunt dissection and pneumodissection.[8] This initial trocar serves as the camera port.

RADICAL PROSTATECTOMY (EXTRAPERITONEAL)
As the peritoneum serves as a natural barrier to prevent the bowel from obscuring the operative field, there is less need for placing the patient in as steep a Trendelenburg's position as for the transperitoneal approach. A 10° to 15° Trendelenburg's position is typically sufficient. In the four-arm technique, after placement of the initial 12-mm trocar, two 8-mm robotic ports are placed along an imaginary line between the anterior superior iliac spine (ASIS) and the umbilicus, approximately 2 cm from the ASIS (Figure 105-4). A third 8-mm robotic port is placed either in the right or left lateral hemiabdomen (depending on surgeon preference), approximately 2.5 cm inferior to the level of the umbilicus and 4 cm medial to one of the previously inserted robotic ports. A 12-mm patient-side assistant port is placed mirror image to the medial robotic port in the contralateral hemiabdomen.[9] The placement of the lateral robotic port and the assistant's port are at the discretion of the surgeon. In the three-arm extraperitoneal approach, the secondary port placement is similar to that of the three-arm transperitoneal approach, with the exception that the ports are placed more caudally on the abdomen. Once the remaining trocars are in place, the procedural steps are similar to those in the transperitoneal approach.

CYSTECTOMY The trocar configuration is similar to that utilized for the three-arm or four-arm transperitoneal robotic-assisted radical prostatectomy. The camera port is placed superior to the umbilicus

such that the urachus is visualized. The patient-side assistant port is placed between the camera port and the right robotic port, approximately 2 to 3 cm superior to umbilicus. This location assures that the port is away from the anterior peritoneal fold that is removed along with bladder.[8]

SACROCOLPOPEXY Robotic surgery has renewed an interest in a minimally invasive approach for the treatment of pelvic floor prolapse as robotic-assisted sacrocolpopexy is gaining popularity among urologists and urogynecologists. Patient positioning and preparation is similar to other transperitoneal pelvic procedures. A 12-mm camera port is placed in a periumbilical location, and two 8-mm robotic ports are placed approximately 2 cm superior to the iliac crest at the lateral margin of each rectus muscle.[10] A 10-mm patient-side assistant trocar is placed in the right subcostal area at the lateral margin of the rectus muscle. An additional 5-mm assistant trocar is placed at the right mid-axillary line slightly inferior to the level of the umbilicus.

UPPER URINARY TRACT SURGERY SETUP

The setup for robotic-assisted renal surgery is similar to that utilized in the conventional laparoscopic approach. The patient's torso rests on a gel pad, and the umbilical region is situated over the break in the operating table. The patient is placed in a modified (45°–60°) lateral decubitus position for the transperitoneal approach, or a full lateral decubitus position for the retroperitoneal approach (Figure 105-5A). An axillary roll is used to protect the dependent brachial plexus, and the arms are generously padded. We prefer to use two large gel rolls to support the patient's back instead of a bean bag (Figure 105-5B). The patient is secured to the table with wide cloth tape at the level of the shoulders and pelvic girdle. The skin is sterilely cleansed and draped from the level of the nipple to the lower abdomen and well across the midline, allowing for possible conversion to an open procedure.

TRANSPERITONEAL APPROACH For transperitoneal procedures, the kidney rest is not elevated, and flexion of the operating table is typically not required. This maneuver, however, may be applied to hyperextend and expose the ipsilateral flank region, if desired. The initial 12-mm camera port is placed periumbilically, and the secondary ports are placed under direct vision after inspection of the peritoneal cavity (Figure 105-6). Unlike pelvic surgery, positioning of ports for upper urinary tract surgery is more variable and is dependent on the patient's anatomy, location of the point of interest (upper or lower pole, ureteropelvic junction, etc), as well as potential distortion of the normal anatomy. After careful planning, two 8-mm robotic trocars are placed 8 to 10 cm away from the camera port.[11] Imaginary lines drawn from the robotic trocars to the camera port should intersect at a right angle. A 12-mm patient-side assistant port is placed

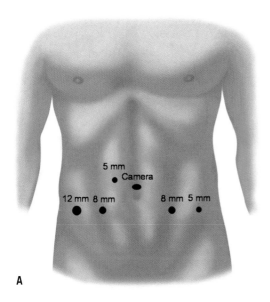

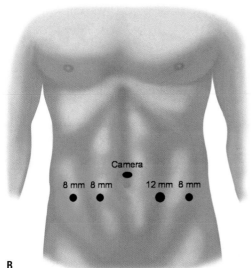

Figure 105-3 Trocar arrangement for robotic-assisted radical prostatectomy. *A*, The three-arm transperitoneal approach. *B*, The four-arm transperitoneal approach.

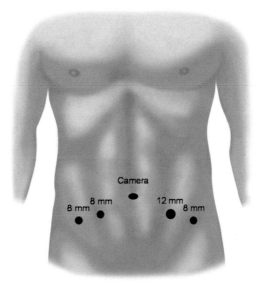

Figure 105-4 Trocar arrangement for robotic-assisted radical prostatectomy: four-arm extraperitoneal approach.

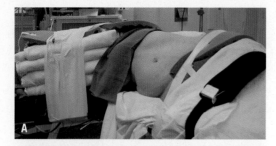

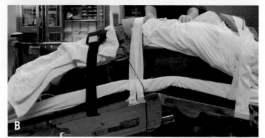

Figure 105-5 Patient positioning for robotic-assisted upper urinary tract surgery. *A*, The anterior view; *B*, the posterior view.

inferior to the camera port in the midline. An additional 5-mm port should be placed just below the sternum for the purpose of liver retraction in the cases of right-sided surgery. For obese patients, the camera port is shifted laterally, and the secondary trocars are adjusted accordingly. Docking of the trocars to the robotic surgical cart is similar to the description provided for pelvic surgery setup.

In robotic-assisted adrenalectomy, the more cephalad anatomic position of the adrenal gland means the 12-mm camera port must be placed supraumbilically. The trocar configuration for secondary ports is similar to that for ipsilateral robotic-assisted renal procedures.[12]

RETROPERITONEAL APPROACH   In the retroperitoneal approach, the kidney rest is elevated for optimal renal displacement. The table is flexed to maximize the space between the costal margin and the iliac crest. The surgical table is tilted slightly anteriorly to allow peritoneal contents to fall away from the retroperitoneal space. There is no consensus regarding sites of trocar placement for retroperitoneoscopic procedures. Due to limited space in the flank, careful planning is necessary to minimize crowding of trocars. Initial trocar placement begins with the creation of a 1.5 cm incision made 2 cm inferior and slightly posterior to the tip of the twelfth rib. The incision is carried through the thoracolumbar fascia and into the retroperitoneal space. The space is developed with blunt digital dissection followed by introduction of a transparent dilating trocar balloon system (PDB 1000, U.S. Surgical). The balloon is directed laterally and posterior to Gerota's fascia. A laparoscope placed through the dissecting balloon allows direct visualization as the retroperitoneal working space is developed. The balloon is then deflated and removed, and a trocar is placed at this site, through which the retroperitoneum is insufflated. Two distinct trocar configurations can be selected based on the surgeon's preference. In one configuration,

the primary port is substituted by a 10-mm assistant port, a 12-mm camera port is placed 2 cm above the iliac crest, and the two 8-mm robotic ports are triangulated from the camera port at a 90° angle toward the costal margin (Figure 105-7A). In an alternative configuration, the primary port is replaced with an 8-mm robotic port, the 12-mm camera port is positioned lateral to the quadratus lumborum, and a second 8-mm robotic port is positioned by triangulating at 90° from the camera port in the direction of the umbilicus. In this situation, the 10-mm assistant port is placed 2 cm above the iliac crest (Figure 105-7B).

PEDIATRIC SURGERY SETUP

Though many pediatric robotic-assisted procedures are similar in setup to their adult counterparts, several basic differences are worth mentioning. Since the working space is limited in children, and the abdominal wall is generally thinner, proper positioning of trocars cannot be overemphasized. The general rule of 8 cm to 10 cm between trocars is not applicable, since in many cases this distance would span the entire abdomen of the patient. Thus, the ports are placed in such a manner as to create a symmetrical array around the camera port, aimed at the site of interest.[13] Furthermore, the small working space poses a higher risk of inadvertent visceral injury with the introduction of trocars and manipulation of instruments. As a result, it is highly important that all manipulation be carried out under direct vision—especially to verify the intended course of each trocar or instrument.

INSTRUMENTATION

Robotic instrumentation varies according to the planned procedure and surgeon preference. The principal difference between instrumentation used for robotic-assisted surgical procedures, compared to conventional laparoscopic procedures, is the implementation of EndoWrist® technology that

allows 7 degrees of freedom in movement of the instruments. This technologic advancement is particularly useful in reconstructive surgery, allowing for complex dissection and suturing as well as permitting the surgeon to manipulate the tip of an instrument in a confined surgical space. New instruments are continually being developed and introduced in order to accommodate the ever-expanding surgical applications for robotic-assisted surgery (Table 105-1). The more common instruments used in robotic-assisted urologic surgical procedures are shown in Figure 105-8.

The majority of robotic urologic surgeons employ a monopolar cautery working instrument

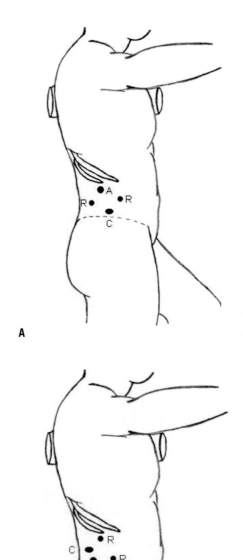

A

B

Figure 105-7 Trocar arrangement for retroperitoneal robotic-assisted renal surgery (right-sided template). *A*, The initial access port converted to a 12-mm assistant port. *B*, The initial access port converted to an 8-mm robotic port. C = 12 mm camera port; R = 8 mm robotic ports; A = 10 mm assistant port.

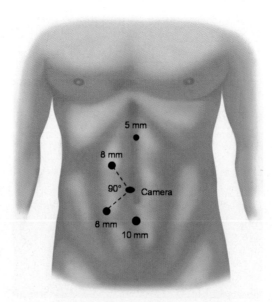

Figure 105-6 Trocar arrangement for transperitoneal robotic-assisted renal surgery (right-sided template).

for dissecting and hemostasis purposes that is controlled by the dominant hand. The earlier forms of these instruments included a spatula or hook tip. Monopolar cautery scissors (Hot Shears) were introduced and are gaining popularity among some surgeons as the dissecting instrument of choice. Another newly developed instrument for robotic-assisted surgery is the Harmonic Curved Shears that offers the benefits of delivering ultrasonic energy.

The non-dominant hand can employ a variety of grasping forceps that are available for selection. Two grasping instruments that incorporate the added benefits of bipolar cautery are the Precise Bipolar forceps and the Maryland Bipolar forceps.

If the fourth robotic arm is employed to assist with surgical exposure, it typically carries forceps used primarily for retraction. The most common forceps are the Cadiere forceps or Pro-Grasp forceps.

When suturing is required, needle holders are employed. While these instruments provide excellent handling of surgical needles, they are inadequate for the purpose of grasping tissues, even for a short period of time. Thus, if tissue handling is required during the placement of a suture, robotic forceps can be controlled with the non-dominant hand, and a needle driver can be manipulated with the dominant hand.

Nearly all adult urological procedures employ 8-mm robotic ports. In the pediatric setting however, 5-mm ports may be implemented. A number of instruments have been developed for these smaller ports, and the range continues to expand (Table 105-2). The EndoWrist® mechanism of the 5-mm instruments differs from the 8-mm counterparts in that the instruments require a longer linear distance to facilitate full angulation (Figure 105-9). This implies that the

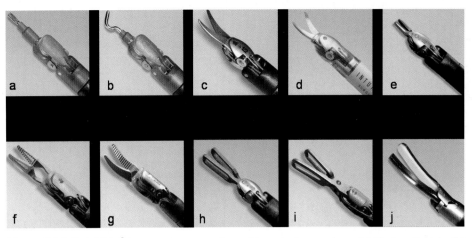

Figure 105-8 EndoWrist® instruments commonly used in urologic procedures: (a) Cautery Spatula; (b) Cautery Hook; (c) Curved Scissors; (d) Hot Shears; (e) Needle Driver; (f) Precise Bipolar; (g) Maryland Bipolar; (h) Cadiere Forceps; (i) ProGrasp Forceps; (j) Harmonic Curved Shears (Photos courtesy of Intuitive Surgical, Inc.).

5-mm instruments protrude through the robotic cannula further and this must be taken into consideration, particularly when working within a confined space.[13]

The InSite Vision System® is capable of providing a 3D view of the operative field. Options for endoscopes include 10-mm 3D endoscopes that offer a 0° or 30° lens. No set rules apply to lens selection for particular steps of urological procedures. The particular lens selected is based on the individual surgeon's preference, patient body habitus, and anatomic variations. In order to avoid disorientation, the camera lens angle must be selected on the keypad of the remote console and should correlate with the endoscope lens used in the patient. It is worthwhile to note that 5-mm endoscopes are also available with 0° or 30° lenses, but these only provide two-dimensional views. These smaller endoscopes may be implemented in select pediatric cases in which reconstructive techniques are not required.

LIMITATIONS AND TROUBLESHOOTING

Limitations of the first-generation da Vinci Surgical System include the bulky design of the surgical arm unit, which limits the working space of the patient-side assistant. The next-generation da Vinci S Surgical System has a smaller profile that is designed to overcome the obstacles associated with its predecessor (Table 105-3).

Another limitation of robotic assistance is the loss of tactile sensation by the surgeon. During conventional laparoscopy, resistance of tissues can be appreciated by using handheld laparoscopic instruments. The current robotic systems, however, operate via telemanipulation, with the absence of both cutaneous sense as well as resistance. Future generations of robotic systems are likely to focus on incorporating sophisticated feedback technology.

As with any new technology, important considerations that can potentially lead to problems during the course of a robotic-assisted procedure must be fully understood in order to appropriately

address and overcome the situation. Some of the more common clinical scenarios will be discussed in the following section.

ROBOTIC INSTRUMENT WORKING LENGTH Instruments attached to each robotic arm are 15 cm in length and can span up to 25 cm when maximally extended. Therefore, it is important for the target area to be less than 25 cm away from the entry point of the instrument. This is the basis behind preoperative planning in terms of optimizing trocar placement. If the full extension of an instrument is inadequate to access the area of interest, the patient-side assistant should manually engage the instrument arm clutch button and insert the instrument as far as the cannula will allow. If this maneuver is unsuccessful in gaining sufficient access, the instrument should be removed from the cannula. The cannula attached to the robotic arm should be securely held by the non-dominant hand of the assistant, while the setup joint release button is engaged with the dominant hand. This maneuver allows the assistant to advance the entire cannula-robotic arm unit further into abdominal cavity under direct vision. A similar technique is used to advance the camera/endoscope port closer to the operative field when it is limited by the trocar-securing cannula mount clip.

Table 105-1 8-mm EndoWrist Instruments for the da Vinci Surgical System	
Needle Holders	**Monopolar Cautery Instruments**
Large Needle Driver	Hot Shears
Black Diamond Micro Forceps	Permanent Cautery Hook
	Permanent Cautery Spatula
Graspers	**Delivery Instruments**
Round Tooth Forceps	EndoPass Delivery Instrument
DeBakey Forceps	
Long Tip Forceps	**Bipolar Cautery Instruments**
Cadiere Forceps	
ProGrasp Forceps	Precise Bipolar
Fine Tissue Forceps	Micro Bipolar
Bowel Grasper	Maryland Bipolar
Resano Forceps	
Double Fenestrated Grasper	Valve Hook
Cobra Grasper	Valve Hook
Scissors	**Scalpels**
Potts Scissors	Snap Fit Instrument
Round Tip Scissors	With Snap-Fit Blue Blade
Curved Scissors	With Snap-Fit Paddle Blade
Clip Applier	**Ultrasonic Energy Instruments**
Small Clip Applier	Ultrasonic Shears
	Harmonic Curved Shears

Table 105-2 5-mm EndoWrist Instruments for the da Vinci Surgical System	
Scissors	**Needle Holders**
Round Scissors	Needle Driver
Curved Scissors	
Graspers	**Monopolar Cautery Instruments**
Schertel Grasper – 20 mm Jaw	Monopolar Cautery with Hook Tip
	Monopolar Cautery with Spatula Tip
Maryland Dissector	
DeBakey Forceps	**Ultrasonic Energy Instruments**
Bullet Nose Dissector	
Bowel Grasper – 30 mm Jaw	Ultrasonic Shears
	Harmonic Curved Shears

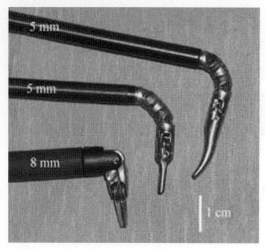

Figure 105-9 EndoWrist® mechanism comparing 8-mm and 5-mm instruments (Photos courtesy of Intuitive Surgical, Inc.).

TROCAR INTERFERENCE It is of paramount importance to position robotic ports so as to avoid the likelihood of collision of the robotic arms with each other or with the bony pelvis. Significant interference between the arms can occur in instances where emphasis is not placed on the distances between trocars or the contour of the pelvis. In order to prevent this situation, once the camera port is inserted and peritoneoscopy is performed, the contours of the bony pelvis should be assessed. The working ports are then placed at least 8 cm to 10 cm away from the camera port, which will ensure an adequate distance and minimize interference. It is also important to keep in mind that the angle of triangulation between the working ports and the camera should be no less than 90° to further avoid port-to-port interference. If a circumstance arises that prevents surgical progression due to colliding robotic arms, two options can be entertained. The robotic trocar in question can be removed, the fascia and peritoneum closed, and the port can be repositioned; alternatively, another robotic port can be placed, and the problematic port can be left unattended or used as an assistant port during portions of the procedure.

When the fourth robotic arm is used, it is common to observe collision between the two closest robotic arms. This can be circumvented by abducting the most lateral robotic arm after the setup joint release is engaged. As this maneuver is performed, the trocar-arm unit should once again be immobilized by the assistant's non-dominant hand in order to prevent inadvertent trocar dislodgement. If a robotic cannula becomes dislodged during manual manipulation, it should be replaced under direct vision with the assistance of a blunt obturator.

PATIENT HABITUS AND TROCAR PLACEMENT The optimal port placement varies slightly, depending on the patient's body habitus. It has been suggested by some authors to move the camera port infraumbilically in shorter patients. One report mentions 172 cm as an arbitrary patient height cut-off for infraumbilical camera

	da Vinci Surgical System (4th arm optional)	da Vinci Surgical System (4th arm integrated)
High-Resolution 3D Video		
InSite vision system	+	+
Dual 3-chip camera system	+	+
Stereo endoscopes 0°/30°	+	+
High-intensity xenon light source	+	+
Immersive stereo display	+	+
Robotic Interface		
Patented Intuitive movement	+	+
Motion scaling	+	+
Tremor filtration	+	+
EndoWrist® Instruments		
7° of freedom	+	+
180° articulation	+	+
540° rotation	+	+
8-mm and 5-mm platforms	+	+
>40 instrument types	+	+
Fast, Foolproof Setup		
Motorized patient cart		+
High-speed fiberoptic connection		+
Quick-click cannula attachment		+
Rapid instrument exchange		+
Multi-Quadrant Access		
Extended reach instruments		+
Large range of motion		+
Interactive Video Displays		
TilePro multi-image stereo viewer		+
Integrated patient cart touch screen		+

Table 105-3 Comparison of da Vinci Surgical System and da Vinci S Surgical System

port placement.[8] In a patient with a wide abdominal cavity or a wide pelvis, it is beneficial to place ports farther apart laterally in order to minimize the potential for robotic arm or instrument collision. Placing ports too far laterally, however, can also be problematic, as this may result in the instruments colliding with the pelvic side wall.

Obesity poses a certain challenge to robotic-assisted surgery. Surgeon experience with laparoscopic surgery can assist in altering the placement of the primary and secondary ports, as similar steps are followed for conventional laparoscopic procedures. In morbidly obese patients, ports should be placed perpendicular to the fascia, in order to prevent oblique port placement and loss of instrument length within the subcutaneous fat. Moreover, extra-long robotic cannulas are available to circumvent difficult access in patients with thick abdominal walls. In performing robotic-assisted renal surgery in obese patients, it is useful to shift all of the ports laterally. The usefulness of the umbilicus as an anatomic landmark is significantly decreased in obese patients.

TRANSPERITONEAL VERSUS EXTRAPERITONEAL/RETROPERITONEAL SURGERY The major limitation of the extraperitoneal or retroperitoneal approach is the reduced working space compared to the transperitoneal approach. This is especially relevant when a well-meaning assistant attempts to clear the operative field of blood or smoke. Suctioning can evacuate gas and rapidly collapse the limited working space. The only solutions for this include the use of a high-flow insufflation system that is connected to a 10-mm or 12-mm trocar, as well as being mindful of the rate of suctioning.

CONCLUSION

Since the introduction of the da Vinci Surgical System to the urological field, robotic-assisted surgery has gained increasing popularity. Advances in technology and instrumentation have allowed for extirpative procedures as well as complex reconstructive procedures via transperitoneal or extra/retroperitoneal approaches. Clinical reports have demonstrated that robotic-assisted surgery is a safe, feasible, and effective technique for managing a variety of urologic conditions. It is evident that the morbidity from a robotic-assisted approach resembles that seen with a conventional laparoscopic approach, and is substantially less than that of open surgery. Robotic-assistance provides improved surgical dexterity and has made minimally invasive procedures more readily available for surgeons of all skill levels. Robotic technology has tremendous potential and may play a major role in enabling the achievement of improved outcomes in the future.

REFERENCES

1. Himpens J, Leman G, Cadiere G. Telesurgical laparoscopic cholecystectomy [Letter]. Surg Endosc 1998;12:1091.
2. Intuitive Surgical Inc. Intuitive Surgical - FDA Clearance; [2 screens]. Available at: http://www.intuitivesurgical.com/products/fdaclearance/index.aspx (accessed February 28, 2006).
3. Ahlering T. Robotic versus laparoscopic radical prostatectomy. Nat Clin Pract Urol 2004;1:58–9.
4. Binder J, Kramer W. Robotically assisted laparoscopic radical prostatectomy. BJU Int 2001;87:408–10.
5. Menon M, Tewari A, Peabody J. The VIP Team: Vattikuti Institute prostatectomy: technique. J Urol 2003;169:2289–92.
6. Sundaram C, Koch M, Gardner T, Bernie J. Utility of the fourth arm to facilitate robot-assisted laparoscopic radical prostatectomy. BJU Int 2005;95:183–6.
7. Hemal A, Eun D, Tewari A, Menon M. Nuances in the optimum placement of ports in pelvic and upper urinary tract surgery using the da Vinci robot. Urol Clin North Am 2004;31:683–92.
8. Gettman M, Hoznek A, Salomon L, et al. Laparoscopic radical prostatectomy: description of the extraperitoneal approach using the da Vinci robotic system. J Urol 2003; 170(2 Pt 1):416–9.
9. Esposito M, Ilbeigi P, Ahmed M, Lanteri V. Use of forth arm in da Vinci robot-assisted extraperitoneal laparoscopic prostatectomy: novel technique. Urology 2005;66:649–52.
10. DiMarco D, Chow G, Gettman M, Elliott D. Robotic sacrocolpopexy [Educational Video]. Mayo Foundation for Medical Education and Research; 2002.
11. Patel V. Robotic-assisted laparoscopic dismembered pyeloplasty. Urology 2005;66:45–9.
12. Desai M, Gill I, Kaouk J, et al. Robotic assisted laparoscopic adrenalectomy. Urology 2002;60:1104–7.
13. Peters C. Robotically assisted surgery in pediatric urology. Urol Clin North Am 2004;31:743–52.

106

Robotic Radical Prostatectomy for Localized Cancer of the Prostate: Vattikuti Institute Prostatectomy (VIP) Technique

Sanjeev Kaul, MD, MCh (Urol)
Mani Menon, MD, FACS

Carcinoma of the prostate is a difficult enemy to combat. In battling this disease, medicine has evolved from being able to diagnose the problem only after the war was lost, to having the tools to win the war but often at great collateral costs for the patient. Despite the technological advances in medicine, prostate cancer remains the most common solid organ malignancy in men in the United States and the second leading cause of cancer death. It was estimated that prostate cancer alone accounted for 33% (232,090) of all new cases of cancer in men, and that 30,350 would die of this disease in 2005.[1] Medical science has made great strides and won many battles, but as these statistics clearly show, the war continues. The widespread use of prostate-specific antigen (PSA) screening has resulted in the majority of patients being diagnosed at an earlier age and with asymptomatic (T1c) disease. In these patients with organ-confined disease,10-year survival approaches 95%, and quality-of-life (QOL) issues assume additional importance. Realizing that radical prostatectomy has become primarily a preventive procedure, we endeavored to develop a minimally invasive technique of radical prostatectomy that offers the curative benefits of open surgery, but with minimal morbidity and impact on QOL(pain, hospital stay, incontinence, or impotence). This journey, with its travails and tribulations, resulted in the birth of robotically assisted radical prostatectomy, or the Vattikuti Institute Prostatectomy (VIP).

BACKGROUND

Radical prostatectomy has been the surgical treatment of choice for localized prostate cancer for over a century. Radical prostatectomy by the perineal approach was first performed by Billroth in 1867.[2] In 1904, Hugh Hampton Young standardized this technique, reporting his preliminary results based on a series of 40 patients.[3] In 1947, Millin introduced the retropubic approach, yet the complications of this operation, such as hemorrhage, impotence, and incontinence, were noteworthy.[4] The retropubic approach did not gain popularity until the description of the anatomy of the dorsal vein complex, and a technique for the preservation of the neurovascular bundles by Walsh and colleagues.[5] Currently, the anatomic radical retropubic prostatectomy is the standard to which all other treatment modalities must measure up.

Surgical treatment of prostate cancer has now entered into the minimally invasive era. Schuessler and colleagues described laparoscopic radical prostatectomy in 1992.[6] Their procedure proved to be technically challenging and time-consuming; the most difficult part being the urethrovesical anastomosis, and for these reasons, the technique was abandoned. A group of French surgeons (Gaston, Guillonneau, and Vallancien) made an attempt to efficiently standardize laparoscopic prostatectomy in a reproducible manner. It is now well accepted that the laparoscopic approach, being less invasive, translates into shorter hospital stay, less pain, and earlier resumption of normal activities.[7] Laparoscopy does have limitations, such as the lack of three-dimensional visualization, a limitation on the degrees of freedom of movement, and poor ergonomics secondary to the use of rigid instruments, which can make dissection and anastomosis technically demanding.[8] It is advantageous for the patient, but tough for the surgeon, and learning curves as high as 50 to 100 cases have been suggested for laparoscopic radical prostatectomy.

Robotics is a recent addition to the armamentarium of minimally invasive urology. It has evolved from a single robotic arm (AESOP) that merely held the camera to newer systems (ZEUS and the da Vinci Surgical System, Intuitive Surgical, Inc., Sunnyvale, CA) which have three or four arms acting as extensions of the surgeon's hands and eyes. The principle advantages of the robot are in its endo-wristed instruments, which are precise, stable and dexterous, and in its magnified stereoscopic vision. The da Vinci system provides three-dimensional visualization and wrist-like movements, which facilitate performance of complex laparoscopic surgery. Thus, many of the disadvantages of laparoscopic techniques can be overcome with robotic technology.[9]

There are several published reports of robotic radical prostatectomy available in the world literature, with the largest experience coming from our institution. Surgeons report that the ergonomics of laparoscopic prostatectomy are improved because the surgeon does not need to be an amateur contortionist to perform the procedure.[10–14] Several authors have detailed improvements in visualization, freedom of movement of camera and instruments, and improved ability to dissect, suture and tie knots through the use of endowristed instruments. This chapter will focus on a step-by-step description of the Vattikuti Institute Prostatectomy technique of robotic radical prostatectomy developed by us. The chapter will also cover various modifications incorporated by our team and will discuss operative data, complications, and functional outcomes of robotic radical prostatectomy, comparing these to perineal, radical retropubic, and laparoscopic prostatectomy.

DEVELOPMENT OF CURRENT TECHNIQUE

The VIP technique evolved from case to case as we learned the abilities and limitations of the da Vinci system and as we became more adept in our use of the robot. As with open radical prostatectomy, the technique continues to evolve with experience. We started the robotic prostatectomy program in October 2000 with Guillonneau and Vallancien training us in laparoscopic radical prostatectomy using the AESOP camera holder. One author learned quite quickly that he was hopeless at laparoscopic surgery. Enter the da Vinci. We started by gaining familiarity with the movements of the robot, so our initial cases were done with the classic Montsouris approach, with the French team standing by for emergency bailout.[15] After 18 cases, we felt comfortable enough with the surgical robot to start developing our own unique approach, one that mimics the steps of open prostatectomy. We then moved on to the completely extraperitoneal approach, but found that this compromised the working space by hampering the smooth movement of the robotic arms. Subsequently, others have performed this technique extraperitoneally by modifying the port placement template.[16–18]

In an effort to combine the benefits of intraperitoneal port placement (wide exposure and more room for the insufflation of CO_2 with the benefits of a predominantly extraperitoneal dissection—ie, more familiar anatomic orientation and less ileus), we developed the Vattikuti Institute Prostatectomy. In this procedure, the ports are placed intraperitoneally as with the transperitoneal approach of laparoscopic radical prostatectomy. The rest of the operation, however, is done extraperitoneally, after entering the Retzius' space. The bowels are kept out of the operative field by placing the patient in a steep Trendelenburg's position and using extraperitoneal dissection. After the procedure, the peritoneal flap falls and re-establishes the integrity of the peritoneal cavity. This chapter provides a detailed description of VIP, based on our experience of over 2,200 cases.

INDICATIONS

Any patient who is a candidate for conventional radical prostatectomy is, with a few exceptions, a candidate for VIP. The operation is more difficult in the very obese (BMI > 35), in people who have had multiple lower abdominal operations, or in patients with a history of peritonitis. Previous herniorrhaphy, even with mesh, is not a contraindication: approximately one-third of our patients have had previous abdominal surgery. Patients with a history of prostatitis, preoperative hormonal therapy, or repeated prostatic biopsies may have obliterated periprostatic planes, making dissection somewhat more difficult. The assistants find the procedure more difficult in the very thin, muscular patient in whom the operative space within the peritoneal cavity may be small.

TECHNIQUE OF ROBOTIC RADICAL PROSTATECTOMY (VIP)

PREOPERATIVE PREPARATION Antibiotic and DVT prophylaxis are given according to hospital protocol. Sequential compression devices are placed routinely during surgery, and the patient should wear compression stockings while in the hospital. Subcutaneous injection of 5,000 units of heparin should be given before surgery and continued postoperatively. Bowel preparation is not necessary, but it is preferable to give a laxative the night before surgery.

PATIENT POSITIONING AND PREPARATION The patient is placed in supine, modified lithotomy position with the arms by the sides of the body to avoid the risk of brachial plexus injury (Figure 106-1). Shoulder support should be avoided because long hours may lead to postoperative pain so, in its place, a thoracic wrap is applied which is more comfortable and supports the patient thoroughly. The legs are separated in flexion and abduction because the length of the robotic arms necessitates bringing the robot in between the legs. Care is taken to adequately pad the pressure points and lower extremities. The table is set in extreme Trendelenburg's position. The abdomen, genitalia, and upper thighs are cleansed with an iodine-based preparation and

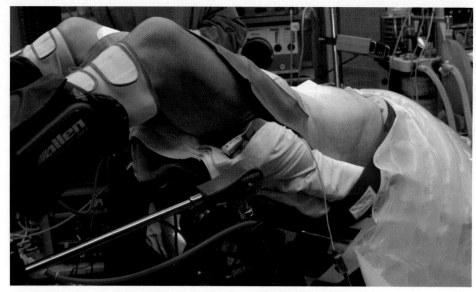

Figure 106-1 Position of the patient to avoid injury to the brachial plexus.

draped. An 18 French Foley catheter is inserted in the sterile field, and the bladder is drained.

ANESTHESIA The procedure is done under standard general endotracheal anesthesia.

PLACEMENT OF LAPAROSCOPIC PORTS Accurate port placement is imperative for successful execution of VIP. Three ports are required for the robotic arms, and three ports for assistance. In most of our cases, we use right and left assistants. The left assistant is inducted as a part of our structured training program, which allows them to observe closely from the patient's side and provides an opportunity for maneuvering robotic arms and instruments. The surgery can, however, be performed with only a single assistant. Pneumoperitoneum is established with a Veress needle. We prefer placing the primary port at the

umbilicus; we utilize this incision for retrieval of specimens, and it provides excellent cosmesis. Initial pressure is raised up to 20 mm Hg for the placement of ports (Figure 106-2). The pressure is reduced to 15 mm Hg for rest of the operation. The Veress needle is replaced with 12-mm trocar, and a 30° laparoscope is inserted to transilluminate the abdominal wall. The rest of the secondary trocars are placed under laparoscopic vision with a 30° laparoscope directed upward to prevent intra-abdominal visceral injuries. Two 8-mm metal trocars for robotic arms are placed 3 to 5 cm below the level of the umbilicus, lateral to the rectus muscle on either side. A 12-mm port is placed in the mid axillary line 2.5 cm above the right anterior superior iliac spine. The 12-mm port is required for passing and removing needles, and removing biopsy tissue material. A 5-mm port is placed on the left side as a mirror image of the

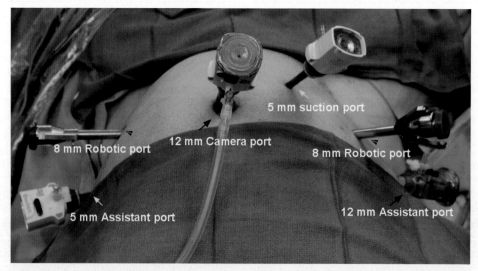

Figure 106-2 One 12-mm port (*black arrow*) is placed at the level of the umbilicus for a camera port (*arrow*); and another 12-mm port (*black arrow*) is placed in the mid-axillary line 2.5 cm above the right superior iliac crest. Two 8-mm robotic ports (*arrowhead*) for robotic arms are placed 3 to 5 cm below the level of the umbilicus, lateral to the rectus muscle on either side. A 5-mm port (*yellow arrow*) is placed in the left iliac fossa 5 cm above and lateral to the anterior superior iliac spine for assistance, and the other 5-mm port (*yellow arrow*) is placed on right side in between the camera port and the right robotic port for the suction cannula.

right assistant port, and another 5-mm port is placed in the right iliac fossa 5 cm above and medial to the anterior superior iliac spine.

PERITONEOSCOPY AND MOBILIZATION OF THE BLADDER
This step is performed with a 30° lens directed upward. First, inspection of the abdomen is done to see the various abdominal organs. Patients with previous intra-abdominal operations may have adhesions, which must be divided to make room for placement of the ports. Since the patient is in an extreme Trendelenburg's position, the small bowel usually falls away. On the left side, the attachment of the sigmoid colon to the retroperitoneum must be transected to allow unimpeded passage of the left-side assistant's instruments and for subsequent lymphadenectomy. An inverted U incision is then made such that the horizontal part of the incision is high enough on the anterior wall of the abdomen to preclude injury to the bladder (Figure 106-3). The vertical limb of the U incision is located lateral to the medial umbilical ligament. This dissection is performed in the avascular plane involving the dissection of adipose and loose areolar tissue. The first landmark visualized is the pubic bone, and dissection is completed laterally on either side anteriorly and completely exposing the endopelvic fascia bilaterally.

LYMPHADENECTOMY
Pelvic lymphadenectomy is done in the following situations: Gleason score 7 or above, PSA > 10, > 50% of cores positive, or a palpable nodule. In our series, over 50% of patients underwent lymphadenectomy, but nodal disease was present in less than 1%. This step is performed with a 30° lens directed downward. The internal inguinal ring can be seen, though the external iliac vessels are hidden in the lateral fold of the peritoneum. The vertical limbs of the peritoneal incision are extended to the vas deferens. The vas deferens is seen coursing obliquely across the incision and can be retracted out of the operating field or divided prior to further dissection. We prefer to perform this dissection using the da Vinci bipolar forceps in the non-dominant hand and the articulated scissors in the dominant hand. Retroperitoneal fat

is cleared off the anterior surface of the external iliac vein. The obturator nerve is identified and preserved. Because of recent information that implies that pelvic lymphadenectomy may be therapeutic in some patients, we remove nodal tissue from the true pelvis, posterior to the obturator vessels.[19] Beginning at the pubic ramus, the lymph nodes and fatty tissues are cleaned out of the obturator fossa. Aberrant obturator veins should be avoided and are clipped or cauterized if encountered. The packet of fibro-fatty and nodal tissue is dissected toward the intersection of the external iliac vein, the obturator nerve, and the umbilical ligament. The nodal package usually has two components—one containing tissue anterior to the plane of the obturator nerves, and one posterior to it (Figure 106-4).

DIVISION OF ENDOPELVIC FASCIA AND CONTROL OF DORSAL VENOUS COMPLEX
Once the anterior surface of the bladder is exposed the camera is changed to a 30° lens facing down, and dissection continues with division and coagulation of the superficial dorsal vein over the prostate (Figure 106-5). The fat over the prostate is then swept cephalad and laterally and endopelvic fascia is incised on either side through the semilunar gaps distally. The levator muscle and fascia is swept off the surface of the prostate. Proximally, identification of a tongue of fat defines the location of the bladder neck, and distally, the puboperinealis muscle is swept off to define the apex of the prostate and the urethra At the apex of the prostate, the closely applied neurovascular bundle is swept laterally on both sides using blunt dissection. We do not divide the puboprostatic ligaments. A 0 Vicryl stitch on a CT-1 needle is used to place a figure-of-eight stitch over the deep dorsal vein (Figure 106-6).

DISSECTION AND DIVISION OF THE BLADDER NECK
The bladder neck dissection is done with a 30° angled lens directed downward. Accurate identification of the bladder neck is crucial; high division of the bladder results in a large bladder opening and the need for bladder neck recon-

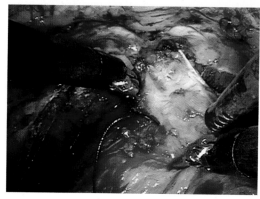

Figure 106-5 Control of deep dorsal vein complex.

struction, and low dissection may cause incision into the prostatic substance and compromise oncologic principles. The assistant grasps the bladder at 12 o'clock and, by lifting the anterior bladder wall superiorly, exposes the junction of the bladder and prostate. Note that we start the bladder neck dissection laterally on either side, and then extend the incision to the midline. The reason for this is that identification of the plane between the bladder and the prostate is much easier laterally than in the midline. The lateral incisions are joined horizontally in the midline, dividing the anterior bladder neck and delivering the tip of the Foley catheter through this opening (Figure 106-7). The assistant pulls the Foley catheter inside the pelvis in an upward direction. This helps in identifying the posterior wall of the bladder neck, which is transected with the electrocautery, ensuring that the ureteral openings are not damaged and maintaining a clean detrusor margin for subsequent vesicourethral anastomosis. In patients with a large median lobe and those with prior transurethral resection of the prostate, additional precaution is taken to protect the ureteral orifices as these are commonly retracted close to the prostate.

DISSECTION OF VAS DEFERENS, SEMINAL VESICLES, AND INCISION OF DENONVILLIERS' FASCIA
Division of the posterior bladder neck leads to the anterior layer of Denonvilliers' fascia, which covers the vasa and the seminal vesicles (Figure 106-8).

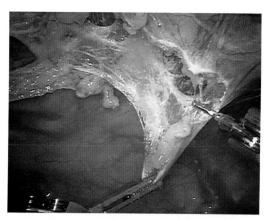

Figure 106-3 The bladder is being dissected off from anterior abdominal wall to enter into Retzius' space.

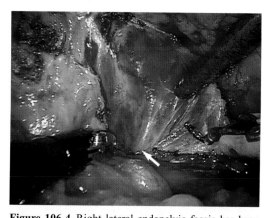

Figure 106-4 Right lateral endopelvic fascia has been incised, the prostate is being dissected off the perineal muscles, and proximal dissection is extended up to delineate smooth glistening fat as a mark of the prostate-vesical junction (*arrow*).

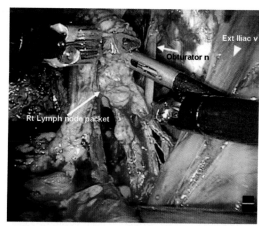

Figure 106-6 Stay suture on the posterior part of the port.

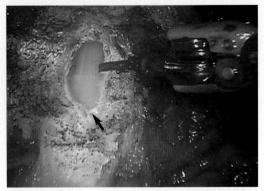

Figure 106-7 Division of anterior wall of bladder neck (*arrow*) and Foley catheter can be seen through the window.

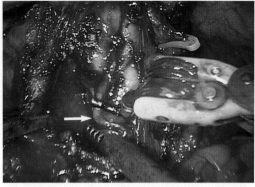

Figure 106-9 Artery to seminal vesicle is being cauterized (*arrow*)

sors so as to preserve a good stump of urethra. The catheter is pulled anteriorly, and the posterior wall of the urethra, the posterior striated sphincter, and the rectourethralis are divided sharply. Bleeding from the dorsal venous complex may be controlled by placing another stitch (2-0 Vicryl, RB-1 needle). After the division of the urethra, the prostate is free, and the specimen is transferred to a 10-mm Endocatch bag (U.S. Surgical, Norwalk, CT) and placed in the left upper quadrant of the abdomen until the end of the procedure.

EXCISION OF PERIAPICAL COLLAR OF TISSUE
Our technique of apical dissection preserves maximum urethral length and leads to early continence. It may, however, result in a higher rate of positive margins, especially at the anterior apex where the distinction between prostate and periurethral fibromuscular tissue is difficult to make visually, even with the magnification offered by the da Vinci lenses. To ensure completeness of removal of the prostatic apex, a 5- to 8-mm collar of tissue is excised from the periurethral area and analyzed by frozen section. In the rare event (< 5% in our series) of residual prostatic tissue being identified, more tissue is removed distally.

VESICOURETHRAL ANASTOMOSIS   In our early experience, the anastomosis was performed with 8 to 18 interrupted sutures. As we became lazier, we have developed a technique of vesicourethral anastomosis, which is a modification of the technique described by van Velthoven and colleagues.[21] The Menon, van Velthoven, Ahlering, Clayman (MVAC) suture is rigged by tying the tails of 7 inches of dyed and undyed 3-0 Monocryl suture on a 17-mm round body (RB-1) needle (Ethicon), to make a single 14-inch suture with a knot in the center and a needle at either end. The anastomosis begins with the dyed suture, starting outside in, at the 5 o'clock position of the bladder neck. The needle is then passed inside out at the corresponding site in the urethra. We apply a continuous suture in a clockwise fashion to 9 o'clock, where the suture is turned inside out in the bladder, and then continued to the 12 o'clock position. At this point, the assistant holds the suture taut, pulling cranially. Then anastomosis is continued with the undyed end of the suture, passing it outside in on the urethra at the 4 o'clock position and then inside out on the bladder neck. The suture is run counterclockwise to 12 o'clock. A new urethral catheter is advanced into the bladder. The needles are cut off, and the two ends are tied together with multiple knots to complete the anastomosis. If the opening in the bladder neck is too large and disproportionate to the urethral opening, the bladder neck may be reconstructed with 2-0 Vicryl sutures placed in a figure-of-eight fashion at the 3 and 9 o'clock positions. This MVAC modification has allowed us to complete the vesicourethral anastomosis with a single intracorporeal knot.

This layer is transected to the plane of the vasa. The Foley catheter is then removed and the left assistant grasps the cut leaf of fascia with firm traction upwards. The vas deferens and seminal vesicles can be dissected and pulled up. The artery to the vas deferens that passes between the vas and the seminal vesicle should be controlled. The seminal vesicles are traced by following the vas back to its junction with the seminal vesicle, and both seminal vesicles are freed circumferentially, taking care to control small arterioles that supply the vesicles laterally and posteriorly. With traction on the divided vas deferens and seminal vesicles, the prostatic pedicles can be dissected on either side, as these are now covered with thin adipose tissue (Figure 106-9). Seminal vesicles are lifted up anteriorly to demonstrate the longitudinal fibers of Denonvilliers' fascia near the apex of the prostate, and a transverse incision is made deep enough to appreciate the prerectal fat posteriorly. We avoid using electrocautery for the entire posterior dissection so as to protect the neurovascular bundles. The prostate is then dissected away from the rectum, leaving a layer of Denonvilliers' fascia over the rectum (Figure 106-10).

CONTROL OF PROSTATIC PEDICLES AND DISSECTION OF THE NEUROVASCULAR BUNDLE (CONVENTIONAL NERVE SPARING)   This step is performed with a 30° lens directed downward. The

lateral pedicles at the prostate vesical junction are controlled using Hem-o-lock clips and bipolar coagulation. The clips are applied close to the prostate, and the pedicle is divided between them. Once the dissection enters the plane between the prostatic fascia medially and the levator fascia laterally, electrocautery is avoided and the anterior nerve-sparing dissection proceeds using sharp cutting with scissors and bipolar coagulation as necessary. Small arterioles entering the substance of the prostate are coagulated with bipolar forceps and divided with scissors. This dissection proceeds to the apex of the prostate distally. One needs to stay close to the surface of the prostate to prevent damage to the neurovascular bundles that are closely related.

APICAL DISSECTION AND URETHRAL TRANSECTION   The camera is now changed to a 0° lens. The anterior prostate is grasped with cephalad traction, making the dorsal venous complex and urethra prominent and taut. The superficial attachments of the puboprostatic ligament are divided, and the dorsal venous complex is divided and gently teased away from the prostate, much as described by Meyers and colleagues for open radical prostatectomy.[20] Rotational retraction by the assistant facilitates dissection of the prostatic apices laterally and posteriorly. Once the apex is dissected circumferentially, the urethra is divided at the apex of the prostate using articulated scis-

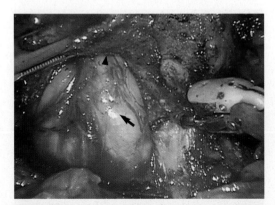

Figure 106-8 Division of posterior bladder neck and Denonvilliers' fascia (*arrowhead*) leads to the vas deferens and seminal vesicle (*arrow*).

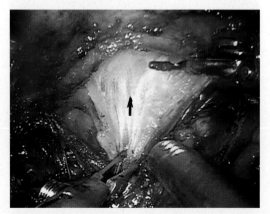

Figure 106-10 Dissection (*arrow*) through layers of Denonvilliers' fascia behind the prostate.

RETRIEVAL OF SPECIMEN AND CLOSURE OF PORTS   A 15F Jackson Pratt drain is introduced through the lateral 5-mm port and placed within the pelvis. The specimen is extracted through the extension of semicircular umbilical incision. The fascia at the umbilical incision is closed with absorbable suture, whereas the other port sites are closed with subcuticular sutures because of the use of non-cutting trocars.

POSTOPERATIVE MANAGEMENT Patients are encouraged to drink fluids immediately and walk on the evening of surgery. Antibiotics are administered for 24 hours and Toradol and Tylenol are administered for control of pain. Patients are discharged within 24 hours, and in the absence of significant drainage, the Jackson Pratt drain is removed prior to discharge. A cystogram is performed on postoperative day 7, and in the absence of contrast leak, the catheter is removed.

TECHNICAL MODIFICATIONS

As our experience with the VIP procedure increased, we incorporated several modifications to our technique; these were designed to make the operation easier to perform and also to improve upon the functional outcomes, especially sexual function and urinary control.

PROSTATIC FASCIA PRESERVATION (VEIL OF APHRODITE) NERVE-SPARING Several investigators have shown that the traditional anatomic concept of neurovascular bundles may not be accurate in all patients.[14,22,23] Both anatomic dissections and physiologic experiments in rats have shown that accessory cavernosal nerves are present within the prostatic fascia, and these play a significant role in erectile function.[24,25] Our dissections in cadavers have supported these findings. We modified the technique of nerve-sparing during robotic radical prostatectomy to preserve these accessory nerves and called this technique the Veil of Aphrodite[26] after the Greek goddess of Love (Figure 106-11). The prostatic fascia is preserved from the bladder neck to the puboprosta-

tic ligaments on either side and hangs much like a veil; hence the name. The technique is described in brief. Following division of the bladder neck and dissection of the vasa and seminal vesicles, the posterior layer of Denonvilliers' fascia is exposed. An inverted U incision is made in this fascia, and a plane is developed between the posterior prostate and Denonvilliers' fascia. Dissection is extended as far distally as possible. Subsequently, the base of the seminal vesicle is retracted superomedially by the assistant, and the prostatic pedicle is delineated and divided. This pedicle lies anterior to the pelvic plexus and neurovascular bundle and includes only prostatic blood supply. Under the magnification of the robotic camera, several arterial branches can be seen. These are coagulated individually or controlled with clips. The pedicle is divided sharply with the "cold" da Vinci scissors (Figure 106-12). The neurovascular bundle runs along the posterolateral aspect of the prostate encircled by the inner (prostatic) and outer (levator) layers of the prostatic fascia and the posterior layer of Denonvilliers' fascia. After dividing the pedicle, the plane between the prostatic capsule and inner leaf of the prostatic fascia is developed at its cranial extent. Once this has been done, the assistants provide superomedial prostate retraction and lateral retraction on tissues adjacent to the neurovascular bundle. This allows the surgeon to enter a plane between the prostatic fascia and the prostatic capsule. This plane, which is deep to the venous sinuses of Santorini's plexus, is developed with blunt dissection with the articulated scissors, using bipolar coagulation only as necessary. In some patients, the plane is developed easier at this location, rather than at the pedicle. Careful sharp and blunt dissection of the neurovascular bundle and contiguous prostatic fascia is performed until the entire prostatic fascia, up to and including the ipsilateral pubourethral ligament, is mobilized in continuity off the lateral aspect of the prostatic apex. This plane is mostly avascular, except anteriorly where the fascia is fused with the puboprostatic ligament, capsule, and venous plexus. The wristed instrumentation facilitates this dissection, especially near the prostatic apex.

When performed correctly, an intact veil of tissue hangs from the pubourethral ligament. The thickness and vascularity of the veil is variable: in men with large prostates, the veil is delicate; in men with small prostates, the veil is robust and vascular. The results of the procedure are discussed below (see "Results").

PRESERVATION OF THE ENDOPELVIC FASCIA Even though incision of the endopelvic fascia provides better visualization of the prostate, the resultant loss of support to the neurovascular bundles and excessive traction on the nerves during nerve-sparing may be responsible for delayed return of erections. By not incising the endopelvic fascia, especially during the Veil of Aphrodite procedure, the cavernous and accessory cavernous nerves are subjected to less traction-induced injury, and this may play a role in better return of erections. A disadvantage of this modification is that the dorsal venous complex cannot be controlled until after the nerve-sparing has been completed, and blood loss from Santorini's plexus may be increased in vascular prostates. The dorsal vein is controlled either immediately prior to or after transaction of the urethra (Figure 106-13).

ATHERMAL TECHNIQUE The pelvic plexus is closely related to the tips of the seminal vesicles, and the cavernous nerves to the posterolateral margin of the prostate. Concern has been raised that the use of monopolar or bipolar coagulation may injure the delicate nerves and hamper return of erections. In young patients with low volume disease and excellent preoperative erections, the VIP procedure may be performed without any electrocautery whatsoever. Five-millimeter titanium and Weck clips are used to control the vasal and vesicular arteries. The nerve-sparing proceeds with careful dissection of the arterioles and individual control with clips. Lack of electrocautery makes the procedure more challenging and time-consuming, taking us 22 minutes longer

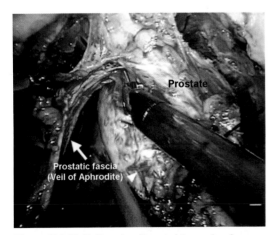

Figure 106-11 Delineating dissected (*arrowhead*) accessory nerves (Veil of Aphrodite) on left side from anterolateral surface (*arrow*) of the prostate, in addition to preservation of the posterior neurovascular bundles with the help of articulated scissor.

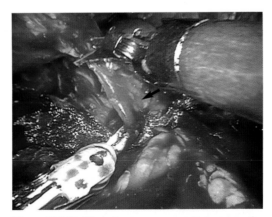

Figure 106-12 Dissection to preserve right neurovascular bundles (*arrow*) from the posterolateral surface of the prostate in same patient with the help of articulated scissor.

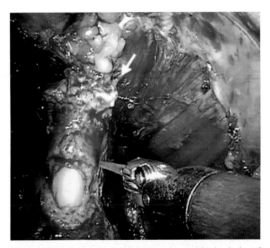

Figure 106-13 Division of the urethra with the help of articulated scissor, tip of Foley catheter can be seen emerging from the urethra and rectourethralis muscle is last to be severed to completely detach urethra from the prostate.

on average. Data about whether this approach results in improved return of erectile function are awaited (Figure 106-14).

RESULTS

Consensus does not exist about how to grade an operation and identify which technique is superior to the others. When the 14 attending surgeons and 12 residents (part of the Vattikuti Urology Institute) were asked to grade the quality of radical prostatectomy, they felt that operative time, blood loss, duration of hospitalization, lack of complications, negative margins, continence, and potency were important considerations (in that order). To confirm the surgeons' perspective on the quality of an operation, all patients over a 1-month period were polled preoperatively about desired outcomes. Patients ranked operations on the basis of completeness of cancer removal, continence, potency, safety (lack of complications), ease of recuperation, and lack of blood transfusion. Interestingly, two factors that were important to the surgeon, operative time and duration of hospitalization, were not considered important to the patients. Based on our own experience, we compared arbitrarily relative advantages of various approaches for radical prostatectomy: perineal, retropubic, laparoscopic, and robotically assisted (Table-106-1). The measures (using the same variables or parameters) for different approaches were size of prostate gland, visualization of operative field, lymph-node dissection, blood loss and need for transfusion, fatigue, operation time, apical exposure, posterior and lateral exposure, nerve sparing, vesicourethral anastomosis, obesity, tactile sensation, incisional pain, morbidity, recovery, ergonomics, cost, and learning curve. The last row of the table gives a total score for each type of surgery. This score allows one to compare the various operative techniques based on the different factors listed. These scores were calculated on what patients considered important and what we considered important in performing these techniques (Figure 106-15). The best possible score for each variable is four stars. Thus, if any technique is found perfect it would have four stars for all 18 variables, scoring

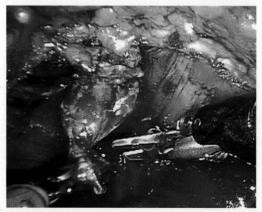

Figure 106-14 Soft tissue biopsy is being taken from apex of urethra for frozen section.

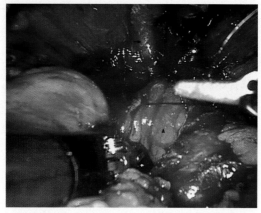

Figure 106-15 Vesicourethral anastomosis is in progress. A single suture (length may vary from 10 to 14 inches, which is guided by the diameter of bladder neck) is prepared by tying dyed and undyed 3-0 monofilament suture on an RB-1 needle. The third throw of dyed suture is being passed through the bladder neck outside-in (*arrowhead*) and the arrow indicates the left lateral margin of the urethra.

72 stars (100%). The possible score in terms of number of stars and percentage is reflected in the last column of Table 106-1.

OPERATIVE DATA

In our initial experience, operative times were between 2 and 3 hours. As of this writing, however, we had performed over 2,200 VIPs, and in the most recent 100 cases, the mean operative time was 97 minutes. The mean robotic setup time is 6 minutes, 96% patients were discharged within 24 hours, and mean duration of catheterization was 7.2 days. Comparison of different series of laparoscopic radical prostatectomies with robotic radical prostatectomy (VIP) in the

context of various variables (eg, operative parameter) is described in Table 106-2.

CANCER REMOVAL

Completeness of cancer removal can be measured by the incidence of negative margins. Negative margins, however, are functions of both surgical technique and the biological characteristics of the cancers removed. Centers that operate on low-volume, low-grade disease can be expected to have a higher likelihood of negative margins than centers that operate on more locally advanced disease.[27] Thus, a mere detailing of the percentage of negative margins is meaningless without understanding the grade and volume of the tumor. The average prostate volume in the VIP patients was 55 cc, mean percent tumor was 19, and the median Gleason grade was 7.[28] Positive margins were seen in 21 of the first 210 patients operated on (10%). By comparison, in a review of 53 studies of open radical prostatectomy, the reported incidences of positive margins ranged from 5 to 53%, with an overall rate of 28%.[29] In our own series of open radical prostatectomies, positive margins were seen in 24% of patients.[30] The positive margin rate for laparoscopic radical prostatectomy ranges from 15 to 28%,[31–33] and from 16 to 24% for perineal prostatectomy.[33–37]

URINARY CONTINENCE

Urinary continence is high, no matter which approach is used for radical prostatectomy. In our own patients undergoing open radical retropubic prostatectomy, 60% were pad-free at 6 months, and 90% were pad-free at 12 months.[30] For the first 200 VIPs, 96% of patients were pad-free at

Table 106-1 Relative Advantages of Perineal, Retropubic, Laparoscopic and Robot Assisted (VIP) Prostatectomies				
Measure for Various Approach	Perineal Radical Prostatectomy	Retropubic Radical Prostatectomy	Laparoscopic Radical Prostatectomy	Vattikuti Institute Prostatectomy (Robotically Assisted)
Size of glands	* to **	***	**	***
Visualisation of operative field	*	**	***	****
Lymph-node dissection	Not possible	***	****	****
Blood loss and need for transfusion	**	*	***	****
Fatigue	****	*	****	****
Operation time	****	**	*	***
Apical exposure	****	**	***	****
Posterior and lateral exposure	****	***	***	****
Nerve sparing	*	***	**	****
Vesicourethral anastomosis	****	**	* to **	****
Obesity	***	**	*	***
Tactile sensation	***	****	**	*
Incisional pain	*	**	***	****
Morbidity	**	*	***	****
Recovery	***	**	***	****
Ergonomics	**	***	*	****
Cost	****	***	**	*
Learning curve	***	***	*	****
Total score	47/72 (65.27%)	42/72 (58.33%)	43/72 (59.72%)	63/72 (87.5%)

* = lowest; **** = highest.

Table 106-2 Comparison of Contemporary Series of Laparoscopic Radical Prostatectomy with Robotic Radical Prostatectomy (VIP)

Series	No. of Patients	Approach	OR Time (hr)	Blood Loss (cc)	Transfusion Rate (%)	Conversion Rate (%)
Guillonneau[49]	350	TP	3.6	354	5.7	2
Turk[52]	125	TP	4.25	185	2	0
Abbou[10]	137	TP	4.75	NA	2.9	NA
Rassweiler[53]	180	TP	4.5	1230	31	4.4
Gill[32]	100	TP/EP	4.5	322	2	1
Menon[28]	530	VIP	2.75	153	0	0
Bhayani[55]	36	TP	5.8	533	NA	3
Dahl[56]	70	TP	4.25	449	5.7	1
GLWG[58]	5824	TP+EP	3.25	NA	4.1	2.4

EP = extraperitoneal; GLWG = German Laparoscopic Working Group; NA = not available; OR = operating room; TP = transperitoneal; VIP = Vattikuti Institute Prostatectomy (a hybrid of EP and TP approaches).

6 months, with the median time for return of continence being 42 days.[13] In this analysis, urinary continence was measured by a validated questionnaire (EPIC). More recently (300 cases), 50% of patients are continent within 24 hours of removal of the catheter. By comparison, Weldon and Tavel reported that continence returned in patients undergoing perineal prostatectomy at the following rates: 23% by 1 month, 56% by 3 months, 90% by 6 months, and 95% by 10 months.[38] For laparoscopic radical prostatectomy, Abbou and colleagues found continence in 78% of their patients at 1 year.[33] Guillonneau and colleagues found a 72% continence rate in the first 60 patients at 6 months , and an 85.5% continence rate at 1 year.[39]

POTENCY

The incidence of potency following radical prostatectomy appears to depend on four main factors: the age of the patient, preoperative quality of erections, whether both neurovascular bundles were preserved, and the cut-off value for preservation of potency.[40] Although unproven, it is reasonable to assume that the surgeon's expertise may also be a factor in this outcome. Quinlan and associates demonstrated that recovery of potency was quantitatively related to preservation of nerves.[41] In our own series, men were polled using the EPIC questionnaire. At 6 months after surgery, 33% of patients undergoing open radical retropubic prostatectomy and 66% of men undergoing VIP were potent as defined by having had sexual intercourse within 4 weeks of answering the questionnaire.[28,30] The frequency of sexual intercourse, however, decreased from 3.4 (more than once a week) to 2.3 (less than once a week), and only 40% of men claimed to have the same quality of erections as before surgery (only measured in the VIP patients). Having developed the Veil of Aphrodite nerve-sparing, we compared sexual function outcomes following conventional nerve-sparing and the Veil of Aphrodite using a standardized QOL questionnaire: the Sexual Health Inventory for Men (SHIM). Ninety-seven percent of patients undergoing the Veil of Aphrodite procedure had erections satisfactory for intercourse at 1 year post-surgery compared to 74% undergoing conventional nerve-sparing. What was more striking was that 86% of the Veil of Aphrodite patients reported that the erections were as good qualitatively as before surgery, compared to only 26% undergoing the conventional nerve-sparing.[42] In a follow-up study of 154 patients undergoing the Veil of Aphrodite procedure the results were similar; a testament to the durability of the procedure. Weldon and co-workers reported potency results in a prospective study of 220 patients undergoing radical perineal prostatectomy.[43] In this group, 70% remained potent, defined as having an erection satisfactory for vaginal penetration. Abbou and colleagues reported that, overall at a 1-year follow-up of a series of laparoscopic radical prostatectomies, 53.8% of patients had postoperative erections.[44] For open radical retropubic prostatectomy, Catalona and Bigg reported potency in 63% of patients when both nerves were preserved, and only 39% when one nerve was spared.[45] A recent report by Walsh and colleagues, however, records an 86% rate of recovered potency at 18 months in a small series of patients.[46]

COMPLICATIONS

Radical retropubic prostatectomy is a safe operation. The overall complication rates with open surgery range from 6 to 15%.[47,48] Guillonneau and colleagues reported that 97 of 567 patients (17.1 %) had complications following laparoscopic radical prostatectomy.[49] In our own series, the complication rate was 15% in patients undergoing radical retropubic prostatectomy and 1.3% in patients undergoing VIP.[30] In a series of 1,508 patients followed for 12 months, 1,453 patients (96.3%) had an ideal postoperative course. Ninety-two percent of patients were discharged in 1 day, 4.3% observed for 1 additional day for social reasons, and 23 (2.5%) stayed more than 3 days (mean for open RRP = 3.4 days). Overall, 37 patients (2.5%) had a Clavien grade II complication. There were 10 reoperations (0.67%): three resection anastomoses for bowel injury, one colostomy, two operations for postoperative bleeding, and one for disrupted anastomosis (Figure 106-16).

POSTOPERATIVE PAIN The average pain score, based on the visual analog scale, was 7 of 10 at 24 hours following open prostatectomy, and 3 of 10 at 24 hours following VIP in our patients.

BLOOD LOSS Transfusion rates are low following radical prostatectomy. Smith and colleagues have reported a transfusion rate of 4.5%.[4] In our own series of open radical prostatectomy, the transfusion rate was 11% for homologous blood, although another 56% utilized autologous blood or the cell saver. Transfusion rates for laparoscopic prostatectomy range from 4 to 31%, and for perineal prostatectomy from 10 to 20%.[16–18,33–39] The lowest reported blood loss of retropubic prostatectomy is 300 cc, and for perineal prostatectomy, 550 cc,[50,51] although patients do ooze in the pelvis following surgery. Thus, a more accurate indicator of blood loss may be the discharge hematocrit. For several series of open radical prostatectomies, the discharge hematocrit is around 32%. Indeed, this has been the average discharge hematocrit of our patients undergoing open prostatectomy. In contrast, the average blood loss for a VIP is less than 100 cc; no patient has required an inoperative transfusion, and the average discharge hematocrit is 37%. Perhaps because of this, patients do not feel fatigued after a VIP, and are able to resume activities sooner than with open surgery.

THE FUTURE (DA VINCI S SYSTEM)

In February 2006, Intuitive Surgical launched a second-generation surgical robotic system called the da Vinci S Surgical System. This system incorporates several modifications designed to make it more user-friendly and also more versatile, as compared to the older systems. Some of the more useful are elaborated upon.

PATIENT SIDE CART The patient side surgical cart has been extensively redesigned. It now incorporates a motorized system for easy movement and also has an assistant monitor attached to the cart (Figure 106-17). The monitor incorporates a touch screen with which the assistant sees,

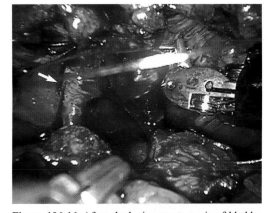

Figure 106-16 After clockwise anastomosis of bladder (*arrowhead*) and urethra (*arrow*) with dyed suture up to 1 or 12-o'clock; counterclockwise anastomosis is started with undyed suture from 4 o'clock off the urethra outside-in.

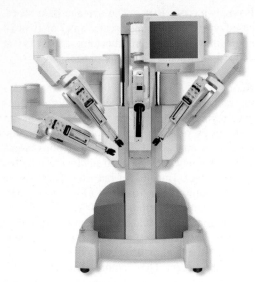

Figure 106-17 A patient side cart is new for the da Vinci S Surgical System.

in real time, additional windows depicting radiographic images. It also depicts error messages clearly, which helps the patient side assistants. A similar system has been incorporated into the surgical console. The robotic arms have disposable sterile adapters incorporated within the drapes; changing instruments is smoother, with fewer errors. The robotic arms also have a set of colored lights at the tips. These lights (white, blue, and red) facilitate detection of instrument lives, instrument insertion errors, and reversible faults. The robotic instruments themselves are 2.5 inches longer, and the entire robotic arm telescopes as the instrument is moved in and out.

SURGICAL CONSOLE The design of the console remains essentially the same except for minor cosmetic changes to the console controls (Figure 106-18). The vision on the console is sharper and less pixilated than in previous generation systems, providing superior visual definition.

We performed 15 VIPs with the new system and found the new system more user-friendly and less complicated to master. The setup times were longer in the initial few cases, but not significantly so. Overall, we believe the new system is a step forward.

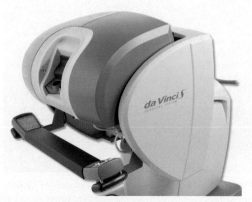

Figure 106-18 A close up of the console in the da Vinci S Surgical System, which has minor cosmetic changes.

COMMENTS

The goals of minimally invasive surgery in the management of prostate cancer are many, but the most important are the need to provide long-term cancer control and to develop a procedure that is associated with minimal morbidity. In performing robotically assisted radical prostatectomy, the intentions are to remove the cancer while maintaining continence and potency. Laparoscopic radical prostatectomy is well-established and effective. Laparoscopy is a demanding technique with a steep learning curve and, therefore, the skills are difficult to transfer to surgeons trained in conventional surgery. It requires the interpretation of laparoscopic pelvic anatomy, hand-to-eye dissociation, the ability to deal with a lack of tactile and visual feedback, and the loss of freedom of movement. These restrictions need to be overcome to make more surgeons comfortable with the idea of attempting robotic laparoscopic surgery. However, the exact role of laparoscopic radical prostatectomy in the treatment of localized prostate cancer still needs to be defined.

Robotics has been embraced with open arms by both urologists and patients alike. The number of VIPs performed has increased exponentially; 17,000 robotic radical prostatectomies were performed worldwide in 2004, and it is estimated that 35,000 will be performed in 2005. VIP may well be considered the new gold standard for surgical treatment of localized prostate cancer. As of this writing, robotically assisted radical prostatectomy compares favorably with open radical retropubic prostatectomy or non-robotic laparoscopic radical prostatectomy. The sub–two-hour operative times, the low positive margin rate, the early return of continence, the easy recuperation, all contribute to the high degree of patient satisfaction with this procedure. As robotic technology improves and more surgeons develop their robotic skills, these results should improve even farther.

REFERENCES

1. Jemal A, Murray T, Samuels A, et al. Cancer statistics, 2003. CA Cancer J Clin 2003;53:5–26.
2. Weyrauch HM. Perineal prostatectomy. In: Weyrauch HM, editor. Surgery of the prostate. Philadelphia: W.B.Saunders; 1959. p. 172–228.
3. Young HH. The early diagnosis and radical cure of carcinoma of the prostate: a study of 40 cases and presentation of radical operation which was carried out in 4 cases. John Hopkins Hosp Bull 1905;16:315–21.
4. Millin T. Retropubic prostatectomy: a new extravesical technique. Lancet 1945;2:693–6.
5. Walsh PC, Lepor H, Eggleston JC. Radical prostatectomy with preservation of sexual function: anatomical and pathological consideration. Prostate 1983;4:473.
6. Schuessler WW, Schulam PG, Clayman RV, et al. Laparoscopic radical prostatectomy: initial short term experience. Urology 1997;50:854–7.
7. Guillonneau B, Vallancien G. Laparoscopic radical prostatectomy: the Montsouris experience. J Urol 2000;163:418–22.
8. Rassweiler J, Frede T. Robotics, telesurgery and telementoring—their position in modern urological laparoscopy. Arch Esp Urol 2002;55:610–28.
9. Menon M, Shrivastava A, Tewari A, et al. Laparoscopic and robot assisted radical prostatectomy: establishment of a structured program and preliminary analysis of outcomes. J Urol 2002;168:945–9.
10. Abbou CC, Hoznek A, Salomon L, et al. Laparoscopic radical prostatectomy with a remote controlled robot. J Urol 2001;165:1964–6.
11. Binder J, Kramer W. Robotically assisted laparoscopic radical prostatectomy. BJU Int 2001;87:408–10.
12. Pasticier G, Reitbergen JBW, Guillonneau B, et al. Robotically assisted laparoscopic radical prostatectomy: Feasibility study in men. Eur Urol 2001;40:70–4.
13. Menon M. Robotic radical retropubic prostatectomy. BJU Int 2003;91:175–6.
14. Tewari A, Peabody JO, Fischer M, et al. An operative and anatomic study to help in nerve sparing during laparoscopic and robotic radical prostatectomy. Eur Urol 2003; 43:444–54.
15. Tewari A, Peabody J, Sarle R, et al. Technique of da Vinci robot – assisted anatomic radical prostatectomy. Urology 2002;60:569–72.
16. Raboy A, Ferzli G, Albert P. Initial experience with extraperitoneal endoscopic radical retropubic prostatectomy. Urology 1997;50:849–53.
17. Bollens R, Bossche MV, Roumeguere, et al. Extraperitoneal laparoscopic radical prostatectomy. Eur Urol 2001;40: 65–69.
18. Stolzenburg M Do, Rabenalt R, Pfeiffer H, et al. Endoscopic extraperitoneal radical prostatectomy: initial experience after 70 cases. J Urol 2003;169:2066–71.
19. Studer U. Lymph node dissection plays expanding role in urology. Urology times 2003;31:1–27.
20. Myers RP, Cahill DR, Devine RM, et al. Anatomy of radical prostatectomy as defined by magnetic resonance imaging. J Urol 1998;159:2148–58.
21. Van Velthoven RF, Ahlering TE, Peltier A, et al. Technique for laparoscopic running urethrovesical anastomosis: the single knot method. Urology 2003;61:699–702.
22. Kiyoshima K, Yokomizo A, Yoshida T, et al. Anatomical features of periprostatic tissue and its surroundings: a histological analysis of 79 radical retropubic prostatectomy specimens. Jpn J Clin Oncol 2004;34:463–6.
23. Savera A, Kaul S, Badani K, Menon M. Robotic radical prostatectomy with the "Veil of Aphrodite" technique: histologic evidence of enhanced nerve sparing. BJU Int.[In Press]
24. Zvara P, Spiess PE, Merlin SL, et al. Neurogenic erectile dysfunction: the course of nicotinamide adenine dinucleotide phosphate diaphorase—positive nerve fibers on the surface of the prostate. Urology 1996;47:146.
25. Sato Y, Rehman J, Santizo C, et al. Significant physiological roles of ancillary penile nerves on increase in intracavernous pressure in rats: experiments using electrical stimulation of the medial preoptic area. Int J Impot Res 2001;13:82–4.
26. Kaul S, Bhandari A, Hemal A, et al. Robotic radical prostatectomy with preservation of the prostatic fascia: a feasibility study. Urology 2005;66:1261–5.
27. Epstein JI. Incidence and significance of positive surgical margins in radical prostatectomy specimen. UCNA 1996;23:651–63.
28. Menon M, Tewari A, members of the Vattikuti Urology Institute prostatectomy team. Robotic radical prostatectomy and the Vattikuti Urology Institute technique: An interim analysis of results and technical points. Urology 2003; 61:15–20.
29. Wieder JA, Soloway MS. Incidence, etiology, location, prevention and treatment of positive surgical margins after radical prostatectomy for prostate cancer. J Urol 1998; 160:299–315.
30. Tewari A, Shrivastava A, Menon M, members of VIP Team. A prospective comparison of radical retropubic prostatectomy and robot assisted Vattikuti Institute prostatectomy: a single institution experience. BJU Int 2003;205–10.
31. Guillonneau B, El-Fettouh, Baumert X. Laparoscopic radical prostatectomy: oncological evaluation after 1,000 cases at Montsouris Institute. J Urol 2003;169:1261–6.
32. Gill IS, Zippe CD. Laparoscopic radical prostatectomy: technique. UCNA 2001;28:423–36.
33. Salomon L, Levrel O, Taille A, et al. Radical prostatectomy by the retropubic, perineal and laparoscopic approach: 12 years of experience in one center. Eur Urol 2002;42: 104–111.
34. Bundrick WS, Gibbon RP, Weissman RM, et al. The long term efficacy of radical prostatectomy in the management of localized prostate cancer. J Urol 1996;155 Suppl: 558A.
35. Trapasso JG, Weiss JP, Blaivas JG, et al. Nerve-sparing radical perineal prostatectomy: effect on margin status [Abstract]. J Urol 2000;163 Suppl:356.
36. Boccon-Gibod L, Ravery V, Vordos D, et al. Radical prostatectomy for prostate cancer: perineal approach increases

risk of surgically induced positive margins and capsular incisions. J Urol 1998;160:1383–5.

37. Iselin CE, Robertson JE, Paulson DF. Radical perineal prostatectomy: oncological outcome during a 20 year period. J Urol 1999;161:163–8.

38. Weldon VE, Tavel FR. Potency sparing radical perineal prostatectomy: anatomy, surgical technique and initial results. J Urol 1988;140:559–62.

39. Guillonneau B, Cathelineau X, Doublet JD, Vallancien G. Laparoscopic radical prostatectomy: the lessons learned. J Endourol 2001;15:441–5.

40. Steineck G, Helgesen F, Adolfsson J, et al. Scandinavian Prostatic Cancer Group study number 4. Quality of life after radical prostatectomy or watchful waiting. N Engl J Med 2002;347:790–6.

41. Quinlan DM, Epstien JI, Carter BS, Walsh PC. Sexual function following radical prostatectomy: influence of preservation of neurovascular bundles. J Urol 1991;145:998–1002.

42. Kaul S, Savera A, Badani K, et al. Functional outcomes and oncological efficacy of Vattikuti Institute prostatectomy with Veil of Aphrodite nerve-sparing: an analysis of 154 consecutive patients. BJU Int 2006;97:467–72.

43. Weldon VE, Tavel FR, Neuwirth H. Continence, potency and morbidity after radical perineal prostatectomy. J Urol 1997;158:1470–5.

44. Katz R, Salomon L, Hoznek A, et al. Patient reported sexual function following laparoscopic radical prostatectomy. J Urol 2002;168:2078–82.

45. Catalona WJ, Bigg SW. Nerve-sparing radical prostatectomy: evaluations of results after 250 patients. J Urol 1990;143:538–43.

46. Walsh PC, Marschke P, Ricker D, et al. Patient-reported urinary continence and sexual function after anatomic radical prostatectomy. Urology 2000;55:58–61.

47. Leandri P, Rossignol G, Gautier JR, et al. Radical retropubic prostatectomy: morbidity and quality of life. Experience with 620 consecutive cases. J Urol 1992;147:883–7.

48. Andriole GL, Smith DS, Rao G, et al. Early complications of contemporary anatomical radical retropubic prostatectomy. J Urol 1994;152:1858–60.

49. Guillonneau B, Rozet F, Cathelineau X, et al. Perioperative complications of laparoscopic radical prostatectomy: the Montsouris 3-year experience. J Urol 2002;167:51–6.

50. Smith JA Jr. Outcome after radical prostatectomy depends on surgical technique but not approach. Curr Urol Rep 2002;3:179–81.

51. Zippe CD, Rackley RR. Non nerve sparing radical prostatectomy in the elderly patient: perineal vs. retropubic approach [Abstract]. J Urol 1996;155:400.

52. Turk I, Serdar D, Winkelmann B, et al. Laparoscopic radical prostatectomy. Eur Urol 2001;40:46–53.

53. Rassweiler J, Sentker L, Seemann O, et al. Laparoscopic radical prostatectomy with the Heilbronn technique: an analysis of first 180 cases. J Urol 2001;166:2101–8.

54. Farouk A, Gill I, Kaouk J, et al. 150 laparoscopic radical prostatectomy (LRP): learning curve in the United States. J Endourol 2002;16 Suppl 1:A33:P9–2.

55. Bhayani SB, Pavlovich CP, Hsu TS, et al. Prospective comparison of short-term convalescence: laparoscopic radical prostatectomy versus open radical retropubic prostatectomy. Urology 2003;61:612–6.

56. Dahl DM, L'esperance JO, Trainer AF, et al. Laparoscopic radical prostatectomy: initial 70 cases at a U.S. university medical center. Urology 2002;60:859–63.

57. Rassweiler J, Stolzenberg J, Sulser T, et al. Laparoscopic radical prostatectomy—the experience of the German Laparoscopic Working Group. Eur Urol 2006;174:113–9.

58. Tewari A, Kaul S, Menon M. Robotic Radical prostatectomy. A minimally invasive therapy for prostate cancer. Curr Urol Rep 2005;6:46–8.

107

Nerve-Sparing Robotic Prostatectomy

Louis Eichel

Douglas Skarecky

Anthony J. Costello

Thomas E. Ahlering, MD

With the advent of laparoscopic radical prostatectomy popularized by Vallencien and Guilloneau and others during the late 1990s, it has been necessary to apply the developed principles of open, retrograde, nerve-sparing surgery to an antegrade laparoscopic approach. During this period of methodological development, additional breakthroughs were occurring in the field of robotically assisted radical prostatectomy, cavernous nerve mapping, and sural nerve grafting following wide excision of the neurovascular bundle (NVB). Advances in these areas led to important discoveries of the anatomy and physiology of the cavernous nerves and has enhanced our ability to preserve erectile function. Although far from complete, our knowledge regarding the neuroanatomy of the male pelvis has increased immensely. This chapter attempts to summarize current knowledge regarding anatomic principles and technique of cavernous nerve preservation during robotically assisted radical prostatectomy.

ANATOMIC STUDIES OF THE CAVERNOUS NERVES

The anatomic basis for erectile function[1] and the subsequent technique for nerve sparing radical retropubic prostatectomy was described by Walsh and associates in 1983.[2] The authors described the tortuous path of the parasympathetic nerves that run from the pelvic plexus past the seminal vesicles alongside the rectum and then along the posterolateral aspect of the prostate between the true capsule and the lateral prostatic fascia, finally piercing the urogenital diaphragm just posterior and lateral to the urethra. With the widespread popularization of this knowledge, a major emphasis has been placed on cavernous nerve preservation in appropriately selected patients. Since this landmark study that involved fetal and neonatal cadavers, other studies in adult male cadavers led to the discovery of additional findings pertinent to preservation of erectile function.

Takenaka and associates have contributed several papers regarding the pelvic neuroanatomy of the adult male. In two studies, they performed gross and histologic dissections of male cadavers defining the cranial and caudal paths of the cavernous nerves.[3,4] With regard to the origin of the

nerves, they determined that, in most individuals, the traditional neurovascular bundles contain few parasympathetic nerve components proximal to the bladder prostate junction. Instead, parasympathetic nerve branches configured in a "spray-like" distribution approach the dorsolateral prostate at least 20 mm below the bladder-prostate junction. Interestingly, they noted that, in some individuals, the cavernous nerves appear to be located deep to the traditional NVB. This might account for the occasional man who retains sexual function following non–nerve-sparing surgery.

In another paper, Takenaka and associates describe the presence of pelvic autonomic ganglion cells, which lack the capacity for regeneration and hence may have detrimental effects on return of potency.[5] Ganglion cells were found throughout the surfaces of the pelvic viscera including the pelvic plexus, the seminal vesicles, the levator ani muscle, the bladder, and the prostate. The NVB also contained many ganglion cells. The number and distribution varied a great deal, and the authors' speculated that this vari-

ability might contribute to susceptibility or resistance to impotence.

Interestingly, similar studies by Tewari and colleagues have also shown that the pelvic plexus is located on the lateral wall of the rectum.[6,7] The midpoint of the plexus (proximal neurovascular plate) was found to correspond approximately to the tip of the seminal vesicle (Figure 107-1). These authors, like Takenaka, also described the appearance of multiple autonomic ganglia in the vicinity of the cavernous nerves. Both describe interconnections between the left and right cavernous nerves along the anterior rectal wall within Denonvilliers' fascia. Unlike Takenaka however, Tewari and associates describe cavernous branches of the pelvic plexus coalescing to form a more traditional "bundle" that runs within a triangular area (the neurovascular triangle) between the inner and outer layers of the periprostatic fascia and Denonvilliers' fascia. The inner layer of periprostatic fascia (also called the prostatic fascia) forms the medial vertical wall of this triangle; the outer layer of periprostatic fas-

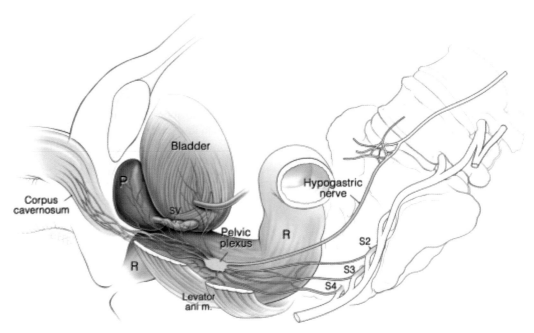

Figure 107-1 Graphic depiction of the neuroanatomy of the male pelvis based on cadaveric dissection. Reproduced with permission from Costello et al.[8]

cia (also called as lateral pelvic fascia) forms the lateral wall, and the posterior wall of this triangle is formed by the anterior layer of Denonvilliers' fascia. This triangular space is wide near the base of the prostate and becomes narrower near the apex. Menon described a belief that additional nerves important for sexual function exist within the periprostatic fascia that covers the lateral and anterior surface of the prostate (aptly named the Veil of Aphrodite). The authors acknowledge they have not traced these nerves to the corpora cavernosa. They also hypothesize that because the plane of dissection is away from the cavernosal nerves, other factors such as decreased traction, avoidance of thermal injury, and preservation of extra blood supply may play a role in preservation of nerve function.

In 2005, Costello and associates reported a detailed description of the plexus of nerves running within the NVB.[8] They found multiple nerve branches (6 to 16 in number) that emanated from the pelvic plexus and spread significantly, with up to 3 cm separating the anterior and posterior nerves, much like the findings of Takenaka and associates (see Figure 107-1). Similar to Menon, Costello noted that the NVB courses along the posterolateral border of the prostate within the bounds of lateral pelvic fascia, the pararectal fascia, and Denonvilliers' fascia. However, in distinction to Menon and associates, they feel that the nerves located within the veil of Aphrodite innervate the prostate only. Similar to Takenaka, Costello found that the nerves converge mid-prostate forming a more condensed bundle and then diverge again when approaching the prostatic apex, where they divide into numerous small branches that descend along the posterolateral aspect of the membranous urethra before penetrating the corpora cavernosa.

PREOPERATIVE CONSIDERATIONS

Preservation of sexual function hinges not only on preservation of the physical structure (ie, the cavernous nerve) but also on traumatic factors such as traction, thermal injury, electrical injury, or inflammatory injury. It has never been suggested, however, nor is it logical that a nerve-sparing radical prostatectomy will make impotent men potent or, for that matter, improve erectile function in men with preoperative diminution of their sexual function. It is impossible and inappropriate to evaluate the presence of preoperative sexual function by asking the patient, "Are you potent?" It is mandatory to have a quantitative assessment of potency, and it should be acquired in an unbiased manner via validated questionnaire. There are a number of validated questionnaires that assess sexual function, and it is our opinion that the International Index of Erectile Function (IIEF) is a reliable means to assess preoperative sexual function. It has also been our experience that shorter forms are more practical than longer forms, simply because men are more likely to fully fill out the shorter forms. Hence, we recommend use of the abbreviated, 5-item questionnaire known as IIEF-5 (see Appendix), also identified

as Sexual Health Inventory for Men (SHIM). Using the IIEF-5 a score of 22-25 is considered normal; 17-21 mild; 12-16 mild to moderate; 8-11 moderate and 1-7 severe dysfunction. It is also recognized that age, especially over age 65, has a deleterious effect on return of sexual function. Lastly, medical conditions and associated medications (eg, anti-hypertensives) can have a significant negative impact on return of sexual function.

It is very important to evaluate and decide preoperatively which patients are candidates for bilateral versus unilateral nerve preservation based on factors that assess risk for extra capsular extension. From a clinical basis, most surgeons assess risk based on the clinical T stage, Gleason score, the number of cores, and the volume of disease on prostate needle biopsy. Some surgeons will assess risk of ECE based on endorectal magnetic resonance imaging or other such findings. It is also necessary for surgeons to know their own pattern of positive margin locations in order to guide and counsel patients. The important point, however, is that it is indeed a risk assessment. With adequate risk assessment, patients can and should play a most definitive role in the decision process of sparing or excising a NVB. We recommend wide excision with abnormal digital findings and/or higher volume disease (> 30 to 40% cores involvement) and higher-grade disease (Gleason Score 4 + 3 and higher).

ANATOMIC FACTORS AFFECTING OPERATIVE TECHNIQUE

It is our belief that, with robotically assisted radical prostatectomy, an antegrade approach to preservation of the neurovascular bundle is preferable to the retrograde approach. First, geometrically speaking, the use of long straight instruments makes the antegrade approach more practical because it is easier to see (especially with 0° and 30° lenses) and dissect in a forward direction towards the penis, as compared to trying to see around the prostate and dissect back towards the bladder. Second, the vascular pedicle to the prostate, in our opinion, is the most important factor to successful nerve preservation with the antegrade approach. There are multiple reasons, including the fact that the vascular pedicle is a very reliable and easy to identify landmark. It always enters the prostate laterally at the base and is a very sturdy structure that cannot be dissected bluntly, requiring sharp transection. Transection of the vascular pedicle is optimized when accomplished with minimal bleeding, and there is growing evidence of the crucial role of no—or minimal—thermal energy in this process. These vessels can be controlled with small laparoscopic hemoclips, or temporarily occluded with a vascular bulldog clamp and oversewn later. After the vascular pedicle has been transected, identification of the plane between the prostatic capsule and the NVB is reliably simple to identify and enter (Figure 107-2). At this point, the texture of the tissue dramatically changes allow-

ing gentle sweeping of the NVB off of the prostatic capsule. As the sweeping process continues towards the apex, smaller but sturdy vessels that resist the gentle sweeping are nerves and vessels that innervate the prostate. These structures require sharp transection in order to avoid entering the prostatic capsule and potentially inducing a surgical margin. The antegrade approach also facilitates the difficult task of separating the NVB from the urethra until last, when the prostate is completely mobilized.

Controversy exists regarding the presence of nerve tissue responsible for erectile function adjacent to the lateral edge of the seminal vesical (SV). In our experience, it is difficult to anatomically picture how cavernosal nerves could course along the length of the SVs and then traverse the prostatic vascular pedicle (see Figure 107-2) and not be transected in conjunction with the vascular pedicle. We agree with the findings of Costello and associates that these nerves innervate the SVs, bladder neck and prostate.[8]

OPERATIVE TECHNICAL ISSUES

VISION Regardless of the surgical task at hand, a clear view of the operative field is the key to successful dissection, and conversely, poor exposure is a recipe for failure. Whether the surgical approach is open, laparoscopic, or robotically assisted, vision is the combined result of hemostasis and retraction.

HEMOSTASIS The most obvious method for maintaining hemostasis during robotically assisted radical prostatectomy is to stay in an avascular plane whenever possible. With regard to cavernous nerve preservation, the plane between the periprostatic fascia and the levator muscles, between the undersurface of the prostate and the rectum, and between the majority of the neurovascular bundle and the prostatic capsule is for the most part avascular. The structure that requires modalities such as cautery, clips, or sutures is the prostatic vascular pedicle.

To avoid cavernosal nerve injury while transecting the prostatic vascular pedicle and dissecting the NVB, it is advisable to avoid electrical and/or thermal injury. The landmark paper by Ong and associates describing the effects of injury on cavernous nerves was performed in a canine model.[9] In this study, monopolar electrocautery, bipolar electrocautery, and harmonic shears were compared to standard suture ligatures for unilateral NVB dissection. The contralateral bundle was not dissected and acted as an internal control. Upon cavernous nerve stimulation, only the energy-free (suture ligature) group maintained similar-to-baseline intracavernosal pressure responses immediately after dissection and two weeks later. The other modalities using electrical energy, heat, or both all resulted in a > 95% decrease in cavernosal pressures. Histologic studies comparing the individual groups confirmed an increased amount of inflammation associated with the use of heat and/or electrocautery.

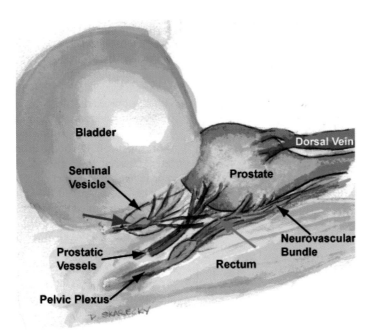

Figure 107-2 Sagittal view of the prostate depicting the relationship of the vascular pedicle of the prostate to the cavernosal nerves. The nerves coursing alongside the seminal vesicle (yellow arrow) would be transected coursing through or around the vascular pedicle on their path to the penis. After transecting the vascular pedicle (red arrow) the texture changes as one engages the neurovascular bundle.

upward, out of the pelvis, and medially. The suction irrigator is used to gently retract the bundle laterally, which accentuates the proper plane of dissection between the bundle and the prostatic capsule (see Figure 107-3C). If the side holes on the suction irrigator are pointed at this plane, irrigation can be applied toward the area of dissection without obstructing or losing exposure (see "title of video" on the accompanying CD-ROM).

The fourth arm can also be used for fixed retraction of the prostate or to retract the bladder if necessary. Another important maneuver is to exchange the scissors to the left for dissection of the left NVB (or to the right for left-handed surgeons). This allows the surgeon to avoid crossing instruments and facilitates the apical dissection (see "title of video" on the accompanying CD-ROM).

POTENCY OUTCOMES WITH CAUTERY-FREE TECHNIQUE

In 2005, we reported outcomes of early three-month return of sexual function in 23 men, comparing our cautery-free technique to our bipolar technique.[11] In Table 107-1, we expanded our experience to 55 men culled from a total of 150 consecutive cases. These 55 represent the men age 65 or less with preoperative IIEF-5 scores of 22 to 25. As illustrated, the groups have nearly identical preoperative clinical data and, as our experience has grown, our results with the cautery-free technique remain stable (43% vs. 42%, p = not significant).

Because of these findings, transection of the vascular pedicles should be accomplished without thermal energy. Commercially available metal or polymer vascular clips are an option for controlling these vessels, but the disadvantage is the potential for clipping over previously placed clips or slipping off. Both Gill and associates and Eichel and associates advocated the use of a temporary vascular clamp (bulldog clamp) to occlude the vascular pedicle of the prostate.[10,11]

In this technique, (see "title of video" on the accompanying CD-ROM) the prostate is sharply dissected from the urogenital diaphragm, the bladder and the rectum. Cautery is used judiciously. The prostate is then retracted upward, and the thick posterior vascular pedicle of the prostate is placed on gentle traction. A straight or curved bulldog clamp (30 mm) is placed on the pedicle at least 10 to 15 mm from the prostate (Figure 107-3A). Sharp scissors are used to divide the pedicle close to the base of the prostate (Figure 107-3B). Once this thick posterior pedicle is divided, the prostate is more mobile and an obvious change in texture occurs signifying the transition to the NVB. The gland can be retracted medially and the NVB can be gently teased off the prostatic capsule (Figure 107-3C). The bundle is freed from the prostate completely to the level of the urethra (Figure 107-3D). During the dissection, no thermal energy is applied to small bleeders because these vessels often simply clot prior to performing the vesicourethral anastomosis. If arterial bleeding persists after the prostate is completely freed, however, the vessel is precisely ligated with absorbable 4-0 suture on an RB needle. Similarly, the bulldog clamps are removed, and the pedicles controlled with suture ligation.

Another important instrument in terms of exposure and keeping the field clear is the suction irrigator. During dissection of the NVB, the assistant uses a grasper to retract the prostate

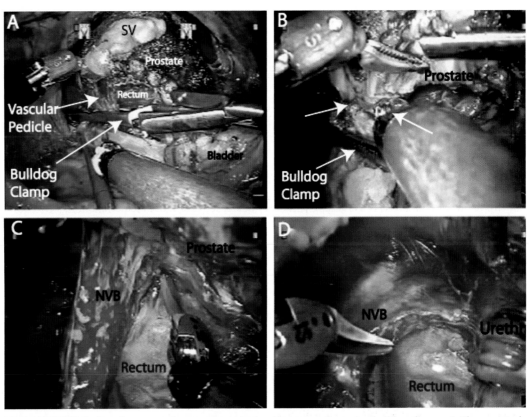

Figure 107-3 Technique for cautery-free neurovascular bundle preservation using bulldog clamps. *A,* The prostate is retracted upward by the assistant, and a bulldog clamp is applied to the prostatic vascular pedicle. *B,* The appropriate starting point for cold division of the vascular pedicle of the prostate. *C,* Lateral retraction of the neurovascular bundle at the mid prostatic level. *D,* Lateral retraction of the neurovascular bundle at the apical level.

Table 107-1 Comparison of Potency Outcomes at 3 Months, Group1 versus Group 2				
Clinical Factor (mean)	Initial* (CFT)	Group 1 (CFT)	Group 2 (Bipolar)	p-value
Number of Patients	23	55	36	
Age	55.7 (48–65)	56.7 (48–65)	56.5 (43–65)	NS
Preoperative SHIMa	24.3	24.4 (22–25)	24.3 (22–25)	NS
PSA ng/mL	5.9 (1.2–16.8)	5.5 (0.5–16.8)	6.6 (1.2–23.0)	NS
Mean Gleason Score	6.4	6.4	6.4	NS
EBL cc	107 (50–225)	107 (50–225)	86 (25–250)	.07
Positive Margins	5 (21.7%)	6 (11.8%)	6(16.7%)	NS
Length of Stay (days)	1.1 (1–2)	1.1 (1–2)	1.1 (1–5)	NS
Complications	0	1 (2.0%)	1(2.7%)	NS
Nerve Sparing				
Bilateral	17 (74%)	42 (76%)	28 (78%)	NS
Unilateral	6 (26%)	13 (24%)	8 (22%)	NS
Potency @ 3 mos:				
All NS	10/23 (43%)	23/55 (42%)	3/36 (8.3%)	<.001†
Bilateral NS	8/17 (47%)	17/42 (41%)	3/28 (11%)	.008†
Unilateral NS	2/6 (33%)	6/13 (46%)	0/8	.05†
AVE SHIM (Potent Men)	15.7	17.6	17.0	NS
Potency @ 9 mos:				
All NS	NA	26/34 (77%)	6/30 (20%)	<.001*
Bilateral NS	NA	20/25 (80%)	5/22 (23%)	<.001**
Unilateral NS	NA	6/9 (67%)	1/8 (13%)	.05**
AVE SHIM (Potent Men)	NA	18.9	14.4	NS

Adapted from Eichel et al.[11]
*Initial refers to the 23 men published previously
†Fisher exact T-test, 2-sided

The expanded group of 55 patients increases the statistical power of the nearly sixfold increase in return of sexual potency (42% vs. 8.3%, $p < .001$) within 3 months. In addition to our three-month data, we now have 34 patients (of the initial 55) who have follow-up data at nine months. The rate of erections adequate for vaginal penetration is approximately 80% with an average IIEF-5 score of 18.9. As noted in Table 107-1, successful "vaginal penetration" is accompanied with more global sexual satisfaction. At 3 months, "potent" men had an average IIEF-5 of 17.6 (range 12 to 25) compared to impotent men at 2.3 (range 1 to 7).

At this writing, there were no established means to measure partial recovery of erectile function in "impotent" men. We have attempted to qualitatively address partial recovery by asking patients about erectile fullness. Assessing partial recovery (ie, 25 to 75% fullness) versus no recovery (0%) arguably presents at least some qualitative assessment of erectile blood flow. Again, in men reporting erections inadequate for vaginal penetration, 33% of the CFT group reported zero fullness, versus 60% of the bipolar group at 3 months following surgery.

A finding of interest is the relatively high rate of potency preservation in patients undergoing unilateral nerve preservation. A possible explanation for this finding is cross-coverage and regenerative compensation. Although the numbers are relatively small, it has been a consistent finding that unilateral nerve preservation has not resulted in significant (ie, 50% of our bilateral nerve-sparing) potency results. Time will tell if these findings are simply a result of an inadequate sample size.

POSTOPERATIVE PROPHYLAXIS FOR ERECTILE DYSFUNCTION

In experimental models, it has been shown that injury to cavernous nerves in rats leads to endothelial cell apoptosis, decreased nitric oxide levels, and hypoxia leading to fibrosis and loss of smooth muscle in the corpora cavernosa.[12–15] In humans, there is clear evidence that fibrosis and loss of smooth muscle occurs and that vasculogenic effects occur as a result. Mulhall and associates first noted that arterial insufficiency occurs in approximately 50% of patients following RP and does not improve within a year of surgery. In addition, approximately 50% of patients developed a venous leak one year following surgery, which was also associated with a decreased return of erectile function.[16] Montorsi and associates reported that 6 months following surgery spontaneous erection occurred in 67% of patients who performed self injection with prostaglandin E_1 (PGE$_1$), compared to 20% in patients that did not use injection therapy. Only 17% of patients who injected PGE$_1$ developed venous leak by Doppler ultrasound criteria, versus 53% of patients who did not.[17] Similar findings have been reported both for PGE$_1$ urethral suppositories[18] (Alprostadil, Vivus) and vacuum devices.[19]

In 2003, Padma-Nathan and associates in a randomized prospective study reported that 27% of 51 patients who were potent prior to bilateral nerve-sparing radical retropubic prostatectomy who took sildenafil citrate at bedtime for 9 months regained full potency, versus only 4%

of patients that did not.[20,21] In order to be considered potent and included in this study, men had to score 8 to 10 on Question 3 and Question 4 of the IIEF-5 and pass a nocturnal penile tumescence examination. The men took either 50 mg or 100 mg of sildenafil or a placebo starting one month after surgery and continuing for 9 months. Then, at 10 months following surgery, the men were taken off of medication and two months later retested with the IIEF-5 questions and repeat penile tumescence. These findings may possibly be explained by Schwartz and associates, who examined the effect of sildenafil citrate on the smooth muscle content of the corporal bodies after RRP.[22] In this study, patients were divided into 2 groups; one receiving 50 mg every other night for 6 months following surgery and the other 100 mg. The higher dose group had a statistically significant increase in smooth muscle present on postoperative biopsy.

Although the cumulative knowledge regarding novel prophylactic treatments to hasten the return of erectile function in men following RRP is encouraging, there is no regimen that is clearly superior. Further, there is no consensus amongst experts with regard to the most effective agent or combination of agents to use. We currently recommend 25 mg of sildenafil citrate nightly, starting on the first postoperative day.

CONCLUSION

Great strides have been made in the last quarter century with regard to our current understanding of the neuroanatomy of the male pelvis. This knowledge has enabled us to make great progress in preserving the cavernosal nerves during radical prostatectomy. Robotically assisted technology offers several advantages, including antegrade dissection of the neurovascular bundle without excessive traction. Great care should be taken to avoid electrocautery and excessive heat application in the area housing the cavernous nerves. Our results using a cautery-free technique seem to hasten the return of erectile function. Novel therapies to hasten the return of erectile function following RRP are forthcoming.

REFERENCES

1. Walsh PC, Donker PJ. Impotence following radical prostatectomy: insight into etiology and prevention. J Urol 1982; 128:492.
2. Walsh PC, Lepor H, Eggleston JC. Radical prostatectomy with preservation of sexual function: anatomical and pathological considerations. Prostate 1983;4:473.
3. Takenaka A, Murakami G, Matsubara A, et al. Variation in course of cavernous nerve with special reference to details of topographic relationships near prostatic apex: histologic study using male cadavers. Urology 2005;65:136.
4. Takenaka A, Murakami G, Soga H, et al. Anatomical analysis of the neurovascular bundle supplying penile cavernous tissue to ensure a reliable nerve graft after radical prostatectomy. J Urol 2004;172:1032.
5. Takenaka A, Kawada M, Murakami G, et al. Interindividual variation in distribution of extramural ganglion cells in the male pelvis: a semi-quantitative and immunohistochemical study concerning nerve-sparing pelvic surgery. Eur Urol 2005;48:46.
6. Tewari A, Peabody JO, Fischer M, et al. An operative and anatomic study to help in nerve sparing during laparo-

scopic and robotic radical prostatectomy. Eur Urol 2003;43:444.

7. Tewari A, El-Hakim A, Horninger W, et al. Nerve-sparing during robotic radical prostatectomy: use of computer modeling and anatomic data to establish critical steps and maneuvers. Curr Urol Rep 2005;6:126.

8. Costello AJ, Brooks M, Cole OJ. Anatomical studies of the neurovascular bundle and cavernosal nerves. BJU Int 2004;94:1071.

9. Ong AM, Su LM, Varkarakis I, et al. Nerve sparing radical prostatectomy: effects of hemostatic energy sources on the recovery of cavernous nerve function in a canine model. J Urol 2004;172:1318.

10. Gill IS, Ukimura O, Rubinstein M, et al. Lateral pedicle control during laparoscopic radical prostatectomy: refined technique. Urology 2005;65:23.

11. Eichel L, Ahlering TE, Chou D, et al. Feasibility study for robotic radical prostatectomy cautery-free neurovascular bundle preservation. Urology 2005;65:994.

12. Klein LT, Miller MI, Buttyan R, et al. Apoptosis in the rat penis after penile denervation. J Urol 1997;158:626.

13. Rehman J, Christ GJ, Kaynan A, et al. Intraoperative electrical stimulation of cavernosal nerves with monitoring of intracorporeal pressure in patients undergoing nerve sparing radical prostatectomy. BJU Int 1999;84:305.

14. User HM, Hairston JH, Zelner DJ, et al. Penile weight and cell subtype specific changes in a post-radical prostatectomy model of erectile dysfunction. J Urol 2003;169:1175.

15. Leungwattanakij S, Bivalacqua TJ, Usta MF, et al. Cavernous neurotomy causes hypoxia and fibrosis in rat corpus cavernosum. J Androl 2003;24:239.

16. Mulhall JP, Slovick R, Hotaling J, et al. Erectile dysfunction after radical prostatectomy: hemodynamic profiles and their correlation with the recovery of erectile function. J Urol 2002;167:1371.

17. Montorsi F, Guazzoni G, Strambi LF, et al. Recovery of spontaneous erectile function after nerve-sparing radical retropubic prostatectomy with and without early intracavernous injections of alprostadil: results of a prospective, randomized trial. J Urol 1997;158:1408.

18. Zippe C. Early use of MUSE following radical prostatectomy facilitates earlier return of erectile function and successful sexual activity. Edited by A. R. T. Symposium. Irvine, CA, 2006.

19. Raina R, Agarwal A, Ausmundson S, et al. Early use of vacuum constriction device following radical prostatectomy facilitates early sexual activity and potentially earlier return of erectile function. Int J Impot Res 2006;18:77.

20. Padma-Nathan H, et al. Postoperative nightly administration of sildenafil citrate significantly improves the return of normal spontaneous erectile function after bilateral nerve sparing radical prostatectomy. J Urol 2003;169:1402.

21. Padma-Nathan H, McCullough A, Forest C. Erectile dysfunction secondary to nerve-sparing radical retropubic prostatectomy: comparative phosphodiesterase-5 inhibitor efficacy for therapy and novel prevention strategies. Curr Urol Rep 2004;5:467.

22. Schwartz EJ, Wong P, Graydon RJ. Sildenafil preserves intracorporeal smooth muscle after radical retropubic prostatectomy. J Urol 2004;171:771.

23. Cappelleri JC, Rosen RC. The Sexual Health Inventory for Men (SHIM): a five year review of research and clinical experience. Int J Impot Res 2005;17:307.

Appendix 107-1

The five-item Sexual Health Inventory for Men (SHIM),[23] also known as the International Index of Erectile Function (IIEF)-5.

Question 1

How do you rate your <u>confidence</u> that you could get and keep and erection?
1. Very low
2. Low
3. Moderate
4. High
5. Very High

Question 2

When you had erections with sexual stimulation, <u>how often</u> were your erections hard enough for penetration (entering your partner)?
0. No sexual activity
1. Almost never or never
2. A few times (much less than half the time)
3. Sometimes (about half the time)
4. Most times (much more than half the time)
5. Almost always or always

Question 3

During sexual intercourse, <u>how often</u> were you able to maintain your erection after you had penetrated (entered) your partner?
0. Did not attempt intercourse
1. Almost never or never
2. A few times (much less than half the time)
3. Sometimes (about half the time)
4. Most times (much more than half the time)
5. Almost always or always

Question 4

During sexual intercourse, <u>how difficult</u> was it to maintain your erection to completion of intercourse?
0. Did not attempt intercourse
1. Extremely Difficult
2. Very Difficult
3. Difficult
4. Slightly Difficult
5. Not Difficult

Question 5

When you attempted sexual intercourse, <u>how often</u> was it satisfactory to you?
0. Did not attempt intercourse
1. Almost never or never
2. A few times (much less than half the time)
3. Sometimes (about half the time)
4. Most times (much more than half the time)
5. Almost always or always

108

Pediatric Robotic-Assisted Antireflux Surgery

Hillary L. Copp, MD
Craig A. Peters, MD, FAAP, FACS

Robotic-assisted laparoscopic surgery emerged within the adult urology community over the last decade.[1] It has facilitated the acquisition of laparoscopic skills for the non-laparoscopically trained surgeon and permitted the maintenance of these skills without a rigorous case-load. Gradually, there has been limited application of this approach to the pediatric urologic patient population due to its potential for enhancement of general and reconstructive laparoscopic skills.[2–4] Robotic-assisted surgery in pediatric urology may have the ability to diminish the learning curve required of laparoscopy while still providing the benefits of minimally invasive surgery. These benefits potentially include reduced incision size, decreased morbidity, shorter hospital stay, and a less painful and more rapid recovery. Furthermore, it may be able to improve the outcomes of the experienced laparoscopist.

There have been various applications of robotic-assisted surgery within pediatric urology. Many of the initial experiences have involved renal surgery.[5–7] As surgeons have adopted this technology, however, they have expanded its application to other areas where standard laparoscopic surgery has been used, including pelvic and bladder surgery.[4,8,9] Specifically, with the demonstration of successful laparoscopic antireflux surgery, the robotic-assisted approach has been applied to ureteral reimplantation.[4,10,11] This chapter will address the general principles and specific surgical approaches of pediatric robotic-assisted antireflux surgery. Complications, limitations, and future advancements of robotic-assisted antireflux surgery in the pediatric urologic population will be covered.

GENERAL PRINCIPLES AND TECHNIQUES

Specific indications as to whether a patient should undergo an extravesical or intravesical robotic reimplantation are the same as that for open or laparoscopic surgery. That said, if a patient has bilateral reflux, an intravesical approach is preferred, secondary to the potential for postoperative urinary retention with bilateral extravesical reimplantation. Although there is a report that the incidence of postoperative urinary retention with bilateral reimplantation is less with a laparoscopic approach,[12] there appears to be some risk of urinary retention, although the significance is unclear. At present, robotic-

assisted extravesical reimplantation is pursued mostly when unilateral reflux is present.

Furthermore, general patient selection for robotic-assisted surgery is equivalent to that of standard laparoscopic surgery. Most contraindications are relative and may vary depending on the surgeon's experience and comfort level. Common relative contraindications include obesity or previous intraperitoneal surgery, but there are a handful of absolute contraindications. These include uncorrectable coagulopathy, intestinal obstruction, abdominal wall infection, massive hemoperitoneum, generalized peritonitis, and suspected malignant ascites,[13] few of which would apply to elective antireflux surgery.

Furthermore, baseline patient issues may be exacerbated by the physiologic effects of pneumoperitoneum. Therefore, patients with conditions such as obstructive airway disease or cardiac issues may not be able to tolerate this type of surgery and should be screened accordingly.[14,15] Additionally, the physiologic effects of carbon dioxide pneumovesicum associated with the transvesical approach are yet to be determined.

Initially, it was thought that lack of tactile feedback with robotic-assisted surgery would be problematic in smaller patients. With appropriate training and experience, however, this issue is less significant and has not seemed to disqualify pediatric patients from undergoing robotic surgery.[6] Patients as young as 0.2 years have successfully undergone robotic-assisted laparoscopic urologic surgery.[5] That said, specific to the intravesical approach, some concern has been voiced in regard to adequate closure of cystotomies owing to the relatively large size of the cannulae versus the small bladder capacity in the young child.[2,4,11]

PATIENT PREPARATION AND POSITIONING

Bowel preparation begins 24 hours before surgery with a clear liquid diet and a glycerin suppository the night before surgery. After anesthesia is induced, a rectal tube is placed for decompression of the rectosigmoid. The bladder catheter is introduced on the sterile field.

For both of the reimplantation approaches, the patient is placed in the supine position with the feet at the end of the operating room table. The robot will be brought in from the patient's feet (Figure 108-1). The bed is kept flat for intravesical reimplantation, while the patient is placed

in Trendelenburg's position for the extravesical approach. No flexion in the table is necessary. All patient positioning and table adjustments must be done prior to engaging the robot.

PORT SITE SELECTION

Basic principles of laparoscopic port placement apply to both approaches in robotic-assisted reimplantation. Importantly, the ports must be placed symmetrically in relation to the site of operation. The central port is reserved for the camera. It is in line with the operative site creating the central axis. The two lateral working ports are placed equidistantly along a line that is perpendicular to the central axis and in closer proximity to the operative site.

A 30-degree, 12-mm telescope is used. A standard laparoscopic cannula will accommodate this scope. The DeBakey forceps or the 5-mm Maryland dissectors are used for tissue handling, manipulation and dissection. The 5-mm hook cautery is a versatile tool not only for hemostasis, but also for tissue dissection. It is the only electrified instrument used. For dissection, it performs better when the elbow of the instrument is pushed against the tissue rather than pulling at the tissue with the hook. The 8-mm needle driver can be used for suturing and is available in both large and fine-tip sizes. The fine needle driver is used for suture smaller than 3-0. Both 8- and 5-mm, non-electrified straight scissors are used for cutting suture. The 8-mm curved electrified scissors are used when larger ports are in place. Due to the design of the instruments, the 5-mm devices require more working space to move the tip of the instrument in a right angle versus the 8-mm instruments.

SPECIFIC APPROACHES TO ROBOTIC-ASSISTED URETERAL REIMPLANTATION

The first reported description of laparoscopic correction of vesicoureteral reflux (VUR) was reported by Atala and colleagues using a modification of the Lich technique in a porcine model in 1993.[16] Less than a year later, the laparoscopic application of the Lich-Gregoir technique was described in humans by Ehrlich and colleagues[17] and has been reproduced and reported by others in the literature.[18,19] In 2005, laparoscopic cross-trigonal ureteral reimplantation with carbon dioxide pneumovesicum was reported as well.[20]

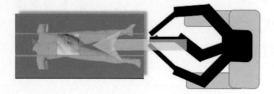

Figure 108-1 Positioning of the robotic system for both extravesical and intravesical antireflux procedures.

Laparoscopic ureteral reimplantation, however, has not become common practice, likely secondary to the technical challenge of the procedure.

In contrast, robotic-assisted laparoscopic surgery appears more technically feasible and potentially applicable to a larger number of surgeons without extensive laparoscopic training. The increased feasibility of this approach is likely due to a number of characteristics afforded by the robot. These include magnification, three-dimensional vision, tremor-filtered instrument control, movement scaling, and wrist-like articulation of the instruments. Accordingly, robotic-assisted vesicoureteral reimplantation surgery utilizing both approaches has materialized over the last few years. The initial report of robotic-assisted pneumovesical ureteral reimplantation was performed in a porcine model by Olsen and colleagues in 2003.[10] Both robotic-assisted extravesical and transvesical ureteral reimplantation were performed and reported in the pediatric population within the next year.[4,11]

EXTRAVESICAL URETERAL REIMPLANTATION

PORT PLACEMENT Access for extravesical robotic-assisted reimplantation is transperitoneal using a modified Lich-Gregoir extravesical reimplant technique.[21] The patient is placed in Trendelenburg's position. The central camera port is placed in the inferior portion of the umbilicus using the Bailez technique.[22] Pneumoperitoneum is established with insufflation of carbon dioxide at a rate of 4 liters per minute up to a pressure of 12 mm Hg. The 5- or 8-mm robotic working ports are positioned just below the level of the umbilicus in the manner previously described (Figure 108-2). They are placed under direct visualization through the fascia with the sharp obturator. Prior to insertion of all cannulae, fascial sutures in a box stitch fashion are placed.[23] This not only helps with later closure of the fascia, but also assists in securing the ports to the abdominal wall. Once the ports are placed and the surgeon is satisfied with the access, the robot is engaged.

DESCRIPTION OF THE OPERATION The obliterated umbilical artery is traced down along the abdominal wall and bladder side wall into the pelvis. The ureter is identified passing under and medial to the obliterated umbilical artery. The peritoneum over the ureter is then incised. In boys the vas deferens is identified and mobilized superiorly. Similarly, in girls the uterine ligament and pedicle are swept posteriorly. The ureter is mobi-

lized adjacent to the bladder for 4 to 5 cm down to the ureterovesical junction. A bladder hitch stitch can be placed to draw the bladder up and over to the contralateral side to improve exposure of the operative site.[4] With the bladder partially filled, a 2.5- to 3-cm incision in the detrusor muscle down to the underlying the mucosa is made. The detrusor muscle is then peeled away laterally creating flaps of muscle that will later be used to wrap the ureter to create its tunnel (Figure 108-3). The ureteral hiatus is mobilized in a Y-shaped fashion. All dissection is performed close to the ureter and careful attention is paid to not extend the dissection dorsomedially along the distal ureter.[24] The detrusor flaps are then wrapped around the ureter and approximated with 3-0 or 4-0 polydioxanone or Vicryl suture (Figure 108-4). No bladder catheter postoperatively is necessary if mucosal injury does not occur.

RESULTS Table 108-1 illustrates the outcomes of the author's experience with robotic-assisted extravesical reimplantation. A total of 24 patients had robotic-assisted antireflux surgery performed. The mean age was 6.5 years (range, 4.6 months to 11.3 years). Twenty-one patients had a unilateral reimplant, whereas three had bilateral reimplants. One patient was lost to follow-up. Persistent reflux was noted in three of 23 patients. In two of those patients, reflux was reduced to grade 1 or 2 reflux, whereas the third patient had stable grade 2 reflux.

One patient's postoperative course was complicated by a bladder leak requiring catheterization and increased hospital stay. In addition, transient postoperative urinary retention occurred in one patient following bilateral reimplantation.

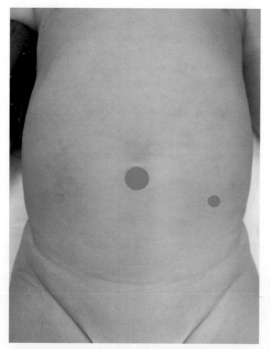

Figure 108-2 Port site placement for extravesical reflux correction. The camera is in the umbilicus while the working ports are placed in the mid-clavicular line, just below the level of the umbilicus.

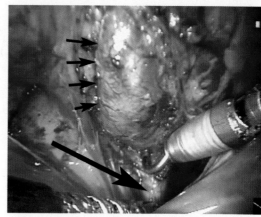

Figure 108-3 Operative image of the creation of the detrusor flaps after incision of the muscularis of the bladder. The mucosa is visible, bulging from the detrusor trough, and the left edge is indicated (*small arrows*). The ureteral hiatus is at the base of the tunnel (*large arrow*).

Lastly, one child who underwent unilateral nephrectomy with contralateral extravesical ureteroneocystostomy required a stent after developing hydronephrosis and a rising creatinine. One month after stent removal, the child had no hydronephrosis, resolved reflux, and a normal creatinine. This case led the author to place a ureteral stent in patients with solitary kidneys undergoing laparoscopic antireflux procedures.

Comparative results with open extravesical reimplantation are shown in Table 108-1. Operative time is longer than that of open surgery, but this would likely improve as the learning curve is tackled. In fact, the author's operative time is now equivalent to that of open surgery. Length of stay and analgesia requirements are significantly less with robotic surgery.

The reflux cessation rate for robotic extravesical reimplantation is 87%. The success rates quoted in the literature for open extravesical reimplantation range between 92.5 and 98%.[25] Although this is better than the initial robotic-assisted extravesical reimplant series, a larger robotic-assisted surgery sample size is needed to soundly evaluate this. Moreover, the author's

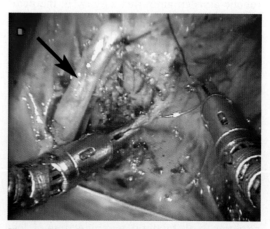

Figure 108-4 Closure of the detrusor tunnel with interrupted braided absorbable sutures. The initial suture at the most proximal end of the tunnel brings the ureter (*arrow*) into the tunnel, and the detrusor flaps are then closed over it.

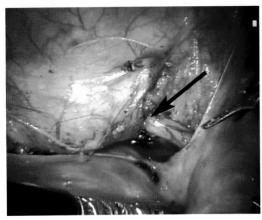

Figure 108-5 Appearance of a completed extravesical right ureteral reconstruction. The ureter can be seen entering its tunnel (*arrow*).

Table 108-1 Robotic and Open Extravesical Antireflux Procedures (Age-Matched Patients)			
	Robotic	Open	*p* Value (paired t-test)
Operative time (min)	179	134	< .001
LOS (hr)	38	61	< .001
First PO intake (hr)	6.5	9.0	NSS (.165)
Analgesia (MSO$_4$ equivalents mg/kg)	1.00	1.38	< .02

LOS = length of stay; MSO$_4$ = morphine equivalent; NSS = not statistically significant; PO = oral.

comparative results in a contemporary, age-matched analysis showed no statistically significant difference in reflux cessation rates between the robotic and open extravesical reimplants. Furthermore, these differences may be reflective of the learning curve, and we may find that the success rate is falsely lowered owing to initial lack of mastery of the technology. That said, the early results clearly underscore the importance of ensuring good tissue quality and adequate length of the tunnel, just as in the open procedure.

INTRAVESICAL URETERAL REIMPLANTATION

PORT PLACEMENT   The robotic-assisted intravesical reimplant is performed via a transvesical approach using the established cross-trigonal Cohen technique.[26] Prior to placement of the cannulae, an 8 French catheter is positioned in the urethra, and the bladder is filled with saline. This not only helps access with the camera, but is also important in facilitating the placement of the two working ports. The urethral catheter is used to evacuate urine and blood that accumulates during the procedure. Suction may be applied intermittently to the catheter to clear the operative field. The central camera port is placed into the dome of the bladder. A 12-mm transverse suprapubic incision is made and then, through blunt dissection, Retzius' space is entered, and the bladder dome is identified. A 3-0 Vicryl suture is used to place a box stitch in the detrusor muscle. This delivers the bladder dome up into the incision and aides with cannula placement. The stitch also functions to hold the bladder wall up during the surgery and to facilitate closure of the cystotomy at completion of the operation. The Veress needle is then used to place the 12-mm VersaStep sheath and cannula. The camera is introduced through the cannula into the bladder. Cannulae can be placed using cystoscopic guidance, as well, to ensure optimal positioning at the dome of the bladder.

Next, the sites for the working ports are selected halfway between the umbilicus and the pubis (Figure 108-5). Purse string sutures are placed, as with the camera port. Under direct visualization, the Veress needle is used to place the VersaStep sheath. Subsequently the 8-mm robotic cannulae are introduced with the blunt-tip obturator. The bladder is then insufflated with carbon dioxide to a pressure of 8 to 10 mm Hg, displacing the saline (Figure 108-6). The ports are secured, and the bladder wall is lifted out of the field using the previously placed detrusor box stitch sutures. The robot is brought in from the foot of the bed and docked.

Yeung described a technique of passing sutures through two angiocatheters, one with a loop snare, which may be particularly useful in patients with more subcutaneous fat (Figure 108-7).[20] Two such sutures would function like a purse-string suture.

DESCRIPTION OF THE OPERATION   Now that the set-up is complete, the operation proceeds in a manner similar to that of the open operation. First, the ureters are stented with a 6-cm segment of a 5F feeding tube. The stent is secured to the ureteral meatus with a 4-0 Vicryl suture and can be used to place traction on the ureter to aid with

dissection. The ureters are mobilized using cautery and blunt dissection in a manner similar to that used in open surgery. Assessment of adequate ureteral mobilization is through visual inspection since normal tactile feedback is not present (Figure 108-8). Each original ureteral muscular hiatus is reduced in size with 4-0 Vicryl suture as needed. The submucosal tunnels are then created using sharp dissection starting in the area of the original hiatus and working to the opposite side of the trigone (Figure 108-9). A new mucosal opening for the ureter is formed by making a small incision in the overlying mucosa. Typically, the lower ureter may exit at the prior mucosal hiatus of the contralateral ureter. Each ureter is grasped by its stent and led through its respective tunnel to its new contralateral mucosal hiatus. The feeding tubes are then removed so the ureters can be sewn into place. Three anchoring 4-0 Monocryl sutures secure each ureter to the mucosa and underlying detrusor muscle. The remainder of the ureteral cuff is sutured into position with 5-0 Monocryl. The mucosal defects at each ureteral hiatus is closed with 5-0 Monocryl. To assess patency a 5F feeding tube is again passed up the ureter (Figure 108-10).

The bladder is irrigated and evaluated for hemostasis. Next, the working ports are removed, and the pneumovesicum is evacuated. The pre-placed detrusor box stitch sutures are tied down and then inspected visually with the telescope to assess for adequate closure of the bladder wall. The suture ends are not cut until it is confirmed that satisfactory closure of the port sites has been achieved. If necessary, this allows the port site to be lifted up into the wound for exposure if

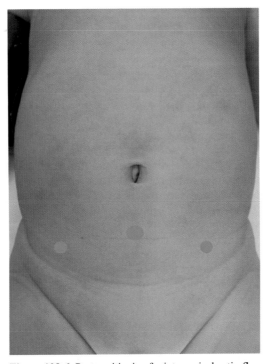

Figure 108-6 Port positioning for intravesical antireflux procedure. The camera port is in the midline below the umbilicus at the dome of the bladder by palpation. Lateral ports are placed where the bladder edge is palpable with distension.

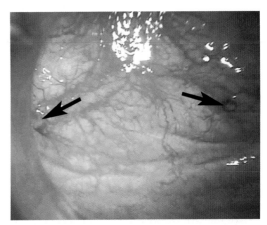

Figure 108-7 View of the trigone at the time of an intravesical antireflux procedure. The gapping ureteral orifices are visible (*arrows*) and will be cannulated and mobilized.

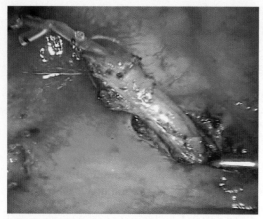

Figure 108-8 Mobilization of the left ureter using intravesical robotic-assisted system. There is excellent visualization of the tissues and complete control of the ureter. Visual clues are used to assess tension and the point of satisfactory mobilization.

another stitch needs to be placed. After this, the telescope is removed and its port site is closed in a similar fashion. The fascial defects are closed in the standard fashion. The subcutaneous tissue and skin are approximated with a 4-0 Vicryl and a 4-0 subcuticular Monocryl suture, respectively. The urethral catheter is left in place for 24 hours.

RESULTS This technique has been applied in eight children with ages ranging between 5 to 15 years.[11] All operations were completed robotically without the need to convert to open surgery. The operative time was longer than open surgery, but with experience, this has decreased. Length of hospital stay was between 2 and 4 days.

Five of six patients with follow-up had cessation of reflux. One patient had persistent lowgrade reflux on initial follow-up. His 6-month voiding cystourethrogram demonstrated grade 2 VUR, improved from grade 3. There were no patients with obstruction. One girl had a urine leak postoperatively from inadequate port-site closure and required prolonged catheterization. The catheter was removed after 1 week and sub-

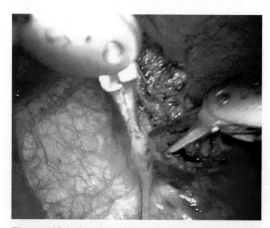

Figure 108-9 Creation of the submucosal tunnel is performed with sharp dissection from the original hiatus to the opposite side of the trigone and into the hiatus of the opposite ureter. Each hiatus has been slightly closed using absorbable suture.

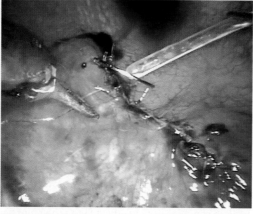

Figure 108-10 Passing a 5 French feeding tube through the reimplanted ureter to confirm patency following completion of the procedure

sequent cystogram demonstrated resolution of urine leak and reflux.

Throughout the development of this approach, there have been modifications to our technique that bear mentioning. First, waiting to transition to pneumovesicum until after the working ports have been placed has proven more effective than placing the working ports after insufflation. The bladder is less likely to collapse if filled with saline versus carbon dioxide when high intravesical pressures are induced from an external source, such as with port placement. Also, a good seal around the port sites to avoid leakage and accumulation of carbon dioxide in the retroperitoneum is crucial. This is obtained by a combination of avoidance of an overly large cystotomy with initial access and placement of a functioning box stitch to cinch the detrusor muscle around the port. In addition, closure of the port sites can be difficult. The pre-placed sutures help dramatically, but in older individuals with more subcutaneous tissue, this can still be challenging. If the closure does not appear adequate, a second stitch may be placed by lifting the puncture site into the wound and placing an additional figure-of-eight suture.

Although the intravesical robotic-assisted reimplantation technique is still evolving, an advantage to this approach was clear early on. The development of the submucosal tunnel is more efficient and facile due to the articulation capabilities of the robot. This allows the scissors to be completely parallel to the trigone and greatly facilitates submucosal tunnel formation. It is not possible to achieve this angle of approach with either open or pure laparoscopic surgery.

We used this technique to perform a ureterocele excision and common sheath reimplantation in a child, suggesting the potentially wide applicability of this approach.

SUMMARY

While robotic-assisted ureteral reimplantation does have its challenges, it has the potential to provide significant benefit. The possibility for decreased morbidity exists with decreased postoperative pain, shorter hospital stays, and smaller

incisions. However, the already high success rates, good postoperative pain management, short hospital stays, and small surgical scars with the open antireflux procedures will make its advantages over open surgery difficult to establish.[27–30] As technology continues to evolve, we can expect smaller working instruments and improved tissue handling devices for the robot that may make the described techniques more efficient in the pediatric population. We should also expect to see a decrease in cost for purchasing and maintaining robots, as their usage becomes more widespread. Furthermore, if the demand for minimally invasive surgery continues to grow, the ability for more surgeons to acquire and use these skills will be augmented by the robot's ability to facilitate typically difficult, standard laparoscopic tasks. Robotic assistance makes remote surgery a possibility, thereby affording a patient, who would otherwise not have access to an experienced surgeon, the ability to have an equivalent level of care.[31] In conclusion, the results of the initial experiences with robotic-assisted antireflux surgery are encouraging and certainly merit further investigation.

REFERENCES

1. Partin AW, Adams JB, Moore RG, Kavoussi LR. Complete robot-assisted laparoscopic urologic surgery: a preliminary report. J Am Coll Surg 1995;181:552–7.
2. Olsen LH. Robotics in paediatric urology. J Ped Urol 2006; 2:40–5.
3. Woo R, Le D, Krummel TM, Albanese C. Robot-assisted pediatric surgery. Am J Surg 2004;188:27S–37S.
4. Peters CA. Robotically assisted surgery in pediatric urology. Urol Clin North Am 2004;31:743–52.
5. Lee RS, Retik AB, Borer JG, Peters CA. Pediatric robot assisted laparoscopic dismembered pyeloplasty: comparison with a cohort of open surgery. J Urol 2006;175: 683–7.
6. Olsen LH, Jorgensen TM. Computer assisted pyeloplasty in children: the retroperitoneal approach. J Urol 2004;171: 2629–31.
7. Yee DS, Shanberg AM, Duel BP, et al. Initial comparison of robotic-assisted laparoscopic versus open pyeloplasty in children. Urology 2006;67:599–602.
8. Pedraza R, Palmer L, Moss V, Franco I. Bilateral robotic assisted laparoscopic heminephroureterectomy. J Urol 2004;171:2394–5.
9. Pedraza R, Weiser A, Franco I. Laparoscopic appendicovesicostomy (Mitrofanoff procedure) in a child using the da Vinci robotic system. J Urol 2004;171:1652–3.
10. Olsen LH, Deding D, Yeung CK, Jorgensen TM. Computer assisted laparoscopic pneumovesical ureter reimplantation a.m. Cohen: initial experience in a pig model. APMIS 2003;Suppl:23–5.
11. Peters CA, Woo R. Intravesical robotically assisted bilateral ureteral reimplantation. J Endourol 2005;19:618–22.
12. Lakshmanan Y, Fung LC. Laparoscopic extravesicular ureteral reimplantation for vesicoureteral reflux: recent technical advances. J Endourol 2000;14:589–94.
13. Gill IS, Kerbl K, Meraney AM, Clayman RV. Basics of laparoscopic urologic surgery. In: Campbell's urology. W.B. Saunders; 2002. p. 3456.
14. Lorenzo AJ, Karsli C, Halachmi S, et al. Hemodynamic and respiratory effects of pediatric urological retroperitoneal laparoscopic surgery: a prospective study. J Urol 2006; 175:1461–5.
15. Halachmi S, El-Ghoneimi A, Bissonnette B, et al. Hemodynamic and respiratory effect of pediatric urological laparoscopic surgery: a retrospective study. J Urol 2003; 170:1651–4.
16. Atala A, Kavoussi LR, Goldstein DS, et al. Laparoscopic correction of vesicoureteral reflux. J Urol 1993;150:748–51.
17. Ehrlich RM, Gershman A, Fuchs G. Laparoscopic vesicoureteroplasty in children: initial case reports. Urology 1994;43:255–61.

18. Sakamoto W, Nakatani T, Sakakura T, et al. Extraperitoneal laparoscopic Lich-Gregoir antireflux plasty for primary vesicoureteral reflux. Int J Urol 2003;10:94–8.
19. Kawauchi A, Fujito A, Soh J, et al. Laparoscopic correction of vesicoureteral reflux using the Lich-Gregoir technique: initial experience and technical aspects. Int J Urol 2003; 10:90–3.
20. Yeung CK, Sihoe JD, Borzi PA. Endoscopic cross-trigonal ureteral reimplantation under carbon dioxide bladder insufflation: a novel technique. J Endourol 2005;19:295–9.
21. Gregoir W. Lich-Gregoir operation. In: Surgical pediatric urology. W.B. Saunders Company; 1977. p. 265–8.
22. Franc-Guimond J, Kryger J, Gonzalez R. Experience with the Bailez technique for laparoscopic access in children. J Urol 2003;170:936–8.
23. Poppas DP, Bleustein CB, Peters CA. Box stitch modification of Hasson technique for pediatric laparoscopy. J Endourol 1999;13:447–50.
24. Leissner J, Allhoff EP, Wolff W, et al. The pelvic plexus and antireflux surgery: topographical findings and clinical consequences. J Urol 2001;165:1652–5.
25. Heidenreich A, Ozgur E, Becker T, Haupt G. Surgical management of vesicoureteral reflux in pediatric patients. World J Urol 2004;22:96–106.
26. Cohen SJ. The Cohen technique of ureteroneocystostomy. In: Surgical pediatric urology. W.B. Saunders Company; 1977. p. 269–71.
27. Chen HW, Yuan SS, Lin CJ. Ureteral reimplantation for vesicoureteral reflux: comparison of minimally invasive extravesical with transvesical and conventional extravesical techniques. Urology 2004;63:364–8.
28. Duong DT, Parekh DJ, Pope JCT, et al. Ureteroneocystostomy without urethral catheterization shortens hospital stay without compromising postoperative success. J Urol 2003;170:1570–3.
29. Miller OF, Bloom TL, Smith LJ, et al. Early hospital discharge for intravesical ureteroneocystostomy. J Urol 2002;167:2556–9.
30. Sprunger JK, Reese CT, Decter RM. Can standard open pediatric urological procedures be performed on an outpatient basis? J Urol 2001;166:1062–4.
31. Challacombe B, Patriciu A, Glass J, et al. A randomized controlled trial of human versus robotic and telerobotic access to the kidney as the first step in percutaneous nephrolithotomy. Comput Aided Surg 2005;10:165–71.

109

Robotic Pyeloplasty

Fatih Atug, MD
Raju Thomas, MD, FACS, MHA

Open pyeloplasty is accepted worldwide as the gold standard therapy for ureteropelvic junction (UPJ) obstruction with success rates exceeding 90%.[1] Open repair, however, is associated with increased hospital stay, postoperative pain, potential disfiguring, scarring, and flank bulge. Various minimally invasive endourologic techniques have been introduced for management of UPJ obstruction as alternative approaches to open surgery.

Endopyelotomy, both percutaneous nephroscopic, and retrograde ureteroscopic/Acucise have been widely used as minimally invasive techniques to manage UPJ obstruction.[2] Results of endopyelotomy did not compete with open surgical pyeloplasty results, but the procedure was acceptable because of its less invasive nature.

With introduction of laparoscopic techniques into urologic surgery in the early to mid-1990s, laparoscopic ablative and reconstructive procedures gained a foothold in treating obstructive uropathy. Laparoscopic pyeloplasty has shown results and success rates comparable to that of open surgical pyeloplasty,[3-9] although it is a technically challenging procedure; it requires advanced intracorporeal suturing skills, and thus, laparoscopic pyeloplasty is limited to certain referral centers. Despite limitations, in skilled hands, laparoscopic pyeloplasty is a preferred minimally invasive treatment option for UPJ obstruction.

Rapid technological developments have produced new inventions such as robots and incorporated them into our daily lives. Today, robots perform vital functions in homes, outer space, hospitals, and on military installations. The development and introduction of robotic surgery has given hospitals and surgeons a valuable tool that is making a profound impact on delivery of hi-tech surgical procedures. The da Vinci Surgical System (Intuitive Surgical, Inc., Sunnyvale, CA) is the most technologically advanced addition to the urologic surgical armamentarium. The advantages of the robot include tremor control, 1:5 motion scaling, 6 degrees of freedom within 1 cm of the tip of the end effector, and three-dimensional vision resulting in simplified suturing and improved operative precision. By incorporating computer-augmented robotic technologies with the technical aptitude of the surgeon, the goals of advanced robotic systems are to improve operative technique, simplify intracorporeal suturing, and increase applicability and disseminated use of advanced surgical techniques such as pyeloplasty.

PREOPERATIVE PATIENT EVALUATION

Patient presentation (signs and symptoms) are similar to any patient with UPJ obstruction. A combination of studies such as intravenous urogram (IVU), computed tomography (CT) scans and/or diuretic renal scans are needed for definitive diagnosis. With changing imaging patterns in settings such as the emergency room, CT scans are increasingly being used for diagnosis of UPJ obstruction. The diagnosis of crossing vessels should be established using CT angiography or color Doppler ultrasonography, as indicated. Preoperatively, all patients should preferably undergo mercaptotriglycylglycine (MAG-3) diuretic renography to assess the degree of obstruction and status of renal function. Retrograde pyelography (RGP) prior to surgical intervention should confirm the diagnosis. RGP also helps assess the length of the obstructing segment, which is critical in management.

The indications for robotically assisted pyeloplasty (RAP) are essentially the same as those for laparoscopic and other described techniques for UPJ obstruction. Moreover, pediatric and failed pyeloplasty patients can be successfully managed with the da Vinci robot.[10,11] Concomitant management of renal calculi with UPJ obstruction using RAP techniques have also been reported.[12] Relative contraindications include previous abdominal surgery with intestinal adhesions, patient size (too small and too large), bleeding disorders and active untreated urinary tract infection.

PREPARATION FOR SURGERY

Informed consent is obtained after explaining the advantages and disadvantages of RAP. Various techniques have been described to manage intraoperative stenting, both antegrade and retrograde.[13] Some patients have a pre-placed ureteral stent to start.[14] We prefer placement of a 5 French open-ended ureteral catheter after performing RGP, just distal to the UPJ obstruction.[11] This technique causes passive dilatation of the renal pelvis since it is not being continuously drained, and the dilated renal pelvis facilitates easy identification and dissection of the renal pelvis (pelviolysis) and the UPJ area. This ureteral catheter is anchored to a Foley catheter which drains the bladder.

PATIENT POSITIONING AND PORT PLACEMENT

Patients are then placed in a modified 45° lateral decubitus position. The ureteral and Foley catheters are prepped into the sterile surgical field (Figure 109-1). A standard 12-mm umbilical port is placed, and the remaining two 8-mm robotic ports are placed under direct laparoscopic vision. A 12-mm port is placed in a subxiphoid position for use by the bedside surgeon (Figure 109-2). The robot is placed on the ipsilateral side of the kidney being operated on and the transperitoneal approach is preferred.

SURGICAL TECHNIQUE

All types of pyeloplasty procedures can be performed using the da Vinci robot, including Anderson-Hynes dismembered pyeloplasty, Y–V-plasty, and non-dismembered pyeloplasty.[15,16] Anderson-Hynes pyeloplasty, however, is the preferred reconstructive technique for RAP. Especially in the presence of a crossing vessel (Figure 109-3) and a patulous renal pelvis, an Anderson-Hynes dismembered pyeloplasty is recommended, since the patulous renal pelvis can be trimmed.

For robotically assisted pyeloplasty, the accessory robotic instruments usually used are: hook electrocautery, Cadiere grasping forceps, needle holders, round-tipped scissors, and bipolar forceps. For patients who have right-sided UPJ obstruction, the line of Toldt is incised and the hepatic flexure retracted medially to identify

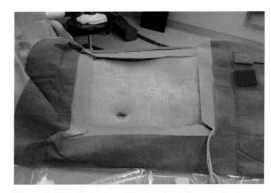

Figure 109-1 Patient positioning for left pyeloplasty.

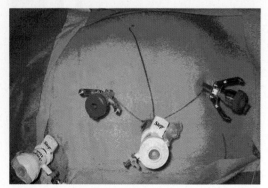

Figure 109-2 Trocar positioning for left-sided robotic pyeloplasty.

Gerota's fascia. For patients who have left-sided UPJ obstruction, the standard approach similarly involves incision of the line of Toldt and medial mobilization of the descending colon to expose Gerota's fascia. For thin patients who have a left-sided UPJ obstruction, an alternative transmesenteric approach can be judiciously used.

The colon is mobilized medially, followed by isolation of the ureter; which is dissected up to the area of the UPJ obstruction. The distended renal pelvis facilitates the dissection. Stay sutures, using 4-0 polyglactin 910 sutures on an RB-1 needle are placed on the ureter and renal pelvis for traction and for maintaining orientation (Figure 109-4). Meticulous pelviolysis is then performed. This will excise any and all fibrous tissue and dissect the renal pelvis and UPJ distally and away from any obstructing vessels. The UPJ obstruction is then transected, the ureter spatulated, and any redundant renal pelvis excised. If any redundant renal pelvis is trimmed, these edges are sutured closed first, using 4-0 polyglactin 910 sutures. The posterior UPJ anastomosis is then completed using running 4-0 polyglactin 910 sutures. Prior to completing the anterior UPJ anastomosis, the bedside surgeon places a double pigtail stent over a super-stiff guidewire, which is passed retrograde through the 5F open-ended catheter in the ureter. The accurate placement of this stent is visualized robotically. The pyeloplasty is then completed using running 4-0 polyglactin 910 sutures for the anterior anastomosis. The proximal ureter and

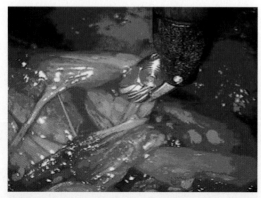

Figure 109-3 Dissection of left ureteropelvic junction area showing crossing vessel.

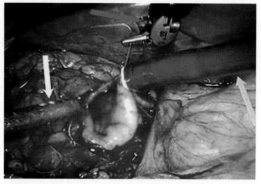

Figure 109-4 Right ureteropelvic junction and concomitant calculus removal. Placement of flexible nephroscope (*yellow arrow*) through one of the robotic ports. The orientation suture was held on traction with the robotic arm (*red arrow*) to facilitate the placement of the flexible nephroscope into the renal pelvis. Suction-irrigator is marked with *white arrow*.

pelvis are inspected to ensure there's no kinking before desufflating the abdominal cavity. The stay sutures should maintain orientation. In most patients with a crossing vessel, the reconstructed UPJ can be repositioned distal to the crossing vessel if adequate pelviolysis is performed. A closed surgical drain is then placed through one of the trocar sites. The trocar site fascia and skin are closed in a standard fashion.

POSTOPERATIVE CARE AND FOLLOW-UP

Most patients are discharged on the first postoperative day. The Foley catheter is left indwelling for 48 hours. The closed suction drain is removed next, usually in the next 24 to 48 hours, and the ureteral stent is left indwelling for approximately 6 weeks. At 3 months follow-up, objective assessment of the repair is performed and compared with the same imaging as performed preoperatively, including diuretic renography, excretory urography, ultrasound, and/or CT scan.

RESULTS AND DISCUSSION

Robotic surgery is being successfully applied to reconstructive procedures such as pyeloplasty. The main advantage of robotics over standard laparoscopy is ease of intracorporeal suturing. The first RAP was performed by Sung and colleagues in 1999 in a porcine model.[17] They performed a pyeloplasty with the Zeus robotic system and concluded that RAP is a feasible and effective procedure that may enhance surgical dexterity and precision.

Following this initial animal feasibility study, several clinical publications emerged.[18–20] Gettman and colleagues compared laparoscopic pyeloplasty performed with the daVinci robotic system versus traditional laparoscopic techniques.[20] They reported shorter overall operative and anastomotic times with the robotic approach. Bentas and colleagues also reported their initial experience of robotically assisted laparoscopic

Anderson-Hynes pyeloplasty.[21] Among the cohort of 11 adult patients, they reported a mean operative time of 197 minutes with no intraoperative complications, no open conversions, minimal blood loss, and a 100% success rate at 1-year follow-up. Moreover, Yohannes and colleagues demonstrated that the learning curve associated with intracorporeal suturing is shorter with the daVinci robotic system than with conventional laparoscopy.[22] Consequently, according to the reported studies, RAP can be performed safely with results comparable to open pyeloplasty.[17–22]

In addition, high success rates are reported with RAP. Siddiq and colleagues reported their experience in 26 patients with RAP. The overall clinical success rate was 95%, with a median follow-up of 6 months.[23] In another study, Palese and colleagues reported 94% success in 35 patients with a mean follow-up of 7.9 months.[24] Of late, Patel reported unobstructed drainage in 48 of 50 patients with a mean follow-up of 11.7 months.[14]

RAP can be successfully utilized in unique situations. In pediatric patients, especially in children over 4 years of age, this technique has been successfully applied.[10] When UPJ obstruction is associated with concomitant renal calculi, intraoperative use of flexible nephroscope during RAP has been reported (see Figure 109-4 and Figure 109-5).[11] In such patients, the cephalad arm of the robot is undocked to pass the flexible nephroscope. The bedside surgeon's trocar is usually used to place a suction-irrigator to manage the irrigation fluid. Moreover, secondary UPJ obstruction is also amenable to RAP. Though this can be technically challenging, with associated longer operative times, RAP has proven to be versatile in a variety of clinically presenting UPJ obstruction situations.[12]

The technically demanding aspect of intracorporeal laparoscopic suturing is minimized with the robotic interface. RAP may prove to be one of the applications that demonstrates a clear advantage of robotics being applied to a minimally invasive approach. The outcomes of RAP can easily be compared to the open and laparoscopic counterparts as objective studies can confirm success rates.[20–22] The one obstacle to overcome in such analyses is to standardize pre- and postoperative studies.

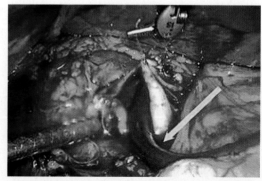

Figure 109-5 Concomittant calculus removal. Advancement of the flexible nephroscope (*yellow arrow*) into the calices to perform nephroscopy.

CONCLUSION

Using the open surgical technique as the gold standard, alternative methods to treat UPJ obstruction have evolved. Reconstructive classic laparoscopy is different from ablative laparoscopic procedures (eg, radical nephrectomy) because it requires intracorporeal suturing skills, which require considerable experience for proficiency. Surgeons who have moved from classic laparoscopy to robotically assisted surgery, however, have shown that the ease of dissection, transection, and suturing is greatly facilitated by the da Vinci robot, which has a freedom of movement similar to that of the human wrist. RAP can be performed safely with results comparable to open pyeloplasty.

We must await long-term results on these robotic procedures. A major drawback of the da Vinci robotic system is the cost of the initial investment, and the costs of continued maintenance and disposable instrumentation. Moreover, additional training is required for physicians and for hospital personnel. Open surgical pyeloplasty will continue to be dominant in pyeloplasty because of the limited worldwide application of advanced laparoscopic techniques and the limited availability of robotic technology. Hopefully, in the not-too-distant future, the proliferation of technology, together with a decrease in costs and improved training of urological surgeons, will make RAP more widely available to correct lesions such as UPJ obstruction.

REFERENCES

1. Scardino PT, Scardino PL. Obstruction at the ureteropelvic junction. In: Bergman H, editor. The ureter. 2nd ed. New York: Springer-Verlag; 1981. p. 697.
2. Meretyk I, Meretyk S, Clayman RV. Endopyelotomy: comparison of ureteroscopic retrograde and antegrade percutaneous techniques. J Urol 1992;148:775–82.
3. Janetschek G, Peschel R, Frauscher F, et al. Laparoscopic pyeloplasty. Urol Clin North Am 2000;27:695–704.
4. Moore RG, Averch TD, Schulam PG, et al. Laparoscopic pyeloplasty: experience with the initial 30 cases. J Urol 1997;157:459–462.
5. Slama MR, Salomon L, Hoznek A, et al. Extraperitoneal laparoscopic repair of ureteropelvic junction obstruction: initial experience in 15 cases. Urology 2000;56:45–8.
6. Soulie M, Salomon L, Patard JJ, et al. Extraperitoneal laparoscopic pyeloplasty: a multicenter study of 55 procedures. J Urol 2001;166:48–50.
7. Janetschek G, Peschel R, Frauscher F, et al. Laparoscopic and retroperitoneoscopic repair of ureteropelvic junction obstruction. Urology 1996;47:311–6.
8. Eden CG, Cahill D, Allen JD. Laparoscopic dismembered pyeloplasty: 50 consecutive cases. Br J Urol 2001;88: 526–31.
9. Bauer JJ, Bishoff JT, Moore RG. Laparoscopic versus open pyeloplasty: assessment of objective and subjective outcome. J Urol 1999;162:692–5.
10. Atug F, Woods M, Burgess S, et al. Robotic pyeloplasty in children. J Urol 2005;174:1440–2.
11. Atug F, Burgess SV, Castle EP, Thomas R. Role of robotics in the management of secondary ureteropelvic junction obstruction. Int J Clin Pract 2006;60:9–11.
12. Atug F, Castle EP, Burgess SV, Thomas R. Concomitant management of renal calculi and pelvi-ureteric junction obstruction with robotic laparoscopic surgery. BJU Int 2005;96:1365–8.
13. Mandhani A, Goel S, Bhandari M. Is antegrade stenting superior to retrograde stenting in laparoscopic pyeloplasty? J Urol 2004;171:1440–2.
14. Patel V. Robotic-assisted laparoscopic dismembered pyeloplasty. Urology 2005;66:45–9.
15. Jarrett TW, Chan DY, Charambura TC, et al. Laparoscopic pyeloplasty: the first 100 cases. J Urol 2002;167:1253–6.
16. Frauscher F, Janetschek G, Klauser A, et al. Effect of crossing vessels on successful laparoscopic pyeloplasty using contrast-enhanced color Doppler imaging. Urology 2002; 59:500–5.
17. Sung GT, Gill IS, Hsu TH. Robotic-assisted laparoscopic pyeloplasty: a pilot study. Urology 1999;53:1099–103.
18. Sung GT, Gill IS. Robotic laparoscopic surgery: a comparison of the da Vinci and Zeus systems. Urology 2001;58:893–8.
19. Gettman MT, Neururer R, Bartsch G, Peschel R. Anderson-Hynes dismembered pyeloplasty performed using the da Vinci robotic system. Urology 2002;60:509–13.
20. Gettman MT, Peschel R, Neururer R, Bartsch G. Laparoscopic pyeloplasty: comparison of procedures performed with the da Vinci robotic system versus standard techniques. Eur Urol 2002;42:453–8.
21. Bentas W, Wolfram M, Brautigam R, et al. Da Vinci robot assisted Anderson-Hynes dismembered pyeloplasty: technique and 1 year follow-up. World J Urol 2003;21:133–8.
22. Yohannes P, Rotariu P, Pinto P, et al. Comparison of robotic versus laparoscopic skills: is there a difference in the learning curve? Urology 2002;60:39–45.
23. Siddiq FM, Leveillee RJ, Villicana P, Bird VG. Computer-assisted laparoscopic pyeloplasty: University of Miami experience with the da Vinci surgical system. J Endourol 2005;19:387–92.
24. Palese MA, Stifelman MD, Munver R, et al. Robot-assisted laparoscopic dismembered pyeloplasty: a combined experience. J Endourol 2005;19:382–6.

110

Laparoscopic Techniques for Pelvic Organ Prolapse

Michael A. Aleman, MD

Raymond R. Rackley, MD

Abdominal surgery for pelvic organ prolapse has a long history, beginning with procedures to secure the uterus to the anterior abdominal wall (Mayo procedure). Eventually, attempts to create a more natural vaginal axis and to prevent enterocele formation led to the suturing of the vaginal apex directly to the anterior longitudinal ligament of the sacrum. The subsequent addition of a piece of material (usually synthetic) between the vaginal apex and the sacrum led to the contemporary version of the abdominal sacrocolpopexy. In patients desiring a uterine-sparing approach, modifications of the abdominal sacrocolpopexy or uterosacral ligament plication procedures have been proposed. While these procedures have documented efficacy and are applicable to a wide variety of patients, their use has been limited due to their invasiveness and prolonged recovery times. These factors and others, such as innovations in vaginal surgery, have led to the development of vaginal approaches to prolapse, most notably the sacrospinous colpopexy. While this procedure is less invasive and has a shorter recovery time than abdominal approaches, it requires a high level of training, and comfort with operating in a field with minimal exposure. Furthermore, it requires sufficient vaginal length to reach the sacrospinous ligament, which may not be the case in patients who have previously undergone failed pelvic organ prolapse repairs or hysterectomy.

With the advent of laparoscopic techniques in urology, there has been a surge in interest in the laparoscopic approach to prolapse repair, as this may combine the success, versatility, and durability of the traditional abdominal repairs with the minimal invasiveness and quick recovery provided by vaginal approaches. In this chapter, we present a review of the experience with laparoscopic uterosacral ligament suspension, laparoscopic sacrocolpopexy, robotically assisted laparoscopic sacrocolpopexy, and an innovative technique of a laparoscopic-assisted percutaneous vaginal tape vault suspension.

LAPAROSCOPIC UTEROSACRAL LIGAMENT SUSPENSION

The use of the uterosacral ligaments in the repair of vault prolapse is well-established.[1–4] Typically, these structures are identified and secured during a vaginal or abdominal hysterectomy, and then secured to the vaginal apex to prevent recurrent prolapse. In the laparoscopic technique as described by Lin and colleagues, the uterosacral ligaments are identified laparoscopically.[5] The ureters are dissected out from the level of the pelvic brim to the level of the cervix, with relaxing incisions made in the peritoneum to prevent ureteral kinking when the uterosacral ligament sutures are tied. To plicate the uterosacral ligament, a double bite of permanent suture is placed through the uterosacral ligament at the level of the ischial spine and then at the vaginal apex before tying. This is performed bilaterally, and concomitant repairs may then also be performed.

Wu reported a series of seven patients undergoing this procedure in 1997, with no recurrences noted at a follow-up of 9 to 17 months.[6] A larger series was reported by Maher in 2001.[7] A Moschowitz culdoplasty was performed in all 43 patients in this series, which reported a subjective success rate of 81% and subjective success rate of 79% at a mean follow-up of 1 year. Mean total operating room time was 99 minutes. Two women in this series subsequently completed term pregnancies and did not develop recurrent prolapse after caesarian delivery. Lin and colleagues reported a retrospective series of 133 cases using the technique described above; at a mean follow-up of 3.2 years (range 2 to 7.3 years), the anatomic success rate was 87.2%.[5] Complications (suburethral sling mesh erosion, DVT, and pelvic pain) developed in only three patients.

While the literature on laparoscopic uterosacral ligament suspension contains no large-scale, prospective, comparative trials, the results from the above case series, combined with the proven history of uterosacral vault suspension via the vaginal approach, suggest that this may be a promising addition to the array of procedures used to address pelvic organ prolapse. It may have a specific role in patients who wish to preserve the uterus and in patients wishing to avoid the use of synthetic mesh. The authors of one review article suggest anecdotally that this procedure may not be successful in women with cervical elongation, who may continue to feel a symptomatic bulge[8]; we would add that, in our observation, the uterosacral ligaments can be difficult to identify in some patients, especially those with a history of prior prolapse repairs.

LAPAROSCOPIC SACROCOLPOPEXY

A recent comprehensive review of the literature on abdominal sacrocolpopexy showed that 39 of 46 published studies yielded success rates of greater than 90%.[9] The first cases of laparoscopic sacrocolpopexy were reported in 1994 by Nezhat and colleagues[10] and Dorsey and Cundiff.[11] These and other early reports typically used a single piece of mesh attached to the posterior vaginal apex; we prefer to use a Y-shaped mesh, which provides both anterior and posterior fixation at the apex and better recapitulates the open technique. Both techniques seem to be effective; at 16 months follow-up, only 1 case in a series of 10 patients using the single-strip technique developed a recurrence,[12] whereas, at 5 years follow-up, only 3 cases out of 51 patients developed recurrence with a Y-shaped mesh technique.[13]

A comparative cohort study from our institution of 61 patients treated with open sacrocolpopexy and 56 treated laparoscopically revealed similar reoperation rates (11% laparoscopic versus 5% open) and similar complication rates.[14] The laparoscopic group had a trend toward higher complications of sutures in the bladder or enterotomy, but this was not statistically significant. The mean total operative time was longer for the laparoscopic group (269 vs. 218 minutes), but hospital stay was shorter in the laparoscopic group (1.8 vs. 4.0 days).

Most described techniques for laparoscopic sacrocolpopexy involve the same initial steps. Four or five ports are used (Figure 110-1), with access obtained at the umbilicus using either an open Hasson technique or with a Veress needle. At the umbilicus and for the two ports at the lateral borders of the rectus muscle, 10- to 12-mm ports are used. The far lateral ports can usually be 5-mm ports that are placed 2 to 3 cm cephalad and 2 to 3 cm medial to the anterior superior iliac spines. The left lower port is utilized to retract the sigmoid colon to the left and cephalad. This port can be eliminated with the use of a 1-0 monofilament suture on a large (CT-X) needle, passed percutaneously through the left lower quadrant port site, which is then threaded through an omental appendage of the sigmoid colon, passed back out through the left lower quadrant, and tied or clamped at the skin level to retract the sigmoid colon. Usually, lysis of adhesions between the

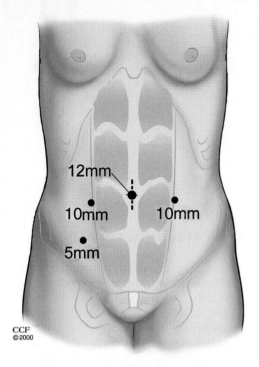

Figure 110–1 Typical port placements for laparoscopic pelvic organ prolapse surgery. A fifth port (5 mm) may be placed in the left lower quadrant, or a suture may be used to retract the sigmoid colon.

sigmoid colon and the vaginal apex is necessary before the colon can be adequately retracted.

After the sigmoid is retracted, the sacral promontory, right common iliac artery, and right ureter are readily visible. The posterior peritoneum over the sacral promontory is incised, and this peritoneal opening is continued toward the apex of the vagina. An endoanal sizer or bivalve speculum can be used to reduce the prolapse while performing this step.

The peritoneum over the vaginal apex is then incised, and this dissection is continued anteriorly along the vaginal wall in an attempt to dissect the plane between the bladder and vagina. The bladder can be filled to help demarcate this plane as well as to facilitate the introduction of a cystoscope light into the bladder. This plane is dissected at least 3 cm distal to the vaginal apex to allow space for placement of the anchoring sutures. The lack of tactile feedback makes this dissection challenging; in a recent study of this technique, cystotomy or sutures thrown into the bladder were noted in 10.7% of cases.[14] Similar dissection is performed on the posterior vaginal wall to de-peritonealize this area and separate the vagina from the rectum posteriorly. The mesh, either in two strips or pre-fashioned in a Y-configuration, is passed into the field and sutured with non-absorbable suture to the posterior wall and then the anterior wall (Figure 110-2). At least four sutures are required on either side to fully anchor the mesh. With the prolapse reduced via an instrument in the vagina, the proximal end of the mesh is anchored to the anterior longitudinal ligament of the sacrum with 2 or more permanent sutures. Excess mesh is trimmed

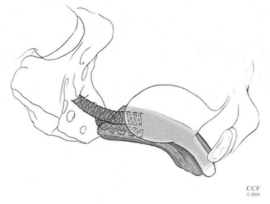

Figure 110–2 Traditional laparoscopic sacrocolpopexy: support is placed anterior and posterior on the vagina.

and the peritoneum is then closed over the mesh for completing the case.

Laparoscopic sacrocolpopexy appears to successfully recapitulate an open technique that has demonstrated durable results for several decades. A comparative study with the open technique suggests similar outcomes in the short term, though there may be an increase in bladder or bowel injury. Operative times appear longer with the laparoscopic approach, although this difference decreases with experience.

ROBOTIC LAPAROSCOPIC SACROCOLPOPEXY

This modification of the laparoscopic sacrocolpopexy utilizes the robotic system to facilitate three-dimensional visualization of the operative field, placement of sutures, and tying of the sutures. Five ports are typically utilized: an umbilical port is used for the camera; two 8-mm ports placed at the lateral edge of the rectus abdominal muscles at the level of the umbilicus are used for the robotic arms, and a 5- or 10-mm port is placed on each side 3 cm medial and cephalad to the anterior superior iliac spine to allow an assistant to retract the sigmoid colon and small bowel. At least one of these ports should be 10 mm to allow passage of the mesh strips and needles as needed. Once access is obtained and the robotic arms positioned, the technique is identical to that described for laparoscopic sacrocolpopexy.

Two small studies (5 and 12 patients) have demonstrated the feasibility of this technique and excellent short term results (4 months and 6 months).[15,16] This technique has a few theoretical advantages over the traditional laparoscopic technique: it allows for very precise dissection and suture placement, and it allows surgeons without extensive laparoscopic experience to perform the case. Practically, however, it also has a few drawbacks—the robotic equipment is expensive, and the instruments must be replaced after a few uses; the bulk of the robotic equipment makes it difficult for the assistant to manipulate instruments in two non-robotic ports, and the positioning of the equipment makes it difficult to access the vagina and urethra (to reduce

the prolapse with a sound or sponge stick, or to perform cystoscopy to assess for bladder sutures). Furthermore, there is a lack of tactile feedback for critical tissue dissection or suture placement. Finally, although centers with extensive robotic volume can reduce the operative times to an acceptable level,[15] in other centers, the robotic setup seems to increase operative times.[17] At our institution, the mean total operating room time for robotic sacrocolpopexy is 317 minutes, compared to 269 for traditional laparoscopic sacrocolpopexy, and 234 minutes for the laparoscopic assisted percutaneous vaginal tape vault suspension.[18]

LAPAROSCOPIC-ASSISTED PERCUTANEOUS VAGINAL TAPE VAULT SUSPENSION AND UTERINE SUSPENSION PROCEDURES

Besides the obvious benefits in recovery time and incision size, one of the benefits of laparoscopy in pelvic surgery is the ability to visualize internal anatomy while working on an external structure. This principle was utilized in creating the laparoscopic-assisted percutaneous vaginal tape vault suspension (Lap PVT-VS), shown in Figure 110-3, and subsequently, the uterine suspension procedure (Lap PVT-US) in Figure 110-4. In these novel procedures, the surgeon, operating vaginally, passes a strip of synthetic mesh percutaneously under the lateral walls of the vagina using angled trocar needles while monitoring the needle's passage both with vaginal inspection and laparoscopic visualization. In order to avoid bladder and bowel injury, as well as to allow use of the technique in a uterine-sparing fashion, the mesh strips are passed along the lateral walls of the vagina. This allows the mesh to provide support along the full length of the vagina, rather then just supporting the apex as in other sacrocolpopexy procedures; consequently, fewer concomitant transvaginal procedures (perineal body repairs, rectocele repairs) are required.[18]

The initial steps of this procedure are identical to the laparoscopic sacrocolpopexy. After the peritoneum over the sacral promontory down toward the vaginal apex has been incised, the prolapse is reduced with a bivalve speculum. Two small stab incisions are made in the labial folds just lateral to the vagina at the 4 o'clock and 8 o'clock positions (see Figure 110-3). Strips of polypropylene mesh, cut 20 cm long and 15 mm wide, are passed using trocar needles with a suture tied to the mesh. Care is taken to pass these in the submucosal plane of the vagina; button-holing the vaginal wall may easily be managed by pulling back and redirecting the needle. The laparoscopic view is used to help direct the mesh toward the area just lateral to the vaginal apex, where the trocar needles are passed into the abdomen. The mesh is then grasped laparoscopically and pulled into the laparoscopic field. The mesh strips are left along the entire length of the vagina, and trimmed at the level of the labial skin. Each

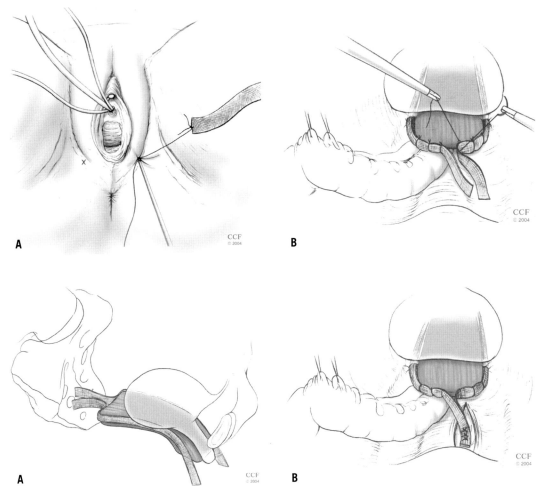

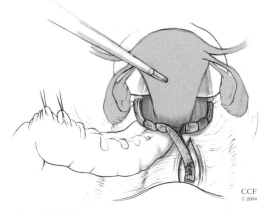

Figure 110–4 Laparoscopic percutaneous vaginal uterine suspension procedure (Lap PVT-US)

Figure 110–3 Laparoscopic percutaneous vaginal vault suspension procedure (Lap PVT-VS).

mesh strip then requires only one stitch to hold it in place, as local tissue reaction to the mesh will fix it in place within 2 weeks, similar to sling fixations for urethral support procedures (see Figure 110-3). A third stitch is thrown near the apex, joining both mesh strips to each other and to the vaginal muscularis. With the prolapse reduced, the proximal end of the mesh is fixed to the anterior longitudinal ligament of the sacrum, as in the traditional approach. Figure 110-4 shows the proper placement of the mesh along the lateral vaginal walls, noting the relation to the cervix in a uterine-sparing case.

We performed this procedure on 58 patients, and analysis of the first 32 cases with a mean follow-up of 10 months revealed a mean total operating room time of 234 minutes. Concomitant repairs were infrequent, with 7 patients undergoing transvaginal posterior colporrhaphy or perineorrhaphy. No bowel or bladder injuries were noted; complications consisted of a DVT in one patient and a port site hernia in one patient. Two patients (6.25%) required a transvaginal anterior colporrhaphy for recurrent anterior wall prolapse.[18] We are currently collecting long-term follow-up data including POP-Q scores and sexual function questionnaires. The initial results are very promising for this technique as a minimally invasive, safe, and easily learned technique with post-hysterectomy and uterine-sparing applications.

SUMMARY

A variety of laparoscopic techniques for the repair of pelvic organ prolapse are available to the urologist. All of these techniques aim to recapitulate the durable success of the traditional open abdominal techniques while avoiding the invasive open approach incision. The laparoscopic sacrocolpopexy (traditional or robotic) should aim to recreate the same technique of its open counterpart approach and thus, the success of open abdominal sacrocolpopexy. The uterosacral ligament suspension and the Lap PVT-US have special appeal to the patient desiring a uterine-sparing approach. Novel techniques like the Lap PVT-VS and Lap PVT-US represent the latest innovative challenge in laparoscopic surgery, which is not to simply recreate the open procedure, but to use the unique advantages of laparoscopy to create improved procedures.

REFERENCES

1. Barber MD, Visco AG, Weidner AC, et al. Bilateral uterosacral ligament vaginal vault suspension with site-specific endopelvic fascia defect repair for treatment of pelvic organ prolapse. Am J Obstet Gynecol 2000;183:1402–11.
2. Karram M, Goldwasser S, Kleeman S, et al. High uterosacral vaginal vault suspension with fascial reconstruction for vaginal repair of enterocele and vaginal vault prolapse. Am J Obstet Gynecol 2001;185:1339–43.
3. Shull BL, Bachofen C, Coates KW, Kuehl TJ. A transvaginal approach to repair of apical and other associated sites of pelvic organ prolapse with uterosacral ligaments. Am J Obstet Gynecol 2000;183:1365–74.
4. Webb MJ, Aronson MP, Ferguson LK, Lee RA. Posthysterectomy vaginal vault prolapse: primary repair in 693 patients. Obstet Gynecol 1998;92:281–5.
5. Lin LL, Phelps JY, Liu CY. Laparoscopic vaginal vault suspension using uterosacral ligaments: a review of 133 cases. J Minim Invasive Gynecol 2005;12:216–20.
6. Wu MP. Laparoscopic uterine suspension for the treatment of uterovaginal prolapse. Int J Gynaecol Obstet 1997;59:259–60.
7. Maher CF, Carey MP, Murray CJ. Laparoscopic suture hysteropexy for uterine prolapse. Obstet Gynecol 2001;97:1010–4.
8. Lin LL, Ho MH, Haessler AL, et al. A review of laparoscopic uterine suspension procedures for uterine preservation. Curr Opin Obstet Gynecol 2005;17:541–6.
9. Nygaard IE, McCreery R, Brubaker L, et al. Abdominal sacrocolpopexy: a comprehensive review. Obstet Gynecol 2004;104:805–23.
10. Nezhat CH, Nezhat F, Nezhat C. Laparoscopic sacral colpopexy for vaginal vault prolapse. Obstet Gynecol 1994;84:885–8.
11. Dorsey JH, Cundiff G. Laparoscopic procedures for incontinence and prolapse. Curr Opin Obstet Gynecol 1994;6:3:223–30.
12. Sundaram CP, Venkatesh R, Landman J, Klutke CG. Laparoscopic sacrocolpopexy for the correction of vaginal vault prolapse. J Endourol 2004;18:620–4.
13. Ross JW, Preston M. Laparoscopic sacrocolpopexy for severe vaginal vault prolapse: five-year outcome. J Minim Invasive Gynecol 2005;12:221–6.
14. Paraiso MF, Walters MD, Rackley RR, et al. Laparoscopic and abdominal sacral colpopexies: a comparative cohort study. Am J Obstet Gynecol 2005;192:1752–8.
15. Ayav A, Bresler L, Hubert J, et al. Robotic-assisted pelvic organ prolapse surgery. Surg.Endosc 2005;19:1200–3.
16. Di Marco DS, Chow GK, Gettman MT, Elliott DS. Robotic-assisted laparoscopic sacrocolpopexy for treatment of vaginal vault prolapse. Urology 2004;63:373–6.
17. Hsiao KC, Kobashi KC, Govier FE, Kozlowski PM. Comparison of laparoscopic and open abdominal sacrocolpopexy. J Urol 2005;173:234–234.
18. Aleman M, Rackley RR, Vasavada S, et al. A comparative cohort study of laparoscopic assisted percutaneous vaginal vault suspension to traditional laparoscopic or open abdominal sacral colpopexies. J Urol 2005;173:235–235.

111

Robotic Assisted Radical Cystectomy

Erik P. Castle, MD

Michael Woods, MD

Benjamin H. Lowentritt, MD

Fatih Atug, MD

Rodney Davis, MD

The standard treatment of muscle invasive bladder cancer is radical cystectomy and urinary diversion. Radical cystectomy can be a challenging operation with significant patient morbidity and mortality.[1] The urologic community has embraced laparoscopy to help decrease operative morbidity, which has been clearly seen by the widespread use of laparoscopic radical and donor nephrectomy. The first laparoscopic simple cystectomy was reported in 1992 by Parra and colleagues describing the removal of a benign retained bladder.[2] Since that publication, there have been several reports of laparoscopic radical cystectomy for malignant disease with various methods of urinary diversion.[3–28] With the introduction of the da Vinci Surgical System (Intuitive Surgical, Inc., Sunnyvale, CA) the prevalence of laparoscopic radical prostatectomies has seen a sharp increase, as this tool has helped surgeons overcome some of the technical challenges of laparoscopic pelvic surgery. It did not take long for surgeons to apply the technology of the da Vinci system to performing laparoscopic cystectomies. In 2003, Menon and colleagues published the first series of robotic-assisted radical cystectomy (RARC) and urinary diversion.[29] The goal of this chapter is to discuss the patient preparation, technique, and available results for robotic-assisted radical cystectomy and urinary diversion with pelvic lymphadenectomy.

INDICATIONS

The indication for radical cystectomy include tumor invasion of muscularis propria, carcinoma in-situ refractory to intravesical therapy, and recurrent multifocal, superficial disease refractory to repeat transurethral resection, with or without intravesical therapy. The importance of performing a pelvic lymphadenectomy was been well established, as approximately 25% of patients will have node positive disease at the time of cystectomy.[30] Pelvic lymphadenectomy provides important prognostic information that may guide adjuvant therapy, as it has been shown that node-positive patients have decreased survival.[30] Although there is little debate about the need for pelvic lymphadenectomy for bladder cancer, there

does exist some debate over the extent. There are no prospective studies to evaluate this issue, but there are several retrospective studies that lend support to the benefit of extending the standard template above the bifurcation of the common iliac vessels and increasing the number of lymph nodes removed.[30–32] These reports demonstrate significant survival benefits with increasing node counts in both node-positive and node-negative patients.[31,32] In addition, it was recognized that node-positive patients with fewer than five positive lymph nodes had improved survival over patients with five or more positive lymph nodes.[7,9] These findings suggest pelvic lymphadenectomy for bladder cancer may be curative in patients with micrometastatic and low-volume metastatic disease. At this time, the recommendation is to perform an extended pelvic lymphadenectomy concurrently with RARC.

The feasibility of RARC has been demonstrated by several groups.[29,33,34] The argument for the use of RARC is to decrease patient morbidity. By eliminating a large midline incision and decreasing the manipulation of the bowel, patients should ambulate and resume a diet sooner, which should decrease perioperative complications and hospital stay. Based on large series of open radical cystectomy, the overall early complication rate is 28 to 30%, with approximately 30% requiring blood transfusion, 17% developing an ileus, and an average hospital stay longer than 8 days.[30,35]

There are no absolute preoperative contraindications specific to patients being considered for RARC. There are two intraoperative situations that are absolute contraindications to proceeding with RARC. The first situation is hypotension or compromised ventilation with positioning and abdominal insufflation. The second is CO_2 retention with insufflation, resulting in unmanageable acidosis. Relative contraindications include abnormal anatomy (eg, ectopic kidney, vascular aneurysm), morbid obesity, prior radiation, and prior abdominal or pelvic surgery. As with all laparoscopic oncologic surgery, the principles of open surgery must be followed with RARC. If there is concern that these oncologic principles will be compromised, a robotic-assisted approach should not be used.

PATIENT AND PREOPERATIVE PREPARATION

Patients being considered for RARC should undergo complete metastatic and staging evaluation. Particular attention needs to be paid to an abdominal and pelvic computed tomography (CT) or magnetic resonance imaging (MRI) scan to evaluate for lymphadenopathy, local extension of tumor, and anatomic abnormalities. Patients with extravesical disease or lymph node involvement should be considered for neoadjuvant chemotherapy.[36] Patients need to undergo full mechanical and chemical bowel preparation. It is recommended that patients be placed on a clear liquid diet the day prior to surgery and take either 4L GoLytely (Braintree Laboratories, Braintree, MA) or one bottle of Fleet Phospho-soda (C.B. Fleet Co. Inc., Lynchburg, VA) and oral antibiotics. All patients should be strategically marked immediately prior to surgery for the potential urostomy site. All patients are educated preoperatively regarding care and maintenance of a urostomy or neobladder based on choice of urinary diversion.

Preoperative Preparation/Checklist
- Laboratory:
  - Basic Metabolic Panel
  - Liver Transaminases
  - Complete Blood Count

- Radiologic Imaging:
  - Chest radiograph
  - CT or MRI of abdomen and pelvis

- Additional:
  - Electrocardiogram
  - Anesthesia and/or Cardiac clearance

ANESTHESIA AND PATIENT POSITIONING RARC is performed under general endotracheal anesthesia. Broad-spectrum antibiotics covering gram-negative, gram-positive, and anaerobic organisms are administered prior to arriving in the operating room. Sequential compression stockings are placed on the lower extremities. A nasogastric tube is placed for decompression of the stomach. An arterial line may be inserted in order to monitor blood gases for developing potential acidosis and hypercarbia. The Foley catheter is placed after the patient is prepped and positioned.

The patient is placed in low lithotomy position with arms tucked to the side. Care must be taken to assure the patient's hands and elbows are adequately padded as they often lie between the patient's thigh and attachment of the stirrup. This will allow access to the abdomen and perineum. The patient will be placed in extreme/maximal Trendelenburg's position during the case, and this must be tested prior to prepping and draping the patient. A chest strap may be employed, but patients rarely move on the bed with the arms tucked and the legs in low lithotomy stirrups. Shoulder harnesses are not needed and may actually cause impingement complications.

POSITIONING OF OPERATING ROOM EQUIPMENT AND PERSONNEL   A da Vinci three- or four-arm system may be used (a four-arm unit may be beneficial by providing additional bowel retraction during lymphadenectomy). The required robotic instruments are as follows: hook electrode, Maryland bipolar, Cadiere forceps, robotic scissors, two camera lenses (0° and 30° and two needle drivers. In addition, an endovascular GIA stapler, Hem-o-lok clips (Weck Closure Systems, Research Triangle Park, NC), a suction-irrigator, and an atraumatic grasper are needed. The da Vinci system is docked between the patient's legs with the robotic arms oriented in a cephalad direction. The primary assistant operates from the patient's right. The robotic fourth arm is positioned on the patient's left side. If a three-arm system is being used, then a second assistant must be on the left side in order to assist with retraction of the bowel and other pelvic contents. The control tower for the da Vinci system is placed just left of the patient's left leg. Adjacent to the control tower is the instrument table. This leaves ample room for the scrub nurse and a second assistant, if needed, on the left side of the patient. A viewing monitor is located on top of the control tower, and one is to the left of the patient's left shoulder for the first assistant (it is preferable if this second monitor is on a ceiling boom). The surgeon console may be placed according to surgeon preference.

TECHNIQUE

Note: In female patients undergoing a cystourethrectomy, periurethral incision should be performed prior to the laparoscopic/robotic portion of the procedure.

1. Port Placement
   • A total of six ports are utilized during the operation. One 12-mm camera port, two 8-mm robotic arm ports, 12-mm and 5-mm assistant ports on the right, and one additional 5-mm assistant port on the left. If a four-arm robotic system is used, then an 8-mm robotic port can be used in place of the left assistant port.
   • The ports are arranged in an "inverted-V" fashion as diagrammed (Figure 111-1).

The camera port is placed in the midline, cephalad to the umbilicus. The port is 4 cm cephalad for ilial conduits, and lowered slightly to 3 cm for neobladder diversions. The two 8-mm robotic ports are placed 8 to 9 cm lateral from the midline and approximately 1 cm above the superior aspect of the umbilicus. In cases where a neobladder is planned, the robotic ports are placed in line with the umbilicus to facilitate suturing. The two assistant ports on the right are placed lateral and caudad to the right robotic port. The left assistant port or fourth-arm port is placed directly lateral to the left robotic port. Access and establishment of the pneumoperitoneum can be performed with a Veress or Hassan technique.

2. Mobilization of the Sigmoid and Left Colon
   • Once ports are in place and the robot is docked, the surgeon should orient himself/herself to the pelvic anatomy by identifying specific landmarks. A 30° lens is used at the outset of the procedure. This will be changed to a 0° lens once the posterior and lateral portions of the bladder are dissected. Identification of the urachus and its relationship to the internal inguinal ring is helpful. By following the peritoneal fold of the medial umbilical ligaments posteriorly, the lateral aspect of the bladder and the umbilical ligaments become apparent. The relationship of the iliac vessels to the internal ring and umbilical ligaments is initially easier on the right because the sigmoid colon obscures the left iliac vessels. The procedure is begun by incising peritoneum lateral to the left colon. The left colon and sigmoid colon should be released from the left side wall to allow access to the left iliac vessels and left ureter.

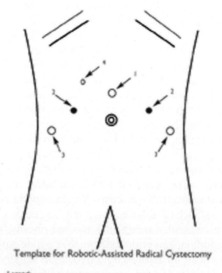

Template for Robotic-Assisted Radical Cystectomy

Legend:
(1) 12 mm camera trocar
(2) 8 mm robotic trocars
(3) 12 mm assistant trocars
(4) 5 mm assistant trocar

Figure 111-1 Template for port placement.

3. Development of the Left Perivesical Space
   • With the left medial umbilical ligament identified, the peritoneum just lateral to the ligament and medial to the left iliac vessels should be incised. Blunt dissection can be employed to develop the left perivesical space. The dissection can often be carried caudad to expose the endopelvic fascia. In male patients, dividing the vas deferens can be helpful by allowing the bladder to be retracted medially. During this maneuver, the left assistant can retract the sigmoid colon medially.

4. Identification, Mobilization and Division of the Left Ureter
   • The left ureter is identified crossing over the iliac vessels. The ureter should be dissected free of its underlying structures while preserving as much periureteral tissue as possible. The distal end can be dissected down to its insertion into the bladder. The left umbilical artery or left superior vesical artery should be seen just lateral to the insertion of the ureter into the bladder. The ureter can be clipped with a locking clip and then divided sharply (clip 1). A margin is sent for frozen section. The ureter should be dissected free of its attachment as far cephalad as possible. Once again, the surrounding periureteral tissue should be preserved. At this point, the distal ureter can be tagged with an 8- to 10-cm 2-0 Vicryl suture. This step can be delayed until the ileum is tagged to avoid an extra instrument change.

5. Identification of the Left Iliac Vessels
   • Optimal visualization of the left iliac vessels is achieved with medial retraction of the sigmoid colon and the bladder. The surgeon should be oriented by the lateral aspect of the bladder and umbilical artery, which have already been identified.

6. Performing the Left Pelvic Lymphadenectomy
   • The left pelvic lymphadenectomy can be performed with a variety of instruments. The authors currently use a Maryland bipolar in one hand and a hook electrode in the other hand. The dissection is begun on the left external iliac artery. A "split-and-roll" technique is utilized. The dissection should be carried proximally along the common iliac artery up to the bifurcation of the aorta (clip 2). Great care should be taken during dissection along the external and common iliac veins due to the collapsed nature of the veins from the pressure of the pneumoperitoneum. Blunt dissection with the back side of the hook electrode is often helpful. The obturator nerve is easily identified by orienting oneself with the pubic ramus. By following a line directly posterior to the point where the external iliac vein crosses the pubic ramus, one can find the obturator nerve and vessels. The hypogastric artery can be

skeletonized down to the take-off of the umbilical artery. Lymph nodes can be removed in separate packets with 10-mm specimen retrieval bags.

7. Development of the Right Perivesical Space
   • Once the left pelvic lymphadenectomy is completed, attention is directed to the right hemipelvis. The right perivesical space is developed similar to the left perivesical space. The peritoneum is incised between the right medial umbilical ligament and right iliac vessels.

8. The Right Ureter and Right Pelvic Lymphadenectomy
   • The right iliac vessels and ureter are easier to identify and dissect owing to less intrusion of the colon. The peritoneum covering the iliac vessels and right ureter is incised. The ureter is dissected free of its surrounding attachments and the distal end is clipped and divided at its insertion into the bladder (clip 3). The right pelvic lymphadenectomy should be performed in fashion similar to the left side. It should be noted that the right common iliac artery crosses over the right common iliac vein. This is important to remember when performing the "split-and-roll" along the common iliac artery as the common iliac vein will be encountered. Dissection proximally up to the aortic bifurcation is easier on this side (clip 4).

9. Identification, Ligation, and Division of the Superior Vesical Arteries
   • The umbilical and superior vesical arteries are clearly seen at the completion of the lymphadenectomy. These vessels can be clipped with a locking clip or taken with an endovascular staple load. The bipolar instrument will often provide adequate coagulation to allow division with the cautery hook.

10. Tagging Both Ureters with 8- to 10-inch 2-0 Vicryl Suture
    • If the ureters have not already been tagged, then one should switch instruments to needle drivers. A 2-0 Vicryl suture on an SH needle can be used to tag the distal ends of both ureters. The suture should be a minimum of 8 to 10 cm in length to facilitate delivery into the extraction incision.

11. Transferring the Left Ureter through the Sigmoid Mesentery
    • The left ureter can be transposed behind the sigmoid mesentery with the help of the right-side assistant. The anterior aspect of the aortic bifurcation should already be visible due to the right extended lymphadenectomy. The peritoneum overlying the sigmoid mesentery can be incised if the window is not large enough. The right-side assistant should gently and bluntly advance a blunt-tipped instrument through the mesentery. The left-side assistant and the operative surgeon can then retract the sigmoid to the right, and the advanced instrument tip should be visualized. The tag on the left ureter can be grasped, and the ureter should easily pass through the mesenteric window. The surgeon may opt to place a locking clip onto both ureteral tags to facilitate delivery of the ureters into the abdominal incision.

12. Tagging the Distal Ileum with 8- to 10-inch 2-0 Vicryl Suture
    • The ileum should be tagged with a 2-0 Vicryl suture. This, too, should be left at least 8 to 10 cm in length. It is often helpful to mobilize the lateral attachments of the cecum so as to make delivery of the ileum into the abdominal incision easier and make identification of the distal portion of the ileum easier.

13. Development of the Prerectal and Posterior Vesical Space
    • The camera lens can be changed to a 0° lens for optimal visualization. The peritoneum extending from the posterior bladder to the anterior sigmoid should be incised. Using blunt and careful cautery dissection, the prerectal space is developed. One must employ the assistant(s) to retract the bladder and its posterior structures anteriorly. In male patients, Denovilliers' fascia needs to be incised to carry the dissection as far caudad as possible. The dissection should be carried down to the rectourethralis muscle.
    • In female patients, the dissection is carried along the anterior vaginal mucosa in a vaginal sparing procedure. If the anterior vaginal wall will not be spared then a sponge-stick in the vagina allows identification of the vaginal cuff. Incision of the vaginal apex can be performed with the hook electrode. Although some gas may escape through vaginal opening, a sponge-stick seems to occlude the vagina sufficiently. The dissection is then carried down to the posterior aspect of the periurethral incision made at the beginning of the operation. In a nerve-sparing procedure for women, the incision of the vagina should be as anterolateral as possible. Lateral vaginal tissue should be preserved to spare any neurovascular tissue coursing along the anterolateral aspect of the vagina.

14. Division of the Remaining Inferior Vesical Vessels
    • Once the limits of dissection are reached along the posterior aspect of the bladder, the lateral attachments of the bladder can be divided. In a non–nerve-sparing procedure, this can be done with a combination of the bipolar instrument and the hook electrode. An endovascular stapler can be used on both sides as well. It should be remembered that the dissection should be carried caudad through the endopelvic fascia, thereby completely mobilizing the bladder from its lateral attachments and the rectum. A combination of lateral and posterior dissection is often used in an alternating fashion to complete the dissection.

15. Preservation of the Neurovascular Bundles
    • In nerve-sparing procedures, the neurovascular bundles are encountered as they project off the posterolateral aspects of the prostate and vagina down to the anterior surface of the colon. The bundles can be mobilized by releasing lateral fascia anterior to the bundles along the surface of the prostate or vagina. The inferior vesical pedicles and prostate pedicles should be clipped and divided with cold scissors to avoid neurovascular injury. The nerve-sparing should be carried down to the genitourinary diaphragm to prevent injury during the apical and urethral dissection (clip 5). Once the nerves are mobilized posterolateral, the remaining posterior and lateral attachments of the bladder and/or prostate can be completed. At this point, the remaining bladder attachments should only be the urachus, anterior attachments, prostate, and urethra.

16. Mobilize the Urachus
    • The medial and median umbilical ligaments should be divided as far proximally as possible with electrocautery. The dissection and peritoneal incision is carried lateral to the medial umbilical ligaments caudad to the anterior surface of the bladder.

17. Complete the Apical Dissection
    • If not already done, the endopelvic fascia should be incised bilaterally. The apical dissection of the prostate or vagina is then completed. At this point, the dorsal venous complex is ligated with a 1 Vicryl suture in a figure-of-eight fashion (clip 6). Although an endovascular stapler can be employed for this step, the authors feel the suture ligation allows for better visualization and identification of the urethra.

18. Dissection, Ligation and Division of the Urethra
    • It is very important to dissect a generous urethral stump—even in cases without a planned neobladder. A generous urethral stump allows for easier application of a locking clip or suture ligation to prevent tumor spillage during division (clip 7). If the previous posterior dissection was adequate, there should be minimal posterior tissue other than some minor remnants of rectourethralis. A frozen section can be taken from the proximal portion of the divided urethra prior to creation of a neobladder.

19. Specimen Extraction
    - The entire specimen can be entrapped in a 15-mm specimen retrieval bag. It will be extracted though a 5- to 6-cm infraumbilical or periumbilical incision. Prior to extraction, the tags on the ureters and the ileum should be grasped in a locking grasper to allow delivery into and through the extraction incision.

20. Creation of Ileal Conduit/Neobladder Urinary Diversion
    - The urinary diversion can be created through the extraction incision (Figure 111-2). The choice of diversion is based on surgeon preference and patient characteristics. If an orthotopic neobladder is created, a urethral catheter should be passed through the urethra and delivered through the extraction incision. The distal portion of the catheter can then be inserted into the anticipated urethral anastomotic site and the balloon inflated (Figure 111-3). Anastomotic sutures can be pre-placed in the posterior lip of the anticipated anastomotic site of the neobladder (Figure 111-4). The authors use two separate 2-0 Monocryl sutures with UR-6 needles tied together and cut at a length of 7 cm. Gentle traction of the urethral catheter will allow for easier downward traction on the neobladder into the pelvis and down to the urethral stump. In some cases, the urinary diversion stents can be sutured to the distal tip of the urethral catheter to allow for removal of the stents with the catheter during postoperative follow-up.

21. Closure of the Fascia and Reestablishing the Pneumoperitoneum
    - The fascia of the extraction incision can be closed and the pneumoperitoneum reestablished. During the remaining portion of the operation, less extreme Trendelenburg's position should be used to decrease tension during suturing of the urethroneovesical anastomosis.

22. Completion of the Urethroneovesical Anastomosis
    - The anastomosis is completed in a running fashion starting at the six o'clock position (clip 8). The balloon of the urethral catheter may be deflated during the anastomosis, and the catheter moved as needed. Once completed, the anastomosis is checked with irrigation.

23. Placement of Abdominal Drains and/or Suprapubic Tube
    - One or two abdominal drains can be placed through one or more port sites. If the surgeon chooses to place a suprapubic tube, the urethral catheter should be withdrawn into the urethra to prevent damage to the balloon of the catheter. Ports should be closed based on surgeon preference.

POSTOPERATIVE CARE

A nasogastric tube is not routinely left in place. The patients are maintained on broad-spectrum antibiotics for at least 48 hours and can be transitioned to oral regimens based on surgeon preference. Epidural catheters are not used. Intravenous morphine and/or ketorolac is usually adequate for pain management and can be promptly switched to oral narcotics once the patient is tolerating a diet.

It is important to increase patient activity as early as the day of surgery. Patients are encouraged to sit in a chair the same night of surgery. They are ambulated on the first postoperative day. Bisacodyl suppositories are administered each morning starting on the first postoperative day until bowel function returns. A liquid diet is started once bowel function returns, which may be as early as the second or third postoperative day. Daily serum chemistry and hematocrit may be followed until discharge, based on surgeon preference. Most patients do not seem to have significant third spacing, and will rarely require additional fluid replacement other than standard maintenance fluids. Although postoperative hemorrhage and delayed bowel injury have not been

an issue to date, patients need to be monitored closely for these complications, as the incidence with RARC is unknown.

Ureteral stents and abdominal drains should be managed according to surgeon preference. The authors remove stents from a urostomy at 7 days. Foley catheters are removed from neobladders in 10 to 14 days. If the stents were not secured to the Foley catheter during creation of the neobladder, then they are removed cystoscopically at the time of Foley catheter removal in the office. The decision to perform a cystogram at the time of Foley catheter removal is based on surgeon preference and can be decided on an individual case basis.

It should be noted that patients can be discharged rather quickly, which may require leaving drains or stents in place until the first office follow-up. The authors have found that some patients may have a continued leak of lymphatic fluid through a drain site up through the fifth or sixth postoperative day. We believe this is because patients are discharged before their lymphatic channels have completely sealed. Whether this is due to the use of cautery and/or bipolar dissection during lymphadenectomy remains to be seen. Consequently, the abdominal drain may be left in place until their first postoperative follow-up, which is on postoperative day seven. If the drain is removed before discharge, then a urostomy appliance can be placed over the drain site to collect the fluid until the incision heals and drainage ceases. We have found this drainage to be self-limited and uniformly resolves spontaneously as the lymphatic fluid is absorbed intraperitoneally. If there is any concern of a urine leak, the fluid may be sent for creatinine analysis.

RESULTS

There is limited information available for this procedure, given its recent development, although there are several small series worth reviewing. The first RARC series was published in 2003 by Menon and colleagues, in which they reported on their first 17 patients.[29] This was subsequently updated in 2004 when the group reported on

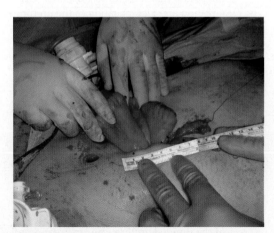

Figure 111-2 Neobladder creation through extraction incision.

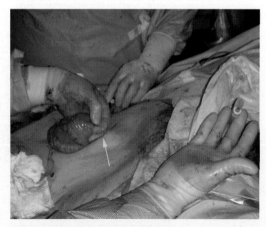

Figure 111-3 Catheter in neobladder.

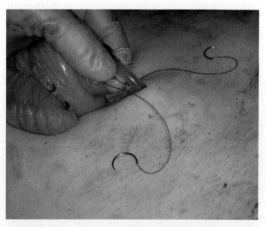

Figure 111-4 Pre-placement of anastomotic sutures.

24 patients, which is the largest series to date.[37] They used a five- to six- port technique. They did not report total operative time, but averaged 110 to 170 minutes for the robotic cystectomy and 120 to 180 minutes for construction of the urinary diversion, which is performed extracorporeally. An extended pelvic lymph node dissection was performed, which yielded 3 to 27 lymph nodes. The blood loss ranged from 100 to 300 cc, and it was stated that most patients were discharged within 4 to 5 days. There were no positive surgical margins, intraoperative complications, or open conversions, although the Menon group did report that one patient needed to be reexplored postoperatively for hemorrhage.[29] In a separate report, this same group reported on the feasibility of robotic cystectomy in female patients with preservation of the uterus, ovaries, and vagina with acceptable oncologic outcomes and comparable operative times.[38]

The second largest series is from the authors at Tulane University, consisting of 18 patients. The technique is as previously described in this chapter (see "Technique"). This experience consists of 14 males and 4 females, with 9 patients receiving ileal conduits and 9 receiving neobladders. Approximately 70% of the male patients underwent a nerve-sparing procedure. The total median operative time for the series was 410 minutes (390 minutes for ileal conduit, 415 minutes for neobladder). Operative time was calculated from incision to last stitch tied. The mean and median blood loss was 230 cc and 150 cc respectively (range 150 to 600 cc). There were no intraoperative complications or open conversions. Four postoperative complications occurred: deep venous thromboses in 2 patients, a urine leak in one patient, and a pulmonary embolus in one patient. The median length of stay in this series was 4 days. With an extended lymphadenectomy including obturator, hypogastric, external iliac, and common iliac lymph nodes (proximal extent being the bifurcation of aorta) a mean of 11 lymph nodes were removed (range 7 to 18). Six patients (30%) were found to have node-positive disease. All surgical margins were negative.

There are two other case reports further demonstrating the feasibility of RARC. Yohannes and colleagues reported their experience with two patients, in which an intracorporeal ileal conduit was created.[34] The operative time was 10 and 12 hours, with estimated blood loss of 435 and 1,800 cc. The average hospital stay was 6 days. A bilateral pelvic lymph node dissection was performed, although the boundaries and number of lymph nodes removed were not stated. They did not experience any intraoperative complications or open conversions. Lastly, Beecken and colleagues reported on one patient who underwent a successful RARC with an intracorporeally constructed neobladder.[33] The operative time was 8.5 hours and blood loss was 200 cc. They achieved negative surgical margins and performed a bilateral pelvic lymphadenectomy, but did not state the number of lymph nodes removed.

As with all laparoscopic cancer surgery, the goal is to duplicate the steps of open surgery, which form the current principles of cancer control. A concern unique to laparoscopy, despite duplicating open surgery, is the potential for port site recurrence. This is of particular concern for transitional cell carcinoma, given its locally aggressive nature. The reality of port site recurrence for TCC was reported in a series of laparoscopic staging pelvic lymphadenectomy for bladder cancer, in which a 4% port site recurrence was seen.[39] To date, one case of port site metastasis has been reported following a RARC, which was discovered 10 months postoperatively.[40] There is encouraging data from Cathelineau and colleagues, in which they have performed 84 pure laparoscopic cystectomies, with a mean follow-up of 18 months, with no port site recurrences.[41] This potential adverse outcome will have to be closely monitored as the follow-up of patients undergoing RARC increases.

Another concern over this approach is the ability to perform an adequate lymphadenectomy, the importance of which cannot be overstated given the potential survival benefit of extended lymphadenectomy in bladder cancer. Menon and colleagues removed 3-27 lymph nodes and the Tulane group removed 7-18 lymph nodes. This number of lymph nodes is in line with the recommendations of a multi-institutional study, which states the removal of 10 to 14 lymph nodes is adequate during a radical cystectomy,[42] although other authors have reported greater lymph node yields with extended lymphadenectomy.[43,44] There are several obstacles to comparing lymph node counts among different institutions,[42] thus further emphasizing the need to adhere to an extended lymphadenectomy template. With the Tulane approach, the bifurcation of the aorta was the proximal extent of the lymph node dissection. The above reported series demonstrate some of the advantages and disadvantages of RARC. First, there is significantly decreased blood loss and need for blood transfusion. The average blood loss for the two larger series is less then 300 cc. The average hospital stay for patients undergoing RARC was 4 to 5 days. These results appear favorable when compared to a contemporary open cystectomy series with blood loss around 700 cc, 30% transfusion rate, and hospital stay of 8 days.[35]

At this time, there are some clear disadvantages to RARC. RARC has, on average, longer operative times.[35] This difference will continue to narrow as more RARCs are performed, as techniques are further refined, and as surgeons become more efficient. The cost of RARC is high. Shorter patient hospital stays will hopefully offset some of this cost. As technology improves, the cost of robotic systems may drop, and as more specialties use these devices, the cost may become less prohibitive for an institution.

CONCLUSIONS

The results of current published reports of laparoscopic and robotic-assisted radical cystectomy are encouraging and demonstrate the technical feasibility of managing muscle-invasive bladder cancer with minimally invasive surgery. Early results suggest that an adequate resection can be performed along with an extended pelvic lymphadenectomy. All forms of urinary diversions can be created and offered to patients. There are several steps in performing this procedure that can be mastered by any surgeon skilled in laparoscopic and robotic surgery. With advantages such as decreased morbidity, decreased blood loss, and decreased convalescence robotic surgery is well suited for radical cystectomy. Once long-term oncologic efficacy is confirmed, urologists will be able to add robotic-assisted radical cystectomy to the armamentarium of treatment modalities for bladder cancer.

REFERENCES

1. Konety BR, Dhawan V, Allareddy V, Joslyn SA. Impact of hospital volume and surgeon volume on in-hospital mortality from radical cystectomy: data from the health care utilization project. J Urol 2005;173:1695–700.
2. Parra RO, Andrus CH, Jones JP. Laparoscopic cystectomy: initial report on a new treatment for the retained bladder. J Urol 1992;148:1140–4.
3. Hemal AK, Singh I, Kumar R. Laparoscopic radical cystectomy and ileal conduit reconstruction: preliminary experience. J Endourol 2003;17:911–6.
4. Gill IS, Kaouk JH, Meraney AM, et al. Laparoscopic radical cystectomy and continent orthotopic ileal neobladder performed completely intracorporeally: the initial experience. J Urol 2002;168:13–8.
5. Basillote JB, Abdelshehid C, Ahlering TE, Shanberg AM. Laparoscopic assisted radical cystectomy with ileal neobladder: a comparison with the open approach. J Urol 2004;172:489–93.
6. Berglund RK, Matin SF, Desai M, et al. Laparoscopic radical cystoprostatectomy with bilateral nephroureterectomy: initial report. BJU Int 2006 ;97:37–41.
7. Hong SH, Seo SI, Kim JC, Hwang TK. Laparoscopic radical cystectomy with extracorporeal urinary diversion: preliminary experience. Int J Urol 2005;12:869–74.
8. Abreu SC, Fonseca GN, Cerqueira JB, et al. Laparoscopic radical cystectomy with intracorporeally constructed Y-shaped orthotopic ileal neobladder using nonabsorbable titanium staples exclusively. Urology 2005;66:657e15–17.
9. Abreu SC, Silveira RA, Cerqueira JB, et al. Stapleless laparoscopic assisted radical cystectomy with ileal neobladder in a male and with ileal loop in a female: initial report from Brazil. Int Braz J Urol 2005;31:214–20.
10. Simonato A, Gregori A, Lissiani A, et al. Laparoscopic radical cystoprostatectomy: our experience in a consecutive series of 10 patients with a 3 years follow-up. Eur Urol 2005;47:785–90.
11. Moinzadeh A, Gill IS, Desai M, et al. Laparoscopic radical cystectomy in the female. J Urol 2005;173:1912–7.
12. Yang S, Huang YH, Ou Yang CM, et al. Clinical experience of laparoscopic-assisted radical cystectomy with continent ileal reservoir. Urol Int 2005;74:240–5.
13. Mariano MB, Tefilli MV. Laparoscopic partial cystectomy in bladder cancer—initial experience. Int Braz J Urol 2004; 30:192–8.
14. Huang J, Xu KW, Yao YS, et al. Laparoscopic radical cystectomy with orthotopic ileal neobladder: report of 33 cases. Chin Med J (Engl) 2005;118:27–33.
15. DeGer S, Peters R, Roigas J, et al. Laparoscopic radical cystectomy with continent urinary diversion (rectosigmoid pouch) performed completely intracorporeally: an intermediate functional and oncologic analysis. Urology 2004; 64:935–9.
16. McGinnis DE, Hubosky SG, Bergmann LS. Hand-assisted laparoscopic cystoprostatectomy and urinary diversion. J Endourol 2004;18:383–6.
17. Hemal AK, Kumar R, Seth A, Gupta NP. Complications of laparoscopic radical cystectomy during the initial experience. Int J Urol 2004;11:483–8.
18. Sorcini A, Tuerk I. Laparoscopic radical cystectomy with ileal conduit urinary diversion. Urol Oncol 2004;22:149–52.
19. Simonato A, Gregori A, Lissiani A, et al. Laparoscopic radical cystoprostatectomy: a technique illustrated step by step. Eur Urol 2003;44:132–8.

20. Peterson AC, Lance RS, Ahuja S. Laparoscopic hand assisted radical cystectomy with ileal conduit urinary diversion. J Urol 2002;168:2103–5.

21. Abdel-Hakim AM, Bassiouny F, Abdel Azim MS, et al. Laparoscopic radical cystectomy with orthotopic neobladder. J Endourol 2002;16:377–81.

22. Matin SF, Gill IS. Laparoscopic radical cystectomy with urinary diversion: completely intracorporeal technique. J Endourol 2002;16:335–41.

23. Gaboardi F, Simonato A, Galli S, et al. Minimally invasive laparoscopic neobladder. J Urol 2002;168:1080–3.

24. Gupta NP, Gill IS, Fergany A, Nabi G. Laparoscopic radical cystectomy with intracorporeal ileal conduit diversion: five cases with a 2-year follow-up. BJU Int 2002;90:391–6.

25. Turk I, Deger S, Winkelmann B, et al. Laparoscopic radical cystectomy with continent urinary diversion (rectal sigmoid pouch) performed completely intracorporeally: the initial 5 cases. J Urol 2001;165(6 Pt 1):1863–6.

26. Kaouk JH, Gill IS, Desai MM, et al. Laparoscopic orthotopic ileal neobladder. J Endourol 2001;15:131–42.

27. Denewer A, Kotb S, Hussein O, El-Maadawy M. Laparoscopic assisted cystectomy and lymphadenectomy for bladder cancer: initial experience. World J Surg 1999;23:608–11.

28. Sanchez de Badajoz E, Gallego Perales JL, Reche Rosado A, et al. Laparoscopic cystectomy and ileal conduit: case report. J Endourol 1995;9:59–62.

29. Menon M, Hemal AK, Tewari A, et al. Nerve-sparing robot-assisted radical cystoprostatectomy and urinary diversion. BJU Int 2003;92:232–36.

30. Stein JP, Lieskovsky G, Cote R, et al. Radical cystectomy in the treatment of invasive bladder cancer: long-term results in 1,054 patients. J Clin Onc 2001;19:666–75.

31. Konety BR, Joslyn SA, O'Donnell MA. Extent of pelvic lymphadenectomy and its impact on outcome in patients diagnosed with bladder cancer: analysis of data from the surveillance, epidemiology and end results program data base. J Urol 2003;169:946–50.

32. Leissner J, Hohenfellner R, Thuroff JW, Wolf HK. Lymphadenectomy in patients with transitional cell carcinoma of the urinary bladder; significance for staging and prognosis. BJU Int 2000;85:817–23.

33. Beecken WD, Wolfram M, Engl T, et al. Robotic-assisted laparoscopic radical cystectomy and intra-abdominal formation of an orthotopic ileal neobladder. Eur Urol 2003;44:337–39.

34. Yohannes P, Puri V, Yi B, et al. Laparoscopy-assisted robotic radical cystoprostatectomy with ileal conduit urinary for muscle-invasive bladder cancer: initial two cases. J Endourol 2003;17:729–32.

35. Cookson MS, Chang SS, Wells N, et al. Complications of radical cystectomy for nonmuscle invasive disease: comparison with muscle invasive disease. J Urol 2003;169:101–4.

36. Advanced bladder cancer meta-analysis collaboration: neoadjuvant chemotherapy in invasive bladder cancer: a systematic review and meta-analysis. Lancet 2003;361:1927–34.

37. Hemal AK, Abol-Enein H, Tewari A, et al. Robotic radical cystectomy and urinary diversion in the management of bladder cancer. Urol Clin N Am 2004;31:719–29.

38. Menon M, Hemal AK, Tewari A, et al. Robot-assisted radical cystectomy and urinary diversion in female patients: technique with preservation of the uterus and vagina. J Am Coll Surg 2004;198:386–93.

39. Elbahnasy AM, Hoenig DM, Shalhav A, et al. Laparoscopic staging of bladder tumor: concerns about port site metastases. J Endourol 1998;12:55–9.

40. El-Tabey N, Shoma AM. Port site metastases after robot-assisted laparoscopic radical cystectomy. Urology 2005;66:1110e1–3.

41. Cathelineau X, Arroyo C, Rozet F, et al. Laparoscopic assisted radical cystectomy: the montsouris experience after 84 cases. Eur Urol 2005;47:780–84.

42. Herr H, Lee C, Chang S, Lerner S, for the bladder cancer collaborative group. Standardization of radical cystectomy and pelvic lymph node dissection for bladder cancer: a collaborative group report. J Urol 2004;171:1823–28.

43. Bochner BH, Cho D, Herr H, et al. Prospectively packaged lymph node dissections with radical cystectomy: evaluation of node count variability and node mapping. J Urol 2004;172:1286–90.

44. Leissner J, Ghoneim MA, Abol-Enein H, et al. Extended radical lymphadenectomy in patients with urothelial bladder cancer: results of a prospective multicenter study. J Urol 2004;171:139–44.

Robotic Mitrofanoff Procedure (Appendicovesicostomy)

Lane S. Palmer, MD, FACS, FAAP
Israel Franco, MD, FACS, FAAP

There have been several landmark advances in the management of the neurogenic bladder. The first of these was the proven efficacy of clean intermittent catheterization as introduced by Lapides and colleagues.[1] The second advance was the acceptance of augmentation cystoplasty with its goal of increasing bladder capacity while reducing storage pressures, thus creating a functional reservoir that would protect renal function.[2] The third advance was the advent of the appendicovesicostomy as described by Mitrofanoff in 1980.[3] This operation facilitated intermittent catheterization so that patients could bypass the urethra, thus providing a technically easier path for catheterization, avoiding trauma to the urethra, and averting the perception of stigma associated with passing a catheter through the genitals. It also provided a mode of catheterization for children with normal sensation where urethral catheterization caused significant pain. While most appendicovesicostomies are performed in conjunction with augmentation cystoplasty, many patients have adequate storage parameters and only need an alternative passage for catheterization.

The progressive evolution of minimally invasive techniques, particularly laparoscopy, has led to many complex surgeries being performed without the need for large incisions. The literature provides the evidence of the steady progression towards a completely minimally invasive appendicovesicostomy. In 1997, Strand and colleagues reported a laparoscopic ureterovesicostomy performed as part of an extirpative procedure.[4] Jordan and Winslow and Van Salvage and Slaughenhoupt reported initial experiences with laparoscopic assisted appendicovesicostomy[5,6]; Docimo, however, who has the largest series with long-term follow up, reported excellent results of laparoscopically assisted appendicovesicostomy (17 cases) and of catheterizable channels using other bowel segments (8 cases).[7] In these cases, laparoscopy is used to mobilize the bowel or appendix, with the remainder of the surgery performed through a Pfannenstiel incision, obviating the need for the usual larger midline incision. In 1997, Lorenzo and colleagues reported on four patients who underwent a modified laparoscopic appendicovesicostomy that was performed without a submucosal tunnel.[8]

The proper appendicovesicostomy was performed completely laparoscopically by two groups in 2004.[9,10] The first report included the use of the da Vinci Surgical System (Intuitive Surgical, Inc., Sunnyvale, CA) to facilitate the more technically challenging anastomosis.

PATIENT EVALUATION AND SELECTION

This discussion will focus on the choice of candidate for an appendicovesicostomy that is coupled to either an augmentation cystoplasty or a continent diversion. The indications for these operations include bladder loss due to malignancy (eg, rhabdomyosarcoma) or noncompliance of the bladder due to neurogenic causes (eg, myelodysplasia) or some non-neurogenic causes (eg, posterior urethral valves) that have failed medical therapy. The available options for accessing the bladders are via catheter passed per the urethra or per catheterizable stoma. Patients with sensate urethras, such as those with posterior urethral valves, are poor candidates for urethral catheterization because of the discomfort experienced with catheterization and are thus ideal candidates for an appendicovesicostomy. Other candidates for whom the urethra is a poor choice include those who are obese and may have difficulty reaching the perineum, patients with poor manual dexterity, and patients who are wheelchair bound, in whom accessing the abdomen is readily achievable.

The appendix is an excellent option for the construction of the catheterizable channel. The blood supply to the appendix from the distal end of the ileocolic artery is very predictable. Once the appendix is mobilized and amputated from the cecum, it usually has ample mobility to be placed comfortably to the abdominal wall. The length of the appendix becomes the limiting factor; for most patients, however, the appendix is sufficiently long to reach the umbilicus, where the best cosmetic result is achieved. Of course, if the umbilicus cannot be reached without undo tension on the blood supply or adequate stomal construction, then it should be placed anywhere on the abdomen where these criteria can be met. The location of alternative sites should be evaluated preoperatively, with the patient standing and sitting to avoid the waistline. The diameter of the

appendix also allows for passage of an 8 French to 10F catheter in most patients.

For some patients, an alternative to the appendix is needed. Prior appendectomy, intraoperative accident, and loss of the appendix (or an inadequate or stenotic appendix) require the use of a bowel segment. The bowel segment used will be that used for the larger reconstruction; ileum or sigmoid. If the Mitrofanoff is the only procedure, however, then the ileum is the better candidate. The Monti technique is best suited for creating a reliable catheterizable channel under these circumstances.[11]

Finally, patient and familial compliance is paramount. Compliance and success with a catheterization program must be proven prior to surgery, otherwise the appendicovesicostomy will be wasted. The commitment must be made before undertaking reconstructive surgery, especially if augmentation cystoplasty or bladder substitution is planned. Preoperative education of stomal care and appropriate catheterization technique is also mandatory.

OPERATIVE PROCEDURE

The patient is brought into the operating theater after informed consent is obtained, which must include consent for possible conversion of the surgery to an open procedure. The patient undergoes general endotracheal anesthesia, passage of a nasogastric tube, pressure point padding and placement of a Foley catheter. The Foley catheter needs to be accessible during the case so that the bladder can be filled and emptied as needed.

Four ports are placed transperitoneally. A 12-mm laparoscopic camera port is placed at the umbilicus and secured. Two 10-mm robotic laparoscopic ports are placed in the left lower quadrant and in the right mid-axillary line at the level of the umbilicus. A fourth port is placed in the left mid-axillary line at the level of the umbilicus.

The dissection begins by mobilizing the appendix and right hemicolon along the line of Toldt up to the hepatic flexure. The mesoappendix is identified and mobilized to obtain adequate length. A gastrointestinal anastomosis stapler is used to divide the appendix at its base. If there is no bleeding from the suture line, then there is no need to use a second layer. After filling the bladder with saline, a 5-cm vertical seromuscular incision is made in the right posterior wall of the bladder down to the mucosa. The mucosa is then incised, and the appendix anastomosed to the bladder using 4-0 Vicryl interrupted sutures. The anastomosis is performed using the da Vinci robotic system. The seromuscular layer of the bladder is then closed using interrupted 4-0 polyglactin 910 sutures, creating a tunnel for the appendix.

The appendix is brought up to the umbilicus and a catheterizable stoma is created where the camera port was placed. The subsequent portion of the operation occurs extracorporeally. The appendix is brought through the fascial defect. A 5-mm laparoscopic lens is used to ascertain that there is no pressure on the appendix or its blood supply. An incision is made on the antimesenteric border of the appendix, and a matching V incision is made from the skin. The V flap from the skin is inserted and approximated to the appendix with interrupted polyglycolic suture. The stoma and appendicovesicostomy are tested by catheterization through the appendix with both a full pneumoperitoneum and with the pneumoperitoneum released. This is repeated with the bladder filled and then with the bladder emptied. The patient is left with the largest Foley that can be passed in the bladder and an 8F catheter left through the appendix. The abdomen is desufflated, and the ports are closed in the standard fashion. A Jackson-Pratt drain is placed in the peritoneal cavity and removed at the earliest possible time.

POSTOPERATIVE CARE

The postoperative course will be shorter and better tolerated when the surgery is performed laparoscopically when compared with open reconstruction. This is true whether the appendicovesicostomy is performed in isolation or as part of a greater reconstructive effort. When appendicovesicostomy is performed alone, patients may be ready for clear liquids that evening. The diet should advance rapidly; slower when a bowel anastomosis is performed. Analgesic requirements are also reduced when the surgery is performed laparoscopically. Ketorolac tromethamine is an excellent choice because there is no gastrointestinal effect, and bladder spasms are not a significant problem. The return to usual activity can be expected within two weeks. The channel will remain catheterized for about three weeks before being used for routine catheterization. Other considerations should be made when bladder substitution or augmentation cystoplasty is performed.

REFERENCES

1. Lapides J, Diokno AC, Silber SJ, Lowe BS. Clean, intermittent self-catheterization in the treatment of urinary tract disease. Trans Am Assoc Genitourin Surg 1971;63:92–6.
2. Smith RB, van Cangh P, Skinner DG, et al. Augmentation enterocystoplasty: a critical review. J Urol 1977;118:35–9.
3. Mitrofanoff P. Cystostomic continente trans-appendiculane dans le traitement des vesse neurologiques. Chir Pediatr 1980;21:297–305.
4. Strand WR, McDougall EM, Leach FS, et al. Laparoscopic creation of a catheterizable cutaneous ureterovesicostomy. Urology 1997;49:272–5.
5. Jordan GH, Winslow BH. Laparoscopic-assisted continent catheterizable cutaneous appendicovesicostomy. J Endourol 1993;7:517.
6. Van Savage JG, Slaughenhoupt BL. Laparoscopic-assisted continent urinary diversion in obese patients. J Endourol 1999;13:571–3.
7. Chung SY, Meldrum K, Docimo SG. Laparoscopic assisted reconstructive surgery: a 7-year experience. J Urol 2004;171:372–5.
8. Lorenzo JL, Castillo A, Serrano EA, et al. Urodynamically based modification of Mitrofanoff procedure. J Endourol 1997;11:77–81.
9. Pedraza R, Weiser A, Franco I. Laparoscopic appendicovesicostomy (Mitrofanoff procedure) in a child using the da Vinci robotic system. J Urol 2004;171:1652–3.
10. Hsu TH, Shortliffe LD. Laparoscopic Mitrofanoff appendicovesicostomy. Urology 2004;64:802–4.
11. Cain MP, Casale AJ, King SJ, Rink RC. Appendicovesicostomy and newer alternatives for the Mitrofanoff procedure: results in the last 100 patients at Riley Children's Hospital. J Urol 1999;162:1749–52.

Index